Respiratory Medicine

Third Edition

Volume 1

Multimedia CD-ROM
Single User License Agreement

1. NOTICE. WE ARE WILLING TO LICENSE THE MULTI-MEDIA PROGRAM PRODUCT TITLED Respiratory Medicine 3e ("MULTIMEDIA PROGRAM") TO YOU ONLY ON THE CONDITION THAT YOU ACCEPT ALL OF THE TERMS CONTAINED IN THIS LICENSE AGREEMENT. PLEASE READ THIS LICENSE AGREEMENT CAREFULLY BEFORE OPENING THE SEALED DISK PACKAGE. BY OPENING THAT PACKAGE YOU AGREE TO BE BOUND BY THE TERMS OF THIS AGREEMENT. IF YOU DO NOT AGREE TO THESE TERMS WE ARE UNWILLING TO LICENSE THE MULTIMEDIA PROGRAM TO YOU, AND YOU SHOULD NOT OPEN THE DISK PACKAGE. IN SUCH CASE, PROMPTLY RETURN THE UNOPENED DISK PACKAGE AND ALL OTHER MATERIAL IN THIS PACKAGE, ALONG WITH PROOF OF PAYMENT, TO THE AUTHORISED DEALER FROM WHOM YOU OBTAINED IT FOR A FULL REFUND OF THE PRICE YOU PAID.

2. **Ownership and License.** This is a license agreement and NOT an agreement for sale. It permits you to use one copy of the MULTIMEDIA PROGRAM on a single computer. The MULTIMEDIA PROGRAM and its contents are owned by us or our licensors, and are protected by U.S. and international copyright laws. Your rights to use the MULTIMEDIA PROGRAM are specified in this Agreement, and we retain all rights not expressly granted to you in this Agreement.

- You may use one copy of the MULTIMEDIA PROGRAM on a single computer
- After you have installed the MULTIMEDIA PROGRAM on your computer, you may use the MULTIMEDIA PROGRAM on a different computer only if you first delete the files installed by the installation program from the first computer.
- You may not copy any portion of the MULTIMEDIA PROGRAM to your computer hard disk or any other media other than printing out or downloading non-substantial portions of the text and images in the MULTIMEDIA PROGRAM for your own internal informational use.
- Your may not copy any of the documentation or other printed materials accompanying the MULTIMEDIA PROGRAM.

Neither concurrent use on two or more computers nor use in a local area network or other network is permitted without separate authorisation and the payment of additional license fees.

3. **Transfer and Other Restrictions.** You may not rent, lend, or lease this MULTIMEDIA PROGRAM. Save as permitted by law, you may not and you may not permit others to (a) disassemble, decompile, or otherwise derive source code from the software included in the MULTIMEDIA PROGRAM (the "Software"), (b) reverse engineer the Software, (c) modify or prepare derivative works of the MULTIMEDIA PROGRAM (d) use the Software in an on-line system, or (e) use the MULTIMEDIA PROGRAM in any manner that infringes on the intellectual property or other rights of another party.

However, you may transfer this license to use the MULTIMEDIA PROGRAM to another party on a permanent basis by transferring this copy of the License Agreement, the MULTIMEDIA PROGRAM, and all documentation. Such transfer of possession terminates your license from us. Such other party shall be licensed under the terms of this Agreement upon its acceptance of this Agreement by its initial use of the MULTIMEDIA PROGRAM. If you transfer the MULTIMEDIA PROGRAM, you must remove the installation files from your hard disk and you may not retain any copies of those files for your own use.

4. **Limited Warranty and Limitation of Liability.** For a period of sixty (60) days from the date your acquired the MULTIMEDIA PROGRAM from us or our authorised dealer, we warrant that the media containing the MULTIMEDIA PROGRAM will be free from defects that prevent you from installing the MULTIMEDIA PROGRAM on your computer. If the disk fails to conform to this warranty you may as your sole and exclusive remedy, obtain a replacement free of charge if you return the defective disk to us with a dated proof of purchase. Otherwise the MULTIMEDIA PROGRAM is licensed to you on an "AS IS" basis without any warranty of any nature.

WE DO NOT WARRANT THAT THE MULTIMEDIA PROGRAM WILL MEET YOUR REQUIREMENTS OR THAT ITS OPERATION WILL BE UNINTERRUPTED OR ERROR-FREE. THE EXPRESS TERMS OF THIS AGREEMENT ARE IN LIEU OF ALL WARRANTIES, CONDITIONS, UNDERTAKINGS, TERMS AND OBLIGATIONS IMPLIED BY STATUTE, COMMON LAW, TRADE USAGE, COURSE OF DEALING OR OTHERWISE ALL OF WHICH ARE HEREBY EXCLUDED TO THE FULLEST EXTENT PERMITTED BY LAW, INCLUDING THE IMPLIED WARRANTIES OF SATISFACTORY QUALITY AND FITNESS FOR A PARTICULAR PURPOSE.

WE SHALL NOT BE LIABLE FOR ANY DAMAGE OR LOSS OF ANY KIND (EXCEPT PERSONAL INJURY OR DEATH RESULTING FROM OUR NEGLIGENCE) ARISING OUT OF OR RESULTING FROM YOUR POSSESSION OR USE OF THE MULTIMEDIA PROGRAM (INCLUDING DATA LOSS OR CORRUPTION), REGARDLESS OF WHETHER SUCH LIABILITY IS BASED IN TORT, CONTRACT OR OTHERWISE AND INCLUDING, BUT NOT LIMITED TO, ACTUAL, SPECIAL, INDIRECT, INCIDENTAL OR CONSEQUENTIAL DAMAGES. IF THE FOREGOING LIMITATION IS HELD TO BE UNENFORCEABLE OUR MAXIMUM LIABILITY TO YOU SHALL NOT EXCEED THE AMOUNT OF THE LICENSE FEE PAID BY YOU FOR THE MULTIMEDIA PROGRAM. THE REMEDIES AVAILABLE TO YOU AGAINST US AND THE LICENSORS OF MATERIALS INCLUDED IN THE MULTIMEDIA PROGRAM ARE EXCLUSIVE.

5. **Termination**. This license and your right to use this MULTIMEDIA PROGRAM automatically terminate if you fail to comply with any provisions of this Agreement, destroy the copy of the MULTIMEDIA PROGRAM in your possession, or voluntarily return the MULTIMEDIA PROGRAM to us. Upon termination you will destroy all copies of the MULTIMEDIA PROGRAM and documentation.

6. **Miscellaneous Provisions**. This Agreement will be governed by and construed in accordance with English law and you hereby submit to the non-exclusive jurisdiction of the English Courts. This is the entire agreement between us relating to the MULTIMEDIA PROGRAM, and supersedes any prior purchase order, communications, advertising or representations concerning the contents of this package, No change or modification of this Agreement will be valid unless it is in writing and is signed by us.

Respiratory Medicine

Third Edition

Volume 1

Edited by

G John Gibson BSc MD FRCP FRCPE

Professor of Respiratory Medicine, University of Newcastle upon Tyne and Consultant Physician, Freeman Hospital, Newcastle upon Tyne, UK

Duncan M Geddes MD FRCP

Consultant Physician, Department of Respiratory Medicine, Royal Brompton Hospital, London, UK

Ulrich Costabel MD FCCP

Professor of Medicine and Chief, Department of Pneumology & Allergy, Ruhrlandklinik, Essen, Germany

Peter J Sterk MD PhD

Professor of Respiratory Physiology, Department of Pulmonary Medicine, Leiden University Medical Centre, Leiden, The Netherlands

Bryan Corrin MD FRCPath

Emeritus Professor of Histopathology, Imperial College Medical School, Royal Brompton Hospital, London, UK

SAUNDERS

SAUNDERS
An imprint of Elsevier Science Limited

© 2003, Elsevier Science Limited. All rights reserved.

© Illustrations, chapter 53, Dr N S L Goh and Dr R M du Bois.

First edition 1990
Second edition 1995
Third edition 2003

ISBN 0 7020 2613 1

British Library Cataloguing in Publication Data
A catalogue record for this book is available from the British Library

Library of Congress Cataloging in Publication Data
A catalog record for this book is available from the Library of Congress

Note
Medical knowledge is constantly changing. As new information becomes available, changes in treatment, procedures, equipment and the use of drugs become necessary. The contributors and the publishers have taken care to ensure that the information given in this text is accurate and up to date. However, readers are strongly advised to confirm that the information, especially with regard to drug usage, complies with the latest legislation and standards of practice.

 your source for books, journals and multimedia in the health sciences
www.elsevierhealth.com

Commissioning Editor: *Cathy Carroll*
Project Development Manager: *Louise Cook*
Project Manager: *Rory MacDonald*
Illustration Manager: *Mick Ruddy*
Designers: *Andy Chapman & Jayne Jones*
Illustrators: *Linda Payne & Tim Loughhead*

The publisher's policy is to use **paper manufactured from sustainable forests**

Printed in China by the RDC Group Ltd

Contents

Contributors

Carlo Agostini MD
Associate Professor of Internal Medicine
Department of Clinical and Experimental Medicine
(Immunology)
Padua University School of Medicine
Padua, Italy

Nicolino Ambrosino MD FCCP
Professor
Pulmonary Department
Scientific Institute of Gussago
Gussago, Italy

Wasif Anees MBBS MRCP
Consultant Respiratory Physician
Department of Respiratory Medicine
Good Hope Hospital
Birmingham, UK

Richard L Attanoos BSc MBBS FRCPath
Consultant Histopathologist
Department of Histopathology
Llandough Hospital
South Glamorgan, UK

Peter J Barnes MA DM DSc FRCP
Professor of Respiratory Medicine
Department of Thoracic Medicine
National Heart and Lung Institute, Imperial College
London, UK

Caroline J Bateman MB BS FRCA
Consultant Anaesthetist
St George's Hospital
London, UK

Richard Beasley MBChB FRACP DM(Southampton)
FAAAAI
Professor of Medicine and Director
Medical Research Institute of New Zealand
Wellington
New Zealand

Elisabeth H D Bel MD PhD
Associate Professor
Department of Pulmonary Medicine
Leiden University Medical Centre
Leiden, The Netherlands

Peter G Blain BMedSci MB BS PhD FIBiol FFOM
FRCP
Professor of Environmental Medicine
Department of Environmental and Occupational
Medicine Medical School
Newcastle upon Tyne, UK

Anders Blomberg MD PhD
Consultant
Department of Respiratory Medicine and Allergy
University Hospital
Umea, Sweden

Chris T Bolliger MD
Professor
Department of Internal Medicine
University of Stellenbosch
Cape Town, South Africa

Jacques Bourbon PhD
Research Director at CNRS
INSERM U492
Faculté de Médecine - Université Paris XII
Creteil, France

Elisabeth Brambilla MD PhD
Professor of Medicine
Laboratoire de Pathologie Cellulaire
CHU Albert Michallon
Grenoble, France

R Alistair L Brewis MD FRCP
Emeritus Consultant Physician
Department of Respiratory Medicine
Royal Victoria Infirmary
Newcastle upon Tyne, UK

Vito Brusasco MD
Professor of Respiratory Medicine
Dipartimento di Medicina Interna
Universita di Genova
Genova, Italy

P Sherwood Burge MD MSc FRCP FRCPE FFDM
MAIAS Dirl
Director of Occupational Lung Disease Unit and
Consultant Physician
Birmingham Heartlands Hospital
Birmingham, UK

Otto C Burghuber MD FACCP
Professor of Medicine
Department of Respiratory and Critical Care Medicine
Pulmonary Centre Vienna
Vienna, Austria

Peter Burney MA MD FRCP FFPHM
Professor of Public Health Medicine
Department of Public Health Services
London, UK

Andrew Bush MD FRCP FRCPCH
Reader in Paediatric Respirology
Department of Paediatrics
Royal Brompton Hospital
London, UK

Elisa Busi Rizzi MD
Department of Radiology
National Institute for Infectious Disease
Rome, Italy

Peter M A Calverley MBChB FRCP FRCPE
Professor of Medicine
Clinical Science Centre
University Hospital Aintree
Liverpool, UK

Ian A Campbell BSc MD FRCP (Edin & Lond)
Consultant Chest Physician
Department of Chest Medicine
Llandough Hospital
Cardiff, UK

Philippe Camus MD
Professor of Pulmonary Medicine
Service de Pneumologie et de Reanimation
Respiratoire
University Medical Centre and Medical School
Dijon, France

Rachel C Chambers PhD
Senior Lecturer
Centre for Respiratory Research
The Rayne Institute
London, UK

Marco Chilosi MD
Professor of Anatomic Pathology
Instituto di Anatomia Patologicà
Universita di Verona
Verona, Italy

Stewart Clarke MD MRCP
Formerly Consultant Physician
Department of Thoracic Medicine
Royal Free Hospital
London, UK

Jean-François Cordier MD
Professor of Medicine
Service de Pneumologie
Hôpital Louis Pradel
Lyon, France

John Corless MB ChB MRCP(UK)
Consultant in Respiratory Medicine
Medical Unit
Whiston Hospital
Prescot, UK

Bryan Corrin MD FRCPath
Emeritus Professor of Histopathology
Imperial College Medical School
Royal Brompton Hospital
London, UK

Paul A Corris MBBS FRCP
Professor of Thoracic Medicine
Department of Respiratory Medicine
Regional Cardiothoracic Centre, Freeman Hospital
Newcastle upon Tyne, UK

Ulrich Costabel MD FCCP
Professor of Medicine and Chief
Department of Pneumology and Allergy
Ruhrlandklinik
Essen, Germany

Vincent Cottin MD PhD
Physician
Service de Pneumologie
Hôpital Louis Pradel
Lyon, France

Adnan Custovic MD PhD
Reader in Allergy
North West Lung Centre
Wythenshawe Hospital
Manchester, UK

John H Dark FRCS FRCP
Consultant Cardiothoracic Surgeon
Department of Cardiothoracic Surgery
Freeman Hospital
Newcastle upon Tyne, UK

Peter D O Davies MA DM FRCP
Consultant Respiratory Physician
Cardiothoracic Centre
Liverpool, UK

Jane C Davies MBChB MD(Hons) MRCP MRCPCH
Senior Lecturer in Gene Therapy and Honorary
Consultant Paediatric Chest Physician
Department of Paediatric Respiratory Medicine
Royal Brompton Hospital
London, UK

Wilfried De Backer MD PhD
Professor of Respiratory Medicine
Department of Respiratory Medicine
University of Antwerp (UIA)
Antwerp, Belgium

Sophie de Bentzmann PhD
INSERM Researcher
UPR 9027 LISM
Marseille, France

André de Troyer MD PhD
Professor of Medicine & Physiology
Chest Service
Erasme University Hospital
Brussels, Belgium

Maurits Demedts MD PhD
Professor of Medicine and Head
Pulmonary Division
University Hospital Gasthuisberg
Leuven, Belgium

David M Denison PhD FRCP
Emeritus Professor of Clinical Physiology
Royal Brompton Hospital
London, UK

Eric Derom MD PhD
Associate Professor
Department of Internal Medicine
University Hospital
Ghent, Belgium

Ratko Djukanovic MD DM FRCP
Senior Lecturer in Medicine
Division of Infection, Inflammation and Repair
Respiratory Cell and Molecular Biology
Southampton General Hospital
Southampton, UK

Gerd Döring PhD
Professor of Experimental Hygiene
and Experimental Microbiology
Department of General and Environmental Hygiene
University of Tübingen
Tübingen, Germany

Roland M du Bois MA MD FRCP
Consultant Physician
Interstitial Lung Disease Unit
Royal Brompton Hospital
London, UK

Sarah E Dunsmore PhD
Honorary Lecturer
Centre for Respiratory Research
The Rayne Institute
London, UK

Stephen R Durham MA MD FRCP
Professor of Allergy and Respiratory Medicine
National Heart & Lung Institute
Imperial College School of Medicine
London, UK

John Earis MD FRCP
Consultant Physician
Aintree Chest Centre
University Hospital Aintree
Liverpool, UK

Anders Eklund MD PhD
Professor of Respiratory Medicine
Department of Respiratory Medicine
Karolinska Hospital
Stockholm, Sweden

J Stuart Elborn MD FRCP
Professor of Respiratory Medicine
Faculty of Medicine and Health Science
Queen's University
Belfast, UK

Peter C Elmes BM BCh FRCP FFOM
Retired Consultant in Occupational Lung Disease
Vale of Glamorgan, UK

Mark W Elliott MA MD FRCP(UK)
Consultant Respiratory Physician
Department of Respiratory Medicine
St James's University Hospital
Leeds, UK

Timothy W Evans BSc MD PhD FRCP DSc EDICM
FMedSci
Consultant in Thoracic and Intensive Care Medicine
Adult Intensive Care Unit
Royal Brompton Hospital
London, UK

Christopher C Evans MD FRCP FRCPI
Consultant Physician
Cardiothoracic Centre
Royal Liverpool University Hospital
Liverpool, UK

Susannah J Eykyn FRCP FRCPath
Honorary Consultant in Clinical Microbiology
United Medical and Dental Schools
St Thomas' Hospital
London, UK

Penny Fitzharris MB ChB MD FRACP FRCP
Associate Professor of Medicine
Department of Medicine
Wellington School of Medicine
Wellington, New Zealand

Patrick Flood-Page MBChB MRCP
Clinical Research Fellow
Department of Allergy and Clinical Immunology
National Heart and Lung Institute
London, UK

Hans Folgering MD PhD
Professor of Respiratory Physiology
Department of Pulmonology Dekkerswald
Univerisity of Nijmegen
Gruesbeek, The Netherlands

Wolfgang Frank MD
Chief Physician
Pneumologischen Klinik III
Johanniterkrankenhaus
Treuenbrietzen, Germany

Roger Freeman MBChB FRCPath
Consultant Medical Microbiologist and Professor of
Public Health Microbiology
Public Health Laboratory
Newcastle General Hospital
Newcastle upon Tyne, UK

Claude Gaultier MD PhD
Professor of Medicine
Service de Physiologie-Exploration Functionnelles
Hôpital Robert Debre
Paris, France

Duncan M Geddes MD FRCP
Consultant Physician
Department of Respiratory Medicine
Royal Brompton Hospital
London, UK

Allen R Gibbs MB BS FRCPath
Consultant Histopathologist
Department of Histopathology
Llandough Hospital
South Glamorgan, UK

G John Gibson BSc MD FRCP FRCPE
Professor of Respiratory Medicine (University of
Newcastle upon Tyne)
Consultant Physician
Freeman Hospital
Newcastle upon Tyne, UK

Carlo Giuntini MD
Professor of Respiratory Medicine
Division of Pneumology and Respiratory
Pathophysiology
Cardiac and Thoracic Department
Università di Pisa
Pisa, Italy

Fergus Gleeson FRCR FRCP
Consultant Radiologist
Department of Radiology
The Churchill Hospital
Oxford, UK

Nicole S L Goh MBBS FRACP
Clinical Fellow
Interstitial Lung Disease Unit
Royal Brompton Hospital
London, UK

John F Golding BA (Biochem) BA (Expt Psychol) MA
DPhil CPsychol
Senior Lecturer in Psychology
Department of Psychology
University of Westminster
London, UK

Peter Goldstraw MB ChB FRCS
Consultant Thoracic Surgeon, Honorary Senior
Lecturer,
Civil Consultant to Navy and Civil Consultant to RAF
Department of Thoracic Surgery
Royal Brompton Hospital
London, UK

Rik Gosselink PhD PT
Professor of Respiratory Rehabilitation
Respiratory Rehabilitation Division
University Hospital Leuven
Leuven, Belgium

Alistair N J Graham MB BCh MD FRCS(C-Th)
Consultant Cardiothoracic Surgeon
Northern Ireland Regional Thoracic Surgical
Department
Royal Victoria Hospital
Belfast, UK

Anne Greenough MD FRCP FRCPCH DCH
Children Nationwide Professor of Neonatology and
Clinical Respiratory Physiology
Department of Child Health
King's College Hospital
London, UK

Mark J D Griffiths MRCP PhD EDICM BDICM
Honorary Consultant Physician
Adult Intensive Care Unit
Royal Brompton Hospital
London, UK

Johan Grunewald MD
Associate Professor of Immunology
Department of Respiratory Medicine
Karolinska Hospital
Stockholm, Sweden

Giovanni Guaraldi MD
Centre for Diagnosis of Viral Diseases
University Hospital of Modena
Modena, Italy

Josune Guzman MD
Professor of Pathology
General and Experimental Pathology
Ruhr-Universitat Bochum
Bochum, Germany

David M Hansell MD FRCP FRCR
Consultant Radiologist
Department of Diagnostic Imaging
Royal Brompton Hospital
London, UK

Mark Harries MD FRCP
Consultant Physician
Northwick Park and St Mark's Hospital
Harrow, UK

Brian D W Harrison MA MB BChir FRCP (Lond)
FRCP (Edin) FCCP
Consultant Physician
Department of Respiratory Medicine
Norfolk & Norwich University Hospital
Norwich, UK

Timothy W Harrison MD MBBS MSC MRCP
Consultant Respiratory Physician
Department of Respiratory Medicine
University of Nottingham
Nottingham, UK

Christopher Haslett FRCP FRCP(E)
Consultant in Respiratory Medicine
Department of Medicine
The Royal Infirmary of Edinburgh
Edinburgh, UK

Karl Häussinger MD
Chief, Professor of Medicine
Zentrum für Pneumologie und Thoraxchirurgie
Asklepios Fachklinik München-Gauting
Gauting, Germany

Roderick J Hay DM FRCP FRCPath
Professor of Medicine
Faculty of Medicine and Health Sciences
Queen's University
Belfast, UK

Ragnberth Helleday MD PhD
Specialist Physician
Department of Respiratory Medicine & Allergy
University Hospital
Umea, Sweden

David J Hendrick MD FRCP FFOM
Professor of Occupational Respiratory Medicine and
Consultant Physician
Department of Respiratory Medicine
Royal Victoria Infirmary
Newcastle upon Tyne, UK

Alexandra Henrion-Caude PhD
Chargee de Recherche Inserm
Unité de Biologie Moléculaire
Hôpital Armand-Trousseau
Paris, France

Martin R Hetzel MD FRCP
Consultant Physician and Senior Clinical Lecturer
Department of Respiratory Medicine
Bristol Royal Infirmary
Bristol, UK

Alison A Hislop BSc PhD
Senior Lecturer
Unit of Vascular Biology & Pharmacology
Institute of Child Health
London, UK

Jens M Hohlfeld MD
Assistant Professor of Medicine
Department of Respiratory Medicine
Hannover Medical School
Hannover, Germany

Stephen T Holgate BSc MD DSc FRCP FRCPath
FIBiol FMedSci
MRC Clinical Professor of Immunopharmacology
Division of Infection, Inflammation and Repair
Respiratory Cell and Molecular Biology
Southampton General Hospital
Southampton, UK

Gerard Huchon MD
Professor of Medicine
Service de Pneumologie et Reanimation
Hôpital de l'Hotel Dieu
Paris, France

James E Jackson MRCP FRCR
Consultant Radiologist
Department of Imaging, Imperial College
Hammersmith Hospital
London, UK

Jacky Jacquot PhD
INSERM Researcher
Laboratoire de Biologie Moléculaire
Hôpital d'Enfants Armand-Trousseau
Paris, France

Peter K Jeffery DSc PhD MSc BSc FRCPath
Professor of Lung Pathology
Lung Pathology Unit
Royal Brompton Hospital
London, UK

Peter A Jenkins PhD
Formerly Head of Mycobacterium Reference Unit
University Hospital of Wales
Cardiff, UK

Simon Johnson BSc(Hons) MBBS DM MRCP
Senior Lecturer and Honorary Consultant Physician
Division of Therapeutics
Queens Medical Centre
Nottingham, UK

Sebastian L Johnston MB BS MRCP
Professorial Fellow in Respiratory Medicine
Department of Respiratory Medicine
National Heart & Lung Institute
London, UK

Paul W Jones BSc MBBS PhD FRCP
Professor of Respiratory Medicine
Division of Physiological Medicine
St George's Hospital Medical School
London, UK

Brian F Keogh MB BS FRCA
Consultant Anaesthetist
Department of Anaesthesia and Adult Intensive Care
Royal Brompton Hospital
London, UK

Huib A M Kerstjens MD PhD
Pulmonologist
Department of Pulmonary Medicine
University Hospital Groningen
Groningen, The Netherlands

Malcolm King PhD FCCP
Professor of Medicine
Pulmonary Research Group
University of Alberta
Edmonton AB, Canada

Martin Kohlhäufl MD
Physician in Respiratory Medicine
Zentrum für Pneumologie und Thoraxchirurgie
Asklepios Fachklinik München-Gauting
Gauting, Germany

Nikolaus Konietzko MD PhD
Ärztlicher Direktor
Department of Pneumology
Ruhrlandklinik
Essen, Germany

Claus Kroegel MD PhD FCCP
Professor of Internal Medicine, Senior Consultant and
Head of Department
Department of Pneumology and Allergy/Immunology
Friedrich-Schiller University
Jena, Germany

Carol A Langford MD MHS
Senior Investigator
Laboratory of Immunoregulation
National Institute of Allergy and Infectious Diseases
Bethesda MD, USA

Geoffrey J Laurent PhD
Professor and Centre Director
Centre for Respiratory Research
The Rayne Institute
London, UK

Patrick Levy MD PhD
Senior Lecturer in Physiology
Laboratoire d'EFCR
CHU Michallon
Grenoble, France

Robert Loddenkemper MD FCCP
Professor of Internal Medicine
Department of Pneumology II
Lungenklinik Heckeshorn
Berlin, Germany

John T Macfarlane MA DM FRCP MRCGP
Consultant Physician
Respiratory Medicine Unit
Nottingham City Hospital
Nottingham, UK

Ian S Mackay FRCS
Consultant ENT Surgeon
The Nose Clinic
Royal Brompton Hospital
London, UK

Joseph MacMahon FRCP
Consultant Physician
Department of Respiratory Medicine
Belfast City Hospital Trust
Belfast, UK

William MacNee MBChB MD (Hons) FRCP(G)
FRCP(E)
Professor of Respiratory and Environmental Medicine
ELEGI, Colt Research Labs
The University of Edinburgh Medical School
Edinburgh, UK

Lorcan McGarvey MD MRCP
Consultant Physician
Department of Respiratory Medicine
Craigavon Area Hospital
Craigavon, UK

James A McGuigan MB BCh FRCS
Consultant Thoracic Surgeon
Northern Ireland Regional Thoracic Surgery Unit
Royal Victoria Hospital
Belfast, UK

Kieran G McManus BMedSc MBBS FRCS(I)
Consultant Thoracic Surgeon
Northern Ireland Regional Thoracic Surgery Unit
Royal Victoria Hospital
Belfast, UK

Bettina Mock MD
Department of Pneumology and Allergy/Immunology
Friedrich-Schiller University
Jena, Germany

John Moore-Gillon MA MD FRCP
Consultant Physician
Department of Respiratory Medicine
St Bartholomew's Hospital
London, UK

Martin F Muers MA DPhil FRCP
Consultant Physician
Respiratory Unit
The General Infirmary at Leeds
Leeds, UK

Robert Naeije MD
Professor of Respiratory Physician
Laboratory of Cardiorespiratory Physiology
Erasme Univeristy Hospital
Brussels, Belgium

Benoît Nemery MD PhD
Professor of Toxicology and Occupational Medicine
Laboratorium Voor Pneumologie
KU Leuven
Leuven, Belgium

Andrew G Nicholson MA MBBS DM FRCPath
Consultant Histopathologist
Department of Histopathology
Royal Brompton Hospital
London, UK

Jorgen H Olsen MD, DMSc
Head of Research Department
Institute of Cancer Epidemiology
Danish Cancer Society
Copenhagen, Denmark

L Peter Ormerod BSc MBChB (Hons) MD DSc
(Med) FRCP
Professor of Medicine
Chest Clinic
Blackburn Royal Infirmary
Blackburn, UK

Antonio Palla MD
Associate Professor of Respiratory Medicine
Division of Pneumology and Respiratory
Pathophysiology
Cardiac and Thoracic Department
Università di Pisa
Pisa, Italy

Martyn R Partridge MD FRCP
Professor of Respiratory Medicine
Faculty of Medicine, NHLI Division
Imperial College of Science, Technology and Medicine
London, UK

Romain Pauwels MD PhD
Professor of Medicine
Department of Respiratory Medicine
University Hospital
Ghent, Belgium

Andrew J Peacock BSc MPhil MD FRCP
Director and Consultant Physician
Scottish Pulmonary Vascular Unit
Western Infirmary
Glasgow, UK

Michael G Pearson MA MB FRCP
Consultant Physician in Respiratory Medicine
Aintree Chest Centre
Fazakerley Hospital
Liverpool, UK

Riccardo Pellegrino MD
Consultant in Respiratory Medicine
Fisiopatologia Respiratoria
Azienda Ospedaliera S.Croce e Carle
Cuneo, Italy

Jean-Louis Pépin MD
Consultant Physician in Respiratory Medicine
Laboratoire d'EFCR
CHU Michallon
Grenoble, France

Venerino Poletti MD
Chief, Clinical Professor of Respiratory Medicine
Dipartimento di Malatti e dell'Apparato Respiratorio e
del Torace
Ospedale G.B. Morgangni
Forli, Italy

Michael I Polkey MRCP PhD
Consultant Physician
Department of Respiratory Medicine
Royal Brompton Hospital
London, UK

Dirkje S Postma MD PhD
Professor of Pulmonology
Department of Pulmonary Medicine
University Hospital Groningen
Groningen, The Netherlands

John Price MD FRCP FRCPCH
Professor of Paediatric Respiratory Medicine
Department of Child Health
King's College Hospital
London, UK

Neil B Pride MA MD FRCP
Professor of Respiratory Medicine
Department of Thoracic Medicine
National Heart and Lung Institute
London, UK

Edith Puchelle PhD
INSERM Director of Research
Head of UMRS 514 INSERM
Reims, France

Klaus F Rabe MD PhD
Professor of Medicine
Department of Pulmonology
Leiden University Medical Centre
Leiden, The Netherlands

Roberto A Rabinovich MD
Research Fellow
Laboratorio de Funcionalismo Pulmonar
Hospital Clinic Provincial
Barcelona, Spain

Angelika Reissig MD
Consultant
Department of Pneumology and Allergy/Immunology
Friedrich-Schiller University
Jena, Germany

Martin Riedel MD FESC
Associate Professor of Medicine
German Heart Center
Technische Universität München
Munich, Germany

Hans L Rieder MD MPH
Tuberculosis Division
International Union Against Tuberculosis and Lung
Disease
Paris, France

Douglas Robinson MBBChir MA MD FRCP
Senior Lecturer in Allergy and Clinical Immunology
Department of Allergy and Clinical Immunology
National Heart and Lung Institute
London, UK

Josep Roca MD
Associate Professor
Laboratorio de Funcionalismo Pulmonar
Hospital Clinic Provincial
Barcelona, Spain

Nicolas Roche MD
Assistant
Service de Pneumologie et Reanimation
Hôpital de L'Hôtel-Dieu
Paris, France

Roberto Rodriguez-Roisin MD FRCP(Ed)
Professor of Medicine
Servei de Pneumologia
Universitat de Barcelona
Barcelona, Spain

Charis S Roussos MD MSc PhD MRS FRCP(C)
Professor of Critical Care and Pulminary Medicine
Athens (Greece) and McGill (Canada) Medical Schools
Critical Care Department
Evangelismos Hospital
Athens, Greece

Robin M Rudd MA MD FRCP
Consultant Physician
Department of Respiratory Medicine
London Chest Hospital
London, UK

Marina Saetta MD
Department of Clinical and Experimental Medicine
Respiratory Medicine Branch
Padua University School of Medicine
Padua, Italy

Cesare Saltini MD
Professor of Respiratory Medicine and Director
Divisione Clinicizzata di Malattie Respiratorie
Istituto Nazionale Malattie Infettive
Rome, Italy

Thomas Sandström MD PhD
Professor of Respiratory Medicine
Department of Respiratory Medicine & Allergy
University Hospital
Umea, Sweden

Dunja T Schmidt MD PhD
Clinical Researcher
Department of Pulmonology
Leiden University Medical Centre
Leiden, The Netherlands

Gianpietro Semenzato MD
Chief of Clinical Immunology
Department of Clinical and Experimental Medicine
(Immunology)
Padua University School of Medicine
Padua, Italy

Pallav L Shah MBBS MD MRCP
Consultant Physician
Department of Respiratory Medicine
Royal Brompton Hospital
London, UK

Dennis J Shale MD FRCP
David Davies Chair of Respiratory and Communicable
Diseases
Section of Respiratory and Communicable Diseases
University of Wales College of Medicine
Vale of Glamorgan, UK

John Shneerson MA DM FRCP
Director of Respiratory Support and Sleep Centre
Department of Respiratory Medicine
Papworth Hospital
Cambridge, UK

Claire L Shovlin PhD MA FRCP
Senior Lecturer and Honorary Consultant in
Respiratory Medicine
National Heart and Lung Institute
Imperial College Faculty of Medicine
London, UK

Halla Skuladottir MD
Research Fellow
Institute of Cancer Epidemiology
Danish Cancer Society
Copenhagen, Denmark

Ulrich Specks MD
Associate Professor of Medicine
Division of Pulmonary and Critical Care Medicine
Mayo Clinic
Rochester, MN, USA

Rudolf Speich MD FCCP
Professor of Medicine
Department of Internal Medicine
University Hospital
Zurich, Switzerland

Stephen G Spiro BSc MD FRCP
Professor of Respiratory Medicine and Medical
Director of University College London Hospitals NHS
Trust
London, UK

Dan C Stănescu MD PhD FCCP
Emeritus Professor of Medicine
Division of Pneumology
Université Catholique de Louvain
Brussels, Belgium

Peter J Sterk MD PhD
Professor of Respiratory Physiology
Department of Pulmonary Medicine
Leiden University Medical Centre
Leiden, The Netherlands

Robert A Stockley MB ChB MRCP MD DSc FRCP
Professor of Medicine
Head of Department of Respiratory Medicine
Queen Elizabeth Hospital
Birmingham, UK

John Stradling MD FRCP
Professor of Respiratory Medicine
Oxford Centre for Respiratory Medicine
Churchill Hospital
Oxford, UK

Christopher R Swinburn MD FRCP
Consultant Physician
Taunton and Somerset Hospital
Taunton, Somerset

Anne E Tattersfield MD
Consultant in Respiratory Medicine
Division of Respiratory Medicine
City Hospital
Nottingham, UK

Paul Taylor BTech MSc MPhil FIBMS
Consultant Clinical Scientist
Microbiology Department
Royal Brompton Hospital
London, UK

Anneke ten Brinke MD PhD
Staff Pulmonologist
Department of Pulmonary Medicine
Medical Center Leeuwarden
Leeuwarden, The Netherlands

Anne Thomson MD FRCP FRCPCH
Consultant in Paediatric Respiratory Medicine
Department of Paediatrics
John Radcliffe Hospital
Oxford, UK

Ian Town MB ChB FRACP DM
Professor of Medicine
Department of Medicine
Christchurch School of Medicine
Christchurch, New Zealand

Paul Vermeire MD
Emeritus Professor of Respiratory Medicine
Department of Respiratory Medicine
University of Antwerp (UIA)
Antwerp, Belgium

Claus Vogelmeier MD
Professor of Medicine and Director
Department of Internal Medicine, Division of
Pulmonary Diseases
University of Marburg
Marburg, Germany

Benoît Wallaert MD
Professor of Medicine
Clinique des Maladies Respiratoires
Hopital A. Calmette - CHRU
Lille, France

F Elizabeth White MB BS MRCP FRCR DMRD
Consultant Radiologist
Department of Radiology
Royal Liverpool Hospital
Liverpool, UK

Robert Wilson MD FRCP
Consultant Physician, Royal Brompton Hospital
Reader, Imperial College of Science, Technology &
Medicine
Host Defence Unit
Royal Brompton Hospital
London, UK

Ashley Woodcock MD FRCP
Professor of Respiratory Medicine
North West Lung Centre
Wythenshawe Hospital
Manchester, UK

Jennifer A Young MA MD FRCPath
Senior Lecturer and Honorary Consultant in
Cytopathology
Department of Pathology
University of Birmingham Medical School
Birmingham, UK

Jean-Marie Zahm PhD
Research Engineer
UMRS 514 INSERM
Reims, France

Spyros G Zakynthinos MD
Assistant Professor of Critical Care Medicine, Athens
Medical School
Critical Care Department
Evangelismos General Hospital
Athens, Greece

Maurizio Zompatori MD
Chief and Clinical Professor of Radiology
Dipartimento di Radiologia Diagnostica
Policlinico S. Orsola-Malpighi
Bologna, Italy

Andrew M Zurek MB BChir MRCP
Specialist Registrar
Department of Respiratory Medicine
Frenchay Hospital
Bristol, UK

Preface to the First Edition

Respiratory medicine is an increasingly popular and rapidly expanding subject so that individual authors no longer have sufficient knowledge and experience to cover the subject in the depth necessary in a post-graduate textbook. Our aim has been to produce a multi-author text which is authoritative and up-to-date, and which reflects the best British traditions by combining applied science with good clinical practice. Many of the 94 contributors are actively practising physicians who were chosen for their expertise in specific fields, but there are also contributions from other specialists including surgeons, radiologists, pathologists and microbiologists as well as experts in biochemistry, morphology and epidemiology. The authors were asked to write for a readership which would be worldwide and which would include both the trainee needing a general account of a particular technique, disease or treatment and the established specialist seeking an entrée to the literature of some rare condition. Such rarities are deliberately represented at lengths disproportionate to their frequency, and pathological and radiographic illustrations have been encouraged.

Some sections of the book merit particular mention. The introductory chapters dealing with structure and function are far from the usual cursory summaries and have dealt with their subjects at a level which we hope will make them useful sources of reference for established specialists. Even traditional thoracic anatomy merits thorough treatment since CT scanning has necessitated the re-learning of relationships from a new angle. Some aspects of managing patients with respiratory disease are not adequately covered in texts that focus on the disease itself, and we have sought to remedy this by commissioning chapters dealing with the principles of surgical treatment, oxygen treatment, mechanical ventilation and inhaled treatment. Other novel chapters include consideration of smoking as a disease and an account of respiratory problems in the adverse environments of altitude and depth.

The scope of the clinical sections of the book is essentially pragmatic, largely reflecting the activities of the clinician practising adult respiratory medicine. We have not included a comprehensive account of paediatric respiratory medicine, but those "paediatric conditions" which are most relevant to adult practice are covered: examples include developmental abnormalities and childhood cystic fibrosis and asthma. Diseases of the upper respiratory tract are not covered in full as many of the relevant conditions fall more appropriately within the ambit of the ENT surgeon: a chapter is, however, included on rhinitis and nasal polyps as these are commonly seen and treated by respiratory physicians. There are also sections on the non-thoracic manifestations of certain diseases such as sarcoidosis, where the respiratory physician is often regarded as the local expert.

We are grateful to all our contributors: they greeted the concept with unexpected enthusiasm and responded positively to editorial amendments and suggestions. We trust that these have not diluted the strength of their contributions.

Preface to the Third Edition

One of the great attractions of the specialty of respiratory medicine is its breadth, encompassing as it does eight or more major disease areas, each of which is becoming a subspecialty in its own right. In addition, respiratory physicians inevitably encounter rarer conditions which enter the differential diagnosis of patients with the common respiratory presentations. Such is the pace of progress in the specialty and in the science which underpins it that we and our publishers agreed that a new edition was needed. To reflect this progress and the diversity of respiratory medicine we have assembled an international expert team of 181 authors (compared with 94 in the first edition and 125 in the second). Our aim, as before, was to produce a comprehensive and scholarly postgraduate text which reviews the basic science relevant, or potentially relevant, to respiratory medicine as well as current clinical practice at a level that we hope will satisfy the established specialist, enlighten the trainee and act as a reference for the generalist seeking an up-to-date expert view.

Most sections have been completely revised and updated but the general format is similar to previous editions, with the first third devoted to basic science, the clinical presentation of respiratory disease and the principles of investigation and treatment, and the remainder organised systematically by disease category. The better understanding of the genetic and molecular mechanisms involved in respiratory disease is particularly emphasised. The new edition also reflects changing clinical practice, with, for example, additional sections on the principles of non-invasive ventilation, pulmonary rehabilitation and respiratory intensive care. New chapters are devoted to each of the common respiratory symptoms and to several rarer respiratory conditions where knowledge has recently increased.

A novel feature of this edition is the inclusion of a CD-ROM of all the illustrations. Although CD-ROM versions of some complete textbooks have been available for a number of years, our perception is that most users still prefer to consult a conventional text. We hope, however, that a CD-ROM of the illustrations will offer a successful compromise between new and traditional technology and will allow ready access to illustrative examples for those preparing lectures, seminars and case presentations.

For the new edition the editorship has expanded to reflect the increasing complexity and more international style of the book. At the same time Alistair Brewis, the senior editor of the first two editions, has stepped down and we extend to him our gratitude and valedictions.

G John Gibson
Duncan M Geddes
Ulrich Costabel
Peter J Sterk
Bryan Corrin

Glossary

Blood flow

$\dot{Q}_S$	shunt flow per minute
$\dot{Q}_T$	total pulmonary blood flow per minute
$\dot{Q}_S/\dot{Q}_T$	shunt fraction

Gas flow

MEF ($\dot{V}_{E\,max}$)	maximum expiratory flow
MEF_{25}, etc.	maximum expiratory flow with 25% of vital capacity remaining in the lung
MEFV	maximum expiratory flow–volume
MIF ($\dot{V}_{Imax}$)	maximum inspiratory flow
MVV	maximum voluntary ventilation
PEF	peak expiratory flow
PIF	peak inspiratory flow
T_E	expiratory time
T_I	inspiratory time
T_{TOT}	total breath duration
$\dot{V}$	ventilation
$\dot{V}_A$	alveolar ventilation (per minute)
$\dot{V}_E$	minute ventilation
V_T/T_I	mean inspiratory flow

Gas exchange

AaP_{O_2}	alveolar–arterial P_{O_2} difference
C_aO_2	arterial blood oxygen content (concentration)
C_cO_2	capillary blood oxygen content (concentration)
$C_{c'}O_2$	end-capillary blood oxygen content (concentration)
$C_{\bar{v}}O_2$	mixed venous blood oxygen content (concentration)
D_LO_2	oxygen diffusing capacity
F_IO_2	fractional concentration of inspired oxygen
K_{CO}	carbon monoxide transfer coefficient
P_{50}	P_{O_2} at 50% oxygen saturation
P_aO_2, P_aCO_2	arterial gas tension
P_AO_2, P_ACO_2, P_ACO	alveolar gas tension
$P_{c'}O_2$, $P_{c'}CO_2$	end-capillary gas tension
P_EO_2, P_ECO_2	mixed expired gas tension
$P_{ET}O_2$, $P_{ET}CO_2$	end-tidal gas tension
P_IO_2	inspired oxygen tension
P_{N_2}	pressure of nitrogen
$P_{tc}O_2$, $P_{tc}CO_2$	transcutaneous gas tension
$P_{\bar{v}}O_2$, $P_{\bar{v}}CO_2$	mixed venous gas tension
S_aO_2	arterial oxygen saturation
T_LCO, (D_LCO)	carbon monoxide transfer factor (diffusing capacity)
$\dot{V}_A/\dot{Q}$	ventilation–perfusion ratio
$\dot{V}CO_2$	carbon dioxide output
$\dot{V}O_2$	oxygen consumption
RQ	respiratory quotient

Lung volumes

FEV_1	forced expiratory volume in 1 second
FIV_1	forced inspiratory volume in 1 second
FRC	functional residual capacity
FVC	forced vital capacity
VC	vital capacity
RV	residual volume
TLC	total lung capacity
V_c	volume of blood in the pulmonary capillaries
V_D	volume of dead space
$V_{D\,anat}$	anatomical dead space
$V_{D\,phys}$	physiological dead space
V_D/V_T	proportion of tidal volume ventilating dead space
V_L	lung volume
V_r	relaxation volume of the lung
V_T	tidal volume

Pressures

$P_{0.1}$	Mouth occlusion pressure 0.1 s after onset of inspiratory effort
P_{ab}	subdiaphragmatic abdominal pressure
P_{Alv}	alveolar gas pressure
P_{atm}	atmospheric pressure

P_c, P_{cap}	capillary pressure
P_B	barometric pressure
P_{di}	transdiaphragmatic pressure
$P_{E\,max}$	maximum expiratory (alveolar) pressure
$P_{I\,max}$	maximum (strictly, minimum) inspiratory (alveolar) pressure
P_{ga}	gastric pressure
P_{H_2O}	pressure of water vapour
$P_{L\,max}$	maximum static lung recoil pressure
P_L	static lung recoil pressure
P_{mo}	mouth pressure
P_{oes}	oesophageal pressure
P_{pl}	pleural surface pressure
P_{pw}	pulmonary artery wedge pressure
P_{rs}	recoil pressure of the respiratory system
P_{tp}	transpulmonary pressure
P_w	chest wall recoil pressure

Resistance and compliance

C_L	lung compliance
C_{rs}	total respiratory system compliance
C_w	chest wall compliance
G_{AW}	airway conductance
R_{AW}	airway resistance (resistance = 1/conductance)
R_L	pulmonary resistance
R_{ti}	tissue resistance
sG_{AW}	specific airway conductance
sR_{AW}	specific airway resistance
X_{rs}	reactance of respiratory system
Z_{rs}	impedance of respiratory system

Miscellaneous

ADP	adenosine diphosphate
AMP	adenosine monophosphate
ATP	adenosine triphosphate
AIDS	acquired immunodeficiency syndrome
a_1-PI	a_1-proteinase inhibitor
ARDS	acute respiratory distress syndrome
BAL	bronchoalveolar lavage
BOOP	bronchiolitis obliterans organising pneumonia
CFTR	cystic fibrosis transmembrane conductance regulator protein
COP	cryptogenic organising pneumonia
COPD	chronic obstructive pulmonary disease
CPAP	continuous positive airway pressure
EGF	epidermal growth factor
HIV	human immunodeficiency virus
HRCT	high resolution CT
IGF	insulin-like growth factor
IPPV	intermittent positive pressure ventilation
MMP	matrix metalloproteinase
NIV	non-invasive ventilation
NSAID	non-steroidal anti-inflammatory drug
PC_{20}	concentration provoking a 20% change in a given index
PD_{20}	dose provoking a 20% change in a given index
PDGF	platelet-derived growth factor
PEEP	positive end-expiratory pressure
TGF	transforming growth factor
TNF	tumour necrosis factor
VEGF	vascular endothelial growth factor

STRUCTURE AND FUNCTION

1 Structure

1.1 Anatomy of the thorax

R Alistair L Brewis and F Elizabeth White

This chapter offers a compact source of reference for the main elements of anatomy relevant to clinical respiratory medicine. A second purpose of the chapter is to draw attention to the appearance of normal anatomical structures in radiographs and computed tomography (CT) images and to indicate ways in which observation of these features can help in interpretation.

Chest wall

Bones

The bones of the thorax comprise the thoracic vertebrae and 12 pairs of ribs, which articulate with them, the manubrium and the sternum.

Thoracic vertebrae

The general arrangement of a thoracic vertebra is indicated in Figure 1.1.1.

The size of the bodies increases regularly from the top to the bottom of the thoracic spine but, paradoxically, the projected radiodensity of the bodies diminishes from above to below when they are viewed in a lateral radiograph. The bodies are slightly shorter anteriorly than posteriorly. The spines of the vertebrae become long and more downward-directed in the mid-thorax so that, with the exception of the first and 12th vertebrae, the tip of the spine is very approximately level with the body of the vertebra below. The intercostal nerve emerges from the intervertebral foramen beneath the notch in the pedicle of the respective vertebra.

Ribs

The upper nine ribs articulate by their heads with a facet on the upper edge of the respective vertebral bodies and with a small facet on the body of the vertebra above. They also articulate at their tubercles with facets on the respective transverse

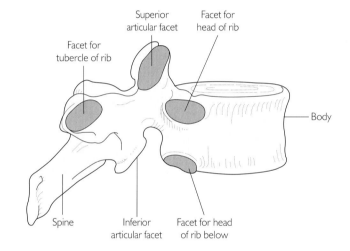

Fig. 1.1.1 Typical thoracic vertebra.

processes. The lower three pairs of ribs are a little different in that the ribs articulate only by their heads and only with a single vertebral body.

Anteriorly, the first rib is connected by a costal cartilage to the manubrium, and the second rib is similarly connected to the manubriosternal junction (sternal angle or angle of Louis). The third to eighth ribs are connected by costal cartilages to the sternum, the ninth and 10th ribs are usually connected to the costal cartilages above, and the last two ribs are generally free at their ends from skeletal connections. Costal cartilages calcify increasingly with age. Calcification starts in the upper cartilages and progresses downwards. In males this begins in the early 20s; males show earlier and more extensive calcification than females.

The cross-section of a typical rib is shown in Figure 1.1.2. The intercostal vessels and nerves run in a groove inferiorly and the lower border of the rib forms a dependent fin outside these structures. This is variably visible in posteroanterior radiographs.

The movement of the ribs is principally that of rotation about the axis of the necks (leaving aside for the moment flexing

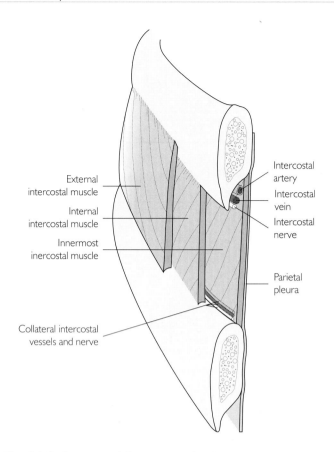

Fig. 1.1.2 Structure of the intercostal space.

External intercostal muscle

Internal intercostal muscle

Innermost inercostal muscle

Collateral intercostal vessels and nerve

Intercostal artery

Intercostal vein

Intercostal nerve

Parietal pleura

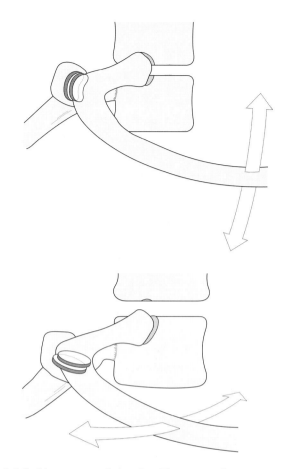

Fig. 1.1.3 Movements of the ribs. The upper ribs move upwards and downwards (arrows in upper panel) rotating about the axis of the neck of the rib. The costotransverse joint surfaces are more or less cylindrical, reflecting this movement. The lower ribs show an increasing component of inward and outward movement (arrows in lower panel) and the costotransverse articular surfaces are flatter, permitting a gliding movement.

movements). The necks of the upper four or five ribs are arranged so that they point medially towards each other. The articular facets on the transverse processes are here curved in cylindrical fashion so that rotation produces upward and forward movement of the rib (so-called pump handle movement). The necks of ribs 6–10 inclusive point forwards[1] so that rotation produces an outward as well as an upward movement[2] (so-called bucket handle movement). In these ribs the articular facets on the transverse processes are flatter and more horizontal so that, as well as rotation, some gliding outward movement of the ribs is permitted (Fig. 1.1.3).

The ribs are flexible in youth and become less so with age. The longest ribs (6–8) are the most pliable and, when stressed, the distal and proximal parts can move simultaneously in different directions even in old age.

Manubrium and sternum

The manubrium articulates with the clavicles and is connected to the first costal cartilages. The second costal cartilage is connected to both the manubrium and the sternum itself at the sternal angle. The connection between manubrium and sternum is by means of a disc of fibrocartilage. The sternum is cartilaginous in early life and has four bony segments, which become united in early adult life. It is connected to the second to sixth costal cartilages; the seventh costal cartilage may join it at the junction with the xiphisternum. There are small synovial joints between the costal cartilages and the sternum. The shape of the

xiphisternum (xiphoid process) is variable but it is frequently leaf-shaped or bifid. It is flexible and cartilaginous in childhood and forms a firm bony union with the sternum in adult life, when it often takes up a forward curve and appears as a sharp protuberance in the epigastrium.

Muscles

Diaphragm

The general arrangement of the diaphragm is shown in Figure 1.1.4. The fibres are arranged into costal, sternal and vertebral groups, which are inserted into the central tendon of the diaphragm. The costal fibres originate from the lower six ribs. The sternal fibres are a few strands arising anteriorly from the xiphisternum and the vertebral fibres arise from the medial and lateral arcuate ligaments and the associated tips of the lateral processes of second and third lumbar vertebrae. The crura of the diaphragm arise below from the fronts of the lumbar vertebral bodies and pass upwards on either side of the aorta joining

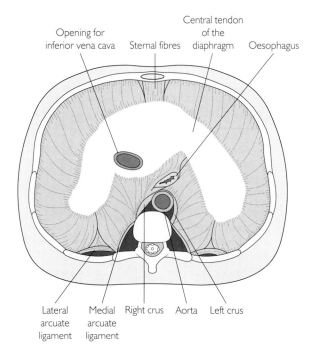

Opening for
inferior vena cava   Sternal fibres   Central tendon
of the
diaphragm   Oesophagus

Lateral   Medial   Right crus   Aorta   Left crus
arcuate   arcuate
ligament   ligament

Fig. 1.1.4 Diagram showing the diaphragm viewed from below. There is considerable individual variation in the arrangement of muscle fibres. Usually the oesophageal opening is invested in fibres derived from the right crus.

together in front of it to form the medial arcuate ligament. The arrangement of the crural fibres higher up is complex. The most common pattern occurring in about 40% of cases is for the right crus to be dominant and enclose the oesophagus, but there is considerable variation.[3] The oesophageal hiatus is formed by the fibres overlapping in the fashion of a closed coat. The anatomical basis of hiatus hernia is outside the scope of this chapter but the subject has been well reviewed by Spencer.[4]

There may be a deficiency in the diaphragm anteriorly between the sternal fibres and the first slips of costal muscle attached to the seventh costal cartilage – the foramen of Morgagni (or between the sternal fibres themselves). This may be the basis of rare anterior herniae, which are usually discovered radiologically and are more common on the right side. There is almost always a peritoneal sac in any herniation and direct communication between peritoneum and pleural cavities is unusual.

A deficiency in the diaphragmatic muscle fibres arising posteriorly from the lower ribs or arcuate ligaments may be referred to as the foramen of Bochdalek. The defect can be of any size and large deficiencies generally represent a failure of separation of pleural and peritoneal cavities, which occurs early in fetal life, so that there may be persistent direct communication between the two cavities.

Minute communications between peritoneal and pleural cavities occur in a substantial proportion of normal individuals. These are very much more common on the right and account for the association between right-sided pleural effusion and ascites (for example in Meigs's syndrome and during peritoneal dialysis) and for the almost invariably right-sided involvement in ectopic endometriosis of the pleural cavity.[5]

The diaphragm is innervated by the right and left phrenic nerves, which have slightly different courses through the mediastinum (see below). The nerves arise from the spinal roots of the third, fourth and fifth cervical nerves. The sensory dermatomes corresponding to these segments lie over the crown of the shoulder, accounting for such phenomena as referred diaphragmatic pain to the shoulder and the occasional paralysis of the phrenic nerve in patients with herpes zoster erupting over the shoulder area. The phrenic nerve carries motor fibres to the diaphragm and sensory fibres that relay pain. The diaphragm has long been known to have relatively few proprioceptive receptors compared with other muscles and relatively few muscle spindle receptors compared with tendon organ afferents.[6]

Intercostal muscles

The arrangement of the intercostal muscles is shown in Figure 1.1.2. The external intercostal muscles have their fibres aligned downwards and forwards and are thicker than the internal intercostals, in which the fibres are aligned downwards and backwards. A thinner innermost intercostal layer lies immediately against the pleura. The intercostal muscles are supplied by their respective intercostal nerves and are known to be well-supplied with proprioceptors.

Anatomy of the intercostal space

The structure of the intercostal space is shown in Figure 1.1.2. The principal intercostal nerves and vessels in each intercostal space lie beneath and deep to the lower edges of the ribs – a point of some relevance to the technique of pleural biopsy. A very small collateral artery, vein and nerve run close to the upper border of each rib. The intercostal arteries arise directly from the thoracic aorta. The intercostal veins drain into the azygos venous system on the right side and the hemiazygos system on the left (see below).

Other muscles

A number of other muscles are important in respiration. The scalene muscles were at one time regarded as accessory muscles of respiration but are now accepted as contributing to the elevation of the upper chest during ordinary breathing. There are three scalene muscles. Scalenus anterior and scalenus medius arise from the lateral processes of the cervical vertebrae and are inserted into the anterior end of the first rib. Scalenus posterior is smaller and arises from the fourth to sixth lateral processes and is inserted into the second rib. The nerve supply of the scalene muscles is derived from nerve roots related to the vertebrae from which the muscles take their tendinous origins. The sternomastoid is more of a true accessory muscle of inspiration, being brought into play only during breathing at high lung volumes or with unusual effort. It is attached above to the skull at the mastoid process of the temporal bone and below by two heads to the manubrium and to the medial quarter of the clavicle. It is innervated by the accessory (XIth) cranial nerve and by small nerves from the second and third cervical nerve roots.

Pleural cavity

Parietal pleura

The parietal pleura is closely applied to the inner surfaces of the ribs and the innermost intercostal muscles. There is, however, a very thin layer of connective tissue separating the pleural membrane from the periosteum of the ribs and this is demonstrated when the pleura is stripped in surgical pleurectomy. A small amount of fat may be present in the same layer, particularly in obese individuals, and this may be visible on plain radiographs as a thin shadow accompanying the ribs (companion shadow). The usual limits of reflection of the pleura are shown in Figure 1.1.5.

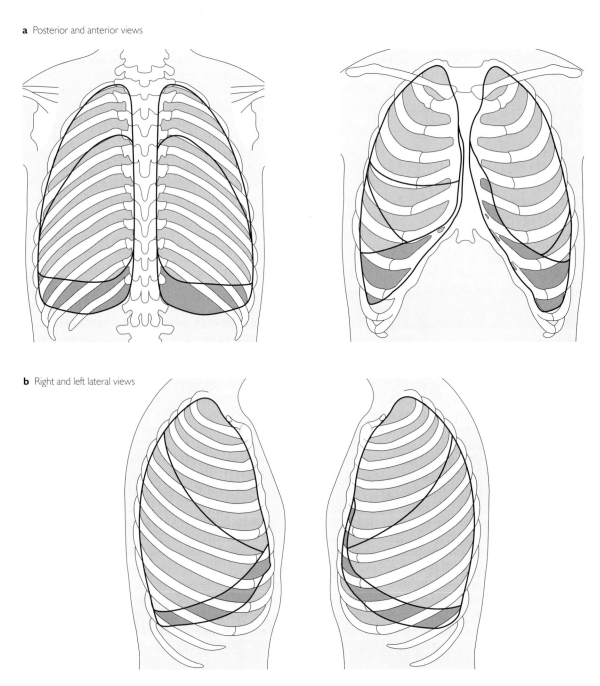

a Posterior and anterior views

b Right and left lateral views

Fig. 1.1.5 Diagram showing the usual limits of the pleural reflections and the positions of the principal fissures. (a) Posterior and anterior view. (b) Right and left lateral view. The dark stippled areas indicate the inferior pleural recess, where parietal pleural surfaces are in contact and are only separated by lung on full inspiration. There is substantial variation in the course of the anterior pleural reflection of the left pleural cavity near the left sternal edge and in the extent to which lung fills this space during quiet breathing.[8]

The dome of the pleural cavity

The pleural cavity extends well above the clavicles up to the level of the neck of the first rib. The structures related to the dome are shown in Figure 1.1.6. The subclavian vessels pass in front of the pleural apex, the artery lying posterior to the vein. The relationship of the vein to the lung apex is nevertheless close, so that it is very easy for the lung to be punctured inadvertently during attempted cannulation. The sympathetic inferior cervical ganglion is also closely related to the pleural apex. The sympathetic nervous supply to the whole of one side of the head, neck and arm passes through this ganglion, which explains why Horner's syndrome is a regular accompaniment of a carcinoma of the lung apex (Pancoast's tumour). The lower components of the brachial plexus are closely related to the pleural dome lying above, anterior and then lateral to it. These nerves may also be involved in Pancoast's tumour.

The costophrenic recess

The parietal pleura is applied to the upper surface of the diaphragm and the lateral surface of the mediastinum. During quiet breathing in normal individuals the diaphragmatic pleura and the costal pleura are in contact in the lower part of the pleural cavity (see Fig. 1.1.5).

The inferior lines of reflection of the parietal pleura and the extent to which the lungs at rest intrude into the costo-diaphragmatic recess show some variation between individuals. The lines indicated on Figure 1.1.5 are derived from the careful work of Lachman.[7] It will be noted that the line of pleural

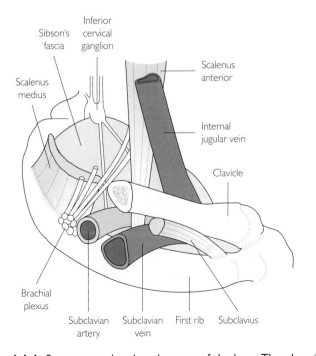

Fig. 1.1.6 Structures related to the apex of the lung. The phrenic nerve (not shown) lies on the front of scalenus anterior and enters the thorax by passing between the subclavian artery and subclavian vein.

reflection marking the lower recess of the pleural cavity runs almost horizontally posteriorly and curves upwards further forwards, and that the line is not closely related to readily perceived rib landmarks except anteriorly. Inexperienced clinicians sometimes imagine that the pleural cavity extends to a line joining the tips of all the ribs, so that attempts to aspirate pleural fluid may be made too low.

Anterior pleural reflection

Anteriorly the line of pleural reflection on the right ascends behind the sternum, sloping gradually left to right towards the right sternal border to a point behind the right sternoclavicular joint. This line of pleural reflection may sometimes be detected on an anteroposterior (AP) radiograph. On the left, the line of reflection in the upper chest lies very close to that of the right but in the third to the fifth intercostal spaces anteriorly it takes a variable detour laterally (see Fig. 1.1.5), exposing a 'cardiac window' of pericardium. This is not always present, however. The most constant site of the window (sometimes referred to as the cardiac incisura) is in the fourth interspace and here the line of cardiac reflection can occur anywhere between 1.5 cm to the left of the left sternal edge and 3 cm to the right of the left sternal edge (i.e. behind the sternum).[8]

Mediastinal surface

Medially, the parietal pleura is applied to the pericardium and the structures of the mediastinum. The pleura of the two sides may come into contact with each other anteriorly in front of the heart, particularly when the lungs are overinflated in disease. This gives rise to a fine line shadow, which is visible on the PA radiograph and is known as the anterior junctional line (see below). There is a further area in the retro-oesophageal space in which the two layers of parietal pleura may be in contact and this is responsible for the occasional identification of a posterior junctional line. Again, it is more often seen when the lungs are abnormally overinflated.

The pleura invests the structures of the hila loosely in the manner of a sleeve. The empty dependent part of the sleeve is sometimes referred to as the hilar ligament and it seems to have the effect of steadying the lower lobe with reference to the hilum itself. A lymph node may be present here between the two layers of pleura.

Visceral pleura

The surface of the lungs is covered by visceral pleura, which is separated from the outer limiting fibroelastic membrane by loose connective tissue. This layer permits the visceral pleura to be surgically stripped from the underlying lung (pleurectomy), a procedure occasionally undertaken for the release of restrictive fibrothorax or in order to achieve pleurodesis in recurrent pneumothorax.

Oblique and horizontal fissures

The visceral pleura extends into the major fissures of the lungs, which separate lobes. The depth of the fissures is variable. The

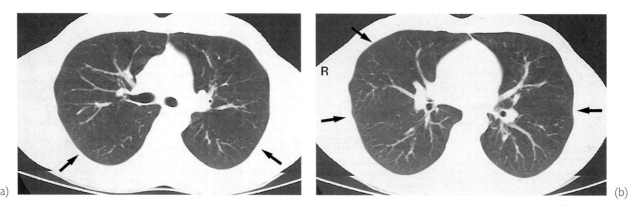

(a)   (b)

Fig. 1.1.7 Orientation of the oblique fissures. (a) Computed tomography (CT) section just below the level of the carina. Arrows indicate the avascular zones representing the oblique fissures, which at this level face outwards and forwards. (b) CT section 4.3 cm lower than (a), showing the oblique fissure in a lateral position orientated in the coronal plane (facing forwards – lower arrows). The upper arrow shows part of the horizontal fissure, which has entered the plane of the section. Lower in the chest the oblique fissures face forwards and inwards.

oblique fissure is quite commonly incomplete medially, so that it may not reach the mediastinal surface of the lungs or may extend only a short way towards the hilum. The oblique fissure on the right extends from the level of the fourth rib posteriorly to a point 2–3 cm behind the anterior end of the diaphragm. Although the plane of the fissure is broadly facing forwards and upwards, the left and the right oblique fissures face slightly away from each other above the hilum and slightly towards each other lower down. This feature is reflected in the changing orientation of the line of avascularity which marks the oblique fissure on CT sections (Fig. 1.1.7).

Accessory fissures

In addition to the oblique fissures and the horizontal fissure between the right upper and middle lobes, occasional accessory fissures are seen. The most common of these is the azygos fissure (Fig. 1.1.8), which is formed by the azygos vein coming forwards from the posterior thoracic wall to drain into the back of the superior vena cava by way of an arched route lateral to the apex of the pleural cavity instead of medial to it. It effectively takes a 'short cut' across the upper part of the pleural cavity but remains an extrapleural structure carrying with it a 'mesentery' of parietal pleura and invaginating the visceral pleura of the right upper lobe so that it runs in the depth of a slit-like fissure (Fig. 1.1.9). Normally the azygos vein comes forwards to drain into the back of the superior vena cava entirely medial to the right upper lobe. The part of the right upper lobe that is tucked medially under the azygos vein is sometimes referred to as the azygos lobe. An azygos lobe or fissure may be identified radiologically in a small proportion of normal individuals (generally accepted as less than 1%).

Two other less common accessory fissures are seen on the right side. The first is a fissure curving vertically upwards from the right diaphragmatic surface near its medial end and then curving slightly medially. This represents a cleft in the posterior surface of the right lower lobe, which may partially separate the medial basal segment from the remainder of the lobe.[9] The second fissure is uncommon and represents a horizontal cleft separating the apical segment of the right lower lobe from the remainder of the right

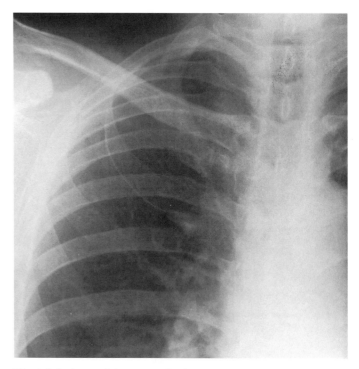

Fig. 1.1.8 Azygos lobe: view of right apical region showing the characteristic appearance of the azygos fissure. This extends inferiorly from the apex of the lung to surround the arch of the azygos vein.

lower lobe. The appearance on the PA radiograph is of a second horizontal fissure a few centimetres below the true one.

Mediastinum

The mediastinum extends from the thoracic inlet above to the diaphragm below and is bounded in front by the sternum, behind by the bodies of the thoracic vertebrae and laterally by the parietal pleura reflected back from the medial surfaces of

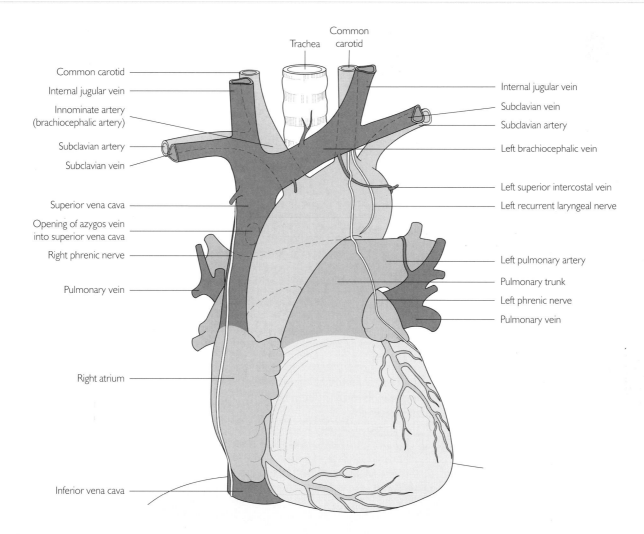

Fig. 1.1.10 The mediastinum, anterior view 1. Turning this page and the following two pages will reveal figures that show progressively more posterior views of the principal mediastinal structures.

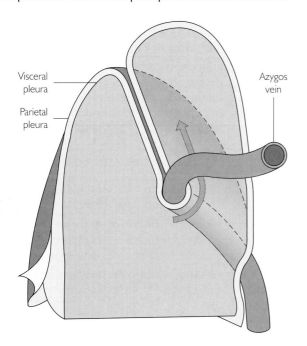

Fig. 1.1.9 Azygos lobe: diagrammatic view of the apex of the right lung to show the extrapleural position of the azygos vein as it arches forwards, cutting across the apex of the lung and drawing a 'mesentery' comprising both visceral and parietal pleural layers. A tongue of upper lobe is tucked medially under the edge of this mesentery.

the lungs. The mediastinum has traditionally been divided up into compartments – superior and inferior – and the inferior compartment is further subdivided into anterior, middle and posterior compartments. Other subdivisions have been recommended. There is in truth no strict natural compartmentalisation and it may be more convenient when describing normal structures or disease to consider anterior, middle and posterior compartments, and to make separate reference to vertical level. The anterior mediastinum extends from the sternum anteriorly to the pericardium, ascending aorta and brachiocephalic vessels posteriorly. It normally contains a variable amount of fat and the thymus gland. The middle mediastinal compartment contains the heart and immediately adjacent major vessels. It extends from the pericardium anteriorly to the vertebral bodies posteriorly. The principal structures contained in the posterior mediastinum are: descending aorta, oesophagus, thoracic duct and the azygos and hemiazygos venous systems.

General arrangement of structures

Some of the principal structures of the mediastinum viewed from the front are shown in Figures 1.1.10, 1.1.11, 1.1.14 and 1.1.15 and are so arranged that they appear as though structures were being peeled off. Lateral views of the mediastinum are shown in Figures 1.1.12 and 1.1.13. The relationship between different structures in the mediastinum is best displayed by computed tomography and an annotated series of CT sections is shown in Figures 1.1.16–1.1.23.

Aorta

The aorta is closely related to the pulmonary trunk and the right pulmonary artery, which passes beneath the aortic arch. The ascending aorta is in contact with pleura over the right lung. The arch of the aorta lies close to the left side of the trachea and the left main bronchus passes closely beneath it. Once across the midline, the aorta is in contact with pleura over the medial surface of the left lung throughout its intrathoracic course; excised lungs show a prominent aortic groove.

The arrangement of the major arteries of the aortic arch is shown in Figure 1.1.10. The position of the subclavian vessels in front of the apices of the lungs is illustrated in Figure 1.1.6. The substernal tissues and the anterior ends of the intercostal spaces are supplied by the internal thoracic artery (also known as the internal mammary artery), which continues into the anterior abdominal wall as the superior epigastric artery.

There are usually nine pairs of intercostal arteries arising from the aorta; the upper two intercostal spaces are usually supplied by a distinct artery, the superior intercostal artery. The intercostal arteries give off small spinal branches supplying vertebrae, meninges and the spinal cord itself.

Superior vena cava

The superior vena cava is formed by the convergence of the left brachiocephalic vein, as it crosses the thoracic inlet behind the manubrium, and the short right brachiocephalic vein (Fig. 1.1.10). It is in contact with the pleura over the right lung throughout its course. It passes downwards to the right and a little in front of the trachea and then in front of the right main bronchus, where it is adjacent to a lymph node (or nodes) related to the azygos vein. These close relations underlie the association of superior vena caval obstruction and carcinoma arising in the right upper lobe. The ascending aorta and arch are closely related (Figs 1.1.8–1.1.20).

The venous drainage of the anterior mediastinum and anterior parts of the intercostal spaces is by internal thoracic veins, which enter brachiocephalic or subclavian veins. The drainage of the posterior thoracic wall and posterior mediastinum is by the azygos and hemiazygos venous system illustrated in Figure 1.1.15. The upper two intercostal spaces are drained by the superior intercostal veins, which take different courses on the two sides (Figs 1.1.12, 1.1.13 & 1.1.15).

The inferior vena cava has only a short intrathoracic section just above the diaphragm.

Oesophagus

From its position behind the trachea in the neck (Fig. 1.1.14), the oesophagus maintains a prevertebral position to the right of the aortic arch, but in the lower mediastinum it lies increasingly anteriorly passing from right to left in front of the aorta (Figs 1.1.14, 1.1.22 & 1.1.23). It may have close relations with the pleura of both lungs throughout most of its course (Figs 1.1.16–1.1.23).

Vagus nerves

On the left side the vagus enters the thorax on the lateral surface of the common carotid artery and on reaching the aortic arch gives off the recurrent laryngeal nerve which loops under the arch and ascends on the left side of the trachea towards the larynx (Fig. 1.1.10 and see below). The main trunk of the left vagus then passes behind the left hilum and forms a plexus from which pulmonary nerves derive. Lower in the mediastinum the vagus lies in front of the oesophagus and divides into a plexus containing fibres from both sides to envelop the oesophagus before it passes through the diaphragmatic hiatus (Figs 1.1.12 & 1.1.13).

On the right side the vagus lies lateral to the right common carotid and passes over the right subclavian artery to enter the thorax. As it does so it gives off the right recurrent laryngeal nerve, which loops backwards under the subclavian artery to ascend on the right of the trachea towards the larynx. The right recurrent laryngeal nerve scarcely enters the thorax and is rarely involved by malignant disease. The main trunk of the vagus continues lateral to the trachea and then adjacent to the oesophagus. As on the left side it forms a pulmonary plexus behind the right hilum and, lower down, an oesophageal network.

Phrenic nerves

The phrenic nerves are derived from the third, fourth and fifth cervical nerves (the same roots that supply the deltoid and the skin over the shoulder tip). The phrenic nerves form on the anterior surface of scalenus anterior and enter the thorax by passing in front of the subclavian artery and behind the subclavian vein (Fig. 1.1.6). The subsequent courses of the two phrenic nerves are shown in Figures 1.1.12 & 1.1.13. The right phrenic nerve passes quite close to front of the right hilum and is more frequently involved by malignant disease than the left, which passes more anteriorly. At the diaphragm the phrenic nerves penetrate the muscular layer and are distributed by branches spreading over the inferior surface.

Sympathetic nerves

There are usually 12 sympathetic ganglia, which comprise the sympathetic chain, lying in front of the head of the ribs (Figs 1.1.12 & 1.1.13). The ganglia are connected to the correspond-

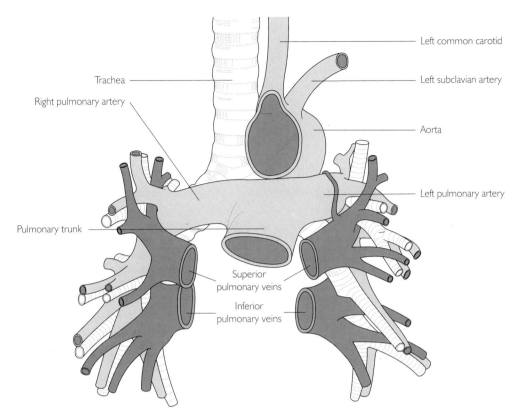

Left common carotid

Trachea

Left subclavian artery

Right pulmonary artery

Aorta

Left pulmonary artery

Pulmonary trunk

Superior
pulmonary veins

Inferior
pulmonary veins

Fig. 1.1.11 Mediastinum, anterior view 2. The arrangement of the pulmonary arteries, pulmonary veins and bronchi represents the most common relationship; there is individual variation. Note that on the right the arrangement of the structures from front to back runs: vein, artery, bronchus. On the left the sequence is vein, bronchus, artery. The pulmonary artery and the bronchi run close to each other in the same connective tissue sheath whereas the pulmonary vein is almost everywhere separate in its course through the lung.

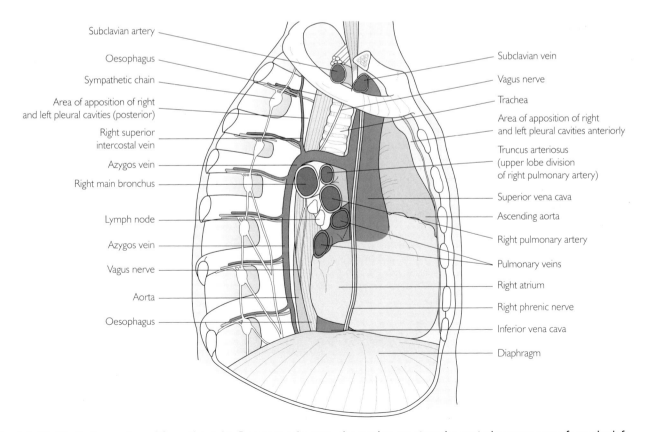

Subclavian artery

Oesophagus

Sympathetic chain

Area of apposition of right
and left pleural cavities (posterior)

Right superior
intercostal vein

Azygos vein

Right main bronchus

Lymph node

Azygos vein

Vagus nerve

Aorta

Oesophagus

Subclavian vein

Vagus nerve

Trachea

Area of apposition of right
and left pleural cavities anteriorly

Truncus arteriosus
(upper lobe division
of right pulmonary artery)

Superior vena cava

Ascending aorta

Right pulmonary artery

Pulmonary veins

Right atrium

Right phrenic nerve

Inferior vena cava

Diaphragm

Fig. 1.1.12 Mediastinum viewed from the right. By turning the page the reader can view the equivalent structures from the left.

ing spinal nerves by grey and white rami communicantes. The white rami of the thoracic sympathetic ganglia are the source of all efferent sympathetic fibres. From midthoracic level downward filaments derived from the sympathetic ganglia coalesce to form greater, lesser and lowest splanchnic nerves. The upper end of the sympathetic chain terminates in the inferior cervical ganglion, which lies close to the neck of the first rib and in relation to the pleura over the apex of the lung (see Fig. 1.1.6). This may represent fused upper thoracic or thoracic and lower cervical ganglia; the fused ganglion is sometimes referred to as the stellate ganglion. Sympathetic nerve supply to the head, neck and most of the arm is transmitted through the inferior cervical ganglion.

Mediastinal lymph nodes

Lymph draining from the lung passes to intrapulmonary and hilar lymph nodes (see below) and then enters the mediastinum to be received by groups of tracheobronchial lymph nodes (Fig. 1.1.24). Right and left tracheobronchial nodes may lie all round the bronchi but there are generally prominent nodes above and below. Inferiorly, a central tracheobronchial lymph node or group of nodes is referred to as the subcarinal node. The superior tracheobronchial node on the left often lies close to the remnant of the ductus arteriosus and hence the recurrent laryngeal nerve. It may be referred to as the subaortic node and enlargement of this commonly leads to recurrent laryngeal nerve paralysis.

There are prominent lymph nodes on either side of the lower end of the trachea, referred to as right and left paratracheal glands. The node in this position on the right is close to the termination of the azygos vein and the term 'azygos node' is sometimes used. Anterior mediastinal lymph nodes situated adjacent to the pericardium sometimes receive lymph from the lungs. A chain of lymph nodes in the posterior mediastinum encircles the oesophagus and this too may receive lymph from the lung. The paratracheal chain of lymph nodes drains into the thoracic duct on the left and the right thoracic duct on the right. These pass upwards behind the subclavian veins and arch forwards to open into the veins near their termination.

Lymphatic drainage from different parts of the lungs follows roughly predictable patterns. Lymph from the upper lobes is likely to drain via bronchopulmonary nodes to the paratracheal nodes of the same side. Lymph from the lower zones passes via bronchopulmonary nodes and is more likely to pass to the inferior tracheobronchial nodes (especially from the right side) before draining to paratracheal nodes. For many years it was believed that the left lower lobe lymphatics drained to the hilar and mediastinal nodes of the right side. Large studies of the distribution of lymphatic metastases from bronchial carcinomas have shown that drainage to the other side is unusual[10] but occurs occasionally in both directions. Involvement of the inferior cervical lymph nodes is common in lung carcinoma. Here again, the usual pattern is for node involvement to reflect the side of origin of the tumour, although occasional cases of contralateral involvement are seen.[10]

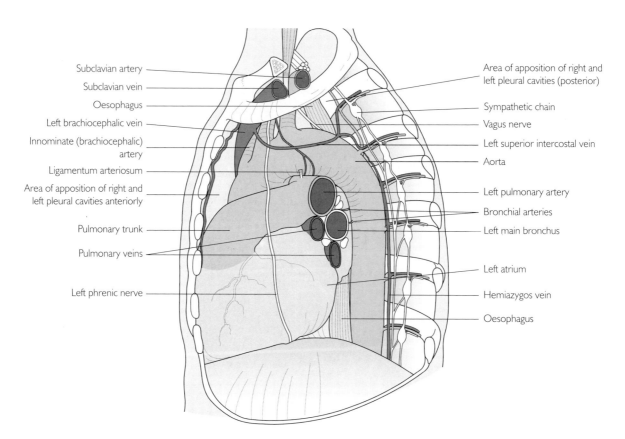

Fig. 1.1.13 Mediastinum viewed from the left.

Subclavian artery

Subclavian vein

Oesophagus

Left brachiocephalic vein

Innominate (brachiocephalic) artery

Ligamentum arteriosum

Area of apposition of right and left pleural cavities anteriorly

Pulmonary trunk

Pulmonary veins

Left phrenic nerve

Area of apposition of right and left pleural cavities (posterior)

Sympathetic chain

Vagus nerve

Left superior intercostal vein

Aorta

Left pulmonary artery

Bronchial arteries

Left main bronchus

Left atrium

Hemiazygos vein

Oesophagus

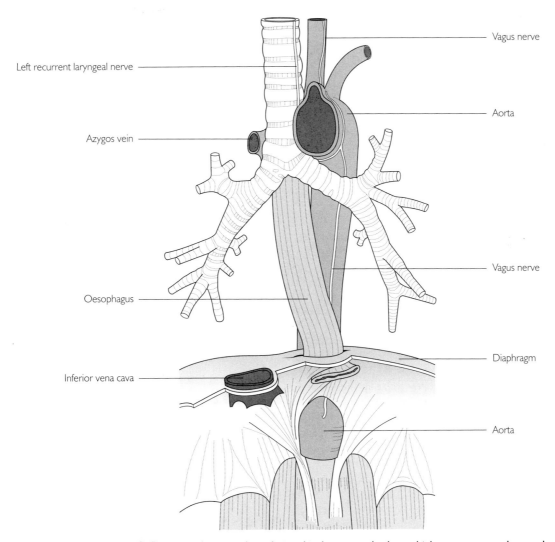

Left recurrent laryngeal nerve

Azygos vein

Oesophagus

Inferior vena cava

Vagus nerve

Aorta

Vagus nerve

Diaphragm

Aorta

Fig. 1.1.14 Mediastinum anterior view 3. Diagram showing the relationship between the bronchial tree, aorta and oesophagus.

Lymphatic drainage of the parietal pleura is by lymph channels and nodes related to intercostal vessels leading posteriorly to a chain of nodes related to the heads of ribs and the thoracic vertebral bodies. This chain communicates with the posterior mediastinal nodes around the oesophagus. More anteriorly, the pleura drains to the internal mammary chain.

Thoracic duct

The thoracic duct courses through the whole of the posterior mediastinum. It originates below the diaphragm in the cisterna chyli and enters the thorax through the aortic opening immediately in front of the vertebral bodies. It passes upwards a little to the right of the midline, situated between aorta and azygos vein. At the level of the aortic arch it passes forwards close to the aorta and medially behind the origin of the left subclavian artery. It then ascends close to the left side of the oesophagus and finally curves forwards to end in the subclavian vein in the angle between it and the jugular vein.[11] It is rather like a vein in structure and usually possesses valves at intervals along its

course.[12] On the right side the right lymphatic duct (which is analogous to but smaller than the thoracic duct) may develop from tributaries from the posterior intercostal chain. It is very variable and the opening of this duct and of other lymphatic channels into the veins on the right is also variable.

Structure of the airways

Upper airways

The anatomy of the nose and paranasal sinuses is reviewed in Chapter 43.

Larynx

Structure of the larynx

The larynx has a complex structure and a full description is outside the scope of this book. Nevertheless, as the clinician engaged in respiratory medicine frequently has opportunity to observe the larynx in the course of bronchoscopy and as laryngeal competence is crucial to the health of the lungs, a brief review of laryngeal anatomy is offered here.

The internal appearance of the larynx from above is shown in Figure 1.1.25. The arytenoid cartilages are three-cornered pyramidal structures seated on the upper rim of the posterior part of the cricoid cartilage. The vocal folds take their origin from the tips of the vocal process anteriorly. As well as an anterior vocal process, each arytenoid cartilage has a lateral muscular process and a superior process on which sits a small cartilage, the cuneiform cartilage, which is readily visible from above. The lateral muscular process acts as a lever rotating the arytenoid cartilage about a vertical axis, varying the aperture of the larynx.

Action of the muscles of the larynx

The posterior arytenoid muscles open the glottis by pulling the lateral processes backwards towards each other; the lateral cricoarytenoid muscles close the glottis by pulling the lateral processes forwards. Tensing of the vocal folds is achieved primarily by contraction of the cricothyroid muscle, which pulls the anterior end of the cricoid up towards the thyroid cartilage so that the posterior edge of the cricoid bearing the arytenoid cartilages is rocked backwards. Vocales is a small muscular slip lying close beneath the surface of the laryngeal epithelium in the edge of the vocal fold. Contraction tenses the anterior part of the vocal fold while at the same time slackening the posterior part resulting in an elevation in pitch. Other muscles related to the epiglottis and the aryepiglottic fold are responsible for constriction of the upper part of the larynx. The larynx is conventionally regarded as having three lines of defence: the aryepiglottic inlet zone, the false vocal folds (vestibular folds) and the true vocal folds.

Innervation of the larynx

All the muscles of the larynx with the exception of the cricothyroid are innervated by the recurrent laryngeal nerve derived from the vagus nerve. The superior laryngeal nerve, which is also a branch of the vagus nerve, supplies motor fibres to the cricothyroid muscle and sensory fibres for the whole of the interior of the larynx at least down to the level of the vocal folds themselves. Interruption of the recurrent laryngeal nerve causes paralysis of one vocal fold, which is either motionless or moves very poorly and fails to reach the midline. Varying degrees of alteration of the voice may result from this but, because of the ability of the opposite fold to reach across the midline, there is scope for compensation and in some individuals there may be little or no disturbance of voice production. Interruption of a superior laryngeal nerve causes anaesthesia of half of the larynx and slackening of one vocal fold. Bilateral lesions produce slackening of both vocal folds, resulting in a lower pitch, which is inevitably accompanied by dangerous laryngeal incompetence because of the sensory loss.

Trachea

Position and course of trachea

The trachea extends downwards from the lower border of the cricoid cartilage to the bifurcation into two main bronchi and is about 10–11 cm long in an average adult. It is angled backwards by up to 30° or even more in the supine position – a point often overlooked by novice rigid bronchoscopists. In normal individuals about half of the course of the trachea is extrathoracic and half intrathoracic – depending on the position of the head and the depth of inspiration. The upper end of the trachea is in the midline provided that the head is pointing forwards; the lower end is either in the midline or slightly to the right. It tends to be further to the right in older individuals in whom there is shortening of the thoracic spine and unfolding of the aorta. The bifurcation of the trachea is situated approximately at the level of the fifth thoracic vertebra posteriorly and the manubriosternal junction anteriorly. The position of the trachea alters with breathing, the lower end moving downwards and forwards by about 1–2 cm during ordinary inspiration.

Structure of trachea

The trachea is lined with ciliated columnar epithelium, which overlies a glandular vascular submucosa. Outside this there are about 15–20 horseshoe-shaped cartilaginous rings, which are incomplete posteriorly. The cartilaginous rings show some variation in shape and some are branched. They are joined together vertically by strong connective tissue (the intercartilaginous ligaments) and the tips of the horseshoes are joined together horizontally posteriorly by a band of transverse muscle. The posterior wall is mobile and elastic; the mucosa here has a longitudinally ridged appearance due to bundles of elastic tissue that lie quite close to the surface. At rest the trachea has a D-shaped section with the flat section directed posteriorly. CT shows, however, that there is considerable variation in the shape. During coughing the elastic posterior wall of the trachea billows briefly forwards so that it almost touches the anterior wall, narrowing the tracheal orifice to a U-shaped slit. Its inherent elasticity achieves almost instantaneous return to the resting position.

Bronchi

The structure of the extrapulmonary section of the bronchial tree (the main bronchi and the lower lobe bronchi) is similar to that of the trachea. The airway is supported by cartilaginous plates except posteriorly.

Main bronchi

Right main bronchus
The right main bronchus is shorter than the left main bronchus (about 2.5 cm in an average man compared with about 5 cm) and it is slightly wider in transverse diameter. In adults the right main bronchus may have its axis displaced only 20–30° from that of the trachea, whereas the left main bronchus makes an

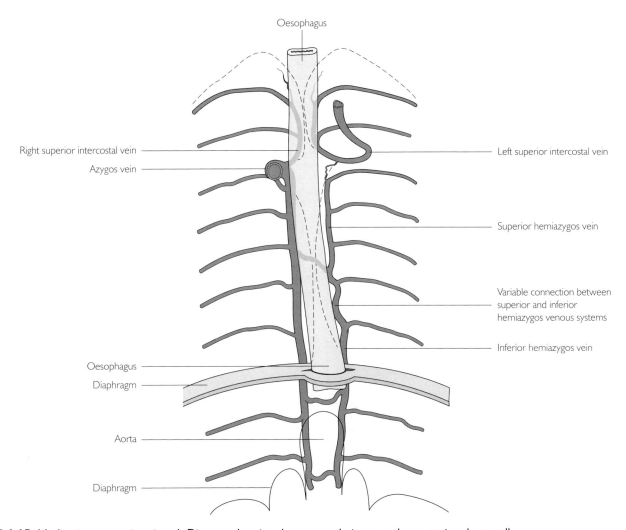

Fig. 1.1.15 Mediastinum anterior view 4. Diagram showing the venous drainage to the posterior chest wall.

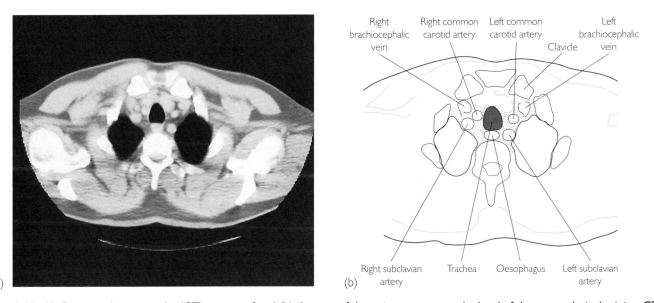

Fig. 1.1.16 (a) Computed tomography (CT) section of and (b) diagram of thoracic structures at the level of the sternoclavicular joint. CT sections are conventionally represented with the anterior surface uppermost and with the subject's right at the left of the viewed image. The viewer should imagine, therefore, that each slice is being viewed from further down the body. At this level six large vessels are visible.

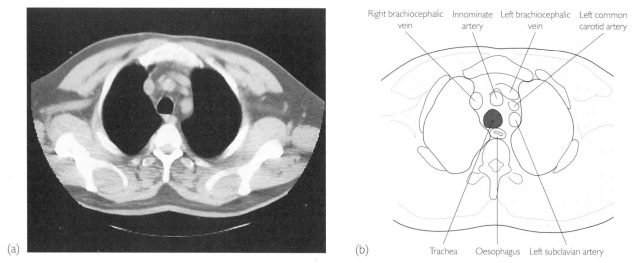

(a)

(b)

Right brachiocephalic vein   Innominate artery   Left brachiocephalic vein   Left common carotid artery

Trachea   Oesophagus   Left subclavian artery

Fig. 1.1.17 (a) Computed tomography section and (b) diagram 2 cm below the section in Figure 1.1.16 at the level of the brachiocephalic vein. Compare with Figure 1.1.10.

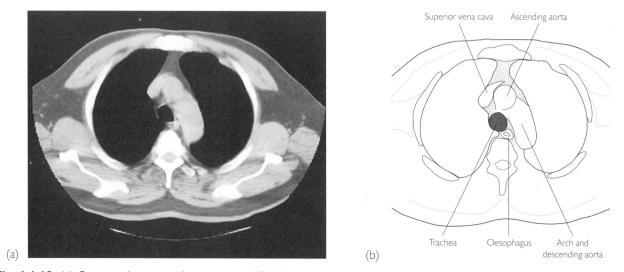

(a)

(b)

Superior vena cava   Ascending aorta

Trachea   Oesophagus   Arch and descending aorta

Fig. 1.1.18 (a) Computed tomography section and (b) diagram at the level of the aortic arch. At this level the veins have resolved into the superior vena cava and the arteries into the aortic arch.

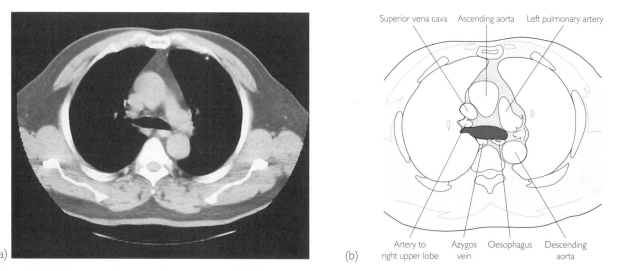

(a)

(b)

Superior vena cava   Ascending aorta   Left pulmonary artery

Artery to right upper lobe   Azygos vein   Oesophagus   Descending aorta

Fig. 1.1.19 (a) Computed tomography section and (b) diagram at the level of the left pulmonary artery and just above the main carina (bifurcation of the trachea). The left pulmonary artery lies higher than the right, which is not visible in this section.

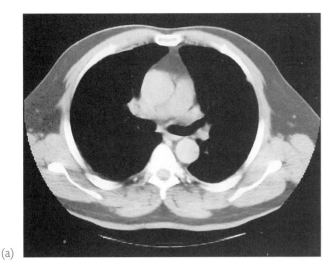

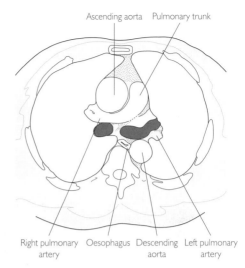

(a)   (b)

Fig. 1.1.20 (a) Computed tomography section and (b) diagram at the level of the right pulmonary artery. At this level the left pulmonary artery has passed over and behind the left upper lobe bronchus. The recess behind the intermediate bronchus and beneath the azygos venous arch is the azygo-oesophageal recess. This zone is difficult to visualise in posteroanterior radiographs. Compare with Figures 1.1.10 & 1.1.11.

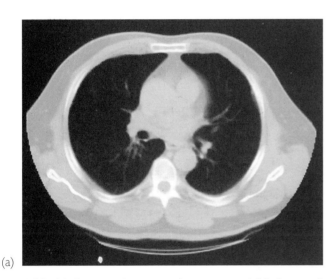

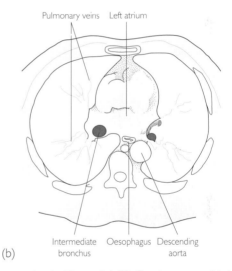

(a)   (b)

Fig. 1.1.21 (a) Computed tomography section and (b) diagram 2 cm below the section in Figure 1.1.20. Sections near this level show superior pulmonary veins and then inferior pulmonary veins converging on the left atrium. Compare with Figure 1.1.30(b).

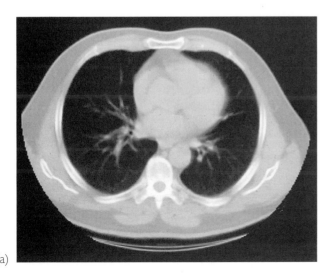

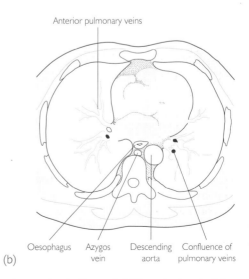

(a)   (b)

Fig. 1.1.22 (a) Computed tomography section and (b) diagram 2 cm below the section in Figure 1.1.21 at the level of the confluence of pulmonary veins. Compare with Figure 1.1.30(b).

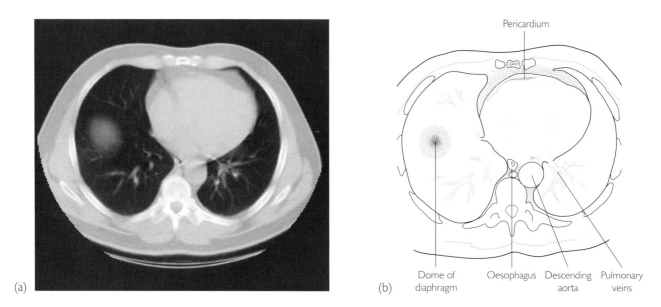

(a)

(b)

Pericardium

Dome of diaphragm   Oesophagus   Descending aorta   Pulmonary veins

Fig. 1.1.23 (a) Computed tomography section and (b) diagram at a lower level, at which the dome of the diaphragm is just appearing on the right. The pericardium is visible anteriorly, where it is outlined by surrounding fat.

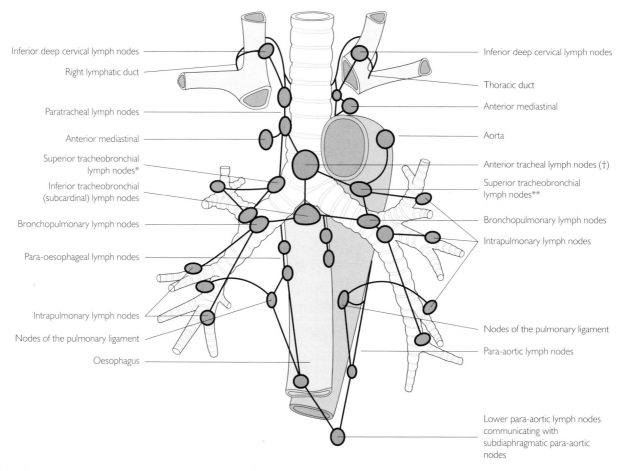

Inferior deep cervical lymph nodes

Right lymphatic duct

Paratracheal lymph nodes

Anterior mediastinal

Superior tracheobronchial lymph nodes*

Inferior tracheobronchial (subcardinal) lymph nodes

Bronchopulmonary lymph nodes

Para-oesophageal lymph nodes

Intrapulmonary lymph nodes

Nodes of the pulmonary ligament

Oesophagus

Inferior deep cervical lymph nodes

Thoracic duct

Anterior mediastinal

Aorta

Anterior tracheal lymph nodes (†)

Superior tracheobronchial lymph nodes**

Bronchopulmonary lymph nodes

Intrapulmonary lymph nodes

Nodes of the pulmonary ligament

Para-aortic lymph nodes

Lower para-aortic lymph nodes communicating with subdiaphragmatic para-aortic nodes

Fig. 1.1.24 Diagram of pulmonary and mediastinal lymph drainage and its relationship to the bronchial tree, aorta and oesophagus. The principal direction of drainage is centrally towards the mediastinum and upwards towards either the thoracic duct or the right lymphatic duct . On the right (*) a prominent superior tracheobronchial lymph node is sometimes referred to as the azygos lymph node and may be visible on the chest radiograph when enlarged. On the left (**) a superior tracheobronchial lymph node is commonly located under the aortic node and may be referred to as the subaortic node or the node of the recurrent laryngeal nerve palsy when it is enlarged because of malignancy. In addition to anterior tracheal lymph nodes (†), there are other, not shown, lying anterior to the aortic arch.

Fig. 1.1.25 View of larynx from above.

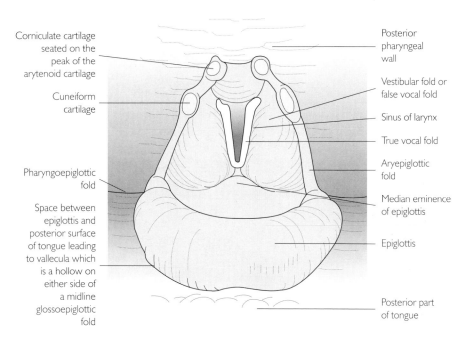

Corniculate cartilage seated on the peak of the arytenoid cartilage

Cuneiform cartilage

Pharyngoepiglottic fold

Space between epiglottis and posterior surface of tongue leading to vallecula which is a hollow on either side of a midline glossoepiglottic fold

Posterior pharyngeal wall

Vestibular fold or false vocal fold

Sinus of larynx

True vocal fold

Aryepiglottic fold

Median eminence of epiglottis

Epiglottis

Posterior part of tongue

angle of about 70° – a relationship usually put forward to explain the higher incidence of inhaled foreign bodies lodging in the right bronchial tree. The right main bronchus, after giving off the right upper lobe bronchus, continues downwards as the intermediate bronchus (intermediate, that is, between the upper lobe above and the middle and lower lobes below); there is no analogous bronchus on the left side.

The right upper lobe bronchus comes off the right main bronchus only a few centimetres from its origin. The level of the upper lobe orifice may be close to that of the carina. The position of the right upper lobe shows some variation and there is a continuum from arrangements in which the lobe opens off the trachea itself (tracheal bronchus) to one in which the right upper lobe arises at the end of a right main bronchus that is longer than usual.

Left main bronchus

The left main bronchus passes under the arch of the aorta and divides into upper and lower lobe bronchi. The upper lobe bronchus almost immediately gives off the lingular bronchus, which is almost in a straight line with the main bronchus, and the superior division of the left upper lobe.

Segmental anatomy

The most common pattern of division of the bronchi into lobar and segmental bronchi is shown in Figure 1.1.26. The nomenclature shown is that in widest use in the UK and derives from Foster Carter.[13] Considerable minor variation occurs, the most common forms of which amount to reduplication of the upper-lobe bronchi or aberrant opening of segmental bronchi proximally from the right or left main bronchus or from the intermediate bronchus.[14,15] Such variation is more common on the right than the left and more common in the upper lobes than in the lower lobes. For detailed descriptions of the more peripheral branching of airways and blood vessels the reader is referred to accounts, based on patient systematic dissections of large numbers of lungs, offered by Appleton[16] and Boyden.[17]

Figure 1.1.27 shows diagrammatic views of the approximate distribution of the pulmonary segments as they impinge on the surface of the lung. Each area indicates the base of a more or less pyramidal volume of the lung, which has the segmental bronchus at its apex.

Smaller bronchi and bronchioles

The horseshoe-shaped cartilaginous hoops of large bronchi give way to irregular plates of cartilage in the medium-sized bronchi. The muscle layer is more prominent and circular fibres surround more and more of the circumference as cartilage becomes more sparse in smaller bronchi. In bronchi of about 1 mm in diameter, all traces of cartilage disappear and the airway becomes by definition a bronchiole. Layers of muscle fibres now completely surround the airway in a circular and spiral arrangement. Smaller bronchioles become thin-walled and, at the point where an alveolus appears in the wall, the airway is termed a 'respiratory bronchiole'. The bronchiole proximal to the point where the respiratory bronchiole begins is referred to as a terminal bronchiole. Terminal bronchioles have a diameter of about 0.5 mm. Each terminal bronchiole supplies a small, self-contained standard unit of peripheral lung anatomy – the acinus.

Branching

The branching of the bronchi resembles that of a tree, large branches giving successively smaller branches, all gracefully tapering towards the periphery (Fig. 1.1.28). Branching is dichotomous, i.e. by division into two at each step. The process is, however, irregular in that the subdivisions of parent airways are usually of different length and calibre. The difference in size is often considerable. There seems to be a complex but standard relationship between the respective sizes of the two branches at any division and the length of the pathway in each and also between the sizes of the two branches and the angle at which

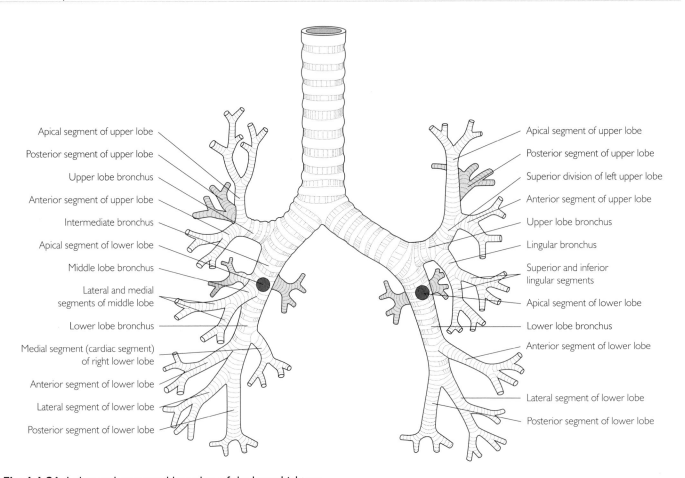

Apical segment of upper lobe
Posterior segment of upper lobe
Upper lobe bronchus
Anterior segment of upper lobe
Intermediate bronchus
Apical segment of lower lobe
Middle lobe bronchus
Lateral and medial segments of middle lobe
Lower lobe bronchus
Medial segment (cardiac segment) of right lower lobe
Anterior segment of lower lobe
Lateral segment of lower lobe
Posterior segment of lower lobe

Apical segment of upper lobe
Posterior segment of upper lobe
Superior division of left upper lobe
Anterior segment of upper lobe
Upper lobe bronchus
Lingular bronchus
Superior and inferior lingular segments
Apical segment of lower lobe
Lower lobe bronchus
Anterior segment of lower lobe
Lateral segment of lower lobe
Posterior segment of lower lobe

Fig. 1.1.26 Lobar and segmental branches of the bronchial tree.

they come off the parent airways. It seems possible that this relationship may give the branches aerodynamic and resistive properties that adjust the airflow to an appropriate degree. At times the airways divide not into two but into three or four divisions at once. These are conventionally regarded as dichotomous branchings that occur close together.

The number of divisions of the airways below the carina to the point where a terminal bronchiole is reached varies between seven or eight in the case of some lung units near the hilum to 24 in the case of lung units furthest from the hilum. It has been estimated from sampling techniques on fixed lungs that there are about 20 000–30 000 terminal bronchioles (and therefore the same number of acini) in the lungs.[18] Within the acinus there are on average three further dichotomous subdivisions of respiratory bronchioles, each being more completely enveloped by alveolar sacs and alveoli.

The total cross-sectional area of the airways increases with each subdivision from about 2 cm² in the trachea to about 80 cm² at terminal bronchiole level and nearly 300 cm² after three orders of respiratory bronchiole. After a further three to nine divisions of alveolar ducts, the cross-sectional area of the airway has increased, according to one authority, to several thousand square centimetres. This classic trumpet-shaped concept of the increase in cross-sectional area with each branching carries with it the implication that within the lobule itself linear velocity of airflow must be very slow indeed relative to the rate in the

trachea. So slow is the airflow that it is necessary to postulate gas transfer by a process of diffusion in the air spaces to account for normal gas exchange. The classic trumpet model may overestimate the peripheral cross-sectional area by failing to take into account the highly asymmetrical nature of the dichotomous branching. The whole subject of the branching of the human airway has been elegantly reviewed by Horsfield.[19]

Lung parenchyma

The microscopic anatomy of the components of the lung parenchyma is outlined in Chapter 1.2. The most convenient basic unit is the *acinus* – the peripheral airways and related blood vessels distal to the terminal bronchiole (see above). The acinus has a diameter of about 7 mm.[20] Other subunits of the lung that have been used in describing parenchymal anatomy and pathology are the primary and secondary lobules. The *primary lobule* is the lung distal to the last respiratory bronchiole. There are therefore about eight primary lobules within an acinus. The *secondary lobule* is the smallest subsection of the lung that is surrounded by a defined layer of connective tissue.

The secondary lobule contains about five or six terminal bronchioles, which have their origins from the more proximal bronchi very close together. The distribution of the connective tissue

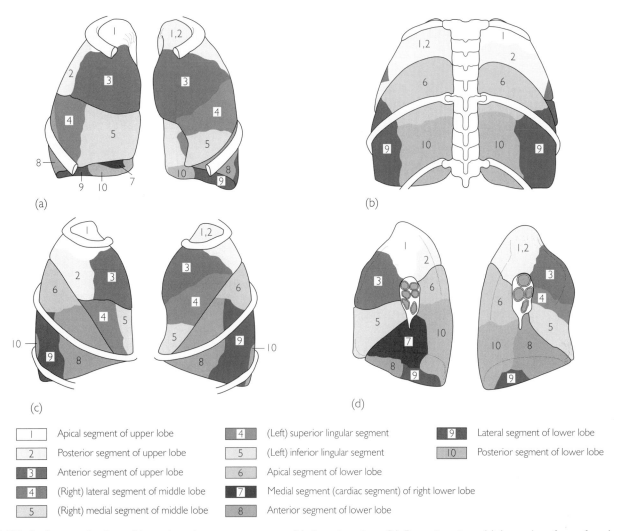

(a)

(b)

(c)

(d)

1 Apical segment of upper lobe	4 (Left) superior lingular segment	9 Lateral segment of lower lobe
2 Posterior segment of upper lobe	5 (Left) inferior lingular segment	10 Posterior segment of lower lobe
3 Anterior segment of upper lobe	6 Apical segment of lower lobe	
4 (Right) lateral segment of middle lobe	7 Medial segment (cardiac segment) of right lower lobe	
5 (Right) medial segment of middle lobe	8 Anterior segment of lower lobe	

Fig. 1.1.27 Surface projection of bronchopulmonary segments. (a) Anterior view. (b) Posterior view. (c) Lateral surface of each lung. (d) Medial surface of each lung.

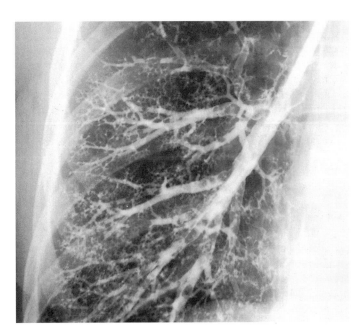

septa that demarcate secondary lobules is, however, very uneven because the lung is quite well-developed laterally in the lower lobes (where the septa appear as Kerley B lines when thickened by distended lymphatic channels) and poorly developed medially and deep in the lungs. Secondary lobules have been found to be of varying size (around 1–2.5 cm in diameter) and, moreover, difficult to recognise. The acinus has become the most used unit of peripheral lung for purposes of pathological description and it is probably the smallest lung unit that is reliably identifiable on the chest radiograph when lung parenchyma is abnormally opacified.[21]

Anatomy of the acinus

The general arrangement of the acinus is indicated in Figure 1.1.29. The respiratory bronchiole divides into an average of three further orders of respiratory bronchioles by asymmetrical

Fig. 1.1.28 Bronchogram showing normal branching pattern. (Courtesy of Dr W. Simpson.)

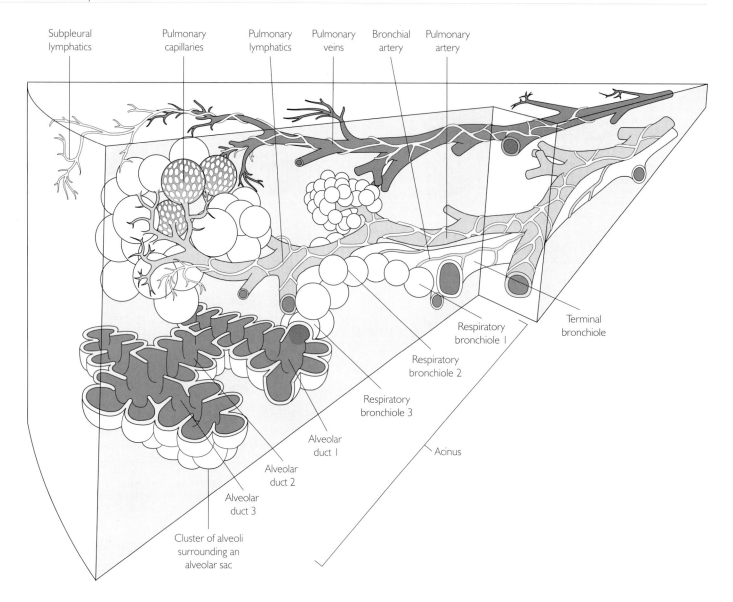

Subpleural lymphatics · Pulmonary capillaries · Pulmonary lymphatics · Pulmonary veins · Bronchial artery · Pulmonary artery

Terminal bronchiole

Respiratory bronchiole 1

Respiratory bronchiole 2

Respiratory bronchiole 3

Alveolar duct 1

Alveolar duct 2

Alveolar duct 3

Acinus

Cluster of alveoli surrounding an alveolar sac

Fig. 1.1.29 Peripheral lung structure. Schematic representation of a wedge of peripheral lung tissue with the pleural surface to the left; only a few of the branches are shown. Bronchioles are shown dividing, closely accompanied by corresponding branches of the pulmonary artery. The terminal bronchiole is the most peripheral bronchiole not to have alveoli in its wall. Fine radicles of the bronchial artery are present in its wall. The structures distal to the terminal bronchiole make up the acinus. Three or more orders of respiratory bronchioles 1, 2, 3, which have alveoli in their walls, give rise to three to eight orders of alveolar ducts (alveolar ducts 1, 2, 3, etc.), in which the wall of the airways is completely made up by the mouths of alveoli or alveolar sacs. An alveolar sac is a terminal air space approximately equivalent to an alveolus in size that is completely made up by the mouths of a cluster of alveoli and the supplying alveolar duct. Alveoli take up complex polyhedral shapes but are shown as rounded shapes in this simplified representation. Pulmonary capillaries drain into pulmonary veins, which take a course through the lung separate from that of the pulmonary artery and airway. Pulmonary capillary blood from an acinus may drain into several adjacent pulmonary venules (only one pulmonary venule is shown in the diagram). Pulmonary venules accept blood from several adjacent acini. Subpleural lymphatics drain centrally into lymphatic channels surrounding pulmonary veins, some forming a network that lies in tissue planes between lobules (see text). Lymphatics derived from alveolar tissue drain partly into these channels and partly into other lymphatics, which drain medially via a network that envelops the pulmonary artery. The term 'pulmonary lobule' is now used less often than 'acinus' in describing peripheral lung structure. The primary lobule comprises the structures distal to (and including) the first order of alveolar ducts. The secondary lobule comprises the peripheral lung bounded by connective tissue septa. These septa are very variable in distribution and difficult to discern but a typical secondary lobule could be considered as occupying a volume about four times that of the wedge of tissue shown in the diagram.

dichotomous division. Each of these bears alveolar ducts made up completely of alveoli off which open alveolar sacs – clusters of alveoli. There are about 800 alveolar ducts in each acinus.[22] The supplying terminal bronchiole and the accompanying pulmonary arteriole enter the acinus from the apex. The pulmonary venules form from capillaries draining towards the outer border of the acinus.

The pulmonary circulation

Principal pulmonary arteries

The main pulmonary artery (or pulmonary trunk) begins at the pulmonary valve and curves upwards, to the left and backwards as shown in Figure 1.1.11. Just before it divides it constitutes part of the left border of the cardiac silhouette on the PA radiograph. The *right pulmonary artery* passes under the arch of the aorta more or less horizontally and before entering the hilum divides into a superior division (which supplies the upper lobe) and the continuation of the main trunk. The superior division, which is quite prominent and is sometimes referred to as the truncus anterior, lies in front of the right upper lobe bronchi and its branches follow those of the airways. The lower division proceeds downwards, lying in front of the intermediate and lower lobe bronchi passing outside the middle lobe bronchus.

The *left pulmonary artery* takes a backward and upward course and contributes to the pulmonary artery silhouette on the PA radiograph. It lies about 1 cm higher than the right pulmonary artery (Fig. 1.1.30a). The remains of the ductus arteriosus of the neonate connects the left pulmonary artery to the

arch of the aorta above. The artery divides into a short superior division, which promptly divides into branches supplying the upper lobe. The inferior division hooks backwards over the top of the upper lobe bronchus and continues downwards and backwards lateral to and a little behind the lower lobe bronchus (see Fig. 1.1.11). In doing so it forms a vascular arch, which is seen on a lateral radiograph as a smaller curved shadow lying below that of the aorta (see Fig. 1.1.42).

The distribution of the pulmonary arteries within the lobes of the lungs, although broadly following the branching pattern of the bronchi, shows considerable variation.

Structure of the pulmonary blood vessels

The large pulmonary arteries have prominent concentric elastic laminae in their walls, although the walls are strikingly thinner than systemic arteries of similar diameter. Elastic arteries are found down to vessels of 1 mm diameter, after which the elastic laminae become limited to internal and external laminae and between these circular muscle is found. These small arteries are referred to as muscular arteries although the amount of muscle is slight compared with analogous systemic vessels. Vessels smaller than $100\,\mu m$ lose their muscular layer and have only a single elastic lamina. Pulmonary venules resemble arterioles in structure. Larger pulmonary veins have an irregular muscular layer and a more prominent fibrous adventitial coat.

Pulmonary veins

The four pulmonary veins drain into the left atrium; the upper pair drain the upper lobes (and the middle lobe on the right) and the lower pair the lower lobes. In the hila and central portion of

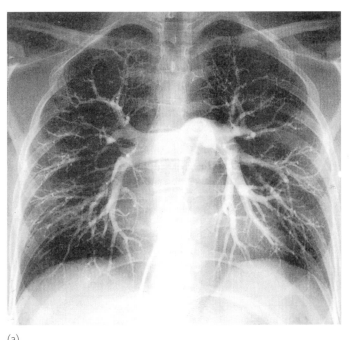

(a)

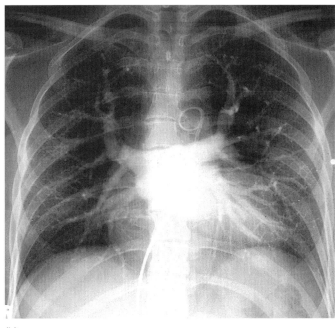

(b)

Fig. 1.1.30 Normal pulmonary angiogram: (a) arterial phase; (b) venous phase. The contrast medium has been injected through a pigtail catheter in the main pulmonary artery. (Courtesy of Dr W. Simpson.)

the lungs the veins are applied to the front of the arteries and airways (see Fig. 1.1.11). From front to back the structures on the right are: vein, artery, bronchus. On the left, because the artery passes backwards over the top of the left upper lobe bronchus, the order approximates to: vein, bronchus, artery. The central veins have a fan-shaped arrangement that focuses on a point well below the origin of the pulmonary arteries (Fig. 1.1.30b, and see Fig. 1.1.11). This often allows distinction between arteries and veins on the radiograph. In particular, the upper lobe veins and the inferior divisions of the pulmonary arteries are often clearly seen crossing each other.

Intrapulmonary venous drainage

The pulmonary veins and pulmonary arteries pursue different courses both peripherally and centrally. The venules draining each pulmonary acinus are arranged around the periphery of the acinus (see Fig. 1.1.29) whereas the arteries penetrate the centre of the acinus alongside the supplying airway. This separation of veins from arteries in the lungs is preserved more centrally. Small veins drain towards larger ones, which are situated around the periphery of lung segments and travel in the connective tissue planes that separate them. The arteries, on the other hand, accompany the airways in the centre of the segment. The intersegmental veins here are not dedicated to particular segments but drain any adjacent segments. The separate distribution of veins and arteries in the hila of the lungs has already been referred to above.

Bronchial circulation

The bronchi, the bronchioles and the walls of the intrapulmonary arteries and veins are supplied by the bronchial arteries. This lesser bronchial circulation in the lungs communicates freely with the pulmonary circulation far out in the lung parenchyma and part of the blood passing through the bronchial arteries returns to the left side of the heart via the pulmonary veins. The overall relationship between the two circulations is represented in Figure 1.1.31.[23] The bronchial arteries are responsible for the blood supply to the airways down to the level of the terminal bronchiole and are also responsible for the supply to the visceral pleura, the lymphoid tissue of the lung and the walls of the intrapulmonary vessels. The bronchial circulation also supplies abnormal tissue in diseased lung such as tumours and abscesses. The bronchial circulation can make an important contribution to gas exchange in certain conditions where there is drastic interference with pulmonary blood supply. This may arise in some forms of congenital heart disease and there is also evidence from animal experimental work that bronchial circulation can increase to take over from severely reduced pulmonary blood flow in advanced chronic pulmonary thromboembolic disease. The structure and function of the bronchial circulation has been well reviewed by Deffebach et al.[24]

Bronchial arteries

The right bronchial artery usually arises from the third or fourth right intercostal artery but occasionally it arises as a branch of

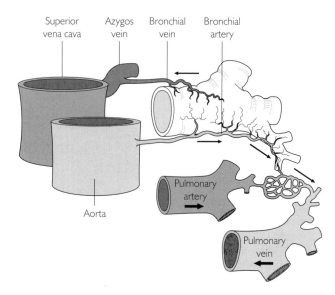

Fig. 1.1.31 Schematic diagram of bronchial circulation. (Reproduced with permission from Brewis.[23])

the left bronchial artery, which springs directly from the aorta itself. The branch passes to the right behind or below the carina and lies along the posterior surface of the right main bronchus, dividing with each branching of the airways. On the left side the bronchial artery arises from the aorta either just above the level of the left main bronchus near the end of the aortic arch or just below the bronchus at the beginning of the descending aorta. The pattern of supply varies considerably and very often there are multiple bronchial arteries, particularly on the left. Occasionally, the right bronchial artery arises as a long branch of the subclavian artery. This may have importance when bronchial artery embolisation is attempted in the management of heavy haemoptysis. The bronchial arteries give off branches that surround the bronchi and supply the outer structures and related adventitial tissue, and other branches that penetrate the muscular coat of the bronchi to supply a delicate but rich submucosal network of small vessels.

Bronchial veins

Blood from the bronchial circulation in the proximal bronchial tree returns by small bronchial veins to drain into the azygos vein on the right or hemiazygos vein on the left. Venous blood from smaller bronchi drains through communications with the pulmonary circulation.

Non-bronchial systemic vessels

The lung receives some systemic blood supply from tiny branches of the pericardiophrenic artery. This is derived from the internal mammary artery and runs close to the phrenic nerve. The importance of this supply is uncertain but it is thought that the walls of the pulmonary veins are supplied by it. Deep in the lung there may be anastomoses with the pulmonary circulation in the septal planes occupied by veins on the outside of acini.[25]

Lymphatic drainage of the lung

The lung has a lymphatic system that drains the parenchyma, air passages and pleura. Lymphatics draining the pleura pass medially in interlobular and then intersegmental planes accompanying the veins (see Fig. 1.1.29). In the lateral parts of the lower lobes the interlobular planes are arranged remarkably horizontally so that, when the lymphatics are greatly distended because of venous congestion, the alignment of the lymphatic vessels with a horizontal X-ray beam results in the casting of small horizontal linear shadows (Kerley B lines). No lymphatics are present in the walls of alveoli themselves. Lymphatic channels draining the parenchyma and airways begin in the centre of acini at alveolar duct or respiratory bronchiolar level and tend to accompany the airways and the arteries centrally. There is some communication between the network accompanying veins and that accompanying arteries.

Hilar lymph nodes

Lymph nodes may be found within the substance of the lung 1–2 cm from the hilum in about one in six normal individuals if careful dissection is undertaken.[26] These are usually small but occasionally cast a small, rounded shadow on the chest radiograph. The lymph nodes of the hilum comprise the bronchopulmonary nodes, which lie in relation to the main bronchi, and small nodes that may lie inferiorly in the hilar ligament (see Fig. 1.1.24). The mediastinal lymph nodes and thoracic duct are described above.

Nerve supply to the lung

The innervation of the lung remains incompletely understood. The subject has been reviewed by Richardson.[27,28] The lung derives a parasympathetic supply from the vagus and a sympathetic supply from the neighbouring sympathetic chain. On entering the lung root the two basic nerve sources become entwined in a plexus, which resolves into a network accompanying the pulmonary arteries and another which accompanies the airways. Microscopic aspects of the nerve supply of the lung are discussed in Chapter 1.2. The smooth muscle of the airways appears to have innervation of three types: vagal afferent; postganglionic, non-cholinergic vagal efferent; and non-adrenergic, non-cholinergic, which may also be derived from the vagus.[29] The smooth muscle appears to receive no direct sympathetic innervation. The innervation of the parietal pleura is derived from intercostal and phrenic nerves. The visceral pleura appears to have no sensory innervation.

Radiographic anatomy

The posteroanterior radiograph

The mediastinum

The mediastinal outline is determined by the air in the lungs, trachea or bronchi, delineating the boundaries of adjacent mediastinal soft tissues. Unlike CT, with its superior contrast resolution, the plain radiograph does not permit detection of the boundaries between mediastinal fat and other soft tissues, except occasionally around the heart. The position of interfaces between fat, soft tissue and air is clearly seen on the cross-sectional images provided by CT.

The right and left mediastinal borders

On the right, a small segment of the brachiocephalic vein can be seen as it emerges from the soft tissues of the neck at the level of the clavicle. Inferiorly, it merges with the superior vena cava, which, with the right atrium, forms the remaining right heart border. The azygos vein may be seen as an added density superimposed on the superior vena cava and, if large, may produce a bulge just above the origin of the right main bronchus. This should not be confused with the enlarged tracheobronchial node. The azygos vein is normally less than 1 cm in diameter, may be considerably larger, e.g. when there is thrombosis or congenital absence of the inferior vena cava. In elderly people an ectatic brachiocephalic artery may produce a convex right border instead of the concave outline of the superior vena cava. On the left, the upper border of the mediastinum starts with the subclavian artery. Like the right brachiocephalic vein, this fades out at the level of the clavicles, where it merges with the soft tissues of the neck and has a concave border to the lung. Situated inferiorly is the aortic arch or knuckle.

Occasionally, the superior intercostal vein projects as a nipple on the outline of the knuckle as it runs forwards to join the left brachiocephalic vein (see Figs 1.1.13 & 1.1.17). Below the aortic arch the main pulmonary artery forms a slight bulge at the level of the hilum. The space between the two forms the lateral border of the aortopulmonary window, often a site of lymph node enlargement. The left atrial appendage occupies the space below the pulmonary trunk but unless enlarged is not usually recognisable as a discrete structure. The left ventricle forms the remainder of the left border.

Quite frequently, on the left side, there is extrapleural fat adjacent to the left ventricle and filling in the cardiophrenic angle. In this situation the fat rather than the left ventricle forms the left border. On the right side, fat is usually confined to the cardiophrenic angle, where it produces an additional bulge between the right atrium and the diaphragm. It is important to recognise the presence of these fat pads when measuring the heart. The true border of the heart can usually be identified as a slightly denser inner structure, since ventricular muscle attenuates X-rays more than fat (Fig. 1.1.32).

Mediastinal lines. In addition to the air–soft-tissue interface that forms the mediastinal outline, the lung contacts the mediastinum at numerous other points. If parallel to the X-ray beam, these interfaces may be detectable on a plain radiograph as lines or stripes. Only those most commonly seen will be described. A diagrammatic summary of these lines is shown in Figure 1.1.33.

Junctional lines. The junctional lines are formed where the right and left lung are separated from each other by four layers of pleura only. These are the points where a lung can potentially herniate to the opposite side. Unless there is a large amount of mediastinal fat, the lungs are usually in contact between the

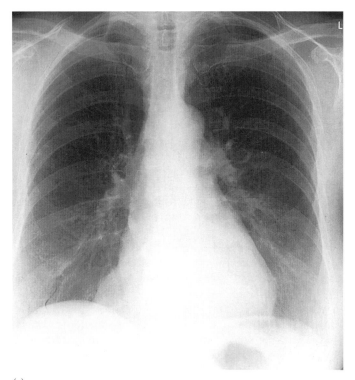

(a)

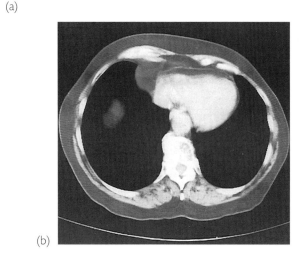

(b)

Fig. 1.1.32 Mediastinal fat. (a) Plain radiograph showing fat in the right cardiophrenic angle and parallel to the left heart border in an obese subject. (b) Computed tomography section from the same patient demonstrating the cardiophrenic fat and also the pericardium as a thin line within the fat anterior to the heart.

sternum and the ascending aorta or great vessels (see Figs 1.1.12 & 1.1.13), forming the anterior junctional line. Seen in cross-section (see Fig. 1.1.20) the line tends to pass from the right posteriorly to the left anteriorly and is therefore not usually parallel to the X-ray beam. When it is parallel, a line will be seen on the plain PA film (Fig. 1.1.34). Superiorly, the line cannot be seen above the sternal notch where the pleura is reflected laterally over the great vessels. Inferiorly, the line is limited by the pleurae separating over the right ventricle (see Fig. 1.1.22b). The posterior junctional line is formed by the lungs contacting

behind the oesophagus (see Figs 1.1.12 & 1.1.13). It is not continuous, as the pleurae separate at the level of the azygos and aortic arches. Superiorly, it may extend up to the apices but inferiorly it is often not seen below the aortic arch (Fig. 1.1.35). Visualisation of a junctional line excludes a mass in that region but the lines are inconstant and their absence does not necessarily indicate disease.

Para-oesophageal lines. Both lungs are potentially in contact with the oesophagus except at the level of the aortic and azygos arches. This results in four potential air–soft-tissue interfaces: between the lungs and the lateral borders of the oesophagus and between the inner borders of the oesophagus and air in the lumen. The para-oesophageal lines are more commonly seen than the posterior junctional line but it may be difficult or impossible to distinguish between them.

Right paratracheal line. The trachea is normally in contact with right lung throughout its intrathoracic course. As the inner wall is outlined by air in the tracheal lumen, a line or stripe is produced that represents the right wall of the trachea, the pleura and any interposed fat (Fig. 1.1.36). This line should be smooth and less than 4 mm in thickness. The line widens where the pleura is reflected over the azygos arch and below this continues as the upper border of the right main bronchus.

Paravertebral lines. Both lungs border the paraspinal soft tissues potentially producing lines (see Fig. 1.1.32). On the right the interface is oblique whereas on the left the descending aorta causes the interface to be sagittal and therefore parallel to the beam. The line is therefore more frequently seen on the left unless there is a right-sided descending aorta. Superiorly, the line curves sharply medially above the aortic arch. Widening of the line may be caused by a soft tissue mass usually secondary to spinal disease, enlarged retro-oesophageal nodes or dilated azygos and hemiazygos veins. The line may also be widened in the elderly because of aortic dilatation or spinal osteophyte formation and, in the obese, by fat deposition. A localised bulge is, however, usually pathological.

The Mach effect

The paraspinal line may be seen as a white line between two areas of radiolucency rather than as an interface. This may be caused by low-density lung and paraspinal fat outlining the interposed pleura but often it is spurious and caused by the Mach effect. Ernst Mach described an optical illusion which may be seen at the border between a dark and light image where a thin line appears at the boundary. This may appear either as a dark or a light line. If the light side is covered and the mask is moved to the edge of the boundary, the line disappears, confirming that it is an optical illusion (Fig. 1.1.37). The aorta (convex to the lung) always produces a dark Mach band whereas the left paraspinal line (concave to the lung) produces a light one. The Mach effect enables them to be differentiated from one another.

Azygo-oesophageal recess

Pleura reflected off the azygos arch passes medially and inferiorly to contact the right border of the oesophagus. This produces a line that is concave towards the right lung and inferiorly continues as the para-oesophageal line. The space behind the heart bordered medially by this line is called the azygo-oesophageal recess. It is easily appreciated on CT (see Fig. 1.1.21) but abnormalities

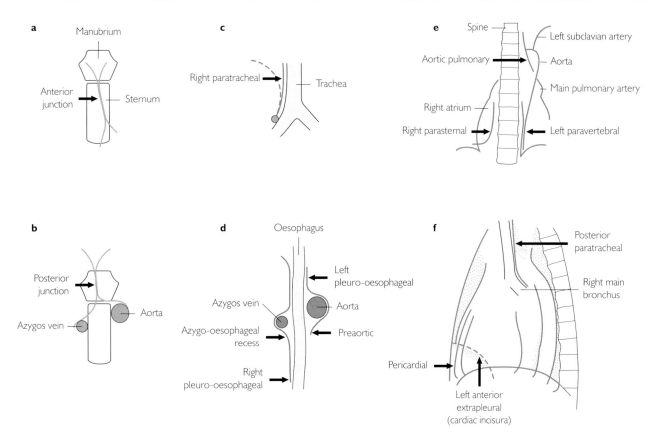

Fig. 1.1.33 Mediastinal lines. (a–e) Posteroanterior (PA) views. (a) The anterior junctional line formed by contact between the right and left pleural layers behind the sternum usually runs slightly obliquely as shown. It is best seen in the left anterior oblique view and never extends above the sternum. (b) The posterior junctional line is formed by contact between right and left pleural layers behind the oesophagus in the upper mediastinum. The line is straight or convex to the left and extends above the manubrium in the PA view. (c) The right paratracheal line ends below at the azygos vein. The dotted line in the diagram represents the right subclavian vessels and the superior vena cava. (d) Right and left pleuro-oesophageal lines. Below the aorta a pre-aortic line may be visible; below the azygos vein the right pleuro-oesophageal line marks the azygo-oesophageal recess. (e) An aortic pulmonary line may be visible on the left anterior to the left subclavian artery and the aorta. A left paravertebral line may be visible as pleura is reflected behind the descending aorta on to the sides of the vertebral bodies. A right parasternal line is sometimes visible representing the pleural reflection behind the costal cartilages. (f) Lateral view of the mediastinum. The posterior paratracheal line continues below along the posterior surface of the right main bronchus. A pericardial line may be visible parallel with the cardiac outline anteriorly. The reflection of the pleura at the cardiac incisura may be visible as a left anterior extrapleural line, which appears curved convex posteriorly in this view.

in this area such as enlarged subcarinal nodes are easily missed on a PA film. Pleural deflections over the posterior part of the azygos arch can be projected over the lower trachea and be mistaken for tracheal stenosis.

Aortopulmonary window

This recess is situated between the aortic arch and the left pulmonary artery and is bordered laterally by the pleural reflection between these structures (see Fig. 1.1.19). The aortopulmonary window is very variable in depth and in its plain radiographic appearance.

The hila

In strict anatomical usage, the hilum of the lung contains all of the structures passing into the lung from the mediastinum. On the PA radiograph the hilum consists of the shadows cast by the central pulmonary arteries. The pulmonary veins enter the left atrium at a lower level.

As the hilar shadow is made up of several arteries branching in different directions, its boundary is only intermittently defined by the edges of the vessels that happen to be tangential to the X-ray beam. Consistently shown are the upper edge of the main left pulmonary artery and the lateral edges of the right intermediate pulmonary artery.

The extent to which the hila protrude beyond the edge of the mediastinum is variable, depending upon several factors. These include the amount of mediastinal fat, the size of the thymus in a child, unfolding of the aorta, positional rotation for the straight PA and the size of the hila. Several attempts have been made to establish normal values for the size of the hila and the individual pulmonary arteries contributing to the hilar shadow. None has been widely used and all suffer from the difficulty of defining end-points for measurement. The right hilum lies at a slightly

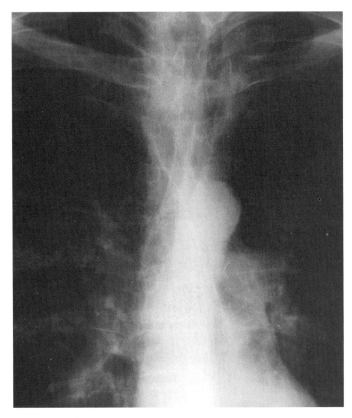

Fig. 1.1.34 Anterior junctional line. This passes obliquely upwards from left to right splitting and fading out at its upper limit below the level of the sternoclavicular joints. (Courtesy of Dr W. Simpson.)

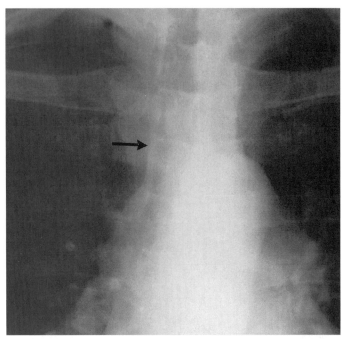

Fig. 1.1.36 Right paratracheal line. The line represents paratracheal tissues outlined by tracheal lumen medially and lung laterally. Normally this consists of the tracheal wall only. Caudally it splits around the azygos arch at the junction of the trachea and right main bronchus. (Courtesy of Dr W. Simpson.)

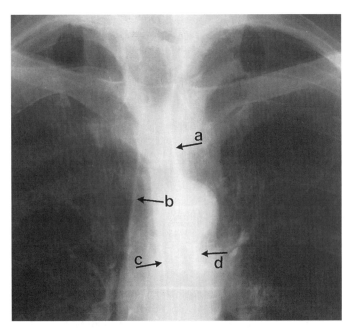

Fig. 1.1.35 Mediastinal lines. Posteroanterior radiograph showing (a) upper posterior junctional line; (b) right paratracheal line; (c) anterior junctional line; (d) lower posterior junctional line. (Courtesy of Dr W. Simpson.)

lower level than the left. A marked difference in the relative position of the hila should always raise the suspicion of lobar collapse. When the two hila lie at the same level this can be normal, but it may be the result of a congenital anomaly. For example, there may be duplication of the right lung. The hila will then appear symmetrical, with the upper lobe bronchus above the artery on both sides, the main bronchi equal in length on the two sides (normally the left is longer than the right) and horizontal fissures on both sides.

The pulmonary vessels

The pulmonary arteries emerge from the hila like shadows of the branches of a leafless tree. Some lying at right angles to the X-ray beam are identifiable as tapering branching structures. Others lying parallel to the beam are seen as rounded shadows – the so-called end-on appearance. It is important not to mistake central end-on arteries for pulmonary nodules and more peripheral ones for diffuse micronodular shadowing. The distinction can at times be very difficult if not impossible.

The pulmonary veins are indistinguishable from arteries in the periphery of the lungs. More centrally they diverge from the arteries as they approach the mediastinum. Below the hila they can be identified as separate structures as they converge to enter the left atrium (Fig. 1.1.38). Sometimes veins can be identified in the upper lobes, where they have a larger distance between branches and a more vertical orientation than arteries. In the upright position, gravity influences the distension of pulmonary veins. They are more distended in the lower lobes than in the

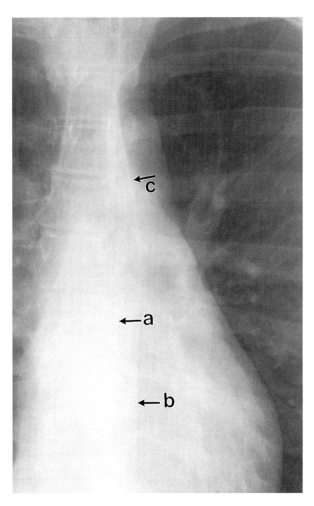

Fig. 1.1.37 Mediastinal lines and Mach bands. a, left paravertebral line; b, edge of descending aorta; c, paravertebral line behind the aortic arch. A Mach band is an optical illusion seen at the boundary between light and dark. It appears as a light or dark band, which will disappear when the light or dark adjacent area is masked out. It is most obvious at c. If the adjacent lung up to the line is covered with a piece of card the bright band will disappear. (Courtesy of Dr W. Simpson.)

upper lobes. Normally pulmonary vessels are not prominent in the upper lobes. In the supine position the vessels are equally prominent throughout the lungs. Reversal of this normal distribution can be seen in heart failure, where there is increased pulmonary venous pressure, perhaps with vasoconstriction in the lower lobes. It may also be seen in chronic obstructive pulmonary disease (COPD) as a consequence of vascular obliteration in the lower lobes and in any condition associated with pulmonary hypertension where the distribution of pulmonary blood flow is relatively less dependent on gravity.

The bronchi

Very little can be seen of the bronchi on a normal chest radiograph. They can be seen in the mediastinum at and close to the hila as darker band-like structures when they are surrounded by

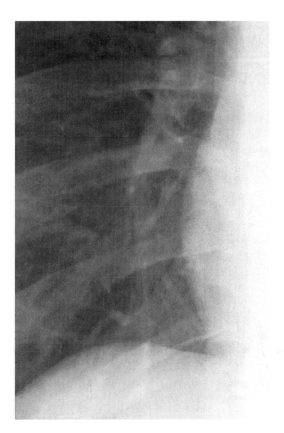

Fig. 1.1.38 The pulmonary veins converge towards the left atrium below the hilum, crossing branches of the pulmonary artery.

vessels. Near the hilum end-on bronchi appear as light rings with dark centres. The ring shadow cast by the bronchial wall is only a fraction of a millimetre thick. Prominence of the bronchial walls is always abnormal – a sign of a variety of diseases that can cause thickening of the bronchial walls or the surrounding interstitial tissues.

The fissures

Only the horizontal fissure is normally detectable on the PA radiograph as a fine horizontal line just below the level of the right hilum. Its height and orientation are variable. Although a change in position can be an indication of a change in volume of the adjacent lobes, this variability should be borne in mind. Rarely, the upper end of the oblique fissure can be seen on a PA radiograph as indrawing of the pleura just below the apex of the lung. The azygos fissure (see Fig. 1.1.8) is the most frequently seen accessory fissure. Others may be seen in the lower lobes (see above).

The diaphragm

In spite of the fact that anatomically and physiologically the diaphragm is a single unit, it has become conventional to refer to right and left diaphragms when discussing the PA radiograph. The diaphragms should be visible from the lateral chest wall to the mediastinum on both sides. On the left side this depends on the highest aspect of the diaphragm lying posterior to the heart and on adequate penetration of the film. Failure to see the medial part of the left diaphragm should raise the possibility of disease in the lower lobe or medial basal pleura.

The intersection of the diaphragm with the lateral chest wall is known as the costophrenic angle, recess or sulcus. The surfaces of the diaphragm normally appear smoothly convex towards the lung. Flattening can occur with overinflation of the lungs. In these circumstances the sharpness of the costophrenic angle may be lost and the attachments of the diaphragm to the chest wall may be visible as angular shadows on its upper margin. The upper surface of the right diaphragm is projected between the anterior ends of the fifth and seventh ribs in most normal individuals. The height of the diaphragm is related to the patient's build, tending to be higher in short, obese, broad-chested individuals than in those with the opposite characteristics. The fact that the right diaphragm is at a higher level than the left is well known. It is less well known that this does not depend on the position of the liver. Review of patients with complex congenital heart diseases and visceral heterotaxy has shown that the lower diaphragm is found on the side of the functional left ventricle irrespective of the position of the liver.[30]

The chest wall

Companion shadows
Shadows cast by extrapleural soft tissues and running parallel either to the chest wall or to the lower margins of ribs are known as companion shadows. The presence of fat in the extrapleural space can produce an appearance simulating pleural thickening (Fig. 1.1.39). This is particularly liable to occur in obese individuals. When present it will usually be symmetrical, uniform and predominantly over the upper lobes. Individual shadows of this sort are particularly likely to accompany the lower borders of the second and third ribs and have been shown to be due to the projection of soft tissues, including intercostal vessels and fat, below the ribs because of the relatively lower trajectory of the X-ray beam relative to the blade of the rib in the upper chest.[31] There is a close relationship between the thickness of the shadows and the degree of obesity and it has been shown that in any individual they become thinner with weight reduction. Lower in the chest the muscles of the chest wall – serratus anterior and the intercostals – together with accompanying fat can produce companion shadows running parallel to the lateral parts of the ribs (Fig. 1.1.40). These tend to be symmetrical and should not be mistaken for pleural plaques.

The lateral chest radiograph

The mediastinum

Anterior and posterior mediastinal borders
The lower part of the anterior border of the mediastinum is formed by the right ventricle. The clarity and extent to which this is visualised depends on the size of the thymus and the amount of lung tissue between the anterior border and the sternum. In infants the normal large thymus fills most of this space and is indistinguishable from the heart. In adults the thymus is not detectable unless abnormal. The extent to which the lungs meet in front of the heart depends on the habitus and the amount of fat in the anterior mediastinum. In most normal persons the lowest part of the right ventricle will contact the retrosternal soft tissues with no intervening lung. Above the right ventricle the anterior border is formed sequentially by the main pulmonary artery, ascending aorta and superior vena cava. The contribution made by the anterior edge of the ascending aorta depends on its unfolding. It therefore increases with age. The back of the left ventricle forms the lower part of the posterior border. Passing cranially, this merges imperceptibly with the back of the left hilum. Above the left hilum the border is interrupted by vessels and bronchi emerging from the posterior part of the hila. The upper part of the posterior border is completed by the back of the trachea or oesophagus.

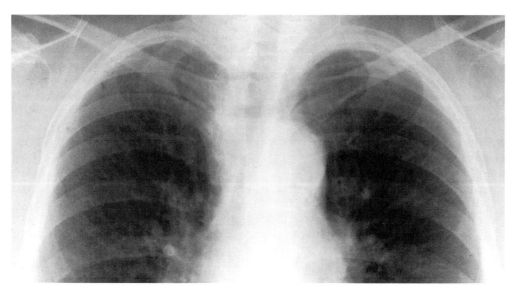

Fig. 1.1.39 Extrapleural fat. The thin layer of tissue between the lung and ribs is normal extrapleural fat, not abnormal pleural thickening. Note the symmetry and even distribution. The appearances are commonly found in obese individuals.

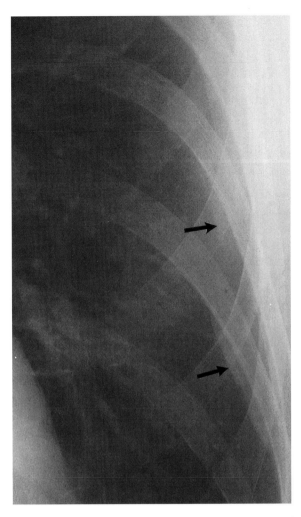

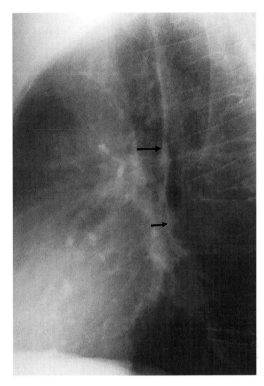

Fig. 1.1.41 Posterior paratracheal line: lateral radiograph showing the posterior paratracheal line (upper arrow) which is continuous inferiorly with the line caused by the main and intermediate bronchi contacting lung posteriorly (lower arrow).

Fig. 1.1.40 Companion shadows. Soft-tissue densities are shown running parallel to the ribs. They are caused by internal bulging of the intercostal tissues.

Mediastinal lines

The posterior paratracheal line is formed by the tissue between the lumen of the trachea and the right lung lying posterior to it (Fig. 1.1.41). Usually, this is simply the posterior wall of the trachea. Sometimes the oesophagus contributes to a thickening of this line. Inferiorly it may be interrupted by the azygos arch, below which it continues as the posterior wall of the right main bronchus. This feature distinguishes the right and left main bronchi on the lateral film.

The pericardial line represents the two layers of the pericardium, anterior to the right ventricle, sandwiched between epicardial fat and mediastinal fat. It is not invariably seen but its identification can be useful in excluding a pericardial effusion. It should be no thicker than the line of an interlobar fissure. The cardiac incisura or left anterior extrapleural line is the anterior edge of the left upper lobe where it reflects over the left ventricle. The shape of this varies considerably. The important point to remember is that the heart prevents the lower part of the left lung from reaching the anterior chest wall. This should reduce the risk of mistaking the normal appearance for abnormalities in the lower anterior part of the chest.

The hila

The different anatomical configurations of the two hila lead to a characteristic appearance of each on the lateral film (Fig. 1.1.42). The left pulmonary artery loops over the left upper lobe bronchus and is passed from front to back. The artery can be seen as a horn-shaped opacity with the black disc of the left upper lobe bronchus below its neck and the tapering lower lobe artery forming its lower descending part. The right pulmonary artery is projected as an end-on oval structure in the lateral radiograph. It lies anterior to the right bronchus intermedius which is easily identified by its posterior margin being the inferior continuation of the posterior paratracheal line. The left hilum lies above and behind the right hilum. This ability to identify and localise the two hila can be very useful when there is a suggestion of a hilar mass on the PA film.

The diaphragms

Both diaphragms are higher anteriorly than posteriorly. Their intersection with the chest wall produces a sharp costophrenic angle posteriorly. This is likely to be the lowest part of the pleural space. As a result, pleural fluid is detectable as a blunting of this angle before it is detectable on a PA film. The heart sits on the anterior part of the left diaphragm, being visualised on a lateral film. As the right diaphragm is visualised from front to back the difference is the most useful feature in distinguishing between the two diaphragms. The pleural reflection over the inferior vena cava as it passes between the diaphragm and right hilum can usually be

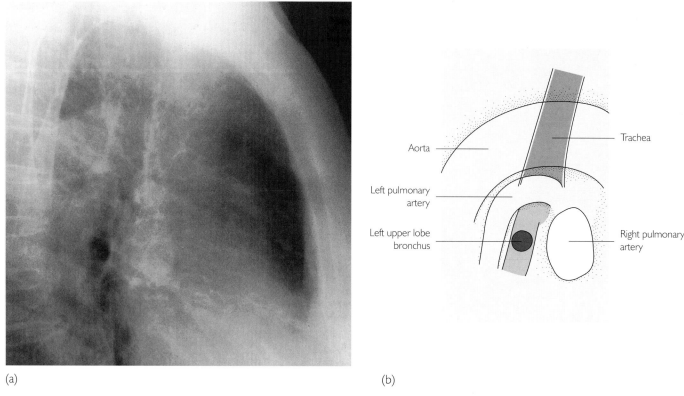

(a)   (b)

Fig. 1.1.42a, b Lateral view of hilum: the right pulmonary artery viewed end-on appears as an oval opacity anterior to and below the left pulmonary artery which is horn shaped and passes over the left upper lobe bronchus seen end-on as a round radiolucency. This is commonly misinterpreted as the left main bronchus at the carina. The carina is higher at the level of the left pulmonary arch.

seen as a 1–2 cm curvilinear shadow crossing the anterior part of the right diaphragm. Other useful features that help to distinguish the diaphragms on a lateral chest radiograph include:

- the gastric air bubble under the left diaphragm
- identification of the right oblique fissure by its continuity with the horizontal fissure and its intersection with the right diaphragm
- identification of the right and left posterior costophrenic angles.

This last feature depends on the greater magnification of the ribs on the side furthest from the film.

The lateral film is conventionally labelled as the side that is nearest the film. Thus on a left lateral film the left ribs posteriorly will appear to be slightly smaller than those on the right. For ordinary clinical purposes it does not matter which lateral view is taken or from which side the film is viewed; the amount of information available to the viewer is the same.

References

1. Von Hayek H. The human lung. New York: Hafner; 1960.
2. Jordanoglou J. Rib movement in health, kyphoscoliosis and ankylosing spondylosis. Thorax 1969; 24: 407.
3. Leigh Collis J, Kelly TD, Wiley AM. Anatomy of the crura of the diaphragm and the surgery of hiatus hernia. Thorax 1954; 9: 175.
4. Spencer J. Diaphragmatic hernia. In: Bouchier IAD, Allan RN, Hodgson JF, Keighley MRB, ed. Textbook of gastroenterology. London: Baillière Tindall; 1984: 75.
5. Davies R. Recurring spontaneous pneumothorax concomitant with menstruation. Thorax 1968; 23: 370.
6. Von Euler C. The control of respiratory movement. In: Howell JBL, Campbell EJM, ed. Breathlessness. Oxford: Blackwell Scientific; 1966: 19.
7. Lachman E. A comparison of the posterior boundaries of lungs and pleura as demonstrated on the cadaver and on roentgenograms of the living. Anat Record 1942; 83: 521.
8. Woodbourne RT. The costomedial border of the left pleura in the praecordial area. Anat Record 1947; 97: 197.
9. Trapnell DH. The differential diagnosis of linear shadows in chest radiographs. Radiol Clin North Am 1973; 11: 77.
10. Baird JA. The pathways of lymphatic spread of carcinoma of the lung. Br J Surg 1965; 52: 868.
11. Rosenberger A, Abrams HL. Radiology of the thoracic duct. AJR 1971; 111: 807.
12. Celis A, Porter JK. Lymphatics of the thorax – an anatomic and radiologic study. Acta Radiol 1952; 38: 461.
13. Foster Carter AF. The anatomy of the bronchial tree. Br J Tuberculosis 1942; 36: 19.
14. Laforet EG, Starkey WB, Scheff. Anomalies of upper lobe distribution. J Thorac Cardiovasc Surg 1962; 43: 595.
15. Atwell SW. Major anomalies of the tracheobronchial tree with a list of minor anomalies. Dis Chest 1967; 52: 611.
16. Appleton AB. Segments and blood vessels of the lungs. Lancet 1944; 2: 592.
17. Boyden EA. The intrahilar and related segmental anatomy of the lung. Surgery 1945; 18: 706.
18. Horsfield K, Cumming G. Morphology of the bronchial tree in man. J Appl Physiol 1968; 24: 373.
19. Horsfield K. The structure of the tracheobronchial tree. In: Scadding JG, Cumming G, ed. Scientific foundations of respiratory medicine. London: Heinemann; 1981: 54.
20. Pump KK. The morphology of the finer branches of the bronchial tree of the human lung. Dis Chest 1964; 46: 379.

21. Fraser RG, Paré PAG. Diagnosis of diseases of the chest, 2nd ed. Philadelphia, PA: WB Saunders; 1978: 52.
22. Parker H, Horsfield K, Cumming G. Morphology of distal airways in the human lung. J Appl Physiol 1971; 31: 386.
23. Brewis RAL. Lecture notes in respiratory disease, 4th ed. Oxford: Blackwell Scientific; 1991.
24. Deffebach ME, Charan NB, Lakshminaryan S, Butler J. The bronchial circulation; small but a vital attribute of the lung. Am Rev Respir Dis 1987; 135: 463.
25. Parke WW, Nichels NA. The nonbronchial systemic arteries of the lung. J Thorac Cardiovasc Surg 1965; 49: 694.

26. Trapnell DH. Recognition and incidence of intrapulmonary lymph nodes. Thorax 1964; 44: 50.
27. Richardson JB. Nerve supply to the lungs. Am Rev Respir Dis 1979; 119: 785.
28. Richardson JB. Recent progress in pulmonary innervation. Am Rev Respir Dis 1983; 128: S65.
29. Barnes PJ. The third nervous system in the lung: physiology and clinical perspectives. Thorax 1084; 39: 561.
30. Wittenborg MH, Aviad I. Organ influence on the normal posture of the diaphragm: a radiological study of inversions and heterotaxies. Br J Radiol 1972; 36: 280.
31. Gluk MC, Twigg HL, Ball MF, Rhodes PG. Shadows bordering the lung on radiographs of normal and obese persons. Thorax 1972; 267: 232.

1.2 Microscopic structure of the lung

Peter K Jeffery

Key points

- The airways perform many functions beyond gas conduction.
- At least eight different surface epithelial cell types have now been delineated.
- Immune cells (lymphocytes, dendritic cells, macrophages and mast cells) migrate into and through the lining epithelium.
- Cilia move mucus by their tips, the interaction being facilitated by minute terminal hooklets.
- The mucous cell is capable of division and may show stem cell multipotentiality.
- Submucosal glands are the major source of tracheobronchial mucus.
- The Clara cell is the principal stem cell of small airways.
- Basal cells are proliferative and reparative and may help adhesion of superficial cells to the basement membrane in large airways.
- The basement membrane acts as an extracellular scaffold and may influence the differentiation of the overlying epithelial cells.
- There is considerable reserve in the pulmonary vascular bed and lymphatics may increase their load up to tenfold when pulmonary oedema threatens.
- Apart from the classic sympathetic (adrenergic) and parasympathetic (cholinergic) nerve supply to the lung, there is a third component that is neither adrenergic nor cholinergic.
- Adult human lungs contain about 300 million alveoli, each measuring about 250 μm in diameter when expanded. Their expansion is facilitated by surface-tension-reducing lipids secreted by alveolar lining cells and collectively known as pulmonary surfactant.
- The alveolar epithelium consists of two principal cell types, known as type I and type II or squamous and granular cells respectively: the type II cell is the stem/reparative cell for the alveolus.

The epithelial lining of the entire respiratory tract is continuous with the skin and with the lining of the alimentary tract, from which the lower respiratory tract develops in utero (see Chapter 1.1). In resting humans, the volume of air entering the nares each day is about 10 000–15 000 litres. The delicate nature of the respiratory lining and the way ambient air moves frequently and freely over its surface make it particularly susceptible to inhaled irritants, infective agents and allergenic substances. The conducting airways condition the inspired air and free it of many of these pollutants before it reaches the respiratory portion of the lung. The effectiveness of the airways in this respect depends, in part, on their branching pattern, the composition and integrity of their structural components and the dynamic interaction of their diverse structural, immunocompetent and neural elements. Although air moves in two directions, airway secretions, together with any foreign material that may have impacted on the airway wall, in general move cranially and, in the upright position, against gravity.

The larynx is conventionally considered to be the boundary between the upper and lower respiratory tracts: the upper extends from the external nares to the larynx and the lower from the larynx to the visceral pleura as a system of airways that branch dichotomously and asymmetrically.[1] The airways of the respiratory tract may be conveniently considered as either conductive or respiratory, with the respiratory bronchioles forming a transitional zone.

Airways are usually designated by structure and order of division: those distal to the trachea with cartilage in their walls are by definition *bronchi*. In the trachea, supportive cartilage is present in the form of irregular, sometimes branching, crescentic rings (16–20 in humans), all of which are incomplete dorsally, where they are bridged by connective tissue and bands of smooth muscle. In large bronchi the cartilages are irregular in shape but frequent enough to be found in any plane. In small bronchi they are less frequent and may be missed in transverse section. Airways distal to the last cartilage plate are *bronchioles*. The last bronchiolar divisions have their ciliated lining epithelium interrupted by alveoli and are referred to as *respiratory bronchioles*: the generation proximal to the first-order respiratory bronchioles consists of *terminal bronchioles*. The terminal bronchioles form the last purely conductive airways and the respiratory bronchiole is the site where gaseous exchange begins. There are generally three orders of respiratory bronchiole. A single terminal bronchiole with its succeeding respiratory bronchioles, two to nine orders of alveolar ducts and alveolar sacs together form the *respiratory acinus*, which is about 1 cm in diameter and forms the basic respiratory unit of the lung.

Conducting airways

These perform many functions beyond gas conduction, e.g. warming, humidification and cleansing of the inhaled air of potentially harmful dust particles, gases and microorganisms. The more distal respiratory zone is kept free of pollution and infection by defence mechanisms that include:

- nervous reflexes causing bronchoconstriction and cough
- ciliary activity
- secretion of mucus, lysozyme, lactoferrin and IgA
- cellular immune reactions.

Figure 1.2.1 shows that the airway wall comprises epithelial, muscular and vascular elements interspersed in a pliable connective tissue support arranged as: (1) a lining mucosa of surface epithelium, basement membrane and supporting elastic lamina propria; (2) a submucosa, in which lie glands, muscle and cartilage; and (3) a relatively thin adventitial coat. There are also lymphoid elements and nerves.

Surface epithelium

Airway epithelium includes the surface lining and the lining that forms the submucosal glands. With the exception of the anterior nares, which are lined by stratified, keratinising, squamous epithelium, much of the epithelium of the upper respiratory tract is formed of pseudostratified, ciliated, columnar cells and occasional mucus-secreting cells. Patches of non-keratinising squamous epithelium are found in the pharynx, whereas in the larynx such epithelium is found over the anterior surface of the epiglottis, the upper half of its posterior surface, the upper part of the aryepiglottic folds and the vocal folds. The stratified squamous epithelium lining much of the larynx gives way, in the trachea, to a pseudostratified, ciliated, columnar epithelium, the term 'pseudostratified' implying that all cells rest on the basement membrane but that not all reach the airway lumen. In humans this type of epithelium extends throughout the major airways, becoming simple cuboidal more peripherally. In other species (such as the rat) the transition to simple cuboidal occurs

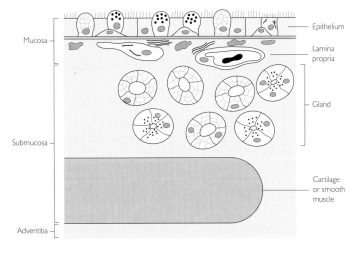

(a)

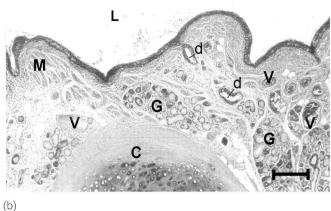

(b)

Fig. 1.2.1 The airway wall. (a) Diagrammatic representation of the structure. (b) Light micrograph of human bronchial inner wall showing the airway lumen (L), surface epithelium, submucosal glands (G) with sections through gland ducts (d), bronchial smooth muscle (M) and bronchial vessels (V) surrounded by connective tissue and supported by cartilage (C). Haematoxylin and eosin stain. Scale bar = 150 μm.

more proximally. In humans, mucus-secreting cells are regularly found in the tracheobronchial tree but are sparse in bronchioles of less than 1 mm diameter. Again, there are species differences: mucus-secreting cells are numerous in the trachea and bronchi of the guinea pig and cat, but few are found in these regions in the rat, mouse, hamster and rabbit. In the cat, mucus-secreting cells are found as far distally as the bronchioles.

At least seven different surface epithelial cell types have now been delineated (Table 1.2.1).[2-4] In addition, cells involved in the immune response may migrate through the epithelial basement membrane: some of these remain within the surface epithelium whereas others pass into the airway lumen. The terminal processes of nerve fibres whose cell bodies lie deep to the epithelium, most being outside the lung, also pierce the epithelial basement membrane and are thought to initiate airway reflexes such as bronchoconstriction and cough.[5] Many but not all of the eight surface epithelial cell types are represented in humans. Ciliated, mucous, Clara and basal cells are consistently identified in all mammals but there is controversy about the occurrence of 'brush' cells and the migratory 'globule leukocyte' in human airways. The structure of some of these cells will now be considered in more detail.

Ciliated cell

The surface of the ciliated cell (Fig. 1.2.2) is covered by 200–300 cilia, each normally beating at about 1000 times per minute with its effective stroke generally in the cranial direction and co-ordinated with those on adjacent cells.[6] In disease there may be widespread loss of cilia, particularly at sites of airway branching, where air-borne pollutants often impact. Each ciliated cell has an abundance of apically placed mitochondria and a moderately well-developed Golgi apparatus. Lysosomes and lamellar bodies are often present in the supranuclear zone. Cilia are thought to beat in a periciliary layer of low viscosity, the origin of which is as yet unknown. Cilia move the overlying mucous sheet only by their tips, the interaction of the ciliary tips and mucus being facilitated by minute terminal hooklets (Fig. 1.2.3).[7] Long, slender microvilli project between the cilia and are associated with an acidic surface mucosubstance, probably a glycosaminoglycan.[8] The rich microvillous border and

associated pinocytotic vesicles may play a role in fluid absorption and thereby control the depth of the periciliary fluid layer in which the cilia beat. Cilia are approximately 6 mm long in the trachea and gradually shorten to about 4–5 mm in distal bronchioles. Cilia extend distally to the junction of respiratory bronchiole and alveolus. Each cilium has a characteristic axoneme consisting of an internal arrangement that in cross-section comprises nine peripheral doublets surrounding two central tubules (Fig. 1.2.4). Genetically determined defects in this arrangement or their cross-linkage via radial spokes may lead to dyskinetic or immotile cilia and impairment of mucociliary transport. The ciliated cell is considered an end-stage cell formed by differentiation and maturation of basal or secretory cells.[9]

Mucous cell

In human trachea the mean density of surface mucous cells is estimated at between 6000 and 7000 cells/mm² surface epithelium. Electron microscopy shows that the mucous cell contains electron-lucent, confluent granules of about 800 nm diameter (Fig. 1.2.5). Most contain mucin, which is acidic as a result of sialic acid or sulphate groups located at the ends of oligosaccharide side chains (which branch from the protein core of high-molecular-weight glycoprotein molecules).[8,10] Secretion of the correct amount of mucus with an optimum viscoelastic profile is important in the maintenance of mucociliary clearance. The acidity of the mucus and the extent to which it complexes with other molecules contributes to its flow properties and hence the ease with which it may be moved by cilia or sheared by cough. Alterations in the histochemical type of mucus have been associated with irritation and carcinogenesis (see Chapter 48.3). The number of mucous cells increases in diseases such as chronic bronchitis[11] and, experimentally, following inhalation of sulphur dioxide or tobacco smoke (see Chapter 48.3). The increase is effected by a combination of other cells undergoing metaplasia and mucous cell division: the mucous cell is clearly capable of division and may show stem-cell multipotentiality.[9,12,13] A number of genes encode the peptide core structure of mucins[14,15] and these are 'switched on' in response to irritants and bacterial lipopolysaccharide.[16]

Serous cell

Serous cells have a lot of rough endoplasmic reticulum and, in contrast to mucous cells, contain discrete, electron-dense granules of about 600 nm diameter. Morphologically, serous cells of the surface epithelium resemble those in the submucosal glands. They are found in the surface epithelium of many species, including humans.[7,17] Some serous cells contain neutral mucin and there is evidence that some may also contain a non-mucoid substance, probably lipid. In the healthy rat the serous cell comprises 20–30% of the dividing bronchial epithelial population[9] and becomes mucous following exposure to cigarette smoke.[12]

Clara (non-ciliated bronchiolar) cell

Clara cells in humans and rabbits are usually restricted to the terminal bronchioles: in other species such as the mouse they

Table 1.2.1 Cells found in the epithelium of the conducting airways

Epithelial cells	Basal
	Ciliated
	Mucous
	Serous
	Clara
	Neuroendocrine
	Brush (non-human species)
Migratory cells	Lymphocyte
	Dendritic cell
	Macrophage
	Mast cell
Neural elements	

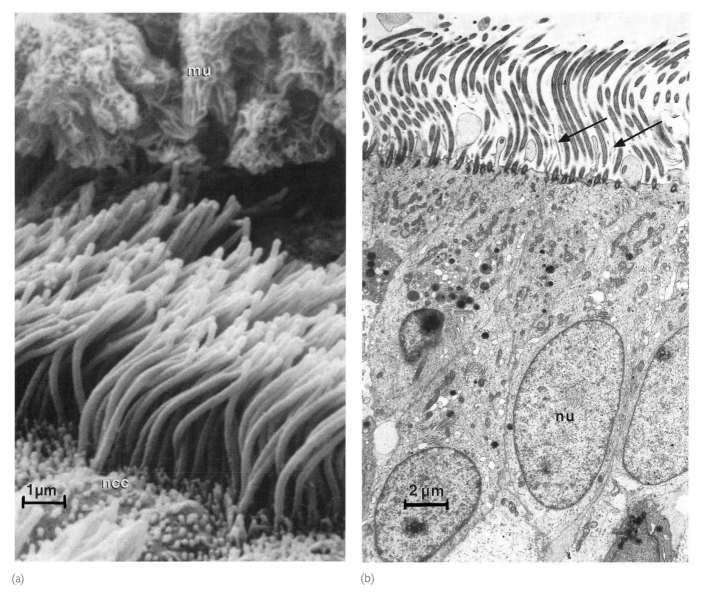

(a)   (b)

Fig. 1.2.2 (a) Scanning and (b) transmission electron micrographs of ciliated cells in the surface epithelium. (a) Cilia beat in a low viscosity periciliary fluid layer and move an overlying gel-like layer of mucus (mu). Non-ciliated cells (ncc) lie in the foreground of the illustration. Scale bar = 1.0 μm. (b) Filiform microvilli are present between the cilia (arrows). nu, nucleus. Scale bar = 2.0 μm.

may be present as far proximally as the nose. They typically bulge into the airway lumen and contain electron-dense granules of about 500–600 nm diameter (Fig. 1.2.6). The function of this cell is as yet undetermined. It may produce a hypophase component of surfactant[18] and an antiprotease.[19] Furthermore, the Clara cell acts as the principal stem cell of small airways, where basal and mucous cells are normally sparse; both ciliated and mucous cells may develop from the Clara cell subsequent to its division and differentiation.[20–22] Clara cells also show cytochrome-P450-dependent mixed-function oxidase activity and are therefore likely to metabolise certain environmental chemicals, including carcinogens that require mixed-function activation.[23]

Neuroendocrine cell

These cells (Synonyms: dense core-granulated, Kultchitsky and Feyrter cells) are argyrophilic and show paraformalde-hydeinduced fluorescence, particularly if the tissue is preincubated with 5-hydroxytryptophan or dihydroxy-pheny-lalanine. Neuroendocrine cells are generally basal in position but often have a thin cytoplasmic projection reaching the airway lumen.[24,25] Single cells and clusters of these cells may be associated with nerve fibres in so-called neuroepithelial bodies or neurite–receptor complexes (Fig. 1.2.7).[26,27] The cytoplasm of neuroendocrine cells usually contains large numbers of small (70–150 nm) spherical granules, each with an electron-dense

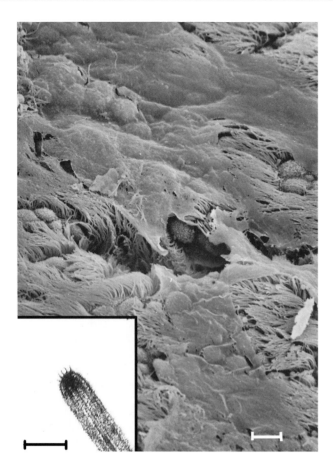

Fig. 1.2.3 Mucus is considered to form a continuous sheet only in the large (proximal) airways, where it is moved by the tips of the cilia. Scale bar = 0.4 μm. Inset: the interaction of the ciliary tip and the mucus is facilitated by minute terminal hooklets, which are shown at higher magnification. Scale bar = 10 μm.

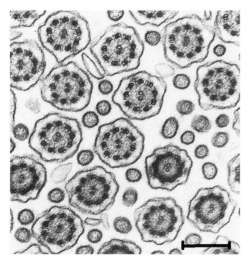

Fig. 1.2.4 Transmission electron micrograph showing cross-sections of the cilia interspersed by more numerous microvilli, which lie between the cilia and close to the cell surface. Each cilium normally has a characteristic internal pattern of nine peripherally placed doublets surrounding two single central microtubules. Scale bar = 0.2 μm.

core surrounded by an electron-lucent halo (Fig. 1.2.7, inset). Granule subtypes have been described.[25] Neuroendocrine cells may contain biogenic amines or peptides such as bombesin,[28] which, when released, may influence vascular and bronchial smooth muscle tone, mucous secretion and ciliary activity. The location of the cell in the surface epithelium and its cytoplasmic content make it a prime candidate for sensing hypoxia in the airway lumen. It is likely that, as a consequence, vasoactive substances are released, which are likely to cause local vasoconstriction and shunting of blood to better ventilated zones of the lung. Hyperplasia of neuroendocrine cells has been described in experimental asbestosis, infantile bronchopulmonary dysplasia, bronchiectasis associated with tumourlets and in bronchi associated with carcinomas of all types.

Basal cell

It is the presence of a basal cell layer in the large bronchi and trachea that contributes to the pseudostratified appearance of the epithelium. The basal cell has sparse cytoplasm containing bundles of monofilaments immunoreactive for cytokeratin. The basal cell is considered by many to be the major stem cell from which the more superficial mucus-secreting and ciliated cells derive.[29]

Airway surface epithelium is replaced only slowly. Normally, less than 1% of its cells is in division at any one time. However, the mitotic index increases in response to irritation by noxious agents such as tobacco smoke (see Chapter 47.3). In these situations, the basal cells play a proliferative role in concert with secretory cells, which are also capable of division. When there is epithelial shedding in response to injury, basal cells often remain as a reparative layer that promptly flattens within 20 minutes of the injury to establish cell-to-cell contact and a continuous barrier that covers the otherwise denuded basement membrane.[30] Apart from their proliferative and reparative role it has been suggested that the prevalence of basal cells in large (proximal) airways may relate to their role in strengthening the adhesion of overlying columnar cells to the epithelial basement membrane.[31]

Indeterminate and transitional forms

Many non-ciliated cells fall into the category of 'indeterminate', a category comprising a mixture of cells, none of which is clearly classifiable. In addition, normal epithelium may show a number of cells, each of which shows features transitional to two or more well-defined cell types. These cells form an interesting group that may be relevant to studies of carcinogenesis.[32]

Migratory cells

In health, polymorphonuclear leukocytes are rarely found in the airways but they are rapidly recruited in inflammatory states. In contrast, lymphocytes, dendritic cells, macrophages and mast cells are normally present within airway epithelium. The intra-epithelial lymphocyte may occur singly or in groups organised into a 'lymphoepithelium' (see below).[33] A major function of intra-epithelial lymphocytes is to remove allergenic particles

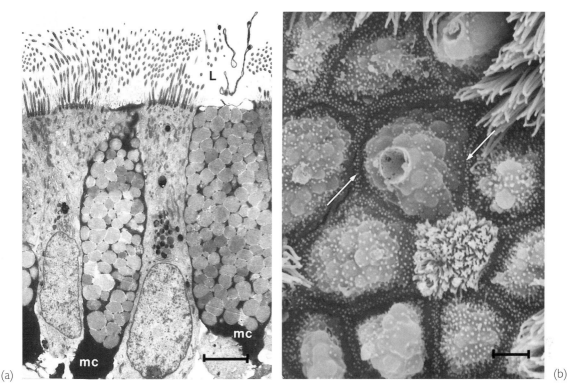

(a)   (b)

Fig. 1.2.5 (a) Transmission electron micrograph and (b) scanning electron micrograph images of mucous cells. (a) Two epithelial mucous or goblet cells (mc), each filled with usually confluent electron-lucent secretory granules. L, airway lumen; Scale bar = 5 μm. (b) En face view of goblet cells showing intracellular secretory granules pressing against the internal aspect of the apical plasma membrane. In the centre a granule appears to have been lost, leaving a crater at the cell apex. The borders of each cell are outlined by increased numbers of bright apical microvilli (arrows). Scale bar = 2.0 μm.

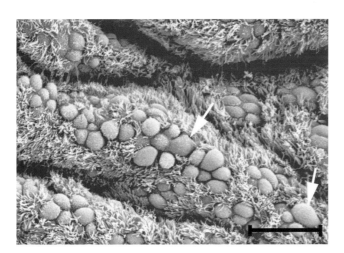

Fig. 1.2.6 Scanning electron micrograph of the lining epithelium of a human bronchiole illustrating the bulging apices of Clara cells (arrows). The intervening ciliated cells have few cilia and they are shorter than those of the larger, more proximal, bronchi. Scale bar = 20 μm.

from the airways. They may be either T or B cells. T-cell surface markers normally identified include CD3, CD4 (helper) and particularly CD8 (suppressor/cytotoxic). CD8+ cells are increased in numbers in chronic obstructive pulmonary disease.[34] Immunostimulation of resting T lymphocytes is thought to require initial presentation of antigen in association with class II major histocompatibility complex (MHC) Ia molecules expressed by dendritic cells. Dendritic cells are also present normally and migrate frequently between the surface epithelium and regional lymph nodes.[35] Also identified in airway digests are macrophages, which inhibit dendritic-cell-induced T-lymphocyte activation in vitro. It appears, therefore, that T-cell immunity is regulated by a balance of signals from resident Ia-positive dendritic cells and macrophages.[36] The surface density of dendritic cells in the laboratory rat is 50–600 cells/mm², decreasing peripherally.

The intra-epithelial and subepithelial (so-called 'mucosal') mast cell is morphologically and functionally distinct from the mast cell present in deep connective tissue.[37] However, both are capable of releasing a wide variety of mediators of inflammation that affect epithelial and vascular permeability, smooth muscle function and other important functional responses. In non-smokers, mast cells form up to 2% of surface epithelial cells but a higher proportion is reported in smokers.[38,39]

Intercellular junctions and cell adhesion

Surface epithelial cells make contact by three types of junction:[40]

- **adhering junctions**, which include the zonula adherens (forming a belt-like structure encircling the cell), maculae adherentes ('spot' desmosomes) and hemidesmosomes,

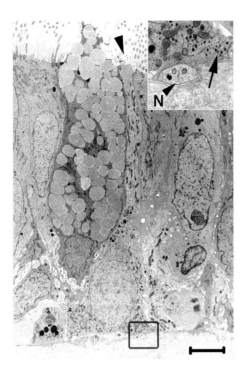

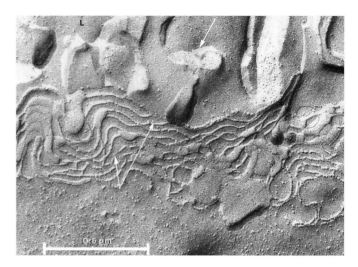

Fig. 1.2.7 Transmission electron micrograph of a neuroendocrine cell. Most of these cells are found at the base of the epithelium. This one has an extended process that reaches the airway lumen (arrowhead). The cytoplasm contains relatively small, electron-dense granules (arrows), each showing a characteristic electron-lucent halo (see inset). Intraepithelial nerve fibres (curved arrows) are often present in close association with the plasma membrane of the neuroendocrine cell (N) Scale bar = 4 μm.

Fig. 1.2.8 The apicolateral tight junction of an epithelial ciliated cell as it appears by the technique of freeze-fracture and transmission electron micrograph. The junction is composed of a series of sealing strands and cross-bridges (arrows) that act as a selectively permeable barrier to the passage of water, ions and macromolecules. The airway lumen is indicated by L and luminal edge of the cell by the arrowhead. (Reproduced by permission of RWA Godfrey, NJ Severs and PK Jeffery). Scale bar = 0.5 μm.

which join cells to their basal lamina; these junctions are linked to the cell cytoskeleton via actin-rich filaments

- **tight junctions**, which form a belt around the apicolateral borders of the epithelial cells and form a selectively permeable/resistive barrier to the paracellular movement of ions, macromolecules and water
- **gap ('nexus') junctions**, which allow cells to communicate directly, e.g. in the co-ordination of ciliary activity.[41]

Normally impermeable, the zonula occludens prevents excessive fluid movement across the epithelium but, following irritation, it may become permeable to markers of molecular weight 40 000–69 000.[42] Transport from lumen to submucosa of potentially antigenic molecules with molecular weights in excess of 69 000 may also involve epithelial cell transport. Tight junctions in normal human epithelium are 0.45–0.48 μm deep in extrapulmonary bronchi and comprise some 11 strands/complementary grooves interconnected along their length at approximately 1 μm intervals (Fig. 1.2.8).[43] Tight junctions are highly labile structures whose formation and architecture can be altered rapidly experimentally in vitro and in disease.[44] The disruption of tight junctions in asthma is of interest with regard to the fragility of the surface epithelium that characterises this disease.[45]

In addition to these adhering junctions, there are cell surface adhesion molecules, which aid epithelial cell-to-cell adhesion and may also enhance the retention of inflammatory cells in the epithelial compartment. The epithelial expression of E-cadherin and intercellular adhesion molecule-1 have been of particular interest.[46] These adhesion molecules may be increased by inflammatory cytokines such as tumour necrosis factor (TNF)-α and interferon (IFN)-γ.

Basement membrane

The epithelial basement membrane is a region specialised for the attachment of the epithelium to the underlying matrix. The basement membrane acts as an extracellular scaffold and, by virtue of its composition, may also influence spatial interrelationships and the differentiation status of its overlying epithelial cells. The so-called 'true' basement membrane consists of a lamina rara (lucida) and a lamina densa (basal lamina); each of these is 40–60 nm thick and much below the resolution of the light microscope. The principal components are type IV collagen, proteoglycans, laminin, entactin, nidogen and fibronectin, present in both soluble and insoluble forms.[47] It has a negative charge, created by sulphate and carboxyl moieties; it is the negative charge that appears to determine, in part, its permeability and capacity for filtration. In the adult, but not in fetal human airway (at least up to 18 weeks of gestation), there is an additional characteristic reticular lamina beneath (external to) the basal lamina, the so-called lamina reticularis (synonym: fibroreticularis), consisting of fine fibrillary reticular collagen. In the laboratory rat, the structural proteins appear to be arranged as a mat of relatively large fibres orientated along the longitudinal axis of the airway. These fibres immunostain for collagen III with some collagen I and V. In addition, there are cross-linking microfibrils of elastin.[48] It is the lamina reticularis, not the basal lamina, that is thickened in asthma (see Chapter 47.3).

As a structural boundary, the reticular basement membrane acts only as a partial barrier to the passage of macromolecules and cells. Inflammatory cells are considered to secrete proteases that facilitate their passage through the basement membrane to enter the epithelium. Recent observations indicate that, like the intestinal and glomerular basement membranes, there may be fenestrations or pores also in the airway reticular basement membrane that act as a conduit for the transmigration of inflammatory cells into the epithelium. In human bronchial mucosa collected at surgery for tumour, these are reported to be present as oval-shaped pores 0.75–3.9 μm in diameter at a density of 863 pores/mm^2.[49] These channels may facilitate bidirectional communication between epithelial and closely apposed mesenchymal cells, an interaction that is probably important during development and repair, in homeostasis and in the regulation of inflammatory conditions of the airways. Indeed the flattened shape of the adjacent fibroblasts/myofibroblasts (as distinct from the more fusiform shape of fibroblasts elsewhere) and their proximity to the basement membrane has led to the application of the term 'attenuated fibroblast sheath' to encompass both the epithelium and the closely apposed mesenchymal cells as one functional unit. Thus the concept of an 'epithelial–mesenchymal trophic unit' extending from the large to the most distal conducting airways has been proposed.[50]

Submucosal glands

The volume, distribution and histochemical composition of the submucosal glands show considerable species variation. In humans the glands are relatively numerous and, in the lower respiratory tract, they are found wherever there is supportive cartilage in the airway wall, i.e. from the larynx to small bronchi. It has been estimated that some 4000 glands are present in the human trachea.[51] Each gland unit is of the tubuloalveolar type and in humans it may be composed of four regions, the lumina of which are continuous (Fig. 1.2.9):[52]

- a relatively narrow ciliated duct continuous with the surface epithelium
- an expanded collecting duct of cells of indeterminate morphology or of eosinophilic cells (also referred to as degenerative cells or 'oncocytes') packed with mitochondria
- mucous tubules and acini
- serous acini.

Although mucins of both acidic and neutral types are produced, other secretions such as lysozyme, lactoferrin, a secretory component of IgA and a low-molecular-weight antiprotease[53] are also found in the submucosal glands, particularly in serous acini. It is suggested that watery, serous secretions pass from the outermost regions of each gland into the mucous tubules and that the ionic balance of this mixed secretion may be adjusted in the collecting duct before its discharge through the ciliated duct to the bronchial lumen.[54] Discharge is aided by contractile myoepithelial cells, which form a basket-like structure around the acinus. Both synthesis and discharge of secretion are influenced by nerves whose terminals lie adjacent to (in humans) or pierce

(in cats) the secretory unit.[5] There is evidence that both parasympathetic and sympathetic agonists stimulate secretion, although the quantity and quality of the resulting secretion from each differ. Submucosal glands are probably the major source of tracheobronchial mucus. Submucosal gland mass increases in chronic bronchitis and, to a lesser extent, in asthma; the increase is the result of cell proliferation within each secretory acinus rather than of increase in the number of gland units.[55] Dense-core granulated cells and intra-epithelial lymphocytes similar to those of surface epithelium are found in the submucosal glands.[56]

Lymphoid tissue

Airway lymphoid tissue comprises:

- lymph nodes
- bronchus-associated lymphoid tissue
- lymphoreticular aggregates.

In addition to these discrete collections of immunoresponsive cells, occasional free lymphocytes and plasma cells may be found scattered throughout the walls of the bronchi. Many of these are T lymphocytes. The plasma cells that secrete IgA are concentrated around the bronchial glands.[57] The secretory component of the IgA found in airway secretions is produced within the serous cells of the glands;[58] it protects the IgA molecule from destruction by the proteases normally present in respiratory tract fluid.

Large numbers of mast cells are normally present in subepithelial tissues of the airways. Their number progressively increases distally so that, in the small bronchioles, total mast cell numbers are 100- to 150-fold greater than in the trachea. Of the 10–100 million mast cells in a monkey's lungs, 83% are associated with the conductive airways.[59] The suggestion that there may be distinct subpopulations of 'mucosal' and connective tissue mast cells in humans, as in rats, is of potential importance and has been the subject of intensive study.[60]

Lymph nodes

Encapsulated lymph nodes increase in prominence in the first year of life. In the adult they are situated mainly in the hilar peribronchial tissues and do not come into direct contact with respiratory epithelium. Although mainly associated with bronchi of the first three or four generations, they may rarely be found in the peripheral lung, even as far out as the pleura.[61]

Bronchus-associated lymphoid tissue

Lymphoid nodules, intimately associated with bronchial epithelium, have been described mainly in non-human species. Because of their resemblance to Peyer's patches (gut-associated lymphoid tissue) they have been termed 'bronchus-associated lymphoid tissue' (BALT). Although BALT may be found anywhere within the bronchial mucosa, it is especially obvious at airway bifurcations, where inhaled antigens impinge in greatest concentrations. Its presence in humans has recently been reviewed.[62]

Bronchus-associated lymphoid tissue is formed of follicular lymphoid tissue, which may complex with overlying epithelium to

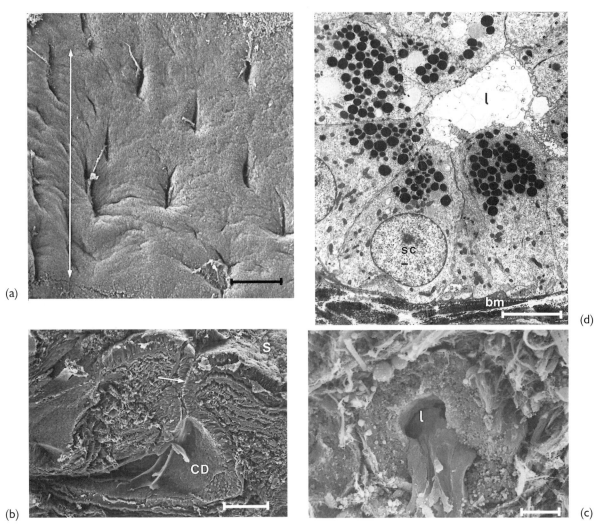

Fig. 1.2.9 (a) Scanning electron micrograph appearance of the epithelial lining to a human bronchus showing the slit-like openings of the underlying submucosal mucus-secreting glands. Arrows denote long axis of the airway. Scale bar = 300 μm. (b) A fortuitous fracture across the mucosa and its surface (S), exposes in section the ciliated duct (arrow) and an expanded region known as the collecting duct (CD). Scale bar = 100 μm. (c) A mucous tubule cut in transverse section with an abundance of secretion spilling from its lumen. Scale bar = 10 μm. (d) Transmission electron micrograph appearance of a serous acinus composed of wedge-shaped serous cells (sc), each cell containing electron-dense secretory granules. Scale bar = 100 μm. l, acinar lumen; bm, basement membrane.

form a 'lymphoepithelium' devoid of cilia and mucus and heavily infiltrated by lymphocytes. Although the follicular aggregate may itself be of considerable size, its contact with the epithelium may be small. High endothelial 'postcapillary' venules are found in the parafollicular region.[63] On scanning electron microscopy there is an obvious lack of cilia on the overlying epithelium but characteristic microvillous projections may be seen.

Lymphoreticular aggregates

These consist of small collections of lymphocytes together with a few plasma cells and eosinophils. The sinusoidal and nodal architecture of a lymph node is lacking. The aggregates may be found around bronchi or within interlobular septa, alveolar tissue or the pleura. In alveolar tissue they are usually located between the respiratory bronchiole and its accompanying artery at a site where

lymphatics start. Interstitial fluid from the alveolar septum, together with dust-laden macrophages, is transported to where the lymphatics start and then by further transport to the lymph nodes and beyond. With heavy atmospheric pollution, the interstitial macrophages accumulate beside lymphoreticular aggregates and form what Macklin termed 'pulmonary dust sumps'.[64]

Airway smooth muscle

Smooth muscle, present only in the intercartilaginous gaps of the trachea and extrapulmonary bronchi, completely encircles the intrapulmonary bronchi internal to their supportive cartilage plates. Two sets of fibres wind along the bronchial tree as opposing spirals – such a geodesic arrangement that, as the muscle contracts, the airway both shortens and constricts. There are species differences in the overall arrangement: muscle fibres are separated from each other in guinea-pig and dog airways, whereas frequent connections of the nexus (gap junction) type are seen in humans. The nexus type of junction provides electrical coupling and allows simultaneous contraction of blocks of muscle fibres; in this respect, the arrangement is similar to that found in the gastrointestinal tract. The proportion of the airway wall occupied by smooth muscle increases in both large and small airways in asthma and in small airways in chronic obstructive pulmonary disease (see Chapters 47.3 and 48.3 respectively).

Arteries, veins and lymphatics

In humans, the trachea receives systemic blood through branches of the inferior thyroid and bronchial arteries, which anastomose with each other. The walls of the bronchi and bronchioles are supplied with systemic blood through the bronchial arteries, which in humans are derived from the descending aorta and the intercostal and internal mammary arteries.[65] Microvascular injection techniques demonstrate an extremely rich vascular network supplying the airway wall. This system nourishes the mucosa, participates in gas exchange via bronchopulmonary anastomoses, contributes transudate to airway secretions and helps to control heat exchange.

Each airway is accompanied by a branch of the pulmonary artery. In fact, the pulmonary arteries divide with the airways and also send off supernumerary branches that do not accompany airways.[66] There is considerable reserve in the pulmonary vascular bed and many vessels may be lost without significantly affecting pulmonary vascular resistance. Most small pulmonary arteries enter the respiratory acinus with the bronchiole and are therefore found at the centre of the acinus. In the alveolar wall the capillaries form a meshwork of short segments in close contact with the alveolar space (Fig. 1.2.10); they converge at the periphery of the acinus to form the pulmonary veins.

The veins run initially in the interlobular septa, separate from the artery and bronchus in the centre of the lobule. Blood drains from the trachea via the thyroid venous plexus and middle and inferior thyroid veins, and from the bronchi via the hilar bronchial veins or pulmonary veins deep in the lung. However, marked species variations exist in this overall anatomical arrangement.[67]

Pulmonary lymphatics provide a unidirectional drainage system that serves to maintain homoeostasis of the interstitium by transporting excess tissue fluid back to the blood stream and by preventing excessive fluid and protein leak across alveolar and conducting-airway epithelium. Pulmonary lymphatics are wide in relation to their wall thickness and are attached to adjacent connective tissues fibres by special anchoring filaments, which hold them open when interstitial fluid accumulates.[68]

There is considerable reserve in the clearance capability of the pulmonary lymphatics, which may increase their load up to 10-fold when pulmonary oedema threatens.[69] Pulmonary lymphatics are valved structures and their endothelium has poorly developed junctions; adjacent lymphatic endothelial cells often merely overlap and their basal lamina is discontinuous. Although lymphatics are not found at the alveolar level, the fact that they start in the regions of respiratory and terminal bronchioles means that no part of the lung is further from a lymphatic

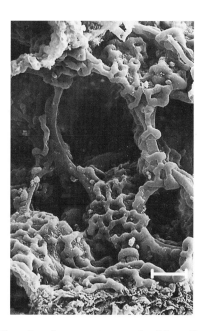

Fig. 1.2.10 Scanning electron micrograph of three/four alveoli. The child has a ventricular-septal defect that has resulted in higher than normal pulmonary vascular pressure, expanded the alveolar pulmonary vessels and demonstrates that their arrangement is as short, interconnecting segments. Scale bar = 20 μm.

vessel than about 2 mm. The lymphatics drain outwards to the visceral pleura and inwards to the hilum. Lymph from both the pleural and pulmonary lymphatics passes through hilar, tracheal and mediastinal lymph nodes to join the systemic circulation via the thoracic duct and the great veins at the base of the neck.

Innervation

Nerve bundles and ganglia are found mainly in the posterior membranous portion of the trachea and main bronchus.[5] On entering the lung, the nerve bundles divide to form distinct peribronchial and perivascular plexus. The peribronchial plexus further divides to form extrachondral and subepithelial plexus. Bronchioles have a single plexus that contains fewer fibres and ganglia than the plexus of more proximal airway generations and early reports of alveolar innervation have now been confirmed by electron microscopy.

The efferent (motor) innervation has excitatory and inhibitory components supplying submucosal glands, bronchial smooth muscle and blood vessels. Apart from the classic sympathetic (adrenergic) and parasympathetic (cholinergic) nerve supply to the lung, a third component that is neither adrenergic nor cholinergic (non-adrenergic, non-cholinergic, NANC) is present.[70,71] Thus pulmonary innervation appears to be more complex than originally proposed and involves previously unrecognised neurotransmitters (peptides and purines) that may prove to be of major biological significance.

Afferent (sensory) endings are present in both the surface epithelium and the underlying submucosa (Fig. 1.2.11). Three types are distinguished on the basis of their position, pattern of firing, adaptation to maintained stimulus and axonal myelination:[72]

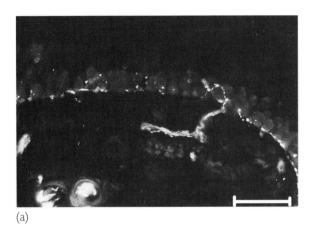

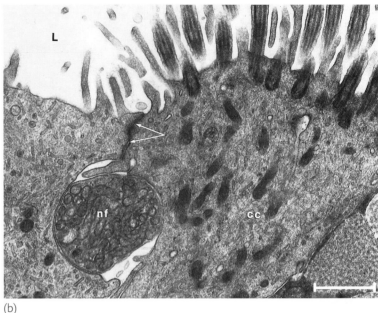

(a)   (b)

Fig. 1.2.11 (a) Immunofluorescence preparation of human bronchial mucosa and of PGP-9.5-positive nerve bundles in the subepithelium. Branches enter the surface epithelium, where they branch further to run between the epithelial cells towards the airway lumen as varicose nerve terminals. Scale bar = 50 μm. (b) Intra-epithelial nerve fibres (nf) may occasionally be found in human bronchi examined by transmission electron micrograph. They have an abundance of characteristically thin mitochondria and the fibres often lie close to the airway lumen (L), immediately beneath the tight junctions of the epithelial cells (arrows). Scale bar = 1.0 μm. cc, ciliated cell.

- type I receptors are rapidly adapting and comprise cough and 'irritant'' receptors
- type II are the slowly adapting pulmonary stretch receptors thought to give rise to the Hering–Breuer reflex
- type III are pulmonary (so-called juxtacapillary) receptors, present deep in the lung.

Respiratory zone

The last of the purely conductive airways is known as the terminal bronchiole, beyond which are further generations of respiratory bronchioles; these bronchioles are transitional because they both conduct gas and participate in gas exchange (Fig. 1.2.12). The transitional zone comprises about three generations of respiratory bronchioles, after which there are two to nine generations of alveolar ducts, terminating in alveolar sacs. All these structures have increasing numbers of alveoli opening off their walls.

The walls of the alveolar ducts consist of only thin spiral bands of collagen and elastin separating the mouths of the alveoli; these act like coils of a spring (Fig. 1.2.13a), lengthening on inspiration and closing on expiration.[73] Adult human lungs contain about 300 million alveoli,[74] each measuring about 250 mm in diameter when expanded. Gravitational forces result in their being bigger in the upper than in the lower parts of the lung. Small openings, the pores of Kohn, are found in the alveolar walls of many species, including humans (Fig. 1.2.13b). There are from one to seven pores in each alveolus and their diameter ranges from 2 mm to 13 mm. The pores are not

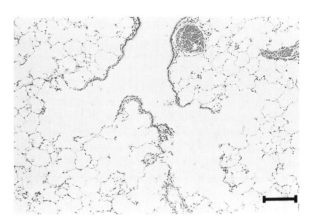

Fig. 1.2.12 A terminal bronchiole with accompanying artery (top) divides into successive generations of respiratory bronchioles, alveolar ducts and alveoli. Moving distally, the respiratory bronchiole is the first airway generation from which alveoli open directly and this marks the beginning of the respiratory zone of the lung. Scale bar = 500 μm.

present at birth and only develop after the first year of life, when they form an alternative route for gas entry by collateral ventilation. The elastic recoil force developed in the lung is proportional to alveolar surface tension and inversely proportional to alveolar size. Expansion of the lung is facilitated by surface-tension-reducing lipids secreted by alveolar lining cells and collectively known as pulmonary surfactant. The structure–function

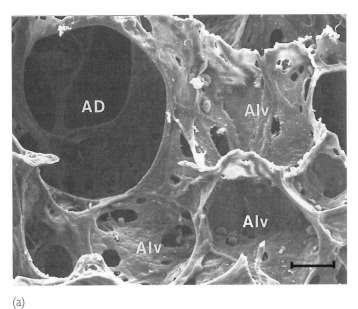

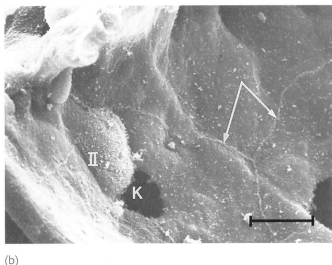

(a)   (b)

Fig. 1.2.13 (a) Scanning electron micrograph showing 'coil spring like' arrangement of an alveolar duct (AD) with alveoli (Alv) budding from it. Scale bar = 30 μm. (b) Scanning electron micrograph of the alveolar wall showing the junctions of adjacent type I cells (arrows) and a type II cell in the corner of the alveolus adjacent to a pore of Kohn. Scale bar = 10 μm.

relationship of the alveolar lining layer is complex but has been usefully reviewed recently.[75]

Alveolar epithelium

Electron microscopy demonstrates a complete simple squamous epithelium lining all alveoli that is in continuity with the columnar epithelium of the conductive airways. The alveolar lining epithelium is separated from the underlying connective tissue and capillaries of the interstitium by its basement membrane. So-called 'thin' and 'thick' aspects of the air–blood barrier are recognised (Fig. 1.2.14). On one side of the alveolar wall the capillary is closely applied to the alveolar epithelium and the endothelial and epithelial basement membranes fuse; here the air–blood barrier is at its thinnest. On the opposite side of the alveolar wall, interstitial tissue separates endothelium from epithelium.

The alveolar epithelium consists of two principal cell types, known as type I and type II or squamous and granular cells respectively. A type III pneumocyte has been described in rats[76] and other species but has not been found in humans.

Type I cells

Type I cells contain few cytoplasmic organelles but have long cytoplasmic extensions (Fig. 1.2.15a). Each cell contributes to the lining of more than one alveolus. The processes of each type I cell cover up to 5000 mm² of the alveolar surface[77] but they measure only about 0.2 mm in thickness. Their function is to provide a complete but thin covering, preventing fluid loss while facilitating rapid gas exchange. However, their thinness makes

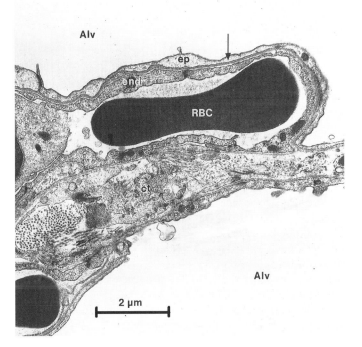

Fig. 1.2.14 Transmission electron micrograph appearance of the blood–gas barrier, illustrating 'thin' regions composed of alveolar epithelium (ep), capillary endothelium (end) and their shared basement membrane (arrow) and a relatively 'thick' portion where connective tissue (ct) and interstitial cells intervene, increasing its thickness. (Courtesy of Ann Dewar, Imperial College, London.) Scale bar = 2 μm.

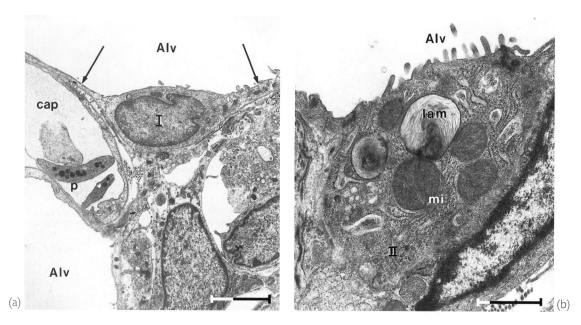

Fig. 1.2.15 (a) Type I and type II cells of the alveolar wall as they appear on a transmission electron micrograph. (a) A type I cell (I indicates the nucleus) covers a large surface area by virtue of its thin cytoplasmic extensions (arrows). Scale bar = 3.0 μm. (b) A cuboidal type II cell (II) with two lamellar bodies (lam) and characteristic large mitochondria. Microvilli extend into the alveolar space (Alv). cap, capillary lumen; p, platelet. Scale bar = 1.0 μm.

them extremely sensitive to injury. As with conducting airways, type I epithelial cells are connected to each other and to type II cells by tight junctions, which provide a selectively permeable barrier to fluid, molecular and ion movements into and out of the alveolus. In addition, macromolecules and very fine particles may reach the interstitium from the alveolar lumen by pinocytosis, from where they may be removed together with interstitial fluid to the lymphatics of the respiratory and terminal bronchioles.

Type II cells

Type II cells are taller and twice as numerous as the type I cells but as a result of their cuboidal shape they cover only about 7% of the alveolar surface.[77] They often occupy the corners of alveoli and their surface has abundant microvilli (Fig. 1.2.15b and see Fig. 1.2.13). Their cytoplasm contains large mitochondria with well-developed cristae, rough endoplasmic reticulum, a Golgi apparatus and characteristic osmiophilic lamellar structures that represent the secretory vacuoles of pulmonary surfactant (Fig. 1.2.15b). Their role in surfactant secretion has been established by ultrastructural autoradiographic studies tracing the incorporation of surfactant precursors.[78] Cell separation techniques, enabling pure type II cell suspensions to be studied in vitro, confirm that these cells secrete surfactant.[79] The extracellular surfactant layer normally lines the entire alveolus. Perfusion fixation shows that it is normally smooth and continuous. Immersion fixation breaks it up into irregular fragments of osmiophilic material (Fig. 1.2.16). The surfactant lining is relatively thick in the corners of the alveoli and thin over the extensions of type I cells. It consists of an aqueous hypophase and a

thin surface latticework of osmiophilic material, which probably represents the surface-active phospholipid component.

Type II cells are the stem cells from which replacements for damaged type I cells differentiate.[80] With chronic damage, type II cells multiply, but initially they do not differentiate and the alveolar wall becomes lined by a cuboidal epithelium that is recognisable with the light microscope. Animal studies have shown that, in the normal lung, the turnover time of type II cells is about 25 days and transformation of type II to type I cells may take as little as 2 days.[81]

Capillaries

The walls of alveolar capillaries consist of an endothelium resting on basement membrane (see Fig.1.2.14). The endothelial cell is similar to the type I alveolar epithelial cell in its thinness but covers only one-third of the area; thus the alveolar wall contains many more endothelial than type I epithelial cells. In contrast to the alveolar epithelium, the endothelial cell junctions readily permit the passage of low-molecular-weight proteins (relative molecular mass 70 000), including the α_1-protease inhibitor.[82] Larger molecules such as albumin are retained by the intercellular junctions, although small amounts of albumin may cross the endothelium to reach the interstitium by pinocytotic transport.

Alveolar capillaries are partially surrounded by pericytes, which are elongated contractile cells rich in cytoplasmic filaments and enclosed by endothelial cell basement membrane.[83] The capillary endothelial cell subserves a number of important metabolic functions, which may take place either on the surface or within the cytoplasm of the endothelial cell, e.g. metabolism of bradykinin, angiotensin I, 5-hydroxytryptamine,

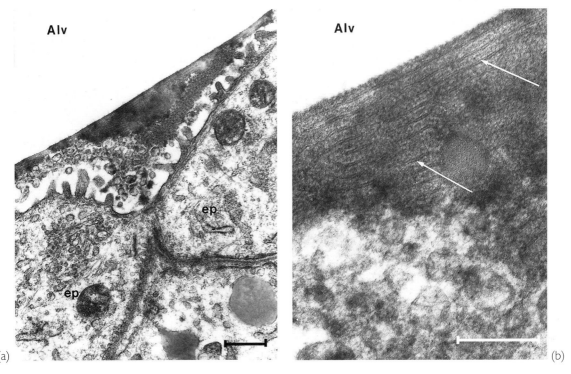

Fig. 1.2.16 (a) Transmission electron micrograph morphology of the surfactant (surface tension reducing) lining of a portion of the human alveolar wall. Scale bar = 0.5 μm. (b) A higher power (Scale bar = 0.25 μm) shows its tubular sub-structure (arrows). Alv, alveolus; ep, epithelial lining cells. (Courtesy of Ann Dewar, Imperial College, London.)

noradrenaline (norepinephrine), prostaglandins of both the E and F series, and the generation of prostacyclin.[84,85]

Interstitium

Between the basement membranes of the alveolar epithelium and capillary endothelium the 'thick' portion of the alveolar interstitium contains collagen and elastic fibres, interstitial cells and nerves (see Fig. 1.2.14). The interstitium is continuous with peribronchial connective tissue and that of the interlobular septa and pleura. Some interstitial cells are free fibroblasts but others lie close to capillaries, contain myofilaments, are contractile and may control alveolar perfusion. Other interstitial cells may represent transitional stages of blood-derived monocytes as they mature into alveolar macrophages.[86] In disease states marked by an increase in alveolar macrophages, these poorly differentiated interstitial cells are increased in number and a minority may divide before passing quickly into the alveolus. Mitoses are also occasionally seen among macrophages free in the alveolar space. The number of alveolar macrophages may therefore increase by enhanced migration from the blood and by division in both the interstitium and the alveolar space.

Alveolar macrophages

Alveolar macrophages are irregular in outline and have prominent pseudopodia (Fig. 1.2.17). The cytoplasm contains many lysosomes, phagosomes and phagolysosomes. In smokers, the

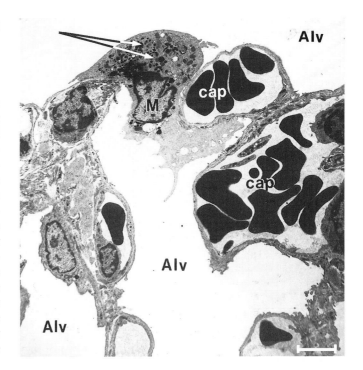

Fig. 1.2.17 Transmission electron micrograph of an alveolar macrophage (M), the normal resident phagocyte of the alveolar space (Alv). These cells are often adherent to the alveolar surface. The cell cytoplasm has an abundance of lysosomes and phagolysosomes (arrows). Some of the ingested material may represent the remains of ingested apoptotic cells. cap, capillary; Scale bar = 5.0 μm.

phagolysosomal inclusions are particularly plentiful and contain characteristic 'tar bodies' and fine kaolinite crystals.[87] Alveolar macrophages, or their interstitial precursors, interact with pulmonary lymphocytes. As well as responding to lymphokines released by antigen-stimulated T lymphocytes, they also play a part in presenting antigen to lymphocytes and they regulate their response to antigen, acting via surface immunoglobulin and complement receptors.[88]

The alveolar macrophage is a normal resident of the alveolus and is avidly phagocytic.[89] As such it forms an important defence mechanism against inhaled bacteria and a major means of clearing the alveolus of inhaled dust. Although primarily concerned with intracellular digestion, lysosomal enzymes (e.g. plasminogen activator, collagenase and elastases) are known to be released during phagocytosis and these, particularly the elastases, may damage lung tissue if the normal antiprotease screen (α_1-antiprotease) is compromised (see Chapter 47.3). In contrast, the bulk of the lysozyme within macrophages is destined for active secretion to the exterior of the cell and its release is therefore independent of phagocytic activity. Other substances secreted by macrophages include matrix metalloproteinases, interferon and fibroblast-stimulating factor.

Under basal conditions the normal life of an alveolar macrophage is approximately 7 days.[90] It appears that the vast majority are drawn to the terminal bronchiole along with the alveolar lining fluid. The fluid moves centrally to join the bronchiolar film, which is then removed to the throat along with the macrophage by the action of cilia.

Pleura

The pleura is covered by a simple layer of flattened mesothelial cells, which are joined by tight junctions and desmosomes. The mesothelium rests on a continuous basement membrane, beneath which there is collagen and a discontinuous elastic lamina. Mesothelial cells contain pinocytotic vesicles, rough endoplasmic reticulum and bundles of fine filaments. From their surface, long slender microvilli extend that measure up to 3 mm in length and 0.1 mm in width. The number of microvilli increases towards the base of the lung. They are more numerous on the visceral than the parietal pleura and are sparse over the ribs. The microvilli may serve an absorptive function and their surface mucopolysaccharide may reduce friction. Mesothelial cells may also have a scavenging role because they have been shown to be phagocytic in culture.[91]

? **Unresolved questions**

- Cilia are thought to beat in a periciliary layer of low viscosity; what is its origin?

- What are the relationships between the genes encoding the peptide core structure of mucins and mucus volume and viscosity and which of these are 'switched on' in response to irritants, bacteria and viruses?

- By what mechanism(s) does the basement membrane influence the differentiation status of its overlying epithelial cells? What is the function and how labile are the pores recently described in this layer?

- We need to understand more about the interaction and trafficking of immune cells to and from the airway epithelium and how this relates to the defence of the lung and host and how alterations may lead to disease

- Relatively little is known about the role of the airway and alveolar epithelium in both repair and inflammation.

- Apart from its surface tension reducing role, surfactant plays an immuno-modulatory role; what implications does this have in homeostasis and inflammatory conditions of the lung?

References

1. Phalen RF, Oldham MI. Tracheobronchial airway structure as revealed by casting techniques. Am Rev Respir Dis 1983; 128: SI.

2. Jeffery PK. Morphology of airway surface epithelial cells and glands. Am Rev Respir Dis 1983; 128: S14–S20.

3. Jeffery PK, Reid L. The respiratory mucous membrane. In: Brain JD, Proctor DF, Reid L, ed. Respiratory defence mechanisms. Lung biology in health and disease, vol. 3. New York: Marcel Dekker; 1977: 193–246.

4. Breeze RG, Wheeldon EB. The cells of the pulmonary airways. State of the art. Am Rev Respir Dis 1977; 116: 705–777.

5. Jeffery PK. Innervation of the airway mucosa: structure, function and changes in airway disease. In: Immunopharmacology of epithelial barriers. London: Academic Press ; 1994: 85–118.

6. Sleigh HA. The nature and action of respiratory tract cilia. In: Brain JD, Proctor DF, Reid L, ed. Respiratory defence mechanisms. Lung biology in health and disease, vol. 3. New York: Marcel Dekker; 1977.

7. Jeffery PK, Reid L. New observations of rat airway epithelium: a quantitative electron microscopic study. J Anat 1975; 120: 295–320.

8. Spicer SS, Schulte BA, Thomopoulos GN. Histochemical properties of the respiratory tract epithelium in different species. Am Rev Respir Dis 1983; 128: S20–S26.

9. Ayers MM, Jeffery PK. Proliferation and differentiation in mammalian airway epithelium. Eur Respir J 1988; 1: 58–80.

10. Carlstedt I, Sheehan JK. Structure and macromolecular properties of mucous glycoproteins. Monogr Allergy 1988; 24: 16.

11. Saetta M, Turato G, Baraldo S et al. Goblet cell hyperplasia and epithelial inflammation in peripheral airways of smokers with both symptoms of chronic bronchitis and chronic airflow limitation. Am J Respir Crit Care Med 2000; 161: 1016–21.

12. Jeffery PK, Reid L. The effect of tobacco smoke with or without phenylmethyloxadiazole (PMO) on rat bronchial epithelium: a light and electron microscopic study. J Pathol 1981; 133: 341–359.

13. McDowell EM, Trump BF. Conceptual review: histogenesis of preneoplastic and neoplastic lesions in tracheobronchial epithelium. Surv Synth Pathol Res 1983; 2: 235–279.

14. Audie JP, Janin A, Porchet N et al. Expression of human mucin genes in respiratory, digestive, and reproductive tracts ascertained by in situ hybridization. J Histochem Cytochem 1993; 41: 1479–1485.

15. Jeffery PK, Li D. Airway mucosa: secretory cells, mucus and mucin genes. Eur Respir J 1997; 10: 1655–1662.

16. Jany B, Basbaum CB. Mucin in disease. Modification of mucin gene expression in airway disease. Am Rev Respir Dis 1991; 144: S38–S41.

17. Rogers AV, Dewar A, Corrin B, Jeffery PK. Identification of serous-like cells in the surface epithelium of human bronchioles. Eur Respir J 1993; 6: 498–504.

18. Gil J, Weibel E. Extracellular lining of bronchioles after perfusion-fixation of rat lungs for electron microscopy. Anat Rec 1971; 169: 185–200.

19. De Water R, Willems LNA, van Muijen GNP et al. Ultrastructural localization of bronchial antileukoprotease in central and peripheral human airways by a gold-labeling technique using monoclonal antibodies. Am Rev Respir Dis 1986; 133: 882–890.

20. Jeffery PK. Goblet cell increase in rat bronchial epithelium following irritation and drug administration: an experimental and electron microscopic study. London University, PhD thesis, 1973.

21. Evans MJ, Cabral-Anderson LJ, Freeman G. Role of the Clara cell in renewal of bronchiolar epithelium. Lab Invest 1978; 38: 648–655.

22. Plopper CG, Hill LH, Mariassy AT. Comparative ultrastructure of the nonciliated bronchiolar epithelial (Clara) cell of the mammalian lung. III. A study of man with comparison of 15 mammalian species. Exp Lung Res 1980; 1: 171–180.

23. Boyd MR. Evidence for the Clara cell as a site of cytochrome P450-dependent mixed-function oxidase activity in lung. Nature 1977; 269: 713–715.

24. Hage E. Electron microscopic identification of several types of endocrine cells in bronchial epithelium of human foetuses. Z Zellforsch Mikrosk Anat 1973; 141: 401–412.

25. Capella C, Hage E, Solicia E, Usellini L. Ultrastructural similarity of endocrine-like cells of the human lung and some related cells of the gut. Cell Tissue Res 1987; 186: 25–37.

26. Lauweryns JM, De Bock V, Verhofstad AAJ, Steinbusch HWM. Immunohistochemical localization of serotonin in intrapulmonary neuro-epithelial bodies. Cell Tissue Res 1982; 226: 215–223.

27. Lauweryns JM, van Ranst L. Protein gene product 9.5 expression in the lungs of humans and other mammals. Immunocytochemical detection in neuroepithelial bodies, neuroendocrine cells and nerves. Neurosci Lett 1988; 85: 311–316.

28. Wharton J, Polak JM, Bloom SR et al. Bombesin-like immunoreactivity in the lung. Nature 1978; 273: 769–770.

29. Ayers M, Jeffery PK. Proliferation and differentiation in adult mammalian airway epithelium: a review. Eur Respir J 1988; 1: 58–80.

30. Erjefalt JS, Erjefalt I, Sundler F, Persson CGA. In vivo restitution of airway epithelium. Cell Tissue Res 1995; 281: 305–316.

31. Evans MJ, Plopper CG. The role of basal cells in adhesion of columnar epithelium to airway basement membrane. Am Rev Respir Dis 1988; 138: 481–483.

32. Jeffery PK. Structure and function of adult tracheo-bronchial epithelium. In: McDowell EM, ed. Lung carcinomas. Edinburgh: Churchill Livingstone; 1987: 42–73.

33. McDermott MR, Befus AD, Bienenstock J. The structural basis for immunity in the respiratory tract. Int Rev Exp Pathol 1982; 23: 47.

34. O'Shaughnessy T, Ansari TW, Barnes NC, Jeffery PK. Inflammation in bronchial biopsies of subjects with chronic bronchitis: inverse relationship of CD8+ T lymphocytes with FEV$_1$. Am J Respir Crit Care Med 1997; 155: 852–857.

35. Holt PG. Regulation of antigen-presenting cell function(s) in lung and airway tissues. Eur Respir J 1993; 6: 120–129.

36. Holt PG, Schon-Hegrad MA, Oliver J et al. A contiguous network of dendritic antigen-presenting cells within the respiratory epithelium. Int Arch Allergy Appl Immunol 1990; 91: 155–159.

37. Enerback L. Mast cell heterogeneity: the evolution of the concept of a specific mucosal mast cell. In: Befus AD, Bienenstock J, Denburg JA, ed. Mast cell differentiation and heterogeneity. New York: Raven Press; 1986: 1.

38. Lamb D, Lumsden A. Intra-epithelial mast cells in human airway epithelium: evidence for smoking-induced changes in their frequency. Thorax 1982; 37: 334–342.

39. Grashoff WF, Sont JK, Sterk PJ et al. Chronic obstructive pulmonary disease: role of bronchiolar mast cells and macrophages. Am J Pathol 1997; 151: 1785–1790.

40. Godfrey RWA. Human airway epithelial tight junctions (Review). Microsc Res Tech 1997; 38: 488–499.

41. Sanderson MJ, Charles AC, Dirksen ER. Mechanical stimulation and intercellular communication increases intracellular Ca^{2+} in epithelial cells. Cell Reg 1990; 1: 585–596.

42. Hulbert WC, Walker DC, Jackson A, Hogg JC. Airway permeability to horseradish peroxidase in guinea pigs: the repair phase after injury by cigarette smoke. Am Rev Respir Dis 1981; 123: 320–326.

43. Godfrey RWA, Severs NJ, Jeffery PK. Freeze-fracture morphology and quantification of human bronchial epithelial tight junctions. Am J Respir Cell Mol Biol 1992; 6: 453–458.

44. Godfrey RWA, Severs NJ, Jeffery PK. Structural alterations of airway epithelial tight junctions in cystic fibrosis: Comparison of transplant and post-mortem tissue. Am J Respir Cell Mol Biol 1993; 9: 148–156.

45. Elia C, Bucca C, Rolla G et al. A freeze-fracture study of tight junctions in human bronchial epithelium in normal, bronchitic and asthmatic subjects. J Submicrosc Cytol Pathol 1988; 20: 509–517.

46. Montefort S, Holgate ST, Howarth PH. Leucocyte endothelial adhesion molecules and their role in bronchial asthma and allergic rhinitis. Eur Respir J 1993; 6: 1044–1054.

47. Abrahamson DR. Recent studies on the structure and pathology of basement membranes. J Pathol 1986; 149: 257–278.

48. Evans MJ, Van Winkle LS, Fanucchi MV et al. Three-dimensional organization of the lamina reticularis in the rat tracheal basement membrane zone. Am J Respir Cell Mol Biol 2000; 22: 393–397.

49. Howat WJ, Holmes JA, Holgate ST, Lackie PM. Basement membrane pores in human bronchial epithelium: a conduit for infiltrating cells? Am J Pathol 2001; 158: 673–680.

50. Evans MJ, Van Winkle LS, Fanucchi MV, Plopper CG. The attenuated fibroblast sheath of the respiratory tract epithelial-mesenchymal trophic unit. Am J Respir Cell Mol Biol 1999; 21: 655–765.

51. Tos M. Mucous glands of the trachea in children: quantitative studies. Anat Anz 1970; 126S: 146–160.

52. Meyrick B, Reid L. Ultrastructure of cells in the human bronchial submucosal glands. J Anat 1970; 107: 281–299.

53. Kramps JA, Franken C, Meijer CJLM et al. Localization of low molecular weight protease inhibitor in serous secretory cells of the respiratory tract. J Histochem Cytochem 1981; 29: 712–719.

54. Meyrick B, Sturgess J, Reid L. Reconstruction of the duct system and secretory tubules of the human bronchial submucosal gland. Thorax 1969; 24: 729–736.

55. Douglas AN. Quantitative study of bronchial mucous gland enlargement. Thorax 1980; 35: 198–201.

56. Bensch KG, Gordon GB, Miller LR. Studies on the bronchial counterpart of the Kultschitzky (argentaffin) cell and innervation of bronchial glands. J Ultrastruct Res 1965; 12: 668–686.

57. Soutar CA. Distribution of plasma cells and other cells containing immunoglobulin in the respiratory tract of normal man and class of immunoglobulin contained therein. Thorax 1976; 31: 158–166.

58. Goodman JR, Link DW, Brown WR, Nakane PK. Ultrastructural evidence of transport of secretory IgA across bronchial epithelium. Am Rev Respir Dis 1981; 18: 115–119.

59. Guerzon GM, Pare PD, Michoud M-C, et al. The number and distribution of mast cells in monkey lungs. Am Rev Respir Dis 1979; 119: 59–66.

60. Befus AD; Bienenstock J; Denberg JA. Mast cell differentiation and heterogeneity. New York: Raven Press; 1986.

61. Trapnell DH. Recognition and incidence of intrapulmonary lymph nodes. Thorax 1964; 19: 44–50.

62. Richmond I, Pritchard GE, Ashcroft T et al. Bronchus associated lymphoid tissue (BALT) in human lung: its distribution in smokers and non-smokers. Thorax 1993; 48: 1130–1139.

63. Chamberlain DW, Nopjaroonsri C, Simon GT. Ultrastructure of the pulmonary lymphoid tissue. Am Rev Respir Dis 1973; 108: 621–631.

64. Macklin CS. Pulmonary sumps, dust accumulations, alveolar fluid and lymph vessels. Acta Anat 1955; 23: 1–33.

65. Laitinen LA, Laitinen A, Widdicombe J. Effects of inflammatory and other mediators on airway vascular beds. Am J Respir Crit Care Med 1987; 135: S67–S70.

66. Hislop A, Reid LM. Formation of the pulmonary vasculature. In: Hodson WA, ed. Development of the lung, vol. 6. New York: Marcel Dekker; 1977: 37–86.

67. McLaughlin MF. Bronchial artery distribution in various mammals and in humans. Am Rev Respir Dis 1983; 128: S57.

68. Lauweryns JM. The blood and lymphatic microcirculation of the lung. In: Sommers SC, ed. Pathology annual, vol. 6. New York: Appleton-Century-Crofts; 1971: 365–415.

69. Staub NC. The pathophysiology of pulmonary edema. Human Pathol 1970; 1: 419–432.

70. Barnes PJ. Neural control of human airways in health and disease. Am Rev Respir Dis 1986; 134: 1289–1314.

71. Barnes PJ, Baraniuk J, Belvisi MG. Neuropeptides in the respiratory tract (part 1). Am Rev Respir Dis 1991; 144: 1187–1198.

72. Widdicombe JG. Nervous receptors in the respiratory tract and lungs. In: Hornbeim T, ed. Regulation of breathing (part 1). Lung biology in health and disease, vol. 17. New York: Marcel Dekker; 1981: 429.

73. Whimster WF. The microanatomy of the alveolar duct system. Thorax 1970; 25: 141.

74. Dunnill MS. Postnatal growth of the lung. Thorax 1962; 17: 329.

75. Bachofen H, Schurch S. Review: alveolar forces and lung architecture. Comp Biochem Physiol A 2001; 129: 183–193.

76. Meyrick B, Reid L. The alveolar brush cell in rat lung a third pneumocyte. J Ultrastruct Res 1968; 23: 71–80.

77. Crapo JD, Barry BE, Cehr P et al. Cell characteristics of the normal lung. Am Rev Respir Dis 1982; 125: 740.

78. Chevalier G, Collet AJ. In vivo incorporation of choline-^{3}H and galactose ^{3}H in alveolar type II pneumocytes in relation to surfactant synthesis. A quantitative radioautographic study in mouse by electron microscopy. Anat Rec 1972; 174: 289.

79. Kikkawa Y, Yoneda K, Smith F et al. The type II epithelial cells of the lung. II chemical composition and phospholipid synthesis. Lab Invest 1975; 32: 295.

80. Evans MJ, Cabral-Anderson LJ, Stephens RJ et al. Renewal of alveolar epithelium in the rat following exposure to NO_2. Am J Pathol 1973; 70: 175–198.

81. Evans MJ, Cabral LJ, Stephens RJ et al. Transformation of alveolar type 2 cells to type 1 cells following exposure to NO_2. Exp Mol Pathol 1975; 22: 142–150.

82. Schneeberger-Keeley EE, Karnovsky MJ. The ultrastructural basis of alveolar–capillary membrane permeability to peroxidase used as a tracer. J Cell Biol 1968; 37: 78.

83. Weibel ER. On pericytes, particularly their existence on lung capillaries. Microvasc Res 1974; 8: 218.

84. Nicholas TE, Strum JM, Angelo LA, Junod AE. Site and mechanism of uptake of ^{3}H-L norepinephrine by isolated perfused rat lungs. Circ Res 1974; 35: 670.

85. Gryglewski RJ. The lung as a generator of prostacyclin. Metabolic activities of the lung. Ciba Found Symp 1980; 78: 147.

86. Kapanci Y, Assimacopoulos A, Irle C et al. 'Contractile interstitial cells' in pulmonary alveolar septa: a possible role of ventilation/perfusion ratio ? J Cell Biol 1974; 60: 375–392.

87. Brody AR, Craighead JE. Cytoplasmic inclusions in pulmonary macrophages of cigarette smokers. Lab Invest 1975; 32: 125.

88. Kaltreider HB. Alveolar macrophages enhancers or suppressors of pulmonary immune reactivity? Chest 1982; 82: 261–262.

89. Brody AR, Hill LH, Adkins B et al. Chrysotile asbestos inhalation in rats: deposition pattern and reaction of alveolar epithelium and pulmonary macrophages. Am Rev Respir Dis 1981; 123: 670–678.

90. Bowden DH, Adamson IYR. Role of monocytes and interstitial cells in the generation of alveolar macrophages. I. Kinetic studies of normal mice. Lab Invest 1980; 42: 511.

91. Jaurand M-C, Kaplan H, Thiollet J. Phagocytosis of chrysotile fibers by pleural mesothelial cells in culture. Am J Pathol 1979; 94: 529–538.

1.3 Embryology and growth

Peter K Jeffery and Alison A Hislop

During development, the lungs must:

- establish communication with the exterior
- fill the chest cavity but remain separated from its wall by a narrow, fluid-filled pleural space bounded by mesothelium
- establish appropriate vascular connections with the heart
- make neural connections with the central nervous system.

The first of these is achieved by the airway primordia, which derive directly from the foregut. The second results from the lateral growth and branching of the lung buds pushing outwards into the splanchnopleural mesenchyme. The third is achieved through modification of the vessels supplying the embryonic branchial arches. Less is known about the development of the pulmonary innervation.

The end-point for lung development and maturation is a gas-exchanging organ in which air and blood come into intimate contact over a large surface area. An oxygen uptake of up to 3 litres per minute (l/min) is facilitated by an area of air–blood contact that is approximately 70 m^2, a little less than half the size of a tennis court, and a barrier separating air and blood that is only 0.2 mm thick – about 50 times thinner than a sheet of airmail paper. Furthermore, ventilation and perfusion need to be carefully matched over this large surface area. The problems inherent in these demands and constraints have been resolved during development by dividing the exchange barrier into a large number of small units, all suspended on a strong, three-dimensional fibre system surrounding three highly branched interdigitating 'trees', one each for air, arterial and venous blood; these converge at their end branches in the gas-exchange units.[1]

Phases of lung development

Following the embryonic period (Fig. 1.3.1), which in humans is the first few weeks following fertilization, four overlapping phases of lung development are recognized:

1. **Pseudoglandular** (5 to about 17 weeks' gestation), during which the preacinar branching pattern of airways and blood vessels is established (Fig. 1.3.2).

2. **Canalicular** (16–26 weeks' gestation), when vascularization of peripheral mesenchyme rapidly increases and the respiratory portion of the lung begins to develop (Fig. 1.3.3).
3. **Saccular** (from about 24 to 36 weeks), when additional respiratory airways develop and the future respiratory units differentiate. These are the acini, which each comprise a single terminal bronchiole and its subsequent divisions of respiratory bronchioles, alveolar ducts and alveoli.
4. **Alveolar** (from about 36 weeks to term and continuing for the first 3 years of infancy). There is great variability in the onset of alveolar formation and in their numbers at birth (Fig. 1.3.4).

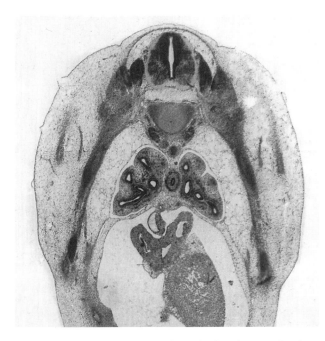

Fig. 1.3.1 Transverse section through the thorax of a human embryo (15 mm, 6 weeks) showing spinal cord and vertebral arch extending to form the rib cage. The lungs lie in the pleural cavity dorsal to the relatively large heart and pericardium. Small fissural depressions show the lobes of the lung; airways within the mesenchyme are lined by columnar epithelium. The oesophagus lies between the two lungs. H&E stain.

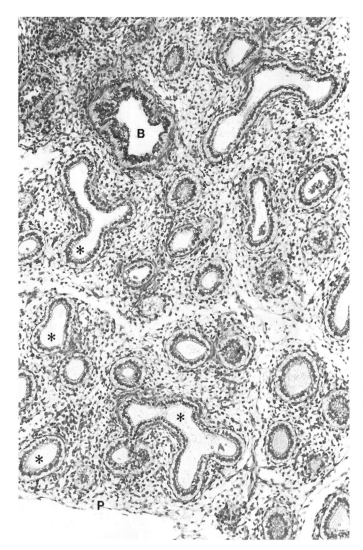

Fig. 1.3.2 Fetal lung at 16 weeks' gestation showing a pseudoglandar pattern. Differentiating bronchi (B), peripheral airway branches (*) and pleura (P). H&E stain.

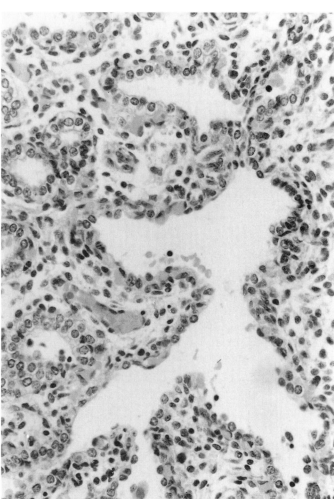

Fig. 1.3.3 Lung from a fetus of 23 weeks' gestation in the canalicular phase of development. A terminal air space has epithelial cells that are thinning with small capillaries immediately under them. There is still a considerable amount of mesenchymal tissue around the air space. H&E stain.

Airway branching

The airways begin their development 22–26 days postfertilization as a ventral diverticulum budding from the foregut and lined by epithelium of endodermal origin. In humans the diverticulum forms two ventrolateral buds (the lung primordia) during the fourth week of gestation. The trachea then progressively separates from the oesophagus by the rostral extension of a septum, which forms by fusion of epithelial ridges at the root of the lung buds until only a small connection remains. The larynx forms after completion of the septum. Incomplete fusion of the ridges results in tracheo-oesophageal fistulas (see Chapter 20). As the two ventrolateral buds grow, they become invested by mesenchyme derived from splanchnic mesoderm. This later condenses and differentiates around the growing bronchial tree to form cartilage, muscle, blood, vessels, lymphatics and other connective tissue elements (see Fig. 1.3.1). These primitive airways divide to form two branches on the left and three on the right (Fig. 1.3.5). By this stage the fissures between the lobes are present and the lung buds have a plexus of capillaries around them connected to the aortic sac by two pulmonary arteries and to the sinus venosus by a pulmonary vein.[2] As the hollow bronchial tubes branch repeatedly, the numerous blind-ending tubules give the lung the pseudoglandular appearances characteristic of the first postembryonic phase (see Fig. 1.3.2).

Normal airway branching requires both epithelium and mesenchyme. If the mesenchyme is stripped away the airway tube will elongate but not divide.[3] Conversely, mesenchymal tissue taken from an area of active branching will promote branching of epithelial tubes from an area where branching was previously complete. Branching is dependent on interactions among cell substrate adhesion molecules, intercellular adhesion molecules and the extracellular matrix proteins, particularly proteoglycans and glycosaminoglycans. The branching is probably brought about by allowing some cells to migrate whereas others remain stationary and therefore form a cleft.[4]

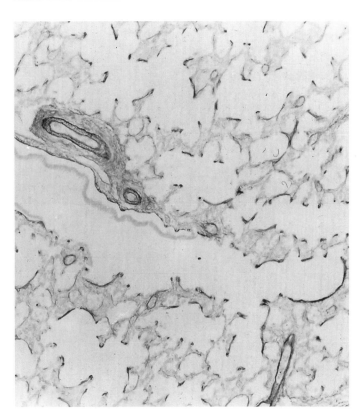

Fig. 1.3.4 Lung from an infant at term in the final alveolar phase of development. An alveolar duct is lined by relatively shallow alveoli. A terminal bronchiole leads into a respiratory bronchiole; alveolar ducts are lined by alveoli. At the tips of each alveolar septum there is an accumulation of elastic fibres. Pulmonary arteries accompany the airways. Miller's elastin/van Gieson stain.

The pattern of conducting airway branching is complete by about the 16th week of intrauterine life. Thus, although airway size obviously changes after birth, the pattern of branching does not and the airways of the newborn lung are essentially those of the adult in miniature.[5]

Airway number

In humans, the lobar and segmental bronchi appear at about the fifth week. At this stage variations in segmental and subsegmental bronchi may occur. Division of intrasegmental airways is fastest between the 10th and 14th weeks. By this time about 70% of the airway generations present at birth have formed.[6] The general pattern of growth is similar in all lung segments, although, in those with a longer axis, more divisions occur and take longer to complete.

The extension of the airways is the result of rapid proliferation of their epithelial lining cells: cell division occurs particularly at the ends of the tubes, the so-called bronchial buds. Branching is determined by interactions with surrounding mesenchyme and is usually by 'irregular dichotomy'. The branching appears to

follow strict physical rules and results in an organ that is 'space-filling' with few gaps between the units. The pattern has been likened to a 'fractal tree',[1] a mathematical abstraction that, in reality, has been modified by space and shape constraints, resulting in the irregular dichotomous bronchial tree with pathways of differing length but whose divisions finally become smaller in logarithmic fashion with each subsequent generation, although at the time of branching they were of similar size. Airway branching and lung growth are influenced by a variety of factors. Several transcription factors, including hepatocyte nuclear factor-3β, thyroid transcript factor and Gli proteins, control early branching morphogenesis, while later the interaction of mesenchyme and epithelium is mediated by various growth factors and their receptors, with a balance being reached between those causing multiplication of epithelial cells (e.g. insulin-like growth factor and epidermal growth factor) and those (such as transforming growth factor-β) that are powerful inhibitors of epithelial cell multiplication but enhance protein synthesis.[7–11]

Physical factors are also implicated in controlling lung growth. Restricted space availability, as in congenital diaphragmatic hernia, leads to a reduction in airway number.[12] Fluid produced within the airway lumen is controlled by the epithelial cells and is vital to normal airway development. Drainage of fluid, either experimentally or as a result of premature rupture of membranes,[13] leads to hypoplastic lungs, whereas tracheal ligation in experimental animals or in cases with laryngeal atresia causes an increase in lung size.[14,15] Changes in the amount of amniotic fluid, as seen in oligohydramnios as a result of renal agenesis and after amniocentesis in experimental animals, leads to a reduced airway number.[16,17] Fetal breathing movements also influence the development of airways.[18,19] The human fetal airway smooth muscle contracts spontaneously in the first trimester and also responds to pharmacological manipulation.[20] Such contractions maintain positive intraluminal pressure and assist airway growth. Blocking spontaneous contractions leads to lung hypoplasia in vitro.[21] Stretch is known to promote protein synthesis and may also influence lung growth.[20] Maternal smoking during pregnancy leads to low birth weight; it is also associated with diminished airflows, which are evident in preterm babies as young as 33 weeks of gestation.[22] Smoking studies in monkeys have shown hypoplastic lungs with increased collagen around airways and an upregulation of nicotinic receptors.[23]

Once airway branching is complete the airways continue to increase in size as lung volume increases. From 22 weeks of gestation to birth there is a linear increase in diameter in all airways from the bronchus to the terminal bronchiole. This continues after birth: airways increase in diameter and length by two to three times between birth and adulthood.[24] The ultimate size of the airways does not appear to be affected by premature birth. The number of terminal bronchioles, which form the last purely conductive airways, is estimated at 25 000 in the adult. Peripheral conducting airways are relatively large in diameter at 1–3 months of age, attaining their normal adult size after 1 year.[25] Gender also affects lung growth. Tracheal size does not differ between sexes during early life but adult males have wider tracheas while the peripheral airways of boys are relatively narrow and predispose to wheeze.[26, 27]

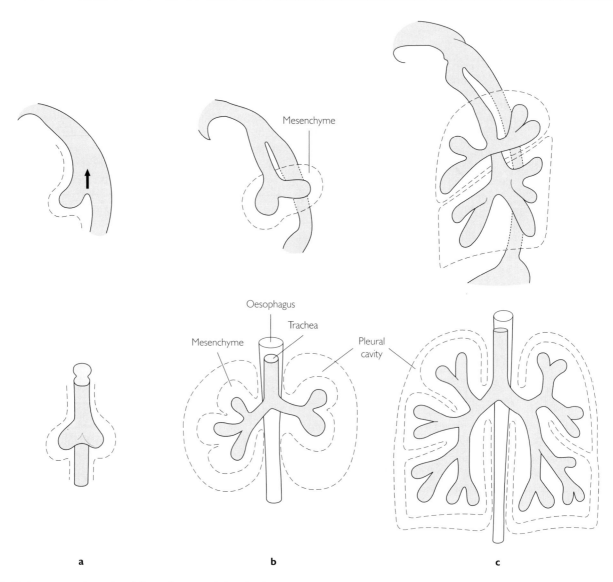

Fig. 1.3.5 Diagrammatic lateral and frontal views of the developing human lung during the (a) fourth, (b) fifth and (c) sixth fetal week. (With permission from Weibel.[1])

Conducting airways

Surface epithelium

Four cell types comprise the surface epithelium of the main conducting airways: (1) ciliated, (2) mucus-secreting (goblet), (3) indeterminate and (4) basal cells. In the terminal bronchioles, a fifth cell is found – the Clara cell. The ciliated cells are present throughout the respiratory tract, as far peripherally as the respiratory bronchioles. (For details of epithelial cells see Chapter 1.2.) In addition, peptide-producing neuroendocrine cells with characteristic dense-core granules occur singly or in groups, and are often innervated. Their number and predominant location vary with lung development and growth. All respiratory epithelial cells developed by differentiation and maturation of primitive endodermal cells. With advancing gesta-

tion the process of differentiation follows a centrifugal pattern, i.e. maturation begins in proximal airways and progressively spreads distally. The major events are shown in Figure 1.3.6.

In both the proximal and distal airways, epithelial thickness steadily decreases from early fetal to postnatal life, whereas airway diameter increases.[28]

The primitive fetal cell

During the late embryonic/early pseudoglandular phase, the epithelial lining is stratified and consists of vertically oriented cells with the thinner cells extending between more basally situated cells.[28–30] At this early stage the tracheal lining closely resembles that of the developing oesophagus. The primitive surface cells are all similar, each having a large vesicular nucleus, prominent nucleoli and electron-lucent cytoplasm with large areas occupied by glycogen and apical microvilli. Single primary

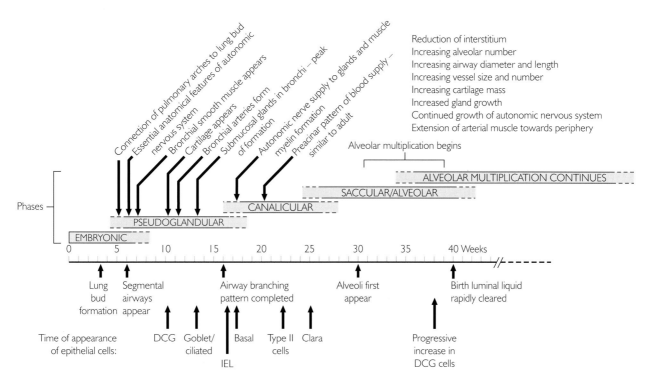

Fig. 1.3.6 Scheme of major events during lung development. DCG, dense-core granule cell; IEL, intraepithelial lymphocyte.

(rudimentary) cilia may be present at all stages during the development of many diverse cell types, both normal and neoplastic. Unlike the motile cilia of the ciliated border, primary cilia lack central microtubules and are immotile. At this time, well-developed cell junctional complexes, the zonula occludens and desmosomes, join adjacent cells; the zona occludens affords a selective permeability barrier to transepithelial movements of ions, molecules and fluid. The cells rest on a predominantly continuous basement membrane with occasional gaps at the ends of the terminal buds that allow contact between epithelial and mesenchymal cells. The epithelial basement membrane in the fetus is thin and consists of basal lamina devoid of the reticular lamina characteristic of the adult human, which appears to thicken with age and in disease (e.g. asthma).

The ciliated cell and ciliogenesis

Differentiation of a ciliated epithelium is apparent between 11 and 16 weeks' gestation in humans, at the end of the pseudoglandular phase when the number of bronchi increases significantly and mesenchyme differentiates into cartilage and bronchial smooth muscle. Cilia develop from centrioles, which arise either directly by division of pre-existing centrioles (as in the formation of primary or rudimentary cilia) or indirectly by a sequence of events initiated in the Golgi region, starting with fibrogranular aggregates from which deuterosomes and a generatic complex of precentrioles arise.[28,31,32] In the formation of the ciliated cell border, the newly formed and maturing precentrioles migrate to the apex of the cell and initiate ciliary outgrowth.

A ciliary bud is formed first and growth of the cilium then proceeds at its tip.[28,33] Initially, there appears to be some lag in the development of the internal microtubules characteristic of the ciliary shaft, but by the time the cilium is one-third its adult length, the microtubules extend throughout the shaft and ciliary beating commences. As with the early centriole, the microtubules of the ciliary shaft first appear to be single and later develop into the doublets typical of the adult cilium. At what stage during growth of the cilium the beat becomes coordinated is not known. Individual cilia develop at different rates, even within a single cell.[33–35] Sorokin[34] has observed that a cell that has developed cilia may still contain ciliary precursors; this suggests that a cell's full complement of cilia does not develop simultaneously but that several waves of ciliogenesis pass along the airways until, within any one cell, the adult number of about 200–300 per cell is reached.[32]

Mucus-secreting cells

The presence of intracellular mucus has been demonstrated histochemically in human fetal lung at 13 weeks' gestation;[6,30] such cells are sparse and located within crypts of corrugated surface epithelium or in newly forming submucosal glands. Presecretory cells appear at about the same time as preciliated cells. Two types of secretory granule may be identified by electron microscopy: electron dense and electron lucent. However, three types of cell may be found:

• those with only electron-dense serous granules
• those with only electron-lucent mucous granules
• those with a mixture of the two.

The three cell types probably correspond to the three histo-chemically distinct types seen by light microscopy after Alcian blue (pH 2.5):periodic-acid–Schiff (PAS) staining:

- PAS-positive (pink)
- Alcian-blue-positive (blue)
- heliotrope (mixed).

By 22 weeks of gestation, goblet cells are found as far as the distal ends of large bronchi. The number of goblet cells peaks at mid-gestation, when they represent 30–35% of cells lining the luminal surface. Towards the end of gestation there is a relative decrease in their number so that they are less frequent than in the adult.[36] With increasing gestational age goblet cells extend more peripherally and by term are present in bronchioles.[24] The proportion of goblet to ciliated cells increases rapidly in the first 4 weeks after birth. In preterm babies the number of goblet cells increases immediately after birth so that they have more than normal for their postconceptional age.[24] After birth, the secretory cells appear to be predominantly mucous in type, as in the adult trachea,[37,38] producing mainly acidic (sulphated) mucin. The 'serous' secretory cells of the surface epithelium do not appear to contain lysozyme, in contrast to the submucosal glands[39] (see below).

Clara cells

Clara cells are thought to develop during the second half of gestation from primitive glycogen-containing non-ciliated cells of the terminal airways (see Fig. 1.1.8). They are thought to be the progenitors of ciliated cells in the bronchioli.[40] By 16–17 weeks' gestation, the dome-like apical protrusion characteristic of the mature cell has formed. Maturation involves gradual loss of cytoplasmic glycogen, increasing ribosomal content and the appearance of electron-dense secretory granules, which may become numerous by 24 weeks' gestation.[39] In the adult human lung, a low-molecular-weight antileukoprotease can be localized to serous cells of submucosal glands, surface goblet cells and bronchiolar Clara cells.[41] This antiprotease has been identified in the human trachea, in submucosal glands, as early as the 16th week of fetal life, and has been shown to be present in bronchiolar epithelium by week 36 of gestation.[42] These data argue for the early appearance of a protective antiprotease and the maturation of Clara cells before parturition.

Neuroendocrine cells

Neuroendocrine or dense-core granulated (DCG) cells are reported to be the first 'mature' type to differentiate within primitive airway epithelium. Distributed singly or in pairs, they are identified at 8 weeks' gestation.[43,44] They are weakly argyrophilic, show immunoreactivity for serotonin and neurone-specific enolase[45] but not, as yet, for bombesin and other peptides. Bombesin-like immunoreactivity and serotonin positivity are found at about 10 weeks' gestation, at a time when submucosal nerves and ganglia are reactive to neuron-specific enolase.[44] The frequency of bombesin and serotonin-immunoreactive DCG cells increases significantly towards term, resulting primarily from an increase in neuroepithelial

bodies in peripheral airways.[44] Associated with this, bombesin-like immunoreactivity in lung tissue extracts is highest during the late fetal/neonatal period and decreases post-partum.[46] Calcitonin and leu-enkephalin are detected only late during fetal development and are identified postnatally.[44,47]

The function of the DCG cell is debated. Among other functions it may, through its amine secretion, affect lobule growth and differentiation.[48] With age, there is a decrease in cell number, in the number of granules per cell and in the electron density of each granule. The number of DCG cells increases in babies recovering from hyaline membrane disease and in those with bronchopulmonary dysplasia.[47] In hypoxic conditions, there are intracellular changes in the bronchial DCG cell of the young rat, similar to those seen in carotid-body chief cells, which suggests that the DCG cell might have a role in the response of the young lung to hypoxia.[49,50] Rare nerve endings in contact with DCG cells have been demonstrated in fetal lung.[51]

Basal cells

The basal cell is the last major cell type to differentiate in large airways. By light microscopy, basal cells have been reported in the trachea of 10-week-old fetuses.[30] However, by electron microscopy and immunocytochemistry, the only basally located cells identified are DCG cells and undifferentiated cells rich in glycogen. By 12 weeks' gestation the immunoreactivity of epidermal keratin (a marker of maturation for the basal cell type) is weakly positive (with a patchy distribution), and electron microscopy shows some basally located cells containing tonofilaments, well-developed desmosomes and some hemidesmosomes, attaching basal cells to basement membrane.[40] Fully mature basal cells are identified during the canalicular and saccular stages of development. For some time, the basal cell has been regarded as the main progenitor cell for the more superficial columnar cells.[52] Recently it has been suggested that the distribution and prevalence of the basal cell in large airways may relate to its role in strengthening adhesion of the tall columnar cells to their basement membrane.[53] The exclusivity of their proliferative and pluripotential stem cell role in squamous and mucous cell metaplasia has also been challenged.[54,55]

Submucosal glands

In the adult trachea and bronchi, there are numerous glands, which are responsible for producing most of the mucus found in the airways. They are present wherever there is a cartilage, located in the submucosa between the cartilage and the surface epithelium. Each gland is tubuloacinar, with a duct opening into and continuous with the airway lumen (see Chapter 1.2).

Submucosal glands first appear in the human trachea as early as 10 weeks' gestation. They develop progressively more peripherally and reach the main carina some 7 days later.[56] In bronchi, they are present by the fourth month of fetal life, in greatest concentration proximally, decreasing peripherally and especially concentrated at airway bifurcations.[57] Their appearance in the membranous wall precedes that in the cartilaginous wall in both bronchus and trachea, and in the case of the trachea by some 9 days.[56,58] In the main extrapulmonary bronchi, the rate of gland formation reaches a peak during fetal week 12–14, decreasing after this and terminating during the middle of week. It has been estimated that, at this time, some 4000 glands are present in the trachea, the highest density being in the cartilaginous wall.[56,57] Few new glands are formed in childhood, and an increase in gland area is the result of an increase in gland complexity. The shape of the gland mass varies and is determined by the space available during development.

One study suggested that there are no sex differences in the density during development,[56] whereas another found a male superiority in gland number, resulting from a higher concentration of glands rather than from a difference in absolute size of the trachea.[57] The proportion of the wall occupied by gland (i.e. the gland : wall ratio or 'Reid index') reaches the adult norm in late fetal life; during childhood, however, mucous glands form a larger proportion of the walls (major bronchi) than in the adult.[59] Thus, gland hyperplasia in response to irritation might be a more significant problem in young children than in adults. A positive correlation has been shown between a high Reid index and atelectasis in infants.[60]

Each gland starts its development within the surface epithelium, by division of basal cells, to form a sharply defined cluster of cells.[30,56] Growth then proceeds radially into the lamina propria as a solid cylinder, still enclosed in basement membrane, which maintains continuity with its surface epithelium. Soon, mucus is secreted into an intercellular space, which expands into a canal. Subsequent widening of the canal pushes the epithelial cells apart, thus forming an opening to the airway lumen.[58] Following radial penetration of the muscle layer, there is continued growth and division but in a tangential or longitudinal direction (either cranially or caudally).[29]

With age, the human gland becomes more complex, although the gland does not approach the form of the adult until 13 years of age, and even then growth continues until 28 years of age. A weakly eosinophilic ductal region is present as early as 24 weeks' gestation. Throughout development, mucous tubules arise from the collecting duct region, with serous acini usually at their distal ends. The number of lysozyme-containing cells in the serous acini increases as term approaches.[40] Low-molecular-weight antileukoprotease is another marker for maturation of glandular serous cells and can be detected from 16 weeks' gestation.[42]

Interstitial elements

While the basal lamina on which the epithelium rests develops at the same time as the epithelium, the underlying lamina reticularis does not develop until 18 weeks of gestation. This layer, which is so characteristically thickened in asthma, develops at a later stage in utero or postnatally.

Little is known about the development of collagen and elastic fibres in the conducting airways. In the rat, the early mesenchymal mass is made up of scattered multiple-branched cells that appear to be in partial continuity with the somatopleural mesothelium. Numerous mitotic figures are seen. Collagen fibrils are detected towards the end of the glandular phase (i.e.

day 18 in the rat) and increase in amount during the canalicular phase. Cartilage first appears in the fourth gestation week in the trachea, in the 10th week in the main bronchi and in the 12th week in segmental bronchi. Cartilage continues to form peripherally until about 2 months after birth. After this time there is little further extension, but a progressive increase in the total cartilage mass is seen through infancy and childhood.

At 6–8 weeks' gestation, smooth muscle is present in the trachea and the main and lobar bronchi. Muscle develops sequentially along the airways as they branch as far as the terminal and respiratory bronchioles and alveolar ducts. During fetal life and childhood, there is an increase in the amount of bronchial smooth muscle relative to the size of the airways. Examination of airways of term and preterm babies suggests that there is a more rapid increase in the amount of bronchial smooth muscle immediately after birth, probably as a result of transition to air breathing. This means that preterm babies have a greater amount of muscle than normal for both their postconceptional age and their airway size. Babies who are ventilated artificially after birth have an even greater amount of muscle.[24] The bronchial smooth muscle at birth has a mature structure, is innervated[61] and has been shown to contract. Airway reactivity to methacholine, reversible with metaproterenol, is demonstrable in normal infants.[62]

Innervation

From the ectoderm, neural plate and associated neural crest develop autonomic nerves that migrate to supply pulmonary effector structures.[63] Migrating neural-crest cells take up position in the walls of the future trachea and lung buds at a stage before separation of the trachea from the oesophagus (i.e. at 4–5 weeks' gestation). By 6 weeks the essential anatomical features of the sympathetic and parasympathetic systems are established.

Ganglia appear in extrachondrial tissue of the trachea by 7 weeks' gestation and extend to the second-generation bronchi, formed by this time. Innervation of major arteries and veins begins at 10 weeks' gestation. By 16 weeks, growth in the trachea results in a well-defined posterior plexus and an inner plexus between cartilage and epithelium, with nerve fibres extending to submucosal glands and tracheal muscle. At this time, ganglia are seen along the extrachondrial and inner plexus at bronchial bifurcations and adventitia down to small bronchi. By this time nerves are present in all but the most peripheral airways, arteries and veins.[64]

The process of myelin formation also begins at about 16 weeks. By 8 months' gestation, nerve cells are reported to be multipolar and highly branched, with processes terminating on bronchial smooth muscle and penetrating the surface epithelium. At birth the distribution and number of nerves to all airway structures is similar to that in the adult, with sympathetic and parasympathetic nerve fibres extending as far as the alveolar ducts. The number and type of neuropeptides within the nerves change with age. The total number of neuropeptide-containing nerves, mainly bronchodilator, decreases in the respiratory region after 3 years of age.[61] The bronchoconstrictor response to histamine and methacholine also decreases with age.

Nerve trunks also supply the preacinar blood vessels running in the vascular adventitia. Nerve fibres do not extend into the muscular walls of arteries but are found as far internally as the endothelium of pulmonary veins. Nerve fibres are only found accompanying pulmonary arteries with muscular walls and, as small peripheral arteries grow and become muscular in structure, there is, in parallel, an extension of the nerve fibres. The neuropeptides in these nerves may have a trophic effect on the muscle cells.[65] In infants with pulmonary hypertension, the increase in arterial smooth muscle is accompanied by an increase in the number of nerve fibres. The vasoactive peptides in the nerves supplying the arteries are mainly vasoconstrictor.[65]

Although little is known of the neuroreceptors in the developing human lung, there is evidence that they change with age.[66] There are fewer β-receptors (bronchodilator) in fetal than in adult rabbits.[67] In rats there is a progressive increase in number with age from newborn to young adults.[68] Conversely, numbers of muscarinic receptors (bronchoconstrictor) decrease with age in the rat.[69] In human fetal lung, β-adrenoceptors are present at 14 weeks' gestation, increasing thereafter.[70] They are found in the surface epithelium, terminal tubules and pulmonary arteries, α₁-adrenoceptors and muscarinic receptors are not detected up to 23 weeks of gestation. Functional studies in humans suggest a drop in muscarinic receptors, with an increase in β-adrenoceptors in the first year of life.[62]

Respiratory zone

Alveolar buds

Although the branching pattern of the conductive airways is complete by 16 weeks' gestation, proliferation of its end buds continues until week 24, laying down the future respiratory portions of the airway tree.[71] At 17 weeks, the acinar boundaries are still incomplete;[72] in the developing respiratory portion of the lung, three processes occur:

- the tall epithelial lining of the terminal buds is reduced
- capillaries move into close contact with the surface epithelium
- connective tissue components are reduced at 17 weeks.

The primitive peripheral lung buds of the pseudoglandular phase (see Fig. 1.1.2) comprise a columnar epithelium with nuclei of variable size and shape, with frequent mitotic figures. With continued branching to form first the prospective respiratory bronchioli and then the alveolar ducts, the epithelial thickness is gradually reduced, giving rise to a cuboidal lining with spherical nuclei. Large amounts of glycogen are present, together with occasional droplets of fat, small mitochondria, many free ribosomes and sparse endoplasmic reticulum. Tight junctions and desmosomes are present, as is a well-defined but occasionally patchy basal lamina.

The gradual flattening of the lining epithelium and consequent widening of tubule lumina gives rise to the spaces that characterize the canalicular phase (see Fig. 1.3.3). The loose network of capillaries around the peripheral airways within the mesenchyme gradually becomes more dense and moves close to the airway epithelium – the process of vascularization. The close apposition and further thinning of overlying epithelium results in the formation of large primitive alveoli or 'saccules' (see Fig. 1.3.4). The lining epithelium differentiates and matures into thin squamous (type I) and the early cuboidal (type II) secretory cells, which will soon synthesize and secrete the phospholipid-rich, surface-tension-reducing substance called 'surfactant'. The type II cell is not only the source of alveolar surfactant but also the progenitor (stem) cell from which the type I alveolar cells differentiate.

The metabolism and turnover of lung surfactant in the adult, and its changes during development, are reviewed in Chapter 2.2. Dipalmitoyl lecithin is an important surface-active component of the alveolar lining layer, and lung lecithin levels rise slowly during the first three-quarters of pregnancy. As the alveolar lining cells mature, there is a sharp rise in total lecithin, which is reflected in its concentration within amniotic fluid. Normally, there is a dramatic rise in the concentration of 'surface-active' lipid during the last 30 days of gestation, in preparation for lung expansion. It is well known that surfactant deficiency at this critical time is associated with the respiratory distress syndrome (see Chapter 22).[73]

Alveolar sacs and alveoli

There is a rapid decrease in average air space wall thickness between 19 and 30 weeks' gestation. The terminal sac/alveolar stage of lung appearance in humans is evident at about 25 weeks' gestation. At 26 weeks' gestation 50% of babies will survive birth, although modern treatment has allowed survival of some babies from 23 weeks' gestation. At the beginning of this phase each adjacent saccule is surrounded by its own closely apposed capillary network; the separating septum between saccules therefore contains two adjacent capillary networks as well as mesenchyme.[1,74,75] Saccule-to-alveolar transformation is made by subdivision of the saccules involving the formation of new (secondary) septa on 'anchoring' points defined by elastic tissue[74] (Fig. 1.3.7, and see Fig. 1.3.4). During the transformation of 'saccular' to 'alveolar' lung, the network of elastic and collagen fibres appears to be the key to initiation of new septal formation and is maximal at points from which the future alveolar septa will protrude. In these septa, there is a central core of fibroblasts and collagenous connective tissue. The process is complex and appears to involve a combination of interstitial thinning and capillary fusion.[76] The increase in alveoli has three phases:

1. early lung expansion
2. a marked increase in tissue proliferation with a diurnal variation that reaches its peak of cell division during the night
3. a phase of proportionate growth involving enlargement of existing structures and capillary remodelling.

In the rat these changes occur entirely after birth. In humans, alveoli can first be identified subdividing the walls of the saccules at about 28 weeks' gestation, when saucer-shaped indentations are delineated by crests containing elastin. Between 28 and 32 weeks' gestation these crests elongate sufficiently to form cup-shaped alveoli lining the saccules, which can now be identified as alveolar ducts.[71]

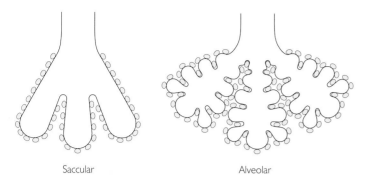

Saccular   Alveolar

Fig. 1.3.7 Simplified diagrammatic model to show how a saccular lung is transformed into its final alveolar phase. (With permission from Weibel.[1])

At first, the walls of the alveoli are still relatively thick and have a double capillary supply. With time, the alveolar walls thin and increase in length, and the capillaries fuse to give the single capillary system of the normal adult lung. At term, elastin is found only at the mouths of alveoli (see Figs 1.3.4 and 1.3.7); by 5 years, elastin is still only at the mouths but, by 12 years, elastic fibres are found around the alveolar walls and, by 18 years, many are present throughout the wall. The relative lack of elastin in the growing lung facilitates increase in size of the alveoli. Factors that prevent cross-linking of elastin and collagen severely reduce alveolar multiplication.[74,77]

By 34–35 weeks' gestation, the alveolar region appears very similar to that seen postnatally (see Fig. 1.3.4). By this time thin-walled alveoli can also be identified in the walls of respiratory bronchioli, which have part of their wall lined by cuboidal epithelium. Counts of alveoli in lungs from fetuses aged from 29 weeks' gestation to term show an increase from 30 million to around 150 million. The number at term varies but is around one-third to one-half the adult number, with a total surface area one-20th of that of the adult. Following birth, there continues to be a period of alveolar multiplication, the length of which is debated.[73,78]

Postnatal alveolar multiplication

The conductive and respiratory airways are filled with fluid throughout fetal development, the fluid being formed by a combination of active ion secretion by the lining epithelium and vascular transudation.[79] In the fetus, lung fluid communicates directly with amniotic fluid; it can be sampled by amniocentesis and analysed for phospholipid content to assess lung maturity. With the first breath, much of the liquid is cleared. Most of it is absorbed rapidly into the interstitium, and the rest more slowly into the circulation and lymphatics during the first 4–6 hours after birth. This clearance increases lung compliance and lung volume, and decreases the work of breathing.

With the tying of the umbilical cord and the closure of the ductus arteriosus and the foramen ovale, the pulmonary circulation becomes fully established and gas exchange begins. In humans, alveolar multiplication and parenchymal maturation continue after birth, particularly in the first 18 months of life,

with the normally regarded adult number of about 300 million alveoli being reached by the age of 2–4 years.[80-82] Other investigators suggest that alveolar multiplication may continue until somatic growth ceases.[77] The final number may depend upon body length and may be as high as 600 million.[83] Males generally have a greater number of alveoli than females at all ages over 1 year, independent of size as well as age.[84] The air–tissue interface at birth has been estimated to be 2.8 m^2, at 1 year 12 m^2, at 4 years 22 m^2, and at 8 years 32 m^2.[44] The average adult human lung is usually considered to have an alveolar surface area of about 70 m^2, varying between 40 and 120 m^2.[1,80,81]

After birth the conductive airways increase in diameter by two to three times up to adulthood, a ninefold increase in area. By comparison, the alveolar area increases over 20-fold. Alveolar development may be affected by a number of factors in utero and postnatally. Malnutrition in utero and postnatally reduces alveolar multiplication in rats, though re-feeding leads to catch-up growth.[85] Vitamin A (retinoic acid) has also been shown to be essential for normal alveolar development and supplementation will lead to increased alveolar septation.[86] In utero infection and maternal smoking have also been shown to affect alveolar development.[87-89] Postnatally, high and low oxygen tensions prevent alveolar multiplication[90,91] and glucocorticoids, although initially enhancing alveolar maturation, may eventually lead to reduced alveolar multiplication.[92-94]

Pulmonary and bronchial vasculature

The development of pulmonary arteries and veins is closely related to that of the bronchial tree: before birth they relate to the dividing airways and following birth to the rapidly multiplying alveoli. The adult lung has a double arterial supply and also a double venous drainage. Pulmonary arteries supply the alveolar capillaries and most of the pleura, whereas systemic bronchial arteries supply the airway wall, pleura at the hilum and large blood vessel walls. Draining from the hilum to the azygos vein are the bronchial veins; pulmonary veins drain most structures within the lung, even many of those supplied by the bronchial arteries.

From 28 days' gestation, pulmonary arteries from the primitive aortic sac connect with a vascular plexus in the mesenchyme surrounding the two lung buds. Between 28 and 35 days' gestation the main pulmonary veins connect between the lung bud hilum and the left atrium. By 37 days the main pulmonary artery has separated from the aorta. During fetal life, connection with the systemic circulation is maintained via the ductus arteriosus, which is derived from the embryonic sixth arch and connects the pulmonary artery to the ascending aorta. A second shunt, the foramen ovale, is preserved in the form of an opening in the atrial septum, allowing right atrial blood to be shunted directly into the left atrium. From 5 weeks' gestation the airways branch into the surrounding mesenchyme and around the edge of each bud endothelial tubules form by vasculogenesis. These tubules coalesce by angiogenic remodelling to form the artery accompanying the airway and an accompanying vein growing in the interairway plane.[2] Thus the pulmonary arteries and veins form at the same time as the airways, which act as a template. After the vessels have coalesced to form an artery or vein the wall becomes invested in muscle cells which increase in number as the vessel increases in size. By 20 weeks' gestation, the preacinar branching pattern of arteries and veins is essentially the same as that seen in the adult. Later in fetal development, the vessels continue to increase in size and new vessels form in the respiratory region as the airways divide. After birth, new vessels in the alveolar region lead to the appearance of a dense 'background haze' of small vessels seen throughout the lung arteriogram (Fig. 1.3.8).

Arteries that run alongside and branch with airways are termed 'conventional'. In addition, there are 'supernumerary' vessels (particularly at the periphery) which do not branch with the airway and supply the adjacent alveoli directly. During development, supernumerary arteries appear at the same time as the conventional arteries,[93] and by 12 weeks' gestation they are present in roughly their adult proportions, even though the full complement of airways has yet to appear and

the alveoli that they will supply are not yet present. Veins develop at the same time as arteries, conventional veins being in similar numbers to conventional arteries; supernumerary veins in greater numbers than supernumerary arteries have also been identified.[94] The total adult number of preacinar conventional vessels is present by the fifth month of intrauterine life. In later fetal life intra-acinar arteries develop; these accompany respiratory airways and alveoli. The vessels grow in size and length, the main branches increasing more rapidly during fetal life and infancy than in childhood (i.e. after 18 months of age).

The systemic bronchial supply appears at the end of the first trimester and extends down the airway wall as the cartilage and glands differentiate. In the adult the bronchial arteries extend to a level a few generations proximal to the terminal bronchioles. They divide into a capillary network, which drains into the pulmonary veins either directly or via adjacent alveoli.[95,96] True bronchial veins drain the trachea and upper bronchi and return blood to the left atrium.

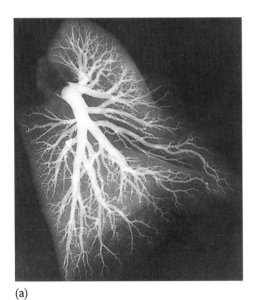
(a)

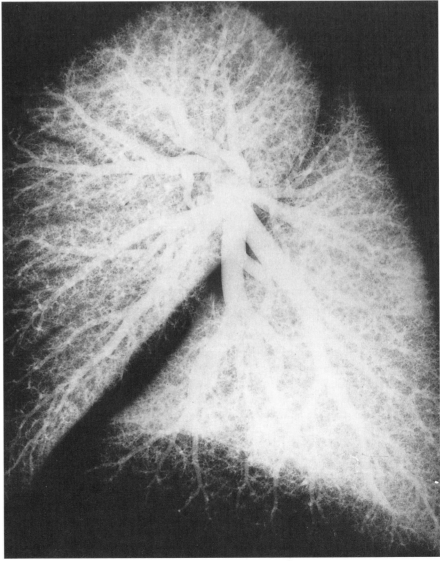
(b)

Fig. 1.3.8 (a) Pulmonary arteriogram (actual size) of the left lung of a baby at term. The branching pattern of the arteries to each segment is complete. There is little background haze obscuring the pattern of preacinar branching as there are few peripheral arteries. (b) Pulmonary arteriogram (actual size) of the left lung of an infant aged 18 months. The branching pattern of the arteries is similar to that seen at birth but there is a dense background haze made up of a large number of arteries too small to be identified as individual lines – arteries that have grown in the alveolar region of the lung after birth.

During childhood, when new alveolar ducts and alveoli appear, additional arteries and veins also appear, mostly of the supernumerary type, which supply the alveoli of the child and adult directly.[96] After the newborn period, the ratio of arteries to alveoli is similar at all ages. With increasing alveolar size in childhood, mean arterial size also increases. The number of veins per unit area of alveolar tissue is greater than that of the arteries.

Intravascular pressure influences the structure of the arterial wall.[97] During fetal life, intrapulmonary pressure is high and the main pulmonary artery wall structure consequently resembles that of the aorta. Changes that probably begin at birth are apparent at 6 months; by 2 years the adult structure is present (i.e. irregular elastic tissue and a wall that is 40–70% as thick as that of the aorta). Many congenital abnormalities can affect this transition (e.g. severe pulmonary hypertension, pulmonary atresia and hypoplastic left heart syndrome). The main pulmonary veins of the human fetus lack elastic tissue and their media are thin; with increasing age the media thickens.

The intrapulmonary arterial wall structure progressively changes peripherally with decreasing external diameter. The arteries are classified as elastic, transitional, muscular, partially muscular and non-muscular, depending on the structure of their media. Although the sequence of structural transition is the same in the fetus and adult, the relationships of size and structure change with development and age. In the developing fetus there is a gradual extension of the elastic component in the arterial wall towards the periphery until, by 19 weeks, it has reached the seventh generation – the adult level. Thus, as arteries increase in size with age, the lower limit for size of an elastic artery becomes larger. The change from muscular to partially muscular and then to a non-muscular structure occurs at a similar diameter in the fetus and the adult and, therefore, at a more proximal level in the small fetal lung. In terms of wall thickness, fetal arteries are more muscular than in the adult, as reflected by their relatively greater (i.e. about twofold) wall thickness for a vessel of similar external diameter. Unlike the arteries, the vein walls are thin throughout fetal life. The relative wall thickness remains the same in the fetus, child and adult.

At birth the blood flow to the lung increases as pulmonary vascular resistance falls, the latter being associated with lung expansion, changes in gas tension and neurohumoral factors. Kinin release by DCG cells may also play a role. Pulmonary arterial pressure falls to about half the systemic value within 3 days of birth, and pressures equivalent to those of the adult are reached by 6 months.[98] These changes result in part from arterial dilatation, and also from a gradual reduction in wall thickness.[99] The adult arterial wall thickness of all vessels is reached by 3 months of age.[100]

Ultrastructural studies on the normal pig lung have shown that at birth, as in the fetus, the peripheral arteries have a wall of chunky, overlapping, smooth muscle cells with relatively small quantities of myofilaments; thus they apparently have less ability to constrict than has been supposed. The endothelial cells are also chunky in shape and protrude into the lumen, leaving a relatively small area for blood to pass. In the first hours after birth there is rapid remodelling of the wall by thinning and spreading of the smooth muscle cells and the endothelial cells, leading to an increase in diameter of the lumen without any loss of muscle cell volume. At this stage the vessel walls contain very little collagen or elastin, which might restrict the dilatation.[101] This dilatation is probably facilitated in part by the stimulation of production of the endothelium-derived relaxation factor nitric oxide.[102] The presence of hypoxia after birth prevents this adaptation taking place.

Although the most dramatic changes are in the small peripheral arteries, there is also thinning of the large elastic arteries; however, the reduction in the adult wall thickness takes longer in the larger vessels. After the initial dilatation, there is smooth muscle cell maturation with an increase in myofilaments and perhaps of contractility. There is an increase in the amount of connective tissue in the vessel walls.[101] Later, as the vessels increase in size with lung growth, there is an increase in muscle cell diameter and extension of muscle into the more peripheral vessels. In the fetus, vessels supplying the respiratory acinus have very little muscle in their walls. With age there is a gradual extension into the acinar region until, in the adult, muscular arteries are found within the alveolar region of the lung (Fig. 1.3.9). Medial thickness may also vary with associated disease (e.g. ventricular septal defect, anomalous pulmonary venous drainage and mitral stenosis).[103]

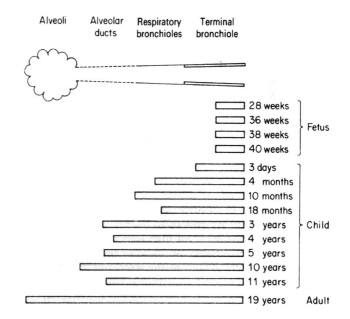

Fig. 1.3.9 Diagram illustrating the extension of muscle in the walls of arteries within the acinus. The extent of the muscular region is shown by the bars. There is little muscle within the acinus in the fetus. With age there is a gradual extension into the acinar region but, even at 11 years, fewer muscular arteries are present in the alveolar wall as compared with the adult. (With permission from Hislop & Reid 1973.[96])

References

1. Weibel ER. Design and development of the mammalian lung. In: The pathway of oxygen. London: Harvard University Press; 1984: 211.

2. Hall SM, Hislop AA, Pierce C, Haworth SG. Prenatal origins of human intrapulmonary arteries: formation and maturation. Am J Respir Cell Mol Biol 2000; 23: 194–203.

3. Masters JRW. Epithelial–mesenchymal interaction during lung development: the effect of mesenchymal mass. Dev Biol 1976; 51: 98.

4. McGowan SE. Extracellular matrix and the regulation of lung development and repair. FASEB J 1992; 6: 2895.

5. Hislop A, Muir DCF, Jacobsen M et al. Postnatal growth and function of the pre-acinar airways. Thorax 1972; 27: 265.

6. Bucher U, Reid LM. Development of the intrasegmental bronchial tree: the pattern of branching and development of cartilage at various stages of intrauterine life. Thorax 1961; 16: 207.

7. Ang S-L, Rossan J. HNF-3β is essential for node and notochord development in mouse development. Cell 1994; 78: 561–574.

8. Minoo P, Hamdan H, Bu D et al. TTF-1 regulates lung epithelial morphogenesis. Dev Biol 1995l 172: 694–698.

9. Whitsett, J. A lungful of transcription factors. Nat Genet 1998; 20: 7–8.

10. Jetten AM. Growth and differentiation factors in tracheobronchial epithelium. Am J Physiol 1991; 260: L361.

11. Warburton D, Zhao J, Berberich MA, Bernfield M. Molecular embryology of the lung: then, now, and in the future. Am J Physiol 1999; 276: L697.

12. Kitagawa M, Hislop AA, Boyden EA, Reid L. Lung hypoplasia in congenital diaphragmatic hernia. A quantitative study of airway, artery and alveolar development. Br J Surg 1971; 58: 342.

13. Perlman M, Williams J, Hirsch M. Neonatal pulmonary hypoplasia after prolonged leakage of amniotic fluid. Arch Dis Child 1976; 51: 349.

14. Wigglesworth JS, Hislop A, Desai R. Fetal lung growth in congenital laryngeal atresia. Pediatr Pathol 1987; 7: 515.

15. Alcorn D, Adamson TM, Lambert TE et al. Morphological effects of chronic tracheal ligation and drainage in the fetal lamb lung. J Anat 1977; 123: 649.

16. Hislop A, Hey E, Reid L. The lungs in congenital bilateral renal agenesis and dysplasia. Arch Dis Child 1979; 54: 32.

17. Hislop A, Fairweather DVI, Blackwell RJ, Howard S. The effect of amniocentesis and drainage of amniotic fluid on lung development in *Macaca fascicularis*. Br J Obstet Gynaecol 1984; 91: 835.

18. Wigglesworth JS, Desai R. Is fetal respiratory function a major determinant of perinatal survival? Lancet 1982; 1: 264.

19. Fewell JE, Hislop AA, Kitterman JA, Johnson P. Effect of tracheostomy on lung development in fetal lambs. J Appl Physiol 1983; 55: 578.

20. McCray PB. Spontaneous contractility of human fetal airway smooth muscle. Am J Respir Cell Mol Biol 1993; 8: 573.

21. Roman, J. 1995. Effects of calcium channel blockade on mammalian lung branching morphogenesis. Exp. Lung. Res 21: 489–502.

22. Hoo, A. F., M. Henschen, C. Dezateux, K. Costeloe, and J. Stocks. 1998. Respiratory function among preterm infants whose mothers smoked during pregnancy. Am J Respir Crit Care Med 158: 700–705.

23. Sekhon, H. S., Y. Jia, R. Raab, A. Kuryatov, J. F. Pankow, and J. A. Whitsett. 1999. Prenatal nicotine increases pulmonary a7 nicotine receptor expression and alters fetal lung development in monkeys. J Clin Invest 103: 637–647.

24. Hislop AA, Haworth SG. Airway size and structure in the normal fetal and infant lung and the effect of premature delivery and artificial ventilation. Am Rev Respir Dis 1989; 140: 1717.

25. Horsfield K, Cordon WI, Kemp W, Phillips S. Growth of bronchial tree in man. Thorax 1987; 42: 383.

26. Dezáteux, C. A. and J. Stocks. 1997. Lung development and early origins of childhood respiratory illness. Br Med Bull 53: 40–57.

27. Martin, T. R., R. G. Castile, J. J. Fredberg, B. Wohl, and J. Mead. 1987. Airway size is related to sex but not lung size in normal adults. J Appl Physio 63: 2042–2047.

28. Jeffery PK, Reid L. The ultrastructure of the airway lining and its development. In: Hodson WA (ed) The Development of the Lung. New York, Marcel Dekker, 1977, 87.

29. Bucher U, Reid L. Development of the mucus secreting elements in human lung. Thorax 1961; 16: 219.

30. De Haller R. Development of mucus-secreting elements. In: Anatomy of the Developing Lung, ed. J. Emmery. Oxford: Heinemann. 1969; 94. delete

31. Sorokin SP. Reconstruction of centriole formation and ciliogenesis in mammalian lungs. J Cell Sci 1968; 3: 207.

32. Fawcett DW. The Cell. Philadelphia: WB Saunders, 1981; 551.

33. Moscoso JG, Nandra K, Driver M. Ciliogenesis and ciliation of the respiratory epithelium in the human fetal cartilagenous trachea. Pathol Res Pract 1989; 184: 161.

34. Sorokin SP. The study of development in organ cultures of mammalian lungs. Dev Biol 1961; 3: 60.

35. Gaillard DA, Lallemand AV, Petit AF, Puchelle ES. In vivo ciliogenesis in human fetal tracheal epithelium. Am J Anat 1989; 185: 415.

36. Jeffery PK, Gaillard D, Moret T. Human airway secretory cells during development and in mature epithelium. Eur Respir J 1991; 5: 93.

37. Rhodin J. ultrastructure and function of the human tracheal mucosa. Am Rev Respir Dis 1966; 93: 1.

38. Kondova V. Ultrastructure of tracheal epithelium in children. Cesk Pediatr 1967; 22: 25.

39. Cutz E. Cytomorphology and differentiation of airway epithelium in developing human lung. In: McDowell EM, ed. Lung carcinomas. Edinburgh: Churchill Livingstone; 1987: 1.

40. Hermans, C, Bernard A. 1999. Lung epithelium-specific proteins – characteristics and potential applications as markers. Am J Respir Crit Care Med 159: 646–678.

41. Water de R, Williams LNA, van Muijen GND et al. Ultrastructural localization of bronchial antileukoproteinase in central and peripheral airways by a gold-labelled technique using monoclobal antibodies. Am Rev Respir Dis 1986; 133: 882.

42. Willems LNA, Kramps JA, Jeffery PK, Dijkman JH. Detection of antileukoprotease in the developing fetal lung. Thorax 1988; 43: 784.

43. Cutz E. Neuroendocrine cells of the lung. An overview of morphologic characteristics and development. Exp Lung Res 1982; 3: 185.

44. Cutz E, Gillan JE, Track MS. Pulmonary endocrine cells in developing human lung and during neonatal adaptation. In: Becker KL, Gazdar AF, ed. Endocrine lung in health and disease. Philadelphia, PA: WB Saunders; 1984; 210.

45. Sheppard MN, Marangos PJ, Bloom SR, Polak JM. Neuron specific enolase: a market for the early development of nerves and endocrine cells in the human lung. Life Sci 1984; 34: 264.

46. Track NS, Cutz E. Bombesin-like immunoreactivity in developing human lung. Life Sci 1982; 30: 1553.

47. Stahlman MT, Castleburg AG, Orth DN, Gray NM. Ontogeny of neuroendocrine cells in human fetal lung. An immunohistochemical study. Lab Invest 1985; 52: 52.

48. Rosan RC, Lauweryns JM. Secretory cells in the premature human lung lobule. Nature (Lond) 1971; 232: 61–61.

49. Moosavi H, Smith P, Heath D. The Feyrter cell in hypoxia. Thorax 1973; 28: 792.

50. Lauweryns JM, Cokelaere M. Hypoxia-sensitive neuro-epithelial bodies: Intrapulmonary secretory neuro-receptors modulated by the CNS. Z Microskop Anat Forsch 1973; 145: 521.

51. Stahlman MT, Gray ME. Ontogeny of neuroendocrine cells in human fetal lung. I. An electron microscopic study. Lab Invest 1984; 51: 449.

52. Inayama Y, Hook GER, Brody AR et al. The differentiation potential of tracheal basal cells. Lab Invest 1988; 58: 706.

53. Evans MJ, Plopper CG. The role of basal cells in adhesion of columnar epithelium to airway basement membrane. Am Rev Respir Dis 1988; 138: 481.

54. McDowell EM, Trump BF. Conceptual review: histogenesis of preneoplastic and neoplastic lesions in tracheobronchial epithelium. Surv Sym Pathol Res 1984; 2: 235.

55. Ayers M, Jeffery PK. Proliferation and differentiation in adult mammalian airway epithelium: a review. Eur Respir J 1988: 1: 58.

56. Tos M. Development of the mucous glands in the human main bronchus. Anat Anz 1968; 123: 376.

57. Thurlbeck WM, Benjamin B, Reid LM. Development and distribution of mucous glands in the fetal human trachea. Br J Dis Chest 1961; 55: 54.

58. Tos M. Development of the tracheal glands in man. Acta Pathol Microbiol Scand 1966: 185.1.

59. Matsuba K., Thurlbeck WM. Amorphometric study of bronchial and bronchiolar walls in children. Am Res Respir Dis 1972; 105: 908.

60. Field W. Mucous gland hypertrophy in babies and children aged 15 years or less. Br J Dis Chest 1968; 62: 11.

61. Hislop A, Wharton J, Allen K et al. Immunohistochemical localisation of peptide-containing nerves in the airways of normal young children. Am J Respir Cell Mol Biol 1990; 3: 191–198.

62. Tepper RS. Airway reactivity in infants: a positive response to methacholine and metaprotererol. J Appl Physiol 1987; 62: 1155.

63. Loosli CG, Hung K-S. Development of pulmonary innervation. In: Hodson WA, ed. Development of the lung, vol. 6: Lung biology in health and disease. New York: Marcel Dekker; 1977: 269.

64. Sparrow MP, Weichselbaum M, McCray PB. Development of the innervation and airway smooth muscle in human fetal lung. Am J Resp Cell Mol Biol 1999; 20: 550–560.

65. Allen KM, Wharton J, Polak JM, Haworth SG. A study of nerves containing peptides in the pulmonary vasculature of healthy infants and children and of those with pulmonary hypertension. Br Heart J 1989; 62: 353.
66. Schocken DD, Roth GS. Reduced beta-adrenoceptor concentrations in ageing man. Nature 1977; 267: 856.
67. Barnes P, Jacobs M, Roberts JM. Glucocorticoids preferentially increase fetal alveolar β-adrenoreceptors: autoradiographic evidence. Pediatr Res 1954; 18: 1191.
68. Schell DN, Durham D, Murphee SS et al. Ontogeny of β-adrenergic receptors in pulmonary arterial smooth muscle, bronchial smooth muscle and alveolar lining cells in the rat. Am J Respir Cell Mol Biol 1992; 7: 317.
69. Pulera N, Bernard P, Carrara M et al. Muscarinic cholinergic receptors in lung of developing rats. Dev Pharmacol Ther 1988; 11: 142.
70. Sharma RK, Jeffery PK. Adrenoceptors and muscarinic receptors in developing and adult human lung. Eur Respir J 1989; 2: 281S.
71. Hislop A, Wigglesworth JS, Desai R. Alveolar development in the human foetus and infant. Early Hum Dev 1986; 13: 1.
72. Boyden EA. Development and growth of the airways. In: Hodson WA, ed. Development of the lung, vol. 6: Lung biology in health and disease: New York: Marcel Dekker, 1977: 3.
73. Clements JA, Avery ME. Lung surfactant and neonatal respiratory distress syndrome. Am J Respir Crit Care Med 1998; 157: S59–S66.
74. Burri PH. Lung development and pulmonary angiogenesis. In: Gaultier C, Bourbon JR, Post M, ed. Lung development. New York: Oxford University Press; 1999: 122–151.
75. Caduff JH, Fischer LC, Burri PH. Scanning electron microscope study of the developing microvasculature in the postnatal rat lung. Anat Rec 1986; 216: 154.
76. Burri PH. Structural aspects of prenatal and postnatal development and growth of the lung. In: MacDonald JA, ed. Lung growth and development. New York: Marcel Dekker; 1997: 1–35.
77. Langston C, Thurlbeck WM. Lung growth and development in late gestation and early post natal life. In: Rosenberg HS, Burnstein J, ed. Pathology, vol. 7. Chicago, IL: Year Book; 1982: 203.
78. Zeltner TD, Caduff JH, Pfenninger J, Burri PH. The post-natal development of growth of the human lung. I. Morphometry. Respir Physiol 1987; 67: 247.
79. Olver RE. Solute and water transfer in fetal and newborn lungs. In: Hodson WA, ed. Development of the lung, vol. 6: Lung biology in health and disease. New York: Marcel Dekker; 1977: 525.
80. Angus GE, Thurlbeck WM. Number of alveoli in the human lung. J Appl Physiol 1972; 32: 2483.
81. Thurlbeck WM. Postnatal growth and development of the lung. Am Rev Respir Dis 1975; 3: 803–844.
82. Dunmill MS. Postnatal growth of the lung. Thorax 1962; 17: 329.
83. Weibel ER. Morphometry of the human lung. Heidelberg: Springer Verlag; 1963.
84. Kalenga M, Tschanz SA, Burri PH. Protein deficiency and the growing rat lung. II. Morphometric analysis and morphology. Pediatr Res 1995; 37: 789–795.
85. Massaro GD, Massaro D. Retinoic acid treatment partially rescues failed septation in rats and mice. Am J Physiol 2000; 278 L955–L960.
86. Watts DH, Krohn MA, Hillier SL, Echenbach DA. The association of occult amniotic fluid infection with gestational age and neonatal outcome among women in preterm labor. Obstet Gynecol 1992; 79: 351–357.
87. Lobe AH, Newnham JP, Willet KE et al. Effects of antenatal endotoxin and glucocorticoids on the lungs of preterm lambs. Am J Obstet Gynecol 2000; 182: 401–408.
88. Massaro GD, Massaro D. Formation of pulmonary alveoli and gas exchange surface area: quantitation and regulation. Annu Rev Physiol 1996; 58: 73–92.
89. Coalson JL, Winter VT, Gerstman DR et al. Pathophysiologic, morphometric and biochemical studies of the premature baboon with bronchopulmonary dysplasia. Am Rev Respir Dis 1992; 145: 872–881.
90. Pinkerton KE, Willet KE, Peake JL et al. Prenatal glucocorticoid and T4 effects on lung morphology in preterm lambs. Am J Respir Crit Care Med 1997; 156: 624–630.
91. Tschanz SA, Damke BM, Burri PH. Influence of postnatally administered glucocorticoids on rat lung growth. Biol Neonate 1995; 68: 229–245.
92. Burri PH, Hislop AA. Structural considerations. Eur Resp J 1998; 12: 59S–65S.
93. Hislop A, Reid LM. Intrapulmonary arterial development during fetal life: branching pattern and structure. J Anat 1972; 113: 35.
94. Hislop A, Reid L. Fetal and childhood development of the intrapulmonary veins in main-branching pattern and structure. Thorax 1973; 28: 313.
95. Pump KK. Distribution of bronchial arteries in human lung. Chest 1973; 62: 447.
96. Hislop A, Reid L. Pulmonary arterial development during childhood: branching pattern and structure. Thorax 1973; 28: 129.
97. Heath D, Dushane JW, Wood EM, Edwards JE. The structure of the pulmonary trunk at different ages and in cases of pulmonary hypertension and pulmonary stenosis. J Pathol 1959; 77: 443.
98. Rudolph AM. The changes in the circulation after birth: their importance in congenital heart disease. Circulation 1970; 41: 343.
99. Wagenvoort CA, Neufeld HM, Edwards JE. The structure of the pulmonary arterial tree in fetal and early ante-natal life. Lab Invest 1961; 10: 751.
100. Haworth SG, Hislop AA. Pulmonary vascular development: normal values of peripheral vascular structure. Am J Cardiol 1983; 52: 578.
101. Haworth SG. Pulmonary vascular remodelling in neonatal hypertension: state of the art. Chest 1988; 93: 1335.
102. Abman SH, Chatfield BA, Hall SL, McMurtry IP. Role of endothelial-derived relaxing factor during transition of pulmonary circulation at birth. Am J Physiol 1990; 259: 1921.
103. Hislop A, Reid LM. Formation of the pulmonary vasculature. In Hodson WA, ed. Development of the lung, vol 6. New York: Marcel Dekker; 1977: 37.

1.4 Molecular basis of lung development

Jacques Bourbon, Alexandra Henrion-Caude and Claude Gaultier

 Key points

- Lung-tissue specificity and the expression control of lung molecular markers results from the simultaneous expression of the homeodomain protein Nkx2.1 (TTF-1) and of various members of the forkhead-homologue hepatocyte nuclear factor 3 family.

- Nkx2.1 is essential to lung morphogenesis and epithelial cell differentiation, whereas HNF-3β is required for the formation of the foregut endoderm and derivative organs, including the lung.

- Growth, morphogenesis and differential cytodifferentiation of lung epithelium along the proximal–distal axis of the organ are driven by lung mesenchyme.

- Branching lung morphogenesis proceeds through reciprocal interactions between embryonic lung epithelium and mesenchyme. These interactions involve the interplay of a

- number of secreted signal molecules and receptors, as well as remodelling of extracellular matrix. FGF-10 produced by the mesenchyme and FGF-R2 expressed in the epithelium play a key role in the process in driving the elongation of epithelial tubes.

- Alveolarisation, i.e. the formation of secondary alveolar septa, requires the presence of PDGF-A, which controls elastin deposition and is enhanced by retinoids.

- The asymmetric pattern of right and left lung lobe formation is genetically determined. Several genes involved in the determinism of left–right asymmetry, including lung lobe formation, have been identified.

- Pre- and postnatal lung maturation, particularly surfactant storage, is submitted to a multifactorial hormonal control in which glucocorticoids play the central role.

Mammalian lung development proceeds through dichotomous branching, which leads to the establishment of an extended and attenuated epithelium. This achieves the large surface area required for optimal gas exchanges. The process of pulmonary morphogenesis has been well documented for a long time. By contrast, the underlying molecular mechanisms have only begun to be explored in recent years. Although recent breakthroughs have allowed a better understanding of some crucial events, particularly as regards mechanisms of branching morphogenesis or determinism of left–right asymmetry, a comprehensive view remains some way off. Lung organogenesis appears to be controlled by the integrated play of various key determinants. These include: cell-selective nuclear proteins (transcription factors); growth factors and growth factor receptors, which mediate paracrine signalling; and extracellular matrix components and integrins, which mediate cell–matrix interaction.

The primitive embryonic lung epithelium is made up of morphologically undifferentiated cells that coexpress various lung cell markers. These markers subsequently segregate and become restricted to separate cell lineages characteristic of either airway or alveolar epithelium. The primitive lung epithelium is therefore multipotential, although it is already assigned to a pulmonary identity. It is striking that the same transcription factors are involved in the control of lung morphogenesis and of the expression of marker proteins specific to the mature lung. Moreover, reciprocal interactions between mesenchyme and epithelium play a crucial role both in branching morphogenesis and in cell differentiation, including the establishment of different cellular subsets along the proximal–distal axis of the lung. This stresses the unity of the molecular mechanisms at work during lung development. These mechanisms are reviewed in this chapter, along with hormonal control, which is especially important for the maturational events that precede birth. Lastly, recent transgenic models in mice that have clinical relevance for humans are analysed.

Lung tissue specificity: role of transcription factors in expression of lung markers and in lung development

Lung cell markers and the pulmonary set of transcription factors

The airways share various cell phenotypes with other organs, including ciliated, mucous and neuroendocrine cells. The lung nevertheless contains several specific epithelial cell types that express lung-specific markers, particularly in the distal part of the bronchiolar tree and in alveoli. Thus, bronchiolar Clara cells express Clara-cell secretory protein (or CC10), a marker that has as a unique counterpart the endometrial uteroglobin. Alveolar type II cells produce the phospholipid-rich alveolar lining material known as pulmonary surfactant, which contains four characteristic proteins (the surfactant proteins, SPs) of which two, SP-B and SP-C, appear to be lung-specific. Lastly, the attenuated cells designated alveolar type I cells, which perform air-blood gas exchanges, have no equivalent in the rest of the organism. The study of the 5′–flanking region of CC10 and SP genes has led to the identification of sequences that confer lung-epithelium-specific expression,[1] as well as several transcription factors involved in lung-specific expression of these proteins. The same transcription factors have been revealed to be essential to lung morphogenesis. Lung tissue identity seems to result from the expression of a particular set of transcription factors the combination of which appears to be unique to the lung. These include the homeodomain protein

Nkx2.1, proteins of the forkhead-homologue hepatocyte nuclear factor 3 family (HNF-3/HFH) also known as Fox factors and characterised by a winged-helix DNA-binding motif, and the GATA and Gli families of zinc finger transcription factors.

Expression control of lung markers

Our knowledge regarding the control of lung marker transcription results from a variety of experimental approaches, including footprinting, gel shift, transfection in cell lines and targeted mutation in mice. Nkx2.1, also known as thyroid transcription factor-1 (TTF-1) or thyroid enhancer binding protein (T/ebp), is essential to the expression of SP-A, SP-B, SP-C, SP-D and CC10.[2] Several functional binding sites for this factor have been discovered in the enhancer/promoter elements of their gene (see Fig. 1.4.1 for an example). These sites are in close proximity to *cis*-active element(s) that bind HNF-3 or its related family members, HFHs.[2] Nkx2.1 and HNF-3/HFH proteins bind DNA as monomers and enhance the transcriptional machinery. GATA-6 has also been reported to regulate SP-A and SP-C gene expression.

Involvement in the lung developmental process

Classically, pulmonary development is divided into five stages (see Chapter 1.3). The lung primordium separates from the oesophagus during the embryonal stage. Branching morphogenesis of the complete airway tree, right to the terminal bronchioles, takes place during the pseudoglandular stage. Respiratory areas, including air–blood barriers, form during the canalicular and saccular stages. All these phases are achieved during intrauterine life in all mammals. The formation of definitive alveoli, i.e. the alveolar stage, may occur before or after birth; in humans, it is mostly a postnatal process.

Nkx2.1/TTF-1 is required for complete induction of embryonic lung organogenesis. Targeted disruption of the gene

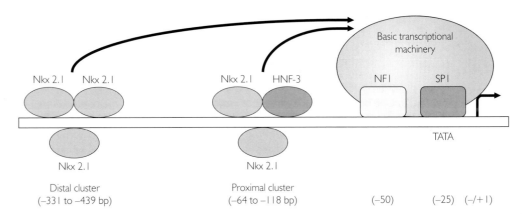

Fig. 1.4.1 Schematic representation of the regulatory elements of the human *SP-B* gene showing the location of transcription factor binding sites. Ubiquitous transcription factors are represented as rectangular blocks and tissue-specific transcription factors as oval blocks. A proximal regulatory element submitted to the combined influence of Nkx2.1 (TTF-1) and HNF-3 activates the transcriptional machinery. A distal element that binds only Nkx2.1 further enhances the activity driven by the proximal element.

in the mouse prevented the separation of trachea from oesophagus, and the paired lung primordia that arose failed to undergo branching morphogenesis.[3] Consistent with data relative to lung marker expression control, SP and CC10 gene expression was turned off in this model. Moreover, the expression of α integrins, collagen IV and vascular endothelium factor 3 were significantly reduced or absent.[3] Nkx2.1 is expressed throughout the embryonic lung at early stages of development (i.e. during the pseudoglandular stage) when the epithelium is still morphologically undifferentiated and multipotent, but at later stages (i.e. beyond the canalicular stage), it becomes restricted to distal areas (bronchioli and alveoli) as cell differentiation progresses (Fig. 1.4.2). Inhibition of Nkx2.1 translation by antisense oligodeoxynucleotide in the cultured embryonic mouse lung consistently not only reduced branching but also prevented the tall columnar immature epithelial cells from becoming cuboidal and displaying morphological and biochemical differentiation at the periphery of the explant.[4]

HNF-3α and β, but not γ, and various HFHs are expressed in the lung. Similar to Nkx2.1, HNF-3β is widely expressed at the pseudoglandular stage in lung epithelium, including in the trachea and bronchial tree, becoming restricted to bronchioloalveolar

portals and type II cells in the mature lung (Figs 1.4.2 & 1.4.3). Targeted disruption of the HNF-3β gene has evidenced the role of this factor in the formation of the foregut endoderm[5] from which the lung epithelium derives, although early arrest of embryonic development before lung budding meant that its role in subsequent lung development could not be determined more precisely. Importantly, HNF-3 forkhead family members may represent upstream regulators of Nkx2.1 (Fig. 1.4.2a). Moreover, HFH-4 has been shown to be essential to ciliogenesis and to ciliated cell differentiation in the lung as well as in other organs;[6] this factor is also involved in the specification of laterality (see below).

Murine Gli1, 2 and 3 proteins have been implicated in transduction of sonic hedgehog (Shh) signal, a key element in branching morphogenesis and specification of left–right asymmetry (see below). Whereas Gli2 and Gli3 null mutations led only to moderate lung defects, *Gli2/Gli3⁻/⁻* double null mutants displayed lowered HNF-3β immunoreactivity and either tracheooesophageal fistula or complete absence of lungs (Fig. 1.4.4).[7]

Temporal–spatial changes in the expression of Nkx2.1 and forkhead factors that occur during development are likely to be involved in differentiation of cell subsets along the proximal–distal axis of the organ. Thus, their expression precedes, then coincides with that of distal lung markers (Fig. 1.4.5). Most

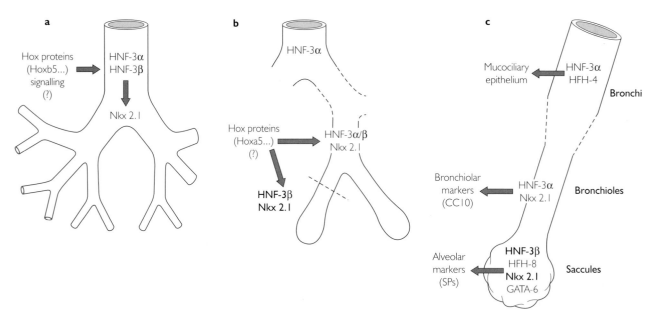

Fig. 1.4.2 Transcription factors involved in lung organogenesis and temporospatial changes in their expression during the different phases of the process. (a) Branching morphogenesis of the airway tree. During this pseudoglandular stage of development, HNF-3β and Nkx2.1 (TTF-1) are strongly expressed throughout the growing epithelium. Nkx2.1 is indispensable to branching morphogenesis and is submitted to positive control by HNF-3β. (b) Demarcation between proximal and distal areas. In the canalicular stage, when the future airways (which retain tall columnar epithelium) demarcate from the presumptive respiratory areas (which develop cuboidal epithelium), changes occur in the distribution of transcription factor expression. Nkx2.1 and HNF-3β disappear from the trachea, which still expresses HNF-3α. They continue to be expressed in the bronchobronchiolar tree and are prominent in cells at the tips of the growing buds. (c) When alveolar sacs develop and epithelial cell differentiation progresses (saccular stage), HNF-3β and Nkx2.1 expression becomes restricted to the most distal areas (bronchioli and saccules). HFH-4, which is involved in ciliogenesis, is expressed in the bronchial tree, whereas HFH-8 is expressed only in saccules. Hox genes, the expression of which appears to be restricted to the mesenchyme, also display changes in their relative level and site of expression. They are likely to be involved in control of the expression of transcription factors located in the epithelium and in the fate of epithelial cells along the proximal–distal axis of the organ, but their mode of action remains unknown.

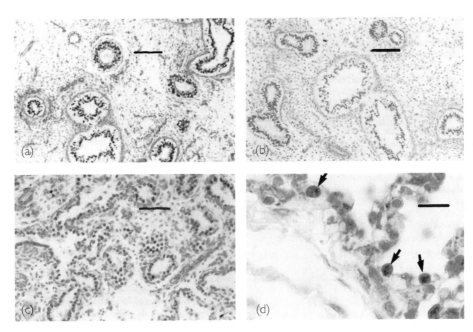

Fig. 1.4.3 Immunostaining for transcription factors HNF-3β and Nkx2.1 (TTF-1) in the developing human fetal lung. (a) Lung of a fetus of 10 weeks' gestation immunostained for HNF-3β. The nuclei of a majority of the lung cells lining conducting and luminal airways are immunolabelled (peroxidase-conjugated streptavidin and nuclear fast red; scale bar = 80 μm. (b) Lung of the same fetus immunostained for Nkx2.1. Nuclei in cells of the same generations of airways as those immunolabelled for HNF-3β are also immunolabelled for Nkx2.1 (peroxidase-conjugated streptavidin and haematoxylin; scale bar = 80 μm). (c) Lung of a fetus of 20 weeks' gestation immunostained for HNF-3β. The nuclei of cells lining the airways are immunolabelled (peroxidase-conjugated streptavidin and nuclear fast red; scale bar = 50 μm.) (d) Lung of a fetus of 36 weeks' gestation immunostained for HNF-3β. Nuclei of type II cells (arrows) are immunolabelled (peroxidase-conjugated streptavidin and nuclear fast red; scale bar = 12 μm). (Reproduced with permission from Stahlman MT, Gray ME, Whitsett JA. Temporal–spatial distribution of hepatocyte nuclear factor-3beta in developing human lung and other foregut derivatives. *Journal of Histochemistry and Cytochemistry* 1998; 46: 955–962.)

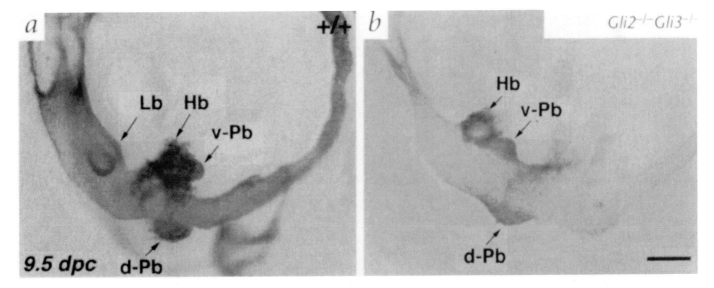

Fig. 1.4.4 Oesophagus, trachea and lung primordia fail to form in *Gli2⁻/⁻ Gli3⁻/⁻* mouse embryos. Whole mount immunostaining of wild-type (a) and *Gli2⁻/⁻Gli3⁻/⁻* embryos (b) on gestational day 9.5 (E9.5) with anti-HNF-3β. HNF-3 immunoreactivity in the *Gli2⁻/⁻ Gli3⁻/⁻* endoderm (b) is weaker than that of wild type (a). Although the hepatic and pancreatic buds are present, lung buds are absent in *Gli2⁻/⁻ Gli3⁻/⁻* embryos (b). Haematoxylin–eosin staining of transverse sections of E10.5 wild type (c–f) and *Gli2⁻/⁻Gli3⁻/⁻* (g–j) embryos at four different levels. In *Gli2⁻/⁻Gli3⁻/⁻* embryos there is no foregut differentiation into oesophagus, trachea and lung (arrows). b, bronchial buds; dpc, days post-conception; e, oesophageal component of the foregut; Hb, hepatic bud; Lb, lung buds; p, pharynx; S, presumptive stomach; t, trachea; d-Pb, dorsal pancreatic bud; v-Pb, ventral pancreatic bud. Scale bar: 500μm. (Reproduced with permission from Motoyama et al.[7])

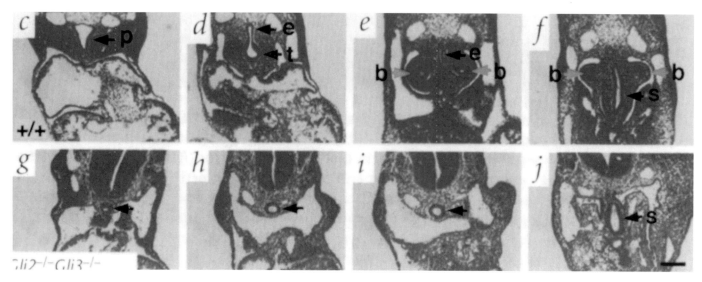

Fig. 1.4.4 (continued)

probably, taking into account the role of homeotic genes in anteroposterior specification, the induction of the endodermal territory destined to give rise to the lung and, later in development, the local expression of cell-specific transcription factors and markers, are determined by the expression of particular sets of homeotic genes. Thus, Hoxb-5 distribution in the developing mouse lung suggests a role in branching morphogenesis and epithelial cell fate[8] (Fig. 1.4.2a), whereas Hoxa-5 may control HNF-3β, Nkx2.1 and surfactant protein gene expression in lung epithelium[9] (Fig. 1.4.2b). Lastly, developmental changes in retinoic acid signalling in the fetal lung[10] may control changes in *hox* gene expression,[11] thus modifying their pattern of expression during the course of development.

Epithelial–mesenchymal interactions in lung development

Fetal lung mesenchyme controls both lung morphogenesis and epithelial cytodifferentiation

At early stages of development, epithelium and mesenchyme of the lung anlage can be separated. Taking advantage of this possibility, a number of in vitro experiments of the last 40 years have demonstrated the crucial role of fetal lung mesenchyme in pulmonary organogenesis. In particular, they established that the epithelium could survive, proliferate and branch only in the presence of mesenchyme. Moreover, through the use of heterologous recombination, they showed that the branching pattern was specified by the mesenchyme, i.e. the epithelium adopted the pattern of the organ from which the mesenchyme originated. More recently, elegant grafting experiments in isolated fetal rat lung explant have clearly and more precisely established the dual role of mesenchyme (Fig. 1.4.6). Grafting

distal (peripheral) lung mesenchyme on to denuded tracheal epithelium forced the latter to branch and elicited the expression of alveolar markers, namely lamellar bodies and SP-C.[12] Grafting mesenchyme from mainstem bronchus on to tracheal epithelium only elicited non-branching supernumerary buds. Reciprocally, grafting proximal (tracheal) mesenchyme on to distal epithelial tubules destined to give rise to acinar areas inhibited the branching process and induced cell-type differentiation typical of tracheal–bronchial epithelium, with production of mucins.[12] These results confirm that epithelial cells display pluripotency and plasticity, at least until a given developmental stage, since tracheal epithelium becomes refractory to distal mesenchyme beyond the pseudoglandular stage of development. Most importantly, they indicate that mesenchyme of the developing lung is 'regionalised', i.e. the mesenchyme gives rise to signalling that differs along the proximal axis of the developing organ and that dictates different fates for the primitive epithelium according to the position of the cell in the air tree. Since most *hox* genes expressed in the lung are expressed in the mesenchyme only, the assumption that *hox* genes are involved in the determination of local development is reinforced.

Molecular mechanisms of lung branching morphogenesis

This aspect of lung development is the one of which we have recently gained the clearest and the most complete picture. To support development of the epithelium, once freed from the mesenchyme, mesenchymal action can be replaced by a combination of a reconstituted basement membrane matrix (EHS matrix) and various soluble growth factors.[13] This suggests that the interaction between epithelium and mesenchyme involves interplay among components of the extracellular matrix and diffusible mediators.

The use of in vitro approaches,[14,15] together with in vivo genetic techniques, including gene inactivation[16] and the dominant-negative transgenesis strategy,[17] has highlighted the central

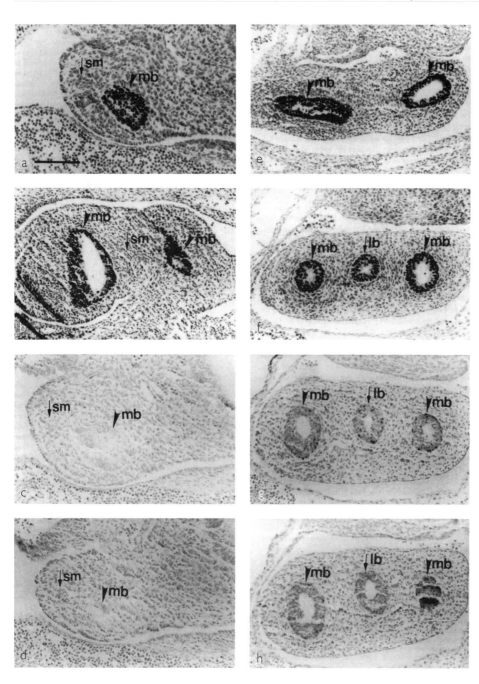

Fig. 1.4.5 Expression of transcription factors HNF-3β and Nkx2.1 (TTF-1) precedes, then colocalises with that of lung protein markers in the embryonic mouse lung. Immunohistochemical staining of NKx2.1 (a & e), HNF-3β (b & f), pro-SP-B (c and g), and pro-SP-C (d and h) in sections of lungs from mouse embryos at gestational days 10 (a–d) and 11 (e–h). Staining with antibodies against Nkx2.1 and HNF-3β was detected at high levels in the epithelial cells lining main bronchi (arrowheads) at gestational day 10, and in main bronchi (arrowheads) and lobar bronchi (arrows) at gestational day 11, being localised to the nuclei of lung epithelial cells. By contrast, pro-SP-B and pro-SP-C were not detected on gestational day 10 but were detected at low levels in the cytoplasm of epithelial cells lining main bronchi (arrowheads) and lobar bronchi (arrows) on gestational day 11. lb, lobar bronchus; mb, main bronchus; sm, splanchnic mesenchyme, scale bar = 64 μm. (Reproduced with permission from Zhou L, Lim L, Costa RH, Whitsett JA. Thyroid transcription factor 1, hepatocyte nuclear factor-3beta, surfactant protein B, C, and Clara cell secretory protein in developing mouse lung. *Journal of Histochemistry and Cytochemistry* 1996; 44:1183–1193.)

role of fibroblast growth factor (FGF)-10 and FGF receptor (FGFR)-2. Other secreted mediators – sonic hedgehog (Shh), sprouty-4 (a mammalian counterpart of the *Drosophila* protein sprouty), transforming growth factor (TGF)-β and bone morphogenetic protein (BMP)-4 – have also been shown to be involved in reciprocal mesenchymal–epithelial influences in the cultured mouse lung.[18] Shh has been reported to be essential to normal lung development; in Shh[−/−] mouse embryos, the lungs are reduced to dilated sacs and cell growth is considerably reduced (Fig. 1.4.7). An integrated mechanistic model of lung branching morphogenesis has recently been proposed.[15,18] FGF-10 production in focal points of the mesenchyme appears to exert a chemotactic attraction on the epithelial tubule, which grows toward the source of FGF-10 (Fig. 1.4.8). The FGF-10 effect is transduced by FGFR-2, the expression of which is restricted to epithelial cells. However, FGF-10 seems to have no or little mitogenic effect on epithelial cells.

Epithelial cell proliferation could be controlled by other factors, possibly FGF-1, FGF-7, epidermal growth factor (EGF), TGFα or hepatocyte growth factor (HGF). Additionally, Shh, which is produced by epithelial cells in the vicinity of branching points (Fig 1.4.9) and acts through a mesenchymal receptor, together with sprouty-4, inhibits FGF-10 production and stops the growth of tubules. Shh signalling appears to act through activation of Gli protein production in mesenchymal cells. Simultaneously, TGFβ and BMP-4 inhibit epithelial growth at the

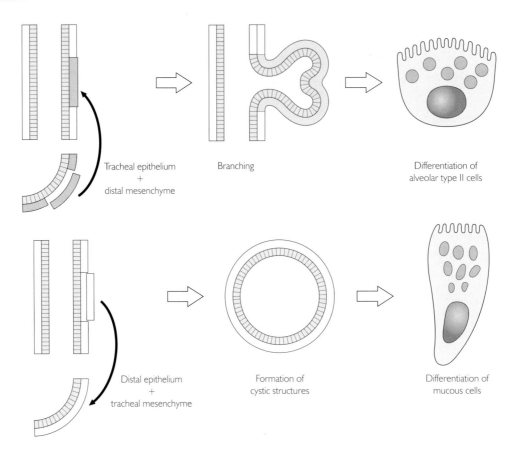

Fig. 1.4.6 Demonstration of the differential roles of proximal and distal fetal lung mesenchyme in epithelial morphogenesis and cyto-differentiation through ex vivo reciprocal grafting experiments (see Shannon et al[12]). (Upper panel) denudation of tracheal epithelium and grafting of distal mesenchyme. The distal mesenchyme forces the tracheal epithelium to branch and induces the differentiation of alveolar type II cells (appearance of lamellar bodies, expression of surfactant protein SP-C). (Lower panel) Distal epithelium is separated from its mesenchyme and associated with tracheal mesenchyme. The latter prevents distal epithelium (which would have branched in the presence of distal epithelium) from branching and induces the formation of cysts. Moreover, tracheal epithelium elicits the differentiation of mucous cells characteristic of airways, containing copious amounts of mucins.

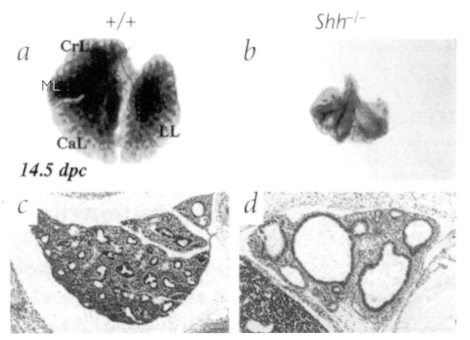

Fig. 1.4.7 Sonic hedgehog (Shh) is essential in lung development, as evidenced by gene targeting in the mouse. Whole-mount view (a, b) and haema-toxylin–eosin-stained sections (c, d) of lungs at gestational day 14.5 in wild-type (a, c) and Shh[−/−] (b, d) embryos. Wild-type lungs show characteristic lobulation (CaL, caudal lobe; CrL, cranial lobe; LL, left lobe; ML, middle lobe), which is not present in the mutant. Histology shows reduction of lung tissue to dilated sacs in which epithelial and mesenchymal cell growth is considerably reduced, as evidenced by BrdU-labelling. (Reproduced with permission from Litingtung Y, Lei L, Westphal H, Chiang C. Sonic hedgehog is essential to foregut development. *Nat Genet* 1998; 20: 58–61.)

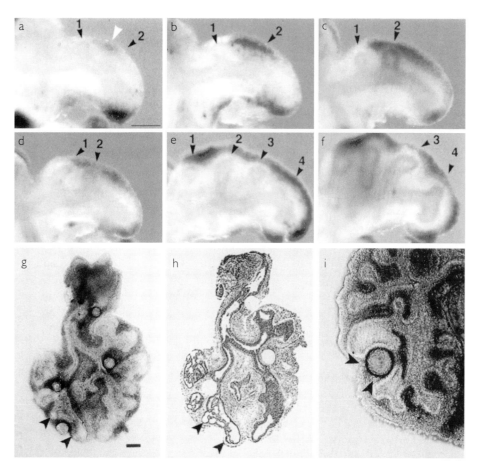

Fig. 1.4.8 Dynamic pattern of expression of fibroblast growth factor 10 (FGF-10) in embryonic mouse lung between gestational ages 11.5 (E11.5) and 12.5 (E12.5) days, and effect of exogenous FGF-10 beads in cultured E11.5 whole-lung explants. (a–f) Whole-mount in situ hybridisation showing *FGF-10* expression at representative stages between E11.5 and E12.5 with (a) being the youngest and (f) the oldest. (a) At E11.5, *FGF-10* is expressed between buds 1 and 2 (white arrowhead), and at high levels at the distal tip of the lobe. (b) *FGF-10* levels increase in the lateral mesoderm and expand caudally as bud 2 grows. (c, d) *FGF-10* expression is restricted to the mesenchyme in between bud 1 and 2, and caudad to bud 2, overlying the region where buds have yet to form. Note that in (d) the main branch of bud 1 is growing toward the *FGF-10* expression domain. (e, f) Branching of lateral buds is observed and the bronchus undergoes bifurcation at the distal tip. Note that *FGF-10* expression is downregulated in the mesenchyme immediately adjacent to the distal endoderm, where *Shh* expression is prominent (compare bud 2 in (c–e) and see Fig. 1.4.9). Scale bar (a–f) = 90 μm. (Reproduced from Bellusci et al[14] with permission from the Company of Biologists.) (g–i) FGF-10-soaked beads implanted on isolated and cultured left lung and trachea are chemoattractant for the lung epithelium. One day after implantation, distal epithelial buds grow toward (arrowheads, g & h) and start encircling the FGF-10 bead (i). Scale bar = 140 μm. (Reproduced with permission from Park WY, Miranda B, Lebeche D et al. FGF-10 is a chemotactic factor for distal epithelial buds during lung development. *Dev Biol* 1998; 201:125–134.)

tip of the tubule. The surge of new points of FGF-10 production, combined with the appearance of a focal point of matrix resistance (see below), induces the tubule to grow in other directions and establishes a cleft that divides the initial tubule into two new ones. Repetition of this sequence of events allows branching morphogenesis of the bronchial tree to occur (Fig. 1.4.10).

The relative role of the various TGFβ isoforms is not clear. Both TGFβ1 and TGFβ2 inhibit branching morphogenesis in culture although TGFβ2 is much more potent than β1. Whereas TGFβ1 gene disruption has little effect on lung development, disruption of the TGFβ2 gene, among a variety of developmental defects, causes fatal respiratory distress without obvious morphological alteration of the lung,[19] and that of the TGFβ3

gene leads to arrest of lung development at the precocious pseudoglandular stage.[20] The abrogation of TGFβ type II receptor signalling stimulates lung morphogenesis and increases Nkx2.1 expression,[18] indicating that this receptor mediates the inhibiting effects of TGFβ.

The role of matrix components is complex and not fully understood. Disruption of collagen synthesis or secretion in the cultured fetal mouse lung severely affects branching morphogenesis[21] but the nature of the involved collagen form(s) is unclear. Laminin is required for branching and mediates epithelial cell proliferation, polarisation and basement membrane assembly,[22] whereas proteoglycans appear to play a crucial role in alveolar maturation and alveolar type II cell differentiation.[23]

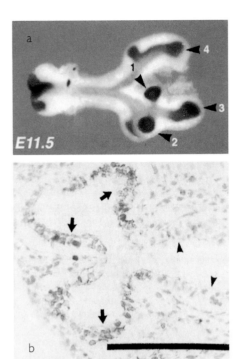

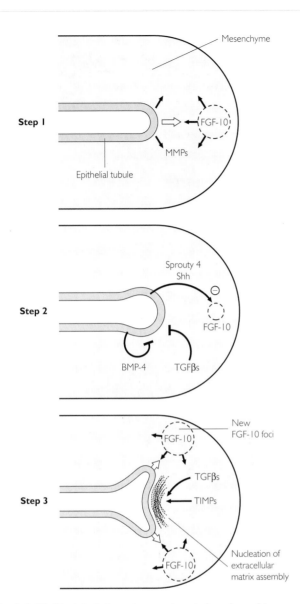

Fig. 1.4.9 Localisation of sonic hedgehog (Shh) expression in the developing embryonic lung. (a) Whole-mount in situ hybridisation showing *Shh* expression in the mouse lung at gestational age 11.5 days. Most prominent expression is seen at the tips of budding epithelial tubules. Lobes indicated by: 1, accessory; 2, right middle, 3; right caudal; 4, left. (Reproduced from Bellusci et al[14], with permission from the Company of Biologists.) (b) Immunostaining of Shh protein in the lung of the 15.5-day rat embryo. Shh is intensely positive in the apical side of epithelium at the branching points (arrows). Scale bar = 100 μm. (Reproduced with permission from Urase K, Mukasa T, Igarashi H et al. Spatial expression of Sonic hedgehog in the lung epithelium during branching morphogenesis. *Biochem Biophys Res Commun* 1996; 225:161–166).

Moreover, production of matrix metalloproteinases (MMPs) by epithelial tubules appears to facilitate their progression through the stroma. Reciprocally, TGFβ induces condensation of matrix components at the points of cleft formation. Thus, abrogation of TGFβ type I receptor signalling reduces the formation of new branch points in the cultured embryonic mouse lung, with failure of fibronectin-rich matrix to condense.[18] The production of tissue inhibitors of MMPs (TIMPs) by mesenchymal cells contributes to stabilisation of the matrix at branching points (Fig. 1.4.10).

Molecular control of epithelial cell differentiation

This aspect of developmental control is less well documented. Clearly, FGFs are involved in the differentiation of distal epithelial lung cells. FGF-7 stimulated the synthesis of all surfactant components in isolated immature epithelial lung cells cultured

Fig. 1.4.10 Model of tissue interactions in lung branching morphogenesis. Step 1: Focal production of fibroblast growth factor (FGF)-10 by mesenchymal cells exerts a chemoattraction upon epithelial tubules, which progress through the mesenchyme. Production of metalloproteinases (MMPs) facilitates progression through the degradation of extracellular matrix components. Step 2: Production of sonic hedgehog (Shh) and sprouty 4 by epithelial cells downregulates FGF-10 production in the vicinity of the tip of epithelial buds. Bone morphogenetic protein (BMP)-4 produced by epithelial cells and TGFβs produced by various cells stop epithelial cell proliferation. These mechanisms lead to tip arrest. Step 3: New foci of FGF-10 production exert lateral attraction on epithelial cells, initiating the formation of a cleft. Simultaneously, TGFβs stimulate the production of extracellular matrix components (particularly collagen fibres and fibronectin), and production of tissue inhibitors of metalloproteinases (TIMPs) by the mesenchyme stabilises the deposition of matrix components at the branching points. The repetition of this sequence of events leads to branching morphogenesis of the bronchial tree. The determinism of domains of *FGF-10* expression is either 'prepatterned' or due to a release from inhibitory influences exerted by epithelial tips as the tips progress.

on EHS matrix.[24] Mesenchyme-free tracheal epithelium from the rat fetus embedded in the same matrix and cultured in the presence of various growth factors extensively proliferated and similarly expressed a type II epithelial cell phenotype.[13,25] Whereas single deletion had no effect, the simultaneous deletion of both FGF-1 and FGF-7 from the medium was sufficient to inhibit growth and to prevent SP-C expression, although FGF-1 and FGF-7 were unable on their own to elicit SP-C expression in the absence of the other components of the medium.[25] Lung development is altered in EGF-receptor (EGFR)-deficient mice,[26] with collapsed alveoli, thickening of septa (Fig. 1.4.11) and reduced immunoreactivity to various surfactant components. This argues for important roles of EGF and/or TGFα in distal lung development also.

The nature of the mediators that determine bronchial and bronchiolar epithelial cell differentiation is unknown. EGF was shown to enhance mucus production and to accelerate the differentiation of tracheal mucous cells in vivo,[27] but this effect is not specific, since EGF also stimulates alveolar cell maturation

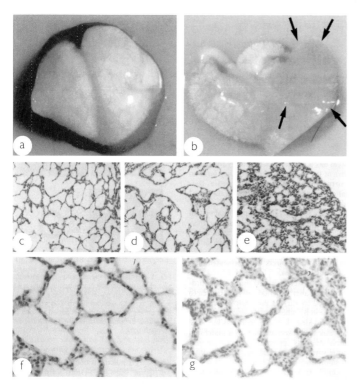

Fig. 1.4.11 Altered lung morphology and histology in newborn epidermal growth factor receptor (EGF-R)[−/−] mice. (a, b) Macroscopically, a newborn wild-type lung (a) has a smooth surface full of air-filled alveoli, whereas the EGFR[−/−] lung (b) is atelectatic, with airless lung parenchyma (arrows). (c–e) Histological examination (haematoxylin–eosin-stained sections) shows symmetrical alveoli in a wild-type newborn mouse (c), whereas, in the EGF-R[−/−] newborn animal, large airways are close to the pleural surface (d) and collapsed, poorly air-filled alveoli are visible (e). At postnatal day 4, the alveoli of wild-type animals have a thin wall (f) as compared with thick-walled EGF-R[−/−] alveoli (g). Scale bars = 50 μm (c–e) and 25 μm (f, g). (Reproduced with permission from *Nature* (Mietttinen et al[26]). Copyright 1996 Macmillan Magazines Limited.)

and surfactant production. Similarly, the paracrine influences that dictate a proximal (airway) or distal (alveolar) fate for epithelial cells are not understood. Proximal–distal differences in Bmp4 signalling may be involved.[18] Retinoids, i.e. vitamin A and its active metabolite retinoic acid, are likely to be involved since, as already stated, retinoic acid alters the pattern of expression of the *hox*-gene.[11] Moreover, in vitro, submitting the developing lung primordium to high doses of retinoic acid inhibited distal lung development and led to 'proximalisation' of airways.[28] Local changes in retinoic acid production during development and local differences in retinoic acid concentration may therefore influence the orientation of the developing epithelium. Last, the double-null mutation of the genes for the retinoic acid receptors (RAR) α and β results, among a variety of defects, in lung abnormalities that vary from simple growth retardation to agenesis.[29]

Retinoids also appear to play an important role in the later stages of development. Interestingly, the fetal lung mesenchyme stores vitamin A, which is used perinatally to produce retinoic acid. Retinoic acid is involved in the control of alveologenesis (see below), but also influences cell maturation. Thus, an excess of retinoic acid downregulates surfactant proteins in the isolated fetal rat lung[28] but, as shown by studies on vitamin A deprivation in the pregnant rat, retinoid availability below a certain threshold becomes a limiting factor for surfactant synthesis, including surfactant proteins.[30] Moreover, premature infants who develop bronchopulmonary dysplasia as a consequence of their initial respiratory distress syndrome have been reported to be vitamin-A-deficient.[31]

Alveolarisation

The formation of alveoli through secondary septation of primitive alveolar sacs is mostly a postnatal process in humans, since newborns have few definitive alveoli. Retinoic acid appears to be a potent stimulus of both alveolar epithelial cell growth in vitro[32] and of saccular septation in the rat in vivo (Fig. 1.4.12).[33] Its mechanism of action in this process is not fully described but it clearly involves stimulation of elastin synthesis and deposition, which is crucial for the formation of secondary septa.[33]

Postnatal alveolarisation is totally impaired in platelet-derived growth factor A (PDGF-A)-null mice.[34] PDGF-A, which is produced by epithelial cells, is essential for differentiation of alveolar myofibroblasts from mesenchymal cells and for elastin fibre deposition.[33] Retinoic acid stimulates alveolar fibroblast proliferation through a PDGF-mediated autocrine mechanism. Lastly, alveolar septation is prevented in mice double null-mutant for FGFR3 and FGFR4 (see Table 1.4.1).

Determinism of left–right asymmetry

In order to acquire a three-dimensional structure, there must be developmental mechanisms that coordinate the left–right axis with the anteroposterior and dorsoventral axes. This left–right axis is actually the last to become morphologically apparent.

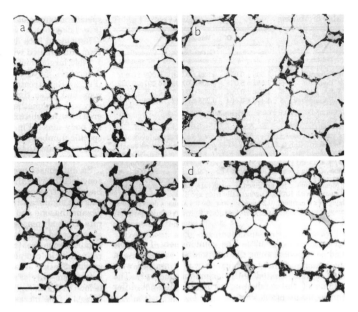

Fig. 1.4.12 Effect of retinoic acid treatment on alveolar formation in postnatal rats. Histological sections of lung from rats that were injected daily from day 3 to 13 with (a) vehicle (control), (b) dexamethasone 0.25 μg/day, (c) retinoic acid 500 μg/kg/day or (d) both dexamethasone and retinoic acid. All rats were killed at 14 days for histological examination. Dexamethasone-treated rats had fewer enlarged alveoli ((b) versus (a)). Retinoic acid treatment of otherwise untreated rats resulted in a 50% increase in the number of alveoli, although alveolar size was smaller ((c) versus (a)). In rats given both drugs, retinoic acid compensated for the effects of dexamethasone (reduced size and increased number of alveoli, (d) versus (b)). Scale bars = 50 μm. (Reproduced with permission from Massaro GD, Massaro, D. Postnatal treatment with retinoic acid increases the number of pulmonary alveoli in rats. *Am J Physiol* 1996; 270: L305–L310.)

During vertebrate embryogenesis, anatomical asymmetry emerges from underlying symmetry. The lungs, although paired, manifest left–right anatomical differences from their earliest stages of development. Asymmetrical development results in characteristic left–right differences, illustrated in the lung by more lobes on the right than on the left. Recently, there has been increasing effort in the attempt to address several questions, such as the genetic events that follow the first split determining left–right asymmetry and the mechanisms that translate the initial left–right signals into left–right patterning of the tissues and the organs. Some recent discoveries at the molecular and cellular levels regarding the establishment of left–right asymmetry during embryogenesis are reviewed here.

Establishment of left–right asymmetry

Lung buds are derivatives of the gut that form different numbers of lung lobes on the left and right sides. As a result, lung anatomy is a good indicator of left–right identity. Unpaired organs of the chest and abdomen begin development in the midline and subsequently lateralise to their adult positions. The lungs, although paired, exhibit conserved left–right anatomical differences that give them the character of an unpaired organ. However, the left and right bronchial trees of the lungs are formed using a different mechanism to create their left–right asymmetry from other unpaired visceral organs. This left–right asymmetry begins and ends in an asymmetrical outgrowth of lung buds towards the left and right side. The initial clue for left–right asymmetry is most probably a break of symmetry in the body that results in the creation of left–right asymmetry, which must subsequently be amplified and stabilised. Several signal transductions and signalling pathways could mediate positional information in this process. The left–right positional information must then be translated into an appropriate morphogenetic response to build up the left–right differences in the organ.

Left–right axis malformations

Although the evolutionary reasons for the lungs' intricate left–right asymmetry are still obscure, it has been observed that disruption of the normal pattern may result in left–right axis malformations with significant associated morbidity and mortality. The significant incidence of human disease conditions associated with left–right laterality defects, particularly those of the cardiovascular system, underscores the importance of understanding how left–right asymmetries become established in the embryo. The association between midline defects and left–right anomalies is also observed in a number of mutations in mouse, zebrafish and experimentally manipulated *Xenopus* embryos. In humans, rough estimates place the incidence of left–right malformations at 1/5000 births. In addition, cases that involve no detriment to the individual, such as complete left–right reversal, most probably escape attention.

The normal left–right anatomical arrangement is called *situs solitus*. Mirror-image reversal of all asymmetrical structures is commonly called *situs inversus*. Heterotaxy or *situs ambiguus* refers to an anatomy that is neither normal nor mirror-image-reversed. Mouse models such as homozygous mutant *iv* (*inversus viscerum*) mice demonstrate random determination of situs.[35] Targeted mutation of *left–right dynein*, the gene mutated in the *iv* mouse, also results in left–right malformations. In the inversion of embryonic turning (*inv*) mouse, homozygous mutants demonstrate *situs inversus*.[36]

Molecular basis of left–right determinism

More than 20 genes have already been implicated in vertebrate left–right asymmetry. Some human genes have been described in association with left–right axis malformations. Developmental biology in other vertebrates has pointed the way to other genes, such as *nodal*, *lefty-1* and *lefty-2*, *gdf-1* and *Pitx2*.

Asymmetrical expression of TGFβ family member genes and targeted mutation of signal pathway components have demonstrated the importance of this TGFβ family signal-transduction pathway in left–right axis formation. Recently, one member of this family, growth/differentiation factor-1 (Gdf-1), of unknown function, was inactivated in mice.[37] Gdf1−/− mice exhibited a spectrum of defects related to left–right axis formation, including visceral situs inversus, right pulmonary isomerism and

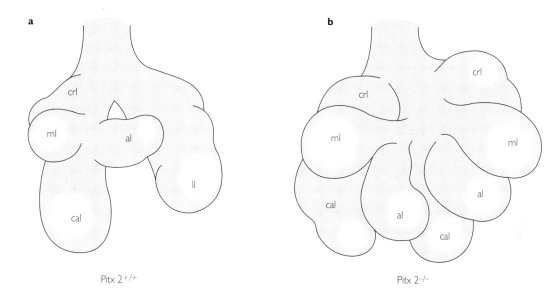

Fig. 1.4.13 Right pulmonary isomerism induced by *Pitx2* null mutation in mouse embryo. Aspect of the embryonic mouse lung at 13.5 days postcoitum in the wild-type (*Pitx2*$^{+/+}$) embryo (a) and in the *Pitx2*$^{-/-}$ embryo (b). In normal development of the wild-type embryo, the right lung has four lobes (crl, cranial lobe; ml, middle lobe; cal, caudal lobe; al, accessory lobe), whereas the left lung has only one (ll, left lobe). In the *Pitx2*$^{-/-}$ embryo, the right lung develops four lobes with a pattern similar to that in normal lung but the left lung also presents four lobes, symmetrical to those of the right lung. (Drawn from data in Kitamura et al.[40])

a range of cardiac anomalies. In most Gdf1$^{-/-}$ embryos, the expression of other members such as *lefty-1* and *-2*, *nodal* and *Pitx2* was absent, suggesting that Gdf-1 acts early in the pathway of gene activation that leads to the establishment of left–right asymmetry. Targeted mutation of the mouse *lefty-1* results in left thoracic isomerism with bilateral anterior expression of genes normally expressed on the left side of the embryo, including *lefty-2*, *nodal* and *Pitx2*.[38] This phenotype suggests that lefty-1, although expressed on the left side of the embryo, does not act as a signal for left-sidedness but prevents left-sided signals from crossing the midline of the embryo.

In the chick, left–right asymmetries are first detected around Hensen's node. Sonic hedgehog (Shh) which is expressed to the left of the node induces *nodal* expression to the left of the node and subsequently in the left lateral plate mesoderm. In turn, Nodal induces expression of *Pitx2*, a homeobox gene. Targeted mutation of *Pitx2*, normally expressed on the left side of the embryo, results in right pulmonary isomerism and cardiac defects[39,40] (Fig. 1.4.13). Thus, Pitx2 seems likely to serve as a critical downstream transcription target that is activated by the left-side-specific signals and mediates left–right asymmetry in vertebrates. Although Shh expression in the mouse is symmetrical, targeted mutation of the mouse gene results in left pulmonary isomerism (Fig. 1.4.7) and heart defects.[41] In contrast to Shh, mice that are compound heterozygotes for *FGF-8* mutations demonstrate right pulmonary isomerism and heart defects.[42]

Another factor required in TGFβ signalling is Cryptic, a member of the *EGF–CFC* gene family. The latter encodes extracellular proteins containing a divergent EGF-like motif and a novel cysteine-rich CFC motif. Once more, although *cryptic* expression is symmetrical, targeted mutation of the mouse gene results in complete right pulmonary isomerism.[43,44] As assessed

by disruption of the asymmetrical expression of *nodal*, *lefty-1*, *lefty-2* and *Pitx2* in *cryptic*$^{-/-}$ embryos, Cryptic seems essential for correct transfer of left–right signals from the node to more peripheral regions of the embryo.

Nodal and lefty are expressed asymmetrically in the left or right lateral mesoderm prior to any organ formation. Yet they initiate a coordinated left–right asymmetry of lung, heart and gut development. Among the downstream mediators of the signalling pathway that control left–right asymmetry within an organ, motor protein genes are likely to be involved. In fact, targeted mutation of the mouse winged-helix transcription factor gene *hfh-4* results not only in the absence of cilia but also in left–right axis malformations including heterotaxy and *situs inversus*, thus reproducing in the mouse the abnormality known as Kartagener's syndrome in man.[6]

Hormonal control

In addition to local organ-specific mechanisms, lung development is also subject to hormonal control, which plays crucial role in the last stages of the process. An aspect that has received particular attention is alveolar epithelial maturation, which leads to surfactant ontogeny during the last third of pregnancy. This has been reviewed a number of times and only a brief summary will be given here. A recent and complete overview can be found in Odom and Ballard.[45]

Glucocorticoids

Glucocorticoids play a major role in lung development. The fact that they are necessary has been directly demonstrated by the development of two gene disruption models in the mouse, of corticotropin-releasing hormone (CRH)[46] and glucocorticoid receptor (GR).[47] In the former, homozygous CRH-deficient fetuses developed normally when the mother was heterozygous, which indicates that hormones of maternal origin were sufficient to support development, whereas those born to homozygous deficient mothers died postnatally because of pulmonary dysplasia with delayed morphological and biochemical maturation. In the second model, homozygous GR-deficient mice developed normally in utero but died of neonatal respiratory distress because their lung development had been arrested at the pseudoglandular stage.

With regard to maturation of lung architecture,[33] the major role of glucocorticoids appears to be to control septal thinning, with involution of interstitial tissue and fusion of the primitive double capillary network into a mature single capillary network. Glucocorticoids appear to drive termination of pulmonary morphogenetic process. Thus, exogenous administration of a glucocorticoid to rat pups in the postnatal period induces precocious arrest of alveolarisation, with a deficit in the number of definitive alveoli. Retinoic acid antagonises this effect, which indicates that the normal process of alveolar septation requires a balance between retinoid and glucocorticoid influences.

With regard to biochemical maturation,[45] glucocorticoids have been shown to enhance the synthesis of all phospholipid and protein components of surfactant in vivo. Enhanced accumulation of phospholipids appears to result mainly from enhanced synthesis of their fatty-acid precursors.

Glucocorticoids appear to directly control transcription of SP-B, SP-C and SP-D genes, but their effects on SP-A gene expression are complex and depend, at least in some experimental systems, on dose and duration of exposure. A practical therapeutical application has been the now generalised use of glucocorticoids for accelerating lung maturation in human fetuses at risk of premature delivery. Numerous multicentric randomised investigations have established the benefit of this practice for the prevention of neonatal respiratory distress syndrome.[48]

Thyroid hormone

Thyroid hormone is also involved in alveolar maturation, as evidenced by the presence of septal thickening and surfactant deficiency in lambs thyroidectomised in utero.[49] In contrast to glucocorticoids, however, it appears to control only the synthesis of the phospholipid moiety of surfactant.[45]

Other hormones

Cyclic adenosine monophosphate (cAMP) agonists and mediators that enhance cAMP, including catecholamines, play an important role in alveolar adaptation at birth through stimulation of surfactant secretion and reabsorption of fetal lung fluid. In addition, they also stimulate the synthesis of several surfactant components, including phospholipids, SP-A and SP-B.[45] Androgens appear to have a delaying effect on alveolar cell maturation, which would account for a relative delay in male lung development as compared with female lung, and for a higher incidence of respiratory distress syndrome in premature male infants than in female infants of same gestational age.[45] Excessive insulin also delays lung maturation, which accounts at least partly for the increased risk of respiratory distress in the hyperinsulinaemic infants of diabetic mothers.[45]

Clinical relevance: the lessons from transgenic mouse models

Transgenic mouse models with abnormal respiratory phenotypes

Recent transgenic techniques capable of producing either gain or loss of function of a gene can be used to obtain mice with abnormal respiratory phenotypes. In addition to illuminating the mechanisms of lung development, certain of these models reproduce features encountered in human syndromes and bring new insights into their aetiology. Lung features in various mouse models are listed in Table 1.4.1. Only those that have obvious clinical relevance are described in more detail here. As stated above, a more or less precocious arrest of lung branching and epithelial development has been reported in mice with targeted deletions of genes involved in lung-branching morphogenesis, including FGF-10,[16] FGFR 2,[17] TGFβ3,[20] and Nkx2.1/TTF-1,[3] whereas targeted deletion of HFH-4 results in absence of cilia.[6] Other targeted deletions produce mouse models of neonatal respiratory distress syndrome (RDS); for instance, alveolar epithelial development is abnormal and leads to postnatal death in EGFR-null mutant mice,[26] and surfactant homeostasis and function are impaired in SP-B-null mutant newborn mice.[50] Interestingly, rescue of SP-B knockout mice with a truncated SP-B proprotein has shown that the C-terminal propeptide of SP-B is not required for the normal structure and function of extracellular surfactant, which the portion of the gene encoding for mature SP-B is sufficient to ensure. Abnormalities persist in these mice, however, which points to a role for the C-terminal propeptide of SP-B in SP-C proprotein processing, maintenance of the size of the lamellar body and control of the size of the intracellular surfactant pool.[51] Targeted SP-D gene deletion also alters alveolar surfactant pool size and clearance, and causes postnatal chronic inflammation and emphysema.[52] Lastly, postnatal alveologenesis is altered in PDGF-A-[34] or retinoic-acid-receptor-γ-null mutant newborn mice.[53]

Investigation of the respiratory phenotypes of these genetically engineered newborn mice may help in the understanding of neonatal respiratory disorders in humans. Severe neonatal respiratory disorders include RDS in premature infants[54] and congenital malformations.[55] Recent insights into the pathways involved in lung development may provide a framework for elucidating both the pathogenesis of genetic disorders such as hereditary SP-B deficiency and the mechanisms underlying lung malformations such as congenital cystic adenomatoid malformation (CCAM) and lung hypoplasia associated with congenital diaphragmatic hernia (CDH).

Table 1.4.1 Lung developmental defects in various transgenic mouse models (loss or gain of function)

Gene	Model	Lung features	References
BMP-4	SP-C/BMP-4 transgene	Reduced lung size, inhibition of epithelial proliferation, cystic alveoli	Bellusci S et al, 1996
Calmodulin inhibitor (*CI*)	SP-C/CI transgene	Impaired branching morphogenesis, lungs lack epithelium	Wang J et al, 1996
C/EBP-α	Null mutation (–/–)	Hyperproliferation and immaturity of alveolar type II cells	Floodby P et al, 1996
EGF-R	Null mutation (–/–)	Thickening of alveolar walls, extended bronchioles. Undifferentiated epithelium in bronchioli and alveoli	Miettinen PJ et al, 1995. Sibilia M et al, 1995
FGFR2	SPC/dominant negative FGFR2 transgene	No branching morphogenesis, lungs reduced to two unbranched tubes	Peters K et al, 1994
FGFR3/4	Double null mutation	Absence of lung phenotype for each individual mutation. No alveologenesis in the double null mutant, no secondary septation	Weinstein M et al, 1998
FGF-10	Null mutation (–/–)	Absence of lung formation beyond the trachea	Min H et al, 1998, Sekine K et al, 1999
Gdf1	Null mutation (–/–)	Right lung isomerism	Rankin CT et al, 2000
Gli2–Gli3	Double null mutation	Variable from tracheo-oesophageal fistula to absence of lungs	Motoyama J et al, 1998
Glucocorticoid receptor	Null mutation (–/–)	Arrested lung development at pseudoglandular stage, surfactant deficiency, death at birth from respiratory failure	Cole TJ et al, 1995.
GM-CSF	Null mutation (–/–)	Alveolar proteinosis, progressive accumulation of surfactant	Dranoff G et al, 1994
HFH-4	Null mutation (–/–)	Absence of cilia, Kartagener syndrome	Chen J et al, 1998
IGF type I-R	Null mutation (–/–)	Death at birth from respiratory failure	Liu JP et al, 1993
IGF type II-R	Null mutation (–/–)	Retarded lung development, alveoli poorly formed	Wang Z-Q et al, 1994
Integrin α3	Null mutation (–/–)	Absence of bronchiolar development, bronchi extend to periphery but alveoli form	Kreidberg JA et al, 1994
KGF (FGF-7)	SP-C/KGF transgene	Cystic lungs with dilated saccules, reduced branching, lethal E15.5–E17.5	Simonet WS et al, 1995
KGF (FGF-7)	ApoE/KGF transgene	Hyperproliferation of alveolar type II cells	Nguyen HQ et al, 1996
lefty 1	Null mutation (–/–)	Left lung isomerism	Meno C et al, 1998
N-myc	Null mutation (–/–)	Death in utero at E11.5, no lung branching	Stanton BR et al, 1992
N-myc	Partial inactivation ("leaky mutation")	Defect in distal airway and airspace development	Moens CB et al, 1992
Ngat1	Null mutation (–/–) (–/+)	Lethal at E9.5. Absence of distinct epithelial layer in the lung anlage	Ioffe E et al, 1996
PDGF-A	Null mutation (–/–)	No myofibroblast differentiation. Absence of elastogenesis and alveolar septation	Boström H et al, 1996
Pitx2	Null mutation (–/–)	Right lung isomerism, Rieger syndrome	Kitamura K et al, 1999
Pod1	Null mutation (–/–)	Perinatal death, pulmonary hypoplasia, defects in branching, alveologenesis, and cell differentiation	Quaggin SE et al, 1999
SP-B	Null mutation (–/–)	Death from respiratory distress, abnormal traffic, storage and function of surfactant	Clark JC et al, 1995
SP-D	Null mutation (–/–)	Inflammation, macrophage hypertrophy, emphysema, accumulation of surfactant phospholipids in airspaces and tissue	Wert SE et al, 2000
TGFα	SP-C/TGFα transgene	Fibrotic lesions, disrupted alveolar architecture	Korfhagen TR et al, 1994

(continued)

Table 1.4.1 (cont'd)

Gene	Model	Lung features	References
TGFβ1	SP-C/TGFβ-1 transgene	Arrested lung development at end of pseudoglandular stage	Zhou L et al, 1996
TGFβ3	Null mutation (–/–)	Reduced branching, thickened mesenchyme, cystic alveoli	Kaartinen V et al, 1995
TTF-1	Null mutation (–/–)	Precocious arrest of branching, distal structures replaced by dilated saccules, impaired alveolar cell differentiation	Kimura S et al, 1996

For null mutations (homologous recombination), (–/–) designates the homozygous state, (–/+) the heterozygous state
For transgenes (expression vectors), the first term designates the regulatory elements used for targeting the transgene and the second term designates the transgenic coding sequence

Congenital malformations

Congenital cystic adenomatoid malformation is a relatively rare disease characterised by expansion of terminal respiratory structures into variable-sized cysts.[56] The pathogenesis of CCAM is unknown but may involve an arrest in lung development resulting in abnormal branching morphogenesis.[56] The large cystic lesions in infants with CCAM are histologically similar to those of the lungs of transgenic mice expressing human KGF in the lung (Fig. 1.4.14).[57] These similarities raise the possibility that disruption of KGF-dependent interactions between epithelium and mesenchyme may be involved in the pathogenesis of CCAM in humans. The role played by Nkx2.1/TTF-1 in the development of CCAM is unclear.[58]

Congenital diaphragmatic hernia occurs in 1/3000 births.[59] Abnormal lung development with lung hypoplasia is associated with the condition. The lungs of patients with CDH are not only small but also immature and exhibit vascular abnormalities.[59] The abnormal number of airways generated in the lungs of CDH patients suggests a disturbance in the pattern of branching morphogenesis. The herbicide nitrofen induces experimental CDH with lung hypoplasia in mice.[60] In situ hybridisation reveals profound disturbances in the temporospatial expression of *FGF-10* (Fig. 1.4.15) and *Bmp4*, two genes involved in lung morphogenesis.[60] Furthermore, a decrease in the expression of vascular endothelial growth factor (VEGF) has been demonstrated in the

lungs of rats with CDH and may explain the abnormal endothelial growth characteristic of this disorder.[61]

SP-B deficiency

Deficiencies in SP-B and other surfactant components are associated with RDS in newborn infants with mutations in the *SP-B* gene.[62] Hereditary SP-B deficiency is an autosomal recessive disorder that typically causes RDS in full-term neonates shortly after birth.[63] The human gene for SP-B contains 11 exons spanning 9.5 kb on the short arm of chromosome 2. The most common mutation causing SP-B deficiency is an insertion in exon 4 (121ins2).[63] However, allelic variation has been identified recently in hereditary SP-B deficiency in newborn infants.[63] The respiratory phenotype of infants with hereditary SP-B deficiency shares similarities with that of homozygous SP-B-deficient newborn mice, which die of respiratory failure at birth.[50] Alveolar type II cells from SP-B-deficient infants and mice lack lamellar bodies and fail to produce tubular myelin. SP-B deficiency is associated with a marked decrease in SP-B mRNA and with complete absence of proSP-B and mature SP-B proteins. Abnormalities in SP-C have also been detected.

With aggressive respiratory support, SP-B-deficient infants have survived beyond the neonatal period but in the absence of lung transplantation the disease has been consistently lethal in the first year of life. However, a recent report described

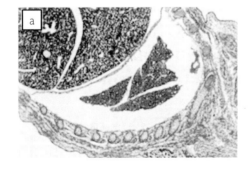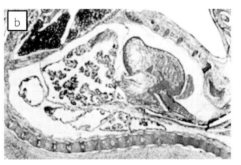

Fig. 1.4.14 Histological aspect of lungs from gestational day 15.5 SP-C–hKGF transgenic and control nontransgenic littermate embryos. Sagittal sections of nontransgenic control embryo (a) and littermate SP-C–hKGF transgenic embryo (b) were stained with haematoxylin and eosin and photographed under bright-field microscopy. Enlarged luminal airways resembling papillary cystadenomas were observed in transgenic embryos. SP-C, surfactant protein C; hKGF, human keratinocyte growth factor (FGF-7). (Reproduced with permission from Simonet et al., Proceedings of the National Academy of Sciences vol. 92, Copyright [1995] National Academy of Sciences, USA[57])

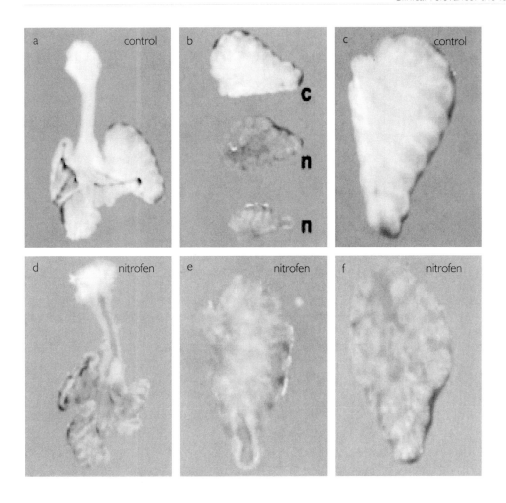

Fig. 1.4.15 FGF-10 expression in control and nitrofen-exposed mouse embryonic lung detected by whole-mount in situ hybridisation at 13.5 days gestation. Note characteristic high levels of *FGF-10* expression present in the mesenchyme adjacent to the distal epithelial buds of control lungs (a) and at higher magnification in the left lobe of a control lung (c), correlating with the sites of future dichotomous branching. The hypoplastic nitrofen-exposed lung (b, d–f) shows profound disturbances in the spatio-temporal expression of *FGF-10*. (f) *FGF-10* transcripts are detected only in the caudal part of the left lobe. (e) *FGF-10* expression was nearly totally abolished in a more severe hypoplastic left lobe. (Reproduced with permission from Acosta et al.[60])

prolonged survival in two children with hereditary SP-B deficiency associated with a novel splicing mutation.[64] It remains unclear why the condition was less severe in these infants. Nevertheless, hereditary SP-B deficiency may cause lung disorders in older children.

Mice genetically engineered to be heterozygous for an SP-B-null allele(SP-B[+/−]) do not have respiratory symptoms at birth and survive to adulthood. However, these mice have a 50% reduction in lung tissue SP-B, an abnormality associated with changes in pulmonary mechanics, decreased pulmonary compliance (Fig. 1.4.16), and mild air trapping.[65] In addition, hetero-

zygous SP-B adult mice are abnormally susceptible to hyperoxic lung injury.[66] The functional abnormalities in heterozygous SP-B adult mice have prompted investigations of lung function in the parents of infants with SP-B deficiency.[67] Lung function tests, including an assessment of lung mechanics, were normal in these adult carriers of the 121ins2 mutation. Nevertheless, it is still unknown whether SP-B heterozygosity in human adults is associated with increased susceptibility to pulmonary injury, as it is in heterozygous SP-B mice. Clearly, there is a need for longitudinal studies of heterozygous humans to determine how advancing age and environmental exposures affect lung function.

Clinical relevance

- Investigation of the respiratory phenotype of certain genetically engineered newborn mice may help to understand neonatal respiratory disorders in humans.

- Pathogenesis of congenital cystic adenomatoid malformation may involve disruption of KGF-dependent epithelial–mesenchymal interactions.

- Disturbances in the pattern of branching morphogenesis in congenital diaphragmatic hernia may involve abnormal temporal–spatial expression of FGF-10 and Bmp4 during morphogenesis.

- The respiratory phenotype of infants with hereditary SP-B deficiency shares similarities with that of homozygous SP-B-deficient newborn mice.

- Nevertheless, increased susceptibility to pulmonary injury evidenced in mice heterozygous for the SP-B null-mutation has not yet been demonstrated in human subjects with a single abnormal SP-B allele.

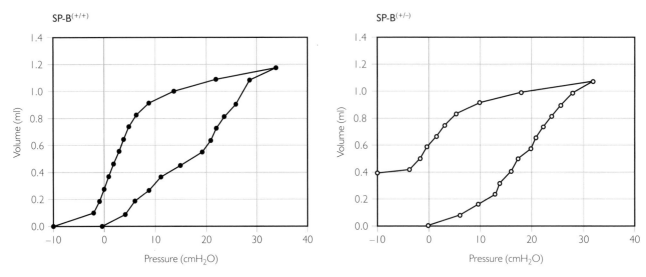

Fig. 1.4.16 Pulmonary compliance as measured by static pressure/volume curves of surfactant protein B (SP-B)$^{+/+}$ and SP-B$^{+/-}$ mouse lungs. Inflation curves were generated from paired littermates in adult mice. The curves presented are representative of data from nine pairs of lungs after normalisation to body weight. Although lung volumes were similar, on inflation and at high pressure, compliance (slope of the curves) was reduced in the lungs of SP-B$^{+/-}$ mice compared with control littermates. (Reproduced with permission from Clark et al.[65])

? Unresolved questions

■ What are the mechanisms through which the fetal lung mesenchyme induces the differentiation of different sets of epithelial cell types along the proximal–distal axis of the airway tree?

■ Obviously, proximal and distal lung mesenchymes are distinct in their ability to induce epithelial cell differentiation, as evidenced in reciprocal grafting experiments. The fate of the primitive epithelium, i.e. its differentiation into tracheobronchial, bronchiolar or alveolar epithelium, is determined through mesenchymal influence and depends on the position of the cells along the proximal–distal axis of the organ.

■ Effects of various exogenous mediators on expression of epithelial cell phenotypes have been reported. For instance, retinoic acid induces a 'proximalisation' of epithelial tubules in the cultured lung

anlage, as evidenced by enhanced development of large bronchi and reduced expression of distal markers. Also, fibroblast growth factors 1 and 7 are both necessary for eliciting alveolar type II cell differentiation in the embryonic epithelium cultured in the absence of mesenchyme.

■ It is nevertheless unknown whether these and/or other mediators are effectively involved in the induction of the various epithelial cell types in vivo, and whether there are local differences in the production of these mediators by the mesenchyme.

■ Similarly, the molecular mechanisms that give instruction for proximal–distal differences in mesenchymal-cell signalling are unknown, although involvement of *hox* genes is a likely hypothesis.

References

1. Glasser SW, Burhans MS, Eszterhas SK et al. Human *SP*-C gene sequences that confer lung epithelium-specific expression in transgenic mice. Am J Physiol Lung Cell Mol Physiol 2000; 278: L933–945.

2. Mendelson CR. Role of transcription factors in fetal lung development and surfactant protein expression. Annu Rev Physiol 2000; 62: 875–915.

3. Minoo P, Su G, Drum H et al. Defects in tracheoesophageal and lung morphogenesis in Nkx2.1 (–/–) mouse embryos. Dev Biol 1999; 209: 60–71.

4. Minoo P, Hamdan H, Bu D et al. TTF-1 regulates lung epithelial morphogenesis. Dev Biol 1995; 172: 694–698.

5. Ang SL, Rossant J. HNF-3 beta is essential for node and notochord formation in mouse development. Cell 1994; 78: 561–574.

6. Chen J, Knowles HJ, Hebert JL, Hackett BP. Mutation of the mouse hepatocyte nuclear factor/forkhead homologue 4 gene results in an absence of cilia and random left-right asymmetry. J Clin Invest 1998; 102: 1077–1082.

7. Motoyama J, Liu J, Mo R et al. Essential function of Gli2 and Gli3 in the formation of lung, trachea and esophagus. Nat Genet 1998; 20: 54–57.

8. Volpe MV, Martin A, Vosatka RJ et al. Hox-b5 expression in the developing mouse lung suggests a role in branching morphogenesis and epithelial cell fate. Histochem Cell Biol 1997; 108: 495–504.

9. Aubin J, Lemieux M, Tremblay M et al. Early postnatal lethality in Hoxa-5 mutant mice is attributable to respiratory tract defects. Dev Biol 1997; 192: 432–445.

10. Malpel S, Mendelsohn C, Cardoso WV. Regulation of retinoic acid signaling during lung morphogenesis. Development 2000; 127:3057–3067.

11. Cardoso WV, Mitsialis SA, Brody JS, Williams MC. Retinoic acid alters the expression of pattern-related genes in the developing lung. Dev Dyn 1996; 207: 47–59.

12. Shannon JM, Nielsen ND, Gebb SA, Randell SH. Mesenchyme specifies epithelial differentiation in reciprocal recombinants of embryonic lung and trachea. Dev Dyn 1998; 212: 482–494.

13. Deterding RR, Shannon JM. Proliferation and differentiation of fetal rat pulmonary epithelium in the absence of mesenchyme. J Clin Invest 1995; 96: 2963–2972.

14. Bellusci S, Grindley J, Emoto N et al. Fibroblast growth factor 10 (FGF 10) and branching morphogenesis in the embryonic mouse lung. Development 1997; 124: 4867–4878.

15. Lebeche D, Malpel S, Cardoso WV. Fibroblast growth factor interactions in the developing lung. Mech Dev 1999; 86:125–136.

16. Min H, Danilenko DM, Scully SA et al. Fgf-10 is required for both limb and lung development and exhibits striking functional similarity to *Drosophila* branchless. Genes Dev 1998; 12:3156–3161.

17. Peters K, Werner S, Liao X et al. Targeted expression of a dominant negative FGF receptor blocks branching morphogenesis and differentiation of the mouse lung. EMBO J 1994; 13:3296–3301.

18. Warburton D, Schwarz M, Tefft D et al. The molecular basis of lung morphogenesis. Mech Dev 2000; 92: 55–81.

19. Sandford LP, Ormsby I, Gittenberg-de Groot AC et al. TGFβ2 knockout mice have multiple developmental defects that are non-overlapping with other TGFβ knockout phenotypes. Development 1997; 124: 2659–2670.

20. Kaartinen V, Voncken J W, Shuler C et al. Abnormal lung development and cleft palate in mice lacking TGFβ3 indicates defects of epithelial–mesenchymal interaction. Nature Genet 1995; 11: 415–421.

21. Spooner B, Faubion J. Collagen involvement in branching morphogenesis of embryonic lung and salivary gland. Dev Biol 1980; 77: 84–102.

22. Schuger L, Skubitz APN, De Las Morenas A, Gilbride K. Two separate domains of laminin promote lung organogenesis by different mechanisms of action. Dev Biol 1995; 169: 520–532.

23. Smith C, Hilfer S, Searls R et al. Effects of β-D-xyloside on differentiation of the respiratory epithelium in the fetal mouse lung. Dev Biol 1990; 138: 42–52.

24. Chelly N, Mouhieddine-Gueddiche OB, Barlier-Mur AM et al. Keratinocyte growth factor enhances maturation of fetal rat lung type II cells. Am J Respir Cell Mol Biol 1999; 20: 423–432.

25. Shannon JM, Gebb SA, Nielsen LD. Induction of alveolar type II cell differentiation in embryonic tracheal epithelium in mesenchyme-free culture. Development 1999; 126: 1675–1688.

26. Miettinen PJ, Berger JE, Meneses J et al. Epithelial immaturity and multiorgan failure in mice lacking epidermal growth factor receptor. Nature 1996; 376: 337–341.

27. St George JA, Read LC, Cranz DL et al. Effect of epidermal growth factor on the fetal development of the tracheo-bronchial secretory apparatus in rhesus monkey. Am J Respir Cell Mol Biol 1991; 4: 95–101.

28. Cardoso WV, Williams MC, Mitsialis SA et al. Retinoic acid induces changes in the pattern of airway branching and alters epithelial cell differentiation in the developing lung in vitro. Am J Respir Cell Mol Biol 1995; 12: 464–476.

29. Mendelsohn C, Lohnes D, Decimo D et al. Function of retinoic acid receptors (RARs) during development. II. Multiple abnormalities at various stages of organogenesis in RAR double mutants. Development 1994; 120: 2749–2771.

30. Chailley-Heu B, Chelly N, Lelievre-Pegorier M et al. Mild vitamin A deficiency delays fetal lung maturation in the rat. Am J Respir Cell Mol Biol 1999; 21: 89–96.

31. Shenai JP, Chytil F, Stahlman MT. Vitamin A status of neonates with bronchopulmonary dysplasia. Pediatr Res 1985; 19: 185–188.

32. Nabeyrat E, Besnard V, Corroyer S et al. Retinoic acid-induced proliferation of lung alveolar epithelial cells: relation with the IGF system. Am J Physiol Lung Cell Mol Physiol 1998; 275: L71–79.

33. Massaro GD, Massaro D. Formation of pulmonary alveoli and gas-exchange surface area: quantification and regulation. Annu Rev Physiol 1996; 58: 73–92.

34. Boström H, Willetts K, Pekny M et al. PDGF-A signaling is a critical event in lung alveolar myofibroblast development and alveogenesis. Cell 1996; 85: 863–873.

35. Supp DM, Witte DP, Potter SS, Brueckner M. Mutation of an axonemal dynein affects left-right asymmetry in inversus viscerum mice. Nature 1997; 389: 963–966.

36. Okada Y, Nonaka S, Tanaka Y et al. Abnormal nodal flow precedes situs inversus in iv and inv mice. Mol Cell 1999; 4:459–468.

37. Rankin CT, Bunton T, Lawler AM, Lee SJ. Regulation of left–right patterning in mice by growth/differentiation factor-1. Nat Genet 2000; 24: 262–265.

38. Meno C, Shimono A, Saijoh Y et al. lefty-1 is required for left–right determination as a regulator of lefty-2 and nodal. Cell 1998; 94: 287–297.

39. Lin CR, Kioussi C, O'Connell S et al. Pitx2 regulates lung asymmetry, cardiac positioning and pituitary and tooth morphogenesis. Nature 1999; 401: 279–282.

40. Kitamura K, Miura H, Miyagawa-Tomita S et al. Mouse Pitx2 deficiency leads to anomalies of the ventral body wall, heart, extra- and periocular mesoderm and right pulmonary isomerism. Development 1999; 126: 5749–5758.

41. Tsukui T, Capdevila J, Tamura K et al. Multiple left–right asymmetry defects in Shh(–/–) mutant mice unveil a convergence of the shh and retinoic acid pathways in the control of Lefty-1. Proc Natl Acad Sci USA 1999; 96: 11376–11381.

42. Meyers EN, Martin GR. Differences in left–right axis pathways in mouse and chick: functions of FGF8 and SHH. Science 1999; 285: 403–406.

43. Gaio U, Schweickert A, Fischer A et al. A role of the cryptic gene in the correct establishment of the left–right axis. Curr Biol 1999; 9:1339–1342.

44. Yan YT, Gritsman K, Ding J et al. Conserved requirement for EGF–CFC genes in vertebrate left–right axis formation. Genes Dev 1999; 13: 2527–2537.

45. Odom MW, Ballard P. Development and hormonal regulation of the surfactant system. In: McDonald JA, ed. Lung growth and development. New York: Marcel Dekker, 1997: 495–575.

46. Muglia LL, Jacobson L, Dikkes P, Majzoub JA. Corticotropin-releasing hormone deficiency reveals major fetal but not adult glucocorticoid need. Nature 1995; 327: 427–432.

47. Cole TJ, Blendy JA, Monhagan AP et al. Targeted disruption of the glucocorticoid receptor gene blocks chromaffin cell development and severely retards lung maturation. Genes Dev 1995; 9: 1608–1621.

48. Kattner E, Metze B, Waiss E, Obladen M. Accelerated lung maturation following maternal steroid treatment in infants born before 30 weeks gestation. J Perinat Med 1992; 20: 449–457.

49. Erenberg A, Rhodes ML, Weinstein MM, Kennedy RL. The effect of fetal thyroidectomy on ovine fetal lung maturation. Pediatr Res 1979; 13: 230–235.

50. Clark JC, Wert SE, Bachurski CJ et al. Targeted disruption of the surfactant protein B gene disrupts surfactant homeostasis, causing respiratory failure in newborn mice. Proc Natl Acad Sci USA 1995; 92: 7794–7798.

51. Akinbi H, Breslin JS, Ikegami M et al. Rescue of SP-B knockout mice with a truncated SP-B proprotein. Function of the C-terminal propeptide. J Biol Chem 1997; 272: 9640–9647.

52. Wert SE, Yoshida M, LeVine A M et al. Increased metalloproteinase activity, oxidant production, and emphysema in surfactant protein D gene-inactivated mice. Proc Natl Acad Sci USA 2000; 97: 5972–5977.

53. McGowan S, Jackson SK, Jenkins-Moore M et al. Mice bearing deletions of retinoid acid receptors demonstrate reduced lung elastin and alveolar numbers. Am J Respir Cell Mol Biol 2000; 23: 162–167.

54. Clements BS. Congenital malformations of the lungs and airways. In: Taussig LM, Landau LI, ed. Pediatric respiratory medicine. St Louis, MO: Mosby, 1998: 1106–1136.

55. Bancalari E, Bidegain M. Respiratory disorders of the newborn. In: Taussig LM, Landau LI, ed. Pediatric respiratory medicine. St Louis, MO: Mosby, 1998: 464–488.

56. Morotti RA, Cangiarella J, Gutierrez MC et al. Congenital cystic adenomatoid malformation of the lung (CCAM): evaluation of the cellular components. Hum Pathol 1999; 30: 618–625.

57. Simonet W S, DeRose ML, Bucay N et al. Pulmonary malformation in transgenic mice expressing human keratinocyte growth factor in the lung. Proc Natl Acad Sci USA 1995; 92: 12461–12465.

58. Morotti RA, Gutierrez MC, Askin F et al. Expression of thyroid transcription factor-1 in congenital cystic adenomatoid malformation of the lung. Pediatr Dev Pathol 2000; 3: 455–461.

59. Ijsselstijn H, Tibboel D. The lungs in congenital diaphragmatic hernia: do we understand? Pediatr Pulmonol 1998; 26: 204–218.

60. Acosta JM, Thébaud B, Castillo C et al. Novel mechanisms in murine Nitrofen-induced pulmonary hypoplasia: FGF10 rescue in culture. Am J Physiol (Lung Cell Mol Physiol) 2001; 281: 250–257.

61. Okazaki T, Sharma H S, Aikawa M et al. Pulmonary expression of vascular endothelial growth factor and myosin isoforms in rats with congenital diaphragmatic hernia in utero. J Pediatr Surg 1997; 32: 391–394.

62. Nogee LM, Garnier G, Dietz H C, et al. A mutation in the surfactant protein B gene responsible for fatal neonatal respiratory disease in multiple kindreds. J Clin Invest 1994; 93: 1860–1863.

63. Nogee LM, Wert SE, Proffit SA et al. Allelic heterogeneity in hereditary surfactant protein B (SP-B) deficiency. Am J Respir Crit Care Med 2000; 161: 973–981.

64. Dunbar AE III, Wert SE, Ikegami M et al. Prolonged survival in hereditary surfactant protein deficiency associated with a novel splicing mutation. Pediatr Res 2000; 48: 275–282.

65. Clark JC, Weaver TE, Iwamoto HS et al. Decreased lung compliance and air trapping in heterozygous SP-B-deficient mice. Am J Respir Cell Mol Biol 1997; 16: 46–52.

66. Tokieda K, Iwatomo HS, Bachurski C et al. Surfactant protein-B-deficient mice are susceptible to hyperoxic lung injury. Am J Respir Cell Mol Biol 1999; 21: 463–472.

67. Yusen RD, Cohen H, Hamvas A. Normal lung function in subjects heterozygous for surfactant protein-B deficiency. Am J Respir Crit Care Med 1999; 159: 411–414.

2 Function

2.1 Matrix proteins

Sarah E Dunsmore, Rachel C Chambers and Geoffrey J Laurent

 Key points

- The structural integrity of the lung is dependent on matrix protein organisation.

- Individual matrix proteins can direct cell behaviour via interactions with cell surface receptors.

- Alterations in matrix protein turnover and deposition can lead to devastating lung pathology.

- Treatment for lung diseases involving matrix remodelling is limited. Novel approaches need to be explored.

In this chapter, the structure and function of the proteins that comprise the lung extracellular matrix are described. The extracellular matrix of the lung encompasses components of the basement membrane and interstitial connective tissue. Fundamental physical properties, such as the intrinsic recoil of the lung, are governed by matrix proteins. Furthermore, normal lung morphogenesis is dependent on the extracellular matrix and alterations in its composition following injury have devastating consequences.

Matrix proteins are found in basement membranes, in the pulmonary interstitium, in provisional matrices such as fibrin clots and in the cartilaginous rings encircling the trachea and large bronchi. Each of these structures is uniquely organised to play a distinct role in normal lung function, which is discussed in the first section of this chapter. In the next section, the characteristic structures and specific functions of individual matrix proteins are outlined. The final section focuses on lung pathology associated with aberrant matrix protein turnover and structure.

Organisation of matrix proteins

Matrix proteins are assembled into three dimensional structures that play a key role in determining the physical and mechanical properties of an organ. Although the matrix proteins that comprise these structures are not solely found in the lung, the organisation of matrix proteins in the lung is unique and highly specialised to facilitate gas exchange.

Basement membranes

Basement membranes are found wherever parenchymal cells directly appose connective tissue. Physically, they serve as a mechanical support structure and diffusion barrier. Biologically, matrix proteins can regulate cell phenotype through direct interactions with cell surface receptors. Integrins are the best characterised cell surface receptors for matrix proteins and mediate both mechanical and chemical signals. These stimuli activate a variety of intracellular signalling pathways to affect cell proliferation, survival and differentiation.[1]

In the lung, basement membranes are present underneath both airway and alveolar epithelial cells, as well as surrounding the vascular endothelium. The structure of the lung basement membrane is highly specialised to facilitate gas exchange. In many areas of the alveoli, the alveolar epithelial and capillary endothelial basement membranes are fused, thus providing a minimal barrier for gas diffusion of about 200 nm at the narrowest junction (Fig. 2.1.1). Matrix proteins located in the basement membrane provide signals that regulate airway branching and are thought to determine the localisation of type I and type II alveolar epithelial cells.

Electron microscopic studies initially defined the structure and nomenclature of the basement membrane. In most tissues, three component layers of the basement membrane can be visualised: the lamina lucida or rara, the lamina densa and the lamina fibroreticularis (Fig. 2.1.2). The approaches of immunohistochemistry and molecular biology have led to better understanding of basement membrane structure. Using these approaches, types IV and V collagen, laminin, entactin, fibronectin and proteoglycans have been defined as components of the lung basement membrane.[2]

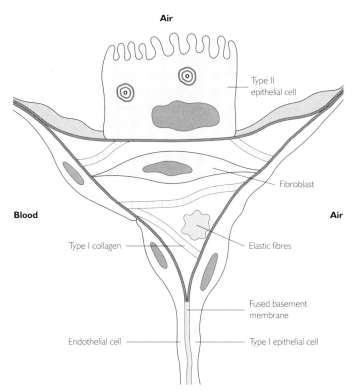

Fig. 2.1.1 Localisation of matrix proteins in the alveolus. In the alveolus, matrix proteins are found in the basement membrane underneath type I epithelial cells, type II epithelial cells and endothelial cells. Basement membranes of type I epithelial cell and endothelial cells are fused to provide a minimal barrier for gas diffusion. Collagen fibrils and elastic fibres are the major components of the alveolar interstitium.

The pulmonary interstitium

The pulmonary interstitium is a key determinant of lung function. It is the mechanical scaffold that maintains structural integrity during ventilation. Fibres of the matrix proteins collagen and elastin form this scaffold (Fig. 2.1.1). It has long been recognised that lung injury is often associated with changes in synthesis or turnover of interstitial matrix proteins. Pulmonary fibrosis is a consequence of increased extracellular matrix synthesis and deposition, particularly of types I and III collagen. In this disease, gas exchange is adversely affected by the loss of capillary beds and increased regional compliance resulting from the thickening of the pulmonary interstitium. Conversely, degradation of elastin is a characteristic of pulmonary emphysema. The reduction in elastin content of the pulmonary interstitium adversely affects ventilation by decreasing the intrinsic recoil of the lung. The role of matrix proteins in lung pathology is discussed in detail in the final section of this chapter. Clinical aspects of chronic obstructive pulmonary disease (COPD) and interstitial lung disease are described in Volume 2.

Provisional matrices

Provisional matrices are assembled during development or wound repair and are degraded when normal tissue architecture is achieved. The most common and best characterised provisional matrix components are fibronectin and fibrin. Thrombospondin, tenascin and SPARC are also present in the lung extracellular matrix during development and following injury. In the lung, fibronectin matrices are important in airway branching morphogenesis.[3] Fibrin matrices and associated

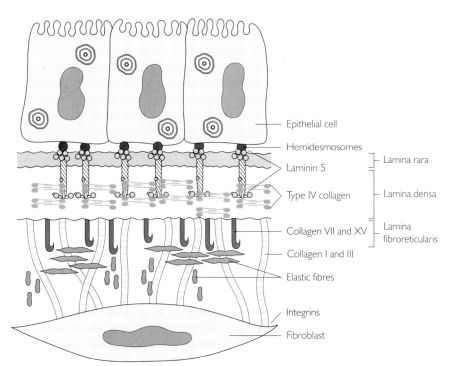

Fig. 2.1.2 Schematic depiction of the layers of the basement membrane. The basement membrane is composed of three layers: the lamina rara, the lamina densa and the lamina fibroreticularis. Laminin 5 connects hemidesmosomes on the basal surface of epithelial cells to the type IV collagen network in the lamina densa. Anchoring fibrils composed of type VII and type XV collagen link the basement membrane to the interstitial matrix where type I collagen, type III collagen and elastic fibres are found. Integrins located on the fibroblast cell surface interact with many matrix proteins including type I collagen.

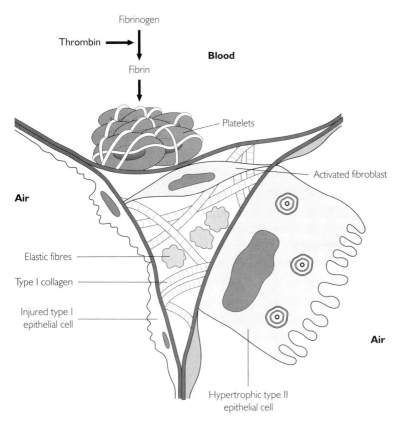

Fig. 2.1.3 Provisional matrix proteins in an injured alveolus. Disruption of the blood–gas barrier results from injury to type I epithelial cells. In this setting, thrombin catalyses the formation of fibrin which interacts with red blood cells to produce a clot in the injured alveolus. Thrombin and associated products of the coagulation cascade stimulate fibroblasts to proliferate and increase matrix production.

products of the coagulation cascade (Fig. 2.1.3) are not only important in pulmonary haemostasis but also play a key role in modulating collagen deposition following acute lung injury.[4]

Cartilage

Cartilage lines the walls of the trachea and large bronchi and is responsible for keeping these airways open despite changes in intrathoracic pressure during breathing. Hyaluronan, collagen types II, VI, IX, X, XI and XII,[5] and aggrecan[6] are the major matrix proteins found in cartilage. In one model of cartilage function, collagen fibres in the outer layers oppose tensile forces, and proteoglycans in the central zone resist compression forces.[7]

Hyaluronan is also present in the lung parenchyma, where it accumulates following lung injury. Since it is capable of immobilising water, hyaluronan is thought to contribute to the alveolar and interstitial oedema observed following acute lung injury. In this setting, hyaluronan and hyaluronan fragments interact with cell surface receptors to activate signal transduction pathways that influence cell adhesion, motility, proliferation and gene expression.[8]

Structure and function of matrix proteins

Matrix proteins have characteristic structures and functions. In most organs, collagens, laminins and proteoglycans are compo-nents of the extracellular matrix. Elastic fibres, on the other hand, are specialised structures only found in tissues subject to mechanical stress. General aspects of the biology of the major classes of matrix proteins are briefly reviewed in this section, which focuses on the localisation and function of individual matrix proteins in the lung.

Collagens

Collagens consist of three polypeptide chains containing the amino acid sequence Gly–x–y. Although x and y may be any amino acid, proline and hydroxyproline predominate in these positions such that approximately every third x is proline and every third y is hydroxyproline. Hydroxyproline is not unique to collagen; however, concentrations present in collagen are much higher than for other proteins, so that this amino acid is used as a specific index of collagen synthesis and concentration. The three polypeptide chains associate via the Gly–x–y sequences to form triple helices. All collagens contain at least one triple helix region. In this conformation, peptide bonds linking adjacent amino acids are buried within the interior of the molecule, rendering the triple helix region highly resistant to proteolysis. The pattern of collagen synthesis is tissue-specific and is regulated at both the transcriptional and translational levels. Collagens are also subject to numerous post-translational modifications.

Collagens may be divided into two classes, fibrillar and non-fibrillar. Fibrillar collagens (types I, II, III, V and XI) are the major structural components of connective tissues and are the most abundant proteins in the lung, accounting for about

15–20% of the dry weight of the tissue. Their primary function is to confer tensile strength to all distensible components of the lung such as the large airways, blood vessels and alveolar interstitium. Types I and III collagen (in a ratio of 2:1) represent approximately 90% of the collagens in the adult human lung. These collagens are located throughout the alveolar interstitium, in pulmonary blood vessels, the visceral pleura and the connective tissue sheaths that surround the tracheobronchial tree. Type I collagen confers tensile strength and rigidity to tissues; whereas type III, which forms a more reticular network of fibres, is probably more important in bestowing compliance.[9] The tensile strength of bronchial and tracheal cartilage is largely determined by types II and XI collagen. Small amounts of type V collagen are present in basement membranes. It is also found in association with type I collagen in the interstitium, alveolar walls and blood vessels.

Type IV collagen is the most abundant non-fibrillar collagen found in the lung, constituting approximately 5% of parenchymal collagen. Instead of forming fibrils, the amino and carboxy terminal regions of the type IV collagen molecule laterally associate to form open-network structures that are thought to play a role in the structural and barrier functions of the basement membrane. Type IV collagen is responsible for the tensile strength of the blood–gas barrier and plays a large part in preventing stress failure of the pulmonary capillaries under normal conditions.[10]

Many other non-fibrillar collagens are present in the lung. Type VI collagen is found in the pulmonary interstitium and vasculature, as fine filaments associated with types I and III collagen. Pulmonary arterioles and venules contain type VIII collagen. Although information on localisation is lacking, expression of types IX and XII collagen in the lung has been documented. Collagen types XV and XVIII, which are also proteoglycans, are components of the lung basement membrane. Although it has been speculated that these other non-fibrillar collagens may play a role in determining tensile strength or in facilitating collagen fibril assembly, their specific functions in the lung are not known.

Elastic fibres

Elastic fibres are responsible for the intrinsic recoil of the heart, lungs and arterial blood vessels and also contribute to resiliency of the skin. The fibres consist of two major components, microfibrils and elastin, which comprises 90% of the mature elastic fibre. In the lung, elastic fibres are predominately found in the parenchyma where, together with collagen fibrils, an integral fibre network that comprises the architectural skeleton of the lung is formed. This fibre network is a key determinant of the mechanical properties of the lung. Elastic fibres encircle respiratory bronchioles and alveolar ducts in a helical fashion and appear as a fine mesh in alveolar walls. In the walls of the pulmonary artery and arterioles, elastic fibres are organised into concentric sheets or lamellae.

Elastin is a unique matrix protein that is capable of being stretched several times its resting length under tension, with a rapid recovery to its original size when the force is released. It is an insoluble protein composed mainly of hydrophobic amino acids (44%), glycine (33%) and proline (10–13%). Two pentapeptides, Val–Pro–Gly–Val–Gly and Pro–Gly–Val–Gly–Val, repeat frequently in the molecule and are thought to form large spiral regions that contribute to the distensibility of the protein (Fig. 2.1.4). Elastin is formed by lysyl-oxidase-catalysed cross-linking of lysine residues on its soluble precursor, tropoelastin. Tropoelastin is transcribed from a single gene; transcripts are subject to alternative splicing. Variant tropoelastin isoforms have been described. Their functional significance is not clear.

The microfibrillar component of elastic fibres forms small, 10–12 nm diameter fibrils at the periphery of amorphous elastin and is thought to act as an organising scaffold in the formation of the elastin network. When examined by rotary shadowing electron microscopy, microfibrils appear as linear arrays of electron-dense 'beads' separated by approximately 50 nm with filamentous 'strings'. Fibrillin-1 and fibrillin-2 are the major structural components of microfibrils. Tropoelastin has been shown to bind to sequences in the amino termini of both fibrillins. Other molecules such as microfibril-associated glycoprotein (MAGP-1) and proteoglycans may be associated with microfibrils.

Elastic fibres are very stable structures: some may last for the life-span of the organism. The relative proportion of microfibrils to elastin, however, declines with increasing age. Thus, the scaffold for elastic fibre assembly is only present for a limited period of time and degradation of elastin in the adult leads to irreversible pathology.

Proteoglycans

Proteoglycans are a diverse family of large molecules in which a core protein is covalently linked to sulphated polysaccharides or glycosaminoglycans (GAGs). GAGs may be divided into three classes: chondroitin sulphate/dermatan sulphate, heparan sulphate/heparin and keratan sulphate; a proteoglycan may be comprised of GAGs from more than one class. Hyaluronan, a non-sulphated GAG, is not a true proteoglycan because of its lack of a core protein. Proteoglycans are synthesised by a variety of cell types and are multifunctional components of most extracellular matrices and plasma membranes.

Because of their large hydrodynamic volumes and charge characteristics, hyaluronan and proteoglycans exert a profound influence on lung compliance and fluid balance. Early studies used cationic dyes, which react with negatively charged regions of carbohydrates and GAGs, to demonstrate the presence of proteoglycans in the lung. Results of these and other studies have demonstrated that proteoglycans are asymmetrically distributed within the alveolar basement membrane.[2] It has been proposed that this asymmetrical distribution of proteoglycans may be important in determining the phenotype of the overlying epithelium.

More recent studies have used antibodies and cDNA probes obtained from molecular cloning of various proteoglycans. These studies have demonstrated that the matrix proteoglycans[11] – versican, perlecan, agrin, decorin, biglycan, PRELP, lumican and fibromodulin – are components of the lung extracellular matrix. Versican is a member of the hyalectan gene family, which contains proteoglycans that interact with hyaluronan and lectins. In pulmonary fibrotic disorders, versican, a chondroitin/dermatan-

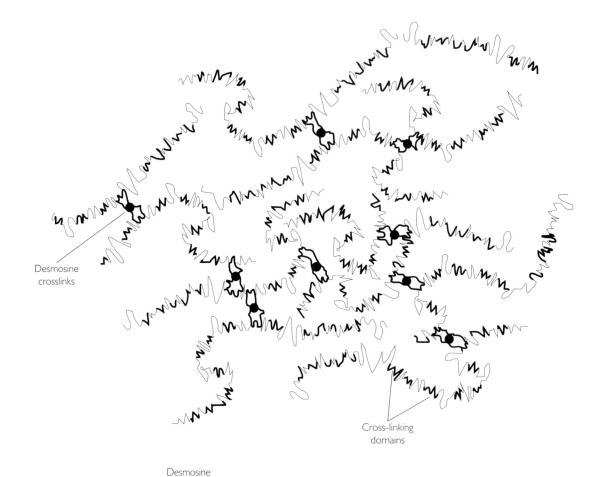

Desmosine
crosslinks

Cross-linking
domains

(a) Relaxed.

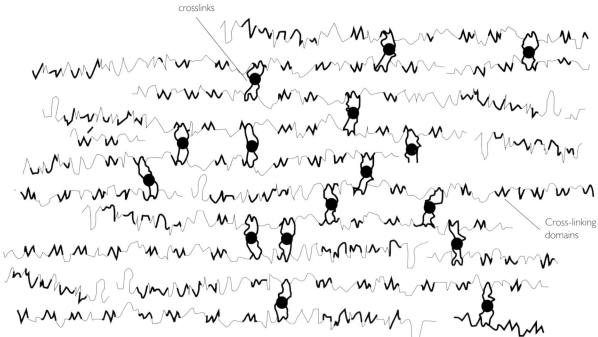

Desmosine
crosslinks

Cross-linking
domains

(b) Stretched.

Fig. 2.1.4 Diagrammatic representation of cross-linked elastin in (a) relaxed and (b) stretched states. Cross-linking domains, some of which are likely in an α-helical conformation, are in bold. For clarity, only a portion of the actual cross-links are depicted. Stretching brings the chains of the molecule into alignment and limits their conformational freedom. (Modified from Rosenbloom J, Abrams WR, Mecham R. Extracellular matrix 4: the elastic fiber. FASEB J 1993; 7:1208–1218.)

sulphate proteoglycan, appears to form a provisional matrix in which myofibroblasts synthesise type I collagen.[12]

Perlecan and agrin are referred to as basement membrane proteoglycans and are predicted to function in determining the filtration properties of the alveolar basement membrane.[13, 14] Both are heparan-sulphate proteoglycans and are also likely to function in sequestering growth factors. Agrin, because of its structural similarity to Kazal-type serine protease inhibitors, may play a role in protecting proteins from degradation.[15]

Decorin, biglycan, PRELP, lumican and fibromodulin are part of the family of small leucine-rich proteoglycans. This family is divided into three distinct subclasses based on genomic and protein organisation. Decorin and biglycan, which contain chondroitin/dermatan-sulphate GAGs, form one subclass. Both are primarily found in the pulmonary interstitium. Levels of decorin and biglycan are increased in pulmonary fibrosis and decreased in pulmonary emphysema. Decorin and biglycan are hypothesised to function by sequestering growth factors and by facilitating collagen fibril assembly. Exogenously administered decorin is antifibrotic. This antifibrotic effect is attributed to binding and inactivation of transforming growth factor (TGF)-β.

PRELP, lumican and fibromodulin, which contain keratan-sulphate GAGs, are part of another subclass of the small leucine-rich proteoglycan family. In the lung, PRELP has only been detected at the mRNA level. The walls of the pulmonary vasculature contain lumican. Expression of fibromodulin is observed in animal models of lung injury. Lumican and fibromodulin appear to be important in collagen fibril assembly.[16,17] Specific functions of these proteoglycans in the lung, however, are not known.

Laminins

Laminins consist of three polypeptide chains (α, β, γ) and are the major non-collagenous components of basement membranes.[18] At present, 5 α, 3 β and 3 γ chains have been identified. These subunits combine to form at least 12 different laminin heterotrimers. All laminin isoforms consist of one α, one β and one γ chain, which associate via their carboxy ends to form a triple-stranded coiled-coil structure. In laminins 1–4 and laminin 12, the amino-terminal regions of the three chains extend to form a cruciform structure. The upper region of this cruciform structure varies such that the arms of the cross are truncated in laminin 5, laminins 6–9 appear 'topless' and the amino terminal of the α chain extends further in laminins 10 and 11 (Fig. 2.1.5). Many laminins (2, 4, 5, 6, 7, 10 and 11) undergo proteolytic modifications that, at least in the case of laminin 5, alter integrin-mediated cell migration.[19]

At both the structural and functional levels, laminin 1 is the best characterised isoform. Laminin 1 was originally identified as a component of the Engelbreth-Holm-Swarm (EHS) sarcoma, a tumour that secretes large amounts of basement membrane, and is the source of the commercial preparation matrigel. It is thought to be essential for basement membrane assembly and binds with high affinity to entactin, which forms a bridge between laminin and the type IV collagen network. Studies with proteolytic fragments, synthetic peptides and domain-specific antibodies have elucidated the regions of the laminin 1 molecule that mediate cell adhesion, spreading and migration, as well as lung alveolarisation and neurite outgrowth.[2]

Laminin 1 is the major laminin expressed during early embryogenesis and plays a role in organogenesis of the lung, kidney and

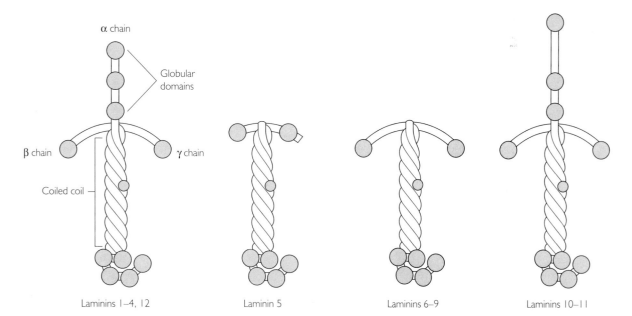

Fig. 2.1.5 Laminin isoforms. At present, 12 laminin isoforms consisting of various combinations of α, β and γ chains have been identified. All laminins consist of one α, one β and one γ chain, which combine to form a triple-stranded coiled-coil structure. Globular domains are found throughout the molecule. Various combinations of α, β and γ chains associate to produce four basic structures. The classical cruciform structure is characteristic of laminins 1–4 and 12. The arms of the β and γ chain are truncated in laminin-5. Laminins 6–9 appear 'topless'. In laminins 10 and 11, the α chain is longer than in the other laminins. (Modified from Colognato & Yurchenco.[18])

gut. In the lung, expression of laminin 1 is restricted to the pseudoglandular stage of development.[20,21] It is unlikely that laminin 1 is present in the basement membrane of adult lungs.[20-23] Antibodies used in earlier studies that reported this observation were reacting with other laminin isoforms.[22] Laminin 1 and matrigel, however, do have profound effects on the phenotype of cultured adult alveolar epithelial cells.[2] Effects of other laminin isoforms on alveolar epithelial cell function have not been studied but are likely to be similar to those of laminin 1 if the same alveolar epithelial cell integrins are involved.

All laminin subunits are expressed to some extent in the lung. Expression of the laminin α_2 chain is also confined to development.[24] Although complete immunohistochemical data is lacking, it is possible that laminins 5–12 may be present in the lung basement membrane. Information on laminin isoform expression in the lung under pathological conditions is lacking and is crucial for understanding the mechanisms of basement membrane reassembly following lung injury.

Provisional matrix proteins

Fibronectin[25] is a dimeric glycoprotein that is ubiquitously present in the lung extracellular matrix. Although at least 10 different forms of fibronectin may result from differential splicing of pre-mRNA, two major forms, plasma fibronectin and cellular fibronectin, predominate in vivo. Fibronectin is encoded by a single gene, which is composed of three distinct homologous repeat sequences, type I, type II and type III (Fig. 2.1.6). Each repeat sequence is the product of a separate exon. Two regions within the type III repeat, EDA and EDB (originally referred to as EIIIA and EIIIB), and another region IIICS (originally referred to as V, for 'variable'), are subject to internal splicing. Plasma fibronectin is synthesised in the liver

and does not contain the EDA or EDB domains. Cellular fibronectin is produced by a variety of cell types and contains the EDA domain. The functional significance of fibronectin splicing variants is not known, although differential expression of splice variants has been observed in fibroblasts isolated from varying tissues. Fibronectin gene polymorphisms are associated with the development of pulmonary fibrosis,[26] suggesting that fibronectin isoforms may play a role in disease processes.

Fibronectin's biological effects on cell adhesion, morphology, migration, proliferation and differentiation are particularly evident during development and wound repair. In the developing lung, fibronectin plays a role in branching morphogenesis[3] and alveolar epithelial cell differentiation.[27] Although fibronectin's precise role in lung repair in vivo has not been elucidated, effects of fibronectin on alveolar epithelial cell phenotype[2] and wound repair in vitro are well documented. Both plasma and cellular fibronectin are incorporated into the extracellular matrix of injured lungs in vivo. Immunostaining for cellular fibronectin is prominent in active fibroblastic foci of fibrotic lungs.[28]

Fibrinogen[29] is a soluble circulating glycoprotein synthesised by hepatocytes. It is composed of three pairs of different polypeptide chains, Aα, Bβ and γ. The molecule is highly heterogeneous, as a result of polymorphic variation in the Aα and Bβ chains, alternative splicing, extensive post-translational modification and proteolytic degradation. Fibrinogen is cleaved by thrombin to form fibrin, the most abundant component of blood clots. The fibrin matrix serves as a scaffold for platelet aggregation and is degraded by plasmin when haemostasis is achieved. Both fibrinogen and fibrin degradation products have biological effects on cell proliferation and migration.

The fibrin matrix is a rich depository for growth factors, matrix proteins, proteases and protease inhibitors. During tissue repair, it provides the framework for re-epithelialization and

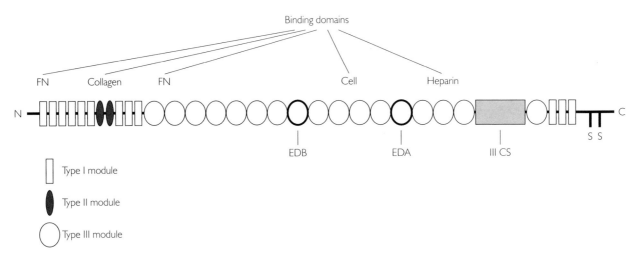

Fig. 2.1.6 Domain structure of fibronectin. The fibronectin dimer is formed through interchain disulphide bonds (S S) at the carboxyl terminus (C). Subunits consist of type I (open rectangles), type II (solid ovals) and type III (open circles) modules. Bold circles represent the EDA and EDB domains, which are not present in plasma fibronectin. These domains, as well as the III CS region (crosshatched rectangle), are subject to internal splicing. Domains that interact with fibronectin (FN), collagen, cells and heparin are indicated. (Modified from Schwarzbauer J, Sechler JL. Fibronectin fibrillogenesis: a paradigm for extracellular matrix assembly. Curr Opin Cell Biol 1999; 11:622–627.)

vascularization. Intra-alveolar and intravascular fibrin deposition is common in acute lung injury. In this setting, procoagulant activity is enhanced and fibrinolytic activity is impaired. The persistent presence of the fibrin matrix and of associated proteases of the coagulation cascade is important in the progression of acute respiratory distress syndrome to pulmonary fibrosis.[4]

Thrombospondins, tenascins and SPARC[30-32] have been termed antiadhesive matrix proteins because they inhibit the spreading of cells. At present, five thrombospondin isoforms have been identified. In the developing lung, thrombospondins 1 and 3 are expressed. Thrombospondin-1 is also found in patients with organising pneumonia.[33] Interestingly, many characteristics of pneumonia are present in the lungs of thrombospondin-1-null mice.[34] Thrombospondin-1 plays a role in the activation of TGF-β[35] but it is not clear how this function relates to the pathogenesis of organising pneumonia. In pulmonary fibrotic disorders, tenascin has been localised to fibroblastic foci and is also found in the basement membrane underneath hypertrophic epithelial cells.[33] The specific tenascin isoforms present in the developing or injured lung have not been precisely identified, however. In development, SPARC plays a role in airway branching.[36] Its function following lung injury has not been fully investigated. Its expression in fibrotic lung disorders, however, is minimal.[33]

Matrix proteins in lung pathology

Devastating pathological consequences result from alterations in matrix protein structure and organisation. Diseases involving matrix proteins in the lung are typified by the pulmonary fibrotic disorders, diseases of excess matrix protein deposition, and pulmonary emphysema, which results from proteolytic destruction of matrix proteins. Although interstitial collagen deposition predominates in most fibrotic lung disorders, it appears that the general increase in matrix protein deposition is responsible for the pathophysiology of these diseases. In contrast, the matrix-related pathophysiology of pulmonary emphysema is largely due to the destruction of elastin fibres.

Fibrosis

Excess matrix protein deposition may occur in the lung interstitium, airways or vasculature. Fibrotic interstitial lung diseases include bronchopulmonary dysplasia, idiopathic pulmonary fibrosis, sarcoidosis and asbestos related diseases. Additionally, areas of interstitial fibrosis are often found in patients with acute or toxic lung injury. Changes in matrix protein deposition are perhaps best characterised in idiopathic pulmonary fibrosis, where increases in the production of types I and III collagen, elastin, proteoglycans and fibronectin have been reported.[37] In idiopathic pulmonary fibrosis and most other fibrotic interstitial lung diseases, fibroblasts are responsible for most of the increased matrix production. Although the factors that initiate the interstitial fibrotic disorders differ, the functional consequences of excess interstitial matrix deposition are similar. Abnormal gas exchange results from the loss of capillary beds and decreased ventilation in affected areas of the lung.

In asthmatics, excess matrix protein deposition is observed in the airways. Increases in types III and V collagen, lumican, biglycan, versican, fibronectin and tenascin in the subepithelial basement membrane or lamina fibroreticularis are observed.[38-40] Myofibroblasts are reported to be the source of the majority of these matrix proteins. Although the functional consequences of matrix protein deposition in the airways are not completely understood,[41] excessive deposition of collagens and other molecules will have profound effects on mechanical properties, metabolism, cell function and transport properties of airways. It is possible that matrix protein deposition in asthma is a teleological response to prevent airway collapse. Excess matrix protein deposition, however, may contribute to the overall narrowing of the airway lumen and thus, in the long term, limit ventilation. In asthmatic airways, deposition of collagenous and non-collagenous matrix proteins is part of a larger remodelling process that also includes changes in smooth muscle and mucus glands.

Remodelling of the pulmonary vasculature occurs in infants and adults. In infants, excess matrix protein deposition is initiated by hypoxia resulting from development abnormalities such as congenital heart disease, diaphragmatic hernia or bronchopulmonary dysplasia.[42] Levels of elastin, type I collagen, fibronectin and tenascin[43] are increased in the vessel walls. Smooth-muscle cells and fibroblasts in the outer medial and adventitial layers of the blood vessels are responsible for most of the excess matrix protein production. In adults, pulmonary vascular remodelling may occur secondary to other disease processes or as a result of genetic mutations,[44] infection, or injury. In contrast to hypoxic pulmonary vascular remodelling in infants, excess matrix deposition occurs in the neointima of the vessel wall in adults, where deposition of elastin, type I collagen, fibronectin and thrombospondin is observed.[45]

Emphysema

Destruction of elastic fibres in the lung interstitium is the pathologic hallmark of emphysema. This destruction results in decreased lung recoil and impaired ventilation. There are two major forms of emphysema, panacinar and centrilobular. Panacinar emphysema predominates in the lower lung zones and occurs in people deficient in α_1-proteinase inhibitor, the serpin that blocks the activity of neutrophil elastase. Uniform destruction of the alveolar walls and permanent enlargement of the alveoli are observed. As the disease progresses, all respiratory airspaces distal to a terminal bronchiole are affected. Centrilobular emphysema predominates in the upper lung zones and begins with inflammation in the terminal and respiratory bronchioles with subsequent enlargement of the alveoli and more distal respiratory airspaces. It is thought to result as a consequence of prolonged exposure to cigarette smoke. Data obtained from using mice deficient in macrophage elastase indicate that this enzyme may be the key protease in centrilobular emphysema.[46] Other proteases such as collagenase and the 92 kDa gelatinase are present in COPD patients and probably contribute to the remodelling of the lung architecture observed in this disease.[47] In animal models of emphysema, alveolar function and architecture can be restored by retinoic acid treatment. In humans, it remains irreversible.

Pulmonary complications of diseases of altered matrix protein structure

Although the consequences of mutations in the genes encoding matrix proteins are most often manifested in the skeletal system, pulmonary complications are not uncommon. Patients with the Marfan mutation in fibrillin-1 may present with pneumothorax and emphysema. Fibrillin-1 mutations also result in Shprintzen–Goldberg craniosynostosis syndrome. Obstructive apnoea is apparent in this disease. Cutis laxa, a disease caused by deletions in the elastin gene, is characterised by skin hyperextensibility and emphysema.

Mutations in collagen genes most often result in osteogenesis imperfecta or in Ehlers–Danlos syndrome. In osteogenesis imperfecta, type I collagen is the altered matrix protein. Pulmonary compromise is the leading cause of death in this disease, and approximately 60% of patients have severe chestwall deformities. Ehlers–Danlos syndrome is a heterogeneous disorder in which several types of collagen may be affected. Pulmonary complications are rare, although cavitary lesions, pneumothorax and pulmonary haemorrhage are occasionally observed in patients with the type IV subtype, in which the gene encoding type III collagen is mutated. Pulmonary haemorrhage is also present in patients with Goodpasture's syndrome, which is characterised by the production of autoantibodies to type IV collagen.

Treatment of matrix-related lung diseases

The lung extracellular matrix is a dynamic structure. Some components, such as recently synthesised collagens and proteoglycans, are turned over quite rapidly. Other components, such as elastic fibres, are very stable. Initial attempts to understand the role of matrix proteins in pulmonary fibrosis and emphysema focused on regulation of matrix turnover and on identification of the enzymes responsible for matrix destruction. Information gathered over the past 20 years indicates that global inhibition of matrix synthesis or of proteolytic activity is impractical and that treatments for pulmonary fibrosis and emphysema must target specific molecules.

To treat pulmonary fibrosis, excessive accumulation of collagen must be prevented. In simplistic terms, this could be achieved by increasing degradation of type I collagen or by decreasing its synthesis or deposition. Drug design is complicated, however, by the multiple cascades that lead to fibroblast activation and collagen production (Fig. 2.1.7). Targeting common mediators such as TGF-β or connective-tissue growth factor[48] may prove efficacious in this respect. Many molecules have been shown to be effective in blocking collagen synthesis, assembly and turnover in animals and should be assessed in clinical trials. Degradation of fibrillar collagen occurs at specific sites in the molecule and is mediated by collagenases, members of the matrix metalloproteinase family. Targeted gene delivery[49] of these proteases may be a possible strategy for the treatment of pulmonary fibrosis.

Emphysema treatment may be viewed from two perspectives. One strategy would depend on assembly of new elastic fibres to replace those damaged by proteolytic attack. Mechanisms of elastic fibre assembly are not well understood but it appears that the microfibrillar proteins that serve as an assembly scaffold are not present in the adult lung. A better understanding of the regulation of microfibril synthesis and turnover and of the interactions of tropoelastin with matrix proteins is necessary before therapeutic restoration of elastic fibres is possible. Another potential emphysema treatment is inhibition of elastolytic proteases. Specific neutrophil elastase inhibitors are available and design of macrophage elastase inhibitors is being actively pursued. For this treatment to be successful, however, patients must be identified and protease inhibitors administered before elastic fibres are destroyed.

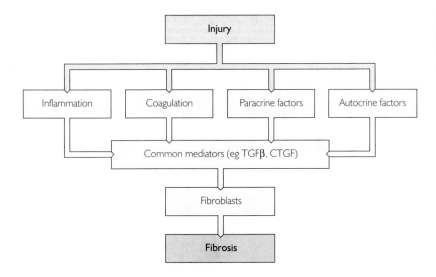

Fig. 2.1.7 Multiple cascades that lead to fibroblast activation. Following injury, many signalling cascades and factors increase production of mediators that stimulate synthesis of matrix proteins by fibroblasts.

Summary

It has long been recognised that matrix proteins are organised into three-dimensional structures that determine the fundamental physical properties of the lung. More recently, it has been appreciated that matrix proteins interact directly with receptors on the cell surface to initiate signalling cascades with the capacity to regulate the majority of cellular functions including proliferation, migration and differentiation. Despite this knowledge, matrix-related lung diseases remain virtually untreatable and none of the present clinical strategies for treating fibrosis or emphysema directly target matrix proteins. A better understanding of matrix protein biology and new approaches for treating matrix-related diseases are still needed.

At the basic level, detailed knowledge of the interactions of matrix proteins with cells, with other matrix proteins and with other molecules is necessary. Advances in molecular biology have led to the cloning and structural characterisation of most matrix proteins. The early lethality of fibronectin and laminin-1 'knockouts' have demonstrated the critical importance of matrix proteins in development. The challenge for the future is to dissect the molecular pathways by which matrix proteins govern cell behaviour and influence lung function. Development of animals in which matrix protein expression is controlled by inducible and lung-cell-specific promoter elements will be useful tools for analysis of these pathways. Increased application of transgenic animals to models of lung injury will also provide valuable information.

One long-term goal in treating matrix-related lung diseases is the development of strategies that will enable regeneration of normal lung in damaged areas. The recent finding that retinoic acid treatment restores alveolar architecture in rats treated with elastase to induce emphysema provides evidence that extensive matrix damage can be repaired. The identification of pluripotent embryonic cells and stem cells in the central nervous system, a tissue previously thought to undergo limited self-repair, implies that various types of precursor cells may be potentially useful in repopulating damaged areas of the lung. Continual application of cutting-edge science to current issues in pulmonary medicine is our best hope for development of better treatments for lung disease and eventual realisation of the goal of lung regeneration.

? Unresolved questions

- Do matrix proteins determine the localisation of type I and type II alveolar epithelial cells?
- How is an elastic fibre assembled?
- Which cell-surface receptors interact with matrix proteoglycans?
- What are the roles of antiadhesive matrix proteins (thrombospondins, tenascins, SPARC) in the lung?
- Why are matrix proteins deposited in the asthmatic airway?
- Can connective tissue metabolism be therapeutically modulated to treat interstitial lung disease?

Clinical relevance

- Matrix proteins play critical roles in lung development. Bronchopulmonary dysplasia is one example of a neonatal disease where an imbalance in matrix metabolism occurs.
- Intrinsic lung recoil is dependent on matrix proteins.
- Matrix protein-related pathology may present in the airways (asthma), alveoli (interstitial lung disease) or vasculature (pulmonary hypertension).
- Matrix proteins are valid targets for therapeutic intervention.
- Common clinical interventions such as oxygen therapy and ventilatory support may lead to matrix protein damage if not properly regulated.
- New evidence suggests that matrix-related changes in interstitial lung disease may be partially reversible.

References

1. Giancotti FG, Ruoslahti E. Integrin signaling. Science 1999; 285: 1028–1032.
2. Dunsmore SE, Rannels DE. Extracellular matrix biology in the lung. Am J Physiol 1996; 270: L3–L27.
3. Roman J, McDonald JA. Expression of fibronectin, the integrin alpha 5, and alpha-smooth muscle actin in heart and lung development. Am J Respir Cell Mol Biol 1992; 6: 472–480.
4. Dabbagh K, Chambers RC, Laurent GJ. From clot to collagen: coagulation peptides in interstitial lung disease. Eur Respir J 1998; 11: 1102–1005.
5. Cremer MA, Rosloniec EF, Kang AH. The cartilage collagens: a review of their structure, organization, and role in the pathogenesis of experimental arthritis in animals and in human rheumatic disease. J Mol Med 1998; 76: 275–288.
6. Watanabe H, Yamada Y, Kimata K. Roles of aggrecan, a large chondroitin sulfate proteoglycan, in cartilage structure and function. J Biochem (Tokyo) 1998; 124: 687–693.
7. Roberts CR, Rains JK, Pare PD et al. Ultrastructure and tensile properties of human tracheal cartilage. J Biomech 1998; 31: 81–86.
8. Entwistle J, Hall CL, Turley EA. HA receptors: receptors of signalling to the cytoskeleton. J Cell Biochem 1996; 61: 569–577.
9. Mays PK, Bishop JE, Laurent GJ. Age-related changes in the proportion of types I and III collagen. Mech Ageing Dev 1988; 45: 203–212.
10. West JB, Mathieu-Costello O. Structure, strength, failure, and remodeling of the pulmonary blood–gas barrier. Annu Rev Physiol 1999; 61: 543–572.
11. Iozzo RV. Matrix proteoglycans: from molecular design to cellular function. Annu Rev Biochem 1998; 67: 609–652.
12. Bensadoun ES, Burke AK, Hogg JC, Roberts CR. Proteoglycan deposition in pulmonary fibrosis. Am J Respir Crit Care Med 1996; 154: 1819–1828.
13. Belknap JK, Weiser-Evans MC, Grieshaber SS et al. Relationship between perlecan and tropoelastin gene expression and cell replication in the developing rat pulmonary vasculature. Am J Respir Cell Mol Biol 1999; 20: 24–34.
14. Groffen AJ, Buskens CA, van Kuppevelt TH et al. Primary structure and high expression of human agrin in basement membranes of adult lung and kidney. Eur J Biochem 1998; 254: 123–128.
15. Verbeek MM, Otte-Holler I, van den Born J et al. Agrin is a major heparan sulfate proteoglycan accumulating in Alzheimer's disease brain. Am J Pathol 1999; 155: 2115–2125.
16. Chakravarti S, Magnuson T, Lass JH et al. Lumican regulates collagen fibril assembly: skin fragility and corneal opacity in the absence of lumican. J Cell Biol 1998; 141: 1277–1286.
17. Svensson L, Aszodi A, Reinholt FP et al Fibromodulin-null mice have abnormal collagen fibrils, tissue organization, and altered lumican deposition in tendon. J Biol Chem 199; 274: 9636–9648.
18. Colognato H, Yurchenco PD. Form and function: the laminin family of heterotrimers. Dev Dyn 2000; 218: 213–234.

19. Giannelli G, Falk-Marziller J, Schiraldi O et al. Induction of cell migration by matrix metalloproteinase-2 cleavage of laminin. Science 1997; 277: 225–228.

20. Virtanen I, Gullberg D, Rissanen J et al. Laminin alpha1-chain shows a restricted distribution in epithelial basement membranes of fetal and adult human tissues. Exp Cell Res 2000; 257: 298–309.

21. Pierce RA, Griffin GL, Miner JH, Senior RM. Expression patterns of laminin α1 and α5 in human lung during development. Am J Resp Cell Mol Biol 2000; 23: 742–747.

22. Miner JH, Patton BL, Lentz SI et al. The laminin α chains: expression, developmental transitions, and chromosomal locations of α1-5, identification of heterotrimeric laminins 8–11, and cloning of a novel α3 isoform. J Cell Biol 1997; 137: 685–701.

23. Falk M, Ferletta M, Forsberg E, Ekblom P. Restricted distribution of laminin alpha1 chain in normal adult mouse tissues. Matrix Biol 1999; 18: 557–568.

24. Virtanen I, Laitinen A, Tani T et al. Differential expression of laminins and their integrin receptors in developing and adult human lungs. Am J Respir Cell Mol Biol 1996; 15: 184–196.

25. Romberger DJ. Fibronectin. Int J Biochem Cell Biol 1997; 29: 939–943.

26. Avila JJ, Lympany PA, Pantelidis P et al. Fibronectin gene polymorphisms associated with fibrosing alveolitis in systemic sclerosis. Am J Respir Cell Mol Biol 1999; 20: 106–112.

27. Arai H, Hirano H, Mushiake S et al. Loss of EDB⁺ fibronectin isoform is associated with differentiation of alveolar epithelial cells in human fetal lung. Am J Pathol 1997; 151: 403–412.

28. Kuhn C III, Boldt J, King TE Jr et al. An immunohistochemical study of architectural remodeling and connective tissue synthesis in pulmonary fibrosis. Am Rev Respir Dis 1989; 140: 1693–1703.

29. Herrick S, Blanc-Brude O, Gray A, Laurent G. Fibrinogen. Int J Biochem Cell Biol 1999; 31: 741–746.

30. Lawler J. Thrombospondin. In: Kreis T, Vale R, ed. Guidebook to the extracellular matrix, anchor, and adhesion proteins. New York: Oxford University Press; 1999: 489–492.

31. Jones FS, Jones PL. The tenascin family of ECM glycoproteins: structure, function, and regulation during embryonic development and tissue remodeling. Dev Dyn 2000; 218: 235–259.

32. Motamed K. SPARC (osteonectin/BM-40). Int J Biochem Cell Biol 1999; 31: 1363–1366.

33. Kuhn C, Mason RJ. Immunolocalization of SPARC, tenascin, and thrombospondin in pulmonary fibrosis. Am J Pathol 1995; 147: 1759–1769.

34. Lawler J, Sunday M, Thibert V et al. Thrombospondin-1 is required for normal murine pulmonary homeostasis and its absence causes pneumonia. J Clin Invest 1998; 101: 982–992.

35. Crawford SE, Stellmach V, Murphy-Ullrich JE et al. Thrombospondin-1 is a major activator of TGF-β1 in vivo. Cell 1998; 93: 1159–1170.

36. Standjord TP, Sage EH, Clark JG. SPARC participates in the branching morphogenesis of developing fetal rat lungs. Am J Respir Cell Mol Biol 1995; 13: 279–287.

37. Chambers RC, Laurent GJ. The lung. In: Comper WD, ed. Extracellular matrix. Amsterdam: Harwood Academic; 1996: 378–409.

38. Roberts CR. Is asthma a fibrotic disease? Chest 1995; 107: 111S–117S.

39. Laitinen A, Altraja A, Kampe M et al. Tenascin is increased in airway basement membrane of asthmatics and decreased by an inhaled steroid. Am J Respir Crit Care Med 1997; 156: 951–958.

40. Huang J, Olivenstein R, Taha R et al. Enhanced proteoglycan deposition in the airway wall of atopic asthmatics. Am J Respir Crit Care Med 1999; 160: 725–729.

41. Pare OD, Roberts CR, Bai TR, Wiggs BJ. The functional consequences of airway remodeling in asthma. Monaldi Arch Chest Dis 1997; 52: 589–596.

42. Durmowicz AG, Stenmark KR. Mechanisms of structural remodeling in chronic pulmonary hypertension. Pediatr Rev 1999; 20: e91–e102.

43. Jones PL, Cowan KN, Rabinovitch M. Tenascin-C, proliferation and subendothelial fibronectin in progressive pulmonary vascular disease. Am J Pathol 1997; 150: 1349–1360.

44. Deng, Z, Morse JH, Slager SL et al. Familial primary pulmonary hypertension (gene PPH1) is caused by mutations in the bone morphogenetic protein receptor-II gene. Am J Hum Genet 2000; 67: 737–744.

45. Botney MD, Kaiser LR, Cooper JD et al. Extracellular matrix protein gene expression in atherosclerotic hypertensive pulmonary arteries. Am J Pathol 1992; 140: 357–364.

46. Hautamaki RD, Kobayashi DK, Senior RM, Shapiro SD. Requirement for macrophage elastase for cigarette smoke-induced emphysema in mice. Science 1997; 277: 2002–2004.

47. Finlay GA, Russell KJ, McMahon KJ et al. Elevated levels of matrix metalloproteinases in bronchoalveolar lavage fluid of emphysematous patients. Thorax 1997; 52: 502–506.

48. Chambers RC, Leoni P, Blanc-Brude OP et al. Thrombin is a potent inducer of connective tissue growth factor production via proteolytic activation of protease-activated receptor-1. J Biol Chem 2000; 274: 35584–35591.

49. Jenkins RG, Herrick SE, Meng QH et al. An integrin-targeted non-viral vector for pulmonary gene therapy. Gene Ther 2000; 7: 393–400.

2 Function

2.2 Pulmonary surfactant and lung fluid balance

Jens M Hohlfeld

Key points

- Pulmonary surfactant is a unique mixture of phospholipids and specific apoproteins covering the entire internal surface of the lung

- Surfactant components are synthesised in alveolar type II cells, secreted into the epithelial lining layer and metabolised either by reuptake into type II cells or by phagocytosis and degradation by alveolar macrophages

- Besides reduction of surface tension at the air–liquid interface, its major biophysical function, pulmonary surfactant possesses immunomodulatory effects and plays a role in the innate immune system

- In the alveolar compartment pulmonary surfactant is important for lung fluid balance because of its high surface pressure

- The principal forces responsible for transcapillary fluid movement from the vascular to the interstitial compartment are best described by Starling's equation of fluid exchange

The lung has an enormous internal surface, where the inspired air comes into close contact with the pulmonary microcirculation. Here the distance between the inspired air and the circulating blood is only $0.35\,\mu m$, which is an important prerequisite for sufficient gas exchange. On the other hand, inhaled gases and particles from the environment are potentially hazardous to the lung tissue and the systemic circulation because of the narrowness of the alveolar–blood barrier. The alveolar epithelial surface is covered by a thin liquid layer. At this air–liquid interface surface forces occur that play a major role in the pressure–volume characteristics of the lung. Pulmonary surfactant forms a layer at the surface of the alveolar lining fluid and regulates the surface tension, depending on the alveolar surface area. Dynamic changes of surface tension with very low values at end-expiration are necessary for normal ventilation of the lung. This chapter summarises the biochemical composition of pulmonary surfactant, its synthesis, metabolism and regulation, and describes the various functions of this unique material that covers the entire internal surface of the lung. In addition, the basic principles important for lung fluid balance are reviewed.

Pulmonary surfactant

History

The existence of a surface-active substance in the lung was first postulated by von Neergaard as early as 1929.[1] However, it was not until the mid 1950s that Pattle[2] and Clements[3] found a substance in lung oedema fluid and lung extracts that did indeed lower surface tension dramatically. The material was found to be composed of a phospholipid and a protein fraction and was termed surfactant (surface active agent). In 1959, Avery and Mead[4] established the role of a surfactant deficit in hyaline membrane disease of premature infants, now commonly called infant respiratory distress syndrome (IRDS). Since this pioneering work, understanding of the pulmonary surfactant system has grown exponentially. The alveolar type II cell has been identified as the site of alveolar surfactant synthesis. The precise composition of the material is now known, down to the genetic codes of surfactant-specific proteins. Many details concerning surfactant synthesis and secretion and its regulation and metabolism have been elucidated. Surfactant replacement therapy is established as a routine life-saving therapy in IRDS. Cumulative evidence strongly suggests that surfactant dysfunction contributes to the morbidity and mortality of the adult respiratory distress syndrome (ARDS) and might probably be ameliorated by substitution therapy.[5,6] In recent years, surfactant functions other than the maintenance of normal lung function have been uncovered. Perhaps most important among these findings is that surfactant seems to play a role in pulmonary defence mechanisms and local immunomodulation.[7] Therefore, the role of surfactant in various lung diseases is attracting growing attention.

Surfactant composition

Surfactant is a unique and complex mixture of lipids and proteins (Fig. 2.2.1). Its extracellular pool size has been investigated in animals and seems to range from 10–15 mg·kg^{-1} body weight in adults. Mature newborns have five- to 10-fold higher values.[8] Assuming similar values in humans, a 70 kg person would thus have an estimated alveolar surfactant pool of approximately 0.7–1.0 g. The calculated surfactant concentration of the alveolar lining layer in the normal adult lung is approximately 120 mg·ml^{-1}. Assuming an alveolar surface area of 100 m^2 with a surfactant hypophase of 50 μl·m^{-2}, the total alveolar surfactant volume would thus approximate 5 ml, or 600 mg.

Surfactant lipids

Lipids are the major surfactant component by weight. The term 'lipids' refers broadly to a functionally heterogenous group of compounds that share a physical property – that of solubility in organic solvents. They can be subdivided into polar and non-polar lipids according to their extractability in various solvents. Lipids make up about 85–90% of whole isolated surfactant.[9] Approximately 90% of this lipid fraction consists of a mixture of phospholipids. The remaining 10% is composed of other lipids, mainly cholesterol. Phospholipids are amphipathic molecules that combine lipophilic and hydrophilic properties. They have a polar head group linked to a glycerol backbone, to which are attached acyl chains of variable length and degree of saturation (Fig. 2.2.2). Because of their amphipathic character they possess the ability to achieve a low surface tension when lining air–liquid interfaces because of the low energy required to stay at the interface.

The phospholipid composition of human lung surfactant is shown in Figure 2.2.1. None of these phospholipids is unique to surfactant, but the composition differs from phospholipid profiles in other organs; for example, the relative concentrations of phosphatidylcholine and phosphatidylglycerol are higher. Phosphatidylcholine accounts for approximately 80% of total surfactant phospholipids and for about two-thirds of whole surfactant. Approximately 70% of its fatty acids are saturated under normal conditions, the most common saturated acid being palmitic acid. Dipalmitoyl-phosphatidylcholine (DPPC) is the surfactant component that is predominantly responsible for reducing alveolar surface tension.[10] Its hydrophilic (choline) residue associates with the alveolar liquid phase while the hydrophobic (palmitic acid) residue reaches into the air phase.

Phospholipid mixtures will spontaneously form a surface film at the air–fluid interface. This process of film formation is called adsorption. By this means, the surface tension of water at 37°C is lowered from 72 mN·m^{-1} to approximately 25 mN·m^{-1}. Adsorption is an important process in the physiology of pulmonary surfactant. This is presumably the mechanism by which the alveolar lining film is formed after the surfactant material has been secreted from the type II cells into the alveolar hypophase. Under compression, as it occurs during the breathing cycle, the phospholipids in the surface film will be packed even more tightly. Surface area compression will lead to enrichment of the surface lining layer with surface-active phospholipid molecules such as DPPC and selective squeezing out of less active non-DPPC molecules (Fig. 2.2.3).

Surfactant proteins

By weight, the total protein portion accounts for approximately 10% of whole isolated surfactant. Only 20% of these proteins are surfactant-specific – roughly 80% are contaminating serum proteins. Four surfactant-specific proteins (SP) have been

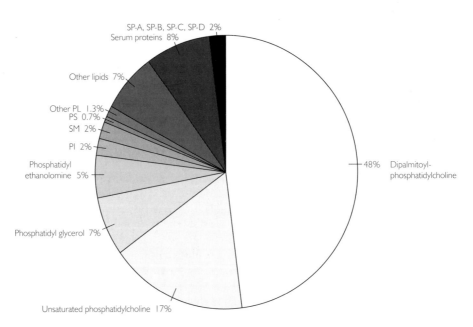

Fig. 2.2.1 Surfactant composition. Surfactant is composed mainly of lipids (90%) and 10% proteins, of which about 2% are surfactant-specific. This pie chart summarises the composition of intra-alveolar surfactant from human bronchoalveolar lavage. PI, phosphatidylinositol; PL, phospholipids; PS, phosphatidylserine; SM, sphingomyelin; SP, surfactant protein.

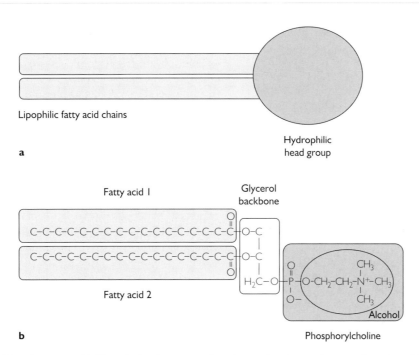

Fig. 2.2.2 Phospholipid biochemistry. (a) Phospholipids are amphipathic molecules as they combine lipophilic and hydrophilic properties. They have a polar head group linked to a glycerol backbone, to which are attached acyl chains of variable length and degree of saturation. (b) Biochemical structure of dipalmitoylphosphatidylcholine, with phosphorylcholine as the hydrophilic part and two saturated fatty acid chains of 16 carbon atoms as the lipophilic tail, both linked to the central glycerol molecule.

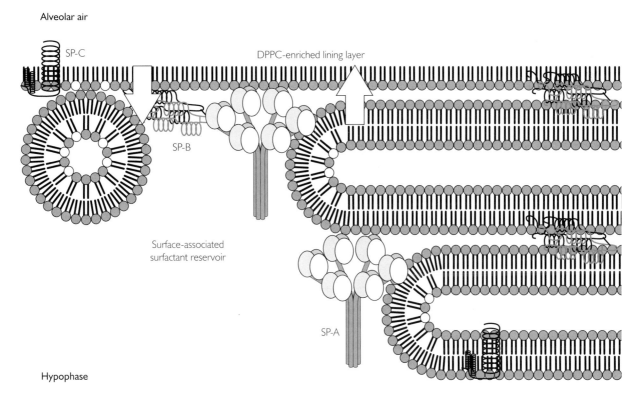

Fig. 2.2.3 The surfactant layer at the air–liquid interface. Selective insertion of dipalmitoylphosphatidylcholine (DPPC) into the lining layer under compression (upward arrow) and selective squeezing out of non-DPPC molecules into the hypophase (downward arrow). (Modified from Perez-Gil and Keough.[65])

identified to date. They are simply termed surfactant protein A, B, C and D.

Surfactant protein A

Surfactant protein A (SP-A) is the most abundant surfactant protein in the alveolar space. In vivo, it is found as a group of isoforms with a molecular weight ranging from approximately 26 kDa to 38 kDa in the reduced state, depending on the extent of post-translational modifications.[11] Its C-terminal domain has structural and functional homologies with C-type lectins. In addition, SP-A contains a collagen-like domain, which is the probable association site of SP-A monomers. After alveolar secretion, native SP-A is predominantly found as a hexamer with trimeric subunits of polypeptide chains, thus forming an 18-meric structure resembling a 'bouquet of flowers' (Fig. 2.2.4).[12]

Surfactant protein A seems to play an important role in the formation of tubular myelin, a transitory surfactant structure that is found immediately after alveolar secretion.[13] In concert with SP-B and SP-C, SP-A probably enhances the surface activity of the mature surfactant layer. However, the importance of SP-A in this seems small and is still a matter of debate.[14]

The structural homologies between SP-A and lectins stimulated investigation into possible common biological functions of these proteins. Indeed, it could be demonstrated that the presence of SP-A enhances the phagocytosis of opsonised sheep erythrocytes by macrophages and monocytes in a concentration-dependent manner. Furthermore, SP-A is able to increase the phagocytosis of *Staphylococcus aureus*, *Escherichia coli*, *Pseudomonas aeruginosa*, herpes simplex virus type 1 and colloidal gold particles.[7] It has also been shown that SP-A binds to influenza A virus via its sialic acid residues and has the ability to neutralise it.[15] Moreover, SP-A also binds to cells infected by herpes simplex virus type 1.[16]

Interestingly, a 120 kDa glycoprotein covering the surface of *Pneumocystis carinii* has been identified that is a ligand for the carbohydrate-binding domain of SP-A.[17] The SP-A binding capacity of *P. carinii* may possibly interfere with the recognition and phagocytosis of this microorganism by alveolar macrophages. Recently, it has also been shown that SP-A promotes attachment of *Mycobacterium tuberculosis* to alveolar macrophages during HIV infection.[18]

Another function of SP-A is to maintain the homeostasis between intracellular and extracellular surfactant pools. In vitro, SP-A blocks the secretion of phosphatidylcholine from cultured alveolar type II cells by feedback inhibition.[19] It also enhances the uptake by type II cells of surfactant lipids. These effects are probably mediated by a SP-A receptor in type II cells. Recently, an SP-A recognition protein (SPAR) has been identified in the membrane of type II cells, which is believed to serve as such a receptor, or at least to represent a portion of it.[20]

Surfactant protein B

Surfactant protein B (SP-B) is a small protein with a molecular weight of approximately 8–9 kDa under reducing conditions.[21] Although it is very hydrophobic, it remains soluble in aqueous solutions to some extent. SP-B forms thiol-dependent oligomers of different sizes, the dimer being the most common form in vivo.[22] It possesses no known immunomodulatory or regulatory function but seems to be a key protein for the formation of a functionally optimal and stable surfactant layer on the alveolar surface, as well as for the formation of tubular myelin.[23] Congenital lack of SP-B expression leads to severe impairment of lung function and subsequently to respiratory failure,[24] demonstrating the vital importance of this protein. The amino acid sequence of SP-B contains high amounts of cysteine, and intramolecular disulphide bridges contribute to the structural properties of the SP-B polypeptide chain. An intermolecular disulphide link explains the frequent natural occurrence of SP-B dimers. Furthermore, SP-B has a strong positive net charge (at physiological pH), which seems to be important to the interaction between SP-B and the anionic phospholipids.[22,23] However, the structural interaction between SP-B and other surfactant components is very complex and has still to be more clearly defined.

Surfactant protein C

Surfactant protein C (SP-C) is a very small protein with a molecular weight of approximately 4–5 kDa (reduced). It is extremely

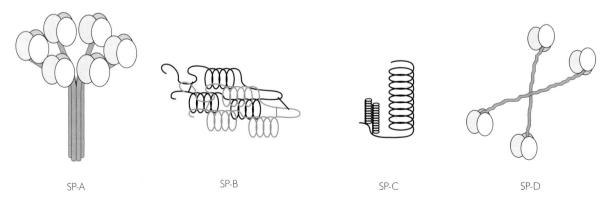

SP-A SP-B SP-C SP-D

Fig. 2.2.4 Schematic diagram of the basic structure of the surfactant proteins A, B, C and D (not to scale). Surfactant protein A (SP-A) monomers of 26–38 kDa and SP-D monomers (43 kDa) assemble to trimers and form a quaternary structure of octadecamers or dodecamers, respectively. SP-B (8.7 kDa) exists in dimeric form. SP-C occurs as a monomer (4.2 kDa).

hydrophobic, in part because it has a high content of the hydrophobic amino acid valine and is therefore only soluble in organic solvents. SP-C probably has no role in tubular myelin formation.[25] As far as its functional role in the surfactant complex is presently understood, it contributes to the formation and stabilisation of the alveolar surfactant monolayer in conjunction with SP-B.[14] Post-translational palmitoylation of SP-C appears to be important both for its optimal function and for its contribution to the resistance of the surfactant complex against potential surfactant inhibitors.[26] The molecular structure and most of the properties of SP-C are substantially different from SP-B, suggesting that the proteins have separate roles in the surfactant complex. Indeed, in vitro studies indicate that SP-C may be more important to the adsorption of phospholipids while SP-B supports the reduction of surface tension more effectively.[27] There seem to be no structural similarities of SP-C to other proteins of known functions that would suggest an additional role for it.

Surfactant protein D

Surfactant protein D (SP-D) is a collagenous glycoprotein that is synthesised by alveolar type II cells but has also been identified in Clara cells.[28] There is an ongoing debate as to whether this protein is a true component of surfactant or a protein that is only loosely and functionally associated with the surfactant complex. In rat bronchoalveolar lavage (BAL) fluid, the total SP-D content was found to be approximately 12% of that of SP-A.[29] SP-D has a molecular size of approximately 43 kDa (reduced) and appears to aggregate to 12-meric complexes in vivo. It has certain structural and biophysical similarities to SP-A, but it is probably even more readily soluble in the aqueous alveolar milieu.

Like SP-A, SP-D does not seem to have a relevant role in the surface activity of the surfactant layer and, as with SP-A, is probably involved in stimulating alveolar macrophages. Structural analogies to C-type lectins such as mannose-binding protein, conglutinin and SP-A suggest just such a role in local host defence. Recently, for example, it has been shown that SP-D binds to *E. coli* in a time- and dose-dependent manner.[30] Furthermore, SP-D enhances the production of oxygen radicals by alveolar macrophages.[31] Another recent study indicates that SP-D may have a regulatory function for alveolar type II cells by counteracting the inhibitory effects of SP-A on phospholipid secretion.[32] Recently, a potential role for the hydrophilic surfactant proteins SP-A and SP-D as modulators of allergic reactions, by binding allergens and inhibiting specific IgE binding and subsequently cellular responses, has been highlighted.[33-35] Finally, it has been shown that SP-D knock-out mice have hypertrophic and activated alveolar macrophages, leading to chronic pulmonary inflammation, and that these animals subsequently develop lung emphysema.[36] Therefore, SP-D seems to play a critical role in the suppression of alveolar macrophage activation.

Morphology and ultrastructure

The site of alveolar surfactant synthesis and secretion is the cuboidal alveolar type II cell, which covers less than 10% of the alveolar surface but comprises about 15% of the total number of cells found in the adult human lung.[37] There is evidence to suggest that surfactant synthesis and secretion in the respiratory tract is not exclusively restricted to the alveolar type II cell but that it may to a small extent also take place in higher airways, e.g. in Clara cells and possibly even in tracheal epithelium.[38,39]

The alveolar surfactant components are synthesised and assembled in the endoplasmic reticulum of type II cells and are then transferred to the Golgi apparatus prior to forming so-called lamellar bodies in the cytoplasm (Figs 2.2.5 & 2.2.6). Immunocytochemistry and autoradiography techniques allow detailed examination of these processes. Mature lamellar bodies are eventually transported into the alveolar space by merocrine secretion. Here, they are rapidly transformed into tubular myelin, a short-lived structure composed of a lattice of highly ordered tubules. SP-A plays a role in the formation of tubular myelin and has been located at the corners of the tubular framework by immune electron microscopic techniques. An in-vitro study suggests that, in addition to SP-A, the presence of SP-B is necessary for tubular myelin formation.[25] Finally, the material is spread on the alveolar surface to form the mature surfactant layer (Fig. 2.2.7).

Synthesis, metabolism and regulation

Pulmonary surfactant undergoes a continuous dynamic process of synthesis and degradation. Basically, all phospholipid components of surfactant are synthesised and incorporated into the lamellar bodies within the alveolar type II cell. DPPC is the phospholipid whose role in intracellular synthesis pathways has been best studied. It is synthesised de novo from blood-derived phospholipid precursors and from recycled material after re-entry from the alveolar space.[40]

Lipids reaching the lung via the circulation are generally in one of two forms: triacylglycerols (triglycerides) complexed to proteins, or fatty acids bound to albumin. The two groups of so-called lipoproteins that are quantitatively most important are chylomicrons and very-low-density lipoproteins (VLDL). They are not taken up directly by the tissue but are first hydrolysed to free fatty acids and glycerol via lipoprotein lipase, which is contained in the outer membrane of lung endothelial cells.

The unique location of the lung in receiving the entire cardiac output means that it could play an important role in lipid balance. Fatty acids may be derived from plasma but they may also be synthesised de novo in the lungs. Two enzyme complexes are important: a biotin-containing multienzyme, acetyl-CoA carboxylase, and a multifunctional enzyme, fatty acid synthase. Every cycle leads to the addition of two carbons from acetyl coenzyme A (acetyl-CoA), forming fatty acids of variable length. Metabolism of fatty acids occurs via β-oxidation, with progressive removal of two-carbon units from the carboxyl end of acetyl-CoA, finally producing acetyl-CoA. Phosphatidylcholine is synthesised by the classic choline incorporation pathway. Although some DPPC is synthesised de novo, most newly synthesised phosphatidylcholine is monoenoic and is converted to DPPC by a deacylation–reacylation mechanism. Although choline-phosphatidic cytidyltransferase is generally considered to be the enzyme that catalyses the rate-limiting step in PC synthesis in type II cells in adult lung, several other enzymes could have regulatory roles under certain conditions. Other phospholipids

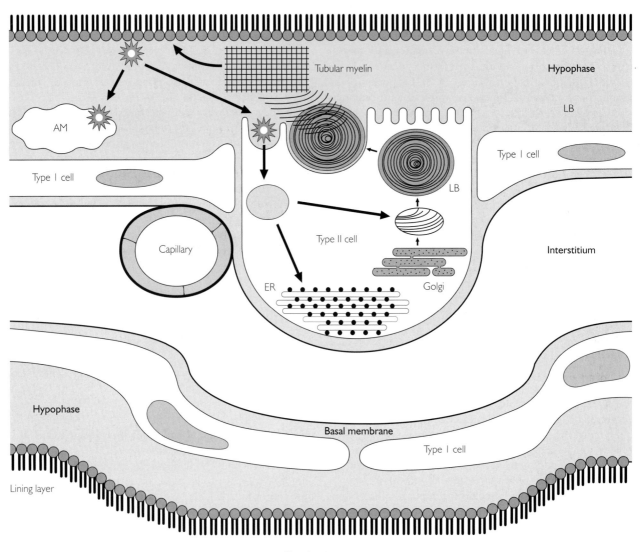

Fig. 2.2.5 Surfactant metabolism. Surfactant lipids and proteins are synthesised in the endoplasmic reticulum (ER). Via the Golgi apparatus, they form multilamellar vesicles and lamellar bodies (LB). After secretion into the alveolar hypophase, surfactant is partly degraded by alveolar macrophages (AM) or taken up into the type II cell for recycling.

use precursors from the PC synthesis pathway to build, for example, phosphatidylglycerol or phosphatidylinositol.

Surfactant synthesis has been found to be influenced by a number of different stimuli.[41] Glucocorticoids, adrenergic stimuli, cyclic adenosine monophosphate (cAMP), oestrogens and thyroid hormones have been reported to enhance surfactant synthesis. However, the in-vivo role and importance of these factors is not clearly determined. Some of these stimuli, e.g. glucocorticoids, may vary in their effects depending on dose and time, and there may be different pathways for the regulation of surfactant phospholipid and protein synthesis.[42] Recent evidence has demonstrated that exogenous glucocorticoids enhance surfactant protein synthesis and suggests that these hormones may have a role in the pulmonary response to stress.[43] On the other

hand, endogenous steroids, under normal conditions, do not seem to be important to baseline surfactant protein synthesis on the mRNA level but may, to a minor extent, contribute to translational or post-translational processing.

Secretion of surfactant into the alveolar space is accomplished by exocytosis of lamellar bodies. However, it appears that they do not transport the whole amount of all alveolar surfactant components. It seems likely that secretion of surfactant-specific proteins such as SP-A partially occurs via independent pathways.[44] Experimental data suggest that various stimuli, including high-volume lung inflation and increased ventilation rate, adrenergic agents, oestrogens and thyroid hormones, may enhance surfactant secretion, while β-receptor-blockade and an SP-A-dependent feedback circuit have inhibitory effects.[45] SP-D

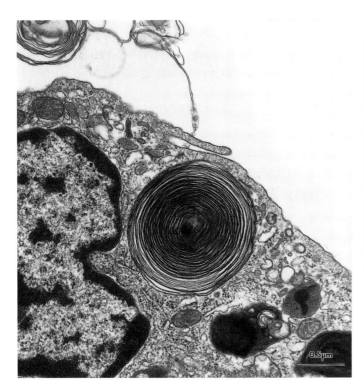

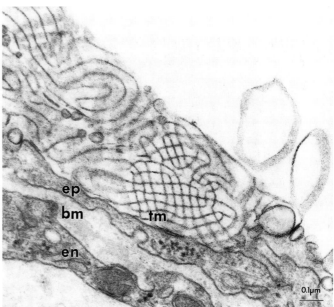

Fig. 2.2.6 Electron micrograph showing a lamellar body within the cytoplasm of a type II pneumocyte. Because of their high levels of synthetic and secretory activity, type II cells are rich in endoplasmic reticulum and mitochondria. The phospholipid lamellae of lamellar bodies are concentrically arranged and surrounded by a limiting membrane. In another case, the lamellae might also appear as densely packed parallel stacks with a periodicity of 4–6 nm. Within the alveolar lumen, multilamellar surfactant material is visible. (Courtesy of Dr M. Ochs, Department of Anatomy, University of Göttingen, Germany.)

Fig. 2.2.7 Intra-alveolar surfactant. The electron micrograph shows the blood–air barrier of an alveolar septum with alveolar epithelium (ep), fused epithelial and endothelial basement membranes (bm) and capillary endothelium (en). Intra-alveolar surfactant covers the alveolar epithelial surface as a thin and continuous lining layer. After secretion into the hypophase of the alveolar lining layer via exocytosis, lamellar body material forms regular lattice-like structures termed tubular myelin (tm), which can spread on to the surface layer. Other intra-alveolar surfactant forms include lamellar-body-like structures, multilamellar and unilamellar vesicles. (Courtesy of Dr M. Ochs, Department of Anatomy, University of Göttingen, Germany.)

seems to counteract the inhibitory effect of SP-A on surfactant secretion.[32]

Turnover studies with labelled surfactant phospholipids have demonstrated alveolar half-lives between 15 and 30 hours. The fate of secreted surfactant material is determined by four mechanisms: first, recycling into the alveolar type II cell and other surrounding tissue; second, phagocytosis and degradation by alveolar macrophages (Fig. 2.2.8); third, intra-alveolar catabolism; and finally, removal by the mucociliary escalator.[40] Clearance studies in rabbits have shown that approximately 7% of radiolabelled phosphatidylcholine is removed via the upper airways within 24 hours, suggesting that this pathway is only of minor importance.[46] Further work by the same group provides evidence that most surfactant material is probably redistributed into the surrounding tissue or recycled into alveolar type II cells.

While surfactant phospholipid synthesis and metabolism is quite well understood, knowledge of surfactant apoproteins is at present fragmentary. It has been shown that gene expression for SP-A and SP-D is found in alveolar type II cells and Clara cells, whereas expression of SP-B and SP-C is restricted to the type II cells, as shown by immunohistochemistry and in-situ hybridisa-

tion. SP-A is synthesised as a preprotein, followed by a variety of post-translational modifications like sialylation, acetylation and sulphation. SP-A monomers are oligomerised to 18-meric 'bouquet-like' structures. The site where SP-A and phospholipids are first assembled is unknown but it has been shown that SP-A is a component of lamellar bodies.

Surfactant and lung function

The tendency of the lung to reduce its volume is due not only to the elasticity of the lung parenchyma but, to a larger extent, to the surface tension at the air–liquid interface in the alveoli.[1,47] Surface tension may be defined as the energy that is necessary to overcome the attractive forces of molecules at an interface in order to increase a surface area, and is expressed in millinewtons per metre ($mN \cdot m^{-1}$). The surface tension in the alveolar space tends to reduce the alveolar surface area, i.e. it tends to keep the alveolar spaces small. Thus, it counteracts alveolar expansion during inspiration and supports alveolar retraction during expiration. The intra-alveolar pressure (P) is proportional to the surface tension (γ) and inversely proportional to the alveolar radius (r). This is expressed by the law of Laplace:

$$P = 2\gamma \cdot r^{-1}.$$

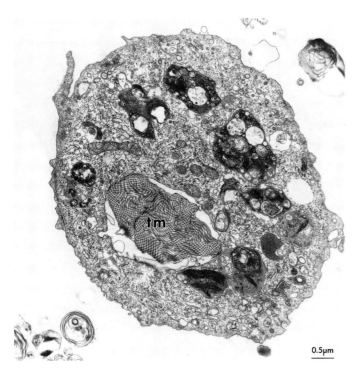

Fig. 2.2.8 Uptake of surfactant by an alveolar macrophage. Alveolar macrophages are situated within the alveolar lumen, usually directly on the alveolar surface. The macrophage shown in this electron micrograph contains a large phagolysosome filled with tubular myelin (tm), evidence of the fact that these cells are involved in removal of intra-alveolar surfactant material. (Courtesy of Dr M. Ochs, Department of Anatomy, University of Göttingen, Germany.)

The law allows the understanding of a number of dynamic changes throughout the ventilatory cycle. As an example, it demonstrates that the alveolar pressure increases when reducing the alveolar radius at constant surface tension. Thus, the workload for alveolar expansion is increased in smaller alveoli.

The surface tension at an ordinary water–air interface is approximately $72\ mN\cdot m^{-1}$. Surfactant reduces the surface tension at the air–liquid interface, but not in a static, detergent-like manner. It is a unique property of this material that it influences the surface tension dynamically, i.e. the degree of surface tension reduction is closely tuned to the alveolar radius. The surface tension is dynamically reduced with the expiratory decrease of the alveolar radius until it reaches values near $0\ mN\cdot m^{-1}$, and then rises again with the next inspiratory expansion. A glance at Laplace's law shows that this surfactant effect is necessary to keep the alveolar pressure constant throughout the ventilatory cycle.

The most important surfactant component in accomplishing the reduction of surface tension is saturated phosphatidylcholine. Other surfactant components, such as SP-A and, more importantly, SP-B and SP-C, enhance the surface activity of this phospholipid. The hydrophobic saturated fatty acids of saturated phosphatidylcholine are aligned in parallel and rise out of the liquid phase into the alveolar air. The hydrophilic choline residues are packed in the aqueous phase of the alveolus. This arrangement remains stable throughout compression and exten-

sion of the alveolus and reduces the strong alveolar cohesive forces. Thus, the respiratory work load is reduced throughout the respiratory cycle, lung compliance is improved and alveolar collapse and atelectasis are prevented.

Surfactant and pulmonary defence mechanisms

Surfactant material may contribute to pulmonary defence mechanisms and local immunomodulation in four different ways:

- support of non-specific defence mechanisms
- direct host defence effects of surfactant components
- immunomodulatory action on lymphocytes
- augmentation of alveolar macrophage activities.

Non-specific defence mechanisms

Surfactant is part of the alveolar and bronchial epithelial lining fluid, which is thought to act as a non-specific barrier against invasion and adhesion of microorganisms. Also, surfactant has antioxidant activity, which may contribute to the protection of the alveolar epithelium by scavenging toxic (reduced) oxygen species.[48]

Direct host defence effects of surfactant components

A number of reports have addressed possible antibacterial properties of surfactant material. Recently, it has been shown in vitro that SP-A binds to influenza A virus via its sialic acid residues and, thereby, neutralises it.[15] Another recent report suggests that SP-A promotes the attachment of *M. tuberculosis* to alveolar macrophages during HIV infection.[18] However, this may be interpreted as an important early step towards the infection of host cells rather than a contribution to local host defence. Furthermore, SP-A binds with high affinity to a 120 kDa glycoprotein on the surface of *P. carinii*.[17] This SP-A binding capacity of *P. carinii* may possibly interfere with the recognition and phagocytosis of this microorganism by alveolar macrophages that normally use this ligand. Thus, it seems that SP-A binding to microorganisms does not effectively contribute to host defence mechanisms in all cases. Knock-out mouse models for the surfactant proteins A and D have demonstrated impaired clearance of various bacteria and viruses from the lung,[49] suggesting a potential role of these surfactant proteins in host defence.

Surfactant and lymphocyte activity

Surfactant suppresses the activation and proliferative response of lymphocytes to various stimuli in a dose-dependent manner. This suppressor activity is contained in the lipid fraction of surfactant.[50] The major surfactant phospholipids phosphatidylcholine, phosphatidylglycerol and phosphatidylinositol were shown to be responsible for this immunoregulatory effect. Its nature has not yet been clarified but may be related to changes in lymphocyte cell membrane dynamics.[51] Surfactant exerts its effects only on dormant lymphocytes or during the early stages of lymphocyte activation. Activated lymphocytes are not affected. The suppression appears to be largely irreversible, even after removal of surfactant material from the medium. These effects have been shown for a variety of lymphocyte activities such as proliferation, differentiation, immunoglobulin synthesis and natural killer cell activity. Inhibitory effects on lymphocyte proliferation and their cytokine production have also been shown for SP-A.[7,52] It may be hypothesised that these surfactant effects protect the lungs from inappropriate immune reactions.

Surfactant and alveolar macrophage activity

Nearly all studies on the influence of surfactant on alveolar macrophage activity report enhancement of macrophage functions. In detail, it has been shown that surfactant material supports phagocytosis and intracellular killing of *S. aureus* and the phagocytosis of herpes simplex virus type 1. It may also enhance the migration of alveolar macrophages and their cytotoxicity against tumour cells.[53]

Several studies have shown that SP-A is responsible for the enhancement of alveolar macrophage functions.[54-56] Probably, this effect is mediated by a macrophage receptor that binds SP-A. The specific binding and uptake of SP-A by macrophages has been demonstrated by electron microscopy. SP-A has also been shown to interact with *M. tuberculosis* and *P. carinii*. However, it seems doubtful whether these phenomena effectively contribute to the clearance of these organisms by alveolar macrophages.

Interestingly, surfactant preparations that lack SP-A inhibit production of proinflammatory cytokines such as interleukin-1β and tumour necrosis factor-α by alveolar macrophages when stimulated by endotoxin or heat-killed *S. aureus* in vitro.[53] In contrast to some of the findings outlined above, this study suggests immunosuppressive properties of SP-A-free surfactants on alveolar macrophages. Thus, the net effect of whole surfactant on alveolar macrophages in vivo is still debatable.

Lung fluid balance

The alveolar blood–gas barrier is optimised for gas exchange as it permits rapid transfer of gases but limits the movement of solutes and water. Any accumulation of fluid within the airspaces would considerably disturb gas exchange. Therefore, efficient mechanisms are necessary to regulate and balance vascular, interstitial and alveolar fluid homeostasis. The preceding section summarised the intra-alveolar compartment, with pulmonary surfactant as the lining layer between inspired air and the intra-alveolar fluid that covers the entire lung. In the following section, the mechanisms by which lung fluids in the vascular and interstitial compartment are regulated will be described.

Structural aspects

The majority of fluid exchange in the lung occurs in the pulmonary capillaries, which are located near to or surrounding the alveolar walls. The capillary endothelium has many pores and is therefore permeable for fluids and plasma proteins. In contrast, alveolar epithelial cells are in close contact, substantially limit-

ing fluid flux across the epithelium. Alveolar epithelial type I cells are flat cells that line most of the alveolar surface. They are closely associated with pulmonary capillaries. Type II pneumocytes are cuboidal in shape and are predominantly located in the corners of the alveoli. Although they are twice as numerous as type I cells they cover less than 10% of the alveoli. The surface area of the 700 billion adult human lung capillaries is thought to be about $100\,m^2$, whereas the combined surface area of arteries, arterioles, veins and venules is only about $5\,m^2$. Because of the large surface area in the capillaries, fluid has a greater tendency to leave the microcirculation and enter the interstitium at this level. In healthy lungs, excess fluid that has reached the interstitium is removed via the lymphatic system. At the alveolar level, the high surface pressure of pulmonary surfactant lining the alveolar surface area counteracts fluid influx into the alveoli.

The following sections describe the forces responsible for fluid movement between the pulmonary microcirculation and the alveoli.

Starling's equation of fluid exchange

The principle forces responsible for transcapillary fluid exchange were first described by Starling in 1896. The following equation summarises the average forces acting across the pulmonary microcirculation which influence fluid filtration and absorption:

$$\dot{Q} = K[(P_c - P_i) - \sigma(\pi_p - \pi_t)],$$

where $\dot{Q}$ is the net fluid filtration rate, K is the filtration coefficient across the pulmonary capillary wall, P is the hydrostatic pressure in the capillary (c) and interstitial fluid (i) compartments respectively, σ is the osmotic reflection coefficient as a measure of solute permeability of the capillary wall and π is the protein osmotic pressure in the plasma (p) and tissue (t). The major force that alters fluid balance in the lung is capillary pressure. Although this equation is extremely helpful in describing oedema formation in the lungs, one has to keep in mind that the forces and coefficients can change considerably depending on the actual position within the lung. Therefore, the Starling equation, using average forces and coefficients, can only estimate overall lung fluid balance. In that equation three major factors occur. One is 'filtration pressure' $(P_c - P_i)$, the second is 'protein absorption force' $(\pi_p - \pi_t)$ and the third is 'membrane parameters' (K, σ).

Filtration pressure

Filtration of fluid in the lung is determined by hydrostatic forces in the vascular and the interstitial compartment. Some 50% of the filtration into the interstitium occurs at the level of the alveolar capillaries, with an additional 50% occurring equally in the pre- and postcapillary vessels. The total precapillary resistance normally contains 50–60% of the total pulmonary vascular resistance, and the total postcapillary resistance is 40–50% of the total vascular resistance. Therefore, the average pulmonary vascular pressure decreases from about 16 mmHg to an alveolar capillary pressure of 10 mmHg across the precapillary resistance, and the pulmonary pressure decreases an additional 5 mmHg across the postcapillary resistance.

Alveolar interstitial hydrostatic pressure is known to be sub-atmospheric and is estimated to range between –3 and –4 mmHg.[57] This pressure promotes fluid flux into the interstitium. However, much more important than absolute values of interstitial hydrostatic pressure is the change of this pressure when fluid enters the interstitium. Results from several studies, which showed an increase of interstitial fluid pressure as fluid filtered into the interstitium,[58] have indicated that the interstitial space surrounding the filtrating vessels has a very low compliance. Higher interstitial fluid pressure at the site of fluid filtration, however, would induce a longitudinal interstitial pressure gradient from the alveolar level towards the perivascular space, promoting fluid flux in this direction and perhaps facilitating lymphatic drainage.

Taken together with a hydrostatic pressure in the capillaries of 10 mmHg and an interstitial hydrostatic pressure of –3 to –4 mmHg, this results in a filtration pressure across the pulmonary capillaries that ranges between 13 mmHg and 14 mmHg under normal conditions.

Protein absorption force

Proteins are large molecules that bind water and therefore exert an osmotic pressure. Two different protein absorption forces are relevant for lung fluid balance. On the one hand there is the protein osmotic pressure in the plasma (π_p) and on the other hand there is the protein osmotic pressure in the interstitium/tissue (π_t). In the plasma, proteins such as albumin and globulins that do not leave easily the pulmonary vessels exert an osmotic pressure across the pulmonary capillary wall. The total osmotic pressure of human plasma is about 28 mmHg,[59] mainly caused by albumin (accounting for about 78% of total osmotic pressure), globulins (21%) and fibrinogen (1%). Changes in the plasma concentration of albumin and globulins affect the total plasma protein osmotic pressure, leading to diminished protein absorption forces.

In the interstitium, a considerable quantity of proteins are present, although the pulmonary microcirculation is not permeable to plasma proteins. However, because of the huge surface area of the pulmonary capillaries, there is always a leakage of plasma proteins through pores and other sites at which they can escape into the interstitium. Besides permeability, the quantity of interstitial proteins is also dependent on the fluid filtration rate occurring across the pulmonary capillaries. The more fluid is filtered the less plasma proteins are in the filtrate.[60] Another mechanism by which interstitial protein concentration is determined is the removal of proteins from the interstitium via the lymphatic system. As stated above, because of differences between pressures and forces in different areas of the lung, the scenario of interstitial protein accumulation is much more complex than is summarised here.

Membrane parameters

The filtration coefficient across the pulmonary capillary wall, K, is a measure of the size and number of 'pores' in the pulmonary capillary vasculature. It is defined as the amount of fluid that will filter across the pulmonary capillaries for every unit change in capillary pressure, time and lung weight. It has been estimated that K ranges between 0.1 and 0.3 ml·min^{-1}·mmHg^{-1}·100 g^{-1}. As the number of capillaries per unit of weight is much higher than in other organs, the K of the lung is very high compared to other organs. However, the filtration properties of a given capillary are similar.

Another membrane parameter is the osmotic reflection coefficient, σ. It is a measure of the solute permeability of the capillary wall. This constant describes the selectivity of the pulmonary microcirculation for a particular protein and is a function of the pore size relative to the protein size. The osmotic reflection coefficient is inversely proportional to the protein leakiness of the microvascular barrier and varies from 0 to 1.0. Whereas small molecules diffuse extremely rapid, large plasma proteins leak across the pulmonary capillary very slowly. Thus, this parameter relates the calculated osmotic pressure of a given protein across an impermeable membrane to the actual osmotic pressure, depending on the solute permeability at the capillary wall. The osmotic reflection coefficient varies at different locations in the pulmonary vasculature. As in other organs, the postcapillary venous sites are more permeable to proteins than the capillaries. Again, this may depend on the position in the lung. Compared to peripheral capillaries, the pulmonary vasculature might become less permeable to plasma proteins at higher vascular pressures, i.e. in the more dependent areas of the lung.

The pulmonary lymphatic system

Besides the forces regulating lung fluid balance that are covered by the Starling's equation, drainage of fluid via the lymphatic system is another important factor in the homeostasis of pulmonary fluid balance. The lung has a very extensive lymphatic system. This provides a pathway for removal of fluid and protein that has been filtered from the vascular compartment. It is probably the most important safety factor in preventing fluid and protein accumulation in the pulmonary tissue and hence pulmonary oedema formation. Protein removal via the lymphatic system is the major mechanism by which accumulation of protein in the tissue is prevented. Otherwise, protein concentration in the tissue would rise to equal that in the plasma.

The second major function of the lymphatics is to remove the fluid that has filtered across the pulmonary microcirculation. Transcapillary fluid exchange according to the Starling equation results in a small amount of fluid filtration into the interstitium of 10–20 ml·h^{-1} at rest. This fluid moves down a pressure gradient into the peribronchovascular interstitium and is then efficiently removed by the lymphatics. Lymph flow can increase 10–15 times normal for large increases in capillary pressure.[61] Thus, the lymphatic system of the lung can drain up to 300 ml·h^{-1}, but greater amounts of fluid accumulate as pulmonary oedema.

Alveolar fluid clearance

The primary mechanism of alveolar fluid clearance is transport of sodium from the air spaces to the lung interstitium. Sodium is taken up by channels on the apical membrane of alveolar type II cells, followed by extrusion of sodium on the basolateral surface by Na$^+$/K$^+$-ATPase.[62] Catecholamine-dependent and catecholamine-independent regulatory mechanisms have been identified that modulate fluid transport, probably acting on uptake by the apical sodium channel or the activity of the Na$^+$/K$^+$-ATPase pumps.[63] Recently, a family of molecular water channels (aquaporins) has been identified that are small (approximately 30 kDa) integral membrane proteins expressed widely in fluid-transporting epithelia and endothelia.[64] Lung phenotype analysis of transgenic mice lacking these aquaporins has been informative. Although some aquaporins play a major role in lung osmotic water permeability, they have little or no effect on physiologically important lung functions such as clearance of alveolar fluid and accumulation of oedema in injured lungs.

Fluid balance in disease

In heart failure, the pulmonary microvascular hydrostatic pressure rises as a result of increases of left atrial pressure and pulmonary capillary wedge pressure. Membrane parameters such as the filtration coefficient and the osmotic reflection coefficient remain constant. The major goal for treatment of cardiac lung oedema is therefore to improve left ventricular performance and, by inducing diuresis, to lower the increased pulmonary hydrostatic pressure. In contrast, in acute lung injury the barrier function of the alveolar–capillary membrane is impaired, leading to changes of both membrane parameters, K and σ, whereas the filtration pressure is basically unchanged. Because there is no direct way of treating altered membrane parameters except to try to achieve control of the underlying disease (e.g. sepsis), treatment for non-cardiac lung oedema again includes reduction of the microvascular filtration pressure by inducing diuresis and improving left ventricular function.

In summary, lung fluid balance in health and disease can best be described by the Starling equation, although it is much more complex and complicated than a simple formula suggests. However, the understanding of the basic forces and coefficients relevant to fluid balance in the lung is a prerequisite for the proper treatment of lung diseases accompanied by oedema.

Clinical relevance

- Exogenous surfactant therapy for premature neonates has become a routine and lifesaving treatment for infant respiratory distress syndrome
- Inflammatory pulmonary diseases such as acute respiratory distress syndrome, idiopathic pulmonary fibrosis, pneumonia, ischaemia–reperfusion injury and asthma are associated with disturbed surfactant function and composition
- Restoration of disturbed surfactant function and composition in these lung disorders, by exogenous surfactant treatment or pharmacological stimulation of the endogenous surfactant system, might be a novel therapeutic option
- Understanding of the basic forces and coefficients relevant for lung fluid balance is a prerequisite for proper treatment of lung diseases accompanied by oedema formation

? Unresolved questions

- Is there a genetic predisposition to various lung diseases as a result of polymorphisms of genes encoding for surfactant proteins?
- Can we find more potent pharmacological agents that stimulate surfactant synthesis and secretion to a degree that is of clinical relevance?
- Which lung diseases other than infant respiratory distress syndrome benefit from exogenous surfactant therapy to a degree that justifies its enormous cost?
- Can we use exogenous surfactant or new synthetic surfactant components to improve pulmonary antimicrobial activity?

References

1. Von Neergaard K. Neue Auffassungen über einen Grundbegriff der Atemmechanik. Die Retraktionskraft der Lunge, abhängig von der Oberflächenspannung in den Alveolen. Z Ges Exp Med 1929; 66: 373–394.
2. Pattle RE. Properties, function and origin of the alveolar lining layer. Nature 1955; 175: 1125–1126.
3. Clements JA. Surface tension of lung extracts. Proc Soc Exp Biol Med 1957; 95: 170–172.
4. Avery ME, Mead J. Surface properties in relation to atelectasis and hyaline membrane disease. Am J Dis Child 1959; 97: 517–523.
5. Walmrath D, Günther A, Ghofrani HA et al. Bronchoscopic surfactant administration in patients with severe adult respiratory distress syndrome and sepsis. Am J Respir Crit Care Med 1996; 154: 57–62.
6. Gregory TJ, Steinberg KP, Spragg R et al. Bovine surfactant therapy for patients with acute respiratory distress syndrome. Am J Respir Crit Care Med 1997; 155: 1309–1315.
7. Wright JR. Immunomodulatory functions of surfactant. Physiol Rev 1997; 77: 931–962.
8. Jobe A, Ikegami M. Surfactant for the treatment of respiratory distress syndrome. Am Rev Respir Dis 1987; 136: 1256–1275.
9. Hamm H, Fabel H, Bartsch W. The surfactant system of the adult lung: physiology and clinical perspectives. Clin Invest 1992; 70: 637–657.
10. Barrow RE, Hills BA. Surface tension induced by dipalmitoyl lecithin in vitro under physiological conditions. J Physiol 1979; 297: 217–227.
11. Hawgood S. Pulmonary surfactant apoproteins: a review of protein and genomic structure. Am J Physiol 1989; 257: L13–L22.
12. Voss T, Schäfer KP, Nielsen PF et al. Primary structure differences of human surfactant-associated proteins isolated from normal and proteinosis lung. Biochim Biophys Acta 1992; 1138: 261–267.
13. Voorhout WF, Veenendaal T, Haagsman HP et al. Surfactant protein A is localized at the corners of the pulmonary tubular myelin lattice. J Histochem Cytochem 1991; 39: 1331–1336.
14. Possmayer F. The role of surfactant-associated proteins. Am Rev Respir Dis 1990; 142: 749–752.
15. Benne CA, Kraaijeveld CA, van Strijp JA et al. Interactions of pulmonary surfactant protein A (SP-A) with influenza A viruses: binding and neutralization. J Infect Dis 1995; 171: 335–341.
16. Van Iwaarden JF, van Strijp JAG, Visser H et al. Binding of surfactant protein A (SP-A) to herpes simplex virus type-1 infected cells is mediated by the carbohydrate moiety of SP-A. J Biol Chem 1992; 267: 25039–25043.
17. Zimmerman PE, Voelker DR, McCormack FX et al. 120-kD surface glycoprotein of P. carinii is a ligand for surfactant protein. Am J Clin Invest 1992; 89: 143–149.
18. Downing JF, Pasula R, Wright JR et al. Surfactant protein A promotes attachment of Mycobacterium tuberculosis to alveolar macrophages during infection with human immunodeficiency virus. Proc Natl Acad Sci USA 1995; 92: 4848–4852.
19. Dobbs LG, Wright JR, Hawgood S et al. Pulmonary surfactant and its components inhibit secretion of phosphatidylcholine from cultured rat alveolar type II cells. Proc Natl Acad Sci USA 1987; 84: 1010–1014.

20. Strayer DS, Yang S, Jerng HH. Surfactant protein A-binding proteins. J Biol Chem 1993; 268: 18679–18684.
21. Weaver TE, Sarin VK, Sawtell N et al. Identification of surfactant proteolipid SP-B in human surfactant and fetal lung. J Appl Physiol 1988; 65: 982–987.
22. Johansson J, Curstedt T, Jörnvall H. Surfactant protein B: disulfide bridges, structural properties, and kringle similarities. Biochemistry 1991; 30: 6917–6921.
23. Cochrane CG, Revak SD. Pulmonary surfactant protein B (SP-B): structure–function relationships. Science 1991; 254: 566–568.
24. Nogee LM, deMello DM, Dehner LP, Colten HR. Deficiency of pulmonary surfactant protein B in congenital alveolar proteinosis. N Engl J Med 1993; 328: 406–410.
25. Williams MC, Hawgood S, Hamilton RL. Changes in lipid structure produced by surfactant proteins SP-A, SP-B, and SP-C. Am J Respir Cell Mol Biol 1991; 5: 41–50.
26. Seeger W, Thede C, Günther A, Grube C. Surface properties and sensitivity to protein-inhibition of a recombinant apoprotein C-based phospholipid mixture in vitro: comparison to natural surfactant. Biochim Biophys Acta 1991; 1081: 45–52.
27. Yu SH, Possmayer F. Role of bovine pulmonary surfactant-associated proteins in the surface-active property of phospholipid mixtures. Biochim Biophys Acta 1990; 1046: 233–241.
28. Crouch E, Parghi D, Kuan SF, Persson A. Surfactant protein D: subcellular localization in nonciliated bronchiolar epithelial cells. Am J Physiol 1992; 263: L60–L66.
29. Kuroki Y, Shiratori M, Ogasawara Y et al. Characterization of pulmonary surfactant protein D: its copurification with lipids. Biochim Biophys Acta 1991; 1086: 185–190.
30. Kuan SF, Rust K, Crouch E. Interactions of surfactant protein D with bacterial lipopolysaccharides. Surfactant protein D is an Escherichia coli-binding protein in bronchoalveolar lavage. J Clin Invest 1992; 90: 97–106.
31. Van Iwaarden JF, Shimizu H, van Golde PHM et al. Rat surfactant protein D enhances the production of oxygen radicals by rat alveolar macrophages. Biochem J 1992; 286: 5–8.
32. Kuroki Y, Shiratori M, Murata Y, Akino T. Surfactant protein D (SP-D) counteracts the inhibitory effect of surfactant protein A (SP-A) on phospholipid secretion by alveolar type II cells. Interaction of native SP-D with SP-A. Biochem J 1991; 279: 115–119.
33. Wang JY, Kishore U, Lim BL et al. Interaction of human lung surfactant proteins A and D with mite (Dermatophagoides pteronyssinus) allergens. Clin Exp Immunol 1996; 106: 367–373.
34. Madan T, Kishore U, Shah A et al. Lung surfactant proteins A and D can inhibit specific IgE binding to the allergens of Aspergillus fumigatus and block allergen-induced histamine release from human basophils. Clin Exp Immunol 1997; 110: 241–249.
35. Wang JY, Shieh CC, You PF et al. Inhibitory effect of pulmonary surfactant proteins A and D on allergen-induced lymphocyte proliferation and histamine release in children with asthma. Am J Respir Crit Care Med 1998; 158: 510–518.
36. Wert SE, Yoshida M, LeVine AM et al. Increased metalloproteinase activity, oxidant production, and emphysema in surfactant protein D gene-inactivated mice. Proc Natl Acad Sci 2000; 97: 5972–5977.
37. Crapo JD, Barry BE, Gehr P et al. Cell number and cell characteristics of the normal human lung. Am Rev Respir Dis 1982; 126: 332–337.
38. Auten RL, Watkins RH, Shapiro DL, Horowitz S. Surfactant apoprotein A (SP-A) is synthetized in airway cells. Am J Respir Cell Mol Biol 1990; 3: 491–496.
39. Wohlford-Lenane CL, Snyder JM. Localization of surfactant-associated proteins SP-A and SP-B mRNA in rabbit fetal tissue by in situ hybridization. Am J Respir Cell Mol Biol 1992; 7: 335–343.
40. Wright JR. Clearance and recycling of pulmonary surfactant. Am J Physiol 1990; 259: L1–L12.
41. Ballard PL. Hormonal regulation of pulmonary surfactant. Endocr Rev 1989; 10: 165–181.
42. Haagsman HP, van Golde LMG. Synthesis and assembly of lung surfactant. Annu Rev Physiol 1991; 53: 441–464.
43. Fisher JH, McCormack F, Park SS et al. In vivo regulation of surfactant proteins by glucocorticoids. Am J Respir Cell Mol Biol 1991; 5: 63–70.
44. Doyle IR, Barr HA, Nicholas TE. Distribution of surfactant protein A in rat lung. Am J Respir Cell Mol Biol 1994; 11: 405–415.
45. Wirtz H, Schmidt M. Ventilation and secretion of pulmonary surfactant. Clin Invest 1992; 70: 3–13.
46. Pettenazzo A, Jobe A, Humme J et al. Clearance of surfactant phosphatidylcholine via the upper airways in rabbits. J Appl Physiol 1988; 65: 2151–2155.
47. Goerke J. Surfactant and lung mechanics. In: Robertson B, van Golde LMG, Batenburg JJ ed. Pulmonary surfactant. From molecular biology to clinical practice. Amsterdam: Elsevier; 1992: 165–192.
48. Matalon S, Holm BA, Baker RR et al. Characterization of antioxidant activities of pulmonary surfactant mixtures. Biochim Biophys Acta 1990; 1035: 121–127.
49. LeVine AM, Bruno MD, Huelsman KM et al. Surfactant protein A-deficient mice are susceptible to group B streptococcal infection. J Immunol 1997; 158: 4336–4340.
50. Catanzaro A, Richman P, Batcher S, Hallman M. Immunomodulation by pulmonary surfactant. J Lab Clin Med 1988; 112: 727–734.
51. Wilsher ML, Parker DJ, Haslam PL. Immunosuppression by pulmonary surfactant: mechanisms of action. Thorax 1990; 45: 3–8.
52. Borron P, Veldhuizen RAW, Lewis JF et al. Surfactant associated protein-A inhibits human lymphocyte proliferation and IL-2 production. Am J Respir Cell Mol Biol 1996; 15: 115–121.
53. Allen JN, Moore SA, Pope-Harman AL et al. Immunosuppressive properties of surfactant and plasma on alveolar macrophages. J Lab Clin Med 1995; 125: 356–69.
54. Tenner AJ, Robinson SL, Borchelt J, Wright JR. Human pulmonary surfactant protein (SP-A), a protein structurally homologous to C1q, can enhance FcR- and CR1-mediated phagocytosis. J Biol Chem 1989; 264: 13923–13928.
55. Van Iwaarden F, Welmers B, Verhoef J et al. Pulmonary surfactant protein A enhances the host-defense mechanism of rat alveolar macrophages. Am J Respir Cell Mol Biol 1990; 2: 91–98.
56. Van Iwaarden JF, van Strijp JA, Ebskamp MJ et al. Surfactant protein A is opsonin in phagocytosis of herpes simplex virus type 1 by rat alveolar macrophages. Am J Physiol 1991; 261: L204–L209.
57. Parker JC, Guyton AC, Taylor AE. Pulmonary interstitial and capillary pressures estimated from intra-alveolar fluid pressures. J Appl Physiol 1978; 44: 267–276.
58. Mitzner W, Robatham JL. Distribution of interstitial compliance and filtration coefficient in canine lung. Lymphology 1979; 12: 140–148.
59. Guyton AC, Taylor AE, Granger HJ. Circulatory physiology. II. Dynamics and control of body fluids. Philadelphia, PA: WB Saunders; 1975.
60. Granger HG, Laine GA, Barnes GE, Lewis RE. Dynamics and control of transmicrovascular fluid exchange. In: Staub NC, Taylor AE, ed. Edema. New York: Raven Press; 1984: 189–228.
61. Yoffey JM, Courtice FC. Lymphatics, lymph and the lymphomyeloid complex. New York: Academic Press; 1970.
62. O'Brodovich HM. The role of active Na+ transport by lung epithelium in the clearance of airspace fluid. N Horiz 1995; 3: 240–247.
63. Matthay MA, Folkesson HG, Verkman AS. Salt and water transport across the alveolar and distal airway epithelia in the adult lung. Am J Physiol 1996; 270: L487–L503.
64. Verkman AS, Matthay MA, Song Y. Aquaporin water channels and lung physiology. Am J Physiol (Lung Cell Mol Physiol) 2000; 278: L867–L879.
65. Perez-Gil J, Keough KMW. Interfacial properties of surfactant proteins. Biochim Biophys Acta 1998; 1408: 203–217.

2.3 Mechanics of ventilation

Vito Brusasco and Riccardo Pellegrino

The fundamental function of the respiratory system is to move air in and out of the lung. The ability to accomplish this task is constrained by the mechanical properties of all components of the respiratory system itself, i.e. airways, lung and chest wall. Knowledge of their static and dynamic characteristics is therefore central to understanding the changes in lung function which occur in disease.

Elastic properties of the respiratory system

The respiratory system exhibits elastic properties that determine its anatomical configuration and maintain patency of its airways and vessels.[1,2] Elasticity originates at a microstructural

level and is modulated by complex interactions between lung and chest wall tissues.

Lung elastic recoil and hysteresis

When excised, the lung tends to achieve a minimum volume at zero (atmospheric) pressure. If a positive pressure sufficient to counteract its elastic recoil is applied at the airway opening, the lung inflates fairly linearly with pressure up to about two-thirds of its maximum volume and then non-linearly until a plateau of volume is achieved (Fig. 2.3.1). The pressure necessary to expand the normal lung fully is about 30 cmH$_2$O, which roughly corresponds to total lung capacity (TLC) measured in vivo. The non-linear part of the pressure–volume relationship is presumably due

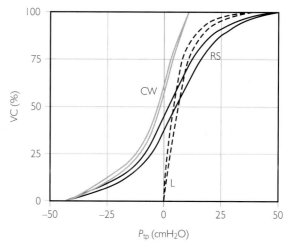

Fig 2.3.1 Quasi-static pressure–volume curves of the lung (L), chest wall (CW), and respiratory system (RS) during inflation and deflation. The hysteresis (area enclosed in the loop) of the lung is greater than that of the chest wall. Volume is expressed as a percentage of vital capacity (VC). P_{tp}, transpulmonary pressure. (Modified from Agostoni & Hyatt.[2])

to the high surface tension of alveoli and the stiffness of connective tissue, which protect the lung from rupture. During deflation from TLC, the pressure–volume curve is shifted to the left of the inflation curve, thus forming a loop (Fig. 2.3.1). The enclosed area is called hysteresis and describes the pressure losses during volume cycling.[1-3] There are a number of mechanisms responsible for lung hysteresis. First, alveolar fluid molecules move from the deepest parts of the surfactant layer to the surface during a large inflation. During the following deflation, however, the film may buckle, causing a decrease in surface tension.[4] Second, during cycling, energy is dissipated in the connective tissue matrix, which deforms like nylon stockings after stretching.[5] Third, contractile elements exhibit energy dissipation, due to detachment of actin–myosin cross-bridges and cytoskeletal deformation with elongation.[6] This mechanism may be responsible for the greater hysteresis in bronchial asthma and chronic obstructive pulmonary disease (COPD) than in normal lungs, because of the substantial involvement of the contractile apparatus of the airways and lung parenchyma (alveolar entrance rings and interstitial Kapanci cells) in disease. Finally, hysteresis may result from the different pressures at which the airways close and open and the alveoli are recruited and derecruited.[7,8]

Chest wall elastic recoil

In contrast to the lung, the chest wall expands after exposing the thoracic cavity to atmospheric pressure,[2] attaining its relaxation volume at about 60% of TLC. A positive pressure of about 10 cmH$_2$O is necessary to further expand it to TLC, whereas a negative pressure of about 40 cmH$_2$O is required to decrease it to residual volume (RV). The chest wall also shows hysteresis, although less than the lung (Fig. 2.3.1).

Measurement of elastic recoil

The elastic recoil of the lung can be fairly easily measured and provides useful clinical information. Elastic recoil of the chest wall is difficult to measure, as it requires complete relaxation of the respiratory muscles, and is of little clinical interest. Elastic recoil of the lung is generally measured during expiration, as it is an estimate of the passive force driving flow out of the lung. The relevant pressure signal is the transpulmonary pressure (P_{tp}), i.e. the difference between oesophageal pressure (P_{oes}), which is an estimate of pleural pressure, and mouth pressure (P_{mo}), which is an estimate of the alveolar pressure when expiration is briefly interrupted and airways are open. P_{tp} is conventionally assumed to be positive and is plotted against lung volume to obtain the 'quasi-static' pressure–volume curve.

The following parameters may be derived from the analysis of the quasi-static pressure–volume curve. First, the slope of the straight part of the curve between functional residual capacity (FRC) and 0.5 litres above it gives an estimate of static lung compliance (C_L). In healthy humans aged 20–30 years C_L is about 0.2 L/cmH$_2$O and increases to about 0.35 L/cmH$_2$O at age of 70–80 years. As it is correlated with height, C_L may be expressed as a percentage of predicted TLC. Second, the shape of the whole pressure–volume curve may be described by an exponential function:[9,10]

$$V = A - Be^{-kP},$$

where V is volume, A is the volume asymptote for infinite P_{tp}, B is the difference between A and the volume at which P_{tp} is zero, and K is the rate of change of curvature. A small value of K denotes a flat curve, as in pulmonary fibrosis; a large value of K denotes a more right-angled curve, as in emphysema.

Third, absolute values of P_{tp} at TLC and at 90%, 80%, 70%, 60% and 50% of TLC can be recorded and compared to predicted values.[11]

The respiratory system under static conditions

Lung volumes: definitions and determinants

Total lung capacity

Total lung capacity is defined as the volume of gas contained in the lungs at maximal inspiration (Fig. 2.3.2). It is determined by the maximum force exerted by the inspiratory muscles necessary to balance the recoil of the lungs and chest wall[2,12] (Fig. 2.3.3). TLC does not vary substantially with ageing, probably because the normal age-related decrease in lung elastic recoil is balanced by a proportional decrease in the force of the inspiratory muscles and/or an increase in chest-wall stiffness. An increase in TLC is generally associated with COPD (especially emphysema) and asthma.[13] Under these conditions, the decrease in lung elastic recoil seems to be the major mechanism for the increase in TLC, although an increased force of inspiratory muscles and chest wall remodelling may also play a role. In severe asthma attacks the increase in TLC may be partially reversed by bronchodilator treatment. TLC decreases in all conditions that are associated with an increased lung elastic recoil (e.g. pulmonary fibrosis,

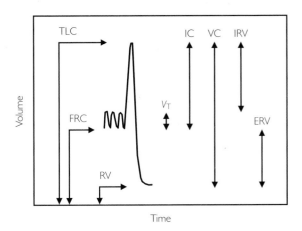

Fig 2.3.2 Subdivisions of lung volume obtained during tidal breathing and maximal inspiration and expiration. FRC, functional residual capacity; TLC, total lung capacity; RV, residual volume. On the right, the double-arrow bars show V_T (tidal volume), inspiratory capacity (IC), vital capacity (VC) and inspiratory and expiratory reserve volumes (IRV and ERV, respectively).

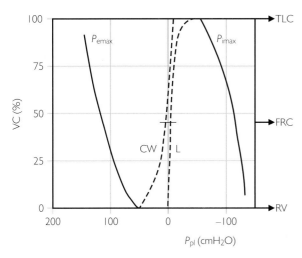

Fig 2.3.3 Quasi-static pressure–volume curves of the chest wall (CW) and the lung (L) related to pleural pressures generated during maximum inspiratory and expiratory static efforts (P_{imax} and P_{emax}, respectively). P_{pl}, pleural pressure. Volume is expressed as a percentage of vital capacity (VC). Total lung capacity (TLC) is the volume at which P_{imax} (pleural) equals the sum of the inward elastic recoil of the lung and chest wall. Residual volume (RV) is the volume at which P_{emax} overcomes the outward elastic recoil of the chest wall. Functional residual capacity (FRC) is the volume at which inward lung recoil equals outward chest wall recoil. (Modified from Rodarte & Rehder.[12])

Table 2.3.1 Definitions of vital capacity

EVC	Expiratory vital capacity recorded during a slow expiration from TLC to RV
IVC	Inspiratory vital capacity recorded during an inspiration from RV to TLC. Values depend on how (slowly or rapidly) RV is attained
FVC	Forced vital capacity recorded during a forced expiration from TLC to RV. It may differ considerably from EVC and IVC, depending on disease conditions

RV, residual volume; TLC, total lung capacity.

cardiac failure), chest wall weakness or stiffness (e.g. neuromuscular diseases, ascites and pregnancy) or pleural space competition (e.g. pleural effusions, pneumothorax).[13]

Residual volume

Residual volume is the volume of gas remaining in the lungs after a maximal expiration (Fig. 2.3.2). In young, healthy subjects, RV is determined by the force exerted by the expiratory muscles when balanced by the outward recoil of the chest wall (Fig. 2.3.3), as can be demonstrated by an increase in air flow at the mouth upon rapid squeezing of the chest wall at the end of a maximal expiration.[14] In older individuals, squeezing the chest wall does not result in an increase in mouth flow, suggesting that airway closure contributes to the determination of RV. In obstructive pulmonary diseases, where premature airway closure may occur because of intrinsic airway disease, loss of lung elastic recoil, stiffness of the chest wall and effects of previous volume history,[13,15,16] the RV tends to increase proportionally to the severity of the disease. Decrease in RV may be observed in some restrictive respiratory diseases, such as pulmonary fibrosis, and after lung resection.

Vital capacity

Vital capacity (VC) is the maximum volume of gas that can be moved in or out of the lungs in a single manoeuvre, thus representing the difference between TLC and RV (Fig. 2.3.2). Although the fact is often underemphasised, VC is highly dependent on the type of respiratory manoeuvre from which it is derived (Table 2.3.1) and the underlying disease.[16] VC was the first lung volume used clinically[17] and reduction in VC is regarded as a sign of respiratory disease. However, a decrease in VC does not allow differentiation between restriction and obstruction, as it may be the result of a decrease in TLC as well as of an increase in RV.

Functional residual capacity

Functional residual capacity is the volume of gas remaining in the lungs at end-tidal expiration in the seated or upright position (Fig. 2.3.2). In young, healthy subjects it is determined by the balance of the inward elastic recoil of the lung and the outward recoil of the chest wall[2] (Fig. 2.3.3). Under these conditions, FRC corresponds to the relaxation volume (V_r) of the respiratory system. In the supine position or during water submersion, the abdominal contents are displaced towards the chest cavity, thus reducing FRC. During speech, singing, laughing and exercise also, FRC tends to decrease to comply with and favour these activities. In contrast, an increase in FRC is generally associated with disease conditions.

In theory, any increase in FRC might be due to an increase in tidal volume (V_T) if the expiratory time (T_E) is not long enough to allow the larger V_T to be fully expired.[18] Alternatively, a rise in FRC could be due to an increase in breathing frequency if T_E is less than the time necessary for the respiratory system to empty, as determined by the product of its resistance and compliance (time constant, τ). Both mechanisms may operate under a variety of conditions associated with alteration of breathing pattern or, in mechanically ventilated patients, when the ventilator setting does not match τ. More often, however, it is an increase of τ relative to T_E that is responsible for premature termination of expiration at lung volume larger than V_r.

A body of evidence has accumulated in the past few years suggesting that limitation of expiratory flow may cause FRC to increase because of premature initiation of tidal inspiration at a lung volume where flow limitation is minimal.[19,20] Decrease in FRC frequently occurs in restrictive respiratory diseases due to increased lung elastic recoil (e.g. in pulmonary fibrosis, atelectasis, lung resection, alveolar liquid filling, cardiac diseases) or reduced chest wall compliance (e.g. in chest wall and pleural diseases, respiratory muscle weakness or obesity).[13]

Inspiratory capacity

Inspiratory capacity (IC) is the volume difference between FRC and TLC (Fig. 2.3.2). Although little used in the past, this measurement has lately attracted interest as a means of detecting changes in FRC during acute interventions affecting airway calibre, such as bronchoprovocation or reversibility tests, when TLC can reasonably be assumed to remain constant.[20,21]

Tidal volume

Tidal volume is the volume of gas inspired and expired during each breath (Fig. 2.3.2). In healthy subjects, its extremes are attained with minimal energy expenditure. This is achieved by neural mechanisms that switch-off inspiration and prevent V_T from occurring over the less compliant part of the pressure–volume curve, and by terminating expiration close to V_r. At rest, V_T is generated mainly by the inspiratory action of the diaphragm, with the other inspiratory muscles preventing the chest wall from distortion, and by the inward recoil pressure of the respiratory system during expiration.

Normally, tidal expiration is slightly longer than inspiration, as a result of glottic narrowing and postinspiratory activity of the inspiratory muscles.[12] When greater ventilation is required, as during exercise, V_T increases by increasing end-inspiratory lung volume and decreasing FRC. This allows V_T to be kept in the linear part of the pressure–volume curve, thus minimising the increase in the work of breathing. Other than during exercise, where a lack of increase in V_T is a sign of ventilatory limitation, and perhaps in patients undergoing assisted ventilation, there is no clear interest in measuring V_T in clinical practice.

Expiratory and inspiratory reserve volumes

These are the volumes available to V_T to expand when necessary (Fig. 2.3.2). Although of no importance at rest, they play a critical role during exercise.

Measurement of lung volumes

Only VC and its subdivisions are measurable by simple spirometry. Absolute lung volumes (TLC, RV and FRC) can be obtained by different methods, the principles and limitations of which are briefly outlined below.

Gas dilution method

Gas dilution methods (nitrogen washout and helium dilution) are based on the principle of the conservation of mass, by which the amount of gas resident in the lungs at the beginning of the test (usually the FRC) can be calculated as the product of concentration times volume of eliminated nitrogen or diluted helium. Both methods yield measurements of gas that communicates with open airways only.[22] Corrections for nitrogen eliminated from body tissues and helium dissolved in blood during the tests must be applied. In patients with severe airways obstruction some lung compartments may have a long τ. Even if the test is usually prolonged in these patients, an underestima-

tion of the true lung volume may result. These techniques are time-consuming and cannot be used to measure rapidly occurring changes of lung volumes.

Body plethysmography

Body plethysmography allows rapid and reproducible measurement of absolute lung volumes.[23] The technique is based on Boyle's law, by which the product of pressure and volume is constant under isothermic conditions. Lung volume is calculated during panting against a closed shutter from the relationship between changes in mouth pressure (assumed in this situation to equal alveolar pressure) and box pressure (constant-volume plethysmograph) or volume (constant-pressure plethysmograph). In contrast to gas dilution techniques, plethysmography measures all intrathoracic gas, thus including non-ventilated and poorly ventilated lung regions. This method may overestimate lung volumes when airflow obstruction is severe, as alveolar pressure does not equilibrate promptly with mouth pressure. This problem may be avoided by panting at a frequency below 1 Hz.[24]

Radiographic techniques

Both standard chest radiographs (planimetry or ellipsoid method) and 3D computed tomography scans (dynamic spatial reconstruction) allow measurement of absolute lung volumes with an accuracy that is close to that of body plethysmography.[25,26]

New methods

New methods have been introduced to measure changes in lung volumes, based on changes in chest wall dimensions. These include inductive plethysmography,[27] optical mapping[28] and optoelectronic plethysmography.[29] The last is based on a 3D analysis of the movements of several markers positioned on the rib cage and abdominal surfaces. This method is highly accurate in detecting lung volume changes and has been successfully applied in different settings, such as exercise[30] and induced bronchoconstriction.[31]

The respiratory system under dynamic conditions

Flow and pressure losses during tidal breathing

The movement of gas through the respiratory system depends on the dimensions of each bronchial generation, flow direction and velocity, lung volume and volume history.[12] To understand the mechanisms of gas motion along the airways, pressure losses across the lung during ventilation may be considered as related to flow (the drop in pressure between the airway opening and the alveoli) and volume (the difference in pressure between alveoli and the pleural surface).

Laminar flow

When gas moves along a tube at low speed, the velocity profile is parabolic, as the molecules close to the tube wall are essentially stationary while in each concentric circular ring the velocity of the molecules increases to reach a maximum in the centre. Pressure decreases along the tube because the 'rings' slide over each other as fluid velocity increases with distance from the wall. Pressure loss (ΔP) under these conditions is proportional to flow ($\dot{V}$) and gas viscosity (μ), but independent of gas density. Thus,

$$\Delta P \propto \mu \dot{V}.$$

Laminar flow dominates in the periphery of the lung, where flow is low; even though the calibre of the airways is small, the total cross-sectional area is large.

Turbulent flow

At higher flow, fluid particles collide with each other and the velocity profile becomes blunted.[12] ΔP under these conditions is dependent on gas density (ρ) and is proportional to the square of flow. Thus,

$$\Delta P \propto \rho \dot{V}^2.$$

Turbulent flow dominates in the more central airways, where flow is high because the total cross-sectional area is small even though the calibre of individual airways is large.

Convective acceleration

During expiration, energy is required to accelerate the gas moving from the large cross-sectional area near the alveoli to the much smaller cross-sectional area of trachea. ΔP due to convective acceleration is described by the Bernoulli equation:

$$\Delta P = \frac{1}{2}\rho\left(\frac{\dot{V}}{A}\right)^2$$

Partitioning of airflow resistance

Pulmonary resistance

Pulmonary resistance (R_L) is defined by the ratio of transpulmonary pressure to flow and includes both airway and tissue resistance (see below). Its measurement in vivo requires the positioning of an oesophageal balloon to estimate P_{tp}. According to the classic equation of motion, P_{tp} during tidal breathing is:[12]

$$P_{tp} = P_{FRC} + EV + R_L\dot{V}$$

where P_{FRC} is the pressure at FRC, V is tidal volume, E is dynamic elastance (i.e. the pressure necessary to increase volume), $\dot{V}$ is flow and R_L is lung resistance (i.e. the pressure required to drive flow). The relationships between these entities are illustrated in Figure 2.3.4, where flow and pressure are plotted against volume. The straight line connecting the extremes of volume on the pressure–volume plot shows the

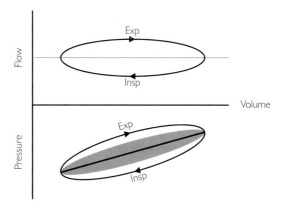

Fig 2.3.4 Diagrammatic representation of flow (upper panel) and pressure (lower panel) plotted against volume ($\dot{V}$–V) and P–V loops, respectively) during quiet breathing. Arrows indicate inspiration (Insp) and expiration (Exp). The slope of the straight line connecting the extremes of the P–V loop is lung elastance (reciprocal of compliance). The heavy external line of the P–V loop is transpulmonary pressure, i.e. the difference between pleural and mouth pressures. The thin internal line within this loop enclosing the shaded area is alveolar pressure related to pleural pressure. The total P–V area divided by the $\dot{V}$–V area is lung resistance (R_L). The shaded area of the P–V loop divided by the $\dot{V}$–V area is tissue resistance (R_{ti}). The small area of the P–V loop external to the shaded area divided by the $\dot{V}$–V loop is airway resistance (R_{AW}).

$P_{FRC} + EV$ term in the above equation. Tidal volume divided by the difference in P_{tp} at the points of zero flow is known as dynamic compliance (C_{dyn}).

During inspiration, P_{tp} is greater than the pressure required to expand the lung by an amount necessary to overcome flow resistance in the airways. The effect of this is shown by the area of the pressure–volume loop below the straight line in Figure 2.3.4. During expiration, the dynamic pressure–volume loop lies above the elastic pressure–volume relationship. The area between the dynamic expiratory pressure–volume curve and the elastance line reflects the stored elastic energy utilised to overcome airway resistance during expiration.

This model assumes that the relationship between pressure and volume is linear, independent of tidal volume amplitude and frequency. However the static pressure–volume relationship of the lung is curvilinear[1,2] and therefore the linear approximation of EV applies only for small-volume excursions and the value of E depends on the initial volume, with the lung becoming stiffer at higher volumes. In addition, the alveolar-to-pleural pressure–volume relationship exhibits hysteresis,[1,2] because of energy losses during cycling. The area of the total pleural pressure loop is attributed to resistance, so that the alveolar pressure–volume loop also contributes to R_L.

Normal values of pulmonary resistance in humans are slightly less during inspiration than expiration. Dynamic compliance is normally slightly less than C_L because of quasi-static lung hysteresis. Pulmonary resistance decreases with breathing frequency, because tissue resistance depends on frequency (see below).

Airway resistance

Airway resistance (R_{AW}) is the ratio of the difference between alveolar and airway opening pressure ($P_A - P_{ao}$) to flow. During tidal breathing, R_{AW} is mostly due to the nose and larynx, whose contributions variably comprise about 40–60% of the total.[32] There is large variability in upper airway resistance between and within individuals, probably because of anatomical differences. The larynx contributes to resistance more on expiration than inspiration, as its calibre increases during inspiration. The nose contributes to resistance more during inspiration than expiration, because intraluminal pressure decreases in inspiration.

In excised lungs, R_{AW} can be measured by the alveolar capsule technique,[33] which yields a direct estimate of alveolar pressure. In living humans, alveolar pressure can be estimated by body plethysmography[23] or by the interrupter method.[34] Using body plethysmography, R_{AW} is calculated from the relation between mouth flow and changes in either box pressure or volume, which, depending on the type of plethysmograph, is related to changes in alveolar pressure. Laryngeal resistance can be minimised by having the subject pant at a frequency slightly greater than 1 Hz, during which the vocal cords are maximally abducted. By the interrupter technique, R_{AW} is computed from the ratio of the sudden pressure drop occurring at the mouth during rapid airway occlusion to the flow recorded immediately before it. The method is based on the assumption that pressure at the mouth during the interruption is equal to alveolar pressure. The method may, however, overestimate R_{AW} because of the damping effect of the tissues of the lung and chest wall on the pressure signal.

Under normal conditions, R_{AW} is virtually independent of breathing frequency but highly dependent on lung volume. This is because the dimensions of intraparenchymal airways vary approximately with the cube root of the volume,[12] because of the three-dimensional traction exerted by pleural pressure on their wall. For each airway, resistance is proportional to its length and inversely proportional to the fourth power of its radius. Therefore, if airway dimensions change in direct proportion to lung volume, resistance will vary in inverse proportion to lung volume. In normal individuals, the product of R_{AW} and absolute volume at FRC is relatively constant (specific resistance, sR_{AW}). To correct for the dependence of R_{AW} on lung volume, its inverse ratio to lung volume (airway specific conductance, $sG_{AW} = 1/sR_{AW}$) is generally used.

Tissue resistance

Tissue resistance (R_{ti}) is the ratio of the pressure dissipated in the parenchymal structures to flow and reflects the hysteretic behaviour of the lung. Figure 2.3.4 illustrates the concept. If both alveolar and transpulmonary pressures are plotted against volume during a breathing cycle, two concentric loops are obtained. The total area included in the external loop (P_{tp}), divided by flow, yields total pulmonary resistance. The area of the internal pressure–volume loop is the pressure difference across lung tissue, which divided by flow yields tissue resistance.

Tissue resistance is independent of the physical properties of gas and is mostly affected by the amplitude of lung excursions rather than their frequency.[35] Thus, if breathing frequency

increases, the width of the loop remains fairly constant whereas, if flow increases, R_{ti} decreases.[36] According to the literature, tissue resistance is a major component of total resistance during tidal breathing.[12,36] It increases during airway narrowing induced by different agonists[37] but whether this is due to a contractile response of lung parenchyma or to its deformation during bronchoconstriction is debated.

Chest wall resistance

Chest wall resistance is the ratio of pressure drop across the chest wall to flow. During quiet breathing it is about one-third of lung resistance.[38] Chest wall resistance is difficult to measure and has little clinical interest.

Respiratory system resistance

Respiratory system resistance (R_{rs}) is the sum of lung and chest wall resistance. It can be measured by relating pressure at the airway opening to flow during sinusoidal oscillations[39] or rapid interruption of flow.[40] At low frequencies, i.e. up to 1–2 Hz, the effect of inertia can be ignored and data can be analysed using the classical equation of motion. However, at higher frequencies, the inertia of the respiratory system and gas are no longer negligible and must be taken into account.

If sinusoidal oscillations or a random-noise excitation signal are superimposed on spontaneous breathing, the relation between pressure and flow can be analysed in the frequency domain by calculating the impedance of the respiratory system, Z_{rs}, as:

$$Z_{rs} = \left[R_{rs}^2 + \left(\frac{1}{\omega C} - \omega I \right)^2 \right]^{\frac{1}{2}},$$

where C is compliance, I is inertance and $\omega = 2\pi f$ is angular frequency. R_{rs} reflects the pressure component in phase with flow and the term $1/\omega C - \omega I$ reflects the reactance of the respiratory system (X_{rs}), which is the pressure component in phase with volume. In this 'lumped' model, R_{rs} is assumed to be independent of frequency, but this may not be the case with non-uniform distribution of mechanical properties and/or large differences between upper and lower airway impedance.

Because of the frequency dependence of compliance and inertance, there is a frequency (resonant frequency) at which they cancel out so that $X_{rs} = 0$ and the system is purely resistive. At low frequencies X_{rs} is dominated by compliance and at high frequencies by inertance. This method is easy to apply in clinical settings and does not require patient cooperation, which makes it particularly useful in small children. However, the data are not always easy to interpret because of the frequency dependence of R_{rs}.

The rapid occlusion method has been particularly used in mechanically ventilated patients and yields values of C_{rs} and R_{rs}, also allowing the latter to be partitioned into two components, the first change in pressure being related to airway resistance and the second to tissue viscoelasticity and/or redistribution of air between parallel units (*pendelluft*).

Work of breathing

During inspiration, the work of breathing has two components, one required to overcome the elastic properties of the respiratory system, the other to overcome flow resistance.[12] The former is generally much greater than the latter in healthy subjects breathing quietly. During exercise, resistive work increases because of the increased flow. In patients with dynamic lung hyperinflation, the elastic work increases because the respiratory system operates over the upper part of the pressure–volume curve. The work required to overcome inertia is small and can be ignored for practical purposes. During expiration, the work exerted by the respiratory muscles is minimal. It may, however, increase to a varying extent in severe airflow obstruction because of activation of the expiratory muscles.

Flow during forced expiration

Concept of expiratory airflow limitation

Expiratory flow limitation is a typical characteristic of all mammals.[12,41,42] The concept is shown in Figure 2.3.5, where flow is plotted against transpulmonary pressure for efforts of different magnitude. At a particular lung volume, flow increases during an expiratory manoeuvre initiated from TLC fairly linearly with pressure until a plateau of flow occurs. The subsequent lack of increase in flow with increasing driving pressure is evidence of flow limitation. This phenomenon occurs with expiratory efforts of greater intensity and higher flow over about 75% of VC above RV. Expiratory flow limitation has been explained in terms of the equal pressure point (EPP) theory[43] or by the analogy of a waterfall.[44]

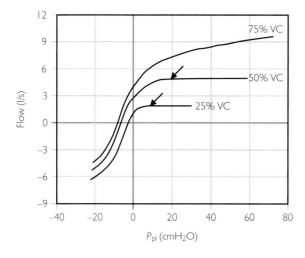

Fig 2.3.5 Isovolume pressure–flow curves of the lung. Flow and pleural pressure (P_{pl}) are plotted during a series of expiratory manoeuvres performed with increasing effort (from right to left). At low-to-mid lung volumes (25% VC, 50% VC), flow first increases with the lowest levels of effort and then plateaus. The arrows indicate the critical pressure associated with maximum flow at a given lung volume. At high lung volume (75% VC), flow is not limited. The graph proves the existence of expiratory flow limitation.

Equal pressure point theory

The EPP theory is illustrated in Figure 2.3.6. Under static conditions (upper panel), the alveoli (balloon) are distended by the negative pleural pressure. The difference between alveolar and pleural pressure is equal to lung elastic recoil. If pleural pressure is increased by an expiratory effort (middle panel), the increase in alveolar relative to the outlet pressure initiates flow. Because of pressure losses, a gradient occurs in the collapsible airways and intraluminal pressure decreases relative to pleural pressure. The equal pressure point is defined as the point at which transmural pressure becomes zero. Downstream from the EPP the airways tend to collapse. Increasing driving pressure does not increase flow because it would further decrease airway calibre at the EPP (lower panel).

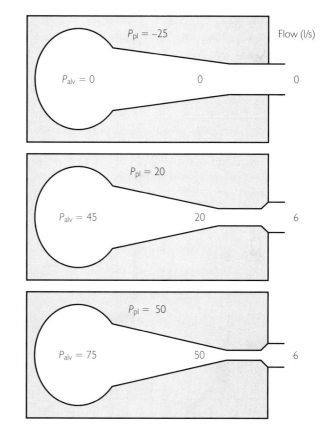

Fig 2.3.6 Schematic representation of the equal pressure point theory. The respiratory system is represented by a box (chest wall), balloon (alveolar compartment) and collapsible tube of gradually decreasing size towards the outlet (airways). The space around balloon and tube represents the pleural space. In the top panel the system is under static conditions. In the middle and lower panels, alveolar pressure (P_{Alv}) at the same lung volume increases due to increase in pleural pressure (P_{pl}). The fall in P_{Alv} along the airways is due mostly to convective acceleration. The tube tends to collapse at the point where internal and external pressures are equal. Flow remains constant at the outlet of the box no matter how much the effort is increased.

The waterfall theory

The mechanism is represented schematically in Figure 2.3.7. A tap fills a container that empties through a hole at the bottom of one side, the size of which is controlled by a shutter connected to a float. The container does not empty until the fluid reaches the float, which then slightly opens the outlet. If inflow increases, the float will be pushed up and the size of the hole will decrease; the outflow will necessarily remain the same. If inflow decreases, the float will descend, thus increasing the size of the hole and once again keeping the outflow constant. The similarity of expiratory flow limitation to a waterfall is based on the independence of outflow and inflow.

Determinants of maximum flow

These can be understood by starting from a simple model (Fig. 2.3.8). The static pressure–area curve of the airway shows that airway wall is stiffer at the extremes (TLC and RV) than at mid lung volumes. If there is no flow, transmural pressure in this airway is lung elastic recoil because external pressure is P_{pl} and intraluminal pressure is alveolar pressure (P_{Alv}). When gas flows at increasing speed, the intraluminal pressure is less than P_{Alv} because of convective acceleration ΔP. This is described in terms of Bernoulli equation (see above) by a family of iso-flow curves superimposed on the pressure–area curve of the airway. The combination of the airway pressure–area curve and Bernoulli isoflow curves represents the mechanical constraints imposed by the static characteristics of the airways to flow. Maximum flow carried by the airway will be that flow at which the tangents of the two curves intersect. Solving the Bernoulli equation

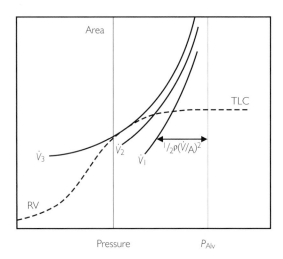

Fig 2.3.8 Area–pressure curve of a hypothetical airway (dashed line) distending with the lung from residual volume (RV) to total lung capacity (TLC). The airway wall is stiffer at the extremes. The continuous lines are isoflow curves derived from the Bernoulli equation, assuming that the pressure drop is due mainly to convective acceleration (see text). P_{Alv} is alveolar pressure. Maximum flow carried by the airway is given by the intersection of the flow and tube laws.

for maximum flow where the pressure–area curve is a tangent to the Bernoulli equation yields:

$$\dot{V}_{max} = A \left(\frac{A}{\rho} \cdot \frac{\Delta P}{\Delta A} \right)^{\frac{1}{2}}$$

Thus, the determinants of maximum flow at the flow-limiting point are the internal airway area and airway wall elastance ($\Delta P / \Delta A$), and gas density.[12,41,42]

The wave speed theory and the choke point

In 1977 Dawson & Elliott[45] recognised that the maximum flow of a fluid passing through a collapsible tube corresponds to the product of the speed (c) of a pressure wave propagating along the tube and the cross-sectional area (A) of the tube. Thus:

$$\frac{\dot{V}_{max}}{A} = c = \left(\frac{A}{\rho} \cdot \frac{\Delta P}{\Delta A} \right)^{\frac{1}{2}}$$

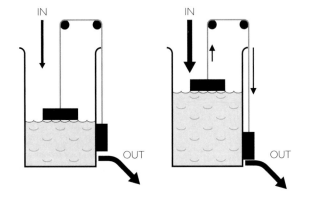

Fig 2.3.7 The waterfall theory. Containers are filled with water and empty through a side hole, the size of which is regulated by a shutter moving up and down, depending on a float on the water level to which it is connected. Inflow (IN) on the left is less than on the right and so is the level of water. However, outflow (OUT) on the right is the same as the left because, even if the pressure drop across the hole is greater because of the higher column of water, the size of the hole is smaller because the float rises as the shutter falls. The analogy of the waterfall to expiratory airflow limitation is based on the fact that both the outflow of the container and forced expiratory flow at the mouth are independent of the magnitude of the pressure drop across the hole or pleural pressures, respectively.

They introduced the concept of wave speed to explain why decreasing airway opening pressure or increasing pleural pressure does not increase flow when this is already maximal. If flow is maximum in an airway, i.e. if $\dot{V}_{max}/A = c$, its velocity must be the same as the speed of a disturbance travelling in the airway wall itself $(A/\rho \cdot \Delta P/\Delta A)^{1/2}$. Thus, if pressure is lowered at the airway opening, the disturbance is stalled and cannot progress upstream. The same occurs if pleural pressure increases. The point along the airway at which this occurs is called the *choke point*. In a model of two or more generations of airways arranged in series with different wall elastance, maximum flow is greater in the stiffer airway. However, as elastic pressure decreases during expiration, the other more compliant airways move to the steepest part of their pressure–area curves, so that mechanical collapse occurs. Overall flow is thus determined by the airway segments that permit the smallest flow. The weakest link of a chain is a relevant comparison. Shift of the limiting segment from the trachea, where it is initially located during a forced expiration, to the intraparenchymal airways is suggested by sudden drops in flow followed by a less rapid decrease.

Effects of upstream frictional losses

So far in modelling maximum flow, convective acceleration has been considered as the only cause of pressure loss. However, in obstructive lung disease upstream frictional losses may account for an additional pressure drop so that the isoflow curves are shifted to the left.[12,41,42] The net effect is that the tangent to the pressure–area curve is a new isopleth with less flow. An analogous effect on maximum flow is obtained by a decrease in lung elastic recoil.

Viscous flow limitation

At low lung volumes, flow is limited by gas viscosity (μ) well before pressure losses due to convective acceleration can cause it.[41,42] In circular tubes of small size the pressure drop (ΔP) is defined by Poiseuille's law:

$$\Delta P = -\frac{a\mu\dot{V}}{A^2}$$

where a is a constant. The equation shows that flow increases as pressure drops at the outlet of the tube, but if cross-sectional area A approaches zero fast enough, then flow becomes limited by μ. The wave-speed limit would occur with a higher ΔP.

Effects of gas physical properties

Decreasing gas density by two-thirds, as when breathing a mixture of 80% helium and 20% oxygen (heliox) may help to identify the site of airflow obstruction.[46,47] This is because ΔP at mid to high lung volumes depends mainly on convective acceleration and thus on gas density. In clinical practice this test may help to identify the site of obstruction in the airways. If narrowing is located mainly in the central airways, decreasing gas density necessarily increases flow. In contrast, if obstruction is predominantly in the peripheral airways, decreasing density in the airways where flow is laminar will be quite ineffective. Although breathing a low-density gas may seem promising as a method of early detection of airflow obstruction in the 'silent zone' of the lung, there are technical problems limiting its clinical application. These are caused by the time necessary for the gas to equilibrate in the lungs, the calibration of flowmeters, the smaller thoracic gas compression volume with heliox than with air, and the frequent differences in vital capacity.

The flow–volume curve

In 1958 Hyatt et al[48] introduced the maximum expiratory flow–volume (MEFV) curve to pulmonary function testing. The interest in this approach is that it shows the maximal flow that

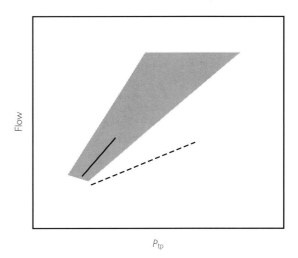

Fig 2.3.9 Schematic representation of maximum expiratory flow plotted against transpulmonary pressure (P_{tp}) at a given absolute lung volume. The shadowed area is the range of normal values. Decrease in flow may be due to intrinsic airway disease (dashed line) or loss of elastic recoil (continuous line).

can be generated at all lung volumes. Furthermore, measurements of expiratory flow and elastic recoil pressure at isovolume in principle distinguish whether flow limitation is due to intrinsic airway disease (as in asthma or chronic bronchitis) or to loss of elastic recoil (as in pulmonary emphysema; Fig. 2.3.9).

Effects of volume history and time on the maximum expiratory flow–volume curve

In 1961, Nadel & Tierney first reported that deep inhalation affected airway calibre[49] because airways and lung parenchyma are interdependent systems. Because the hysteresis of airways and lung parenchyma may differ, the time required for airway calibre to be re-established after stretching to TLC may be different from the time required for re-establishment of lung elastic recoil. Therefore the distending force acting on the airways at a given lung volume may be different before and after a deep inhalation. According to Froeb & Mead,[50] airway hysteresis prevailing over parenchymal hysteresis will cause the external elastic load on the airways to exceed airway smooth muscle tone, thus leading to transient bronchodilatation after deep inspiration. The opposite will happen when parenchymal hysteresis prevails over airway hysteresis. The effect of volume history on airway calibre can easily be inferred by comparing the MEFV curve with the partial expiratory flow–volume (PEFV) curve, i.e. from an expiratory manoeuvre started from a lung volume below TLC, or by measuring airway resistance before and after a deep inhalation.[51,52] The concept is illustrated in Figure 2.3.10.

When the lung is kept at a constant volume over time, a reduction in its elastic recoil pressure occurs, a phenomenon known as *stress relaxation*. The largest effect is seen at high lung volumes and is manifest in the first few seconds.[1] As elastic recoil is one of the most important determinants of maximum flow, the time spent on inhalation to TLC before forced expiration may be critical in this respect.[53] Consequently, maximum expiratory flow is less after a slow than a fast inspiration and is also less if the breath is held for a few seconds before expiration.

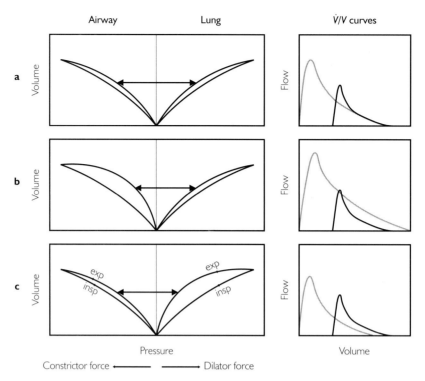

Fig 2.3.10 Schematic representation of the relative hysteresis theory. On the left are three sets of pressure–volume curves of the airways and lung parenchyma during maximum inflation and deflation. The area inside the loop is hysteresis. Bronchial size depends on the balance between airway and lung pressures, which have constrictor and dilating effects respectively. On the right are expiratory flow–volume curves before (partial loop, thick lines) and after a deep breath (maximal loop, thin lines). Case (a) Airway and parenchymal hysteresis are the same, so that, at a given lung volume, airway and lung recoil are the same on both inflation and deflation limbs. If forced expiratory flow is a unique function of airway calibre, partial and maximal flows should be the same. Case (b) Airway hysteresis is greater than parenchymal hysteresis. During deflation lung elastic recoil is greater than bronchial pressure (horizontal arrows), which leads to an increase in airway calibre and thus in maximal flow after a deep breath. Case (c) Parenchymal hysteresis is greater than airway hysteresis. Lung recoil is now less than airway pressure during deflation. Thus, airway size decreases after a deep breath and maximum flow is less than after partial inspiration.

Effects of thoracic gas compression

In clinical practice, the MEFV curve is generally displayed as flow plotted against expired volume. Because intrathoracic gas is compressed during forced expiration, changes in expired volume may lag behind changes in lung volume.[12] As illustrated in Figure 2.3.11, ignoring the effect of gas compression can result in underestimation of flow at any given lung volume above RV. This effect may be particularly important in patients with severe airway obstruction, in whom MEFV curves should ideally be displayed as flow against change in thoracic volume measured by plethysmography. A practical consequence of thoracic gas compression is that instantaneous flows at a given expired volume and, by inference, the forced expiratory volume in 1 second (FEV$_1$) are not truly effort-independent, as they tend to be greater with submaximal rather than maximal efforts[54] especially in patients with airway obstruction.

Clinical application of forced expiration

Recommendations for standardisation of spirometry have been issued by both the European Respiratory Society[55] and American Thoracic Society[56] and will not be discussed in this chapter. Among the many parameters that may be derived from

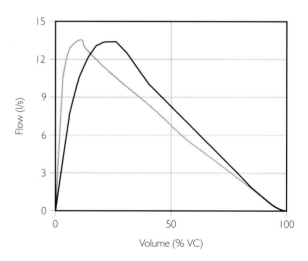

Fig 2.3.11 Flow–volume curve during a maximum forced expiratory manoeuvre. Flow is measured at the mouth by a pneumotachograph. Volume is expressed as a percentage of vital capacity (VC) and is either integrated from the flow signal (dashed line) or measured in a volume-compensated body plethysmograph (continuous line). At any given flow the volume difference between the two curves represents the thoracic gas compression volume.

the forced expiratory manoeuvre, some merit specific consideration. In general, the FEV_1 and FVC are the most important and reproducible and are recommended as a first approach to assess lung function. Because of dependence on age, height, gender and race, they should be related to predicted values. As the scatter of normal values is constant over the whole range, errors may occur if percentages of predicted values are used. Expressing results as standardised residuals is therefore more appropriate.[55] The within-subject variability of the parameters is mostly due to the inspiratory manoeuvre and breath-holding time preceding the forced expiration, the volume history effect of the manoeuvre, and the effort generated during expiration. The ratio of the FEV_1 to FVC (FEV_1/FVC) is an index of airway function. Any decrease in flow (or FEV_1) below the predicted value with less or no change in FVC is consistent with airflow obstruction (Fig. 2.3.12a). In theory a normal FEV_1/FVC with similar proportional decrements in FEV_1 and FVC may also occur with airway disease if this is characterised mainly by airway closure and a consequent increase in RV (Fig. 2.3.12b). In practice, most patients show both a reduced FEV_1/FVC and increased RV.

Peak expiratory flow is a very popular index, which is used as a surrogate for FEV_1. Its variability is much greater than that of FEV_1 even apart from any problems related to the accuracy of peak flow meters. It is not among the indices recommended for the functional diagnosis of disease.[56] Instantaneous maximum expiratory flows at specific volumes below TLC are of some help in describing the shape of the flow–volume curve, although their variability is very high because of dependence on the preceding inspiratory manoeuvre, breath-holding time, volume history, expiratory effort and size of FVC. Reductions in flow at low lung volumes may be due to intrinsic disease of the small airways, to a decrease in elastic recoil or to associated central airway narrowing. Therefore, it is unrealistic to assume that flows at low lung volumes necessarily represent small-airway function.

Flow during forced inspiration

Maximum inspiratory flows depend mainly on the force and velocity of shortening of the inspiratory muscles. Flow reaches a maximum around 50% of vital capacity. In subjects with extra-thoracic airway obstruction, maximum inspiratory flow decreases in proportion to the degree of narrowing. Comparison of maximum expiratory and inspiratory flow may help to distinguish fixed from variable extrathoracic obstruction.[42] In the latter case only forced inspiratory flows are markedly reduced, because the airway wall collapses when subjected to negative intraluminal pressure. In fixed extrathoracic lesions, inspiratory and expiratory flows are decreased to a similar degree because of the high resistance of the lesion independent of transmural pressure changes.

Flow limitation during tidal breathing

Healthy humans hardly ever generate maximal flow during tidal breathing except on strenuous exercise. In contrast, patients with respiratory disease may attain maximum flow during tidal breathing if the lung disease is sufficiently severe to decrease maximum flow near FRC to values similar to tidal flow.[13] Under such conditions, FRC tends to increase, thus avoiding collapse of the airways downstream from the flow-limiting segment,[13,19,20] but this manoeuvre results in increased elastic work of breathing.

The traditional method of identifying flow limitation during tidal breathing is to plot flow and P_{pl} as in Figure 2.3.5 during expirations of increasing effort. Flow limitation is recognised by no increase in tidal expiratory flow with increase in P_{pl}. Non-invasive variants have been proposed, one of which is to compare tidal and forced expiratory flow–volume loops. Flow limitation is assumed to be present when forced and tidal flows are the same over a portion of the expiratory time. This method is not free of pitfalls, however, mostly due to tidal breathing irregularities and also the various factors affecting the MEFV curve (effort, volume history, etc.; see above). These can be minimised with certain precautions (Table 2.3.2). Alternatively, flow limitation can easily be recognised by comparison of tidal expiratory flow before and after applying a negative expiratory pressure at the mouth. This method avoids most of the problems mentioned above (except the irregularity of tidal breathing) and may also be applied to mechanically ventilated patients[57] but collapse of the upper airways may limit its clinical application.[58]

Other, less usual methods of identifying expiratory flow limitation are based on analysis of the pressure–flow relationship by

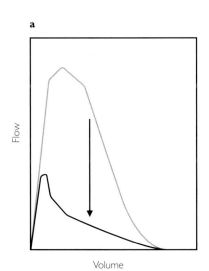
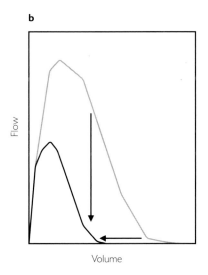

Fig 2.3.12 Theoretical representation of extreme patterns of decrease in flow with airway narrowing. The thin curves are the predicted flow–volume curves. (a) Airway narrowing is associated with a decrease in flow (heavy line) with no change in vital capacity (decrease in slope). (b) Decrease in flow is associated with an increase in residual volume (heavy line) with total lung capacity remaining constant (parallel shift). Arrows indicate decrease in flow and volume.

Table 2.3.2 Recommendations for assessment of expiratory flow limitation using flow–volume curves

Problem	Recommendations to solve
Irregular tidal breathing	Wait for regular breathing. Correct for volume drift
Volume history effects	Initiate forced expiration from end-tidal volume
Time history effects	No breath hold at end-inspiration
Thoracic gas compression artefacts	Use pressure-compensated or flow-type plethysmographs or submaximal expiratory efforts

body plethysmography,[59] the time course of airway pressure during rapid airway occlusion,[60] a reduction of respiratory reactance during expiration[61] and modelling of the tidal pressure–volume relationship by the equation of motion.[62]

For practical purposes, because of the close association between flow limitation and dynamic lung hyperinflation,[19,20] its occurrence during tidal breathing following changes induced in airway calibre (e.g. bronchial challenge or reversibility test) or during exercise may simply be inferred from changes in inspiratory capacity, assuming that TLC remains constant.

Distribution of ventilation

Mechanical determinants

Ventilation is non-uniformly distributed even in normal lungs,[63] because of gravitational forces and pressures exerted by the heart, mediastinal structure and chest wall. These forces, which make the shape of the lung conform to the chest cavity, conspire to generate a pleural pressure gradient that distends the upper (non-gravity-dependent) lung regions more than the lower (gravity-dependent) regions. As airway dimensions change with the cube root of lung volume, airway resistance is correspondingly higher in the lower than in the upper lung regions.

Lung inhomogeneity during tidal breathing

During tidal breathing, the lower lung regions inflate more than the upper lung regions, even although airflow resistance is higher. The reason is that, for a given increase in pleural pressure, lung volume increases more where the pressure–volume curve is steep (lower regions) than where it is flat (upper regions). If inspiratory flow increases, however, the greater resistance in the lower regions counterbalances their greater compliance and ventilation becomes more uniformly distributed. Other causes of inhomogeneous ventilation are non-uniformities in regional compliance[64] and redistribution between parallel lung units (*pendelluft*).[65]

Parallel and serial lung inhomogeneities during tidal breathing lead to frequency dependence of R_L and C_{dyn}.[66] This phenomenon is observed in older healthy individuals, asymptomatic

smokers, subjects with viral infections and patients with manifest airway obstruction.[22]

Lung inhomogeneities and maximum expiratory flow

Serial inhomogeneities may affect flow depending on the site at which they occur.[67] For example, narrowing of the trachea is associated with a decrease in maximum expiratory flow at high lung volumes and a shift of the choke point to lower lung volume. In contrast, increased resistance of the intrathoracic airways decreases maximum flow, both at high and low lung volumes, as a result of the increased frictional losses, which, together with convective acceleration losses, decrease transmural pressure and cross-sectional area at the choke point. In addition, the transition of the choke point from the trachea to the bronchi occurs at higher volumes, because of a premature decrease in P_{tp}. FVC may decrease because of collapse of the airways at higher lung volumes. An increase in elastic recoil leads to a decrease in absolute lung volume due to inability of the inspiratory muscles to overcome the greater lung stiffness. Flows at high and low lung volumes increase because of increased transmural pressure and cross-sectional area. The latter is due to increased tethering forces on the airway wall. The choke point is shifted to lower volumes and RV is decreased as a result of delayed airway closure.

Parallel inhomogeneities due to increased flow resistance in large airways close to the trachea determine a net decrease in flow at high volume and shift of the choke point to low volumes. In contrast, an asymmetrical increase in resistance in the smaller bronchi is associated with a variable decrease in flow both at high and low lung volumes, shift of the choke point to higher volumes and a variable increase in RV. The mechanisms are the same as those discussed above.[67] Lung units with short time constants empty first during forced expiration, independent of the volume at which expiration starts. Under these conditions flow recorded during a PEFV curve is higher than flow recorded at the same volume during a MEFV manoeuvre and is relatively unaffected by a preceding deep breath.[68] In contrast to maximal flow, changes in parameters recorded during tidal breathing (which minimise differences in emptying times) such as lung or airway resistance, are relatively trivial.

? Unresolved questions

- Is maximum flow always a reliable index in obstructive lung disease?
- Should inspiratory capacity be used as a simple index of lung inflation?
- Is oscillatory resistance useful in clinical practice?
- Is there a reliable way to identify small-airway obstruction?
- What is the clinical relevance of regional expiratory flow limitation?

References

1. Hoppin FG Jr, Stothert JC Jr, Greaves IA et al. Lung recoil: elastic and rheological properties. In: Macklem PT, Mead J, ed. Handbook of physiology. The respiratory system. Mechanics of breathing. Section 3, Vol. III, part 1. Bethesda, MD: American Physiological Society; 1986: 195–215.
2. Agostoni E, Hyatt RE. Static behavior of the respiratory system. In: Macklem PT, Mead J, ed. Handbook of physiology. The respiratory system. Mechanics of breathing. Section 3, Vol. III, part 1. Bethesda, MD: American Physiological Society; 1986: 113–130.
3. Hildebrandt J. Dynamic properties of air-filled excised cat lung determined by liquid plethysmograph. J Appl Physiol 1969; 27: 246–250.
4. Adamson AW. Physical chemistry of surfaces. New York: John Wiley; 1982.
5. Bull HB. Protein structure and elasticity. In: Remmington JW, ed. Tissue elasticity. Washington, DC: American Physiological Society; 1957: 33–42.
6. Alexander RS. Viscoplasticity of smooth muscle of urinary bladder. Am J Physiol 1973; 224: 618–622.
7. Mead J, Whittenberger JL, Radford EP Jr. Surface tension as a factor in pulmonary volume-pressure hysteresis. J Appl Physiol 1957; 10: 191–196.
8. Frazer DG, Franz GN. Trapped gas and lung hysteresis. Respir Physiol 1981; 46: 237–246.
9. Salazar E, Knowles JH. An analysis of pressure–volume characteristics of the lungs. J Appl Physiol 1964; 19: 97–104.
10. Colebatch HJH, Ng CKY, Nikov N. Use of an exponential function for elastic recoil. J Appl Physiol 1979; 46: 387–393.
11. Quanjer PhH, ed. Standardized lung function testing. Lung mechanics I: Lung elasticity. Report of the Working Party Standardization of Lung Function Tests, European Community for Coal and Steel. Bull Eur Physiopathol Respir 1983; 19(suppl 5): 28–32.
12. Rodarte JR, Rehder K. Dynamics of respiration. In: Macklem PT, Mead J, ed. Handbook of physiology. The respiratory system. Mechanics of breathing. Section 3, Vol. III, part 1. Bethesda, MD: American Physiological Society; 1986: 131–144.
13. Pride NB, Macklem PT. Lung mechanics in disease. In: Macklem PT, Mead J, ed. Handbook of physiology. The respiratory system. Mechanics of breathing. Section 3, Vol. III, part II. Bethesda, MD: American Physiological Society; 1986: 659–692.
14. Leith DE, Mead J. Mechanisms determining residual volume of the lungs in normal subjects. J Appl Physiol 1967; 23: 221–227.
15. Pellegrino R, Violante B, Selleri R, Brusasco V. Changes in residual volume during induced bronchoconstriction in healthy and asthmatic subjects. Am J Respir Crit Care Med 1994; 150: 363–368.
16. Brusasco V, Pellegrino R, Rodarte JR. Vital capacities during acute and chronic bronchoconstriction. Dependence on flow and volume histories. Eur Respir J 1997; 10: 1316–1320.
17. Hutchinson J. On the capacity of the lungs, and on the respiratory movements, with the view of establishing a precise and easy method of detecting disease by the spirometer. Lancet 1846; 1: 630–632.
18. Vinegar A, Sinnett EE, Leith DE. Dynamic mechanisms determine functional residual capacity in mice, Mus musculus. J Appl Physiol 1979; 46: 867–871.
19. Pellegrino R, Brusasco V, Rodarte JR, Babb TG. Expiratory flow limitation and regulation of end-expiratory lung volume during exercise. J Appl Physiol 1979; 74: 2552–2558.
20. Pellegrino R, Violante B, Nava S et al. Relationship between expiratory airflow limitation and hyperinflation during methacholine-induced bronchoconstriction. J Appl Physiol 1993; 75: 1720–1727.
21. Eliasson O, Degraff AC Jr. The use of criteria for reversibility and obstruction to define patient groups for bronchodilator trials: influence of clinical diagnosis, spirometric, and anthropometric variables. Am Rev Respir Dis 1985; 132: 858–864.
22. Anthonisen NR. Tests of mechanical function. In: Macklem PT, Mead J, ed. Handbook of physiology. The respiratory system. Mechanics of breathing. Section 3, Vol. III, part II. Bethesda, MD: American Physiological Society; 1986: 753–784.
23. DuBois AB, Botelho SY, Comroe JH Jr. A new method for measuring airway resistance in man using a body plethysmograph: values in normal subjects and in patients with respiratory disease. J Clin Invest 1956; 35: 327–335.
24. Shore SA, Huk O, Mannix S, Martin JG. Effect of panting frequency on the plethysmographic determination of thoracic gas volume in chronic obstructive pulmonary disease. Am Rev Respir Dis 1983; 128: 54–59.
25. Miller RD, Offord KP, Roentgenologic determination of total lung capacity. Mayo Clin Proc 1980; 55: 694–699.
26. Krayer S, Rehder K, Beck KC et al. Quantification of thoracic volumes by three-dimensional imaging. J Appl Physiol 1987; 62: 591–598.
27. Gonzales H, Haller B, Watson HL, Sackner MA. Accuracy of respiratory inductive plethysmograph over wide range of rib cage and abdominal contribution to tidal volume in normal subjects and in patients with chronic obstructive pulmonary disease. Am Rev Respir Dis 1984; 130: 171–174.
28. Peacock AJ, Morgan MDL, Gourlay S et al. Optical mapping of the thoraco-abdominal wall. Thorax 1984; 39: 93–100.
29. Cala SJ, Kenyon CM, Ferrigno G et al. Chest wall and lung volume estimation by optical reflectance motion analysis. J Appl Physiol 1996; 81: 2680–2689.
30. Aliverti A, Cala SJ, Duranti R et al. Human respiratory muscle actions and control during exercise. J Appl Physiol 1997; 83: 1256–1269.
31. Gorini M, Iandelli I, Misuri G et al. Chest wall hyperinflation during acute bronchoconstriction in asthma. Am J Respir Crit Care Med 1999; 160: 808–816.
32. Hyatt RE, Wilcox RE. Extrathoracic airway resistance in man. J Appl Physiol 1961; 16: 326–330.
33. Fredberg JJ, Keefe DH, Glass GM et al. Alveolar pressure nonhomogeneity during small amplitude high-frequency oscillation. J Appl Physiol 1984; 57: 788–800.
34. Mead J, Whittenberger JL. Evaluation of airway interruption technique as a method for measuring pulmonary air-flow resistance. J Appl Physiol 1954; 6: 408–416.
35. Stamenovic D, Glass GM, Barnas GM, Fredberg JJ. Viscoplasticity of respiratory tissues. J Appl Physiol 1990; 69: 973–988.
36. Brusasco V, Warner DO, Beck KC et al. Partitioning of pulmonary resistance in dogs: effect of tidal volume and frequency. J Appl Physiol 1989; 66: 1190–1196.
37. Nagase T, Moretto A, Ludwig MS. Airway and tissue behavior during induced constriction in rats: intravenous vs. aerosol administration. J Appl Physiol 1994; 76: 830–838.
38. Ferris BG Jr, Mead J, Opie LH. Partitioning of respiratory flow resistance in man. J Appl Physiol 1964; 19: 653–658.
39. Peslin R, Fredberg JJ. Oscillation mechanics of the respiratory system. In: Macklem PT, Mead J, ed. Handbook of physiology. The respiratory system. Mechanics of breathing. Section 3, Vol. III, part 1. Bethesda, MD: American Physiological Society; 1986: 145–177.
40. Bates JHT, Ludwig MS, Sly PD et al. Interrupter resistance elucidated by alveolar pressure measurement in open-chest normal dogs. J Appl Physiol 1988; 65: 408–414.
41. Wilson TA, Rodarte JR, Butler JP. Wave-speed and viscous flow limitation. In: Macklem PT, Mead J, ed. Handbook of physiology. The respiratory system. Mechanics of breathing. Section 3, Vol. III, part 1. Bethesda, MD: American Physiological Society; 1986: 55–61.
42. Hyatt RE. Forced expiration. In: Macklem PT, Mead J, ed. Handbook of physiology. The respiratory system. Mechanics of breathing. Section 3, Vol. III, part 1. Bethesda, MD: American Physiological Society; 1986: 295–314.
43. Mead J, Turner JM, Macklem PT, Little JB. Significance of the relationship between lung recoil and maximum expiratory flow. J Appl Physiol 1967; 22: 95–108.
44. Permutt S, Riley RL. Hemodynamics of collapsible vessels with tone: the vascular waterfall. J Appl Physiol 1963; 18: 924–932.
45. Dawson SV, Elliott EA. Wave-speed limitation on expiratory flow – a unifying concept. J Appl Physiol 1977; 43: 498–515.

46. Schilder DP, Roberts A, Fry DL. Effects of gas density and viscosity on the maximal expiratory flow–volume relationships. J Clin Invest 1963; 42: 1705–1713.

47. Despas PJ, Leroux M, Macklem PT. Site of airway obstruction in asthma as determined by measuring maximal expiratory flow breathing air and a helium–oxygen mixture. J Clin Invest 1972; 51: 3235–3243.

48. Hyatt RE, Schilder DP, Fry DL. Relationship between maximum expiratory flow and degree of lung inflation. J Appl Physiol 1958; 13: 331–336.

49. Nadel JA, Thierney DF. Effect of a previous deep inspiration on airway resistance in man. J Appl Physiol 1961; 16: 717–719.

50. Froeb HF, Mead J. Relative hysteresis of the dead space and lung in vivo. J Appl Physiol 1968; 25: 244–248.

51. Ingram RH Jr. Physiological assessment of inflammation in the peripheral lung of asthmatic patients. Lung. 1990; 168: 237–247.

52. Pellegrino R, Sterk P, Sont JK, Brusasco V. Assessing the effect of deep inhalation on airway calibre. A novel approach to lung function in bronchial asthma and COPD. Eur Respir J 1998; 12: 1219–1227.

53. D'Angelo E, Prandi E, Milic-Emili J. Dependence of maximal flow–volume curves on time-course of preceding inspiration. J Appl Physiol 1993; 75: 1155–1159.

54. Krowka MJ, Enright P, Rodarte JR, Hyatt RE. Effects of effort on measurement of forced expiratory volume in one second. Am Rev Respir Dis 1987; 136: 829–833.

55. Quanjer PH, Tammeling GJ, Cotes JE et al. Standardized lung function testing. Eur Respir J 1993; 6: 1–99.

56. American Thoracic Society. Lung function testing: selection of reference values and interpretative strategies. Am Rev Respir Dis 1991; 144: 1202–1218.

57. Koulouris NG, Valta P, Lavoie A et al. A simple method to detect expiratory flow limitation during spontaneous breathing. Eur Respir J 1995; 8: 306–313.

58. Tantucci C, Duguet A, Ferretti A et al. Effect of negative expiratory pressure on respiratory system flow resistance in awake snorers and nonsnorers. J Appl Physiol 1999; 87: 969–976.

59. Hage R, Aerts JGJV, Verbraak AFM et al. Detection of flow limitation during tidal breathing by the interruptor technique. Eur Resp J 1995; 11: 1910–1914.

60. Gottfried SF, Rossi A, Higgs BD et al. Noninvasive determination of respiratory system mechanics during mechanical ventilation for acute respiratory failure. Am Rev Respir Dis 1985; 131: 414–420.

61. Vassiliou M, Peslin R, Saunier C, Duvivier C. Expiratory flow limitation during mechanical ventilation detected by the forced oscillation method. Eur Respir J 1996; 9: 779–786.

62. Officer TM, Pellegrino R, Brusasco V, Rodarte JR. Measurement of pulmonary resistance and dynamic compliance with airway obstruction. J Appl Physiol 1998; 85: 1982–1988.

63. Milic-Emili J. Static distribution of lung volumes. In: Macklem PT, Mead J, ed. Handbook of physiology. The respiratory system. Mechanics of breathing. Section 3, Vol. III, part II. Bethesda, MD: American Physiological Society; 1986: 561–574.

64. Rodarte JR, Chaniotakis M, Wilson TA. Variability of parenchymal expansion measured by computed tomography. J Appl Physiol 1989; 67: 226–231.

65. Paiva M, Engel LA. Model analysis of gas distribution within human lung acinus. J Appl Physiol 1984; 56: 418–425.

66. Mead J. Contribution of compliance of airways to frequency-dependent behavior of the lung. J Appl Physiol 1969; 26: 670–673.

67. Pedersen OF, Ingram RH Jr. Configuration of maximum expiratory flow–volume curve: model experiments with physiological implications. J Appl Physiol 1985; 58: 1305–1313.

68. Melissinos CG, Webster P, Tien YK, Mead J. Time dependence of maximum flow as an index of non-uniform emptying. J Appl Physiol 1979; 47: 1043–1050.

2.4 Respiratory muscle function

André De Troyer

The so-called respiratory muscles are those muscles that provide the motive power for the act of breathing. Although many of these muscles are involved in a variety of other activities, such as speech production, cough, vomiting and trunk motion, their primary task is to displace the chest wall rhythmically to pump gas in and out of the lungs. Depending on whether their contraction expands or deflates the lungs, they are customarily divided into inspiratory and expiratory muscles.

The diaphragm is the main respiratory muscle in humans, but moving the chest wall during breathing is an integrated process that involves many muscles. During spontaneous quiet breathing in healthy individuals, groups of intercostal and neck muscles contract in concert with the diaphragm to expand the chest wall and to inflate the lungs, and relaxation of these muscles at end-inspiration allows the respiratory system to return, through its passive elastic properties, to its neutral (resting) position.

During exercise, as the production of CO_2 by the locomotor muscles increases, the regulation of chest wall muscle activation becomes even more complex, involving not only increased activation of the muscles already active during resting breathing but also recruitment of additional muscles that augment chest wall expansion (the so-called 'accessory' muscles). In addition, exercise hyperpnoea is associated with phasic contraction of muscles that increase expiratory airflow and rhythmically bring the respiratory system below its resting volume. Although these muscles have an expiratory action on the lungs, their relaxation at end-expiration during exercise causes an increase in lung volume; in so doing, they therefore reduce the load on the inspiratory muscles and help them meet the increased ventilatory requirements.

Breathing is primarily an automatic process and the pattern of respiratory muscle activation is to a large extent 'hard-wired' to the central respiratory controller. Thus, essentially similar adaptations take place when the work of breathing is increased by disease. When some respiratory muscle groups are weak or paralysed, the remaining muscles have to overcome the entire resistive and elastic load associated with breathing and the strain imposed on them is consequently greater than normal. Similarly, when airflow resistance is abnormally elevated or when dynamic pulmonary and/or chest wall compliance is abnormally reduced, the inspiratory muscles have to generate a greater reduction in pleural pressure to inflate the lungs. The presence of static or dynamic hyperinflation also places an additional load on these muscles by making them operate at shorter than normal lengths and by reducing their ability to lower intrathoracic pressure. When breathing at rest, patients with severe obstructive or restrictive pulmonary impairment therefore use their muscles in much the same way as normal subjects do during exercise. In such patients, however, as in patients with respiratory muscle paralysis, some of the contracting muscles may have little or no beneficial effect on the act of breathing.

The respiratory muscles are structurally and functionally skeletal muscles. As with any skeletal muscle, their actions are therefore essentially determined by their anatomy and by the structures they have to displace when they contract. Consequently, the present chapter starts with a discussion of the basic mechanical structure of the chest wall in humans. It next analyses the action of each group of muscles. For the sake of clarity, the functions of the diaphragm, the intercostal muscles and the muscles of the neck, abdominal wall and upper airway are examined sequentially, but the most critical aspects of the interactions between these muscle groups are emphasised. Finally, some specific disorders are considered in which the respiratory displacements of the chest wall are abnormal as a result of either a particular distribution of muscle weakness or chronic lung disease.

The chest wall

The chest wall can be thought of as consisting of two compartments – the rib cage and the abdomen – separated from each other by a thin musculotendinous structure, the diaphragm[1] (Fig. 2.4.1). These two compartments are arranged in parallel. Expansion of the lungs, therefore, is accommodated by expansion of either the rib cage or the abdomen or of both compartments simultaneously.

The displacements of the rib cage during breathing are essentially related to the motion of the ribs. Each rib articulates by its head with the bodies of its own vertebra and of the vertebra above, and by its tubercle with the transverse process of its own vertebra. The head of the rib is very closely connected to the vertebral bodies by radiate and intra-articular ligaments, such that

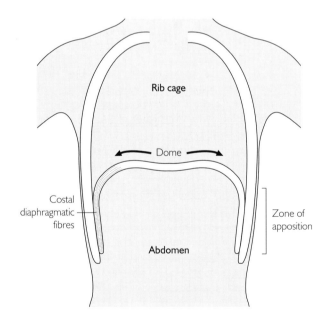

Fig. 2.4.1 Functional anatomy of the human chest wall at end-expiration (frontal section). Note the cranial orientation of the costal diaphragmatic fibres and their apposition to the inner aspect of the lower rib cage (zone of apposition). (Reproduced with permission from De Troyer A, Loring SH. Actions of the respiratory muscles. In: Roussos C, ed. The thorax, vol. 85, 2nd ed. New York: Marcel Dekker; 1995: 535–563.)

only slight gliding movements of the articular surfaces on one another can take place. Also, the neck and tubercle of the rib are bound to the transverse process of the vertebra by short, strong ligaments that limit the movements of the costotransverse joint to slight cranial and caudal gliding. As a result, the costovertebral and costotransverse joints together form a hinge, and the respiratory displacements of the rib occur primarily through a rotation around the long axis of its neck, as shown in Figure 2.4.2(a). However, this axis is oriented laterally, dorsally and caudally. In addition, the ribs are curved and slope caudally and ventrally from their costotransverse articulations, such that their ventral ends and the costal cartilages are more caudal than their dorsal part (Fig. 2.4.2(b&c)). When the ribs are displaced in the cranial direction, therefore, their ventral ends move laterally and ventrally as well as cranially, the cartilages rotate cranially around the chondrosternal junctions, and the sternum is displaced ventrally. Consequently, there is usually an increase in both the lateral and the dorsoventral diameter of the rib cage (Fig. 2.4.2(b&c)). Conversely, a displacement of the ribs in the caudal direction is usually associated with a decrease in rib-cage diameters. As a corollary, the muscles that elevate the ribs as their primary action have an inspiratory effect on the rib cage, whereas the muscles that lower the ribs have an expiratory effect on the rib cage.

It is notable, however, that, although all the ribs move predominantly by rotation around the long axis of their neck, the costovertebral joints of ribs 7–10 have less constraint on their motion than the costovertebral joints of ribs 1–6. The long cartilages of ribs 8–10 also articulate with one another by little synovial cavities, rather than with the sternum. Hence, whereas the upper ribs tend to move as a unit with the sternum, the lower ribs have some freedom to move independently. Both in animals and in humans, deformations of the rib cage may therefore occur under the influence of muscle contraction or other forces.

The respiratory displacements of the abdominal compartment are more straightforward than those of the rib cage because, setting aside the 100–300 ml of abdominal gas, its contents are virtually incompressible. This implies that any local inward displacement of its boundaries results in an equal outward displacement elsewhere. Furthermore, many of these boundaries, such as the spine dorsally, the pelvis caudally and the iliac crests laterally, are virtually fixed. The parts of the abdominal container that can be displaced are thus largely limited to the ventral abdominal wall and the diaphragm. When the diaphragm contracts during inspiration (see below), therefore, its descent usually results in an outward displacement of the ventral abdominal wall; conversely, when the abdominal muscles contract, they cause in general an inward displacement of the belly wall resulting in cranial motion of the diaphragm into the thoracic cavity.

Diaphragm

Functional anatomy

Anatomically, the diaphragm is unique among skeletal muscles in that its muscle fibres radiate from a central tendon to insert peripherally into skeletal structures. The crural (or vertebral)

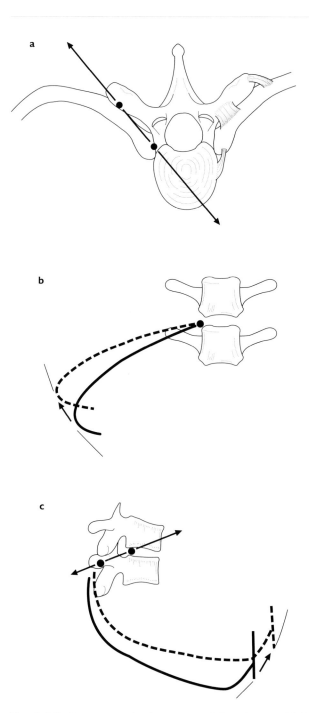

portion of the diaphragmatic muscle inserts on to the ventro-lateral aspect of the first three lumbar vertebrae and on the aponeurotic arcuate ligaments, and the costal portion inserts on to the xiphoid process of the sternum and the upper margins of the lower six ribs. From their insertions, the costal fibres run cranially so that they are directly apposed to the inner aspect of the lower rib cage (Figure 2.4.1); this is the so-called 'zone of apposition' of the diaphragm to the rib cage.[2] Although the older literature suggested the possibility of intercostal motor innervation of some portions of the diaphragm, it is now clearly established that its only motor supply is through the phrenic nerves, which, in humans, originate in the third, fourth and fifth cervical segments.

Actions of the diaphragm

As the muscle fibres of the diaphragm are activated during inspiration, they develop tension and shorten. As a result, the axial length of the apposed diaphragm diminishes and the dome of the diaphragm, which corresponds primarily to the central tendon, descends relative to the costal insertions of the muscle. The dome of the diaphragm remains relatively constant in size and shape during breathing, but its descent has two effects. First, it expands the thoracic cavity along its craniocaudal axis. Hence, pleural pressure falls and, depending on whether the airways are open or closed, lung volume increases or alveolar pressure falls. Second, it produces caudal displacement of the abdominal viscera and an increase in abdominal pressure, which in turn pushes the ventral abdominal wall outwards.

In addition, because the muscle fibres of the costal diaphragm are inserted along the upper margins of the lower six ribs, they also apply a force on these ribs when they contract, and the cranial orientation of these fibres is such that this force is directed cranially. Diaphragmatic contraction therefore has the effect of lifting the ribs and rotating them outwards (Fig. 2.4.3). The fall in pleural pressure and the rise in abdominal pressure that result from diaphragmatic contraction, however, act simultaneously on the rib cage, which probably explains why the action of the diaphragm on the rib cage has been controversial for so long.

Action of the diaphragm on the rib cage

When the diaphragm in anaesthetised dogs is activated selectively by electrical stimulation of the phrenic nerves, the upper ribs move caudally and the cross-sectional area of the upper portion of the rib cage decreases.[3] In contrast, the cross-sectional area of the lower portion of the rib cage increases. If a bilateral pneumothorax is subsequently introduced so that the fall in pleural pressure is eliminated, isolated contraction of the diaphragm causes a greater expansion of the lower rib cage, but the dimensions of the upper rib cage now remain unchanged.[3] It therefore appears that the diaphragm has two opposing effects on the rib cage when it contracts: on the one hand, it has an expiratory action on the upper rib cage, and the fact that this action is abolished by a pneumothorax indicates that it is the result of the fall in pleural pressure; on the other hand, the diaphragm also has an inspiratory action on the lower rib cage. Measurements of chest wall motion during phrenic nerve pacing

Fig. 2.4.2 Respiratory displacements of the rib cage. (a) Diagram of a typical thoracic vertebra and a pair of ribs (viewed from above). Each rib articulates with the body and the transverse process of the vertebra and is bound to it by strong ligaments (right). The motion of the rib occurs therefore primarily by rotation around the axis defined by these articulations (solid line and double arrow-head). From these articulations, however, the rib slopes caudally and ventrally (b & c). Therefore, when it becomes more horizontal in inspiration (dotted line), it causes an increase in both the transverse (b) and the anteroposterior (c) diameter of the rib cage (small arrows). (Reproduced with permission from De Troyer A. Respiratory muscle function. In: Shoemaker WC, Ayres SM, Grenvik A, Holbrook PR, ed. Textbook of critical care. Philadelphia, PA: WB Saunders; 2000: 1172–1184.)

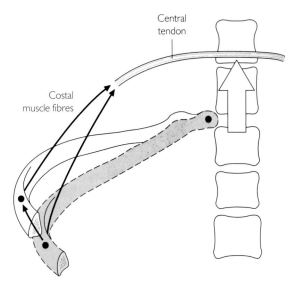

Central
tendon

Costal
muscle fibres

Fig. 2.4.3 Insertional component of diaphragmatic action. During inspiration, as the fibres of the costal diaphragm contract, they exert a force on the lower ribs (arrow). If the abdominal visceral mass effectively opposes the descent of the diaphragmatic dome (open arrow), this force is oriented cranially. As a result, the lower ribs are lifted and rotate outwards. (Reproduced with permission from De Troyer A. Mechanics of the chest wall muscles. In: Miller AD, Bishop B, Bianchi AL, ed. Neural control of the respiratory muscles. Boca Raton, FL: CRC Press; 1996: 59–73.)

in patients with transection of the upper cervical cord[4] and during spontaneous breathing in patients with traumatic transection of the lower cervical cord (in whom the diaphragm is often the only muscle active during quiet breathing)[5] have shown that, as in the dog, the diaphragm in humans has both an expiratory action on the upper rib cage and an inspiratory action on the lower rib cage.

Theoretical and experimental studies have confirmed that the inspiratory action of the diaphragm on the lower rib cage results, in part, from the force the muscle applies on the ribs by way of its insertions; this force is conventionally referred to as the 'insertional' force.[6,7] This inspiratory action of the diaphragm, however, is also related to its apposition to the rib cage. The zone of apposition, in effect, makes the lower rib cage part of the abdominal container, and measurements in animals have established that, during breathing, the changes in pressure in the pleural recess between the apposed diaphragm and the rib cage are almost equal to the changes in abdominal pressure. Pressure in this pleural recess rises, rather than falls, during inspiration, thus indicating that the rise in abdominal pressure is truly transmitted through the apposed diaphragm to expand the lower rib cage. This mechanism of diaphragmatic action has been called the 'appositional' force.

Although the insertional and appositional forces cause the normal diaphragm to expand the lower rib cage, it should be appreciated that this action of the diaphragm is determined largely by the resistance provided by the abdominal contents to diaphragmatic descent. If this resistance is high (i.e. if abdominal compliance is low), the dome of the diaphragm descends

less, so that the zone of apposition remains significant throughout inspiration and the rise in abdominal pressure is greater. Therefore, for a given diaphragmatic activation, the appositional force tending to expand the lower rib cage is increased. Conversely, if the resistance provided by the abdominal contents is small (i.e. if the abdomen is very compliant), the dome of the diaphragm descends more easily, the zone of apposition decreases more and the rise in abdominal pressure is smaller. Consequently, the inspiratory action of the diaphragm on the rib cage is decreased. Should the resistance provided by the abdominal contents be eliminated, the zone of apposition would disappear in the course of inspiration but, in addition, the contracting diaphragmatic muscle fibres would become oriented transversely inwards at their insertions on to the ribs. The insertional force would then have an expiratory rather than an inspiratory action on the lower rib cage. Indeed, when a dog is eviscerated, the diaphragm causes a decrease, rather than an increase, in lower rib-cage dimensions.[3,6]

Influence of lung volume

The balance between pleural pressure and the insertional and appositional forces of the diaphragm is also markedly affected by changes in lung volume. As lung volume decreases below functional residual capacity, the zone of apposition increases and the proportion of the rib cage exposed to pleural pressure decreases. As a result, the appositional force increases while the effect of pleural pressure diminishes, so that the inspiratory action of the diaphragm on the rib cage is enhanced. Conversely, as lung volume increases above functional residual capacity, the zone of apposition decreases and a larger fraction of the rib cage becomes exposed to pleural pressure. The inspiratory action of the diaphragm on the rib cage is therefore diminished.[3,6,7] When lung volume approaches total lung capacity, the zone of apposition all but disappears and the diaphragmatic muscle fibres become oriented transversely inwards as well as cranially. As in the eviscerated animal, the insertional force of the diaphragm is then expiratory rather than inspiratory in direction.

The muscles of the rib cage

The intercostal muscles

The intercostal muscles are two thin muscle layers occupying each of the intercostal spaces. The external intercostals extend from the tubercles of the ribs dorsally to the costochondral junctions ventrally, with their fibres oriented obliquely caudad and ventrally from the rib above to the rib below. In contrast, the internal intercostals extend from the angles of the ribs dorsally to the sternocostal junctions ventrally, with their fibres running caudad and dorsally from the rib above to the rib below. Thus, although the intercostal spaces contain two layers of intercostal muscle in their lateral portion, they contain a single layer in their ventral and dorsal portions. Dorsally, from the angles of the ribs to the vertebrae, the only fibres come from the external intercostal muscles, whereas ventrally, between the sternum and the chondrocostal junctions, the only fibres are those of the internal intercostal muscles; because of its location and particular function (see below), this portion of the internal intercostals is usually called the 'parasternal intercostals'. All the intercostal muscles are innervated by the intercostal nerves.

The actions of the intercostal muscles are conventionally regarded according to the theory proposed by Hamberger in the mid-1700s.[8] As illustrated in Figure 2.4.4, when an intercostal muscle contracts in one interspace, it pulls the upper rib down and the lower rib up. However, as the fibres of the external intercostal slope caudad and ventrally from the rib above to the rib below, their lower insertion is more distant from the centre of rotation of the ribs (the costovertebral articulations) than their upper insertion. Consequently, when this muscle contracts, the torque acting on the lower rib is greater than that acting on the upper rib. The net effect of the muscle, therefore, would be to raise the ribs and to inflate the lung. In contrast, as the fibres of the internal intercostals slope caudad and dorsally from the rib above to the rib below, their lower insertion is less distant from the centre of rotation of the ribs than the upper one. As a result, when this muscle contracts, the torque acting on the lower rib is less than that acting on the upper rib, so that its net effect would be to lower the ribs and to deflate the lung. The parasternal intercostals are part of the internal intercostal layer, but their action should be referred to the sternum rather than to the vertebral column; their contraction would therefore raise the ribs and inflate the lung.

Although this theory is based on a simple, two-dimensional model of the rib cage, several of its conclusions have been confirmed experimentally. When the parasternal intercostals in the dog are selectively activated by electrical stimulation, they produce cranial displacement of the ribs into which they insert

and an increase in lung volume.[9] Also, a number of electromyographic studies in animals[9] and in humans[10] have clearly established that the parasternal intercostals invariably contract during the inspiratory phase of the breathing cycle. These muscles, therefore, have a clear-cut inspiratory action. In the dog, the external intercostals in the dorsal portion of the upper interspaces also have a definite inspiratory effect on the lung, whereas the internal interosseous intercostals in the lower interspaces have a large expiratory effect.[11] However, the inspiratory effect of the external intercostals decreases rapidly both toward the costo-chondral junctions and toward the base of the rib cage, as shown in Figure 2.4.5. As a result, this inspiratory effect is reversed to an expiratory effect in the lower interspaces. Similarly, the expiratory effect of the internal interosseous intercostals decreases ventrally and dorsally, such that it is reversed to an inspiratory effect in the first and second interspaces. Such topographical differences imply that the actions of these muscles during breathing are determined primarily by the topographical distribution of neural drive.

Detailed electrical recordings from intercostal muscles and nerves in cats and dogs have demonstrated that, as with the parasternal intercostals, the external intercostals are active only during inspiration whereas the internal interosseous intercostals are active only during expiration.[12,13] Inspiratory activity in the external intercostals, in fact, is greatest in the dorsal portion of the upper interspaces and declines gradually in the caudal and the ventral directions. On the other hand, expiratory activity in the internal interosseous intercostals is greatest in the dorsal portion of the lower interspaces and decreases progressively in the cranial and ventral directions.[13] The external intercostals in the ventral portion of the lower interspaces and the internal interosseous intercostals in the ventral portion of the upper interspaces are

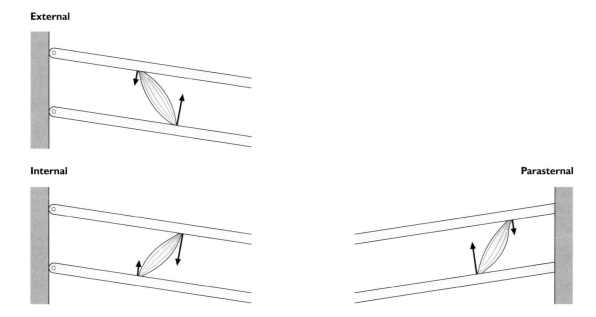

Fig. 2.4.4 Diagram illustrating the actions of the intercostal muscles, as proposed by Hamberger.[8] The dark area in the left panels represents the spine (dorsal view), and the dark area in the lower right panel represents the sternum (ventral view). The two bars oriented obliquely represent two adjacent ribs. The external and internal intercostal muscles are depicted as single bundles, and the torque acting on the ribs during contraction of these muscles is represented by arrows.

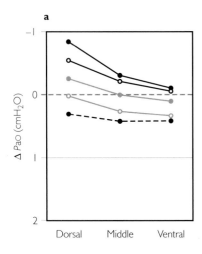

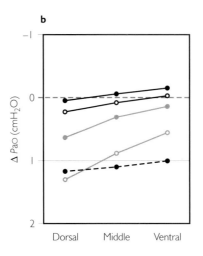

Fig. 2.4.5 Actions of the canine external (a) and internal interosseous (b) intercostal muscles on the lung. These data are the maximal changes in airway pressure (ΔPaO) that the muscles in the dorsal, middle, and ventral portions of the second (●), fourth (○), sixth (●), eighth (○) and tenth (●) interspace can generate when contracting against a closed airway. A negative ΔPaO indicates an inspiratory effect while a positive ΔPaO indicates an expiratory effect. (Reproduced with permission from De Troyer et al.[11])

never active during breathing, even when the demand placed on the respiratory muscle pump is increased by CO_2-enriched gas mixtures or by external mechanical loads. In view of the topographical distributions of respiratory effect among the muscles, such topographical distributions of neural drive confer on the external intercostals an inspiratory action on the lung during breathing and on the internal interosseous intercostals an expiratory action. Although the precise distribution of activity among the external and internal intercostals in humans remains to be assessed, in particular in the dorsal aspect of the upper interspaces, the muscles appear to have similar actions as in the dog;[14] in fact, whereas the inspiratory action of the parasternal intercostals in the dog is greater than that of the external intercostals, in humans the inspiratory action of the external intercostals is predominant.

The external and internal interosseous intercostals are also involved in postural movements, and electromyographic studies in normal subjects have shown that the external intercostals on the right side of the chest are activated when the trunk is rotated to the left but remain silent when the trunk is rotated to the right; conversely, the internal intercostals on the right side contract only when the trunk is rotated to the right.[15] Indeed, the insertions and orientations of these muscles make them ideally suited to twist the rib cage. Contraction of the external intercostals on one side of the sternum rotates the ribs in a transverse plane, so that the upper ribs move forwards while the lower ribs move backwards. Contraction of the internal intercostals on one side has the opposite effect, moving the upper ribs backwards and the lower ribs forwards.

The scalene muscles

The scalenes in humans comprise three muscle heads that run from the transverse processes of the lower five cervical vertebrae to the upper surface of the first two ribs. In dogs, when these muscles are activated selectively by electrical stimulation, they produce marked cranial displacement of the ribs and sternum and cause an increase in rib cage anteroposterior diameter. Although the scalenes have traditionally been considered as 'accessory' muscles of inspiration, electromyographic studies with needle electrodes have established that, in normal humans, they invariably contract in concert with the

diaphragm and the parasternal intercostals during inspiration[16,17] (Fig. 2.4.6).

There is no clinical setting that causes paralysis of all the inspiratory muscles without also affecting the scalenes. Therefore, the isolated action of these muscles on the human rib cage cannot be defined precisely. Two observations, however, indicate that contraction of the scalenes is an important determinant of the expansion of the upper rib cage during breathing. First, when normal subjects attempt to inspire with the diaphragm alone, there is a marked, selective decrease in scalene activity associated with either less inspiratory increase or a paradoxical decrease in anteroposterior diameter of the upper rib cage.[16] Second, the inspiratory inward displacement of the upper rib cage characteristic of quadriplegia is usually not observed when scalene function is preserved after lower cervical cord transection.[5] As the scalenes are innervated from the lower five cervical segments, persistent inspiratory contraction is frequently seen in subjects with a transection at the C7 level or below. In such subjects, the anteroposterior diameter of the upper rib cage tends to remain constant or to increase slightly during inspiration.

The sternocleidomastoids and other accessory muscles of inspiration

Many additional muscles, such as pectoralis minor, trapezius, erector spinae, the serrati and sternocleidomastoids, can elevate the ribs when they contract. These muscles, however, run between the shoulder girdle and the rib cage, between the spine and the shoulder girdle, or between the head and the rib cage. Therefore, they have primarily postural functions. In healthy individuals, they contract only during increased inspiratory efforts; in contrast to the scalenes, therefore, they are true 'accessory' muscles of inspiration.

Of all these muscles, only the sternocleidomastoids have been thoroughly studied. These descend from the mastoid process to the ventral surface of the manubrium sterni and the medial third of the clavicle. Their action in humans has been inferred from measurements of chest wall motion in patients with transection of the upper cervical cord. Indeed, in such patients, the diaphragm, intercostals, scalenes and abdominal muscles are paralysed, although the sternocleidomastoids (the

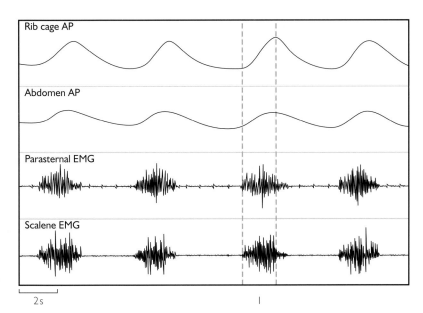

Fig. 2.4.6 Pattern of electrical activation of the scalene and parasternal intercostal (third interspace) muscles in normal humans. The subject shown is breathing quietly in the seated position. The inspiratory phase of the breathing cycle (I) is indicated by an increase in the anteroposterior (AP) diameter of the rib-cage and abdomen.

motor innervation of which largely depends on the XIth cranial nerve) are spared and contract forcefully during unassisted inspiration. When breathing spontaneously, these patients show marked inspiratory cranial displacement of the sternum and large inspiratory expansion of the upper rib cage, particularly in its anteroposterior diameter. There is, however, a decrease in the transverse diameter of the lower rib cage.[4]

The triangularis sterni

The triangularis sterni, also called transversus thoracis, is a thin flat muscle that lies deep to the sternum and the parasternal intercostals. Its fibres originate from the dorsal aspect of the caudal half of the sternum and insert into the inner surface of the costal cartilages of the third to seventh ribs. The motor supply of the muscle comes from the intercostal nerves.

In quadrupeds, the triangularis sterni invariably contracts during the expiratory phase of the breathing cycle. In so doing, it pulls the ribs caudally and deflates the rib cage below its neutral position.[18] Consequently, when the muscle relaxes at the end of expiration, there is passive rib cage expansion and an increase in lung volume that precedes the onset of inspiratory muscle contraction. In these animals, the triangularis sterni thus helps the parasternal and external intercostals to produce the rhythmic inspiratory expansion of the rib cage.[18] In normal humans, however, the muscle contracts only during voluntary or involuntary expiratory efforts such as coughing, laughing and speech. Presumably, the muscle then acts in concert with the internal interosseous intercostals to deflate the rib cage and increase pleural pressure.

The abdominal muscles

Functional anatomy

The four abdominal muscles with significant respiratory function in humans make up the ventrolateral wall of the abdomen. The rectus abdominis is the most ventral of these muscles. It originates from the ventral aspect of the sternum and the fifth, sixth and seventh costal cartilages, and it runs caudally along the whole length of the abdominal wall to insert into the pubis. The muscle is enclosed in a sheath formed by the aponeuroses of the three muscles situated laterally. The most superficial of these is the **external oblique**, which originates by fleshy digitations from the external surface of the lower eight ribs, well above the costal margin, and directly covers the lower ribs and intercostal muscles. Its fibres radiate caudally to the iliac crest and inguinal ligament and medially to the linea alba. The **internal oblique** lies deep to the external oblique. Its fibres arise from the iliac crest and inguinal ligament and diverge to insert on the costal margin and an aponeurosis contributing to the rectus sheath down to the pubis. The **transversus abdominis** is the deepest of the muscles of the lateral abdominal wall. It arises from the inner surface of the lower six ribs, where it interdigitates with the costal insertions of the diaphragm. From this origin, and from the lumbar fascia, the iliac crest and the inguinal ligament, its fibres run circumferentially around the abdominal visceral mass and terminate ventrally in the rectus sheath.

Actions of the abdominal muscles

These four muscles have important functions as flexors (rectus abdominis) and rotators (external oblique, internal oblique) of the trunk, but as respiratory muscles, they have two principal actions. First, as they contract, they pull the abdominal wall inwards and produce an increase in abdominal pressure; this causes the diaphragm to move cranially into the thoracic cavity, which, in turn, results in an increase in pleural pressure and a decrease in lung volume. Second, these four muscles displace the rib cage through their insertions on the ribs. These insertions would suggest that the action of all abdominal muscles is to pull the ribs caudally and to deflate the rib cage. Measurements of rib-cage motion during stimulation of the individual muscles in dogs have shown, however, that the rise in abdominal pressure also confers on them an inspiratory action on the rib cage.[19] The zone of apposition of the diaphragm to the rib cage (Fig. 2.4.1) allows abdominal pressure to be transmitted to the lower rib cage. In addition, by forcing the diaphragm cranially and stretching it, the rise in abdominal pressure induces passive diaphragmatic tension. This passive tension tends to raise the lower ribs and to expand the lower rib cage in the same way as does an active diaphragmatic contraction ('insertional' force).

The action of the abdominal muscles on the rib cage is thus determined by the balance between the insertional, expiratory force of the muscles and the inspiratory force related to the rise in abdominal pressure. Isolated contraction of the external oblique in humans produces a small caudal displacement of the sternum and a large decrease in the transverse diameter of the rib cage, although the rectus abdominis, while causing marked caudal displacement of the sternum and a large decrease in the anteroposterior diameter of the rib cage, also produces a small increase in the transverse diameter. The isolated actions of the internal oblique and transversus abdominis muscles on the human rib cage are not known. The anatomical arrangement of the transversus, however, would suggest that, among the abdominal muscles, this muscle has the smallest insertional expiratory action on the ribs and the greatest effect on abdominal pressure. Isolated contraction of the transversus should therefore produce little or no expiratory rib cage displacement.

Respiratory function of the abdominal muscles

Irrespective of their actions on the rib cage, the abdominal muscles are primarily expiratory muscles through their action on the diaphragm and lungs, and they play important roles in activities such as coughing and speaking. However, when these muscles contract rhythmically in phase with expiration so as to reduce lung volume below the neutral position of the respiratory system, their relaxation at end-expiration promotes passive descent of the diaphragm and induces an increase in lung volume before the onset of inspiratory muscle contraction.

This inspiratory action of the abdominal muscles takes place all the time in quadrupeds; in dogs placed in the head-up or the prone posture, the relaxation of the abdominal muscles at end-expiration accounts for up to 40–60% of the tidal volume. Healthy humans do not use such a breathing strategy at rest. However, phasic expiratory contraction of the abdominal muscles does occur in healthy subjects whenever the demand placed on the inspiratory muscles is increased, such as during exercise or when breathing carbon-dioxide-enriched gas mixtures. It is noteworthy that, in these conditions, the transversus muscle is recruited well before activity can be recorded from either the rectus or the external oblique.[20] In view of the actions of these muscles, this preferential recruitment of the transversus also supports the notion that the effect of the abdominal muscles on abdominal pressure is more important to the act of breathing than is their action on the rib cage.

There is a second mechanism by which the abdominal muscles can assist inspiration. Most normal human subjects, when standing, develop tonic abdominal muscle activity unrelated to the phase of the breathing cycle, and studies in patients with transection of the upper cervical cord, in whom bilateral pacing of the phrenic nerves allows the degree of diaphragmatic activation to be kept constant, clearly illustrate the effect of this tonic abdominal contraction on inspiration.[4] When such patients are supine, the unassisted paced diaphragm can generate an adequate tidal volume. However, when they are tilted head-up or moved to the seated posture, the weight of the abdominal viscera and the absence of abdominal muscle activity cause the belly wall to protrude. The tidal volume produced by pacing in this posture is markedly reduced relative to the supine posture, but this reduction is significantly diminished if a pneumatic cuff is inflated around the abdomen to mimic the tonic abdominal muscle contraction. Thus, by contracting throughout the breathing cycle in the standing posture, the abdominal muscles make the diaphragm longer at the onset of inspiration and prevent it from shortening excessively during inspiration; in accordance with the length–tension characteristics of the muscle, its ability to generate pressure is therefore increased.

The upper airway muscles

The muscles of the upper airway comprise those of the external nares, soft palate, pharynx and larynx. Although they do not have any direct effect on the chest wall, they promote patency of the upper airway during breathing; they are, therefore, a primary determinant of inspiratory flow and contribute to the maintenance of normal ventilation.[21]

The anatomy of these muscles is complex and the mechanical interactions between them are not completely understood. Several muscles, however, contract during inspiration and may, in fact, display phasic inspiratory activity during resting breathing in healthy individuals. These include the **alae nasi**, which dilate the nasal passage by elevating the mobile alar cartilages; the **genioglossus**, a fan-shaped muscle that runs dorsally from the ventral portion of the mandible to the tongue and protrudes the tongue when it contracts; and the **posterior cricoarytenoid** muscles, which abduct the vocal cords by rotating the arytenoid cartilages.

The pattern of activity of these three muscles, however, is strikingly different from the pattern of activity of the diaphragm, inspiratory intercostals and scalene muscles.[22] Whereas activity in these chest-wall muscles increases progressively during inspiration and reaches its peak at or near the cessation of inspiratory flow, activity in the alae nasi, genioglossus and posterior cricoarytenoid starts rather abruptly, reaches its peak early after the onset of inspiration and declines well before cessation of inspiratory flow. Furthermore, the onset of activity in these muscles usually precedes the onset of diaphragmatic activity and, when negative pressure is applied selectively to the upper airway in anaesthetised animals, they show a reflex increase in peak inspiratory activity and a greater lead time relative to the onset of diaphragmatic activity.[22] This pattern of contraction allows the upper airway to stabilise or dilate (and upper airway resistance to decrease) throughout the period when it is subjected to the negative intraluminal pressure produced by contraction of the inspiratory chest wall muscles. If the forces generated by the upper airway dilating muscles are not sufficient to oppose the negative intraluminal pressure, the upper airway decreases in size and may, in fact, collapse; inappropriate reduction in activity of the upper airway dilating muscles during sleep, in particular the genioglossus, combined with anatomical narrowing of the pharynx, is a key feature in most patients with the obstructive sleep apnoea syndrome (see Chapter 45).

The chest wall and respiratory muscles in specific disorders

Quadriplegia

As pointed out above, the particular distribution of muscle paralysis in patients with traumatic transection of the lower cervical cord causes distinct abnormalities in the pattern of chest-wall motion during breathing (Fig. 2.4.7). Because diaphragmatic function in such patients is preserved, the expansion of the abdomen during inspiration is associated with expansion of the lower rib cage. However, whereas the rib cage in healthy subjects expands uniformly, in quadriplegic patients the lower rib cage expands predominantly over its lateral walls, where the area of apposed diaphragm is greater (greater appositional force).[5] In addition, the paralysis of the inspiratory intercostal muscles is such that many quadriplegic patients at rest have an inspiratory decrease (paradoxical motion) of the anteroposterior diameter of the upper rib cage.

Quadriplegic patients also have complete paralysis of all the well recognised muscles of expiration (abdominal muscles, internal intercostals, triangularis sterni). As a result, the expiratory reserve volume is markedly reduced and residual volume is greater than normal. The peak pleural pressures developed during cough are also less than normal, such that the clearance

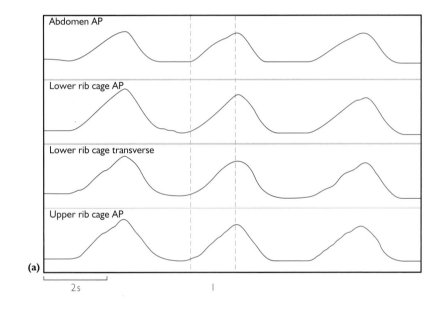

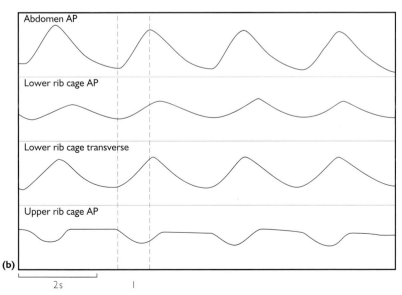

Fig. 2.4.7 Pattern of chest wall motion in a healthy subject (a) and a C_5 quadriplegic patient (b) breathing at rest in the seated posture. The respiratory changes in anteroposterior (AP) diameter of the abdomen, lower rib cage and upper rib cage are shown, as well as the changes in transverse diameter of the lower rib cage. In all traces, an upward deflection corresponds to an increase in diameter and a downward deflection corresponds to a decrease in diameter; I indicates the duration of inspiration. (Reproduced with permission from De Troyer A, Estenne, M. The respiratory system in neuromuscular disorders. In: Roussos C, ed. The thorax, vol. 85, 2nd ed. New York: Marcel Dekker; 1995: 2177–2212.)

of bronchial secretions is severely impaired. Most quadriplegic patients, however, contract the clavicular portion of the pectoralis major during voluntary expiration and during coughing.[23] The insertions of this muscle bundle on the humerus and the medial half of the clavicle make it displace the manubrium sterni and the upper ribs in the caudal direction when it contracts on both sides of the chest. In so doing, it causes collapse of the upper rib cage and produces partial emptying of the lung. In a number of patients, the clavicular portion of the pectoralis major may even induce dynamic compression of the intrathoracic airways,[24] thus indicating that cough in this setting is really an active, rather than a passive phenomenon.

Diaphragmatic paralysis

Paralysis or severe weakness of both hemidiaphragms is usually seen in the context of generalised respiratory muscle weakness, but in occasional patients the diaphragm is specifically or disproportionately affected (see Chapter 77.5). Selective paralysis of the diaphragm results in a compensatory increase in activation of the inspiratory rib cage muscles, so that inspiratory expansion of the rib cage compartment of the chest wall is accentuated.[9] In addition, whereas in healthy subjects simultaneous contraction of the diaphragm and rib cage inspiratory muscles causes a rise in abdominal pressure associated with a fall in pleural pressure, with diaphragmatic paralysis the fall in pleural pressure is transmitted through the flaccid diaphragm so that abdominal pressure falls as well. As a result, the abdomen moves paradoxically inwards, opposing the inflation of the lung.[9]

Some patients also compensate for diaphragmatic paralysis by contracting the abdominal muscles during expiration, thus displacing the abdomen inwards and the diaphragm cranially into the thorax. Relaxation of the abdominal muscles at the onset of inspiration may therefore result in outward abdominal motion and passive descent of the diaphragm. Such a contraction of the abdominal muscles during expiration seems to be particularly frequent in the erect patient, and when present it may negate the inspiratory inward motion of the abdomen that is the cardinal sign of diaphragmatic paralysis on clinical examination. This compensation does not, however, occur in the supine posture, where the abdominal muscles usually remain relaxed during the whole respiratory cycle.

Chronic obstructive pulmonary disease

Measurements of thoracoabdominal motion during breathing have shown that patients with chronic obstructive pulmonary disease (COPD) and hyperinflation have relatively greater expansion of the rib cage and less expansion of the abdomen than healthy subjects.[25] The normal inspiratory positive swing of abdominal pressure is also attenuated, while the fall in pleural pressure is greater than normal because of the increased airflow resistance and reduced dynamic pulmonary compliance. In patients with severe disease, abdominal pressure may even become negative during inspiration and the abdomen may move paradoxically inwards, as though the diaphragm were paralysed.[25] This altered pattern has led to the widespread belief that these patients have more use of the rib-cage inspiratory muscles

and less use of the diaphragm than healthy subjects, possibly as a result of diaphragmatic fatigue.

In agreement with this idea, in many patients the scalenes and parasternal intercostals feel tense on palpation during inspiration. Electromyographic studies using concentric needle electrodes have also shown that, when breathing at rest, patients with severe COPD have increased firing frequencies in the parasternal intercostal and scalene motor units compared with normal subjects.[26] The patients also have a greater number of active motor units in these two muscles. However, motor units in the diaphragm also show substantial increases in firing frequency during resting breathing (Fig. 2.4.8), indicating that COPD is associated with an increase in neural drive not only to the rib-cage inspiratory muscles but also to the diaphragm.[27] The altered thoracoabdominal motion on inspiration results, therefore, from mechanical factors alone. Indeed, the diaphragm in such patients is characteristically flat and low compared with that of normal subjects and the zone of apposition is reduced in size. Consequently, for the same neural activation, the ability of the diaphragmatic dome to descend is impaired, such that the rise in abdominal pressure and the outward displacement of the abdominal wall are reduced. In some patients with severe hyperinflation, the zone of apposition has virtually disappeared, and the normal curvature of the diaphragm is even reversed, with its concavity facing upward rather than downward. The muscle fibres at their insertions on the ribs then run transversely inward rather than cranially, so that the dome cannot descend at all. Instead, the vigorous contraction of the rib cage inspiratory muscles, resulting in a greater than normal elevation of the ribs, tends to pull the diaphragm cranially and to displace the ventral abdominal wall inwards. Contraction of this flat diaphragm, however, produces an inspiratory decrease in the transverse diameter of the lower rib cage (Hoover's sign).

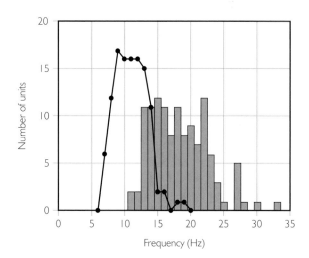

Fig. 2.4.8 Histograms of the peak discharge frequencies of diaphragmatic motor units recorded in eight patients with severe COPD (solid bars) and in six control healthy subjects (closed circles) during resting breathing in the seated posture. The discharge frequencies in the patients averaged 17.9 ± 4.3 Hz (mean ± SD) and were substantially higher than in the control subjects (10.5 ± 2.4 Hz; $P < 0.001$). (Reproduced with permission from De Troyer et al.[27])

In contrast to normal subjects, many resting patients with severe COPD also have phasic expiratory contraction of the abdominal muscles, in particular the transversus abdominis.[28] The neural drive to the expiratory muscles is therefore also increased, and abdominal pressure is commonly observed to increase, rather than to decrease, during expiration. The expiratory contraction of the transversus is thus mechanically significant, yet its benefit to the act of breathing is probably negligible. As previously pointed out, contraction of the abdominal muscles during expiration is a natural component of the response of the normal respiratory system to increased stimulation to breathe. In both healthy individuals and patients with diaphragmatic paralysis, this expiratory muscle contraction is appropriate because it allows the work of breathing to be shared between the inspiratory and expiratory muscles. Most patients with severe COPD, however, have airflow limitation even at rest. In this situation, expiratory contraction of the transversus abdominis is unlikely to achieve a significant increase in expiratory airflow or significant deflation of the respiratory system below its neutral position.[28]

? Unresolved questions

- The topographic distribution of activity among the external and internal intercostals in humans remains uncertain, so the actions of these muscles cannot be precisely defined.

- Whether the actions of the different inspiratory muscle groups on the lung are additive, synergistic or antagonistic is unknown.

- Although several muscles of the pharynx and larynx are known to contract during inspiration to stabilise or dilate the upper airway, the mechanical interactions between them are not completely understood.

- Patients with severe chronic obstructive pulmonary disease and hyperinflation have a greater than normal neural drive to the diaphragm and abdominal muscles but whether these muscles usefully contribute to the act of breathing has not yet been determined.

Clinical relevance

- Hyperinflation reduces the mechanical advantage of the inspiratory muscles, particularly the diaphragm. In severe hyperinflation, diaphragmatic contraction causes indrawing rather than expansion of the lower ribs.

- Patients with severe airway obstruction or lung restriction use their respiratory muscles in similar ways to healthy subjects during exercise.

- Relaxation of the abdominal muscles aids inspiration in healthy subjects during exercise and in patients with diaphragmatic paralysis.

- Ineffective activity of the upper airway muscles results in obstructive sleep apnoea.

References

1. Konno K, Mead J. Measurement of the separate volume changes of rib cage and abdomen during breathing. J Appl Physiol 1967; 22: 407.
2. Mead J. Functional significance of the area of apposition of diaphragm to rib cage. Am Rev Respir Dis 1979; 119: 31.
3. D'Angelo E, Sant'Ambrogio G. Direct action of contracting diaphragm on the rib cage in rabbits and dogs. J Appl Physiol 1974; 36: 715.
4. Danon J, Druz WS, Goldberg NB, Sharp JT. Function of the isolated paced diaphragm and the cervical accessory muscles in C$_1$ quadriplegics. Am Rev Respir Dis 1979; 119: 909.
5. Estenne M, De Troyer A. Relationship between respiratory muscle electromyogram and rib cage motion in tetraplegia. Am Rev Respir Dis 1985; 132: 53.
6. De Troyer A, Sampson M, Sigrist S, Macklem PT. Action of costal and crural parts of the diaphragm on the rib cage in dog. J Appl Physiol 1982; 53: 30.
7. Loring SH, Mead J. Action of the diaphragm on the rib cage inferred from a force-balance analysis. J Appl Physiol 1982; 53: 756.
8. Hamberger GE. De respirationis mechanismo et usu genuino. Jena, 1749.
9. De Troyer A, Kelly S. Chest wall mechanics in dogs with acute diaphragm paralysis. J Appl Physiol 1982; 53: 373
10. Taylor A. The contribution of the intercostal muscles to the effort of respiration in man. J Physiol 1960; 151: 390.
11. De Troyer A, Legrand A, Wilson TA. Respiratory mechanical advantage of the canine external and internal intercostal muscles. J Physiol 1999; 518: 283.
12. Sears TA. Efferent discharges in alpha and fusimotor fibres of intercostal nerves of the cat. J Physiol 1964; 174: 295.
13. Legrand A, De Troyer A. Spatial distribution of external and internal intercostal activity in dogs. J Physiol 1999; 518: 291.
14. Wilson TA, Legrand A, Gevenois PA, De Troyer A. Respiratory effect of the external and internal intercostal muscles in humans. J Physiol 2001; 530: 319.
15. Whitelaw WA, Ford GT, Rimmer KP, De Troyer A. Intercostal muscles are used during rotation of the thorax in humans. J Appl Physiol 1992; 72: 1940.
16. De Troyer A, Estenne M. Coordination between rib cage muscles and diaphragm during quiet breathing in humans. J Appl Physiol 1984; 57: 899.
17. Raper AJ, Thompson WT Jr, Shapiro W, Patterson JL Jr. Scalene and sternomastoid muscle function. J Appl Physiol 1966; 21: 497.
18. De Troyer A, Ninane V. Triangularis sterni: a primary muscle of breathing in the dog. J Appl Physiol 1986; 60: 14.
19. De Troyer A, Sampson M, Sigrist S, Kelly S. How the abdominal muscles act on the rib cage. J Appl Physiol 1983; 54: 465.
20. De Troyer A, Estenne M, Ninane V et al. Transversus abdominis muscle function in humans. J Appl Physiol 1990; 68: 1010.
20. Van Lunteren E, Strohl KP. The muscles of the upper airways. Clin Chest Med 1986; 7: 171.
22. Van Lunteren E, Van de Graaf WB, Parker DM. Nasal and laryngeal reflex responses to negative upper airway pressure. J Appl Physiol 1984; 56: 746.
23. De Troyer A, Estenne M, Heilporn A. Mechanism of active expiration in tetraplegic subjects. N Engl J Med 1986; 314: 740.
24. Estenne M, Van Muylem A, Gorini M et al. Evidence of dynamic airway compression during cough in tetraplegic patients. Am J Respir Crit Care Med 1994; 150: 1081.
25. Sharp JT, Goldberg NB, Druz WS et al. Thoracoabdominal motion in chronic obstructive pulmonary disease. Am Rev Respir Dis 1977; 115: 47.
26. Gandevia SC, Leeper JB, McKenzie DK, De Troyer A. Discharge frequencies of parasternal intercostal and scalene motor units during breathing in normal and COPD subjects. Am J Respir Crit Care Med 1996; 153: 22.
27. De Troyer A, Leeper JB, McKenzie DK, Gandevia SC. Neural drive to the diaphragm in patients with severe COPD. Am J Respir Crit Care Med 1997; 155: 1335.
28. Ninane V, Yernault JC, De Troyer A. Intrinsic PEEP in patients with chronic obstructive pulmonary disease. Role of expiratory muscles. Am Rev Respir Dis 1993; 148: 1037.

2 Function

2.5 Pulmonary gas exchange

Roberto Rodríguez-Roisin

 Key points

- In the process of alveolar ventilation, there is permanent balance between continuous addition of oxygen molecules to the alveoli and continuous removal by the pulmonary capillary blood exiting the lungs.

- The relationship between alveolar P_{CO_2} and alveolar ventilation is set out by the alveolar gas equation for carbon dioxide.

- In a perfect lung, alveolar P_{O_2} and P_{CO_2}, and hence arterial P_{O_2} and P_{CO_2}, are related through the ideal alveolar gas equation for oxygen.

- Hypoventilation occurs when alveolar ventilation is inadequately reduced relative to carbon dioxide production and the alveolar P_{CO_2} settles out at a higher level than the physiological range.

- Under normal conditions, in any single alveolar unit the rate of equilibration for oxygen and carbon dioxide between alveolar gas and the pulmonary capillary are the $\dot{V}_A/\dot{Q}$ ratio, the composition of the inspired gas and the composition of the mixed venous blood.

- The multiple inert gas elimination technique (MIGET) represents a major conceptual breakthrough in our understanding of the pathophysiology of pulmonary gas exchange in disease states.

- The molecules of oxygen are carried in two forms in blood. The most relevant component carried is combined with haemoglobin within the red blood cell, while a small amount is simply dissolved in the blood.

- Carbon dioxide is transported in the blood in three different forms: dissolved, as bicarbonate ions and in combination with proteins as carbamino compounds.

The most critical function of the lung in health and disease is pulmonary gas exchange.[1] Pulmonary gas exchange requires adequate ventilation and pulmonary perfusion within the alveoli to match oxygen (O_2) uptake ($\dot{V}_{O_2}$) and carbon dioxide (CO_2)

elimination ($\dot{V}_{CO_2}$) to the whole-body metabolic oxygen consumption and carbon dioxide production respectively, whatever the levels of these two gases in the arterial blood are.[2] When the lung fails as a gas-exchange organ, either arterial hypoxaemia or hypercapnia, or both, appear and respiratory insufficiency or failure ensues. To physiologically exchange the respiratory gases the lung needs to thoroughly integrate the processes of pulmonary ventilation, alveolar to end-capillary diffusion, alveolar ventilation to blood flow relationships and, finally, their proper systemic transport to peripheral tissues[3] (Fig. 2.5.1).

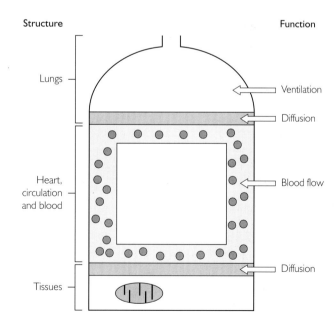

Figure 2.5.1 Schematic representation of the major processes involved in the oxygen transport pathway. Oxygen is moved from atmospheric air to the mitochondria through the integrated participation of several tissues and organs. (With permission from Roca et al 2000.[3]).

Over the past half-century, we have witnessed an impressive explosion of knowledge about the pathophysiology of pulmonary gas exchange in both acute and chronic respiratory conditions. More specifically, the heterogeneity of ventilation–perfusion ($\dot{V}_A/\dot{Q}$) units within the lung was identified as the principal factor causing arterial hypoxaemia.[4] In addition to the key role played by alveolar hypoventilation in the development of hypercapnia, the relevance of $\dot{V}_A/\dot{Q}$ inequality as a key determinant of hypercapnia in chronic obstructive airway diseases was also highlighted.[5,6]

In the middle 1950s, a crucial step toward a better understanding of the physiological determinants of pulmonary gas exchange was the development of the three-compartment model of the lung, illuminated almost simultaneously by the early work of Rahn & Fenn and Riley & Cournand[7] (Fig. 2.5.1). Indeed, the graphical analysis of this representation of the lung provided the conceptual basis for the traditional interpretation of arterial blood gas measurements in the clinical set-up, namely the mixed venous admixture ratio, so-called physiological shunt, and the physiologic dead space. During the 1960s, progress in the mathematical description of the behaviour of oxygen and carbon dioxide in the blood facilitated substantial contributions to the numerical analysis of pulmonary gas exchange. We now know that traditional parameters measured from physiological gases (oxygen and carbon dioxide partial pressures (P) in arterial blood) or calculated (e.g. the alveolar–arterial P_{O_2} difference, AaP_{O_2}, mixed venous admixture ratio and physiological dead space), were conditioned by $\dot{V}_A/\dot{Q}$ imbalance. Furthermore, it was also learned that variations in total lung indices, such as minute ventilation, cardiac output,[8] oxygen consumption[9] and inspired oxygen fraction[10] lead to frequent misinterpretations in the clinical setting.[11,12]

The multiple inert gas elimination technique (MIGET) was developed in the early 1970s by Wagner and coworkers[13–17] as a tool to obtain the most extensive information about the entire spectrum of $\dot{V}_A/\dot{Q}$ ratio distributions in the lung. Its principle is based on the observation that the retention of any inert gas is dependent on the solubility of that gas and the $\dot{V}_A/\dot{Q}$ distribution (Fig. 2.5.2). Over the last quarter-century, the use of the MIGET by several groups around the world has been crucial to produce a substantial amount of experimental and clinical research that has achieved a full understanding of pulmonary gas exchange in different clinical conditions.[11,12,17–22] This inert gas approach has been shown to be one of the most robust tools for understanding the basic mechanisms of physiological gas abnormalities and the effects of therapeutic interventions as well. Along with its ability to estimate $\dot{V}_A/\dot{Q}$ ratio distributions in real lungs, MIGET provides information on another intrapulmonary factor governing hypoxaemia and hypercapnia, i.e. alveolar–capillary diffusion limitation.[2,23–25] This technique provides more information concerning the role of the $\dot{V}_A/\dot{Q}$ relationships on pulmonary gas exchange than any other one measurement previously available, such as topographical radioactive-tracer-based techniques, which have more limited resolution and thus underestimate the underlying degree of $\dot{V}_A/\dot{Q}$ imbalance.

A practical way to clinically classify respiratory failure may be based on the major processes involved in abnormalities in arterial blood gases and subdivide abnormality into hypercapnia and hypoxaemia[26] (Fig. 2.5.3). Hypercapnic respiratory failure

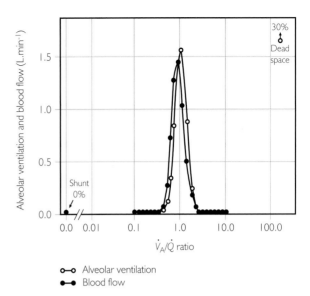

Figure 2.5.2 Distributions (each individual point represents a particular amount of ventilation and blood flow) of $\dot{V}_A/\dot{Q}$ ratios in a healthy individual, at rest, breathing room air, assessed with the multiple inert gas elimination technique (MIGET). Ventilation (open symbols) and perfusion (closed symbols) are plotted against a logarithmic scale of $\dot{V}_A/\dot{Q}$ ratios. Both distributions are symmetrical, well centred at a $\dot{V}_A/\dot{Q}$ ratio of 1.0, and narrow. Intrapulmonary shunt (left, bottom, closed symbol) is absent.

can be present in patients with 'normal lungs', in which the major component is alveolar hypoventilation, or with abnormal, structurally disrupted, lungs, where the principal alteration is $\dot{V}_A/\dot{Q}$ imbalance.[5,6] Hypoxaemic respiratory failure can be observed either in acute conditions, in which increased intrapulmonary shunt remains the pivotal mechanism, or in the context of a chronic respiratory condition, in which $\dot{V}_A/\dot{Q}$ inequality is the main pathophysiological disturbance. Depending on the individual clinical conditions, these four major pathophysiological abnormalities may be present alone or in combination.

Composition of ambient, inspired, and expired gases

In assessing the function of the lung as a gas exchanger, it is useful to first consider the physical properties of all the gases involved in the process. Atmospheric air is composed of a mixture of oxygen, nitrogen, argon and trace amounts of other gases, such as carbon dioxide (Table 2.5.1). The total sum of the dry gas fractions or concentrations (F_G) must equal 1.0. The composition of a gas mixture can be described in terms of either the gas concentrations or the corresponding partial pressures (P). Although classically partial pressures are expressed in millimetres of mercury or torr units, during the last few years the European scientific community has recommended using the Système Internationale (SI) units and express partial

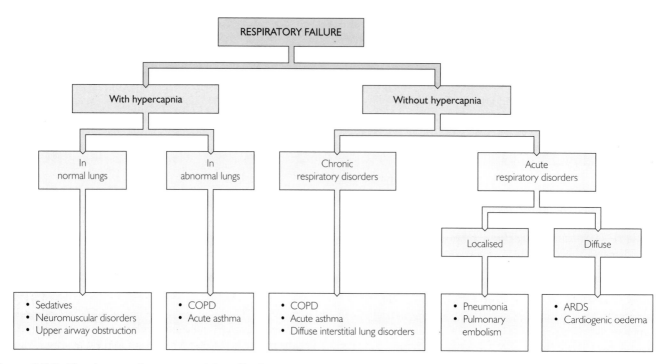

Figure 2.5.3 Classification of respiratory failure (for further explanation, see text). Note that the third row includes four subgroups that reflect the underlying major pathophysiological changes. Thus hypercapnic respiratory failure is subclassified into that shown in conditions with normal lungs (due to alveolar hypoventilation) and in those types found with abnormal lungs (due to ventilation–perfusion mismatch); hypoxaemic respiratory failure includes conditions observed in chronic (due to ventilation–perfusion imbalance) and in acute respiratory disorders (due to increased intrapulmonary shunt). Diffusion limitation is only slightly abnormal in diffuse interstitial lung disorders. (Modified from Rodríguez-Roisin 2000.[26])

Table 2.5.1 Partial pressures of the principal physiological gases (mmHg)

Gas (fraction)	Dry ambient air	Inspired tracheal air*	Alveolar gas
Oxygen (0.2093)	159.1	149.2	105
Carbon dioxide (0.0003)	0.23	0.21	40
Water (0)	0	47	47
Nitrogen (0.7904)	600.7	563.6	572.9
Total (1.00)	760	760	760

* Body temperature, 37°C; barometric pressure, 760 mmHg.

pressures in kilopascals (kPa) (1 torr = 1 mmHg = 0.133 kPa; 1 kPa = 7.5006 mmHg).

Accordingly, the partial pressure of each gas corresponds to the product of its dry gas (F_G) concentration (e.g. dry air has 0.2093 oxygen) and the total ambient, or atmospheric (P_{atm}), pressure at sea level (total pressure 760 mmHg):

$$P_G = F_G \times P_{atm} \qquad \text{(Equation 1)}$$

such that, at sea level, the ambient oxygen partial pressure would be:

$$P_{O_2}\,(air) = 760 \times 0.2093 = 159\,\text{mmHg}. \qquad \text{(Equation 2)}$$

Since each of the gases present contributes to the total atmospheric pressure, the sum of the partial pressures of all the gases equals barometric pressure (P_B). At high altitude, i.e. at 8000 m, the gas concentrations of ambient air are the same as at sea level, yet the barometric pressure is substantially reduced, such that the partial pressure of each gas is also decreased even although its concentration is the same.

However, as dry air is inspired it comes into contact with the moist, warm upper and lower airways and becomes humidified and warmed by body temperature. Thus, inhaled gas is saturated with water vapour, hence taking up as much water as it can hold at that temperature. Gas saturated with water has a water-vapour partial pressure (P_{H_2O}) that depends on that at body temperature (37°C), 47 mmHg. By adding P_{H_2O} to the total barometric pressure, the addition of water effectively reduces the partial pressures of other gases present, even before they reach the alveoli. Under these circumstances, the total dry gas pressure is only $760 - 47 = 713$ mmHg, such that the process of saturating dry ambient air during inspiration provokes a reduction of approximately 10 mmHg in the Po_2 of a gas. Accordingly, the Po_2 of moist inspired air is:

$$Po_2 = (P_B - PH_2O) \times F_G = 713 \times 0.2093 = 149 \text{ mmHg.}$$
(Equation 3)

Although, in practice, ambient air also contains some moisture, the PH_2O is usually small (at 20°C = 17.5 mmHg or even less if the relative humidity of the air is less than 100%) and therefore practically negligible.

In a study of 64 healthy subjects,[27] arterial Po_2 fell with age as expected, but only slightly. The slope of regression indicated a mean decrease of about 6 mmHg, from a mean of 102.3 mmHg at age 20 years to 96.5 mmHg at age 70 years. Likewise, arterial Pco_2 also fell with age, by almost 4 mmHg, from a mean of 38.0 mmHg to 34.3 mmHg over the same range of age, while $AaPo_2$ (see below) ranged from 4 mmHg to 8 mmHg, respectively. An earlier study on arterial blood gases in healthy individuals[28] reported a linear decay between the ages of 40 and 70 years, but no further fall in arterial Po_2 was observed in people up to 90 years old. In the most recent study,[29] a set of reference equations of arterial blood gas measurements and carbon-monoxide analytes studied in several laboratories and based on a population of 369 healthy lifetime non-smokers at sea level and at an altitude of 1400 m has been reported. The mean decline of arterial Po_2 with age (– 0.245 mmHg/year) was consistent with previous studies.[30] At sea level, mean arterial Po_2 and mean $AaPo_2$ at age 20 years were 100 ± 5.3 mmHg and 2.0 ± 5.7 mmHg, respectively; the corresponding figures at age 70 years and above were 88.7 ± 10.7 mmHg and 14.8 ± 8.8 mmHg.

Oxygen cascade and carbon dioxide elimination

By the time the oxygen molecules reach the alveoli, Po_2 has fallen by about 50 mmHg (from 149 mmHg in ambient air to nearly 100 mmHg). This is essentially because of the process of alveolar ventilation itself (see below), in which there is a permanent balance between continuous addition of oxygen molecules to the alveoli and their continuous removal by the pulmonary capillary blood leaving the lungs. The alveolar Po_2 and systemic (arterial) blood Po_2 have almost the same value. Nevertheless, by the time the oxygen molecules reach the peripheral tissues at the mitochondrial level there has been a remarkable fall in Po_2 values, a movement basically driven by passive diffusion.

The tissue cells perform a wide spectrum of metabolic activities, including those necessary for cell integrity, an active process that requires the expenditure of a lot of energy. These energy demands are met by oxidative metabolism, which produces adenosine triphosphate (ATP) in the mitochondrial electron transport system as molecular oxygen is consumed. At rest, the cells consume about 250 ml of oxygen per minute (oxygen consumption or uptake, $\dot{V}o_2$). The cellular rate of ATP

formation depends therefore on these metabolic demands and not on the local availability of oxygen molecules. At this cellular level, the oxygen concentration is usually far greater than that required for electron transport and the mitochondrial Po_2 is considerably lower than that in arterial and mixed venous blood. The values of Po_2 in the mitochondria may vary considerably according to the specific tissue of the body and its oxygen consumption.

For carbon dioxide molecules, the process is inverted as there is essentially no carbon dioxide in ambient air. The Pco_2 may also vary quite considerably throughout the body and will depend ultimately on the metabolic state of the tissues. At rest, the cells continuously produce approximately 200 ml of carbon dioxide per minute (carbon dioxide production, $\dot{V}co_2$). To prevent its retention in the tissues, carbon dioxide is carried out to the lungs, where it is continuously eliminated. As the Pco_2 within the cells is greater than in arterial blood entering the tissue capillaries, carbon dioxide diffuses initially from the mitochondria directly into the capillary blood, where Pco_2 increases. Then it is transported by peripheral venous blood to mixed venous blood (pulmonary artery) into the lungs, where carbon dioxide (range, 45–47 mmHg) leaves the blood by passive diffusion down its partial pressure gradient into the alveolar gas. Under normal resting conditions, the Pco_2 on both the alveolar and arterial sides is nearly identical (about 38–40 mmHg), slightly lower than in mixed venous blood.

Alveolar ventilation

Because the main achievement of the lung is pulmonary gas exchange, it has to facilitate oxygen movement from ambient air into the blood and to allow the excess of carbon dioxide produced by cellular metabolism to be eliminated from the blood. It is universally accepted that the process of movement of gas throughout the bronchial tree, and ultimately across the blood–gas interface, is passive diffusion from a zone of high partial pressure to one of low pressure. In this regard, both the thickness and wide surface of the blood–gas interface are very well suited for the purposes of gas exchange. *Fick's principle of diffusion* (see Diffusion, below) states that the amount of gas transferred across a tissue is directly proportional to the area and inversely proportional to the thickness.

The process of pulmonary ventilation is not continuous, as it is accomplished intermittently with each breath; similarly, the process of pulmonary capillary perfusion is not continuous either, as it is pulsatile, accelerating during systole and slowing during diastole. However, for the purposes of analysis it is useful to assume that the volume of gas in the lung at functional residual capacity is sufficiently large to cope with these oscillations such that alveolar ventilation and capillary blood flow can be regarded as if they were continuous.

At functional residual capacity, most of the gas volume, approximately 3 litres, is contained in the alveoli and only about 150 ml is contained in the conducting airways, those involved only in conducting air between the mouth and the periphery of the lung. During inspiration, the alveolar volume increases by an amount equal to tidal volume (V_T), nearly 500 ml, as the volume in the conducting airways remains essentially unchanged during quiet breathing. Yet the amount of fresh gas entering the alveoli during quiet breathing is only two-thirds of V_T, approximately 350 ml or 12% of total alveolar volume, since the first gas to enter the alveoli is the gas already located in the conducting airways. The product of V_T and respiratory frequency (f, usually 15 breaths · min⁻¹) is known as minute ventilation or total ventilation ($\dot{V}_E$, average 7500 ml · min⁻¹). Alveolar ventilation ($\dot{V}_A$) is the component of total ventilation that goes to ventilate alveoli, is part of gas exchange properly speaking and averages nearly 5250 ml · min⁻¹; anatomical dead space ventilation ($\dot{V}_D$) is the remainder portion of $\dot{V}_E$ that does not take part in gas exchange (approximately 2250 ml · min⁻¹).

As discussed, alveolar PO_2 is determined by a balance imposed by the continuous addition of oxygen by alveolar ventilation and its removal by the pulmonary blood flow. Blood returning to the lungs from the body carries carbon dioxide produced metabolically in the cells. Only a small part of this gas exits the blood as it transfers to alveolar gas to be eliminated to ambient air. The majority of the carbon dioxide remains in blood and passes into capillary blood. Accordingly, under steady-state conditions (i.e. stable ventilatory and haemodynamic conditions and stability in oxygen and carbon dioxide elimination), the volume of carbon dioxide eliminated from the lungs by alveolar ventilation ($\dot{V}CO_2$) is equal to that produced by the cells of the body.

The relationship between alveolar PCO_2 and alveolar ventilation is set out by the *ideal alveolar gas ventilation equation for carbon dioxide*, in which K is a constant:

$$\dot{V}_A = \frac{\dot{V}CO_2}{P_ACO_2} \cdot K \qquad \text{(Equation 4)}$$

Thus,

$$PCO_2 = \frac{\dot{V}CO_2}{\dot{V}_A} \cdot K \qquad \text{(Equation 5)}$$

Since blood leaving the alveoli will normally have the same PCO_2 as alveolar gas, the PCO_2 in arterial blood is almost identical to alveolar PCO_2 and can replace it in the equation. The significance of this relationship is a very important one, since it establishes that alveolar PCO_2 is set by the ratio of carbon dioxide production to the alveolar ventilation such that, for a given metabolic production of this gas, changes in alveolar ventilation provoke reciprocal changes in alveolar PCO_2. For example, if the alveolar ventilation is halved, the PCO_2 shows a twofold increase; conversely, if the former is doubled, the latter is halved. It is of note, however, that this relationship is true only if a steady state has been re-established and the carbon dioxide production ($\dot{V}CO_2$) has been reset as before.[5,31,32]

Alveolar PO_2 and PCO_2, and hence arterial PO_2 and PCO_2 in a perfect, homogeneous lung, are related through a very important relationship, the *ideal alveolar gas equation for oxygen*:

$$P_AO_2 = P_IO_2 - \frac{P_ACO_2}{R} + \left[[P_ACO_2 \cdot F_IO_2] \cdot \frac{[1-R]}{R} \right]$$

$$\text{(Equation 6)}$$

where R is the respiratory exchange ratio or $\dot{V}CO_2/\dot{V}O_2$, often assumed (at about 0.8), since it is not considered worth measuring as it requires expired gases. Under steady-state conditions, R is equal to the metabolic respiratory quotient (RQ), defined as the number of carbon dioxide molecules produced relative to oxygen molecules consumed by intermediary metabolism.

This equation can be also expressed more simply as:

$$P_AO_2 = P_IO_2 - \frac{P_ACO_2}{R} \qquad \text{(Equation 7)}$$

since the term in brackets is a correction factor for the difference between inspired and expired volumes, being quantitatively negligible during quiet breathing (1–3 mmHg), and can be disregarded in most clinical conditions. The value of alveolar PO_2 calculated with this equation is then nearly that value expected if the lung was ideally perfect. This difference is termed *alveolar–arterial PO_2 difference or gradient* and is given by the following relationship:

$$AaPO_2 = \left[P_IO_2 - \frac{P_aCO_2}{R} \right] - P_aO_2 \qquad \text{(Equation 8)}$$

where P_IO_2 during quiet breathing, at ambient air and sea level, is in the range of 148–150 mmHg. Under air-breathing conditions, this equation is in practice very useful for estimating the degree of alveolar hypoventilation. Normally, there is always a small $AaPO_2$ in the range of 4–8 mmHg due to gravitational topographical $\dot{V}_A/\dot{Q}$ differences and to the admixture of small amounts of venous blood to arterial blood (see Ventilation–perfusion relationships, below). Therefore, any difference greater than that physiologically expected between the calculated P_AO_2 and the directly measured P_aO_2 becomes a rough estimate of $\dot{V}_A/\dot{Q}$ mismatch, increased intrapulmonary shunt and/or diffusion limitation, alone or in combination; and conversely, a normal $AaPO_2$ will preferentially reflect a condition of alveolar hypoventilation (Table 2.5.2). However, the $AaPO_2$ can be markedly affected by the lack of steady-state conditions, the level of inspired oxygen, changes in mixed venous blood and the shape of the oxyhaemoglobin dissociation curve.[33] From a clinical viewpoint, it is important to point out a characteristic feature of alveolar hypoventilation, i.e. the response to supplementary oxygen provided that minute ventilation remains unchanged. It follows from the alveolar gas equation alluded to that any small increase in the inspiratory PO_2 will optimise substantially the levels of alveolar PO_2 (Table 2.5.2).

Hypoventilation occurs when alveolar ventilation is inadequately reduced relative to $\dot{V}CO_2$ and the alveolar PCO_2 settles out at a lower level than the physiological range. In practice, the hypoxaemia is usually of less importance than the level of hypercapnia. In general, for any increase in P_ACO_2 there is a commensurate fall in P_AO_2, with only a smaller lower difference in P_aO_2. The respiratory control centres in the brain stem regulate minute ventilation in accordance with the level of carbon dioxide production. An increase in arterial PCO_2 induces a reduced pH, or respiratory acidosis, whereas a decrease in arterial PCO_2 produces an increased pH, or respiratory alkalosis. The

Table 2.5.2 Behaviour of arterial P_{O_2} and P_{CO_2} and of the alveolar–arterial P_{O_2} difference in alveolar hypoventilation, alveolar–capillary diffusion impairment, increased intrapulmonary shunt and ventilation–perfusion imbalance

	Alveolar hypoventilation	Abnormal diffusion	Intrapulmonary shunt	Ventilation–perfusion inequality
Arterial P_{O_2}	↓	↓	↓	↓
Arterial P_{CO_2}	↑	↓	↓	↓–↑
Alveolar–arterial P_{O_2} difference	–	↑	↑	↑
Effects of 100% O_2 on P_aO_2	+++	+++	–	+++

–, unchanged; ↓, decreased; ↑, increased; +++, markedly increased ($P_aO_2 \geq 400$ mmHg).

body controls changes in pH by regulating the alveolar P_{CO_2}, in order to offset enzymatic and cellular disruptions provoked by acid–base disturbances.

The most common clinical conditions related to hypoxaemia and hypercapnia due to alveolar hypoventilation include any depression of respiratory centres induced either spontaneously or by drugs, disorders involving anterior horn cells, respiratory muscle fatigue or weakness, myoneural junctions, thoracic cage deformities, sleep apnoea syndrome, upper airway obstruction and metabolic alkalosis. Yet, as a mechanism of abnormal arterial blood gases it is less relevant, less common, in the clinical set-up, than $\dot{V}_A/\dot{Q}$ mismatching or increased intrapulmonary shunt. Moreover, it is often present in conjunction with $\dot{V}_A/\dot{Q}$ imbalance.[26] Thus, respiratory muscle fatigue or weakness is commonly demonstrated in the context of widespread obstructive airway diseases, such as chronic obstructive pulmonary disease (COPD). Likewise, several chronic neuromuscular and sleep apnoea conditions, including morbid obesity, can facilitate the coexistence of $\dot{V}_A/\dot{Q}$ inequalities with or without some degree of increased intrapulmonary shunt, as the original process ultimately alters the normal physiology of the airways and the lung parenchyma.

There is only a single clinical condition in which alveolar hypoventilation is not associated with arterial hypercapnia, so-called *hypopnea*, observed during the routine application of haemodialysis.[34] This essentially happens because of a decrease in carbon dioxide production secondary to continuous carbon dioxide losses through the membrane dialyser during this specific therapeutic procedure. It follows from the alveolar gas equation (see Equation 4) that a decrease in carbon dioxide production may produce a reduction in alveolar ventilation without any accompanying changes in the levels of alveolar (arterial) P_{CO_2}.

Diffusion

In the air spaces of the lung, diffusion is the primary mechanism responsible for transport of oxygen (and other gases) from the most peripheral airways to and through the alveolar–capillary interface that separates alveolar gas from capillary blood. Diffusion also involves the process by which gases, notably oxygen, move from capillary blood into the interior of the cells and by which carbon dioxide produced in the cell moves out into the blood.

Oxygen and carbon dioxide diffuse simply passively from regions of higher partial pressure to lower partial pressure, without expending energy expenditure, following *Fick's law of diffusion*. This equation states that the rate of diffusion (or transfer) of a gas (V_G, in ml · min⁻¹) through the liquid barrier is directly proportional to the available surface area for diffusion (A, in cm²), the diffusion coefficient (D, in cm² · mmHg⁻¹ · min⁻¹), and the partial pressure difference across the alveolar to end-capillary interface ($P_1 - P_2$, in mmHg), and inversely proportional to its thickness (T):

$$\dot{V}_G = \frac{A}{T} \cdot D \cdot (P_1 - P_2). \qquad \text{(Equation 9)}$$

The available surface area for gas exchange between alveolar gas and pulmonary capillary blood is ideally suited for passive diffusion. It is extensive, as it ranges between 50 m² and 100 m², contains approximately 300 million alveoli and has a blood–gas interface up to 0.3 μm thick. The rate of diffusion is also proportional to a diffusion coefficient (D) that depends on the physical and chemical properties of the tissue and of the specific gas. Moreover, this diffusion constant is a direct function of the solubility of the gas (Sol) in the interface (or barrier) liquid and inversely proportional to the square root of the molecular weight (mol. wt) of that gas:

$$D \propto \frac{\text{Sol}}{\sqrt{\text{mol. wt}}}. \qquad \text{(Equation 10)}$$

The solubility is defined as the volume of gas (in millilitres) that must be dissolved in 100 ml of the interface liquid to raise the partial pressure in it by 1 mmHg. When the solubility of a gas in the tissue (membrane) is large, gas will diffuse at a faster rate through the interface such that, if the gas is highly soluble in the membrane, it will become dissolved more readily than an insoluble gas.

The dependence of diffusion on molecular weight relates to the velocity of the molecular motion in a gas, such that the heavier the molecular weight of a gas the slower its rate of diffusion. Because carbon dioxide has a much higher solubility (24:1) than oxygen but the square root of the molecular weight is very much the same, carbon dioxide diffuses through tissue 20 times more rapidly than oxygen.

Oxygen, carbon dioxide and carbon monoxide all combine chemically with blood, resulting in non-linear relationships

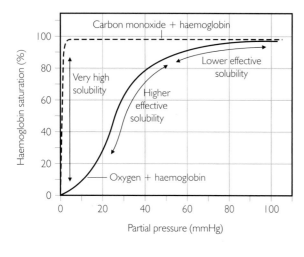

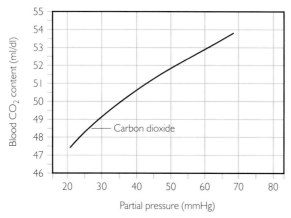

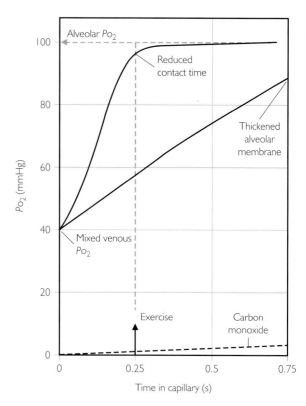

Figure 2.5.4 Oxygen, carbon monoxide and carbon dioxide contents plotted against their own partial pressures in arterial blood. The slope of the line at any point corresponds to the effective solubility of each gas. Oxygen is highly soluble at partial pressures of 20–60 mmHg but relatively insoluble above 100 mmHg. Compared to oxygen, carbon dioxide is much more soluble in blood, with a steeper slope, and its solubility is relatively constant as a function of partial pressure. Effective carbon monoxide solubility is very high at partial pressures below 1 mmHg; above 1 mmHg, carbon monoxide content increases by adding dissolved carbon monoxide only and solubility is low. (With permission from Leff & Schumacker 1993.[35])

Figure 2.5.5 Characteristic time courses of partial pressures of oxygen along the pulmonary capillary under normal diffusion conditions, at rest and during exercise, and also when the blood–gas interface is pathologically thickened (for further explanation, see text). (With permission from West 1998.[36])

between their partial pressures and contents (millilitres of dissolved gas per decilitre of liquid)[35] (Figure 2.5.4; see Oxygen and carbon dioxide transport in blood, below). The slope of this relationship corresponds to its effective solubility. Thus, the effective solubility of oxygen in blood is low at high partial pressures (above 100 mmHg) where it is quite flat but becomes markedly increased at low partial pressures (below 60 mmHg) because of the lower, straighter shape of the oxygen dissociation curve. Because the solubility of carbon dioxide is much greater than oxygen, as we have seen, its slope is much steeper, although this relationship is more linear because the solubility varies less. As carbon monoxide shows a much steeper slope at partial pressures below 1 mmHg, its solubility in blood is extremely great; by contrast, at partial pressures above 1 mmHg carbon monox-

ide content increases by adding its dissolved component in blood only, resulting in little solubility.

The time spent by the blood in the pulmonary capillary under normal conditions at rest is approximately 0.75 s[36,37] (Fig. 2.5.5). At approximately a third of the available time in the capillary, the P_{O_2} and P_{CO_2} of pulmonary capillary blood almost reach that of the alveolar gas.[38] Both oxygen and carbon dioxide equilibrate at about the same rate, even though carbon dioxide diffuses through water about 20 times faster than oxygen, because the larger diffusion coefficient of carbon dioxide is offset by its lower membrane–blood solubility ratio.[39] In other words, there is usually ample time in the capillary for complete equilibration of the blood with alveolar gas for both physiological gases, such that the normal lung has substantial diffusion reserves. Under most normal conditions oxygen and carbon dioxide transfer are perfusion-limited, and only under very special or abnormal situations is oxygen transfer diffusion-limited.[40] Figure 2.5.4 also illustrates the fact that the transfer of carbon monoxide by the lung is diffusion-limited because of the very steep shape of its dissociation curve with blood. In fact, the avidity of carbon monoxide for haemoglobin is so high (approximately 300 times greater than that of oxygen) that its partial pressure in the blood of the pulmonary capillary is almost flat. In other words, the amount of carbon monoxide is taken up completely in the diffusion characteristics of the blood–gas barrier.

Why is gas exchange perfusion- or diffusion-limited? Gas transfer entering or leaving blood, is perfusion- or diffusion-limited as a function of the slope of the solubility of the blood dissociation curve to the solubility of the gas in the blood–gas barrier. To further understand the diffusion process across the blood–gas interface it is worth considering the behaviour of inert gases such as nitrogen, helium or sulphur hexafluoride. An inert gas is a gas that does not combine chemically with blood, so that its blood concentration is directly proportional to partial pressure, thus obeying *Henry's law of solubility*. Inert gases exhibit an almost identical solubility in blood and in the blood–gas membrane and have a rapid rate of equilibration along the pulmonary capillary, such that they are completely perfusion-limited in their transfer. By contrast, gases that combine chemically with blood, such as the physiological gases and carbon monoxide, have a much higher solubility in blood than in the membrane, resulting in a much slower rate of equilibration along the capillary. In the case of oxygen, under hypoxic conditions, the transfer is in part diffusion-limited because the lung is working low on the oxygen dissociation curve; by contrast, under hyperoxic conditions the transfer of oxygen is perfusion-limited because its blood concentration is high on the oxygen dissociation curve.[40]

During very intense exercise, the normal exchange of oxygen and carbon dioxide faces a marked reduction of the capillary transit time, to less than 0.25 s, such that blood leaves the capillary before the equilibration with alveolar gas has been fully completed. If this occurs, the exchange of the two physiological gases becomes diffusion-limited and arterial blood contains both a P_{O_2} that is lower and a P_{CO_2} that is slightly higher than alveolar gas, an effect only observed at extreme, strenuous exercise conditions.[41]

A similar situation can be detected at extremely high altitudes, i.e. on Mount Everest, where the inspired and alveolar P_{O_2} are reduced, both at rest and during exercise, because of the decrease in barometric pressure. On the summit of Mount Everest, atmospheric pressure is about a third of that at sea level. Under these extreme hypoxic conditions, the effective solubility of oxygen is increased whereas that of the blood–gas barrier remains unchanged, thus slowing the rate of oxygen equilibration along the pulmonary capillary and causing oxygen transfer to be limited by diffusion.

In interstitial lung disorders, the structural derangement at the interstitial space level should provoke a diffusion limitation to both oxygen and carbon dioxide. Indeed, oxygen and carbon dioxide are diffusion-limited both at rest and during exercise but this contributes only in part to the prevalent levels of hypoxaemia.[23] Yet this only represents a small proportion of the increased AaP_{O_2} observed at rest and slightly more during exercise. It is the degree of underlying $\dot{V}_A/\dot{Q}$ mismatch that is mostly responsible for the abnormally low $P_{a}O_2$ shown in fibrotic patients. By contrast, in patients with COPD whose predominant emphysematous component causes widespread destruction of alveolar walls and capillaries and marked reduction of diffusion surface, both oxygen and carbon dioxide remain perfusion-limited.[42] However, the conventional measurement of diffusing capacity for carbon monoxide is characteristically reduced in these two pathologically distinct entities.

In patients with arterial hypoxaemia caused by severe hepatopulmonary syndrome there can be a *diffusion–perfusion defect*, which represents less than 20% of increased AaP_{O_2} and aggravates the underlying degree of arterial deoxygenation.[25] Presumably, the distance is too great for adequate equilibration of oxygen with haemoglobin in the centre stream of the markedly dilated pulmonary capillary, a mechanism that is commonly exaggerated by a high cardiac output, resulting in a shorter transit time of the red blood cell.[24] This diffusion–perfusion defect was originally described in patients with multiple large arteriovenous fistulae (Rendu–Osler).[43]

In all these clinical conditions with diffusion limitation, in which the predominant process that causes arterial hypoxaemia is always the coexistence of $\dot{V}_A/\dot{Q}$ abnormalities, there is hypocapnia since patients commonly hyperventilate (Table 2.5.2). In addition, the levels of AaP_{O_2} are abnormally increased. The amount of arterial hypoxaemia is easily corrected with the administration of high levels of inspired oxygen.

Diffusing capacity

From Fick's law of diffusion (see Equation 9), it follows that the term $[A \cdot D/T]$ represents an effective conductance (or the inverse of resistance) for gas transfer from alveolus to blood. Because it is not possible to determine the surface area nor the thickness of the barrier, this equation can be rewritten combining its three components into one single constant, named D_L or diffusing capacity of the lung, as follows:

$$\dot{V}_G = D_L \cdot (P_1 - P_2). \qquad \text{(Equation 11)}$$

Because this equation is so complex for oxygen, as the P_{O_2} into the pulmonary capillary can never be measured, it can be reformulated taking advantage of the carbon monoxide properties such that the diffusing capacity for carbon monoxide after rearrangement of this equation is given by:

$$D_L = \frac{\dot{V}_{CO}}{P_1 - P_2} \qquad \text{(Equation 12)}$$

where P_1 and P_2 are the partial pressures of carbon monoxide in alveolar gas and pulmonary capillary blood respectively. Since the partial pressure of this gas is almost negligible in the pulmonary capillary blood, the equation can be rewritten as:

$$D_L CO = \frac{\dot{V}_{CO}}{P_A CO} \qquad \text{(Equation 13)}$$

where $P_A CO$ corresponds to the alveolar partial pressure of carbon monoxide. This equation states that the conductance (1/resistance) of carbon monoxide into blood, or diffusing capacity of the lung for carbon monoxide, equals the rate (in $ml \cdot min^{-1}$) at which carbon monoxide is taken up divided by the average alveolar partial pressure of CO (in mmHg).

The amount of oxygen or carbon monoxide taken up by the lungs per unit time ($ml \cdot min^{-1}$) depends on the resistance to gas uptake by the alveolar–capillary interface and also by that offered by the red blood cell and its rate of combination with haemoglobin. In other words, the total resistance to gas uptake ($1/D_L CO$) is made up of these two components as follows:

$$1/D_L CO = 1/D_M + 1/\theta V_C \qquad \text{(Equation 14)}$$

where l/D_M is the membrane resistance and $1/\theta V_C$ is the resistance to uptake into the red blood cell in combining with haemoglobin.[44] These two resistances are arranged in series and contribute almost in the same proportion to the total resistance to gas uptake. The term $1/\theta V_C$ is a function of the volume of blood in the pulmonary capillaries (V_C) and the rate at which the gas can combine with haemoglobin (θ). The latter varies with haemoglobin saturation and the haemoglobin concentration in blood. (See also Chapter 6.)

Ventilation–perfusion relationships

The alveolar-to-end-capillary diffusion equilibration is completed because of the partial pressure difference between alveolar gas and the capillary blood, a gradient that is maintained by alveolar ventilation to pulmonary blood flow balance. The alveolar ventilation–perfusion $\dot{V}_A/\dot{Q}$ ratio is defined as the ratio of its ventilation to pulmonary capillary blood flow, which is the most pivotal determinant of alveolar PO_2 and PCO_2. For the whole lung, the overall $\dot{V}_A/\dot{Q}$ ratio is the total alveolar ventilation $(\dot{V}_A)$ divided by the cardiac output $(\dot{Q}_T)$. However, this overall $\dot{V}_A/\dot{Q}$ ratio tells us very little about the entire gas exchange of the lung.

Under normal conditions, in any single alveolar unit the rate of equilibration for oxygen and carbon dioxide between alveolar gas and the pulmonary capillary are determined by the $\dot{V}_A/\dot{Q}$ ratio, the composition of the inspired gas and the composition of the mixed venous blood.[2] It is important to appreciate the key role played by these three components governing the respiratory gases in any single gas exchange unit. Figure 2.5.6 illustrates the behaviour of the end-capillary PO_2 and PCO_2 in a single functional unit of the lung, as the $\dot{V}_A/\dot{Q}$ ratio is increased. Note that, as the $\dot{V}_A/\dot{Q}$ ratio rises above 0.1, P_aO_2 increases sharply but there is still little change in P_aCO_2 until a $\dot{V}_A/\dot{Q}$ ratio of 1.0 is approached. Note that, if the overall $\dot{V}_A/\dot{Q}$ ratio increases (right-shifted), because overall ventilation is increased and/or cardiac

output is decreased, a situation commonly observed when mechanical ventilation is applied, this will tend to increase PO_2 and decrease PCO_2. And conversely, if ventilation is disturbed or decreased and/or cardiac output is increased, i.e. during weaning from the ventilator or while using vasodilators, then gas exchange worsens and respiratory gases become abnormal or further deteriorate. In a homogeneous lung, the ideal, perfect alveolar PO_2 can be calculated from the ideal alveolar gas equation (see Equation 6), while that of alveolar PCO_2 will be set by the level of carbon dioxide production relative to alveolar ventilation, or the ideal alveolar gas equation for carbon dioxide (see Equation 4). In addition, we know that the amount of carbon dioxide lost into alveolar gas from capillary blood per minute is given by:

$$\dot{V}CO_2 = \dot{Q} \cdot (C_{\bar{v}}CO_2 - C_{c'}CO_2) \qquad \text{(Equation 15)}$$

where $\dot{Q}$ is blood flow and C is the content of carbon dioxide in mixed venous blood $(\bar{v})$ and end-capillary blood flow (c′) respectively. Under steady-state conditions, both the amount of carbon dioxide exhaled from the alveoli and that lost from the pulmonary capillary blood flow must be equal, such that Equations 4 and 15 can be equated as follows:

$$\dot{V}_A \cdot P_A O_2 \cdot K = \dot{Q} \cdot (C_{\bar{v}}CO_2 - C_{c'}CO_2) \qquad \text{(Equation 16)}$$

and by rearrangement,

$$\dot{V}_A/\dot{Q} = \frac{C_{\bar{v}}CO_2 - C_{c'}CO_2}{P_A O_2} \cdot K \qquad \text{(Equation 17)}$$

In other words, the $P_A O_2$ and its corresponding end-capillary carbon dioxide content are determined by the $\dot{V}_A/\dot{Q}$ ratio. Although this equation appears to be relatively simple, this is not the case, as the alveolar PO_2 is an implicit variable to be considered: it increases when the $\dot{V}_A/\dot{Q}$ ratio rises. Moreover, the relationships between PCO_2 and content are not linear. Thus, it was only possible to solve the equation graphically using the *oxygen–carbon-dioxide diagram* designed by Riley & Cournand[45] and Rahn & Fenn[46] almost simultaneously. It was not until the introduction of numerical analysis by computer that the calculation of the specific distributions of $\dot{V}_A/\dot{Q}$ ratios became easier.

Figure 2.5.7 depicts an oxygen–carbon-dioxide diagram in which the composition of inspired and mixed venous PO_2 are constrained to a single line termed the ventilation–perfusion ratio line. In this scheme, diffusion between alveolar gas and end-capillary blood flow for respiratory gases is assumed to be complete.[36]

Intrapulmonary shunt

This term refers to an extreme end-spectrum of $\dot{V}_A/\dot{Q}$ inequality, by which there is continuous blood flow but no ventilation through non-ventilated areas of the lung. It is of note, however, that, under physiological conditions, there is always a small amount of shunt that reaches less than 1% of cardiac output. This normal or *physiological shunt*, also known as *postpulmonary shunt*,[12] essentially includes a small amount of venous blood that drains directly into the arterial pulmonary circulation (part of the venous drainage of the bronchial veins) and the systemic circulation (coronary thebesian veins drawing to the left ventricle).

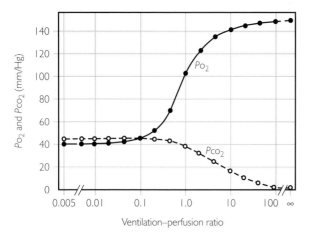

Figure 2.5.6 Variations in partial pressures of oxygen and carbon dioxide in a gas exchange alveolar unit modelled as a function of ventilation–perfusion ratio (for further explanation, see text). (Modified from West 1977.[2])

From a pathophysiological viewpoint, it is always useful to calculate the amount of venous blood flow that exits non-ventilated alveoli, namely intrapulmonary shunt, in relation to normal blood flow that is properly oxygenated. In its calculation it is stated that the total amount of oxygen that exits the system corresponds to the total blood flow, or cardiac output ($\dot{Q}_T$), times the oxygen concentration (or content, C) in the systemic arterial blood. This must be equal to the sum of the amount of oxygen in the shunted blood ($\dot{Q}_S \cdot C_{\bar{V}}O_2$) and that in the end-capillary blood ($[\dot{Q}_T - \dot{Q}_S] \cdot C_{C'}O_2$):

$$\dot{Q}_T \cdot C_aO_2 = (\dot{Q}_S \cdot C_{\bar{V}}O_2) + ([\dot{Q}_T - \dot{Q}_S] \times C_{C'}O_2)$$

(Equation 18)

The re-arrangement of this equation can solve the fraction of blood flow perfusion to the shunt fraction, giving:

$$\frac{\dot{Q}_S}{\dot{Q}_T} = \frac{C_{c'}O_2 - C_aO_2}{C_{c'}O_2 - C_{\bar{V}}O_2}$$

(Equation 19)

where $C_{C'}O_2$ is calculated from the ideal alveolar gas equation and the oxygen dissociation curve. The term $\dot{Q}_S/\dot{Q}_T$ is also known as *mixed venous admixture ratio*.

In this situation, there is usually no carbon dioxide retention even although this gas is not exchanged in the non-ventilated areas (Table 2.5.2). This is because the control of ventilation resets and increases minute ventilation to eliminate the excess of carbon dioxide through ventilated alveolar units. The calculation of the $AaPO_2$ will always provide abnormally increased values. Finally, breathing 100% oxygen will have little influence on the levels of baseline arterial PO_2 because the mixed venous blood of non-ventilated alveoli is never exposed to these levels of oxygen enrichment. Thus, it will continue to maintain a low arterial PO_2. Nevertheless, there can be some improvement in arterial PO_2 essentially motivated by the added oxygen from the dissolved component. The latter is the product of arterial PO_2 times the oxygen solubility in plasma that, added to the haemoglobin-bound oxygen component, will make up the total oxygen content of the arterial blood (C_aO_2; see below).

The presence of an increased intrapulmonary shunt can be observed in the setting of catastrophic, acute respiratory failure, when alveoli are completely filled with water (oedema), blood and/or purulent secretions (acute respiratory distress syndrome, ARDS,[48–51] acute lung injury, ALI,[52] cardiogenic oedema or life-threatening pneumonia[53]). This also occurs when ventilation in a specific lung region is totally abolished because of complete bronchial occlusion (atelectasis) or complete collapse of the lung (massive pneumothorax or pleural effusion[54]). Moreover, congenital or acquired cardiac or pulmonary vascular disorders (arteriovenous fistulae; hepatopulmonary syndrome[24]) can be an important source of increased intrapulmonary shunting, by developing defects between the right and left sides of the cardiovascular system respectively. This situation can be viewed as a dramatic, unique, pattern of $\dot{V}_A/\dot{Q}$ inequality, i.e. zero $\dot{V}_A/\dot{Q}$ ratio, in that the process of arterial hypoxaemia responds very poorly, if at all, to 100% oxygen breathing.

Nevertheless, it is important to note that the response of gas exchange abnormalities to the administration of 100% oxygen

may differ between ARDS/ALI and severe pneumonia.[52] Thus, we know that, in patients with ARDS/ALI, the baseline levels of intrapulmonary shunt will increase by about 25% owing to the development of resorption atelectasis, whereas there is no inhibition or release of hypoxic pulmonary vasoconstriction. The latter phenomenon is evidenced by a significant further worsening in $\dot{V}_A/\dot{Q}$, essentially indicated by an increase in the areas with a low $\dot{V}_A/\dot{Q}$ ratio.[52] By contrast, in patients with life-threatening pneumonia with similar volumes of basal increased intrapulmonary shunt, breathing 100% oxygen further deteriorates $\dot{V}_A/\dot{Q}$ mismatch because of hypoxic vasoconstriction attenuation without influencing the pre-existing levels of shunt.[53] As a consequence of this oxygen response, arterial PO_2 in patients with ARDS/ALI remains nearly unchanged while breathing 100% oxygen, whereas it increases markedly in those with life-threatening pneumonia.

Ventilation–perfusion mismatch

As alluded to, one of the most influential determinants of alveolar PO_2 and PCO_2 is $\dot{V}_A/\dot{Q}$ inequality. It is of note that, under physiological conditions, there is always some $\dot{V}_A/\dot{Q}$ imbalance owing to topographic inequality induced by gravitational differences. Because of the influence of gravity on pleural and transpulmonary pressures, alveoli are better ventilated near the bottom than at the top of the lungs;[54] by the same token, perfusion is more prominent in the alveoli located at the bottom than in those at the top.[55] Thus, both alveolar ventilation and blood flow per unit volume increase from top to bottom of the lung.[56]

Nevertheless, these changes do not run in parallel. The gravitational changes in the distribution in alveolar ventilation are less noticeable than those in blood flow. Accordingly, the $\dot{V}_A/\dot{Q}$ ratio is substantially increased at the top and markedly decreased at the bottom of the lungs.[56] Under normal conditions, this physiological heterogeneity of the distribution of the $\dot{V}_A/\dot{Q}$ ratio makes the overall gas exchange of the lung less efficient. Thus, the arterial blood exiting the apex of the lung, where areas with a high $\dot{V}_A/\dot{Q}$ ratio predominate, will have a much higher PO_2 and a much lower PCO_2 than that leaving from the alveoli located at the bases, where areas with a low $\dot{V}_A/\dot{Q}$ ratio are widespread. These natural differences in the heterogeneity of the $\dot{V}_A/\dot{Q}$ distribution form the basis of the abnormalities observed during clinical conditions, in that they are overall accentuated and spread more unpredictably and chaotically through the lung parenchyma. As mentioned, abnormal alveolar ventilation to pulmonary perfusion balance is the most common cause of altered respiratory physiological gases, including carbon dioxide retention, in respiratory medicine. This inefficiency, however, applies to any gas that can be transferred by the lung and ultimately depends on the solubility or slope of the blood dissociation curve of each gas.

Traditionally, one of the most common approaches for assessing the extent of $\dot{V}_A/\dot{Q}$ imbalance has been through the three-compartment model of the lung originally introduced in the middle 1950s.[44,45] This has been, and it still is, a particularly useful way of interpreting $\dot{V}_A/\dot{Q}$ mismatch in the setting of acute lung problems. This model is made up of three populations or compartments of alveoli[46] (Fig. 2.5.7). The first com-

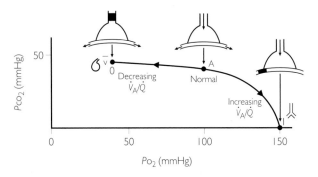

Figure 2.5.7 Schematic representation of the three-compartment lung model. Oxygen–carbon dioxide diagram showing a $\dot{V}_A/\dot{Q}$ ratio line. Both the oxygen and carbon dioxide partial pressures of an alveolar unit move along this line from the mixed venous point ($\bar{v}$), to the inspired gas point (I), through the alveolar gas point (A – alveolar gas for a lung unit with a normal $\dot{V}_A/\dot{Q}$ ratio). For further explanation, see text. (With permission from West 1998.[47])

partment is a hypothetical subset that is not ventilated but receives perfusion ($\dot{V}_A/\dot{Q} = 0$) and represents the *shunt compartment*. Under clinical conditions, its relevance can be calculated by means of the mixed venous admixture ratio ($\dot{Q}_S/\dot{Q}_T$) (see Equation 19). Normally, it does not exceed 1% of cardiac output. The second compartment corresponds to the *ideal* lung, in which the matching of ventilation and blood flow is perfect and homogeneous and where all the possible compositions of alveolar gas and arterial blood are consistent with the overall metabolic needs. The $\dot{V}_A/\dot{Q}$ ratio in this population of alveoli is usually within a normal range, located between 0.3 and 10, and the ideal alveolar P_{O_2} is calculated from the ideal alveolar gas equation (see Equation 6). The third population of alveoli receives ventilation but no perfusion such that the balance of ventilation to perfusion is infinite ($\dot{V}_A/\dot{Q}$ ratio = ∞). This third compartment matches perfectly with the traditional index or descriptor of physiological dead space, which refers to the total amount of wasted ventilation, including that due to the anatomical dead space (see Alveolar

ventilation, above) as well as any other wasted in excessively ventilated alveoli. In healthy individuals, the normal value of the physiological dead space represents about 20–25% of minute ventilation. The physiological dead space (V_{Dphys}) can be calculated from *Bohr's dead space equation*, as follows:

$$\frac{V_{Dphys}}{V_T} = \frac{P_aCO_2 - P_ECO_2}{P_aCO_2} \qquad \text{(Equation 20)}$$

where V_T is tidal volume and P_ECO_2 is expired P_{CO_2}, while it is assumed that ideal P_{CO_2} in alveolar gas and arterial P_{CO_2} are almost equal.

All in all, this three-compartment model approach has proved to be very useful in clinical practice to assess the underlying degree of $\dot{V}_A/\dot{Q}$ imbalance. Accordingly, areas with predominant intrapulmonary shunt, i.e. non-ventilated or very poorly ventilated but well-perfused alveoli, and/or physiological dead space, including non-perfused or poorly perfused but well-ventilated alveoli, could be calculated by using the equations given by the mixed venous admixture ratio (Equation 19) and the physiological dead space (Equation 20).

A new approach, based on the principles governing inert gas elimination or the multiple inert gas elimination technique (MIGET), represents a major conceptual breakthrough in our understanding of the pathophysiology of pulmonary gas exchange in disease states.[14-18] The basic principles and technical details of MIGET have been extensively addressed in other publications, to which the reader is referred for further information. Suffice to say that MIGET affords three major advantages over the previously reported traditional tools. First, it estimates the pattern of pulmonary blood flow and alveolar ventilation and calculates the mismatch of $\dot{V}_A/\dot{Q}$ relationships. Second, it partitions the AaP_{O_2} gradient into components of increased intrapulmonary shunt, $\dot{V}_A/\dot{Q}$ inequality and diffusion limitation to oxygen. And lastly, it apportions and unravels arterial P_{O_2} and P_{CO_2} changes into intrapulmonary and extrapulmonary (or systemic) determinants[12,13] (Table 2.5.3). An additional advantage is that measurements can be made at any inspired P_{O_2} without perturbing the vascular or bronchial wall tone, as inspired oxygen fraction needs not be altered.

Table 2.5.3 Intra- and extrapulmonary V factors determining hypoxaemia or hypercapnia.

Intrapulmonary	Extrapulmonary (systemic)	
Factors determining hypoxaemia		
$\dot{V}_A/\dot{Q}$ mismatch	Primary factors:	Decreased ventilation
Intrapulmonary shunt		Decreased cardiac output
Diffusion limitation		Decreased inspired P_{O_2}
		Increased O_2 uptake
	Secondary factors:	Decreased P_{50}
		Decreased haemoglobin
		Increased pH
Factors determining hypercapnia		
$\dot{V}_A/\dot{Q}$ mismatch	Primary factors:	Decreased ventilation
	Secondary factors:	Increased CO_2 production
		Metabolic alkalosis

When an inert gas dissolved in saline is steadily infused into the venous circulation, the proportion of gas that is eliminated by ventilation from the blood of a given lung unit is a function of the solubility of the gas and the ventilation–perfusion ratio.[14–18] In essence, this is the simple physiological principle behind MIGET. This relationship is expressed as:

$$\frac{P_{C'}}{P_{\bar{v}}} = \frac{\lambda}{\lambda + \dot{V}_A/\dot{Q}}$$ (Equation 21)

where $P_{c'}$ is the partial pressure of the gas in end-capillary blood, and λ is the blood–gas coefficient partition. The ratio of $P_{c'}$ to $P_{\bar{v}}$ is known as the *retention*.

Figure 2.5.2 illustrates a characteristic representative distribution of a healthy, young individual breathing room air at rest, obtained with MIGET. Each data point represents a particular value for blood flow or alveolar ventilation, while overall pulmonary perfusion and total ventilation corresponds to the sum of each data point (the lines have been drawn for clarity only). These quantities (distributions) are plotted against a wide range of $\dot{V}_A/\dot{Q}$ ratios, from zero (shunt) to infinity (dead space) on a log scale. The unimodal pattern of each distribution has three main characteristics: symmetry, location around a $\dot{V}_A/\dot{Q}$ ratio of 1.0 and narrowness (very little dispersion). Note that there is no inert gas shunt (compared to the concept of mixed venous admixture ratio), as the tracer nature of inert gases used for MIGET are insensitive to the presence of postpulmonary shunt (i.e. the bronchial–pulmonary communications and thebesian circulations). Inert gas physiological dead space is also slightly lower than Bohr's dead space because it does not include all those alveolar areas whose alveolar P_{CO_2} is lower than arterial.

Ventilation–perfusion mismatching is the principal determinant governing abnormal arterial blood gases in respiratory medicine either alone or in conjunction with increased intrapulmonary shunt. In general, most of the spectrum of chronic respiratory conditions – COPD,[42,58] bronchial asthma[59] and interstitial lung disorders[60] – show major or minor degrees of $\dot{V}_A/\dot{Q}$ imbalance both in stable and acute (exacerbations) conditions (Fig. 2.5.8). Under conditions of $\dot{V}_A/\dot{Q}$ inequality, arterial hypoxaemia, with or without hypercapnia, and increased AaP_{O_2} are common traits of abnormal pulmonary gas exchange (Table 2.5.2) The response to high levels of enriched inspired fractions of oxygen is commonly very positive, with substantial increases in arterial P_{O_2}, a finding that is also accompanied by a small increase in arterial P_{CO_2}.[52] As inspired oxygen will reach all the alveolar units of the lung, even those with the most modest low $\dot{V}_A/\dot{Q}$ relationship, alveolar P_{O_2} can always be improved. This benefit is sufficiently efficient to fully oxygenate the blood exiting the lung. Despite the significant increase in arterial P_{O_2} during 100% oxygen breathing, the underlying degree of $\dot{V}_A/\dot{Q}$ inequality is further impaired because of the simultaneous mitigation of hypoxic pulmonary vasoconstriction.[61]

Oxygen and carbon dioxide transport in blood

This section deals with the mechanisms involved in carriage of the two respiratory gases, oxygen and carbon dioxide, in blood and with the determinants that modulate the uptake and release of these gases from pulmonary capillary blood through the body tissues. The consumption of oxygen into blood passing through the lung capillaries is interdependently favoured by the elimination of carbon dioxide from the blood to the alveolar gas compartment; and conversely, the release of carbon dioxide is facilitated by the simultaneous uptake of oxygen. In other words, blood is ideally suited to the simultaneous interdependence of the transport of oxygen to the tissues and carbon dioxide to the lungs.

Oxygen

The molecules of oxygen are carried in two forms in blood. The most relevant component is combined with haemoglobin within the red blood cell while a small amount is simply dissolved in the blood. The dissolved portion of oxygen is proportional to the P_{O_2} and is calculated by the product of the partial pressure of oxygen and the solubility of oxygen in plasma, which is very low ($0.003\ ml \cdot dl^{-1} \cdot mmHg$). Thus, for a normal P_aO_2 value of 100 mmHg, the dissolved component must contain $0.3\ ml \cdot dl^{-1}$. The portion of dissolved oxygen, usually very small and negligible, may become slightly relevant when an individual is asked to breathe 100% oxygen. Under normal conditions, this will produce an alveolar P_{O_2} of the order of 600 mmHg, so that the amount of oxygen dissolved in the blood will become nearly $2\ ml \cdot dl^{-1}$.

Haemoglobin (Hb) is a molecule contained in red blood cells that consists of an iron-containing porphyrin compound (haem) and a protein with four polypeptide chains (globin). During intrauterine life, there is a fetal form of haemoglobin (HbF), which is gradually replaced after birth by newly formed red blood cells that contain adult HbA. HbA is composed of two types of polypeptide chain, α and β, whereas in HbF the β chain is replaced by two γ chains. Differences in the amino-acid sequences of haemoglobin produce different subsets of haemoglobin in humans. For instance, HbS (sickle) contains valine instead of glutamic acid in the β chains.

The avidity with which oxygen binds to haemoglobin is clearly modulated by its tertiary molecular structure and the changes in confirmation that it undergoes as oxygen is bound or released. Under these circumstances, the affinity of haemoglobin for oxygen is abnormally reduced, so that oxygen carriage is abnormally jeopardised. Many abnormal varieties of haemoglobin have been reported in the literature. Methaemoglobin is produced when the ferrous ion of normal HbA is oxidised to the ferric form, a situation that occurs in the presence of various drugs and chemicals or when there is deficiency of the enzyme cytochrome b5 reductase within the red blood cell. In addition to not be suitable for an efficient oxygen transport, methaemoglobin increases oxygen affinity of the remaining haemoglobin, hence minimising the unloading of oxygen to the tissues.

Blood carries large quantities of oxygen because its binding to haemoglobin to form oxyhaemoglobin is easily reversible. The molecular weight of haemoglobin is nearly 65 000 and each molecule can potentially bind to four oxygen atoms. When the saturation of haemoglobin is complete (100%), each gram may carry 1.39 ml of oxygen, which corresponds to the theoretical oxygen binding capacity of haemoglobin. Because normal blood has nearly 15 g Hb·dl⁻¹, the oxygen capacity when all the binding sites are

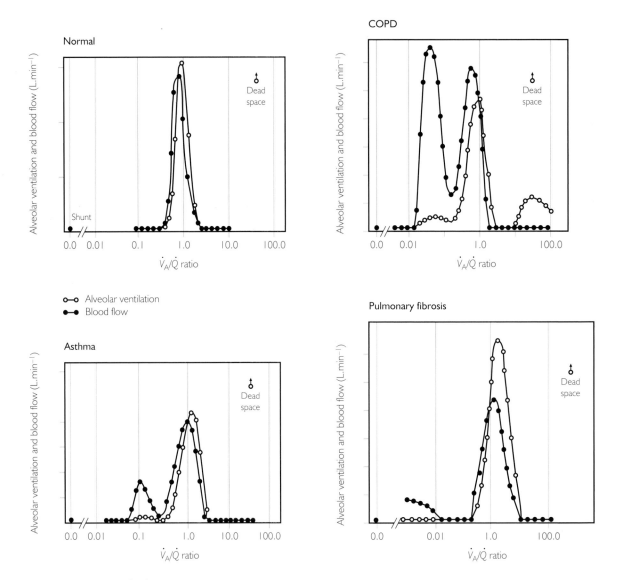

Figure 2.5.8 Distributions of $\dot{V}_A/\dot{Q}$ ratios in a normal individual (for comparison) and in patients with different respiratory diseases. In stable chronic obstructive pulmonary disease (COPD), a bimodal distribution of blood flow and ventilation is shown, reflecting the presence of areas with low and high $\dot{V}_A/\dot{Q}$ units; intrapulmonary shunt (left, bottom, closed symbol) is negligible whereas dead space (right, top, open symbol) is increased. In acute severe asthma, the most characteristic hallmark is a bimodal blood flow distribution, indicating the presence of extensive areas with low $\dot{V}_A/\dot{Q}$ ratios; shunt is also negligible. In stable lung fibrosis, $\dot{V}_A/\dot{Q}$ ratio distributions are moderately abnormal (widened) with a small bimodal blood flow distribution; dead space is increased.

occupied is about 20.8 ml O₂·dl⁻¹ of blood. The total content or concentration of oxygen in blood represents the volume of oxygen contained per unit volume of blood and includes both the combined and dissolved components as follows:

Oxygen content =

$$1.39 \; (ml \cdot g^{-1}) \cdot 14 \; (g \cdot dl^{-1}) \cdot \frac{[\% \; saturation]}{100}$$
$$+ \; 0.003 \; (ml \cdot dl^{-1} \cdot mmHg) \cdot P_{O_2} \; (mmHg)$$

(Equation 22)

A value of 1.34 m·g⁻¹Hb is sometimes used to represent the physiological oxygen binding capacity. The number of molecules bound to haemoglobin is a function of the P_{O_2} in the blood, also known as the *oxygen dissociation curve*. Figure 2.5.9

illustrates the relationship between the P_{O_2} in blood (abscissa) and the percentage of the oxygen binding sites that are occupied by oxygen molecules or haemoglobin saturation (ordinate). The characteristic curvilinear shape of this curve has two important pathophysiological advantages. Firstly, under normal conditions, the upper almost flat portion of the curve means that a marked fall of the normal P_{O_2} value (100 mmHg), of a magnitude of 20–30 mmHg, by accident or disease, is still compatible with a nearly complete haemoglobin saturation. In other words, the flat shape of the oxygen dissociation curve 'protects' against oxygen desaturation resulting from moderate decreases in the P_{O_2} in the arterial side. Secondly, the steep portion of the curve means that, as oxygen diffuses out of the capillary in the body tissues, the P_{O_2} in the plasma is reduced, thus provoking the dissociation of oxygen from haemoglobin inside the red

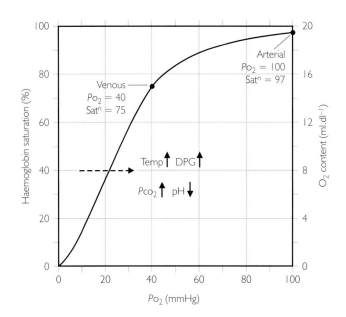

Figure 2.5.9 Oxyhaemoglobin dissociation curve and its modulation by minor extrapulmonary factors (for further explanation, see text). (With permission from West 1998.[47])

blood cells and diffusion into the plasma. In other words, considerable amounts of oxygen can be unloaded to the tissues without minimising the levels of Po_2 in the capillary. Indeed, by the time the red blood cell leaves from the end of the capillary it will have release only a small part of its oxygen content, approximately a quarter (the average mixed venous oxygen saturation is about 75%). This gives rise to a large partial pressure difference between the blood and the tissues, which facilitates diffusion out of the capillaries.

Various factors influence the position of the oxygen dissociation curve. A useful descriptor of the binding affinity of haemoglobin for oxygen is expressed by the Po_2 for 50% oxygen saturation, also known as haemoglobin P_{50} (normal value, about 27 mmHg). A higher P_{50} denotes a lower affinity, because a higher Po_2 is needed to achieve a given oxygen saturation. The curve is shifted to the right because of an increase in temperature, Pco_2 and hydrogen ion concentration (low pH) or an increase in 2,3-diphosphoglycerate (2,3-DPG), thus minimising the affinity of oxygen for haemoglobin. Bohr's effect corresponds to the effect of carbon dioxide on the affinity of haemoglobin for oxygen, part of which is due to the decrease in pH that occurs as Pco_2 increases and part to direct effects of carbon dioxide on the haemoglobin molecule. Moreover, the right shift of the oxygen dissociation curve assists in the unloading of more oxygen at any given Po_2. Conversely, a left shift of the curve is shown with decreases in temperature, Pco_2 and hydrogen ion concentration (high pH), or decreases in 2,3-DPG. This means an increase in the affinity of oxygen for haemoglobin. The compound 2,3-DPG is an end-product of the metabolism of the red blood cell that tends to increase during chronic hypoxaemia whereas it is depleted in blood storage in acid-citrate–dextrose anticoagulant solution.[62,63] However, the physiological relevance of changes in haemoglobin P_{50} caused by 2,3-DPG changes now appears to be relatively slight.

Carbon monoxide is a lipophilic molecule that combines with haemoglobin at the haem sites where oxygen binds. The affinity of haemoglobin for carbon monoxide is nearly 300 times higher than that for oxygen. Thus, with very low values of partial pressure, of the order of 0.5 mmHg, virtually all the binding sites on haemoglobin will become saturated by carbon monoxide (Fig. 2.5.4), hence profoundly minimising the unloading of oxygen in the peripheral tissues.

Systemic oxygen transport

While blood passes through the tissue capillaries and some of the transported molecules of oxygen move to the tissues, the rest stay in the blood and return to the lungs through the venous system. The cardiac output ($\dot{Q}_T$) is the amount of blood volume pumped by the heart to the body tissues. The systemic *oxygen delivery* (O_2D) or the total volume of oxygen carried to the systemic tissues per time unit can be calculated as the product of the cardiac output times the oxygen content of arterial blood (C_aO_2):

$$O_2D = \dot{Q}_T \cdot C_aO_2 \qquad \text{(Equation 23)}$$

A similar equation can be written to calculate the volume of oxygen that returns to the lung by using the oxygen content of mixed venous blood instead the arterial one. Accordingly, oxygen uptake or consumption ($\dot{V}O_2$) will be equal to cardiac output times the difference between arterial and mixed-venous oxygen content ($C_aO_2 - C_vO_2$):

$$\dot{V}O_2 = \dot{Q}_T \cdot (C_aO_2 - C_vO_2). \qquad \text{(Equation 24)}$$

This equation, also known as *Fick's principle*, is based on the principle of body mass conservation.

Carbon dioxide

To prevent the build-up of carbon dioxide, which is produced by the cell tissues at rest, this gas first diffuses into the local capillaries because the tissue Pco_2 is higher than in arterial blood entering the capillaries. Carbon dioxide is transported in the blood in three different forms: dissolved, as bicarbonate ions, the most important component, and in combination with proteins as carbamino compounds.

The dissolved carbon dioxide content is proportional to the Pco_2. Although carbon dioxide is more soluble in plasma than oxygen, but still has some degree of insolubility, relatively less carbon dioxide is carried in this form. Bicarbonate ions are formed directly from the hydroxylation of carbon dioxide by water (H^+OH^-) inside the red blood cells by the following hydration reaction, which is accelerated very rapidly by the enzyme carbonic anhydrase (present within the red blood cells but not in plasma):

$$(H^+OH^-) + CO_2 \leftrightarrow HCO_3^- + H^+. \qquad \text{(Equation 25)}$$

Most of the hydration of carbon dioxide therefore occurs in the red blood cells, so that bicarbonate ions move out of the red blood cell to be replaced by chloride ions to maintain electrical neutrality. This is known as the *chloride shift*. Some of the hydrogen ions formed in the red blood cell during the formation of bicarbonate and carbamino compounds are buffered by deoxygenated haemoglobin. Because the production of reduced haemoglobin is increased as oxygen is unloaded, this enhances the amount of carbon dioxide that can be taken up by the blood at any given P_{CO_2}. The effect of changes in oxyhaemoglobin saturation on the relationship of the carbon dioxide content to P_{CO_2} is called the *Haldane effect*.

The carbon dioxide dissociation curve is much more linear in its working range than the oxygen dissociation curve. As oxygen is released from blood along the tissue capillaries, the dissociation curve is shifted upwards. Thus, the lower the oxygen saturation of haemoglobin, the greater the carbon-dioxide content at any given P_{CO_2}. The shift is mostly caused by an enhanced ability of deoxygenated haemoglobin to form carbamino compounds. The third component is transported in chemical combination with haemoglobin, at a different site from where oxygen is bound. Carbamino compounds are formed when carbon dioxide combines with the terminal amine groups of blood proteins.

Extrapulmonary factors regulating partial pressure of oxygen

These factors are summarised in Table 2.5.3.

Inspired P_{O_2}

The influence of inspired O_2, one of the critical factors conforming P_{O_2} in a single unit, on P_aO_2 depends on the degree of underlying $\dot{V}_A/\dot{Q}$ mismatch. The end-capillary O_2 content rises as inspired O_2 is increased for conditions in which the level of $\dot{V}_A/\dot{Q}$ inequality are mild to moderate; by contrast, as the $\dot{V}_A/\dot{Q}$ imbalance becomes more severe the rise in the end-capillary O_2 content is much slower, reaching similar values to those obtained in moderate conditions but using much higher inspired P_{O_2} (of the order of 400–500 mmHg). By contrast, little change is shown in P_aO_2 at greater levels of shunt.[1]

When assessing the influence of the inspired P_{O_2} on $\dot{V}_A/\dot{Q}$ distributions, it must be borne in mind that this can be determined through two different mechanisms: hypoxic pulmonary vasoconstriction[64] and instability of alveolar units with very low $\dot{V}_A/\dot{Q}$ ratios (critical inspired $\dot{V}_A/\dot{Q}$ ratios).[65]

One of the main adjustments for $\dot{V}_A/\dot{Q}$ mismatch in the normal lung is the ability of the pulmonary vasculature to reduce perfusion and shift blood flow from collapsed areas, where alveolar P_{O_2} values are modest. Other things being equal, this will minimise the amount of $\dot{V}_A/\dot{Q}$ inequality in a diseased lung and limit the fall in P_aO_2. Hypoxic pulmonary vasoconstriction represents a major response of the pulmonary blood vessels that, although variable, is present in many chronic respiratory disorders, such as COPD[42,58] and bronchial asthma,[59] but also in some acute life-threatening conditions (i.e. pneumonia[53]), although its mechanism remains elusive as yet.

A theoretical analysis of the gas exchange factors involved in the development of shunt while breathing 100% O_2[65] showed that low inspired $\dot{V}_A/\dot{Q}$ ratios, termed 'critical', could result in a condition of absent expired ventilation, thus inducing reabsorption atelectasis in the alveoli. By increasing the inspired oxygen, such a critical unit will no longer eliminate gas but may continue gas uptake. Moreover, this unit becomes unstable and may ultimately collapse, leading to the development of reabsorption atelectasis, a classical observation evidenced in patients with ARDS/ALI requiring mechanical ventilation.[51,66]

Oxygen consumption

In a lung model of increased intrapulmonary shunt, P_aO_2 may be fairly sensitive to O_2 consumption changes, such that an increase from 300 ml · min[-1] to 600 ml · min[-1] only would decrease P_aO_2 by 10 mmHg.[10] In contrast, in a model characterised by pure $\dot{V}_A/\dot{Q}$ mismatch a 10% change in oxygen uptake can vary the P_aO_2 by 10 mmHg in either direction. The different results in each model may be related to the different degrees of P_aO_2 in each condition. When P_aO_2 is located in the lower, steeper, linear part of the oxyhaemoglobin dissociation curve in the shunt model, variations in $\dot{V}O_2$ induce fewer P_aO_2 changes. During exacerbations of COPD, $\dot{V}O_2$ is abnormally elevated during the most acute phase,[67] essentially because of increased work of breathing[68] but also because of the overuse of β-selective adrenergic agonists.[69] In these conditions, increased $\dot{V}O_2$ decreases by about 25% the levels of P_aO_2 observed during stable conditions.

Cardiac output

There are three potential ways in which cardiac output may modulate pulmonary gas exchange.[8,12,13,69] The most influential is by means of the effect on the O_2 content of the mixed venous blood, a well-known concept yet too often ignored in the clinical scenario. From Fick's principle (see Equation 24), it follows that:

$$C_{\bar{v}}O_2 = C_aO_2 - \left[\dot{V}O_2/\dot{Q}_T\right] \qquad \text{(Equation 26)}$$

such that mixed venous hypoxemia ($C_{\bar{v}}O_2$) may result from decreased arterial O_2 content, or either from increased O_2 consumption or depressed cardiac output, or both. A second way by which cardiac output may determine pulmonary gas exchange is by modifying the transit time of the red blood cell in the pulmonary capillary. If cardiac output increases, then the transit time decreases, such that abnormal gas exchange due to incomplete alveolar end-capillary equilibration may occur, as has been shown in idiopathic pulmonary fibrosis, both at rest and during exercise.[60] A third way by which cardiac output may influence gas exchange, common in critically sick patients, is by redistributing pulmonary blood flow within the lungs. Alterations in blood flow may be achieved by different means. One is through the well-known, although poorly understood, strong positive 'shunt–cardiac output' association; if shunt fraction increases then cardiac output rises, and vice versa.[8,70] Another way may be through modification of the pulmonary vascular tone, the major determinant of pulmonary vascular resistance; however, $P_{\bar{v}}O_2$ may also influence hypoxic vasoconstriction, at least in part, through an as yet undetermined pathway.[71] Finally, increases and decreases in intracardiac and pulmonary artery pressures may also lead to redistribution of pulmonary blood flow.[70]

Conclusion

In sum, there are several determinants governing Po_2 and Pco_2 in critical care and respiratory medicine[12,13] (Table 2.5.3). The most remarkable intrapulmonary factors are $\dot{V}_A/\dot{Q}$ and intrapulmonary shunt; by contrast, diffusion limitation to O_2 plays a marginal role. Among the extrapulmonary factors, inspired Po_2, overall ventilation, cardiac output and oxygen consumption are viewed as the most influential. Note that the three intrapulmonary factors plus oxygen consumption are not under the direct control of the physician, but the three extrapulmonary factors are. Clinicians may easily control inspired Po_2, the amount and pattern of total ventilation by means of the use of mechanical ventilators; and, to some extent, cardiac output, particularly during vasodilator medication. Arterial Po_2 may fall if inspired Po_2, overall ventilation and/or cardiac output decrease, and/or if oxygen consumption increases, even though the intrapulmonary factors remain unaltered. And conversely, if inspired Po_2, ventilation and/or cardiac output increase, and/or O_2 uptake decreases, P_aO_2 may increase irrespective of the changes that may operate at the level of the intrapulmonary determinants. Notice also that the three intrapulmonary factors, along with overall ventilation, constitute the four classical mechanisms of hypoxaemia and hypercapnia. It is interesting that changes in the minor factors determining the oxyhaemoglobin dissociation (temperature, Pco_2, pH) curve may also minimally modulate P_aO_2, just as

changes in acid–base balance and/or carbon dioxide production, along with alveolar ventilation, may be more influential on the levels of arterial Pco_2.[72,73] This is why P_aO_2 and P_aco_2 are the endpoint outcomes of the interaction of all the intrapulmonary and extrapulmonary determinants of gas exchange. This represents a more novel concept to properly interpret arterial blood gas changes at the bedside.

Clinical relevance

- When the lung fails as a gas-exchange organ, either arterial hypoxaemia and/or hypercapnia, appear and respiratory insufficiency ensues.

- Abnormal alveolar ventilation to pulmonary perfusion ($\dot{V}_A/\dot{Q}$) balance is the most common cause of altered respiratory physiological gases, including carbon dioxide retention, in respiratory medicine.

- In shunt, the breathing of 100% oxygen will have little influence on the levels of arterial Po_2 because the mixed venous blood through non-ventilated alveoli is never exposed to these levels of oxygen enrichment.

- In interstitial lung disorders, oxygen and carbon dioxide are diffusion-limited both at rest and during exercise but this contributes only in part to the current levels of hypoxaemia.

- The oxygen dissociation curve is shifted to the right because of an increase in temperature, Pco_2 and hydrogen ion concentration, or an increase in 2,3-diphosphoglycerate, and decreases the affinity of oxygen for haemoglobin.

- The systemic oxygen delivery can be calculated as the product of the cardiac output times the oxygen content of arterial blood.

- Arterial Po_2 and Pco_2 become the end-point outcomes of the interaction of all the intrapulmonary and extrapulmonary determinants of gas exchange.

References

1. West JB. Ventilation-perfusion inequality and overall gas exchange in computer models of the lung. Respir Physiol 1969; 7: 88–110.
2. West JB. Ventilation-perfusion relationships. Am Rev Respir Dis 1977; 116: 919–943.
3. Roca J, Rodríguez-Roisin R, Wagner PD. Pulmonary and peripheral gas exchange and their interactions. In: Roca J, Rodríguez-Roisin R, Wagner PD, ed. Pulmonary and peripheral gas exchange in health and disease. New York: Marcel Dekker; 2000: 1–27.
4. Roca J, Wagner PD. Contribution of multiple inert gas elimination technique to pulmonary medicine. 1: Principles and information content of the multiple inert gas elimination technique. Thorax 1993; 49: 815–824.
5. West JB. Causes of carbon dioxide retention in lung disease. N Engl J Med 1971; 284: 1232–1236.
6. Weinberger SE, Schwartzstein RM, Weis JW. Hypercapnia. N Engl J Med 1989; 321: 1223–1231.
7. West JB. Ventilation/blood flow and gas exchange, 4th ed. Oxford: Blackwell Scientific Publications; 1985.
8. Dantzker, DR. The influence of cardiovascular function on gas exchange. Clin Chest Med 1983; 4: 149–159.
9. Light RB. Intrapulmonary oxygen consumption in experimental pneumococcal pneumonia. J Appl Physiol 1988; 64: 2490–2495.
10. Wagner PD. Ventilation-perfusion inequality in catastrophic lung disease. In: Prakash O, ed. Applied physiology in clinical respiratory care. The Hague: Martinus Nijhoff; 1982: 363–379.
11. Rodríguez-Roisin R, Wagner PD. Clinical relevance of ventilation-perfusion inequality determined by inert gas elimination. Eur Respir J 1990; 3: 469–482.
12. Wagner PD, Rodríguez-Roisin R. Clinical advances in pulmonary gas exchange (State of the Art/Conference Report). Am Rev Respir Dis 1991; 143: 883–888.
13. Wagner PD, Saltzman HA, West JB. Measurements of continuous distributions of ventilation-perfusion ratios: theory. J Appl Physiol 1974; 36: 588–599.
14. Wagner PD, Naumann PF, Laravuso RB, West JB. Simultaneous measurement of eight foreign gases in blood by gas chromatography. J App Physiol 1974; 36: 600–605.
15. Evans JW, Wagner PD. Limits on $\dot{V}_A/\dot{Q}$ distributions from analysis of experimental inert gas elimination. J Appl Physiol 1977; 36: 600–605.
16. Wagner PD. Susceptibility of different gases to ventilation-perfusion inequality. J Appl Physiol 1979; 46: 372–386.
17. Wagner PD, Laravuso RB, Uhl RR, West JB. Continuous distributions of ventilation-perfusion ratios in normal subjects breathing air and 100% O_2. J Clin Invest 1974; 54: 54–68.
18. West JB, Wagner PD. Pulmonary gas exchange. In: West JB, ed. Bioengineering aspects of the lung. New York: Marcel Dekker; 1977: 361–457.
19. Gale GE, Torre-Bueno J, Moon RE et al. Ventilation-perfusion inequality in normal humans during exercise. J Appl Physiol 1985; 58: 978–988.
20. Wagner PD, Gale GE, Moon RE et al. Pulmonary gas exchange in humans exercising at sea level and simulated altitude. J Appl Physiol 1986; 61: 260–270.
21. Hammond MD, Gale GE, Kapitan KS et al. Pulmonary gas exchange in humans during normobaric hypoxic exercise. J Appl Physiol 1986; 60: 1590–1598.
22. Hammond MD, Gale GE, Kapitan KS et al. Pulmonary gas exchange in humans during normobaric hypoxic exercise. J Appl Physiol 1985; 58: 978–988.
23. Agusti AG, Roca J, Rodríguez-Roisin R et al. Mechanisms of gas exchange impairment in idiopathic pulmonary fibrosis. Am Rev Respir Dis 1991; 143: 219–225.
24. Rodríguez-Roisin R, Agusti AGN, Roca J. The hepatopulmonary syndrome: new name, old complexities (editorial). Thorax 1992; 47: 897–902.
25. Martinez GP, Barberà JA, Visa J et al. Hepatopulmonary syndrome in candidates for liver transplantation. J Hepatol 2001; 34: 651–657.
26. Rodriguez-Roisin R. Insuficiencia respiratoria. In : Farreras P, Rozman C, ed. Medicina interna, 14th ed. Madrid: Ediciones Harcourt SA; 2000: 827–840.

27. Cardús J, Burgos F, Diaz O et al. Increase in pulmonary ventilation-perfusion inequality with age in healthy individuals. Am J Respir Crit Care Med 1997; 156: 648–653.

28. Cerveri I, Zoia MC, Fanfulla F et al. Reference values of arterial oxygen tension in the middle-aged and elderly. Am J Respir Crit Care Med 1995; 152: 934–951.

29. Crapo RO, Jensen RL, Hegewald M, Tashkin DP. Arterial blood gas reference values for sea level and an altitude of 1400 meters. Am J Respir Crit Care Med 1999; 160: 1525–1531.

30. Glenny R, Wagner PD, Roca J, Rodríguez-Roisin R. Gas exchange in health: rest, exercise, and aging. In: Roca J, Rodríguez-Roisin R, Wagner PD, ed. Pulmonary and peripheral gas exchange in health and disease. New York: Marcel Dekker; 2000: 121–148.

31. Fahri LE, Rahn H. Gas stores of the body and the unsteady state. J Appl Physiol 1955; 7: 472–484.

32. West JB, Wagner PD. Ventilation, blood flow, and gas exchange. In: Murray JF, Nadel JA, Mason RJ, Boushey HA, ed. Textbook of respiratory medicine, vol 1, 3rd ed. Philadelphia, PA: WB Saunders; 2000: 55–89.

33. Wagner PD. Mixed venous PO_2 (PvO_2) and arterial PO_2, (PCO_2) and pH. In: Chusid EL, ed. The selective and comprehensive testing of pulmonary function. Mount Kisco, NY: Futura Publishing; 1983: 173–196.

34. Romaldini H, Rodríguez-Roisin R, López FA et al. The mechanisms of arterial hypoxemia during hemodialysis. Am Rev Respir Dis 1984; 129: 780–784.

35. Leff AR, Schumacker PF. Respiratory physiology. Basics and applications. Philadelphia, PA: WB Saunders; 1993.

36. West JB. Pulmonary pathophysiology – the essentials, 5th ed. Baltimore, MD: Lippincott Williams & Wilkins; 1998.

37. Bohr C. Über die spezifische Tätigkeit der Lungen be der respiratorischen Gasaufnahme und ihr Verhalten zu der durch die Alveolarwand stattfindenden Gasdiffusion. Skand Arch Physiol 1909; 22: 221–280.

38. Roughton FJ. Average time spent by blood in human lung capillary and its relation to the rates of CO uptake and elimination in man. Am J Physiol 1945; 143: 621–633.

39. Wagner PD, West JB. Effects of diffusion impairment on O_2 and CO_2 time course in the pulmonary capillaries. J Appl Physiol 1972; 33: 62–71.

40. Scheid P, Piiper J. Diffusion. In: Crystal RG, West JB, Barnes PJ, Weibel, eds. The lung: Scientific foundations, 2nd ed. New York: Raven Press; 1997: 1681–1691.

41. Wagner PD, Sutton JR, Reeves JT et al. Operation Everest II: pulmonary gas exchange during a simulated ascent of Mt Everest. J Appl Physiol 1987; 63: 2348–2359.

42. Barberà JA. Chronic obstructive pulmonary disease. In: Roca J, Rodríguez-Roisin R, Wagner PD, ed. Pulmonary and peripheral gas exchange in health and disease. New York: Marcel Dekker; 2000: 229–262.

43. Genovesi MG, Tierney DF, Taplin GV, Eisenberg H. An intravenous radionuclide method to evaluate hypoxemia caused by abnormal alveolar vessels. Am Rev Respir Dis 1976; 114: 59–65.

44. Roughton FJW, Forster RE. Relative importance of diffusion and chemical reaction rates in determining rate of exchange of gases in the human lung, with special reference to true diffusing capacity of pulmonary membrane and volume of blood in lung capillaries. J Appl Physiol 1957; 11: 290–302.

45. Riley RL, Cournand A. 'Ideal' alveolar air and the analysis of ventilation-perfusion relationships in the lungs. J Appl Physiol 1949; 1: 825–847.

46. Fenn WO, Rahn H, Otis AB. A theoretical study of the composition of alveolar air at altitude. J Appl Physiol 1946; 146: 637–653.

47. West JB. Respiratory Physiology – The Essentials (6th edn). Baltimore: Lippincott Williams & Wilkins; 2000.

48. Dantzker DR, Brook L, DeHart P et al. Ventilation-perfusion distribution in the adult respiratory distress syndrome. Am Rev Respir Dis 1979; 120: 1039–1052.

49. Coffey RL, Albert RK, Robertson HT. Mechanism of physiological dead space response to PEEP after acute oleic acid lung injury. J Appl Physiol Respir Environ Exer Physiol 1983; 55: 1550–1557.

50. Matamis D, Lemaire F, Harf A et al. Redistribution of pulmonary blood flow induced by positive end-expiratory pressure and dopamine infusion in acute respiratory failure. Am Rev Respir Dis 1984; 129: 39–44.

51. Ralph DD, Robertson HT, Weaver U et al. Distribution of ventilation and perfusion during positive end-expiratory pressure in the adult respiratory distress syndrome. Am Rev Respir Dis 1985; 131: 54–60.

52. Santos C, Ferrer M, Roca J et al. Pulmonary gas exchange response to oxygen breathing in acute lung injury. Am J Respir Crit Care Med 2000; 161: 26–31.

53. Gea J, Roca J, Torres A et al. Mechanisms of abnormal gas exchange in patients with pneumonia. Anesthesiology 1991; 75: 782–789.

54. Agusti AGN, Cardús J, Roca J et al. Ventilation–perfusion mismatch in patients with pleural effusion. Effects of thoracocentesis. Am J Respir Crit Care Med 1997; 156: 1205–1209.

55. Milic-Emili J, Henderson JAM, Dolovich MB et al. Regional distribution of inspired gas in the lung. J Appl Physiol 1966; 21: 749–759.

56. West JB, Dollery CT, Naimark A. Distribution of blood flow in isolated lung: relation to vascular and alveolar pressures. J Appl Physiol 1964; 19: 713–724.

57. West JB, Dollery CT, Distribution of blood flow and ventilation–perfusion ratio in the lung, measured with radioactive CO. J Appl Physiol 1960; 15: 405–410.

58. Rodríguez-Roisin R, Roca J. Pulmonary gas exchange. In: Calverley P, Pride NB, ed. Chronic obstructive pulmonary disease. London: Chapman & Hall; 1995: 161–184.

59. Young IH, Crawford ABH. Asthma. In: Roca J, Rodríguez-Roisin R, Wagner PD, ed. New York: Marcel Dekker; 2000: 199–228.

60. Agusti AGN. Interstitial lung diseases. In: Roca J, Rodríguez-Roisin R, Wagner PD, ed. New York: Marcel Dekker; 2000: 263–284.

61. Robinson TC, Freiberg DB, Regnis JA, Young IH. The role of hypoventilation and ventilation–perfusion redistribution in oxygen-induced hypercapnia during acute exacerbations of chronic obstructive pulmonary disease. Am J Respir Crit Care Med 2000; 161: 1524–1529.

62. Benesch R, Benesch RE. Intracellular organic phosphate as regulators of oxygen release by hemoglobin. Nature 1969; 118: 618–622.

63. Chanutin A, Curnish RR. Effect of organic and inorganic phosphates on the oxygen equilibrium of human erythrocytes. Arch Biochem 1967; 121: 96–102.

64. Barer GR, Howard P, Shaw JW. Stimulus–response curves for the pulmonary vascular bed to hypoxia and hypercapnia. J Physiol (London) 1970; 211: 139–155.

65. Dantzker DR, Wagner PD, West JB. Instability of lung units with low $\dot{V}_A/\dot{Q}$ ratios during O_2 breathing. J Appl Physiol 1975; 38: 886–895.

66. Amato MBP, Marini JJ. Barotrauma, Volutrauma, and the ventilation of acute lung injury. In: Marini JJ, Slutsky AS, ed. Physiological basis of ventilatory support. New York: Marcel Dekker; 1998: 1187–1245.

67. Barbera JA, Roca J, Ferrer A et al. Mechanisms of worsening gas exchange during acute exacerbations of chronic obstructive pulmonary disease. Eur Respir J 1997; 1285–1291.

68. Tobin MJ. Respiratory muscles in disease. Clin Chest Med 1988; 9: 263–286.

69. Amoroso P, Wilson SR, Moxham J, Ponte J. Acute effects of inhaled salbutamol on the metabolic rate of normal subjects. Thorax 1993; 48: 882–885.

70. Rodríguez-Roisin R. Effect of mechanical ventilation on gas exchange. In: Tobin MJ, ed. Principles and practice of mechanical ventilation. New York: McGraw-Hill; 1994: 673–693.

71. Sandoval J, Long GR, Skoog C et al. Independent influence of blood flow and mixed venous PO_2 on shunt fraction. J Appl Physiol 1983; 55: 1128–1133.

72. Brimouille S, Kahn RJ. Effects of metabolic acidosis on pulmonary gas exchange. Am Rev Respir Dis 1990; 141: 1185–1189.

73. Brimouille S, Vachiery JL, Lejeune P et al. Acid-base status affects gas exchange in canine oleic acid pulmonary edema. Am J Physiol 1991; 260: 1080–1086.

2 Function

2.6 Pulmonary circulation

Robert Naeije

Key points

- The pulmonary circulation is a high-flow–low-pressure circuit.

- Pulmonary artery pressures increase passively with left atrial pressure and with pulmonary blood flow.

- Pulmonary vascular resistance increases at high and at low pulmonary volumes and is minimal at functional residual capacity.

- Gravity determines an increase in pulmonary blood flow from, non-dependent to dependent lung regions.

- Hypoxic pulmonary vasoconstriction redistributes blood flow to better aerated lung areas, thereby limiting the hypoxaemic effects of local decreases in ventilation/perfusion ratios.

- The most likely mechanism of hypoxic pulmonary vasoconstriction is a hypoxia-induced inhibition of smooth muscle cell voltage-dependent potassium channels, resulting in membrane depolarisation, influx of calcium and cell shortening.

- Hypoxic pulmonary vasoconstriction is modulated by endothelium-dependent vasoconstricting and vasodilating factors.

- Global hypoxic pulmonary vasoconstriction leads to pulmonary hypertension and right heart failure.

- Right ventricular afterload is determined by a complex interplay between pulmonary arterial resistance, compliance and wave reflection.

The pulmonary circulation is a high-flow and low-pressure circuit. Pulmonary arterial pressures are in the range of one-sixth of systemic arterial pressures. This favours pulmonary gas exchange by preventing fluid from moving out of the pulmonary vessels into the interstitial space, and allows the right ventricle to operate at a low energy cost. However, because of the low pressures, the pulmonary circulation is very sensitive to mechanical influences, and the 'flow generator' right ventricle is thin-walled – poorly pre-pared to rapid changes in loading conditions. In addition, the pulsatility of the pulmonary circulation is more important than that of the systemic circulation, which affects the energy transmission from the right ventricle to the pulmonary arteries.

The gold standard for the functional evaluation of the pulmonary circulation still remains a right heart catheterisation with the complex pulmonary artery pressure and flow waves summarised by mean values used for pulmonary vascular resistance (PVR) calculations. Progress in technology now allows refined beat-by-beat non-invasive approaches that improve the understanding of the coupling of the right ventricle to normal and abnormal pulmonary haemodynamic conditions.

Many cardiac and pulmonary diseases are associated with an abnormal increase in pulmonary artery pressures. The most common causes of pulmonary hypertension are left heart failure and chronic hypoxemic lung diseases. Pulmonary hypertension is the third most common cardiovascular condition, after coronary heart disease and systemic hypertension. As the pulmonary circulation is entirely within the thorax, relatively hidden from clinical examination, and symptoms appear only after pulmonary artery pressures have more than doubled from baseline, a sound physiological approach is essential for the diagnosis and treatment of pulmonary hypertension.

Normal pulmonary vascular pressures and flows

The exploration of the pulmonary circulation is normally done with a triple lumen thermodilution catheter inserted into a central vein and placed into the pulmonary artery under constant pressure wave monitoring. The genius of Swan, Ganz and their coworkers, who introduced this technology in 1970, was to tip the catheter with a small 1 ml balloon, allowing for ease of placement into the pulmonary artery without fluoroscopic control, and the estimation of *left* ventricular filling pressures while catheterising the *right* side of the heart.[1]

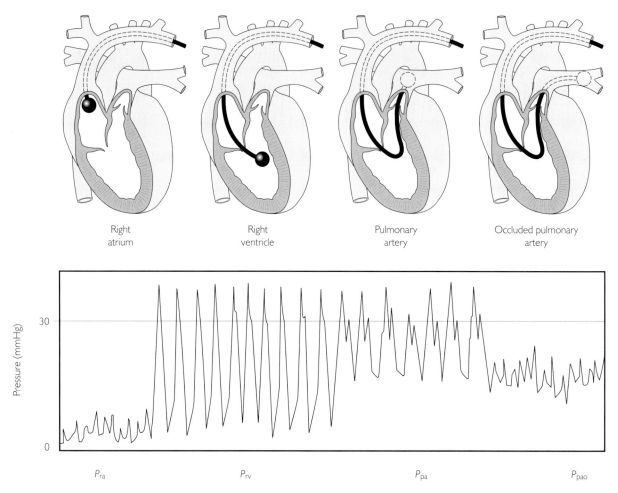

| Right atrium | Right ventricle | Pulmonary artery | Occluded pulmonary artery |

Fig. 2.6.1 A pulmonary artery catheter with the balloon at the tip inflated is passed through the right side of the heart until it impacts in a branch of the pulmonary artery. The continuously monitored pressure signal shows typical aspects of right atrial pressure (P_{ra}), right ventricular pressure (P_{rv}), pulmonary artery pressure (P_{pa}) and occluded P_{pa} (P_{pao}).

Figure 2.6.1 illustrates the pulmonary artery catheter floating through the right heart chambers with measurements successively of right atrial pressure (P_{ra}), right ventricular pressure (P_{rv}), pulmonary artery pressure (P_{pa}) and, at final impact in a peripheral arterial branch, occluded P_{pa} (P_{pao}). A P_{pao} gives a satisfactory estimate of left atrial pressure (P_{la}) provided the pulmonary vessels are fully recruited with a pulmonary capillary pressure (P_{cap}) higher than surrounding alveolar pressure, defining a zone 3 condition according to West's terminology.[2] Lungs of a recumbent normal subject are essentially in a zone 3 condition. With the catheter in place, a proximal lumen located 30 cm from the tip serves to measure P_{ra}, a distal lumen at the tip to measure P_{pa} and an air-filled lumen to inflate the balloon. A thermistor located 4 cm from the catheter tip records small temperature changes in the pulmonary artery induced by the injection of a bolus of cold saline into the right atrium, permitting the calculation of mean pulmonary blood flow ($\dot{Q}$) from a thermodilution curve. To minimise the influence of intrathoracic pressure changes associated with respiratory movements, pulmonary vascular pressures are measured at end-expiration, when the lungs are at functional residual capacity.

In a streamlined steady-flow haemodynamic system, it is possible to calculate resistance as a pressure drop versus flow ratio. The pulmonary circulation is markedly pulsatile, but a PVR can be estimated as the difference between mean P_{pa}, taken as the inflow pressure, and mean P_{la}, taken as the outflow pressure, divided by $\dot{Q}$:

$$\text{PVR} = \frac{(P_{pa} - P_{la}) \cdot}{\dot{Q}}$$

A resistance calculation derives from a simple physical law, which governs laminar flows of newtonian fluids through thin, non-distensible circular tubes. This law, initially formulated by the French physicist Poiseuille, states that resistance (R) to flow, defined as the ratio of pressure drop (ΔP) to flow ($\dot{Q}$), is equal to the product of the length (l) of the tube by a viscosity constant (η) divided by the product of fourth power of the internal radius r by π:

$$R = \frac{\Delta P}{\dot{Q}} = \frac{8 \cdot l \cdot \eta \cdot}{\pi \cdot r^4}$$

Table 2.6.1 Limits of normal of pulmonary blood flow and vascular pressures

Variables	Mean	Limits of normal
$\dot{Q}$ (l.min^{-1})	6.5	4–8.3
Heart rate (bpm)	69	40–100
P_{pa} systolic (mmHg)	19	13–31
P_{pa} diastolic (mmHg)	10	6–15
P_{pa}, mean (mmHg)	13	8–20
P_{pao} (mmHg)	9	5–14
Pra (mmHg)	5	2–11
PVR (dyne.s.cm^{-5})	48	20–110

Table 2.6.2 Influence of gender on pulmonary blood flow and vascular pressures

Variables, mean + SE	Men (n = 19)	Women (n = 13)
$\dot{Q}$ (l.min^{-1})	6.8 ± 0.2	6.0 ± 0.3
$\dot{Q}$ (l.min^{-1}.m^{-2})	3.6 ± 0.2	3.6 ± 0.2
P_{pa} (mmHg)	13 ± 1	13 ± 1
P_{pao} (mmHg)	9 ± 1	9 ± 1

Table 2.6.3 Influence of age on pulmonary blood flow and vascular pressures

Age (years)	16–28	61–83
n	22	16
$\dot{Q}$ (l.min^{-1})	7.6 ± 0.3	5.6 ± 0.3
P_{pa} (mmHg)	13 ± 1	16 ± 1
P_{pao} (mmHg)	8 ± 1	9 ± 1
PVR (dyn.s.cm^{-5})	54 ± 6	96 ± 7

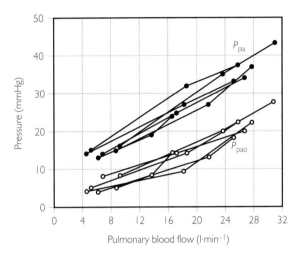

Fig. 2.6.2 Pulmonary artery pressures (P_{pa}) (closed circles) and occluded P_{pa} (P_{pao}; open circles) as a function of pulmonary blood flow in athletes at rest and at two levels of exercise. The highest level of exercise is associated with marked increases in P_{pa} and P_{pao}. (After Naeije et al[11].)

The fact that r in the equation is at the fourth power explains why R is exquisitely sensitive to small changes in radius. Accordingly, PVR is a good indicator of the state of constriction or dilatation of pulmonary resistive vessels, and helpful for monitoring disease-induced pulmonary vascular remodelling and/or changes in tone.

The limits of normal of resting pulmonary vascular pressures and flows as derived from measurements obtained in a total of 32 healthy resting supine young adult healthy volunteers[3,4] are shown in Table 2.6.1. From that study population it is apparent that there are no gender differences in pulmonary haemodynamics after a correction of flow for body dimensions (Table 2.6.2). Earlier studies have shown that ageing is associated with an increase in P_{pa} and a decrease in $\dot{Q}$, leading to a doubling of PVR over a five-decade life-span[5–8] (Table 2.6.3)

Effects of exercise

Mild to moderate levels of exercise do not normally much increase P_{pa}, which reaches no more than the upper limit of normal of 20 mmHg, while P_{pao} (or P_{la}) remains unchanged.[9] Exercise increases cardiac output proportionally more than the pulmonary vascular pressure gradient, and therefore PVR is calculated to decrease.[9,10] However, high levels of exercise may markedly increase P_{pa}, partly in relation to an upstream transmission of increased P_{la}.[10] This is illustrated in Figure 2.6.2, which represents measurements of P_{pa} and P_{pao} in six athletes at

a progressively increased workload, up to oxygen consumptions between 3.5 and 4 l.min^{-1} and cardiac outputs ranging from 24 to 32 l.min^{-1}.[11] It is interesting to note that athletes at high levels of exercise commonly present with P_{pa} higher than 30 mmHg, which defines pulmonary hypertension, and with P_{pao} reaching or even exceeding a value around 20 mmHg, generally considered as being the capillary pressure threshold for the onset of hydrostatic lung oedema.

As mentioned above, PVR increases with ageing, so that the slope of $P_{pa}/\dot{Q}$ plots during exercise averages 1 mmHg.l^{-1}.min^{-1} in young adults, but more than doubles, up to 2.5 mmHg.l^{-1}.min^{-1} in old subjects, who also present with an earlier and more important increase in P_{pao} (or P_{la}).[10]

Pulmonary capillary pressure

Pulmonary artery occluded pressure is not the same as pulmonary artery wedge pressure (P_{pw}), which is obtained by wedging a pulmonary catheter with a deflated balloon into a small branch of the pulmonary artery. As illustrated in Figure 2.6.3, arterial occlusion creates a stop-flow condition that extends the catheter lumen down to veins of the same diameter, so that an increase in small-vein resistance can conceivably increase P_{pw} but not P_{pao}.[12] It has been shown that P_{pw} exceeds P_{pao} by an average of 3–4 mmHg in patients with congestive heart failure or with the acute respiratory distress syndrome (ARDS).[13]

Because of the resistance of the smallest veins, which do not contribute to P_{pw}, being narrower than the pulmonary artery catheter, and a low but significant capillary resistance, pulmonary capillary pressure (P_{cap}) is necessarily higher than P_{pw}. A value for P_{cap} can be obtained by the analysis of a P_{pa} decay curve after balloon occlusion. As shown in Figure 2.6.4, such a pressure decay curve is made of a first fast component, which corresponds to the obstruction of flow through arterial resistance, and a slower component, which corresponds to the emptying of the compliant capillaries through venous resistance.[14] The transition point between the two components of the curve gives an estimate of P_{cap} that agrees well with the reference isogravimetric method.[15]

Measurements of P_{cap} from analysis of the P_{pa} decay curve after balloon occlusion have recently been reported in young adult volunteers, yielding a mean value of 10 mmHg, range 7–13 mmHg.[16] Assuming a normal longitudinal distribution of resistance within the pulmonary circulation, ascribing 60% PVR to the arterial segment and 40% to the capillary–venous segment,[9] the normal P_{cap} can also calculated as proposed by Gaar et al[17]:

$$P_{cap} = P_{pao} + 0.4(P_{pa} - P_{pao}).$$

The Gaar equation is obviously invalid in disease states associated with variable increases in the arterial, capillary or venous component of PVR.

Pulmonary capillary pressure increases with cardiac output and pulmonary venous pressure. Changes in lung volume affect PVR[18] but associated changes in P_{cap} are not known. Hypoxia increases P_{cap}, albeit normally only slightly,[16] because of a small venous element in hypoxic pulmonary vasoconstriction.[19] Variable increases in P_{cap} have been reported in ARDS, with recorded values higher than 20 mmHg known to be associated with hydrostatic oedema in normal lungs.[20,21] According to one study, P_{cap} is higher than normal in primary pulmonary hypertension, perhaps because venous involvement in these patients is more significant than was previously appreciated.[22] A recent study described markedly increased P_{cap} in early high-altitude pulmonary oedema, suggesting that a hydrostatic mechanism might explain this hitherto mysterious entity.[16]

Pulmonary vascular pressure–flow relationships

The inherent assumption of a PVR calculation is that the $P_{pa}/\dot{Q}$ relationship is linear and crosses the pressure axis at a value equal to P_{pao}, allowing PVR to remain constant whatever the absolute level of pressure of flow. While the $(P_{pa} - P_{pao})/\dot{Q}$ relationship has indeed been shown to be reasonably well described by a linear approximation over a limited range of physiological flows, the zero-crossing assumption holds good only for well oxygenated lungs in supine resting subjects, suggesting complete recruitment and minimal distension. Hypoxia and a number of cardiac and respiratory diseases increase both the slope and the extrapolated intercepts of multipoint $(P_{pa} - P_{pao})/\dot{Q}$ plots.[23]

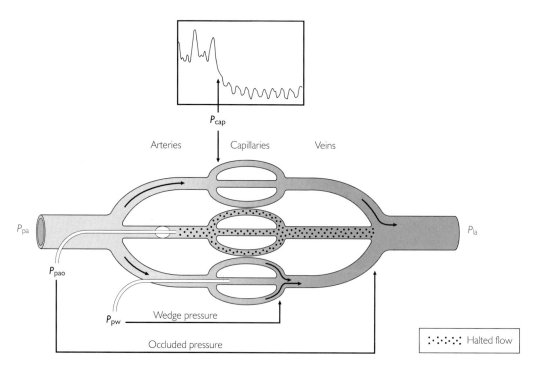

Fig. 2.6.3 Occluded pulmonary artery pressure (P_{pao}) is not pulmonary artery wedge pressure (P_{pw}), which is not pulmonary capillary pressure (P_{cap}). Stippled areas indicate halted flow.

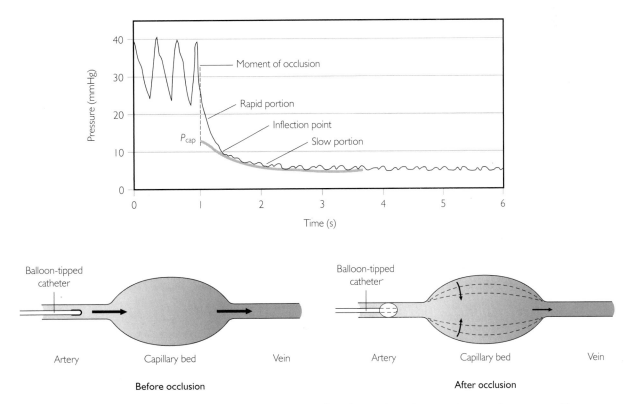

Fig. 2.6.4 Analysis of the transient pressure after pulmonary arterial occlusion, in order to estimate pulmonary capillary pressure (P_{cap}). This can be calculated either from the transition point between the fast and slow components of the pressure decay curve or by extrapolating the slow component of the pressure decay curve to the moment of occlusion. (After Perret et al[14].)

While an increase in the slope of a $P_{pa}/\dot{Q}$ plot is easily understood as being caused by a decrease in the cumulative surface area of the vessels contributing to pulmonary resistance, the positive extrapolated pressure intercept has inspired various explanatory models. Permutt et al conceived a vascular waterfall model made of parallel collapsible vessels with a distribution of closing pressures.[24] At low flow, these vessels would be progressively derecruited, accounting for a low-flow $P_{pa}/\dot{Q}$ curve that is concave to the flow axis and intercepts the pressure axis at the lowest closing pressure that must be overcome to generate a flow. At higher flow, completed recruitment and negligible distension account for a linear $P_{pa}/\dot{Q}$ curve with an extrapolated pressure intercept representing a weighted mean of closing pressures. In this model, the mean closing pressure is the effective outflow pressure of the pulmonary circulation. A left atrial pressure lower than the mean closing pressure is then only apparent downstream, as irrelevant to flow as is the height of a waterfall. Resistance calculations remain applicable for the evaluation of the functional state of the pulmonary circulation, provided the apparent downstream pressure is replaced by the effective one.[24]

However, distensible vessel models have been developed that explain the shape of $P_{pa}/\dot{Q}$ curves as the result of changes in resistance and compliance.[25–27] In fact, as illustrated in Figure 2.6.5, $P_{pa}/\dot{Q}$ curves can always be shown to be curvilinear with concavity to flow axis provided a large enough number of coordinates are generated and that they are submitted to an adequate fitting procedure. On the other hand, derecruitment can be directly

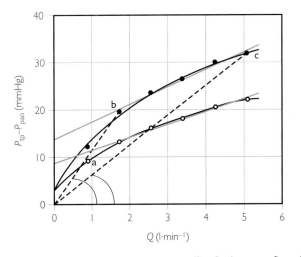

Fig. 2.6.5 The pulmonary artery pressure(P_{pa}–P_{pao}) versus flow ($\dot{Q}$) coordinates at two levels (open and closed circles) of pulmonary hypertension are correctly described by a linear approximation over a physiological range of flows. The extrapolated pressure intercepts of these linearised pressure/flow relationships are positive, suggesting a closing pressure higher than left atrial pressure. However, the pressure/flow coordinates are better described by a curvilinear shape, which makes better allowance for the natural distensibility of the pulmonary vessels. In both situations, pulmonary vascular resistance (PVR) calculations are misleading: in the presence of aggravated pulmonary hypertension (as assessed by higher pressures at a given flow), PVR does not change from a to b and PVR decreases from a to c.

observed at low pressures and flows.[28] Together, recruitment and distension probably explain most $P_{pa}/\dot{Q}$ curves. According to this integrated view, at low inflow pressure, many pulmonary vessels are closed as an effect of their intrinsic tone and surrounding alveolar pressure, and those that are open are relatively narrow. As inflow pressure increases, previously closed vessels progressively open (recruitment), and previously narrow vessels progressively dilate (distension). Together, these mechanisms explain a progressive decrease in the slope of pulmonary vascular pressure/flow relationships with increasing flow or pressure.

The practical consequence is that single PVR determinations cannot be used to evaluate reliably the functional state of the pulmonary circulation at variable flow (Fig. 2.6.5). A better description of the resistive properties of the pulmonary circulation requires measurements of pulmonary vascular pressure at several levels of flow. The problem is to alter flow without affecting vascular tone. This could be achieved with low-dose dobutamine.[22] Exercise to alter flow may lead to a spuriously increased slope of $P_{pa}/\dot{Q}$, plotting exercise-induced pulmonary vasoconstriction[22] due to a decrease in mixed venous P_{O_2}, sympathetic nervous system activation and an exercise-associated increase in left atrial pressure.

Passive regulation of the pulmonary circulation

Left atrial pressure and cardiac output

At a given $\dot{Q}$, an increase in P_{la} is transmitted upstream to P_{pa} in a ratio of less than 1:1, depending on the state of arterial distension and the presence or absence of a closing pressure higher than P_{la}.[27] As discussed above, an increase in $\dot{Q}$ at a given P_{la} increases P_{pa} but decreases PVR because of a variable combination of pulmonary vascular recruitment and distension.

Lung volume

An increase in lung volume above functional residual capacity increases the resistance of alveolar vessels, which are the vessels exposed to alveolar pressure, but decreases the resistance of extra-alveolar vessels, which are those exposed to interstitial pressure. A decrease in lung volume below functional residual capacity has the opposite effects. It has been shown that the combination of alveolar and extra-alveolar vessel resistance that gives the lowest resultant PVR is observed at functional residual capacity.[18,28]

Gravity

Pulmonary blood flow increases almost linearly from non-dependent to dependent lung regions. This inequality of pulmonary perfusion is best demonstrated in an upright lung.[2] The vertical height of a lung is on average about 30 cm. The difference in pressure between the extremities of a vertical column of blood of the same height amounts to 23 mmHg, which is quite a large variation compared to the mean perfusion pressure of the

pulmonary circulation. Accordingly, the physiological inequality of the distribution of perfusion of a normal lung can be explained by a gravity-dependent interplay between arterial, venous and alveolar pressures.[2] At the top of the lung, alveolar pressure (P_A) is higher than mean P_{pa} and pulmonary venous pressure (P_{pv}). In this *zone 1*, flow may be present only during systole, or not at all. Zone 1 is extended in clinical situations of low flow, such as hypovolaemic shock, or increased alveolar pressure such as during ventilation with a positive end expiratory pressure (PEEP). Further down the lung there is a *zone 2* where $P_{pa} > P_A > P_{pv}$. In this zone 2, alveolar pressure is an effective closing pressure and the driving pressure for flow is the gradient between mean P_{pa} and P_A. As mentioned above, such a flow condition can be likened to a waterfall since P_{pv}, the apparent outflow pressure, is irrelevant to flow. In *zone 3*, P_{pv} is higher than P_A, so that the driving pressure for flow is $P_{pa}-P_{pv}$.

At the most dependent regions of upright lung, there is an additional region where flow decreases.[29] This *zone 4* has been attributed to an increase in the resistance of extra-alveolar vessels, because it expands when lung volume is reduced or in the presence of lung oedema. Active tone may be an additional explanation for zone 4 as it is also reduced by the administration of vasodilators.

The vertical height of lung tissue in a supine subject is of course much reduced and, accordingly, almost all the lung is then normally in zone 3, but with persistence of a still measurable increase in flow from non-dependent to dependent lung regions (Fig. 2.6.6).

While gravity is the major determinant of regional changes in blood flow in the normal pulmonary circulation, three-dimensional reconstructions using single photon emission tomography (SPET) have shown that there is also a decrease in blood flow from the centre of the lung to the periphery.[30] This may reflect an intrinsic effect of the pulmonary vascular geometry, and has not been shown to be relevant to gas exchange.

Active hypoxic regulation of the pulmonary circulation

There is an active intrapulmonary control mechanism able to some extent to correct the passive gravity-dependent distribution of pulmonary blood flow: a decrease in P_{O_2} increases pulmonary vascular tone. Hypoxic pulmonary vasoconstriction was first reported by von Euler and Liljestrand,[31] who proposed a functional interpretation that can still be considered valid. In lung tissue, P_{O_2} is determined by a ratio between O_2 carried to the lung by alveolar ventilation ($\dot{V}_A$) and O_2 carried away from the lung by blood flow ($\dot{Q}$):

$$P_{O_2} = \frac{\dot{V}_A}{\dot{Q}}.$$

In contrast with hypoxic vasodilation in systemic tissue, where local P_{O_2} is accordingly determined by the ratio between the flow of O_2 carried to the tissues ($\dot{Q}$) and local O_2 consumption ($\dot{V}_{O_2}$):

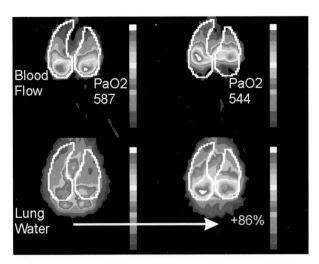
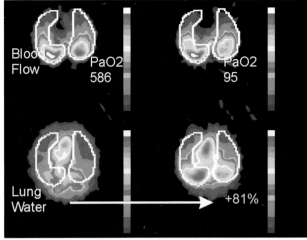

Fig. 2.6.6 Positron emission tomography measurements of regional blood flow and lung water in a supine dog ventilated with pure oxygen, before and after induction of oleic acid lung injury, with intact (left) or ablated (right) hypoxic pulmonary vasoconstriction. Lung injury is associated with a significant increase in lung water. Pulmonary blood flow is redistributed upwards by hypoxic pulmonary vasoconstriction, and this is associated with preserved arterial P_{O_2}.

$$P_{O_2} = \frac{\dot{Q}}{\dot{V}_{O_2}}.$$

The hypoxic pulmonary pressor response is universal in mammals and in birds but with considerable interspecies and interindividual variability.[9,32] The attributes of hypoxic pulmonary vasoconstriction can be summarised as follows.[9,32,33] The response is vigorous in cattle and in pigs, moderate in humans, dogs and camelids (including the llama) and almost absent in guinea pigs and rabbits. It is turned on in a few seconds, fully developed after 1–3 min and more or less stable thereafter according to the experimental conditions. It is reversed in less than a minute. It is observed in lungs devoid of nervous connections, and indeed also in isolated pulmonary arterial smooth muscle cells. Hypoxic pulmonary vasoconstriction is enhanced by acidosis, a decrease in mixed venous P_{O_2}, repeated hypoxic exposure (in some experimental models), perinatal hypoxia, decreased lung segment size, cyclooxygenase inhibition, nitric oxide inhibition and certain drugs or mediators, which include almitrine and low-dose 5-HT. Hypoxic pulmonary vasoconstriction is inhibited by alkalosis, hypercapnia, an increase in pulmonary vascular or alveolar pressures, vasodilating prostaglandins, nitric oxide, complement activation, low-dose endotoxin, calcium-channel blockers, β_2 stimulants, nitroprusside and, paradoxically, peripheral chemoreceptor stimulation. The hypoxic pressor response is biphasic, with a progressive increase as P_{O_2} is progressively decreased to approximately 35–40 mmHg, followed by a decrease ('hypoxic vasodilatation') in more profound hypoxia.

The hypoxia-induced increase in PVR is mainly caused by a constriction of precapillary small arterioles.[9,32,33] Small pulmonary veins also constrict in response to hypoxia but this should not normally contribute to more than 20% of the total change in PVR.[19] An exaggerated hypoxic pulmonary venoconstriction may explain high-altitude pulmonary oedema.[16]

While hypoxic pulmonary vasoconstriction has been shown by sophisticated modelling to be only a moderately efficient

feedback mechanism,[4,34] it may still produce substantial improvements in arterial oxygenation of patients with inhomogeneous lungs, as occurs in COPD or ARDS.[35] This is illustrated in Figure 2.6.6 as applied to an experimental ARDS preparation, where changes in blood flow distribution and arterial P_{O_2} conform to the expected functional effects of hypoxic pulmonary vasoconstriction.[36]

The biochemical mechanism of hypoxic pulmonary vasoconstriction remains incompletely understood. Current thought is that a decrease in P_{O_2} inhibits smooth-muscle-cell voltage-dependent potassium channels, resulting in membrane depolarisation, influx of calcium and cell shortening.[33] Two such channels, $Kv_{2.1}$ and $Kv_{1.5}$, have been identified in rat pulmonary arteries.[37] However, the nature of the low-P_{O_2}-sensing mechanism remains elusive.[33] Inhibition of voltage-dependent potassium channels has been observed in isolated pulmonary artery smooth muscle cells of patients with primary pulmonary hypertension, and might thus be a universal pathway to enhanced pulmonary vascular reactivity and subsequent remodelling.[38] The reversal of hypoxic vasoconstriction by profound hypoxia is caused by activation of ATP-dependent potassium channels.[33]

Normal as well as abnormal pulmonary vascular tone has been shown to be modulated by a series of endothelium-derived and circulating mediators.[39] Endothelium-derived relaxing factors include nitric oxide, prostacyclin and the endothelium-derived hyperpolarising factor. The major endothelium-derived contracting factor is endothelin. These observations form the basis of current attempts to treat pulmonary hypertension with inhaled nitric oxide, intravenous prostacyclin or oral antiendothelins. It is interesting to note that the pulmonary vasodilating effects of nitric oxide and prostacyclin are mediated by the cyclic guanylic acid (cGMP) and the cyclic adenosine monophosphate (cAMP) pathways respectively, suggesting the possibility that the effects are additive.

The pulmonary circulation is richly innervated by the autonomic nervous system, which includes adrenergic, cholinergic and nonadrenergic noncholinergic (NANC) elements.[9,32,39] However, the role played by the autonomic nervous system in the control of pulmonary vascular tone appears to be a minor one. In fact, autonomic innervation of the pulmonary arterial tree is predominantly proximal, suggesting a more important effect in the modulation of proximal compliance.[40]

Pulsatile flow pulmonary haemodynamics

The study of the pulmonary circulation as a steady flow system is a simplification, since pulmonary arterial pulse pressure, or the difference between systolic and diastolic P_{pa}, is in the order of 40–50% of mean pressure, and instantaneous flow varies from its maximum at mid-systole to around zero in diastole.[9,41] While pulmonary artery pressure and flow waves are superposable in normal subjects, they become markedly different in aspect and desynchronised in patients with pulmonary hypertension.[41]

In patients with severe pulmonary hypertension, the right ventricular pressure wave is characterised by a sharp initial upstroke followed by a short plateau and then a late systolic peak, and the pulmonary artery pressure wave is characterised by a huge pulse pressure and again a late systolic peak. In fact, in the most severe forms of pulmonary hypertension the pulmonary artery pressure wave looks 'ventricularised'. On the other hand, the pulmonary blood flow wave shows late systolic deceleration, or even midsystolic deceleration.

These morphological aspects of pulmonary artery pressure and flow waves in pulmonary hypertension are completely explained by decreases in pulmonary arterial compliance and earlier return of reflected waves on forward waves. It can be shown experimentally that right ventricular output decreases because of an increased afterload if, at a given resistance, pulmonary arterial compliance decreases and/or wave reflection increases.[42,43]

Pulmonary artery pressure and flow waves can be decomposed into their constituent harmonic oscillations by an application of the Fourier theorem.[9,41] This analysis is possible because the pulmonary circulation acts as a linear system; in other words, that a purely sinusoidal flow oscillation produces a purely sinusoidal pressure oscillation of the same frequency. From the spectral analysis of the pulmonary arterial pressure and flow waves, pulmonary arterial impedance (PVZ) can be calculated.[9,41] Pulmonary arterial impedance is the ratio of pressure oscillations to flow oscillations. It is graphically represented as a pressure/flow ratio and a phase angle, both as a function of frequency. A typical PVZ spectrum is illustrated in Figure 2.6.7.

Pulmonary arterial impedance at 0 Hz (Z_0) corresponds to PVR calculated as $P_{pa}/\dot{Q}$. Normally, the ratio of pressure to flow decreases rapidly to a first minimum at 2–3 Hz and increases again to a first maximum at 5–6 Hz. At low frequencies, the phase angle is negative, indicating that flow is greater than pressure.

An increase in the pressure/flow ratio at all frequencies indicates decreased pulmonary arterial distensibility. A shift of the first minimum and maximum values to higher frequencies indicates an increased wave velocity or a change in the dominant reflection site.

The PVZ spectrum allows the quantification of characteristic impedance (Z_c), defined as PVZ without wave reflection. Characteristic impedance is measured as the average pressure/flow ratio at the highest frequencies. It can also be measured as the linearised slope of the early systolic pulmonary artery pressure/flow relationship (Fig. 2.6.7).

Characteristic impedance is dependent on the ratio between inertia and compliance in the pulmonary circulation, and can be approximated by the equation:

$$Z_c = \left[\frac{(\rho/\pi r^4)}{(\Delta \pi r^2/\Delta P)}\right],$$

where ρ is the density of blood, r the mean internal radius, $\rho/\pi r^4$ the inertia and $\Delta \pi r^2/\Delta P$ the compliance of the pulmonary arterial tree.

The extent of the difference between Z_0 and Z_c can be used to calculate an index of wave reflection:

$$Z_c = \frac{(1 - Z_c/Z_0)}{(1 + Z_c/Z_0)}.$$

It is thus apparent that a PVZ calculation makes it possible to quantify the forces that oppose right ventricular ejection, or

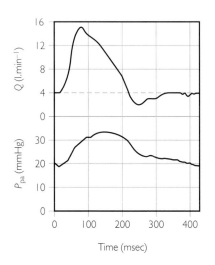

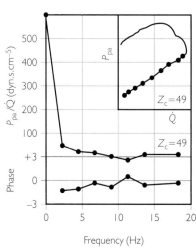

Fig. 2.6.7 Pulmonary artery pressure and flow waves and the derived pulmonary arterial impedance (PVZ) spectrum in experimental embolic pulmonary hypertension. The pressure and flow waves are desynchronised, the first minimum of the pressure/flow ratio is shifted to a higher frequency and the phase angle is negative at low frequencies, indicating that flow is greater than pressure. There is a good correlation between the value obtained for characteristic impedance (Z_c) in the frequency domain and that obtained by measuring directly on the instantaneous pressure/flow curve (inset).

afterload, as a dynamic interplay between resistance, compliance and wave reflection.

The pulsatile hydraulic power is most important in the proximal pulmonary arterial tree[9,41] and, accordingly, PVZ calculations are relatively insensitive to peripheral physiological or pathological changes. The spectrum of PVZ is little affected by normal breathing[44] or by disease processes limited to alveolar or juxta-alveolar vessels.[43,45] In contrast, proximal pulmonary arterial obstruction markedly affects pressure and flow wave morphology and the PVZ spectrum, and, at any given PVR, has a more important depressant effect on right ventricular output.[43,46]

Non-invasive evaluation of the pulmonary circulation

Non-invasive methods of evaluating the pulmonary circulation have made a lot of progress in recent years. Doppler echocardiography has already entered routine cardiology practice, permitting easy measurement of instantaneous pulmonary arterial flow velocity and satisfactory recalculation of instantaneous pulmonary artery pressures[47–50] (Fig. 2.6.8).

Pulmonary flow velocity measured by the pulsed Doppler technique normally exhibits a dome-like contour, with a peak in the middle of systole.[47,48] Pulmonary hypertension is associated with a decrease in the acceleration time (from start to peak velocity of flow) and with late systolic deceleration of flow. Severe pulmonary hypertension is associated with extreme shortening of acceleration time and a midsystolic deceleration of flow, with eventually a late systolic reversal of flow.[47,48] These aspects were previously observed using electromagnetic volume flow measurements.[41] Acceleration time is affected by heart rate and it is therefore reasonable to correct the measurement according to ejection time.[48] Acceleration time normally exceeds 100 ms. The limits of normal of acceleration time corrected for ejection time vary from 0.35 s to 0.47 s. Acceleration time is inversely correlated to invasively measured P_{pa} and PVR but, in spite of the fact that correlation coefficients are reported to be in the range of 0.8–0.9 in many studies, acceleration time is usually a poor predictor of P_{pa} or PVR on an individual basis.[47,48] This is explained by the operator-dependent variability of the measurement, the insufficient frequency response of fluid-filled pulmonary catheters and the fact that, as discussed above, a flow measurement cannot be considered physiologically identical to a pressure or resistance calculation.[49]

The detection of tricuspid regurgitation by continuous Doppler measurement allows the calculation of transtricuspid pressure gradient using the simplified form of the Bernouilli equation:

$$\Delta P = 4 \times v^2,$$

where ΔP is the pressure gradient and v the velocity of flow.

In general, a systolic pulmonary artery pressure is calculated from the maximum velocity of the regurgitant flow and estimated or measured right atrial pressure.[48–50] Tricuspid regurgitant flow can be recorded in about 60% of normal subjects and in most patients with pulmonary hypertension. Inflation of the chest decreases the recovery of satisfactory signals.[51] There is a good correlation between systolic pulmonary artery pressure

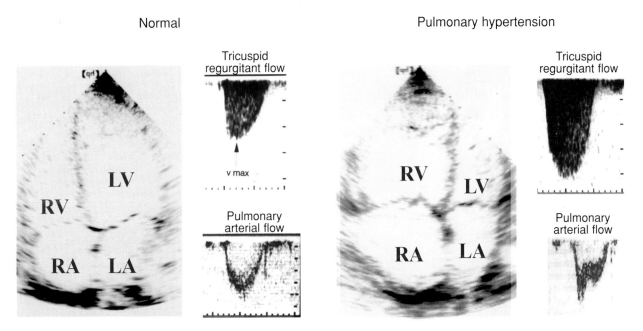

Fig. 2.6.8 Doppler pulmonary flow–velocity waves and tricuspid regurgitant flows in a normal subject (left) and a patient with severe pulmonary hypertension (right). Pulmonary artery pressures (P_{pa}) measured invasively were 21/9 mmHg and 62/24 mmHg respectively. Pulmonary hypertension is associated with shortened acceleration time and late systolic deceleration of the pulmonary arterial flow ($\dot{Q}$) wave, and with increased velocity of the tricuspid regurgitant jet.

directly measured during right heart catheterisation and pressure predicted from the tricuspid regurgitant jets.[48,50] However, the prediction of invasive from non-invasive measurements can be disappointing on an individual basis because of the assumptions of the pressure gradient calculation and also because of the limited frequency response of fluid-filled catheters when measuring right ventricular pressure.[49] The shape of the tricuspid regurgitant jet is interesting to analyse as it shows a late systolic peak in patients with severe pulmonary hypertension – like the directly measured pulmonary artery pressure curve.[48]

It is possible to apply the Bernouilli equation to the tricuspid and pulmonary regurgitant jets to recalculate complete pulmonary artery pressure curves.[48] This method has been reported to be as accurate as direct invasive measurements in showing significant differences in the morphology of pulmonary artery pressure curves in patients with primary pulmonary hypertension, a disease process that mainly involves small peripheral arterioles rather than proximal thromboembolic obstruction of the pulmonary arteries.[52]

Clinical relevance

- Pulmonary hypertension is defined by a mean pulmonary artery pressure higher than 25 mmHg at rest and 30 mmHg at exercise.

- Pulmonary hypertension is a frequent complication of cardiac and pulmonary diseases.

- Pulmonary hypertension may be associated with an increase in pulmonary capillary filtration pressure, which is estimated from the analysis of the pulmonary arterial pressure decay curve after balloon occlusion, or by adding to left atrial pressure 40% of the difference between mean pulmonary artery pressure and left atrial pressure.

- Pulmonary vascular resistance is unreliable for the evaluation of the functional state of the pulmonary circulation at variable flow, and better defined by pulmonary vascular pressure measurements at several levels of flow.

- Hypoxic pulmonary vasoconstriction is an important protective mechanism to limit hypoxaemia associated with acute lung diseases.

- Recent advances in the treatment of pulmonary hypertension have been achieved with exogenous administration of endothelium-derived vasodilators, prostacyclin and nitric oxide.

- The evaluation of right ventricular afterload requires the determination of pulmonary arterial impedance.

- Pulmonary arterial impedance can be estimated using echo-Doppler cardiography for the measurement of tricuspid regurgitant and pulmonary arterial flows.

References

1. Swan HJC, Ganz W, Forrester JS et al. Catheterization of the heart in man with use of a flow-directed catheter. N Engl J Med 1970; 283: 447–451.
2. West JB, Dollery CT, Naimark A. Distribution of blood flow in isolated lung: relation to vascular and alveolar pressures. J Appl Physiol 1964; 19: 713–724.
3. Naeije R, Mélot C, Mols P, Hallemans R. Effects of vasodilators on hypoxic pulmonary vasoconstriction in normal man. Chest 1982; 82: 404–410.
4. Mélot C, Naeije R, Hallemans R et al. Hypoxic pulmonary vasoconstriction and pulmonary gas exchange in normal man. Respir Physiol 1987; 68: 11–27.
5. Holmgren A, Jonsson B, Sjostrand T. Circulatory data in normal subjects at rest and during exercise in the recumbent position, with special reference to the stroke volume at different working intensities. Acta Physiol Scand 1960; 49: 343–363.
6. Granath A, Strandell T. Relationships between cardiac output, stroke volume, and intracardiac pressures at rest and during exercise in supine position and some anthropometric data in healthy old men. Acta Med Scand 1964; 176: 447–466.
7. Granath A, Jonsson B, Strandell T. Circulation in healthy old men, studied by right heart catheterization at rest and during exercise in supine and sitting position. Acta Med Scand 1964; 176: 425–446.
8. Bevegaard S, Holmgren A, Jonsson B. Circulatory studies in well trained athletes at rest and during heavy exercise, with special reference to stroke volume and the influence of body position. Acta Physiol Scand 1963; 57: 26–50.
9. Fishman AP. Pulmonary circulation. In: Handbook of physiology. The respiratory system. Circulation and nonrespiratory functions. Bethesda, MD: American Physiology Society; 1985; s 3, vol 1, ch 3: 93–166.
10. Reeves JT, Dempsey JA, Grover RF. Pulmonary circulation during exercise. In: Weir EK, Reeves JT, ed. Pulmonary vascular physiology and physiopathology. New York: Marcel Dekker; 1989; ch 4: 107–133.
11. Naeije R, Mélot C, Niset G et al. Improved arterial oxygenation by a pharmacological increase in chemosensitivity during hypoxic exercise in normal subjects. J Appl Physiol 1993; 74: 1666–71.
12. Zidulka A, Hakim TS. Wedge pressure in large vs small pulmonary arteries to detect pulmonary venoconstriction. J Appl Physiol 1985; 59: 1329–1332.
13. Teboul JL, Andrivet P, Ansquer M et al. Bedside evaluation of the resistance of large and medium pulmonary veins in various lung diseases. J Appl Physiol 1992; 72: 998–1003.
14. Perret C, Tagan D, Feihl F, Marini JJ. The pulmonary artery catheter in critical care. Oxford: Blackwell Science; 1996.
15. Cope DK, Grimbert F, Downey JM, Taylor AE. Pulmonary capillary pressure: a review. Crit Care Med 1992; 20: 1043–1056.
16. Maggiorini M, Mélot C, Pierre S et al. High altitude pulmonary edema is initially caused by an increased capillary pressure. Circulation 2001; 24; 103: 2078–2083.
17. Gaar KA Jr, Taylor AE, Owens LJ, Guyton AC. Pulmonary capillary pressure and filtration coefficient in the isolated perfused lung. Am J Physiol 1967; 213: 910–914.
18. Howell JBL, Permutt S, Proctor DF, Riley RL. Effect of inflation of the lung on different parts of the pulmonary vascular bed. J Appl Physiol 1961; 16: 71–76.
19. Hillier SC, Graham JA, Hanger CC et al. Hypoxic vasoconstriction in pulmonary arterioles and venules. J Appl Physiol 1997; 82: 1084–1090.
20. Collee CG, Lynch KE, Hill D, Zapol WM. Bedside measurements of pulmonary capillary pressure in patients with acute respiratory failure. Anesthesiology 1987; 66: 614–620.
21. Rossetti M, Guenard H, Gabinski C. Effects of nitric oxide on pulmonary serial resistances in ARDS. Am J Respir Crit Care Med 1996; 154: 1375–1381.
22. Abdel Kafi S, Mélot C, Vachiéry JL et al. Partitioning of pulmonary vascular resistance in primary pulmonary hypertension. J Am Coll Cardiol 1998, 31: 1372–1376.
23. McGregor M, Sniderman A. On pulmonary vascular resistance: the need for more precise definition. Am J Cardiol 1985; 55: 217–221.
24. Permutt S, Bromberger-Barnea B, Bane HN. Alveolar pressure, pulmonary venous pressure and the vascular waterfall. Med Thorac 1962; 19: 239–260.
25. Zhuang FY, Fung YC, Yen RT. Analysis of blood flow in cat's lung with detailed anatomical and elasticity data. J Appl Physiol 1983; 55: 1341–1348.
26. Nelin LD, Krenz GS, Rickaby DA et al. A distensible vessel model applied to hypoxic pulmonary vasoconstriction in the neonatal pig. J Appl Physiol 1992; 73: 987–994.
27. Mélot C, Delcroix M, Lejeune P et al. Starling resistor versus viscoelastic models for embolic pulmonary hypertension. Am J Physiol 1995; 267 (Heart Circ Physiol 36): H817–27.
28. Glazier JB, Hughes JMB, Maloney JE, West JB. Measurements of capillary dimensions and blood volume in rapidly frozen lungs. J Appl Physiol 1969; 26: 65–76.
29. Hughes JM, Glazier JB, Maloney JR, West JB. Effect of lung volume on the distribution of pulmonary blood flow in man. Respir Physiol 1968; 4: 58–72.

30. Hakim TS, Lisbona R, Michel RP, Dean GW. Role of vasoconstriction in gravity-nondependent central–peripheral gradient in pulmonary blood flow. J Appl Physiol 1993; 63: 1114–1121.

31. Von Euler US, Liljestrand G. Observations on the pulmonary arterial blood pressure in the cat. Acta Physiol Scand 1946; 12: 301–320.

32. Grover RF, Wagner WW, McMurtry IF, Reeves JT. Pulmonary circulation. In: Handbook of physiology. The cardiovascular system. Peripheral circulation and organ blood flow. Bethesda, MD: American Physiology Society; 1983; s 2, vol 3, part 1, chap 4: 103–136.

33. Weir EK, Archer SL. The mechanism of acute hypoxic pulmonary vasoconstriction: the tale of two channels. FASEB J 1995; 9: 183–189.

34. Grant BJB. Effect of local pulmonary blood flow control on gas exchange: theory. J Appl Physiol: Respirat Environ Exercise Physiol 1982; 53: 1100–1109.

35. Brimioulle S, Lejeune P, Naeije R. Effects of hypoxic pulmonary vasoconstriction on gas exchange. J Appl Physiol 1996; 81: 1535–1543.

36. Gust R, Kozlowski J, Stephenson AH, Schuster DP. Synergistic hemodynamic effects of low-dose endotoxin in acute lung injury. Am J Respir Crit Care Med 1998; 157: 1919–1926.

37. Archer SL, Souil E, Dinh-Xuan AT et al. Molecular identification of the role of voltage-gated K^+ channels, Kv1.5 and Kv2.1, in hypoxic pulmonary vasoconstriction and control of resting membrane potential in rat pulmonary artery myocytes. J Clin Incest 1998; 101: 2319–2330.

38. Yuan XJ, Aldinger AM, Juhaszova M et al. Dysfunctional voltage-gated K^+ channels in pulmonary artery smooth cells of patients with primary pulmonary hypertension. Circulation 1998; 1400–1406.

39. Barnes PJ, Liu SF. Regulation of pulmonary vascular tone. Pharmacol Rev 1995; 47: 87–131.

40. Downing SE, Lee JC. Nervous control of the pulmonary circulation. Annu Rev Physiol 1980; 42: 199–210.

41. Nichols WW, O'Rourke MF. In: McDonald's blood flow in arteries, 4th ed. London: Edward Arnold; 1998.

42. Elzinga G, Piene H, de Jong JP. Left and right ventricular pump function and consequences of having two pumps in one heart. Circ Res 1980; 46: 564–574.

43. Furuno Y, Nagamoto Y, Fujita M et al. Reflection as a cause of mid-systolic deceleration of pulmonary flow wave in dogs with acute pulmonary hypertension: comparison of pulmonary artery constriction with pulmonary embolisation. Cardiovasc Res 1991; 25: 118–124.

44. Murgo JP, Westerhof N. Input impedance of the pulmonary arterial system in normal man: effects of respiration and comparison to systemic impedance. Circ Res 1984; 54: 666–673.

45. Pagnamenta A, Bouckaert Y, Wauthy P et al. Continuous versus pulsatile pulmonary hemodynamics in oleic acid lung injury. Am J Respir Crit Care Med 2000; 162: 936–940.

46. Fitzpatrick JM, Grant BJB. Effects of pulmonary vascular obstruction on right ventricular afterload. Am Rev Respir Dis 1990; 141: 944–952.

47. Kitabatake A, Inoue M, Asao M et al. Noninvasive evaluation of pulmonary hypertension by a pulsed Doppler technique. Circulation 1983; 68: 302–309.

48. Hatle J, Angelsen B. In: Doppler ultrasound in cardiology: physical principles and clinical applications, 2nd ed. Philadelphia, PA: Lea & Febiger; 1985.

49. Naeije R, Torbicki A. More on the noninvasive diagnosis of pulmonary hypertension: Doppler echocardiography revisited. Eur Respir J 1995; 8: 1445–1449.

50. Yock P, Popp R. Noninvasive estimation of right ventricular systolic pressure by Doppler ultrasound in patients with tricuspid regurgitation. Circulation 1984; 70: 657–662.

51. Torbicki A, Skwarski K, Hawrylkiewicz I et al. Attemps at measuring pulmonary arterial pressure by means of Doppler echocardiography in patients with chronic lung disease. Eur Respir J 1989; 2: 856–860.

52. Nakayama Y, Sugimachi M, Nakanishi N et al. Noninvasive differential diagnosis between chronic pulmonary thromboembolism and primary pulmonary hypertension by means of Doppler ultrasound measurement. J Am Coll Cardiol 1998; 31: 1367–1371.

2 Function

2.7 Respiratory function during exercise

Josep Roca and Roberto A Rabinovich

Key concepts

- The integrity of the different pathways governing cellular oxygen transport and oxygen utilisation, and their functional integration, are pivotal determinants of exercise capacity.

- In healthy humans, ventilation and cardiac output increase markedly during exercise to match O_2 transport to augmented cellular O_2 requirements. At moderate levels of exercise, the efficiency of the lung as O_2 and CO_2 exchanger improves. At extreme exercise, however, the efficiency of the lung as O_2 exchanger decreases because of:
  - ventilation–perfusion mismatching
  - alveolar–end capillary O_2 diffusion limitation.

- Response to exercise in disease may result in:
  - low performance limits (low peak levels of both O_2 uptake and work rate) and/or
  - abnormal specific response(s) of heart, pulmonary or muscle function to a given exercise load.

- The amount of $\dot{V}O_2$ achieved during exercise by a given patient is not only set by the intrinsic characteristics of the system, it also depends on:
  - environmental factors (altitude above sea level, F_1O_2)
  - cellular O_2 requirements determined by the amount of exercising muscle mass (cycling, walking, etc.) and the type of exercise
    protocol (incremental test, 6-min walking test, etc.).

- Identification of a plateau in $\dot{V}O_2$ despite further increases in work rate indicates that maximum O_2 uptake ($\dot{V}O_{2\,max}$) of the

system has been achieved. In this circumstance, $\dot{V}O_{2\,max}$ can be the result of:
  - having reached the limits of O_2 supply (O_2 uptake will further increase by experimentally augmenting any one of the components of O_2 transport) or
  - having reached mitochondrial oxidative capacity (increase in O_2 supply will not lead to any further raise in $\dot{V}O_{2\,max}$)

- Incremental exercise testing in disease usually identifies peak $\dot{V}O_2$ (at exhaustion) without evidence of plateau. In this circumstance, whether peak is limited by O_2 supply, mitochondrial oxidative capacity or other factors (symptom-limited exercise) can not be properly identified.

- Exercise tolerance ($\dot{V}O_{2\,max}$) is determined by the capacity of the O_2 transport/O_2 utilisation system rather than by the muscle's contractile machinery. Two physiological muscle properties (muscle strength and muscle fatigability) may, however, modulate functional performance of the patient's activities of daily life as well as during clinical exercise testing.

- Muscle strength is defined as the force generated by a muscle. It is determined by the number and type of motor units recruited; whereas muscle fatigue has been defined as a loss of contractile functions caused by prolonged exercise and reversible by rest. Factors involved in muscle fatigue are complex:
  - contractile machinery
  - muscle respiratory capacity
  - redox status of the skeletal muscle.

Survival depends on the availability of oxygen to all body tissues and cells. During steady-state conditions, oxygen consumption ($\dot{V}O_2$) matches the turnover of adenosine triphosphate (ATP), the high-energy phosphate needed to fulfil the bioenergetic requirements of the cells. It is well-known that ATP is efficiently generated by oxidative phosphorylation into the mitochondria. Within the inner mitochondrial matrix, pyruvate is converted to acetyl coenzyme A (CoA) and metabolised aerobically via the tricarboxylic acid cycle to yield water and carbon dioxide (CO_2) as residual products to be subsequently eliminated.

Alternative pathways of energy production not requiring oxygen constitute rapid but only transient solutions to fulfil the bioenergetic requirements. That is, anaerobic reduction of pyruvate to lactate in the cytosol is inefficient in terms of ATP production. Moreover, increased lactate levels provoke a marked fall in intracellular pH that may alter mitochondrial function. Likewise, skeletal muscle contains high levels of phosphocreatine (PCr) compared to other tissues, but the breakdown of muscle PCr stores can supply cellular needs of ATP for only few seconds of strenuous contraction. Compared to anaerobic glycolysis, aerobic metabolism requires longer to be activated. Energy utilisation during the first 2–3 min of exercise requires more ATP than can be synthesised from aerobic pathways in the muscle. This phenomenon causes an 'oxygen debt' that must be repaid after exercise. Aerobic metabolism, in turn, is more efficient in terms of ATP production and enables the cell to use stored lipids as fuel via fatty-acid metabolism.[1] Consequently, the integrity of the different pathways governing cellular O_2 transport/O_2 utilisation are pivotal determinants of exercise capacity both in health and disease (Fig. 2.7.1).

This chapter examines the interactions among the different steps influencing O_2 transport and cellular respiration during exercise. Attention is paid to the analysis of exercise responses close to exhaustion, but more importantly we emphasise the interest of assessing the system responses during submaximal exercise. Finally, the role of exercise testing in the evaluation of functional performance in healthy subjects and in patients with chronic disorders is examined.

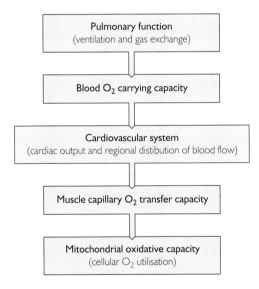

Fig. 2.7.1 Major elements of the O_2 transport/O_2 utilisation pathway. Integrated effects of all steps involved to move oxygen from air to mitochondria are essential to determine maximum capacity of the system. In disease, non-uniformity of ventilation/perfusion ratios in the lung and/or metabolism/perfusion ratios in the peripheral tissues may be of considerable importance.

Responses to exercise in health and disease

There is nothing intrinsically different in the direction of the overall system response to exercise comparing normal subjects and patients with lung disease. Thus, as a patient exercises harder, O_2 consumption, CO_2 production, ventilation and cardiac output all increase to fulfil increased muscle bioenergetic requirements, as they do in the normal subject,[2] but peak levels attained are less, more so with increasing severity of disease. Differences in lung diseases from the normal situation with regard to exercise response include:

- resting cardiopulmonary function
- physical deconditioning
- the intensity and duration of exercise that can be performed, and the relationship between intensity/duration and symptom development
- the specific responses of the heart and lungs/chest wall to a given exercise load in terms of rate, magnitude and performance limits
- the relative importance of each part of the O_2 and CO_2 transport pathway in contributing to any limitation of exercise that is found
- the relative importance of locomotor and respiratory muscle fatigue
- metabolic accompaniments of exercise, in particular lactate release and accumulation, and high energy phosphate levels.

Pulmonary response to exercise in healthy humans

It is well known that ventilation and cardiac output markedly increase during exercise to match O_2 transport with augmented cellular O_2 requirements.[3] Since ventilation increases to a relatively higher extent than pulmonary blood flow, the ratio of total alveolar ventilation to blood flow (overall $\dot{V}_A/\dot{Q}$ ratio) rises rather substantially. At moderate levels of exercise, the dispersion of the $\dot{V}_A/\dot{Q}$ distributions does not change[4-6] but the $\dot{V}_A/\dot{Q}$ ratios at the mean of both ventilation and perfusion distributions increase markedly because of the higher overall $\dot{V}_A/\dot{Q}$ ratio. Consequently, the efficiency of the lung as an O_2 and CO_2 exchanger improves at these exercise levels. Mixed venous P_{O_2} falls dramatically during exercise because the relative increase in $\dot{V}_{O_2}$ is considerably greater than that of cardiac output, and mixed venous P_{CO_2} levels rise equally remarkably. Arterial P_{O_2} levels generally remain unchanged until extremely high levels of exercise are undertaken. Arterial P_{CO_2} levels are also relatively stable until the appearance of high blood lactate levels generates acidosis, even more ventilation, and thus a fall in P_{CO_2} levels.

The alveolar–arterial O_2 gradient (AaP_{O_2}), however, progressively increases with the level of exercise, reaching values of 20–30 mmHg close to maximal exercise ($\dot{V}_{O_2}$ peak) in average subjects, and even greater (up to 40 mmHg or more) in some elite athletes.[7] Such an increase in AaP_{O_2} indicates inefficiency of pulmonary gas exchange during heavy exercise that is even more apparent in other animal species such as horse.[8] It has been shown that the increase in the AaPo$_2$ during exercise is due, in part, to $\dot{V}_A/\dot{Q}$ mismatching[4-6] but it is mostly explained by limitation of alveolar–end-capillary O$_2$ diffusion.[5,9]

Abnormalities of pulmonary gas exchange during heavy exercise in well-trained healthy subjects are clearly accentuated if exercise is carried out during hypoxia produced either by breathing a low inspired O$_2$ fraction[9] or simulating altitude in a hypobaric chamber.[4,5,10,11] The increase in the dispersion of the perfusion distribution (log SD$_Q$) during heavy exercise is not associated with altered spirometry but shows a significant correlation with the increase in mean pulmonary artery pressure. Experimental studies suggest that development of subclinical pulmonary oedema[5,11] may explain the deterioration of pulmonary gas exchange during heavy exercise.

Pulmonary response in lung diseases

In patients with chronic obstructive pulmonary disease (COPD), resting levels of minute ventilation ($\dot{V}_E$) are abnormally high but, during exercise, the slope between $\dot{V}_E$ and work rate is normal. For a given level of $\dot{V}_E$ during exercise, tidal volume (V_T) tends to be lower and respiratory rate (f) higher in patients than in healthy subjects.[12,13] Moreover, the O$_2$ cost of breathing per unit ventilation is higher in COPD patients than in healthy subjects. Impaired respiratory mechanics requires more effort to move a given volume of air.

Peak exercise V_T is strongly related to vital capacity in these patients.[14] They adopt two strategies during exercise to increase $\dot{V}_E$:[12]

- end-expiratory lung volume increases, allowing higher maximum expiratory flow rates (Fig. 2.7.2). This dynamic hyperinflation does not occur in normal humans, who show a fall in end-expiratory lung volume during exercise[12]
- inspiratory flow rate increases, so that inspiratory time decreases and more time is available for expiration.[12]

Impaired respiratory mechanics (dynamic hyperinflation) seems to play a major role-limiting exercise tolerance in these patients. During exercise in COPD, a balance is struck between the need for ventilation and the high cost of breathing. The most common end-result is a small rise in arterial PCO$_2$ and similar fall in P_aO$_2$. However, unless pulmonary CO transfer capacity (DLCO) is severely impaired (< 50% predicted value), P_aO$_2$ does not fall during exercise, and may even increase in some subjects. Studies using the multiple inert gas elimination technique in COPD show that $\dot{V}_A/\dot{Q}$ mismatch is usually unaltered from that at rest, that shunts do not develop and that diffusion limitation also does not occur.[15] This is even the case when COPD is severe.[15] In milder disease, there is evidence that small improvements in $\dot{V}_A/\dot{Q}$ relationships may occur on exercise,[16,17] providing a partial reason for improvement in arterial PO$_2$. However, it is not infrequently observed that, when the patient with COPD is encouraged to maximal effort, sudden hypoxaemia and hypercapnia can develop just before the patient stops exercising.[15]

In a variety of chronic respiratory disorders such as interstitial lung diseases and pulmonary vascular diseases, abnormally high resting levels of minute ventilation ($\dot{V}_E$) and normal slope

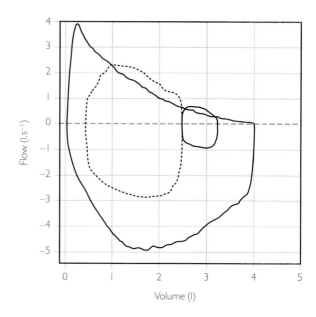

Fig. 2.7.2 The resting maximal flow-volume curve from a patient with chronic obstructive pulmonary disease is represented by the solid line. The smallest solid loop corresponds to tidal volume at rest and the dashed curve indicates tidal volume at maximal exercise. During exercise, end-inspiratory and end-expiratory lung volumes are increased (dynamic hyperinflation) and expiratory flow limitation is seen over most of expiration. (Redrawn with permission from Roca & Whipp 1997.[65])

between $\dot{V}_E$ and work rate during exercise are commonly observed, but not dynamic hyperinflation as seen in COPD patients. They do not change end-expiratory lung volume significantly during exercise.[18] Oxygen cost of breathing per unit ventilation is increased in patients with interstitial lung disease because the increased elastic recoil requires more inspiratory muscle activity. They show a strong linear relationship between peak exercise V_T and vital capacity,[18] suggesting that differences in peak V_T are mainly due to abnormal respiratory mechanics.

During exercise, patients with interstitial lung disease generally show typical and substantial blood-gas changes, even at moderate effort. While arterial PCO$_2$ is generally unaffected,[18] P_aO$_2$ falls in almost all patients,[19-21] sometimes severely, as does mixed venous PO$_2$. It is mainly this profound degree of arterial hypoxaemia (and not respiratory mechanics) that limits exercise tolerance in interstitial lung disease.[22-25] Worsening of $\dot{V}_A/\dot{Q}$ mismatching and shunt does not play a relevant role in the exercise-induced hypoxaemia seen in these patients.[19] Therefore, the blood-gas changes on exercise in interstitial lung disease are mostly the consequence of:

- insufficient increase of alveolar ventilation relative to the raise in $\dot{V}$O$_2$ and $\dot{V}$CO$_2$
- secondary effects from the fall in mixed venous PO$_2$ causing a fall in arterial PO$_2$.[26]

Also, O$_2$ diffusion limitation is seen during exercise in most patients with interstitial lung disease, further adding to the hypoxaemia.[19] The presence of O$_2$ diffusion limitation in these patients despite the relatively low cardiac output at peak exercise ($< 10\,L\,min^{-1}$) is likely related to the combination of:

- an abnormally low mixed venous P_{O_2}
- a short capillary transit time
- some increased interstitial resistance for the diffusion of O_2 from the alveolar gas to the capillary blood caused by the large collagen deposits there.

Exercise-induced hypoxaemia in patients with interstitial lung disease is found to be largely due to the fall in venous P_{O_2}, because there is no systematic change in $\dot{V}_A/\dot{Q}$ relationships nor does diffusion limitation develop.[19]

Haemodynamic responses to exercise in health and disease

In healthy subjects, cardiac output ($\dot{Q}_T$) shows a linear increase in relation to O_2 uptake during exercise. Likewise, both stroke volume and heart rate (HR) also increase as $\dot{V}_{O_2}$ rises. In well-trained subjects, an increase of up to fivefold (approximately $25\,l\cdot min^{-1}$) in $\dot{Q}_T$ at peak exercise can often be seen. Systolic pulmonary pressure increases during exercise, but pulmonary vascular resistance falls because of vascular recruitment. At systemic levels, systolic pressure increases, but not diastolic pressure.

It is of note, however, that elite athletes at peak exercise show a potent sympathetic vasoconstriction at systemic level inducing massive redistribution of cardiac output, which ensures preferential perfusion to active skeletal muscle (due to local exercise-induced vasodilator effects) while preserving blood flow and O_2 delivery to essential organs such as the brain.[27] It has been reported that, in well-trained cyclists during maximal exercise, respiratory muscles subvert blood flow that otherwise would have been directed to limb muscles. In these subjects, unloading the respiratory system with proportional assist ventilation resulted in an increase in both leg blood flow and leg vascular conductance.[28,29] This phenomenon is not seen in chronic respiratory patients because they are unable to reach such extreme levels of O_2 uptake during exercise, although they may show increased O_2 cost of breathing per unit ventilation.[30]

In chronic respiratory disease, pulmonary vascular abnormalities are present well before frank heart failure occurs. There is pulmonary hypertension, often evident even at rest and usually during exercise. The increase in pressure per unit increase in cardiac output is some three times greater in these patients than in normal subjects.

In contrast to normal subjects, in whom pulmonary vascular resistance normally falls during exercise because of a combination of vascular recruitment and distension in the lungs, in COPD, vascular resistance remains constant or may even rise. The vascular destruction or obstruction that is well-known to occur in these diseases, together with some distortion and also hypoxic vasoconstriction, are the reasons underlying these physiological abnormalities. Eventually, as disease progresses, the right heart will hypertrophy and ultimately fail, and clinically significant cor pulmonale will be present. Despite the two- to threefold increase in vascular resistance and high pulmonary

artery pressures, it is remarkable that, even in advanced lung disease, the heart can pump essentially normally as a function of filling pressure, as shown from the limited data available.

At peak exercise, systemic O_2 delivery is clearly below normal level in patients with COPD.[12] While the obvious culprit is impaired pulmonary function, it is not always through a reduction in S_aO_2 that systemic O_2 delivery is primarily reduced, since, despite $\dot{V}_A/\dot{Q}$ inequality and reduced effective alveolar ventilation, hypoxaemia may not necessarily provoke a marked fall in arterial O_2 content.[12] It is accepted that cardiac output at peak exercise is always well below normal levels. However, in COPD patients, as in normal subjects, cardiac output increases linearly in relation to oxygen uptake as work rate increases during incremental exercise, such that cardiac output at a given submaximal O_2 uptake[31] is close to the expected normal value. It should be noted, however, that the rise in cardiac output during exercise is usually achieved by means of a higher heart rate and lower stroke volume than are found in healthy subjects.

Since total ventilation, cardiac output and exercise intensity remain closely coupled in COPD as in health, the inability to raise ventilation appears to be the principal governor of the O_2 transport process: a low ceiling on ventilation means a low ceiling on cardiac output and thus on systemic O_2 delivery. It should be mentioned that the mechanisms that couple ventilation to cardiac output during exercise are still not well understood. Montes de Oca et al[32] proposed that the large pleural pressure swings observed during exercise can be paramount in constraining left ventricular function, thus limiting both peak cardiac output and exercise tolerance in patients with very severe COPD. The coupling between whole-body O_2 uptake and cardiac output during exercise implies that the O_2 difference between arterial and mixed venous blood and the fractional O_2 extraction are normal or near normal.[33,34]

Femoral venous blood flow ($\dot{Q}_{leg}$) measurements by thermodilution in patients with moderate to severe airflow limitation[34,35] have recently shown, as for cardiac output, a marked reduction in peak $\dot{Q}_{leg}$. Leg blood flow (and leg O_2 delivery)[35] at a given submaximal whole-body O_2 uptake is normal in these patients.

The cardiac response to exercise in patients with interstitial lung disease is similar to that described for COPD patients. In contrast, patients with pulmonary vascular disease show different cardiac response to exercise. Certainly, at peak exercise cardiac output is lower. More importantly, however, the slope of the relationship between $\dot{V}_{O_2}$ and cardiac output is different. This suggests that for any given degree of exercise (i.e. $\dot{V}_{O_2}$), cardiac output in patients with pulmonary vascular disease does not increase as much as in controls or in patients with COPD or interstitial lung disease. This abnormal behaviour is probably related to the increased afterload of the right ventricle.[36–38] As expected, at rest, patients with pulmonary vascular disease have pulmonary artery hypertension and increased pulmonary vascular resistance. Compared to patients with COPD and interstitial lung disease, patients with pulmonary vascular disease show by far the worst haemodynamic situation. During exercise, pulmonary artery pressure increases in direct proportion to the increase in cardiac output and reaches extremely high values.

This indicates the lack of pulmonary vascular reserve. In fact, the pathologically elevated pulmonary vascular resistance seen at rest does not change substantially during exercise.

Peripheral O₂ transfer

Normal delivery of oxygen to muscle (muscle blood flow × arterial O_2 content) does not necessarily ensure adequate oxygenation of cells. A proper O_2 transfer capacity from muscle capillary to mitochondrion, a phenomenon that encompasses several steps, is required:

- O_2 unloading from haemoglobin (Hb)
- diffusion through the red cell wall, the plasma and the capillary wall
- diffusion through the myocyte and its binding to myoglobin, which greatly facilitates the intramuscular diffusion pathway.

Muscle P_{O_2} is quite homogeneous throughout the myocyte. It is of note that almost all the impedance to O_2 diffusion is located in the initial part of the pathway from Hb ($P_{O_2} \approx 40$ mmHg) to the sarcolemma ($P_{O_2} \approx 3$ mmHg), which represents only few microns of approximately a total of $50\,\mu m$ until the mitochondrion. From a morphometric standpoint, the ability to transfer oxygen from Hb to mitochondria is a function of how many capillaries surround each muscle fibre (surface available for O_2 transfer) rather than the distance from capillary to mitochondrion. Different studies[39-41] have identified the fact that impedance to peripheral O_2 diffusion may constitute a relevant factor contributing to set maximum O_2 uptake in well-trained subjects[39,40] and in patients with chronic renal failure.[42] In COPD patients, two indirect factors – low number of capillaries per muscle fiber[41] and O_2 supply dependency – seem to suggest that low peripheral O_2 diffusion capacity may also contribute to exercise-induced cell hypoxia, even in the absence of arterial hypoxaemia.

Utilisation of O₂ by muscles in health and disease

It has been reported that in, well-trained humans, maximum O_2 uptake depends on O_2 supply,[40] indicating that mitochondrial capacity does not constitute the rate-limiting factor for maximum exercise performance. In contrast, data from healthy sedentary subjects[39,43] strongly suggest that muscle mitochondrial function is a limiting step for maximum O_2 uptake in sedentary humans. A recent study including direct measurements of cell P_{O_2} saturation during exercise breathing different concentrations of O_2 further indicates that sedentary subjects does not exhibit dependency of maximum $\dot{V}_{O_2}$ on O_2 supply.[42] The plasticity of skeletal muscle during high-intensity physical training programmes[44] fully accounts for the differences alluded to between athletes and sedentary subjects.

The scenario is far more complex in patients with COPD. Since leg blood flow during submaximal exercise is preserved in moderate to severe COPD patients,[34,35] and early increase in blood lactate levels indicates an increased net lactate output across the leg.[34,35,45] The increased lactate production is responsible for the fall in muscle pH, which, in turn, may play a role

determining exercise intolerance in these patients.[35] Premature lactic acidosis during exercise in COPD patients has been associated with reduced oxidative enzyme concentrations in the lower limb muscles,[45,46] which can be at least partly reversed by physical training. This biochemical abnormality has been considered a hallmark of muscle dysfunction in COPD.

Several studies[34,47,48] exercising different muscle groups in heterogeneous groups of COPD patients have consistently shown lower cellular bioenergetic status, as indicated by a low ratio of phosphocreatine (PCr) to total intracellular phosphate (Pi) and lower intracellular pH (pHi) than those seen in healthy sedentary controls at equivalent levels of exercise. Also, a slow half-time of PCr recovery, measured after a constant-work rate protocol keeping pHi unchanged, has been observed in COPD patients.[34] These results are consistent with the low citrate synthase concentration in the quadriceps described by Maltais et al.[45,46] Recently, however, increased activity of cytochrome oxidase (COX) and upregulated mitochondrial gene expression of COX in the skeletal muscle of COPD patients with hypoxaemia requiring continuous oxygen therapy has been reported.[49] Since COX is the last enzyme of the oxidative phosphorylation chain, it can be speculated that upregulation of COX in these patients might reflect a compensatory phenomenon in the face of cellular hypoxia similar to that seen in peripheral vascular disease.[50,51]

Recent lines of evidence suggest that intrinsic skeletal muscle dysfunction may be present in patients with COPD as well as in other chronic disorders such as congestive heart failure. It is of note, however, that identification of skeletal muscle dysfunction in COPD can be obscured by several confounding factors, such as:

- impaired convective O_2 transport
- hypercapnia
- electrolyte abnormalities
- steroid therapy or other treatments
- (mainly) muscle deconditioning as a result of physical inactivity.

Analysis of intrinsic skeletal muscle dysfunction and quantitation of the relative contribution of peripheral factors in the limitation of peak O_2 uptake requires further studies, assessing:

- the impact of potential confounding factors on O_2 uptake, physical detraining being one of the key issues
- regional exercise performance (quadriceps exercise) unloading, at least partly, the central (pulmonary function) limiting factors.

It should be recognised that reduced mitochondrial capacity in these patients does not necessarily imply intrinsic muscle dysfunction due to COPD. There is evidence[34] suggesting that muscle deconditioning plays a major role in explaining the disturbances of skeletal muscle bioenergetics in COPD patients. Interestingly, a recent study[52] has demonstrated clear-cut differences in training-induced adaptations of muscle redox status between COPD patients and controls. While healthy sedentary subjects had increased muscle levels of the antioxidant glutathione after training, COPD patients had reduced redox potential. The phenomenon was even more accentuated in those patients with low body mass index ($< 20\,kg \cdot m^{-2}$). This study highlight the importance of training-induced peripheral adaptation and its relevance in the assessment of training outcomes in COPD patients. Whether oxidative stress is a central factor prompting muscle mass wasting, particularly in susceptible subsets of COPD patients in whom muscle apoptosis[53] can be observed, remains to be elucidated.

Engelen et al.[54,55] have speculated on a causal relationship between abnormally low muscle redox potential at rest and the alterations of cysteine-amino-acid metabolism observed in COPD patients.[54] There is increasing evidence that mitochondria are not only pivotal in the energy production process but also play a central role in cell survival and apoptosis control,[56] which appears to be a characteristic consistent with the myopathy associated with chronic diseases such as COPD and congestive heart failure. In this scenario, it can be speculated that susceptible COPD patients with a low body mass index may favour the induction of cytokines such as tumour necrosis factor-α (TNF-α) through activation of oxidative-sensitive transcription factors such as nuclear factor-κB (NF-κB), Upregulation of TNF-α and its targeting to mitochondria may establish a vicious cycle promoting muscle wasting and apoptosis in susceptible COPD patients. Further studies, however, are needed to shed light on the complex relationships between tissue hypoxia, abnormalities in the redox system, inflammatory cytokines and the phenomenon of weight loss in COPD patients.[57–59]

Factors determining exercise performance: integrated response

The preceding section set out the physiological responses to exercise at the different steps of oxygen transport and utilisation in healthy humans (well-trained and sedentary subjects) and in patients with common lung diseases. It is presently well accepted that the level of exercise tolerance is set by the integrity of each of the functions involved in the O_2 transport/O_2 utilisation system as well as by proper interactions among all of the physiological responses alluded to above.[60]

Complex integrative pathways both at whole body level and at cellular level have been identified. Since not only intracellular pH[61] but also cell P_{O_2}[62] has been shown to modulate mitochondrial function, O_2 transport (cell P_{O_2}) and O_2 utilisation (mitochondrial capacity) can not be analysed as separate systems.

Also of major interest are the events surrounding peak or maximal $\dot{V}_{O_2}$ and the physiological reason why peak or maximal $\dot{V}_{O_2}$ is reduced, as it almost always is, in disease. In this regard, it must be noted that the amount of $\dot{V}_{O_2}$ achieved by a given patient is not only set by the intrinsic characteristics of the system, it also depends on several other factors that modulate the physiological response of the whole body, such as:

- environmental conditions (altitude above sea level, fraction of inspired oxygen)
- amount of exercising muscle mass (cycling, walking, localised quadriceps exercise)
- type of exercise protocol (incremental, endurance test, 6-minute walking distance, shuttle test, etc.).

Since the catabolic capacity of the myosin ATPase is such that it outstrips by far the capacity of the respiratory system to deliver energy aerobically, exercise tolerance (maximum $\dot{V}_{O_2}$) is determined by the capacity of the O_2 transport/O_2 utilisation system rather than by the muscle's contractile machinery.

Two physiological muscle properties (muscle strength and muscle fatigability) may modulate functional performance of the patient in activities of daily life as well as during clinical exercise testing. Muscle strength is defined as the force generated by a muscle. It is determined by the number and type of motor units recruited; whereas muscle fatigue has been defined as a loss of contractile functions (force, velocity, power or work) caused by prolonged exercise and is reversible by rest. Factors involved in muscle fatigue are complex, but it mainly depend on:

- contractile machinery
- muscle respiratory capacity
- redox status of the muscle.

In practical terms, it may be useful to consider two different scenarios (peak $\dot{V}_{O_2}$ and maximum $\dot{V}_{O_2}$; Fig. 2.7.3). These are the following:

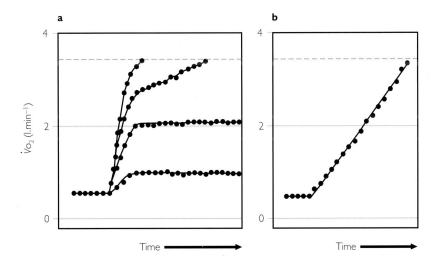

Fig. 2.7.3 Response of oxygen uptake to (a) a series of constant-work rate exercise tests, from moderate to heavy exercise and (b) a ramp-incremental test. Note that peak oxygen uptake (dashed horizontal line) does not differ between the protocols (a & b). There was no evidence of a plateau in oxygen uptake response (maximum O_2 uptake). Steady-state oxygen uptake was observed at moderate intensity constant-work rate exercise (a). (Redrawn with permission from Roca & Whipp 1997.[65])

1. A peak $\dot{V}_{O_2}$ has been reached without evidence of $\dot{V}_{O_2}$ plateauing. This is perhaps the commonest outcome in the clinical setting. Taken as it is, one cannot say whether this peak $\dot{V}_{O_2}$ is limited by O_2 supply, mitochondrial oxidative capacity or perhaps neither (i.e. symptoms are so severe that neither O_2 supply nor mitochondrial function have been fully exploited). In these circumstances, it will be useful to identify the $\dot{V}_{O_2}$ at which the transition from moderate to heavy exercise took place (lactate threshold, LT) and evaluate the organ system responses (ventilation, gas exchange, heart rate, etc.) during submaximal exercise and at peak $\dot{V}_{O_2}$. Despite not having information about the capacity of the system (a plateau of O_2 uptake was not identified), we will know about:

- the physiological burden imposed by exercise
- the reserve of the system depending upon the location of the transition from moderate to heavy exercise.

2. A plateau in $\dot{V}_{O_2}$ at maximal exercise is clearly identified such that the subject has achieved his/her maximum exercise (maximum O_2 uptake) capacity in that particular setting or there is physiological evidence that we are very close to maximum. In this circumstance, we may face two situations:

- maximum $\dot{V}_{O_2}$ ($\dot{V}_{O_{2max}}$) is the result of having reached mitochondrial oxidative capacity. In this scenario, the key concept is that acute increases in O_2 supply to the mitochondria would not lead to any further increase in maximum $\dot{V}_{O_2}$. In other words, no O_2 supply dependency can be observed by giving 100% O_2 to breathe or by blood transfusion (Fig. 2.7.4).
- maximum $\dot{V}_{O_2}$ is the result of having reached limits to the supply of O_2. In this circumstance, one or more components of the integrated O_2 transport system (the lungs, heart and blood vessels, blood and muscles) has reached maximum capacity for the given conditions, and this can be tested experimentally by augmenting any one of the components alluded to above (Fig. 2.7.4).

Exercise testing

Cardiopulmonary exercise testing is a unique tool to assess the limits and mechanisms of exercise tolerance. It also provides indices of the functional reserve of the organ systems involved in the exercise response, with inferences for system limitation at peak exercise. Moreover, cardiopulmonary exercise testing is useful for establishing the profiles and adequacy of the system responses at submaximal exercise. Several studies[63,64] have shown that the functional reserve (i.e. aerobic capacity) of patients with COPD and interstitial lung disease is not accurately predicted from indices of resting lung function. This section examines the protocols recommended for clinical exercise testing.

Exercise protocols

The goal of protocols for cardiopulmonary exercise testing is to stress the organ systems involved in the exercise response in a

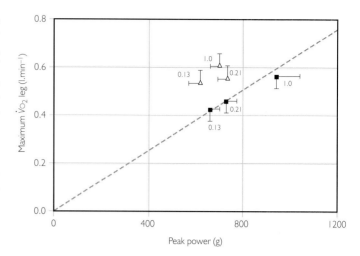

Fig. 2.7.4 Quadriceps maximum $\dot{V}_{O_2}$ (y axis) plotted against maximum work rate (x-axis; mean ± SEM) in healthy sedentary subjects (open triangles) and in chronic renal patients (filled squares) breathing 130%, 21% and 100% inspired O_2 concentrations (F_iO_2 0.13, 0.21 and 1.0 respectively). While chronic renal patients increased $\dot{V}_{O_{2max}}$ and W_{max} proportionally to the F_iO_2 increase, indicating dependency of $\dot{V}_{O_{2max}}$ on O_2 supply, healthy sedentary subjects did not show any relationship between exercise performance and changes in O_2 transport (and in cell oxygenation), suggesting that mitochondrial capacity, not O_2 transport, was limiting $\dot{V}_{O_{2max}}$. (Redrawn with permission from Sala et al 2001.[42])

controlled manner. For this reason the testing generally involves exercising large muscle groups, usually the muscles of the lower extremities. A key requirement is that exercise stimulus be quantifiable in terms of the external work and power performed. The appropriateness of the integrated systemic responses to the tolerable range of work rates is best studied using incremental exercise testing. This provides a smooth incremental stress to the subject so that the entire range of exercise intensities can be spanned in a short period of time.

The recommended incremental exercise testing protocol, usually electronically-braked cycle ergometry with a constant pedalling frequency of 60 rpm, is recommended. Equivalent results are obtained when the work rate is either increased continuously (ramp test) or by a uniform amount each minute (1-minute incremental test) until the patient is limited by symptoms (he/she can not cycle at more than 40 rpm) or is not able to continue safely. The increment size should be set according to the characteristics of the patient in order to achieve approximately 10 minutes duration of the incremental part of the protocol. This may represent incremental rates of 10–20 W · min⁻¹ in a healthy sedentary subject, or less in a patient.

Standard non-invasive cardiopulmonary exercise testing carried out breathing room air ($F_iO_2 = 0.21$) involves acquisition of expired O_2 and CO_2 concentrations (F_EO_2 and F_ECO_2 respectively), work rate (W), expired airflow, heart rate (HR) and systemic arterial pressure as primary variables.

Electrocardiogram (ECG) and pulse oximetry should be continuously monitored during the test. It is useful to establish a sense of the patient's exercise-related perceptions during the exercise test and at the point when he/she discontinues exercise. This includes exertion, dyspnoea, chest pain and skeletal muscle effort. Quantifying these perceptions should be done using standardised rating procedures (Borg scale, visual analogue scale, etc.). Proper evaluation of pulmonary gas exchange in patients with lung disease requires assessment of arterial respiratory blood gases. Alternative protocols can be considered for specific purposes.[65]

The greatest diagnostic potential and impact on the clinical decision-making process of exercise testing should rely not on the utility of any one individual measurement, although some are obviously more important than others, but rather on their integrated use. Identification of a cluster of responses characteristic of different diseases is often useful. The major portion of the interpretation strategy is focused on results generated during maximal, symptom-limited, incremental exercise testing. This is currently the most popular, albeit not the exclusive protocol. Often, insufficient attention is paid to trending phenomena as the work rate progresses from submaximal to peak levels. To facilitate this type of analysis, the results should be formatted in an appropriate manner. Figure 2.7.5 displays data obtained in a normal subject performing cycle ergometry – using an ergometer that employs an 'assist' to provide an actual 0 W work rate at 'unloaded' pedalling. The four plots in the left column of this figure provide, in addition to the peak $\dot{V}O_2$, the variables commonly used to provide an indirect estimation of the lactate threshold, i.e. identification of the O_2 uptake at which the transition between moderate- and heavy-intensity exercise occurs.

The plot on the top of the right column (O_2 uptake versus work rate) reflects the exercise efficiency and the limits of exercise tolerance of the subject. The plot immediately below (ventilation versus CO_2 output) and the one on the bottom (tidal volume versus ventilation) characterise aspects of the ventilatory response during submaximal and peak exercise. However, some investigators find the relationship between $\dot{V}_E$ and $\dot{V}O_2$ during such tests to be useful. Finally, the plot between heart rate (and O_2 pulse) versus O_2 uptake is informative with respect to the characteristics of the haemodynamic response to exercise.

The next step is to choose adequate reference values to establish patterns of normal or abnormal response. Available reference values and present limitations in this particular issue are discussed in Roca & Whipp 1997.[65] Relatively few studies have evaluated the sensitivity, specificity and predictive value of patterns of measurements in distinguishing among different clinical entities. Even more importantly, the precise role of clusters of variables commonly used in the decision-making process in well-identified diseases (i.e. evaluation of interstitial lung disease, preoperative evaluation for resection lung cancer surgery, etc.) is insufficiently known. In the future, studies addressing the use of likelihood ratios might be even more useful to clinicians than sensitivity/specificity, since likelihood ratios refer to actual test results before disease status is known. This shift to an evidence-based approach for interpretation of cardiopulmonary exercise

testing will hopefully provide important answers to clinically relevant questions that are not immediately available.

The timed walking tests have been extensively used in the clinical evaluation of patients with chronic cardiopulmonary disorders, mainly because of their simplicity. A present, these tests are acknowledged to add prognostic information useful to the staging of patients with COPD,[66,67] primary pulmonary hypertension[68] and heart failure.[69] Timed walking tests have shown to be sensitive to changes after interventions such as inhaled bronchodilators,[70] volume reduction surgery[71] and, pulmonary rehabilitation.[72,73] The 6-minute walking test, for example, is currently performed in a large number of rehabilitation programmes. Recent studies[74] suggest that the encouraged 6-minute walking test is a strenuous protocol that evaluates sustainable exercise performance. The two tests (6-minute walking and incremental cycling protocols) clearly measure different aspects of exercise tolerance and should be considered to be complementary.

Detailed recommendations on the indications, standardisation and interpretation of clinical exercise testing in patients with lung disease have recently been published by a Task Force of the European respiratory Society.[65,75]

Clinical relevance

- Cardiopulmonary exercise testing is a unique tool for assessing the limits and mechanisms of exercise tolerance. It also provides indices of the functional reserve of the organ systems involved in the exercise response, with inferences for system limitation at peak exercise. The subject's functional performance can not be inferred from resting pulmonary function tests.

- Exercise tolerance in chronic respiratory diseases is a predictor of both mortality and use of health-care resources, independent of resting pulmonary function.

- Important aspects in the evaluation of exercise testing in patients are:
  - assessment of exercise tolerance (peak $\dot{V}O_2$ and peak work rate)
  - identification of the $\dot{V}O_2$ at which the transition from moderate to heavy exercise takes place (lactate threshold, LT)
  - evaluation of the organ system responses at a given submaximal work rate and at peak exercise.

- Clinical exercise testing should be performed according to a validated and standardised protocol, including all safety precautions. Incremental cycling protocols are recommended to assess the physiological response to a range of exercise stimulus properly quantified in terms of external work rate.

- Timed-walking tests are extensively used in the clinical evaluation of patients with chronic cardiopulmonary disorders mainly because of their simplicity. These tests are recognised to add valuable prognostic information useful to the staging of patients with chronic obstructive pulmonary disease, pulmonary vascular diseases and heart failure, as well as to assess changes after interventions.

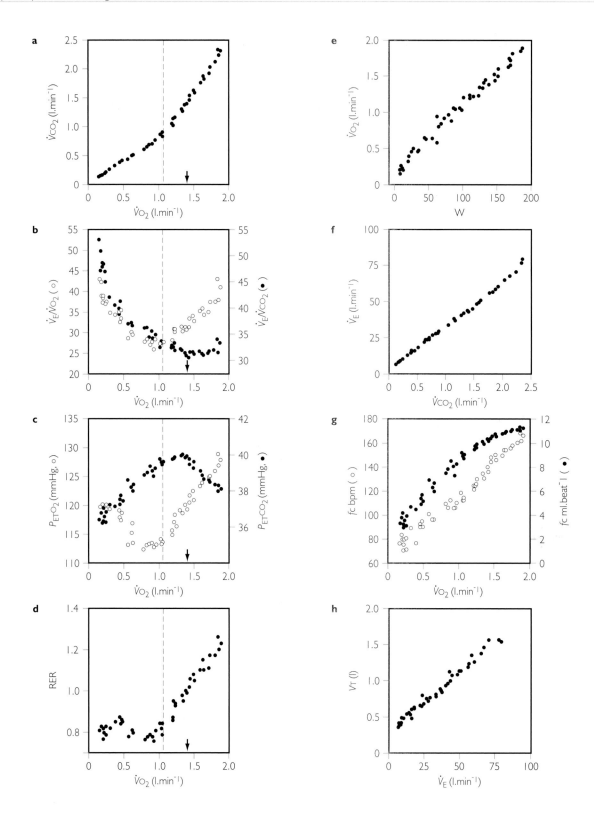

Fig. 2.7.5 Exercise performance in a healthy sedentary male subject. The basic plots for the interpretation of cardiopulmonary exercise testing are reported. In a–d, in addition to peak $\dot{V}O_2$, the variables commonly used to indirectly estimate lactic threshold (LT) are given. That is, the $\dot{V}O_2$ at which the transition from moderate- to high-intensity exercise occurs is identified (vertical dashed line). The expected LT for a healthy subject (55% of predicted peak $\dot{V}O_2$) is indicated in a–d by a small arrow (continuous line). Predicted peak $\dot{V}O_2$ is indicated in a by an arrow (dashed line). In e, $\dot{V}O_2$ versus work rate reflects the exercise efficiency and limits of exercise tolerance of the subject; with the expected peak exercise performance represented by the asterisk. f & h indicate ventilation versus $\dot{V}CO_2$ and tidal volume (V_T) versus ventilation, respectively; these two plots describe the characteristics of the ventilatory response during submaximal and peak exercise. Finally g presents characteristics of the haemodynamic response to exercise with estimated peak heart rate (HR) represented by the asterisk and predicted peak O_2 pulse by the arrow. $\dot{V}O_2$, oxygen uptake; $\dot{V}CO_2$, carbon dioxide production; $\dot{V}_E$, minute ventilation; PET_1O_2, end-tidal oxygen pressure; PET_1CO_2, end-tidal carbon dioxide pressure; RER, respiratory exchange ratio ($\dot{V}CO_2/\dot{V}O_2$); f_c = cardiac frequency; $\dot{V}_T$ = tidal volume; W = work rate. (Redrawn with permission from Roca et al 1997.[75])

←

? Unresolved questions

■ Recent lines of evidence suggest that skeletal muscle dysfunction may be present in patients with chronic respiratory diseases, particularly in chronic obstructive pulmonary disease with muscle wasting. However, identification of the problem is obscured by several confounding factors:
  – impaired O_2 flow
  – hypercapnia
  – electrolyte abnormalities
  – steroid therapy or other treatments and, mainly,
  – muscle deconditioning due to physical inactivity.

■ Further studies are needed to shed light on the systemic abnormalities in chronic obstructive pulmonary disease (COPD), particularly the complex relationships among tissue hypoxia, abnormalities in the redox system, inflammatory cytokines and the phenomenon of weight loss in COPD patients. Response to exercise and physical training constitute proper scenarios for examining the phenomenon.

■ Uniform reference values for standardised exercise testing are needed to improve the clinical interpretation of these tests.

Preferred guidelines

■ Astrand PO, Rodahl K. Textbook of work physiology. Physiological basis of exercise, 3rd ed. New York: McGraw-Hill; 1986.

■ ERS Task Force on 'Standardization of clinical exercise testing'. Clinical exercise testing with reference to lung disease: indications, standardization and interpretation strategies. Eur Respir J 1997; 10: 2662–2689.

■ Task Force on Practice Guidelines. ACC/AHA guidelines for exercise testing: a report of the American College of Cardiology/American Heart Association. J Am Coll Cardiol 1997; 30: 260–311.

■ Jones NL. Clinical exercise testing, 4th ed. Philadelphia: WB Saunders; 1997.

■ Wasserman K, Hansen JE, Sue DY et al. Principles of exercise testing and interpretation, 3rd ed. Philadelphia: Lippincott Williams & Wilkins; 1999.

■ American College of Sports Medicine. ACSM's guidelines for exercise testing and prescription, 6th ed. Philadelphia: Lippincott Williams & Wilkins; 2000.

References

1. Westerblad H, Lee JA, Lännergren J, Allen DC. Cellular mechanisms of fatigue in skeletal muscle. Am J Physiol 1991; 261: C195–C209.
2. Wasserman K, Hansen JE, Sue DY et al. Principles of exercise testing and interpretation, 2nd ed. Philadelphia, PA: Lea & Febiger; 1994.
3. Agusti A, Cotes J, Wagner PD. Responses to exercise in lung diseases. In: Roca J, Whipp B, ed. Clinical exercise testing. European Respiratory Monograph. Sheffield, UK: European Respiratory Society; 1997: 32–50.
4. Gale GE, Torre-Bueno J, Moon RE et al. Ventilation-perfusion inequality in normal humans during exercise. J Appl Physiol 1985; 58: 978–988.
5. Wagner PD, Gale GE, Moon RE et al. Pulmonary gas exchange in humans exercising at sea level and simulated altitude. J Appl Physiol 1986; 61: 260–270.
6. Hammond MD, Gale GE, Kapitan KS et al. Pulmonary gas exchange in humans during exercise at sea level. J Appl Physiol 1986; 60: 1590–1598.
7. Dempsey JA, Hanson PG, Henderson KS. Exercise-induced arterial hypoxemia in healthy subjects at sea level. J Physiol (Lond) 1984; 355: 161–175.
8. Wagner PD. A comparison of man and horse during heavy exercise. In: Hypoxia: the adaptations. Sutton JR, Coates G, Remmers JE, eds. Toronto: BC Decker Inc; 1999: 142–147.
9. Hammond MD, Gale GE, Kapitan KS et al. Pulmonary gas exchange in humans during normobaric hypoxic exercise. J Appl Physiol 1985; 58: 978–988.
10. Torre-Bueno J, Wagner PD, Saltzman HA et al. Diffusion limitation in normal humans during exercise at sea level and simulated altitude. J Appl Physiol 1985; 58: 989–995.
11. Wagner PD, Sutton JR, Peeves JT et al. Operation Everest II: pulmonary gas exchange during a simulated ascent of Mt Everest. J Appl Physiol 1987; 63: 2348–2359.
12. Gallagher CG. Exercise limitation and clinical exercise testing in chronic obstructive pulmonary disease. Clin Chest Med 1994; 15: 305–326.
13. Casaburi R, Petty TL. Ventilatory control in lung disease. In: Barstow TJ, Casaburi R, ed. Principles and practice of pulmonary rehabilitation. Philadelphia, PA: Publisher; 1993: 50–65.
14. Gowda KS, Zintel T, McParland C et al. Diagnostic value of maximal exercise tidal volume Chest 1990; 98: 1351–1354.
15. Dantzker DR, D'Alonzo GE. The effect of exercise on pulmonary gas exchange in patients with severe chronic obstructive pulmonary disease. Am Rev Respir Dis 1986; 134: 1135–1139.
16. Agusti AGN, Barbera JA, Roca J et al. Hypoxic pulmonary vasoconstriction and gas exchange during exercise in chronic obstructive pulmonary disease. Chest 1990; 97: 268–275.
17. Barberà JA, Roca J, Ramirez et al. Gas exchange during exercise in mild chronic obstructive pulmonary disease. Am Rev Respir Dis 1991; 144: 520–525.

18. Marciniuk DD, Gallagher CG. Clinical exercise testing in interstitial lung disease. Clin Chest Med 1994; 15: 287–303.
19. Agusti AG-N, Roca J, Rodriguez-Roisin P et al Mechanisms of gas exchange impairment in idiopathic pulmonary fibrosis. Am Rev Respir Dis 1991; 143: 219–225.
20. Cherniack RM, Colby TV, Flint A et al. Correlation of structure and function in idiopathic pulmonary fibrosis. Am J Respir Crit Care Med 1995; 151: 1180–1188.
21. Agusti C, Xaubet A, Agusti AG-N et al. Clinical and functional assessment of patients with idiopathic pulmonary fibrosis: results of a 3 years follow-up. Eur Respir J 1994; 7: 643–650.
22. Harris-Eze AO, Sridhar G, Clemens RE et al. Pole of hypoxemia and pulmonary mechanics in exercise limitation in interstitial lung disease. Am J Respir Crit Care Med 1996; 154: 994–1001.
23. Marciniuk DD, Sridhar G, Clements RE et al. Lung volumes and expiratory flow limitation during exercise in interstitial lung disease. J Appl Physiol 1994; 77: 963–973.
24. Marciniuk DD, Watts RE, Gallagher CG. Dead space loading and exercise limitation in patients with interstitial lung disease. Chest 1994; 105: 183–189.
25. Harris-Eze AC, Sridhar G, Clemens RE et al. Oxygen improves maximal exercise performance in interstitial lung disease. Am J Respir Crit Care Med 1994; 150: 1616–1622.
26. Wagner PD. Ventilation-perfusion inequality and gas exchange during exercise in lung disease In: Dempsey JA, Reed CE, ed. Muscular exercise and the lung Madison, WI: University of Wisconsin Press; 1977: 345–356.
27. Rowell LB. Human cardiovascular control. New York: Oxford University Press; 1993.
28. Harms CA, Babcock MA, McClaran SR et al. Respiratory muscle work compromises leg blood flow during maximal exercise. J Appl Physiol 1997; 82: 1573–1583.
29. Harms CA, Wetter TJ, McClaran SR et al. Effects of respiratory muscle work on cardiac output and its distribution during maximal exercise. J Appl Physiol 1998; 85: 609–618.
30. Onorati P, Rabinovich R A, Mancini M et al. Effects of proportional assist ventilation (PAV) on limb exercise in COPD (abstract). Am J Respir Crit Care Med 2000; 161: A228.
31. Light RW, Mintz HM, Linden GS, Brown SE. Hemodynamics of patients with severe chronic obstructive pulmonary disease during progressive upright exercise. Am Rev Respir Dis 1984; 130: 391–395.
32. Montes de Oca M, Rassullo J, Celli BR. Respiratory muscle and cardiopulmonary function during exercise in very severe COPD. Am J Respir Crit Care Med 1996; 154: 1284–1289.
33. Raffestin B, Escourrou P, Legrand A et al. Circulatory transport of oxygen in patients with chronic airflow obstruction exercising maximally. Am Rev Respir Dis 1982; 125: 426–431.
34. Sala E, Roca J, Marrades RM et al. Effects of endurance training on skeletal muscle bioenergetics in chronic obstructive pulmonary disease. Am J Respir Crit Care Med 1999; 159: 1726–1734.
35. Maltais F, Jobin J, Sullivan MJ et al. Lower limb metabolic and hemodynamic responses during exercise in normal subjects and in COPD. J Appl Physiol 1998; 84: 1573–1580.
36. D'Alonzo GE, Gianotti LA, Pohil RL. Comparison of progressive exercise performance of normal subjects and patients with primary pulmonary hypertension. Chest 1987; 92: 57–62.
37. Mèlot Ch, Naeije R, Mols P et al. Effects of nifedipine on ventilation/perfusion matching in primary pulmonary hypertension. Chest 1983; 83: 203–207.
38. Rubin LJ, Peter RH. Oral hydralazine therapy for primary pulmonary hypertension. N Engl J Med 1980; 302: 69–73.
39. Roca J, Agusti AG-N, Alonso A et al. Effects of training on muscle O_2 transport at $\dot{V}O_2$max. J Appl Physiol 1992; 73: 1067–1076.
40. Richardson RS, Noyszewski EA, Kendrick KF et al. Myoglobin O_2 desaturation during exercise: evidence of limited O_2 transport. J Clin Invest 1995; 96: 1916–1926.
41. Jobin J, Maltais F, Doyon JF et al. Chronic obstructive pulmonary disease: capillarity and fiber characteristics of skeletal muscle. J Cardiopulmon Rehab 1998; 18: 432–437.
42. Sala E, Noyszewski EA, Campistol JM et al. Impaired muscle oxygen transfer in patients with chronic renal failure. Am J Physiol 2001; 280: R1240–R1248.
43. Cardus J, Marrades RM, Roca J. Effects of F_IO_2 on leg $\dot{V}O_2$ during cycle ergometry in sedentary subjects. Med Sci Sports 1998; 30: 697–703.
44. Saltin B, Gollnick PD. Skeletal muscle adaptability: significance for metabolism and performance. In: Peachey LD, ed. Handbook of physiology, sect. 10: Skeletal muscle. Washington DC: American Physiological Society; 1983: 555.
45. Maltais F, Simard AA, Simard C et al. Oxidative capacity of the skeletal muscle and lactic acid kinetics during exercise in normal subjects and in patients with COPD. Am J Respir Crit Care Med 1996; 153: 288–293.
46. Maltais F, Leblanc P, Simard C et al. Skeletal muscle adaptation to endurance training in patients with Chronic Obstructive Pulmonary Disease. Am J Respir Crit Care Med 1996; 154: 442–447.
47. Payen JF, Wuyam B, Levy P et al. Muscular metabolism during oxygen supplementation in patients with chronic hypoxemia. Am Rev Respir Dis 1993; 147: 592–598.
48. Mannix ET, Boska MD, Galassetti P et al. Modulation of ATP production by oxygen in obstructive lung disease as assessed by ^{31}P-MRS. J Appl Physiol 1995; 78: 2218–2227.
49. Sauleda J, García-Palmer F, Wiesner RJ et al. Cytochrome oxidase activity and mitochondrial gene expression in skeletal muscle of patients with chronic obstructive pulmonary disease. Am J Respir Crit Care Med 1998; 157: 1413–1417.
50. Jansson E, Johansson J, Sylven C, Kaijser L. Calf muscle adaptation in intermittent claudication. Side-differences in muscle metabolic characteristics in patients with unilateral arterial disease. Clin Physiol 1988; 8: 17–29.
51. Lundgren F, Dahllof A-G, Schersten T, Bylund-Fellenius A-C. Muscle enzyme adaptation in patients with peripheral insufficiency: spontaneous adaptation, effect of different treatment and consequences on walking performance. Clin Sci 1989; 77: 485–493.
52. Rabinovich RA, Ardite E, Troosters T et al. Reduced muscle redox capacity after endurance training in COPD patients. Am J Respir Crit Care Med 2001; in press.
53. Agusti AGN, Sauleda J, Batle S et al. Skeletal muscle apoptosis in COPD (abstract). Eur Respir J 2000; 16(suppl 31): 575.
54. Engelen MPKJ, Schols AMWJ, Does JD et al. Altered glutamate metabolism is associated with reduced muscle glutathione levels in patients with emphysema. Am J Respir Crit Care Med 2000; 161: 98–103.
55. Engelen MPKJ. Muscle wasting in COPD: a metabolic and functional perspective. Doctoral thesis, University Hospital Maastricht, 2001.
56. Brenner C, Kroemer G. Mitochondria – the death signal integrator. Science 2000; 289: 1150–1151.
57. Di Francia M, Barbier D, Mege J, Orehek J. Tumor necrosis factor-alpha and weight loss in chronic obstructive pulmonary disease. Am J Respir Crit Care Med 1994; 150: 1453–1455.
58. Sridhar MK. Why do patients with emphysema lose weight? Lancet 1995; 345: 1190–1191.
59. De Godoy I, Donahoe M, Calhoun WJ et al. Elevated TNF-α production by peripheral blood monocytes of weight-losing COPD patients. Am J Respir Crit Care Med 1996; 153: 633–637.
60. Wagner PD, Hoppeler H, Saltin B. Determinants of maximal oxygen uptake. In: Crystal RG, West JB, ed. The lung: scientific foundations. Philadelphia, PA: Lippincott-Raven; 1997: 2033–2041.
61. McCully K, Vanderborne K, Posner JD, Leigh JS. Muscle metabolism in track athletes, using ^{31}P magnetic resonance spectroscopy. Can J Physiol Pharmacol 1992; 70: 1353–1359.
62. Haseler LJ, Richardson RS, Videen JS, Hogan MC. Phosphocreatine hydrolysis during submaximal exercise: the effect of FIO_2. J Appl Physiol 1998; 85: 1463.
63. Weisman IM, Zeballos RJ. Cardiopulmonary exercise testing. Pulmon Crit Care Update 1995; 11: 1–9.
64. Sue DY. Exercise testing in the evaluation of impairment and disability. Clin Chest Med 1994; 15: 369–387.
65. Roca J, Whipp BJ, ed. Clinical exercise testing. European Respiratory Monograph. Lausanne, Sheffield. European Respiratory Society Journals; 1997.
66. Celli BR, Cote CG, Marin JM et al. Combining 6MWD, FEV$_1$, MRC dyspnea and BMI is better predictor of mortality than FEV$_1$ (abstract). Am J Respir Crit Care Med 2001; 163(suppl): A504.
67. Kessler R, Faller M, Fourgaut G et al. Predictive factors of hospitalization for acute exacerbation in a series of 64 patients with chronic obstructive pulmonary disease. Am J Respir Crit Care Med 1999; 159: 158–164.
68. Miyamoto S, Nagaya N, Satoh T et al. Clinical correlates and prognostic significance of six-minute walk test in patients with primary pulmonary hypertension. Comparison with cardiopulmonary exercise testing. Am J Respir Crit Care Med 2000; 161: 487–492.
69. Willenheimer R, Erhardt LR. Value of 6-min-walk test for assessment of severity and prognosis of heart failure. Lancet 2000; 355: 515–516.
70. Blosser SA, Maxwell SL, Reeves-Hoche MK et al. Is an anticholinergic agent superior to a β$_2$-agonist in improving dyspnea and exercise limitation in COPD? Chest 1995; 108: 730–735.
71. Wilkens H, Demertzis S, Konig J et al. Lung volume reduction surgery versus conservative treatment in severe emphysema. Eur Respir J 2000; 16: 1043–1049.

72. Troosters T, Gosselink R, Decramer M. Short- and long-term effects of outpatient rehabilitation in patients with chronic obstructive pulmonary disease: a randomized trial. Am J Med 2000; 109: 207–212.

73. Lacasse Y, Wong E, Guyatt GH et al. Meta-analysis of respiratory rehabilitation in chronic obstructive pulmonary disease. Lancet 1996; 348: 1115–1119.

74. Troosters T, Vilaro J, Capitán A et al. Organ system responses during the six minute walking test (abstract). Am J Respir Crit Care Med 2001; 163: A268.

75. Roca J, Whipp BJ, Agusti AGN et al. Clinical exercise testing with reference to lung disease: indications, standardization and interpretation strategies. Eur Respir J 1997; 10: 2662–2689

2.8 Control of breathing

Hans Folgering

Key points

- The ventilatory control system finds a 'working point' at the intersection of the ventilatory response curve to CO_2 and the metabolic hyperbola.

- The ventilatory sensitivity to CO_2 shows a very wide interindividual range in normal subjects.

- Quiet breathing in normal subjects is mainly controlled by the wakefulness drive and the arterial P_{CO_2}.

- The hypercapnic and hypoxic stimuli for breathing show mutual interaction: the effect of hypercapnia is augmented by hypoxia and vice versa.

The respiratory control system has to regulate a number of functions related to breathing, including:

- Intake of oxygen and excretion of carbon dioxide
- Control of the pH of the internal environment
- Behavioural mechanisms such as speech
- Thermoregulation (mostly in animals; weakly in humans).

These functions have a mutual hierarchy. This means that, when one is activated, other functions are overruled. When, for instance, breathing is being used for speech, most people hyperventilate, and thus the function of controlling the pH of the internal environment is made subordinate to the behavioural function.

Control systems

Maintaining homeostasis of pH, P_{CO_2} and P_{O_2} requires a control system where chemoreceptors, 'respiratory centres', respiratory muscles and lungs are functionally coupled. Figure 2.8.1 shows a diagram of this control system. Gas exchange in the lungs results in certain blood gas values in the arterial blood, which are detected by the peripheral chemoreceptors in the carotid and aortic bodies. Signals from these receptors are transmitted via the carotid sinus nerve (a branch of the glossopharyngeal nerve) and the vagus nerve respectively to the medullary respiratory 'centres'. In addition, the pH and P_{CO_2} of the cerebrospinal fluid is sensed by the central chemoreceptors on the ventral surface of the medulla, near the root of the hypoglossal nerve. Signals from both groups of chemoreceptors converge on the 'respiratory centres' in the pons and medulla. Peripheral chemoreceptors contribute approximately 30% of the total chemical drive; central chemoreceptors contribute approximately 70% of this drive.

The 'respiratory centres' are part of the brainstem reticular formation, which also mediates alertness and blood pressure (vasomotor centres) The respiratory centres consist of a ventral respiratory group and a dorsal respiratory group. Their efferent neuronal traffic goes to the spinal motoneurones of the phrenic nerves (C3–6) and to the intercostal muscle motoneurones (T1–12).

The activity of the respiratory muscles generates pleural pressure variations that are modified by the compliance of the thorax and of the lungs and eventually cause displacement of air. The actual amount of air displaced depends on the activity of these muscles, the elastic properties of the thorax and lungs and the resistance to airflow in the airways. Thus in patients with restrictive or obstructive diseases, the minute ventilation may be an inadequate index of the output from the 'respiratory centres'. In obstructive disease, this problem of measuring the output of the controlling system can be partially overcome by using a breathing circuit with a valve in the inspiratory pathway. When the valve is closed, the pressure in the occluded mouthpiece, in the first 0.1 s of inspiration ($P_{0.1}$) is a better index of the output of the 'respiratory centres' than minute ventilation.[1] Other methods for quantifying the output of the respiratory controller are pleural pressure or electromyographic activity of the respiratory muscles.

In the respiratory control system of Figure 2.8.1, the upper half, above the broken line, comprises the controlling system, or

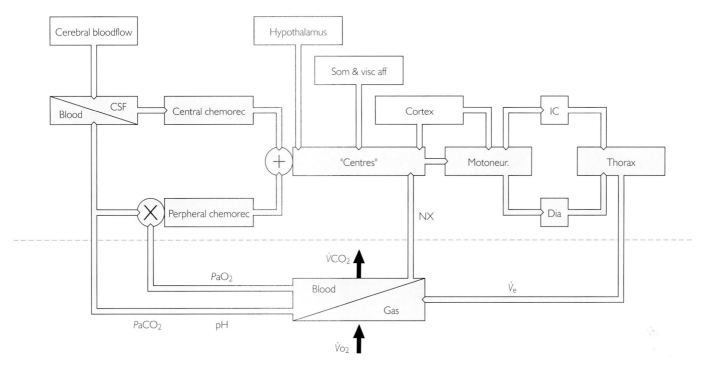

Fig. 2.8.1 Diagram of the ventilatory control system. The lower box is the lung, where gas exchange between alveolar air and blood takes place. Below the broken horizontal line is the controlled system, with input ventilation and output blood gas values. Above the broken line is the controlling system, with input blood gas values and output minute ventilation. IC, intercostal muscles; Dia, diaphragm; Motoneur, spinal motoneurones of the respiratory muscles; NX: vagus nerve; Som & visc aff, somatic and visceral afferents; +, additive effect of inputs of central and peripheral chemoreceptors to the 'respiratory centres'; X, interaction (multiplicative effect) of hypoxic and hypercapnic stimuli at the peripheral chemoreceptors.

controller. The input to this system is the arterial blood gas values; the output can be minute ventilation, $P_{0.1}$ or respiratory muscle electromyogram. The relation between the input and the output of the controller is the *ventilatory response curve* to hypercapnia or hypoxia. The lower half of Figure 2.8.1, below the broken line, is the controlled system. Its input is minute ventilation; the output is the blood gas values. This describes the situation when a patient is being ventilated artificially: high ventilator settings cause hypocapnia and vice versa. The position of this hyperbolic relationship depends on the level of CO_2 production and thus on the metabolism; it is therefore called the *metabolic hyperbola* (Fig. 2.8.2).

Unlike technical control systems (e.g. central heating systems in our homes), there is no evidence of a 'set point' for the respiratory control system. In spontaneously breathing humans, the control loop is closed. This means that the input of the controller (blood gas values) is the output of the controlled system and vice versa. The *working point* of the control system is at the intersection of the ventilatory response curve and the metabolic hyperbola. When one of the characteristics changes, there will usually be a change in position of this working point and this will lead to different blood gas values. Sedatives, for instance, change the slope of the ventilatory response curve to CO_2 and thus also change blood gas values. Figure 2.8.2 shows a ventilatory response curve and the metabolic hyperbola in two different metabolic states.

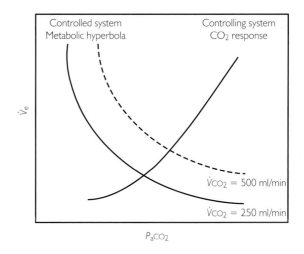

Fig. 2.8.2 Relationship between minute ventilation ($\dot{V}_E$) and arterial P_{CO_2} values. The characteristic of the controlled system is described by the hyperbolic relationship as it exists in a ventilated patient: ventilation is the independent variable and the arterial P_{CO_2} is the result of this ventilation. The position of this hyperbola depends on the metabolic CO_2 production ('metabolic hyperbola'). The CO_2 response curve describes the properties of the controlling system. During spontaneous breathing, the input of one system is the output of the other. Therefore the control system works at the intersection of the CO_2 response curve with the metabolic hyperbola.

The above control mechanism is a *feedback system*: the effect of ventilation is fed back via chemoreceptors to the respiratory centres. This is in contrast to a number of *non-feedback stimuli*, such as sympathetic activity, hypothalamic stimuli (emotion and thermoregulatory stimuli), cortical stimuli, somatic and visceral afferents, and airway afferents. Hormones also affect ventilation in a non-feedback manner. Thyroxine increases the gain of the controller. On the other hand, it also increases the metabolism and CO_2 production. The net effect is hyperventilation and low $P\text{CO}_2$. Progesterone also stimulates ventilation. This can be seen in females in the second half of the menstrual cycle or in pregnancy; both situations are characterised by hyperventilation. This hormone is sometimes used therapeutically in situations of hypoventilation.

The control of breathing during *exercise* 'is the best kept secret in physiology'.[2] In light to moderate exercise, the ventilation increases proportionally to the increase in CO_2 production. The arterial $P\text{CO}_2$ remains at resting levels and thus cannot be the stimulus for chemoreceptors to maintain an elevated exercise ventilation. Hypotheses about 'cortical irradiation' of motor signals, hypothalamic motor centre stimulation, afferent activity of proprioceptors in the moving limbs, increased production of endogenous catecholamines and an increase in the amplitude of respiratory oscillations of blood gas values have all been invoked to explain exercise hyperpnoea but have failed to account for it convincingly. Hypothetical sensors measuring the flux of CO_2 in the pulmonary artery have also never been demonstrated.

Peripheral chemoreceptors

Peripheral chemoreceptors are located at the bifurcation of the carotid arteries and on the aortic arch, where they are known as the glomus caroticum (carotid bodies) and glomus aorticum (aortic bodies) respectively. The latter generate a minor contribution to the chemical drive to breathing (approximately 5%), while the carotid bodies contribute about 20–25% of the total chemical drive.[3] Two types of cell have been described in the

receptors: type I glomus cells and type II sustentacular cells. Both contain neurotransmitter granules. It is hypothesised that the chemoreceptive mechanism is located at the synapses between the two types of cell.

All peripheral chemoreceptors have a very high blood flow, by far exceeding the metabolic needs of these organelles. Both groups of peripheral chemoreceptors sense arterial pH, $P\text{O}_2$ and $P\text{CO}_2$ values. Their discharge frequency depends on the combination of these blood gas values. At low $P\text{O}_2$, sensitivity to $P\text{CO}_2$ is high. At high $P\text{CO}_2$, sensitivity to hypoxia is high, because of *interaction of stimuli* (Fig. 2.8.3). There is still discussion whether the peripheral chemoreceptors are 'silent' in hyperoxia, e.g. when breathing very high oxygen mixtures. There are indications that the receptors may not be sensitive to CO_2 in hyperoxia. Peripheral chemoreceptors respond very quickly to changes in blood gas values (within seconds) and consequently also cause rapid ventilatory reactions to hypercapnia and hypoxia. Potassium and adrenaline (epinephrine) positively modulate the activity of the receptors. Carbonic anhydrase inhibitors depress the chemosensitivity of the peripheral chemoreceptors.

Afferent signals from the carotid body are transmitted via the carotid sinus nerve and glossopharyngeal nerve to the brain stem. Aortic body signals are transmitted by the vagus nerve. The carotid sinus nerve also carries afferent signals from baroreceptors in the wall of the carotid artery. Sudden increases in systemic blood pressure lead to ventilatory depression.

Central chemoreceptors

The central chemoreceptors are located at the ventral side of the medulla oblongata, medial to the hypoglossal root. They 'sense' the pH/$P\text{CO}_2$ of the extracellular fluid of the brain and/or of the cerebrospinal fluid (CSF) produced by the choroid plexus of the fourth ventricle. They are located on the CSF side of the blood–brain barrier, and hardly 'sense' any metabolic changes in blood pH. As CO_2 readily passes the blood–brain barrier, this is the primary stimulus for the central chemoreceptors. CO_2 is

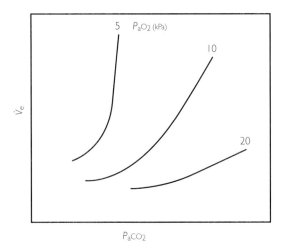
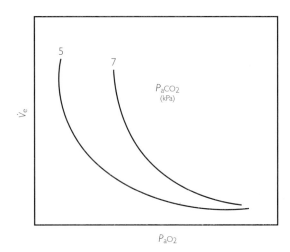

Fig. 2.8.3 Ventilatory response curves to hypercapnia and hypoxia. Both responses are shown at different levels of P_aO_2 and P_aCO_2 respectively, demonstrating the interaction between both stimuli.

converted in the brain extracellular fluid into H^+ and HCO_3^- ions. The H^+ ions also stimulate the central chemoreceptors. These receptors generate approximately 70–80% of the total chemical drive to breathing. The chemoreceptive cells have not yet been identified with certainty.[4] Signals from the central and peripheral chemoreceptors act additively on the 'respiratory centres'.

Cerebral blood flow

As the cerebral blood flow carries the metabolically produced CO_2 away from the brain tissue, it also influences the PCO_2 of the CSF and consequently also ventilation.[5] This most vulnerable of all tissues apparently has an extra control loop for maintaining homeostasis of PCO_2 and pH. Hypocapnia causes cerebral vasoconstriction, which in extreme conditions may even be detrimental to the oxygen supply to the cortex. Thus extreme hyperventilation may lead to fainting and collapse. In patients with COPD, (nocturnal) hypercapnia causes cerebral vasodilatation and subsequent headaches.

Hypoxaemia also leads to some cerebral vasodilatation, thus compensating for the diminished oxygen delivery to the brain tissue. This happens, for example, in acclimatisation to altitude. The initial hypoxic hyperventilation mediated by peripheral chemoreceptor stimulation is attenuated, after 1–2 days, as a result of the increased central washout of CO_2 and consequently lowered central chemoreceptor stimulation.

Rostral central nervous system inputs

Hypothalamic structures such as thermoregulatory nuclei, locomotor nuclei and parts of the emotional brain are connected to the brain-stem 'respiratory centres'.

Thermoregulating nuclei in the preoptic and posterior hypothalamic regions project to the medullary respiratory centres. Effects of this connection can be seen in animals (dogs, cattle) that pant with (very) high respiratory frequencies during thermal stress. In humans this type of thermoregulation is still present rudimentarily, so that ventilation increases in humans during heat stress. It may be relevant that many patients with the hyperventilation syndrome report that their first attack occurred in a car in a traffic jam on a hot summer day, or when taking a hot bath.

The infundibular area of the hypothalamus contains progesterone receptors,[6] stimulation of which with progesterone also causes hyperventilation. This effect has been used in stimulating ventilation in hypercapnic COPD patients with medroxy-progesterone acetate. 'Priming' of these progesterone receptors with oestrogens enhances the ventilatory effects of progesterone. Hypothalamic locomotor centres also project to the pontomedullary respiratory centres. According to some authors, this contributes to exercise hyperpnoea. Cortical motor areas presumably also radiate activity to the brainstem respiratory centres. Such 'cortical irradiation' has been invoked as one of the explanations for exercise hyperpnoea. On the other hand, some cortical areas have an inhibitory effect on breathing, with the result that hyperventilation may be observed after a stroke.

The motor cortex of the prefrontal gyrus also projects directly, via the pyramidal tract, to the motor neurones of the respiratory muscles at the spinal levels of C3–5 for the diaphragm and T1–12 for the intercostals. This pathway mediates voluntary breathing movements, e.g. during lung function testing, and allows voluntary breath-holding. This tract is an independent descending respiratory tract, mediating voluntary breathing manoeuvres, and is separate from the bulbospinal tract that mediates 'automatic' breathing.[7] Either descending pathway can be interrupted separately. Partial spinal cord lesions that only interrupt the corticospinal tract make voluntary breathing manoeuvres such as speech difficult. Lesions of the bulbospinal tract interrupt the automatic pathways and affected patients have to breathe voluntarily. Consequently, breathing ceases during sleep, when such patients require artificial ventilation ('Ondine's curse').

Vagal afferents

The vagal nerve contains afferent fibres from three types of pulmonary receptor: stretch receptors (slowly adapting receptors), irritant receptors (rapidly adapting), and J receptors (juxtacapillary pulmonary).

The slowly adapting receptors are located in the smaller airways, and are excited by stretching of these airways during inspiration. A deep inspiration generates so much afferent traffic in these fibres that medullary inspiratory neurones are inhibited and inspiration is stopped (Breuer–Hering reflex). Presumably this reflex is not active in quietly breathing normal subjects.

Stimulation of irritant receptors causes hyperventilation and tonic inspiratory activity of the inspiratory muscles ((i.e. during the expiratory phase also).[7,8] This phenomenon contributes to the hyperinflation and hyperventilation seen during acute episodes of asthma. Stronger irritant receptor stimulation mediates a cough reflex and bronchoconstriction.

J receptors sense the amount of water in the interstitial space of the lung. Overfilling of the interstitium in situations such as cardiac failure, pulmonary oedema or pneumonia results in rapid shallow breathing.

Brain-stem respiratory neuronal organisation

The involuntary respiratory rhythm is generated in the medullary respiratory neuronal organisation, often referred to as 'respiratory centres'. However, these are not 'centres' in the strict sense of a morphologically recognisable nucleus of cells with only one function. This respiratory organisation also mediates reflex effects from chemoreceptors, hypothalamic pathways, vagal afferents, somatic afferents and cortical projections. It is located in the medulla oblongata and pons. The neurones show bursts of activity with trains of impulses, synchronously with inspiration, expiration and with all transitional phases (in-expiratory, ex-inspiratory, early or late in- or expiratory). Neurophysiological mapping shows a *dorsal respiratory group* that possibly processes visceral sensory input and vagal input from slowly adapting receptors (Fig. 2.8.4). These are mostly inspiratory neurones. Many neurones of the dorsal respiratory group project monosy-

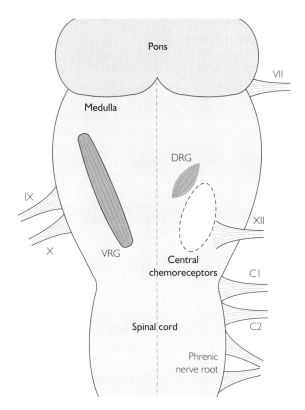

Fig. 2.8.4 Schematic representation of the pons and medulla oblongata, seen from the ventral side. All structures shown are present at both sides of the midline (drawn unilaterally for clarity). Roman numerals indicate the roots of the cranial nerves. C1, C2, roots of first and second cervical nerves; DRG, dorsal respiratory group; VRG, ventral respiratory group.

naptically to contralateral spinal motoneurones of the phrenic nerve. Dorsal respiratory group inspiratory neurone activity is inhibited by afferent vagal input from slowly adapting receptors, and thus may mediate the Breuer–Hering reflex. The *ventral respiratory group* contains both inspiratory and expiratory neurones, and is possibly associated with the nucleus ambiguus. Rostrally of the dorsal and ventral respiratory groups lies the *Bötzinger complex*, which is regarded by some investigators, as the 'pacemaker' for the respiratory rhythm. The pons contains the *pontine respiratory group* of neurones. Lesions of this pontine structure in patients result in an 'apneustic breathing' pattern with tonic inspiration and occasional short expirations.

Testing the control system

The function of control systems can be tested in two basically different ways:

- The control loop is kept intact and one measures whether the system is able to maintain homeostasis of pH, P_{CO_2} and/or P_{O_2} in the presence of external disturbing factors such as drugs, altitude, hormones, high temperatures etc.
- The control loop can be 'opened' so that the action of the controlled system cannot affect the controlling system, or

viceversa. This situation occurs, for instance, when a CO_2 response curve is obtained by adding CO_2 to the inspiratory air, or when a patient is paralysed and ventilated by a ventilator.

When measuring ventilatory response to hypercapnia or hypoxia, one tests the properties of the controller. In the situation of the paralysed and ventilated patient, the properties of the controlled system can be evaluated. In such situations it is essential to define clearly what are being used as input and output parameters. In normal subjects, it is quite acceptable to use end-tidal P_{CO_2} as the input parameter in a CO_2 response, but in patients with COPD it is better to use arterial P_{CO_2} as the input parameter, as this more closely approximates the actual stimulus to the chemoreceptors. Similarly, minute ventilation is an adequate output parameter for the controlling system in normal subjects, whereas in patients with severe obstructive disease the measurement of $P_{0.1}$ may better reflect the reaction of the respiratory centres to increases in chemoreceptor stimulation. Depending on which input and output parameters are measured, one can obtain different values for chemosensitivity of the controlling system and consequently one can assess whether or not a response is normal.

Ventilatory responses to CO_2

The ventilatory response to hypercapnia can be measured in three ways: as a steady-state response, during rebreathing, or dynamic end-tidal forcing.

When measuring steady-state responses to increased CO_2, a constant low percentage of CO_2 is added to the inspiratory air until full equilibration in the arterial blood and cerebrospinal fluid is achieved, and until the cerebral blood flow is fully adapted to the new increased level of P_{CO_2}. A constant level of minute ventilation will indicate this equilibration, which takes about 6–10 min in normal subjects.

In the rebreathing method, the subject rebreathes from a bag (in a box), filled with 7% CO_2 in oxygen. The P_{CO_2} in the bag approximately equals or exceeds the value in mixed venous blood. Thus all CO_2 excretion stops and the arterial P_{CO_2} rises linearly with time. During this time the minute ventilation is measured. The test is completed when the subject cannot tolerate higher P_{CO_2} levels or when the end-tidal P_{CO_2} is about 9 kPa (68 mmHg)

In the dynamic end-tidal forcing method, a computer-controlled system of mass-flow controllers mixes the inspiratory air from three cylinders containing nitrogen, oxygen and carbon dioxide. The computer measures minute ventilation, and calculates the amount of CO_2 that is to be given in the next breath, in order to attain a desired level of end-tidal P_{CO_2}. Thus the end-tidal P_{CO_2} can be changed abruptly to any desired level. Two time-constants of the ventilatory response to such a step-change in P_aCO_2 are calculated: a fast one related to the peripheral chemoreceptor response and a slower one related to the central chemoreceptor reflex.

Ventilatory response curves to CO_2 are usually quantified as a linear relationship according to the equation:

$$\dot{V}_E = S(P\text{CO}_2 - B),$$

where S is the slope of the response line ($1 . \text{min}^{-1} . \text{kPa}^{-1}$) and B is the (extrapolated) intercept where ventilation would be zero.

Normal values for S show a wide interindividual range: in males $23.3 \pm 6.8\,1 . \text{min}^{-1} . \text{kPa}^{-1}$ ($3.1 \pm 0.9\,1 . \text{min}^{-1} . \text{mmHg}^{-1}$) and in females $13.5 \pm 5.3\,1 . \text{min}^{-1} . \text{kPa}^{-1}$ ($1.8 \pm 0.7\,1 . \text{min}^{-1} . \text{mmHg}^{-1}$).[10] In females, the response is modulated by levels of progesterone. Consequently, when more than one response is obtained in a female, this should be done at the same point in the menstrual cycle.

The hypoxic ventilatory response

As the peripheral chemoreceptors in the carotid and aortic bodies are the only ones active in detecting hypoxia, there is no need to wait many minutes for equilibration with central compartments as with CO_2 responses. Rebreathing hypoxic ventilatory response curves are quite adequate. Carotid bodies are responsible for about 95% of the hypoxic drive, the aortic bodies hardly contributing to the hypoxic response in mammals.

As hypoxia is potentially hazardous, monitoring both pulse oximetry and electrocardiogram is recommended.

During hypoxic hyperventilation, CO_2 is blown off. Consequently, the subject becomes hypocapnic. Because of the interaction of chemical stimuli at the peripheral chemoreceptors, this hypocapnia alters the hypoxic ventilatory response. Thus, some CO_2 should be added to the inspired air in order to keep arterial $P\text{CO}_2$ constant.

The $\dot{V}_E/P_a\text{O}_2$ relationship is hyperbolic and can be quantified by the equation:

$$\dot{V}_E = \dot{V}_o + \frac{A}{\left(P_a\text{O}_2 - C\right)}$$

where $\dot{V}_o$ is the horizontal asymptote, i.e. ventilation at very high $P_a\text{O}_2$ levels, C is the vertical asymptote where $\dot{V}_E$ reaches infinity (usually the value of 4.3 kPa – 32 mmHg – is taken for C) and A is the shape constant of the hyperbola.[11]

When plotting the ventilatory response to hypoxia in terms of minute ventilation versus arterial oxygen saturation, the ventilatory response is a straight line and can consequently be described by a very simple equation:

$$\dot{V}_E = \dot{V}_o - a . S\text{O}_2.$$

$\dot{V}_o$ in this equation is the minute ventilation at $S_a\text{O}_2 = 100\%$ and a is the slope of the ventilatory response: the 'hypoxic sensitivity'.

The mean normal hypoxic response in normocapnia is $1.55 \pm 0.98\,1 . \text{min}^{-1}$ divided by the percentage desaturation (Fig. 2.8.5).

Interaction between hypoxic and hypercapnic responses.

The peripheral chemoreceptors sense both hypoxia and hypercapnia. Because of interaction between these stimuli, the sensitivity of the peripheral chemoreceptors for CO_2 is substantially

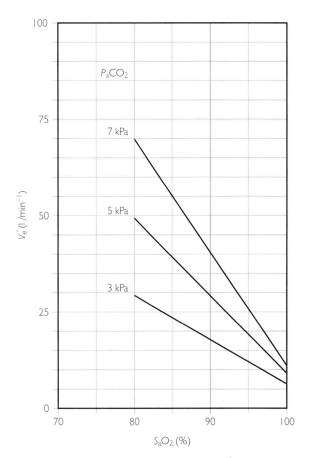

Fig. 2.8.5 Ventilatory response curves to hypoxia, expressed as $\dot{V}_E$ versus $S_a\text{O}_2$. Due to the curvilinear relationship between $P_a\text{O}_2$ and $S_a\text{O}_2$, these response lines are straight lines. The true stimulus for the chemoreceptors, however, is the $P_a\text{O}_2$. The different levels of $P_a\text{CO}_2$ illustrate the interaction (multiplication) of stimuli at the peripheral chemoreceptors.

reduced at very high levels of arterial $P\text{O}_2$. Hyperoxia thus removes some of the ventilatory drive in, for example, COPD patients on long-term oxygen treatment, and consequently contributes a little to the increase in $P\text{CO}_2$ seen in these patients. However, the major cause of hypercapnia during oxygen treatment is ventilation–perfusion inhomogeneities.

Disturbances in the control of breathing

A disturbance in the control of breathing results from an anomaly in either the controller or the controlling system. Irrespective of the cause, the net result is always abnormal blood gas values. However in certain physiological conditions, such as exercise, stress/emotion, sleep, medication, and body temperature, ventilation is modified and consequently the blood gas values deviate from normality.[12] Thus when testing the control of breathing, these conditions should be kept as constant as possible, both within subjects when doing repeated measurements and between subjects when making a cross-sectional survey. The effects of changes in sleep–wake status on ventilatory responses are shown in Figure 2.8.6.

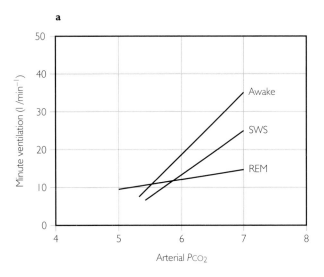

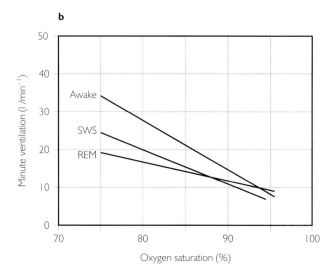

Fig. 2.8.6 Ventilatory responses to (a) hypercapnia and (b) hypoxia in various sleep stages, showing the effects of loss of the 'wakefulness drive'. REM, rapid-eye-movement sleep; SWS, slow wave sleep.

Disturbances in the controlling system

As the elimination of CO_2 from the body depends mainly on alveolar ventilation, changes in ventilatory drive express themselves in changes in arterial P_{CO_2} values: hypercapnia and hypocapnia. Hypoxaemia can result from at least four mechanisms:

- low inspiratory P_{O_2}
- diffusion problems
- ventilation/perfusion mismatching
- hypoventilation.

Therefore, hypocapnia or hypercapnia rather than hypoxaemia are the most appropriate parameters for assessing aberrant ventilatory control in spontaneously breathing subjects.

Cheyne–Stokes breathing

Many neurological and neuromuscular diseases are associated with abnormal control of breathing.[7] A distinct pattern of alternating hyper- and hypoventilation is seen in Cheyne–Stokes breathing (Fig. 2.8.7). The cycle of one episode of this type of breathing is about 40–60 s. It can be observed in patients with severe cardiac disease (forward failure). It has been hypothesised that the respiratory oscillations in blood gas values arriving at the peripheral chemoreceptors are so delayed, that the oscillating afferent neuronal input from these peripheral chemoreceptors becomes out of phase with the rhythm of the respiratory centres. Changes in either direction in the 'gain' of the controller might also cause the waxing and waning in breathing.[13] Thus, stage 1 non-REM sleep, sojourn at high altitudes and severe COPD can all induce instabilities in the breathing pattern. Giving as little as 1–2% CO_2 in the inspiratory air will stabilise the ventilatory control system and make the Cheyne Stokes pattern disappear. An extreme form of episodic breathing is Biot breathing where groups of four to eight breaths alternate with periods of complete apnoea. This is usually seen in preterminal patients.

Hypoventilation

Hypoventilation occurs in the obesity hypoventilation syndrome, hypothyroidism, various conditions associated with respiratory muscle weakness, Prader–Willi syndrome, after medication with sedatives or loop diuretics (metabolic alkalosis) and during REM sleep in various conditions.

The **obesity–hypoventilation syndrome** is characterised by hypoxaemia, hypercapnia, very low or absent ventilatory responses to hypercapnia and/or absent responses to hypoxia. It is not clear whether to begin with the obesity as such causes the hypoventilation. In spite of the fact that the work of breathing, and the oxygen cost of breathing are substantially increased, most obese persons are normocapnic.[14,15] Tracheostomy greatly reduces the hypoventilation in the obesity hypoventilation syndrome, suggesting that a high resistance in the upper airway is an important contributor to the hypoventilation. The obesity hypoventilation syndrome is not necessarily accompanied by obstructive sleep apnoea. Treatment of obesity hypoventilation consists of weight loss, treatment of cor pulmonale, pharmacological stimulation of ventilation and sometimes nocturnal ventilatory support.

Hyperventilation

Hyperventilation is seen in conditions such as hyperthyroidism, after strokes involving the cortex, in cirrhosis of the liver, in metabolic acidosis (e.g. diabetic acidosis with Kussmaul breathing; Fig. 2.8.7), during withdrawal from morphine and alcohol addiction and in situations of anxiety or psychological stress. This last is often referred to as the hyperventilation syndrome.[16] Activity from the reticular activating system, the sympathetic adrenergic system and 'emotional centres' drive the ventilation, overruling the normal chemoreflex drives. Breathing is characterised by irregular breathing at high frequency (Fig. 2.8.7). The ventilatory response to CO_2 is inverted in about half of patients with this syndrome: adding CO_2 to the inspired air by rebreathing from a plastic bag causes ventilation to decrease instead of

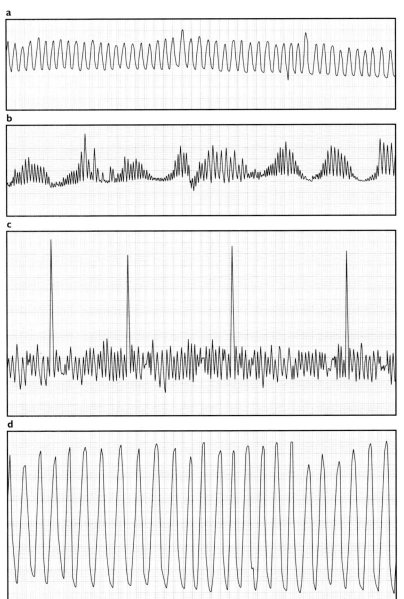

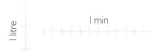

Fig. 2.8.7 Breathing patterns in (a) normals, (b) Cheyne–Stokes breathing, (c) idiopathic hyperventilation and (d) diabetic acidosis (Kussmaul breathing).

increase. Symptoms associated with this syndrome are extremely diverse, the main ones being dizziness, tingling of fingers and lips, palpitations and derealisation. Therapy consists of relaxation and breathing exercises to achieve low-frequency breathing, sedatives and psychotherapy for some extreme cases.

Disturbances in the controlled system

Failure of the ventilatory pump is diagnosed from (relative) hypoventilation with hypercapnia and results from a negative balance between the working capacity of the respiratory muscles versus the load on these muscles. The load is determined by the metabolic CO_2 production (exercise), the flow resistance in the airways (FEV_1) and the elastic resistance of the lungs and thorax (compliance). The working capacity of the ventilatory pump depends on the central ventilatory drive, the

strength (P_{Imax}, P_{Emax}) and endurance of the respiratory muscles, blood gas values, medication and the degree of hyperinflation (FRC, RV). Hyperinflation adversely affects the position of the muscles on their length–strength relationship, and shifts the thorax and the lungs towards a less compliant part of their pressure–volume curves. Intrinsic positive end-expiratory pressure (PEEP) develops with hyperinflation and further increases the work of breathing. Consequently respiratory failure is more likely to occur in situations of hyperinflation, chronically in severe COPD and acutely in asthma attacks and during exercise in patients with moderate and severe obstructive disease. Patients then show a high-frequency breathing pattern, with inefficient high dead-space ventilation.

With respiratory pump failure in COPD, the first signs usually occur during REM sleep, when intercostal muscles are 'paralysed', and the diaphragm is the only active respiratory muscle.[17] Training of the inspiratory muscles may be considered in these patients (see Chapter 16). Patients with deformity of the thoracic wall, such as kyphoscoliosis, or with neuromuscular disease may also eventually show ventilatory pump, and thus respiratory, failure.[18]

Control of breathing in pulmonary diseases

Asthma

Stimulation of irritant receptors in patients with asthma reflexly causes hyperventilation, as shown by their characteristically low P_aCO_2.[19,20] At the same time, irritant receptor stimulation also causes airway narrowing. Only when the bronchoconstriction is very severe, e.g. at levels of FEV_1 of 20% of the reference value or less, can hyperventilation no longer be sustained, and the patient becomes hypercapnic. The hypocapnia during hyperventilation also increases the contractility of the smooth muscle of the bronchial wall and thus contributes to the bronchoconstriction.[21,22] This direct effect of hypocapnia is also demonstrated in preparations of isolated bronchial smooth muscle in a tissue bath. Consequently, it is most probably a direct effect of hypocapnia on the muscle. This effect is greater in patients with bronchial hyper-responsiveness than in normal subjects.

Physiotherapeutic interventions such as breathing exercises aimed at preventing hyperventilation in the early stages of an asthma attack may help overcome or ameliorate the attack.

COPD

Two types of disturbance occur in patients with COPD:

- defects in the controlled system: ventilatory pump and respiratory mechanics
- possibly, in some patients, a defect in the controlling system, contributing to hypoventilation and to hypercapnia.[23]

By definition, these patients suffer from a chronic airway obstruction. Hyperinflation occurs secondary to this obstruction, leading to chronic shortening of inspiratory muscles, shifting their position to an unfavourable point on the length–strength curve. Animal experiments suggest that long-term shortening of the diaphragm may cause loss of sarcomeres and a shift of the length–strength curve to the left. The maximal force or maximal inspiratory pressure that COPD patients can generate will be lower than in normal subjects.

The hyperinflation also results in intrinsic PEEP. At FRC the outward elastic force of the chest wall is in equilibrium with the inward elastic retractional force of the lungs. In hyperinflation, the thoracic wall will have a tendency to recoil inward, more or less 'compressing' the lungs, especially when these have diminished recoil, as in emphysema. With every inspiration this intrinsic PEEP has to be overcome before the thoracic wall will move outward at all. Thus the inspiratory muscles are already performing a lot of work before the actual start of inspiratory airflow. At higher end-expiratory volumes, the pressure–volume curves of both the thorax and the lungs become shallower, i.e. the thorax and lungs become 'stiffer'. Thus the inspiratory muscles have to expend more energy for inhalation of the same amount of air than they would at lower end-expiratory lung volumes.

The chronic inflammation and the increased work of breathing also increase metabolism and more CO_2 is produced. Energy intake in food will not always match this increased metabolism, thus leading to muscle wasting. In addition, steroid treatment during exacerbations of COPD may result in steroid myopathy, which also affects the respiratory muscles.

Thus in COPD, the function of the ventilatory pump is jeopardised by chronic shortening of the respiratory muscles, intrinsic PEEP, muscle wasting, sometimes steroid myopathy and having to work over the stiffer part of the pressure–volume curve of the thorax and lungs.

In patients with severe COPD, two extreme forms of control of breathing can be observed: some patients remain normocapnic whereas others with the same degree of airflow obstruction hypoventilate and become hypercapnic. These subtypes of COPD patients used to be called 'pink puffers' and 'blue bloaters' respectively. Between these extremes, all intermediate stages can be observed.[24,25] Why is one group normocapnic, and the other hypercapnic? Studies suggest that chemosensitivity to CO_2, as well as respiratory mechanics, contribute to the hypercapnia in the blue and bloating type of COPD patient (see Chapter 47.4).

Incipient respiratory failure in COPD first manifests itself as nocturnal hypoventilation, especially during REM sleep. In all non-REM-sleep stages, the respiratory drive is lowered because of the absence of a 'wakefulness' drive. This results in slight hypoventilation. During REM sleep, there is virtual abolition of activity in muscles that contain spindles. These include the intercostal muscles, whereas the diaphragm hardly has any. Therefore, during REM sleep, the diaphragm is required to maintain ventilation on its own. However, in COPD the diaphragm is shortened and less effective and may be unable to maintain normal ventilation. Furthermore, CO_2 sensitivity is very low during REM sleep (Fig. 2.8.6). Thus hypoventilation and hypoxaemia will first and mainly occur during REM episodes.[17] The importance of the resulting bouts of about 30–45 min of hypoxaemia for clinical prognosis, is unclear. The accompanying hypercapnia may cause morning headaches in these patients.

Interstitial pulmonary diseases

Restrictive lung diseases, such as pulmonary fibrosis, are characterised by a high-frequency breathing pattern. Characteristically the resting respiratory rate is about 20 per minute. This is not necessarily accompanied by hypocapnia as dead-space ventilation is substantially increased because of the small tidal volume, which in turn reflects the reduced compliance of the lungs. Therefore the organism 'chooses' to breathe with an increased respiratory frequency and small tidal volume. Only when the interstitial disease is so severe and the diffusion capacity of the alveolar membranes so low that they lead to hypoxaemia does alveolar hyperventilation occur, leading to hypocapnia.

Respiratory stimulants

Hypoventilation and chronic hypoxaemia and hypercapnia may be detrimental for life expectancy. The MRC and NOTT trials in the UK and USA respectively showed that adding supplemental oxygen to the inspiratory air for at least 15 h per day improved the survival of hypoxaemic patients. Adding oxygen aggravates hypercapnia to different extents in different patients. Increasing hypercapnia is only partly due to lowering of the hypoxic drive to peripheral chemoreceptors, and is made worse by ventilation–perfusion inequality. Evidence is accumulating that hypercapnia, as such, is a determinant of poor prognosis, independently of hypoxaemia. Thus, it may become desirable to treat not only the hypoxaemia but also the hypercapnia. The ultimate treatment is, of course, mechanical ventilatory support.

Pharmacological stimulation of ventilation may be an attractive alternative, especially in the early stages of respiratory failure.[26] Respiratory stimulant drugs exert their influence directly or indirectly on the brain-stem respiratory centres. The resulting increased respiratory drive has to be effected by the respiratory muscles. Therefore, such treatment is appropriate only if the respiratory pump is able to increase its performance: 'Don't whip a tired horse'. It may be helpful to evaluate whether the patient has any ventilatory reserves. One method is to use a capnograph to sample expired air while the patient is asked to try and hyperventilate. If he/she is able to lower the end-tidal P_{CO_2} by voluntary overbreathing, this indicates that the ventilatory pump still has some reserves, at least in the short term. If the patient cannot lower the end-tidal P_{CO_2}, respiratory stimulants should not be prescribed.

Doxapram

This is a respiratory stimulant that can only be given intravenously.[27,28] When starting this therapy, a loading method is used, e.g. starting with 3 mg/min for the first 15 min, then 2 mg/min for the second 15 min, followed by 1.5 mg/min for the next half hour. The maintenance dose is usually between 0.5 and 1.5 mg/min. The drug acts mainly on the peripheral chemoreceptors, and hardly at all on the respiratory centres. It has analeptic properties.

Theophylline

Methylxanthines such as theophylline have respiratory stimulant properties, in addition to bronchodilator effects and probably positive inotropic effects on (respiratory) muscles.[29] The therapeutic range is rather narrow. Therefore, the plasma levels of this drug should be checked regularly. Plasma levels of 3–5 mg/l are adequate for ventilatory stimulation.

Progesterone

The hypothalamus has progesterone receptors. The infundibular hypothalamic centres project to the brainstem respiratory centres and can thus mediate ventilatory stimulation. A daily dose of 100 mg medroxyprogesterone acetate or chlormadinone acetate will reduce the P_aCO_2 by about 1 kPa (7.5 mmHg).[30,31] Not all COPD patients seem to respond to this therapy. Male patients should be warned about impotence. Progesterone also increases the metabolic rate. However, the ventilatory stimulant effect is greater than the metabolic effect, resulting in a lower P_aCO_2.

Acetazolamide

The carbonic anhydrase inhibitor acetazolamide causes metabolic acidosis. It has a stimulatory effect on central chemoreceptor mechanisms and a small inhibitory effect on the peripheral chemoreceptors.[32,33] The net effect on ventilation is

stimulatory. The oral dose is 500–1000 mg daily. Side effects include paraesthesiae and nausea. It is a weak diuretic, much less effective than loop diuretics but, on the other hand, loop diuretics such as furosemide (frusemide) cause metabolic alkalosis and thus depress ventilation.

Almitrine

This drug stimulates peripheral chemoreceptors and thus ventilation. It is not available in a number of countries because of a peripheral neuropathy allegedly caused by the drug.[34] Early studies were performed with rather high doses, and many patients with COPD have a neuropathy without this drug, so the risk may have been overestimated. Pulmonary hypertension is also one of the side effects ascribed to this drug. The adequate oral dose is 50 mg once or twice daily.

Protriptyline

The antidepressant drug protriptyline is also occasionally used as a respiratory stimulant in an oral dose of 20 mg daily.

Prethcamide

This analeptic drug is given intravenously in acute respiratory insufficiency. It has a wide therapeutic range between 75 and 450 mg once to thrice daily. It is not available in a number of countries.

Caffeine

This methylxanthine preparation is sometimes used as respiratory stimulant in neonates subject to apnoea. The dose is 1 mg/kg/day

---

? Unresolved questions

- It is still unclear why some patients with severe COPD hypoventilate and others who have the same degree of airway obstruction do not.

- The mechanism of hyperpnoea during exercise is most probably multifactorial; the interaction between all possible stimuli is clear.

- The clinical relevance of chronic hypercapnia (independently of significant hypoxaemia) and the need for its treatment remain to be established.

Clinical relevance

- In quiet breathing in normal subjects, more than 75% of the ventilation is generated by the diaphragm.

- The sensation of dyspnoea is mediated by multiple mechanisms: the receptors playing a role in this sensation include chemoreceptors, mechanoreceptors in respiratory muscles, mechanoreceptors in other working muscles, pulmonary receptors with vagal afferents and probably several more.

- The hyperventilation syndrome is a complex mechanism of abnormal breathing and diffuse complaints. The mechanism of the symptoms is not exclusively hypocapnia.

References

1. Whitelaw WA, Derenne JP, Milic-Emili J. Occlusion pressure as a measure of respiratory centre output in conscious man. Respir Physiol 1975; 23: 181–199.
2. Wasserman K, Hansen JE, Sue DY et al. Principles of exercise testing and interpretation, 2nd ed. Philadelphia, PA: Lea & Febiger; 1994: 42–53.
3. Whipp BJ. Carotid bodies and breathing in humans. Thorax 1994; 49: 1081–1084.
4. Bruce EN, Cherniack NS. Central chemoreceptors. J Appl Physiol 1987; 62: 389–402.
5. Poulin MJ, Robins PA. Influence of cerebral blood flow on the ventilatory response to hypoxia in humans. Exp Physiol 1998; 83: 95–106.
6. Bayliss DA, Millhorn D. Central neural mechanisms of progesterone action: application to the respiratory system. J Appl Physiol 1992; 73: 393–404.
7. Colice GL, Bernat JL. Neurologic disorders and respiration. Clin Chest Med 1989; 10: 521–543.
8. Meessen NEL, van den Grinten C, Luijendijk S, Folgering H. Breathing pattern during bronchial challenge in humans. Eur Respir J 1997; 10: 1058–1063.
9. Meessen NEL, van den Grinten CPM, Luijendijk SCM, Folgering HThM. Histamine induced bronchoconstriction and end-tidal inspiratory activity in man. Thorax 1996; 51: 1192–1198.
10. Brodovsky D, MacDonnell LA, Cherniack RM. The respiratory response to carbon dioxide in health and in emphysema. J Clin Invest 1960; 39: 724–729.
11. Weil JV, Byrne-Quinn E, Sodal IE et al. Hypoxic ventilatory drive in normal man. J Clin Invest 1970; 49: 1061–1072.
12. Caruana-Montaldo B, Gleeson K, Zwillich CW. The control of breathing in clinical practice. Chest 2000; 117: 205–225.
13. Gibson GJ. Neuromuscular diseases. In: Clinical tests of respiratory function. London: Chapman & Hall; 1996: 267–291.
14. Zwillich CW, Sutton FD, Pierson DJ et al. Decreased hypoxic ventilatory drive in patients with the obesity hypoventilation syndrome. Am J Med 1975; 59: 343–348.
15. Burki NK, Baker W. Ventilatory regulation in eucapnic morbid obesity. Am Rev Respir Dis 1984; 129: 538–543.
16. Folgering H. The hyperventilation syndrome. In: Altose MD, Kawakami Y, ed. Control of breathing in health and disease. New York: Marcel Dekker; 1999: 633–660.
17. Vos PJE, Folgering H, van Herwaarden CLA. Predictors for nocturnal hypoxaemia (mean SaO$_2$, <90%) in normoxic and mildly hypoxic patients with COPD. Eur Respir J 1995; 8: 74–77.
18. Bergofsky E. Respiratory failure in disorders of the thoracic cage. State of the art. Am Rev Respir Dis 1979; 119: 643–669.
19. McFadden ER, Lyons HA. Arterial blood gas tension in asthma. N Engl J Med 1968; 278: 1027–1032.
20. Demeter SL, Cordasco EM. Hyperventilation syndrome and asthma. Am J Med 1986; 81: 989–994.
21. Kesten S, Maleki-Yazdi R, Sanders BR et al. Respiratory rate during acute asthma. Chest 1990; 97: 58–62.
22. Van den Elshout F, van Herwaarden C, Folgering H. Effects of hypercapnia and hypocapnia on pulmonary resistance in normals and asthmatics. Thorax 1991; 46: 28–32.
23. Gorini M, Misuri G, Corrado A et al. Breathing pattern and carbon dioxide retention in severe chronic obstructive pulmonary disease. Thorax 1996; 51: 677–683.
24. Scano G, Spinelli A, Duranti R et al. Carbon dioxide responsiveness in COPD patients with and without chronic hypercapnia. Eur Respir J 1995; 8: 75–85.
25. Tardif C, Bonmarchand G, Gibon J-F et al. Respiratory response to CO$_2$ in patients with chronic obstructive pulmonary disease in acute respiratory failure. Eur Respir J 1993; 6: 619–624.
26. Bardsley PA. Chronic respiratory failure in COPD. Is there a place for a respiratory stimulant? Thorax 1993; 48: 781–784.
27. Riordan JF, Sillett RW, McNicol MW. A controlled trial of doxapram in acute respiratory failure. Br J Dis Chest 1975; 69: 57–62.
28. Lugliani R, Whipp BJ, Wassermann K. Doxapram hydrochloride: a respiratory stimulant for patients with primary alveolar hypoventilation. Chest 1979; 76: 414–419.
29. De Backer W. Central sleep apnea, pathogenesis and treatment: an overview and perspective. Eur Respir J 1995; 8: 1372–1383.
30. Vos PJE, von Herwaarden CLA, de Boo Th et al. Effects of acetazolamide, chlormadinone acetate, and oxygen on awake and asleep gas exchange in COPD patients. Eur Respir J 1994; 7: 850–855.
31. Tatsumi K, Kimura H, Kunimoto F et al. Effects of chlormadinone acetate on ventilatory control in patients with chronic obstructive pulmonary disease. Am Rev Respir Dis 1986; 133: 552–557.
32. Swenson ER, Hughes JMB. Effects of acute and chronic acetazolamide on resting ventilation and ventilatory responses in men. J Appl Physiol 1993; 74: 230–237.
33. Skatrud JB, Dempsey JA. Relative effectiveness of acetazolamide versus medroxyprogesterone acetate in correction of chronic carbon dioxide retention. Am Rev Respir Dis 1983; 127: 405–412.
34. Tweney J. Almetrine bismesylate: current status. Clin Respir Physiol 1987; 23(suppl. 11): 153S–163S.

3 Respiratory defences

3.1 Physical defences

Stewart Clarke and Malcolm King

 Key points

- The respiratory system is exposed to a myriad of particles suspended in air, which may be inhaled with potentially injurious effects to the lung.

- With high flows in central airways, inertial impaction of large particles predominates; small particles reach the terminal ventilatory units, where they are deposited by sedimentation.

- Clearance of airway secretions takes place by two principal means, mucociliary action and coughing, the latter being essentially a reserve mechanism.

- The mucociliary system serves the tracheobronchial tree from the larynx to about the 16th bronchial division.

- The efficiency of mucociliary clearance depends on the integrity of the ciliated epithelium, the ciliary beat frequency and coordination, the consistency and depth of the sol and gel layers and the viscoelasticity of the latter.

- Cough clearance derives from the high-velocity interaction between airflow and mucus, leading to wave formation in the mucus layer and ultimately to shearing and forward propulsion of the mucus.

- The volume of mucus and the airflow linear velocity are critical determinants of cough clearance. Mucus physical properties that impact on cough clearance are viscosity, elastic recoil and adhesivity.

- Alveolar clearance for insoluble particles is slow (more than 24 h and often much longer), and usually involves alveolar macrophages and both pulmonary and extrapulmonary lymphatics.

- In health, much of the tracheobronchial tree is cleared within 6 h and virtually all within 24 h. A variety of diseases, including acute and chronic bronchitis, asthma, bronchiectasis and cystic fibrosis, cause abnormally slow clearance and retention of mucus. This faulty clearance is partially compensated for by cough clearance.

- The shortcomings of cough as a clearance mechanism are its limitation to the central airways and its inefficiency in chronic airflow obstruction. In practice, coughing from a high lung volume should be encouraged, and clearance augmented by the forced expiration technique, by gravity and by various physiotherapy devices.

- Many agents are claimed to modify mucus and aid in expectoration but few have been assessed adequately. Combined mucokinetic therapies aim to address more than one mechanism involved in the control of airway mucus secretion and clearance.

The average person is exposed to a myriad of particles suspended in air, which may be inhaled with potentially injurious effects to the tracheobronchial tree and lung. Each day a surface as large as a tennis court, the area of the alveolar capillary membrane, is exposed to a volume of air and contaminants that would fill an average swimming pool.[1] Inhaled tobacco smoke causes chronic obstructive pulmonary disease (COPD) and lung cancer, inhaled microorganisms cause pneumonia and tuberculosis, inhaled allergens such as house dust and mites, pollens, feathers and pet dander precipitate bronchial asthma, and spores cause extrinsic allergic alveolitis (e.g. farmer's lung). Inhaled particles cause pneumoconiosis in miners and asbestosis in those exposed to asbestos particles. This merely gives some examples of the importance of inhaled particles in the induction of lung disease.

Aerosols are used extensively for the management of lung diseases; examples include long-acting beta-agonists and anticholinergics in asthma and COPD, antibiotics and mucolytics in cystic fibrosis and pentamidine in *Pneumocystis carinii* pneumonia.

This is a field that has expanded considerably in recent years (see Chapter 19).

The importance of physical respiratory defences is self-evident. By the same token, knowledge of these defences enables therapeutic aerosols to be targeted to the requisite site of drug action.

Upper airways

The respired air is subjected to considerable modification in the upper airways, which may be defined as those airways lying between the nose or mouth and the lower border of the cricoid cartilage. Not only do the upper airways conduct air, they also take part in air conditioning by warming and humidification, as well as swallowing, speech and smell.[2]

The nose

The nose is normally the first barrier to the ingress of inhaled particles and toxins. The nostrils lead via the vestibule to the start of the ciliated mucosa at the anterior aspect of the nasal septum and the turbinates. In this region lies the smallest total cross-sectional area in the respiratory tract. The main channel sweeps back some 6–8 cm to the posterior end of the turbinates and septum, the turbinates dividing the airway into the inferior, middle and superior meati. The vestibule is lined by skin with sebaceous glands and contains many coarse hairs, which act as an initial filter to the air stream. The mucous membrane of the nasal cavities is ciliated, highly vascular, provided with abundant mucous glands and goblet cells, and closely applied to the periosteum. In the nasopharynx, where the septum ends, there is a transition from columnar ciliated to squamous epithelium, which extends to the larynx, except for a partially ciliated surface posteriorly. The nasopharynx ends at the lower border of the soft palate, from where the oropharynx extends to the larynx.

The upper airways can be considered as a series of fine aerodynamic filters, removing most particles from the inspired air. First the nasal hairs act as a coarse filter. Particle impaction commences there and continues where there is narrowing, and then there is expansion between the nasal vestibule and middle meatus; this then increases as the airflow changes direction by

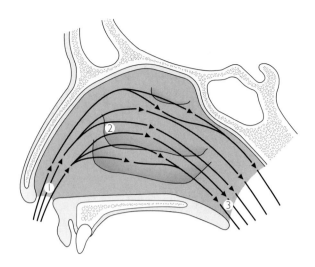

Fig. 3.1.1 Nasal airflow, with sites of particle deposition indicated: 1 where the airway narrows and 2 and 3 where the air stream bends.

60–130°. In the nasopharynx this airflow bends by a further 90° and at any of these sites inertial impaction of particles is enhanced by turbulence (Fig. 3.1.1).

Clearance of secretions, debris and particles from the nose is chiefly by mucociliary action, which sweeps the secretions backwards at a mean rate of about 6 mm/min, usually to be swallowed or cleared from the throat. In a small region that lies anterior to the inferior turbinates, motion is forward to the anterior nares, from which point the secretions are blown or wiped away. Sometimes sneezing clears the nose by two-phase air–liquid interaction at high flows (Fig. 3.1.2; see Cough clearance, below).

Mouth

The aerodynamic filter with mouth breathing is provided by inertial impaction round the 90° bend of the oropharynx, combined with that encouraged by the variable cross-sectional area of the larynx. Any impaction is increased at higher flows.

The larynx extends from the pharynx to the beginning of the trachea at the lower border of the cricoid cartilage.[3] The vocal

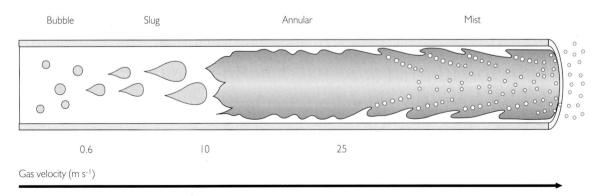

Bubble   Slug   Annular   Mist

0.6   10   25

Gas velocity (m s⁻¹)

Fig. 3.1.2 Two-phase air–liquid interaction through a tube, showing the four types with increasing air velocity, culminating in mist flow with aerosol production (and the potential for the spread of infection during coughing).

folds are covered by closely attached stratified squamous epithelium. The functions of the larynx are:

- to act as a respiratory channel and flow regulator
- to act as a sphincter during cough and expiration
- to protect the lower airways during swallowing and vomiting
- to act as a focus for reflexes, e.g. the cough reflex
- to initiate phonation in speech
- to exert a circulatory function in controlling venous return, e.g. in the Valsalva manoeuvre.

The variable cross-sectional area of the larynx and glottis contributes significantly to airway resistance, the onset of turbulence and inertial impaction of particles. In patients with airflow obstruction, the glottis may be narrowed on expiration, even on maximal effort, suggesting that this may play a part in controlling airflow.[4]

Lower airways

Tracheobronchial anatomy

The trachea extends from the larynx to the carina, is D-shaped and has 16–20 cartilaginous rings that are joined posteriorly by longitudinal smooth muscle.[5] The mucosa is lined by pseudostratified ciliated columnar epithelium with occasional goblet cells and submucosal glands, which contribute to the mucous blanket overlying the cilia. The cartilaginous rings support the trachea and extrapulmonary bronchi which, in contrast to the intrapulmonary airways, have no support from the lung parenchyma. The C-shaped cartilage extends to the origin of the apical lower bronchus on each side, becoming progressively discontinuous and absent from bronchioles less than 0.8 mm in diameter. Inside the cartilage, circular and diagonal muscle fibres are so arranged that on contraction they constrict and shorten the airways.

The lobar bronchi are 7–12 mm in diameter and divide progressively into segmental (4–7 mm) and subsegmental bronchi, and eventually into the bronchioles.[6] The bronchioles lead to the terminal bronchiole, which divides into three generations of respiratory bronchioles about 0.5 mm in diameter, initially lined by ciliated pseudocolumnar epithelium with Clara cells but changing to non-ciliated low cuboidal epithelium thereafter. They divide further into about four generations of alveolar ducts opening on to numerous alveolar sacs.

Alveolar anatomy

The alveolar capillary membrane is composed of three layers: epithelium (0.1 μm thick), basement membrane plus interstitial substance, and capillary endothelium with a total thickness of about 0.8 μm. The pores of Kohn interrupt the continuity of the alveolar walls and allow collateral ventilation and the migration of cells. The area of the alveoli is about 143 m², the capillary surface 120–150 m² and the blood capillary volume 150–200 ml.[7]

Lung models

For the purpose of describing flow patterns within the human lung, which profoundly influence particle deposition, two models are often used, those of Weibel[8] and Horsfield et al.[9] The models have been used to predict the frequency distribution of pathway lengths in the lung and to calculate fluid flow in the airways and mucociliary clearance. Other studies have taken into account the variability in airway dimensions, as well as branching angles and angles of inclination to gravity, which are also important for deposition.

Airflow patterns[10]

During the breathing cycle, the tidal volume of air, usually containing a mixture of particles, is inhaled through the nose or mouth and pharynx to mix with the air in the anatomical dead space, the front penetrating deeply into the lung. Secondary motions (also known as vortices or eddies) form at bifurcations and accentuate deposition, but turbulence is minimal, the majority of flow being laminar or streamline (Fig. 3.1.3). This is not the case at higher flow rates during exercise or rapid breathing, when secondary motions and turbulence are generated at airway bifurcations and the airways are too short to allow smooth flow to develop before the next bifurcation. Linear velocity falls as the cross-sectional area of the airways increases with increasing divisions of the airways (Fig. 3.1.4), so that in the terminal ventilatory units the linear velocity of the inspired gas is only a fraction of a millimetre per second. Similar but reversed patterns are seen on inspiration and expiration.

It is important to realise that a large part of the airway resistance lies in the upper respiratory tract, that flow is not entirely laminar and thus cannot be predicted by Poiseuille's law (because of the secondary eddies), and that the resistance of the peripheral airways is only a small proportion of the total. Thus respired air can be said to move by three processes: the first is convective flow in the conducting airways with non-laminar conditions favouring particle deposition centrally; the second is axial molecular diffusion in the respiratory airways, where forward flow is low; and the third is molecular diffusion across the alveolar capillary membrane. The interaction between convective flow and simultaneous molecular diffusion is known as Taylor dispersion.

Particle deposition

Some of the above information has been used to predict the deposition of inspired particles within the tracheobronchial tree. With high flows in central airways, inertial impaction of large particles predominates; small particles reach the terminal ventilatory units where they are deposited by sedimentation (see Chapter 19). Deposition is irregular, with localised increases at the carina and further downstream, consistent with localised variation in airflow. Deposition at bifurcations may be as much as 100 times more than elsewhere, being increased by turbulence and high local flow rates. At such sites[11] inhaled particles in tobacco smoke may be deposited in high concentrations and most lung tumours are located there.

Although the theoretical models have their limitations, they permit predictions of deposition under a variety of conditions such as different initial lung volumes, inspired volumes, flow rate, breath-holding pauses, particle sizes (Fig. 3.1.5) and patterns of bronchoconstriction.[12]

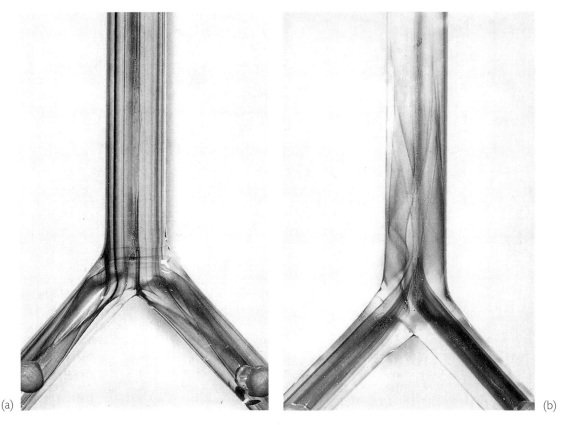

Fig. 3.1.3 Laminar (or streamline) flow in a glass model of the trachea showing secondary motions induced by the carina (a) on inspiration and (b) on expiration.

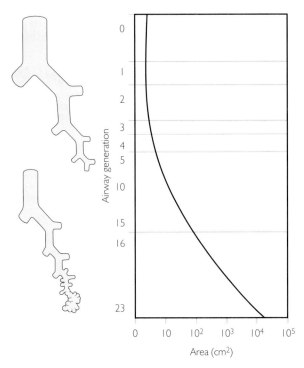

Fig. 3.1.4 The increase in the cross-sectional area of the peripheral airways. With permission from Clarke SW, Pavia D, eds. Aerosols and the lung. London: Butterworths; 1984.)

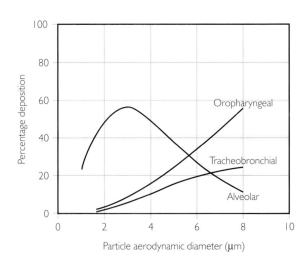

Fig. 3.1.5 Deposition within the tracheobronchial tree of different-sized aerosol particles.

Airway clearance

Clearance of airway secretions takes place by two principal means, mucociliary action and coughing, the latter being essentially a reverse mechanism. A third means, alveolar clearance, may also deal with a certain amount of the peripheral airway secretions but is less important to the airways.

Mucociliary clearance

Most of the tracheobronchial tree is swept clear by this system,[13] which extends from the larynx proximally to about the 16th bronchial division distally. The cilia are described in Chapter 1.2. The shaft of each cilium is composed of longitudinal fibres with a highly characteristic structure of nine outer double and two central single microtubules. The outer doublet consists of two microtubules, one complete and one incomplete, which are attached laterally. They are composed of the contractile protein tubulin; dynein arms connect the microtubules to the adjacent doublet, dynein being an ATPase protein that is the major protein component of the axoneme; it derives energy from ATP distributed along the length of the cilium and provides the motive force. At the tip of the cilium a crown of claws has been identified, which may penetrate into the overlying mucus and aid propulsion.

The ciliary beat cycle consists of an effective and a recovery stroke. During the effective stroke the cilium is fully extended, penetrates the mucus by $0.5\,\mu m$ and sweeps cephalad. In the recovery phase it is bent and flexed (Fig. 3.1.6). The duration of the recovery stroke is twice that of the effective stroke, namely about 29 ms and 15 ms respectively. The ciliated cells are found in groups, within which the cilia beat in a coordinated fashion, probably as a result of mechanochemical coupling with the overlying mucus.[14] The beating is independent of nervous control and appears to arise spontaneously. Ciliary beating is activated by calcium release from internal stores and sustained by the influx of calcium from the extracellular environment. The latter can be triggered by extracellular adenosine 5'-triphosphate (ATP).[15] Coordinated ciliary action is developed through cell-to-cell signalling mechanisms.[16]

Ciliary beat frequency is normally 12–14 beats per second but is modified by physical and chemical factors, temperature, pH and the viscoelastic properties of mucus, as well as by disease. The cilia can transport secretions against gravity and carry weights of up to 10 g/cm without slowing.[17] Furthermore, they can survive freezing for up to a month and then resume normal beating after re-warming.[18] This permits mucosal biopsies to be examined at will long after sampling. Finally, they may beat for several hours after death.

Assessment of ciliary function

Ciliated epithelium can be obtained by direct nasal brushing or by bronchial brushing or biopsy at fibreoptic bronchoscopy. The specimen must be handled carefully, with rapid immersion in tissue culture medium and maintenance of the temperature at 37°C. A motility index may be devised, from examination of the specimen on a graticule slide under high magnification, and classification of a given number of graticule squares as containing either motile or immotile cilia. The motility index is the ratio of 'motile' squares to the total number examined.

Ciliary beat frequency is usually measured by a photometric technique and has a mean value in normal human subjects of 13–14 cycles/s. The rate slows with cooling and speeds up with acetylcholine and extracellular ATP. Although beta-agonists increase ciliary beat frequency in human airway epithelial cells in vitro,[19] they may inhibit the calcium-dependent mechanism that controls intrinsic beat frequency.[20] Azelastine may stimulate ciliary motility and hence mucociliary transport, and also protect against sulphur-dioxide-induced ciliary dysfunction, probably by inhibiting intracellular cyclic adenosine monophosphate (cAMP) loss.[21] Acute exposure to inhaled bradykinin accelerates tracheobronchial clearance in normal human airways.[22]

A variety of ciliary defects has been described.[23-27] In certain patients there may be little coherent ciliary movement, although the cilia are by no means 'immotile'; hence the name 'immotile cilia syndrome' has been replaced by the term 'primary ciliary dyskinesia'.[25] Ultrastructural studies combined with measurements of ciliary beat frequency and motility patterns are critical in diagnosing primary ciliary dyskinesia.[26] Microtubular abnormalities with deviation from the usual 9 + 2 arrangement, compound cilia, loss of dynein arms (outer, inner or both) and radial spokes can be assessed, providing a standardised technique is used and sampling errors avoided.[27]

As nasal and bronchial cilia are morphologically similar in health and disease, clearance studies have been undertaken on the nose for simplicity. The most popular method is the saccharine test, in which a small particle of saccharin (or aspartame) is placed on the inferior nasal turbinate. The time taken for the dissolved saccharin to cause a sweet taste on the pharynx is noted, the normal value being less than 30 min.[28] Other methods have used a dye droplet to give a visual representation of nasal

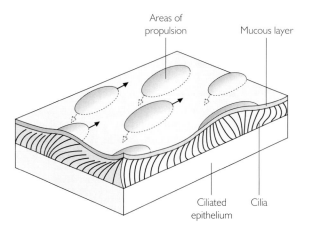

Fig. 3.1.6 Ciliated epithelium and the mucous layer. Cilia recover in periciliary fluid beneath the mucus but propel mucus during erect effective strokes, lifting it up in these areas of propulsion. Mucus is propelled in the direction of the solid arrows, but metachronal waves move in the direction of the dotted arrows. (With permission from Sleigh MA. Ciliary function in mucus transport. Chest 1981; 80: 79.).

clearance, a radiolabelled resin particle or radiographic contrast. However, the saccharin test is probably the simplest and it continues to be widely employed.[29]

Airway mucus[30-35]

Airway secretions originate from four main sources:

- the submucosal glands located chiefly in the cartilaginous airways
- the goblet cells – also lining the central airways
- Clara cells
- tissue fluid transudate.

Of these, the first is the most important. With a density of one submucosal gland per square millimetre of epithelium, the gland volume is 40 times that of the goblet cells. The gland has a ciliated duct opening on to the surface epithelium, a collecting duct, and mucous and serous tubules. Both mucous fluid and serous fluid pass into the collecting duct where ionic and water adjustment takes place before discharge. Chemical mediators and regulatory peptides influence secretion, there are vagal efferents ending in the glands, and both vagal stimulation and acetylcholine cause discharge. The role of sympathetic nerves is not clear, nor is that of the non-adrenergic, non-cholinergic inhibitory nerves. Several biologically active peptides, such as substance P, bombesin and vasoactive intestinal peptide (VIP), have been isolated from nerve endings in human airways. This complex has been called a diffuse neuroendocrine system. By contrast, secretion from the goblet cells is controlled mainly by local mechanical and chemical stimulation (e.g. smoking).

Airway mucus in health is composed of water (95%), glycoproteins (2%), proteins including immunoglobulins, lysozyme and lactoferrin (1%), lipids (1%) and inorganic salts (1%). The mucus behaves as a non-newtonian fluid (i.e. shear stress versus shear strain is non-linear) and has viscoelastic properties that are suitable for optimal clearance. Viscosity and elasticity vary over a wide range, exerting a negative effect on clearance beyond the optimum. Changes in viscosity/elasticity ratio, though smaller, exert a more important effect in model studies; too high a ratio means that ciliary energy is dissipated as friction instead of transformed into forward motion. Surface tension and adhesivity are other properties that may affect clearance.

Mucus viscoelasticity is dependent upon a number of types of interaction.

- **Disulphide bonds**. These covalent links are mainly intramolecular, and join glycoprotein subunits into extended macromolecular chains known as mucins.
- **Entanglements**. Because of their extended size, these mucin polymers readily form entanglements with neighbouring macromolecules, which act as time-dependent crosslinks, susceptible to mechanical degradation.
- **Hydrogen bonds**. The sugar units that make up the oligosaccharide side-chains (about 80% of the mucin weight), form hydrogen bonds with complementary units on neighbouring mucins. Although each bond is weak and readily dissociates, the vast numbers of bond sites give importance to this type of bonding.

- **Ionisation**. Mucins are also ionised, containing both positively charged amino acid residues and negatively charged sugar units, principally sialic acid and sulphated residues. The latter increase in airway disease in general, and in cystic fibrosis the proportion of sulphated residues is further elevated, possibly because of alterations in glycosyl transferase activities within the Golgi apparatus.
- **Ionic interactions**. The ionic interactions between fixed negative charges result in a stiffer, more extended macromolecular conformation, effectively increasing the polymer size and adding to the numbers of entanglements.
- Added to this, in airway diseases characterised by infection and inflammation, especially cystic fibrosis, are extra networks of high-molecular-weight DNA and actin filaments released by dying leukocytes, and exopolysaccharides secreted by bacteria.

Airway epithelial cells have the potential for both Cl^- secretion and Na^+ absorption. This active ion transport is believed to cause water to pass along both paracellular (through epithelial tight junctions) and transcellular pathways.

The mucous blanket that lies on the cilia is divided into a watery periciliary layer of liquid on which viscous mucus, the gel layer, floats. These layers have also been termed the 'hypophase' (sol) and 'epiphase' (gel), the same terminology as applied to alveolar surfactant. The sol layer may originate from ciliated cells and from Clara cells. The gel layer forms a three-dimensional fibrous network with a thickness of 8–12 μm in the trachea, becoming thinner in subsequent airway generations, amounting to 2–5 μm in the lobar bronchi. The daily volume of this transported mucus has been estimated to be about 10 ml in health. In chronic bronchitis and particularly during exacerbations the volume may be as high as 200–300 ml per day. The flow rate of this mucus in the trachea is about 10 mm/min, decreasing to about half this figure in the main bronchus and slowing further distally. The function of this mucus is to trap and clear particles, lubricate the airways, humidify the air and dilute toxic substances. Cells such as neutrophils and macrophages are present and act as scavengers. Lysin, bronchotransferrin and antiproteases are also found in mucus and have antimicrobial and antiproteolytic effects. Inhaled insoluble particles and cellular debris are transported on this escalator to the larynx, where they may be swallowed imperceptibly or cleared by coughing. In summary, the efficiency of mucociliary clearance depends on the integrity of the ciliated epithelium, the ciliary beat frequency and coordination, the consistency and depth of the sol and gel layers, and the viscoelasticity of the latter.

Methods for measuring mucociliary clearance

In health, much of the tracheobronchial tree is cleared within 6 h and virtually all within 24 h. In chronic bronchitis and a variety of other endobronchial diseases, however, this clearance time may be delayed. There are three main techniques for measuring clearance.

- **Cinebronchofibrescopic technique**. This uses small polytetrafluoroethylene (Teflon®) discs insufflated into the trachea via the channel of the fibreoptic bronchoscope.[36] The subsequent cephalad motion of 20–30 of these discs is filmed over a given time and tracheal mucus velocity (TMV) is estimated as mean distance over time. The mean rate is 21.5 ± 5.5 mm/min by this method.

■ **Radiographic technique.** This is a modification of the above, again using Teflon® discs coated with bismuth and introduced through a fibreoptic bronchoscope.[37] Motion is monitored by fluoroscope and an image intensifier attached to a television monitor and video tape. Up to 10 tracheal radiographs are taken at intervals of 1 min, and the movement of identified discs at a given time is measured. This gives a TMV of 11.4 ± 3.8 mm/min.

■ **Radioaerosol bolus technique.** By using rapid inhalation, near-total lung-capacity-localised radioaerosol particle deposition is achieved in the trachea or central airways.[38] The movement of this bolus in a given time can be monitored by gamma camera or special probe. This has yielded figures of 4.4 ± 1.3 mm/min.

It will be noted that there is a wide discrepancy between the above values, which is probably related to the invasiveness of the technique. In the first method, the bronchoscope is inserted into the tracheobronchial tree, in the second method only to the level of vocal folds, whereas the third method is totally non-invasive. It does, however, cast some doubt on the accuracy of the first two techniques, although they require only short observation periods, which minimises cough artefact and enables rapid repeat measurement to be made to test the effect of drugs.

Radioaerosol method. This older method for measuring lung mucociliary clearance was first used in 1955.[39] A radioactive aerosol is inhaled by the subject under strictly controlled conditions (i.e. particle size, inspiratory flow rate and lung volume) and subsequent chest radioactivity is monitored by external counters or a gamma camera. An immediate reading gives the initial deposition and distribution in the lungs. Further counts are taken over a period of 6 h, giving the biological clearance of radioaerosol after correction for isotopic decay. The results are plotted as clearance (or retention) of radioactivity, as a percentage of the initial count, against time. This lung clearance curve comprises mucociliary clearance, cough, which can be corrected for,[40] and alveolar clearance, although the last is of course slow (Fig. 3.1.7).

This curve is usually divided into two phases: an early fast phase (phase 1) caused by mucociliary clearance (plus cough if present), which is normally 80–85% complete within 6 h; and a later slow phase (phase 2), which reflects alveolar clearance, with a biological half-life of several months. Subtracting a 24-hour estimate of alveolar deposition from the whole lung clearance curve yields a tracheobronchial clearance curve.

The curve can be assessed by retention or clearance at say 2 and 6 h after inhalation, or the time taken to clear 50% radioactivity. Over short periods, clearance may be plotted as a linear regression and its slope measured; the area under the curve may also be measured; and finally the shape of the curve may give useful information. Regional clearance can be determined on the gamma camera, although lack of a three-dimensional image means that the accuracy of this method is low. Attempts have been made to use different-sized particles labelled with differ-

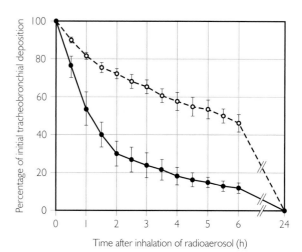

Fig. 3.1.7 Clearance curve showing the reduction of radioaerosol with time and comparing chronic bronchitis (open circles; n = 9) with healthy controls (closed circles; n = 9).

ent radionuclides to compare clearance from larger and smaller airways, with limited success.

Changes in mucociliary clearance

The variability in the measurement of mucociliary transport by the radioaerosol method has been assessed in a large number of subjects.[40] Clearance may be affected by a variety of factors, including physiological, environmental (pollutants), disease states and drugs.

Physiological factors

Several studies have demonstrated that mucociliary clearance slows with age by as much as 60%. However, there appears to be no difference between the sexes. Posture may enhance clearance of the lung secretions, e.g. in patients with cystic fibrosis. However, in normal subjects there is no such effect. No circadian rhythm of clearance has been found, but sleep is associated with a significant slowing,[41] both in health and disease (asthma); this may contribute to the early morning cough, sputum and wheeze in such patients. Brisk exercise is thought to enhance clearance and has been used for such in cystic fibrosis.

Environmental pollutants

Environmental pollutants that may disturb clearance include sulphuric acid mist, which, depending on dose, either decreases or increases clearance. The effect of tobacco smoke has yielded various results ranging from increasing to slowing clearance but in the long term there is undoubted depression.[42] Chronically slowed clearance (mucus retention) is in part related to altered mucus properties.

Disease states

A variety of diseases, including acute and chronic bronchitis, asthma even when mild, bronchiectasis and cystic fibrosis, cause abnormally slow clearance. Similar abnormalities can be seen, particularly in primary ciliary dyskinesia where there are defects in the ultrastructure of the cilia, with male infertility, and chronic infection of the upper and lower respiratory tracts.[43] Kartagener's syndrome with situs inversus is included in this group. Patients with Young's syndrome, which combines bronchitis and bronchiectasis in men with obstructive azoospermia but no situs inversus, also have depressed clearance.[44]

Mucolytics and expectorants[35, 45–54]

Many agents are claimed to modify mucus and aid expectoration but few have been assessed adequately. This field has recently been reviewed.[35] Treatment with rhDNase is based on the fact that the major factor involved in the elevated viscoelasticity of cystic fibrosis sputum is largely attributable to the presence of naked DNA released into the airway surface fluid from bacteria, leukocytes and other cellular debris. Enzymatic digestion of these DNA macromolecules effectively decreases mucus viscoelasticity and spinnability and enhances the clearability of airway secretions. Other direct-acting mucolytic treatments, such as N-acetylcysteine derivatives, gelsolin and hypertonic saline, are effective in vitro but may not necessarily show clinical efficacy. Indirect mucolysis, such as with inhaled amiloride, which blocks the uptake of salt and water across the airway epithelium, is a strategy aimed at enhancing the degree of hydration and diluting the macromolecular component of the airway surface fluid. Combined mucokinetic therapies aim to address more than one mechanism involved in the control of airway mucus secretion and clearance.

Nebulised water and physiological saline have only a minor effect on clearance, whereas hypertonic saline (7.1%) doubles the clearance rate. Low-molecular-weight oligosaccharides such as dextran are potentially capable of reducing the crosslink density of airway mucus through disruption of hydrogen bonds between mucin molecules. Substitution of low-molecular-weight saccharide moieties provided by dextran in place of the oligosaccharide moieties linked to the high-molecular-weight mucin peptides can reduce the number of load-bearing crosslink points at any given moment, making the mucus more easily deformable under the stresses applied by ciliary action and airflow.

Respiratory drugs

Beta-agonists are effective bronchodilators given by inhalation and they also stimulate clearance, particularly at higher doses. Conversely, beta-blockers in healthy subjects seem to reduce clearance. Oral methylxanthines enhance clearance, as well as causing bronchodilatation in patients with airway obstruction. Likewise, in asthma, even when airway obstruction is mild, corticosteroids appear to improve both obstruction and clearance.[55] Cholinergic drugs (e.g. acetylcholine) increase clearance whereas the anticholinergics atropine and hyoscine appear to slow clearance. Ipratropium bromide, a synthetic anticholinergic drug, had no slowing effect on clearance even in high dosage.[56] Aspirin, 100% oxygen therapy and general anaesthesia have all been suggested to cause slowing of clearance, which may contribute to postoperative lung collapse.

Cough clearance

Cough is a common accompaniment of respiratory infection, chronic bronchitis and asthma. It helps to clear airways down to the seventh to eighth division, augmenting mucociliary clearance when the latter is overwhelmed by copious secretions, as occurs in chronic bronchitis.[57] Cough is a reflex mechanism (often termed the watchdog of the lung) and may be a reflection of bronchial irritability or hyper-reactivity and asthma as well as bronchopulmonary infection and localised endobronchial obstruction.

Coughing starts with a brief rapid inspiration usually greater than the resting tidal volume, which is followed by glottal closure for about 200 ms accompanied by an abrupt rise in pleural (and abdominal) pressure to 50–100 mmHg (6.6–13.3 kPa) resulting from expiratory muscle (and diaphragmatic) contraction.[58] Subsequent glottal opening is accompanied by the typical explosive cough, which has an accelerative peak of expiratory flow reached within 20–50 ms and may well exceed 12 l/s; this is about the same as the peak expiratory flow and is considerably lower in patients with COPD. Oscillation in the air stream and of the airway walls may contribute to the 'scrubbing' action of the cough and help expectoration of mucus at this stage. The trachea and central airways then collapse and lead to an important postpeak phase of flow, which is well demonstrated on cough flow–volume curves and follows the forced expiratory envelope (Fig. 3.1.8). Linear airflow velocities in excess of 5 m/s may occur down to the seventh to eighth airway generation. At the peak of cough linear velocities of 160–240 m/s may be achieved. The cough lasts for about 0.5 s, during which up to 1 litre of air is expelled; it is terminated by either glottal closure or respiratory muscle relaxation, with a consequent fall in pleural pressure. Often there are subsequent small coughs, which diminish in intensity as lung volume declines towards residual volume.

These high linear flows interact with bronchial secretions to cause 'two-phase air–liquid flow' by which energy is transferred from the air to the liquid, thereby shearing the liquid secretions

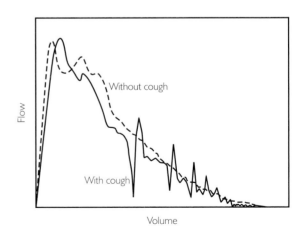

Fig. 3.1.8 Superimposed maximal expiratory flow–volume and cough curves, the latter showing a typical sequence of six coughs diminishing towards residual volume. Note the postpeak flow plateau, particularly marked after the first cough.

and finally producing expectoration of sputum.[59] A linear velocity of 10–25 m/s is required for the annular type of two-phase flow; with rates over 25 m/s mist flow with aerosol formation occurs (see Fig. 3.1.2). In health, these limits are vastly exceeded but this may not happen when there is airflow obstruction. Shearing and expectoration are affected by the viscosity, elasticity and surface tension of the bronchial secretions in a complex fashion.[60] Furthermore, the thickness of the secretions is of crucial importance because the air–liquid interaction with energy loss occurs more readily where there is narrowing with a local increase in resistance. Model studies have shown that, in addition to the airflow rate and the thickness of mucus layer, the main physical variables relating to cough clearance are mucus viscosity, elasticity (recoil) and surface properties[61] (Fig. 3.1.9).

Through use of radiographic methods to measure flow and tracheal cross-section during coughing, an index of 'scrubbing action' has been derived.[62] With the first cough the majority – about 59% – of the scrubbing action occurs whereas a lesser amount, 26% for the second cough and 16% for the third in a typical cough sequence, was found in healthy subjects. It seems reasonable to assume therefore that (1) coughs initiated from lower lung volumes may be relatively ineffective, and (2) patients with severe airflow obstruction and low flows have an inefficient cough – although energy-consuming and tiresome for the patient.

Copious bronchial secretions that overwhelm mucociliary clearance can best be cleared by coughing. Such secretions may increase flow resistance in the lung by up to one-third.[63] In a healthy subject, cough adds little to tracheobronchial clearance, whereas in chronic bronchitis it may account for about 50% of clearance, compensating for deficient mucociliary transport.[64]

The shortcomings of cough as a clearance mechanism are first its limitation to the central airways and second its inefficiency in chronic airflow obstruction. In this situation there may be insufficient linear velocity to mobilise secretions; furthermore, airways may close intermittently. In practice, coughing from a high lung volume should be encouraged and clearance should be augmented by the forced expiration technique, i.e. huffing from mid-lung volume,[65] and by gravity.

Viscosity

Viscosity is the primary variable governing cough clearance. For purely viscous materials, the mucus velocity profiles follow Newton's law.

Spinnability

Spinnability or thread formation is a measure of large deformation elasticity. A high degree of spinnability inhibits viscous deformation by creating recoil in the mucus

Adhesivity

High surface tension increases the work of adhesion of the mucus to the underlying surface, and inhibits wave formation in the mucus layer, reducing air–mucus interaction

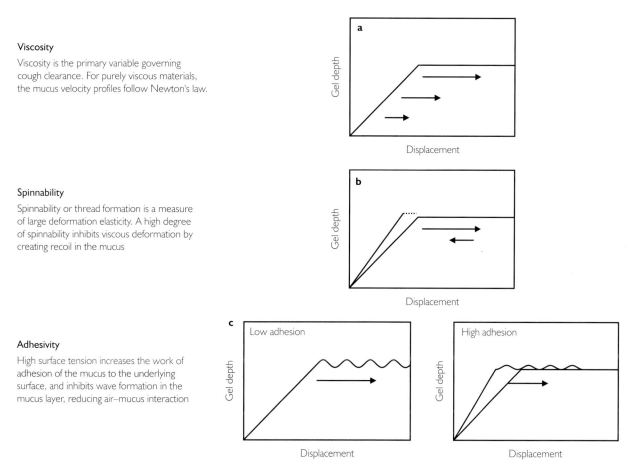

Fig. 3.1.9 Primary mucus variables related to cough-type clearance. (a) Viscosity is the primary variable governing cough clearance. For purely viscous materials, the mucus velocity profiles follow Newton's law. (b) Spinnability or thread formation is a measure of large deformation elasticity. A high degree of spinnability inhibits viscous deformation by creating recoil in the mucus. (c) Adhesivity – high surface tension increases the work of adhesion of the mucus to the underlying surface and inhibits wave formation in the mucus layer, reducing air–mucus interaction.

Alveolar clearance

For over a century it has been known that the bronchial walls are far less permeable than are the alveolar walls to the passage of soluble compounds. Alveolar clearance for insoluble particles is slow (more than 24 h and often much longer) and usually involves alveolar macrophages and both pulmonary and extra-pulmonary lymphatics.

Anatomy and physiology

The advent of electron microscopy enabled fine detail of the alveoli to be visualised.[58] The capillaries lie slightly asymmetrically within the alveolar walls so that on one side the alveolar–capillary membrane is thin and is capable of rapid gas transfer (see Fig. 1.2.13). On the other, thicker side of the capillary there is an interstitial space between the capillary and alveolar basement membranes, which is drained by lymphatics. The epithelium undergoes a transition from the flattened alveolar epithelial cells to the pseudocolumnar ciliated epithelium of the mucociliary escalator at the respiratory bronchiole. Type I and type II alveolar epithelial cells are joined by tight junctions, giving the epithelium a 10-fold greater resistance to the permeation of small hydrophilic molecules than the vascular endothelium.[66]

Freeze-fracture electron microscopy has shown that the epithelial tight junction consists of a network of sealing strands made up of interdigitating rows of protein molecules like a zipper (see Fig. 1.2.8).[67] By partial or selective unzipping of strands, cells may enter or leave the air space without there being a large leak of solute or water. Active transport of salt and water takes place across the epithelium itself. In contrast, the basement membrane does not appear to be a functional barrier to micromolecules.

Clearance mechanisms

Inhaled particles of 2.5 mm diameter or less may be deposited in the alveolar region of the lungs in considerable quantities (50% of inhaled dose) depending on the mode of breathing.

Finer particles (0.1–0.5 mm) show less tendency for deposition (20%) and may be respired like an insoluble gas.

Alveolar clearance (Fig. 3.1.10) may be divided as follows:[68]

- **Non-absorptive**: involving transport of particles from alveoli by surfactant or macrophages to the ciliated airways for removal by mucociliary clearance – this involves a very small proportion of particles
- **Absorptive**:
  - by direct penetration into the epithelial cells with subsequent cell death followed by transport of the cell debris to the mucociliary escalator or the interstitial space
  - transport through the epithelial wall via the transcellular or paracellular pathway
  - by phagocytosis and destruction within the phagocytic system or transport to lymphatics.

Transcellular transport

Macromolecules of different size and chemical composition are handled in different ways. For instance, ferritin and carbon particles are both endocytosed by the alveolar type I cells. Some ferritin is subsequently released into the interstitial space but large numbers of particles are digested by dense secondary lysosomes within the cells. In contrast, carbon is released into the interstitial space, with little appearing in epithelium lysosomes. Retention of carbon in these cells leads to desquamation and shedding into the alveolar lumen. Furthermore, alveolar macrophages absorb much larger amounts of carbon than ferritin.

Paracellular transport[68]

This involves the passage of hydrophilic substances through the intercellular tight junction by passive diffusion. The permeability of the alveolar epithelium is some 10 times less than the pulmonary vascular endothelium for hydrophilic solutes ranging in molecular weight from 50 000 to 100 000. This is related to the effective pore radius of the alveolar epithelium, which is about 1 nm, and of the endothelium, 4–8 nm. In several disease processes the permeability of the epithelial barrier may increase

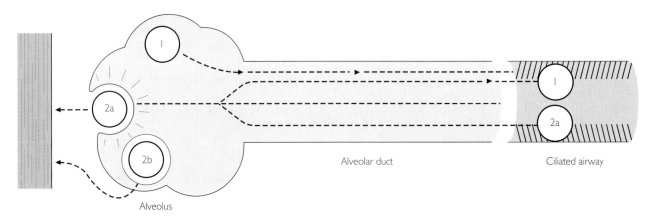

Fig. 3.1.10 Diagrammatic representation of alveolar clearance. 1 is cleared by surfactant motion; 2a is cleared by direct penetration into the epithelial cells and removal of cell debris either by route 1 or by penetration into the interstitial space and clearance by blood or lymphatic flow; and 2b is cleared by phagocytosis and destruction or transport to lymphatics to subpleural and paraseptal sites centrifugally.

Table 3.1.1 Factors associated with increased alveolar permeability. (After Jones.[68])

Inhalation	Infection	Emboli	Drugs/poisons	Miscellaneous
100% oxygen	Viral	Fat	Aspirin	Uraemia
Nitrogen dioxide	*Pneumocystis* spp.	Air	Bleomycin	Neurogenic pancreatitis
Ozone	*Legionella* spp.	Amniotic fluid	Busulfan	Cardiopulmonary bypass
Fire smoke	Gram-negative bacteria		Nitrofurantoin	Trauma
Gastric contents			Heroin	
Acrolein			Alloxan	
			Paraquat	

considerably (Table 3.1.1). The evidence for this increase is based on the albumin concentration in pulmonary oedema in many of these conditions. As albumin has a molecular radius of approximately 4 nm it is clear that the leakiness of the epithelial layer is quite marked.

More recently, lesser degrees of defective permeability have been shown in the human alveolar epithelium in the absence of pulmonary oedema by the use of low-molecular-weight solutes as probes of epithelial permeability. In particular, diethylenetri-aminepentaacetic acid (DTPA), with a molecular weight of 492 and an approximate molecular radius of 0.57 nm, has been used as a probe molecule to derive an index of permeability of the paracellular pathway in the human lung. It may be inhaled as a radiolabelled aerosol and its rate of transfer from alveoli to blood is measured either with a gamma camera or with twin scintillation detectors. It is principally a test of the alveolar epithelium, which accounts for more than 90% of the resistance to paracellular transport, large changes in endothelial permeability having only a small effect on the results. Taking account of mucociliary clearance,[69] possibly as a result of binding of ^{99m}Tc-DTPA to mucus, the index of pulmonary epithelial permeability is expressed as the half-time clearance rate of technetium from the lung into blood (TLG). Background radioactivity in vascular tissue within the field of the lung detectors must be corrected for, otherwise the results are unreliable.[70]

Increased clearance has been noted in various interstitial lung diseases as well as in cigarette smokers and in firemen chronically exposed to smoke. By contrast, non-smokers with asthma or COPD have no evidence of increased clearance. Patients with pulmonary infections, e.g. pneumonia caused by *Pneumocystis carinii* and adult respiratory distress syndrome, also have increased clearance.

Phagocytosis

Phagocytosis by the alveolar macrophages is the fate of most particles deposited in the alveoli. A proportion may be transported from the alveolar region to the ciliated airways, there to undergo mucociliary clearance. Alternatively, the macrophage may migrate through the epithelial wall into the interstitial space and either enter the lymphatics or re-enter the airways and ciliated zone. The optimum particle size for phagocytosis appears to be about 2–3 mm. Uptake may also be a function of the mass of particles: with Teflon®-coated particles 4–5 mm in diameter, carbon is phagocytosed faster than aluminium and chromium, which in turn are faster than silver, manganese and uranium. Alveolar macrophages may be damaged by relatively insoluble gases such as ozone and nitrogen dioxide, thereby reducing phagocyte and bactericidal activity and increasing the susceptibility to bacterial infection. They may also be damaged by nickel, cadmium, manganese, chromium and vanadium – emphysema after cadmium exposure may ensue from such damage with release of proteases. Damage from silicon or asbestos may be from direct cytotoxic effects coupled with release of proteases.

Operation of alveolar clearance

In summary, alveolar clearance is slow,[70,71] may be subdivided into three stages and is principally by alveolar macrophages and both pulmonary and extrapulmonary lymphatics. Particles are isolated and detoxified by phagocytosis, following which the macrophage (with a cell life of 1–5 weeks) acts as a vehicle for transport of such material through the lung.

- The initial fast phase lasts about 24 h. Some particle-laden cells are carried by surfactant or macrophages from the alveolar surface to the mucociliary escalator directly or via the pores of Kohn and rapidly cleared, accounting for a small amount of the initial 24-hour clearance curve of the lung.
- The intermediate phase lasts 3–20 days, when laden macrophages may migrate into the interstitium and then either re-enter the airways via lymphoid nodules at the bronchoalveolar junction or pass along lymph vessels to bronchial and hilar nodes, the thoracic duct and the systemic circulation.[72]
- The prolonged slow phase lasts 100 days or more, during which particle-laden cells may be transported by lymphatic flow to subpleural and paraseptal sites from which there is no exit.

The pulmonary lymphatic system

The pulmonary lymphatic system is composed of a pleural and a peribronchial plexus which drain to the hilar lymph nodes. Lymphatics are thin-walled structures that start in the centre of the acini and in the interlobular septa. They consist of collecting channels composed of endothelial cells with relatively tight junctions, smooth muscle and valves, and lymphatic capillaries lined by endothelial cells with loose junctions and frequent gaps, consistent with a very high permeability to macromolecules. This permeability of the lymphatic capillaries results in a highly efficient lymphatic clearance of macromolecules introduced into the alveoli; the amount of albumin (molecular radius 4 nm) placed in the alveoli and cleared by lymphatics is 37 times greater than that cleared by capillaries, in spite of the average lymph flow being 400 times slower than pulmonary blood flow.[73]

Surfactant

Surfactant (see Chapter 2.2) provides alveolar stability, maintains the patency of small airways, and is instrumental in transporting particles from the alveolar surface to the small airways.[74]

Clinical aspects

Primary ciliary dyskinesia

Primary ciliary dyskinesia (see Chapter 49) includes a mixed group of conditions, some inherited, causing impairment of mucociliary transport in the respiratory tract, e.g. Kartagener's syndrome. Males are usually infertile as a result of sperm immotility because the sperm tail is similar to a cilium and has the same defect. The cardinal features are chronic sinusitis, chronic bronchitis and eventually bronchiectasis, often serous otitis media and, in 50% of patients, situs inversus. There is up to a 50% decrease in ciliary beat frequency and the cilia beat in an abnormal incoordinated fashion. Several structural defects, including absence of dynein arms, radial spokes or microtubules, have been described. Studies of mucociliary clearance have shown virtual absence of activity. These patients are dependent on coughing for clearance.

Infection

Acute bronchitis or pneumonia (see Chapter 35) may cause epithelial damage and stripping; in particular, influenza and mycoplasmal infection have been implicated. Similar damage has been seen in children with recurrent respiratory tract infections, all suggesting an abnormality in mucociliary function; this is supported by clearance studies. Clearance may take 2–3 months to recover completely and, particularly in the case of influenza, this may be the cause of superadded infection.

Cystic fibrosis

In cystic fibrosis (see Chapter 50), bronchial secretions are increased in volume and viscosity and they are often purulent. Mucociliary transport may be decreased in severe disease but ciliary structure and function appear normal. Although mucociliary dysfunction is probably important in cystic fibrosis, it is likely to be secondary to airway damage and sputum purulence. Bioelectric potentials across the nasal and tracheobronchial epithelium of cystic fibrosis patients are increased about twofold compared with non-cystic-fibrosis patients and normals.

This bioelectric abnormality is characteristic of the disease and relates to the lack of chloride-ion channel activity, combined with hyperabsorption of sodium, leading to underhydration of the airway surface fluid.

Asthma

Bronchial asthma is another condition in which mucociliary clearance is impaired even when the condition is in remission.[75] There is mounting evidence that this impairment increases as asthma deteriorates, culminating in the plugging seen in acute severe asthma attacks and sudden death. There is copious cellular debris as well as a variety of mediators in the sputum, and frequently mucosal stripping, which adds to the problem.

? Unresolved questions

- Mucociliary clearance and clearance by airflow mechanisms depend on different mechanisms. How can these two processes be mutually optimised?

- The stickiness (adhesivity) of mucus in trapping particles is not well studied. How does this work? Can adhesivity be improved without compromising clearance?

- Are there practical approaches to improving alveolar clearance?

- Can we design better techniques to assess the efficacy of mucus clearance treatments?

References

1. Green GM, Jakab GJ, Low RB, Davis GS. Defense mechanisms of the respiratory membrane. Am Rev Respir Dis 1977; 115: 479.
2. Proctor DF. The upper airways. I. Nasal physiology and defense of the lungs. Am Rev Respir Dis 1977; 115: 97.
3. Proctor DF. The upper airways. II. The larynx and trachea. Am Rev Respir Dis 1977; 115: 315.
4. Higgenbottam T, Payne J. Glottis narrowing in lung disease. Am Rev Respir Dis 1982; 125: 746.
5. Clarke SW. Anatomy and physiology of the human lung: aspects relevant to aerosols. In: Clarke SW, Pavia D, ed. Aerosols and the lung. London: Butterworths; 1984: 1.
6. Horsfield K. The relation between structure and function in the airways of the lung. Br J Dis Chest 1974; 68: 145.
7. Weibel ER. Morphometry of the human lung: the state of the art after two decades. Bull Eur Physiopathol Respir 1979; 15: 999.
8. Weibal ER. Morphometry of the human lung. Berlin: Springer Verlag; 1963.
9. Horsfield K, Dart G, Olson DE et al. Models of the human bronchial tree. J Appl Physiol 1971; 31: 207.
10. Schroter RC, Sudlow MF. Flow patterns in models of the human bronchial airways. Respir Physiol 1969; 9: 341.
11. Schlesinger RB, Gurman JL, Lippmann M. Particle deposition within bronchial airways. Ann Occup Hyg 1982; 26: 47.
12. Agnew JE. Physical properties and mechanisms of deposition of aerosols. In: Clarke SW, Pavia D, eds. Aerosols and the lung. London: Butterworths; 1984: 49.
13. Wanner A, Salathé M, O'Riordan TG. Mucociliary clearance in the airways. Am J Respir Crit Care Med 1996; 154: 1868.
14. Gheber L, Priel Z. Ciliary activity under normal conditions and under viscous load. Biorheology 1990; 27: 547.
15. Korngreen A, Priel Z. Purinergic stimulation of rabbit ciliated airway epithelia: control by multiple calcium sources. J Physiol (Lond) 1996; 497: 53.

16. Dirksen ER. Intercellular communication in mammalian airway ciliated epithelia. In: Baum GL, Priel Z, Roth Y et al, ed. Cilia, mucus, and mucociliary interactions. New York: Marcel Dekker, 1998: 59.

17. Lucas AM, Douglas LC. Principles underlying ciliary activity in the respiratory tract. Arch Otolaryngol 1934; 20: 518.

18. Di Benedetto G, Gill J, Lopez-Vidriero MT, Clarke SW. Preservation of human respiratory ciliated epithelium at −196°C: effect on ciliary beat frequency. Clin Sci 1988; 74: 35.

19. Devalia JL, Sapsford RJ, Rusnak C et al. The effects of salmeterol and salbutamol in ciliary beat frequency of cultured human bronchial epithelial cells in vitro. Pulm Pharmacol 1992; 5: 257.

20. Honeyman G, Kemp PJ, Cobain C et al. Beta-agonist terbutaline makes the ciliary beta frequency of freshly isolated human airway cells refractory to calcium signaling. In: Baum GL, Priel Z, Roth Y et al, ed. Cilia, mucus, and mucociliary interactions. New York: Marcel Dekker, 1998: 71.

21. Tamaoki J, Chiyotani A, Sakai N et al. Effect of azelastine on sulphur dioxide impairment of ciliary motility in airway epithelium. Thorax 1993; 48: 542.

22. Polosa R, Hussain A, Babiya D et al. Acute effect of inhaled bradykinin on tracheo-bronchial clearance in normal humans. Thorax, 1992; 47: 952.

23. De Iongh RU, Ing A, Rutland J. Mucociliary function, ciliary ultrasound, and ciliary orientation in Young's syndrome. Thorax, 1992; 47: 184.

24. Rutman A, Cullinan P, Woodhead M et al. Ciliary disorientation: a possible variant of primary ciliary dyskinesia. Thorax 1993; 48: 770.

25. Greenstone M, Rutman A, Dewar A et al. Primary ciliary dyskinesia; cytological and clinical features. Q J Med 1988; 67: 405.

26. Rutland J, Morgan L, Waters KA et al. Diagnosis of primary ciliary dyskinesia. In: Baum GL, Priel Z, Roth Y et al, ed. Cilia, mucus, and mucociliary interactions. New York: Marcel Dekker, 1998: 407.

27. Fox B, Bull TB, Makey AR, Rawbone R. The significance of ultrastructural abnormalities of human cilia. Chest 1981; 805: 796.

28. Stanley P, MacMillan L, Greenstone M et al. Efficacy of a saccharin test for screening to detect abnormal mucociliary clearance. Br J Dis Chest 1984; 78: 62.

29. Newhouse MT. Ciliary beat frequency, ultrastructural abnormalities, and mucus clearance in primary ciliary dyskinesia. In: Baum GL, Priel Z, Roth Y et al, ed. Cilia, mucus, and mucociliary interactions. New York: Marcel Dekker, 1998: 399.

30. Leff AR. Endogenous regulation of bronchomotor tone. Am Rev Respir Dis 1988; 137: 1198.

31. Supplement: airway neuropeptides. Am Rev Respir Dis 1987; 136: S1.

32. King M. Mucus, mucociliary clearance and coughing. In: Bates DV Respiratory function in disease, 3rd ed. Philadelphia, PA: WB Saunders; 1989: 69.

33. Dasgupta B, King M. Molecular basis for mucolytic therapy. Can Respir J 1995; 2: 223.

34. Zayas JG, Man GCW, King M. Tracheal mucus rheology in patients undergoing diagnostic bronchoscopy: interrelations with smoking and cancer. Am Rev Respir Dis 1990; 141: 1107.

35. King M, Rubin BK. Mucus-controlling agents: past and present. Respir Care Clin North Am 1999; 5: 575–594.

36. Sackner MA, Rosen MJ, Wanner A. Estimation of tracheal mucus velocity by bronchofiberoscopy. J Appl Physiol 1973; 34: 495.

37. Friedman M, Stott FD, Poole DO et al. A new roentgenographic method for estimating mucous velocity in airways. Am Rev Respir Dis 1977; 115: 67.

38. Yeates DB, Aspin N, Levison H et al. Mucociliary tracheal transport rates in man. J Appl Physiol 1975; 30: 487.

39. Albert RE, Arnett LC. Clearance of radioactive dust from the lung. Arch Environ Health 1955; 12: 99.

40. Del Donno M, Pavia D, Agnew JE et al. Variability and reproducibility in the measurement of tracheobronchial clearance in healthy subjects and patients with different obstructive lung diseases. Eur Respir J 1988; 1: 613.

41. Bateman JRM, Pavia D, Clarke SW. The retention of lung secretions during the night in normal subjects. Clin Sci Mol Med 1978; 55: 523.

42. Camner P. Clearance of particles from the human tracheobronchial tree. Clin Sci 1980; 59: 79.

43. Mossburg M. The immotile cilia syndrome: ultrastructurally heterogeneous and clinically homogeneous. Eur J Respir Dis 1985; 65: 161.

44. Pavia D, Agnew JE, Bateman JRM et al. Lung mucociliary clearance in patients with Young's syndrome. Chest 1981; 80: 892.

45. Pavia D. Effects of pharmacologic agents on the clearance of airway secretions. Semin Respir Med 1984; 5: 345.

46. Shak S, Capon DJ, Hellmiss R et al. Recombinant human DNase I reduces the viscosity of cystic fibrosis sputum. Proc Natl Acad Sci USA 1990; 87: 9188–9192.

47. Dasgupta B, Tomkiewicz RP, Boyd WA et al. Effects of combined treatment with rhDNase and airflow oscillations on spinnability of cystic fibrosis sputum in vitro. Pediatr Pulmonol 1995; 20: 78–82.

48. Dasgupta B, King M. Reduction in viscoelasticity in cystic fibrosis sputum in vitro using combined treatment with nacystelyn and rhDNase. Pediatr Pulmonol 1996; 22: 161–166.

49. Vasconcellos CA, Allen PG, Wohl ME et al. Reduction in viscosity of cystic fibrosis sputum in vitro by gelsolin. Science 1994; 263: 969–971.

50. Wills PJ, Hall RL, Chan W, Cole PJ. Sodium chloride increases the ciliary transportability of cystic fibrosis and bronchiectasis sputum on the mucus-depleted bovine trachea. J Clin Invest 1997; 99: 9–13.

51. Tomkiewicz RP, App EM, Zayas JG et al. Amiloride inhalation therapy in cystic fibrosis. Influence on ion content, hydration, and rheology of sputum. Am Rev Respir Dis 1993; 148: 1002–1007.

52. King M, Dasgupta B, Tomkiewicz RP, Brown NE. Rheology of cystic fibrosis sputum after in vitro treatment with hypertonic saline alone and in combination with recombinant human deoxyribonuclease. Am J Respir Crit Care Med 1997; 156: 173–177.

53. Pavia D, Thompson ML, Clarke SW. Enhanced clearance of secretions from the human lung after the administration of hypertonic saline aerosol. Am Rev Respir Dis 1978; 117: 199.

54. Feng W, Garrett H, Speert DP, King M. Improved clearability of cystic fibrosis sputum with dextran treatment in vitro. Am J Respir Crit Care Med 1998; 57: 710–714.

55. Agnew JE, Bateman JRM, Sheahan NF et al. Effect of oral corticosteroids on mucus clearance by cough and mucociliary transport in stable asthma. Bull Eur Physiopathol Respir 1983; 19: 37.

56. Taylor RG, Pavia D, Agnew JE et al. Effects of four weeks' high dose ipratropium bromide treatment on lung mucociliary clearance. Thorax 1986; 41: 295.

57. Leith DE. Cough. In: Brain JD, Proctor DF, Reid LM, ed. Respiratory defense mechanisms, Part II. New York: Marcel Dekker, 1977; 545.

58. Weibel ER. The pathway of oxygen. Structure and function in the mammalian respiratory system. Cambridge, MA: Harvard University Press; 1984.

59. Clarke SW, Jones JG, Oliver DR. Resistance to two-phase gas-liquid flow in airways. J Appl Physiol 1970; 29: 464.

60. Scherer PW. Mucus transport by cough. Chest 1981; 805: 830.

61. King M, Zahm JM, Pierrot D et al. The role of mucus gel viscosity, spinnability, and adhesive properties in clearance by simulated cough. Biorheology 1989; 26: 737.

62. Harris RS, Lawson TV. The relative mechanical effectiveness and efficiency of successive voluntary coughs in healthy young adults. Clin Sci 1968; 34: 569.

63. Cochrane GM, Webber BA, Clarke SW. Effects of sputum on pulmonary function. Br Med J 1977; 2: 1180.

64. Puchelle E, Zahm JM, Girard F et al. Relationships to sputum properties in chronic bronchitis. Eur J Respir Dis 1980; 61: 254.

65. Sutton PP. Chest physiotherapy: time for reappraisal. Br J Dis Chest 1988; 82: 127.

66. Barrowcliffe MP, Jones JG. Solute permeability of the alveolar capillary barrier. Thorax 1987; 42: 1.

67. Staehelin LA, Hull BE. Junctions between living cells. Sci Am 1978; 238: 140.

68. Jones JG. Clearance of inhaled particles from the alveoli. In: Clarke SW, Pavia D, ed. Aerosols and the lung. London: Butterworths; 1984: 170.

69. Barrowcliffe MP, Jones JG. Agnew JE et al. The relative permeabilities of human conducting and terminal airways to ^{99m}TcDTPA. Eur J Respir Dis 1987; 71(suppl 153): 68.

70. Bailey MR, Fry FA, James AC. The long term clearance kinetics of insoluble particles from the human lung. Ann Occup Hyg 1982; 26: 273–290.

71. Bohning DE, Atkins HL, Cohn SH. Long-term particle clearance in man: normal and impaired. Ann Occup Hyg 1982; 26: 259–271.

72. Lauweryns JM, Baert JH. Alveolar clearance and the role of the pulmonary lymphatics. Am Rev Respir Dis 1977; 115: 625.

73. Meyer EC, Dominsuez EA, Bensch KG. Pulmonary lymphatic and blood absorption of albumin from alveoli. A comparison. Lab Invest 1969; 20: 1.

74. Mason RJ. Surfactant synthesis, secretion and function on alveoli and small airways. Respiration 1987; 51(suppl): 3.

75. Bateman JRM, Pavia D, Sheahan NF et al. Impaired tracheobronchial clearance in patients with mild stable asthma. Thorax 1983; 38: 463.

3.2 Defence properties of airway surface liquid

Edith Puchelle, Sophie de Bentzmann, Jean-Marie Zahm and Jacky Jacquot

Key points

- Airway surface liquid contains critical molecules of the innate airway defence that are required to maintain sterility of the airways by exerting antimicrobial activities

- The volume and composition of the airway surface liquid are mainly determined by active Na^+ and/or Cl^- ion transport and by passive water permeability through the respiratory epithelium

- The integrity of the fluid balance controls the efficacy of mucociliary transport by maintaining the optimal physical properties of the airway surface liquid

- The airway surface liquid may regulate inflammation of the airway

During breathing of ambient air, the airways are exposed to a multitude of potential pathogens and pollutants. The concentration of airborne organisms can vary from 10^3 to $10^7/m^3$ according to the environmental milieu, which represents a major infective risk. Airway defences against inhaled bacteria include physical barriers and a diversity of biochemical defence molecules.

Airway surface liquid (ASL) contains critical molecules of the innate airway defence required to maintain sterility of the airways. All along the respiratory tract, the integrity of fluid balance and optimal physical properties of the airway secretions allow the mucociliary transport of inhaled particles and the maintenance of a protective interface between the external environment and the underlying cells.

This chapter will consider the origin of ASL, the techniques allowing its collection, the ion composition, regulation and biochemical and related physical properties of ASL. We will also describe the innate defence molecules of ASL. They include enzymes, peptides, antioxidants and antiproteases, which exert antimicrobial activities via direct mechanisms or by facilitating interactions between phagocytes and pathogens. We will also consider molecules released by the airway epithelial cells, which can regulate the immune inflammatory response.

Origin

Airway surface liquid covering the mucociliary epithelium is generally described as a biphasic layer subdivided into a periciliary 'sol' layer surrounding the cilia and a more superficial 'gel' layer. The thickness of the sol layer is about the same as the length of the cilia (7 μm), whereas the overlying gel layer has a thickness ranging between 0.5 μm and 50 μm. This two-phase layer, originally proposed by Lucas and Douglas,[1] has been revealed by electron microscopic observation in rapidly frozen samples.[2] The ASL is 25–50 times thinner (0.2–2 μm) in the distal airways than in the proximal airways. The continuity of the gel layer in these distal airways is debated. Under transmission electron microscopy, the periciliary sol layer where the cilia beat is electron-lucent whereas the gel layer is electron-dense and is mainly composed of high-molecular-weight mucous glycoproteins. The normal volume of tracheobronchial secretions is estimated to range from 10 ml to 100 ml per day.

The ASL is a mixture of water, ions, proteins, lipids and mucous glycoproteins. Several secretory cell types contribute to ASL, including:

- mucous goblet cells in the surface epithelium and submucosal glands
- serous cells in submucosal glands in human adults
- the ciliated cells along the surface epithelium of the upper (nose), proximal (bronchi) and lower (bronchioles) airways
- the brush border cells, mainly in the upper airways.

The gel phase of ASL is mainly composed of mucins and proteins, which are secreted by surface mucous cells and submucosal glandular cells (mucous, serous and mixed mucous/serous). Submucous glandular cells outnumber goblet cells by a ratio of 40:1 in the normal tracheobronchial tree.

The ASL secreted by the glands reaches the luminal surface of the airways by a series of ducts. The mucin (MUC) products of ASL originate from mucous goblet cells in the surface epithelium and from mucous and serous cells in the submucosal glands. Among the nine human MUC genes and MUC products, seven are expressed in the upper (nasal) and lower (bronchial) respiratory tract tissue. There is a cell-specific expression of MUC genes along the tracheobronchial tree.[3] The secretions are packed inside intracellular secretory granules ranging in size from 100 nm to 1800 nm. The serous cells of human glands, contrary to their initial definition (which refers to cells containing serum proteins), secrete most of the locally synthesised antibacterial, antiprotease and antioxidant molecules contained in the ASL (lysozyme, lactoferrin, secretory leukocyte protease inhibitor, peroxidase) but also show a strong reaction to mucins, especially sulphated mucins. These cells are frequently referred to as seromucous, because of their apparently large carbohydrate content.

Although these cells represent the main source of nasal and tracheobronchial ASL, ciliated cells and brush border cells are also involved in the secretion of ions and water. The brush border cells, identified by their microvilli, are mainly located at the upper nasal level or can be observed during the process of airway epithelium maturation and differentiation and play an important role in the regulation and homeostasis of the periciliary layer.

Ion and water transport is regulated through the cystic fibrosis transmembrane conductance regulator (CFTR) protein, located at the apical domain of ciliated cells and serous glandular cells. Apart from their mechanical role in mucociliary transport, the ciliated cells produce glycoconjugates and transport them to the surface. The ciliated cell therefore represents the most efficient cell in airway defence, since it is capable of regulating the water content of ASL, secreting glycoconjugates and maintaining sterility of the airways by ciliary beating (Table 3.2.1). The columnar epithelial cells of the collecting duct may also contribute to regulation of the ion and water concentration of the ASL.

The Clara cell in the distal airways is characterised by discrete electron-dense granules and secretes a bronchiolar lining fluid that contains CC10 protein as well as surfactant apoproteins (SP-A and SP-B).

Table 3.2.1 Main functional properties of airway surface liquid

- Physical barrier to inhaled pathogens, pollutants and irritants
- Recognition and entrapment of inhaled pathogens then transported by mucociliary activity
- Provision of a 'waterproof' layer protecting the airway epithelium from dehydration
- Humidification of inspired gas
- Rheological properties optimal to mucous transport by mucociliary activity and coughing
- Antibacterial, antioxidant and antiprotease defence of the airways
- pH buffering capacity
- Regulation of airway inflammation

Some major questions asked by Widdicombe and Widdicombe[4] have not as yet been answered: to what extent do the volume and the composition of the ASL vary during their progression along the respiratory tract? What is the total output of ASL at the larynx and the contribution of the different cells? In particular, what is the respective contribution of surface epithelial cells and glandular cells to the water content of the ASL?

Collection methods

In many disease situations characterised by hypersecretion, particularly in cystic fibrosis (CF), it is of importance to evaluate the rheological, biochemical and antibacterial properties of well-collected samples of ASL. Whereas the ASL can be easily collected in hypersecreting patients, it is more difficult to collect in healthy control subjects. In humans, ASL can be collected by both non-invasive and invasive methods. Recently developed humanised animal models are powerful tools for studying the diverse properties of ASL with some advantages over the many animals previously used.

Methods in humans

Non-invasive

Spontaneous expectoration after coughing is the simplest way to collect ASL. However, these secretions may be contaminated by salivary secretions, thereby significantly altering the ASL analysis. An alternative is to perform protected expectoration associated with physiotherapy. Dental cotton-wool swabs are used to absorb saliva thus minimising salivary contamination.[5] Before the swabs are placed, the patients are prepared to expectorate with the help of a physiotherapist, who controls the quality of the expectoration.

Over the past few years, sputum induction has been developed to assess airway inflammation. Holz et al[6] have recently reviewed this technique. In most of the studies, hypertonic saline (3–5%) is aerosolised; isotonic saline is better tolerated in patients with severe asthma and is often sufficient to induce sputum. The samples collected are mainly used for analysing cellular sputum composition, identifying cellular subtypes and cellular activation. The potential application of this technique to full analysis of sputum composition needs to be determined.

Invasive

The upper airways, specifically the nasal epithelium, share many properties with the lower airways and are easily accessible. Therefore, the collection of nasal ASL is attractive for repetitive analysis. It may be collected by nasopharyngeal aspiration or by instilling saline into the nasal cavity. Secretions can also be collected via absorption by cotton strips, filter paper, rubber foam samplers[7] or after gently scraping the nasal mucosa with a blunt curette[8].

In intubated patients, ASL can be collected by aspiration through the endotracheal tube. The material is collected into a tube connected to the suction apparatus. ASL coating the endotracheal tube during short surgical procedures in patients with no clinical evidence of respiratory disease can also be analysed.[9] Large bronchofibrescopes have a 2–2.6 mm inner channel through which one can collect ASL samples either by aspiration or by using different tools such as a cytology brush or filter paper.

The filter paper technique has been used to collect ASL for ion concentration determination.[10] A small sealed Teflon catheter containing a small strip of ashless filter paper is passed through the suction channel; the tip of the filter is then extended out of the catheter and, under visual inspection, briefly touches the mucosa (less than 5 s), enabling the paper to become wetted with ASL by capillary action. The paper is thereafter drawn up into the catheter, removed from the bronchofibrescope, immersed in water-saturated mineral oil and stored at –20°C until analysis.

A cytological brush technique has been developed to collect and measure the viscoelastic properties of ASL.[11] The brush is introduced into the channel of a bronchofibroscope placed in the trachea and left in contact with the bronchial mucosa for 20–30 s to allow ASL to be collected. The brush is then withdrawn and the ASL sample is scraped from the brush and immediately covered with paraffin oil.

These collection techniques do not allow collection of large volumes of samples, which limits the range of possible analysis.

Methods in animals

Many laboratory animals have been used to collect ASL under physiological conditions, either in vivo or ex vivo.

In-vivo techniques

Acute ASL collection often requires the laboratory animal to be anaesthetised. The method of Perry and Boyd[12] has been extensively used and modified. A T-cannula is inserted into the trachea half opened along the cartilage and connected to a collection tube.

In intubated dogs, it is possible to collect ASL accumulating at the outer part of an endotracheal tube.[13] A similar technique has also been adapted for small animals such as mice:[14] a small polyethylene catheter is introduced through a tracheotomy retrogradely toward the larynx. The catheter is left in place for 1.5 h and the ASL adhering to the catheter is thereafter scraped off for analysis. Collection with a cytological brush through a bronchofibroscope has also been used for studying the physical properties of ASL.[11]

For rats or mice, a sampling technique has been developed by Cowley et al.[15] Submicrolitre volumes of ASL are collected in a sampling capillary, which is passed through the intubation tubing left in the trachea for a period of 2 min before being pulled out. The composition of the ASL is then determined by capillary electrophoresis.

A cryotechnique to collect ASL for X-ray microanalysis, using a cryoprobe adapted to the internal curvature of the longitudinally open mouse trachea, has been recently developed.[16] The cryoprobe is cooled in liquid nitrogen and placed at controlled pressure for 15 s on the trachea, allowing the collection of ASL without damaging the surface epithelium. In these sampling conditions, native ASL can be collected without contamination by cellular debris or secretion induced by mechanical stimulation.

Ex-vivo techniques

This method consists of mounting the whole trachea of a ferret, laryngeal end downward, in an organ bath. The trachea remains air-filled and undiluted mucus can be collected over a 15–30 min period.[17]

Methods in humanised animal models

A model of human fetal trachea implanted under the skin of severe combined immunodeficiency (SCID) mice allows full histological maturation from immature human fetal tracheas.[16] These human fetal tracheal xenografts can be maintained for several months and ASL accumulating within the xenograft can be easily collected by micropipetting. Another xenograft model in immunodeficient nude mice is extensively used to perform studies on fully differentiated airway epithelium.[18,19] Rat tracheas denuded of their surface epithelium by repeated cycles of freezing and thawing are seeded with adult airway epithelial cells (from animal or human origin) and subcutaneously implanted in nude mice. The connection of polyethylene tubes at both sides of the grafted trachea allows repeated collection of ASL.

Method of collection from specific sources

Most of the mucus overlying the airway epithelium originates from submucosal glands. A method based on the use of a micropipette, either in vivo or in vitro, allows ASL collection from this specific source.[20] After anaesthetising the animal, the cervical trachea is opened and water-saturated oil is placed on the mucosal surface. Duct orifices are identified under a dissecting microscope and a glass micropipette is adjusted by a micromanipulator so that its tip surrounds the orifice. The glandular secretion is withdrawn for 1–10 min under negative pressure. An alternative is to remove the trachea from the animal and to mount a portion in a chamber, bathing the under surface in physiological solution and collecting ASL by micropipette.[21]

Ion composition and regulation

The volume and composition of ASL are mainly determined by active Na^+ and/or Cl^- ion transport and the passive water permeability through the respiratory epithelium. The absorption of water keeps mucus in close contact with the cilia.[22] Directional transport of ions requires the presence of different proteins in the apical and basolateral membranes. On the apical (luminal) membrane, there is a predominant Cl^- channel, a Na^+ channel and a K^+ channel with a negligible conductance. The airway basolateral membrane, which is K^+-selective, contains the Na^+/K^+-ATPase and $Na^+/K^+/2Cl^-$ co-transporters. The absorption of Na^+ occurs in a two-step process: Na^+ enters the cell down an electrochemical gradient through a selective apical Na$^+$ channel and is removed from the cell by the basolateral Na$^+$/K$^+$-ATPase (Fig. 3.2.1). Philips et al[24] suggest that the hydration of the periciliary fluid layer in tracheal epithelium is mainly regulated by luminal-to-basolateral water transport coupled to active transepithelial sodium transport via the active Na$^+$,K$^+$-ATPase pump. The accompanying absorptive movement of Cl$^-$ and water occurs through cellular and paracellular pathways. Under resting conditions, there is no net Cl$^-$ flux in normal human airways, and active ion transport is dominated by Na$^+$ absorption from lumen to submucosa (Fig. 3.2.1).

According to Boucher et al,[25] in proximal and distal airways, active Na$^+$ absorption dominates. At alveolar level, active and passive salt transport regulates liquid movement. A driving force that regulates ASL axial flow from alveolar and distal regions to proximal airways may be related to surfactant concentrations (Fig. 3.2.2).

However, as a result of the relative inaccessibility and small volume of ASL, its ion composition in healthy subjects is still debated. In human lung tissues, the highest levels of CFTR protein are observed in serous cells of airway submucosal glands.[26,27] Animal and cell culture models of the serous gland cell-type have indicated that CFTR protein is critical for glandular fluid secretion driven by Cl$^-$ and HCO$_3^-$.[28,29] It is suggested that bicarbonate secretion stimulated by cyclic adenosine monophosphate (cAMP) is mediated by the apical membrane exit of bicarbonate via CFTR and that the influx of bicarbonate across the basolateral membrane is mediated by a disulphonic stilbene-sensitive electrogenic sodium bicarbonate cotransporter. Studies on nasal epithelial cells revealed that there is a small net secretory driving force for bicarbonate in non-CF cells compared to a net absorptive driving force for bicarbonate in CF cells.[23]

Other data suggest that impaired Cl$^-$ secretion and increased Na$^+$ absorption in CF airway epithelia impair mucociliary clearance,[30] thereby making the CF airways susceptible to infection. Pharmacological modulation of ion transport across CF bronchial epithelia, using benzimidizalones, psoralens or isoflavones, restores transepithelial Cl$^-$ secretion.[31] By restoring Cl$^-$ permeability, these compounds may increase ASL volume and thereby improve mucociliary transport. A direct coupling exists between the level of cellular adenosine 5′ triphosphate (ATP) and Cl$^-$ channel activity.

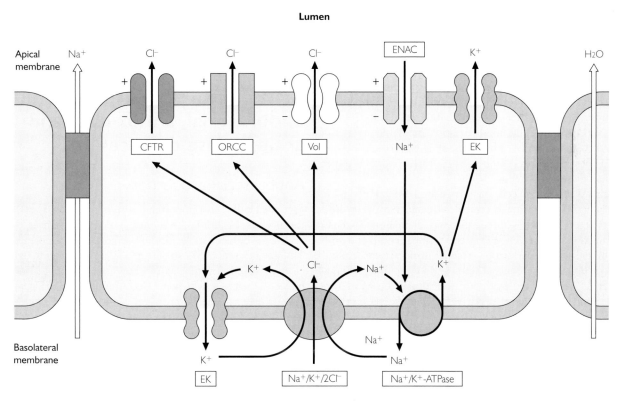

Fig. 3.2.1 The volume and composition of airway surface liquid is mainly determined by active ion transport (driven by Na$^+$ and/or Cl$^-$ transport) and the passive permeability of the respiratory epithelium to water. The absorption of water by the epithelium keeps mucus in close contact with the cilia.[23] Directional transport of ions by the airway epithelium requires the presence of different proteins in the apical and basolateral membranes. On the apical (luminal) membrane, there is a predominant Cl$^-$ channel, a Na$^+$ channel and a K$^+$ channel with negligible conductance. The airway basolateral membrane. which is K$^+$-selective, contains the Na$^+$/K$^+$-ATPase and Na$^+$/K$^+$/2Cl co-transporters. The absorption of Na occurs in a two-step process: Na$^+$ enters the cell down an electrochemical gradient through a selective apical Na$^+$ channel and is removed from the cell by the basolateral Na$^+$/K$^+$-ATPase. CFTR, cystic fibrosis transmembrane conductance regulator; EK, Epithelial potassium channel; ENAC, Epithelial sodium channel; ORCC, Outwardly rectifying chloride channel; Vol, Volume - regulated chloride channel.

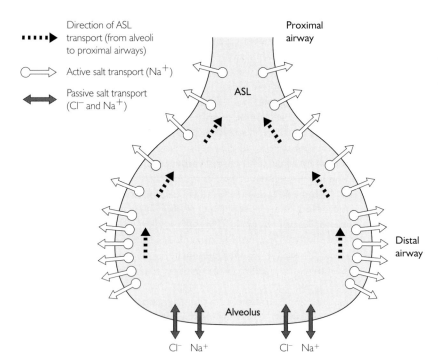

Direction of ASL
transport (from alveoli
to proximal airways)

Active salt transport (Na$^+$)

Passive salt transport
(Cl$^-$ and Na$^+$)

Proximal
airway

ASL

Distal
airway

Alveolus

Cl$^-$ Na$^+$ Cl$^-$ Na$^+$

Fig. 3.2.2   In proximal and distal airways, active Na$^+$ absorption dominates. At alveolar level, active and passive salt transport regulates liquid movement. A driving airway surface liquid (ASL) axial flow from alveolar to distal and proximal airways may be related to surfactant concentrations. (Redrawn with permission from Boucher et al.[25])

Extracellular ATP and uridine 5′ triphosphate (UTP) are highly effective secretagogues in human airway epithelium in vivo through interaction with a subclass of nucleotide receptors.[32] The addition of ATP or UTP increases Cl$^-$ secretion and, in parallel, luminal fluid transport, which may be particularly useful in the hydration of mucus.[33] Also, the activation of ciliary motility by ATP can be attenuated by elevated extracellular Na$^+$ content. This modulation is mediated by a P2X receptor.[34] Consequently, inhalation of a hypertonic aerosol that does not contain Na$^+$ could improve mucociliary clearance better than hypertonic saline.

The airway epithelial cells are innervated from a plexus of axons deriving from both the sympathetic and the parasympathetic ganglia.[35] α- and β-adrenergic and cholinergic agonists both stimulate gland secretion, but the result is completely different. β-adrenergic stimulation results in secretions characterised by a high protein concentration and low volume, whereas α-adrenergic stimulation leads to the opposite. Moreover, adrenergic and cholinergic stimulation of gland secretion result in a different pattern of rheological properties.[36] Activation of capsaicin-sensitive sensory nerves induces mucus secretion in human bronchi, substance P being the neurotransmitter. Neuropeptides such as neuropeptide Y and vasoactive intestinal peptide (VIP) are also involved in the regulation of airway secretions. In chronic airway inflammatory diseases such as asthma, chronic bronchitis and CF, a number of locally produced inflammatory mediators, including cyclo-oxygenase products (prostaglandins A$_2$, D$_2$, F$_2$, E$_2$ and their intermediates) and the lipoxygenase products (leukotriene C$_4$, D$_4$, mono-hydroxy-eicosapentaenoic acid), stimulate Cl$^-$ and fluid secretion. Furthermore, the proinflammatory cytokines, interferon-γ (IFN-γ) and tumour necrosis factor-α (TNF-α) can modulate transepithelial ion transport. Human bronchial epithelial cells show an amiloride-sensitive fluid absorption that is inhibited by

IFN-γ but not by TNF-α.[37] The role of ASL in chronic lung disease needs further study.

Biochemical properties: antibacterial, antioxidant and antiprotease defences

Antibacterial properties

Epithelial cells form important barriers to bacterial pathogens in the airways. In addition to serving as a physical barrier, these cells synthesise defence molecules to overcome pathogenic intruders.[38] The gel layer of ASL, mainly made up of mucins, is the first barrier: respiratory mucins represent a large population of high molecular mass, polydisperse glycoproteins exhibiting a considerable diversity at the peptide and at the carbohydrate level. This diversity of O-glycans represents a mosaic of carbohydrate determinants, which are particularly useful in binding inhaled bacteria or viruses. There is a plethora of potential sites in human mucins that can serve as receptors for bacteria. Although mucins cannot be considered as antibacterial components per se, their capacity to bind bacteria and facilitate their clearance allow them to be considered as an important partner in the antibacterial properties of ASL.[39] Antibacterial proteins and peptides are the main means by which bacteria are killed. They include lysozyme, lactoferrin, secretory phospholipase A$_2$, secretory leukoprotease inhibitor and lactoperoxidase (Fig. 3.2.3). Other substances, such as IgA, complement, surfactant proteins (also called collectins) and Clara-cell proteins, also contribute to host defence.

The most abundant airway antimicrobial factors are lysozyme, lactoferrin and secretory leukocyte protease inhibitor (SLPI),

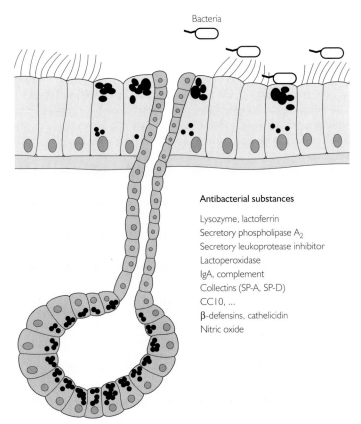

Bacteria

Antibacterial substances

Lysozyme, lactoferrin
Secretory phospholipase A$_2$
Secretory leukoprotease inhibitor
Lactoperoxidase
IgA, complement
Collectins (SP-A, SP-D)
CC10, ...
β-defensins, cathelicidin
Nitric oxide

Fig. 3.2.3 Schematic representation of secreted antimicrobial substances and immunomodulatory mediators involved in host defence mechanisms of human respiratory epithelium.

which are produced by serous cells of airway glands. Other bactericidal molecules include β-defensin and cathelicidin peptides.[40] These peptides act by inducing rapid microbial membrane permeabilisation.[41] Their concentration in ASL is not precisely known – levels are about 1000-fold lower than those of lysozyme.[42] These defensins are cationic cysteine-rich peptides exhibiting broad antimicrobial activity. Synergistic antibacterial activity against *Staphylococcus aureus* has been reported between lysozyme and lactoferrin[40] and changes in the NaCl concentrations of ASL modulate their bactericidal efficacy. It has been proposed that the defect in *CFTR* results in elevated salt concentration, which could be responsible for the particular sensitivity to bacterial infection that is a feature of CF lung disease.

Many other proteins and enzymes may contribute to airway defence, and lysozyme and lactoferrin are the most abundant. They are bactericidal alone for Gram-positive bacteria and in combination for some Gram-negative bacteria.[43] Other potential contributors to the total microbicidal activity of ASL include secretory phospholipase A$_2$, which has Ca^{2+}-dependent antimicrobial activity against both Gram-positive and Gram-negative bacteria.

Human milk lactoferrin, which is structurally very close to human airway lactoferrin, attenuates the pathogenic potential of *Haemophilus influenzae* by selectively inactivating its IgA1 protease and adhesins.[44]

Lactoperoxidase uses hydrogen to oxidise thiocyanate in airway secretions and is active against Gram-positive and Gram-negative bacteria as well as against viruses and fungi.[45] Its inhibition leads to decreased ability to clear inspired bacteria,[46] suggesting significant implications for the chronic airway colonisation seen in respiratory diseases such as CF.

Recently, a wide variety of potential antibacterial defence functions have been reported for surfactant proteins A and D, also called lung collectins.[47] These are structurally homologous members of a family of collagenous, calcium-dependent lectins. They are synthesised by airway epithelial cells lining the larger airways and glands and by bronchiolar and alveolar epithelial cells. The interactions of collectins with bacteria involve binding of microbial lectins. Surfactant protein-A-null transgenic mice[48] demonstrate increased proliferation and decreased phagocytosis of streptococci as well as decreased clearance of *S. aureus* and *Pseudomonas aeruginosa* after tracheal inoculation.

Nitric oxide (NO) is a multifunctional molecule that, at low concentration, has not only an anti-inflammatory activity but is also able to increase ciliary beat frequency[49] and to exert antibacterial properties. Reduced NO production in epithelial cells of CF patients could contribute to their susceptibility to bacterial infection.[50]

Antioxidant properties

The inhalation of allergens, pollutants and microorganisms induces an inflammatory reaction of the airway epithelium, which responds by increasing production of reactive oxygen and nitrogen species. As inflammation in the airways increases, additional infiltrating cells increase the level of these products.[51]

Extracellular glutathione peroxidase is synthesised by airway epithelium and alveolar macrophages and functions as a first line of defence against inhaled reactive oxygen species.[52] NO potentiates the response by reacting with O$_2$ and producing OH radicals.

Glutathione (GSH) is a tripeptide containing a thiol group, and has been shown to be critical to lung antioxidant defence in protecting epithelium from oxidative/free-radical-mediated injury and inflammation.[53] Levels of GSH are decreased in the ASL in idiopathic pulmonary fibrosis[54] and in CF.[55] A low concentration of GSH in the ASL may contribute to an imbalance between oxidants and antioxidants and induce an increased inflammatory response so facilitate airway and lung damage.

The nasal mucosal surface is potentially subjected to a variety of oxidant stresses. Cholinergically induced secretions from the nasal submucosal gland contain a low-molecular-weight antioxidant, uric acid, which has antioxidant activity at concentrations higher than 1.5 μmol/l.[56] The secretion of uric acid correlates closely with the secretion of lactoferrin, suggesting that submucosal glands are involved.[57]

Antiprotease activity

Proteinase inhibitors regulate the extracellular action of proteinases such as leukocyte elastase, which is responsible for airway and lung degradation. They include α$_1$-proteinase inhibitor, which is produced in the liver and reaches the lung by passive diffusion.

The two locally produced proteinase inhibitors are SLPI, also known as antileukoprotease, and elafin.[58] SLPI is produced by serous submucosal glands and by Clara cells and goblet cells. The wide airway distribution of the SLPI suggests that this proteinase inhibitor maintains proteinase–antiproteinase balance in the proximal as well as in the lower airways. Furthermore, SLPI has antibacterial properties against *Escherichia coli* and *S. aureus*, which suggests that it contributes to the host defences against both airway degradation and infection.[59]

Physical properties

Main physical properties

It is difficult to define precisely the biochemical and physical properties of 'normal' ASL because of sampling problems (see above). Therefore, most studies of the rheological, physical and biochemical properties of ASL (including the gel and the sol phases of mucus) are carried out on sputum samples.

Although extrapolation from pathological to normal ASL remains questionable, the large quantities of pathological mucus available can be used to analyse the relationship between physical and biochemical properties.

Different biochemical components are involved in the gel-like properties of airway secretions, where proteins, glycoproteins, proteoglycans and lipids are bound to ions and water (Table 3.2.2). Glycoprotein–protein interactions play a major role in the rheological properties of airway mucus.[60]

Airway surface liquid possesses both flow and deformation (viscoelasticity) properties, characterised by non-linear (non-newtonian viscosity) and time-dependent flow (thixotropy), and surface properties, such as adhesiveness and wettability. These

Table 3.2.2 Relationships between rheological, physical, biochemical and functional properties of airway surface liquid

	Rheological and physical properties	Biochemical components	Functional properties
Rheological properties	Viscoelasticity	Mucins	Airway epithelium
	Thixotropy	Proteins Lipids Ions Water	Hydration Mucociliary and cough transport
	Spinnability	Mucins Proteoglycans Proteins Water	Filtration barrier Mucociliary and cough transport
Physical surface properties	Wettability	Mucins Phospholipids	Hydrophobic barrier Lubrication Mucociliary and cough transport

physical characteristics, which are independent of the viscoelastic properties, determine the capacity of the mucous gel layer to protect, hydrate and lubricate the underlying airway epithelium and, therefore, are probably at least as important as the rheological properties. The gel phase of ASL is a highly non-newtonian viscoelastic material. Under a discontinuous stress, induced by ciliary motion during active ciliary beating or by coughing, the mucus instantaneously deforms and, once the stress is removed, relaxes. Using biopolymers to simulate normal and pathological respiratory mucus, it has been demonstrated that intermediate viscoelastic properties represent an optimal rheological profile for transport of mucus.[61] Adhesivity and wettability contribute markedly to the optimal interface properties between the gel and sol phases of ASL, and therefore contribute directly to the efficiency of ciliary and cough clearance.[62] Wettability characterises the capacity of a fluid or gel-like airway mucus to spread on a solid surface. The interface properties of airway secretions can be analysed in terms of work of adhesion.[63]

Close and significant correlations have been shown between mucin content and the viscoelasticity of airway mucus. Secretory proteins such as IgA and lysozyme are also directly involved in its viscoelastic properties.[64]

Other proteins such as lactoferrin, IgG and IgM may also interfere in the gel network formation of mucus. Mucins concentrated in the gel layer of airway secretions directly interfere with their surface-active properties. It is probable that their association with phospholipids reinforces the surface-active properties of mucus.

The water content, ionic concentration and pH of airway secretions may alter the rheological properties by interfering with the degree of cross-linking of macromolecules. Although lipids make up only 1–2% of the macromolecules in ASL, their contribution to the rheological properties of mucus is unclear. Girod et al[65] have identified phospholipids in the serous and mucous secretory granules of the submucosal glands as well as on the glycocalyx of the microvilli of epithelial cells. These data suggest that the airway mucosa is coated by a layer of phospholipids, which, in association with mucins, may simultaneously lubricate and isolate the epithelium from aggressive agents.

Physical properties in disease

Changes in the physical properties of ASL occur in numerous inflammatory airway diseases and in genetic disorders such as CF.

It has been shown that no significant differences in ion composition, water content and viscoelastic properties exist in ASL collected in a human xenograft model of CF.[16] Other authors demonstrated that, in the absence of infection, increased sulphation of CF glycoproteins contributed per se to abnormal viscoelastic properties[66] in a humanised bronchial epithelial xenograft model and could explain the decrease in mucociliary clearance seen in CF mice compared with control mice raised in pathogen-free conditions.[67] From these results, it is not clear whether the biochemical composition and physical properties of ASL are directly controlled by functional CFTR prior to infection or inflammation. However there is a strong relationship between water content, ion content and viscoelastic properties, and improvement in the viscoelasticity of the tracheal mucus in mice treated with chloride-channel agonists.[68] Altered ionic composition of the ASL could by itself induce changes in the viscoelastic properties[69] and surface properties of ASL.[63]

Acute infectious and inflammatory episodes can contribute to alterations in biochemical physical properties of ASL. In addition to their deleterious action on the structure of the ciliated epithelium, bacterial toxins, in particular those of *P. aeruginosa*, modify epithelial function,[70] either by altering the junctional barrier or by reducing the transcellular flux of Cl⁻. Pneumococcal infection also increases the absorption of Na⁺ and thereby contributes to both the dehydration of the airway mucosa and the hyperviscosity of the mucus.[71] This link between inflammation, infection and ASL is illustrated in the study of Deneuville et al,[72] who showed in a well-documented cohort of CF patients that the *P. aeruginosa* and sputum leukocyte counts were negatively correlated with sputum water content and cough transport.

In chronic airway inflammatory diseases such as CF, chronic bronchitis and asthma, the biochemical composition of airway secretions undergoes marked changes. Mucus hypersecretion is generally accompanied by an increase in serum protein transudate, with a high glycoprotein, protein, proteoglycan and lipid content in association with DNA. During infection, the increase in macromolecule secretion results in a 5–10-fold increase in the dry weight of mucus.[73] These biochemical abnormalities cause marked hyperviscosity, associated with an increase in the adhesiveness and a lowering of wettability. Such a rheological profile is inefficient for mucociliary and cough transport. In CF, it has been shown that there is an imbalance between the surface-active phospholipid fractions such as phosphatidylcholine and phosphatidylglycerol, which are decreased, and rigidifying fractions such as phosphatidylethanolamine and sphingomyelin, which are increased.[74] A parallel increase in cholesterol and glycolipids is responsible for the marked adhesiveness of CF purulent mucus. The increase in glycolipids represents an early marker of irritation[62] and a possible role for lipid–glycoprotein association has been suggested in the formation of airway mucus plugs in cases of status asthmaticus.

Regulation of inflammation by airway surface liquid

Airway epithelial cells play a major role in the lung defence as a mechanical barrier and by mucociliary transport, actively participate in airway mucosal immunity[75,76] and are capable of responding to a wide array of agents including viruses, adherent and invasive bacteria and active lipid. In response to these exogenous agents, airway epithelial cells produce pro- and anti-inflammatory cytokines, particularly chemokines, NO and inflammatory lipid mediators which influence the adjacent immune and mesenchymal mucosal cells by recruiting circulating leukocytes to the airway mucosa (Fig. 3.2.4). In turn, pro-inflammatory molecules such as TNF-α, interleukin (IL)-1β and IFN-γ, produced by recruited inflammatory and immune cells, reciprocally stimulate adjacent airway epithelial cells.[77]

In human airways, the innate immune system has both a recognition function, which detects bacterial products in tissues,

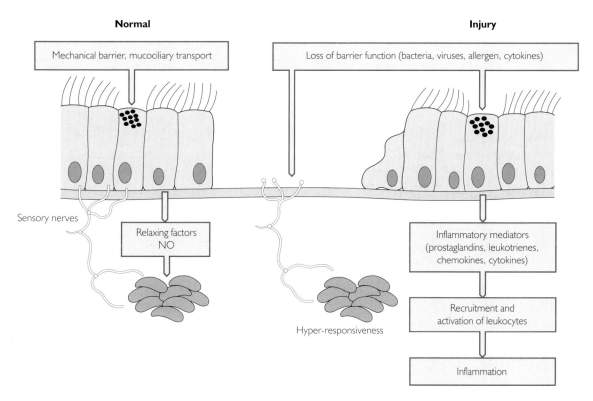

Fig. 3.2.4   Role of normal and injured airway epithelium on modulating airway responsiveness and inflammatory mediators release. NO, nitric oxide. (Redrawn with permission from Van der Velden et al.[76])

and an effector function, which attracts phagocytic leukocytes to sites of bacterial entry into tissues. Bacteria are recognised by surface receptors such as CD14 and toll-like receptors,[78] which include more than 10 members able to mediate responses to different types of stimulus.[79] Toll-like receptor 2 mediates macrophage responses to yeast, mycobacteria and Gram-positive bacteria, whereas toll-like receptor 4 facilitates recognition of Gram-negative lipopolysaccharide (LPS) endotoxin.[80] Airway epithelial cells respond to the presence of microbes and viruses by the induction of two complementary parts of the innate immune response. The first is the increased production of antimicrobial molecules and the second is the induction of a signal network to recruit phagocytic cells to contain infection. This inflammatory response is fundamental in the pathogenesis of many lung diseases, such as asthma, chronic obstructive pulmonary disease, acute respiratory distress syndrome, idiopathic pulmonary fibrosis and CF.

While much is known about the signal transduction mechanisms activating the production of inflammatory mediators by immune cells, little is understood about the production of such mediators by the airway epithelium, especially at the molecular level. Most of the molecules synthesised seem to be the result of a highly integrated complex cascade that includes transmission to the nucleus of key transcription factors such as nuclear factor (NF)-$_k$B and activator protein-1 via activation of a series of protein kinases and phosphatases.[81] The subsequent synthesis and release of chemoattractants and adhesion molecules induce neutrophil and T lymphocyte recruitment as well as their activation and thereby augment the inflammatory response and tissue damage.

The cellular site and the specific characteristics of the inflammatory responses differ in asthma, chronic obstructive pulmonary disease, acute respiratory distress syndrome and CF. Inhalation of air pollutants and particles, and/or modifications in the osmolarity of the ASL resulting from water loss and the alteration of airway temperature, are involved in the pathogenesis of exercise-induced asthma[82] and are a major cause of the lung disease in CF. Although numerous studies suggest a major role of airway epithelial cells in airway inflammation, it is still unclear whether they participate in the initiating phase of inflammation. Hyperosmotic stress is sufficient to rapidly increase IL-8 and RANTES production in airway epithelial cells at the mRNA and protein levels.[83,84] In CF patients, the genetic defect in CFTR may contribute not only to an increased propensity to pulmonary bacterial infection but also to defective regulation of the lung inflammatory response.[85] CFTR gene expression is modulated by extracellular hyperosmolarity[86] and inflammation, as evidenced by high levels of proinflammatory cytokines (IL-8, IL-1β, TNF-α) in bronchoalveolar lavage fluid from CF infants as early as 4 weeks, including some patients without any evidence of detectable infection.[85] Consistently, bronchial epithelial cells isolated from CF patients secrete more IL-8 protein and are deficient in anti-inflammatory cytokine IL-10 production compared to cells cultured from patients without CF.[87,88] In addition, human CF bronchial epithelial cells are hyper-responsive either to *P. aeruginosa*[89] or to TNF-α-dependent stimulation[86] compared to normal

and CF-corrected epithelial cell lines. In a CF mouse model, instillation of *P. aeruginosa* embedded in agar beads resulted in increased inflammation and mortality in CFTR$^{-/-}$ mice compared with similarly treated wild-type controls.[90] Using a model of naive and mature human CF fetal tracheal graft, Tirouvanziam et al[91] demonstrated that, before the first infectious episode, human CF airways are already in a proinflammatory state characterised by a highly increased chemokine IL-8 content in ASL and consistent accumulation of airway subepithelial leukocytes. In contrast, low levels of anti-inflammatory cytokine IL-10 production have been described in both the activated human CF peripheral blood T lymphocytes[92] and human bronchial epithelial cells expressing defective CFTR.[93] Whether altered regulation of pro- and anti-inflammatory genes is a primary abnormality in CF cells as a direct consequence of impaired CFTR function is unknown.

Conclusion

Airway surface liquid represents a complex mixture of secretory molecules that provide a multifaceted defence against the environment. In this chapter, we have listed all the potential host-defence molecules contained in the ASL. Although the list is long, it is certainly incomplete. Moreover all these molecules are synthesised, secreted and regulated at multiple levels in the airways. There is a wide variety of constitutively and inducible glycoproteins, proteins and peptides which are important components of the innate lung immunity. These components are synthesised mainly by airway cells but they can be also synthesised and released by parenchymal cells and resident or recruited leukocytes. By means of the mixture of active airway defence molecules, the ion and water content regulated by the airway epithelial cells and the physical properties optimal to mucociliary clearance, the ASL maintains a protective interface between the airway mucosa and the external environment.

? Unresolved questions

- How should normal human ASL be collected for analysis?

- What is the respective contribution of surface airway epithelium and submucosal glands to the water content of airway surface liquid?

- To what extent do the volume, ion and biochemical composition of airway surface liquid vary along the respiratory tract?

- Do changes in the ion composition of airway surface liquid modulate mucus production?

- What is the role of inflammatory cells in the biochemical and physical properties of airway surface liquid?

- How should the composition of airway surface liquid be pharmacologically modulated in chronic airway disease?

References

1. Lucas AM, Douglas LC. Principles underlying ciliary activity in the respiratory tract. Arch Otolaryngol 1934; 20: 518.
2. Yoneda K. Mucous blanket of rat bronchus: ultrastructural study. Am Rev Respir Dis 1976; 114: 837.
3. Rose MC, Gendler SJ. Airway mucin genes and gene products. In: Rogers DF, Lethem MI, ed. Airway mucus: basic mechanisms and clinical perspectives. Basel: Birkhäuser Verlag; 1997: 41.
4. Widdicombe JH, Widdicombe JG. Regulation of human airway surface liquid. Respir Physiol 1995; 99: 3.
5. Puchelle E, Tournier JM, Zahm JM, Sadoul P. Rheology of sputum collected by a simple technique limiting salivary contamination. J Lab Clin Med 1984; 103: 347.
6. Holz O, Kips J, Magnussen H. Update on sputum methodology. Eur Respir J 2000; 16:150.
7. Frisher T, Baraldi E. Upper airway sampling. Am J Crit Care Med 2000; 162: S28.
8. Lioté H, Zahm JM, Pierrot D, Puchelle E. Role of mucus and cilia in nasal mucociliary clearance in healthy subjects. Am Rev Respir Dis 1989; 140:132.
9. Rubin BK, Ramirez O, Zayas JG et al. Collection and analysis of respiratory mucus from subjects without lung disease. Am Rev Respir Dis 1990; 141: 1040.
10. Joris L, Dab I, Quinton PM. Elemental composition of human airway surface fluid in healthy and diseased airways. Am J Respir Dis 1993; 148: 1633.
11. Jeanneret-Grosjean A, King M, Michoud MC et al. Sampling technique and rheology of human tracheobronchial mucus. Am Rev Respir Dis 1988; 137: 707.
12. Perry WF, Boyd EM. A method for studying expectorant action in animals by direct measurement of output of respiratory tract fluids. J Pharmacol Exp Ther 1941; 73: 65.
13. Puchelle E, Zahm JM, Jacquot J, Pierrot D. Effect of air humidity on spinability and transport capacity of canine airway secretions. Biorheology 1989; 26: 315.
14. Sudo E, Lee MM, Boyd WA, King M. Effects of metacholine and uridine 5'-triphosphate on tracheal mucus rheology in mice. Am J Respir Cell Mol Biol 2000; 22: 373.
15. Cowley EA, Govindaraju K, Lloyd DK, Eidelman H. Airway surface fluid composition in the rat determined by capillary electrophoresis. Am J Physiol Lung Cell Mol Physiol 1997; 17: L895.
16. Baconnais S, Tirouvanziam R, Zahm JM et al. Ion composition and rheology of airway liquid from cystic fibrosis fetal tracheal xenografts. Am J Respir Cell Mol Biol 1999; 20: 605.
17. Robinson N, Widdicombe JG, Xie CC. In vitro collection of mucus from the ferret trachea. J Physiol 1983; 340: 7.
18. Engelhardt JF, Yankaskas JR, Wilson JM. In vivo retroviral gene transfer into human bronchial epithelia of xenografts. J Clin Invest 1992; 90: 2598.
19. Dupuit F, Gaillard D, Hinnrasky J et al. Differentiated and functional human airway epithelium regeneration in tracheal xenografts. Am J Physiol Lung Cell Mol Physiol 2000; 278: L164.
20. Ueki I, German V, Nadel JA. Direct measurement of tracheal mucous gland secretion with micropipettes in cats: Effect of cholinergic and α-adrenergic stimulation. Clin Res 1979; 27: 59A.
21. Quinton PM. Composition and control of secretions from tracheal bronchial submucosal glands. Nature 1979; 279: 551.
22. Wong LB, Yeates DB. Dynamics of the regulation of ciliated epithelial function. Comments Theor Biol 1997; 4: 183.
23. Willumsen NJ, Boucher RC. Intracellular pH and its relationship to regulation of ion transport in normal and cystic fibrosis human nasal epithelia. J Physiol 1992; 445: 247.
24. Phillips JE, Wong LB, Yeates DB. Bidirectional transepithelial water transport: measurement and governing mechanisms. Biophys J 1999; 76: 869.
25. Boucher RC. Human airway ion transport. Am J Respir Crit Care 1994; 150: 271.
26. Engelhardt JF, Yankaskas JR, Ernst SA et al. Submucosal glands are the predominant site of CFTR expression in the human bronchus. Nat Genet 1992; 2: 240.
27. Jacquot J, Puchelle E, Hinnrasky J et al. Localization of the cystic fibrosis transmembrane conductance regulator in airway secretory glands. Eur Respir J 1993; 6: 16.
28. Lee MC, Penland CM, Widdicombe JH, Wine JJ. Evidence that Calu-3 human airway cells secrete bicarbonate. Am J Physiol 1998; 274: L450.
29. Ballard ST, Trout L, Bebök Z et al. CFTR involvement in chloride, bicarbonate, and liquid secretion by airway submucosal glands. Am J Physiol 1999; 277: L694.
30. Matsui H, Grubb BR, Tarran R et al. Evidence for periciliary liquid layer depletion, not abnormal ion composition, in the pathogenesis of cystic fibrosis airways diseases. Cell1998; 95: 1005.
31. Anderson MP, Berger HA, Rich DP et al. Nucleoside triphosphates are required to open the CFTR chloride channel. Cell 1991; 67: 775.
32. Knowles MR, Clarke LL, Boucher RC. Activation by extracellular nucleotides of chloride secretion in the airway epithelium of patients with cystic fibrosis. N Engl J Med 1991; 325: 533.
33. Benali R, Pierrot D, Zahm JM et al. Effect of extracellular ATP and UTP on fluid transport by human nasal epithelial cells in culture. Am J Respir Cell Mol Biol 1994; 10: 363.
34. Ma W, Korngreen A, Uzlaner N et al. Extracellular sodium regulates airway ciliary motility by inhibiting a P2X receptor. Nature 1999; 400: 894.
35. Culp DJ, McBridge RK, Graham LA, Marin MG. α-adrenergic regulation of secretion by tracheal glands. Am J Physiol 1990; 259: L198.
36. Leikauf GD, Ueki IF, Nadel JA. Autonomic regulation of viscoelasticity of cat tracheal gland secretions. J Appl Physiol 1984; 56: 426.
37. Galietta LJ, Folli C, Marchetti C et al. Modification of transepithelial ion transport in human cultured bronchial epithelial cells by interferon-γ. Am J Physiol Lung Cell Mol Physiol 2000; 278: L1186.
38. Agerberth B, Grinewald J, Castanos-Velez E et al. Antibacterial components in bronchoalveolar lavage fluid from healthy individuals and sarcoidosis patients. Am J Respir Crit Care Med 1999; 160: 283.
39. Scharfman A, Van Brussel E, Houdret N et al. Interactions between glycoconjugates from human respiratory airways and Pseudomonas aeruginosa. Am J Respir Crit Care Med 1996; 154: S163.
40. Bals R, Goldman MJ, Wilson JM. Mouse β-defensin 1 is a salt-sensitive antimicrobial peptide present in epithelia of the lung and urogenital tract. Infect Immun 1998; 66: 1225.
41. Hancock REW. Peptide antibiotics. Lancet 1997; 349: 412.
42. Bals R, Weiner DJ, Moscioni AD et al. Augmentation of innate host defense by expression of a cathelicidin antimicrobial peptide. Infect Immun 1999; 67: 6084.
43. Ellison RT and Giehl TJ. Killing of Gram-negative bacteria by lactoferrin and lysozyme. J Clin Invest 1991; 88: 1080.
44. Qui J, Hendrixson DR, Baber EN et al. Human milk lactoferrin inactivates two putative colonization factors expressed by Haemophilus influenzae. Proc Natl Acad Sci USA 1998; 95: 12641.
45. Rather AJ, Prince A. Lactoperoxidase. New recognition of an old enzyme in airway defenses. Am J Respir Cell Mol Biol 1999; 20: 642.
46. Gerson C, Sabater J, Scuri M et al. The lactoperoxidase system functions in bacterial clearance of airways. Am J Respir Cell Mol Biol 2000; 22: 675.
47. Crouch EC. Modulation of host–bacterial interactions by collectins. Am J Respir Cell Mol Biol 1999; 21: 558.
48. Levine AM, Kurak KE, Wright JR et al. Surfactant protein-A binds group B Streptococcus enhancing phagocytosis and clearance from lungs of surfactant protein-A-deficient mice. Am J Respir Cell Mol Biol 1999; 20: 279.
49. Li D, Shirakami G, Zhan X, Johns RA. Regulation of ciliary beat frequency by nitric oxide–cyclic guanosine monophosphate signaling pathway in rat airway epithelial cells. Am J Respir Cell Mol Biol 2000; 23: 175.
50. Kelley T, Drumm M. Inducible nitric oxide synthase expression is reduced in cystic fibrosis murine and human airway epithelial cells. J Clin Invest 1998; 102: 1200.
51. Martin DL, Kiunkosky TM, Voynow JA, Adler KB. The role of reactive oxygen and nitrogen species in airway epithelial gene expression. Environ Health Perspect 1998; 106(suppl 5): 1197.
52. Comhair SA, Thomass MJ, Erzurum SC. Differential induction of extracellular glutathione peroxidase and nitric oxide synthase in airways of healthy individuals exposed to 100% O_2 or cigarette smoke. Am J Respir Cell Mol Biol 2000; 186: 350.
53. Rahmzin I, MacNee W. Oxidative stress and regulation of glutathione in lung inflammation. Eur Respir J 2000; 16: 534.
54. Cantin AN, Hubbard RC, Crystal RG. Glutathione deficiency in the epithelial lining of the lower respiratory tract in idiopathic pulmonary fibrosis. Am Rev Respir Dis 1989; 139: 370.
55. Gao L, Kim KJ, Yankaskas JR, Forman HJ. Abnormal glutathione transport in cystic fibrosis airway epithelia. Am J Physiol Lung Cell Mol Physiol 1999; 277: L113.
56. Peden DB, Hohman R, Brown ME et al. Uric acid is a major antioxidant in human nasal airway secretions. Proc Natl Acad Sci USA 1990; 87: 7638.
57. Peden DB, Swierzz M, Ohkubo K et al. Nasal secretion on the ozone scavenger uric acid. Am Rev Respir Dis 1993; 148: 455.
58. Kramps JA, Klasen EC. Characterization of a low molecular weight anti-elastase isolated from bronchial secretion. Exp Lung Res 1985; 9: 151.
59. Hiemstra PS, Maassen RJ, Stolk J et al. Antibacterial activity of antileukoprotease. Infection and Immunity 1996; 64: 4520.
60. Girod S, Zahm JM, Plotkowski MC et al. Role of the physicochemical properties of mucus in the protection of the respiratory epithelium. Eur Respir J 1992; 5: 447.

61. Puchelle E, Zahm JM, Quemada D. Rheological properties controlling mucociliary frequency and respiratory mucus transport. Biorheology 1987; 24: 557.

62. Girod S, Galabert C, Pierrot D et al. Role of phospholipid lining on respiratory mucus clearance by cough. J Appl Physiol 1991; 71: 2262.

63. Pillai RS, Chandra IF, Miller J et al. Work of adhesion of respiratory tract mucus. J Appl Physiol 1992; 72: 1604.

64. Puchelle E, Jacquot J, Zahm JM. In vitro restructuring effect of human airway immunoglobulins A and lysozyme on airway secretions. Eur J Respir Dis 1987; 71S: 117.

65. Girod S, Fuchey C, Galabert C et al. Identification of phospholipids in secretory granules of human submucosal gland respiratory cells. J Histochem Cytochem 1991; 39: 193.

66. Zhang Y, Yankaskas J, Wilson J, Engelhardt JF. In vivo analysis of fluid transport in cystic fibrosis airway epithelia of bronchial xenografts. Am J Physiol 1996; 270: C1326.

67. Zahm JM, Gaillard D, Dupuit F et al. Early alterations in airway mucociliary clearance and inflammation of the lamina propria in CF mice. Am J Physiol 1997; 272: C853.

68. Tomkiewicz RP, App EM, Zayas JG et al. Amiloride inhalation therapy in cystic fibrosis. Am Rev Respir Dis 1993; 148: 1002.

69. Quinton PM. Viscosity versus composition in airway pathology. Am J Respir Crit Care Med 1994; 149: 6.

70. Stutts MJ, Schwab JH, Chen MG et al. Effects of *Pseudomonas aeruginosa* on bronchial epithelial ion transport. Am Rev Respir Dis 1986; 134: 17.

71. Phipps RJ. The airways mucociliary system. In: Widdicombe JG, ed. International review of physiology III, vol 23. Baltimore, MA: University Park Press; 1981; 213.

72. Deneuville E, Perrot-Minot C, Pennaforte F et al. Revisited physicochemical and transport properties of respiratory mucus in genotyped cystic fibrosis patients. Am J Respir Crit Care Med 1997; 156: 166.

73. Matthews LW, Spector S, Lemm J, Potter J. Studies on pulmonary secretions. 1. The overall chemical composition of pulmonary secretions from patients with cystic fibrosis bronchiectasis and laryngectomy. Am Rev Respir Dis 1963; 88: 199.

74. Girod S, Galabert C, Lecuire A et al. Phospholipid composition and surface-active properties of tracheobronchial secretions from patients with cystic fibrosis and chronic obstructive pulmonary diseases. Pediatric Pulmonol 1992; 13: 22.

75. Martin LD, Rochelle LG, Fischer BM et al. Airway epithelium as an effector of inflammation: molecular regulation of secondary mediators. Eur Respir J 1997; 10: 2139.

76. Van der Velden VHJ, Savelkoul HFJ, Versnel MA. Bronchial epithelium: morphology, function and pathophysiology in asthma. Eur Cytokine Net 1998; 9: 585

77. Larsen GL, Holt PG. The concept of airway inflammation. Am J Respir Cell Mol Biol 2000; 162: S2.

78. Martin TR. Recognition of bacterial endotoxin in the lungs. Am J Respir Cell Mol Biol 2000; 23: 128.

79. Aderem A, Ulevitch RJ. Toll-like receptors in the induction of the innate immune response. Nature 2000; 406: 782.

80. Underhill DM, Ozinsky A, Hajjar M et al. The Toll-like receptor 2 is recruited to macrophage phagosomes and discriminated between pathogens. Nature 1999; 401: 811.

81. Ghost S, May MJ. Signal transduction through NF-kB. Immunol Today 1998; 19: 80.

82. Anderson SD. Exercise-induced asthma and the use of hypertonic saline aerosol as a bronchial challenge. Respiratology 1996; 1: 175.

83. Hashimoto S, Matsumoto K, Gon Y et al. Hyperosmolarity-induced interleukin-8 expression in human bronchial epithelial cells through p38 mitogen-activated protein kinase. Am J Respir Crit Care Med 1999; 159: 634.

84. Loitsch SM, Von Mallinckrodt C, Kippenberger S et al. Reactive oxygen intermediates are involved in IL-8 production induced by hyperosmotic stress in human bronchial epithelial cells. Biochem Biophys Res Commun 2000; 276: 571.

85. Khan TZ, Wagener JS, Bost T et al. Early pulmonary inflammation in infants with cystic fibrosis. Am J Respir Crit Care Med 1995; 151: 1075.

86. Baudouin-Legros M, Brouillard F, Cougnon F et al. Modulation of CFTR gene expression in HT-29 cells by extracellular hyperosmolarity. Am J Physiol 2000; 278: C49.

87. Tabary O, Escotte S, Couetil J et al. High susceptibility for cystic fibrosis human airway gland cells to produce interleukin-8 through the I_kB kinase α pathway in response to extracellular NaCl content. J Immunol 2000; 164: 3377.

88. Bonfield TL, Konstan MW, Burfiend P et al. Normal bronchial epithelial cells constitutively produce the anti-inflammatory cytokine IL-10 which is downregulated in cystic fibrosis. Am J Respir Cell Mol Biol 1995; 113: 257.

89. DiMango E, Ratner AJ, Bryan R et al. Activation of NF-$_k$B by adherent *Pseudomonas aeruginosa* in normal and cystic fibrosis respiratory epithelial cells. J Clin Invest 1998; 101: 2598.

90. Heeckeren AV, Walenga R, Konstan MW et al. Excessive inflammatory response of cystic fibrosis mice to bronchopulmonary infection with *Pseudomonas aeruginosa*. J Clin Invest 1997; 100: 2840.

91. Tirouvanziam R, De Bentzmann S, Hubeau C et al. Inflammation and infection in naive human cystic fibrosis airway grafts. Am J Respir Cell Mol Biol 2000; 23: 121.

92. Moss R, Hsu YP, Olds L. Cytokine dysregulation in activated cystic fibrosis (CF) peripheral lymphocytes. Clin Exp Immunol 2000; 120: 518.

93. Bonfield TL, Konstan MW, Berger M. Altered respiratory epithelial cell cytokine production in cystic fibrosis. J Allergy Clin Immunol 1999; 104: 72.

3 Respiratory defences

3.3 Immunology of the lung

Carlo Agostini and Gianpietro Semenzato

 Key concepts

- T cells account for the great majority of lung lymphocytes. CD4+ T-helper (Th) cells have immunoregulatory functions and govern the magnitude and/or duration of the effector cell responses via the release of cytokines. They can be subdivided into two broad types of cell, called Th1 and Th2, based on the lymphokine production pattern. The balance of Th1 and Th2 cytokine production influences the development of pulmonary inflammatory events.

- Cytotoxic lymphocytes, including natural killer (NK) cells, major-histocompatibility-complex (MHC)-restricted and MHC-unrestricted cytotoxic lymphocytes, are involved in antiviral immunity and are also essential for defence mechanisms against tumours.

- Lung B lymphocytes show functional and phenotypic similarities to peripheral blood B cells. Each type of antibody (IgG, IgA, IgM, IgD, IgB) can be produced in the lung as a circulating molecule or as a stationary molecule.

- Pulmonary macrophages show a wide variety of functions, including regulation of pulmonary immune responses, scavenging of senescent cells, lysis of infected or malignant cells, and repair and remodelling of lung tissues. The major part of this activity is carried out via the release of proinflammatory molecules, chemokines and other cytokines. The lung also has a substantial population of dendritic cells, which are effective antigen-presenting cells.

- Usually, only a few polymorphonuclear neutrophils reside within the alveolar spaces. Whenever there are conditions that require additional phagocytic help, neutrophils are rapidly recruited via the release of chemokines. Under normal conditions, eosinophils, mast cells and basophils are also found in very small numbers in the lung.

The large surface area of the respiratory mucosa, which represents the widest interface between the external environment and the internal milieu, is equipped with an extraordinary repertoire of immunologically competent cells that are capable of undergoing activation, migration and differentiation to specialised effector cells when challenged by foreign antigens. The efficiency of this local defence system is maintained by a continuous influx of cells from the systemic immune system apparatus and from the bone marrow. Furthermore, there is an intriguing network of interactions between cells and soluble mediators of the general immune system and immunocompetent cells associated with the respiratory tract. In other words, the pulmonary immune system is a peculiar immunological organ that can operate both independently and synchronously with the general immune apparatus.

In this chapter we will review the basic elements that regulate the immune system at the lung level and the constituents of in situ pulmonary host defence mechanisms that recognise, destroy and remove potentially harmful inhaled antigenic materials.

The pulmonary defence mechanisms

The internal milieu of the lung is daily exposed to over 10 000 litres of inspired air and mechanical mechanisms are crucial to avoid infection. Most inhaled particles are eliminated via the mucociliary clearance apparatus of the upper respiratory tract, which allows the transport of the majority of particulates to the posterior pharynx, where they are swallowed[1] (see also Chapters 3.1 and 3.2). Nonetheless, small amounts of inhaled agents and antigens elude removal by the mucociliary system, reach the lower respiratory tract and require processing by the immune system of the lung.

As in other organs, there are two different types of response to these antigens: innate and adaptive responses. The innate responses use phagocytic cells (neutrophils and macrophages), basophils, mast cells, eosinophils and natural killer (NK) cells.[2] There are also soluble components of the innate response, which include complement and acute-phase proteins. Acquired (adaptive) responses involve the expansion of antigen-specific B and T cells, which occurs when the surface receptors of these cells bind to antigens presented by specialised cells, called antigen-presenting cells. In the lung, dendritic cells and, more rarely, alveolar macrophages may display the antigen to lymphocytes and collaborate with them in the response to the antigen.[3] As specified later in more detail, pulmonary B cells secrete antigen-specific antibodies responsible for the clearance of extracellular microorganisms. T cells, releasing a wide range of cytokines that help B cells to produce antibody, contribute to the antigenic clearance by activating macrophages and by killing virally infected cells.

Innate and acquired responses usually work together in the lung, indicating that the pulmonary immune system is able to determine whether an antigenic molecule is more dangerous than another through the use of pattern-recognition receptors. Under normal conditions most infectious agents or foreign antigenic material do not usually signal to the host and may be processed without requiring an inflammatory response (innate response). Only when the infectious or antigenic burden becomes dangerous do immunocompetent lung cells release chemokines and cytokines. These mediate the recruitment of inflammatory cells and trigger antigen-specific pulmonary immune responses in the secondary lymphoid tissue or within the alveolar spaces (acquired response).

The bronchus-associated lymphoid tissue

Antigens and microorganisms can be processed and presented to local lymphatic tissues when they reach these compartments. According to their specific properties and discrete functions, human lymphocytes are functionally compartmentalised into primary, secondary and tertiary lymphoid organs. The great majority of organised lymphoid tissue is represented by the so called bronchus-associated lymphoid tissue (BALT) and lymph nodes that drain the nose or lung.[4] Lymphoid follicles are located throughout the bronchial tree as far down as the small bronchioles and are made up of B-cell germinal centres surrounded by T cells, macrophages and dendritic cells. These structures can be considered to be specialised sites for secondary lymphoid differentiation. They share morphological characteristics with Peyer's patches of the intestine and form strict associations with mucosal epithelium. In pulmonary follicles, naive B and T cells localise, differentiate in memory and effector lymphocytes and continuously traffic until they respond to their cognate antigen. In this respect, contiguity between the respiratory epithelium and lymphoid follicles is crucial. It allows antigens to pass across the epithelial barrier and to contact cells with antigen-presenting capacity (i.e. B cells, macrophages, dendritic cells).

Unwanted antigens induce the clonal expansion of intraalveolar precursor effector cells and the migration of memory lymphocytes, leading to local accumulation and differentiation

of antigen-specific T and B lymphocytes with effector specialisations (immunoglobulin secretion, cytotoxic activity, delayed-type hypersensitivity response, immunoregulatory activity, etc.). Another short-term consequence of the recognition of antigen by pulmonary memory B and T cells is their functional activation and up-regulation of the surface expression of several accessory molecules, including activation-dependent integrins of the α4 (CD49d) and β2 classes (CD18/LFA-1) and a member of the hyaluronate-binding receptor family, CD44. Bearing in mind that these molecules assist the interaction of lymphocytes with the cellular and extracellular matrix components, the heightened expression of adhesion molecules allows effector cells to extravasate efficiently from secondary lymphoid tissues to the inflamed pulmonary parenchyma.

In synthesis, we can assume that pulmonary lymphocytes continuously traffic throughout two functionally distinct lymphoid compartments: BALT tissue, i.e. the afferent lymphoid area where antigens first enter the system and initiate an immune response; and the remainder of the lung parenchyma, where differentiated memory T and B cells that have developed in the secondary follicles travel for renewed interaction with inciting antigens. The increase in pulmonary memory T cells seen after antigen challenge may be the consequence either of local proliferation or of migration from secondary lymphoid tissues (BALT and lymph nodes draining the pulmonary parenchyma). Both these functions are probably mediated by the interaction of lymphocytes with accessory cells, including dendritic cells.[5] In fact, pulmonary intra-epithelial and interstitial T cells can recognise antigens with high efficiency when presented by 'professional' dendritic cells expressing major histocompatibility complex (MHC) class II antigens (see later). In turn, as observed in other epithelial systems, pulmonary dendritic cells can capture and transfer antigens from the airway epithelium to BALT and draining lymph nodes. Here, after antigen presentation and activation, resting T cells can proliferate and the repertoire of adhesive and homing receptors necessary for their migration to lung parenchyma is up-modulated.

T and NK cells

T cells account for the great majority of lung lymphocytes found in the lower respiratory tract of normal individuals.[6] Less than 1×10^6 lymphocytes are usually recovered from a normal bronchoalveolar lavage; they are CD45R0 T 'memory' cells, which coexpress the α/β T-cell receptor (TCR). By contrast, only a few normal lung cells (about 5%) stain with the monoclonal antibody TCR-δ₁, which recognises a common epitope of the δ chain apparently expressed by all TCR-γ/δ cells. Some 70–90% of lymphocytes in bronchoalveolar lavage express CD2 related to sheep blood red cells.

In healthy non-smoking individuals both CD4 helper-related and CD8 cytotoxic/suppressor-related cells are present in approximately the same proportions as in the peripheral blood (pulmonary ratio of CD4/CD8 = 2).[7] These cells are located within the airways, alveolar epithelium and interstitium. Interestingly, a discrete decrease in pulmonary CD4/CD8 ratio may be observed in cigarette-smokers. As in the other tissues, pulmonary CD4 and CD8 molecules are functionally associated with the TCR and represent two structures that are involved in cell–cell adhesion and in signal transduction during T-cell activation. In particular, CD4 is a receptor for a monomeric part of MHC class II products (HLA-DR, -DQ and -DP) expressed on pulmonary antigen-presenting cells (such as lung B cells, alveolar and interstitial monocyte/macrophages, dendritic cells, activated T cells, endothelial cells, some epithelial cells), while CD8 binds class I MHC molecules (HLA-A, -B and -C) on the surface membrane of the target cells.

Most functions shown by lung T cells are mediated by the in situ release of biological response modifiers.[8] After antigenic activation, pulmonary CD4 lymphocytes acquire the capacity to produce a broad repertoire of cytokines (see below). These molecules act as critical mediators of cell functions and cell–cell communications by influencing many physiologic cell properties, including proliferation, differentiation and activation of other immunocompetent cells, chemotaxis, connective tissue metabolism, etc.

As in other organs, lymphokine-producing CD4[+] T-helper (Th) cells can be subdivided into two broad types of cell, called Th1 and Th2, on the basis of the lymphokine production pattern. Th1 cells secrete interleukin (IL)-2 , interferon (IFN)-γ and tumour necrosis factor (TNF)-β, while Th2 lymphocytes produce IL-4, IL-5, IL-6, IL-9 and IL-10. Both cell types produce granulocyte–macrophage-colony-stimulating factor (GM-CSF) and IL-3. The two subpopulations differs from a functional point of view. In fact, Th1 lymphocytes elicit a delayed-type hypersensitivity reaction and help in IgG synthesis, but they inhibit cytokine release by Th2 lymphocytes and IgE synthesis through the release of IFN-γ. In contrast, Th2 cells release IL-10, which inhibits the proliferative activity of Th1 lymphocytes.

The respiratory mucosa is equipped with CD8[+] cells that can be activated whenever challenged by foreign antigens.[9] In particular, the pulmonary immune system comprises:

- CD8 cell populations showing suppressor activity on B cells
- antigen-specific cytotoxic T lymphocytes, which recognise target cells via the CD3-Ti complex and require the expression of MHC gene products on targets
- MHC unrestricted cytotoxic T cells, which may lyse certain tumour and viral infected targets without prior sensitisation.

The role of suppressor cells in the modulation of pulmonary immune responses is still poorly understood. In fact, the means by which suppressor CD8 cells control the size and duration of the pulmonary immune activation pathways is not fully characterised.

More data are available on cytotoxic T lymphocytes resident in the respiratory mucosa. They play a central role in antiviral immunity and are also essential for the defence mechanism against tumours and in the allograft rejection (Fig. 3.3.1). Unlike specific cytotoxic T lymphocytes, which increase only during

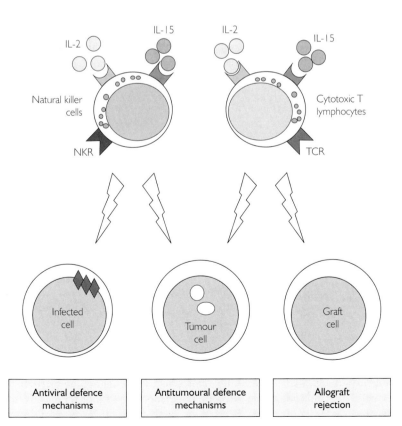

Fig. 3.3.1 Cytotoxic lymphocytes, including natural killer (NK) cells and major-histocompatability-complex (MHC)-restricted and MHC unrestricted cytotoxic lymphocytes, play a central role in antiviral immunity and in allograft rejection, and are also essential for the defence mechanism against tumours. Among different cytokines that are released within the pulmonary microenvironment, interleukin (IL)-2 and IL-15 play a key role in the events leading to the in situ expansion of NK cells and cytotoxic T lymphocytes.

conditions resembling host invasion, non-MHC restricted cells are present in discrete numbers under normal conditions also. While the major part of circulating non-MHC restricted cells are CD3-negative, lung CD56 and CD57 cells coexpress high proportions of CD3 molecules and the α/β TCR, showing the phenotype that characterises T cells with NK-like activity. It is notable that, while the majority of peripheral blood cytotoxic cells with NK activity are large granular lymphocytes that carry CD16 and lack expression of the CD3/TCR, yet there are few CD3-/CD16+ cells in the pulmonary microenvironment under normal conditions. Nonetheless, the number and the functional activity of NK cells may increase during viral infection of the pulmonary microenvironment, under the influx of locally released cytokines, including IL-2 and IL-15. Both IL-2 and IL-15 are also able to trigger the cytotoxic activity of cytotoxic T lymphocytes in the lung.

Under normal conditions the majority of lung T cells are relatively hyporesponsive and appear to be functional only after undergoing an activation process.[7] However, in non-smoking normal subjects also a subset of pulmonary lymphocytes (5%) stains with HLA-DR monoclonal antibody. Moreover, a similar proportion of lung T cells carry activation antigens, such as very-late-activation antigen-1 (VLA-1/CD49) and molecules analogous to the integrins, such as B-ly-7/CD103 and CD69. T cells may proliferate in response to mitogens, such as phytohaemagglutinin and concanavalin A, and in mixed lymphocyte reaction; furthermore, in pathological conditions they cooperate strictly with pulmonary accessory cells in the process of antigenic recognition.

Following activation, several accessory and adhesion molecules are expressed on the surface of pulmonary T lymphocytes.[10] Antigen-dependent activation increases the expression of CD2, CD18, CD29, CD38, CD44, CD45R0, CD54 and CD58, class II MHC antigens and VLA determinants on the cell surface of pulmonary T cells. These structures have been involved in non-antigen-specific homing of primed T cells to the secondary lymphoid tissues, in the process of T-cell activation and in the localisation of T cells to the sites of inflammation. The compartmentalisation of T cells involves the interaction of homing receptors on the surface of 'virgin' lymphocytes (CD44, LFA-1 and VLA antigens) to organ-specific endothelial molecules (known as the vascular addressin) of the secondary lung lymphoid tissues. The conversion of naive CD45RA T cells to memory pulmonary CD45R0 T cells coincides with the increase in the surface expression of adhesion structures (by a factor of 2–5). In turn, CD45R0 T cells express high levels of accessory molecules (CD2, CD11α/ LFA-1, CD58/LFA-3, VLA and CD44) and, as described in the section on the role of chemokines in the lung, acquire the ability to selectively localise within the pulmonary parenchyma via the expression of activated T-cell-specific chemokine receptors (CXCR3).[11]

Cytokines mainly produced by T lymphocytes

Following antigen recognition, discrete B- and T-lymphocyte subpopulations develop functional effector capabilities (immunoglobulin synthesis, cytotoxic activity, etc.), while other T-cell subsets acquire immunoregulatory functions that

govern the magnitude and/or the duration of the effector cell responses. In addition, the interaction between pulmonary lymphocytes and alveolar macrophages results in the generation of a number of biological response modifiers, which are responsible for the recruitment of peripheral blood lymphocytes, monocytes and polymorphonuclear lymphocytes, and for the further activation of surrounding immunocompetent cells. Thus, the effectiveness of the lung immune system is dependent on the ordered differentiation of the lymphocyte subpopulations, which acquire different functional capabilities under antigenic pressure. Furthermore, networks of interacting cytokines are responsible for controlling the state of activation of all local immunocompetent cells, in both hypersensitivity reactions and allergic responses taking place in the lung. This section will focus on the pattern of lymphokine production within the respiratory tract.

Interleukin-2

Actively released by pulmonary Th1 cells, the role of IL-2 in the pulmonary immune system is to expand activated T-cell populations; its receptor is formed by three different chains: α (CD25), β (CD122) and γ (CD132). IL-2 acts as a local growth factor for T lymphocytes infiltrating lung tissues of patients with hypersensitivity reactions. This classic Th1 cytokine is also involved in the regulation of immunoglobulin production and in the enhancement of the potential capabilities of pulmonary cytotoxic T lymphocyte and NK cells (Fig. 3.3.1).

The range of lung cell targets of IL-2 is broader than originally appreciated. Inasmuch as some alveolar macrophages normally express β/γ IL-2R at low density and considering the fact that the addition of IL-2 to activated alveolar macrophages increases GM-CSF expression, it is believed that IL-2 may play a role in the activation of some functional capabilities of activated alveolar macrophages. Binding sites for IL-2 have also been demonstrated on human lung fibroblasts. Addition of IL-2 to fibroblast leads to an enhanced expression of the gene coding for the chemokine monocyte chemoattractant protein-1 (MCP-1/CCL2), which is involved in fibrosis through the regulation of profibrotic cytokine generation and matrix. IL-2 may thus serve to integrate fibroblasts and tissue macrophages into a coordinated response of the connective tissue initiated by Th1 lymphocytes.

Interleukin-4

This lymphokine, released by most cell types, including Th2 cells, eosinophils and mast cells, is a cofactor for proliferation of fibroblasts.[12] Inducing the expression of class II MHC antigens on the surface membrane of accessory cells, it acts in synergism with IL-2 in stimulating the growth of T cells. The IL-4/IL-13 axis is also involved in the triggering and maintaining of the recruitment, homing and activation of inflammatory cells during remodelling process of the airways.[13] Finally, IL-4 induces the release of chemokines from human bronchial epithelial cell, including IL-8/CXCL8. This effect is thought to be of particular importance in attracting neutrophils and monocytes to sites of inflammation.

Interleukin-9

Interleukin-9 is a multifunctional cytokine produced by activated Th2 cells in vitro and during Th2-like T cell responses in vivo. Data obtained in animal models indicate that IL-9 promotes inflammation and airway hyper-responsiveness.[14] Lung expression of IL-9 in transgenic mice causes massive airway inflammation with eosinophils and lymphocytes as predominant infiltrating cell types. An additional striking finding is the presence of increased numbers of mast cells within the airway epithelium. Other impressive pathological changes in the airways are epithelial cell hypertrophy associated with accumulation of mucus-like material within non-ciliated cells and increased subepithelial deposition of collagen. Since human fibroblast express the IL-9 receptor, it is believed that this cytokine is involved in fibroproliferative responses.

Interleukin-10

Interleukin-10 has anti-inflammatory and immunoregulatory properties. It inhibits proinflammatory cytokine and chemokine production in addition to blocking T-cell responses to specific antigens.[15] It acts primarily through inhibition of costimulatory properties of macrophages.

Activated Th2 cells may represent a source for this molecule in the pulmonary microenvironment. Nonetheless, Th0 CD4+ T cells, CD8+ T cells, lipopolysaccharide-activated macrophages and mast cells may also produce IL-10.[16] From a functional point of view, IL-10 shows inhibitory activity on the release of IFN-γ and IL-2 by lung Th1 cells, stimulates mast cell growth and regulates the accessory function of antigen-presenting cells resident in the pulmonary microenvironment.

In the lung, IL-10 has inhibitory activity on local immune response, via its capability of inhibiting dendritic-cell–T-cell interactions. IL-10 can reduce the production of biologically active IL-12 in lung dendritic cells. Furthermore, since IL-10 may induce differentiation of naive Th cells into Th2 cells,[16] this cytokine has been involved in the pathogenesis of pulmonary allergic disorders. There are also data on the involvement of IL-10 in the regulation of fibroproliferative responses in the lung. This cytokine has also partial inhibitory effects on T-cell-mediated immune responses taking place during some hypersensitivity reactions.[17]

Interleukin-13

Interleukin-13 is expressed in activated Th0 cells, Th1-like cells, Th2-like cells and T-cells expressing CD8.[18] This molecule strongly inhibits cytokine secretion induced by lipopolysaccharide in monocyte/macrophages. In particular, the pulmonary release of IL-1, IL-6, TNF-α and IL-8 may be influenced by the local release of IL-13. IL-13 is also a monocyte chemoattractant.

Interleukin-13 is believed to be involved in the regulation of pulmonary inflammatory responses. During lung inflammation endogenous IL-13 regulates NF-κB activation and related cytokine/chemokine generation, determining the intensity of the inflammatory response. IL-13 has also effects on fibrogenesis, since it increases adhesion molecule and inflammatory cytokine expression in human lung fibroblasts and is critical for recruitment of inflammatory cells. IL-13 serves as an important mediator of Th2-mediated inflammation in the lung.[19] In particular, in allergic asthma, a dysregulation of IL-13 production has also been found to be a key factor.[20] The pulmonary expression of IL-13 causes a mononuclear and eosinophilic inflammatory response, mucus cell metaplasia, airway fibrosis, the production of the chemokine eotaxin/CCL15, airways obstruction and non-specific airways hyper-responsiveness.

Interleukin-17

This cytokine is produced by CD4 T cells and is able to induce cytokine expression on target cells, including IL-6 and IL-8. It enhances the surface expression of ICAM-1 on fibroblasts. Recent evidence also indicate that IL-17 can link the activation of certain T-lymphocytes to the recruitment and activation of airway neutrophils.[21] The IL-17-induced neutrophil recruitment is mediated via induced CXC chemokine release through steroid-sensitive mechanisms and is modulated by release of endogenous tachykinins. These effects of IL-17 are potentiated by other proinflammatory cytokines such as IL-1β and TNF-α. Taken together, these findings suggest the potential role of this cytokine in T-cell-driven lung fibrosis.

Interferon-γ

This typical Th1 cytokine is a key factor in the events that favour local immune responses in the lung.[22] IFN-γ enhances the accessory function of alveolar macrophages, increases the cytotoxic function of lung macrophages and lymphocytes, and regulates the secretion of an array of lymphokines, cytokines and chemokines into the surrounding microenvironment. In addition, this Th1 cytokine activates pulmonary macrophages to phagocytose intracellular pathogens. IFN-γ is typically expressed by T cells infiltrating the lung during most interstitial lung diseases, including sarcoidosis, hypersensitivity pneumonitis, tuberculosis and human immunodeficiency virus (HIV) infection. There are data suggesting that monocyte/macrophages may represent a cell source of IFN-γ in the lungs, but the data are debated.

Through its pleiotropic effects on cytokine production, IFN-γ modulates mucosal immune responses in interstitial lung disease.[23] IFN-γ up-regulates the expression of the costimulatory molecules on pulmonary accessory cells, including CD80 and CD86.[24] It influences cell-mediated mechanisms of cytotoxicity and modulates T-cell growth and functional differentiation. However, inducing non-ERL chemokines – CXC chemokines without the Glu–Leu–Arg (ERL) motif before the CXC motif (Mig/CXCL9, IP-10/CXCL10, ITAC/CXCL11) – the cytokine plays a major role in the recruitment of activated CXCR3+ T cells into inflamed tissues of patients with interstitial lung disease (see later). IFN-γ has also crucial antifibrotic effects, since it inhibits the proliferation of endothelial cells and the synthesis of collagens by fibroblasts.

The Th1/Th2 model

The pattern of Th1 and Th2 cytokine production in the lung can be summarised in the context of the Th1/Th2 paradigm[25]

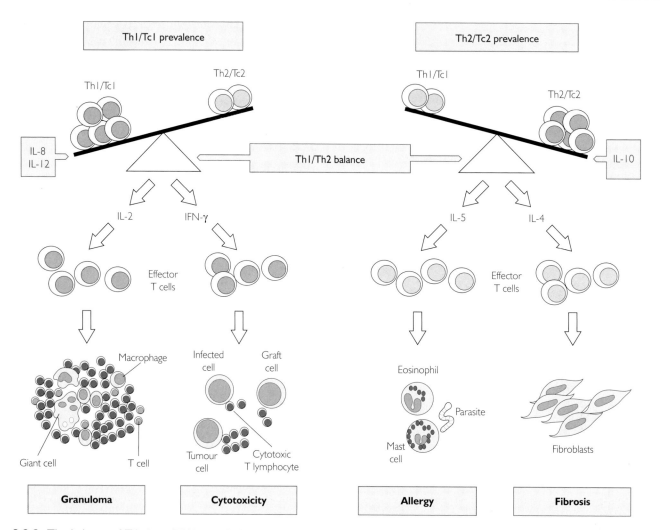

Fig. 3.3.2 The balance of T-helper (Th)1 and Th2 cytokine production influences the development of pulmonary inflammatory events. Th1 cells producing interferon (IFN)-γ or interleukin (IL)-2 are responsible for initiating the alveolitis in the lung of patients with granulomatous disorders or disorders characterised by a massive influx of cytotoxic T lymphocytes while a Th2 type pattern is associated with local activation of allergic mechanisms, fibroproliferative responses or with a reduced resistance to intracellular pathogens.

(Fig. 3.3.2). A Th1 CD4 or Tc1 T-cell profile predominates during the formation of the typical T-cell mediated alveolitis. Th1 cells producing IFN-γ or IL-2 are responsible for initiating the alveolitis in the lung of patients with granulomatous disorders including sarcoidosis or disorders characterised by a massive influx of cytotoxic T lymphocytes, including viral diseases or in the rejection mechanisms to lung allograft. By contrast, the Th2 type pattern is associated with local activation of allergic mechanisms, fibroproliferative responses or a reduced resistance to intracellular pathogens. For instance, a Th2 response with concomitant release of IL-10, IL-6 and IL-4 is involved in the pathogenesis of pulmonary hypersensitivity diseases characterised by eosinophilic pneumonia, (including asthma, allergic bronchopulmonary aspergillosis, Löffler's syndrome, etc.) as well as in patients with interstitial lung disease evolving toward pulmonary fibrosis.[26]

As better specified in other chapters, the natural history of several diffuse lung diseases may be influenced by the Th1/Th2 pattern of cytokine production. Two examples are here provided to outline this possibility. In the lung of patients with HIV infec-

tion the Th1/Th2 shift is associated with a decrease of the cytotoxic activities of HIV-specific cytotoxic T lymphocytes and favour the development of a number of pulmonary opportunistic infections. Again, in patients with sarcoidosis the net effect of the Th1 response is the development of a hypersensitivity reaction (i.e. the granuloma). In general terms, an inhibition of fibrogenetic processes may be observed in this phase. However, depending on the host susceptibility, a switch to Th2 cells may occur in some patients with concomitant release of cytokines, including IL-4, which stimulates the production of extracellular matrix proteins and of chemoattractants for fibroblasts and the consequent evolution towards lung fibrosis.

Pulmonary B cells and the humoral response

As in other secondary lymphoid tissues, highly differentiated B cells largely predominate in the germinal centres of BALT follicu-

while most of the IgA is localised in the proximal bronchial tubes, IgG represents the predominant Ig isotype in the alveolar spaces. IgM is present in the lavage fluid and its concentrations is higher than would be expected for simple diffusion of the molecule into bronchial secretions from serum, suggesting that IgM levels are the result of the active secretion by IgM-expressing B-lymphocytes present in the bronchial mucosa, or of the transport of IgM across epithelial cells into the airway lumen. Levels of bronchoalveolar lavage IgE and cells with intracytoplasmic IgE are detected only in atopic individuals and no detectable IgD have been found in normal individuals.

The synthesis of immunoglobulins by lung B cells plays an important role in the pulmonary immune response (Fig. 3.3.3). IgA immunoglobulins are found principally in their secretory form and are involved in the clearance of microorganisms from the respiratory tract. IgG opsonins specific for bacteria, together with complement factor (C3b), greatly facilitate phagocytosis by alveolar macrophages. Specific IgG is mandatory for the killing of Gram-negative microorganisms, for instance *Pseudomonas aeruginosa* or *Escherichia coli*. In pathological conditions IgG may also induce antibody-dependent cellular cytotoxicity against microorganisms and tumours (Fig. 3.3.3). This activity is mediated by multiple cell types having on their surface membrane the Fc receptors for IgG as a common denominator. They include granular lymphocytes with NK activity, some T cells, macrophages and neutrophils.

Functional assessments of B lymphocytes from bronchoalveolar lavage demonstrate similarities to B cells in peripheral blood. In fact, they are responsive to T-dependent B mitogens, such as pokeweed mitogens, and can be elicited to synthesise immunoglobulins in vitro. By taking advantage of this technique, it has been possible to study the ability of pulmonary B cells to actively produce antibodies. Despite the fact that immunoglobulins are present in bronchoalveolar lavage, it has been shown that immunoglobulin-secreting cells are rare in the alveolar space. In fact, in one comparative study, it has been shown that IgG is actively produced only by B cells of the lung parenchyma, and that intra-epithelial cells do not synthesise IgG de novo. Understandably, it is generally assumed that most of the IgG in the lower respiratory tract results from transudation of IgG molecules from serum to the alveolar space. It is also possible that, following antigenic challenge, immunoglobulins are produced in the pulmonary interstitium by parenchymal B cells and then released within the alveolar space.

Impairment of the pulmonary B-cell system may lead to an increased susceptibility to develop certain kinds of respiratory infection. Examples are the association between a defect in IgG production and recurrent sinopulmonary infections and the high virulence of those pathogenic bacteria able to elaborate IgA protease, which can destroy lung immunoglobulins. Abnormal Ig production has been implicated in the pathogenesis of lung involvement in autoimmune diseases and in allograft rejection mechanisms.

Alveolar macrophages

Under normal conditions more than 90% of the cells within the alveolar spaces are macrophages. Alveolar macrophages, the rep-

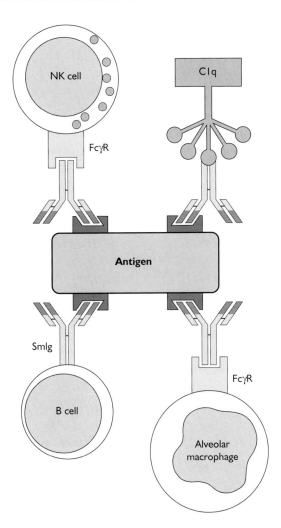

Fig. 3.3.3 In the lung, B cells may act in isolation or in collaboration with other cell types. When antibodies are bound to antigen, multiple Fc regions are exposed. This may lead to the activation of the complement pathway after binding of C1q to Fc and/or to the activation of phagocytosis or antibody-dependent cellular cytotoxicity after the cross-linking of Fc receptors and binding of the Fcγ receptor on the alveolar macrophages (AM) and natural killer (NK) cells respectively.

lar aggregates. In contrast, within alveolar spaces and in the interstitial parenchyma less than 5% of the lymphocytes are B cells. The distribution of B-cell subpopulations in the lung is similar to that in the blood. The majority of pulmonary B cells are CD19- and CD20-positive, showing the phenotype of mature B cells and bearing surface immunoglobulins and, in a small number of cases, plasma cells with intracytoplasmic immunoglobulins.

Although B lymphocytes are able to function as antigen-presenting cells, their primary role in the lung is to produce immunoglobulins (Ig) important for local defence against microbial pathogens. Each type of antibody (IgG, IgA, IgM, IgD, IgE) can be produced in the lung as a circulating molecule or as a stationary molecule. The latter functions as the B-cell receptor for lung 'effector' B cells (Fig. 3.3.3). Immunoglobulins are major mediators of a number of host defence mechanisms. IgA is the predominant Ig isotype detectable in the upper respiratory tract where the ratio of IgA:IgG is approximately 2.5:1. However,

resentatives of the mononuclear phagocyte system in the lung, are unique among macrophages found in particular body compartments because they are strategically located at the air–tissue interface and are regularly exposed to inhaled antigens.[27] These cells are crucial in the defence against invading pathogens and, in addition, have a wide variety of functions in the lung, including regulation of pulmonary immune responses, scavenging of senescent cells, lysis of infected or malignant cells, and repair and remodelling of lung tissues.

Although some alveolar macrophages can replicate in normal lung, the majority arise from circulating monocytes. These latter, originally formed in the bone marrow, pass into the peripheral blood, where they remain for 2–3 days, and then migrate through the alveolar walls to the lungs and other tissues. The events resulting in recruitment of monocytes to the respiratory tract have recently been identified. Expression of molecules involved in leukocyte–endothelial cell recognition (CD11α/CD18, CD49α and CD62L),[28] the consequent binding of monocytes to tissue-specific vascular adhesion molecules and the release of macrophage-specific chemokines are the mechanisms that determine the compartmentalisation of monocytes into the lung (see below). In the pulmonary microenvironment, freshly recruited monocytes differentiate into mature macrophages, under the influence of vitamin D metabolites and other unknown stimuli, to become long-lived phagocytes with a life span of months to years.

Under normal conditions alveolar macrophages are poor antigen-presenting cells.[29] Thus, these end-stage differentiated cells are functionally quiescent and may be considered as mobile scavengers that are attracted to an infected or inflamed focus by many substances, including chemokines, endotoxin, immune complexes, collagen fragments and complement products. Once arrived at the site of inflammation, alveolar macrophages can ingest non-self antigens, bacteria, fungi and viruses, and are also capable of inactivating viable virulent encapsulated and Gram-negative microorganisms. They process and clear antigens that reach the lower respiratory tract without signalling for an inflammatory response to be amplified. The ability to clear antigenic particles or infective agents without evoking an immune response allows the removal of antigens without initiating unnecessary T-cell responses that may damage the alveolar capillary membrane (Fig. 3.3.4)

The reduced capacity of normal alveolar macrophages to initiate T-cell immune response is linked to the fact that, under resting conditions, normal alveolar macrophages carry only low levels of costimulatory molecules, if any.[30] The accessory function of alveolar macrophages depends on the expression of members of the B7 family (CD80 and CD86), CD40 and the CD5 co-ligand CD72. Only in pathological conditions, e.g. when the infectious or antigenic burden is dangerous, do alveolar macrophages express high levels of these co-ligands and function as effective antigen-presenting cells.[31] Under these circumstances, phagocytosis represents the first step for the recognition and process of antigen by T cells. The antigen is ingested by endocytosis, is degraded and part of its molecule is transported to the cell membrane and bound to the class II

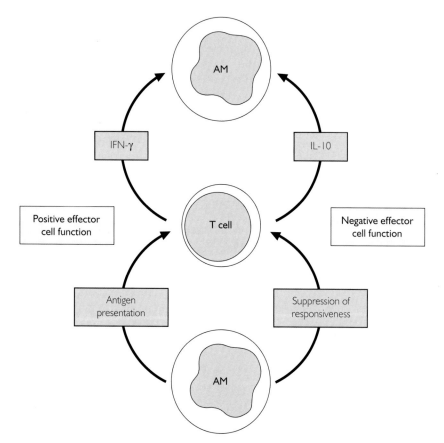

Fig. 3.3.4 The duality of alveolar macrophages in the pulmonary microenvironment. Depending on their context in vivo, they clear antigens without initiating unnecessary T-cell responses that might damage the alveolar capillary membrane or trigger T-cell antigen-specific immune responses activating the surrounding microenvironment. In turn, T cells may further activate or suppress alveolar macrophages via the release of interferon (IFN)-γ and interleukin (IL)-10 respectively.

MHC molecule (HLA-DR), i.e. the structure expressed on the surface membrane of alveolar macrophages that physically presents the antigen to T cells.

Following the interaction of the TCR with the bimolecular complex antigen/HLA-DR, T cells become activated and release a series of immunomodulatory substances, including IFN-γ. In particular, the interaction between IFN-γ and its receptor triggers alveolar macrophages to become 'primed'. This activation state of alveolar macrophages is indicated by an increase in metabolic activity and enhanced secretion of immunomodulatory molecules such as proinflammatory cytokines, chemokines and other cytokines specified below. Pulmonary macrophages are also able to mediate oxygen-dependent and oxygen-independent killing of tumour cells and microorganisms.[32] The oxygen-dependent mechanisms entail the production of hydrogen peroxide, superoxide anion and single oxygen molecules. The oxygen-independent mechanisms require acidification of the phagocytosed material followed by the fusion of vacuoles with lysosomes containing proteinases, hydrolase, complement breakdown products (C3a) and other lytic proteins.

Dendritic cells

The lung has a substantial population of dendritic cells, which derive from peripheral blood monocytes, or partially differentiated, blood-derived dendritic cells that are recruited into lung tissues.[33] Under normal conditions small numbers of dendritic cells may be found around the vessels and in the alveolar walls but not in the alveolar spaces.[34] While normal alveolar macrophages are unresponsive and poor antigen-presenting cells, human lung dendritic cells are considerably more potent in inducing T-cell immune responses.[35] This property is due to the fact that they constitutively bear molecules, including CD54 (ICAM-1), CD58

(LFA-3) and B7 members (CD80/ CD86), that are able to enhance the interaction of antigen-presenting cells with T cells and deliver a second proliferative signal (Fig. 3.3.5).

Although dendritic cells are more effective than alveolar macrophages in presenting antigens, alveolar macrophages may in turn influence dendritic cell function. Depending on the type of inhaled antigen, alveolar macrophages may release anti-inflammatory cytokines that inhibit signalling for the inflammatory responses (IL-10) or proinflammatory mediators that are able to activate surrounding dendritic cells to acquire the ability to phagocytose particles and microbes. The local network of dendritic cells extends from the basement membrane up to the tight junctions between the apical sides of the epithelial cells and is involved in the clearance of antigens.[36]

Once dendritic cells have captured the antigen, they migrate to lymph nodes to trigger antigen-specific immune responses; their trafficking is closely regulated by chemokines, mostly released by local immunocompetent cells[37] (see below). As a consequence, dendritic cells migrate toward the paracortical T-cell zone of the draining lymph nodes of the lung, where they interact with naive T and B cells. Primed, antigen-specific T cells may then migrate to the lung parenchyma, where they release Th1 cytokines, such IFN-γ, which further activate dendritic cells and alveolar macrophages, thus potentiating local immune responses.

Cytokines mainly produced by lung macrophages and dendritic cells

Interleukin-1

Pulmonary macrophages are capable of producing detectable amounts of IL-1α and IL-1β as well as IL-1ra, a specific receptor antagonist of IL-1, in response to several inflammatory

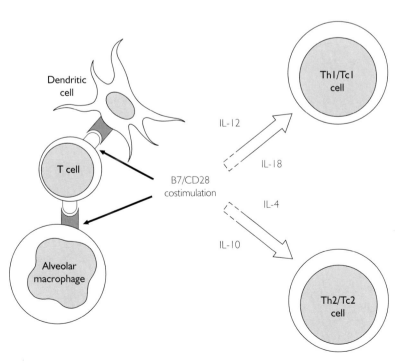

Fig. 3.3.5 The accessory function of dendritic cells and, to a lesser extent, alveolar macrophages depends on the expression of a series of accessory molecules, including members of the B7 family (CD80 and CD86), as shown here. B7 molecules are able to enhance the interaction of antigen presenting cells with T cells via the link with CD28, and deliver a second proliferative signal. Only in pathological conditions characterised by a dangerous antigenic burden do alveolar macrophages express high levels of these co-ligands and function as effective antigen presenting cells.

stimuli. IL-1 is also produced by other cell types that participate to the ongoing inflammatory response, including neutrophils, endothelial cells and fibroblast. Although powerful antigen-presenting cells, lung dendritic cells produce little IL-1.

Interleukin-1 provides accessory growth factor activity for inflammatory lung T cells.[38] In fact, the main biological activity of IL-1 is the stimulation of T-helper cells, which are induced to secrete IL-2 and to express IL-2 receptors. Promoting the adhesion of neutrophils, monocytes and T-cells by enhancing the expression of adhesion molecules such as intercellular adhesion molecule (ICAM)-1/CD54 and endothelial leucocyte adhesion molecule (ELAM)/CD62E, IL-1 regulates the development of alveolar inflammation (alveolitis). Since it promotes the proliferation of fibroblasts and increases collagen production, IL-1 has been involved in the development of lung fibrosis associated with some interstitial lung diseases.

Interleukin-6

Interleukin 6 is a polypeptide mediator regulating the immune response, the acute phase reaction and haematopoiesis.[39] In the lung this proinflammatory factor is mainly produced by alveolar macrophages, but it is known that T cells, endothelial cells and fibroblasts may also produce IL-6. By contrast, dendritic cells appear to be poor producers of IL-6. Dysregulating production of IL-6 was suggested to be involved in a variety of chronic pulmonary inflammatory diseases, including sarcoidosis, tuberculosis, berylliosis, HIV infection and interstitial lung disease associated with autoimmune disorders.

In the lung this cytokine influences antigen-specific immune responses and potentiates inflammatory reactions. IL-6 is also involved in the control of the in situ proliferation of fibroblasts.[40]

Interleukin-12

This cytokine is mainly produced in the lung by macrophages and dendritic cells.[41] It has been also reported that neutrophils may represent a cell source of IL-12.[42] IL-12 is involved in Th1 immune responses and stimulates the proliferation and the lytic activity of activated lung T cells. Specifically, IL-12 induces the Th0 versus Th1 shift and stimulates the proliferation and lytic activity of activated T cells and NK cells. In synergy with IL-15, IL-12 favours the contact between activated T cells and antigen-presenting cells. The cytokine acts by interacting with specific receptors (IL-12Rβ) expressed by lymphocytes accumulating in the lung during most Th1-driven diffuse lung diseases.

Interleukin-15

This pleiotropic lymphokine shares biological activities and components of its receptor with IL-2 (β/γ IL-2R). In the lung, IL-15 is mainly produced by macrophages and dendritic cells. IL-15 is produced by alveolar macrophages and supports the growth and chemotaxis of T cells, favouring the development of T-cell alveolitis. It also behaves as a co-stimulatory factor for the production of other cytokines and chemokines (IL-17, CXCL8/IL-8, CCL2/MCP-1, GM-CSF, IFN-γ and TNF-α) and for the expression of molecules involved in the antigen-pre-

senting capability of resident accessory cells (CD80/CD86). Furthermore, the finding that IL-15 down-regulates the apoptosis rate of lung T cells introduces IL-15 as a possible inhibitor of death-inducing effects of physiological apoptotic stimuli. IL-15 may also regulate neutrophil functions in the lung. In fact, it induces cytoskeletal rearrangements, enhances phagocytosis and delays apoptosis of neutrophils.[43] Moreover, IL-15 has been found to elicit other functional responses in neutrophils, such as chemokine production, that may influence pulmonary host defence mechanisms.

Interleukin-18

Previously known as IFN-γ-inducing factor (IGIF), IL-18 has activity roughly similar to, though distinct from, that of IL-1. Mainly produced by monocytes, macrophages and lung epithelial cells,[44] it induces expression of IFN-γ and colony-stimulating factors while inhibiting production of IL-10. In addition to stimulating IFN-γ synthesis, IL-18 also possesses inflammatory effects by inducing synthesis of the proinflammatory cytokines TNF-α, IL-6 and IL-1β, the chemokines IL-8/CCL8 and macrophage inflammatory protein-1α (MIP-1α/CCL3), nitric oxide synthase and nitric oxide. It is also able to inhibit transforming growth factor (TGF)-β-induced proliferation. Interestingly, IL-18, IL-12 and IL-15 act on Th1 cells synergistically to induce IFN-γ, pointing to the possibility that both cytokines cooperate in the development of Th1-type immune responses.

Colony-stimulating factors

Granulocyte–macrophage-colony-stimulating factor, granulocyte-colony-stimulating factor (G-CSF), monocyte-colony-stimulating factor (M-CSF) and IL-3 are able to induce the growth and differentiation of myeloid progenitors, facilitating the accumulation of macrophages in the lung. Furthermore, GM-CSF modulates cytokine production and enhances the antigen-presenting capacity and growth of alveolar macrophages.

Transforming growth factor-β and related cytokines

Transforming growth factor-β and the family of TGF-related cytokines are secreted by monocyte/macrophages and activated lymphocytes, including pulmonary lymphocytes. TGF-β is a potent immunosuppressive molecule that exerts chemotactic activity on monocytes and modulates the synthesis and effect of several other molecules, including IL-1, IL-2, IL-3, GM-CSF, IFN-γ and TNF-α. TGF-β, which is constitutively released in the respiratory tract, has been implicated in the development of fibrotic processes.

Tumour necrosis factor and other molecules belonging to the TNF-ligand superfamily

Tumour-necrosis factor-α is a pleiotropic factor, predominantly produced by activated cells belonging to the monocyte/macrophage lineage, that activates both neutrophils and macrophages, leading to protease release, stimulation of the respiratory burst and the induction of the vascular adhesion molecule expression essential for cell recruitment at sites of inflammation. In the lung, TNF-α is actively produced by pulmonary macrophages. It plays a critical role in pulmonary injury and in the regulation of fibroblast growth via the induction of IL-6. Furthermore, TNF-α stimulates and regulates the synthesis and release of other lymphokines (IL-1, GM-CSF, platelet activating factor and IL-6) and increases prostaglandin (PG) production (PGE$_2$).

Tumour-necrosis factor-α is a member of an emerging family of soluble molecules with several and complex immunoregulatory properties, which interact with specific receptors (TNF-R). TNF-α and other ligands of the TNF superfamily (TNF-L) have a role in modulating apoptotic mechanisms at sites of inflammation. There are data suggesting that the chronic overexpression of TNF-α and IFN-γ and the dysregulation of TNF-R/TNF-L set the stage for the persistence and progression of inflammatory events during some inflammatory pulmonary diseases. In some circumstances, alteration in the TNF-R/TNF-L balance leads to the chronic recruitment of inflammatory cells, which, once in the inflamed tissue, assemble granulomatous structures. On the other hand, it has been shown that TNF-α is induced in inflammatory cells during the resolution phase of granulomatous processes, rather suggesting a role for the cytokine in recovery from inflammation. Both phenomena are likely to be possible in the lung. TNF-α may be essential or have little impact on the control of apoptotic mechanisms, depending on a combination of genetic factors, previous environmental exposure and local alterations in immunocompetence.

Other macrophage-derived factors

Fibrosing processes taking place in the lung result in the generation of other macrophage-derived molecules, including platelet-derived growth factor (PDGF) and insulin-like growth factor I (IGF-I). These growth factors for fibroblasts and epithelial cells and their receptors are abundantly expressed in fibrotic lung. They cooperate with the TGF family in promoting fibroblast growth and deposition of collagen fibrils.

Another group of mediators whose role in the evolution of fibrosis has recently been investigated are the 5-lypoxigenase metabolites of arachidonic acid (LTB4 and LTC4). The alveolar macrophages of patients with lung fibrosis elaborate significant amounts of leukotrienes. In addition, lung fibroblasts isolated from these subjects show a striking defect in their capacity to synthesise the anti-inflammatory and anti-fibrogenic molecules PGE$_2$ and phospholipase A$_2$. In view of the fact that LTB4 and LTC4 stimulate fibroblast proliferation and chemotaxis and favour collagen deposition, their hyperproduction and the defect in PGE synthesis could be relevant in the pathogenesis of lung fibrosis.

Neutrophils and other polymorphonucleates

Neutrophils are usually marginated along the walls of the microvasculature while only a few polymorphonuclear cells reside within the alveolar spaces (less than 5% of alveolar cells are neutrophils). Polymorphonucleates represent the second line of the scavenger function. In normal non-smokers they are few but whenever there are conditions that require additional phagocytic help they are rapidly recruited via the release of chemokines.[45] For instance, if the inoculum of antigen or microorganisms is too large for the phagocytic capacity of alveolar macrophages, or pathogens are particularly virulent, we can expect a ready supply of polymorphonucleates to be marginated in the blood vessels adjacent to the alveoli.[46] These newly recruited cells are equipped with lysosomal granules containing a large repertoire of enzymes, including lactoferrin, cathepsin G, elastase, myeloperoxidase, hydrolase and bacterial-permeability-inducing proteins. Furthermore, migrating polymorphonucleates are capable of releasing a wide variety of oxygen intermediates with antibacterial activity, such as hydrogen peroxide, superoxide and hydroxyl radicals.

The alveolar macrophage is the key cell that initiates and drives the migration of polymorphonucleates at the site of inflammation.[2] In theory, many products of alveolar macrophages may account for the recruitment of polymorphonucleates. For instance, it has been shown that IL-1, TNF-α and leukotriene B$_4$ are potent chemotactic factors for granulocytes. Furthermore, a recently discovered phagocyte-derived lymphokine, called IL-8/CXCL8, has been implicated in the mechanisms that control neutrophil recruitment. It might also be hypothesised that pulmonary T cells could favour the polymorphonucleates accumulation, by releasing lymphokines such as IL-3 and IL-5, which are important for the differentiation and proliferation of neutrophils and eosinophils respectively.

In recent years, however, it has become obvious that the contribution of neutrophils to host defence and natural immunity extends well beyond their traditional role as professional phagocytes[42] (Fig. 3.3.6). Neutrophils can be induced to express a number of genes whose products lie at the core of inflammatory and immune response. Activated lung neutrophils have the capacity to produce cytokines (TNF-α, IL-1, vascular endothelial growth factor, IL-12)[42] and a number of chemokines (including IL-8/CXCL8, GROα/CXCL1, MIP-1α/CCL3, MIP-1β/CCL4, IP-10/CXCL10, MIG/CXCL9, MIP-3α/CCL20, MIP-3β/CCL19 and I-TAC/CXCL11, see below for further details), further amplifying local inflammatory responses. In particular, since some of these chemokines are primarily chemotactic for dendritic cells and specific lymphocyte subsets, the ability of neutrophils to produce chemokines might be significant in orchestrating the recruitment of other cell types to the inflamed sites and therefore in contributing to the regulation of the immune response.

Under normal conditions eosinophils, mast cells and basophils are also found in very low proportions in the lung.[47] Eosinophils are only weakly phagocytic and, if activated, kill parasites mainly by releasing cationic proteins and reactive oxygen metabolites into the surrounding microenvironment. It is also known that eosinophils also secrete leukotrienes, prostaglandins and various cytokines. In the lung they play important roles in the pathogenesis of pulmonary hypersensitivity diseases, lung parasitic diseases, lung injury and fibrosis. As with that of

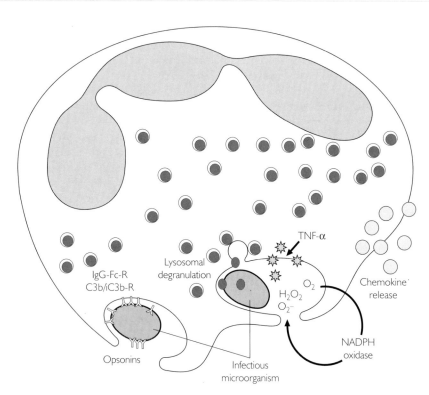

Fig. 3.3.6 The complex contribution of neutrophils to the pulmonary immune system. They participate in the lung host defence by acquiring the ability to phagocytose opsonised particles and microbes and releasing a large repertoire of enzymes (including lactoferrin, cathepsin G, elastase, myeloperoxidase, hydrolase and bacterial-permeability-inducing proteins), oxygen intermediates with antibacterial activity, proinflammatory cytokines – including tumour necrosis factor (TNF)-α and interleukin-1 – and chemokines. Ig, immunoglobulin; NADPH, nicotinamide adenine dinucleotide phosphate.

neutrophils, the recruitment of eosinophils is mediated by chemokines[48] (see below).

Mast cells and basophils possess high-affinity receptors for IgE and thus become coated with IgE antibodies. For this reason, they are crucial in the pathophysiology of asthma, when allergen binding to the IgE cross-links the FcεR. This event triggers the cell to secrete inflammatory mediators, such as histamine, prostaglandins and leukotrienes, that mediate asthma reactions (see Chapter 48).

Chemokines and other chemotactic molecules: major regulators of pulmonary inflammation

The superfamily of chemokines consists of an array of chemoattractant proteins that has been divided into four branches (C, CC, CXC, CXXXC) according to variations in a shared cysteine.[49–51] The current roster approaches 50 related proteins (Table 3.3.1). Structural variations in chemokines have been demonstrated to be associated with differences in their ability to regulate the trafficking of immune cells during inflammation, with a well-defined sequence of events (Fig. 3.3.7)

CC chemokines

Most molecules of this chemokine branch are highly expressed in the lung during inflammatory responses[52] (Table 3.3.1). Monocyte chemoattractant protein 1 (MCP-1/CCL2), monocyte inflammatory protein-1α (MIP-1α/CCL3), MIP-1β/CCL4,

RANTES/CCL5 and eotaxin/CCL11 cooperate to immobilise several leukocyte subpopulations in perivascular foci of inflammation. MCP-1/CCL2 and RANTES/CCL5, interacting with CCR1/CCR2 or CCR1/CCR3/CCR5 respectively, may be chemoattractant for different cell targets that have been involved in the pathogenesis of most lung diseases, including macrophages, T lymphocytes, neutrophils, mast cells and eosinophils.

Furthermore, immature lung dendritic cells respond to many CCs (MIP-1α/CCL3, MIP-1β/CCL4, MIP-3α/CCL20, MIP-5/CCL15, MCP-3/CCL7, MCP-4/CCL14, RANTES/CCL5 and TECK/CCL25) that are inducible upon inflammatory stimuli.[53] Inflammatory chemokines and non-chemokine attractants promote recruitment and localisation of immature dendritic cells at sites of inflammation and infection. Upon exposure to maturation signals, dendritic cells undergo a chemokine receptor switch, with down-regulation of inflammatory chemokine receptors followed by induction of CCR7 (the receptor for 6Ckine/CCL21 and MIP-3β/CCL19). These temporally coordinated events allow dendritic cells to leave tissues and to localise in lymphoid organs by responding to CCR7 agonists.

A positive signal for RANTES/CCL5 has been detected at sites of hypersensitivity reactions.[54] Furthermore, eotaxin/CCL6 has been involved in the recruitment and activation of eosinophils. Other chemokines that may interact with eosinophils are eotaxin-2/CCL24 and eotaxin-3/CCL26.

CXC chemokines

CXC chemokines encompass a number of chemokines that may target T and B lymphocytes, eosinophils, alveolar macro-

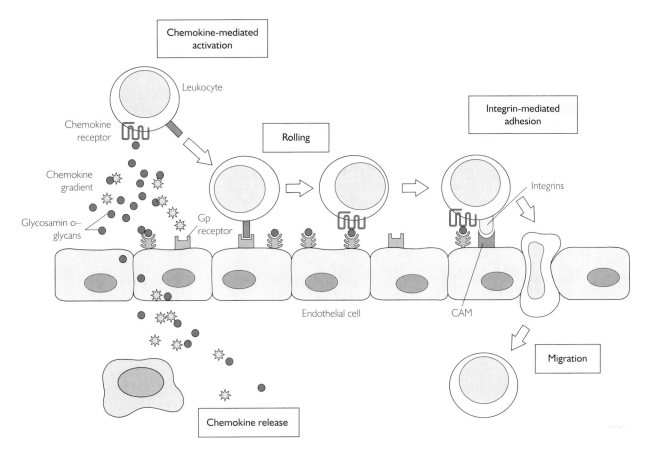

Fig. 3.3.7 Events leading to leukocyte migration into the lung. The secreted chemokine is bound by the extracellular glycosaminoglycan matrix of the endothelial cell and triggers leucocyte rolling along the endothelial wall. The rolling is mediated by lectin selectins that interact with glycoprotein (gp) counter-receptors. During the rolling, chemokines bind to the seven-transmembrane receptors expressed on the surface of the leucocytes, favouring adhesion to the endothelium via upregulation of integrin receptors (cellular adhesion molecule, CAM). The leukocyte migrates into the tissue, where it can secrete inflammatory cytokines and chemokines, facilitating the migration of additional leukocytes to the site of inflammation.

phages and lung dendritic cells (Table 3.3.2). Three lymphocyte-specific CXC chemokines (IP-10/CXCL10, Mig/CXCL9 and I-TAC/CXCL11), which are produced in response to IFN-γ, play an important role in the recruitment of activated T cells into the pulmonary micoenvironment.[11,23] Signalling mediated by these non-ERL CXC-chemokines is mostly directed towards pulmonary activated T lymphocytes. Alveolar macrophages are the main cell source for these molecules; they release large amounts of CXCL10 and CXCL9, which, by interacting with specific receptors expressed by Th1 and Tc1 cells (CXCR3), favours the migration and accumulation of pulmonary T lymphocytes during hypersensitivity reactions, viral infection and response to an allograft.[55,56] Activated bronchial epithelium is another important source of CXCL9, CXCL10 and CXCL11.

Interleukin-8/CXCL8, a chemokine that favours T-cell and neutrophil recruitment, is actively released in the airways during different diffuse lung diseases associated with lung damage.[57] Usually, an elevated percentage of neutrophils in bronchoalveolar lavage fluid, as well as raised levels of the granulocyte activation markers myeloperoxidase and eosinophil cationic protein,

correlates with levels of this chemokine. Immunolocalisation of IL-8 demonstrated that pulmonary fibroblasts in lungs with idiopathic pulmonary fibrosis are the predominant cellular source of IL-8, even if there are data suggesting that macrophages may release this chemokine. Interestingly, pulmonary fibrosis may be associated with increased release of IL-8/CXCL8 and dysregulation of CXCL10/IP-10 production,[58] suggesting that the balance in chemokine production is an important factor in the regulation of local angiogenesis and fibrogenesis. CXC chemokines, as CXCL12/SDF-1, are also able to favour the recruitment and activation of dendritic cells.

CX3C and C chemokines

The fractalkine receptor CX3CR1 is expressed in human CD8+ T lymphocytes, both CD45RO- and CD45RO+ or CD45RO+/CD4+ T cells. Expression of fractalkine/CXC3CL1 has been also detected in endothelial cells of normal human lung, suggesting that CXC3CL1 may contribute to the recruitment of effector Th lymphocytes into the lung.

Table 3.3.1 CC chemokine/receptor family according to the nomenclature of the International Union of Immunological Societies. A name in parentheses indicates that the human homologue has not yet been identified. Note that leukocyte distribution refers to the expression of chemokine receptors by cells involved in pulmonary immunity. The table does not taken into account other cell types that may express CC receptors, including thymocytes and CD34+ cells.

Chemokines		Receptor	Leukocyte distribution
CCL1	I-309	CCR8	B, T, Ma
CCL2	MCP-1/MCAF	CCR2	NK, B, T, Ma, N
CCL3	MIP-1α/ LD78a	CCR1, CCR5	NK, T, DCi, Ma, Ba, E, N
CCL4	MIP-1β	CCR5	B, T, DCm, DCi, Ma
CCL5	RANTES	CCR1,CCR3, CCR5	NK, B, T, DCi, DCm, Ma, Ba, E, N
(CCL6)	Unknown	Unknown	unknown
CCL7	MCP-3	CCR1, CCR2,CCR3	NK, B, T, Ma, N, DCi, B, E
CCL8	MCP-2	CCR2, CCR3	NK, B, T, Ma, N
(CCL9/10)	Unknown	Unknown	Unknown
CCL11	Eotaxin	CCR3	T, Ba, E
(CCL12)	Unknown	CCR2	NK, B, T, Ma, N
CCL13	MCP-4	CCR2, CCR3	NK, B, T, Ma, N
CCL14	HCC-1	CCR1	NK, T, DCi, Ma, Ba, E, N
CCL15	HCC-2/MIP-1δ/Lkn-1	CCR1,CCR3	NK, T, Ba, E, Ma, N
CCL16	HCC-4, LEC	CCR1	NK, T, DCi, Ma, Ba, E, N
CCL17	TARC	CCR4	NK, T, DCi
CCL18	DC-CK1, PARC	Unknown	Unknown
CCL19	MIP-3β/ELC/exodus-3	CCR7	B, T, DCm
CCL20	MIP-3α/exodus-1	CCR6	B, T, DCi, Ma
CCL21	6Ckine/SLC/exodus-2,	CCR7	B, T, DCm
CCL22	MDC, STCP-1	CCR4	NK, T, DCi
CCL23	MPIF-1	CCR1	NK, T, DCi, Ma, Ba, E, N
CCL24	Eotaxin-2/MPIF-2	CCR3	T, Ba, E
CCL25	TECK	CCR9	T
CCL26	Eotaxin-3	CCR3	T, Ba, E
CCL27	CTACK/ALP	CCR10	NK, T

B, B cell; Ba, basophil; DCi, dendritic cell immature; DCm, dendritic cell mature; E, eosinophil; Ma, macrophages; N, neutrophil; NK, natural killer cell; T, T cell.

Concerning C chemokines, there are data from animal models indicating that messages encoding lymphotactin/XCL1 are highly expressed during the development of pneumonitis and fibrosis, together with the message for RANTES/CCL5, IP-10/CXCR3 and MCP-1/CCL2.

Chemokine and lung Th/Th2 cells

Chemokines are believed also to regulate Th1 and Th2 cells, which in turn may influence chemokine release.[59] For instance, MCP-1 favours the formation of the eosinophil-rich type-2 granuloma and also appears to have a broader role in the regulation of Th differentiation and expression at sites of granuloma formation. Two other possible candidates involved in regulating the Th pattern are:

- IL-10, which promotes the Th2-type immune response via the inhibition of Th1-type reactions
- IL-12, which has proinflammatory properties, induces the Th0 versus Th1 shift and stimulates the proliferation and the lytic activity of activated T cells.

In synergy with IL-15, IL-12 also favours contact between activated T cells and antigen-presenting cells. The balance between IL-10 and IL-12 may thus dictate the outcome of pulmonary inflammation. On the other hand, it is also clear that the release of Th1 or Th2 cytokines in the lung tissue polarises lung fibroblasts to produce either RANTES/CCL5 or eotaxin/CCL11 as major eosinophil attractants.[60]

In the last 2 years the challenge to most investigators has been to define and validate therapeutic targets able to inhibit chemokine–chemokine-receptor interactions. A quantity of data has been obtained in the animal model to demonstrate that chemokine blockade impairs inflammatory processes. For instance, using a mouse strain that develops spontaneous, fatal autoimmune disease, it has been shown that deletion of CCR2 or CCL2 attenuates the development of immune disorders in MCP-1-deficient mice.[61] Furthermore, MCP-1−/− mice are deficient in mounting an efficient Th1 polarised response in the antigen-elicited granuloma model. Other data have also clearly shown that neutralising antibodies for CXCR3 ligands have a major effect in attenuating immune responses to foreign antigen. Since, as reported above, CXCR3+ T cells massively

Table 3.3.2 CXC, C and CX3C chemokine/receptor families according to the nomenclature of the International Union of Immunological Societies. A name in parentheses indicates that the human homologue has not yet been identified. Note that leukocyte distribution refers to the expression of chemokine receptors by cells involved in pulmonary immunity. The table does not taken into account other cell types that may express CXC receptors, including platelets, thymocytes and CD34+ cells.

Chemokines		Receptor	Leukocyte distribution
CXC chemokine/receptor family			
CXCL1	GROα, MGSAα	CXCR2>CXCR1	N, Ma, E
CXCL2	GROβ/MIP-2	CXCR2	N, E, Ma
CXCL3	GROγ, MIP-2β	CXCR2	N, E, Ma
CXCL4	PF4	Unknown	Unknown
CXCL5	ENA-78	CXCR2	N, E, Ma
CXCL6	GCP-2	CXCR1, CXCR2	N, Ma, E
CXCL7	NAP-2	CXCR2	N, E, Ma
CXCL8	IL-8	CXCR1, CXCR2	N, E, Ma
CXCL9	Mig	CXCR3	T, B
CXCL10	IP-10	CXCR3	T, B
CXCL11	I-TAC	CXCR3	T, B
CXCL12	SDF-1α/β	CXCR4	N, Ma, DCm, DCi,
CXCL13	BLC, BCA-1	CXCR5	T, B
CXCL14	BRAK/bolekine	Unknown	Unknown
(CXCL15)	Unknown	Unknown	Unknown
C chemokine/receptor family			
XCL1	SCM-1α, ATAC, lymphotactin	XCR1	T, NK
XCL2	SCM-1β	XCR1	T, NK
CX3C chemokine/receptor family			
CX3CL1	Fractalkine	CX3CR1	Ma, T, NK

B, B cell; Ba, basophil; DCi, dendritic cell immature; DCm, dendritic cell mature; E, eosinophil; Ma, macrophages; N, neutrophil; NK, natural killer cell; T, T cell.

infiltrate lung tissue in several diffuse pulmonary inflammatory disorders, it is expected that antibodies to CXCR3 or CXCR3 antagonists might prove to be beneficial in these diseases. In particular, the therapeutic use of molecules selective for chemokine receptors appears to have great potential for all the inflammatory disorders that are characterised by a massive accumulation of T cells within affected organs, including sarcoidosis and other T-cell-mediated diffuse lung diseases.

Other chemotactic molecules

Interleukin-16 is a proinflammatory cytokine produced by CD8 T cells, CD4 T cells, eosinophils, mast cells, fibroblasts and bronchial epithelial cells. This cytokine induces the migratory response of CD4 cells, increases intracellular levels of calcium and inositol 1,4,5-triphosphate, and induces the production of proinflammatory cytokines. IL-16, which is involved in the pathogenesis of hypersensitivity reactions even at the pulmonary level, plays a role in directing lymphocyte emigration from the circulation to sites of inflammation and tissue injury.[62] It has chemoattractant activity for both eosinophils and CD4 T cells and high amounts can be detected in the lung at sites of inflammatory processes where perivascular accumulation of lymphocytes may be demonstrated.

Interleukin-15 is also able to favour the chemotaxis of T cells.[63] It induces migration of lung T cells carrying an effective IL-15 receptor during inflammatory diseases of the lung that are associated with T-cell alveolitis.

Collectively, these data emphasise the role of chemokines and chemotactic molecules in the development of pulmonary inflammation. It is also likely that cell-to-cell and cell-to-matrix interactions modulate the local chemokine expression, contributing to the pathological outcome toward fibrosis of inflammatory lesions.

Conclusions

Several pieces of evidence are emerging on the intriguing maze of the pulmonary host defence mechanisms. This complexity derives from the heterogeneity of the lung effectors spaced along the respiratory tree and from the large repertoire of molecules with pleomorphic activity that are released in situ in a manner that does not interfere with the primary biological functions of the lungs. As we come closer to understanding the pathways that lead to disordered inflammatory and lung immune responses, it is hoped that we will achieve a more efficient approach to the treatment of a variety of idiopathic or progressive and chronic lung diseases that demonstrate impairment or abnormal activity of lung host defences. The availability of new technologies and drugs will provide pharmacological opportunities to achieve control of local immune responses in patients with most inflammatory pulmonary diseases.[64,65]

? Unresolved questions

■ What are the aetiological agents involved in the pathogenesis of diffuse lung disease of unknown aetiology?

■ What mechanisms lead to the perpetuation of the inflammatory response in immune-mediated diffuse lung diseases?

■ Which are the molecules and the molecular mechanisms that regulate the development of lung fibrosis?

■ How useful will chemokine and cytokine antagonists prove to be in the therapy of inflammatory disorders characterised by a massive accumulation of immunocompetent cells within the lung?

References

1. Nicod LP. Pulmonary defence mechanisms. Respiration 1999; 66: 2–11.
2. Zhang P, Summer WR, Bagby GJ, Nelson S. Innate immunity and pulmonary host defense. Immunol Rev 2000; 173: 39–51.
3. Jahnsen FL, Brandtzaeg P. Antigen presentation and stimulation of the immune system in human airways. Allergy 1999; 54: 37–49.
4. Pabst R, Schuster M, Tschernig T. Lymphocyte dynamics in the pulmonary microenvironment: implications for the pathophysiology of pulmonary sarcoidosis. Sarcoidosis Vasc Diffuse Lung Dis 1999; 16: 197–202.
5. Holt PG. Regulation of antigen-presenting cell function(s) in lung and airway tissues. Eur Respir J 1993; 6: 120–129.
6. Semenzato G, Bortolin M, Facco M et al. Lung lymphocytes: origin, biological functions, and laboratory techniques for their study in immune-mediated pulmonary disorders. Crit Rev Clin Lab Sci 1996; 33: 423–455.
7. Agostini C, Chilosi M, Zambello R et al. Pulmonary immune cells in health and disease: lymphocytes. Eur Respir J 1993; 6: 1378–1401.
8. Mehrad B, Standiford TJ. Role of cytokines in pulmonary antimicrobial host defense. Immunol Res 1999; 20: 15–27.
9. Agostini C, Zambello R, Trentin L, Semenzato G. HIV and pulmonary immune responses. Immunol Today 1996; 17: 359–364.
10. Shanley TP, Warner RL, Ward PA. The role of cytokines and adhesion molecules in the development of inflammatory injury. Mol Med Today 1995; 1: 40–45.
11. Loetscher M, Gerber B, Loetscher P et al. Chemokine receptor specific for IP-10 and Mig: structure, function and expression in activated T-lymphocytes. J Exp Med 1996; 184: 963–969.
12. Choi P, Reiser H. IL-4: role in disease and regulation of production. Clin Exp Immunol 1998; 113: 317–319.
13. Striz I, Mio T, Adachi Y et al. IL-4 and IL-13 stimulate human bronchial epithelial cells to release IL-8. Inflammation 1999; 23: 545–555.
14. Temann UA, Geba GP, Rankin JA, Flavell RA. Expression of interleukin 9 in the lungs of transgenic mice causes airway inflammation, mast cell hyperplasia, and bronchial hyperresponsiveness. J Exp Med 1998; 188: 1307–1320.
15. Spits H, de Waal Malefyt R. Functional characterization of human IL-10. Int Arch Allergy Immunol 1992; 99: 8–15.
16. Pretolani M, Goldman M. IL-10: a potential therapy for allergic inflammation? Immunol Today 1997; 18: 277–280.
17. Tinkle SS, Kittle LA, Newman LS. Partial IL-10 inhibition of the cell-mediated immune response in chronic beryllium disease. J Immunol 1999; 163: 2747–2753.
18. De Vries JE. The role of IL-13 and its receptor in allergy and inflammatory responses. J Allergy Clin Immunol 1998; 102: 165–169.
19. Chiaramonte MG, Schopf LR, Neben TY et al. IL-13 is a key regulatory cytokine for Th2 cell-mediated pulmonary granuloma formation and IgE responses induced by Schistosoma mansoni eggs. J Immunol 1999; 162: 920–390.
20. Wills-Karp M. IL-12/IL-13 axis in allergic asthma. J Allergy Clin Immunol 2001; 107: 9–18.
21. Linden A, Hoshino H, Laan M. Airway neutrophils and interleukin-17. Eur Respir J 2000; 15: 973–977.
22. Agostini C, Semenzato G. Cytokines in sarcoidosis. Semin Respir Infect 1998; 13: 184–196.
23. Farber JM. Mig and IP-10: CXC chemokines that target lymphocytes. J Leukocyte Biol 1997; 61: 246–257.
24. Agostini C, Trentin L, Perin A et al. Regulation of alveolar macrophage-T cell interactions during Th1-type sarcoid inflammatory process. Am J Physiol 1999; 277: L240–L250.
25. Romagnani S. The Th1/Th2 paradigm. Immunol Today 1997; 18: 263–266.
26. Romagnani S. T-cell subsets (Th1 versus Th2). Ann Allergy Asthma Immunol 2000; 85: 9–18; quiz 18, 21.
27. Lohmann-Matthes ML, Steinmuller C, Franke-Ullmann G. Pulmonary macrophages. Eur Respir J 1994; 7: 1678–1689.
28. Striz I, Pokorna H, Zheng L et al. Different expression of integrins by mononuclear phagocytes in peripheral blood and bronchoalveolar lavage fluid. Respir Med 1998; 92: 1326–1330.
29. Lyons CR, Ball EJ, Toews GB et al. Inability of human alveolar macrophages to stimulate resting T cells correlates with decreased antigen-specific T cell-macrophage binding. J Immunol 1986; 137: 1173–1180.
30. Chelen CJ, Fang Y, Freeman GJ, et al. Human alveolar macrophages present antigen ineffectively due to defective expression of B7 costimulatory cell surface molecules. J Clin Invest 1995; 95: 1415–1421.
31. Tager AM, Luster AD, Leary CP et al. Accessory cells with immunophenotypic and functional features of monocyte-derived dendritic cells are recruited to the lung during pulmonary inflammation. J Leukocyte Biol 1999; 66: 901–908.
32. Fels AO, Cohn ZA. The alveolar macrophage. J Appl Physiol 1986; 60: 353–369.
33. Holt PG. Pulmonary dendritic cell populations. Adv Exp Med Biol 1993; 329: 557–562.
34. Suda T, McCarthy K, Vu Q et al. Dendritic cell precursors are enriched in the vascular compartment of the lung. Am J Respir Cell Mol Biol 1998; 19: 728–737.
35. Reynolds HY. Advances in understanding pulmonary host defense mechanisms: dendritic cell function and immunomodulation. Curr Opin Pulm Med 2000; 6: 209–216.
36. Lambrecht BN, Pauwels RA, Bullock GR. The dendritic cell: its potent role in the respiratory immune response. Cell Biol Int 1996; 20: 111–120.
37. Sozzani S, Mantovani A, Allavena P. Control of dendritic cell migration by chemokines. Forum (Genoa) 1999; 9: 325–338.
38. Rosenwasser LJ. Biologic activities of IL-1 and its role in human disease. J Allergy Clin Immunol 1998; 102: 344–350.
39. Barton BE. IL-6: insights into novel biological activities. Clin Immunol Immunopathol 1997; 85: 16–20.
40. Shahar I, Fireman E, Topilsky M et al. Effect of IL-6 on alveolar fibroblast proliferation in interstitial lung diseases. Clin Immunol Immunopathol 1996; 79: 244–251.
41. Scott P, Trinchieri G. IL-12 as an adjuvant for cell-mediated immunity. Semin Immunol 1997; 9: 285–291.
42. Scapini P, Lapinet-Vera JA, Gasperini S et al. The neutrophil as a cellular source of chemokines. Immunol Rev 2000; 177: 195–203.
43. Cassatella MA, McDonald PP. Interleukin-15 and its impact on neutrophil function. Curr Opin Hematol 2000; 7: 174–177.
44. Cameron LA, Taha RA, Tsicopoulos A et al. Airway epithelium expresses interleukin-18. Eur Respir J 1999; 14: 553–559.
45. Sibille Y, Marchandise FX. Pulmonary immune cells in health and disease: polymorphonuclear neutrophils. Eur Respir J 1993; 6: 1529–1543.
46. Wagner JG, Roth RA. Neutrophil migration mechanisms, with an emphasis on the pulmonary vasculature. Pharmacol Rev 2000; 52: 349–374.
47. Lane SJ, Lee TH. Mast cell effector mechanisms. J Allergy Clin Immunol 1996; 98: S67–S71.
48. Rothenberg ME. Eotaxin. An essential mediator of eosinophil trafficking into mucosal tissues. Am J Respir Cell Mol Biol 1999; 21: 291–295.
49. Baggiolini M. Chemokines and leukocyte traffic. Nature 1998; 392: 565–568.
50. Luster A. Chemokines – chemotactic cytokines that mediate inflammation. N Engl J Med 1998; 228: 436–445.
51. Kim CH, Broxmeyer HE. Chemokines: signal lamps for trafficking of T and B cells for development and effector function. J Leukocyte Biol 1999; 65: 6–15.
52. Kunkel SL, Lukacs NW, Strieter RM, Chensue SW. The role of chemokines in the immunopathology of pulmonary disease. Forum 1999; 9: 339–355.

53. Sozzani S, Allavena P, Vecchi A, Mantovani A. Chemokines and dendritic cell traffic. J Clin Immunol 2000; 20: 151–160.

54. Devergne O, Marfaing-Koka A, Schall TJ et al. Production of the RANTES chemokine in delayed-type hypersensitivity reactions: involvement of macrophages and endothelial cells. J Exp Med 1994; 179: 1689–1694.

55. Agostini C, Cassatella M, Zambello R et al. Involvement of the IP-10 chemokine in sarcoid granulomatous reactions. J Immunol 1998; 161: 6413–6420.

56. Agostini C, Facco M, Siviero M et al. CXC chemokines IP-10 and mig expression and direct migration of pulmonary CD8+/CXCR3+ T cells in the lung of patients with HIV infection and T-cell alveolitis. Am J Respir Crit Care Med 2000; 162: 1466–1473.

57. Baggiolini M, Moser B, Clark-Lewis I. Interleukin-8 and related chemotactic cytokines. Chest 1994; 105: 95S–98S.

58. Keane MP, Arenberg DA, Lynch JP III et al. The CXC chemokines, IL-8 and IP-10, regulate angiogenic activity in idiopathic pulmonary fibrosis. J Immunol 1997; 159: 1437–1443.

59. Kunkel SL. Th1- and Th2-type cytokines regulate chemokine expression. Biol Signals 1996; 5: 197–202.

60. Teran LM, Mochizuki M, Bartels J et al. Th1- and Th2-type cytokines regulate the expression and production of eotaxin and RANTES by human lung fibroblasts. Am J Respir Cell Mol Biol 1999; 20: 777–786.

61. Tesch GH, Maifert S, Schwarting A et al. Monocyte chemoattractant protein 1-dependent leukocytic infiltrates are responsible for autoimmune disease in MRL-Fas(lpr) mice. J Exp Med 1999; 190: 1813–1824.

62. Yoshimoto T, Wang CR, Yoneto T et al. Role of IL-16 in delayed-type hypersensitivity reaction. Blood 2000; 95: 2869–2874.

63. Waldmann T, Tagaya Y, Bamford R. Interleukin-2, interleukin-15, and their receptors. Int Rev Immunol 1998; 16: 205–226.

64. Standiford TJ, Tsai WC, Mehrad B, Moore TA. Cytokines as targets of immunotherapy in bacterial pneumonia. J Lab Clin Med 2000; 135: 129–138.

65. Semenzato G. Chemotactic cytokines: from the molecular level to clinical use. Sarcoidosis Vasc Diffuse Lung Dis 1998; 15: 131–133.

3 Respiratory defences

3.4 Antiproteinases and antioxidants

Robert A Stockley

 Key points

- Inflammation is central to the pathogenesis of chronic obstructive pulmonary disease

- Proteinases released by inflammatory cells cause tissue damage and many of the pathological features of chronic obstructive pulmonary disease

- Antiproteinases protect lung tissue and limit the area of damage

- Antiproteinases may have other effects, improving tissue repair and contributing to host defences

- Inflammatory cells release a variety of oxidant species when activated

- These oxidants are highly toxic to lung cells

- Antioxidants control the radius of activity of oxidants and thereby protect tissues

- Oxidants have several proinflammatory properties and may perpetuate inflammation

One potential effect of inflammation in the lung is tissue damage that leads to incomplete repair. The ability of inflammatory cells to release proteinases and reactive oxygen species has been implicated in many of the pathological features of chronic obstructive pulmonary disease (COPD). However the lung also has a system of antiproteases and antioxidants that play a critical role in limiting the damaging effects of inflammation. The study of these 'defence' mechanisms has continued over the past 30–40 years, resulting in a clearer understanding of their role in the modulation of lung disease. This chapter provides a general overview of the variety of antiproteinases and antioxidants, together with current knowledge of their function.

Antiproteases

Proteolytic enzymes released from inflammatory cells play a major role in the development of pathological and physiological abnormalities in the lungs because of their ability to digest proteins and damage cells. Experimental studies have shown that these enzymes can disrupt epithelial integrity[1] as well as digesting the cell basement membrane and connective tissues of the lung interstitium. In addition, ciliary beat frequency can be reduced and the presence of these enzymes can lead to other responses, such as mucus gland hyperplasia and mucus secretion.[2] All these processes interrupt the integrity of the lung, thereby reducing both its defences and its ability to move air in and out and exchange gases at the alveolar region. Needless to say, the lung has an equally sophisticated ability to inactivate these enzymes, involving a series of specific protease inhibitors that protect the lung both in health and more specifically during periods of excess inflammation, when the enzymes and their cell sources are present in increased amount and numbers.

Serine proteinase inhibitors

An understanding of the role of proteinases in the pathogenesis of lung disease and the protective influence of antiproteinases dates from a single observation in 1963. Laurell & Eriksson identified five subjects who appeared to have a deficient protein band in the alpha-1 region seen on paper electrophoresis.[3] It was subsequently shown that this protein was the major serum inhibitor of the enzyme trypsin hence it has been known predominantly as alpha-1-antitrypsin (α_1-AT). Of these five patients, three had early-onset severe emphysema. Family studies confirmed that this was an inherited defect and was associated with chronic bronchitis and emphysema being expressed in an autosomal recessive manner.[4]

Shortly after this discovery, animal experiments indicated that the plant proteolytic enzyme papain could produce lesions that were similar to those seen in emphysema in man.[5] These two observations formed the basis of the proteinase/antiproteinase theory of the development of emphysema (and subsequently bronchial disease), because α_1-AT was a major inhibitor of a range of proteolytic enzymes. It was concluded that lung destruction was the results of the release of enzymes in the lung that would normally be inhibited by α_1-AT. Because of the deficiency, the enzymes would be controlled incompletely, leading to excessive tissue destruction. This concept has been extended from emphysema to major airway diseases such as cystic fibrosis,[6] bronchiectasis[7] and acute exacerbations of chronic bronchitis.[8] In these instances it is believed that the inhibitors themselves are not deficient, but excessive release of proteinases overwhelms the protective inhibitory screen, leading once again to pathological change and tissue destruction.

Alpha-1-antitrypsin

For historical reasons α_1-AT has been thought to be the major antiprotease that protects the lung from damage and much of the early work was based on the study of the form and function of this inhibitor, with particular reference to primary or secondary deficiency states.

In early studies, lung lavage data indicated that the concentration of α_1-AT was markedly reduced in the epithelial lining fluid of patients with deficiency.[9] In addition, it was demonstrated that α_1-AT was the predominant inhibitor of the enzyme neutrophil elastase in this fluid. It was concluded that the sequence of events in α_1-AT deficiency related primarily to the lack of an effective elastase inhibitor in the airway and this in turn led to the persistence of neutrophil elastase activity which stimulated macrophages to release LTB4.[10] This subsequently led to further neutrophil recruitment, thereby amplifying the inflammatory process and the defect. The continued release of neutrophil elastase led to connective tissue damage and the development of emphysema in these patients. This sequence of events is summarised in Figure 3.4.1.

On the basis of these studies it seemed logical to prevent the development and progression of emphysema by augmenting the defective levels of α_1-AT both in the blood and the lung. Intravenous replacement therapy[11] and inhaled therapy[12] have been shown to 'normalise' the concentrations of α_1-AT in the lung. This approach and its efficacy will be dealt with in detail below.

Alpha-1-antitrypsin is a 52 kDa glycoprotein consisting of 394 amino acids. The gene is on chromosome 14 at position q32.1 and is transcribed as a 1.6 kilobase messenger RNA. The amino acid at position 358 is methionine, which gives the α_1-AT its enzyme-specificity. During the interaction with the active site of neutrophil elastase, the methionine–serine amino acid sequence is cleaved, resulting in inactivation of the α_1-AT and the elastase, together with the formation of stable enzyme inhibitor complexes.

The protein is made predominantly in the liver but is also expressed in monocytes and macrophages as well as lung epithelial cells (below). Serum α_1-AT has a half-life of approximately 5–6 days, it is produced constitutively with a normal serum concentration of approximately 2 grams per litre. In addition, it demonstrates an 'acute phase' response, which is related to specific response elements in the α_1-AT promoter region. During periods of inflammation the concentration in plasma rises some

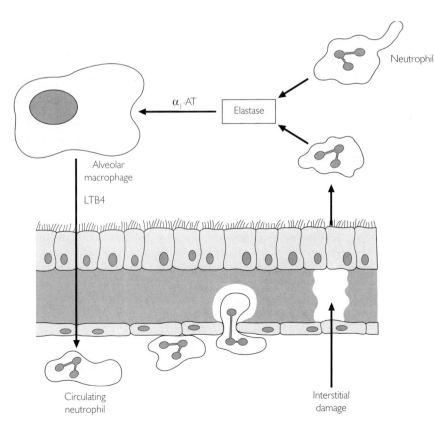

Fig. 3.4.1 Proposed mechanism for perpetuation of inflammation in alpha-1-antitrypsin (α_1-AT) deficiency. Neutrophil recruitment leads to the release of elastase in the lower respiratory tract, which persists because of lack of α_1-AT. The elastase then stimulates alveolar macrophages to release the neutrophil chemoattractant LTB4, leading to neutrophil recruitment. During migration of neutrophils through the lung interstitium, connective tissue damage occurs, leading to the development of progressive emphysema.

two- to fourfold[13] and this, together with endothelial and epithelial leakage as a result of inflammation, leads to markedly increased concentrations within the tissues, thereby increasing its protective role at times when this is particularly necessary. In lung secretions the concentration of α_1-AT increases with infection and the form of α_1-AT is often altered, demonstrating the presence of complexes with neutrophil elastase.[8]

The protein has been called antitrypsin because it was initially demonstrated to be a good inhibitor of trypsin. However, in the lung it has been demonstrated to be a much better inhibitor of neutrophil elastase, and in addition inhibits two other serine proteinases released by the neutrophil (cathepsin G and proteinase 3), both of which have been implicated in the pathological changes of chronic bronchitis and emphysema.[2]

Alpha-1-antitrypsin is transcribed equally from two alleles. The protein itself is polymorphic, with a variety of amino-acid variants, most of which do not influence function. However, these amino-acid substitutions do alter the electrophoretic properties of α_1-AT and it has been customary to describe the variants phenotypically by their isoelectric point. The common variants include the M phenotype (which also has M subsets), the S variant, which is associated with a 40% reduction (approximately) in the circulating concentration of α_1-AT, and the Z variant, which is associated with an 80% reduction in circulating α_1-AT. Heterozygous states lead to intermediate serum concentrations such that the MS heterozygote has approximately 80% of the normal circulating levels, the MZ variant 60% and the SZ variant 30–40%. In addition, there are a variety of other genetic defects that have been described including point mutations, frame shift mutations and major gene deletions,[14] all of which can result in complete absence of production of α_1-AT (null genes). By far the commonest deficiency state, however, is the Z homozygote; the mutation is probably of Scandinavian origin. The prevalence of both the heterozygotes and therefore homozygotes varies geographically, becoming less common further away from Scandinavia.[15]

The α_1-AT variants are inherited in simple autosomal fashion, although the heterozygotes are probably not at an overall increased risk for the development of lung disease.[16] Thus α_1-AT deficiency appears phenotypically to be an autosomal recessive condition. The basic genetic inheritance is shown diagrammatically in Figure 3.4.2.

Risk factors

The Z homozygous state is an accepted risk factor for the development of emphysema. This is almost certainly the case for Znull heterozygotes as well as null patients, although few such patients have been studied or identified through random population screening. However, the SZ heterozygote state is less certain as a risk factor. Large studies of such patients have not been carried out, although the limited data available suggests that there is a low risk of developing lung disease.[17] On the other hand, the MZ heterozygote is almost certainly not a major risk factor, as large epidemiological studies have shown.[16] Nevertheless, it remains a constant observation in several studies that the MZ heterozygote is over-represented in populations of patients with established lung disease.[18-20] On balance, therefore, it is likely that the MZ heterozygote state provides a slightly

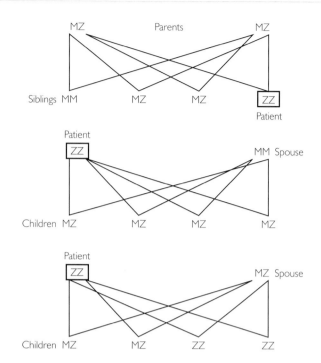

Fig. 3.4.2 Diagrammatic representation of autosomal co-dominant inheritance of common alpha-1-antitrypsin phenotypes (M and Z variant). Identification of a patient with Z deficiency suggests that the parents are likely to be heterozygotes. Screening siblings will identify a significant number of heterozygotes as well as having a 1 in 4 chance of identifying a non-index Z homozygote. The second section indicates the reasons for screening the spouse. A most likely situation is that the spouse will be an M homozygote and all the offspring MZ heterozygotes. However should the spouse be an MZ heterozygote there is a significant chance (1 in 2) of children being homozygous Z (third section).

increased susceptibility to developing disease and perhaps to hospital admission.[21]

However, even Z homozygotes do not invariably develop lung disease. Smoking is clearly an important risk factor and recent studies have also suggested that pollution may play a role.[22] In studies of non-smokers, on the other hand, lung function is often well maintained at least until later in life.[23] A proportion of these never-smokers do subsequently develop lung disease, which may be related to a previous history suggestive of asthma or indeed pollution. Nevertheless, routine population screening can detect healthy individuals with the Z phenotype, suggesting that selection bias may influence our understanding of the impact on disease.

Overall the studies suggest that α_1-AT plays a key role in protecting the lung from damage due to proteolytic enzymes, that there is a threshold level that is relatively protective and finally that the development of protease-mediated lung damage is also dependent upon other factors that lead to or modulate, inflammation.

Clinical features

Patients with α_1-AT deficiency tend to develop respiratory symptoms at a younger age. The emphysema develops rapidly

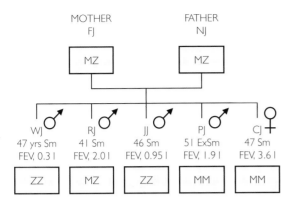

Fig. 3.4.3 Family tree of patient identified with alpha-1-antitrypsin (α_1-AT) deficiency. The index case is a young heavy smoker with severe lung function impairment and one further sibling with severe lung function impairment who is also a Z homozygote. However other siblings of the MZ phenotype who smoke have moderate impairment of lung function and indeed mild impairment is seen in a sibling with a normal α_1-AT. This family suggests that the emphysema trait is genetically inherited, perhaps in a dominant manner, but that the α_1-AT phenotype determines the severity of the condition.

particularly in cigarette smokers. About 40% of the patients develop chronic bronchitis[24] and some patients have clearly reversible airflow obstruction[25] although the relationship between α_1-AT deficiency and asthma remains somewhat contentious. Epidemiological studies have indicated that the lung function of non-index cases is usually better preserved than the index cases[26] and that non-smokers may retain their lung function very well.[23]

Thus, even within families there is some variation and, although cigarette smoke is of major importance, it is likely that other genetic factors are involved. For instance, in the family tree indicated in Figure 3.4.3 it can be seen that airflow obstruction runs through the family although the severity is related to the α_1-AT phenotype.

The protective role of alpha-1-antitrypsin in emphysema

It is generally believed that destruction of lung connective tissue and in particular the integrity of the elastin fibre network, is central to the pathogenesis of emphysema. Connective tissue degradation is believed to occur in the immediate vicinity of migrating neutrophils. α_1-AT inhibits elastase in a 1:1 molecular ratio but elastase release from the azurophil granule produces very high local concentrations approximately 100 times greater than that of serum α_1-AT.[27] Thus, for a period of time and in the immediate vicinity of the granule the concentration of elastase far exceeds even normal α_1-AT levels. The net result would be that any connective tissue that is susceptible to elastase would be degraded in the immediate vicinity of the neutrophil, which may be a critical process to permit neutrophil migration through tight connective tissue matrices. As the elastase diffuses away from the granule the concentration drops exponentially and once the molecular concentration equals that of the surrounding

α_1-AT it will be inactivated.[27] Studies have shown both theoretically[27] and practically[28] that there is a critical concentration of inhibitor (approximately 11 μmol/l) below which the enzyme can diffuse much further before it is inactivated.

The concentration of α_1-AT in the interstitium of the lung, where elastin damage is thought to take place, is largely unknown. However, it is a freely diffusable molecule approximately the same size as albumin and studies have shown that the albumin concentration in the interstitium is approximately 80% of that seen in the circulation because of the relative permeability of the endothelial cells.[29] On the other hand, the epithelial surface of the lung is highly impermeable to protein, leading to a much-reduced concentration of serum protein in the airway. It can therefore be predicted that the concentration of α_1-AT in the interstitium would be approximately 80% of that in plasma. In patients with normal α_1-AT this would be about 24 μmol/l. In those who are heterozygous for α_1-AT deficiency it should be at least 14.4 μmol/l. Whereas, in subjects with severe α_1-AT deficiency (Z homozygote) the predicted concentration would be approximately 4 μmol/l. It can be seen from these data that the concentration of α_1-AT in the interstitium, even in heterozygotes, is above the critical threshold of 11 μmol/l that would limit elastase activity. On the other hand, in homozygous α_1-AT deficiency the concentration is well below this protective level and would result in elastase activity over a wider area before it is dilute enough to be inactivated.

Once elastase is bound to elastin it can continue digesting the substrate and α_1-AT cannot influence this process.[30] It therefore seems likely that the true role of α_1-AT is to provide a significant degree of protection to the interstitium limiting the elastase activity and hence area of damage that can occur as a side effect of neutrophil migration. In α_1-AT deficiency a critically low level can lead to extensive tissue degradation as the enzyme diffuses away before it is dilute enough to be inactivated. These concepts are outlined in Figure 3.4.4.

During periods of inflammation the interstitial concentration of α_1-AT should rise due to a slight increase in vascular leakage but particularly as a result of the acute phase response. This alone may have very little effect on the connective tissue damage that would be produced by the migrating neutrophils (see theory above). Nevertheless, during these episodes the epithelial layer would also become more permeable, permitting diffusion of α_1-AT into the airway where it may now play an additional role protecting the airway from damage due to elastase and other serine proteinases released at this site. This concept will be discussed later.

Implications for augmentation therapy

Studies in the past have shown that intravenous infusion of α_1-AT can lead to an increased concentration in the plasma as well as in the airway.[11] The concentrations achieved have been shown to exceed (for up to a week) the critical threshold for α_1-AT necessary to restrict damage in the airway. Although no clinical trial has yet been carried out that is sufficiently powered to demonstrate the efficacy of such treatment – it can be argued, at least on theoretical grounds, that this approach would be effective.

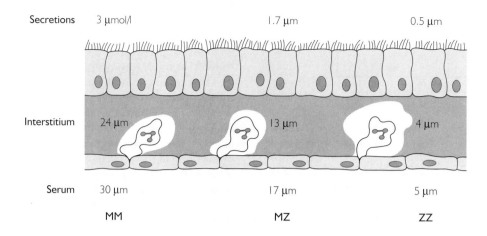

Fig. 3.4.4 Lung alpha-1-antitrypsin (α_1-AT) concentrations. In the normal M homozygote the serum concentration of α_1-AT is approximately 30 µmol/l and the concentration in the interstitium should be approximately 24 µmol/l with a secretion concentration of approximately 3 µmol/l. In MZ heterozygotes the serum concentration is approximately 17 µmol/l leading to 13 µmol/l in the interstitium and 1.7 µmol/l in the airway secretions restricting elastase activity to the near vicinity of the neutrophil limiting tissue damage during cell migration. However in the Z homozygote subjects the serum concentration is 5 µmol/l, that in the interstitium approximately 4 µmol/l and in the airway 0.5 µmol/l. The interstitial concentration is below the critical threshold of 11 µmol/l required to confine elastase activity leading to more extensive connective tissue damage during cell migration and development of emphysema.

Secretory leukoproteinase inhibitor

Secretory leukoproteinase inhibitor (SLPI) is an 11.7 kDa, 107 amino-acid non-glycosylated protein. This enzyme inhibitor is found at many epithelial sites including the parotid glands, in cervical and seminal mucus as well as the lung secretions. In the lung it is produced by tracheal and bronchial cells as well as bronchiolar and type II alveolar cells. In addition, it is produced by Clara cells, serous cells of submucosal glands of the airway, monocytes, macrophages and finally neutrophils. The inhibitor inactivates neutrophil elastase and cathepsin G but, unlike α_1-AT, has no activity again proteinase 3. Again its highest affinity is for neutrophil elastase, suggesting that this is its major target enzyme and, because of its local production, its role is thought to be predominantly at the epithelial surface. However, studies have shown that SLPI can be secreted vectorially by epithelial cells[31] and it has been identified in the lung interstitium associated with lung elastin,[32] suggesting that it plays a role at this site.

Initial studies concluded that SLPI was a non-regulatable protein,[33] although subsequent data has shown that this is not true. Gene transcription can be initiated by TNF-α and IL-1β, as well as neutrophil elastase,[34] although paradoxically the latter leads to a reduction in secretion of SLPI from the cells.[34] More recently, endotoxin, which can increase gene transcription in macrophages,[35] has also been shown to lead to a reduction in secretion of the protein by airway cells.[36] Gene sequence shows the presence of typical five prime TATA and CAAT boxes as well as regulatory sequences for the transcription factors AP1, AP2 and C/EBP.[37]

The protein is thought, conventionally, to be an inhibitor in the airway and certainly at bronchial level it is the major elastase inhibitor even in patients with bronchitis associated with excess mucus production.[38] It is believed to protect the airway from elastase-induced damage and this is supported by animal models.[39] However, in addition, it is a cationic protein that has also been shown to bind to connective tissue, protecting it from enzymes released from activated neutrophils.[40] The inhibitor can also inactivate elastase bound to elastin and hence is more effective than α_1-AT at controlling enzyme at this site.[30]

During periods of inflammation associated with increased neutrophil recruitment to the airway, the concentration of SLPI is decreased in secretions,[41] perhaps as a result of the excess elastase. (The implications of this will be discussed below.) However, the increase in inflammation also permits increased protein transudation from plasma, which results in an associated increase in α_1-AT concentration (Fig. 3.4.5). This may therefore be a protective mechanism in the airway whereby inflammation reduces the local inhibitor while at the same time permitting an increase in the systemic inhibitor to redress the protective anti-elastase role.

At first sight it may seem inappropriate to reduce SLPI concentrations during periods of inflammation when the protease burden may be increased. However, SLPI has been shown to have several other functions that may provide some explanation. Recent data has shown that a serine proteinase is released by the bacterium *Haemophilus influenzae*. This enzyme has been shown to promote adherence and the formation of microcolonies but the enzyme also undergoes autoproteolytic cleavage, which can be prevented by SLPI.[42] Indeed, in the presence of SLPI, adherence and microcolony formation is increased and this would therefore facilitate colonisation of the airway. Clearly, the converse of this situation would be for the host to down-regulate SLPI production and thereby interfere with the adherence and colony formation properties of the bacterium. In addition, studies have shown that endotoxin from *H. influenzae* can equally reduce SLPI in secretions.[36]

However, as indicated previously, during such episodes the serum acute-phase response of α_1-AT and the increased protein leakage into the airway will at least partly redress this balance.

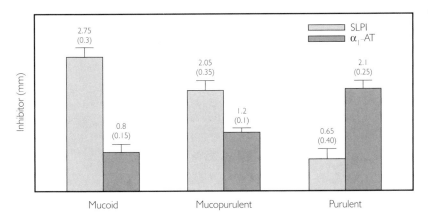

Fig. 3.4.5 This shows the relative concentrations of SLPI and alpha-1-antitrypsin (α_1-AT) in secretions from studies carried out by the author. In mucoid sputum, when inflammation is relatively low, the predominant inhibitor is SLPI with a small contribution from α_1-AT. However, in mucopurulent or purulent secretions, when elastase activity is easily detected, a reduction in SLPI release and the increased diffusion of serum α_1-AT as part of the inflammatory process reverses the relationship of these two inhibitors and α_1-AT predominates.

It is likely, therefore, that these two processes are synergistic. The decrease in SLPI would abrogate bacterial adhesion and microcolony formation while the increase in α_1-AT would protect the airway from enzyme-induced damage. However, it has yet to be demonstrated whether α_1-AT in the airway can have the same effect on bacterial colonisation as SLPI, which would counteract the beneficial effect of reducing the SLPI. These possible interactions are summarised in Figure 3.4.6. These changes have to be weighed against other properties of SLPI, since it has been shown to have specific antiviral and antibacterial properties in its own right.[43]

In addition, to its influence on microorganisms, SLPI also has other anti-inflammatory properties and can reduce the TNF response in macrophages following endotoxin stimulation,[44] which may be mediated through NF-κB, thereby decreasing proinflammatory cytokine production. Furthermore, SLPI has been shown recently to mediate induction of hepatocyte growth factor,[45] thereby acting both as an anti-inflammatory and a regenerative factor. Finally, SLPI may also influence wound healing[46] and can moderate the production of monocyte matrix metalloproteinases,[44] which could influence damage to other lung connective tissue components.

Secretory leukoproteinase inhibitor has also been suggested as an important mediator of the asthma response and animal studies have indicated that SLPI prevents allergen-induced inflammation.[47] The exact mechanisms are unknown, although many allergens are serine proteinases and it may be that the effect is related to its inhibitory properties. Whether this also influences the development of chronic airflow obstruction remains unknown.

Elafin

Studies in the early 1980s suggested that lung secretions contained a further elastase inhibitor and this was subsequently purified and characterised in 1991.[34] The results indicated that the inhibitor was similar to one identified in the skin and referred to as SKALP. The protein is a 9.8 kDa molecule produced by Clara and type 2 cells. Again, the gene has traditional controlling sequences as well as regulatory sequences for AP1 and NF-κB, and transcription can be regulated by the cytokines interleukin 1 and TNF-α as well as elastase.[48] The protein consists of 117 amino acids and at the amino terminus is a sequence that enables protein to form polymers with itself and to adhere to other polypeptides. At present little is known of the role of this protein but its adhesion properties suggest that it may be predominantly a tissue-bound inhibitor. Although elafin has about 40% homology with SLPI, unlike the latter protein it is able to inhibit porcine pancreatic elastase. There have been limited studies of this protein so far; however, its concentration is highest in sputum, where it is approximately 10% of the concentration of SLPI. Its true function at present remains unknown although, as for SLPI, some antibacterial function has been demonstrated in vivo.[49]

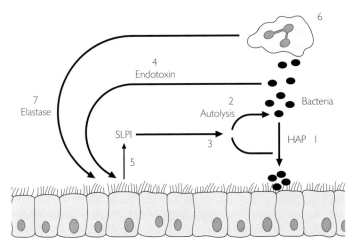

Fig. 3.4.6 The interaction between SLPI and the bacterial proteinase Hap 1. Bacterial Hap leads to adherence and microcolony formation. 2. Hap causes autoproteolysis, preventing this process. 3. SLPI inhibits Hap, preventing autoproteolysis and facilitating adherence and microcolony formation. 4. Endotoxin release by bacteria inhibits SLPI secretions (5.), thereby reducing inhibition of Hap, reducing bacterial adherence and microcolony formation. 6. During inflammation, neutrophils recruited to the airway ingest bacteria and release elastase, which inhibits SLPI release (7.), also preventing microcolony formation and bacterial adherence.

Other serine proteinase inhibitors

Alpha-2-macroglobulin

Alpha-2-macroglobulin is a large protein (780 kDa) that can inhibit a wide range of proteinases, including metalloproteinases. In view of its large size, the concentration of this protein within lung secretions remains low even when inflammation is present. Its role in the protection of the lung, therefore, remains uncertain and deficiency states have not been described.

Alpha-1-antichymotrypsin

Alpha-1-antichymotrypsin, as its name implies, has a greater affinity for chymotrypsin-like enzymes. It is therefore a more efficient inhibitor of cathepsin G than α_1-AT or SLPI. Its concentration in plasma, however, is much lower than that of α_1-AT, although it also shows a rapid acute-phase response.[13] Concentrations of alpha-1-antichymotrypsin in the airway suggest that it is locally produced,[50] although further characterisation suggests that it is present in the latent form rather than functionally active.[51] Alpha-1-antichyotrypsin has been shown to have a major effect on neutrophil chemotactic responses[52] and may therefore play a role in reducing cell migration. In addition, this protein has other effects on the neutrophil that are not dependent upon its enzyme inhibitory properties, including reduction in superoxide anion generation.[53] Both of these functions are likely to protect lung tissue from damage by the relevant mediators.

There have been individual case reports of patients with partial or marked deficiency of alpha-1-antichymotrypsin and there does seem to be an association with lung disease,[54] which suggests that it also plays a role in the modulation of lung damage.

Metalloproteinase inhibitors

The matrix metalloproteinases (MMPs) are becoming increasingly recognised as a family of enzymes capable of degrading a wide variety of connective tissue proteins. Evidence of metalloproteinase activity has been found in the airways of patients with chronic lung disease[55] and the knock-out mouse in which MMP12 has been deleted seems to be protected against the development of cigarette-smoke-induced emphysema.[56] Whether this is a direct result of deletion of the enzyme or a consequence of a reduced inflammatory response remains uncertain. Nevertheless, these studies suggest that the metalloproteinases may be of some relevance to human disease. Metalloproteinases can be inhibited by alpha-2-macroglobulin (see above), although the large size of this protein largely excludes it from the lung, suggesting that it has little role. However, a family of metalloproteinase inhibitors (tissue inhibitors of metalloproteinases; TIMPs) have also been identified, indicating that these enzymes can be regulated at local level.

How these inhibitors influence tissue degradation by their specific enzyme targets is unknown. Recent studies assessing the human MMP9 and its specific inhibitor, TIMP1, have suggested that an imbalance exists between the two in patients with asthma[57] and chronic bronchitis.[58] These results suggest that MMP9 may play a role in the airway in certain situations, which may influence tissue damage and remodelling.

Cysteine proteinase inhibitors

The role of cysteine proteinases in lung disease is also poorly researched. Animal studies have shown that cathepsin B is capable of producing pathological changes in the airway and at alveolar level that are similar to the human conditions bronchitis and emphysema.[59] Cathepsin B activity has been identified in bronchial secretions from patients with lung disease[60] and is thought to be the result of cleavage of the proenzyme to its active form by human neutrophil elastase.[61] Inhibitors of cathepsin B have also been identified in airway secretions,[61] again raising the possibility of an imbalance in some patients that leads to pathological change.

Antioxidants

Reactive oxygen species are highly toxic molecules that are liberated as part of the inflammatory response but by necessity have a short radius of activity.[62] Their conventional role is thought to be in bacterial killing and for this reason patients with a genetic defect of oxidant production (chronic granulomatous disease) are subject to recurrent infections.[63] In contrast, mice that do not express the mitochondrial form of superoxide dismutase (an enzyme that removes oxygen radicals) develop extensive lung damage and do not survive long.[64] Both provide evidence that oxidants and their controls are important in the maintenance of health.

The reactive oxygen species include superoxide anion, hydrogen peroxide, hydroxyl radical and hypochlorous acid. The sources of oxidants in the lung include activation of epithelial cells as well as the inflammatory response and activation of neutrophils and macrophages. Activation of inflammatory cells leads to the generation of superoxide radical from the nicotinamide adenine dinucleotide phosphate (NADPH) oxidase/cytochrome b_{554} system. This reaction can be rapid and 10^6 neutrophils can produce 5 nmol O_2^- in 1 ml in 1 min. Superoxide dismutase can transform superoxide radicals into hydrogen peroxide and hydroxyl radicals can be generated in the presence of ferrous anion. Hydrogen peroxide can be further changed by the presence of myeloperoxidase (MPO), which is an enzyme stored in and released from the azurophil granule of neutrophils. In the presence of chloride ions, MPO activity can lead to the generation of the most toxic reactive species, hypochlorous acid. In addition, interaction of superoxide radicals with nitric oxide can lead to the generation of peroxynitrate, which is also highly toxic to cells. These reactions are shown in Figure 3.4.7.

Thus, there are a variety of situations and chemical events that lead to the generation of these highly toxic species and there is circumstantial evidence that they play a role in the pathogenic processes in acute and chronic lung disease. For instance, cigarette smoke can increase airway resistance via an oxidant-mediated pathway.[65] In addition, treatment of patients with COPD using antioxidants[66–68] can lead to a reduction in the

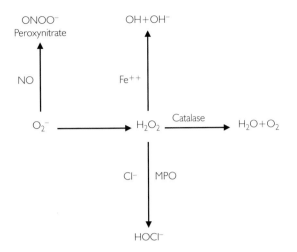

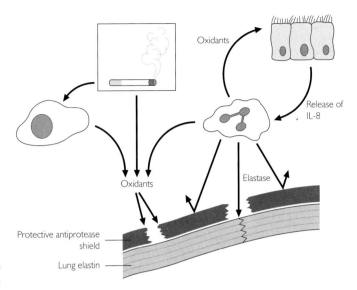

Fig. 3.4.7 Some of the key equations in production of reactive oxygen species are shown. These include the dismutation of oxygen radicals released by inflammatory cells to hydrogen peroxide by the enzyme superoxide dismutase (SOD), the degradation of hydrogen peroxide by catalase and the production of hypochlorous acid from hydrogen peroxide by the enzyme myeloperoxidase (MPO). In addition, in the presence of ferrous anion hydrogen peroxide can generate the hydroxyl radical. Finally, superoxide radicals in the presence of nitric oxide can generate peroxynitrate (see text for details).

Fig. 3.4.8 Proposed mechanisms implicating oxidants in the generation of emphysema. Lung elastin is normally protected from damage by neutrophil elastase by an antiprotease shield. Oxidants released by inflammatory cells and inhaled cigarette smoke inactivate the active site of the inhibitors, leading to a defect in the protective shield. Elastase release from the neutrophils is then able to degrade lung elastin. In addition, oxidants can act on epithelial cells, leading to the release of neutrophil chemoattractants, which results in further recruitment of neutrophils. The process of cell migration in response to this stimulus causes further connective tissue degradation (see text).

number and severity of acute exacerbations (episodes when an oxidant burden results from recruitment and activation of inflammatory cells). Furthermore, a polymorphism of the glutathione S-transferase P1 gene has been shown to be associated with COPD.[69] Enzymes produced by this gene family are thought to be important in the functioning of glutathione, which is a major antioxidant (see below). Finally, epidemiological evidence suggests that a variety of dietary factors known to have antioxidant activity may influence the development and impact of COPD.[70]

Role of reactive oxygen species in chronic lung disease

Because reactive oxygen species have a small radius of activity, their identification either has to be implied or detected by their stabilisation or interaction with appropriate substrates. In the early days it was believed that oxidants either present in inhaled cigarette smoke or from activated inflammatory cells were a major reason for the inactivation of α_1-AT in the lung.[71] The active site of α_1-AT contains methionine, which can be oxidised, leading to a significant reduction in the association rate constant of this inhibitor for its enzyme neutrophil elastase. This mechanism was implicated in the pathogenesis of emphysema in smokers, since it was proposed that it led directly to a functional deficiency of α_1-AT, thereby resulting in emphysema by a similar mechanism to that seen for genetic deficiency (Fig. 3.4.8).

Subsequent studies produced contradictory results and evidence for oxidative inactivation of α_1-AT has been elusive. Nevertheless, there is undoubtedly reactive oxygen species stress, either continually or particularly at times of increased inflammation (such as during exacerbations), in patients with COPD.[72] It is possible that the major influence of reactive oxygen species is indirect via the amplification of inflammation through cell-signalling pathways involving the transcription factors AP1 and NF-κB. For instance, oxidants from cigarette smoke have been shown to influence the neutrophil chemoattractant interleukin-8 production by airway epithelial cells[73] and this in its own right would lead to inflammation via neutrophilic infiltration. Whatever the mechanism, it is clearly important to control the activity of these reactive species and for this reason both cells and lungs have sophisticated mechanisms for their regulation.

Non-enzymatic antioxidants

Free methionine is present in all biological fluids. Because of its small size it is freely diffusible and free methionine has been shown to be highly protective for tissues against oxidants released by inflammatory cells.[62]

Taurine is another amino acid that is distributed widely in both extracellular and intracellular spaces. It is able to react directly with species such as hypochlorous acid to form less reactive molecules and has been shown to limit connective tissue degradation by activated neutrophils, although only partially.[74]

Vitamins have long been considered to be important antioxidants. Vitamin E is lipid-soluble and has been shown to limit oxidant-induced membrane injury in human tissues.[75] It is particularly effective in converting O_2^-, OH• and lipid peroxyl radicals to less reactive oxygen metabolites. Although present in extracellular fluids, vitamin E is localised predominantly in the cell membrane. β-carotene is a metabolic precursor of vitamin A that accumulates in high concentrations in the membranes of certain tissues and can scavenge O_2^- and react directly with peroxyl free radicals. Finally, vitamin C is widely available in both the extracellular and intracellular spaces. Again it can scavenge O_2^- and OH•, forming a semi-dehydroascorbate-free radical that is subsequently reduced by glutathione (see below).

Antioxidant enzyme systems

Catalase is an antioxidant enzyme that is effective in converting hydrogen peroxide to water and is located primarily in peroxisomes, which contain many of the enzymes that generate H_2O_2. Superoxide dismutase is an enzyme that uses superoxide anion as a substrate, although it has variable effects on the overall oxidant/antioxidant balance. For instance, the removal of superoxide anion could be seen to be protective but this is at the expense of generating hydrogen peroxide, which can be used in the presence of ferrous anion to increase the production of the hydroxyl radical. If on the other hand ferrous anion is compartmentalised or unavailable, the hydrogen peroxide can be removed by enzymes such as catalase, therefore providing a protective role.

The glutathione redox cycle

This is perhaps the best studied of all the antioxidant systems. Glutathione (GSH) is a tripeptide (L-γ-glutamyl-L-cysteinyl-glycine) containing a thiol group. GSH is thought to be critical in the lung antioxidant defences, particularly in protecting airspace epithelium from oxidative/free radical mediated injury. GSH levels have been shown to be altered in a variety of inflammatory conditions. For example, GSH is decreased in lung secretions in interstitial pulmonary fibrosis,[76] adult respiratory distress syndrome[77] and cystic fibrosis[78] but increased in patients with mild asthma[79] and chronic smokers.[80]

The glutathione redox cycle is a self-generating cycle in which glutathione becomes oxidised via its interaction with oxygen species to the oxidised form glutathione disulphide. This product can then be transformed by GSH reductase to regenerate active glutathione. GSH synthesis is under the control of a rate limiting enzyme, γ-glutamyl cysteine synthetase. The heavy subunit and light subunit genes for this enzyme contain regulatory sequences, including an antioxidant response element. These regulatory sequences are activated by oxidants and inflammatory and anti-inflammatory agents in a complex interaction. In addition, another enzyme, γ-glutamyl transpeptidase, may cleave extracellular glutathione into its constituent amino acids, resulting in the resynthesis of intracellular glutathione. Thus, glutathione synthesis, oxidation, regeneration and resynthesis are complex processes that can be modulated by the inflammatory milieu as well as the oxidants themselves. Whether defects in this regulation are associated with increased susceptibility to lung disease has yet to be determined. These complex interactions are dealt with in detail in the review article by Rahman & MacNee[81] but further studies will be necessary to clarify their role in the development of lung disease.

In summary the lung can be damaged by several byproducts of the inflammatory process, including proteinases and oxygen radicals. A complex system of protective mechanisms has been evolved to prevent this damage. However the enzymes and oxygen radicals themselves may also play a central role in the generation and modulation of inflammation in the lung. The exact roles of these processes (protective or damaging) will only become known with the development of specific therapeutic probes.

? Unresolved questions

- Do oxidants affect disease progression?
- If so, why, when, how?
- Do enzymes affect disease progression?
- If so, which ones, when, why, how?
- Do specific agonists modify disease progression?

Clinical relevance

- All patients with COPD early-onset emphysema (especially) should be tested for α_1-antitrypsin deficiency
- Strategies to modulate inflammation should be undertaken:
  - Smoking cessation
  - Rapid treatment of exacerbations
  - Balanced diet
- Antioxidant and inhaled corticosteroids should be considered for frequent exacerbations

References

1. Peterson MW, Walter ME, Nygaard SD. Effect of neutrophil mediators on epithelial permeability. Am J Respir Cell Mol Biol 1995; 13: 719–727.
2. Stockley RA. The pathogenesis of chronic obstructive lung diseases: implications for therapy. Q J Med 1995; 88: 141–146.
3. Laurell C, Eriksson S. The electrophoretic α1-globulin pattern of serum in α1-antitrypsin deficiency. Scand J Clin Lab Invest 1963; 15: 132–140.
4. Eriksson S. Studies of α-1 antitrypsin deficiency. Acta Med Scand 1965; 177(suppl. 432): 1–85.
5. Gross P, Pfizer EH, Tolker E et al. Experimental emphysema: its production with papain in normal and silicotic rats. Arch Environ Health 1964; 11:50–58.
6. Jackson AH, Hill SL, Afford SC, Stockley RA. Sputum sol phase proteins and elastase activity in patients with cystic fibrosis. Eur J Respir Dis 1984; 65: 114–124.
7. Stockley RA, Hill SL, Morrison HM. Effect of antibiotic treatment on sputum elastase in bronchiectatic outpatients in a stable clinical state. Thorax 1984; 39: 414–419.
8. Stockley RA, Burnett D. Alpha-1-antitrypsin and leukocyte elastase in infected and non-infected sputum. Am Rev Respir Dis 1979; 120: 1081–1086.

9. Gadek JE, Fells GA, Zimmerman RL et al. Antielastases of the human alveolar structures: implications for the protease–antiprotease theory of emphysema. J Clin Invest 1981; 68: 889–898.

10. Hubbard RC, Fells G, Gadek J et al. Neutrophil accumulation in the lung in alpha-1-antitrypsin deficiency. J Clin Invest 1991; 88: 891–897.

11. Gadek JE, Klein HG, Holland PV, Crystal RG. Replacement therapy of alpha-1-antitrypsin deficiency reversal of protease–anti-protease balance within alveolar structures of PiZ subjects. J Clin Invest 1981; 68: 1158–1165.

12. Hubbard RC, Brantly ML, Sellars SC et al. Anti-neutrophil elastase defences of the lower respiratory tract in α1-antitrypsin deficiency, direct augmentation with aerosol α1-antitrypsin. Ann Intern Med 1989; 111: 206–212.

13. Aronsen KF, Ekelund G, Kindmark CO, Laurell CB. Sequential changes of plasma proteins after surgical trauma. Scand J Clin Lab Invest 1972; 29: 127–136.

14. Brantly M, Nukiwa T, Crystal RG. Molecular basis of alpha-1-antitrysin deficiency. Am J Med 1988; 84: 13–31.

15. Hutchinson DC. Alpha 1-antitrypsin deficiency in Europe: geographical distribution of Pi types S and Z. Respir Med 1998; 92 (3): 367–377.

16. Bruce RM, Cohen BH, Diamond EL et al Collaborative study to assess risk of lung disease in PiMZ phenotype subjects. Am Rev Respir Dis 1984; 130: 386–390.

17. Turino GM, Barker AF, Brantly ML et al. Clinical features of individual with PiSZ phenotype of alpha1-antitrypsin deficiency. Alpha-1-antitrypsin deficiency registry study group. Am J Respir Crit Care Med 1996; 154: 1718–1725.

18. Lieberman J, Winter B, Sastre A. Alpha-1-antitrysin Pi-types in 965 COPD patients. Chest 1986; 89: 370–373.

19. Janus ED. Alpha-1-antitrypsin Pi types in COPD patients. Chest 1988; 92: 446–447.

20. Stockley RA. Alpha-1-antitrypsin phenotypes in cor pulmonale due to chronic obstructive airways disease. Q J Med 1979; 191: 419–428.

21. Seersholm N, Wilcke JTR, Kok-Jensen A, Dirksen A. Risk of hospital admission for obstructive pulmonary disease in alpha-1-antitrypsin heterozygotes of phenotype PiMZ. Am J Respir Crit Care Med 2000; 161: 81–84.

22. Mayers AS, Stoller JK, Bucher Bartelson B et al. Occupational exposure risks in individuals with PI*Z alpha(1)-antitrypsin deficiency. Am J Respir Crit Care Med 2000; 162: 553–558.

23. Janus ED, Phillips NT, Carrell RW. Smoking, lung function, alpha-1-antitrypsin deficiency. Lancet 1985; 1: 152–154.

24. Brantly ML, Paul LD, Miller BH et al. Clinical features and history of the destructive lung disease associated with α1-antitrypsin deficiency of adults with pulmonary symptoms. Am Rev Respir Dis 1988; 138: 327–366.

25. Eden E, Mitchell D, Mehlman B et al. Atopy, asthma and emphysema in patients with severe α-1-antitrypsin deficiency. Am J Respir Crit Care Med 1997; 156: 68–74.

26. Seersholm N, Kok-Jensen A, Dirksen A. Survival of patients with severe alpha-1-antitrypsin deficiency with special reference to non index cases. Thorax 1994; 94: 695–698.

27. Liou TG, Campbell EJ. Nonisotropic enzyme-inhibitor interactions: a novel nonoxidative mechanism for quantum proteolysis by human neutrophils. Biochemistry 1995; 34: 16171–16177.

28. Liou TG, Campbell EJ. Quantum proteolysis resulting from release of single granules by human neutrophils. J Immunol 1996; 2624–2631.

29. Gorin AB, Stuart PA. Differential permeability of endothelial and epithelial barriers to albumin flux. J Appl Physiol 1979; 47: 1315–1324.

30. Morrison HM, Welgus HG, Burnett D et al. Effect of anti-elastases on human leukocyte elastase (HLE) bound to elastin: mechanism of action. Am Rev Respir Dis 1988; 4: 204.

31. Dupuit F, Jacquot J, Spilmont C et al. Vectorial delivery of newly-synthesized secretory proteins by human tracheal gland cells in culture. Epithel Cell Biol 1993; 2: 91–99.

32. Willems LN, Otto-Verberne CJ, Kramps JA et al. Detection of antileukoprotease in connective tissue of lung. Histochemistry 1986; 86: 165–168.

33. Dijkman JH, Kramps JA, Franken C. Antileukoprotease in sputum during bronchial infections. Chest 1986; 89: 731–736.

34. Sallenave JM, Marsden MD, Ryle AP. Isolation of elafin and elastase-specific inhibitor (ESI) from bronchial secretions. Evidence of sequence homology and immunological cross-reactivity. Biol Chem Hoppe-Seyler 1992; 373: 27–33.

35. Jin F-Y, Nathan C, Radzioch D, Ding A. Secretory leukocyte protease inhibitor: a macrophage product induced by and antagonistic to bacterial lipopolysaccharide. Cell 1997; 88: 417–426.

36. Campbell JK, McCann KP, Stewart PM, Stockley RA. Regulation of secretory leukoprotease inhibitor by sputum. Am J Respir Crit Care Med 1999; 159: A192.

37. Kikuchi T, Abe T, Satoh K et al. Cis-acting region associated with lung-cell specific expression of the secretory leukoprotease inhibitor gene. Am J Respir Cell Mol Biol 1997; 17: 361–367.

38. Stockley RA, Morrison HM, Smith S, Tetley T. Low molecular mass bronchial proteinase inhibitor and alpha-1-proteinase inhibitor in sputum and bronchoalveolar lavage. Hoppe-Seylers Z Physiol Chem 1984; 365: 587–595.

39. Rudolphus A, Heinsel-Wieland R, Vincent VAMM et al. Oxidation-resistant variants of recombinant anti-leucoprotease are better inhibitors of human-neutrophil-elastase-induced emphysema in hamsters than natural recombinant antileucoprotease. Clin Sci 1991; 81: 777–784.

40. Llewellyn-Jones CG, Lomas DA, Stockley RA. Potential role of recombinant secretory leucoprotease inhibitor in the prevention of neutrophil mediated matrix degradation. Thorax 1994; 49: 567–572.

41. Hill AT, Bayley D, Stockley RA. The inter-relationship of sputum inflammatory markers in patients with chronic bronchitis. Am J Respir Crit Care Med 1999; 160: 893–898.

42. Hendrixson DR, St Geme JW III. The Haemophilus influenzae Hap serine protease promotes adherence and microcolony formation, potentiated by a soluble host protein. Molec Cell 1998; 2: 841–850.

43. Schalkwijk J, Wiedow O, Hirose S. The trappin gene family: proteins defined by an N-terminal transglutaminase substrate domain and a C-terminal four-disulphide core. Biochem J 1999; 340: 569–577.

44. Zhang Y, DeWitt DL, McNeely TB et al. Secretory leukocyte protease inhibitor suppresses the production of monocyte prostaglandin H synthase-2 prostaglandin E2, and matrix matalloproteinases. J Clin Invest 1997; 199: 894–900.

45. Kikuchi T, Abe T, Yaekashiwa M et al. Secretory leukoprotease inhibitor augments hepatocyte growth factor production in human lung fibroblasts. Am J Respir Cell Mol Biol 2000; 23: 364–370.

46. Ashcroft OS, Lei K, Jin W et al Secretory leukocyte protease inhibitor mediates non-redundant functions necessary for normal wound healing. Nat Med 2000; 6: 1147–1153.

47. Wright CD, Havill AM, Middleton SC et al. Secretory leukocyte protease inhibitor prevents allergen-induced pulmonary responses in animal models of asthma. J Pharmacol Exp Ther 1999; 289: 1007–1014.

48. Sallenave J-M, Silva A. Characterization and gene sequence of the precursor of elafin, an elastase-specific inhibitor in bronchial secretions. Am J Respir Cell Mol Biol 1993; 8: 439–445.

49. Simpson AJ, Maxwell AL, Govan JRW et al. Elafin (elastase-specific inhibitor) has anti-microbial activity against Gram-positive and Gram-negative respiratory pathogens. FEBS Lett 1999; 452: 309–313.

50. Stockley RA, Burnett D. Alpha-1-antichymotrypsin in infected and non-infected sputum. Am Rev Respir Dis 1980; 122(1): 81–88.

51. Chang WS, Lomas DA. Latent α-1-antichymotrypsin. A molecular explanation for the inactivation of alpha-1-antichymotrypsin in chronic bronchitis and emphysema. J Biol Chem 1998; 273: 3695–3701.

52. Lomas DA, Stone SR, Llewellyn-Jones C et al. The control of neutrophil chemotaxis by inhibitors of cathepsin G and chymotrypsin. J Biol Chem 1995; 270: 3437–3443.

53. Kilpatrick L, Johnson JL, Nickbarg EB et al. Inhibition of human neutrophil superoxide generation by alpha 1-antichymotrypsin. J Immunol 1991; 146: 2388–2393.

54. Poller W, Faber J-P, Weidinger S et al. A leucine-to-proline substitution causes a defective α-1-antichymotrypsin allele associated with familial obstructive lung disease. Genomics 1993; 17: 740–743.

55. Finlay GA, Russell KJ, McMahon KJ et al. Elevated levels of matrix metalloproteinases in bronchoalveolar lavage fluid in emphysematous patients. Thorax 1997; 52: 502–506.

56. Hautamaki RD, Kobayashi DK, Senior RM, Shapiro SD. Requirement for macrophage elastase for cigarette smoke-induced emphysema in mice. Science 1997; 277: 2002–2004.

57. Ohno I, Ohtani II, Nitta Y et al. Eosinophils as a source of matrix matalloproteinase-9 in asthmatic airway inflammation. Am J Respir Cell Mol Biol 1997; 16: 212–219.

58. Viguola AM, Riccobono L, Mirabella A et al. Sputum metalloproteinase-9/tissue inhibitor of metalloproteinase-1 ratio correlates with airflow obstruction in asthma and chronic bronchitis. Am J Respir Crit Care Med 1998; 158: 1945–1950.

59. Lesser M, Padilla ML, Cordozo C. Induction of emphysema in hamsters by intra-tracheal installation of cathepsin B. Am Rev Respir Dis 1992; 145: 661–668.

60. Burnett D, Stockley RA. Cathepsin B-like cysteine proteinase activity in sputum and bronchoalveolar lavage samples: relationship to inflammatory cells and effects of corticosteroids and antibiotic treatment. Clin Sci 1985; 68: 469–474.

61. Buttle DJ, Abrahamson M, Burnett D et al. Human sputum cathepsin B degrades proteoglycan, is inhibited alpha-2-macroglobulin and is modulated by neutrophil elastase cleavage of cathepsin B precursor and cystatic. Cell Biochem 1991; 276: 325–331.

62. Weiss SJ. Tissue destruction by neutrophils. N Engl J Med 1989; 320: 365–376.

63. Curnette JT, Whitten DM, Babior BM. Defective superoxide production by granulocytes from patients with chronic granulomatous disease. N Engl J Med 1974; 290: 593–597.
64. Huang TT, Carlson EJ, Raineri I et al. The use of transgenic and mutant mice to study oxygen free radical metabolism. Ann NY Acad Sci 1999; 893: 95–112.
65. Wright JL, Sun JP, Churg A. Cigarette smoke exposure causes constriction of rat lung. Eur Respir J 1999; 14: 1095–1099.
66. Pela R, Calcagni AM, Subiaco S et al. N-acetylcysteine reduces the exacerbation rate in patients with moderate to severe COPD. Respiration 1999; 66: 495–500.
67. Boman G, Backer U, Larsson S et al. Oral acetylcysteine reduces exacerbation rate in chronic bronchitis: report of a trial organized by the Swedish Society of Pulmonary Diseases. Eur J Respir Dis 1983; 64: 405–415.
68. Multicentre Study Group. Long-term oral acetylcysteine in chronic bronchitis. A double-blind controlled study. Eur J Respir Dis 1980; 60(suppl. 111): 93–108.
69. Ishii T, Matsuse T, Teramoto S et al. Glutathione S-transferase P1 (GSTP1) polymorphism in patients with chronic obstructive pulmonary disease. Thorax 1999; 54: 693–696.
70. Britton JR, Pavord ID, Richards KA et al. Dietary antioxidant vitamin intake and lung function in the general population. Am J Respir Crit Care Med 1995; 151: 1383–1387.
71. Carp H, Janoff A. Possible mechanisms of emphysema in smokers. In vitro suppression of serum elastase-inhibitory capacity by fresh cigarette smoke and its prevention by anti-oxidants. Am Rev Respir Dis 1978; 118: 617–621.
72. Rahman I, Skwarska E, MacNee W. Attenuation of oxidant/anti-oxidant imbalance during treatment of exacerbations of chronic obstructive pulmonary disease. Thorax 1997; 52: 565–568.
73. Nishikawa M, Kakemizu N, Ito T et al. Superoxide mediates cigarette smoke-induced infiltration of neutrophils into the airways through nuclear factor-κB activation and IL-8 mRNA expression in guinea pigs in vivo. Am J Respir Cell Mol Biol 1999; 189–198.
74. Weiss SJ, Regiani S. Neutrophil degrade subendothelial matrices in the presence of alpha-2-proteinase inhibitor. J Clin Invest 1984; 73: 1297–1303.
75. Burton GW, Ingold KU. Auto oxidation of biological molecules. 1. The antioxidant activity of vitamin E and related chain-breaking phenolic antioxidants in vitro. J Am Chem Soc 1981; 103: 6472–6477.
76. Cantin AM, Hubbard RC, Crystal RG. Glutathione deficiency in the epithelial lining of the lower respiratory tract in idiopathic pulmonary fibrosis. Am Rev Respir Dis 1989; 139: 370–372.
77. Bunnel E, Pacht ER. Oxidised glutathione is increased in the alveolar fluid of patients with the adult respiratory distress syndrome. Am Rev Respir Dis 1993; 148: 1174–1178.
78. Roum JH, Behl R, McElvaney NG et al. Systemic deficiency of glutathione in cystic fibrosis. J Appl Physiol 1993; 75: 2419–2424.
79. Smith LJ, Houston M, Anderson J. Increased levels of glutathione in bronchoalveolar lavage fluid from patients with asthma. Am Rev Respir Dis 1993; 147: 1461–1464.
80. Morrison D, Rahman I, Lannan S, MacNee W. Epithelial permeability, inflammation and oxidant stress in the airspaces of smokers. Smoking as a cause of oxidative damage. Am J Respir Crit Care Med 1999; 159: 473–479.
81. Rahman I, MacNee W. Oxidative stress and regulation of glutathione in lung inflammation. Eur Respir J 2000; 16: 534–554.

3.5 Lung inflammation and repair

Christopher Haslett

Key points

- Inflammation is a powerful, principally beneficial response to injury or infection.

- The inflammatory response is a precarious balance that can easily be tipped towards excessive and persistent tissue injury, which characterises most inflammatory diseases.

- The dynamics of the interaction between neutrophils and endothelial or epithelial cells are a major determinant of the occurrence of injury.

- Understanding of how inflammation resolves and how repair occurs is critical for the development of successful therapies in inflammatory diseases.

- The degree of injury to the epithelium and its basement membrane during the primary inflammatory damage to the lung is a key factor in excessive scarring.

The biological battlefield

For many centuries inflammation has been recognised as a beneficial response of the host to injury or infection. Metchnikoff, the founder of inflammatory cell biology, described inflammation as 'a salutary response to some injurious influence', early surgeons were reassured by the appearance of 'the noble pus' and, from his experience on the battlefields of Europe, John Hunter asserted that 'inflammation is itself not to be considered as a disease but as a salutary operation consequent either to some violence or to some disease'. Indeed, battlefield analogies are useful to illustrate the cellular events of inflammatory processes generated by bacterial invasion of tissues; lung inflammation is initiated by the responses of a highly sensitive resident 'garrison' (alveolar macrophages and other cells), which calls in large numbers of rapidly mobile, highly responsive and heavily armed 'forward commando troops' (neutrophil granulocytes); these remain under the influence of the newly arrived 'battalion commanders' (monocyte-derived inflammatory macrophages), which sense the need for further troop deployment by calling in more inflammatory cells if required and yet are highly effective killers in their own right. Inflammatory macrophages also act as effective scavengers of dead and injured bacteria. What could be better for the overall efficiency of the operation when, after a successful antibacterial offensive, large numbers of troops conveniently remove themselves from the battlefield in a mass 'altruistic' suicide process (see below)?

Beneficial aspects of inflammation

Perhaps the best example of a 'beneficial' inflammatory response in the lungs is provided by the massive accumulation of inflammatory cells that occurs in the lungs in response to streptococcal invasion during the development of lobar pneumonia. In the preantibiotic era, full-blown streptococcal pneumonia was very common. In one series of patients from the Harlem Hospital, more than 3000 cases were admitted over a 5-year period and lobar pneumonia was found incidentally in more than 20% of all necropsies.[1] At least 70% of patients survived – a clear testament to the effectiveness of the inflammatory response in protecting the host against a potentially lethal invasion of bacteria. The other remarkable feature of lobar pneumonia is its clear potential to resolve completely, leaving no obvious residual tissue injury or scarring.[2] These days, this seems quite remarkable when we consider the enormous potential of neutrophils and macrophages to release agents that can injure tissues, exacerbate inflammation and promote scarring.

This is not to suggest that there is no host tissue injury when the battle is at its most fierce – even modern armies are familiar with the concept of 'friendly fire' and 'bystander injury'. Histological examination of lobar pneumonia during the stage of red hepatisation, when maximal consolidation of the lobe with inflammatory cells is occurring, shows clear evidence of injury to epithelial and endothelial cell layers. However, the injury must not be so severe or extensive as to prevent healing. This leads to the concept of resolution of inflammation, together with the repair of inevitable tissue injury, as important late phases of the inflammatory response. The fact that there is inevitable injury to healthy tissues even in 'beneficial inflammation' suggests that there are phases of the inflammatory response when this powerful process is barely under control and that little further provocation might be required to tip this precarious balance towards the excessive and persistent tissue injury states that characterise most inflammatory diseases.

Although the destructive capacity of inflammation has only been fully recognised in recent decades, the warfare analogy suggests some speculations about the circumstances in which inflammation could become part of a disease process; the foe itself may be impregnable in spite of persistent waves of acute and chronic inflammation, and attempts to 'wall off the problem' by excessive tissue scarring may occur (e.g. asbestosis, silicosis); the attack may be misdirected against host tissues, which themselves have become altered so as to resemble the enemy; or the processes of inflammation and repair may be disordered and uncontrolled, with the troops 'going berserk', killing innocent bystanders indiscriminately and causing an excessive scarring response leading to inappropriate, generalised fibrosis.

Termination of acute inflammation

In the early 18th century, Sir William Cullen[3] recognised that acute inflammation could have more than one outcome, and he described resolution, gangrene (necrosis or tissue destruction) and the formation of 'scirrhus' (scarring). In the intervening years, little attention has been paid to the processes whereby inflammation might terminate but, in his treatise on acute inflammation, Hurley[4] considered that the acute inflammatory response might terminate by resolution, scarring, suppuration or abscess formation, or by the development of chronic inflammation. It is reasonable to suggest that all the alternatives to resolution represent compromises that could contribute to disease processes, particularly in the lung, where function depends critically on the integrity of delicate gas-exchange membranes. Why some bacteria provoke inflammatory processes that resolve (e.g. streptococcal pneumonia), whereas others are associated with persistent inflammation, suppuration and abscess formation (staphylococcal pneumonia) or tissue destruction (*Klebsiella* pneumonia), is a mystery, the solution of which is likely to yield important new insights into the pathogenesis of inflammatory diseases.

The paradox – detrimental effects of inflammation and inflammatory disease

More recently it has become clear that inflammation plays a central role in the pathogenesis of a range of lung diseases:

- chronic bronchitis and emphysema
- bronchial asthma
- adult respiratory distress syndrome (ARDS)
- neonatal respiratory distress syndrome
- fibrosing alveolitis
- extrinsic allergic alveolitis
- pneumoconioses
- bronchiectasis
- cystic fibrosis
- lung injury in bacterial pneumonias
- lung involvement in systemic connective-tissue disorders.

These diseases are characterised by the persistent accumulation of inflammatory cells, which is often accompanied by tissue destruction or a scarring response. Inflammation and its sequelae can interfere with lung function at many levels. Gross thickening of the peripheral lung and pleura with chronic inflammatory tissue and fibrosis interferes with lung inflation and deflation, and the function of the diaphragm and intercostal muscles may be disrupted in polymyositis and other connective-tissue diseases. Inflammation may also interfere with gas exchange by several mechanisms:

- **small-airway inflammation and leakage of fluid and protein**: contributes to the mucous plugging and submucosal oedema that make important contributions to airway obstruction and disordered gas exchange in bronchial asthma
- **major loss of the lung surface area available for gas exchange**: in chronic obstructive pulmonary disease it is thought that smoking causes persistent low-grade inflammation and release of destructive proteolytic enzymes from neutrophils and other inflammatory cells, which over many years destroy the alveolar septa
- **thickening of the interstitial spaces** by inflammatory oedema (e.g. ARDS) or scar tissue (e.g. fibrosing alveolitis): these processes markedly impair oxygen transport in the lung. Unlike some other organs (e.g. skin), where extravascular oedema and even scarring may cause little more than undesirable cosmetic effects, these processes occurring diffusely in the lung cause catastrophic loss of lung function and serious morbidity and mortality.

As a result of these detrimental effects, much research effort has been directed at events involved in the initiation and amplification of acute inflammation. The recent explosion of knowledge about cellular and molecular mechanisms has provided a number of specific therapeutic targets in the earliest phases of acute inflammation, e.g. in the latent phase of ARDS. However, many inflammatory lung diseases present after the early initiation phases, and it is probable that improved understanding of how inflammation resolves, and definition of repair processes, will lead to therapies favouring resolution and repair.

In this chapter, there will be a discussion of the mechanisms underlying the initiation of lung inflammation and processes involved in inflammatory resolution and repair, consideration of how these may go awry in the development of inflammatory and scarring disorders, and a final speculation about the derivation of novel, mechanism-based inflammatory therapies and possible associated pitfalls.

The initiation of inflammation

This section deals with the mechanisms underlying the development of a simple inflammatory stereotype, such as would occur following the deposition of bacteria in the alveoli (Fig. 3.5.1). Neutrophils appear in the air spaces after emigration through the endothelium and alveolar epithelium from about 2 h after an inflammatory stimulus, with a peak of emigration occurring at 4–6 h. Monocyte emigration follows, starting about 6 h after the inflammatory stimulus and reaching a peak 12–18 h later. In most inflammatory reactions there is leakage of fluid and proteins from microvessels during neutrophil emigration. This exudate contains an array of proteins that may assist host defences, including members of the complement and coagulation cascades and immunoglobulins, together with mediators that may aid repair processes. Neutrophils migrate rapidly through tissues to the scene of perturbation, where they ingest and destroy bacteria. Extravasated monocytes mature into inflammatory macrophages in situ. Inflammatory macrophages exert important control functions in the later phases of inflammation and are centrally involved in the processes of scavenging, resolution and repair.

Emigration of neutrophils and monocytes from pulmonary microvessels

In other organs, neutrophils migrate through the postcapillary venules but in the lungs the bulk of neutrophil emigration occurs in the capillaries.[5] Neutrophil emigration involves a complex interplay between resident tissue cells, which generate the mediators driving neutrophil chemotaxis (Table 3.5.1), and the expression and activation of adhesive molecules on the surface of neutrophils and capillary endothelial cells (Fig. 3.5.1). This sets in train neutrophil sequestration in capillaries, adhesion between

Table 3.5.1   Neutrophil chemotactic factors

C-X-C chemokines

- Interleukin 8 (IL-8)
- Neutrophil-activating protein 2 (NAP-2)
- Granulocyte chemotactic protein 2 (GCP-2)
- Epithelial neutrophil-activating protein (ENA-78)
- Growth regulating oncogene-α (GRO-α)
- Growth regulating oncogene-β (GRO-β)
- Growth regulating oncogene-γ (GRO-γ)

Complement cascade

Leukotriene cascade

- Leukotriene B4 (LTB$_4$)

Bacterial peptides

- Formulated peptides (e.g. *N*-formyl-methionyl-leucyl-phenylalanine, f-met-leu-phe, FMLP)

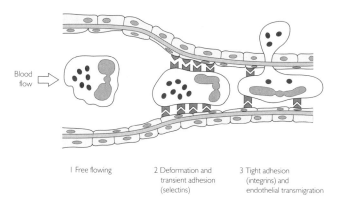

| 1 Free flowing | 2 Deformation and transient adhesion (selectins) | 3 Tight adhesion (integrins) and endothelial transmigration |

Fig. 3.5.2 Neutrophil sequestration and endothelial transmigration in pulmonary capillaries.

the neutrophil and the capillary endothelial cell, and finally neutrophil diapedesis between the endothelial cells and migration through the endothelial basement membrane (Fig. 3.5.2).

Local generation of inflammatory signals

Bacteria release agents, including the formylated peptides (e.g. *N*-formyl-methionyl-leucyl-phenylalanine, f-met-leu-phe, FMLP), that are chemotactic for neutrophils. They may also activate the complement cascade to produce the chemotactic fragment C5a. When injected directly into tissues, a large number of inflammatory agents cause neutrophil extravasation but the number of true chemotaxins, i.e. agents that cause directed cell migration through ligation of specific surface receptors, is likely to be quite restricted. True chemotaxins include complement C5a, leukotriene (LT)B$_4$ and f-met-leu-phe. There has also been much recent interest in a new family of chemoattractant peptides, the 'chemokines', which are likely to be critically important in vivo.[6] The archetype is interleukin(IL)-8, which belongs

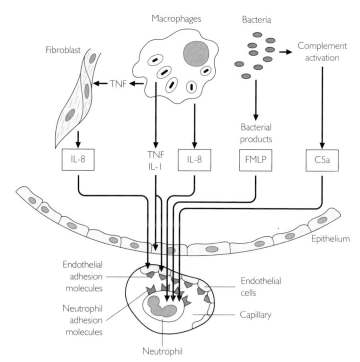

Fig. 3.5.1 Early events in the evolution of lung inflammation: attraction of neutrophils to the lung in the initiation of acute inflammation.

to a family of small, platelet-factor-4-like proteins of molecular
weight 8–19 kDa that contain four cystine residues. Alignment
of these residues determines two groups of peptides; one group
('C–X–C') with the first two cystines separated by one amino
acid and the other with adjacent cystines ('C–C'). The C–X–C
group includes IL-8 and two other closely related peptides, neutrophil activation peptide (NAP)-2 and growth-regulating oncogene (GRO)-α₂, which are also chemotactic for neutrophils
(Table 3.5.1). The C–C group includes macrophage chemotactic
peptide (MCP)-1 and RANTES, eotaxin peptides that are
chemotactic for monocytes and eosinophils. These chemokines
can be generated by a variety of cells and cell lines, including
monocytes, neutrophils, macrophages, epithelial cells and
fibroblasts, although the lung macrophage is an extremely
potent source of IL-8.[7] The IL-8 receptor has been cloned and
functionally expressed. It has 30% sequence homology to f-met-
leu-phe and C5a receptors and is a member of the G-protein
receptor family, which is characterised by seven transmembrane
domains.[8]

Agents such as IL-1 and tumour necrosis factor (TNF)-α,
which themselves are not specifically chemotactic in vitro, exert
indirect chemotaxic effects in vivo by inducing the release of
specific chemoattractants from other cells (see Fig. 3.5.1). The
alveolar macrophage is likely to play a key role by releasing
chemotaxins and other proinflammatory mediators in response
to phagocytosis of bacteria or other tissue perturbations. It can
produce a number of specific chemotactic peptides, including
C5a, IL-8, GRO-α, macrophage inhibitory peptide (MIP)-1α
and the lipid chemotaxin LTB₄, as well as agents such as IL-1 and
TNF, which also act on capillary endothelial cells to induce the
expression of adhesive molecules essential for neutrophil
adhesion and endothelial transmigration. Although alveolar
macrophages are of undoubted importance in recruiting
inflammatory cells, it is now clear that other resident lung cells,
including airway epithelial cells and interstitial fibroblasts, can
generate IL-8, IL-1 and TNF.[9] Thus, local paracrine effects,
including macrophage-derived TNF acting on local fibroblasts
and epithelial cells, which cause them to release IL-8 and other
chemokines (see Fig. 3.5.1), may provide opportunities for rapid
and major amplification of chemotactic signals for neutrophils
and monocytes.

Until recently it was thought that the sequential emigration
of neutrophils, followed by monocytes, was likely to result
simply from differing locomotor responses to a common chemotactic factor, such as C5a. However, the availability of
chemokines that are relatively specific for neutrophils (e.g. IL-8
and GRO-α) or for monocytes (MCP-1) provides a further level
of sophistication whereby differing concentrations or time
profiles of their production by local macrophages probably
provide fine control. Furthermore, it is now clear that the monocyte may use different components of the adhesive molecule
repertoire (see below), with very-late-activation antigen (VLA)-
4 on its surface interacting with the vascular cell adhesion molecule (VCAM)-1 on the endothelium, in contrast with, for
example, CD11b, CD18 on the neutrophil surface interacting
with the intercellular adhesion molecule (ICAM)-1 on the
endothelium (see below). As VCAM-1 is often expressed later
on the surface of stimulated endothelial cells, sequential emi-

gration of leukocytes may also be influenced by the type and
timing of endothelial adhesion molecule expression.

Inflammatory cell sequestration

The arrest of neutrophils in pulmonary capillaries is a necessary
prelude to their transmigration through the endothelium. This
sequestration is likely to result from the combination of a reduction in neutrophil deformability and the expression/activation of
neutrophil surface adhesive molecules, which interact with
counter-receptors on the surface of activated endothelial cells
(Fig. 3.5.2).

The average diameter of a neutrophil is 7–8 μm whereas that
of the pulmonary capillary is 5.5 μm.[10] Therefore, in its passage
through the pulmonary microcirculation, the neutrophil is normally required to 'squeeze' through the capillary, and any reduction in its ability to deform would tend to result in prolonged
sequestration. Agents such as C5a, endotoxic lipopolysaccharide
and cigarette smoke cause marked reduction of neutrophil
deformability in a fashion that correlates directly with its
sequestration.[11-13]

Adhesion between neutrophils and capillary endothelial cells
is a complex process. Under conditions of shear stress during
blood flow in postcapillary venules, it appears that molecules of
the selectin family (particularly L-selectin on the neutrophil
surface) are important in the first phase of transient adhesion
('rolling'),[14] whereas neutrophil surface molecules of the integrin family are involved in the second phase of tight adhesion,[15]
which is required for capillary transmigration (Fig. 3.5.2).
Whether these general observations, made in postcapillary
venules of the systemic circulation, hold true for the pulmonary
capillaries remains to be established.

The in-vivo importance of the leukocyte integrins, and more
recently the selectins, has been highlighted by accidents of nature
in which patients with genetic defects of these receptors have
recurrent infections associated with an inability of neutrophils
to migrate to inflamed and infected lesions (see below).
Furthermore, hints are emerging that inflammatory processes in
different organs and even different bacterial stimuli within the
same organ may make use of different components of the
adhesive molecule repertoire. For example, monoclonal antibodies
directed against the common β chain of the leukocyte integrins,
CD18, will block neutrophil emigration to sites of streptococcal
inflammation in the skin but not in the lung, whereas the same
antibodies will block neutrophil emigration to experimental pneumonia caused by *Escherichia coli* or endotoxin.[16] Thus it may be
possible to block neutrophil emigration to tissues involved in a
particular pathological process, while allowing neutrophils to
enter other organs in defence against infection. A large number of
adhesive molecules have now been identified. They have been
divided broadly into molecules of the integrin, selectin and
immunoglobulin supergene families. Counter-receptors have been
identified for most, but by no means all of these (Table 3.5.2).

The leukocyte integrins
The leukocyte integrins are part of a phylogenetically ancient
family of molecules that have important functions in the morphogenesis and tissue organisation of insects and vertebrates.[17]

Table 3.5.2 Adhesion molecules involved in neutrophil–endothelial adhesion and transmigration

	Receptor	Other names/cluster designation	Distribution	Induced by	Ligand/counter-receptor	Promotes adhesion of
Integrin family	LFA-1	CD11a/CD18	All leukocytes		ICAM-1, ICAM-2, ICAM-3	Endothelial cells
	Mac-1/CR3	CD11b/CD18	Monocytes, granulocytes, NK cells, lymphocytes		ICAM-1, factor X, LPS, C3bi, factor B	Endothelial cells, phagocytic particles
	p150.95	CD11c/CD18	Monocytes, granulocytes		?	Endothelial cells
Immunoglobulin superfamily	ICAM-1	CD54	Endothelial cells, epithelial cells, fibroblasts, mast cells	TNF IL-1 2–4 h LPS	LFA-1 Mac-1 ?CD43	All leukocytes
	ICAM-2		Monocytes, lymphocytes, endothelium	Not induced	LFA-1	All leukocytes
	ICAM-3		All leukocytes – not endothelium			
	VCAM-1	INCAM-1	Activated endothelium	IL-1 TNF 2–4 h IL-4	VLA-4	Monocytes, ?eosinophils
Selectin family	E-selectin	ELAM-1	Endothelium	LPS TNF 2–4 h IL-1	Sialyl Lewis X (CD15) CD66 CD67	Neutrophils, memory T cells
	P-selectin	GMP-140 CD62 PADGEM	Endothelium, platelets	Thrombin PAF 5 min Histamine	Sialyl Lewis X	Neutrophils
	L-selectin	LE-CAM-1 LAM-1 Leu 8; Mel 14 gp90 Dreg 56	Neutrophils, monocytes, lymphocytes	Rapidly shed on activation	?E-Selectin ?P-Selectin Gly-CAM-1	Endothelium

ELAM, endothelial–leukocyte adhesion molecule; ICAM, intercellular adhesion molecule; IL, interleukin; INCAM, intercellular neural cell adhesion molecule; NK, natural killer; LFA, lymphocyte-function-associated antigen; LPS, lipopolysaccharide; Mac-1/CR3, macrophage-1/complement receptor 3; PAF, platelet-activating factor; TNF, tumour necrosis factor; VCAM, vascular cell adhesion molecule; VLA, very-late-activation antigen.

They are heterodimeric transmembrane glycoproteins each with an α and β subunit. At least seven β units have now been cloned and sequenced and it is recognised that single β units have the capacity to associate with different α subunits, the description of subfamilies being based on the subunit associations. Most of the 'β₁' subfamily of integrins are involved with cell–matrix interactions, although VLA-4 is expressed on monocytes and is the ligand for VCAM-1 (a member of the immunoglobulin superfamily on the endothelial surface). Most attention has been focused on members of the β₂ subfamily of leukocyte integrins – lymphocyte-function-associated antigen (LFA-1), complement-receptor factor type III (CR3; Mac-1) and p150.95 – and their role in neutrophil adhesion and endothelial transmigration. The fundamental importance of the leukocyte integrins was confirmed by the discovery of an autosomal recessive trait[18] now, called leukocyte adhesion deficiency, in which recurrent severe infections, delayed umbilical cord separation, destructive skin ulceration and poor wound healing with dystrophic scars[19] are associated with failure of neutrophils to emigrate from blood vessels to inflamed and infected sites (Fig. 3.5.3). This disease is the result of a deficiency of cell-surface glycoproteins now recognised as the leukocyte integrins.

Individual leukocyte integrins may serve a number of functions and may combine with different ligands on endothelial cells (Table 3.5.2):

- LFA-1 is involved in the binding of leukocytes to a variety of cells, including endothelial cells; ICAM-1, a member of the immunoglobulin supergene family, was first demonstrated as a ligand for LFA-1 but subsequent experiments showing that LFA-1-dependent adhesion to endothelial cells was not completely blocked by monoclonal antibodies against ICAM-1 led to the discovery of ICAM-2 and ICAM-3[20,21]
- CR3, as well as being important in the phagocytosis of particles opsonised by the complement fragment iC3b, is

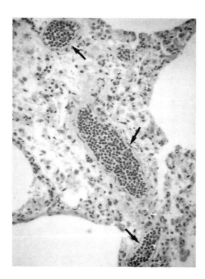

Fig. 3.5.3 Histological section of the lung of a patient with leukocyte adhesion deficiency who developed a fatal pneumonia. Large numbers of neutrophils (arrows) have sequestered in pulmonary vessels but failed to migrate into lung tissue. (With permission from Davies et al. 1991[19])

also involved in neutrophil–endothelial adhesion by binding to a site on endothelial ICAM-1 distinct from the LFA-1 binding site.[22]
- p150.95 has also been implicated in neutrophil–endothelial interactions but the endothelial ligands have not yet been identified.[23]

In the two-stage model of neutrophil binding to microvascular endothelial cells, the leukocyte integrins are critically involved in the 'tight' adhesion second stage that precedes and is necessary for capillary transmigration. The attachment and detachment processes which must occur during capillary transmigration imply regulation of integrin function and 'on/off' switching.[24] This is likely to occur by ligand regulation, e.g. modulation of cell surface expression and redistribution of ICAM-1 by cytokines (see below) and by integrin receptor regulation.[25]

The selectins

E-selectin (previously called ELAM-1) and P-selectin (previously called GMP-140) on the endothelial surface, and L-selectin (previously called LAM-1) on the leukocyte surface, are a family of cell-surface glycoproteins so named because of their amino-terminal C-type lectin domain that appears essential for their adhesive properties. The selectins appear to exert important effects at the earliest stages of leukocyte–endothelial adhesion, during the transient 'rolling' phase. Evidence is now accumulating that P-selectin is an important molecule in the adhesive process necessary for neutrophil-mediated endothelial injury in vivo,[26,27] and a further genetic abnormality has recently been discovered that provides direct evidence for an in-vivo role of the selectin molecules in neutrophil emigration. This clinical syndrome is similar to leukocyte adhesion deficiency, with repeated infections and failure of neutrophil emigration, although with the retention of β₂ integrins and failure of neutrophils to adhere to E-selectin; it is associated with loss of its ligand, sialyl Lewis X (CD15), on the neutrophil surface. It has been suggested that this genetic abnormality should be called 'leukocyte adhesion deficiency type II'.[28]

The immunoglobulin supergene family

This family possesses a common amino-acid chain, originally described in the constant variable regions of the immunoglobulin light and heavy chains, and it now includes a range of surface molecules of diverse function, such as the T-cell receptors – CD4, CD8, major histocompatibility complex (MHC) class I and II – and a range of adhesive molecules such as neural cell adhesion molecule (NCAM).[20] Those of direct relevance for leukocyte–endothelial adhesion are ICAM-1, ICAM-2, ICAM-3 and VCAM-1 on the surface of endothelial cells. ICAM-1 is the major counter-receptor for LFA-1 but lack of complete binding in the presence of anti-ICAM-1 monoclonal antibody led to the discovery of ICAM-2 and, similarly, the failure of a combination of anti-ICAM-1 and anti-ICAM-2 to block CD18-dependent adhesion completely suggested the presence of a third moiety, ICAM-3.

The ICAM-1 molecule is constitutively expressed on the surface of all endothelial cells but is strongly upregulated in the presence of mediators such as TNF-α, IL-1 and platelet-activating factor (PAF).[29] TNF-α causes gradually increasing expression of ICAM-1 with a 50% increase at 6 h, reaching a maximum at 24 h, although with continued expression for 24–72 h. This implies that ICAM-1 may have an important role in the later stages of neutrophil emigration from blood vessels, a concept supported by observations that it is not effective under the conditions of shear stress that are probably involved in the early phases of transient neutrophil adhesion. Thus, it is widely agreed that ICAM-1 is critically involved in the later stages of adhesion and neutrophil–endothelial transmigration, when it interacts with LFA-1 and Mac-1 on the neutrophil surface. The use of anti-ICAM-1 monoclonal antibodies in experimental models of allergic asthma suggests a role of ICAM-1 in eosinophil migration into the lung.

The VCAM-1 molecule is activated by IL-1, TNF-α and endotoxic lipopolysaccharide, with maximum upregulation taking several hours. VCAM-1 binds to monocytes and eosinophils in a CD11/CD18-independent fashion and it is thought that the adhesive interaction is mediated through the β_1 integrin VLA-4.[30] It has been suggested that this may be part of the mechanism accounting for selective eosinophil emigration in allergic conditions such as asthma, but this is by no means established in vivo.

Capillary transmigration

Since Addison's classic light microscopic observations in 1843 and Lord Florey's detailed early electron microscopic work, it became clear that emigrating neutrophils can 'squeeze' between endothelial cells by a process of diapedesis. It is known that adhesive molecules, including ICAM-1 on endothelial cells and the leukocyte integrins on neutrophils, are involved but the complex intercellular signalling processes that must be required are obscure at present.

The next barrier to neutrophil emigration is the capillary basement membrane, the broaching of which might be expected to involve some inevitable degradation of matrix proteins. Although neutrophils contain an impressive repertoire of degradative enzymes (Table 3.5.3 & Fig. 3.5.4), there have been intriguing experiments that suggest that endothelial cells themselves may play a key role in the local degradation and reformation of the capillary basement membrane during neutrophil transmigration.[31]

The final phase of neutrophil emigration from the lung capillary to the alveolus requires transmigration across the epithelium, which, unlike endothelium, is formed by cells attached by a number of complex intercellular adhesive mechanisms, including 'tight junctions'. Neutrophils can be induced in vitro to migrate through intact monolayers of epithelial cells without causing increased permeability of the monolayer, or even loss of electrical resistance across the monolayer.[32] Although there are in-vivo examples of single mediators causing neutrophil migration to the lung without obvious exudate formation or injury, most simple models of inflammation of the lung or other organs, including streptococcal pneumonia, are associated with significant exudation of plasma proteins and a degree of injury to endothelial and epithelial cell layers. This implies that, although mechanisms are available for neutrophil emigration through endothelial and epithelial layers to occur without 'bystander

Table 3.5.3 Neutrophil products with the potential to injure tissues

Reactive oxygen species	Superoxide anion
	Hydrogen peroxide
	Singlet oxygen
	Hydroxyl radical
	Hypohalous acid
Enzymes	Elastase
	Cathepsin G
	Collagenases
	Neuraminidase
	Heparanase
	Myeloperoxidase
Cationic proteins	Defensins
	Cationic antimicrobial proteins
Proinflammatory mediators	Platelet-activating factor
	Leukotrienes
	Cytokines (e.g. IL-1)
	Chemokines (e.g. IL-8)

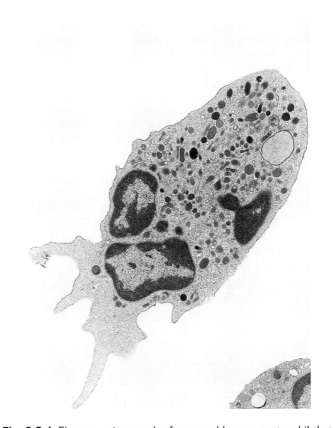

Fig. 3.5.4 Electron micrograph of a normal human neutrophil that has been activated by exposure to a chemotactic peptide. Note the elongation and polarisation of the cell, the granular appearance of the nuclear chromatin and the large numbers of cytoplasmic granules.

injury', even in beneficial inflammation local control mechanisms may be inadequate. It therefore seems likely that this stage of inflammation represents a pivotal point at which any loss of restraining control mechanisms could greatly amplify inflammatory tissue injury, and it may be pertinent that many inflammatory diseases, such as ARDS and fibrosing alveolitis, are characterised in their early stages by excessive endothelial and epithelial injury and persistent microvascular fluid exudation.

Neutrophil chemotaxis, activation and phagocytes

After penetration of endothelial and epithelial cell layers, neutrophils undergo directed migration along a concentration gradient of chemotaxins. Chemotaxins act by binding to specific receptors, which are highly mobile and appear to be swept back from the leading edge of the cell, internalised and then recycled. During this remarkable process neutrophils are able to sense, across their length (5 μm), the tiny differences in chemotaxin levels that form the concentration gradient. The receptors for C5a, f-met-leu-phe and IL-8 have been cloned and sequenced and have been identified as members of the G-protein-linked receptor superfamily.[8] Generalised neutrophil chemotactic responses and activation appear to be mediated through common receptor-linked mechanisms that cause the rapid formation of the intracellular signalling molecules: inositol 1,4,5-trisphosphate, diacylglycerol and markedly increased levels of free intracellular calcium, $[Ca^{2+}]_i$. The modulating effects of guanosine triphosphate (GTP) and the inhibitory effects of certain bacterial toxins indicate a role for a guanine-nucleotide-binding protein (G-protein) in this process (Fig. 3.5.5). Although the same general pathways can be activated by many chemotaxins,[33] there are fine levels of control for specific neu-

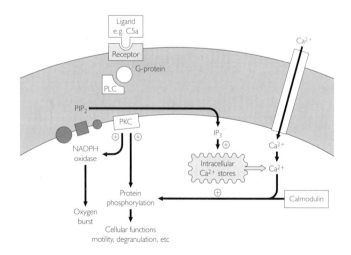

Fig. 3.5.5 Some early events in neutrophil activation following ligation of a chemotaxin receptor (e.g. C5a), showing signal transduction processes in the neutrophil. IP$_3$, inositol trisphosphate; NADPH, nicotinamide adenine dinucleotide phosphate (reduced form); PIP$_2$, phosphatidyl inositol (4,5)-bisphosphate; PKC, phosphokinase C; PLC, phospholipase C.

trophil functions such as degranulation and motility. For example, LTB$_4$ is a good chemotaxin but a poor secretagogue. Similarly, a degree of cell activation and alteration in the cytoskeletal framework is necessary for maximal effect of the adhesive receptors in neutrophil sequestration and capillary transmigration, but the full-blown respiratory burst and maximal secretory response would be undesirable until a much later stage when the neutrophil has ingested bacteria that, when isolated in the phagolysosome, can receive the full force of the neutrophil's destructive armamentarium. The fine details of sensing mechanisms and the discrete motor mechanisms required for the localised protrusive and retractive movements necessary for locomotion through tissues remain obscure.

Cytoskeletal changes

The earliest morphological event in the stimulated neutrophil is a change of shape from its normal spherical state to a polarised form. This is associated with reduction in cell deformability, which may itself make an important contribution to neutrophil sequestration in pulmonary microvessels, an essential prelude to neutrophil emigration (see above). Actin polymerisation plays a key role in these cytoskeletal changes. When neutrophils are at resting state, half of the actin complement is insoluble and forms a branching network under the cell membrane that extends into and controls the formation of microvilli and other surface conformational changes. The network is composed of actin monomers (G-actin), which are polymerised to form actin filaments (F-actin). These are in turn cross-linked into a web-like structure by another protein, actin-binding protein (ABP). The remaining 50% of actin is maintained in soluble form by agents (including profilin and gelsolin) that inhibit polymerisation, thus providing the opportunity for considerable amplification of the actin framework upon cell activation. Profilin and gelsolin are controlled by second messengers and Ca^{2+} generated during neutrophil activation. Once formed, the actin web can be induced to contract by myosin, which is activated locally by the action of a Ca^{2+}–calmodulin-dependent myosin light chain kinase. Thus, the mechanical responses necessary for most neutrophil functions are linked to early events in signal transduction, although the detailed control mechanisms are poorly understood.

The functional state of neutrophils in tissues

Until quite recently the neutrophil was thought of as an unsophisticated cell that migrated to the inflamed site where it killed bacteria and disgorged its enzyme contents before finally disintegrating. However, it is now clear that granulocytes can exist in tissues in relatively quiescent states, that neutrophils are sensitive to different levels of external control and that they can themselves secrete a number of important inflammatory cytokines (Table 3.5.3), including IL-8, IL-1 and granulocyte–monocyte-colony-stimulating factor (GM-CSF).[34] Moreover, not all inflammatory mediators exert identical effects on neutrophils; some important mediators, e.g. IL-8 and C5a, are powerful secretagogues that stimulate neutrophil release of reactive oxygen species and granule enzymes, whereas others, e.g. lipopolysaccharides, TNF and PAF, are only moderately effective secretagogues even at very high concentrations. These latter agents, however, even in very low concentration, may exert important 'priming effects' whereby neutrophil behaviour is modulated such that it releases greatly enhanced quantities of potentially injurious agents upon subsequent simulation with known secretagogues, e.g. C5a.[35-37] Neutrophil-mediated in-vitro endothelial injury[38] requires the combination of priming and triggering agents, as does experimental acute lung injury.[39]

To understand the processes responsible for prolonged or excessive neutrophil secretion, it will be necessary to define the mechanisms of neutrophil priming and activation, particularly because the priming process also alters a number of other neutrophil functions. These include increased adhesiveness, reduced deformability and reduced chemotactic response,[36,40] the combination of which might be expected to promote excessive and prolonged vascular sequestration of actively secreting neutrophils in direct contact with capillary endothelial cells.

Neutrophil phagocytosis

Bacteria and other foreign particles are phagocytosed most effectively when coated with an opsonising IgG or with opsonic components of C3 (C3b, C3bi). Particles coated with IgG are recognised by the Fc receptors of the neutrophil, and particles coated with C3b and C3bi are recognised by complement receptor type I (CR1) and CR3 respectively. Engulfment of particles is accompanied by a movement of granules, or lysosomes, to the site of phagosome formation, where the two structures fuse, forming a phagolysosome, into which granule contents are discharged. Neutrophil granules contain a massive array of antibacterial agents, including defensins and destructive enzymes (see Fig. 3.5.4). Degranulation into the phagosome is probably closely related to the metabolic burst, which generates a range of reactive oxygen species that are also highly toxic to bacteria. The respiratory burst may also have an important role in acidifying the phagolysosomal microenvironment, thus facilitating the action of some of the degradative and hydrolytic enzymes from the azurophil granules, which have a low optimal pH. Some external release of granule enzymes and reactive oxygen intermediates appears to occur inevitably as a result of this process but how quantitatively significant this is in vivo and what its mechanisms and purposes are remains uncertain. Nevertheless, many of these agents are highly toxic to healthy host tissues and it is likely that their excessive secretion contributes to inflammatory disease processes.

Monocyte emigration and maturation into inflammatory macrophages

Compared with resident alveolar macrophages, inflammatory macrophages contain more lysosomes and mitochondria.[41] They display a greatly increased pinocytotic rate and increased phagocytic capacity, as well as a greater capacity to secrete enzymes and reactive oxygen intermediates.[42] Inflammatory macrophages are derived from blood monocytes, which migrate to the inflamed site and therein achieve their full potential by a combination of maturation and activation under the influence of local cytokines. Monocytes in vitro take several days to mature into macrophages and over this time there are major changes in expression of a variety of cell receptors, although in vivo this process occurs over a 24–48 h period. Monocyte emigration from blood vessels is less well understood than neutrophil emigration. It succeeds neutrophil emigration and there is some evidence that monocyte emigration could actually depend on prior neutrophil emigration. This temporal sequence may be explained by the local generation, particularly by alveolar macrophages, of monocyte-specific chemokines (e.g. MCP-1) and the monocyte's use of the VLA-4/VCAM-1 axis of adhesive molecules.

The fully developed inflammatory macrophage is indeed a formidable weapon in host defence. It expresses a vast array of receptors (Table 3.5.4) and is capable of secreting most of the products contained by resident macrophages and performing the bacterial killing, coagulation promotion and antigen presentation roles; it displays enhanced expression of a range of receptors for altered and damaged proteins as well as gaining the capacity to recognise and ingest senescent neutrophils (see below). These last functions are obviously of key importance for its scavenging role in the resolution of inflammation. However, it is also capable of releasing a wide range of cytokines and growth factors that are known to promote fibroblast proliferation and collagen deposition, and can present antigens and release lymphokines that provoke immune responses. Thus it is likely that mechanisms controlling macrophage function in the later stages of inflammation are also critically important in determining whether inflammation resolves, progresses to chronic inflammation or becomes associated with a pathological degree of scarring.

Resolution of inflammation and lung repair

In contrast to the amount of research carried out on the initiation of inflammation, comparatively little attention has been paid to the processes of resolution (Fig. 3.5.6) and repair, in spite of their probable importance for our understanding of the pathogenesis of chronic inflammation and scarring which characterise so many lung diseases.[43] Therefore, some of the following discussion will, of necessity, be somewhat hypothetical.

For lung tissues to return to normal during the resolution of inflammation, all the processes occurring in its evolution must be reversed, including removal of the inciting stimulus and dissipation of mediators, cessation of granulocyte emigration from blood vessels, restoration of normal microvascular permeability, limitation of granulocyte secretion of potentially histotoxic and proinflammatory agents, cessation of monocyte emigration from blood vessels and their maturation into inflammatory macrophages, and finally removal of extravasated fluid, fibrin clot, proteins, bacteria and cellular debris, granulocytes and macrophages. Therefore, during the resolution of inflammation very effective mechanisms must exist for repair and reconstitution of tissues. With the completion of resolution and repair processes, the stage should be set for full recovery of normal architecture and function (Fig. 3.5.6).

Table 3.5.4   Some receptors on and molecules binding to macrophages

Complement components	C1q, C3b, C3bi, C3d, C5a
Immunoglobulins	IgG, IgA, IgE
Growth factors and cytokines	IFN-α/β, IFN-α, CSF-1, GM-CSF, TNF-α
	Interleukins 1, 2, 3, 4, 6
Adhesion molecules and phagocytic receptors	LFA-1, Mac-1, p150/95, ICAM-1, $\alpha v \beta_3$ (VnR), CR1, CR3, FcR
Glycoproteins and carbohydrates	Mannosyl fucosyl receptor
	Mannose 6-phosphate
	Heparin
	Advanced glycosylation end-products
Proteins and hormones	Fibronectin
	Laminin
	Transferrin
	Fibrin
	Lactoferrin
	Calcitonin
	Oestrogen
	Insulin
	Parathyroid hormone
	Progesterone
Peptides and small molecules	Adenosine, bombesin, bradykinin, adrenaline (epinephrine)
	Dexamethasone, glucagon, histamine
	Tachykinins, PAF, serotonin, substance P
	VIP
Lipids and lipoproteins	Leukotrienes C, D_4, B_4, E_2
	LDL; βVLDL; modified LDL

CR, complement receptor; CSF, colony-stimulating factor; FcR, Fc fragment receptor; GM-CSF, granulocyte–macrophage-colony-stimulating factor; ICAM, intercellular adhesion molecule; IFN, interferon; IL, interleukin; LDL, low-density lipoprotein; βVLDL, very-low-density lipoprotein; LFA, lymphocyte-function-associated antigen; Mac-1, macrophage-1; PAF, platelet-activating factor; TNF, tumour necrosis factor; VIP, vasoactive intestinal peptide, $\alpha v \beta_3$, vitronectin receptor.

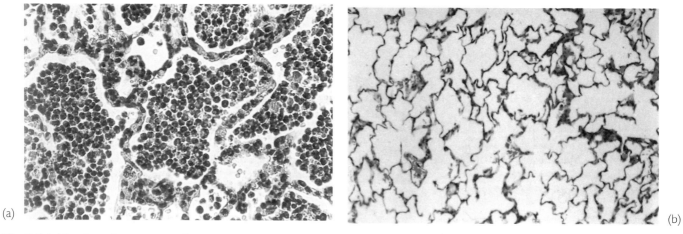

Fig. 3.5.6 Histological appearance of experimental pneumococcal pneumonia. (a) The appearances at 48 h. There is a profound inflammatory response, the alveolar spaces being packed with neutrophils, monocytes and macrophages. (b) Resolution at 7 days. The inflammation has resolved and the lung has returned to a virtually normal appearance. (Reproduced with permission from Haslett C, 1992, Resolution of acute inflammation and the role of apoptosis in the tissue fate of granulocytes. Clinical Science (London), 83(6), 639–48. The Biochemical Society and the Medical Research Society.[43])

Removal of inflammatory mediators

The most powerful mediators initiating the inflammatory response must be removed, inactivated or otherwise rendered impotent. Thromboxane A_2 and endothelial-derived relaxing factor (nitric oxide, NO) are labile factors that are spontaneously unstable. PAF and C5a are inhibited by inactivating enzymes. Reduction of mediator efficacy might also occur by local reduction of their concentration as a consequence of dilution by inflammatory oedema, or by attenuation of target cell receptors, e.g. the downregulation of receptors that occurs during desensitisation of neutrophils to high concentrations of a variety of inflammatory mediators. Recent interest in cytokine biology has been directed largely at agents that initiate or amplify inflammation but, by analogy with the peptides involved in the blood coagulation and complement cascades, the whole system must be kept under tight control by very effective inhibitors or other counteracting influences. Some have been discovered (e.g. the IL-1 receptor antagonist) but the inhibitory partners of the chemokines and other powerful phlogistins have yet to be described. The final requirement for the success of most of the above mechanisms is that the production of mediators at the site must cease.

The control of a complex function such as neutrophil chemotaxis in response to C5a or IL-8 is influenced by the concentration of mediators, the concentration of their inhibitors, possible desensitisation mechanisms and the effects of other locally generated agents that exert negative influences on the process. The redundancy of the inflammatory response in vivo must also be taken into consideration. Not only may single mediators exert multiple effects on various cells under different circumstances but important inflammatory events can be provoked by agents from different mediator families. For example, neutrophil chemotaxis can be driven by members of the complement (C5a), leukotriene (LTB_4) and chemokine (IL-8) families of mediators. To gain a dynamic perspective of the resolution of inflammation it will therefore be necessary to consider how a variety of important mediators may act in concert at the inflamed site and to ascertain the integrated impact of negative and positive stimuli on these dynamic events in situ. Thus the overall propensity for inflammation to persist would be expected to cease when the balance of mediator effects tips towards the inhibitory rather than the stimulatory, presumably as a result of at least some of the mechanisms considered above.

Cessation of neutrophil emigration

The factors controlling cessation of inflammatory cell emigration from microvessels remain obscure. The evolution and resolution of inflammation are both dynamic processes and simple histological observations may inadequately represent these events. As other, poorly understood factors, such as cell removal rates, may also exert major influences on the numbers of cells observed in 'static' histological sections, the study of neutrophil emigration kinetics requires careful monitoring of labelled populations of cells. When intravenous pulses of radiolabelled neutrophils were used to define the emigration patterns of neutrophils into sites of inflammation at various stages of evolution in skin, joints and lungs, it was discovered that neutrophil migration ceased remarkably early,[44-46] by contrast with the greatly prolonged influx that occurred in an inflammatory model, which progresses to chronic tissue injury and scarring.[47] Indeed in experimental streptococcal pneumonia, in which the histological appearance at 48 h shows massive neutrophil accumulation, it was possible to demonstrate that neutrophil emigration to the site had ceased 24 h previously (Fig. 3.5.7). Supporting evidence has also been obtained from human acute lobar pneumonia, in which, by the time of hospital presentation, intravenously injected labelled neutrophils failed to migrate from the blood into the lung. Thus, cessation of neutrophil emigration occurring so soon in the evolution of acute inflammation may represent one of the earliest resolution events.

A number of hypothetical mechanisms could be responsible; these include locally generated chemotactic factor inhibitory agents, deactivation or desensitisation of neutrophils to high concentrations of mediators; negative feedback loops whereby extravasated neutrophils exert influences preventing more neutrophils entering the site – the layers of endothelial and epithelial cells that normally permit neutrophils to emigrate during the initiation of inflammation could alter to form a

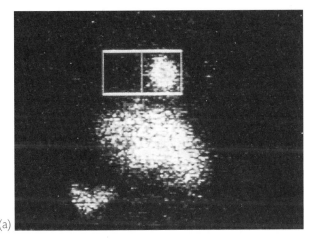 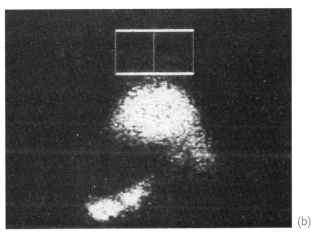

(a) (b)

Fig. 3.5.7 Early cessation of neutrophil emigration in streptococcal pneumonia. External gamma-camera scintigraphy of emigration of intravenously injected indium-[111]I-radiolabelled neutrophils in experimental pneumococcal pneumonia. (a) When a 'pulse' of labelled neutrophils is delivered intravenously 6 h after the initiation of pneumonia, the posterior gamma-camera image taken 24 h thereafter shows neutrophil accumulation in the pneumonic lobe. (b) However, if labelled neutrophils are injected intravenously 24 h after the initiation of pneumonia, no neutrophil emigration is detected, even though large numbers of neutrophils are known to be present in the lung at this stage of pneumonia (see Fig. 3.5.6). (Reproduced with permission from Haslett C, 1992, Resolution of acute inflammation and the role of apoptosis in the tissue fate of granulocytes. Clinical Science (London), 83(6), 639–48. The Biochemical Society and the Medical Research Society.[43])

'barrier' to further neutrophil emigration; or, finally, cessation of neutrophil emigration may simply result from dissipation or removal of chemotaxins from the inflamed site. Which of these possible mechanisms are important in vivo is unclear.

In a skin model of inflammation it appeared that desensitisation mechanisms were operating[44] and in some human diseases involving persistent inflammation it has been suggested that chemotactic-factor-inhibitory agents may be defective. However, in experimental arthritis there was no evidence for either of these mechanisms and cessation of neutrophil emigration coincided with loss of chemoattractants from the joint space.[45] This loss was not dependent on cellular accumulation at the site – evidence against a simple negative feedback mechanism. Although the processes responsible for loss of chemotactic activity were not identified, these observations suggest that the local generation and removal of chemotaxins are likely to be centrally important in determining whether neutrophil emigration ceases or persists. This does not imply that interactions between neutrophils and capillary endothelial cells are unimportant at the stage of cessation of neutrophil emigration, but in experimental arthritis[45] the inflamed site will permit a further wave of neutrophil emigration in response to a second inflammatory stimulus given at the time of the initial cessation of neutrophil emigration. Therefore any 'barriers' to cell adhesion or transmigration existing at the time of cessation of neutrophil emigration must be readily reversible, presumably by the further action of newly generated inflammatory cytokines, which induce renewed expression and/or activation of endothelial surface adhesive molecules, together with parallel effects on neutrophil locomotion and the expression/activation of neutrophil surface adhesive molecules. Thus, it is reasonable to suggest that the detailed definition of mechanisms governing the local generation and dissipation of agents that promote chemotaxis and upregulate and activate adhesive molecules is essential for our ultimate understanding of the termination or persistence of neutrophil emigration in situ.

Factors controlling monocyte emigration are poorly understood but it appears that monocyte emigration in vivo may be dependent on the prior emigration of neutrophils.[48] Although the underlying mechanisms are obscure, it is now known that the neutrophil is capable of secreting a wide range of cytokines,[34] some of which may be involved in the control of monocyte emigration. Similar principles to those discussed above will also apply to the identification of mechanisms responsible for the cessation of monocyte emigration.

Restoration of normal microvascular permeability and restoration, and repair of damaged endothelial and epithelial layers

Conheim deduced that inflammatory blood vessels become more permeable to fluid before structural abnormalities can be demonstrated. In 1961 Majno & Palade demonstrated gaps between endothelial cells at inflamed sites.[49] These were not associated with endothelial injury and it is probable that they represented transient gaps in intercellular junctions that are controlled by the endothelial cytoskeleton and are therefore reversible. This probably occurs by a combination of the recovery of individual cells from sublethal injury and restoration of cell layers by local cellular proliferation. Epithelial cell monolayers in vitro appear to be able to recover from hydrogen-peroxide-mediated injury by a mechanism requiring protein synthesis.[50] Epithelial monolayers also display a remarkable capacity to regenerate, although after extensive epithelial type I cell injury it is the type II alveolar epithelial cells that proliferate at a massive rate (as can be seen in early ARDS) to produce cells that eventually differentiate into type I alveolar cells in an attempt to reconstitute the alveolar epithelium. However, most pathologists agree that the extent of injury to epithelial cells is critical: if it is too extensive, particularly if the basement membrane structural integrity is lost, it is thought that the lesion does not heal by reconstitution of cell layers but rather by an excessive fibrotic response.

It is important to recognise that, even in beneficial inflammation, there are likely to be areas of the lung where a localised or limited scarring response is necessary for effective repair, e.g. to heal tears in basement membranes or localised areas of extensive epithelial injury, particularly if normal alveolar architecture is lost locally. Many of these mechanisms are identical to those fibroproliferative events described below. However, it seems likely that, if this response is too extensive or poorly controlled, rather than the minimal amount of scarring required for adequate tissue repair, potentially catastrophic, generalised lung fibrosis may result.

Control of inflammatory cell secretion

Tight control, and ultimately cessation of neutrophil granule enzyme secretion, are probably important in the limitation of inflammatory tissue injury and in the resolution of inflammation. Although there has been much research into the initiation and amplification of phagocyte secretion in vitro, little is understood of how these processes are controlled in vivo. However, the secretory rate is again likely to be influenced by the balance between stimulatory and inhibitory mediators. The simplest mechanism for the termination of secretion, i.e. the cell exhausting its secretory potential, is unlikely because cells removed from inflamed sites retain their capacity for further secretion upon stimulation ex vivo.[51] Other factors that may contribute to downregulation or termination of secretion are exhaustion of internal energy supplies, receptor downregulation, dissipation of stimuli and, finally, death or removal of the cell itself.

In a short-lived, terminally differentiated cell such as the neutrophil granulocyte, which normally has a circulating half-life of only 6 h, death of the cell could itself be an important mechanism in irreversibly terminating its secretory function. It has recently been shown that granulocytes constitutively undergo apoptosis (programmed cell death, see below). During apoptosis the neutrophil retains its granule enzyme complement, its membranes remain intact (Fig. 3.5.8), but it loses the ability to secrete granule contents in response to external stimulation with inflammatory mediators.[52] Apoptosis could therefore provide a mechanism that renders the neutrophil inert and functionally isolated from the effects of inflammatory mediators, thus greatly limiting its destructive potential during the resolution phase of inflammation.

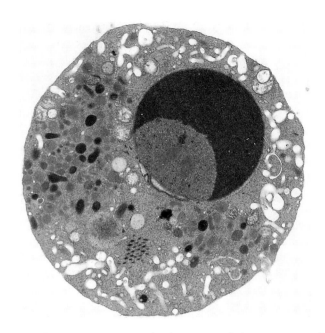

Fig. 3.5.8 Electron micrograph of an apoptotic human neutrophil. Note the smooth outline and membrane retention, the characteristic aggregation of nuclear chromatin, the prominent nucleolus and the dilated endoplasmic reticulum. Note also that large numbers of apparently intact granules remain in the cytoplasm.

The clearance phase of inflammation

Once the extravasated inflammatory cells have completed their tasks in host defence and inciting agents, e.g. bacteria, have been destroyed, the site must be cleared of fluid, fibrin clot, proteins and debris, and finally the (now redundant) cells, particularly granulocytes, inflammatory macrophages and their potentially histotoxic contents, must be removed before the tissues can return to normal.

Clearance of fluid proteins and debris

Most fluid is probably removed via the lymphatic vessels, although reconstitution of normal haemodynamics may contribute by restoring the balance of hydrostatic and osmotic forces in favour of net fluid absorption at the venous end of the capillary. Proteolytic enzymes in plasma exudate and inflammatory cell secretions are likely to break down fibrin strands and clots at the inflamed site, the products of this digestion being drained by lymphatics, which become widely distended as the removal of fluid and proteins increases. The removal of the fibrin strands, which are characteristically seen in lobar pneumonia and acute lung injury, is likely to be a very important phase of resolution, because their retention promotes collapse and fusion of denuded alveolar walls and presents an abnormal surface for deranged re-epithelialisation.[53] Moreover, their partial degradation may generate fragments that not only promote inflammation and scarring but also reduce surfactant production. Macrophages are likely to play a key role by secret-

ing the plasminogen and plasminogen activators necessary for fibrin fragmentation and degradation, as well as providing the phagocytic and pinocytotic functions that contribute to the uptake of fibrin fragments and other proteins, including immunoglobulins. In activated inflammatory macrophages, pinocytosis can occur at a rate such that 25% of the cell surface is reused every minute! Inflammatory macrophages (as discussed above) also have a greatly increased phagocytic potential; they can recognise opsonised and non-opsonised particles and they express cell-surface receptors for a wide variety of altered and damaged cells and proteins. The critical role of macrophages in the clearance phase of inflammation was first appreciated by Metchnikoff more than a century ago and we are now just beginning to define the molecular mechanisms of some of his seminal light-microscopic observations.

Tissue clearance of extravasated granulocytes

There is no evidence that neutrophils return to the blood stream or that lymphatic drainage provides an important disposal route, and it is generally agreed that the bulk of extravasated neutrophils meet their fate at the inflamed site.[4] However, it had been widely assumed that neutrophils inevitably disintegrate in situ before their fragments are removed by local macrophages. If this was the rule, healthy tissues would inevitably be exposed to large quantities of potentially injurious neutrophil contents. Although a number of pathological descriptions have favoured neutrophil necrosis as the major mechanism operating in inflammation, many of these examples have derived from disease states rather than from 'benign' self-limiting inflammation. Moreover, since the classic observations of Metchnikoff, there has been evidence of an alternative fate whereby intact extravasated neutrophils were removed by macrophages.[54] Over the intervening decades there have been a number of sporadic reports, in health and disease, of intact neutrophil phagocytosis by macrophages. Of particular relevance to the resolution of inflammation, is the clinical phenomenon of 'Reiter's cells' – neutrophil-containing macrophages seen on cytological examination of patients with Reiter's disease and other acute arthritides.[55] Also, in experimental peritonitis, where it is possible to sample the inflammatory exudate with ease, macrophage ingestion of apparently intact neutrophils is the dominant mode of neutrophil removal from the inflamed site.[56]

Newman and his colleagues showed that 'aged', but not freshly isolated, neutrophils were ingested by inflammatory macrophages (but not by monocytes), but the time-related process responsible for neutrophil recognition as 'non-self' or 'senescent-self' was not identified.[57] It has since been discovered that ageing granulocytes constitutively undergo apoptosis (programmed cell death).[58] This process is responsible for recognition of intact senescent granulocytes by macrophages[58] and there is evidence from a variety of tissues, including acute lung injury[59] and resolving pneumonia (see below), for its role in acute inflammation.

Necrosis versus apoptosis

From the work of Wyllie and his colleagues it is now recognised that the death of nucleated cells may be classified into at least two distinct types: 'necrosis' or accidental death and 'apoptosis' or programmed cell death.[60,61] Necrosis can be observed where tissues are exposed to gross insults such as high concentrations of toxins or hypoxia. At the cellular level there is rapid loss of membrane function and abnormal permeability of the cell membrane, which can be recognised by failure to exclude vital dyes such as trypan blue, and there is early disruption of organelles, including granule disruption and irreversible mitochondrial damage. Perhaps not surprisingly, significant necrosis may be associated with evidence of local tissue injury and the initiation or amplification of inflammatory responses.

In contrast, apoptosis characteristically occurs in situations where death is predictable or physiological, such as the removal of unwanted cells during embryonic remodelling, thymic involution and a number of other situations in which cell turnover is physiologically rapid, e.g. crypt cells in the gut epithelium. In the many pathophysiological situations where apoptosis is now recognised, the process occurs with remarkably stereotypical cytological and broad biochemical changes, implying a common pattern of underlying molecular mechanisms. During apoptosis, cells shrink and there are major changes in the cell surface, which becomes featureless, with loss of microvilli. However, the membrane remains intact and continues to exclude vital dyes, and intracellular organelles, including granules, remain intact until very late in the process, although the endoplasmic reticulum appears to become markedly dilated, giving the appearance on light microscopy of cytoplasmic vacuolation (Fig. 3.5.8). A prominent biochemical feature of apoptosis is internucleosomal cleavage of chromatin in a pattern indicative of endogenous endonuclease activation. This results in the characteristic ladder pattern of DNA fragments upon the electrophoresis of DNA extracted from apoptotic cells. Final characterisation of the endonucleases responsible remains elusive, although a number of candidates have been proposed.

Fate of apoptotic cells

Apoptotic cells are very rapidly ingested by phagocytes in vivo, such that, in tissue sections of the remodelling embryo,[60] for example, apoptotic cells are usually seen only within macrophages, although other 'semiprofessional' phagocytes, e.g. epithelial cells and fibroblast-like cells, may also participate. The speed and efficiency of this process and the fact that it occurs at random renders this mode of cell death less conspicuous in 'static' histological sections. It is also remarkable that, in embryonic remodelling or in thymic involution, whole tissue tracts can be removed over a few hours by the process without causing local tissue injury or inciting an inflammatory response (which in the developing embryo would presumably have catastrophic effects).

These analogies led to the hypothesis that apoptosis in granulocytes represents an alternative tissue fate to necrosis and one that by contrast would tend to limit inflammatory tissue injury and promote resolution processes.[62,63] 'Programmed' cell death also implies the potential for internal and external controls that modulate the time of tissue residence and function of granulocytes in situ and thereby represent important factors in the control of inflammation itself.

Phagocytosis of apoptotic neutrophils by macrophages

Human neutrophils harvested from peripheral blood or from acutely inflamed joints remain intact, exclude vital dyes such as trypan blue and fail to disgorge their complement of enzymes for up to 24 h in culture. Over this period there is a steadily increasing proportion of cells demonstrating apoptosis (Fig. 3.5.8), and it has been shown that apoptosis is responsible for macrophage recognition of the intact cell.[58] Apoptotic cells are not indestructible and beyond 24 h in culture there is a progressive increase in 'secondary necrosis', indicated by the percentage of cells that fail to exclude trypan blue, together with steadily increasing spontaneous granule enzyme release. However, when these neutrophils are cultured beyond 24 h in the presence of macrophages, the removal of apoptotic cells is so effective that no trypan-blue-positive cells are seen and there is no release of granule enzyme markers into the surrounding medium. Similar results have been obtained with human eosinophilic granulocytes.[64] Although eosinophils appear to demonstrate a slower constitutive rate of apoptosis in culture (which may be consistent with their probable longer tissue existence), this process also determines macrophage recognition of the senescent, intact eosinophil.

There are now numerous histological descriptions demonstrating an in-vivo role for granulocyte apoptosis. These include acute arthritides,[58] neonatal acute lung injury[59] and the resolution phase of experimental bacterial pneumonia (Fig. 3.5.9). Eosinophil apoptosis and the ingestion of apoptotic eosinophils by macrophages is a prominent feature in dexamethasone-treated experimental eosinophilic enteritis.[65]

There are now several additional in-vitro observations that suggest ways in which granulocyte apoptosis provides an injury-limiting clearance mechanism that would tend to promote resolution rather than the persistence of inflammation,

- During apoptosis, marked loss of a number of neutrophil functions is seen.[52] These include chemotaxis, secretion of superoxide anion and secretion of granule enzymes in response to deliberate external neutrophil stimulation. Thus, apoptosis leads to 'functional isolation' of neutrophils from stimuli in the external medium that would otherwise trigger responses with the potential to damage tissue – a

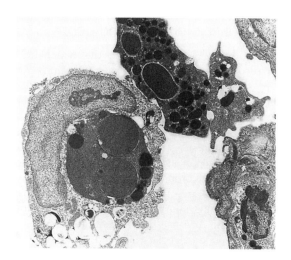

Fig. 3.5.9 Electron micrograph of experimental pneumococcal pneumonia at 72 h (in the early clearance phase), showing a macrophage that has engulfed an apoptotic neutrophil.

mechanism that may assume importance if fully competent phagocytes are not available in the vicinity of neutrophils undergoing apoptosis.

- Neutrophils undergoing apoptosis are ingested while still intact and without leakage of granule enzymes, which would occur should the cell disintegrate before or during uptake. This is emphasised by in-vitro experiments showing that only if macrophage uptake of apoptotic neutrophils is blocked (e.g. by colchicine) do the apoptotic neutrophils eventually disintegrate and release their contents.

- The usual response of macrophages to the ingestion of particles in vitro is to release proinflammatory mediators, e.g. thromboxanes, enzymes and cytokines. However, it has been shown that even maximal macrophage ingestion of apoptotic neutrophils fails to release proinflammatory mediators.[66] When apoptotic neutrophils were deliberately opsonised before their interaction with macrophages, macrophages then responded to the uptake of opsonised apoptotic neutrophils by releasing thromboxane. This also occurred when they were exposed to granulocytes that had been cultured beyond the phase of apoptosis to a point where they failed to exclude trypan blue. These experiments imply that it is recognition of the senescent granulocyte in the apoptotic morphology that determines the lack of a macrophage response and that this lack of response is not a function of the apoptotic particle itself but relates to the mechanisms by which apoptotic cells are normally recognised and ingested. These observations provided considerable impetus for work on the molecular mechanisms responsible for macrophage recognition and ingestion of apoptotic cells.

Mechanisms whereby macrophages recognise apoptotic neutrophils

Earlier work had suggested that macrophages possessed a lectin-like mechanism capable of recognising sugar residues on apoptotic thymocytes, exposed by loss of sialic acid.[67] This process does not appear to be involved in macrophage recognition of apoptotic neutrophils, but work with amino sugars and amino acids suggested a novel charge-sensitive phagocytic mechanism.[68] There is now evidence that this involves the integrin $\alpha v\beta_3$ (the vitronectin receptor)[69] and CD36 (a thrombospondin receptor)[70] on the macrophage surface. These molecules appear to link with thrombospondin, which binds to an as yet unidentified moiety on the apoptotic neutrophil surface. Recent studies on putative ionic sites on apoptotic murine thymocytes suggested that macrophages recognise exposed phosphatidylserine residues on the surface of apoptotic cells,[71] which may have been exposed by 'flipping' of the membrane phospholipid bilayer in a fashion analogous to that which occurs in the sickling of erythrocytes. The in-vivo significance of these observations is as yet uncertain. However, definition of cell-surface molecules used in macrophage uptake of apoptotic neutrophils suggests mechanisms by which this function may be controlled and modulated.

Clearance of apoptotic granulocytes by cells other than macrophages

In embryonic remodelling and in thymic involution it has been observed that, although apoptotic cells are usually removed by local macrophages, they may also be seen within epithelial, endothelial and fibroblast-like cells in the locality. In in-vitro experiments comparing the ability of monolayers of endothelial, epithelial and fibroblasts from various sources, only fibroblasts appeared to recognise and ingest apoptotic neutrophils. The fibroblast has long been recognised as a 'semiprofessional' phagocyte capable of ingesting latex beads, dye particles and mast-cell granules. More recently, it has been shown that the renal mesangial cell, a close relative of the fibroblast and also recognised as a semiprofessional phagocyte, has the capacity to ingest apoptotic neutrophils. The significance of these observations is uncertain. Fibroblasts appear to use a sugar-lectin-type mechanism, in addition to those described for recognition of apoptotic neutrophils, and it is possible that they may serve as a clearance mechanism for neutrophils before macrophages are fully matured from monocytes or should the macrophage system be overwhelmed by massive waves of neutrophil apoptosis. However, as the fibroblast is an inflammatory effector cell in its own right and is responsible for scar tissue matrix secretion, it is possible that this represents an 'undesirable' clearance route.

Modulation of granulocyte apoptosis by inflammatory mediators – a control point for their longevity and function in tissues?

Recent histological observations of resolving pulmonary inflammation suggested that extravasated neutrophils underwent apoptosis at a slower rate than that observed ex vivo in neutrophils derived from peripheral blood. This implied that factors present at the inflamed site might have retarded the inherent rate of neutrophil apoptosis. It has been known for several years that a range of inflammatory mediators, including GM-CSF, are able to prolong cultured neutrophil lifespan[72] in terms of the final necrosis of the cell (assessed by trypan blue positivity). More recently, it has been discovered that the rate of neutrophil apoptosis in vitro is markedly inhibited by a variety of inflammatory mediators, including endotoxic lipopolysaccharide, C5a and GM-CSF,[73,74] suggesting that mechanisms underlying the previous observations may be explained by their modulation of the process of apoptosis, which precedes necrosis in cultured eosinophils and neutrophils (see above). Experiments with eosinophils in vitro demonstrate that GM-CSF inhibits eosinophil apoptosis but IL-5 is also extremely potent in this regard, whereas it has no effect on neutrophil longevity.[64] It has been shown not only that inflammatory mediators such as C5a and GM-CSF prolong the life in tissue culture of neutrophil granulocytes by inhibiting apoptosis but also that this process results in greatly prolonged neutrophil functional longevity, as assessed by a number of in-vitro assays including chemotaxis granule secretion and other locomotor responses.[74]

Intracellular mechanisms governing apoptosis are as yet poorly understood but involve second-messenger signalling, including $[Ca^{2+}]_i$,[75] and a range of oncogene products, including c-*myc*, c-*ras*, *bcl2* and *p53*, have recently been shown to have controlling roles in certain cells under certain circumstances.[76] Ultimately it may be possible to use mechanisms underlying granulocyte apoptosis for therapeutic benefit. It is intriguing that two such closely related cells as the neutrophil and the eosinophil should appear to possess different inherent rates of apoptosis, which are further influenced by different external mediators. These observations suggest that it may be possible specifically to induce eosinophil apoptosis, for example, without influencing neutrophil apoptosis. Presumably this would result in clearance of eosinophils from tissues by the 'mechanisms that nature intended' and offer novel anti-inflammatory therapeutic approaches.

The clearance of macrophages

Although monocytes have the capacity to undergo apoptosis in vitro, the mechanisms involved in the clearance of macrophages that have completed their functions in host defence and clearance of inflammation remains obscure.

The paradox revisited – detrimental effects versus beneficial effects of the inflammatory response

It is reasonable to speculate that, in 'beneficial inflammation', potentially injurious events are tightly controlled so that inflammatory tissue injury is limited, inflammation ceases promptly and repair processes are effected with a minimum of scarring. It would therefore be expected ideally that:

- neutrophil emigration is rapid and contact time between neutrophil and endothelial or epithelial size minimised, possibly with the neutrophils in a non-secretory state during this phase
- essential matrix degradation necessary for cell emigration is localised and highly controlled
- neutrophil release of granule enzymes and reactive oxygen intermediates during phagocytosis and digestion of bacteria is minimal
- neutrophil emigration ceases promptly and extravasated neutrophils are removed rapidly, mostly as intact apoptotic cells
- local injury to epithelial and endothelial cells is minimal and is rapidly repaired
- fibrosis is absent except for the small amounts necessary for effective repair.

In this precariously balanced system it can be seen that even quantitative loss of efficiency at any of a number of important points could tip the balance towards excessive tissue injury and lead to the vicious cycles of persistent inflammation, tissue injury and scarring, that are cardinal features of inflammatory disease. The fact that endothelial and epithelial injury occur even in beneficial self-limiting inflammation implies that endothelial and epithelial cells may be particularly at risk in poorly controlled inflammation – a concept supported by the histological appearances of many inflammatory and allergic diseases.

The mechanisms whereby neutrophils may cause excessive injury to host tissues are now coming under more rigorous scrutiny. Neutrophil-mediated endothelial injury in vitro[38] and acute lung injury in an experimental model[39] both appear to require the combination of priming and activating agents for

injury to occur. It is now clear that very close apposition between the neutrophil and the 'target' cell is also necessary for injury.[77] This may be mediated by surface adhesive molecules but in vascular beds, such as that in the lung, factors reducing neutrophil deformability could also promote cell–cell contact in capillaries. Intercellular adhesion is a dynamic event in vivo and the kinetics of this interaction, as well as the degree of intercellular adhesion, are likely to be important, because prolongation of cell–cell contact would obviously increase the potential for injury by each incoming wave of primed and activated neutrophils.

Close and prolonged contact between actively secreting neutrophils and endothelial cells is thought to favour injury by more than one mechanism; the intracellular microenvironment creates an exclusive domain in which the local concentrations of histotoxic agents would reach very high levels, and inhibitors and scavengers, particularly those of high molecular weight, would tend to be excluded. The highly reactive nature of reactive oxygen species inevitably limits their range of activity in tissues. Their potential for injury may therefore be enhanced in circumscribed areas of very close cell–cell contact. Furthermore, potentially injurious neutrophil enzymes may be presented in very high concentrations locally on the neutrophil surface that makes contact with the endothelial cell.

A difficult problem at present is to identify which of the plethora of potentially injurious inflammatory cell products are involved centrally in mediating tissue injury in disease. Many of these, even if secreted in small amounts, may prove highly toxic if presented on the surface of adherent neutrophils. Much attention in the last decade has been paid to a primary and direct role for reactive oxygen species. However, the most toxic intermediates are so evanescent and reactive that they are likely to be rapidly inactivated and to possess a relatively short effective range in tissues. More recently, it has been suggested that reactive oxygen species could exert an additional important *indirect* role by damaging antiproteinases, some of which are very prone to being rendered ineffective by low concentrations of oxidants.[78]

Neutrophil elastase is now widely believed to play a prominent role in neutrophil-mediated tissue injury. It is capable of digesting a variety of proteins in addition to elastin and is a highly cationic molecule. It is certainly toxic to cells in vitro but whether its toxic effects are mediated by its enzymatic activity or by other properties remains uncertain. From Table 3.5.3 it can be seen that there is a large range of neutrophil and other inflammatory cell products with huge potential to injure tissues, some of which (such as the cationic proteins) have not as yet had in-vivo function attributed to them. Thus, in the future other agents may well assume prominence in the pathogenesis of inflammatory diseases.

Lung inflammation and scarring

Although the inflammatory response in streptococcal pneumonia characteristically resolves completely without scarring, other types of pneumonia, including staphylococcal pneumonia, are often associated with persistent inflammation, tissue destruction and massive scarring responses. In most examples of inflammatory lung disease (even asthma), there is evidence that persistent accumulation of inflammatory cells is associated with at least a degree of local fibrotic tissue reaction.

A causal relationship between inflammation and scarring responses has been suspected for many years. In inflammatory lung diseases, e.g. fibrosing alveolitis, an acute inflammatory phase is thought to precede chronic inflammation, which itself precedes scarring. Although this is probably broadly true, scarring may occur very early (in ARDS, for example), and even in 'end-stage' fibrosing alveolitis there is often clear evidence of continued emigration of acute inflammatory cells, including neutrophils, as well as the monocytes and lymphocytes that characterise chronic inflammation. In experimental models of inflammation and scarring, the phases of acute inflammation, chronic inflammation and fibroblast proliferation and secretion that characterise scarring appear to merge together in a continuum rather than occurring as easily separable phases.

Most pathologists currently hold the view that the degree of injury to the epithelium and its basement membrane in the primary inflammatory damage to the lung is a key factor determining whether excessive scarring occurs. It is thought that the lung can tolerate a certain degree and extent of injury to type I epithelial cells without the necessity for excessive scarring, the gaps in the epithelium being repaired by division of type II epithelial pneumocytes to form a new monolayer of type I cells. However, if there is extensive disruption of the epithelium, and particularly if the basement membrane is severely damaged and loses its architectural integrity, a scarring response appears likely to result. This concept arose from intriguing experiments carried out by Witschi, in which he denuded varying amounts

of the tracheal epithelium and found that there was a critical degree of denudation beyond which repair was effected by fibrosis rather than by re-epithelialisation of the 'wounded area'.

The inflammatory response is likely to impinge on the scarring process at a number of levels (Fig. 3.5.10a), including the degree of primary epithelial injury caused by the inflammatory process itself, and by inflammatory cell-derived agents inducing fibroblasts to proliferate and deposit excessive scar tissue matrix proteins. Again it must be stressed that, although the fibroproliferative response in the controlled formation of granulation tissue (the precursor of scar tissue) is a necessary part of natural repair processes, scarring diseases of the lungs are considered to represent a disordered and excessive fibroproliferative response that leads to a pathological end result.

The fibroproliferative response is characterised by dividing fibroblasts that lay down scar tissue matrix proteins, including collagen. Collagen production by fibroblasts is normally a highly regulated process with internal and external controls being exerted at several levels (Fig. 3.5.10).[79] All but 30% of the extracellularly secreted collagen is normally degraded, mainly by fibroblast-derived collagenase. The effect of collagenase itself is under a further internal control mechanism whereby it is kept in check by enzyme inhibitors including a tissue inhibitor of metalloproteinases (TIMP). Fibroblast activity is also under the control of external factors, including cytokines and growth factors (Fig. 3.5.10b), many of which can be secreted in large quantities by local cells, particularly inflammatory macrophages. Most of these factors, including platelet-derived growth factor (PDGF), transforming growth factor (TGF)-β, fibroblast growth factor (FGF) and insulin-like growth factor (IGF) have

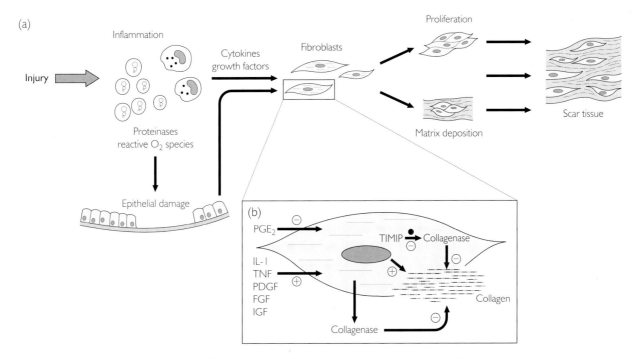

Fig. 3.5.10 (a) Complex interactions between injury, inflammation, repair and lung scarring. (b) The fibroblast – key involvement in the control of inflammation and repair. FGF, fibroblast growth factor; IGF, insulin-like growth factor; PDGF, platelet derived growth factor; PGE₂, prostaglandin E₂; TIMP, tissue inhibitor of metalloproteinase.

been shown to exert permissive or stimulatory effects on fibroblast growth and secretion. External factors exerting negative influences must also exist. Although these have received less attention, prostaglandin E_2 represents an example of an inflammatory mediator with mainly inhibitory effects on fibroblast function.

The fibroblast itself is now recognised to be a complex and multipotent cell that is not only important in the control of tissue architecture and matrix assembly but is also capable of generating a number of important cytokines, including IL-8, IL-1 and TNF, which probably play important roles in the initiation of inflammation. Indeed, it now appears that fibroblast subpopulations exist with different phenotypic features, some of which appear to be important in lung diseases associated with persistent inflammation and scarring.

Prospects for more specific anti-inflammatory therapy

Non-specific anti-inflammatory therapies, including corticosteroids, have been useful in many inflammatory diseases but in examples such as fibrosing alveolitis the results are disappointing or are associated with serious adverse effects from chronic use of the medications themselves. With the recent explosion of knowledge concerning the cellular and molecular mechanisms of the inflammatory process, it is likely that novel and specific therapeutic strategies will become available. These might include:

- agents that specifically inhibit the mediators initiating inflammation
- agents directed against specific cell–cell adhesion molecules
- inhibitors of certain secretory mechanisms
- agents directed against injurious products such as neutrophil elastase or reactive oxygen species.

However, these exciting possibilities should not detract from the knowledge that any really effective anti-inflammatory therapeutic strategy must take account of the paradox of inflammation. Thus mechanisms that appear to be involved in tissue injury in inflammatory diseases may be identical to those used in host defence, and there are many examples of multiplicity and redundancy in these mechanisms. This raises at least two immediate problems.

First, the efficacy of the inflammatory response in host defence lies at least in part in the redundancy of many of its mechanisms. Thus, the inhibition of a single mediator or single cell type is not likely to render the whole response ineffective. For example, several members of the chemokine family of mediators may initiate neutrophil emigration but components of the complement cascade, e.g. C5a and leukotriene mediators (LTB_4), as well as bacterial products themselves, are also chemotactic for neutrophils. The spider's web provides an useful analogy, because unless the 'key strand' can be identified, the removal or loss of other less important strands is not likely to attenuate the overall effectiveness of the response. This redundancy is obviously a great advantage for an effective host

defence but, when the same principle is turned against the host in the pathogenesis of inflammatory diseases, the development of rational therapeutic strategies becomes a formidable challenge. It may be possible, however, to identify certain key groups of mediators that are critically involved at certain phases of the pathogenesis of inflammatory disease and that could be rendered ineffective with limited 'cocktails' of anti-inflammatory mediators.

Second, effective anti-inflammatory strategies are likely to weaken host defences critically, particularly against bacterial infection, and, although it may be possible to identify mainly detrimental mechanisms, the more we learn about inflammatory diseases the clearer it becomes that the cellular and molecular mechanisms are identical to those employed in host defence. It is probable, therefore, that powerful, new, mechanism-based anti-inflammatory strategies will need to be applied during 'windows of opportunity' when the inflammatory mechanisms are more critical to the evolution of the disease process than they are to the general defence of the host; at the same time it will be necessary, however, to employ other approaches to prevent infective complications during therapeutic periods.

Alternatively, it may be possible to promote mechanisms that favour resolution of inflammation rather than progression or to boost local defence mechanisms by, for example, promoting the local genetic expression of antiproteinases, antioxidants or other agents responsible for cytoprotection of healthy host tissues during inflammatory responses.

? Unresolved questions

- Which qualitative or quantitative disturbances of the beneficial inflammatory responses tip the balance towards excessive tissue injury and persistent inflammation?
- What will be the most successful therapeutic targets in the cellular and molecular mechanisms of inflammatory lung diseases:
  - agents that inhibit mediators initiating inflammation?
  - agents directed against specific cell–cell adhesion molecules?
  - agents that inhibit certain secretory mechanisms?
  - agents directed against injurious products?
- Will 'cocktails' of anti-inflammatory interventions be required, because of the multiplicity and redundancy of inflammatory pathways in disease?
- Are there 'windows of opportunity' for successful application of new mechanism-based anti-inflammatory strategies, by which weakening of host defence can be avoided?
- Should interventions be directed towards favouring resolution of inflammation rather than inhibiting progression? Can this be obtained by promoting local genetic expression of endogenous agents for cytoprotection of healthy host tissues?

References

1. Heffron R. Pneumonia: with special reference to pneumococcus lobar pneumonia, vol xvii. Commonwealth Fund, 1939: 1086p.
2. Robertson OH, Uhley CG. Changes occurring in the macrophage system of the lungs in pneumococcus lobar pneumonia. J Clin Invest 1938 15: 115.
3. Cullen Sir William. The practice of physic, 2nd ed. Edinburgh; 1778–84.
4. Hurley JV. Termination of acute inflammation. 1. Resolution. In: Acute inflammation. 2nd edn. Edinburgh: Churchill Livingstone, 1983: 109.
5. Lien D, Haslett C, Henson PM et al. Neutrophil sequestration in the pulmonary circulation: direct visualisation of localisation in capillaries. J Appl Physiol 1987; 1236.
6. Donnelly SC, Strieter RM, Kunkel SL. Chemotactic cytokines in the established adult respiratory distress syndrome and at-risk patients. Chest 1994; 105(Suppl. 3): 988.
7. Kunkel SL, Standiford T, Kasaahara K, Strieter RM. Interleukin-8: the major neutrophil chemotactic factor in the lung. Exp Lung Res 1991; 17: 17.
8. Gerard C, Gerard NP. Molecular biology of human neutrophil chemotactic receptors. In: Helliwell PG, Williams TJ, ed. Immunopharmacology of neutrophils. London: Academic Press; 1994: 115.
9. Streiter RM, Kunkel SL, Showell HJ, Marks RM. Monokine-induced gene expression of a human endothelial cell derived chemotactic factor. Biochem Biophys Res Commun 1988; 156: 1340.
10. Schmid-Schonbein GW, Shih YY, Chion S. Morphometry of human leukocytes. Blood 1985; 56: 866.
11. Worthen GS, Schwab B, Elson EL, Downey GP. Mechanisms of stimulated neutrophils: cell stiffening induces retention on capillaries. Science 1989; 245: 183.
12. Erzurum SC, Downey GP, Worthen GS. Bacterial lipopolysaccharide mediates microfilament-dependent retention of neutrophils in model capillaries. Am Rev Respir Dis 1989; 139: A298.
13. Drost EM, Selby C, Lannan S et al. Changes in neutrophil deformability following in vitro smoke exposure. Am J Respir Cell Mol Biol 1992; 6: 287.
14. Rosen SD. Cell surface lectins in the immune system. Semin Immunol 1993; 5: 237.
15. Lawrence MB, Springer TA. Leukocytes roll on a selectin at physiologic flow rates: distinction form and prerequisite for adhesion through integrins. Cell 1991; 65: 859.
16. Doershuk CM, Winn RK, Coxson H, Harlan JM. CD18-dependent and independent mechanisms of neutrophil emigration in the pulmonary and systemic microcirculation of rabbits. J Immunol 1990; 144: 2327.
17. Springer TA. Adhesion receptors of the immune system. Nature 1990; 346: 425.
18. Arnaout MA. Leukocyte adhesion molecules deficiency: its structural basis, pathophysiology and implications for modulating the inflammatory response. Immunol Rev 1990; 114: 145.
19. Davies KA, Toothill VJ, Savill J et al. A 19-year-old man with leucocyte adhesion deficiency. In vitro and in vivo studies of leucocyte function. Clin Exp Immunol 1991; 84: 223.
20. Williams AF, Barclay AN. The immunoglobin superfamily: domains for cell surface recognition. Annu Rev Immunol 1988; 6: 381.
21. Staunton DE, Dustin ML, Springer TA. Functional cloning of ICAM-2, a cell adhesion ligand for LFA-1 homologous to ICAM-1. Nature 1989; 339: 61.
22. Hogg M, Bates PA, Harvey J. Structure and function of intercellular adhesion molecule-1. In: Hogg M, ed. Integrins and ICAM-1 in immune responses, vol. 50. Basel: S Karger; 1991: 98.
23. Arnaout MA. Structure and function of the leukocyte adhesion molecules CD11/CD18. Blood 1990; 75: 1037.
24. Dransfield I. Regulation of leukocyte integrin function. In: Hogg M, ed. Integrins and ICAM-1 in immune responses, vol. 50. Basel: S Karger; 1991: 13.
25. Hynes RO. Integrins: versatility, modulation and signalling in cell adhesion. Cell 1992; 69: 11.
26. Mulligan MS, Varani J, Dane MK et al. Role of endothelial-leukocyte adhesion molecule 1 (ELAM-1) in neutrophil-mediated lung injury in rats. J Clin Invest 1991; 88: 1396.
27. Mulligan MS, Watson SR, Fennie C, Ward PA. Protective effects of selectin chimeras in neutrophil-mediated lung injury. J Immunol 1993; 131: 6410.
28. Etzioni A, Frydman M, Pollock S et al. Recurrent severe infections caused by a novel leukocyte adhesion deficiency. N Engl J Med 1992; 327: 1789.
29. Pober JS, Cotran RS. Cytokines and endothelial cell biology. Physiol Rev 1990; 70: 427.
30. Norris P, Poston RN, Thomas DS et al. The expression of endothelial leukocyte adhesion molecule-1 (ELAM-1), intercellular adhesion molecule-1 (ICAM-1)

and vascular cell adhesion molecule-1 (VCAM-1) in experimental cutaneous inflammation: a comparison of ultraviolet-B erythema and delayed hypersensitivity. J Invest Dermatol 1991; 96: 763
31. Huber AR, Weiss SJ. Disruption of the subendothelial basement membrane during neutrophil diapedesis in an in vitro construct of a blood vessel wall. J Clin Invest 1989; 83: 1122.
32. Milks L, Cramer E. Transepithelial electrical resistance studies during in vitro neutrophil migration. Fed Proc Fed Am Soc Exp Biol 1984; 43: 477.
33. Cockroft S. Receptor-mediated signal transduction pathways in neutrophils. In: Helliwell PG, Williams TJ, ed. Immunopharmacology of neutrophils. London: Academic Press; 1994: 159.
34. McColl SR, Showall HJ. Neutrophil-derived inflammatory mediators. In: Helliwell PG, Williams TJ, ed. Immunopharmacology of neutrophils. London: Academic Press; 1994: 95.
35. Guthrie LA, McPhail LC, Henson PM, Johnston RB. The priming of neutrophils for enhanced release of oxygen metabolites by bacterial lipopolysaccharide. J Exp Med 1984; 160: 1656.
36. Haslett C, Guthrie LA, Kopaniak MM et al. Modulation of multiple neutrophil functions by preparative methods or trace concentrations of lipopolysaccharide. Am J Pathol 1985; 119: 101.
37. Worthen GS, Seccombe JF, Clay KL et al. The priming of neutrophils by lipopolysaccharide for production of intracellular platelet activating factor. J Immunol 1988; 140: 3553.
38. Smedley LA, Tonnesen MG, Sandhaus RA et al. Neutrophil mediated injury to endothelial cells: enhancement by endotoxin and essential role of neutrophil elastase. J Clin Invest 1986; 77: 1233.
39. Worthen GS, Haslett C, Rees AJ et al. Neutrophil-mediated pulmonary vascular injury. Synergistic effects of trace amounts of lipopolysaccharide in C5a-induced lung injury. Am Rev Respir Dis 1987; 136: 19.
40. Young SK, Worthen GS, Haslett C et al. Interaction between chemoattractants and bacterial lipopolysaccharide in the induction and enhancement of neutrophil adhesion. Am J Respir Cell Mol Biol 1990; 2: 523.
41. Mackaness GB. The monocyte in cellular immunity Semin Haematol 1970; 7: 172.
42. Johnstone RB, Godzik CA, Cohn ZA. Increased superoxide anion production by immunologically activated and chemically-elicited macrophages. J Exp Med 1978; 148: 115.
43. Haslett C. Resolution of acute inflammation and the role of apoptosis in the tissue fate of granulocytes. Clin Sci 1992; 83: 639.
44. Colditz IG, Movat HZ. Desensitisation of acute inflammatory lesions to chemotaxins and endotoxin. J Immunol 1984; 133: 2163.
45. Haslett C, Jose PJ, Giclas PC et al. Cessation of neutrophil influx in C5a-induced acute experimental arthritis is associated with loss of chemoattractant activity from joint spaces. J Immunol 1989; 142: 3510.
46. Clark RJ, Jones HA, Rhodes CG, Haslett C. Non-invasive assessment in self-limited pulmonary inflammation by external scintigraphy of [111]indium-labelled neutrophil influx and by measurement of the local metabolic response with positron emission tomography. Am Rev Respir Dis 1989; 139: A58.
47. Haslett C, Shen AS, Feldsien DC et al. [111]Indium-labelled neutrophil flux into the lungs of bleomycin-treated rabbits assessed non-invasively by external scintigraphy. Am Rev Respir Dis 1989; 140: 756.
48. Doherty DE, Downey GP, Worthen GS et al. Monocyte retention and migration in pulmonary inflammation. Lab Invest 1988; 59: 200.
49. Majno E, Palade GE. Studies on inflammation. 1. The effect of histamine and serotonin on vascular permeability: an electron microscopic study. J Biol Phys Biochem Cytol 1961; 11: 571.
50. Parsons PE, Sugahara K, Cott GR et al. The effect of neutrophil migration and prolonged neutrophil contact on epithelial permeability. Am J Pathol 1987; 129: 302.
51. Zimmerli W, Seligmann B, Gallin JI. Exudation primes human and guinea pig neutrophils for subsequent responsiveness to the chemotactic peptide N-formyl methionyl leucyl phenylalanine and increases complement C3bi receptor expression. J Clin Invest 1986; 77: 925.
52. Whyte MKB, Meagher LC, MacDermot J, Haslett C Impairment of function in aging neutrophils is associated with apoptosis. J Immunol 1993; 150: 5123.
53. Bitterman BP. Pathogenesis of fibrosis in acute lung injury. Am J Med 1992; 92: 395.
54. Metchnikoff E. Lectures on the comparative pathology of inflammation. Lecture VII. Delivered at the Pasteur Institute in 1891, trans. Starling FA, Starling EH. New York: Dover; 1968.
55. Spriggs RS, Biddington MM, Mowat AG. Joint fluid cytology in Reiter's syndrome. Ann Rheum Dis 1978; 37: 557.
56. Chapes SK, Haskill S. Evidence for granulocyte-mediated macrophage activation after C. parvum immunization. Cell Immunol 1983; 75: 367.

57. Newman SL, Henson JE, Henson PM. Phagocytosis of senescent neutrophils by human monocyte-derived macrophages and rabbit inflammatory macrophages. J Exp Med 1982; 156: 430.

58. Savill JS, Henson PM, Haslett C. Phagocytosis of aged human neutrophils by macrophages is mediated by a novel 'charge sensitive' recognition mechanism. J Clin Invest 1989; 84: 1518.

59. Grigg JM, Savill JS, Sarraf C et al. Neutrophil apoptosis and clearance from neonatal lungs. Lancet 1991; 338: 720.

60. Wyllie AH, Kerr JFR, Currie AR. Cell death: the significance of apoptosis. Int Rev Cytol 1980; 68: 251.

61. Arends MJ, Morris RG, Wyllie AH. Apoptosis. The role of the endonuclease. Am J Pathol. 1990; 136:593–608.

62. Haslett C, Savill JS, Whyte MKB et al. Granulocyte apoptosis and the control of inflammation. Philos Trans R Soc Lond B Biol Sci 1994; 345: 327–333.

63. Haslett C, Savill JS, Meagher L The neutrophil. Curr Opin Immunol 1989; 2: 10.

64. Stern M, Meagher L, Savill J, Haslett C. Apoptosis in human eosinophils. Programmed cell death in the eosinophil leads to phagocytosis by macrophages and is modulated by IL-5. J Immunol 1992; 148: 3543.

65. Kawabori S, Soda K, Perdue MH, Bienenstock J. The dynamics of intestinal eosinophil depletion in rats treated with dexamethasone. Lab Invest 1991; 64: 224.

66. Meagher LC, Savill JS, Baker A et al. Phagocytosis of apoptotic neutrophils does not induce macrophage release of thromboxane B_2. J Leukocyte Biol 1992; 52: 269.

67. Duvall E, Wyllie AH, Morris RG. Macrophage recognition of cells undergoing programmed cell death. Immunology 1985; 56: 351.

68. Savill JS, Henson PM, Haslett C. Phagocytosis of aged human neutrophils by macrophages is mediated by a novel charge-sensitive mechanism. J Clin Invest 1989; 84: 1518.

69. Savill JS, Dransfield I, Hogg N, Haslett C. Macrophage recognition of 'senescent self'; the vitronectin receptor mediates phagocytosis of cells undergoing apoptosis. Nature 1990; 342: 170.

70. Savill JS, Hogg N, Haslett C. Thrombospondin co-operates with CD36 and the vitronectin receptor in macrophage recognition of aged neutrophils. J Clin Invest 1992; 90: 1513.

71. Fadok VA, Savill JS, Haslett C et al. Different populations of macrophages use either the vitronectin receptor or the phosphatidylserine receptor to recognise and remove apoptotic cells. J Immunol 1992; 149: 4029.

72. Lopez AF, Williamson DJ, Gamble JR et al. Recombinant human granulocyte-macrophage colony-stimulating factor stimulates in vitro mature human neutrophil and eosinophil function, surface receptor expression, and survival. J Clin Invest 1986; 78: 1220.

73. Brach MA, de Vos S, Gruss H-J, Herrman F. Prolongation of survival of human polymorphonuclear neutrophils by granulocyte–macrophage colony-stimulating factor is caused by inhibition of programmed cell death. Blood 1992; 80: 2920.

74. Lee A, Whyte MKB, Haslett C. Inhibition of apoptosis and prolongation of neutrophil functional longevity by inflammatory mediators. J Leukoc Biol 1993; 54: 283.

75. Whyte MKB, Meagher LC, Hardwick S et al. Transient elevations of cystolic free calcium retard subsequent apoptosis in neutrophils in vitro. J Clin Invest 1993; 92: 446.

76. Evan GI, Wyllie AH, Gilbert CS et al. Induction of apoptosis in fibroblasts by c-*myc* protein. Cell 1992; 69: 119.

77. Campbell EJ, Senior RM, Welgus HG. Extracellular matrix injury during lung inflammation. Chest 1987; 92: 161.

78. Weiss SJ. Tissue destruction by neutrophils. N Engl J Med 1989; 320: 365.

79. Gauldie J, Jordana M, Cox G et al. Fibroblasts and other structural cells in airway inflammation. Am Rev Respir Dis 1992; 145: S14.

SYMPTOMS AND SIGNS OF RESPIRATORY DISEASE

4 Clinical assessment

John Earis

Cough and sputum

- Dry cough is associated with early pneumonia, tumours and the use of angiotensin-converting-enzyme inhibitors; chronic moist cough is characteristic of chronic obstructive pulmonary disease and bronchiectasis.

- Nocturnal cough is characteristic of asthma, gastro-oesophageal reflux, postnasal drip.

- Large quantities of watery sputum may he associated with alveolar-cell tumours.

- Green sputum can be caused by allergy as well as infection.

- Sputum plugs occur with asthma, especially when complicated with bronchopulmonary aspergillosis.

- Haemoptysis in smokers (particularly over 40 years of age) should always be investigated to exclude malignancy.

Chest pain

- Pleurisy can be associated with infection, malignancy, infarction, vasculitis and pneumothorax.

- Pleurisy of the outer diaphragmatic pleura may be referred to the abdomen and pleurisy of the central diaphragmatic pleura to the neck and tip of shoulder.

- Chest wall pain is usually localised but can be mistaken for cardiac pain.

- Oesophageal pain can also mimic cardiac pain and pericardial pain can be mistaken for pleurisy.

Breathlessness

- Breathlessness is the subjective sensation of an uncomfortable need to breathe.

- Very sudden dyspnoea is rare and usually associated with severe disease (e.g. pneumothorax, pulmonary embolism, left ventricular failure or sudden asthma).

- Orthopnoea may be associated with diaphragmatic paralysis as well as pulmonary oedema.

- Nocturnal breathlessness is associated with asthma as well as cardiac disease

- Occasionally, left ventricular failure is also associated with wheeze.

Signs of respiratory disease

- Cyanosis:
  - is an unreliable sign
  - can only be detected when saturation falls to 85%
  - may be absent when associated with severe anaemia
  - is exaggerated when associated polycythemia.

- Central cyanosis can only be diagnosed when the area is warm (e.g. the tongue) and lighting conditions are good.

- Clubbing:
  - is usually bilateral and usually affects both fingers and toes
  - lesser degrees are difficult to identify clinically.

- Hypertrophic osteodystrophy:
  - is associated with clubbing and with increased blood flow but not new vessel formation
  - presents with pain around wrists and ankles and has characteristic X-ray and isotope bone scan appearances
  - is of unknown cause but is thought to be associated with vagal stimulation and/or release of vasoactive substances.

Key points

Chest shape and deformities

- When severe, scoliosis may be associated with cardiorespiratory failure (particularly if it affects the upper spine and/or in the presence of muscle weakness).

- Kyphosis, when not associated with scoliosis, is unlikely to cause significant respiratory impairment.

- Thoracoplasty may result in late onset of cardiorespiratory failure.

- Funnel-shaped sternal deformity does not cause respiratory impairment.

- Pigeon chest is either congenital (as with Harrison's sulcus) or a consequence of childhood airflow obstruction.

Breath sounds at the mouth

- Gasping is associated with fright, intense cold or a deranged respiratory centre, while sighing overcomes alveolar cohesion in normal subjects; excessive sighing is associated with functional breathing disorders.

- Hissing (Kussmaul's breathing) is associated with metabolic disturbances and may not be noticed by the patient.

- Panting respiration is a response to either increase in elastic load (e.g. fibrosis) or resistance (e.g. airflow obstruction).

- Wheezing associated with airflow obstruction is most marked in asthma and may be very quiet and only heard at the end of expiration in emphysema.

- Whistles and grunts are common in emphysema and may induce 'auto-PEEP', while whoops and stridor are associated with laryngeal or major airway narrowing.

- Rattles and loud crackles signify secretions in airways and are prominent during the terminal stages of chest disease.

Percussion

- Percussion is only of clinical value when comparing one hemithorax to the other.

- Stony dull percussion suggests pleural effusion; intermediate grades of dullness can signify consolidation or collapse but need to be taken in association with other physical signs.

- Hyper-resonant percussion is difficult to detect unless very marked (e.g. large pneumothorax or large emphysematous bulla).

Palpation

- Lymph nodes are frequently missed unless palpation of the neck and axillae is undertaken systematically.

- In the absence of chest drainage surgical emphysema suggests a 'mediastinal' air leak (e.g. air tracking down peribronchial tissues or a ruptured oesophagus).

- Mediastinal shift does not occur with consolidation alone and may not occur with a combination of collapse and effusion.

- Chest expansion is better assessed by inspection than palpation.

- Vocal fremitus is only of value if grossly impaired (e.g. large effusion).

Breath sounds at the chest wall

- Breath sounds heard at the chest wall are modified central airway sounds where the higher frequencies have been filtered-out by the lung tissue.

- Tracheal sounds have a wide frequency band (less filtering from lung tissue) and are directly related to airflow.

- Breath-sound intensity at the chest wall depends on airflow and the transmission characteristics of the lung.

- Global airflow obstruction is associated with reduced sound intensity at the chest wall.

- Bronchial breathing occurs because consolidated lung allows higher-frequency sounds to reach the chest wall.

Wheezing

- Wheezing is a dynamic sound that alters in pitch during expiration.

- Airflow obstruction can occur without wheezing and very severe obstruction may be associated with a 'silent' chest.

- Wheeze duration rather than its intensity is associated with FEV_1.

- Three main types of wheezing have been described: fixed monophonic, random monophonic and expiratory polyphonic.

- Low-pitched wheezes (rhonchi) are most commonly cased by secretions or narrowing of large airways.

- Short musical inspiratory sounds (squawks) are associated with interstitial disease, particularly extrinsic allergic alveolitis.

Crackles

- Crackles are most commonly the result of the sudden opening of smaller airways.

- Crackles heard by auscultation are generated within a few centimetres of the stethoscope.

- Fine late crackles are usually associated with interstitial disease or pulmonary oedema.

- Coarse early inspiratory crackles are associated with chronic obstructive pulmonary disease.

A careful and detailed clinical history and examination of patients with respiratory disease is the basis of a logical and focused approach to diagnosis and investigation. To place too much reliance on diagnostic tests leads to unnecessary investigations and a failure to address the patient's main concerns. The assessment of a patient's problem starts as soon as the physician sees them. General features such as their degree of breathlessness, weight loss, anxiety and ability to walk can be observed. Questioning of symptoms has to be logical and detailed with the avoidance, where possible, of leading questions. The classic sequence of first exploring the presenting complaints, followed by past history, systematic review, family and social history, industrial and smoking history has stood the test of time. Making careful observations of the patient while taking their history often elicits many of the physical signs that are analysed in more detail during the physical examination (e.g. clubbing, superior vena cava obstruction, tar-stained fingers, basic breathing pattern). Further aspects of the history may need to be explored if physical signs – scars, skin lesions, etc. – that have hitherto been undisclosed by the patient are found during the physical examination.

It has been shown that there is considerable intraobserver variation in eliciting respiratory physical signs.[1] The most reliable signs are clubbing, wheezes, pleural rub, crackles and percussion note, while there is less agreement about such signs as cyanosis, tracheal deviation, whispering pectoriloquy and tactile vocal fremitus.[2]

This chapter will discuss the clinical assessment of the main symptoms and signs associated with chest disease and provide, where possible, underlying physiological and anatomical explanations, as well as outlining the newer understanding of the acoustics of respiratory sounds. More detailed descriptions of the main respiratory symptoms of cough, haemoptysis, breathlessness and chest pain are found in Chapter 5.

Assessment of respiratory symptoms

General symptoms

As well as the specific symptoms outlined below, respiratory disease may produce a variety of general symptoms of which tiredness, lassitude and weight loss are the commonest. Together with fever, these symptoms are characteristic of infection, especially tuberculosis, and lung cancer. The latter may also give rise to a variety of extrathoracic manifestations due to metastasis (in lymph nodes, brain, bone, liver or other organs) or to the secretion of hormones causing myoneuropathies and endocrine syndromes (Cushing's syndrome, inappropriate antidiuretic hormone secretion, etc.). Respiratory failure alone may lead to weight loss (without the presence of a tumour) and oedema if associated with cor pulmonale. If hypercapnia is also present, particularly if there has been a rapid rise in $P\text{CO}_2$ because of infection, sedation or oxygen therapy, then headaches and confusion (especially on waking), drowsiness and difficulty in concentrating may occur.

Upper respiratory tract symptoms

Chronic nasal obstruction or rhinorrhoea is often due to conditions that can also affect the lower respiratory tract. Allergic rhinitis, with or without polyp formation, is a manifestation of atopy and therefore a common accompaniment of asthma. A persistent purulent nasal discharge with occasional episodes of fever and facial or periorbital pain suggests chronic sinusitis and this may be associated with bronchiectasis. A bloodstained and sometimes offensive nasal discharge can also be the presenting feature of a more widespread granulomatous condition such as Wegener's granulomatosis or sarcoidosis. Malignancy may present with a bloody discharge from either the nose or mouth. The latter may signal postnasal-space malignancy and can be mistaken for haemoptysis.

The main symptoms from the mouth are pain or soreness due to mouth ulcers, gum infections or herpes simplex ulceration around the lips. These conditions may be associated with lower respiratory infections, such as lung abscesses, bronchiectasis and pneumonia. Halitosis is associated with gum/dental disease, particularly in cases of poor oral hygiene, but can also be a manifestation of immunodeficiency or chronic lung sepsis.

The pharynx may be painful on swallowing because of upper respiratory infection, particularly when tonsillitis is present. However, the most important symptom relevant to respiration is the functional airflow obstruction that accompanies snoring. At laryngeal level the main symptoms are hoarse voice, stridor and cough.

Hoarse voice

Normal speech sounds are broadly divided into voiced sounds (e.g. vowels), where the sound is generated by the vocal cords, and non-voiced sounds (e.g. 'p' 't'), where the sound is created by turbulent airflow in the upper airway. Hoarseness is associated with abnormality of voiced sounds due to disorganised movement of the vocal cords. Normally the cords open and close in an orderly and regular fashion but when they are damaged this regular movement breaks down and the pitch period (time between one closure and the next) becomes irregular.[3,4] Any damage to the vocal cords will produce hoarseness; such damage may be caused by laryngitis, tumours or cord paralysis. If the left cord is paralysed the possibility of a bronchial neoplasm invading the left recurrent laryngeal nerve at the level of the hilum has to be considered.

Lower respiratory symptoms

Cough

Cough is a basic protective mechanism of the upper airway designed to eliminate foreign material and clear the airways of secretions. The sound of cough is easily recognised and can be very loud, reaching levels well above 100 dB. Generally, cough has two sounds (energy peaks), which are easily heard by the ear, a first cough sound produced at glottic opening, then a short period (approximately 500 ms) when harmonic structure may be observed followed by a second sound at the time of glottic

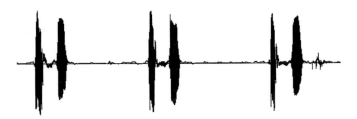

Fig. 4.1 Cough sounds. The time-domain waveform for three separate coughs is shown. Each cough has two sounds: the first occurs with glottic opening and the second at the time of glottic closure.

closure (Fig. 4.1). Some coughs have single or multiple peaks and it has been reported that these are more often associated with disease states.[5] Each individual's cough tends to have particular acoustic characteristics.[6] Coughs may be isolated or multiple within a single breath (peal of coughs), when this happens each cough tends to be quieter than the preceding one.

Two main types of cough are recognised, namely, dry and moist, the latter being associated with increased airway sputum. A short, dry cough, sometimes described as hacking, is characteristic of upper respiratory tract infections and the early stages of pneumonia but, if it is persistent, the possibility of tumour should be excluded. A similar dry cough presents in 10% of patients treated with angiotensin-converting-enzyme inhibitors.[7] A moist productive cough, often prolonged and repetitive, occurs in chronic obstructive pulmonary disease (COPD) and bronchiectasis. A feeble non-explosive 'bovine' cough is heard when vocal cord paralysis is present. Widespread respiratory muscle weakness from any cause has a similar effect. The cough produced by laryngeal inflammation or tumour tends to be harsh and hoarse while the cough associated with tracheal compression is said to have a curious metallic quality ('brassy'). In children especially, violent fits of coughing followed by inspiratory stridor or 'whoop' due to laryngeal spasm suggest pertussis or the inhalation of a foreign body. Children with asthma may present with a 'loose' cough not necessarily accompanied by sputum production. When expiratory airflow is severely reduced, cough may have a muffled quality.

Associate features

The circumstances in which cough occurs may give clues to its cause. Nocturnal cough is a common presenting symptom of asthma in children, while a postnasal drip, oesophageal reflux of gastric contents and pulmonary congestion from left heart failure should be considered among older patients. Patients with chronic bronchitis and asthma often complain of cough that is worse on rising in the morning, in a smoky atmosphere and with changes of temperature, as well as during the winter. Cough during swallowing is an important symptom of neurogenic dysphagia suggesting inhalation of food and fluid; patients with otherwise unexplained cough should be observed while drinking from a glass of water, especially those with known neurological conditions or when a tracheo-oesophageal fistula is suspected. Allergic disorders of the airways and lungs, both asthma and alveolitis, may present with cough during or after exposure to the offending agent.

Sputum

The tracheobronchial tree is protected by a thin layer of visco-elastic mucus, which is constantly wafted to the larynx by the ciliated epithelium (mucociliary escalator). This keeps the mucosa moist and traps particulate matter that enters the main airways. Increased production of sputum is associated with damage to the tracheobronchial tree, particularly damage caused by acute and chronic respiratory infections and bronchial irritation by chemicals or smoke.

The character of expectorated secretions is of fundamental importance in the diagnosis and management of respiratory disorders. It is necessary first to ensure that the material has originated in the lower respiratory tract. The best way of establishing this is to have the patient produce a sample in the presence of the physician, who can readily check that it was coughed up and not simply spat from the mouth, hawked from the nose or throat or regurgitated from the oesophagus. Patients may say that they 'vomit' phlegm when a productive bout of cough concludes with retching, and indeed sputum is sometimes swallowed and subsequently vomited. When a measure of quantity is needed, sputum is collected over a period of 24 hours. The macroscopic examination of the sputum includes quantity, colour, consistency, the shape of any solid constituents and smell.

Quantity

The quantity of sputum produced in chronic bronchitis and acute infections is usually small. The regular production of purulent sputum in large amounts is characteristic of bronchiectasis, although this does sometimes occur in chronic bronchitis. However, if it is a sudden event on a single occasion, the rupture of a lung abscess or empyema into the bronchial tree is the most likely cause. The continuous expectoration of a great quantity of thin watery sputum, often 100 ml or more per day and sometimes with a salty taste, is an occasional symptom of the rare alveolar cell carcinoma; the profuse expectoration of pink frothy sputum in an acutely breathless patient suggests pulmonary oedema.

Colour

The colour of sputum is of diagnostic value. A green colour, imparted by the pigment verdoperoxidase, indicates pus, usually arising from a bacterial infection. Yellow sputum may also be due to pus or to the presence of eosinophils in allergic states such as asthma. A brown colour may result from altered blood or from fungal infections and may rarely also be seen when an amoebic liver abscess ruptures into the lung. Rarely, a greenish-yellow tinge suggests a bronchobiliary fistula. Occasionally, blackened sputum may be seen in coal miners. The presence of blood in the sputum is considered separately.

Consistency

The consistency of sputum has great therapeutic significance because the two extremes of texture can each be life-threatening. Thick, viscid, tenacious sputum is the most typical and dangerous feature of acute severe asthma; it is difficult to expel and the patient may asphyxiate from plugging of the smaller airways. Conversely, the thin watery sputum of acute pulmonary oedema may drown patients in their own secretions.

Appearance and smell

The shape and general appearance of any solid expectorated material should be noted. Viscid secretions sometimes assume the shape of the airway from which they were expectorated. These bronchial casts may appear as string-like strands or short elliptical plugs; they are a characteristic feature of bronchopulmonary aspergillosis, in which they are often golden-brown in colour (Fig. 4.2). Other solid matter that may be recognised in the sputum includes blood clots, portions of necrotic tumour, inhaled foreign material (teeth, food, etc.) and, rarely, parasitic worms as in paragonimiasis. An offensive smell or taste in sputum suggests infection, by anaerobic organisms usually in bronchiectasis, lung abscess or empyema.

Haemoptysis

The coughing of blood (see Chapter 5.2) is one of the most alarming and potentially significant of all respiratory symptoms. The most important causes are bronchial carcinoma (or carcinoid), tuberculosis, bronchiectasis, mitral valve disease and pulmonary infarction.

Pneumonia can also produce haemoptysis in the form of 'rusty' sputum while acute left ventricular failure results in pink frothy sputum. Rarer causes of haemoptysis are mycetoma, vascular malformations, haemorrhagic disorders and Goodpasture's syndrome. Major haemoptysis, which may be life-threatening, is usually associated with tuberculosis, bronchiectasis, abscess, mycetoma or bronchial carcinoma.

Chest pain

Chest pain (see Chapter 5.4) arises in the parietal pleura, chest wall or tracheobronchial tree, or from mediastinal organs such as the heart, pericardium and oesophagus.[8]

Pleuritic pain

In contrast to the lung and visceral pleura the parietal pleura has a rich innervation of sensory fibres. Stimulation of the upper part of the parietal pleura causes a pain localised to the chest itself. The lower portion, including the outer segment of the diaphragmatic pleura, is innervated by the lower six intercostal nerves, which also supply the abdominal wall; pleurisy at this site may therefore give rise to pain in the upper abdomen or loin. The central part of the diaphragmatic pleura is innervated by the phrenic nerve (C3 and C4) so that pain from here is felt in the neck and tip of the shoulder.

Pleuritic pain is typically sharp, stabbing and related to inspiration and is most commonly caused by inflammation of the parietal pleura secondary to infection, malignancy, pulmonary infarction or vasculitis and spontaneous pneumothorax.

Chest-wall pain

Pain arising in the chest wall is very common and is often mistaken for ischaemic cardiac pain or pleurisy. It may vary from the vague discomfort or feeling of tightness common among asthmatic subjects to the acute pain of rib fracture, torn muscle or disc injury induced by violent coughing. A focal traumatic lesion in the chest wall causes pain very similar to pleuritic pain. The main distinguishing features are the sudden onset following violent cough or other trauma and the presence of tenderness localised to the site of the pain.

Tracheobronchial pain

Pain of tracheobronchial origin may accompany acute inflammation due to infections such as influenza or from the inhalation of irritant fumes. It is usually described as a raw, painful, retrosternal discomfort and is distinguished from oesophageal and cardiac pain by its relationship to cough rather than to meals or exertion.

Mediastinal pain

Many of the tissues and structures within the mediastinum can cause pain or discomfort including the heart, pericardium, aorta and oesophagus.

Dyspnoea

The physiological mechanisms and measurement of breathlessness are described in Chapter 5.3. Here only the clinical aspects of dyspnoea will be outlined.

Breathlessness, usually termed dyspnoea when due to disease, is difficult to define. Common descriptions include 'the sense of an uncomfortable need to breathe'; 'the sensation of difficulty in breathing' or 'an undue awareness of breathing'.[9] Clinically important details about breathlessness are the patients' description of the sensation, its time course (mode of onset, development over days, continuous or episodic), related features (nocturnal or orthopnoea), any associated symptoms (wheeziness, pain, etc.) and its severity. If a good and detailed history is taken, the correct diagnosis can be suggested in about two thirds of cases.

Sensation of breathlessness

Patients do not describe breathlessness in terms of the rate, depth or rhythm of breathing and in any case these abnormalities of breathing pattern are not necessarily associated with dyspnoea (e.g. hyperventilation produced by a metabolic acidosis). Common descriptions of the sensation of breathlessness are:

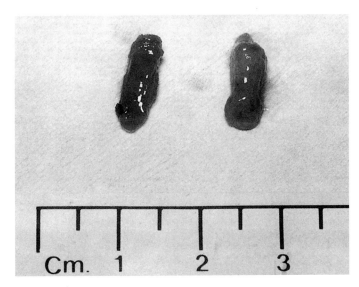

Fig. 4.2 Bronchial casts from a patient with allergic bronchopulmonary aspergillosis.

shortness of breath, feeling puffed, inability to get enough air, suffocation, breathing discomfort, increased breathing effort, sensation of tightness and an increased urge to breathe.

Different disease processes may produce different types of breathlessness sensation but these cannot be relied upon to differentiate between disease processes. Asthma often produces chest tightness while COPD patients report increased effort of breathing; both these conditions are associated with wheezy breathlessness. Patients with pulmonary oedema, massive effusions or central airway occlusion may complain of suffocation. Patients whose dyspnoea is psychogenic feel the need to take occasional deep sighing breaths (and often complain of dyspnoea at rest, especially while talking, rather than on effort).

Time course of dyspnoea

Very sudden onset of dyspnoea is rare, usually severe and associated with potentially serious and sometimes life-threatening disease. Common causes are spontaneous pneumothorax, pulmonary embolism, acute left ventricular failure, occlusion from inhalation of foreign body and rarely a sudden devastating attack of asthma. Dyspnoea developing over hours or a few days may be due to pneumonia, asthma, pleural effusion, acute extrinsic allergic alveolitis, left heart failure or lung collapse due to bronchial carcinoma. In contrast, breathlessness occurring over weeks, months or even years is commonly due to chronic airflow obstruction (COPD or chronic asthma) interstitial lung disease (particularly fibrosing alveolitis), extrinsic allergic alveolitis, sarcoidosis, chronic anaemia, bronchial tumours and chronic cardiac insufficiency.

Associated features of breathlessness

The features that are associated with breathlessness can give important clues to its cause. *Orthopnoea* is a characteristic feature of left ventricular failure and also of diaphragmatic paralysis (particularly if bilateral), but can occur in patients with severe respiratory dysfunction of any cause. *Paroxysmal nocturnal dyspnoea*, although a common symptom of left heart failure, may be wrongly attributed to this cause when an inadequate history is taken. Patients who complain of attacks of breathlessness while in bed at night fall into one of three categories (Table 4.1).

Table 4.1 Nocturnal breathlessness

Breathlessness on first going to bed This is a common complaint among patients with a variety of causes for dyspnoea because the effort of going to bed – climbing the stairs, undressing, washing, etc. – is their chief exertion of the day.
Breathlessness during the night ■ Left heart failure is associated with intense, non-wheezing dyspnoea that compels the patient to sit or get up (occasionally this is also associated with wheezing). ■ Wheezing dyspnoea, often associated with coughing, is usually a feature of nocturnal asthma. Bronchitic patients may also wake with bouts of coughing and wheezing.
Breathlessness on waking This symptom, often associated with expectoration and wheezing, is characteristic of both chronic bronchitis and asthma.

Accompanying symptoms

The symptoms that accompany dyspnoea may give clues to the cause. Dyspnoea of sudden onset associated with pleuritic pain suggests pneumothorax or pulmonary infarction and the latter is often associated with haemoptysis. When the accompanying pain is retrosternal, myocardial infarction or massive pulmonary embolism should be considered and, in both these conditions, syncope may also occur. Wheezing and chest tightness are associated with airflow obstruction of any cause but are not always complained of in these conditions. Cough and sputum may accompany breathlessness associated with COPD and bronchiectasis and a dry cough is often a feature of interstitial disease.

Severity of breathlessness

The subjective severity of effort dyspnoea can roughly be gauged from the amount of exercise needed to induce it. This is most simply achieved by asking how far a patient can walk on the flat, how many stairs can be climbed, if they can get out of the house and do simple shopping or if they are confined to the house. There are many more precise ways of measuring the severity of breathlessness (see Chapter 5.3).

Assessment of the signs of respiratory disease

The first steps are to look and to listen with the unaided ear, then palpate, percuss and finally listen with the stethoscope.

Looking

General inspection of the patient should be undertaken first and may give clues as to the severity of their chest disease. In particular the presence anaemia, cyanosis, clubbing, co-existing cor pulmonale, a flapping tremor and superior vena caval obstruction should be sought. Blistering or scabbed lesions of herpes simplex around the lips is a common accompaniment of respiratory infections, especially when due to *Streptococcus pneumoniae* (Fig. 4.3.)

Jugular veins

Engorgement, sometimes with a prominent V wave of tricuspid incompetence, is seen in cor pulmonale. Occasionally the veins

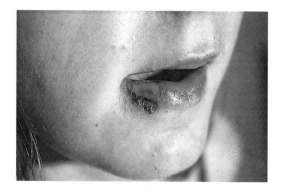

Fig. 4.3 Herpes simplex.

are engorged, with a characteristic rise in inspiration, because of pericardial effusion or constriction. Pulmonary associations include local spread of a bronchial neoplasm to the pericardium or constrictive pericarditis as a result of tuberculosis.

Non-pulsatile engorgement of the jugular veins may signify the presence of superior vena caval obstruction. This is often associated with dilated veins over the upper chest wall and in severe cases with oedema of the head, conjunctivae and the neck. The commonest cause is either a primary upper lobe tumour or malignant glands in the superior mediastinum. Very rarely superior vena caval obstruction can also be due to mediastinal fibrosis, a benign tumour or large aortic aneurysm.

Cyanosis

Cyanosis is an unreliable marker of hypoxaemia as the shape of the oxygen dissociation curve is such that there must be a considerable drop in arterial oxygen tension (to less than 10.6 kPa or 80 mmHg) before the oxygen saturation of haemoglobin starts to fall, and a further drop to less than 7 kPa (53 mmHg) before saturation falls to less than 85% where cyanosis might be detected. Cyanosis may be absent when there is severe anaemia and missed in poor lighting; it may also be intermittent, occurring only on exercise or with changes in posture. Conversely, cyanosis may be exaggerated by polycythaemia and simulated by some forms of artificial lighting and by the formation of met- or sulphaemoglobin after the ingestion of certain drugs. Cyanosis can also result from excessive extraction of oxygen from normally oxygenated blood when the local circulation is sluggish (peripheral cyanosis). It can only be accepted as a sign of hypoxaemia due to lung disease (central cyanosis) when visible in daylight in a warm part (the tongue, or the hand after warming in water) and can be diminished by the administration of oxygen. The failure of cyanosis to improve after breathing oxygen indicates either abnormal haemoglobin or a right-to-left shunt of blood The possibility of hypoxaemia must be considered in any patient with severe lung disease, even in the absence of cyanosis, and oxygen saturation must be measured. Symptoms and signs suggestive of hypoxia include tachycardia (or bradycardia when hypoxaemia is profound), restlessness, mental confusion and irritability.

Finger clubbing and hypertrophic osteodystrophy

Finger clubbing has been known to be associated with chest disease for thousands of years. If all the features of clubbing are present (Table 4.2), the diagnosis is obvious; however, less severe degrees of clubbing are difficult to identify and the diagnosis is subjective and sometimes open to dispute. Clubbing is nearly always bilateral and also affects the toes (Fig. 4.4) unless the cause is a venous malformation or compression of the brachial plexus in one arm.

Clubbing is usually caused by respiratory or cardiac disease (Table 4.3) but may also occur in liver disease and inflammatory bowel conditions. It is occasionally seen as an idiopathic condition but patients do not recognise the gradual onset of clubbing and often say they have always had unusually shaped fingernails. Rare conditions such as thyroid acropachy and the congenital condition idiopathic pachydermoperiostosis[10] have features of clubbing.

Hypertrophic (pulmonary) osteoarthropathy

As there are non-pulmonary causes, this condition is also known simply as hypertrophic osteoarthropathy.[11] It is closely allied to clubbing and probably has an identical underlying aetiology.[12] It can occur with any severity of clubbing and is characterised by marked vascularity with overgrowth of connective tissue in the proximal long bones, which in time is associated with sub-

Table 4.2 Clinical features of clubbing

- Filling in of the angle of the nail bed so that the angle between the nail and the skin of the proximal phalanx is greater than 180°
- Increased curvature of the nail bed
- Increase in the bulk of the nail bed and terminal phalanx (if extreme this gives the appearance of a drumstick)
- Sponginess of the nail bed, which gives the feeling that the nail is floating on its bed
- Periungual erythema

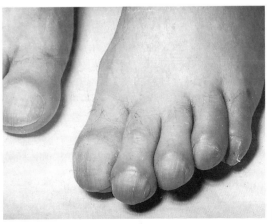

(a)

(b)

Fig, 4.4   Clubbing of fingers and toes.

Table 4.3 Causes of clubbing and hypertrophic osteoarthropathy

Thoracic	Tumours	Carcinoma of the bronchus
		Secondary lung tumours (carcinomas and sarcomas)
		Lymphomas, leukaemia and other tumours
		Mediastinal tumours (thymomas, oesophageal tumours)
	Pulmonary fibrosis	Interstitial fibrosis of any cause (e.g. asbestosis, cryptogenic fibrosing alveolitis)
	Chronic sepsis	Empyema
		Lung abscess
		Bronchiectasis (including cystic fibrosis)
		Chronic tuberculosis
	Vascular	Arteriovenous malformations
	Cardiac	Congenital cyanotic heart disease
		Bacterial endocarditis
		Rare conditions such as atrial myxoma
Non-pulmonary	Liver disease (cirrhosis)	
	Inflammatory bowel disease (ulcerative colitis)	
	Malabsorption (coeliac disease)	
	Congenital (pachydermoperiostosis)	
	Idiopathic without other genetic disease	

periosteal calcification. Clinically it presents as pain and swelling around wrists ankles and knees, simulating arthritis of these joints. The X-ray (Fig. 4.5A) is characteristic and a bone scan shows intense uptake because of the vascularity (Fig. 4.5B). Over 90% of cases of hypertrophic osteoarthropathy are associated with malignancy, particularly lung cancer.

Aetiology of clubbing and hypertrophic osteoarthropathy
Both clubbing and hypertrophic osteoarthropathy are associated with marked increase in vascularity but not new vessel formation.[13] The causes of both are similar and involve disease of visceral organs that are supplied by the vagus or hypoglossal nerves (Table 4.3). This has led to the neurogenic theory, whereby stimulation of the vagus sets up reflex vasodilation of the peripheral limbs. The second main theory is that hormones or other substances are released either by the tumour or vagal stimulation (e.g. oestrogens, growth hormone or vasoactive substances)[14] and result in peripheral vasodilation. It is also possible that vasoactive substances that are normally degraded by the lung are released into the systemic circulation via arteriovenous shunts opened by tumours or cardiac septal defects.

Inspection of the chest shape

The configuration of the chest is determined by the condition of the spine, ribs and sternum, the overlying muscles and soft tissues and the underlying lung and pleura[15].

Scoliosis
Scoliosis – lateral curvature of the spine – is the most important of all the chest deformities because of its potential effect upon cardiorespiratory function. Scoliosis is almost invariably accompanied by rotation of the spine but only rarely by significant kyphosis so that the popular term 'kyphoscoliosis' is often inappropriate. It is the rotation of the spine that causes a posterior

hump comprising ribs and scapula on one side (simulating a kyphosis), and an anterior hump on the other. The rotation is also largely responsible for the reduction in lung volume and impaired mechanical function, which, in severe cases, lead in early middle life to respiratory and then cardiac failure. This complication is more likely to occur if the scoliosis affects the upper part of the spine and is not abolished by forward flexion (Fig. 4.6), occurs early in life, is associated with muscle weakness and the vital capacity is less that 1 to 1.5 litres.

Kyphosis
Kyphosis is the most common cause of a *barrel* chest, which is therefore not a specific sign of emphysema. Kyphosis unaccompanied by scoliosis does not cause any significant impairment of lung function except in extreme cases, which usually result from tuberculosis (Potts disease).

Rib deformity
Abnormalities of the ribs altering the configuration of the chest include those associated with scoliosis (see above), the local flattening of the chest resulting from surgical excision of ribs for tuberculosis (thoracoplasty) or empyema and the phenomenon of Harrison's sulcus. The latter, which consists of a bilateral groove in the rib cage, has been attributed to the effect of diaphragmatic contraction in patients with airway obstruction (from adenoids or asthma) during early childhood when the bones are still malleable. It is particularly common among rachitic children, in whom enlargement of the rib epiphyses ('rickety rosary') may also be seen.

Sternal deformity
Deformities of the sternum are of two kinds: funnel sternum (pectus excavatum), which is a congenital saucer-shaped depression of the sternum and of cosmetic significance only (Fig. 4.7) and pigeon chest (pectus carinatum) with prominence of the

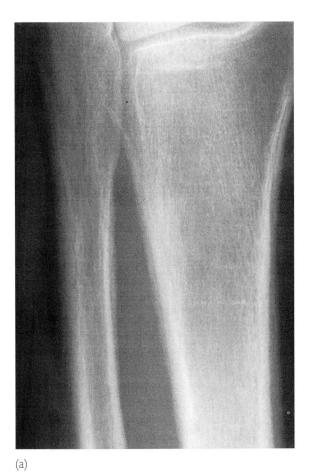

(a)

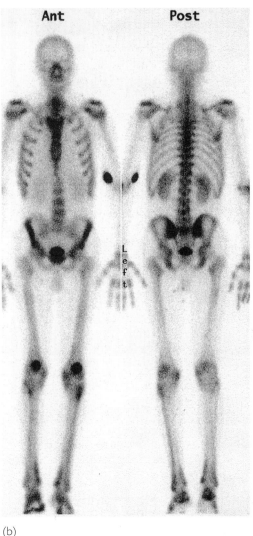

(b)

Fig. 4.5 Hypertrophic osteoarthropathy. a. X-ray of the tibia and fibula. A line of new bone formation is seen running alongside both bones. b. Isotope bone scan. Note the marked increase in the uptake of the isotope at the lower ends of the tibia and fibula. (By courtesy of Dr J Curtis.)

sternum and/or anterior ends of the ribs (Fig. 4.8). Pigeon chest may be congenital or the consequence of airflow obstruction in childhood, as in Harrison's sulcus, but again it does not of itself cause respiratory dysfunction.

Soft tissue deformity

Asymmetry of the chest with either prominence or flattening may result from abnormalities of soft tissues, such as a diffuse lipoma, congenital absence of the pectoralis major or wasting of the scapular muscles. Pleural or pulmonary fibrosis can lead to flattening, contraction and impaired expansion of one hemithorax.

Inspection of breathing movements

Inspection of breathing movements involves not only the chest itself but also respiratory movements of the nose, mouth, neck and abdomen.

Chest movements

Examination of breathing movements of the chest should include the rate, depth, rhythm of breathing, equality of expansion and presence of paradox. At rest normal healthy subjects take between 12 and 15 breaths per minute, expiration being

slightly longer than inspiration. The commonest abnormal breathing pattern is rapid, shallow breathing, which is a response to increased loading whether this is resistive (i.e. due to severe airflow obstruction of any cause) or elastic (i.e. due to reduced lung compliance secondary to consolidation, oedema or diffuse fibrosis).[16] In patients with severe COPD or asthma the expiration becomes a little lengthened and in addition the breathing pattern tends to be somewhat disorganised.[17]

Abnormal slowing of breathing is invariably central in origin (e.g. narcotic drugs or disorders of the central nervous system). Psychogenic causes account for most instances of *irregular* breathing, especially when this is punctuated by deep sighing breaths. *Periodic (Cheyne–Stokes) breathing*, in which spells of hypopnoea or apnoea alternate with hyperpnoea, signifies a cerebral or cardiac disorder and is common following a stroke and in cases of left ventricular failure. Episodes of *apnoea* during sleep may have a respiratory basis, resulting either from the main airway obstruction associated with snoring (obstructive apnoea) or from central depression (central apnoea; see also Chapters 2.7 and 41).

The overall expansion of the chest can be assessed from the end of the bed but of greater significance is *inequality of expan-*

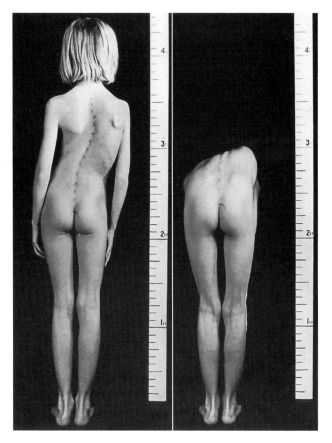

Fig. 4.6 Scoliosis with posterior rib hump not abolished by forward flexion.

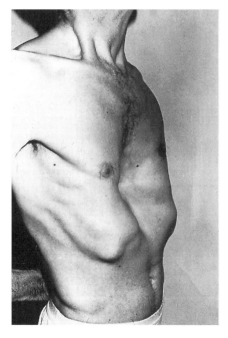

Fig. 4.7 Funnel sternum.

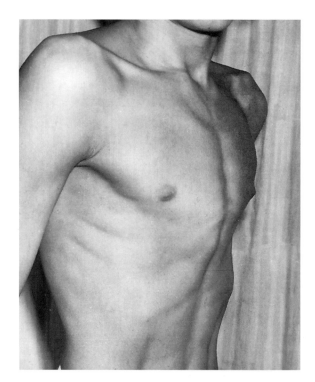

Fig. 4.8 Pigeon chest.

sion, which may occur with any predominantly unilateral disease of the underlying pleura or lung. *Paradoxical movements* of the chest wall are also of potential clinical importance. Inspiratory indrawing of the intercostal spaces is commonly seen in children with respiratory distress from any cause. The distorted action of a depressed and flattened diaphragm in patients with chronic airflow obstruction is probably responsible for the paradoxical motion of the lower ribs during inspiration. Crush injuries of the chest with fractured ribs and sternum can lead to a 'flail' chest with a dangerous degree of paradox.

Nose and mouth

The respiratory movements of the nose and mouth include the dilatation of the nostrils brought about by the contraction of the alae nasi – a common accompaniment to respiratory distress in children – and gasping or pursing movements of the mouth. The latter are characteristic of severe airflow obstruction, especially in patients with emphysema (see below).

Neck

The accessory muscles of respiration in the neck are brought into play when there is laboured breathing from any cause but especially when there is airflow obstruction with overinflation of the lungs. Further inspiratory expansion is then achieved by contraction of the sternomastoid, causing vertical elevation of the thorax through its action on the clavicles. Inspiratory elevation of the shoulders may also occur. The forceful breathing needed to overcome airflow obstruction may give rise to two other respiratory movements in the neck – expiratory engorgement of the jugular veins and paradoxical hollowing of the supraclavicular fossae in inspiration and distension in expiration.

Abdomen

Abdominal respiratory movements may be abolished by peritonitis and be paradoxical in direction when the diaphragm is paralysed or rendered ineffectual by gross overinflation of the lungs; in these cases, the lower chest and upper abdomen are drawn in during inspiration, especially in the supine position.

Listening

Breathing sounds at the mouth

Listening to breath sounds at the mouth yields valuable information about underlying chest disease. Added sounds may be superimposed on to the breath sounds and these can originate from the upper airway (e.g. hissing respiration) or from the intrathoracic airways (e.g. wheezing and crackles). At more than about a foot away from the mouth breathing is inaudible and no added sounds are heard. On exercise breathing becomes noisy because of increased turbulent flow in airways, including the mouth. In disease the breathing pattern may be disorganised, the basic breath sounds altered and added sounds present. The following descriptions encompass sounds that commonly occur in health and/or disease.

Gasps

These are noises of sudden, rapid, deep inspirations. They are most commonly observed as a physiological response to fright. In addition, they are part of an involuntary response to cold particularly when diving into cold water. This reflex is so strong that it cannot be overridden voluntarily and is one of the causes of drowning in cold water. Infrequent, irregular, gasping inspirations are also seen as a terminal event when the respiratory centre is deranged.

Sighs and yawns

These consist of slow, deep inspirations near to vital capacity followed by expirations that may be prolonged and frequently associated with the voiced sound 'ah' produced by apposition of the vocal cords. Sighs and yawns occur in all normal people and are thought necessary to overcome alveolar cohesion from surface tension forces. Prolonged shallow breathing of narcosis or even natural drowsiness can lead to segmental atelectases if not punctuated by occasional deep breaths, sighs or yawns. The plate atelectases seen above a paralysed diaphragm are probably due to the ineffectiveness of yawns and sighs in this circumstance. Frequent sighs and yawns, often accompanied by loud expiratory sounds, are associated with psychogenic functional breathing disorders.

Hisses

Hissing (Kussmaul's) breathing is caused by hyperventilation through opposed teeth. The sound is generated by turbulent airflow in the mouth and surprisingly the patient rarely complains of the subjective sensation of breathlessness. This type of breathing is characteristic of metabolic acidosis particularly when due to salicylate poisoning or uraemia. The cause is unknown but there may be absence of reflex opening of the mouth which occurs in the presence of pulmonary disease. An alternative explanation is that hyperventilation with a partially closed mouth produces less drying of the airway mucosa.

Snores

Snoring is predominantly an inspiratory sound that occurs as a result of vibration of the soft tissues of the pharynx or palate during sleep or in conditions that cause impaired consciousness. Socially embarrassing heavy snoring is estimated to affect at least 15% of the population, with snoring sounds sometimes exceeding 100 dB.[18] Severe snoring is also a feature of obstructive sleep apnoea (see Chapter 45).

Pants

Panting respiration is used to describe the noises of rapid, shallow breathing. Panting is typical of any condition in which there is increased stiffness of the lung tissue resulting in increased elastic work of breathing (i.e. lung compliance is reduced) but studies of breathing patterns have shown similar patterns of breathing in patients with airflow obstruction.[17] Common examples of conditions associated with reduced lung compliance are any cause of interstitial fibrosis (e.g. fibrosing alveolitis or asbestosis), interstitial lung disease (e.g. severe infections, acute respiratory distress syndrome, diffuse malignancy) and pulmonary oedema. In addition, an increased elastic load of breathing also occurs in patients with severe chest-wall deformities and in neuromuscular disease such as the muscular dystrophies. Initially, panting may only be seen when a patient exercises but as the disease progresses panting occurs at minimal exercise and finally even at rest. In the most extreme cases inspiration stops abruptly; this has been described as 'doorstop' breathing.

Wheezes

Any cause of increased airflow obstruction may be accompanied by continuous wheezing sounds at the mouth. Wheezes have a defined tone and are most commonly heard in expiration. Although wheezing is not universally heard with airflow obstruction, the breathing pattern itself may alter, with prolongation occurring in the expiratory phase of the respiratory cycle. In asthma, wheezy breathing can vary markedly throughout the day and may be particularly troublesome during the night. In COPD wheezes tend to be present all the time but are more marked at times of exacerbations. In contrast, the breathing sounds of patients with predominant emphysema are often relatively quiet, wheezing only occurring at the end of a prolonged expiration (thought to be due to passive collapse of the proximal airways by the positive pressure needed to expel air from the inelastic lungs).

Whistles and grunts

Whistles and grunts are heard most commonly in patients suffering from emphysema and were noted by Shakespeare in his sixth age of man, 'the lean and slipper'd pantaloon', who 'pipes and whistles in his sound'. Whistles are caused by breathing out through pursed lips while grunts are caused by opposing the vocal cords. Grunting may occur throughout most of expiration or consist of intermittent cogwheel-like grunts during expiration, only too often interpreted as attention-seeking.

Both lip and laryngeal pursing are thought to have a beneficial physiological effect by raising the intrabronchial pressure and reducing airway collapse by applying 'auto-PEEP'.[19] Lip pursing is also seen in athletes during maximal effort and grunting may occur if breathing is painful for any reason.

Whoops (stridor)

Stridor is caused by narrowing of the main airway or larynx. It has a lower pitch than wheezing and resembles a voiced sound.

It is loudest in inspiration for two main reasons, first because the narrowing is usually in the extrathoracic portion of the trachea and is thus not subject to intrathoracic pressure changes, and second because the obstruction is usually fixed (i.e. due to a tumour or tight benign stricture). In children stridor or 'croup' can be caused by infective laryngitis or, more seriously, epiglottitis. At times it may be difficult to distinguish stridor from the inspiratory wheezing sounds in a patient with asthma and in this circumstance the possibility of a tumour in the trachea or around the main carina has to be considered.

Sniffles
Sniffly nose and nasal discharge or obstruction, in the absence of the common cold, indicated potentially serious upper respiratory disease (See Upper respiratory tract symptoms, above).

Rattles
The Hippocratic 'death rattle' is well named. This is the sound of air passing through fluid, setting mucus into vibration in the main airways during both inspiration and expiration. It is usually a sign that the cough reflex has failed because of either decreased efficacy or excessive demand. The reflex may be impaired by narcosis or extreme weakness, or it may be overwhelmed by a massive transudation of fluid into the airways, as in acute pneumonia, severe pulmonary oedema or aspiration of swallowed or regurgitated fluids.

Crackles
Crackles (see below) are most commonly caused by the sudden opening of smaller airways and are localised to within a few centimetres of their origin; thus they are not usually heard at the mouth. However, similar sounds can be produced by air bubbling through secretions in larger airways, as is a feature of chronic airway obstruction with sputum production. Very loud crackles are also part of the rattles described above.

Breath sounds of chest wall

Breath sounds of chest wall are described in a separate section entitled Auscultation of respiratory sounds at the end of this chapter.

Palpation

The six traditional acts of palpation in examination of the respiratory system are to feel the neck for enlarged nodes, subcutaneous emphysema and tracheal position and the chest for the site of the heart apex, expansion and vocal fremitus. Of these, the findings in the neck are by far the most important.

The cervical (and axillary) lymph nodes

These may be involved by diseases that can also affect the lung – notably tuberculosis, sarcoidosis and lymphoma. With these conditions, any group of nodes may be enlarged; their consistency tends to be firm and rubbery but not hard and, except in some advanced cases of lymphatic tuberculosis, the individual lymph nodes are discrete and unattached to surrounding tissues. Bronchial carcinoma usually reaches the supraclavicular nodes first and it is especially important to palpate with finger and

thumb deep to the sternal head of the sternomastoid. The affected nodes are hard and may become fused together to form a mass, which is fixed to adjacent structures.

Subcutaneous (surgical) emphysema

The chest, and particularly the neck, should be lightly palpated for the characteristic crackly feeling, or crepitus, of air beneath the skin. The crackling can be heard as well as felt and may be confused with lung crackles if it has not first been detected by palpation. A special search should be made for this sign following any episode of severe chest trauma, acute airflow obstruction or violent vomiting. After trauma, it may signify lung injury from a fractured rib or a ruptured bronchus. Acute asthma or transient main airway obstruction (e.g. a difficult intubation) can cause intrapulmonary rupture of air spaces with tracking of air in the peribronchial tissues to the mediastinum and neck. Subcutaneous emphysema in the neck is also an important sign of ruptured oesophagus and should be sought in every patient in whom violent vomiting is accompanied by severe chest pain or followed by a left pleural effusion.

Palpation of the trachea and apex beat of the heart

This may provide information about the position of the mediastinum. It must be remembered, however, that the trachea is sometimes displaced by a mass in the neck such as a goitre and the apex beat by cardiac enlargement. Gross deformity of the spine may also alter the position of the trachea or heart apex. When these causes are excluded, displacement of the trachea from the midsternal line will usually signify disease of the pleura or lung. Deviation away from the abnormal side (as identified by percussion and auscultation) suggests pleural effusion, pneumothorax, bullous emphysema or, rarely, a massive tumour. Deviation towards the abnormal side occurs when there is collapse of the upper lobe or the whole lung and in cases of pleural or pulmonary fibrosis.

Consolidation alone does not affect the position of the trachea. It may also remain in a central position when a carcinoma has caused a combination of collapse and effusion or has infiltrated and fixed the mediastinum. The trachea should be palpated with the patient's head fully extended and the chin in the midline. The observer's finger is gently slid deep into the suprasternal fossa where, in a normal subject, it should meet the centre of the trachea. The site of the heart apex is a less useful guide to the position of the mediastinum, not only because it may be displaced by cardiac enlargement but also because it is more difficult to locate than the cervical trachea. It is chiefly of value for detecting lower lobe collapse, in which the trachea remains central, and for picking up the occasional case of dextrocardia in patients with bronchiectasis (Kartagener's syndrome).

The degree and equality of chest expansion

This is judged as well by inspection from the end of the bed, or looking down from above the patient's head, as by palpation (see under Inspection of the chest shape, above). However, palpation may help to confirm a suspicion that expansion is diminished or unequal. Apical expansion is examined by resting the fingers on the clavicles, drawing the thumbs together in the midline at full expiration and watching the movement of the thumbs during full inspiration. A similar manoeuvre, but with the fingers spread widely in the axillae (anteriorly, then posteriorly), is used for examining the lung bases. It is sometimes useful to measure the total chest wall expansion using a tape measure around the chest at the level of the nipples (or beneath the breasts in women). The diameter should increase by 6–9 cm from full expiration to full inspiration. This measurement is of little clinical value except to demonstrate fusion of the costovertebral joints in ankylosing spondylitis.

Vocal fremitus

Feeling the vibrations of voiced sounds at the chest wall is a crude way of assessing the transmission characteristic of the respiratory system sounds and is dependent on the same acoustic principles described for breath sounds (see below). In normal individuals the transmission of sound (traditionally the number 'ninety-nine' is used) from the larynx to the chest wall can be easily felt as a vibration by the physician's hand. If the transmission of sound is grossly impaired, most commonly by an effusion, then vocal fremitus is reduced; this can be of help in distinguishing effusion from consolidation. Increase in vocal fremitus over consolidation is a very subtle sign and has very limited value.

Percussion

The thorax is a closed conical cavity encased in a semi-rigid chest wall, which acts as a complex acoustic resonant chamber. It is divided by the mediastinum, which turns the chest into two separate chambers that to a large extent can resonate separately. The act of percussion provides an 'impulse' sound source producing a broad frequency band of energy that sets the chest cavity into vibration at its resonant frequency for a short period of time. The most important aspect of percussion is this ability to compare the resonance of the left and right side of the chest.

In order to produce the most effective impulse it has been found that the middle finger of the left hand should be placed in close contact with the chest wall and struck at right angles with the middle finger of the right hand. The striking finger must be lifted clear immediately to make sure that the vibrations are not damped. The resultant resonance is assessed by both the sound and the tactile sensation received by the finger of the left hand. If resonant the sound is clear and ringing and vibrations are felt (resonant percussion), signifying aerated lung, while if the sound is dull, rapidly damped and no vibrations felt (stony, dull percussion) then the structures under the finger are solid or fluid. It is sometimes said that light percussion can give information about structures near the chest wall while heavy percussion is used for deeper structure. However, percussion is never a precise procedure as vibrations can be widely dispersed in the chest.

The percussion note may vary from a stony dullness in cases of pleural effusion to a hyper-resonant, tympanitic sound over a large pneumothorax. Intermediate grades of dullness (as in con-

solidation or collapse) or of hyper-resonance (as in emphysema) can only be regarded as abnormal if there is a clear difference between corresponding parts of the two lungs. Some observers claim that auscultatory percussion can also detect such differences (i.e. by comparing the note over the two lungs while the sternum is percussed).

The chief clinical value of percussion is to locate a pleural effusion, although this can be achieved with much greater accuracy by imaging techniques.[20] The combination of reduced or absent breath sounds with normal or hyper-resonant percussion note is suggestive of pneumothorax or localised emphysema. In all other conditions with altered breath sounds, the percussion note is usually impaired

Auscultation of respiratory sounds

Stethoscope

Modern stethoscopes have a bell and a diaphragm and there has been debate about which should be used for auscultation of the chest. The bell functions as an impedance transformer, 'amplifying' sounds in the range of 40–115 Hz by approximately 5–10 dB. In contrast, the diaphragm tends to attenuate these lower frequencies. The advantage of the bell lies in listening to the heart, particularly low-pitched murmurs. However, these same frequencies will accentuate low-pitched interfering noise from intercostal muscles, chest wall movements and the heart, masking the higher frequencies required for characterisation of lung sounds. Thus it is most appropriate to use the diaphragm to listen to the chest.[21]

The stethoscope should be used to compare the two lungs for the quality and intensity of breath and voice sounds and to detect any added sounds. Combining palpation, percussion and auscultation will provide an indication at the bedside of the presence of consolidation, collapse, fibrosis, effusion and pneumothorax (or bullous emphysema). In hospital practice X-rays are readily available, which allow these conditions to be recognised more precisely, but in primary care and in day-to-day patient assessment the stethoscope still has some utility for these conditions (Table 4.4). Added sounds, on the other hand, often provide additional information even in the presence of a normal or unhelpful radiograph.

Auscultation with the stethoscope has many limitations. It is a subjective process and it is not easy to quantify measurement or produce permanent records. Long-term monitoring or correlation with other physiological signals is difficult. There is now interest in using modern digital signal techniques (intelligent computerised stethoscope) to analyse the sounds from the lungs and monitor patients over time.[22]

Classification

There has been considerable debate and confusion about the classification of respiratory sounds. Many terms originate from those used by Laennec early in the 19th century and it was not until 1984 that a logical system based on the acoustics of the

Table 4.4 Changes in physical signs in five intrathoracic conditions

Observation	Intrathoracic condition				
	Consolidation*	Collapse	Fibrosis	Effusion	Pneumothorax
Mediastinal shift	None	Towards	Towards (with chest wall retraction)	Away	Away
Vocal fremitus	Increased	Decreased	Decreased	Decreased	Decreased
Percussion note	Dull	Dull	Dull	Flat or stony	Tympany
Breath sounds	Bronchial	Absent	Decreased	Decreased (bronchial above)	Decreased or amphoric
Vocal sounds	Bronchophony Whispering pectoriloquy	Decreased	Decreased	Decreased (aegophony may be present)	Decreased

* Similar signs occur when there is collapse or fibrosis with a patent bronchus.

sounds was introduced[23] and later adopted by the International Lung Sounds Association.[24] Table 4.5[25] provides an up-to-date and simple classification, which relates the mechanism of sound production to its origin within the lungs, the acoustics of the sound and its clinical relevance.

Breath sounds heard at the chest wall

There is much evidence that breath sounds originate predominately from broadband-frequency sound produced by turbulent airflow in larger airways (inspiration in lobar airways and expira-tion in larger airways).[26,27] Thus the original idea that breath sounds are vesicular, arising from the lung alveoli, was incorrect, as mass airflow does not occur in this part of the lung. However, despite this, the term vesicular breathing is still used by many physicians to describe normal breath sounds. As sound travels through the airways, into the parenchyma and then to the chest wall, higher frequencies are differentially attenuated (low-pass filtering effect).[23,25,26] This phenomenon occurs in any tissue but is more marked through the 'sponge-like' structure of the lung parenchyma. Moreover, at frequencies below 300 Hz, larger airways vibrate in response to the intra-airway sounds and this

Table 4.5 Categories of respiratory sounds (with permission from Pasterkamp et al, 1997[25])

Respiratory sound	Mechanisms	Origin	Acoustics	Relevance
Basic sounds				
Normal lung sound	Turbulent flow vortices, unknown mechanisms	Central airways (expiration), lobar to segmental airway (inspiration)	Low-pass filtered noise (range < 100 to > 1000 Hz)	Regional ventilation, airway calibre
Normal tracheal sound	Turbulent flow, flow impinging on airway walls	Pharynx, larynx, trachea, large airways	Noise with resonances (range < 100 to > 3000 Hz)	Upper airway configuration
Adventitious sounds				
Wheeze	Airway wall flutter, vortex shedding	Central and lower airways	Sinusoid (range ~ 100 to > 1000 Hz; duration typically > 80 ms)	Airway obstruction, flow limitation
Rhonchus	Rupture of fluid films, airway wall vibrations	Larger airways	Series of rapidly dampened sinusoids (typically < 300 Hz duration > 100 ms)	Secretions, abnormal airway collapsibility
Crackle	Airway wall stress -relaxation	Central and lower airways	Rapidly dampened wave deflection (duration typically < 20 ms)	Airway closure, secretions

This table lists only the major categories of respiratory sounds and does not include other sounds such as squawks, friction rubs, grunting, snoring or cough. Current concepts on sound mechanisms and origin are listed but these concepts may be incomplete and unconfirmed.

lower-frequency energy is then coupled to the parenchyma and the chest wall, further enhancing the low-frequency spectrum of breath sounds.[28] The net effect of these acoustic phenomena is that breath sounds heard at the chest wall have a low-frequency-noise-like quality, with peak energy at about 100 Hz and rapid attenuation above 200 Hz, so that nearly all the energy has disappeared by 1000 Hz. The sound is usually described as 'rustling' in character, the expiratory component being quieter and shorter than the inspiration but continuous with it.

The two main determinants of breath-sound intensity at the chest wall are airflow (intensity varies inversely with the square of airflow at the mouth) and the transmission pathway to the listening site.[29] Thus reduced breath sounds do not always mean 'reduced air entry'. In normal individuals, lung sounds vary at different chest-wall sites and isotope studies suggest that this is mainly due to differences in regional ventilation. However, the situation is complex, with different patterns for inspiration and expiration.[25]

With global airflow obstruction (e.g. asthma or COPD) lung-sound intensity is reduced even when listening with the stethoscope[30] and this can be correlated with the FEV_1. A series of recent experiments using bronchial challenge show that changes in FEV_1 of as little as 20% can be detected by the stethoscope as reduced inspiratory sound.[31] In addition, there are changes in the frequency content of breath sounds even in the absence of wheeze. The situation with emphysema is more complex as the parenchymal damage changes the transmission characteristics of the lung.[32]

Large changes in regional airflow and/or transmission characteristics resulting in reduced breath sounds can occur from pleural effusion (where sound is deflected by the air–fluid interface), local bronchial occlusion with lobar or lung collapse, diaphragmatic paralysis, gross abdominal distension and morbid obesity.

Tracheal breath sounds

Breath sounds heard over the trachea are of higher intensity, expiration and inspiration being separated, and are easily heard. The sound intensity of tracheal sounds is directly related to airflow[33] and this relationship has potential use as a non-invasive index of airflow. The spread of sound frequencies is wide because of the absence of filtering by the lung tissue, components above 1 kHz being easily demonstrated. The main clinical use of tracheal sounds is as an indication of upper airway obstruction. Initially, the sounds become harsh, with greater power at higher frequencies, and then true stridor is heard.

Bronchial breath sounds

Bronchial breathing occurs when the underlying lung parenchyma is airless as a result of pneumonia (consolidated), collapse or dense fibrosis, provided that the bronchus to the diseased area is patent. Such abnormal lung tissue is a good conductor of the higher frequency components of the central airway sounds to the periphery, where they produce the characteristic sound of bronchial breathing. As well as the change in frequency content, bronchial breathing is often louder and has a more prolonged expiratory phase than normal breathing. Even when the upper-lobe bronchus is occluded, a similar sound may be transmitted directly to the apex of the hemithorax This is thought to be due to direct coupling of central airways sound from the trachea into the collapsed/consolidated lung.

In the past, two variations of 'bronchial breathing' have been described. First, when there is a cavity within consolidated lung, particularly associated with tuberculosis, the breath sounds have been described as 'hollow' or cavernous. Second, in some circumstances (e.g. partially deflated lung in the presence of a bronchopulmonary fistula) bronchial breathing with a high-pitched, metallic quality termed 'amphoric breathing' is heard.

Voice sounds

The transmission of voice sounds and the transmission of breath sounds are governed by the same acoustic principles. Normally, lung tissue filters out the high-frequency vowel sounds so that speech heard through the stethoscope is an unintelligible blur of consonants. When the normal filter is lost, the spoken word (e.g. voiced 'ninety-nine') is clear and syllabic. This is termed *bronchophony* and occurs in the same circumstances as bronchial breathing. These changes in filtering characteristics over consolidated lung have also been noted to change the sound of vowels, the spoken 'F' sounding like an 'A'.[34] *Whispering pectoriloquy* has a similar significance: it is heard when the high-frequency sound of whispering (e.g. non-voiced ninety-nine) reaches the stethoscope. *Aegophony* is the term used to describe a high-pitched nasal bleating quality of voice sounds typically heard over the upper limit of a pleural effusion where the thin layer of fluid deflects the low-frequency components of the sound.

Wheezing

Wheezing is the commonest adventitious lung sound. It is a 'musical' sound and was defined by the American Thoracic Society as lasting longer than 250 ms;[24] however, shorter sounds of around 100 ms are also perceived as wheezing. The frequency range varies from below 100 Hz to over 1000 Hz. The cause of wheezing is still debated but fundamental studies of the underlying mechanisms suggest that 'flutter' in bronchi occurring at flow limitation is responsible.[35] Wheeze is a dynamic phenomenon, usually decreasing in frequency during expiration as the tension and stiffness of the involved airway varies.[36] Thus wheeze of many different frequencies can be produced in airways of similar size depending on the physical condition of the airway.

Although many normal individuals produce brief wheezing sounds during forced expiration, wheezing during tidal or deep breathing is nearly always associated with conditions causing airflow obstruction. There is an inverse association between the FEV_1 and the proportion of each expiratory cycle that contains wheeze.[37] However, it must be realised that patients can have airflow obstruction without wheezing and that, even in those who do wheeze, very severe airflow obstruction may be associated with a relatively silent chest. Auscultation of wheezing has been advocated as a useful way of determining endpoint for bronchial challenge in young children.[38]

Listening with a stethoscope and using modern computerised techniques has enabled characterisation of wheeze by the position in the respiratory cycle (inspiration or expiration), frequency and loudness. Forgacs[26] suggested that the ear can distinguish between a number of different wheezing patterns.

- *Fixed monophonic wheeze* is a single musical sound, which tends to be constant in timing and pitch and is associated with a fixed obstruction in a large airway, most usually due to a bronchial neoplasm.
- *Random monophonic wheezes* are where there are a number of monophonic wheezes scattered and overlapping with varying duration timing and pitch. They are most common in expiration but are also heard in inspiration and are associated with widespread airflow limitation in asthma and COPD.
- *Expiratory polyphonic wheezes* are a complex musical sound made up of a number of wheezes all starting at approximately the same time in expiration. They most frequently occur late in expiration and are thought to be due to dynamic compression of airways, most commonly resulting from emphysema.

Low-pitched musical sounds with a duration of greater than 100 ms have been recognised for many years and are sometimes still termed *rhonchi*. They are most commonly caused by airway secretions or narrowing of large, very collapsible airways and have a rapidly damping periodic waveform similar to some snoring waveforms.[25] They are often heard in unconscious or seriously ill patients.

Occasionally, very short musical sounds are heard which are associated with conditions associated with crackles.[39] These sounds are often single (*squawks*; Fig. 4.9) but may be sequential and overlapping. They are associated with pulmonary fibrosis, especially extrinsic allergic alveolitis, and are also heard in bronchiolitis. As a large crackle often precedes a squawk it is thought that the sound is caused by vibration of a smaller airway wall (e.g. a bronchiole) as it snaps open. Interstitial pulmonary fibrosis as well as bronchiolitis is known to affect bronchioles.

Crackles

These are brief, interrupted explosive sounds, which are often termed *discontinuous*. Forgacs[26] suggested that crackles are generated in the lung parenchyma by the sudden opening of smaller airways on inspiration. Physiological experiments in the 1970s[26,40] identified two main types: fine late inspiratory crackles and coarse early inspiratory crackles.[23]

Fine late inspiratory crackles are short (the duration of the first two cycles is less than10 ms (Fig. 4.10) and are thought to result either from explosive equalisation of downstream and upstream pressures or from sudden release of tension as smaller airways snap open.[23,26,41] Any condition associated with airway closure may be associated with fine crackles (e.g. restrictive lung conditions such as interstitial fibrosis or pulmonary oedema) and scanty crackles may occasionally occur in normal individuals when they inspire from residual volume. They tend to be late in

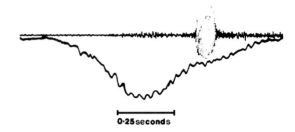

Fig. 4.9 Late inspiratory crackles interrupted by a squawk. The curved line indicates flow rate, inspiration downwards.

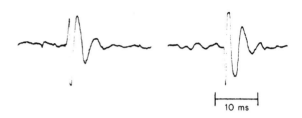

Fig. 4.10 Time-expanded sound amplitude tracing of two crackles. They are less than 10 ms in duration.

inspiration (i.e. when sufficient transpulmonary pressure is present to open closed airways) and are often gravity-dependent. *Fine expiratory crackles* are also recognised and may represent opening and closing of the airway during expiration.[42] Crackles heard by auscultation occur within a few centimetres of the stethoscope head and thus represent local disease.[43] This is in keeping with the known peripheral distribution of diseases such as cryptogenic fibrosing alveolitis and probably explains the paucity of crackles in the more centrally distributed diseases such as sarcoidosis.

Early inspiratory crackles are coarse, with a two-cycle duration of more than 10 ms. They are scanty, not dependent on gravity, often audible at the mouth and also commonly heard in expiration. They are usually present with severe airflow obstruction, particularly when associated with secretions (e.g. severe COPD or bronchiectasis), and are thought to be produced by air passing through secretions or with closure and opening of larger airways.

Pleural rub

Friction between the two inflamed surfaces of the pleura gives rise to a sound that has traditionally been described like that of creaking leather. It may also have a vague musical tone, like the bowing of a violin,[26] or sound like a series of low-pitched crackles. Acoustically its waveform does indeed resemble a 'train' of coarse crackles.[25] The sound tends to recur at the same moment in each respiratory cycle, often in both inspiration and expiration, and may be altered by posture but not by coughing. A pleural rub may last for as little as a few hours in pneumonia to months or even years in patients with more chronic pleurisy.

Conclusion

The use of the clinical assessment of respiratory disease outlined in this chapter is often underestimated within hospital practice where sophisticated diagnostic tests (e.g. X-rays, computed tomography, magnetic resonance imaging and ultrasound scanning) are readily available. In primary care, clinical skills are used to determine a likely diagnosis and decide whether further investigations and specialist help are needed. In hospital, clinical assessment of patients enables more effective and focused investigation and, once a diagnosis is established, the progress of many conditions such as pneumonia, pulmonary oedema, asthma and pleural effusions can be, at least in part, monitored using physical signs, reducing over-reliance on expensive tests. In fact, in most parts of the world, clinical skills are the mainstay of medical practice.

Acknowledgement

I would like to acknowledge the help and support of Dr Colin Ogilvie who wrote this chapter in the last edition. Much of the original material remains in this chapter and his help in reading and commenting on the text was much appreciated.

References

1. Smyllie HC, Blendis LM, Armitage P. Observer disagreement in physical signs of the respiratory system. Lancet 1965; 2: 412.
2. Spiteri MA, Cook DG, Clarke SW. Reliability of eliciting physical signs in examination of the chest. Lancet 1988; 1: 873–875.
3. Plante F, Kessler H, Sun XQ et al. Inverse filtering applied to upper airway sounds. Technol Health Care 1998; 6: 23–32.
4. Jones TM, Plante F, Cheetham BM, Earis JF. Objective assessment of hoarseness by measuring jitter. Otolaryngol 2000; 25: 1–4.
5. Thorpe CW, Toop U, Dawson KP. Towards a quantitative description of asthmatic cough sounds. Eur Respir J 1992; 5: 685–692.
6. Doherty MJ, Wang U, Donague S et al. The acoustic properties of capsaicin-induced cough in healthy subjects. Eur Respir J 1997; 10: 202–207.
7. Tomaki M, Ichinose M, Miura M et al Angiotensin converting enzyme (ACE) inhibitor-induced cough and substance P. Thorax 1996; 51: 199–201.
8. Schneider RR, Seckler SG. Evaluation of acute chest pain. Med Clin North Am 1981; 65: 53–66.
9. Jones PW. Measurement of breathlessness. In: Hughes JBM, Pride NB, ed. Lung function tests: physiological principles and clinical applications. London: WB Saunders; 1999: 121–131.
10. Rimion DL. Pachydermoperiostosis (idiopathic clubbing and periostosis): genetic and physiologic considerations. N Engl J Med 1965; 272: 294.
11. Martinez-Lavin M, Matucci-Cerinic M, Jajic I, Pineda C. Hypertrophic osteoarthropathy: consensus on its definition, classification, assessment and diagnostic criteria. J Rheumatol 1993; 20: 1386–1387.
12. Shneerson JM. Digital Clubbing and hypertrophic osteoarthropathy: the underlying mechanisms. Br J Dis Chest 1981;75: 113.
13. Currie AF, Gallagher PJ. The pathology of clubbing: vascular changes in the nail bed. Br J Dis Chest 1988; 82: 382–385.
14. Gosney JR. Pulmonary endocrine pathology. Oxford: Butterworth-Heinemann, 1992.
15. Shneerson JM. Disorders of the thoracic cage and diaphragm. In: Weatherall DJ, Ledingham GG, Warrell DA, ed. Oxford textbook of medicine. Oxford: Oxford University Press, 1996: 2872–2878.
16 Calverley PMA. Control of breathing. In: Hughes JBM, Pride NB, ed. Lung function tests: physiological principles and clinical applications. London: WB Saunders; 1999: 107–131.
17. Tobin MJ, Chadha TS, Jenouri G et al. Breathing patterns. 2. Diseased subjects. Chest 1983; 84: 286–294.
18. Young T, Palta M, Dempsey J et al. The occurrence of sleep-disordered breathing among middle-aged adults. N Engl J Med 1993; 328: 1230–1235.
19. Mueller RE, Petty TL, Filley GF. Ventilation and arterial blood gas changes induced by pursed lips breathing. J Appl Physiol 1970; 28: 784–789.
20. Bohadana AE, Patel R, Kraman SS. Contour maps of auscultatory percussion in healthy subjects and patients with large intrapulmonary lesions. Lung 1989; 167: 359–372.
21. Welsby PD, Earis JE. Some high pitched thoughts on chest examination. Postgrad Med J 2001, 77: 617–620.
22. Earis JE, Cheetham BM. Perspectives of respiratory sound research. Eur Respir Rev 2000; 10: 641–646.
23. Loudon R, Murphy RL Jr. Lung sounds. Am Rev Respir Dis 1984; 130: 663–673.
24. Mikami R, Murao M, Cugell DW et al. International Symposium on Lung Sounds. Synopsis of proceedings. Chest 1987; 92: 342–345.
25. Pasterkamp H, Kraman SS, Wodicka GR. Respiratory sounds. Advances beyond the stethoscope. Am J Respir Crit Care Med 1997; 15: 6974–987.
26. Forgacs P. Lung sounds. London: Baillière Tindall, 1978.
27. Kraman SS. Determination of the site of production of respiratory sounds by subtraction phonopneumography. Am Rev Respir Dis 1980; 122: 303–309.
28. Pasterkamp H, Patel S, Wodicka GR. Asymmetry of respiratory sounds and thoracic transmission. Med Biol Eng Comput 1997; 35: 103–106.
29. Gavriely N, Nissan M, Rubin AH, Cugell DW. Spectral characteristics of chest wall breath sounds in normal subjects. Thorax 1995; 50: 1292–1300.
30. Pardee NE, Martin CJ, Morgan ET. A test of the practical value of estimating breath sound intensity. Breath sounds related to measured ventilatory function. Chest 1976; 70: 341–344.
31. Purohit A, Bohadana A, Kopferschmitt-Kubler MC et al. Lung auscultation in airway challenge testing. Respir Med 1997; 91: 151–157.
32. Schreur HJ, Sterk PJ, Vanderschoot J et al. Lung sound intensity in patients with emphysema and in normal subjects at standardised airflows. Thorax 1992; 47: 674–679.
33. Charbonneau G, Sudraud M, Soufflet G. Method of the evaluation of flow rate from pulmonary sounds. Bull Eur Physiol-pathol Respir 1987; 23: 265–270.
34. Baughman RP, Loudon RG. Sound spectral analysis of voice-transmitted sound. Am Rev Respir Dis 1986; 134: 167–169.
35. Gavriely N, Grotberg JB. Flow limitation and wheezes in a constant flow and volume lung preparation. J Appl Physiol 1988; 64: 17–20.
36. Spence DP, Graham DR, Jamieson G et al. The relationship between wheezing and lung mechanics during methacholine-induced bronchoconstriction in asthmatic subjects. Am J Respir Crit Care Med 1996; 154: 290–294.
37. Baughman RP, Loudon RG. Quantitation of wheezing in acute asthma. Chest 1984; 86: 718–722.
38. Avital A, Bar-Yishay E, Springer C, Godfrey S. Bronchial provocation tests in young children using tracheal auscultation. J Pediatr 1988; 112: 591–594.
39. Earis JF, Marsh K, Pearson MG, Ogilvie CM. The inspiratory 'squawk' in extrinsic allergic alveolitis and other pulmonary fibroses. Thorax 1982; 37: 923–926.
40. Nath AR, Capel LH. Inspiratory crackles and mechanical events of breathing. Thorax 1974; 29: 695–698.
41. Fredberg JJ, Holford SK. Discrete lung sounds: crackles (rales) as stress-relaxation quadrupoles. J Acoust Soc Am 1983; 73: 1036–1046.
42. Walshaw MJ, Nisar M, Pearson MG et al. Expiratory lung crackles in patients with fibrosing alveolitis. Chest 1990; 97: 407–409.
43. Benedetto G, Dalmasso F, Spagnolo R. Surface distribution of crackling sounds. IEEE Trans Biomed Eng 1988; 35: 406–412.

5.1 Cough

Lorcan McGarvey and Joseph MacMahon

Key points

- Short-term cough is most frequently caused by viral infection

- Smoking is the most common cause of chronic cough

- Postnasal drip syndrome, asthma and gastro-oesophageal reflux are responsible for most causes of persistent cough in non-smokers

- Empirical therapy can be substituted for specific diagnostic testing

- Combination therapy may be required as persistent cough may have more than one cause

Cough is a powerful physiological reflex that prevents inhalation of foreign material into the lungs and ensures that secretions are removed efficiently from the airway. However, cough may become persistent, non-productive and a source of great distress to the individual. Coughing is probably the most common symptom for which patients seek medical attention. It can be so severe as to induce vomiting, incontinence and syncope, and is known to significantly impair quality of life.[1] Cough may be categorised as *acute*, frequently following an upper respiratory tract infection and lasting less than 3 weeks, or *chronic* (lasting more than 3 weeks).[2] Cough may be either *productive* (of more than 30 ml of sputum per day)[3] or *non-productive*.

Epidemiology

The prevalence of chronic cough is strongly associated with smoking.

Up to one-third of current smokers report chronic cough and the rates increase with the number of cigarettes smoked but decrease significantly with smoking cessation. Current smokers have a two- to threefold greater prevalence of chronic cough compared to never-smokers.[4] The prevalence of cough as a sole symptom among non-smokers ranges from 3% to 13% of the general population.[4,5] Viral upper respiratory tract infections account for much of the seasonal variation in acute cough. *Bordetella pertussis* can cause prolonged cough in all age groups. Cough appears to increase with age, particularly in females.[6] Differences in the prevalence of cough between ethnic groups can be explained by cigarette consumption. Air pollution is associated with an increased prevalence of all respiratory symptoms, including cough.[7]

The neurophysiological mechanisms of cough

An effective cough requires the generation of a column of expired air moving at high linear velocity through the airway.[8] The kinetic energy generated applies a high shearing force to the airway wall, ensuring the removal of adherent mucus or foreign material. A cough usually begins with deep inspiration followed by forced expiration, initially against a closed glottis (compressive phase), followed by expulsion of air on glottic opening.

Coughing involves a complex reflex arc, usually initiated by stimulation of afferent structures innervated by the vagus nerve and its branches.[9] These afferent sites are chiefly found in the lower pharynx, larynx and tracheobronchial tree and, via the auricular branch, the tympanic membrane and external auditory meatus. Once an afferent receptor is stimulated, impulses are conducted to the 'cough centre' in the brain stem, probably located in the medulla oblongata. Motor outputs activate the appropriate efferent pathways to the expiratory musculature, including the diaphragm, larynx, pharynx and intercostals. Cough can also be generated voluntarily, indicating some degree of cortical input on the human cough reflex (Fig. 5.1.1).

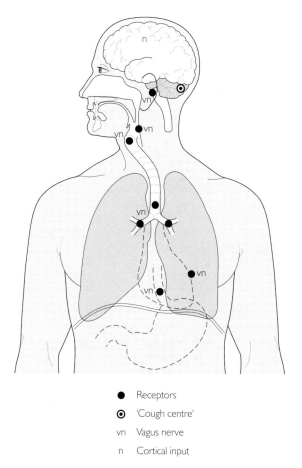

●   Receptors

◉   'Cough centre'

vn   Vagus nerve

n   Cortical input

Fig. 5.1.1 The anatomy of the afferent limb of the cough reflex. (Redrawn with permission from Irwin RS, Madison JM. Anatomical diagnostic protocol in evaluating chronic cough, with specific reference to gastroesophageal reflux disease. Am J Med 2000; 108: 126S–130S.)

In the larynx and tracheobronchial tree, sensory nerves and receptors presumed to mediate cough are present within and under the airway epithelium. Interest has focused on two of these, the thin myelinated rapidly adapting receptors (RARs) and the neuropeptide-containing non-myelinated C-fibre receptors.[10] A third receptor, the slowly adapting pulmonary stretch receptor, may also help to modulate the cough reflex. The RARs and C-fibre receptors respond in varying degrees to mechanical and chemical stimulation and are sensitive to a number of tussive stimuli, including citric acid and capsaicin, a pungent extract from the hot chilli pepper.[11] Evidence from animal studies suggests that stimulation of C fibres may inhibit cough. However their net effect in the lung is most probably to participate with RARs in the afferent component of the cough reflex. When activated, RARs and C fibres may directly initiate a cough and, in addition, when stimulated, C fibres may release neuropeptides that in turn activate RARs and indirectly trigger cough (Fig. 5.1.2).

Patients with chronic cough display an enhanced tussive response to inhaled capsaicin, suggesting an up-regulation in the afferent component of the cough reflex.[12] This cough sensitivity is heightened in females but is independent of atopy and bronchial hyper-reactivity.[13] It has been suggested that airway inflammation may contribute to the sensory hyper-responsiveness.[14]

Aetiology

Acute cough

Acute cough is frequently caused by viral infection and usually resolves within 2 weeks.[15] In adults, a severe cough may follow pertussis infection and persist beyond 3 weeks, with some cases lasting more than 3 months.[16] Acute cough may be the present-

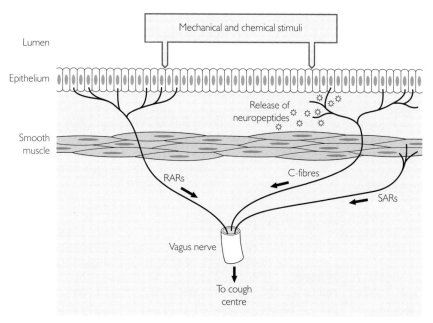

Fig. 5.1.2 Participation of sensory nerves in the afferent limb of the cough reflex. Rapidly-adapting receptors (RARs) and C fibres are activated by mechanical and 'chemical' stimulation and may directly mediate cough. Stimulation of C fibres may also release neuropeptides that in turn activate RARs and indirectly activate cough. Slowly-adapting pulmonary stretch receptors (SARs) may modulate cough centrally by making the expiratory effort more forceful. (Redrawn with permission from Irwin RS, Madison JM, Fraire AE. The cough reflex and its relation to gastroesophageal reflux. Am J Med 2000;108: 73S–78S.)

ing symptom in pneumonia and pulmonary oedema. Cough can also be a prominent symptom in pulmonary embolus, where it has been documented in 11–50% of angiographically proven cases.[17,18] In smokers, the onset of a new cough, a change in cough character or the presence of haemoptysis should raise the suspicion of bronchogenic carcinoma.

Chronic cough

Chronic cough in a smoker is usually due to chronic bronchitis. In non-smokers with a normal chest radiograph and no recent infection, the cause for chronic cough may not be immediately apparent. Prospective studies on the evaluation of such patients in both community and hospital settings consistently show that cough is most likely to be due to postnasal drip syndrome, asthma or gastro-oesophageal reflux disease and in up to a third of cases the cough may be simultaneously due to two or more of these conditions.[19-21] Postnasal drip is the most common cause, identified in up to 40% of cases.[19,20] Asthma may account for cough in up to 35% of cases,[21] with gastro-oesophageal reflux determined to be the third most common cause, occurring in up to 21% of patients.[19] Less common causes of cough include bronchiectasis, angiotensin-converting enzyme (ACE) inhibitors, diffuse parenchymal lung disease, psychogenic cough and inhaled foreign body. No clear cause is found in up to 20% of cases, when the cough is termed 'idiopathic'

Chronic bronchitis

Cough in a smoker that is productive of phlegm on most days for 3 months for 2 consecutive years satisfies the diagnosis of chronic bronchitis.[22] Smoking cessation is associated with resolution or improvement in the cough in over 90% of individuals, most often within 4 weeks,[23] but sometimes taking months.

Postnasal drip syndrome

This is the most common cause of chronic cough among patients referred for specialist advice.[19-21] The diagnosis is based on a combination of history, inspection of the upper airways, radiological imaging of the nasal passages and paranasal sinuses and most critically the resolution of cough after specific treatment.

Postnasal drip is characterised by the sensation of nasal secretions or a 'drip' at the back of the throat (posterior rhinorrhoea), along with frequent throat clearing. The precise underlying cause is not always clear but is often attributed to rhinitis, sinusitis or rhinosinusitis. Rhinitis may lead to one or more of the following symptoms: nasal congestion, rhinorrhoea, sneezing and itching.[24] It may be allergic or non-allergic, seasonal or perennial, secondary to viral infection or vasomotor. The contribution of sinusitis to postnasal drip varies from 8% when the cough is nonproductive[25] up to 64% when the cough is productive.[3] Sinusitis is defined as inflammation in one or more of the paranasal sinuses but usually refers to infection of the sinuses. A history of purulent nasal discharge, fever and headache or facial pains is suggestive of sinusitis. Additional evidence may be provided by radiological imaging of the sinuses.

Cough-variant asthma

Cough, shortness of breath and wheezing form a triad of symptoms characteristic of asthma. Cough may be the only symptom and such patients are described as having 'cough-variant asthma'.[26] Spirometry is normal, there is bronchial hyper-responsiveness and the cough usually responds to bronchodilators and inhaled steroids. Long-term follow-up studies suggest that many adults later develop more typical asthma symptoms, and in children the subsequent development of wheeze may be as high as 75%.[27]

A chronic cough with sputum eosinophilia but no other asthmatic symptoms or hyper-responsiveness has been reported.[28] The term 'eosinophilic bronchitis' has been used to describe this patient group, which may account for up to 15% of patients referred for specialist opinion.[29]

Gastro-oesophageal reflux disease

In gastro-oesophageal reflux disease (GORD), there is retrograde movement of stomach contents into the oesophagus, which may arise as a result of lower oesophageal sphincter dysfunction. The diagnosis of such reflux as the cause of cough can only be made with confidence when the cough improves with specific anti-reflux therapy. The diagnosis is suggested when the cough is associated with meals, worsens at night when lying flat, increases on stooping or is accompanied by dyspepsia. The reflux itself may be clinically silent in up to 75% of patients with associated cough.[30]

Barium studies of the oesophagus, oesophageal manometry and oesophagoscopy have all been used in the diagnosis but the most useful test is 24-hour ambulatory oesophageal pH monitoring, which can quantify the degree of reflux and determine the temporal relationship between cough and episodes of acid reflux.

There are two proposed mechanisms by which reflux may induce coughing:

- First, by macro- or microaspiration of gastric contents into the laryngeal or tracheobronchial tree. However, 24-hour ambulatory oesophageal pH monitoring, using proximal and distal probes, indicates only minor amounts of reflux proximally in patients with cough.[31]
- Second, acid gastric contents in the distal oesophagus may stimulate a vagally mediated oesophageal–tracheobronchial cough reflex.[30]

Irrespective of exactly how reflux causes a cough, increased trans-diaphragmatic pressure during coughing may result in transient lower oesophageal sphincter relaxation, itself resulting in some acid reflux. Therefore, a positive feedback loop exists whereby reflux causes cough, which may worsen reflux, and so on.

ACE-inhibitor therapy

Although ACE inhibitors are usually well-tolerated, a persistent cough is the most common side effect, occurring in around 10% of patients treated.[32] It is a dry tickly cough, more common among women and usually developing within a week but sometimes as long as 6 months after starting therapy.[32] Peptides such as bradykinin and substance P, which are both tussive, are normally degraded by angiotensin-converting enzyme[33] and inhibition of this pathway may potentiate the effects of these peptides in the airways. After stopping the ACE inhibitor, coughing usually subsides within a few days, but may take several weeks.

Bronchiectasis

A daily cough productive of copious amounts of sputum is characteristic although not universal among patients with bronchiectasis. Its prevalence in prospective studies of patients attending specialist cough clinics is low but is higher in general respiratory clinics.[34]

Diffuse parenchymal lung disease

It is not clear why these patients are sometimes troubled with a persistent dry cough. It may result from coexistent disease, in particular gastro-oesophageal reflux, which has an increased prevalence among patients with idiopathic pulmonary fibrosis.[35] Alternatively, the alveolar inflammation may stimulate peripheral cough receptors.

Psychogenic cough

A psychogenic or 'habit' cough has most frequently been reported in children and adolescents.[36] Typically it occurs throughout the day and disappears during sleep. Psychogenic cough should only be considered as the cause of persistent cough in adults when organic causes have been rigorously excluded. In patients with an established organic cause, psychological factors may exacerbate the problem.

Idiopathic cough

In up to 20% of cases, despite extensive investigation and/or empirical therapy, a cause for the cough may not be identified.[21]

Patients with idiopathic cough tend to be middle-aged, female and have marked cough reflex hyper-responsiveness. The pathogenesis is unclear, although an increased density of neuropeptide-containing intra-epithelial nerves in the airways has been reported.[37]

The evaluation of a patient with persistent cough

History

The history may establish a recent respiratory tract infection or the fact that the cough is associated with a postnasal drip, occurs mainly at night or after meals, is made worse by lying flat or is worse with exercise or in cold air. Reliance solely on the characteristics of the cough may be misleading: the symptoms of postnasal drip in a patient may reflect only coexistent rhinitis and the absence of dyspepsia does not rule out reflux as the cause of cough.

Examination

Physical examination may reveal clinical signs of asthma, bronchiectasis, lung cancer, pulmonary fibrosis or heart failure. A careful inspection of the ear, nose and throat may demonstrate evidence of nasal obstruction due to inflamed turbinates, the presence of polyps or the appearance of draining secretions in the posterior pharynx. A 'cobblestone' appearance of the oropharyngeal mucosa has been suggested but is uncommon in the routine examination of patients with chronic cough.[21]

Investigations

Investigations should be organised systematically to evaluate the major causes of persistent cough (Table 5.1.1). The following advice is based on the recommendations of the American College of Chest Physicians.[38] A chest radiograph is essential. Spirometry should be performed in all patients with reversibility testing if airflow obstruction is present. Variable airflow may also be demonstrated by measuring peak expiratory flows morning and evening over 2–4 weeks. Bronchial challenge testing should be considered for patients with normal spirometry and/or no variable airflow on peak flow monitoring. A negative challenge reliably rules out asthma as the cause for cough but may not entirely exclude steroid responsive cough due to eosinophilic bronchitis.[29]

A plain radiograph of the sinuses may reveal evidence of sinus opacity, mucosal thickening and air–fluid levels in individuals with sinusitis. Sinus aspiration and culture offers the most accurate guide to antibiotic therapy for infectious sinusitis. Computed tomography (CT) of the sinuses adds little to the diagnostic yield and should be reserved for patients with persistent symptoms despite sustained therapy.

Twenty-four-hour ambulatory oesophageal pH monitoring is likely to contribute significantly to the evaluation of cough. A negative test is useful in confidently excluding reflux as a cause for cough.

In non-smokers with cough, fibreoptic bronchoscopy should be reserved for diagnostic uncertainty after extensive evaluation and courses of empirical therapy. In this selected group the diagnostic yield is improved and may identify causes such as broncholithiasis, tracheobronchopathia and laryngeal dyskinesia.[39] Thoracic CT scanning is unlikely to add much to the routine evaluation of cough patients. In situations where bronchiectasis is considered, a high-resolution scan may be helpful.

Table 5.1.1 Guidelines for investigations in chronic cough[38]

- Chest radiograph
- Spirometry and reversibility testing
- Peak flow recording
- Bronchial challenge testing
- Paranasal sinus radiograph/CT scan
- 24-hour ambulatory pH monitoring
- Computed tomography of the thorax
- Fibreoptic bronchoscopy

Empirical therapy is sometimes appropriate, e.g. when the relevant investigations are not available. Diagnostic strategies that begin with trials of postnasal drip therapy have been effective.[25] Where postnasal drip and asthma have been excluded, the empirical use of anti-reflux medication has been suggested and may be more cost effective than 24-hour oesophageal pH monitoring in identifying anti-reflux responders.[40]

On the rare occasions when psychogenic cough is likely, and usually after extensive evaluation, psychological or psychiatric referral may be appropriate.

Treatment of chronic cough

Antitussive therapy may be characterised as *specific*, directed at the suspected aetiology or *non-specific*, simply controlling the symptom.

Specific treatment

Specific approaches include smoking cessation or withdrawal of an ACE inhibitor. Alternatively, combinations of one or more of the following regimens may be required.

Postnasal drip syndrome

When rhinitis is prominent, first-generation antihistamines and decongestant combinations are recommended.[38] Non-sedating antihistamines, along with intranasal steroids, are effective in allergic rhinitis but sedating antihistamines may be used if this approach fails. In chronic bacterial sinusitis, antibiotics should be given for at least 3 weeks and should cover *Streptococcus pneumoniae* and *Haemophilus influenzae*. The concurrent use of an antihistamine and decongestant followed by intranasal steroids for 3 months has been suggested.[38] An improvement should be seen within a few weeks but may require longer. Failure to resolve or frequent relapse may necessitate sinus surgery.

Cough-variant asthma

Although the cough may respond to a bronchodilator, inhaled (and sometimes oral) steroids are almost always needed. Cough-variant asthma can be difficult to control and, at 2-year follow up, 80% of one group of patients still required inhaled steroids and 20% were receiving daily oral prednisolone.[41]

Gastro-oesophageal reflux disease

Lifestyle measures, including weight reduction, high-protein/low-fat diet, smoking cessation and reducing alcohol and coffee consumption, should be recommended. Avoidance of stooping and elevation of the head of the bed may help. Adequate acid suppression with either H_2 antagonists or proton-pump inhibitors is the mainstay of treatment. The above measures should result in satisfactory improvement in cough within a month, although it sometimes takes consider-

ably longer.[38] Laparoscopic fundoplication may be effective for patients with persisting reflux and cough despite medical therapy.[42]

Non-specific treatment

Many demulcent syrups, drops and lozenges are marketed as cough suppressants. There is little evidence for their effectiveness. Opiates are centrally acting antitussives but knowledge of their precise mechanism of action is incomplete. The efficacy of codeine has been questioned and it may be no better than placebo in treatment of cough due to the common cold.[43] The long-term use of opiate antitussives is not recommended except for palliative purposes in patients with lung cancer.

Nebulised local anaesthetics give short-term relief for severe cough but cause undesirable inhibition of important upper airway reflexes; they have not been evaluated adequately and cannot be recommended.

Future therapy for cough

The hypothetical role of tachykinins in the pathogenesis of cough has therapeutic implications. Antitussive properties have been consistently demonstrated for tachykinin-receptor antagonists in animal experiments, although evidence of efficacy in humans is limited.[44] γ-aminobutyric acid (GABA) is an inhibitory neurotransmitter found in the central nervous system and in peripheral tissue including the lung. The GABA-agonist baclofen inhibits cough in animal studies via a central mechanism.[45] In pilot human studies, low-dose oral baclofen inhibits cough, possibly via a peripheral mechanism.[46] Understanding the precise central and peripheral neural pathways will provide new targets for drug development.

References

1. French CL, Irwin RS, Curley FJ, Krikorian CJ. Impact of chronic cough on quality of life. Arch Intern Med 1998; 158: 1657–1661.
2. Irwin RS, Corrao WM, Pratter MR. Chronic persistent cough in the adult: the spectrum and frequency of cases and successful outcome of specific therapy. Am Rev Respir Dis 1981; 123: 414–417.
3. Smyrnios NA, Irwin RS, Curley FJ. Chronic cough with a history of excessive sputum production: the spectrum and frequency of causes, key components of the diagnostic evaluation, and outcome of specific therapy. Chest 1995; 108: 991–997.
4. Barbee RA, Halonen M, Kaltenborn WT, Burrows B. A longitudinal study of respiratory symptoms in a community population sample. Correlations with smoking, allergen skin-test reactivity, and serum IgE. Chest 1991; 99: 20–26.
5. Di Pede C, Viegi G, Quackenboss JJ et al. Respiratory symptoms and risk factors in an Arizona population samples of Anglo and Mexican American whites. Chest 1991; 99: 916–922.
6. Gulsvik A. Prevalence of respiratory symptoms in the city of Oslo. Scand J Respir Dis. 1979; 60: 275–289.
7. Krzyzanowski M, Lebowitz MD. Changes in chronic respiratory symptoms in two populations of adults studied longitudinally over 13 years. Eur Respir J 1992; 5: 12–20.
8. McCool FD, Leith DE. Pathophysiology of cough. Clin Chest Med 1987; 8: 189–195.
9. Korpas J, Tomori Z. Cough and other respiratory reflexes, 12th ed. Basel: S Karger; 1979.

10. Widdicombe JG. Neurophysiology of the cough reflex. Eur Respir J 1995; 8: 1193–1202.
11. Coleridge HN, Coleridge JCG. Reflexes evoked from the tracheobronchial tree and lungs. In: Cherniack NS, Widdicombe JG, ed. Handbook of physiology. 3. The respiratory system. Vol. II. Control of breathing. Bethesda, MD: American Physiological Society; 1986; 395–429.
12. Choudry NB, Fuller RW. Sensitivity of the cough reflex in patients with chronic cough. Eur Respir J 1992; 5: 296–300.
13. Fujimura M, Kasahara K, Yasui M et al. Atopy in cough sensitivity to capsaicin and bronchial responsiveness in young females. Eur Respir J 1989; 11: 060–1063.
14. McGarvey LPA, Forsythe P, Heaney LG et al. Bronchoalveolar lavage findings in patients with chronic nonproductive cough. Eur Respir J 1999; 13: 59–65.
15. Curley FJ, Irwin RS, Pratter MR. Cough and the common cold. Am Rev Respir Dis 1988; 138: 305–311.
16. Birkebaek NH, Kristiansen M, Seefeldt T et al. *Bordetella pertussis* and chronic cough in adults. Clin Infect Dis 1999; 29: 1239–1242.
17. Miniata M, Prediletto R, Formichi B et al. Accuracy of clinical assessment in the diagnosis of pulmonary embolism. Am J Respir Crit Care 1999; 159: 864–871.
18. Bell WR, Simon TL, DeMets DL. The clinical features of submassive and massive pulmonary emboli. Am J Med 1977; 62: 355–360.
19. Irwin RS, Curley FJ, French CL. Chronic cough: the spectrum and frequency of causes, key components of the diagnostic evaluation and outcome of specific therapy. Am Rev Resp Dis 1990; 141: 640–647.
20. Poe HR, Harder RV, Israel RH. Chronic persistent cough: experience in diagnosis and outcome using an anatomic diagnostic protocol. Chest 1989; 95: 723–727.
21. McGarvey LPA, Heaney LG, Lawson JT et al. Evaluation and outcome of patients with chronic non-productive cough using a comprehensive diagnostic protocol. Thorax 1998; 53: 738–743.
22. Medical Research Council. Committee report on the aetiology of chronic bronchitis: definition and classification of chronic bronchitis for clinical and epidemiological purposes. Lancet 1965; 1: 775–778.
23. Wynder EL, Kaufman PL, Lesser RL. A short-term follow up study on ex-cigarette smokers. Am Rev Respir Dis 1966; 92: 645–655.
24. Lund VJ, Aaronson DW, Bousquet J et al. International consensus report on the diagnosis and management of rhinitis. Allergy 1994; 49 (suppl 19): 5–34.
25. Pratter MR, Bartter T, Akers S, Dubois J. An algorithmic approach to chronic cough. Ann Intern Med 1993; 119: 977–983.
26. Corrao WM, Braman SS, Irwin RS, Chronic cough as the sole presenting manifestation of bronchial asthma. N Engl J Med 1979; 300: 633–637.
27. Corrao WM. Chronic persistent cough: diagnosis and treatment update. Pediatr Ann 1996; 25: 162–168.
28. Gibson PG, Dolovich J, Denberg J et al. Chronic cough: eosinophilic bronchitis without asthma. Lancet 1989; 17: 1346–1348.
29. Brightling CE, Ward R, Goh KL et al. Eosinophilic bronchitis is an important cause of chronic cough. Am J Respir Crit Care Med 1999; 160: 406–410.
30. Ing AJ, Ngu MC, Breslin ABX. Pathogenesis of chronic persistent cough associated with gastro-oesophageal reflux. Am J Respir Crit Care Med 1994; 149: 160–167.
31. Irwin RS, French CL, Curley FJ et al. Chronic cough due to gastroesophageal reflux. Clinical, diagnostic and pathogenetic aspects. Chest 1993; 104: 1511–1517.
32. Israili ZH, Hall WD. Cough and angioneurotic oedema associated with angiotensin-converting enzyme inhibitor therapy: a review of the literature and pathophysiology. Ann Intern Med 1992; 117: 234–242.
33. Erdos EG, Yang HYT. An enzyme in microsomal fraction of kidney that inactivates bradykinin. Life Sci 1967; 6: 569–574.
34. McGarvey LPA, Heaney LG, MacMahon J. A retrospective survey of diagnosis and management of patients presenting with chronic cough to a general chest clinic. Int J Clin Pract 1998; 52: 158–161.
35. Toboin RW, Pope CE, Pelligrini CA et al. Increased prevalence of gastroesophageal reflux in patients with idiopathic pulmonary fibrosis. Am J Respir Crit Care Med 1998; 158: 1804–1808.
36. Lokshin B, Lindgren S, Weinberger M, Koviach. Outcome of habit cough in children with a brief session of suggestion therapy. Ann Allergy 1991; 67: 579–582.
37. O'Connell F, Springall DR, Moradoghli-Haftvani A et al. Abnormal intraepithelial airway nerve in persistent unexplained cough. Am J Respir Crit Care Med 1995; 152: 2068–2075.
38. Irwin RS, Boulet LP, Cloutier MM et al. Managing cough as a defence mechanism and as a symptom. A consensus panel report of the American College of Chest Physicians. Chest 1998; 114): 133S–181S.
39. Sen RP, Walsh TE. Fibreoptic bronchoscopy for refractory cough. Chest 1991; 99: 33–35.
40. Ours TM, Kavuru MS, Schilz RJ, Richter JE. A prospective evaluation of oesophageal testing and a double blind, randomized study of omeprazole in a diagnostic and therapeutic algorithm for chronic cough. Am J Gastroenterol 1999; 94: 3131–3138.
41. Cheriyan S, Greenberger PA, Patterson R. Outcome of cough variant asthma treated with inhaled steroids. Ann Allergy 1994; 73: 478–480.
42. Allen CJ, Anvari M. Gastro-oesophageal reflux related cough and its response to laparoscopic fundoplication. Thorax 1998; 53: 963–968.
43. Freestone C, Eccles R. Assessment of the antitussive efficacy of codeine in cough associated with the common cold. J Pharm Pharmacol 1997; 49: 1045–1049.
44. Advenier C, Lagente V, Boichot E. The role of tachykinin receptor antagonists in the prevention of bronchial hyperresponsiveness, airway inflammation and cough. Eur Respir J 1997; 10: 1892–1906.
45. Bolser DC, Aziz SM, DeGennaro FC et al. Antitussive effects of GABA agonists in the cat and guinea pig. Br J Pharmacol 1993; 110: 491–495.
46. Dicpingaitis PV, Dobkin JB. Antitussive effect of the GABA-agonist baclofen. Chest 1997; 111: 996–999.

5 An approach to common respiratory symptoms

5.2 Haemoptysis

Michael G Pearson and John Corless

Key points

- The aetiology of haemoptysis varies geographically, influenced by the relative prevalence of tuberculosis/infection and of cigarette smoking.

- The bleeding usually originates from systemic vessels within the lungs.

- Diagnosis depends on first proving that the source of the bleeding is from the lungs – examination of the sputum can yield useful clues.

- If bleeding is not catastrophic then computed tomography is the investigation of first choice, with bronchoscopy when negative or when tumour is suspected.

- Haemoptysis with a clear chest radiograph is unlikely to require investigation in persons aged less than 40 years or in non-smokers.

Haemoptysis is the medical term used to describe the expectoration of blood. It is derived from the Greek *haima* ('blood') and *ptysis* ('a spitting').

Aetiology and epidemiology

A Straining to vomit, to go to Stool, Labour, Running, Fighting, violent Sneezing, a strong inspiration, Shouting aloud, Fencing too hard and long together, carrying of great Loads, or lifting them up, holding one's Breath too long, too great Straining in Coition, Dancing too much and too long, excessive Laughter; hence Wrestlers, Racers, Hunters, Singers, Trumpeters, Dancers, Porters and such like, are subject to Spittings of Blood. Amongst all the Passions of the Mind, Anger is the chief Cause of this Distemper.

An 18th-century list of the causes of haemoptysis from *The Family Companion for Health* (F. Fayram, London, 1929).

In the 17th century, expectoration of blood was often a sign of the 'Black Death'. In the 19th and early 20th century haemoptysis was considered to be almost synonymous with a diagnosis of tuberculosis[1] but then it was shown that one-third of those admitted to sanatoria with haemoptysis did not have tuberculosis.[2] In more modern times a myriad of causes are recognised; a Medline database search produced more than 2000 articles, although many are single case reports. Table 5.2.1 sets out a summary of the better documented causes.

The most likely causes of haemoptysis vary geographically, influenced predominantly by the prevalence of active pulmonary tuberculosis and of cigarette smoking. Some regions have specific causes to consider that may not be seen elsewhere (e.g. paragonimiasis in south-east Asia). There is little reliable epidemiological evidence to indicate how the causes have changed over time. The changing pattern of disease with the decline of tuberculosis in Europe and the USA is illustrated in Table 5.2.2. The scourge of tuberculosis and the ravages of untreated infections (bronchiectasis) have been replaced in developed countries by the problems of cigarette smoking, with bronchitis and cancer becoming the most common causes

All such figures must be interpreted with caution since there is no common denominator. Episodes of haemoptysis seen in hospital practice are usually suspected of being due to serious pathology and actively investigated but in the community many episodes may never being reported to a doctor.[4] Thus the true prevalence of haemoptysis may be much higher. Also surgical series tend to have higher cancer rates than medical series reflecting referral practice.

Even with the increased frequency of lung cancer it is important not to equate haemoptysis with cancer. Most cases of haemoptysis will not prove to have cancer and conversely only 31% of a bronchoscopy series of cancer patients had had haemoptysis before presenting for investigation.[5]

Table 5.2.1 Causes of haemoptysis

Neoplastic
Primary bronchial carcinoma
Pulmonary metastatic disease
Bronchial Adenoma
Kaposi's sarcoma

Infection
Bacterial pneumonia
Tuberculosis
Lung abscess
Aspergillus disease
Parasitic disease
Viral infection (Influenza, varicella)

Pulmonary
Bronchiectasis
Bronchitis
Cystic fibrosis
Cryptogenic organising pneumonia

Vascular
Pulmonary embolism
Pulmonary hypertension
Arteriovenous malformations
Bronchial artery malformations
Congenital vascular abnormalities
Aortic aneurysm
Valvular heart disease
Amniotic fluid embolism
Hepatopulmonary syndromes
Pulmonary venous hypertension/congestive cardiac failure

Haematological
Coagulopathies
Lung transplant rejection
Thrombolysis
Abnormal platelet function

Systemic disease
Vasculitides
Goodpasture's syndrome
Systemic lupus erythematosus
Idiopathic pulmonary haemosiderosis
Diffuse alveolar haemorrhage/capillaritis

Iatrogenic
Bronchoscopy
Percutaneous lung biopsy
Radiotherapy
Swan–Ganz catheters
Implantable cardiac defibrillators

Drugs
Anticoagulants
Aspirin
Amiodarone
Penicillamine
Solvents
Crack cocaine

Miscellaneous
Foreign body inhalation
Pulmonary amyloid
Thoracic endometriosis
Inadvertent or deliberate self-harm (e.g. tongue biting)
Gingival disease
Gastro-oesophageal reflux disease
Pulmonary sequestration
Behçet's syndrome
Pulmonary allograft

Table 5.2.2 Changing causes of haemoptysis. (With permission from Corey & Khin.[3])

	Heller 1946 (416)	Abbott 1948 (497)	Levitt 1951 (683)	Souders 1952 (105)	Moerschi 1952 (200)	Johnston 1956 (324)	Boucot 1959 (395)	Purse 1961 (105)	Soll 1978 (200)	Corey 1984 (120)
Cancer	2	21	12	3	24	4	8	19	13	13
Bronchitis	15	2	3	12	9	17	19	5	55	50
Bronchiectasis	7	21	15	29	27	13	4	24	0	2
Tuberculosis	40	22	50	2	6	10	7	13	3	3
Other	26	34	20	54	30	59	64	40	29	32

Where is the bleeding from?

Anatomy of blood supply to the lung

In a typical adult 5 litres of deoxygenated blood pass through the lungs each minute in the pulmonary circulation at a mean arterial pressure of 20 mmHg. Most of this blood supplies the pulmonary capillary network and the pulmonary arterioles interact with the airway only at the level of the terminal bronchiole. The tissues of the lungs derive their oxygenated blood supply from the bronchial arterial circulation, which usually arises from the proximal descending thoracic aorta. The bronchial arterial circulation runs the entire length of the bronchial tree and, unlike the pulmonary arterial circulation, is at systemic arterial pressure. Small penetrating arteries supply the bronchial mucosa and form an extensive plexus in the submucosa. Given the higher circulating pressure and closer proximity to the airway, haemoptysis is much more likely to arise from the bronchial than from the pulmonary arterial circulation. The anatomy of the bronchial circulation is very variable and recruitment of non-bronchial systemic arteries may occur in some disease processes. There are some anastomotic connections between the two circulations. Bleeding from the pulmonary vessels alone is rare except in the situation of an arteriovenous malformation

Mechanisms of bleeding

The mechanisms by which the bleeding occurs are poorly understood. In tuberculosis, chronic inflammation and damage leads to ectatic arteries (Rasmussen's aneurysm) in the wall of the tuberculous cavity. A further additional insult, such as inflammation or infection, can precipitate bleeding from these abnormal vessels that may be massive. Up to 5% of tuberculosis patients were said to die of massive haemoptysis.[6] Any inflammation such as is associated with chronic infection, e.g. bronchiectasis, aspergillosis or cystic fibrosis, also leads to enlargement and proliferation of the bronchial arteries, which can be shown on bronchial artery angiography[7].

In lung cancer, the tumour has to achieve a supply of oxygenated blood and thus develops connections from the systemic circulation. The vessels in a tumour are often poorly formed and thus prone to bleed. Anything that damages the tumour, e.g. endobronchial radiotherapy (brachytherapy), may cause bleeding from damaged systemic vessels. In addition, a tumour may invade large vessels such as the pulmonary artery or the aorta, leading to massive bleeding.

The mechanism in pulmonary embolism is less clear. By definition the pulmonary circulation is interrupted and therefore should not leak, but why the bronchial circulation should bleed in this situation is not clear. Such bleeding is usually minor. Haemorrhage from large bronchopulmonary collaterals developing in infarcted lung segments has been described.[8]

Arteriovenous malformations may arise from the systemic circulation such as the case of a sequestered segment, in which a segment or lobe achieves its 'pulmonary' supply from the systemic circulation or may develop from pre-existing weaknesses within the pulmonary circulation, e.g. an arteriovenous abnormality. When bleeding occurs it can be substantial but is very likely to be amenable to surgical or embolic therapy because of its localised nature.

A cause of haemoptysis that is now rare in Europe and North America is mitral stenosis. Elevated left atrial pressure results in pulmonary venous hypertension. This in turn can cause a reversal of flow into the bronchial circulation through the anastomotic connections. The engorged, dilated veins lining the airways may then bleed in response to acute rises in the left atrial pressure.[9] The same situation can pertain in chronic congestive cardiac failure, although it is not known why haemoptysis occurs only in a minority of such patients.

Aspects of management of haemoptysis

The specific diagnostic and management issues for each of the various conditions are described elsewhere, so the remainder of this section will address general issues that apply to patients with haemoptysis. These include:

- confirmation that the blood is from the chest
- management of major catastrophic bleeding
- management of lesser degrees of frank haemoptysis
- management of minor haemoptysis or 'streaking' of the sputum
- management of haemoptysis with a normal radiograph.

The evidence base for managing acute haemoptysis is not well defined. A survey of 118 experienced physicians[10] revealed considerable differences of opinion as to the best choice in different situations. Medicolegal concerns and the availability or not of particular techniques may have influenced the views expressed. There is still a lack of trial data to distinguish between many of the options.

Confirming the history of haemoptysis

When there is frank haemoptysis, it can sometimes be difficult to differentiate blood that has been coughed up from haematemesis or blood that originates from the buccal or gingival mucosa, which may discolour saliva. Factors that favour haemoptysis rather than haematemesis include an alkaline pH, blood that is darker in colour and the presence of respiratory epithelial cells or haemosiderin-laden macrophages on microscopy. Resolving whether a patient has haemoptysis or haematemesis may be difficult and it has previously been shown that an upper gastrointestinal haemorrhage can stimulate cough via extrapulmonary cough receptors in the stomach. The same effect can be seen with bleeding from the nose and pharynx.[11]

When the blood is mixed with sputum – whether frothy, clear or purulent – there is little doubt as to its origin and, particularly when there are repeated episodes, it is possible to visually inspect a specimen. The appearance may give clues as to the cause. Frank blood with or without clots points to tumour, an arteriovenous malformation, a pulmonary embolus or a major haemorrhage – from tuberculous or aspergillous disease. Sputum that is frothy or pink suggests heart failure. Sputum that is purulent or rusty-coloured is suggestive of an acute bacterial infection, while blood streaks in white sputum are more likely to indicate tumour. Recurrent bleeding is much more likely to be due to malignancy, especially if it continues for more than a few days.

Overall, the history and sputum inspection will only point to and will not make the diagnosis, or define the cause. It is, however, important to inspect the sputum just to confirm that what the patient has described as blood really is just that and thus to avoid multiple unwarranted investigations.

Management of massive catastrophic haemoptysis

There is no agreement on what constitutes major or massive haemoptysis. It is difficult to estimate blood loss and amounts recorded are often unreliable.[12] The amount of blood coughed up over 24 hours can vary from large volumes of more than a litre to a few streaks mixed with phlegm. Massive haemoptysis is a life-threatening emergency, with reported mortality of up to 85%,[13] and is most often due to malignancy, bronchiectasis or aspergilloma, or following tuberculosis when a major vessel has been invaded or damaged. Investigation of the cause has to take second place to the attempt to resuscitate the patient. However, sometimes, such as when a tumour invades the aorta, bleeding is so rapid and treatment options so limited that there is little that can be done other than to comfort the patient and his/her distressed relatives.

Management of severe but not catastrophic haemoptysis

When the bleeding is rapid but not sufficient to constitute a medical emergency, there is time to consider and investigate the cause with the intention of instituting surgical or embolic therapy where possible. Most series define a loss of 200 ml or more in 24 h as major and larger losses (> 500–1000 ml per day) as massive.[14] The mortality is related to the rate of blood loss and in one study was 71% with a loss of more than 600 ml in 4 h, 45% if the 600 ml was lost over 16 h and 5% if the same 600 ml loss occurred over 16–48 h. There used to be a belief that the only useful therapy was surgical but Cory showed that conservative medical resuscitation was likely to be as effective as urgent surgery.[3] Elective interventions can then be reserved for specific treatable causes, when they have been identified.

Resuscitation is directed at maintaining the airway and circulatory volume. There is a danger that blood will flood the lungs and 'drown' the patient. Bronchoscopy allows direct visualisation of the bronchial tree, although the timing depends on the local facilities and condition of the patient, in particular the estimated rate of bleeding. Rigid bronchoscopy is preferable (although not always practical) as it allows better visualisation and a wider range of therapeutic options to deal with bleeding into an airway.

If bronchoscopy is not available or is contraindicated by the poor clinical status of the patient, endotracheal intubation is often recommended to allow aspiration to clear the airway of clots and blood. If the site of bleeding is known, some would advocate inserting the tube into the contralateral main bronchus, thereby isolating the healthy lung from the bleeding in the other. Others have argued that, unless there is a threat to the patient's oxygenation, it is better to allow the patient to cough the blood naturally while encouraging clearance with postural drainage, with bronchodilators (where needed) and avoidance of sedatives that might depress the cough reflex. This latter course is preferable for lesser degrees of bleeding.

Investigation of the source of the bleeding begins with a chest radiograph, which may help to identify the source of bleeding and guide subsequent investigations. Occasionally, blood that has spilled into areas of the lung distant from the source of bleeding produces misleading radiographic infiltrates.[15] Thereafter the most useful investigation is usually a bronchoscopy to try and localise, and if possible identify, the underlying cause. Only about 30–50% of bronchoscopies find a cause. Given that these patients have not had a massive bleed, there is usually time to perform the procedure electively and several studies have shown that the yield is little different if delayed by up to 48 h.[16] Computed tomography (CT) scanning with contrast media may be helpful in identifying arteriovenous abnormalities and tumours beyond the range of the scope. Spiral CT has the advantage of reliably identifying large to medium-sized pulmonary emboli. Other urgent investigations include assessment of the patient's coagulation status and arterial oxygenation with action to correct deficits as appropriate. Bronchography to identify bronchiectasis used to be a commonly performed procedure with a significant yield in the days when tuberculosis was common. It has largely been replaced by high-resolution CT scanning but there are still some who believe that the yield, especially if performed directly through a bronchoscope, is worthwhile.[17]

Older physicians were taught to bronchoscope every patient with haemoptysis but, given the rather modest yield and the technical improvements in CT scanning, it is probable that for most patients CT is less invasive and more informative. A CT scan may obviate the need for bronchoscopy. However, bronchoscopy will still be required when central tumours are suspected, when bacteriological or similar samples are required or when the source of the bleeding is in doubt. Visualisation of blood in a segment or lobe of the lung confirms the diagnosis of haemoptysis unequivocally and can also localise the source within the lungs.

If bleeding persists and the lobe or segment that the bleeding originates from can be identified, then surgery or angiographic embolisation can be considered. Surgical resection has a certainty of effect when the origin of bleeding is known but many patients will have other lung problems and may not be fit to withstand the effect of a thoracotomy. Bronchial arterial embolisation has been made much more feasible with the recent technical advances in catheters and, when available, may now be the treatment of choice when either bleeding is persistent or causes are identified that carry a high risk of recurrence. Bronchial artery embolisation does, however, carry a risk of paraplegia from inadvertent damage to nearby spinal arteries. As most bleeds arise from systemic vessels, the yield of pulmonary angiography is much lower. It will pick up pulmonary artery aneurysms, pulmonary arteriovenous malformations and some rarer congenital lesions, such as an absent pulmonary artery or branch.

It must not be forgotten that there are other systemic causes of bleeding, such as Goodpasture's syndrome, the leukaemias and the hypocoagulable states, that have to be treated in their own right.

Other investigations are then aimed at treating the primary cause, if known, as described elsewhere in this book. However there remain a significant number of patients with a normal radiograph who have had a significant bleed and been fully investigated without finding a cause. A normal chest radiograph is said to suggest that the origin of the bleeding lies in the tracheobronchial tree rather than in the pulmonary parenchyma.[18] Such causes are considered below.

Management of minor haemoptysis or 'streaking' of the sputum

When blood is mixed with sputum there is little doubt as to its origin but the importance is much less clear. The major concern for both patient and physician is to exclude cancer. A normal radiograph reduces the possibilities considerably but cancer, pulmonary emboli, bronchitis and other minor infective causes remain possible. The history may help in the assessment of possible pulmonary embolism or may point to bronchiectasis, and the chest radiograph will usually localise *Aspergillus* or tuberculosis cavities, as well as tumours. However, simple bronchitis cannot be diagnosed in a positive manner and, if the radiograph is clear, subsequent management depends largely on the estimated risk of lung cancer for that individual.

Unless there is a clear past diagnosis of a known cause of bleeding, e.g. established bronchiectasis or a documented mycetoma, all patients with an abnormal radiograph will require investigation. The CT scan is the most likely investigation to provide an explanation, is less invasive than bronchoscopy and should therefore be the first choice. Bronchoscopy should be reserved for cases where the CT has not provided the answer, where histology is required or where there is doubt about whether the reported bleeding was indeed haemoptysis. The yield from the two investigations is not identical and both can miss some tumours: bronchoscopy cannot detect peripheral lesions and CT may miss endobronchial tumours or may mis-attribute small opacities to other causes.[19]

Diffuse alveolar bleeding/capillaritis[20]

This is a relatively unusual presentation of haemoptysis associated with coagulation disorders, inhaled toxins or infections. The capillaritis is usually caused by systemic autoimmune and vasculitic syndromes. Investigation and management of these rare but potentially life-threatening conditions is difficult and referral to a specialist centre is appropriate. The diagnosis may be suggested by the other manifestation of the systemic disorder. The patchy alveolar shadowing on a CT scan may be hard

Table 5.2.3 Studies after 1980 of patients presenting with haemoptysis and a normal chest radiograph

	n	Mean age	Smokers (%)	Cancers identified	Follow-up if performed
Gong & Salvatierra 1981[16]	47	55		3/43	No follow-up
Ackert et al 1982[24]	259	N/A	N/A	1/259	No follow-up
Peters et al 1984[25]	26	52		0/26	No follow-up
Cory & Khin 1987[3]	59	50		5/59	No follow-up
Jackson et al 1985[26]	48	47	55	2/48	No follow-up
Adelman et al 1985[27]	67	55	72	0/67	Followed for 3 years – 1 tumour at 20 months
Heaton 1987[28]	41	56	66	4/41	Followed for 18 months – 1 tumour at 10 months
Santiago et al 1987[29]	58	56	90	6/58	Followed for 56 months – 2 more tumours and 3 unrelated deaths
Poe et al 1988[30]	196	57	74	12/196	2 tumours in 136 followed for more than 1 year – one of rib at 6 weeks and one of lung at 13 months
Lederle et al 1989[31]	106	62	90	6/106	Followed for 32 months – 6 cancers (all at more than 12 months)
Lee et al 1989[32]	478	44	64	4/478	128 followed for 20 months – no tumours
O'Neil & Lazarus 1991[33]	75	41	69	2/75	No follow-up
Sharma et al 1991[34]	53	37	27	0/53	No follow-up
Set et al 1993[35]	42	63	87	2/42	No follow-up
Totals	1555			47/1555	

to distinguish from various forms of fibrosing alveolitis and a firm diagnosis will usually depend on obtaining a lung biopsy sample – most often by a thoracoscopic technique.

Cryptogenic haemoptysis

If both bronchoscopy and CT are unhelpful and the investigation for other causes considered above is also unproductive, the haemoptysis can be considered as cryptogenic. Some 5–15% of cases may fall into this category[21] and there are two series that have followed such patients for several years. Despite about one-third having repeat episodes of bleeding, the incidence of carcinoma over 5 years was 1/55 cases in one series[22] and none in the other.[23]

Haemoptysis and a normal chest radiograph

The expectoration of blood is always an alarming symptom.

Most serious causes of haemoptysis produce significant radiographic changes that will point the way to subsequent investigations. A normal radiograph reduces the possibilities considerably but cancer, pulmonary emboli, bronchitis and other minor infective causes remain possible. The history may help but there will remain a group of patients with haemoptysis that could be due to cancer or could be due to bronchitis or another non-threatening condition.

There are a number of series that have examined this problem over the past 20 years and these are summarised in Table 5.2.3. The overall incidence of cancer in these studies is only 3% (47/1555). However these are, almost by definition, small 'early' tumours, which are likely to be surgically respectable. A yield of 1 in 33 cases is sufficient to justify active investigation (bronchoscopy and CT scanning). Factors favouring malignancy include:

- age over 40 years (only one case described was aged less than this)
- current smokers (only one non-smoker has been described)
- haemoptysis lasting for more than a week.

Therapeutic principles

- Establish that the blood has definitely originated from the lungs.

- If bleeding is massive, immediate action to resuscitate the circulation is required.

- If bleeding is not catastrophic, treatment is dependent on the underlying diagnosis. The aim is to investigate first with a chest radiograph and if abnormal follow on with computed tomography. Bronchoscopy should be performed if a diagnosis remains unclear or tumour is suspected.

- Attend to underlying systemic disorders, e.g. coagulation deficits. If alveolar haemorrhage is present then consider referral to specialist centre for lung biopsy.

- If investigations are negative and particularly if the chest radiograph is clear then the likelihood of late disease is small. There is little to be gained from routine review.

In the absence of these pointers the indication for invasive procedures is much weaker (0.13% incidence) and many patients may decline to undergo them. In those studies that have included follow-up the number of late tumours is also very low and all but one occurred more than 12 months after the sentinel event, i.e. the initial haemoptysis was probably unrelated. This suggests that if initial investigation is negative there is little justification for routine 3- or 6-monthly radiographic surveillance.

One study stands out from these. It comes from India, where there is a much lower incidence of smoking and a significant proportion of tuberculosis – figures that resemble the situation in Europe and the USA 50 years ago. The investigators found little pathology and concluded that there was little value in bronchoscopy, demonstrating how indications may vary between different regions of the world.

References

1. Wolfe JD, Simmons DH. Hemoptysis: diagnosis and management. West J Med 1977; 127: 383–390.
2. Wurtzen CH, Sjorslev N. Infection et morbidité de la tuberculose parmi les infirmières – notamment, parmi les élèves d'un service hôpital pour les tuberculeux. Acta Tuberc Scand 1936; 10: 310–319.
3. Corey R, Khin MB. Major and massive hemoptysis: reassessment of conservative management. J Am Med Sci 1987; 294: 301.
4. Stewart F M, Harding V, Shum C, Stewart AG. Worrying respiratory symptoms in an urban population. Thorax 1999; 54(suppl 3): A17.
5. Thompson S, Bucknall CE, Pearson G Presenting symptoms and signs of lung cancer - significance and relation to tumour type Am Rev Resp Crit Care Med 1999; 159: A61.
6. Thompson JR. Mechanisms of fatal pulmonary haemorrhage in tuberculosis. Dis Chest 1954; 25: 193.
7. Cohen AM, Doershuk CF, Stern RC. Bronchial artery embolization to control hemoptysis in cystic fibrosis. Radiology 1990; 175: 401–405.
8. Thomas CS, Endrys J, Abul A, Cherian G. Late massive haemoptyses from bronchopulmonary collaterals in infarcted segments following pulmonary embolism. Eur Respir J 1999; 13: 463–464.
9. Braunwald ED. Valvular heart disease. In: Heart disease. A textbook of cardiovascular medicine. Philadelphia, PA: WB Saunders; 1980: 1897–1899.
10. Haponik EF, Chin R. Hemoptysis: clinician's perspective. Chest 1990; 97: 469–475.
11. Moersch HJ. Clinical significance of haemoptysis JAMA 1952; 148: 471–474.
12. Conlan AA, Hurwitz SS, Krige L et al. Massive haemoptysis. J Thorac Cardiovasc Surg 1983; 85: 120.
13. Santiago S, Tobias J, Williams A. A reappraisal of the causes of hemoptysis. Arch Intern Med 1991; 151; 2449–2451.
14. Thompson AB, Teschler H, Rennard SI. Pathogenesis, evaluation and therapy for massive haemoptysis. Clin Chest Med 1992; 13: 75.
15. Bobrowitz ID, Ramakrishna S, Shim Y. Comparison of medical v surgical treatment of major hemoptysis. Arch Intern Med 1983; 143: 1343.
16. Gong H, Salvatierra C. Clinical efficacy of early and delayed fiberoptic bronchoscopy in patients with hemoptysis. Am Rev Respir Dis 1981; 124: 221–225.
17. Jones DK, Cavanagh P, Shneerson JM, Flower CDR. Does bronchography have a role in the assessment of patients with haemoptysis? Thorax 1985; 40: 668–670.
18. Israel RH, Poe RH. Haemoptysis. Clin Chest Med 1987; 8: 197.
19. White CS, Romney BM, Mason AC et al. Primary carcinoma of the lung overlooked at CT: analysis of findings in 14 patients. Radiology 1996; 199: 109–115.
20. Specks U. Diffuse alveolar haemorrhage syndromes. Curr Opin Rheumatol 2001; 13: 12–17.
21. Wolfe ID, Simmons DH. Hemoptysis: diagnosis and management. West J Med 1977; 127: 383–390.
22. Douglass BE, Carr DT. Prognosis in idiopathic hemoptysis. JAMA 1972; 150: 764–765.
23. Barret RJ, Tuttle WM. A study of essential haemoptysis. J Thorac Cardiovasc Surg 1960; 40: 468–474.

24. Ackart RS, Foreman DR, Klayton RJ et al. Fibreoptic bronchoscopy in outpatient facilities 1982. Arch Intern Med 1983; 143: 30–31.

25. Peters J, McClung HC, Teague RB. Evaluation of hemoptysis in patients with a normal chest roentgenogram. West J Med 1984; 141: 624–626.

26. Jackson CL, Savage PJ, Quinn DL Role of fibreoptic bronchoscopy in patients with haemoptysis and a normal chest roentgenogram. Chest 1985,87: 142–145.

27. Adelman M, Haponik EF, Bleecker ER, James Britt E. Cryptogenic haemoptysis. Ann Intern Med 1985; 102: 829–834.

28. Heaton RW. Should patients with haemoptysis and a normal chest X-ray be bronchoscoped? Postgrad Med J 1987; 63: 947–949.

29. Santiago S, Tobias J, Williams AJ. A Reappraisal of the causes of hemoptysis. Arch Intern Med 1991; 151: 2449–2451.

30. Poe RH, Israel RH, Marin MG et al. Utility of fibreoptic bronchoscopy in patients with hemoptysis and a nonlocalising chest roentgenogram. Chest 1988; 92: 70–75.

31. Lederle FA, Nichol KL, Parenti CM. Bronchoscopy to evaluate hemoptysis in older men with nonsuspicious roentgenograms. Chest 1989; 95: 1043–1047.

32. Lee C-J, Lee C-H, Lan R-L. The role of fibreoptic bronchoscopy in patients with hemoptysis and a normal chest roentgenogram. Chang Gung Med J 1989; 12: 136–140.

33. O'Neil KM, Lazarus AA. Hemoptysis. Indications for bronchoscopy. Arch Intern Med 1991; 151: 171–174.

34. Sharma SK, Dey AB, Pande JN, Verma K. Fibreoptic bronchoscopy in patients with haemoptysis and normal chest roentgenograms. Ind J Chest Dis 1991; 33: 15–13.

35. Set PA, Flower CDR, Smith I et al. Hemoptysis: comparative study of the role of CT and fiberoptic bronchoscopy. Radiology 1993; 189: 677–680.

5.3 Breathlessness

Paul W Jones

Key concepts

- Breathlessness is a 'synthetic' sensation.

- There are no specific breathlessness nerves, pathways or centres.

- It involves integration of multiple sources of neuronal information about breathing.

- The words used to describe breathlessness may provide diagnostic clues.

- Breathless correlates with inspiratory events.

- It correlates poorly with FEV_1.

- Measurements of disability due to breathlessness may be made easily in the clinic.

Breathlessness is one of the most important symptoms in lung disease but also the least well understood. It is the subjective experience of discomfort in breathing. Unlike pain, for which clearly defined neural pathways and centres have been identified within the brain, the pathways and systems by which breathlessness is perceived are much more complex.

There are no specific breathlessness receptors or nerves and no area in the brain has been identified as a 'breathlessness centre'.

The difficulty in identifying mechanisms responsible for breathlessness has been matched by the difficulty in defining it. Earlier attempts focused upon those components of the sensation associated with increased respiratory effort, e.g. 'consciousness of the necessity for increased respiratory effort'. More recent definitions include: 'an awareness of respiratory distress'; 'conscious awareness of an unpleasant or noxious sensation associated with breathing'; or 'an unpleasant or uncomfortable awareness of breathing or need to breathe'. These reflect the current view that breathing is a reflex action and that breathlessness is the conscious interpretation of the neural traffic associated with it.

It follows from this that breathlessness is a sensation that can be perceived only by the individual who is experiencing it. It is not a clinical sign that can be assessed by an outside observer and should not be confused with tachypnoea or evidence of laboured breathing. It is argued occasionally that 'dyspnoea' should be used to indicate breathlessness due to disease and that 'breathlessness' should be restricted to the sensation experienced by normal subjects. This distinction implies that dyspnoea and breathlessness have different mechanisms, but there is no evidence that this is the case. Furthermore, it may be difficult to know when 'normal' breathlessness ends and dyspnoea begins. For this reason, the two terms are now used interchangeably.

Mechanism of breathlessness

In the absence of specific pathways or brain centres for breathlessness, it is useful to think of dyspnoea as a 'synthetic' sensation that results from the integration of many different neuronal signals.

Motor command theory

When trying to understand the mechanisms responsible for breathlessness, it is important to distinguish between the level of breathing and the work of breathing since dyspnoea is influenced by both. An increase in ventilation, such as occurs with exercise or a metabolic acidosis, will cause dyspnoea in the absence of lung disease. Most lung diseases associated with breathlessness are characterised by changes in the mechanical properties of the lungs or chest wall, or a change in efficiency of the respiratory apparatus. Such effects all increase the work of breathing, which in turn will demand a reflex increase in level of respiratory motor output if arterial blood gas homeostasis is to be maintained.

Breathlessness is associated largely with inspiratory events, even in patients with airflow limitation.[1,2] Current hypotheses concerning its generation are based around evidence for a corollary discharge from the respiratory motor output that arises in the brain-stem respiratory centres and passes to the cerebral cortex. Within the cortex, this discharge is processed along with afferent information related to breathing and is perceived as breathlessness when there is a mismatch between the outgoing respiratory motor command and incoming afferent sensory traffic. This is often termed the 'motor-command' hypothesis. There is a good association between the level of ventilation or respiratory work and the accompanying sense of dyspnoea, but conclusive proof of the motor command theory is lacking.

Afferent information from chemoreceptors

The role of chemoreceptors in the generation of breathlessness is complex and has proved difficult to disentangle. Hypercapnia and hypoxia both stimulate ventilation, but there is evidence that hypercapnia may induce breathlessness by mechanisms other than simple reflex stimulation of breathing. When ventilation is experimentally suppressed below that required to maintain normal blood gas levels, there is an increase in breathlessness, even though the level of breathing is unchanged.[3] Normal subjects and patients with chronic airflow limitation both experience greater breathlessness with hypercapnia than during normocapnic voluntary overbreathing.[4,5] This occurs even when the overall level of ventilation and pattern of breathing is similar in the two conditions. In paraplegic patients, breathlessness increases when the arterial $P\text{CO}_2$ is allowed to rise above normal.[6] Studies in normal subjects have shown that, when paralysed, they experienced the same sensation during hypercapnia as they experienced when they could breathe normally.[7] Evidence for hypoxia as a direct cause for breathlessness is less complete, but it may also cause breathlessness by mechanisms other than those just due to respiratory stimulation.

Vagal nerve afferents from the lungs

The role of vagally mediated information from the lungs is not clear. An increased drive to breathe occurs with lung disease such as pneumonia, asthma and interstitial lung disease, but it is difficult to distinguish this influence on breathlessness from a direct 'dyspnogenic' effect of vagal neuronal traffic. Furthermore, diseases that cause an increase in the drive to breathe also induce changes in lung mechanics that increase the work of breathing. It is also difficult to distinguish between effects on breathlessness due to changes in lung volume and those arising from movement of the chest wall and diaphragm, since these will change simultaneously with changes in the work of breathing.

The sense of bronchoconstriction induced by histamine is eased by lidocaine (lignocaine) applied topically to the airways; in contrast, the sense of discomfort associated with the application of an external resistive load is not.[8] Indeed, asthmatic subjects rarely describe a sensation of chest tightness with such loads, but they do so during bronchoconstrictor trials. This suggests that the sensation arises from changes within the airways rather than as a result of the physical forces upon them. It is likely that the sensation of constriction is mediated through airway irritant receptors since these are known to respond to histamine.

Vagal afferent traffic may also reduce breathlessness. In patients with high-level quadriplegia (who have intact vagus nerves, but no afferents from the chest wall) air hunger occurs when the tidal volume of their ventilator is reduced, even if the level of CO_2 is unchanged.[6] Thus it is possible that stretch-receptor feedback reduces the mismatch between the outgoing motor command and incoming afferent traffic.

Afferent traffic from chest wall receptors

Tolerance of hypercapnia may be increased if patients are allowed to take larger breaths,[9] although this could be caused by afferent traffic from the lungs. The respiratory apparatus contains a variety of receptors in the joints, tendons and muscles of the chest wall and diaphragm. These could all provide information to the cerebral cortex about the act of breathing. Studies using stimulation of chest wall receptors through vibration have shown that dyspnoea can be influenced without changes in ventilation. For example, vibration of either the inspiratory intercostal muscles during inspiration or the expiratory intercostals during expiration decreases dyspnoea.[10] In contrast, vibration of the expiratory muscles during inspiration increases dyspnoea.[11,12]

Afferent mismatch

Patients with severe lung disease may have difficulty talking and eating. Even normal subjects experience breathlessness if required to stop breathing temporarily at high levels of ventilation. In subjects on ventilators, breathlessness develops if the inspiratory flow rate is set below that desired by the subject. The sensation is described as air hunger[13] and can occur even if the chemoreceptor drive to breathe is unchanged.[5,14] These findings suggest that the brain expects a certain pattern of ventilation (or at least its associated afferent feedback) and deviation from this will cause breathlessness.

Breathlessness due to specific disease

Asthma

A number of mechanisms may cause dyspnoea in asthma. First, there is the increased drive to breathe that causes the fall in arterial $P\text{CO}_2$ characteristic of a mild–moderate acute exacerbation. Second, there is the sense of bronchoconstriction, which can be mimicked by histamine challenge and blocked by aerosolised lidocaine. Third is overinflation of the lungs. This reduces the efficiency of respiratory muscles, leading to a greater motor drive to breathe. Experimental studies using methacholine-induced bronchoconstriction have shown that the increase in breathlessness correlated with an increase in respiratory work and correlated better with the rise in FRC than the fall in FEV_1.[15] During exercise in asthma, the FRC rises still further (dynamic hyperinflation) causing a further increase in breathlessness.[15]

Chronic obstructive pulmonary disease

Mechanisms similar to those that operate in asthma apply in chronic obstructive pulmonary disease (COPD). In this condition, there may be additional effects of internal positive end-expiratory pressure (PEEP). Internal PEEP increases the respiratory work that is needed before inspiratory flow can begin. During exercise in COPD, dynamic hyperinflation places a substantial elastic and inspiratory load on the inspiratory muscles that reduces their ability to generate pressure, causing a compensatory increase in respiratory motor drive and an increase in breathlessness.[16,17] Treatment with a bronchodilator reduces breathlessness during exercise and this improvement correlates better with the reduction in end-inspiratory lung volume and other inspiratory parameters than with changes in FEV_1.[18,19] In essence, the major mechanical consequence of COPD is a restrictive impairment due to dynamic hyperinflation and it is this that causes breathlessness rather than a direct effect of expiratory airflow limitation.

Interstitial lung disease

There appears to be an increased drive to breathe that may be mediated through lung 'c fibres', but evidence for the mechanisms of this is not clear. Otherwise the mechanisms for breathlessness are probably caused by a mismatch between the increased drive and afferent feedback from the lungs and chest wall consequent upon decreased lung compliance (i.e. increased stiffness).

Neuromuscular disease

In myotonic dystrophy and myasthenia gravis there appears to be an increased respiratory motor output, as evidenced by a greater $P_{0.1}$ (the pressure generated in the first 100 ms of inspiration against a resistance).[20,21] If the motor command theory of breathlessness is correct, this should be associated with a higher level of breathlessness. Some of these patients do have more dyspnoea, particularly as their respiratory muscle weakness progresses, but there have been no formal studies of this. Set against this is the clinical observation that patients with Guillain–Barré syndrome may be asymptomatic, despite considerable respiratory weakness.

Pulmonary embolism

In this condition there is minimal disturbance to lung mechanics, but there is often an increased drive to breathe arising from the lungs due to pulmonary 'c fibre' stimulation, as evidenced by the tachypnoea that may occur. Stimulation of these fibres may also cause dyspnoea directly, although there is no experimental evidence for this suggestion.

Language of breathlessness

In recent years, there has been considerable interest in the semantics or language used to describe breathlessness.[22,23] The words and phrases employed show a consistent pattern of descriptions between different clinical conditions (Table 5.3.1). These descriptors can also yield clinically useful information and may help elucidate the cause of breathlessness in patients in whom laboratory investigations have not been helpful.[24]

Air hunger

This includes the descriptions 'urge to breathe', 'cannot get enough air', 'need to breathe', 'out of breath'. This sensation appears to be related to an increased respiratory drive since it occurs with hypoxia, even in the absence of active mechanical contraction.[7]

Effort

The sense of effort is distinct from the urge to breathe.[3] It is believed to be driven by a corollary discharge from the motor drive to breathe to the cerebral cortex. As mechanical impedance increases or the respiratory muscles weaken this discharge goes up.

Chest tightness and asthma

Patients with asthma have different types of breathlessness with different stages of severity of an acute attack. At a mild level, it takes the form of a sense of tightness or constriction.[25] With more severe bronchoconstriction, effort becomes more prevalent.[26] However, during an episode of acute bronchoconstriction, patients may use all of the terms 'chest tightness', 'difficulty breathing', 'breathlessness' and 'laboured breathing' to describe the sensation that they are experiencing.[27]

Table 5.3.1 Descriptors for breathlessness in different conditions

Rapid breathing	Congestive cardiac failure
Incomplete exhalation	Asthma
Shallow breathing	Neuromuscular/chest wall disease
Increased work or effort	Chronic obstructive pulmonary disease, interstitial lung disease, asthma, neuromuscular/chest wall
Suffocation	Congestive cardiac failure
Air hunger	Chronic obstructive pulmonary disease, congestive cardiac failure
Tight chest	Asthma
Heavy breathing	Asthma

Measurement of breathlessness

Breathlessness is measured in two basic ways but only one measures breathlessness directly: the second quantifies the effect of breathlessness on the subject's recent daily activities

Direct measurements of breathlessness

In many clinical situations or studies, an assessment of the impact of breathlessness on a patient's daily physical activity may be the measurement of greatest interest, but there are circumstances where a direct measurement of breathlessness is needed. This applies particularly when investigating causes of breathlessness in an individual patient, but such measurements are also needed when studying mechanisms of dyspnoea or evaluating treatments designed to reduce it.

Visual analogue scale

The visual analogue scale takes the form of a line, which may be vertical or horizontal and has descriptors at either end to provide anchor or reference points between which all intermediate levels of the sensation are scaled.[28] These reference points are often labelled 'none' or 'not at all' and at the severe end: 'extremely breathless' or 'maximum imaginable' or 'as bad as can be'. The repeatability of the scale over time is moderately high in both normal subjects and patients with lung disease.[29]

Borg scale

The version of this scale in widest use is often called the CR-10 scale.[30] It has a series of numbers from 0–10 with descriptors at certain points along its length. The CR-10 scale behaves in a similar way to the visual analogue scale but has the advantage that it is standardised and a range of values for CR-10 scores obtained in normal subjects and patients with chronic airflow limitation has been published.[31]

Reference point for breathlessness measurements

To be meaningful, direct measurements of breathlessness must be related to a reference point; they cannot be made in isolation. Measurements can be made at rest but more usually during an exercise test. In this setting they may be used in two ways. The simplest technique is to record the level of dyspnoea at peak work during an incremental exercise test or at the end of a 6-minute walking test, but care must be taken in the interpretation of such measurements. Treatment may reduce the level of dyspnoea during exercise and thus permit the patient to achieve a higher level of work for the same degree of breathlessness. If the patient exercised to the same level of breathlessness it would appear that their dyspnoea was unchanged, whereas in fact they were able to achieve a higher maximum work rate.

This highlights the need to refer the level of breathlessness to a standardised level of ventilatory or metabolic demand.

Direct measurements of breathlessness have been used quite widely in clinical trials, especially in studies of pulmonary rehabilitation in which it has been shown that the slope of the relationship between breathlessness and work falls following participation in an exercise programme. This observation illustrates the different contributions of indirect and direct measurements of breathlessness to the understanding of dyspnoea. Indirect measurements can show that physical rehabilitation may reduce impairment due to dyspnoea in daily life, but they do not identity the processes by which this happens. In contrast, direct measurement may provide some insights into mechanisms. For example, the finding that exercise training directed to the legs can reduce the level of breathlessness for a given level of work suggests that breathlessness involves more than just the simple processing of respiratory motor activity and its associated sensory feedback.

Indirect measurements of breathlessness (clinical dyspnoea scales)

A number of scales have been developed to measure breathlessness in daily life. They all use a similar approach, based upon the patient's recall of breathlessness during daily activities. These activities are analogous to the work rate or level of ventilation during an exercise test — they provide a means of standardising the measurement conditions.

Medical Research Council (MRC) Dyspnoea Scale

This has appeared in a number of versions and one of the most widely used is illustrated in Table 5.3.2. It is a simple standardised measure that can be completed by the patient themselves. MRC dyspnoea grades provide a useful way of defining impairment of activity due to breathlessness, both in individuals and in populations of patients.[32] Its major limitation is that the inter-

Table 5.3.2 Medical Research Council Dyspnoea Scale. This version is in wide use, although in the USA another common version uses the same descriptions but scales from 0–4.

Grade 1	Breathless with strenuous exercise
Grade 2	Short of breath when hurrying on the level or walking up a slight hill
Grade 3	Walk slower than people of the same age on the level or stop for breath while walking at own pace on the level
Grade 4	Stop for breath after walking about 100 yards or after a few minutes on the level
Grade 5	Too breathless to leave the house or breathless when dressing or undressing

vals between its categories are quite wide, so the scale may be too insensitive to detect small but clinically worthwhile responses to treatment. Despite this theoretical limitation, improvements in MRC scores have been reported following lung volume reduction surgery and surgery for the removal of emphysematous bullae.

Oxygen Cost Diagram

The Oxygen Cost Diagram (OCD) is a visual analogue scale with 13 activities listed along a 100 mm line.[33] The position of these activities along this vertical line corresponds approximately to their oxygen requirements. The patient is asked to indicate the level of activity at which they begin to experience dyspnoea. The OCD score is measured in millimetres. The shorter the distance, the greater the breathlessness. This measure is simple to use and for this reason has been used quite widely.

The Baseline Dyspnoea Index and Transitional Dyspnoea Index

These indices are more sophisticated and complex than the MRC scale or OCD and cannot be completed by the patient themselves. They have three components. One assesses functional impairment due to dyspnoea in a manner similar to other scales for indirect measurement of breathlessness. The other two components are largely unique to these two indices and assess the magnitude of the task and the magnitude of effort as factors that provoke breathlessness.[34] The Baseline Dyspnoea Index (BDI) is designed to discriminate between different levels of breathlessness in different patients at a single point in time whereas the Transitional Dyspnoea Index (TDI) is an evaluative instrument designed to measure changes from the baseline state. In clinical trials, the TDI has been shown to detect changes in breathlessness following pulmonary rehabilitation and lung reduction surgery in patients with emphysema and long-acting bronchodilators in COPD.

Practical application of clinical dyspnoea scales

These rating scales provide valid estimates of breathlessness-induced disability since they tend to measure what patients are unable to do because of breathlessness rather than the amount of breathlessness they experience while they are exercising. Such scores have been shown to correlate well with impaired 6-minute walking distance and impaired health status ('health-related quality of life'). By contrast, they correlate very poorly with FEV_1 measurements (Fig. 5.3.1); thus, it is not possible to predict a patient's level of breathlessness-induced disability from the FEV_1. This is especially important in COPD patients who have relatively mild airways obstruction, many of whom may have a MRC dyspnoea grade of 3 or greater. It is important to identify such patients because they may receive worthwhile benefit from pulmonary rehabilitation.

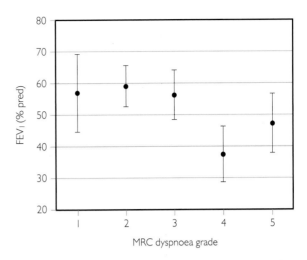

Fig. 5.3.1   Association between postbronchodilator FEV_1 and MRC dyspnoea grade in patients with asthma and chronic obstructive pulmonary disease. The error bars are 95% confidence intervals.

It is clear that these measurements provide information that is complementary to that obtained from spirometric measurements. The MRC scale is quick and easy to use and record in the patient's notes. It is well standardised and moves are afoot to incorporate it into a more comprehensive method of staging COPD than methods based solely on the FEV_1.

Assessment of symptomatic response in individual patients

The relationship between improvement in breathlessness and spirometric changes is too weak to permit the FEV_1 to be used as a surrogate measurement for symptomatic benefit.[35] Unfortunately, none of the clinical rating scales is suitable for assessing whether an individual patient has had a clinically worthwhile symptomatic response to therapy. There is evidence that a patient's simple global estimate of a treatment's efficacy correlates well with a clinically significant improvement in health status.[35] This can be supported by a few further questions:

- In what way are you less breathless?
- Can you do more things without getting breathless?
- Can you do the same amount but are less breathless when you do it?
- Can you do things faster?
- Do you have to stop less often?

Ask the patient to provide examples and believe the answers. Breathlessness is a symptom. Only the patient can judge its severity. If patients provide evidence that they are less breathless, they should be believed, regardless of any change in FEV_1. Reductions in the effects of dynamic hyperinflation during exercise are better correlates of improved breathlessness with bronchodilators in COPD than FEV_1.[18]

References

1. Burns BH, Howell JBL. Disproportionately severe breathlessness in chronic bronchitis. Q J Med 1969; 38: 277–294.
2. Chapman KR, Rebuck AS. Inspiratory and expiratory loading as a model of dyspnea in asthma. Respiration 1983; 44: 425–432.
3. Demediuk BH, Manning H, Lilli J et al. Dissociation between dyspnea and respiratory effort. Am Rev Respir Dis 1992; 146: 1222–1225.
4. Freedman S, Lane R, Guz A. Breathlessness and respiratory mechanics during reflex voluntary hyperventilation in patients with chronic airflow limitation. Clin Sci 1987; 73: 311–318.
5. Chonan T, Mulholland MB, Cerniak NS et al. Effects of voluntary constraining of thoracic displacement during hypercapnia. J Appl Physiol 1987; 1987: 1822–1828.
6. Banzett RB, Lansing RW, Reid MB et al. 'Air hunger' arising from increased P_{CO_2} in mechanically ventilated quadriplegics. Respir Physiol 1989; 76: 53–68.
7. Banzett RB, Lansing RW, Brown R et al. 'Air hunger' from increased P_{CO_2} persists after complete neuromuscular block in humans. Respir Physiol 1990; 81: 1–18.
8. Taguchi O, Kikuchi Y, Hida W et al. Effects of bronchoconstriction and external resistive loading on the sensation of dyspnea. J Appl Physiol 1991; 71: 2183–2190.
9. Remmers JE, Brooks JG, Tenney SM. Effect of controlled ventilation on the tolerable limit of hypercapnia. Respir Physiol 1968; 4: 78–90.
10. Manning HL, Basner R, Ringler J et al. Effect of chest wall vibration on breathlessness in normal subjects. J Appl Physiol 1991; 71:1 75–81.
11. Sibuya M, Yamada M, Kanamaru A et al. Effect of chest wall vibration on dyspnea in patients with chronic respiratory disease. Am J Respir Crit Care Med 1994; 149: 1235–1240.
12. Homma I, Toshihiko O, Sibuya M et al. Gate mechanism in breathlessness caused by chest wall vibration in humans. J Appl Physiol l984; 56: 8–l1.
13. Manning HL, Molinary E, Leiter JC. Effect of inspiratory flow rate on sensory experience. Am J Respir Crit Care Med 1995; 151: 751–757.
14. Schwartzstein RM, Simon PM, Weiss JW et al. Breathlessness induced by dissociation between ventilation and chemical drive. Am Rev Respir Dis 1989; 139: 1231–1237.
15. Lougheed MD, Lam M, Forket L et al. Breathlessness during acute bronchoconstriction in asthma. Pathophysiologic mechanisms. Am Rev Respir Dis 1993; 148: 1452–1459.
16. O'Donnell DE, Webb KA. Breathlessness in patients with severe chronic airflow limitation: physiological correlates. Chest 1992; 102: 824–831.
17. O'Donnell DE, Webb KA. Exertional breathlessness in patients with chronic airflow limitation: the role of hyperinflation. Am Rev Respir Dis 1993; 148: 1351–1357.
18. Belman MJ, Botnick WC, Shin JW. Inhaled bronchodilators reduce dynamic hyperinflation during exercise in patients with chronic obstructive pulmonary disease. Am J Respir Crit Care Med 1996; 153: 967–975.
19. Taube C, Lehnigk B, Paasch K et al. Factor analysis of changes in dyspnea and lung function parameters after bronchodilation in chronic obstructive pulmonary disease. Am Rev Respir Crit Care Med 2000; 162: 216–220.
20. Spinelli A, Marconi A, Gorini M et al. Control of breathing in patients with myasthenia gravis. Am Rev Respir Dis 1992; 145:1359–1366.
21. Begin R, Bureau M, Lupien L et al. Pathogenesis of respiratory insufficiency in myotonic dystrophy. Am Rev Respir Dis 1982; 125: 312–318.
22. Simon PM, Schwartzstein RM, Weiss JW et al. Distinguishable types of dyspnea in patients with shortness of breath. Am J Respir Dis 1990; 1990: 1009–1014.
23. Ellott MW, Adama L, Cockcroft A et al. The language of breathlessness: use by patients of verbal descriptors. Am J Respir Dis 1991; 144: 826–832.
24. Schwartzstein RM. The language of dyspnea. In: Mahler DA, ed. Dyspnea. New York: Marcel Dekker; 1998: 35–62.
25. Moy ML, Weiss JW, Sparrow D et al. Quality of dyspnea in bronchoconstriction differs from external resistive loads. Am J Respir Crit Care Med 2000; 162: 451–455.
26. Moy ML, Lantin ML, Harver A et al. Language of dyspnea in assessment of patients with acute asthma treated with nebulized albuterol. Am J Respir Crit Care Med 1998; 158: 749–753.
27. Killian KJ, Watson R, Otis J et al. Symptom perception during acute bronchoconstriction. Am J Respir Crit Care Med 2000; 162: 490–496.
28. Adams L, Chronos N Lane R et al. The measurement of breathlessness induced in normal subjects: validity of two scaling techniques. Clin Sci 1985; 69: 7–16.
29. Mador MJ, Kufel TJ. Reproducibility of visual analogue scale measurement of dyspnea in patients with chronic obstructive pulmonary disease. Am Rev Respir Dis 1992; 146: 82–87.
30. Schwartzstein RM, Manning HL, Weiss JW et al. Dyspnea: a sensory experience. Lung 1990; 168: 185–199.
31. Killian KJ, Leblanc P, Martin DH et al. Exercise capacity and ventilatory, circulatory, and symptom limitation in patients with chronic airflow limitation. Am Rev Respir Dis 1992; 146: 935–940.
32. Bestall JC, Paul EA, Garrod R et al. Usefulness of the Medical Research Council (MRC) dyspnoea scale as a measure of disability in patients with chronic obstructive pulmonary disease. Thorax 1999; 54: 581–586.
33. McGavin CR, Artvinli M, Naoe H et al. Dyspnoea, disability and distance walked: comparison of estimates of exercise performance in respiratory disease. Br Med J 1978; 2: 241–243.
34. Mahler DA, Weinberg DH, Wells CK et al. Measurements of dyspnea. Contents, interobserver correlates of two new clinical indices. Chest 1984; 85: 751–758.
35. Jones PW, Bosh TK. Changes in quality of life in COPD patients treated with salmeterol. Am J Respir Crit Care Med 1997; 155: 1283–1289.

5.4 Chest pain

Pallav L Shah

Key concepts

Acute presentation with chest pain to the emergency department:

- Rapid clinical assessment
- Immediate electrocardiogram
- Urgent chest radiograph
- Consider life-threatening causes:
  - Myocardial ischaemia
  - Aortic dissection
  - Pulmonary embolism
  - Pneumothorax
  - Oesophageal rupture
- Some patients with life-threatening causes may have no abnormal clinical signs

Chest pain is one of the symptoms most likely to cause patients to seek early medical attention. There is good public awareness that it may signify a potentially life-threatening illness.

Epidemiology

Pain is a very personal experience and varies from individual to individual. The actual prevalence of chest pain is difficult to measure but some series suggests that it affects 10% of the population.[1,2] A survey of chest pain in the USA estimated an average annual rate of 27.7 consultations per 1000 persons. Of these approximately 11% were due to cardiac ischaemia.[3] Pain may be measured by the use of either visual analogue scores or questionnaires.[4] The advantages of questionnaires are that they allow a multidimensional evaluation of pain rather than a simple measure of intensity. The McGill questionnaire is probably the most widely used.[5,6]

Aetiology

The aetiology of chest pain can be classified according to the location of the pain as central, when there is a substernal element, or peripheral. The main aetiological factors are outlined in Table 5.4.1. Central pain is primarily visceral pain originating from the heart, main pulmonary arteries, oesophagus or mediastinum. Peripheral pain consists of pleural, musculoskeletal, neurogenic and some gastrointestinal sources of pain.

Pathophysiology

The development of chest pain is a complex process and involves peripheral nociceptors, the sympathetic nervous system, primary afferent-derived neuropeptide mediators and the spinal dorsal horn. Nociceptors are mainly composed of unmyelinated C fibres. Injury or inflammation leads to the release of arachidonic acid, which is then converted to prostaglandins. These prostaglandins directly sensitise the nociceptors, leading to hyperalgesia and allodynia (conditions where normal stimuli are perceived as painful).[7] Primary afferent nerve terminals release neurotransmitters such as substance P and calcitonin-gene-related peptide into the periphery.[8,9] These contribute to inflammation and increased sensitivity of peripheral nociceptors.[10] Sympathetic nerves also contribute to this process as inflammatory mediators stimulate the release of prostaglandins from their nerve terminals, which again increases the sensitivity of the nociceptors and contributes to hyperalgesia and allodynia.

Referred pain is thought to be due to convergence of visceral and somatic afferent nerves in the spinal dorsal horn. Stimulation from the visceral nerve is often perceived by the brain as having originated from somatic structures.[11] Central sensitisation occurs as a result of increased excitability of spinal cord neurones, which up-regulates inputs from adjacent healthy tissue and leads to secondary allodynia and hyperalgesia.[10,12]

Table 5.4.1 Differential diagnosis based on source of pain

Central	Peripheral
Cardiac	**Pleural**
Myocardial infarction	Pleurisy
Myocardial ischaemia	Infection
Angina	Collagen vascular disorders
Variant angina	Pulmonary embolus
Syndrome X	Pneumothorax
Aortic stenosis	Malignant infiltration of pleura
Hypertrophic obstructive cardiomyopathy	Mesothelioma
Aortic dissection	Pleural fibrosis
Aortitis	
Syphilitic	**Musculoskeletal**
Takayasu's	Fractured ribs
Myocarditis	Tietze's syndrome – costochondritis
	Bornholm disease – Coxsackie B virus infection
Pericardial	Slipping ribs
Pericarditis	Arthritis
Infection	Shoulder
Dressler's syndrome	Spinal
Collagen vascular disorders	Bursitis – subacromial
	Tendinitis
Pulmonary	Biceps
Pulmonary hypertension	Supraspinatus
Pulmonary embolus	Deltoid
Tracheobronchitis	Fibromyalgia
Hyperventilation syndrome	Chest wall tumour
Tumour	
	Neurological
Mediastinal	Neuritis–radiculitis
Mediastinitis	Spinal nerve root compression
Mediastinal emphysema	Herpes zoster infection
Lymphoma	Brachial plexus
	Pancoast's tumour
Oesophageal	Cervical rib
Oesophageal reflux	Shoulder–hand syndrome
Oesophageal dysmotility	Reflex sympathetic dystrophy
Achalasia	
Spasm	**Gastrointestinal**
Oesophageal rupture	Peptic ulcer disease
	Pancreatitis
Gastrointestinal	Cholecystitis
Peptic ulcer disease	Biliary colic
Pancreatitis	Hepatitis
Intestinal spasm	
	Others
Others	Breast inflammation
Hyperventilation syndrome	Mondor's syndrome – thrombophlebitis of superficial thoracic veins
Panic attacks	

This process is mediated by phosphorylation of N-methyl-D-aspartate (NMDA) receptors in the dorsal horn neurones.[13]

Cardiac pain usually occurs when there is an imbalance between myocardial oxygen supply and myocardial oxygen consumption. In ischaemic heart disease this results from narrowing of the coronary arteries by atheroma or clot. Valvular disease also impairs coronary blood flow, either by decreasing mean aortic pressure (e.g. aortic stenosis) or by increasing left ventricular end-diastolic pressures (e.g. mitral valve disease). The C fibres are stimulated by mechanical and biochemical stimuli produced during ischaemia and the adenosine released potentiates the pain.[14] Pain fibres are located in the diaphragmatic portion of the parietal pericardium but the predominant pain in pericardial disease is due to extension of inflammatory processes to the parietal pleura.

Pulmonary pain experienced in pulmonary hypertension and pulmonary emboli is thought to arise from distension of the main pulmonary arteries, but right ventricular ischaemia may contribute. Although the lungs themselves are insensitive to pain there are some C fibres in the mucosa of the trachea and main bronchi that may result in pain when stimulated.[15]

Pleural pain originates from stimulation of nociceptors in the parietal pleura. The pain is localised according to the nerve supply and hence the area supplied by the costal nerves localises to the adjacent chest wall whereas the subdiaphragmatic portion, which is supplied by the phrenic nerve, localises to the shoulder. Musculoskeletal pain is a somatic pain and hence is usually well-localised and occurs as a result of trauma or inflammation of the joints, cartilages, tendons, fascia, bones and muscles of the thoracic cage. Neurological pain is due to stimulation of the thoracic nerve roots or brachial plexus by compression, inflammation or direct invasion by tumour.

Stimulation of the oesophagus by acid reflux and inflammation or strong mechanical stimuli (e.g. oesophageal spasm) leads to both local hypersensitivity and secondary hypersensitivity in the upper oesophagus and anterior chest wall. Primary and secondary allodynia also occur, suggesting that central sensitisation contributes to the development of the chest pain syndrome observed in patients with oesophageal disease.[16]

Clinical assessment

The approach to patients presenting with chest pain varies according to the circumstances. Patients presenting to the accident and emergency department/emergency room acutely and unwell need a rapid assessment of their vital signs, brief clinical history, urgent electrocardiogram and chest radiograph in order to identify a life-threatening illness such as myocardial infarction, dissecting aortic aneurysm, pulmonary embolism or tension pneumothorax. A detailed clinical history can be performed once the patient is clinically stable.

Clinical history

For the majority of patients a detailed history is an essential step. This includes obtaining a clear account of the chest pain; time of onset, duration, character and intensity. Precipitating and relieving factors, including relationship with respiration, posture and movement, should also be evaluated. Specific risk factors such as smoking, hypertension, hypercholesterolaemia, previous history of ischaemic heart disease and family history of ischaemic heart disease should be identified as they predict the risk of a cardiac ischaemic event.

Physical examination

A thorough clinical examination is essential, although many patients with life-threatening conditions have no abnormal clinical signs. The examination should include a complete peripheral examination as well as close attention to the cardiovascular and respiratory system, as clues to the aetiology of the chest pain

may be provided by the presence of signs such as xanthelasma around the eyes.

Cardiac pain

The pain of myocardial ischaemia is classically described as a central, heavy or crushing pain.[17] The pain is usually substernal, or just to the left of the sternum, and may radiate to the neck or the inner aspect of the arm. In stable angina the pain is often precipitated by stress or exertion and relieved by rest or the use of glyceryl trinitrate (GTN). The pain may occur at rest or at a much lower exercise threshold in unstable angina. The intensity of pain during myocardial infarction is considerably greater, not relieved by GTN and usually accompanied by systemic symptoms of nausea, vomiting and sweating. Prinzmetal's (variant) angina has similar characteristics to angina but classically occurs at night or at rest and is usually due to coronary artery vasospasm.[18] Pain similar to that of angina is occasionally observed in patients with valvular heart disease (aortic stenosis, aortic regurgitation, mitral valve stenosis) and hypertrophic obstructive cardiomyopathy.

Dissecting aortic aneurysm

An abrupt, ripping or tearing chest pain that radiates to the intrascapular region of the back is experienced in aortic dissection. Severe chest pain is found in over 90% of patients. The pain may radiate to the neck, jaw, back or abdomen.[19,20] Profound sweating, nausea, vomiting and light-headedness frequently accompany the chest pain. Other features that may occur are painful limbs and neurological symptoms, which range from paraesthesia to paralysis depending on the branch arteries involved. Patients may have a past history of hypertension, Marfan's syndrome, Ehlers–Danlos syndrome or other connective tissue abnormalities.

On examination there may be differential or absent peripheral pulses and unequal upper arm blood pressures. An early diastolic murmur of aortic regurgitation is present in up to 25% of patients. Neurological signs may be present, depending on the vital arteries that are occluded. They vary from sensory loss to weakness of a limb to paraplegia. These signs are often rapidly progressive. Pallor, cold, cyanotic and a pulseless limb may be present if an artery supplying a limb is affected.

Aortitis

Angina-like chest pain may be experienced in aortitis. In Takayasu's disease there may be a prodromal phase with malaise, fever and arthralgia. Erythema nodosum is also observed in some patients. On examination there are often signs of aortic regurgitation.

Myocarditis

Typically in myocarditis, a pain similar to pericarditis (40%) is experienced, but in some cases it may resemble angina (20%). Patients often have systemic symptoms of fever, myalgia, fatigue and evidence of congestive cardiac failure.

Pericardial pain

The pain in pericarditis is often a sharp, constant, substernal chest pain, which is exacerbated by lying back or on to the left side and partially relieved by sitting up or leaning forward. A more specific feature of the pain in pericarditis is radiation to the upper portion of the trapezius muscle. There is often a pleuritic component to the pain. In a few patients the pain mimics angina, but radiation to the ulnar aspect of the arms is rare. A pericardial rub may be audible on clinical examination.

Pulmonary pain

True pulmonary pain is unusual and resembles angina. It is observed in a small proportion of patients with acute pulmonary embolism, pulmonary hypertension, pulmonary artery stenosis, Eisenmenger's syndrome and pulmonary vasculitis. On clinical examination there may be central cyanosis, right ventricular heave and a loud pulmonary component of the second heart sound.

A raw burning pain felt in the midline anteriorly from the larynx to the xiphoid process is observed in tracheobronchitis.[15] Occasionally, the pain can be felt in the anterior chest close to the sternum. The pain is exacerbated on deep breathing. There are usually no abnormal findings on physical examination. Pulmonary tumours usually cause pain when there is pleural or mediastinal involvement. However, there are reports of localised chest pain with reasonable correlation to the site of the tumour in patients with early lung cancer.[21]

Pleural pain

Pleuritic chest pain is described as a sharp, stabbing pain, which is exacerbated by deep inspiration, coughing and movement. It is usually unilateral and tends to be localised to the area involved, but may radiate to the shoulder and neck if the diaphragmatic area is involved, It is usually acute in onset and accompanying symptoms such as a cough, productive sputum and haemoptysis may provide additional clues to the aetiology. A past medical history of chronic obstructive pulmonary disease, asthma or parenchymal lung disease may be relevant in a patient with a possible pneumothorax. The history should again identify any potential risk factors for pulmonary embolism as 80% of these patients have pleuritic chest pain. An occupational history, particularly exposure to asbestos, may be relevant in a patient with mesothelioma.

On clinical examination there may be a pleural rub. The presence of cyanosis or tachypnoea, with or without hypotension, may indicate a life-threatening cause. There may be focal abnormalities, depending on the underlying cause, such as signs of consolidation in a patient with pneumonia. Coexisting arthralgia or skin rashes may be relevant in patients with collagen vascular disease.

Musculoskeletal pain

Musculoskeletal pain is usually a well-localised pain and may be a constant gnawing ache exacerbated by deep inspiration and movement, with palpable tenderness of the affected region. There may be a clear history of preceding trauma. Examination of the patient with chest pain should include thorough palpation of the chest wall, especially the parasternal area, and movement of the arms and shoulders to see if the pain is reproduced or exacerbated. In Tietze's syndrome there is redness and swelling of the costosternal joints with tenderness on palpation localised to these areas. Tietze's syndrome usually affects the second, third and fourth costochondral cartilages but any cartilaginous portion of the anterior thoracic cage may be affected. In Bornholm disease costochondritis is due to infection with Coxsackie B virus. Chest-wall pain is observed in sickle-cell disease during sickling crises as a result of ischaemia or infarction of the bone marrow. Similarly, multiple myeloma and metastatic carcinoma may lead to focal chest pain because of rib involvement.

Neurological pain

The pain of neuritis or radiculitis is a sharp, knife-like pain felt within the thoracic cage in the cutaneous distribution of the involved nerve. It may be exacerbated by coughing, sneezing or deep inspiration (Déjérine's sign) but not by normal breathing. It may also be worse after a period of lying flat. There may be hyperaesthesia or anaesthesia of the skin in the involved area. The pain may be precipitated by rotation of the head to the involved side or to the opposite side, bending forward, hyperextending the upper spine or throwing back the shoulders. In the case of herpetic neuritis there is a characteristic vesicular rash in the dermatomal distribution during the acute phase, but the pain often occurs prior to the vesicular eruption.

Brachial plexus involvement by a Pancoast's tumour causes a deep, unrelenting pain in the scapular and shoulder region and often progresses to involve the arm and forearm. On examination, there may be weakness and sensory loss, depending on the nerve roots involved. Horner's syndrome may be present if the sympathetic chain or the stellate ganglion is involved. Thoracic outlet obstruction by a cervical rib can compress the brachial plexus and the subclavian artery, causing pains in the anterior chest and arms that are similar to angina.

The shoulder–hand syndrome, which was previously associated with myocardial infarction, presents with pain over the shoulder, with radiation to the scapula and neck. It is associated with painful osteoarthritis, and limitation of movement of the shoulder joint may form part of a reflex sympathetic dystrophy.

Oesophageal pain

Oesophageal pain may be a deep, burning, midline discomfort or there may be substernal pain indistinguishable from angina. GTN, calcium antagonists or antacids may relieve it. There may be a history of exacerbation after meals, lying flat or bending forward. Associated features may be odynophagia, dysphagia and regurgitation of acid or undigested food. Oesophageal pain may account for chest pain in up to 30% of patients with angina-like pain but normal coronary arteries .[22]

Oesophageal rupture may present with severe central chest pain with radiation to the back. There is usually a history of oesophageal instrumentation or violent vomiting (Boerhaave's syndrome) prior to the event. On clinical examination there may be surgical emphysema in the neck, Hamman's sign – a crunching sound heard over the anterior chest synchronous with cardiac systole – and, in more severe cases, features of cardiac tamponade.

Gastrointestinal pain

Pain due to cholecystitis, pancreatitis or peptic ulcer disease is usually epigastric but may be felt in the lower chest. In pancreatitis the pain may be similar to pericardial pain and accompanying T-wave changes on the electrocardiogram may be misleading. In peptic ulcer disease the pain may be similar in quality to anginal pain. Collection of gas in the splenic flexure may present with precordial pain. Features that may help to distinguish these from cardiac pain are a history of accompanying gastrointestinal symptoms such as constipation, relationship to meals and bowel function, and lack of response to GTN.

Mediastinal pain

Inflammation of the mediastinum and mediastinal emphysema may cause a persistent heavy substernal chest pain, which may radiate to the back. There may be a pericardial and or pleural element to the pain. It is usually due to iatrogenic oesophageal rupture but some cases may be due to descending pharyngeal infection (Ludwig's angina).

Hyperventilation/psychiatric pain

Hyperventilation may produce chest pain and other symptoms of cardiac disease such as dizziness, palpitations, paraesthesia of the upper extremities and even syncope. Patients with psychiatric disorders may also present with atypical chest pain. They may have inconsistent and atypical features in the history and on examination. However, caution should be exercised, all patients should be appropriately evaluated and the diagnosis should be based on the exclusion of organic diseases.

Other causes of pain

Sharp, superficial chest pain may be associated with thrombophlebitis of the anterior chest wall or breasts (Mondor's disease). The pain is usually superficial, with tenderness in the affected area.[23]

Investigations

Electrocardiography (ECG) is an essential test in the diagnosis of patients with chest pain and should be obtained immediately in patients presenting with acute pain to the emergency department. Patients with acute myocardial infarction will have ST elevation of ≥ 1 mm in two or more leads. Patients with ST depression of ≥ 1 mm or T-wave inversion are likely to have some myocardial ischaemia. In the USA there has been a vogue for developing chest pain units in an effort to improve the

quality of care for patients with suspected myocardial injury.[24] Algorithms and models of computer-assisted decision-making have also been developed that use clinical and biochemical markers to improve the accuracy of diagnosis and also to determine the risk of a significant myocardial event.[25,26] Markers of myocardial damage are now available that are even more specific than CK-MB, such as cardiac troponins T and I.[27] These markers are useful in patients when myocardial ischaemia is suspected but ECG is inconclusive, or where routine cardiac enzyme levels are normal.

Once patients are considered to be stable they are usually assessed by exercise ECG. Urgent angiography is the investigation of choice in patients with unstable angina and it also provides an opportunity for therapeutic intervention by angioplasty and insertion of stents. In selected unstable patients, radionuclide (thallium) scintigraphy is useful in demonstrating both fixed and reversible areas of ischaemia. Alternatively, echocardiography may demonstrate abnormalities in wall motion consistent with infarction or significant ischaemia. The later two modalities may be combined with dipyridamole or dobutamine stress testing.

Echocardiography is also useful in patients suspected of aortic dissection and large pulmonary emboli. It is probably more widely used when valvular disease, myocarditis, pericarditis, hypertrophic obstructive cardiomyopathy or pulmonary hypertension are suspected as the cause of chest pain.

Chest radiographs are an essential early investigation although they can be completely normal in some patients even with life-threatening disease. Patients with ischaemic heart disease may have features of pulmonary oedema. In aortic dissection there may be a widened mediastinum and depression of the left main bronchus so that the angle with the trachea is less than 40°. Other features are:

- deviation of the trachea to the right
- loss of the aortic border
- loss of the angle between the aortic arch and pulmonary artery
- obliteration of the medial aspect of the left lower lobe or left pleural effusion.

Pulmonary conditions such as pneumonia, pneumothorax, pleural effusion, pulmonary neoplasm and mediastinal emphysema are usually evident on the chest radiograph. A chest radiograph may be suggestive in pulmonary embolism. Additional investigations that are required to confirm the diagnosis are ventilation–perfusion scanning and spiral computed tomography (CT) of the thorax with intravenous contrast (these are discussed in appropriate chapters). CT scans of the thorax also have a role in the investigation of dissecting aortic aneurysm, thoracic tumours and oesophageal rupture.

Management

Although precise treatment is dictated by the aetiology of the chest pain, appropriate analgesia is a universal requirement. Morphine is required for the severe pain experienced in myocardial infarction and aortic dissection. Inflammatory conditions involving the pleura, pericardium or musculoskeletal system usually respond to non-steroidal anti-inflammatory drugs. More severe cases may require systemic corticosteroids. Neural pain may require adjunctive therapy with amitriptyline, carbamazepine or gabapentin.

In ischaemic heart disease treatment is directed at reversing the imbalance between myocardial oxygen consumption and oxygen delivery. This is achieved with nitrates, which act as coronary vasodilators, beta-blockers, which reduce myocardial work load, and calcium antagonists and potassium-channel activators, which reduce afterload by arterial vasodilatation. Urgent revascularisation is required in acute myocardial infarction and this can be achieved by the use of thrombolytics, angioplasty with or without stents, or coronary artery bypass grafting. The latter two modalities are useful in patients with angina not controlled on medical therapy, or with critical lesions.

Calcium antagonists or prostacyclin may improve pain due to right ventricular strain.

The specific treatment of chest pain due to pulmonary causes is discussed in detail in the appropriate chapters.

Pain due to reflux oesophagitis and peptic ulcer disease is managed by reducing acid secretion, using either H_2 antagonists or proton-pump inhibitors. In cases where *Helicobacter pylori* is isolated, eradication therapy may be curative.[28] Oesophageal spasm may also improve with calcium antagonists. Oesophageal rupture is treated by broad-spectrum intravenous antibiotics and early surgical intervention.

Therapeutic principles

- Appropriate analgesia
  - Non-steroidal anti-inflammatory drugs for inflammatory conditions
  - Opiates for severe cardiovascular diseases
- Treat underlying condition
- Consider secondary prevention for cardiovascular diseases

References

1. Von Korff M, Dworkin SF, Le Resche L, Kruger A. An epidemiologic comparison of pain complaints. Pain 1988; 32: 173–183.
2. Kroenke K, Mangelsdorff AD. Common symptoms in ambulatory care: incidence, evaluation, therapy, and outcome. Am J Med 1989; 86: 262–266.
3. Burt CW. Summary statistics for acute cardiac ischemia and chest pain visits to United States EDs, 1995–1996. Am J Emerg Med 1999; 17: 552–559.
4. Chapman CR, Casey KL, Dubner R et al. Pain measurement: an overview. Pain 1985; 22: 1–31.
5. Melzack R. The McGill Pain Questionnaire: major properties and scoring methods. Pain 1975; 1: 277–299.
6. Graham C, Bond SS, Gerkovich MM, Cook MR. Use of the McGill pain questionnaire in the assessment of cancer pain: replicability and consistency. Pain 1980; 8: 377–387.
7. Martin HA, Basbaum AI, Kwiat GC et al. Leukotriene and prostaglandin sensitization of cutaneous high-threshold C- and A-delta mechanonociceptors in the hairy skin of rat hindlimbs. Neuroscience 1987; 22: 651–659.
8. Brodin E, Gazelius B, Lundberg JM, Olgart L. Substance P in trigeminal nerve endings: occurrence and release. Acta Physiol Scand 1981; 111: 501–503.
9. Diez Guerra FJ, Zaidi M, Bevis P et al. Evidence for release of calcitonin gene-related peptide and neurokinin A from sensory nerve endings in vivo. Neuroscience 1988; 25: 839–846.
10 Treede RD, Meyer RA, Raja SN, Campbell JN. Peripheral and central mechanisms of cutaneous hyperalgesia. Prog Neurobiol 1992; 38: 397–421.
11. Ruch TC. Visceral sensitisation and referred pain. In: Fulton JF, ed. Howell's textbook of physiology, 15th ed. Philadelphia, PA: WB Saunders; 1946: 385–401.
12. Torebjork HE, Lundberg LE, LaMotte RH. Central changes in processing of mechanoreceptive input in capsaicin-induced secondary hyperalgesia in humans. J Physiol 1992; 448: 765–780.
13. Woolf CJ, Thompson SW. The induction and maintenance of central sensitization is dependent on N-methyl-D-aspartic acid receptor activation: implications for the treatment of post-injury pain hypersensitivity states. Pain 1991; 44: 293–299.
14. Cannon RO. Cardiac pain. In: Gebhart GF, ed. Visceral pain. Seattle, WA: IASP Press; 1995: 373–389.
15. Morton DR, Klassen KP, Curtis GM. The clinical physiology of the human bronchi. I. Pain of tracheobronchial origin. Surgery 2000; 28: 699–704.
16. Sarkar S, Aziz Q, Woolf CJ et al. Contribution of central sensitisation to the development of non-cardiac chest pain. Lancet 2000; 356: 154–159.
17. Jesse RL, Kontos MC. Evaluation of chest pain in the emergency department. Curr Prob Cardiol 1997; 22: 149–236.
18. Prinzmetal M, Kennamer R, Merlis R et al. Angina pectoris: a variant form of angina pectoris. Am J Med 1959; 27: 375–388.
19. Slater EE, DeSanctis RW. Dissection of the aorta. Med Clin North Am 1979; 63: 141–154.
20. Eagle KA, DeSanctis RW. Aortic dissection. Curr Prob Cardiol 1989; 14: 225–278.
21. Marino C, Zoppi M, Morelli F et al. Pain in early cancer of the lungs. Pain 1986; 27: 57–62.
22. Richter JE. Gastroesophageal reflux disease as a cause of chest pain. Med Clin North Am 1991; 75: 1065–1080.
23. Lunn CM, Potter JM. Mondor's disease (subcutaneous phlebitis of the breast region). Br Med J 1954; 1: 1074.
24. Farkouh ME, Smars PA, Reeder GS et al. A clinical trial of a chest-pain observation unit for patients with unstable angina. Chest Pain Evaluation in the Emergency Room (CHEER) Investigators. N Engl J Med 1998; 339: 1882–1888.
25. Goldman L, Cook EF, Brand DA et al. A computer protocol to predict myocardial infarction in emergency department patients with chest pain. N Engl J Med 1988; 318: 797–803.
26. Qamar A, McPherson C, Babb J et al. The Goldman algorithm revisited: prospective evaluation of a computer-derived algorithm versus unaided physician judgment in suspected acute myocardial infarction. Am Heart J 1999; 138: 705–709.
27. Hamm CW, Goldmann BU, Heeschen C, Kreymann G, Berger J, Meinertz T. Emergency room triage of patients with acute chest pain by means of rapid testing for cardiac troponin T or troponin I. New England Journal of Medicine 1997; 337(23): 1648–1653.
28. Danesh J, Pounder RE. Eradication of *Helicobacter pylori* and non-ulcer dyspepsia. Lancet 2000; 355(9206): 766–767.

PRINCIPLES OF DIAGNOSIS AND TREATMENT

6 Respiratory function tests

G John Gibson

Key concepts

- The ratio $FEV_1/(F)VC$ is a good guide to the presence of airway obstruction but a poor guide to its severity.

- In patients with airway obstruction the inert gas dilution technique underestimates lung volume; the plethysmographic technique may overestimate volume unless care is taken.

- CO transfer factor has good sensitivity but poor specificity in assessing the overall gas-exchanging capacity of the lung.

- Results in patients should be compared to the relevant 'normal range' for that individual rather than to a single predicted value.

- Respiratory acid base disturbances are best evaluated using P_aCO_2, pH (or hydrogen ion concentration) and the actual bicarbonate ion concentration.

Scope of respiratory function tests

The main clinical roles of respiratory function tests include diagnosis, assessment of severity, monitoring of treatment and evaluating prognosis. Their diagnostic role is usually supportive rather than definitive. Exceptions are arterial blood gases in respiratory failure (which is defined in terms of P_aO_2 and P_aCO_2) and peak expiratory flow (PEF) or forced expiratory volume in 1 second (FEV_1) in asthma, where the characteristic spontaneous variation or response to bronchial challenge establishes the diagnosis. Otherwise, their diagnostic use is in recognition of particular patterns of abnormality that characterise various diseases and in identifying the likely site of a pathological process, e.g. in the central or peripheral airways with obstructive ventilatory defects, or in the chest wall or alveoli with restrictive defects. In addition, they are frequently used to quantify the severity of the functional disturbance, which is important for assessing whether the symptoms of an individual patient (usually shortness of breath) can be adequately explained, and also for estimating the prognosis.

In general, the most useful clinical information is obtained from the most easily performed and most robust tests, such as those based on forced expiration and arterial blood gases. The commonly used tests are most conveniently classified as those evaluating respiratory mechanics, gas exchange and acid–base balance and exercise.

Performance, standardisation and quality control of respiratory function tests

Recommendations for the performance of respiratory function tests are available in the literature and details are beyond the scope of this chapter. Most laboratories follow the guidelines of either the European Respiratory Society[1,2] or the American Thoracic Society.[3,4] Safety, hygiene and quality control are other important issues. Most respiratory function tests are safe, even for patients with considerable respiratory disability. Routine tests, including spirometry, carbon monoxide transfer factor and lung volumes, can safely be performed by a qualified technician and rarely require a medical presence. However, for exercise testing (other than exercise mimicking a patient's normal activities), appropriate electrocardiographic monitoring and the presence of an experienced medical practitioner is usually necessary. A high standard of hygiene is essential and standard written protocols should be followed for cleaning and disinfecting mouthpieces, tubing and other equipment.[1-4] Quality control of the measurements can be assessed by regular calibration, both physical (e.g. with a calibrating syringe) and 'biological', using healthy subjects whose test results are known to be reproducible.[1-4] Control between laboratories is also desirable but is not practised widely in many countries.

Tests of respiratory mechanics

Static pressure–volume curves

In principle, the mechanical function of the respiratory system can be described in terms of compliance of the lungs and chest wall and resistance of the airway, but in practice none of these is commonly measured directly in clinical laboratories.

Measurement of pulmonary compliance requires estimation of pleural pressure using either a balloon-tipped catheter or a miniature pressure transducer introduced into the oesophagus.[5] The static pressure–volume curve of the lungs can then be constructed (see Chapter 2.3) and lung elasticity can be assessed in various ways. These include measurement of the slope of the assumed linear portion of the curve ('static compliance'), lung recoil pressures at specific percentages of total lung capacity (TLC)[2] and the mathematical fitting of a monoexponential function to the overall curve between TLC and functional residual capacity (FRC).[6] In general, however, lung distensibility in conditions, such as diffuse pulmonary fibrosis, that cause increased stiffness of the lungs is adequately assessed by measuring lung volumes (vital capacity – VC – or TLC). Furthermore, with extrapulmonary restriction (e.g. muscle weakness), secondary changes occur in the elastic behaviour of the lungs, reducing their compliance so that a low value does not necessarily indicate that the increased lung 'stiffness' results from a primary pathological process in the alveoli or alveolar walls. Occasionally, the measurement of maximum static recoil pressure at TLC ($P_{L\,max}$) is of value: it is increased with intrapulmonary volume restriction or diffuse pleural thickening but reduced with extrapulmonary restriction caused by chest-wall deformity or muscle weakness. $P_{L\,max}$ is also diminished in emphysema, where it is associated with an increase in static (but not dynamic) lung compliance.

Lung volumes

Because of its intrinsic variability, tidal volume is rarely measured in the resting awake subject. It is of more value in assessing the response to exercise (see below), in patients receiving ventilatory support (e.g. in intensive care units) and during sleep investigations (see Chapter 45). During exercise testing, tidal volume is usually obtained by electrical integration of airflow measured at the mouth while, for prolonged monitoring (e.g. during sleep), the less intrusive method of measuring external movements of the ribcage and abdomen is used, although estimates of tidal volume and overall ventilation are then at best only semiquantitative.

Total lung capacity and its subdivisions (residual volume – RV, FRC, inspiratory capacity – IC, etc.) can be measured by one of two main techniques: inert gas dilution[7] and whole body plethysmography.[8] The former is time-consuming and the values obtained in patients with airway disease underestimate the actual TLC because of the existence of areas of poor ventilation in which equilibration of the test gas is very slow and often incomplete. Body plethysmography is performed much more rapidly but requires more expensive equipment and

careful attention to technique. The method depends on application of Boyle's law (pressure × volume is constant at constant temperature) and on the assumption that, during gentle breathing manoeuvres against a closed shutter at the mouth, alveolar and mouth pressures are effectively identical. This assumption is justified only if breathing is gentle and shallow ('panting'), at a frequency less than 1 Hz and with the subject's hands supporting the cheeks. The subject seated within the airtight plethysmograph makes gentle breathing efforts against the shutter that closes the airway at the mouth. The alternating inspiratory and expiratory efforts lead to slight rarefaction and compression respectively of thoracic gas. These changes in thoracic gas volume are reflected by increases and decreases respectively in pressure within the rigid plethysmograph. The volume measured is that in the lungs at the point when the shutter is closed (usually FRC). TLC and RV are then derived by full inspiration and expiration via a spirometer or similar device immediately on opening the shutter. Unlike the inert gas method, the plethysmograph measures the volume of any air spaces within or outside the lungs that share the pressure changes occurring during breathing efforts. Thus, for example, poorly ventilated or even totally unventilated areas of lung are included. Consequently either a bulla or a pneumothorax would be included in the volume derived.

The more common causes of abnormal increases and decreases in TLC are listed in Tables 6.1 and 6.2. An increase in TLC is seen in most patients with moderate or severe diffuse airway narrowing, unless there is a complicating coexisting abnormality that prevents this from occurring.

Table 6.1 Causes of increased total lung capacity (TLC)

Generalised airway obstruction*
■ Chronic obstructive pulmonary disease
■ Emphysema (including bullae)
■ Bronchiectasis
■ Asthma
Other
■ Acromegaly

* Elevation of total lung capacity may not be evident if measured by inert gas dilution.

Table 6.2 Causes of reduced total lung capacity (TLC)

Intrapulmonary	**Extrapulmonary**
■ Pneumonectomy	■ Pleural disease
■ Collapsed lung	Effusion
■ Consolidation	Thickening
■ Oedema	Pneumothorax
■ Fibrosis, etc.	■ Rib cage deformity:
	Scoliosis
	Thoracoplasty
	■ Respiratory muscle weakness
	■ Ascites
	■ Obesity (gross)

Although originally proposed as a specific feature of emphysema, it is well-recognised that a marked increase in TLC is not specific for emphysema and is frequently also seen in asthma, even in relative remission.

Conditions causing a reduction in TLC may be primarily intrapulmonary or extrapulmonary (Table 6.2). In general, all are also associated with reduction in VC, but this is less specific as it also occurs in patients with airway obstruction. Residual volume tends to increase with airway obstruction of all causes, and also in conditions where the lung resists deflation (e.g. mitral stenosis or expiratory muscle weakness; Table 6.3). Reduction of RV is seen in most of the conditions that lead to a reduced TLC, but frequently the effect on RV is proportionately less so that the RV/TLC ratio is greater than normal, and in these circumstances it does not necessarily imply airway obstruction. Occasionally, patients are seen with a reduced RV but TLC and VC within normal limits; recognised causes include cardiac failure, sarcoidosis and skeletal deformity.[9]

Respiratory muscle tests

The simplest test of respiratory muscle strength is measurement of pressure at the mouth during forceful inspiratory and expiratory efforts against a closed airway – maximum expiratory ($P_{E\,max}$) and maximum inspiratory ($P_{I\,max}$) pressures. Such measurements are, by definition, effort dependent and subjects require encouragement and several practice efforts to achieve reproducible values.[10] They are also influenced by the lung volume at which they are performed – expiratory (predominantly abdominal) muscles perform most effectively at high lung volumes and inspiratory muscles (predominantly the diaphragm) at lower volumes. $P_{E\,max}$ is therefore usually measured after a full inspiration and $P_{I\,max}$ at either FRC or RV. The measurements are also dependent on the exact details of mouthpiece, noseclip, etc. and some subjects have difficulty performing the tests. An alternative for assessing inspiratory muscle strength, which some find easier, is measurement during a forceful 'sniff' with the pressure measured in an occluded nostril (sniff nasal inspiratory pressure – SNIP).[11]

Maximum respiratory pressures assess the global strength of the inspiratory or expiratory muscles. Occasionally, more specific information on diaphragmatic function is required. This can be obtained during a forceful sniff or sustained inspiratory effort by measuring transdiaphragmatic pressure (P_{di}), with pressure-sensing devices in the oesophagus and stomach. An indirect index of diaphragmatic paralysis or disproportionate weakness is a large (> 25%) reduction in VC in the supine compared to the erect posture. *Isolated* bilateral diaphragmatic paralysis or

severe weakness is, however, very unusual (see Chapter 77.5) and most patients with respiratory muscle weakness have conditions that affect all the muscles. Examples include muscular dystrophies, myopathies, motor neurone disease, myasthenia gravis, corticosteroid treatment, and some endocrine and connective tissue disorders, as well as cachexia from whatever cause. Respiratory muscle weakness also frequently contributes to difficulty weaning from assisted ventilation (see Chapter 14). One disadvantage of the tests of respiratory muscle function discussed above is their dependence on patient cooperation; more specialised non-volitional tests are covered in Chapter 77.5.

Airway resistance

Although the calibre of individual airways becomes progressively smaller towards the alveoli, the overall cross-sectional area at various levels of the tracheobronchial tree increases as the diminishing calibre is outweighed by the effect of an increasing number of parallel airways with each generation. The overall resistance of the normal airway, therefore, is very dependent on the calibre of the central airway (trachea, larynx, nose) and such measurements are poorly sensitive to disease in the more peripheral airways. By the time symptomatic generalised airway obstruction has developed, however, overall airway resistance is measurably increased (i.e. airway conductance, the reciprocal of resistance, is decreased).

Measurement of airway resistance requires estimation of the pressure difference along the airway from the mouth to alveoli. The techniques available for estimating alveolar pressure include oesophageal pressure monitoring (rarely used in clinical practice), body plethysmography[12] and transient interruption of airflow when mouth pressure during occlusion is taken to equal the immediately prior alveolar pressure.[13] None is widely used in clinical testing. An alternative, which is more generally used in some countries, is forced oscillation,[13,14] which involves superimposition on normal tidal breathing of a small oscillating pressure at the mouth, from which the resulting pressure and flow information is used to calculate resistance (see Chapter 2.3). This has the theoretical advantage of giving a more 'physiological' assessment of airway function during tidal breathing and it requires less cooperation than other techniques, being applicable, for example, in children and mechanically ventilated patients.

Measurement of airway resistance by plethysmography[12] uses the same equipment as described above for measurement of lung volumes. The subject seated in the plethysmograph breathes gently via a flow measuring device, while flow and plethysmographic pressure are recorded continuously in x-y mode. As for volume measurements, a shutter at the mouth is then closed and the subject continues to make gentle efforts, during which mouth pressure (now assumed to equal alveolar pressure since no air is flowing) is displayed against plethysmographic pressure. Multiplication of the gradients of these two relationships (box pressure/flow and alveolar pressure/box pressure) gives airway resistance (alveolar pressure/flow). It should be noted that the measurement of resistance is made during airflow and closure of the shutter is merely a calibration device to allow expression of plethysmographic pressure in terms of alveolar pressure. Since closure of the shutter also allows simul-

Table 6.3 Causes of raised residual volume

Generalised airway obstruction	All causes
Pulmonary vascular congestion	Mitral stenosis Atrial septal defect
Expiratory muscle weakness	Spinal injury Myopathies, etc.

taneous calculation of thoracic gas volume (usually FRC), the measured resistance or conductance can be related to lung volume (usually as specific airway conductance, sG_{aw}).

During forced oscillation[14] the imposition of sinusoidal oscillations of flow on normal tidal flow at the mouth gives a pressure and flow profile from which, strictly, respiratory impedance rather than resistance is obtained. This includes functions relating to lung volume and inertia in addition to resistance. Processing techniques are applied to the signal to eliminate the effects of volume and inertia so that only the pressure used to overcome flow is considered and consequently respiratory resistance is calculated; a small proportion of this is tissue resistance, which is measured in addition to airway resistance.

Nasal resistance

Nasal airway resistance is usually distributed unequally between the two nostrils in parallel and, within an individual, this distribution tends to vary over a few hours (the 'nasal cycle'). This intrinsic variability of nasal resistance has limited its application but several techniques are available.[15] The main differences between them relate to whether resistance is measured during normal breathing (*'active' rhinomanometry*) or during breath-holding with a flow applied from an external source (*'passive' rhinomanometry*). In addition, the pressure may be recorded at the back of the nose (*posterior rhinomanometry*) or anteriorly from one otherwise occluded nostril during breathing through the other (*anterior rhinomanometry*). With the latter, the resistance of each unoccluded nostril is measured sequentially, with the pressure within the occluded nostril used to estimate pressure at the back of the nostril through which air flows. The total nasal resistance is obtained by summing the effects of the two nostrils acting in parallel. In posterior rhinomanometry, the pressure is recorded under the palate via a tube introduced through the mouth around which the lips are closed. Although this directly records the resistance of both nostrils in parallel, the technique requires considerable cooperation. Alternative methods for assessing nasal function include measurement of peak nasal inspiratory flow and acoustic rhinometry.[16] In the latter, a sonic pulse is delivered to each nostril and an acoustic image is obtained, from which nasal cross-sectional area at various distances from the nostril can be estimated.

Forced expiratory tests

The factors underlying tests of forced expiration are complex (see Chapter 2.3). Although the FEV_1 is deceptively simple to obtain, its value depends on several factors, which include the size and elastic properties of the lungs, the calibre of the bronchial tree and the collapsibility of the airway walls. The ratio of FEV_1/VC (or FEV_1/FVC) is widely used as an index of the presence or absence of airflow limitation. In young and middle-aged, healthy, non-smoking subjects, this ratio usually exceeds 75%. In childhood it tends to be higher and may approach 100%, while in older normal subjects values between 70% and 75% are often found. Although a good guide to the *presence* of significant airway narrowing, the FEV_1/VC ratio shows a poor correlation with *severity*.[17] As airway disease pro-

gresses, not only does the FEV_1 fall but so also does the VC as forced expiration becomes progressively more prolonged. The manoeuvre is eventually terminated when the patient can no longer sustain the necessary effort.

A traditional spirometer records volume against time. An alternative way of displaying the same information obtained during forced expiration is to plot instantaneous maximum expiratory flow ($\dot{V}_{E\,max}$) against volume throughout the forced vital capacity manoeuvre to give the maximum expiratory flow/volume (MEFV) curve (Fig. 6.1). The greatest flow, which is obtained early during the forced expiration, is effectively equivalent to the PEF recorded with a simple peak-flow meter.

One of the strengths of forced expiratory tests is their relative independence of the effort applied, but they are strictly effort-dependent to the extent that a preliminary full inspiration is required. During the subsequent forced expiration, the larger intrathoracic airways are subjected to dynamic compression by the surrounding positive pleural pressure (see Chapter 2.3). The net result is that, provided a modest effort is applied, increasing the effort merely compresses the airway further without any increase in flow. This effort-independence becomes more marked as forced expiration proceeds and it is also more marked in patients with airway obstruction than in healthy subjects. At higher volumes, i.e. close to full inflation, maximum expiratory flow is more dependent on effort. Consequently, PEF, which is attained rapidly at the start of forced expiration, is more effort-dependent than FEV_1 which integrates maximum expiratory flow over a large proportion of the FVC. PEF does, however, have the advantage of being measurable by a simple device that is easily used by patients at home.

In young healthy subjects, the descending limb of the MEFV curve approximates a straight line, while in older healthy subjects there is a disproportionate reduction at lower lung volumes so that the curve becomes more concave (convex the volume axis). In patients with generalised intrathoracic airway obstruction such as asthma or chronic obstructive pulmonary disease (COPD) this effect is greatly exaggerated and expiratory flow falls more markedly as volume declines with a consequently greater convexity to the volume axis (Fig. 6.1). The shape of the expiratory curve in an individual does not distinguish between different diseases causing diffuse airway narrowing, i.e. it is not useful for distinguishing asthma from COPD or emphysema.

The maximum inspiratory flow volume (MIFV) curve has a more symmetrical appearance than the expiratory curve. In patients with generalised airway narrowing, there is an overall reduction in inspiratory flow, but with no change in shape. Flow volume curves are of most clinical value in recognising patients with narrowing of the central airway (larynx and trachea). Narrowing at this site tends to have the greatest effect on maximum expiratory flows at high lung volumes (where flow is normally more effort-dependent) and also on maximum inspiratory flow, giving a characteristic appearance to the flow volume curves (Fig. 6.1). Often there is virtually a 'plateau' of expiratory flow in the early part of forced expiration. If the central airway is narrowed within the thorax (lower trachea or carina),

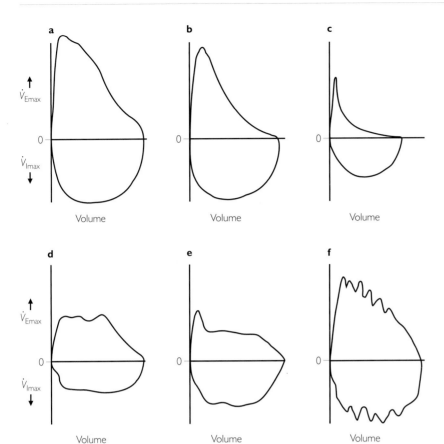

Fig. 6.1 Schematic maximum flow volume curves. a. Young healthy subject. b. Older healthy subject. c. Patient with severe generalised intrathoracic airway obstruction (chronic obstructive pulmonary disease or asthma). d. Narrowing of extrathoracic airway (upper trachea or larynx). e. Narrowing of central intrathoracic airway (e.g. lower trachea). f. 'Saw-tooth' appearance. See text for explanation.

a similar plateau of expiratory flow, often with a small early peak, is seen, but maximum inspiratory flow is less affected than when the extrathoracic airway is narrowed (Fig. 6.1). These patterns of flow volume abnormality may be quantitated as various ratios, such as $\dot{V}_{E\,max}/\dot{V}_{I\,max}$ at 50% FVC or as the ratio of PEF (markedly reduced with upper airway obstruction) to FEV_1 (less severely affected). Often, however, simple visualisation of the curves gives the clue to the likely site of airway narrowing. The sensitivity of the MEFV curve to extrathoracic airway narrowing is reduced by the presence of coexistent generalised airway obstruction (e.g. COPD).[18]

One criticism of forced expiratory tests, particularly in asthma, is that the preliminary full inspiration can alter the calibre of the airways. In healthy subjects, deep inspiration characteristically increases maximum expiratory flow at a specific lung volume through relaxation of bronchial smooth muscle. In asthma, on the other hand. the converse may sometimes be seen, with apparent bronchoconstriction (see Chapters 2.3 & 48.4). The effect of deep inspiration is avoided by recording a partial expiratory flow volume (PEFV) curve, with the forced expiration initiated from a volume less than full inflation, usually near normal end-tidal inspiratory volume. The relation between MEFV and PEFV curves can be expressed as the M/P ratio, i.e. the ratio of maximum expiratory flow at a specific lung volume taken from maximum and partial curves respectively.[19] Similar information is obtained by measuring specific airway conductance before and after deep inspiration.

A further feature sometimes noted on maximum flow–volume curves is oscillation of flow, giving the so-called 'saw-

tooth pattern' (Fig. 6.1). In the earlier literature this appearance was ignored or dismissed as instrumental 'noise' but it is now recognised as having pathophysiological implications. It implies instability of the upper airway resulting in fluctuation of airway calibre and therefore of resistance during forced expiration and/or inspiration. This pattern has been observed in several conditions (Table 6.4).

Sensitive tests of airway function

In the early stages of generalised airway disease, measurements such as FEV_1 may remain relatively normal, whereas maximum expiratory flow at small lung volumes (e.g. $\dot{V}_{E\,max\,25}$) is impaired (Fig. 6.1). Theoretical considerations (Chapter 2.3) show that such measurements reflect the function of the smaller intrathoracic airways, which are particularly affected in the earlier stages of diseases such as COPD. Unfortunately, the normal

Table 6.4 Causes of 'saw-tooth' flow–volume curves

- Obstructive sleep apnoea
- Snoring
- Upper airway stenosis/tracheomalacia
- Thermal airway injury
- Extrapyramidal disorders
- Bulbar muscle weakness

ranges of $\dot{V}_{E\,max}$ at small lung volumes are very large, which limits their value in cross-sectional studies of mild airway dysfunction as the 'signal-to-noise' ratio is considerable. The value of such indices is increased if sequential information is available within an individual, e.g. during short-term challenge testing.

An alternative, sensitive method of measuring airway function is the single-breath nitrogen test, in which the concentration of expired nitrogen is followed during a full expiration after a vital capacity inspiration of pure oxygen. The slope of the alveolar 'plateau' of nitrogen concentration is a sensitive index of uneven ventilation and this has been shown to have prognostic value in recognising cigarette smokers who are more prone subsequently to develop clinically significant COPD.[20]

Obstructive and restrictive defects

Traditionally, abnormalities of mechanical function of the lungs and thorax are classified as either 'obstructive' or 'restrictive'. The former is readily recognisable from the forced expiratory spirogram. With restrictive defects, however, the definition varies, with some authorities using the term to refer to a reduction in vital capacity and others to total lung capacity. Since, in severe airway obstruction, VC is almost always reduced, it is preferable to reserve the term 'restrictive' for the pattern associated with a reduced TLC. Some patients with undoubted mechanical abnormalities of pulmonary function do not fit comfortably into either of these groups, e.g. patients with mitral stenosis may have a relatively normal FEV$_1$/VC ratio, a reduced VC and raised RV, but normal TLC.

Tests of gas exchange

Carbon monoxide transfer

The transfer factor for carbon monoxide (T_LCO) or diffusing capacity is a simple index of the integrity of the alveolar capillary membrane and of the overall gas-exchange function of the lungs. It is sensitive but lacks specificity as reduction can result from several pathological processes (Table 6.5). Almost universally nowadays the single breath technique is used, in which the subject inspires fully a gas mixture containing a very low concentration of CO followed by a breath-hold for 10 seconds during which the rate of uptake of gas is measured. Also incorporated in the test gas is helium, which is used to measure the

Table 6.5 Conditions associated with abnormal CO uptake

	T_LCO*	Kco
Airway obstruction		
COPD/emphysema	↓	↓
Asthma	→ (↑ occasionally) (↓ if airway obstruction severe)	→ or ↑
Interstitial lung disease		
Pulmonary fibrosis	↓	↓ (→ in minority)
Sarcoidosis	↓	→ (↓ with extensive fibrosis)
Pneumonectomy	↓	↑
Extrapulmonary volume restriction		
Muscle weakness	→ (or slightly ↓)	↑
Skeletal deformity	→ (or slightly ↓)	↑
Pleural disease	→ (or slightly ↓)	↑
Cardiovascular diseases		
Cardiac disease (mitral stenosis, left ventricular failure)	↓	↓
Pulmonary vascular disease	↓	↓
Left to right shunts	↑	↑
Right to left shunts	↓	↓
Miscellaneous		
Anaemia	↓	↓
Polycythaemia	↑	↑
Renal failure	↓	↓
Hepatic cirrhosis	↓	↓
Collagen diseases (rheumatoid, SLE, systemic sclerosis)	↓	↓
Pulmonary haemorrhage	↑†	↑†

COPD, chronic obstructive pulmonary disease; SLE, systemic lupus erythematosus.
* Measured by single breath technique using single breath estimate of alveolar volume. † Depending on underlying cause – there may be an increase against background reduced values.

'effective' alveolar volume (V_A) in which the gas has been distributed.[21] In healthy subjects, V_A is close to total lung capacity while in disease, particularly airway disease, V_A is appreciably less than TLC, for the same reason that the helium dilution technique discussed above underestimates TLC in patients with airway disease. The most important factor reducing T_LCO is the effective surface area of alveoli as, for example, after resection of a lung or with generalised emphysema; in the latter, large air spaces replace normal alveoli, with a consequent reduction in surface area of the alveolar capillary membrane. T_LCO is also reduced when there is loss of effective volume (V_A), as with maldistribution of ventilation. The specificity of the measurement is improved a little by examining both T_LCO and transfer coefficient (KCO). This represents the rate of uptake of CO per litre of 'effective' alveolar volume (i.e. $KCO = T_LCO/V_A$). Since the distribution of both CO and helium are affected similarly by the distribution of ventilation, KCO to some extent allows correction for any real or effective reduction of lung volume.[21]

Both T_LCO and KCO are reduced by anaemia (Fig. 6.2) and an appropriate correction may need to be applied, particularly when haemoglobin concentration is less than 10 g/dl[22] (Fig. 6.2). Conversely, T_LCO and KCO are increased in polycythaemia.

Because it is very sensitive to various types of pathological abnormality, measurement of T_LCO is of considerable value as a screening test. Specific clinical situations where its measurement is helpful are in recognising emphysema in patients with airway obstruction and in the assessment of patients with interstitial lung disease. With extrapulmonary restriction and consequent inability to achieve a normal full inspiration (disease of the pleura, ribcage or respiratory muscles), KCO tends to be greater than normal even in the face of some reduction in the overall T_LCO. This pattern is mimicked in normal subjects if measurements are made at volumes below total lung capacity. A frank increase in T_LCO (inevitably associated with an increased KCO; Table 6.5) is seen with an increase in pulmonary capillary blood volume, e.g., with left to right intracardiac shunts and with lung haemorrhage where the extravasated blood retains its avidity for carbon monoxide. T_LCO is also increased in some patients with asthma. The precise cause is not clear; suggested mechanisms include a mild increase in pulmonary arterial pressure, resulting in a more even gravitational distribution of blood flow and blood volume or an increased pulmonary capillary blood volume resulting from the more negative intrathoracic pressure needed to overcome increased airway resistance (see Chapter 48.4).

Arterial blood gases and oximetry

The most common abnormality of blood gases in disease is a reduction in P_aO_2 with normal or reduced P_aCO_2. The general mechanisms of hypoxaemia are discussed in Chapter 2.5. Reduction of P_aO_2 is a very sensitive index of inefficient pulmonary gas exchange; in respiratory disease, ventilation–perfusion ($\dot{V}_A/\dot{Q}$) mismatching is much the most common mechanism and the causes are legion. More precise information on the efficiency of gas exchange is obtained by calculating the alveolar–arterial oxygen tension difference (AaPO_2) using the simplified form of the alveolar air equation to obtain the 'ideal' alveolar PO_2:

$$P_AO_2 = P_IO_2 - P_aCO_2/0.8, \qquad \text{(Equation 1)}$$

(where P_IO_2 is inspired PO_2 and P_AO_2 is the ideal alveolar PO_2).

The normal value for the AaPO_2 is less than 15 mmHg (2 kPa) but it has the disadvantage that for a constant degree of 'physiological shunt' its value varies with the absolute level of alveolar PO_2. This is exemplified by voluntary hyperventilation by a normal subject when P_AO_2 rises and P_ACO_2 falls and the AaPO_2 gradient widens. Conversely, if P_AO_2 is less than normal, e.g. in a patient with hypercapnia, the AaPO_2 will decrease for a given degree of $\dot{V}_A/\dot{Q}$ mismatching, so that in this situation a numerically 'normal' value of AaPO_2 is actually abnormal.[23] The dependence of AaPO_2 on P_AO_2 is due to the shape of the haemoglobin–oxygen dissociation curve. Causes of hypoxaemia other than $\dot{V}_A/\dot{Q}$ mismatching include anatomical right to left shunting, true hypoventilation (where hypoxaemia is accompanied by increased P_aCO_2) and a low inspired oxygen concentration (e.g. at altitude).

One technique used to estimate the 'anatomical' shunt is measurement of blood gases after the subject has breathed 100% oxygen for a period of 10–15 minutes. In principle, during pure oxygen breathing, the effects of $\dot{V}_A/\dot{Q}$ mismatching should be eliminated and the PO_2 rises to very high levels, even in alveoli with relatively little ventilation. Any residual hypoxaemia is then attributed to the 'anatomical' shunt. Although sometimes of clinical value, the results need to be interpreted with caution. Prolonged breathing of pure oxygen is likely to cause alveolar atelectasis, which would itself exaggerate the shunt. The upper limit of normal for the 'anatomical' shunt measured

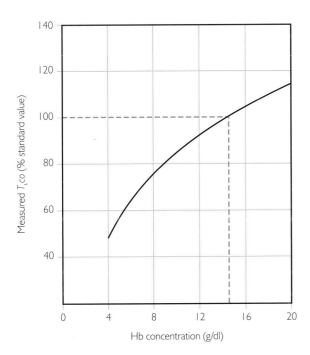

Fig. 6.2 Effect of anaemia on T_LCO, based on equation derived by Cotes et al.[22] T_LCO is expressed in relation to a standardised value at haemoglobin (Hb) 14.6 g/dl. The effect of anaemia becomes progressively more marked as Hb falls below 10 g/dl.

by this technique is about 5% of the cardiac output. A value for P_aO_2 above 500 mmHg (73 kPa) is normally achieved – this represents an $AaPO_2$ of more than 100 mmHg, which, of course, greatly exceeds the normal upper limit breathing room air because of the effect on this index of the prevailing alveolar PO_2. At these high levels of P_aO_2, haemoglobin is effectively fully saturated and increasing P_aO_2 to values above 200–300 mmHg increases oxygen carriage by simple solution only. Consequently, oxygen content (concentration) and PO_2 become linearly related on the 'flat' upper part of the dissociation curve. As an approximate guide, for P_aO_2 above 300 mmHg, each 20 mmHg of $AaPO_2$ represents an 'anatomical' shunt of 1%. It should, however, be noted that 'anatomical' in this sense does not necessarily imply a single structural communication between the right and left sides of the circulation: it may reflect multiple microscopic communications, as is occasionally seen in patients with hepatic cirrhosis, or it may represent shunting through alveoli that are totally unventilated but still perfused, as in the alveolar 'flooding' of the acute respiratory distress syndrome (ARDS).

Alternatives to $AaPO_2$ that are more predictably related to the degree of $\dot{V}_A/\dot{Q}$ mismatching are the ratio of arterial to alveolar PO_2 (a/APO_2) and the ratio of arterial PO_2 to the inspired oxygen fraction (P_aO_2/F_1O_2). The a/APO_2[24] is normally more than 0.75 and changes little as F_1O_2 increases (whereas the more conventional $AaPO_2$ increases). The ratio of P_aO_2/F_1O_2[25] is popular in assessment of patients with severe problems of oxygenation, such as acute lung injury or ARDS, where a value above 300 (P_aO_2 in mmHg, F_1O_2 as a fraction) indicates relatively mild hypoxaemia, while a value below 100 indicates very severe disturbance of gas exchange.

Arterial oxygen saturation is measurable directly by use of an oximeter with a probe attached to either the finger or the earlobe. This has the advantage of allowing continuous monitoring, but self-evidently provides no information on P_aCO_2. The general relation between PO_2 and saturation is defined by the oxygen/haemoglobin dissociation curve (Fig. 6.3). The position of this curve is affected by temperature and by the prevailing PCO_2 and pH. In addition, several genetically determined variants of the haemoglobin molecule have been described that displace the curve, either to the right (reduced oxygen affinity) or left (increased affinity). The position of the curve can be defined by measurement of P_{50}, i.e. PO_2 at a saturation of 50%, which for normal adult haemoglobin is approximately 27 mmHg (3.5 kPa), with higher values representing decreased affinity and lower values increased affinity for oxygen respectively. A more clinically useful 'landmark' on the oxygen dissociation curve is represented by a saturation of 90%,[26] which, with a curve in a normal position, is close to the point of maximum curvature and represents a PO_2 of approximately 60 mmHg (8 kPa).

Respiratory failure

Respiratory failure occurs as a result of defective pulmonary gas exchange leading to hypoxaemia with or without hypercapnia. Arbitrary limits have been set of P_aO_2 less than 60 mmHg (8 kPa) and P_aCO_2 more than 50 mmHg (6.7 kPa); these levels apply at sea level and in the absence of both an anatomical right-to-left shunt and a metabolic alkalosis. Hypoxaemia without CO_2 reten-

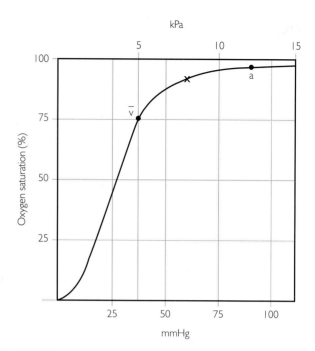

Fig. 6.3 Schematic diagram of normal oxyhaemoglobin dissociation curve, showing: (a) typical arterial values of saturation and PO_2 in a healthy subject; ($\bar{v}$) typical mixed venous values at rest in a healthy subject; (x) PO_2 of 90 mmHg (8 kPa), which corresponds approximately to SO_2 of 90%.

tion is sometimes called 'type 1' respiratory failure and hypoxaemia with hypercapnia 'type 2' respiratory failure or ventilatory failure. The arbitrary defining level of P_aO_2 was chosen because it is close to the critical point on the oxygen dissociation curve below which the curve rapidly becomes much steeper, so that any further relatively small reduction in P_aO_2 is associated with increasingly large falls in blood oxygen content and saturation (Fig. 6.3) and hence in oxygen supply to the metabolising tissues.

Some of the numerous causes of respiratory failure are shown in Figure 6.4. In general, most pulmonary and cardiac causes lead to hypoxaemia without hypercapnia ('type 1' failure). Hypercapnic ('type 2') respiratory failure is seen most commonly in patients with COPD. Although in such individuals the presence of hypercapnia is often attributed to 'alveolar' hypoventilation, such an explanation is tautological. In fact, it has been shown that CO_2 retention in patients with COPD results predominantly from $\dot{V}_A/\dot{Q}$ mismatching[27] and the effect of a small tidal volume and large physiological dead space. The overall ventilation in such patients is typically not reduced and may actually be greater than usual. True hypoventilation, with reductions in both alveolar and total ventilation, is seen with failure of the thoracic bellows, for example, if the neural drive to the respiratory muscles is impaired, the muscles themselves function inadequately or the ribcage is so mechanically deranged that lung expansion is seriously impeded (i.e. sites 1–6 in Fig. 6.4). Two additional types of respiratory failure (III and IV) have recently been added,[28] which represent abnormal gas exchange in specific circumstances relevant particularly to the intensive care environment (see Chapter 14).

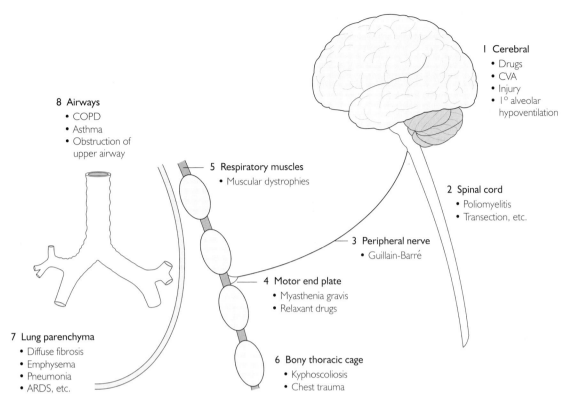

Fig. 6.4 Causes of respiratory failure. ARDS, acute respiratory distress syndrome; COPD, chronic obstructive pulmonary disease; CVA, cerebrovascular accident.

Acid–base balance and ventilatory control

The values of P_{CO_2}, bicarbonate ion concentration ($[HCO_3^-]$) and pH (or hydrogen ion concentration $[H^+]$) are linked inevitably by the carbon dioxide dissociation equation:

$$CO_2 + H_2O \rightleftharpoons H^+ + HCO_3^-. \qquad \text{(Equation 2)}$$

This defines the chemical reaction between the three variables. If two are measured, the third is readily calculated using the Henderson–Hasselbalch equation:

$$pH = 6.1 + \log_{10} \frac{[HCO_3^-]}{0.03\, P_{CO_2}\,(mmHg)}$$

$$\text{or} \quad 6.1 + \log_{10} \frac{[HCO_3^-]}{0.225\, P_{CO_2}\,(kPa)}. \qquad \text{(Equation 3)}$$

Alternatively, hydrogen ion concentration may be expressed arithmetically (rather than logarithmically as pH), when the equation becomes:

$$[H^+]\,(\times 10^{-9}\,mol/l) = \frac{24 \times P_{CO_2}\,(mmHg)}{[HCO_3^-]} \quad \text{or}$$

$$\frac{180 \times P_{CO_2}\,(kPa)}{[HCO_3^-]}.$$

Other derived indices are often quoted, i.e. standard bicarbonate, base excess or deficit, etc., but these often serve to confuse rather than to illuminate. They are generally of more value in assessing primary metabolic than respiratory acid–base disorders. In principle, the use of standard bicarbonate attempts to remove the 'metabolic' component of an acid–base abnormality but, in respiratory disorders, it fails to distinguish between a coexisting primary metabolic alkalosis and the renal retention of bicarbonate that occurs with chronic respiratory acidosis (see below).

Classically, four primary acid–base disorders are recognised (Table 6.6). In respiratory acidosis or alkalosis, the prime event is respectively an increase or reduction in P_{CO_2}. This shifts the dissociation equilibrium (Equation 2), leading to *immediate* changes in $[H^+]$ and $[HCO_3^-]$. Subsequently, over a period of hours or days, further changes in $[HCO_3^-]$ occur as a result of renal retention or excretion and as a result the hydrogen ion concentration reverts towards more normal values. In respiratory acidosis the immediate 'acute' increase in $[HCO_3^-]$ is dictated by the chemical relationship (Equation 2) and not by the physiological response that occurs later ('chronic' respiratory acidosis). The vast majority of hydrogen ions produced in response to changing CO_2 levels are buffered by proteins in the blood and extracellular fluid, with the result that the measured rise in $[HCO_3^-]$ is actually very much greater than the measured increase in hydrogen ion concentration (the logarithmic pH scale conceals the fact that the changes in blood hydrogen ion concentration are extremely small. It should be remembered that a normal hydrogen ion concentration (pH = 7.4) is only 40×10^{-9} mol/l whereas the normal $[HCO_3^-]$ is measured in millimoles per litre

Table 6.6 Types of acid–base disturbance

Condition	Primary disturbance	Immediate (chemical) effects $CO_2 + H_2O \rightleftharpoons H^+ + HCO_3^-$	'Compensatory' effects
Respiratory acidosis	$\uparrow P_{CO_2}$	$\uparrow[H^+]$ $\uparrow[HCO_3^-]$	$\uparrow\uparrow[HCO_3^-]$
Respiratory alkalosis	$\downarrow P_{CO_2}$	$\downarrow[H^+]$ $\downarrow[HCO_3^-]$	$\downarrow\downarrow[HCO_3^-]$
Metabolic acidosis	$\downarrow[HCO_3^-]$	$\uparrow[H^+]$	$\downarrow P_{CO_2}$
Metabolic alkalosis	$\uparrow[HCO_3^-]$	$\downarrow[H^+]$	$\uparrow P_{CO_2}$ (inconsistent)

(10^{-3} mol/l) so that the hydrogen ion concentration is approximately one millionth of the concentration of bicarbonate or other ions that are commonly measured in blood).

In respiratory alkalosis, the increased excretion of CO_2 accompanying increased ventilation is accompanied immediately by a reduction in $[HCO_3^-]$ and in hydrogen ion concentration (pH rises). Again, most of the reduction in hydrogen ion concentration is buffered. In practice, it is less useful to distinguish acute and chronic respiratory alkalosis than with acidosis.

In metabolic disorders, the prime event is loss or increase of bicarbonate ions, accompanied by reciprocal changes in hydrogen ion concentration. In metabolic acidosis, the physiological response (hyperventilation) is so rapid that acute and chronic phases are not distinguishable. With metabolic alkalosis, the bicarbonate excess and falling $[H^+]$ (rise in pH) would be expected to inhibit ventilation, leading to a rise in P_aCO_2. The ventilatory response is, however, variable: in subjects with healthy lungs, a mild or moderate metabolic alkalosis is usually associated with little change in P_aCO_2 but when the alkalosis is severe (classically with the persistent vomiting of pyloric stenosis), marked hypercapnia may be seen.[29] In patients with lung disease and a coexistent metabolic alkalosis, hypoventilation occurs more readily, particularly in those with severe airway obstruction in whom pre-existing hypercapnia may be present.[30] In patients with severe COPD a primary metabolic alkalosis (often in addition to chronic respiratory acidosis) is common. The usual cause is iatrogenic, due to use of diuretics and/or corticosteroids.

The venous concentration of bicarbonate is a relatively crude, but often useful, index of acid–base status, although elevations are seen with both chronic respiratory acidosis and primary metabolic alkalosis. In particular, in a patient who presents with hypercapnia, a previously normal venous bicarbonate is useful in excluding chronic ventilatory failure, while an earlier raised value (which may have passed unremarked at the time) may suggest that the elevation of P_{CO_2} is longstanding. Recognition of the four classic acid–base disorders is relatively straightforward, but not infrequently mixed disorders occur, when analysis becomes more complex. Graphical display of the data can then be very helpful. Of the three acid–base variables (i.e. pH or $[H^+]$, P_aCO_2, $[HCO_3^-]$), any two can be plotted in x–y fashion, with the third represented by a series of isopleths on the graph. Each of the modes of presentation has its advocates. One variant is illustrated in Figure 6.5 with 'confidence bands' for the expected ranges in normal subjects after induction of the appropriate acid–base disorders. The bands for acute respiratory acidosis[31] and alkalosis[32] are based on measurements obtained in healthy subjects, whereas those for chronic respiratory disturbances[33,34] and metabolic disorders[35,36] were obtained from carefully selected patients in an apparent steady state, in whom complicating factors had as far as possible been excluded. An example of the use of this type of analysis is shown in Figure 6.6. The causes of respiratory acidosis are discussed above in the section on Respiratory failure, and the more common causes of the other primary acid–base disturbances are given in Table 6.7.

Tests of ventilatory control

In clinical practice, information about ventilatory control is most readily obtained from measurements of arterial blood gases and acid–base status, as discussed in the previous section. In the great majority of cases, the development of hypercapnia is attributable to disease of the lungs (usually COPD) or to clearly recognisable chest wall or neuromuscular conditions. Although for many years hypercapnia in patients with airway obstruction was assumed to imply an abnormality of central control, it is now clear that in most patients the underlying mechanisms are peripheral and related to a combination of inefficient gas exchange and abnormal ventilatory mechanics and hyperinflation impairing the mechanical efficiency of the inspiratory muscles. Occasional patients have unexpected hypercapnia in the face of relatively mild airway obstruction, and it is assumed that these individuals in their premorbid state had constitutionally lower than average chemosensitivity to CO_2. A further factor complicating interpretation of ventilatory control in this situation is that the raised bicarbonate concentration associated with chronic respiratory acidosis itself has a potential depressant influence on ventilation. Reversal of this compensatory process has been proposed as the explanation for the beneficial effects of nocturnal ventilatory support in patients with chronic hypercapnia caused by chest wall disease or respiratory muscle weakness (see Chapters 73 and 77.5). After a period of ventilatory support at night only, such patients

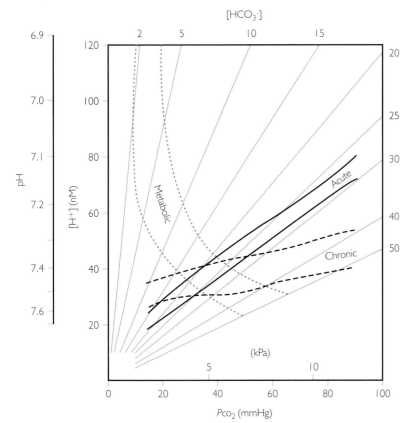

Fig. 6.5 Relationship of [H⁺] (and pH) to P_{CO_2}, in blood with isopleths representing [HCO₃⁻]. The confidence bands represent the expected ranges with uncomplicated primary acid–base disorders (see text for references): Acute = acute respiratory acidosis and alkalosis; Chronic = chronic respiratory acidosis and alkalosis; Metabolic = metabolic acidosis and alkalosis. Values lying between these bands indicate mixed acid–base disturbances.

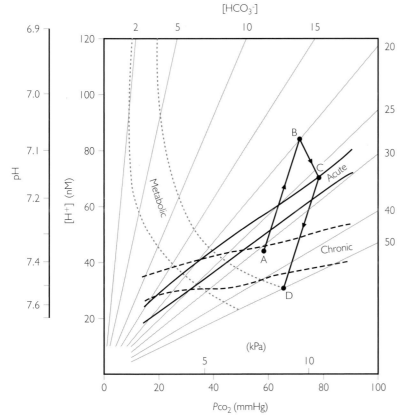

Fig. 6.6 Sequential acid–base data in a patient with respiratory failure displayed as in Fig. 6.5. (A) The patient initially has chronic respiratory failure. (B) A severe exacerbation leads to a combined respiratory and metabolic acidosis (the latter due to severe hypoxaemia and lactic acidosis). (C) With improved oxygenation the metabolic acidosis is corrected but hypercapnia increases. (D) Several days later the patient has improved, but now has a combined respiratory acidosis and metabolic alkalosis (the latter due to diuretic treatment). Actual values are:

	P_aCO_2		[H⁺]	pH	[HCO₃⁻]
	(mmHg)	(kPa)	(10^{-9} mol/l)		(10^{-3} mol/l)
A	58	7.7	44	7.36	32
B	72	9.6	82	7.09	21
C	75	10.0	67	7.18	27
D	65	8.7	31	7.49	50

Table 6.7   Causes of acid–base disturbances

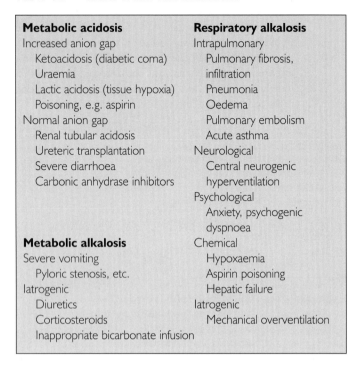

Metabolic acidosis	Respiratory alkalosis
Increased anion gap	Intrapulmonary
Ketoacidosis (diabetic coma)	Pulmonary fibrosis,
Uraemia	infiltration
Lactic acidosis (tissue hypoxia)	Pneumonia
Poisoning, e.g. aspirin	Oedema
Normal anion gap	Pulmonary embolism
Renal tubular acidosis	Acute asthma
Ureteric transplantation	Neurological
Severe diarrhoea	Central neurogenic
Carbonic anhydrase inhibitors	hyperventilation
	Psychological
	Anxiety, psychogenic
	dyspnoea
Metabolic alkalosis	Chemical
Severe vomiting	Hypoxaemia
Pyloric stenosis, etc.	Aspirin poisoning
Iatrogenic	Hepatic failure
Diuretics	Iatrogenic
Corticosteroids	Mechanical overventilation
Inappropriate bicarbonate infusion	

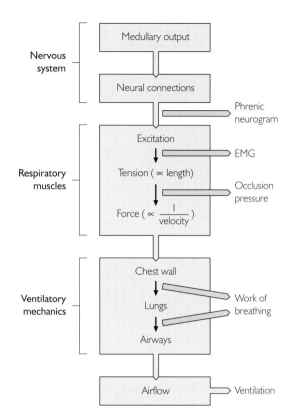

Fig. 6.7   Factors involved in neuromuscular control of ventilation and various indices used to assess respiratory drive.

show a marked improvement in daytime blood gases, often with correction of hypercapnia.

The traditional method of assessing chemosensitivity to CO_2 or oxygen is by measurement of the ventilatory responses to hypercapnia[37] or hypoxia,[38] usually during rebreathing. These techniques have the major disadvantage that the index measured (ventilation) is itself inevitably affected by abnormalities of pulmonary, chest wall or respiratory muscle function. For this reason, other indices that may be less influenced by 'end-organ' function have been proposed. These involve measurements at more proximal levels in the pathway of ventilatory control (Fig. 6.7). The indices used are mainly of research interest but one, the mouth occlusion pressure $(P_{0.1})$ is sometimes used in clinical investigation.[39] This represents the pressure recorded transiently at the mouth during brief occlusion of the airway at the onset of inspiration. It was initially proposed as an index which should be independent of lung and airway mechanics, but it is dependent on respiratory muscle function, and this in turn is affected by alterations in the size and configuration of the thorax, e.g. by the hyperinflation associated with chronic airway obstruction.[40] Measurements of the ventilatory or mouth occlusion pressure responses to hypercapnia are also influenced by the prevailing unstimulated level of P_aCO_2, so that reduction in the slope of the relationship is probable in virtually all patients with hypercapnia. In practice, the use of such measurements is limited to the occasional patient in whom a defect of central control is suspected but in whom there is no significant abnormality of ventilatory mechanics and the resting P_aCO_2 is normal. Mouth occlusion pressure $(P_{0.1})$ is of more value during resting rather than stimulated breathing and it has been used, for example, in intensive care units as an index of respiratory drive.[41]

Exercise tests

Measurements during exercise may be performed for any of several reasons. At the simplest level, exercise has the great advantage of allowing the observer to see the patient at the time when he or she is experiencing the most severe symptoms. This may be helpful in understanding the nature of the symptom because the term 'breathlessness' may be used differently by different patients – to some it implies excessive ventilation, to others difficulty in breathing because of airway narrowing, while to a few it may represent the sensation associated with cardiac ischaemia. In the particular situation of suspected asthma induced by exercise, a simple running test can be diagnostic; this is particularly useful in children, who are more likely than adults to experience exercise-induced asthma.

Quantification of exercise capacity is often desirable, particularly in subjects in whom the reported disability appears to be out of proportion to the objective evidence of abnormality at rest. Some such patients can be shown in formal testing to have normal performance and can then be reassured, whereas in others the general level of performance is poor and a diagnosis of psychogenic dyspnoea may be supported by results showing inconsistency and apparent lack of effort. During progressive exercise testing such patients fail to approach their predicted maximum values of either ventilation or heart rate. They characteristically tend to have low values of P_aCO_2 with high P_aO_2 and normal $AaPO_2$ gradient, both at rest and on exercise.

In a progressive exercise test, the most commonly measured indices are ventilation and heart rate, with results compared to well-established normal data[42] (see also Chapter 2.7). If the subject ceases exercise before the predicted maximum level, the pattern of ventilatory and cardiac responses at submaximal levels may be helpful. A markedly excessive cardiac response with the heart rate reaching its predicted maximum at a low level of exercise may suggest a cardiac cause of dyspnoea, whereas excessive ventilation with values close to the predicted maximum ventilation during mild exercise is more suggestive of pulmonary disease. Interpretation requires caution, however, because in many patients with cardiac disease inadequate tissue perfusion leads to anaerobic metabolism and consequent stimulation of ventilation due to lactic acid production; equally, many patients with significant respiratory disease are relatively unfit and therefore may show an excessive heart rate response. Measurements during exercise are easily combined with assessment by the subject of the severity of breathlessness, using either the Borg scale of perceived exertion or a visual analogue score with the subject grading breathlessness at each workload. The intensity of breathlessness should be interpreted in relation to the measured ventilation.[43] Oximetry or measurement of blood gases during exercise is particularly helpful in patients with suspected or confirmed interstitial lung disease. The $AaPO_2$ difference during exercise is used by some as a sensitive method for assessing and following abnormalities of pulmonary gas exchange in such patients.

Simple timed walk tests (e.g. 6-minute walking distance) are popular and are commonly incorporated in studies of the effects of drugs, particularly bronchodilators, where subjective improvements in exercise tolerance may be reported with very little objective change in spirometric indices. Account should be taken, however, of the well-recognised training effect with such tests; in patients with chronic airway obstruction, it has been shown that as many as five practice walks may be required before adequately reproducible results are achieved.[44] More recently, shuttle tests have been introduced in which the subject increases his walking speed each minute. The results are generally more reproducible and closer to laboratory-based tests of maximum performance than are those of timed walk tests.[45]

Miscellaneous breath tests

Traditionally, analysis of expired air is limited to oxygen and carbon dioxide but recently attention has turned to other gases present in very low concentrations. The concentration of exhaled carbon monoxide is used as a guide to its inhalation and as a valuable method for confirming non-smoking claims. Its expired concentration is directly proportional to the concentration of carboxyhaemoglobin in blood. The measurement can be made very simply with a portable analyser.[46] Breath carbon monoxide is also increased in non-smoking subjects with asthma and cystic fibrosis, where it appears to be released as a result of airway inflammation.[47] Similarly, the concentration of nitric oxide (NO) is increased with airway inflammation and it has been proposed as a non-invasive method of assessing airway inflammation in subjects with asthma.[47] Care needs to be taken to avoid contamination of expired air from the bronchial tree with that from the nose and nasal sinuses, which contain higher concentrations of NO.[48] Measurement of breath concentrations of other substances such as hydrogen peroxide and ethane have also been proposed as indicators of oxidative stress in the lungs but none is yet in regular use.[49]

Well-established uses of breath analysis in non-respiratory conditions include measurements of alcohol concentration in suspected intoxication[50] and of radiolabelled urea in detection of *Helicobacter pylori* infection of the stomach.[51]

Normal variation of test results

Interpretation of lung function tests in patients requires comparison with values obtained in healthy subjects. Several sources of variation are recognised in the normal population, both between and within subjects.[5,52]

Variation between subjects

In healthy subjects, the most obvious source of variation is body size. The total lung capacity can vary as much as threefold in the healthy adult population. There are corresponding (and approximately proportional) variations in all the static and dynamic subdivisions of lung volume. Standardisation of normal data for body size is usually achieved by incorporating a term for height in the appropriate prediction equations. The effect of size-dependent variation in lung volume also affects T_LCO, which is directly dependent on lung size, while KCO is independent of size. Size variation inevitably affects oxygen consumption and carbon dioxide production but it has other more subtle consequences; for example, the normal variations in pulmonary compliance[53] and in ventilatory responses to carbon dioxide[54] and to hypoxia[55] are all reduced by scaling for size. Indices of airway function that are normally expressed after 'correction' for lung volume, e.g. specific airway conductance and FEV_1/VC ratio, show little variation with size in adults, although the latter tends to be a little lower in tall individuals.

Sex differences in normal respiratory function are closely related to size differences, but even after accounting for size, important differences in certain tests remain. In particular, the VC and TLC of men are larger than those of women of similar height, with most of the difference attributable to differences in proportions of the body frame.[56] Similar sex differences are seen in T_LCO, although values of KCO are similar in the two sexes.[57] As with skeletal muscle function generally, maximum respiratory pressures are greater in men than in women.[58] After standardising for height, age and sex, residual variation in spirometric volumes is dependent on both genetic and environmental factors: twin studies have shown closer concordance of FEV_1 and VC in monozygotic than in dizygotic twins[59] and heritable influences are generally greater than environmental factors.[60] Severe pneumonia before the age of 2 years is associated with lower indices of airway function in later life.[61]

Important differences in lung volumes also occur between races, with subjects of European origin generally having values of VC and TLC 10–15% larger than non-Europeans of similar height. Again, differences in body frame and proportions are important in determining the total complement of alveoli, as size-independent estimates of lung distensibility suggest no racial differences.[62] Populations of Chinese origin have spirometric volumes intermediate between white and black races.[62]

When the effects of smoking are considered, differences between the normal and abnormal become blurred. As a group, asymptomatic smokers have lower values of FEV_1, VC, FEV_1/VC and T_LCO than non-smokers.[63] The last is caused in part by increased carboxyhaemoglobin content of blood but there is an additional effect, possibly resulting from a reduction in the volume of blood in the pulmonary capillaries of smokers, with changes demonstrable even after a single cigarette.[64]

Variations within subjects

The most obvious sources of variation within individual subjects are growth and ageing. During childhood, lung volumes, maximum flows and T_LCO generally correlate well with stature. Around puberty there is an accelerated increase in relation to height, especially in boys.[65,66] Indices of function continue to increase after somatic growth has ceased, with maximal values achieved at about 18–20 years.[67] From the age of approximately 25 years there is a gradual but relentless decline. With ageing there is a loss of elastic recoil of the lungs[68] but apparently very little change in TLC, with residual volume increasing at the expense of a declining vital capacity. The RV/TLC ratio increases progressively with age, while FEV_1/VC and maximum expiratory flow, particularly at smaller lung volumes, fall.[69] The overall efficiency of gas exchange declines, with a gradually falling P_aO_2[70] and widening $AaPO_2$.[71] T_LCO and KCO also both fall with age,[57] as does maximum exercise capacity.[72]

Posture has important effects on certain lung volumes, particularly FRC, which is appreciably smaller with the subject supine compared to upright because gravity no longer aids diaphragmatic descent in the supine position. There is a small difference in vital capacity between the erect and supine postures but usually this is less than 15%.[73] Gravity also has important effects on the regional distribution of ventilation and pulmonary perfusion, and in older subjects this results in a lower P_aO_2 and increased $AaPO_2$ in the supine position.[74] Because of the larger volume of blood in the pulmonary capillaries when the subject is lying down, T_LCO and KCO are both greater in the supine than in the erect posture.[75]

Although diurnal variation in lung function is seen most notably in patients with asthma, similar but less marked changes are demonstrable in non-asthmatic subjects, with the airways relatively narrower in the early morning. The variation in PEF over the 24-hour period in normal subjects is usually less than 10%.[76] The important changes in respiratory function that occur during sleep are described in Chapter 45.

Normal reference values

The ideal reference data against which to assess the lung function of a patient would be his/her premorbid function but,

except in short-term challenge tests, such information is not available. For the more common tests, prediction equations based on large series of normal subjects are used.[1,2]

The equations usually incorporate terms for age, sex and height, and sometimes for ethnic origin; some indication of the residual deviation around the mean values is also usually quoted. The usefulness of such reference equations depends critically on the size and comparability of the reference population. Most laboratories in Europe use the summary equations recommended by the European Respiratory Society.[1,2] These are based on the pooled data of several series. The American Thoracic Society[77] recommends that each laboratory should choose equations from the literature that best suit a group of healthy subjects studied in that laboratory. Clearly, whether 'summary' or individual equations are used, it is important to check that they predict values close to those measured in healthy subjects in the same laboratory.

Reference values were previously least reliable in elderly subjects and during the growth spurts of adolescence, but studies in elderly people[78] and detailed measurements throughout childhood and adolescence[65,66] have helped to rectify this. Extrapolation of reference equations beyond the limits of variation of the population studied is potentially unwise, but it does appear that extrapolation to the extremes of stature encountered in otherwise healthy subjects produces valid results.[79]

The level at which the result of an individual test should be considered abnormal is a matter of some contention. In some laboratories, values outside the range 80–120% of mean predicted are regarded as abnormal but this takes no account of the extent of variation of different tests in the reference population. More appropriately, the deviation from the mean reference value should be related to the standard deviation of the results obtained in the healthy population. Normal ranges are variously quoted as ± 1 SD, ± 2 SD or ± 1.65 SD; the last encompasses 90% of the normal population. For most measurements, the abnormality being assessed is in one predictable direction, e.g. reduced, rather than increased, FEV_1. Thus, assuming a normal distribution, a value that is more than 1 SD less than the mean would be expected in the healthy population on 16% of occasions, more than 1.65 SD below the mean on 5% of occasions and more than 2 SD below the mean on only 2.5% of occasions. Expression of results as '% predicted' is often assumed to account for variations in body size but such 'correction' does not completely remove the relation to height.[80] An increasingly popular alternative is to express each result in terms of the number of standard deviations by which it differs from the mean predicted value ('standardised residual' or Z score). A result of –1.65 would then represent a value at the lower 90% confidence limit, –1.96 at the lower 95% confidence limit, etc.

Clinical applications

The choice of a test or group of tests in an individual patient or particular clinical situation depends critically on the information being sought. Additional factors that need to be taken into account are the ease of performance of the test, its acceptability to the patient (e.g. the choice between arterial blood-gas measurements and oximetry), its discriminatory power (e.g. in assessing bronchodilator responses where not only the magnitude of the likely change is important but also the signal-to-noise ratio of the measurement) and finally its cost-effectiveness in relation to the information gained. On all counts, the simpler and best-established tests usually score most highly.

The role of lung function testing in specific diseases and in situations such as preoperative assessment and responses to therapy is detailed in the appropriate chapters. Some broad guidelines are given below.

The patient with breathlessness

Assessment of the severity of airway narrowing on the basis of physical signs is recognised to be poor, and in many patients breathlessness becomes readily explicable once simple spirometric volumes are measured. Although clinical recognition of wheezing is a reliable guide to the presence of airway narrowing, its intensity bears no relation to severity. Measurement of $T_\mathrm{L}CO$ is the next most useful screening test for breathless patients as it is easily performed, usually readily available and has a high sensitivity. If both $T_\mathrm{L}CO$ and spirometric volumes are normal, most primary pulmonary diseases can effectively be excluded as causes of breathlessness; it is, however, important to ensure that a measurement is obtained at a time when the patient is symptomatic and consequently asthma cannot be ruled out by normal spirometric measurements. Pulmonary embolism also may still need to be excluded as small or moderate-sized emboli have no effect on spirometric volumes and little on $T_\mathrm{L}CO$.

The possible value of other tests in the breathless patient depends on the particular clinical suspicions. Measurement of TLC allows identification of a restrictive ventilatory defect but does not indicate whether the primary pathological change is intra- or extrapulmonary; in the face of radiographically clear lung fields and a relatively normal $T_\mathrm{L}CO$ (perhaps with a high KCO), an extrapulmonary cause, e.g. respiratory muscle weakness, is suggested. The most appropriate further measurements would then be of respiratory muscle function. If, however, TLC is increased with relatively normal spirometry, asthma is the most likely diagnosis but early emphysema would also be a possibility and the distinction would be aided by measurement of $T_\mathrm{L}CO$ and KCO. If spirometric volumes are reduced without obvious airway obstruction and the total lung capacity is normal (implying an increase in residual volume), possible explanations would include mitral valve disease and some forms of respiratory muscle weakness.

A common diagnostic dilemma is the distinction between possible cardiac and respiratory causes of exertional dyspnoea. Not infrequently, there is clinical, radiographic or electrocardiographic evidence of abnormality of both heart and lungs so that tests are required to evaluate the dominant cause of symptoms. Apart from the static tests mentioned above, a simple progressive exercise test, together with electrocardiographic monitoring, may then be helpful. Occasionally, progressive dyspnoea is the presenting symptom of patients with multiple recurrent pulmonary emboli; tests of pulmonary mechanics are likely to be relatively normal and $T_\mathrm{L}CO$ may not be greatly reduced. A perfusion lung scan is then the investigation of choice.

The patient with airway obstruction

For the recognition and assessment of diffuse intrathoracic airway narrowing, simple measurements based on the forced expiratory manoeuvre, i.e. FEV_1, and (F)VC give the most useful clinical information and usually suffice. In patients with suspected asthma, domiciliary monitoring of PEF allows evaluation of nocturnal symptoms and identification of the characteristic variation in ventilatory function. $T_\mathrm{L}CO$ and KCO help in the recognition of significant emphysema. In patients with possible asthma with normal or near normal function and perhaps atypical symptoms such as cough, monitoring of FEV_1 or PEF following non-specific bronchial challenge using either exercise (in children) or methacholine may be diagnostic. Although maximum flow–volume curves have become routine in many laboratories and are included in the output of many automated spirometers, in most instances they offer no more useful information than FEV_1 and FEV_1/VC ratio. Their main clinical role is in recognition and assessment of narrowing of the central airway. The 'plateau' of constant maximum expiratory flow at high lung volumes corresponds to the 'straight' appearance of the more easily obtained forced expiratory spirogram from which the presence of central airway obstruction may first be suspected (see Chapter 44).

In assessing responses of patients with airway obstruction to bronchodilator drugs, arguments about the 'best' test to apply are usually sterile and it is doubtful whether other tests of airway function are more useful than FEV_1. Larger proportional changes may be seen in other indices but usually this apparent advantage is outweighed by the innate variability ('noise') of the measurements. In symptomatic patients with airway obstruction the measured response to a bronchodilator is not usually a useful guide to whether such a drug is indicated, as subjective and objective benefits are nearly always demonstrable. Bronchodilator responses may, however, aid the choice of agent and dose. A large short-term improvement can support or confirm a clinical impression of asthma but a small increase is unhelpful diagnostically. The classification of patients with 'reversible' or 'irreversible' airway obstruction on the basis of an arbitrary increase in FEV_1 (e.g. 15%) is clinically valueless and may be counterproductive if such 'irreversibility' is taken as a contraindication to the use of bronchodilator therapy.

The patient with interstitial lung disease

Measurements of vital capacity and $T_\mathrm{L}CO$ are usually sufficient for assessment and follow-up. Although patients with fibrotic lung disease have a reduction in pulmonary compliance, its measurement requires oesophageal intubation and in most cases no further information of clinical value is obtained.

The $AaPO_2$ gradient, especially on exercise, is a sensitive index of interstitial lung disease and is used in some centres. More simply, monitoring S_aO_2 using an ear oximeter allows recognition of clinically important arterial desaturation during exercise. Useful responses to treatment of patients with conditions such as sarcoidosis or fibrosing alveolitis are usually accompanied by measurable changes in VC but, in a few, the changes in pulmonary mechanics are slight and more definite improvements may be seen in $T_\mathrm{L}CO$ or arterial oxygenation.

Clinical relevance

■ The diagnostic role of respiratory function tests is predominantly one of pattern recognition, with results interpreted in the context of appropriate clinical and radiographic information.

■ Other roles include assessment of severity, monitoring treatment and estimating prognosis.

■ Simple spirometric tests, together with CO transfer factor and arterial blood gases, give the most useful clinical information.

■ Maximum flow–volume curves are of most value in recognition and assessment of narrowing of the extrathoracic or central intrathoracic airway.

? Unresolved questions

■ What are the precise mechanisms of reduction of $T_L\text{CO}$ in conditions such as collagen-vascular, hepatic and renal disease?

■ What is the best method for evaluating disordered control of breathing?

■ Can the diagnostic precision of exercise tests be improved?

■ What are the specific clinical uses of measurement of nitric oxide and other substances in expired air?

References

1. Quanjer PH, ed. Standardised lung function testing. Clin Respir Physiol 1983; 19(suppl 5).
2. Quanjer PH, ed. Standardised lung function testing. Eur Respir J 1993; 6(suppl 16).
3. American Thoracic Society. Standardization of spirometry: 1994 update. Am J Respir Crit Care Med 1995; 152: 1107–1136.
4. American Thoracic Society. Single-breath carbon monoxide diffusing capacity (transfer factor). Recommendations for a standard technique – 1995 update. Am J Respir Crit Care Med 1995; 152: 2185–2198.
5. Gibson GJ. Clinical tests of respiratory function, 2nd ed. London: Chapman & Hall; 1996.
6. Gibson GJ, Pride NB, Davis J, Schroter RC. Exponential description of the static pressure–volume curve of normal and diseased lungs. Am Rev Respir Dis 1979; 120: 799–811.
7. Meneely GR, Kaltreider NL. The volume of the lung determined by helium dilution. J Clin Invest 1949; 28: 129–139.
8. DuBois AB, Botelho SY, Bedell GN et al. A rapid plethysmographic method for measuring thoracic gas volume. J Clin Invest 1956; 35: 322–326.
9. Owens MW, Kinasewitz GT, Anderson WM. Clinical significance of an isolated reduction in residual volume. Am Rev Respir Dis 1987; 136: 1377–1380.
10. Koulouris N, Mulvey DA, Laroche CM et al. Comparison of two different mouthpieces for the measurement of $P_I$max and P_E max in normal and weak subjects. Eur Respir J 1988; 1: 863–867.
11. Heritier F, Rahm F, Pasche P, Fitting J-W. Sniff nasal pressure. A non-invasive assessment of inspiratory muscle strength. Am J Respir Crit Care Med 1994; 150: 1678–1683.
12. DuBois AB, Botelho SY, Comroe JH. A new method for measuring airway resistance in man using a body plethysmograph. J Clin Invest 1956; 35: 327–332.
13. Pride NB. Airflow resistance. In: Hughes JMB, Pride NB, eds. Lung function tests: physiological principles and clinical applications. London: WB Saunders, 1999; 27–43.
14. Peslin R. Methods for measuring total respiratory impedance by forced oscillations. Bull Eur Physiopathol Respir 1986; 22: 621–631.
15. Eiser N. The hitch-hiker's guide to nasal potency. Respir Med 1990; 84: 179–183.
16. Hilberg O, Pederson OF. Acoustic rhinometry: recommendations for technical specifications and standard operating procedures. Rhinology 2000; suppl 16: 3–17.
17. Burrows B, Strauss RH, Niden AH. Chronic obstructive lung disease. III Interrelationships of pulmonary function data. Am Rev Respir Dis 1965; 91: 861–868.
18. Robertson DR, Swinburn CR, Stone TN, Gibson GJ. Effects of an external resistance on maximum flow in chronic obstructive lung disease; implications for recognition of coincident upper airway obstruction. Thorax 1989; 44: 461–468.
19. Lim TK, Pride NB, Ingram RH. Effects of volume history during spontaneous and acutely induced airflow obstruction in asthma. Am Rev Respir Dis 1987; 135: 591–596.
20. Stanescu D, Sanna A, Veriter C, Robert A. Identification of smokers susceptible to development of chronic airflow limitation: a 13-year follow-up. Chest 1998; 114: 416–425.
21. Hughes JMB, Pride NB. In defence of the carbon monoxide transfer coefficient $K\text{CO}$ (T_L/V_A). Eur Respir J 2001; 17: 168–174.
22. Cotes JE, Dabbs JM, Elwood PC et al. Iron deficiency anaemia: its effect on transfer factor for the lung (diffusing capacity) and ventilation and cardiac frequency during submaximal exercise. Clin Sci 1972; 42: 325–335.
23. Gray BA, Blalock JM. Interpretation of the alveolar–arterial oxygen difference in patients with hypercapnia. Am Rev Respir Dis 1991; 143: 4–8.
24. Gilbert R, Keighley JF. The arterial/alveolar oxygen tension ratio. An index of gas exchange applicable to varying inspired oxygen concentrations. Am Rev Respir Dis 1974; 109: 142–145.
25. Murray JF, Matthay MA, Luce JM, Flick MR. An expanded definition of the adult respiratory distress syndrome. Am Rev Respir Dis 1988; 138: 720–723.
26. Rebuck AS, Chapman KR. The P_{90} as a clinically relevant landmark on the oxyhaemoglobin dissociation curve. Am Rev Respir Dis 1988; 137: 962–963.
27. West JB. Causes of carbon dioxide retention in lung disease. N Engl J Med 1971; 284: 1232.
28. Wood LDH. The pathophysiology and differential diagnosis of acute respiratory failure. In: Hall JB, Schmidt GA, Good LDH, ed. Principles of critical care. New York: McGraw-Hill; 1998: 499–508.
29. Javahen S, Kazemi H. Metabolic alkalosis and hypoventilation in humans. Am Rev Respir Dis 1987; 136: 1011.
30. Robin ED. Abnormalities of acid–base regulation in chronic pulmonary disease, with special reference to hypercapnia and extracellular alkalosis. N Engl J Med 1963; 268: 917.
31. Brackett NC, Cohen JJ, Schwartz WB. Carbon dioxide titration curve of normal man. N Engl J Med 1865; 272: 6.
32. Arbus GS, Herbert LA, Levesque PR et al. Characterisation and applications of the 'significance band' for acute respiratory alkalosis. N Engl J Med 1969; 280: 117.
33. Brackett NC, Wingo CF, Muren O, Solano JT. Acid–base response to chronic hypercapnia in man. N Engl J Med 1969; 280: 124.
34. Grimbert F, Reynaert M, Perret C. Acid base responses to chronic hypocapnia in man. Bull Eur Physiopathol Respir 1997; 13: 659.
35. Bone JM, Cowie J, Lambie AT, Robson JS. The relationship between arterial PCO_2 and hydrogen ion concentration in chronic metabolic acidosis and alkalosis. Clin Sci 1974; 46: 113.
36. Verdon F, van Melle G, Perret C. Respiratory response to acute metabolic acidosis. Bull Eur Physiopathol Respir 1981; 17: 223.
37. Read DJC. A clinical method for assessing the ventilatory response to CO_2. Austr Ann Med 1976; 16: 20–32.
38. Rebuck AS, Campbell EJM. A clinical method for assessing the ventilatory response to hypoxia. Am Rev Respir Dis 1974; 109: 345–350.
39. Whitelaw WA, Derenne J-P, Milic Emili J. Occlusion pressure as a measure of respiratory centre output in conscious man. Respir Physiol 1975; 23: 181–199.
40. Gribbin HR, Gardiner IT, Heinz GJ et al. Role of impaired inspiratory muscle function in limiting the ventilatory response to carbon dioxide in chronic airflow obstruction. Clin Sci 1983; 64: 487–495.
41. Yang KL, Tobin MJ. A prospective study of indexes predicting the outcome of trials of weaning from mechanical ventilation. N Engl J Med 1991; 324: 1445–1450.
42. Jones NL, Makrides L, Hitchcock C et al. Normal standards for an incremental progressive cycle ergometer test. Am Rev Respir Dis 1985; 131: 700–708.
43. Adams L, Chronos N. Lane R, Guz A. The measurement of breathlessness induced in normal subjects: validity of two scaling techniques. Clin Sci 1985; 69: 7.
44. Knox AJ, Morrison JFJ, Muers MF. Reproducibility of walking test results in chronic obstructive airways disease. Thorax 1988; 43: 388.
45. Singh SJ, Morgan MDL, Hardman AE et al. Comparison of oxygen uptake during conventional treadmill test and shuttle walk test in patients with chronic obstructive pulmonary disease. Eur Respir J 1994; 7: 2016–2020.

46. Jarvis MJ, Belcher M, Vesey C, Hutchinson DCS. Low cost carbon monoxide monitors in smoking assessment. Thorax 1986; 41: 886–887.

47. Kharitonov SA. Exhaled nitric oxide and carbon monoxide in asthma. Eur Respir Rev 1999; 9: 212–218.

48. Kharitonov S, Alving K, Barnes PJ. ERS Task Force Report: exhaled and nasal nitric oxide measurements: recommendations. Eur Respir J 1997; 10: 1683–1693.

49. Kharitonov S, Barnes PJ. Exhaled markers of pulmonary disease. Am J Respir Crit Care Med 2001; 163: 1693–1722.

50. Stephens A, Franklin SDA. Level of lung function required to use the Camic Datamaster breath alcohol testing device. Sci Justice 2001; 41: 49–52.

51. Gisbert JP, Benito LM, Lara S et al. ^{13}C-urea breath test for the diagnosis of *Helicobacter pylori* infection: are basal samples necessary? Eur J Gastroenterol Hepatol 2000; 12: 1201–1205.

52. Cotes JE. Lung function, 5th ed. Oxford: Blackwell Scientific; 1993.

53. Yernault JC, Baran D, Englert M. Effect of growth and ageing on the static mechanical lung properties. Bull Eur Physiopathol Respir 1977; 13, 777–788.

54. Rebuck AS, Rigg JRA, Kangalee M, Pengelley LD. Control of tidal volume during rebreathing. J Appl Physiol 1974; 37: 475–478.

55. Hirshman CA, McCullough RE, Weil JV. Normal values for hypoxic and hypercapnic ventilatory drives in man. J Appl Physiol 1975; 38: 1095–1108.

56. Jacobs DR, Nelson ET, Dontas AS et al. Are race and sex differences in lung function explained by frame size? The CARDIA study. Am Rev Respir Dis 1992; 146: 644–649.

57. Bradley J, Bye C, Hayden SP, Hughes DTD. Normal values of transfer factor and transfer coefficient in healthy males and females. Respiration 1979; 38: 221–226.

58. Wilson SH, Cooke NT, Edwards RHT, Spiro SG. Predicted normal values for maximal respiratory pressures in Caucasian adults and children. Thorax 1984; 39: 535–538.

59. Redline S, Tishler PV, Lewitter FI et al. Assessment of genetic and nongenetic influences on pulmonary function: a twin study. Am Rev Respir Dis 1987; 135: 217–222.

60. Cotch MF, Beaty TH, Cohen BH. Path analysis of familial resemblance of pulmonary function and cigarette smoking. Am Rev Respir Dis 1990; 142: 1337–1343.

61. Gold DR, Tager IB, Weiss ST et al. Acute lower respiratory illness in childhood as a predictor of lung function and chronic respiratory symptoms. Am Rev Respir Dis 1989; 140: 877–884.

62. Donnelly PM, Yang T-S, Peat JK, Woolcock AJ. What factors explain racial differences in lung volumes? Eur Respir J 1991; 4: 829–388.

63. Burrows B, Knudson RJ, Cline MA, Lebowitz MD. Quantitative relationships between cigarette smoking and ventilatory function. Am Rev Respir Dis 1977; 115: 195–205.

64. Sansores RE, Paré P, Abboud RT. Acute effect of cigarette smoking on the carbon monoxide diffusing capacity of the lung. Am Rev Respir Dis 1992; 146: 951–958.

65. Rosenthal M, Bain SH, Cramer D et al. Lung function in white children aged 4–19 years. I. Spirometry. Thorax 1993; 48: 794–802.

66. Rosenthal M, Cramer D, Bain SH et al. Lung function in white children aged 4–19 years. II. Single breath analysis and plethysmography. Thorax 1993; 48: 803–808.

67. Sherrill DL, Camilli A, Lebowitz MD. On the temporal relationships between lung function and somatic growth. Am Rev Respir Dis 1989; 140: 638–644.

68. Gibson GJ, Pride NB, O'Cain C, Quagliato R. Sex and age difference in pulmonary mechanics in normal non-smoking subjects. J Appl Physiol 1976; 41: 20–25.

69. Knudson RJ, Slatin RC, Lebowitz MD, Burrows B. The maximal expiratory flow volume curve. Normal standards, variability and effects of age. Am Rev Respir Dis 1976; 113: 587–600.

70. Cerveri I, Zoia MC, Fanfulla F et al. Reference values of arterial oxygen tension in the middle aged and elderly. Am J Respir Crit Care Med 1995; 152: 934–941.

71. Mellemgaard K. The alveolar–arterial oxygen difference. Acta Physiol Scand 1966; 67: 10–20.

72. Jones NL, Summers E, Killan KJ. Influence of age and stature on exercise capacity during incremental cycle ergometry in men and women. Am Rev Respir Dis 1989; 140: 1373–1380.

73. Allen SM, Hunt B, Green M. Fall in vital capacity with posture. Br J Dis Chest 1985; 79: 267–271.

74. Ward RJ, Rolas AG, Benveniste RJ et al. Effect of posture on normal arterial blood gas tensions in the aged. Geriatrics 1966; 21: 139–143.

75. Hyland RH, Krastins IRB, Astin N et al. Effect of body position on carbon monoxide diffusing capacity in asymptomatic smokers and non-smokers. Am Rev Respir Dis 1978; 117: 1045.

76. Hetzel MR, Clark TJH. Comparison of normal and asthmatic circadian rhythms in peak expiratory flow rate. Thorax 1980; 35: 732–738.

77. American Thoracic Society. Lung function testing: selection of reference values and interpretative strategies. Am Rev Respir Dis 1991; 144: 1202–18.

78. Burr ML, Phillips KM, Hurst DN. Lung function in the elderly. Thorax 1985; 40: 54–59.

79. Aitken ML, Schoene RB, Franklin J, Pierson DJ. Pulmonary function in subjects at the extremes of stature. Am Rev Respir Dis 1985; 131: 166–168.

80. Miller MR, Pincock AC. Predicted values: how should we use them? Thorax 1988; 43: 265–267.

7 Imaging

7.1 Thoracic imaging

David M Hansell

The chest radiograph is justifiably regarded as an integral part of the examination of a patient with suspected lung disease. Despite advances in other imaging techniques, chest radiography remains the cornerstone of thoracic imaging. Because of the wealth of information available from chest radiography, careful interpretation of the chest radiograph remains a necessary skill. Advances in cross-sectional imaging have had a considerable impact on improving the diagnosis of thoracic disease, not only for the assessment of mediastinal pathology but also in the evaluation of patients with suspected diffuse lung disease. Nevertheless, a chest radiograph should always be obtained and scrutinised carefully before submitting a patient to more sophisticated imaging techniques; the expense and, in the case of computed tomography, radiation burden remain important considerations.

Chest radiography is just over 100 years old (Fig. 7.1.1) and continues to provide new insights into thoracic disease. It seems remarkable that it was not until the 1940s, some 50 years after the first radiograph was taken, that it was finally determined that the branching structures seen in the lungs on a chest radiograph were blood-filled vessels rather than bronchi.[1] A further 10 years were to pass before it became recognised that upper lobe blood diversion on a chest radiograph was a sign of mitral stenosis.[2] Given the slow rate at which understanding of the plain chest radiograph has been acquired over many years, it can be anticipated that, with the newer imaging techniques, many fresh insights into chest disease are still to be made.

Techniques

Chest radiography

The technique of chest radiography has changed surprisingly little over the years although digital technology is increasingly being used to overcome some of the shortcomings of conventional film-based radiography.

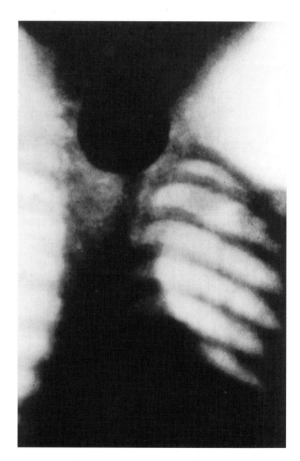

Fig. 7.1.1 One of the earliest surviving chest radiographs, taken in the 1890s. The infant had swallowed a coin. The exposure time was 13 minutes.

Technical considerations

An ideal frontal chest radiograph is taken with the patient standing, suspending respiration at near total lung capacity and with the X-ray beam traversing the thorax from back to front – the

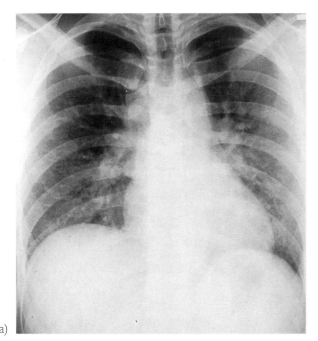

(a)

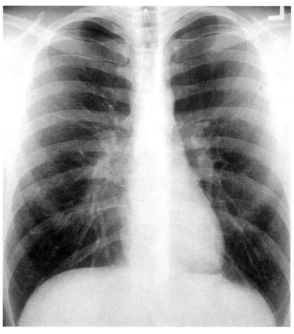

(b)

Fig. 7.1.2 (a) Posteroanterior chest radiograph of a normal 20-year-old male; a poor inspiratory effort has resulted in a deceptive impression of hilar lymphadenopathy and diffuse lung shadowing, mimicking sarcoidosis. (b) A repeat radiograph of the same individual at total lung capacity – the hila and lungs appear normal.

posteroanterior (PA) or frontal view. Because of the wide range of densities within the chest (dense soft tissues of the mediastinum through to aerated lung), perfect exposure of every part of the chest radiograph is impossible. The state of inflation of the lungs can have a profound effect on the appearance of the lungs and mediastinum; underinflation may give a spurious appearance of diffuse lung disease and hilar enlargement (Fig. 7.1.2). The steep S-shaped dose–response (or amount of incident radiation/ film blackening) curve of standard radiographic film makes it impossible to obtain perfect exposure of the densest and most lucent parts of the chest in a single radiograph.

Using modern film/screen combinations, the radiation dose to the patient is, very approximately, equivalent to that received by an individual from background (mostly cosmic) radiation over a 2-month period. High-kV radiographs have several advantages over low-kV films. Because the coefficients of X-ray absorption of bone and soft tissue approach one another at high kilovoltage, the skeletal structures no longer obscure the lungs to the same degree as with low-kV technique. The high-kV radiograph thus demonstrates much more of the lung. Furthermore, the improved penetration of the mediastinum and breast tissues allows greater detail of the airways and lung to be seen through these structures.

However, low-kV radiographs provide excellent detail of the unobscured lung because of the improved contrast between lung vessels and surrounding aerated lung. Moreover, calcified lesions, for example pleural plaques, and small pulmonary nodules[3] are particularly well demonstrated on low-kV films.

Because attenuation of X-rays by the mediastinum is up to 10 times greater than attenuation by the lungs, there have been many attempts to produce a more uniformly exposed chest

radiograph. Exposure equalisation may be achieved by using simple portal 'trough' filters between the patient and incident X-ray beam.[4] Another technique is the advanced multiple beam equalisation radiography (AMBER) system.[5] The AMBER unit uses a horizontally orientated scanning slit beam that is effectively divided into 20 segments, each being modulated by an electronic feedback loop from 20 corresponding detectors on the far side of the patient. Such a system is particularly good at demonstrating lung pathology obscured by the heart and diaphragm[6] (Fig. 7.1.3). There appears to be no clear difference in observer performance in detecting diffuse lung disease[7] or pulmonary consolidation[8] between scanning equalisation radiography and conventional chest radiography. Such techniques, which attempt to overcome the deficiencies of film, are increasingly being replaced by digital technology.

Digital chest radiography

Digital technology is fundamental to techniques such as computed tomography, magnetic resonance imaging and ultrasonography. It has long been recognised that conventional film as a means of image capture, storage and display is not ideal in all respects[9] and it has become apparent that digital image acquisition, transmission, display and storage can, with some advantages, be applied to projectional chest radiography.

Much useful information has been derived from observer performance studies of digitised conventional film to establish the parameters for clinically acceptable digital radiographs.[10,11] The most widely implemented technique for producing digital chest radiographs is phosphor plate computed (or digital) radiography. Considerable clinical experience worldwide has now

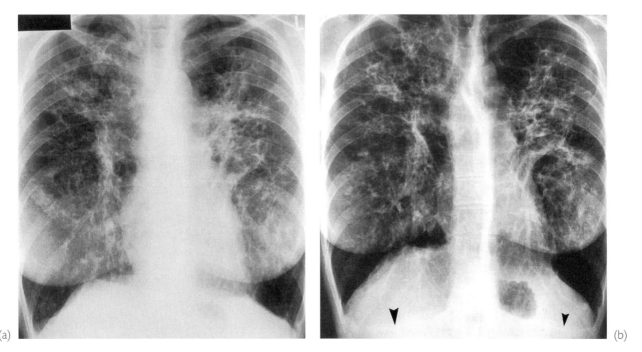

(a)   (b)

Fig. 7.1.3 (a) High-kilovoltage chest radiograph of a patient with cystic fibrosis. (b) AMBER chest radiograph of the same patient at the same kilovoltage. Note the lung detail seen through the mediastinum and diaphragm; the inferior extent of the lung delimited by the costophrenic gutters is also visible (arrowheads).

been gained with these systems, particularly for portable radiography in intensive care units.

A phosphor plate computed radiography system employs conventional radiographic equipment but uses a reusable photo-stimulable phosphor plate[12] instead of a conventional film–screen combination. The phosphor plate is a large-area detector, which is housed in a 'filmless' cassette. The phosphor plate stores some of the energy of the incident X-ray photons as a latent image. On scanning the plate with a focused laser beam, the stored energy is emitted as light, which is detected by a photo multiplier and converted to a digital signal. The digital information can then be manipulated, displayed and stored in whatever format is desired (Fig. 7.1.4). The phosphor plate can be reused once the latent image has been erased by exposure to white light. Most currently available computed radiography systems produce a digital radiograph with a 2 K × 2 K matrix (with a picture element size of 0.2 mm) and a grey scale of up to 1024 discrete levels. Because of the fundamental requirement of segmenting the image into a finite number of pixels, much work has been done to determine the relationship between pixel size, which affects spatial resolution, and lesion detectability.[13,14] Doubts remain about whether digital radiography can match conventional film radiography for

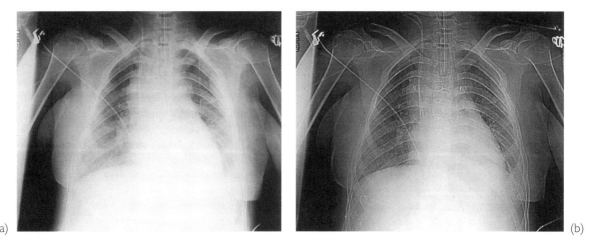

(a)   (b)

Fig. 7.1.4 A portable digital chest radiograph of an intensive care patient. The image pair is minified and laser-printed on to film. (a) This image has been made to resemble a conventional radiograph. (b) This image has been processed to give wider latitude (note the mediastinal detail) and edge enhancement.

the detection of extremely subtle pneumothoraces[15] and early interstitial lung disease.[16] Although it would seem desirable to aim for an image composed of the smallest possible pixels, there is a direct relationship between the pixel size and the cost and ease of data handling of an imaging system. Thus, pixel size is ultimately a practical compromise between image fidelity and ease of data processing and storage.

An unequivocal advantage of phosphor plate computed radiography over conventional film radiography is the ability to retrieve an image of diagnostic quality from a suboptimal exposure that, with conventional film, would have resulted in an uninterpretable radiograph; this has led to the increasing implementation of such systems for portable chest radiography. The move towards 'filmless' radiography has recently accelerated with the development of solid-state, thin-film, transistor flat-panel X-ray detectors, which can be regarded as digital image receptors.[17]

Numerous observer performance studies have shown that digital radiography can equal conventional film radiography in virtually any specific task.[18,19] To do so, however, postprocessing of the digital image has to be used to match the digital radiograph to the task. This is the problem inherent in all forms of digital manipulation – enhancement of the image for one purpose will degrade it for another. Nevertheless, the gradual transition to digitally acquired chest radiographs seems inevitable. Some of the advantages and disadvantages of conventional film versus digital chest radiography are summarised in Table 7.1.1.

Standard radiographic projections

The posteroanterior (PA) projection is the standard view. The patient is positioned with the anterior chest wall against the film cassette and the arms are abducted to rotate the scapulae away from the posterior chest. The X-ray beam traverses the patient from back to front. In a correctly exposed film, most of the lung should be visible (particularly the portions behind the heart) as well as the complex interfaces of the lung with the mediastinum. Many technical factors, notably the kilovoltage and film screen combination used, will determine just how well the lung is demonstrated.

Chest films taken in the anteroposterior (AP) projection are usually taken with mobile equipment when the patient is too ill to stand for a formal PA radiograph. Portable or mobile chest radiography has the obvious and very real advantage that the examination can be done without moving the patient from the ward. In many centres the proportion of portable to departmental chest radiographs has gradually increased over the years. Although this is expedient, the fact that the portable radiograph has many disadvantages is often overlooked.

- The shorter X-ray tube-to-film distance results in undesirable magnification.
- High-kilovolt radiographs cannot be obtained because:
  - portable machines are unable to deliver the high kilovoltage
  - it is difficult to accurately align the X-ray beam with a grid
  - the maximum milliamperage is severely limited so that long exposure times are needed with the risk of significant blurring.
- Positioning of bed-bound patients is difficult, so that the resulting radiographs are often of half-upright or even rotated subjects – even in the so-called erect position with the patient sitting up, the chest is rarely as vertical as it is in a standing patient. More importantly, the patient is unable to take a deep breath when sitting in bed.

Nevertheless, recognising that many patients are unable to be moved to the X-ray department for a formal radiograph, any method of improving the quality of a portable chest radiograph would represent a significant advance. In this particular area, digital chest radiography has proved valuable.

A lateral chest radiograph is often taken in addition to the PA film when a patient first presents with a respiratory problem; at follow-up a lateral film is usually unnecessary. The lateral radiograph is obtained by placing the patient at right angles to the film cassette. In practice, whether the film is a left or right lateral is unimportant. The lateral projection provides the third dimension and helps to determine the site of a lesion identified on the PA projection (although an opacity clearly seen on the PA radiograph is often invisible on the lateral radiograph because of the superimposition of normal structures). As well as allowing the accurate localisation of lesions, the lateral radiograph may reveal cryptic abnormalities that lie behind the heart or diaphragm. Furthermore, evaluation of the hilar structures and major airways is aided by the lateral radiograph.

Table 7.1.1 Advantages and disadvantages of film versus digital chest radiography

	Advantages	Disadvantages
Conventional film radiography (analogue technique)	Readily available Inexpensive	Optimal exposure impossible in a single image Variable quality portable chest radiographs Limited storage life Lost films
Digital radiography	Wide exposure latitude Image processing improves specific details Advantages of archiving and networking digital images hospital-wide Radiation dose reduction possible	Spatial resolution inferior to film High cost Maintenance of complex system

Plain radiographic views, other than the PA and lateral, are less frequently requested with the increasing availability of cross-sectional imaging. Nevertheless, they should not be overlooked since they may solve a specific clinical problem quickly and cheaply. The lateral decubitus view is not, as its name would imply, a lateral view. It is a frontal view taken with a horizontal beam with the patient lying on his/her side. Its main purpose is to demonstrate the movement of fluid in the pleural space. If a pleural effusion is not loculated, it will gravitate, to some extent, to the dependent part of the pleural cavity. If the patient lies on his/her side, the fluid will layer between the chest wall and the lung edge. Because the ribs, unlike the diaphragm, are always identifiable, comparison of a standard frontal view with a lateral decubitus view is a reliable way of diagnosing free pleural fluid. Ultrasonography has largely replaced the need for this view in identifying and characterising pleural effusions.

Oblique views for demonstrating rib and pleural lesions and lordotic views for questionable apical opacities often provide sufficient information to obviate the need for further investigation. The technique of screening the patient with fluoroscopy has the advantage of allowing 'real-time' radiographic examination of the patient. It allows localisation of lesions by the use of unusual oblique projections (spot-films can be taken to document the abnormality), e.g. distinguishing a small pleural plaque from an intrapulmonary nodule. Fluoroscopy is also the quickest method of evaluating diaphragmatic movement and diagnosing air-trapping in a child with suspected inhalation of a foreign body.

Although it is a simple matter to request a medley of non-standard radiographic views in an attempt to clarify the nature and site of a lesion, the interpretation of such views depends largely on how familiar the requester and/or the radiologist is with the analysis of these infrequently performed views; it is a fact that the accurate interpretation of such views is a dying art.

Ultrasonography

Very high-frequency sound waves do not travel effectively through air and are completely reflected at interfaces between soft tissue and air. The use of ultrasonography in the chest is therefore limited because of normal aerated lung. However, fluid collections can readily be detected and the main use of ultrasound in the chest is for the localisation of small or loculated pleural effusions. Furthermore, ultrasound can readily differentiate between pleural fluid and pleural thickening.

Ultrasonography is an extremely useful technique for guiding percutaneous needle biopsy of masses arising from the chest wall,[20] mediastinum[21,22] or pleura,[23] peripheral pulmonary masses[24] or consolidation that abuts the chest wall,[25,26] and for aiding the accurate placement of a chest drain within a pleural collection.[27] Ultrasonography is able to show clearly septations within an exudative pleural effusion (Fig. 7.1.5), which may inform the patient's management in terms of conservative versus surgical intervention or intracavitary fibrinolytic treatment.[28,29]

Computed tomography

Computed tomography (CT) depends on the same basic principle as conventional radiography, namely the differential absorp-

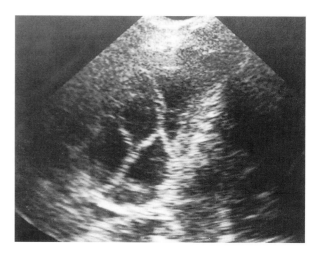

Fig. 7.1.5 Ultrasonographic demonstration of septations within a small parapneumonic pleural effusion.

tion of X-rays by tissues of disparate densities. Using multiple projections and computed calculations of radiographic density, slight differences in X-ray absorption can be displayed in a cross-sectional format.

The basic components of a CT machine are an X-ray tube and an array of X-ray detectors opposite the tube. The number and geometry of these detectors is variable: the latest machines have multiple rows of detectors. Routine scanning is now performed with continuous movement of the patient through the scanner (rather than 'slice by slice'). The speed with which a CT scanner acquires the image depends upon the table speed and the number of detector rows. The signal from the X-ray detectors is reconstructed by a computer and displayed on the computer console. It is then either laser-printed on to film or viewed on a monitor for interpretation.

Variations on CT scanner technology include electron beam ultrafast CT scanners that dispense with a rotating mechanical anode – the patient is surrounded by a tungsten target ring and the X-ray beam is produced by sweeping a focused electron beam around the tungsten ring at high speed. Such machines are capable of acquiring an image in milliseconds and thus 'real-time' studies with images acquired at 17 frames per second at a given level are possible. Rapid-acquisition studies allow the evaluation of normal and abnormal dynamic structural changes, e.g. lung density during the respiratory cycle[30] or the excursion of the tracheal wall during forced respiratory manoeuvres.[31] Spiral (also known as continuous volume or helical) scanning, first described a decade ago, entails continuous scanning while the table feeds into the CT gantry.[32,33] In this way a 'spiral' of information is acquired in a single breath-hold. Software reconstructs the information into axial sections perpendicular to the long axis of the patient, similar to conventional CT sections. The main advantage of spiral CT scanning is that truly contiguous scanning, unaffected by variations in the depth of respiration between sections, is possible so that, for example, small pulmonary nodules are not missed.[34] Because a continuous data set is acquired with spiral scanning, exquisite three-dimensional reconstructions of complex anatomical areas can be produced

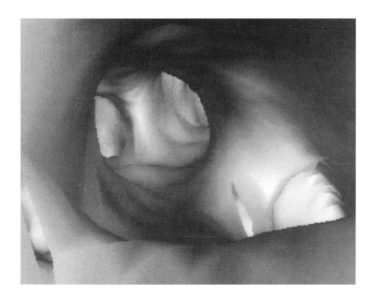

Fig. 7.1.6 Three-dimensional reconstruction of computed tomography data simulating a bronchoscopic view of the segmental bronchi.

(Fig. 7.1.6). It is also possible to tailor examinations so that particular areas are scanned while contrast enhancement is at its maximum, e.g. the pulmonary arteries in patients with suspected pulmonary embolism.[35]

Technical considerations

The CT image is composed of a matrix of picture element (pixels). There is a fixed number of pixels within the picture matrix, so the size of each pixel varies according to the diameter of the circle to be scanned. The smaller the size of the scan circle, the smaller the area represented by a pixel and the higher the spatial resolution of the final image. In practical terms, the size of the field of view should be adjusted to the size of the area of interest, usually the thoracic diameter of the patient. Depending upon the size of the field of view, the pixel size varies between 0.3 mm and 1 mm.

There is often a striking difference between CT scanners in the appearance of the lungs on the final image. This is generally the result of differences in the reconstruction algorithms of the software, which 'smooth' the image to a greater or lesser extent. Smoothing is employed to reduce the apparent image noise but has the drawback that it reduces the definition of fine structures. The lung is a high-contrast environment and such smoothing is undesirable; higher-spatial-resolution algorithms (which make image noise or 'graininess' more conspicuous) are generally preferable.

Section thickness

Although a CT section appears as a two-dimensional image it has a third dimension of depth (i.e. thickness). Thus each pixel has a volume and this three-dimensional element is called a voxel. The computer calculates the average radiographic density of tissue within each voxel and the final CT image consists of an en face representation of the numerous voxels. The single attenu-

ation value of a voxel represents the average of the attenuation values of all the various structures within it. The thicker the section, the greater the chance of different structures being included within the voxel and so the greater the averaging that occurs. This is known as the 'partial volume' effect and can be reduced by using thinner sections.

When the whole thorax is examined, contiguous sections are usually employed (for example, 10 mm thick sections at 10 mm intervals). Thinner sections are infrequently required to clarify partial volume effects or to study areas of anatomy that are orientated obliquely to the plane of section; contiguous 3 mm or 5 mm sections are sometimes preferable when examining the aorto-pulmonary window and subcarinal regions of the mediastinum. Another specific example where narrow sections of about 2 mm may be useful to display differential densities (which would otherwise be lost because of the partial volume effect) is the small deposits of fat or calcium that are sometimes seen within a hamar-toma. Extremely fine sections of 1–2 mm thickness are used to study the fine morphological detail of the lung parenchyma (Fig. 7.1.7). This technique is discussed in more detail in the section on high-resolution computed tomography (HRCT).

Apart from the evaluation of diffuse lung when sampling of a few parts of the lung (with sections taken at 20 mm or 30 mm intervals) is adequate, contiguous section scanning is necessary to allow the accurate interpretation of most thoracic abnormalities. There is a striking reduction in the radiation dose to the patient if an interspaced thin section scanning protocol (e.g. 1.5 mm/10 mm) is used, as opposed to a standard contiguous section (e.g. 10 mm/10 mm) protocol.[36] With the current interest in population screening for lung cancer there are likely to be further developments in reducing the radiation dose of CT while maintaining diagnostic quality.[37]

Window settings

The average density of each voxel is measured in Hounsfield units (HU); these units have been arbitrarily chosen so that 0 is

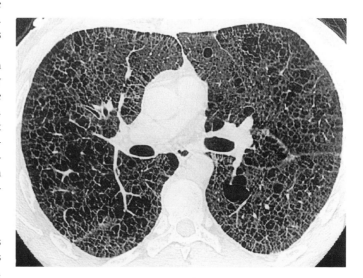

Fig. 7.1.7 High-resolution computed tomography. Thin collimation (1.5 mm thick section) showing exquisite detail of the lung parenchyma in a patient with neurofibromatosis.

water density and –1000 is air density. The range of Hounsfield units encountered in the thorax is wider than in any other part of the body, ranging from aerated lung (–850 HU) to ribs (700 HU). Two variables are employed that allow the operator to select the range of densities to be viewed: window width and window centre.

The window width is the number of Hounsfield units to be displayed. Any densities greater than the upper limit of the window are displayed as white, and any below the limit of the window are displayed as black. Between these two limits, the densities are displayed in shades of grey. The median density of the window chosen is the 'centre' or 'level', and this centre can be moved higher or lower at will, thus moving the window up or down through the range. The narrower the window width the greater the contrast discrimination within it. No single window setting can depict this wide range of densities on a single image. For this reason, thoracic work requires at least two sets of images, usually to demonstrate the lung parenchyma and soft tissues of the mediastinum respectively (Fig. 7.1.8). Furthermore, it is sometimes necessary to customise the window settings to improve the demonstration of a particular abnormality. Standard window widths and centres for thoracic CT vary between institutions but some generalisations can be made:

■ For the soft tissues of the mediastinum and chest wall a window width of 400–600 HU and a centre of +30 HU is appropriate.
■ For the lungs, a wide window of 900 HU or more at a centre of approximately –600 HU is usually satisfactory.
■ For bones the widest possible window setting at a centre of 30 HU is best.

Window settings have a profound influence on the conspicuity of normal and abnormal structures and their apparent size. Nevertheless, it is impossible to prescribe precise window settings since there is an element of observer preference and difference between machines. The most accurate representation of an object appears to be achieved if the value of the window level is half way between the density of the structure to be measured and the density of the surrounding tissue.[38,39] For example, the diameter of a pulmonary nodule, measured on soft tissue settings appropriate for the mediastinum, will be grossly underestimated.[40] It is also important to remember that, when inappropriate window settings are used, smaller structures (e.g. peripheral pulmonary vessels) are proportionately much more affected than larger structures.

Intravenous contrast enhancement

Because of the high contrast on CT between vessels and surrounding air in the lung, and vessels and surrounding fat within the mediastinum, intravenous contrast enhancement only needs to be given in specific instances. An example is the demonstration of emboli within pulmonary arteries. The exact protocol for timing the injection of contrast media depends mainly on the time the CT scanner takes to scan the thorax. With faster scanners, the circulation time of the patient becomes a critical factor. Contrast medium rapidly diffuses out of the vascular space into the extravascular space, so that opacification of the vasculature following a bolus injection will quickly decline and non-vascular structures such as lymph nodes will steadily increase in density. Because of these dynamics, there will be a time at which a solid structure has exactly the same density as an adjacent vessel. The timing and duration of the contrast medium must therefore be taken into account when interpreting a contrast-enhanced CT scan. Rapid-scanning protocols with automated contrast injectors tend to improve contrast enhancement of vascular structures at the expense of the visualisation of solid lesions because of the rapidity of scanning. When examining inflammatory lesions, such as the reaction around an empyema, it may be necessary to delay scanning to allow contrast to diffuse into the extravascular space. Ideally, all CT examinations should be carefully tailored to the clinical

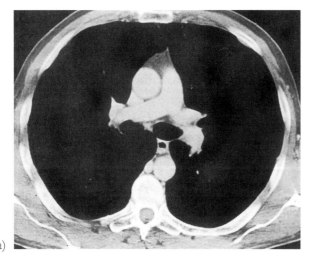

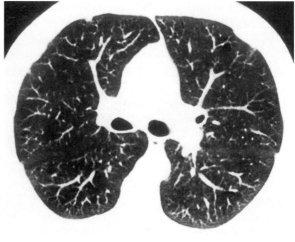

(a)   (b)

Fig. 7.1.8 A single-section CT just below the level of the carina with window settings adjusted for (a) mediastinal detail (level 25 HU, width 550 HU) and (b) lung detail (level –600 HU, width 900 HU). There is a marked difference in the conspicuity of the small bilateral pleural plaques on these two window settings.

problem: the protocol for investigation of a suspected aortic dissection using an ultrafast scanner is very different from that used for the evaluation of an empyema with a conventional scanner.

Indications for computed tomography of the thorax

The indications for CT of the thorax continue to expand, but CT should still be considered to be a second-line study that is only used when other tests have failed to solve the problem. Indications for CT can be broadly divided into those situations in which CT elucidates an abnormality shown on a plain chest radiograph, most frequently abnormalities of the mediastinum or hilar contour, and instances where the chest radiograph appears normal but there is reason to believe that there is cryptic pulmonary or mediastinal disease. The indications for CT when a chest radiograph are normal are rare. Specific instances include:

- the detection of pulmonary metastases in a patient with an extrathoracic malignancy that has a tendency to metastasise to the lung
- the identification of subtle interstitial or airways disease
- patients with endocrinological or biochemical evidence of disease that might be related to a mediastinal or small pulmonary tumour, e.g. a thymoma or parathyroid adenoma
- patients with haemoptysis and no obvious cause, to exclude a peripheral lung tumour or bronchiectasis.

The current indications for CT of the thorax are summarised in Table 7.1.2.

High-resolution computed tomography

The development of HRCT has changed the approach to the imaging of diffuse interstitial lung disease and airways disease. HRCT images of the lung correlate closely with the macroscopic appearances of pathological specimens[41,42] so that, in the context of diffuse lung disease, HRCT represents a substantial improvement over chest radiography in terms of sensitivity,

specificity, diagnostic accuracy and assessment of disease reversibility.[43–45]

Technical considerations

Three factors significantly improve the detail of CT images of the lung: narrow scan collimation, a high spatial reconstruction algorithm and a small field of view.[46] Other aspects that affect the final image, which are properties of the individual CT scanner, include the geometry and array of detectors and the frequency of data sampling.[47]

Section thickness

Narrowing the X-ray beam reduces volume averaging within the section and so increases spatial resolution compared with standard (i.e. 7–10 mm) collimation sections.[48,49] For HRCT work 1 to 1.5 mm collimation is generally regarded as ideal.[48,50] Narrow collimation has a marked effect on the appearance of the lungs, notably the vessels and bronchi: the branching vascular pattern seen particularly in the mid-zones on standard 10 mm sections has a more nodular appearance on narrow sections, because shorter segments of the obliquely running vessels are included in the plane of section. The resulting 'nodular' pattern of the normal lungs can be pronounced on some CT scanners and needs to be taken into account when interpreting HRCT images from an unfamiliar machine.

Reconstruction algorithm

The type of software algorithm used to reconstruct the HRCT image is at least as crucial as narrow-beam collimation. In conventional body CT, images are reconstructed with a 'medium sharpness' algorithm designed to smooth the image and so reduce the visibility of image noise and improve contrast resolution. In HRCT lung work a high-spatial-frequency algorithm is used that takes advantage of the inherently high-contrast environment of the lung. The high-spatial-frequency algorithm (also known as the edge-enhancing, sharp or, formerly, 'bone' algorithm) reduces image smoothing and makes structures visibly sharper, but at the same time it makes image noise more conspicuous[46,48] (Fig. 7.1.9). More than any other manipulation in HRCT technique, it is the combination of section thickness and

Table 7.1.2 Main clinical indications for computed tomography (CT) of the chest

Abnormal chest radiograph	Normal chest radiograph
Further evaluation of mediastinal or pleural mass	Identification of cryptic diffuse lung disease (high-resolution CT)
Lung cancer staging Assessment of thoracic aortic dissection	Detection of pulmonary metastases from known extrathoracic malignancy
Evaluation of patients with severe emphysema considered for lung volume reduction surgery	Investigation of patients with biochemical or endocrinologic evidence of disease that might be related to a small intrathoracic tumour (e.g. thymoma or bronchial carcinoid) Demonstration of pulmonary embolism on contrast-enhanced spiral CT Investigation of haemoptysis (e.g. endobronchial lesion or subtle bronchiectasis)

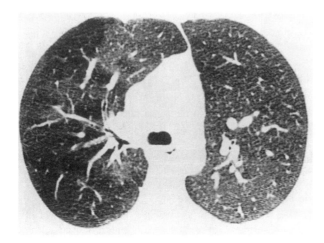

Fig. 7.1.9 An example of severe quantum noise on a CT section of a large patient. This artefact is made more conspicuous by the high-resolution reconstruction algorithm but is rarely severe enough to obscure important detail. The regional inhomogeneity of the lung density was due to constrictive obliterative bronchiolitis.

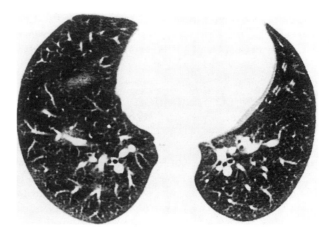

Fig. 7.1.10 Pulsation artefact on CT: cardiac movement has resulted in vessels in the lingula being imaged twice, thus producing short 'tramlines' that resemble bronchiectatic airways.

the unique reconstruction algorithm that determines the final appearance of the lung image.

Targeted reconstruction

High-resolution computed tomography is usually performed using a field of view that encompasses the whole patient in cross-section (approximately 40 cm diameter). After acquiring the image data, it is possible to 'target' the reconstruction to a single lung, thus reducing the pixel size and so increasing spatial resolution. For example, with a matrix of 512 × 512 pixels and a 40 cm field of view the pixel size is 0.78 mm. If the image reconstruction is targeted to a field of view 25 cm in diameter (large enough to encompass a single average-size lung in cross-section) the pixel size is reduced to 0.5 mm and the spatial resolution is correspondingly increased. In practice, of the three factors under operator control that contribute to the high spatial resolution of the image, this is the least frequently employed: the greatest return is from the combination of narrow collimation and a high-spatial-frequency reconstruction algorithm.

Artefacts

Although several artefacts can be consistently identified on HRCT images, they do not usually degrade the diagnostic content. It is useful to be aware of the commonest artefacts, which are caused by patient motion and image noise.

Probably the most frequently encountered artefact on both standard and high-resolution CT images of the lung is a streaky appearance due to motion. When scan acquisition time is less than 3 s, respiratory motion is rarely responsible for significant motion artefact. However, even with millisecond scan acquisition, movement of the lung as a result of cardiac motion sometimes causes degradation of image quality of the adjacent lingula and, to a lesser extent, the right middle lobe. Pulsation artefacts take the form of high-density linear streaks, usually arising from the border of the heart. Another manifestation of movement is

a 'star' pattern centred on pulmonary vessels,[51] which may show a superficial resemblance to bronchiectatic airways in cross-section.[52] Sometimes the oblique fissure may be seen as two fine parallel lines.[53] While the double-fissure artefact is unlikely to cause misdiagnosis, 'double vessels' may convincingly resemble bronchiectasis[52] (Fig. 7.1.10).

The size of the patient has a direct effect on the quality of the lung image: the larger the patient the more conspicuous the noise because of increased X-ray absorption by the patient (i.e. fewer photons, and therefore less signal, reach the detectors). Image noise, or mottle, takes the form of granular streaks arising from high-attenuation structures and is particularly evident in the posterior lung adjacent to the vertebral column (Fig. 7.1.9). Image noise rarely interferes with diagnosis and, while the problem can be counteracted by increasing the kVp and mA settings, the reduction in noise is, except in the largest patients, barely perceptible.

Scanning protocols

An HRCT examination can be varied in terms of:

- the number of sections
- the levels at which the sections are obtained
- the position of the patient
- the phase in which respiration is suspended.

There is no single protocol that can be recommended for every eventuality without being prohibitively time-consuming or excessive in terms of radiation dose to the patient. Early investigators recommended the combination of a conventional CT study of the lungs, using contiguous 10 mm collimation scans, with as few as five HRCT sections at selected levels.[49] This approach provides conventional images that may help in the interpretation of HRCT for those unfamiliar with the technique. The disadvantage of this protocol is that, even given the widespread distribution of most interstitial lung diseases (the usual indication for HRCT), the pathological process is often patchy and so is better assessed using a greater number of fine sections.[50] The simplest protocol is to perform 1 mm collimation sections at 10 mm intervals from apex to lung bases with the patient supine. Clearly, any given scanning protocol may need to be modified: a patient referred with unexplained haemoptysis should ideally be scanned with contiguous standard sections through the major airways (to show a small endobronchial tumour) and interspaced narrow sections through the remainder of the lungs (to identify bronchiectasis).[54]

When early interstitial fibrosis is suspected, particularly in asbestos-exposed individuals, HRCT scans in the prone position are needed to prevent any confusion between subtle interstitial fibrosis and the normal increased opacification seen in the dependent posterobasal segments of many individuals scanned in the supine position. The increased density seen in the posterior dependent lung in the supine position will disappear in normal individuals when the scan is repeated at the same level with the patient in the prone position (Fig. 7.1.11). Patients with obvious diffuse lung disease on chest radiography do not need sections in the prone position.[55]

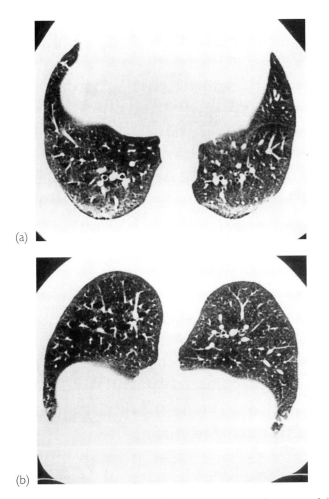

(a)

(b)

Fig. 7.1.11 (a) Increased opacification in the dependent part of the lungs in the supine position in a normal individual. Such increased density may be seen in early fibrosing alveolitis. (b) On turning the patient prone, there is clearing of this opacification, thus excluding a fixed abnormality in the posterobasal segments.

There are a number of conditions (e.g. obliterative bronchiolitis and extrinsic allergic alveolitis) in which small-airways disease may cause patchy air-trapping because of a bronchiolitic component. A limited number of scans taken at full expiration may reveal evidence of air-trapping not detectable on routine inspiratory scans:[56] areas of air-trapping range from a single secondary pulmonary lobule to a cluster of lobules giving a patchwork appearance of low-attenuation areas adjacent to higher-attenuation normal lung parenchyma.

The relatively high radiation dose to the patient inherent in CT scanning needs constant consideration. The radiation burden to the patient is considerably less with interspaced, finely collimated HRCT scans than with conventional contiguous CT scanning.[57] It has been estimated that the mean skin radiation dose delivered with HRCT using 1 mm sections at 20 mm intervals is 6% that of conventional 10 mm contiguous scanning protocols.[36] A further method of reducing the radiation burden to the patient is to decrease the amperage; it is possible to reduce the amperage by a factor of 10 and still obtain comparably diagnostic images.[58] Such a low-dose technique results in a considerable increase in image noise, and subtle parenchymal abnormalities such as early emphysema or ground-glass opacification may be obscured. Nevertheless, this technique should be considered for young patients who are likely to be monitored with HRCT, or for screening purposes (e.g. for population screening for lung cancer).

Clinical application of high-resolution computed tomography

It is difficult to gauge the overall frequency with which HRCT reveals pulmonary abnormalities when chest radiography is normal. Nevertheless, the prevalence of normal chest radiographs in patients with abnormalities on HRCT and confirmed diffuse interstitial lung disease probably ranges from 10% to 30%.[59,60]

The characteristics of HRCT abnormalities likely to be encountered in patients with diffuse lung disease and a normal chest radiograph can be summarised as:

- subtle differences in density of the lung parenchyma (e.g. obliterative bronchiolitis;[61] Fig. 7.1.9)
- parenchymal abnormalities involving a small volume of the lung often obscured by superimposed structures (e.g. the basal subpleural distribution of fibrosing alveolitis;[62] Fig. 7.1.12) – this is of particular relevance in asbestos-exposed individuals in whom there may be considerable pleural thickening obscuring the underlying lung parenchyma on chest radiography[60,63,64]
- structural changes requiring high spatial resolution for their demonstration (e.g. the thin-walled cystic air spaces of lymphangioleiomyomatosis;[65] Fig. 7.1.13).

Diffuse lung disease characterised by well-defined nodules or areas of frank pulmonary consolidation is usually conspicuous on chest radiography. Several studies have confirmed that HRCT predicts the correct histological diagnosis more often, and with a greater degree of confidence, than chest radiography.[66–68]

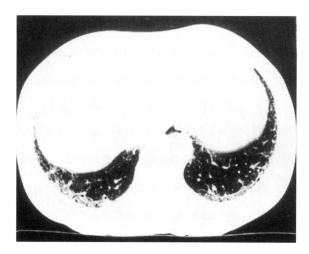

Fig. 7.1.12 A computed tomography scan through the lung bases reveals a subpleural reticular pattern, not visible on a chest radiograph, in a patient with fibrosing alveolitis associated with systemic sclerosis.

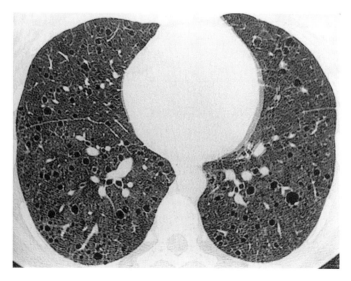

Fig. 7.1.13 High-resolution CT image showing small, thin-walled cystic air spaces in a patient with lymphangioleiomyomatosis. The chest radiograph appeared normal.

In the first study to compare the diagnostic accuracy of chest radiography and CT in the prediction of specific histological diagnoses in patients with diffuse lung disease, Mathieson et al showed that three observers could make a confident diagnosis in 23% of cases on the basis of chest radiographs and 49% using CT; the correct diagnoses were made in 77% and 93% of these readings respectively.[66] In this early study, approximately half of the patients had conventional CT sections only. In another study using HRCT exclusively in 140 consecutive patients with diffuse lung disease, Grenier et al showed that the percentage that were correct of high-confidence diagnoses by each of three observers using chest radiography alone were 29%, 34% and 19%. With HRCT the results were 57%, 55% and 47% respectively.[67] Moreover, the intraobserver agreement for the proposed diagno-

sis was better with HRCT than with chest radiography. These and other studies show that HRCT is useful in the assessment of patients with suspected diffuse lung disease in whom the clinical features and chest radiograph do not allow a confident diagnosis. In some instances the HRCT appearances are virtually pathognomonic of a specific diffuse lung disease and, as experience increases, the need for lung biopsy for diagnostic confirmation may be reduced. The decision of whether or not to confirm a diagnosis of diffuse lung disease by biopsy is often complex, but HRCT may have a decisive role in such decision-making.

There have been many attempts to use non-invasive tests to assess disease reversibility in interstitial lung diseases, particularly fibrosing alveolitis. Chest radiography, lung function tests, bronchoalveolar lavage and radionuclide techniques all have limitations.[69–72] As a result, there has been much interest in defining the role of HRCT. A predominant ground-glass opacification pattern on HRCT in patients with fibrosing alveolitis predicts a good response to treatment[73] and increased actuarial survival[74] over patients with a predominant reticular pattern, which denotes established fibrosis. In other conditions the identification of exclusive ground-glass opacification on HRCT, although non-specific, almost invariably indicates a potentially reversible disease.[75]

Since the HRCT pattern of some diffuse lung diseases indicates disease activity and so predicts the subsequent behaviour of the disease, HRCT can be used to follow up such patients. Anatomically comparable sections should be obtained on follow-up because of the patchy nature of many diffuse lung diseases (which may give a spurious impression of the change in both pattern and extent of disease on serial non-comparable HRCT sections). In practice this may be difficult to achieve and so any judgement about change in extent or pattern of diffuse lung disease needs to take account of the comparability of sections on serial HRCT examinations.

In patients in whom lung biopsy is required, HRCT may be invaluable in indicating which type of biopsy procedure is likely to be successful in obtaining diagnostic material. The broad distinction between peripheral disease versus central and bronchocentric disease is easily made on HRCT and thus disease with a subpleural distribution such as fibrosing alveolitis is most unlikely to be successfully sampled by transbronchial biopsy, whereas bronchocentric disease such as sarcoidosis and lymphangitis carcinomatosa is more readily accessible. In patients in whom an open or thoracoscopic lung biopsy is contemplated, HRCT will assist the surgeon in determining the optimal biopsy site and specifically avoids sampling areas of end-stage interstitial fibrosis.

Magnetic resonance imaging

The physical principles of magnetic resonance imaging (MRI) are very different from those governing CT. An MR image is obtained by placing an individual in a strong magnetic field, which polarises some of the ubiquitous hydrogen protons (which can be thought of as behaving like randomly orientated bar magnets) in the body so that they have the same alignment. The application of radio-frequency wave pulses of specified lengths and repetition (pulse sequences) displace the protons and some of this transmitted energy is absorbed by them. With the cessation of the radio-frequency pulse, the protons return to their initial alignment and in so doing emit, as a weak signal, some of the energy they have absorbed; this signal is received and then amplified and handled in digital form and is subsequently reconstructed into an image.

The most significant advantage of MRI over other cross-sectional imaging is its excellent contrast resolution of soft tissue. A further benefit is its multiplanar imaging capability, which allows a truly three-dimensional appreciation of complex anatomical regions such as the hila and mediastinum (Fig. 7.1.14). This capability is now matched by spiral computed tomography, which allows near-perfect 3-D image reconstructions. There are a few specific instances in which MRI provides additional information about the lung that are not so readily available from CT. These include:

- the identification of mediastinal or chest wall invasion by tumour[76,77]
- the differentiation between solid and vascular hilar masses[78,79]
- the evaluation of posterior and superior mediastinal masses[80]
- the evaluation of flow in vascular abnormalities (more specifically, the use of MR angiography for the detection of pulmonary embolism).[81]

High-spatial-resolution imaging with MRI is technically possible but there is always the trade-off between resolution on one hand and signal-to-noise ratio and acquisition time on the other. This balance is particularly important when considering MRI of the lung parenchyma. The relatively poor spatial resolution of MRI remains a major obstacle to its more widespread clinical use in thoracic imaging. For example, the spurious appearance of small clusters of lymph nodes in the mediastinum, which appear as a single mass, prevents the routine application of MRI to the staging of bronchogenic carcinoma. However, faster spin echo techniques

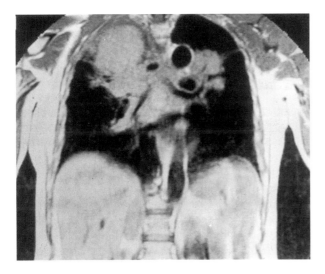

Fig. 7.1.14 Coronal magnetic resonance imaging section showing the relationship of a tumour mass to the hilar and mediastinal structures and its extent. An incidental finding is a metastatic deposit in the right adrenal gland. (Courtesy of Dr P. Goddard.)

have improved contrast and spatial resolution by reducing motion artefact compared with standard T2-weighted images. Further developments of rapid breath-hold imaging and improvements in cardiac and respiratory gating techniques and dedicated chest coils will further improve image quality and promise a wider role for MRI in the investigation of thoracic disease. Imaging sequences and protocols have been developed to evaluate the lung parenchyma.[82–84] However, early studies showed that there are considerable difficulties in obtaining an adequate and reproducible signal,[85–87] and MR is not routinely used for imaging the lung parenchyma. Recent reports of the MR imaging of hyperpolarised noble gases within the airspaces hold the promise of functional imaging with good spatial resolution of regional ventilation.[88]

Technical considerations

The basic physics of MRI[89] will not be considered in detail but factors particularly affecting MR imaging of the thorax will be reviewed. The thorax poses some uniquely difficult challenges for MRI, particularly those of cardiac and respiratory movement and the extremely low proton density of normal lung. The large tissue–air interface in the lung induces susceptibility artefacts, which affect magnetic field homogeneity.[90] Several techniques have been devised to minimise this artefact.[91,92] With the numerous imaging sequences, gating techniques and variety of planes of sections available to the radiologist, no single protocol can be prescribed for a thoracic MRI examination: more than any other imaging investigation in the chest, the protocol needs to be tailored to the clinical question being asked.

Magnetic resonance images are degraded by periodic cardiac and respiratory motion. The result is both blurring of the image and superimposition of ghost images. At higher magnetic fields, degradation of the image by motion is more marked and the ghost images are more obvious. Artefacts from cardiovascular motion can be minimised by synchronising the acquisition of the images to a certain point in the cardiac cycle by ECG triggering. The pulsatile flow of blood in major cardiovascular structures is capable of generating variable amounts of signal and may thus produce artefacts within a vessel lumen.

Artefact from the movement of normal breathing presents a distinct challenge that cannot be countered by simple respiratory gating. Fast scan techniques with single-section acquisition times of a few seconds can be used with the patient breath-holding.[93]

Sequences for thoracic magnetic resonance imaging

Sequences that have a reduced repetition time and a short echo time, so-called T1-weighted sequences, increase the contrast between fat and surrounding tissues and reduce motion and susceptibility artefacts. T2-weighted images have long echo and repetition times and may, with some caveats, allow further characterisation of abnormalities detected on the T1-weighted images.[94,95] The long repetition time is crucial to the quality of T2-weighted scans and must be matched with the heart rate of the patient. If necessary, ECG gating is adjusted to cover every third or fourth heart beat. Cardiac gating is routinely used unless the region of interest is unaffected by cardiac motion, for

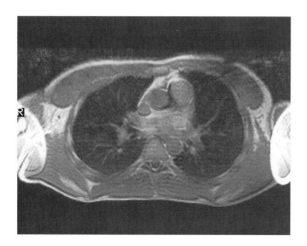

Fig. 7.1.15 Transverse short spin echo (TE 7 ms) magnetic resonance image used to demonstrate some detail in the lungs (invisible with conventional magnetic resonance imaging sequences).

example a Pancoast tumour. When ECG gating is used, the repetition is equal to the R–R wave interval of the cardiac cycle. At a normal heart rate, ECG gating will produce pulse sequences with a repetition of 800–1000 ms.

It has been recommended that the first part of a routine thoracic examination should comprise coronal T1-weighted 10 mm width sections with a 3–5 mm interspace between sections, a 256×192 matrix, one radio frequency excitation and a 42–48 cm field of view.[96] Respiratory compensation and presaturation should be used. Depending upon the information gained from the first sequence, a series of T1-weighted transverse sections can then be planned. In general, if no abnormality is found on these T1-weighted sequences, it is unlikely that further imaging with T2-weighted sequences will reveal additional information that would otherwise be overlooked.[97] The ability of MRI to image parenchymal lung disease with extremely short spin echo sequences has been demonstrated[83,98] (Fig. 7.1.15), but the images do not compare favourably with the anatomical detail of an HRCT image.

Magnetic resonance imaging tissue characteristics

Differences in MR signal intensity between various tissues are due to a complex relationship between proton density and spin–lattice (T1) and spin–spin (T2) relaxation times.[99] Relaxation times are influenced by the size and freedom of molecules in tissues. After excitation by a radio-frequency pulse, the nuclei return to their resting state and in the process there is an exchange of energy; if this process is inefficient the T1 time is long. T1 time is thus an index of the time taken by spins to return to their resting state. Fat has the shortest T1 relaxation time of all human tissues. In contrast, the large collagen macromolecules of fibrous (solid) tissue have much longer T1 relaxation times.

The T2 relaxation time is influenced mainly by interactions between molecules. In basic terms, large molecules that are restricted in motion have a very short T2 time so that the MR

signal is very short-lived and cannot be recorded within the echo time. While the mobile molecules of water and fat generate most signal, it should be remembered that these molecules usually interact with the surrounding macromolecules that comprise the bulk of the soft tissue, and thus their relaxation times are altered. It is this fundamental influence on water (and to a lesser extent fat) molecules by the macromolecular components of different tissues that produces the striking contrast differences on MRI between various tissues. Thus an increase in the concentration of freely mobile water molecules and a decrease in the proportion of macromolecules (particularly protein) capable of interacting with water will give long T1 and T2 relaxation times. Conversely, tissue with a high protein content will produce shorter T1 relaxation times and at the same time have a less predictable effect on T2 relaxation times.

Paramagnetic agents, in the form of blood or a gadolinium-complex contrast medium, will also reduce T1 times; this phenomenon is the result of increasing the range of resonant frequency of protein protons by varying the magnetic field in the immediate vicinity of the paramagnetic material. In this way, a wider range of proton-bearing molecules are recruited. The net result is a greater signal on T1 images with no substantial effect on T2 images at the usual gadolinium concentrations.

The MR signal intensity of a given tissue is an average of the contribution from each constituent. In the same way, different pathological processes will produce different signal intensities depending on the proportions of, for example, fibrosis, oedema and necrosis. As a result, the signal intensity of a lesion cannot be regarded as specific because of the wide overlap due to the many components that contribute to the final signal; different pathologies may produce similar signals. Any change in the various components of a tissue over time will be reflected in the MR signal. For this reason, MR, unlike CT, is sensitive to serial change in pathology; this characteristic has been exploited in monitoring some tumours.

The major naturally occurring contrast agents in the thorax that provide clinically useful information on MRI are fat, flowing blood and air. The high signal intensity of fat on T1-weighted images is of particular value because of its abundance in the mediastinum and in the extrapleural region around the chest wall: demonstration of local invasion by a tumour relies largely on the striking contrast between its signal and that of the adjacent fat.

There are certain pathologies that lend themselves to characterisation by MRI, notably haemorrhagic lesions or haematoma,[100] the proteinaceous contents of some foregut duplication cysts (which may appear as high attenuation solid masses on CT[101]) and alveolar proteinosis, all of which result in a shortening of the T1 relaxation time. Differences in relaxation time in mediastinal lymph nodes containing reactive hyperplasia or metastases have not been shown to be large enough to be clinically useful.[102] Recent work with hyperpolarised gases, notably helium and xenon, suggests that these 'contrast' agents, when inhaled into the lungs, provide unique anatomical and functional information.[103]

Pulmonary arteriography

Pulmonary arteriography was first shown to be an accurate method of diagnosing pulmonary embolus in the early 1960s.[104]

The major indication remains the demonstration of pulmonary embolism; less common indications include the identification of pulmonary arteriovenous malformations or pulmonary artery aneurysms. Pulmonary arteriography should probably be performed more readily, given that it is a relatively safe test; however, in many hospitals the facilities for high-quality pulmonary arteriography are lacking.[106] Furthermore, the increasing use of spiral CT in patients with suspected pulmonary embolism has led to a decrease in the number of centres able to produce high-quality pulmonary arteriograms.

The arteriographic features of a recent large pulmonary embolus are usually obvious: there is a filling defect with at least one surface of the embolus adherent to the vessel wall. If the thrombus in the pulmonary arteries is laminated, the typical arteriographic finding of filling defects may be absent.[107] Complete occlusion of a branch of the pulmonary artery (Fig. 7.1.16) is a less specific sign (this may result, for example, from direct involvement of a pulmonary artery by a neoplasm or fibrotic disease). Furthermore, it is easier to overlook a completely occluded 'absent' vessel than the sign of a filling defect, particularly when there are numerous overlapping pulmonary artery branches. An even less specific sign of pulmonary embolism is an area of delayed opacification of the pulmonary arterial branches (equivalent to a relative perfusion defect seen on radionuclide perfusion scanning). Such a phenomenon occurs in any condition that destroys the lung parenchyma, notably emphysema or any disease that leads to focal hypoxic vasoconstriction of pulmonary vessels. In patients with chronic thromboembolic disease, the central pulmonary arteries are frequently dilated, with rapid distal tapering. Web-like filling defects and pouching of partially or completely occluded pulmonary arteries are sometimes seen in chronic thromboembolic disease.[108]

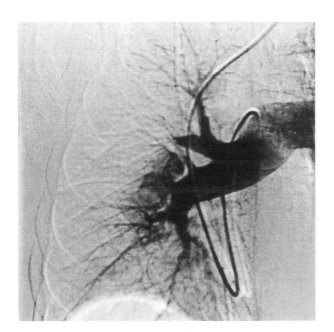

Fig. 7.1.16 Digital subtraction pulmonary arteriogram of a patient with chronic thromboembolic disease. There is marked dilatation of the proximal pulmonary arteries and complete occlusion by an embolus of an artery in the right upper lobe.

Although pulmonary arteriography can be regarded as a relatively safe procedure in experienced hands, it remains an invasive technique with a number of potentially dangerous complications.[109] In one of the largest series to date, there were five deaths (0.5%) out of the 1111 patients who underwent pulmonary arteriography.[110] Pulmonary arterial hypertension is a major predisposing factor for such deaths and there is a significant increase in the mortality rate in patients with right-ventricular end-diastolic pressures greater than 20 mmHg.[110] Of the non-fatal complications, arrhythmias and cardiac perforations are probably the most common. The risk of myocardial perforation has been reduced with the use of pigtail catheters. Low-osmolar contrast agents produce less pulmonary vasoconstriction and thus less increase in pulmonary arterial pressure during arteriography.[111]

Over the years, there have been many guidelines about which patients should be submitted for pulmonary arteriography but in practice these criteria are often not followed. Furthermore, the decline in the availability of the expertise needed to perform pulmonary arteriography and the increasing availability of alternative techniques, notably spiral CT and MR angiography, dictate a decreasing role for it.

Bronchial arteriography and embolisation

The indications for bronchial arteriography have changed over the years and it is now most often performed as a precursor to embolisation to stop a massive haemoptysis in patients unsuitable for surgical management.[112–115] Surgical resection is still regarded as the treatment of choice in patients with massive haemoptysis; without surgical intervention the mortality in such patients is more than 50%.

The commonest causes of bronchial artery hypertrophy and consequent intrapulmonary haemorrhage are suppurative lung diseases (particularly the bronchiectasis of cystic fibrosis[112,115–117]) and post-tuberculous cavities containing mycetomas. Less common causes of haemorrhage from the bronchial circulation include bronchial carcinoma, chronic pulmonary abscess and congenital cyanotic heart disease. In some haemorrhagic pulmonary lesions, the vascular supply is complex and there are contributions from the pulmonary circulation, systemic bronchial arteries and sometimes non-bronchial systemic arteries which transgress the pleura.

There are no contraindications to bronchial artery embolisation, although the patient should be haemodynamically stable and able to lie flat for the duration of the procedure. If a spinal artery arising from a bronchial artery is identified, special care has to be taken if embolisation of that bronchial artery is contemplated. It is theoretically likely that the fast-flowing blood in the hypertrophied bronchial artery will direct embolic material to the abnormal intrapulmonary circulation rather than to the spinal artery.[118]

The number and origins of the bronchial arteries are highly variable. Up to 20% of bronchial arteries arise from vessels other than the descending aorta.[112] The commonest arrangement is one main right bronchial artery from a common intercostobronchial trunk arising from the thoracic aorta at approximately the level of T5, and two left bronchial arteries arising more inferiorly.[119] The wide variation in both the numbers and origins of the bronchial arteries may be a problem for the angiographer when comprehensive bronchial arteriography is contemplated: up to 35% of patients have either multiple vessels or unusual origins.[112,120,121]

Fibreoptic bronchoscopy is sometimes advocated prior to bronchial artery embolisation to establish the site of haemorrhage. However, a large haemoptysis will almost invariably result in vigorous coughing and so spread blood throughout the bronchial tree, making localisation at a lobar level (or indeed, the side) impossible. Embolisation, with particles of polyvinyl alcohol foam, pledgets of absorbable gelatine and sometimes combinations of materials,[115] is directed at the vessels considered most likely to be the source of haemorrhage (Fig. 7.1.17): bronchial arteries with a diameter greater than 3 mm can be considered to be pathologically dilated. Patients may be surprisingly reliable in localising the origin of the haemoptysis (e.g. a gurgling or curious sensation in one part of one lung). In patients with diffuse suppurative lung disease, most commonly cystic fibrosis, an attempt should be made to embolise all significantly enlarged bronchial arteries bilaterally.[112,115,122,123] If no abnormal bronchial arteries are identified, a systematic search has to be made for aberrant ones. When a patient continues to have haemoptysis after embolisation of all suspicious systemic arteries, it may be necessary to investigate the pulmonary circulation for a source of haemorrhage. Such an approach is demanding for both patient and operator. An appreciation of the anatomy and pathophysiology of these complex disorders reduces the likelihood of complications.[124]

Serious complications after bronchial artery embolisation are rare. Most of the reported cases of transverse myelitis have been due to contrast toxicity rather than inadvertent embolisation[118,125–127] and predate the introduction of low-osmolar contrast media. Necrosis of the main stem bronchi is an exceedingly rare complication and has only been reported twice;[113,128] the later development of a broncho-oesophageal fistula has been reported in one patient. Spillover of embolisation material into

the thoracic aorta may cause distant ischaemia or infarction in the legs or abdominal organs.

The aim of bronchial artery embolisation, the immediate control of life-threatening haemoptysis, is achieved in 75–90% of patients.[91,113,115,129,130,131] Failures are due to inability to complete the procedure, failure to identify significant (possibly aberrant) bronchial arteries and inability to maintain the catheter position and proceed to embolisation. Up to 20% of patients will rebleed within 6 months following an initially successful bronchial artery embolisation.[113,127] The reasons for recurrent haemorrhage are recanalisation of previously embolised vessels, incomplete initial embolisation and hypertrophy of small bronchial arteries not initially embolised. Bronchial artery embolisation can usually be successfully repeated in patients who rebleed.

Superior vena cavography and stenting

Superior vena cavography is usually performed to evaluate the exact site of narrowing in patients with symptoms of obstruction of the superior vena cava; it is not generally required to confirm the diagnosis, which is usually evident from the clinical signs alone. Patients with symptoms of superior vena cava obstruction, most frequently due to neoplastic involvement of mediastinal lymph nodes, may be successfully palliated by radiotherapy, and more recently expandable metallic wire stents have been used to treat strictures of the superior vena cava. Reliable and successful palliation of obstruction has been reported with a variety of stent designs.[132-134] A superior vena cavagram is mandatory to identify the length and site of the stenosis and to exclude intraluminal thrombus or tumour (a contraindication to the procedure).

Following balloon dilatation the stent is positioned across the stricture and a postplacement cavagram is performed to confirm patency and free flow of blood into the right atrium. After stent placement (Fig. 7.1.18), relief of symptoms of superior vena cava obstruction is usually rapid and dramatic. Complications, such as rupture of the vessel, seem surprisingly rare.

The role of intravascular stents in non-malignant obstruction of the superior vena cava has not been clearly established. Patients with obstruction due to fibrosing mediastinitis have been successfully treated,[134,135] although the frequency of late recurrence of the stenosis because of progression of the mediastinal fibrosis or endothelial proliferation within the superior vena cava is not documented.

Image-guided percutaneous drainage procedures

The application of percutaneous drainage techniques of fluid collections within the thorax has increased with improved image guidance, particularly ultrasonography and CT (Fig. 7.1.19); a further advantage of these techniques is the ability to identify septations within the pleural collection and distant loculations, respectively. Supplementary techniques include the instillation of fibrinolytic agents for the treatment of loculated empyemas[29,136,137] and sclerotherapy for malignant effusions.[138,139]

The indications for therapeutic percutaneous drainage of an intrathoracic fluid collection range from the relief of symptoms

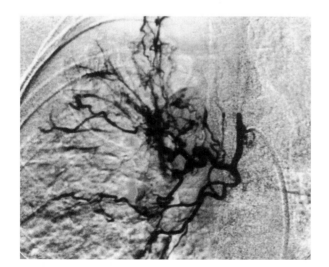

Fig. 7.1.17 Digital subtraction bronchial arteriogram of a patient with cystic fibrosis prior to embolisation. The main right bronchial artery and its branches are considerably hypertrophied.

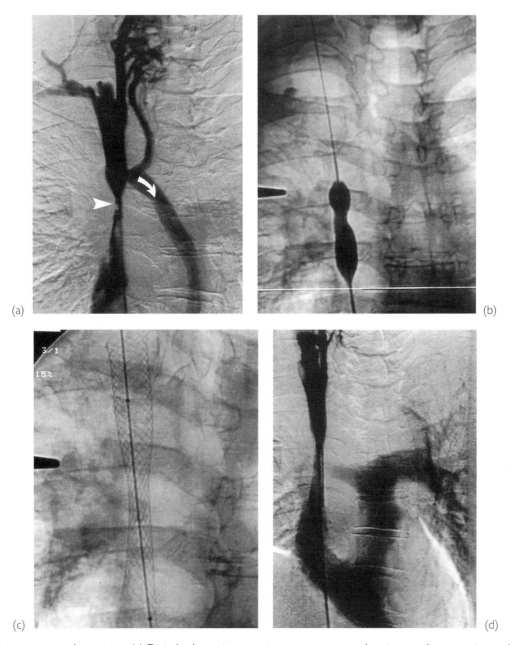

(a)

(b)

(c)

(d)

Fig. 7.1.18 Superior vena cava obstruction. (a) Digital subtraction superior vena cavagram showing a malignant stricture (arrowhead) and retrograde flow down the azygos vein (arrow). (b) Balloon angioplasty of the stricture. (c) Magnified view of the stent traversing the dilated stricture. (d) Post-stenting cavagram showing rapid flow through the superior vena cava into the right heart and pulmonary arteries.

caused by the mass effect of a large effusion to drainage of an empyema or infected bulla, a mediastinal pus collection (e.g. post-sternotomy) or a sterile chronic pleural collection, e.g. a malignant effusion. The indications and technique for the drainage of intrapulmonary abscesses are in most respects similar to those for drainage of a pleural collection. While the indications for drainage of a subacute pleural effusion depend largely on its size, chronicity and aetiology, opinions on the timing and method of drainage are highly variable and usually reflect whether the patient is being managed by a physician or a surgeon.

Patient selection is probably the most important factor in determining the success of percutaneous drainage of a pleural collection. For example, young children usually do not readily tolerate an indwelling chest drainage tube while, conversely, frail or elderly patients may be better served by percutaneous drainage than by undergoing a surgical procedure. There are no absolute contraindications to the percutaneous drainage of intrathoracic fluid collections apart from severely impaired haemostasis or a patient who is unable to co-operate. The choice of imaging guidance lies between ultrasonography or CT and is determined by the site and size of the collection as well as the operator's preference.

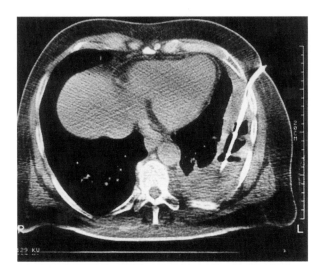

Fig. 7.1.19 CT guidance allowing precise placement of a chest drain in an empyema.

There are many different types of chest drainage catheter, each with its own advocate. One of the most commonly used is a polyethylene nephrostomy-type pigtail catheter (8–10 F). The two design features of a drainage catheter that are most likely to influence successful drainage of a collection are the internal luminal diameter and number of side holes: a larger-bore drainage catheter (14–24 F) is less likely to clog when the collection contains fibrinous material or necrotic debris. Smaller-bore tubes are better tolerated by many patients, especially children, and drainage catheters as small as 8 F are satisfactory in most cases.

It is useful, and generally easy, to establish from the preliminary imaging of the patient whether the fluid collection lies within the pleural space or the lung: in patients with severe bullous emphysema this may be impossible, even with CT. Ultrasonography is a quick and efficient technique for identifying pleural collections, providing there is no subcutaneous air or calcification in the pleural rind to prevent sonographic access. Ultrasonography can also be used for localising intrapulmonary abscesses, again provided there is no aerated lung between the abscess and chest wall.

Fibrinolytic agents have a place in the treatment of multi-loculated empyemas and provide a useful non-surgical alternative for many patients.[28,29]

Patients with malignant pleural effusions that have been drained with small-bore drainage catheters may be treated by instilling sclerosing agents, such as bleomycin or doxycycline, into the pleural space in an attempt to prevent reaccumulation of the effusion.[139–141]

It is difficult to establish the success rate of image-guided drainage of pleural and intrapulmonary collections because of the wide variations in patient selection, technique and aftercare. This last factor is particularly important and is often overlooked by radiologists: in one series, 59% of patients who had had chest or abdominal catheters placed by radiologists were found to have catheter-related problems that were discovered on daily ward rounds following the procedure. At least 30% of these problems required further intervention in the radiology department; the remainder were managed at the bedside. In experienced hands the success rate of image-guided drainage of pleural collections is high.[27,29,142–144] Although fewer, reports of the results of drainage of intrapulmonary abscesses after failed medical management are equally encouraging.[145–147]

Serious complications of percutaneous catheter drainage are rare, the most important being severe haemorrhage. Kinking and blockage of the catheter occur frequently but can often be rectified without replacing it.[148] Inadvertent puncture of major cardiovascular structures or the liver is less frequent with CT guidance and the use of a guide-wire technique. The creation of a bronchopleural fistula is a theoretical possibility when draining a lung abscess but this seems to be an exceedingly rare problem.[142,146,147]

Interpretation of the chest radiograph

Even when there is an obvious radiographic abnormality, there is much to recommend a careful and systematic method of reviewing a chest radiograph. Such an approach will increase the recognition of normal anatomical variations with time. With increasing experience an appreciation of deviation from normal appearances becomes more rapid and this leads quickly to a directed search for related abnormalities. When interpreting a chest radiograph, it is important to establish whether there are any previous radiographs for comparison: the sequence and pattern of radiographic change is often as important as the identification of an abnormality. Information gained from preceding radiographs, particularly the lack of serial change, will often prevent needless further investigation. Demographic details, particularly the age and racial origin of the patient, should be noted, since this information may refine a differential diagnosis based on the radiographic findings alone.

A quick check that the radiograph is of satisfactory quality includes an estimation of the radiographic exposure, depth of inspiration and position of the patient. As a general rule, the intervertebral disc spaces of the entire dorsal spine should be visible on a correctly exposed high-kilovoltage radiograph; the midpoint of the right hemidiaphragm lies at the level of the anterior end of the sixth rib if the patient has taken a satisfactory breath in. The patient is not rotated if the medial ends of the clavicles are equidistant from the spinous process of the cervical vertebral body at that level.

The order in which the structures on a chest radiograph are analysed is unimportant. A suggested sequence is to start with an evaluation of the position of the trachea, the mediastinal contour (which should be clearly outlined in its entirety) and then the position, outline and density of the hilar shadows. Only then are the lungs examined, taking into account their size, the relative transradiancy of each zone, and the position of the horizontal fissure (and any other indirect signs of volume loss – see section on lobar collapse, below). Pulmonary vessels are seen as far as the outer third of the lung and the number of vessels should be symmetrical on the two sides. Next, the position and clarity of the hemidiaphragms should be noted, followed by an assessment of the ribs and soft tissues of the chest wall. Special care should be taken to look for pleural thickening along the lateral chest walls, which may easily be overlooked.

It is useful to become accustomed to viewing a lateral film in the same orientation whether it is a right or left lateral projection. Familiarity with the same orientation improves the viewer's ability to detect deviations from normal. The trachea is angled slightly posteriorly as it runs towards the carina and the posterior wall of the trachea is always visible as a fine stripe. Furthermore, the posterior walls of the right main bronchus and the right intermediate bronchus are outlined by air and are also seen as a continuous stripe on the lateral radiograph. The spines of the scapulae are invariably seen running almost vertically in the upper part of the lateral radiograph and they should not be confused with intrathoracic structures. Further spurious shadows are formed by the soft tissues of the outstretched arms, which are projected over the anterior and superior mediastinum. Although the carina is not visible on the lateral radiograph, the two transradiancies projected over the lower trachea represent the right main bronchus (superiorly) and the left main bronchus (inferiorly).

More lung is obscured by overlying structures on a lateral radiograph than on the frontal view. The unobscured lung in the retrosternal and retrocardiac regions should be of the same transradiancy. Furthermore, as the eye travels down the dorsal spine, the viewer should be aware of a gradual increase in transradiancy. The loss of this phenomenon suggests the presence of disease in the posterobasal segments of the lower lobes (sometimes not visible on the frontal radiograph).

All the branching structures seen within the lungs on a chest radiograph represent either pulmonary arteries or veins. The larger pulmonary vessels can be traced back to the hila and mediastinum. The pulmonary veins can sometimes be differentiated from the pulmonary arteries: the superior pulmonary veins have a characteristically vertical course, but in practice it is often impossible to distinguish arteries from veins in the outer two-thirds of the lung. On a chest radiograph taken in the erect position, there is a gradual increase in the diameter of the vessels, at equidistant points from the hilum, travelling from lung apex to base; this is a gravity-dependent effect and is abolished if the patient is supine or in cardiac failure.

The two major fissures are seen as diagonal lines on a lateral radiograph, often incomplete and of a hair's breadth, running from the upper dorsal spine to the anterior surface of the diaphragm. Care must be taken not to confuse the obliquely running edges of ribs with fissures. The minor fissure extends horizontally from the mid right major fissure. It is often not possible to distinguish the right from the left major fissures with confidence. Similarly, although the two hemidiaphragms may be identified individually (especially if the gastric bubble is visible under the left dome of the diaphragm), the distinction between the right and the left is sometimes impossible. A helpful sign is the relative heights of the two domes: the dome furthest from the film is usually considerably higher because of magnification.

The summation of both hila on the lateral radiograph generates a complex shadow. However, there are some generalisations that aid the interpretation of this difficult area. The right pulmonary artery lies anterior to the trachea and right main bronchus whereas the left pulmonary artery hooks over the left main bronchus so that most of it lies posterior to the major bronchi. As a result, any mass identified on a PA and lateral radiograph that lies anterior to the left hilum or posterior to the right hilum is not vascular in origin and is most likely to represent enlarged hilar lymph nodes. A band-like opacity is often seen along the lower third of the anterior chest wall behind the sternum on the lateral chest radiograph. This represents a normal density and occurs because there is less aerated lung in contact with the chest wall because the space is occupied by the heart; it should not be confused with pleural disease.

Before assigning normality to a chest radiograph, it is worth reviewing areas that are either poorly demonstrated on chest radiography or often misinterpreted. These include:

- the central mediastinum, where even a large mass may be barely visible on the PA view
- the areas behind the heart and hemidiaphragms
- the lung apices, often obscured by overlying clavicle and ribs
- the lung and pleura just inside the chest wall.

Once a radiographic abnormality has been detected it should be considered in terms of gross pathology. Both the site and the radiographic characteristics of the lesion will allow the observer to proceed to, at the very least, a generic diagnosis. A precise histopathological diagnosis can only rarely be achieved from the radiographic appearances alone without knowledge of the clinical context.

Basic radiographic signs of disease

Pulmonary consolidation

Consolidation describes the state of the lungs when the normal air-filled spaces distal to the bronchi are occupied by the products of disease (the most obvious examples being pulmonary oedema or inflammatory exudate). The most important radiographic signs of pulmonary consolidation are:

- an area of increased opacification in the lungs, which obscures the underlying blood vessels and has a poorly defined margin (unless it is bounded by a fissure; Fig. 7.1.20)
- an 'air bronchogram'
- the 'silhouette sign'.

The air bronchogram is seen as a radiolucent branching structure of the bronchi against a more opaque background of airless consolidated lung. It is a distinctive and reliable sign of pulmonary consolidation. However, an air bronchogram may also be present when lung has become collapsed and airless, e.g. because of a large surrounding pleural effusion. The silhouette sign is seen when the normally clear border of a structure is lost because the aerated lung outlining the border is replaced by fluid or a mass (the term is actually a misnomer: it could be more accurately called the 'lost silhouette sign'). Recognition of this sign can help to localise the area of abnormality within the lungs; for example, consolidation in the lingula makes the left heart border indistinct. As with the air bronchogram sign, the silhouette sign may be seen in either pulmonary consolidation or collapse. For example, loss of a clear right heart border may be due to right middle lobe consolidation with or without col-

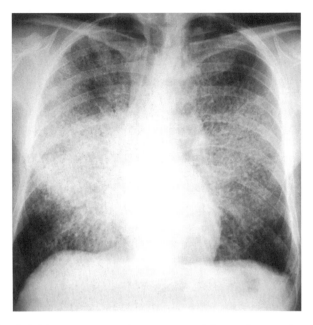

Fig. 7.1.20 Extensive pulmonary consolidation due to alveolar proteinosis. The loss the silhouette of the right heart border indicates that some of the disease involves the right middle lobe.

lapse of the lobe or medial segment; common to collapse and consolidation is loss of normal aeration of the affected lung. The causes of widespread pulmonary consolidation are numerous but may usefully be divided into the broad categories shown in Table 7.1.3.

Table 7.1.3 Causes of widespread pulmonary consolidation

Pulmonary oedema	Cardiogenic oedema/fluid overload Adult respiratory distress syndrome Inhalational injury (noxious gases) Drug abuse Neurogenic (raised intracranial pressure or head injury) Renal disease Fat embolism
Exudate	Infective consolidation Acute extrinsic allergic alveolitis Eosinophilic lung disease Cryptogenic organising pneumonia Radiation pneumonitis
Neoplasm	Bronchioloalveolar cell carcinoma Lymphoproliferative disorders
Blood	Contusion Infarction Idiopathic pulmonary haemorrhage (Goodpasture's syndrome)
Other	Alveolar proteinosis Sarcoidosis

Pulmonary collapse

The word 'collapse' is used to describe loss of aeration, and consequent deflation, of the lung. Depending on the cause, collapse may occur at any level from small, subsegmental areas of lung through to an entire lung. Although used synonymously, the term 'atelectasis' is preferred by some because, unlike 'collapse', it does not imply complete loss of volume.[149] Small areas of subsegmental atelectasis occur very commonly in debilitated and postoperative patients, where they are seen as short, linear, usually horizontal, opacities. At the other end of the spectrum, collapse of an entire lung, most commonly as a result of an endobronchial lesion, has a dramatic radiographic appearance with complete opacification of the affected lung and consequent loss of volume of that hemithorax. At the lobar level, the signs of collapse of an individual lobe are characteristic but, depending on the lobe, may be subtle. Recognition of the collapse of individual lobes is important and merits a detailed description.

Collapse of individual lobes

Right upper lobe (Fig. 7.1.21a). On the frontal radiograph there is elevation of the minor fissure and of the right hilum. If the collapse is complete, the non-aerated lobe is seen as a density alongside the superior mediastinum. On the lateral view the minor fissure moves upwards and the major fissure moves forwards. The retrosternal area becomes progressively more opaque and the anterior margin of the ascending aorta becomes obscured.

Right middle lobe (Fig. 7.1.21b). On the frontal radiograph the lateral part of the minor fissure moves down. There is blurring of the normally sharp right heart border; this may be a subtle abnormality and is easily overlooked. On the lateral view the minor fissure moves downwards and lower half of the major fissure moves forwards, giving rise to a triangular shadow with its apex at the hilum and the base against the lower sternum.

Right lower lobe (Fig. 7.1.21c). There is an increase in density overlying and obscuring the medial portion of the right hemidiaphragm and the right hilum is depressed on the frontal radiograph. In contrast to right middle lobe collapse, the right heart border usually remains sharply defined, since this is in contact with the aerated right middle lobe. On the lateral view the major fissure moves posteriorly and inferiorly; with further collapse there is a loss of definition of the posterior part of the right hemidiaphragm as well as increased density overlying the lower dorsal vertebral column.

Left upper lobe (Fig. 7.1.21d). The characteristic finding on the frontal radiograph is a veil-like increase in density, without a sharp margin (quite unlike right upper lobe collapse), spreading upwards and outwards from the elevated left hilum. The outlines of the aortic knuckle, left hilum and left heart border become ill-defined. As the collapse increases, the lobe moves centrally and the apical segment of the left lower lobe expands to fill the space left by the collapsed upper lobe: this is the cause of the relative transradiancy at the apex of the left lung. With complete left upper lobe collapse, a sharp border may return to the aortic arch because it becomes surrounded by the hyperinflated apical segment of the lower lobe. On the lateral view the major fissure moves superiorly and anteriorly while remaining relatively vertical and roughly parallel to the anterior chest wall.

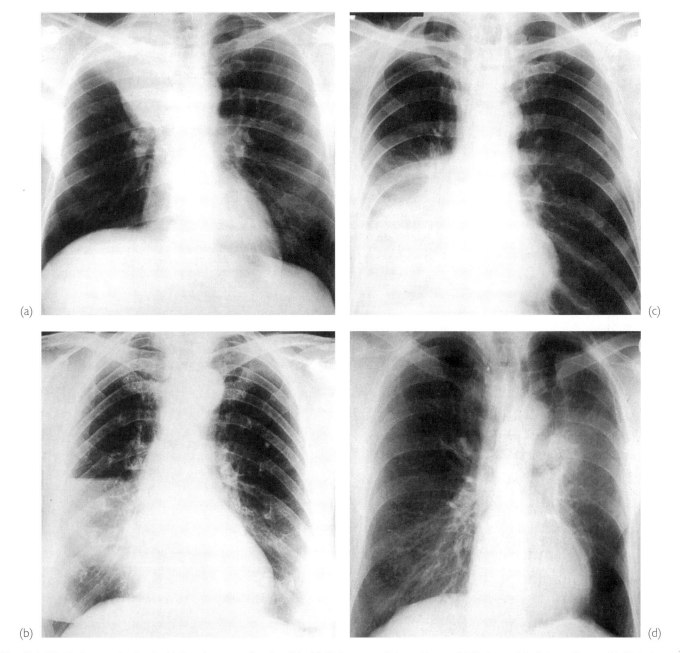

Fig. 7.1.21 Collapse of individual lobes (see text for details). (a) Right upper lobe collapse. (b) Right middle lobe collapse. (c) Right lower lobe collapse. (d) Left upper lobe collapse. (e) Left lower lobe collapse.

Left lower lobe (Fig. 7.1.21e). On the frontal radiograph there is a triangular opacity behind the heart with loss of the medial part of the left hemidiaphragm; even on a properly exposed radiograph it may be difficult to appreciate the collapsed lobe behind the heart. Supplementary signs include inferior displacement of the left hilum, loss of volume and increased transradiancy of the left hemithorax. On the lateral view there is posterior displacement of the major fissure. As with right lower lobe collapse, there is increased density over the lower dorsal vertebral column and the posterior part of the left hemidiaphragm is effaced.

Complete opacification (a 'white-out') of a hemithorax is generally due to either complete collapse of a lung or a large pleural effusion or tumour. Shift of the mediastinum to the affected side implies that volume loss, i.e. collapse of the lung, has occurred. In contrast, a pleural effusion or soft tissue mass that is large enough to cause complete opacification of a hemithorax will almost invariably displace the mediastinum away from the side of the opacified hemithorax. An important exception is an advanced mesothelioma, which may encase one lung and 'freeze' the mediastinum, thus preventing contralateral mediastinal shift. Occasionally, when there is no obvious shift of the mediastinum, it may be surprisingly difficult to differentiate between these two completely different causes of an opacified hemithorax. In these instances, ultrasonography and CT allow

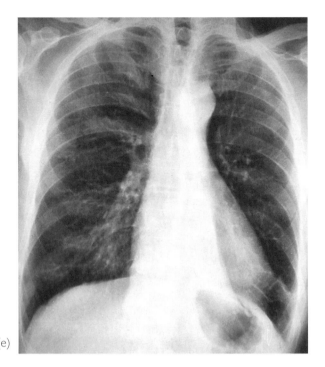

(e)

Fig. 7.1.21 *Continued*

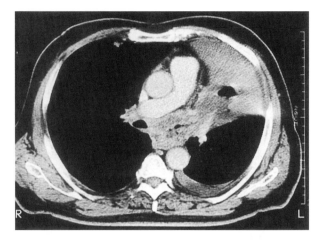

Fig. 7.1.22 Necrotic bronchogenic carcinoma surrounding the left main bronchus and causing left upper lobe collapse. The tumour mass extends centrally between the right pulmonary artery and descending aorta into the subcarinal region.

the distinction to be made with confidence and provide further information about the underlying cause.

The pulmonary nodule or mass

Many pulmonary masses are discovered incidentally on a chest radiograph. Whenever possible, previous films should be obtained so that the growth rate of the lesion can be estimated. The growth rate is a more reliable indicator of the likely nature of a pulmonary mass than any one of its radiographic features. If a lesion doubles in volume (increases in diameter by approximately 25% on serial chest radiographs) in less than 1 week or more than 18 months, it is unlikely to be malignant: the doubling time of most malignant lesions is between 1 and 6 months, although exceptions to this rule do occur.

Over the years much importance has been attached to the radiological characteristics of a solitary pulmonary mass in an attempt to make the crucial distinction between benign and malignant lesions. With the possible exception of heavy calcification within the lesion (most commonly seen in ancient granulomas), no radiological appearance will reliably differentiate a benign from a malignant mass. Although generalisations can be made about the radiographic features of benign and malignant lesions (e.g. bronchial carcinomas have irregular and spiculated margins whereas benign lesions are more likely to have a smooth outline), in a given patient it is not safe to rely on these radiographic features alone. The same applies to the individual morphological features of a nodule detected on computed tomography.[150] However, malignant nodules have been shown to have different contrast enhancement characteristics from benign nodules[151] and this may be useful in determining which patients need incidentally detected nodules to be followed or resected.

After the discovery of a pulmonary mass on chest radiography, the need for further imaging of a patient will depend on the symptomatology, age and smoking history of the patient and results of other investigations. In patients with lung cancer, computed tomography is useful for evaluating extension of a central mass into the mediastinum[152] (Fig. 7.1.22), for demonstrating the presence or absence of enlarged mediastinal lymph nodes which may indicate local tumour spread[153] and for the detection of distant metastases (e.g. to the contralateral lung, adrenal glands or liver). The absolute size of mediastinal lymph nodes identified on a staging CT is not a very reliable indicator of malignant involvement.[154] Although markedly enlarged lymph nodes, greater than 2 cm in diameter, often signify malignant spread, enlargement of lymph nodes may also represent reactive hyperplasia of little clinical significance. Conversely, small-volume lymph nodes or lymph nodes not identified by CT may sometimes contain micrometastases from a distant primary neoplasm, particularly an adenocarcinoma. CT is generally regarded as complementary to mediastinoscopic examination and sampling of lymph nodes in staging patients.[155-157] Positron emission tomography is increasingly being used because of its superior (but not infallible) sensitivity for what may be small-volume (and therefore undetectable by CT) distant metastases.[158,159]

Cavitating pulmonary masses

The radiological definition of cavitation is a lucency, representing air, within a mass or area of consolidation. The cavity may or may not contain a fluid level or an intracavitary body and is surrounded by a wall of variable thickness and irregularity. The two commonest diagnoses in an adult presenting with a cavitating pulmonary mass on chest radiography are bronchial carcinoma (central, large, and often squamous in type; Fig. 7.1.23) or a lung abscess (usually peripheral and often multiple). Cavitation in areas of consolidation is seen in a variety of bacterial pneumonias, particularly those due to tuberculosis, *Staphylococcus* spp., *Klebsiella* spp. and anaerobes. Less commonly, cavitation is seen within pulmonary infarcts, which may be sterile or infected, and

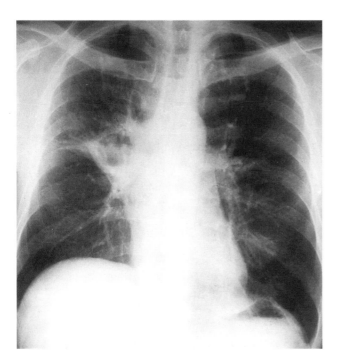

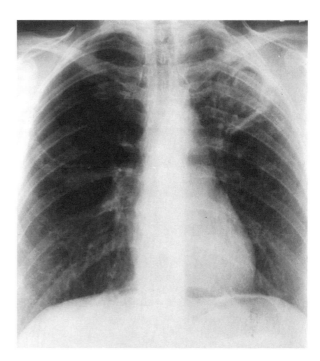

Fig. 7.1.23 Cavitating squamous cell bronchogenic carcinoma. The elevation of the right hemidiaphragm was due to phrenic nerve involvement.

Fig. 7.1.24 The air-crescent sign in the left upper lobe, caused by a fungus ball in a post-tuberculous fibrotic cavity.

in areas of pulmonary contusion due to trauma. Multiple cavitating nodules are a feature of many diseases (including septic emboli, pulmonary metastases and Wegener's granulomatosis) and it is usually the clinical features rather than the radiographic appearances alone that suggest the aetiology. Long-standing cavities in lungs scarred by previous tuberculosis predispose to the formation of mycetomas; once these fungus balls occupy most of the cavity, a characteristic translucent 'air-crescent sign' may be seen between the upper surface of the fungus ball and the margin of the cavity (Fig. 7.1.24).

Multiple pulmonary nodules

Many conditions are characterised by multiple small pulmonary nodules. Only by combining the relevant clinical information with a description of the size and distribution of the nodules can the differential diagnosis be narrowed. In the UK, one of the commonest causes of multiple pulmonary nodules of varying sizes in an adult is disseminated malignancy (Fig. 7.1.25), whereas in some parts of southern USA, where histoplasmosis is endemic, pulmonary granulomas would be a commoner cause. A myriad of small nodules less than 3 mm in diameter produces a pattern that is often described as miliary. A list of causes of fine nodular shadowing is given in Table 7.1.4.

As always, comparison with previous radiographs will give invaluable information about the rate of progression and thus the likely nature of the pulmonary nodules. To a lesser extent the distribution of nodules is a consideration in refining the differential diagnosis of multiple pulmonary nodules: for example, the small nodules of pulmonary sarcoidosis tend to be mid-zone and perihilar, whereas haematogenous metastases are generally of varying sizes and have a predilection for the lower lobes, because of increased blood flow to these regions.

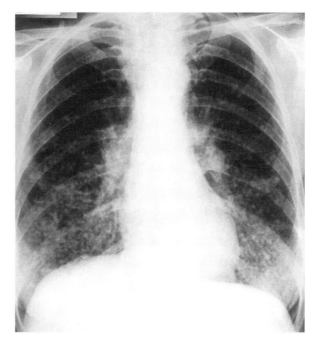

Fig. 7.1.25 Multiple pulmonary metastases varying in size from 3 mm to 6 mm in a patient with a carcinoma of the thyroid.

The density of nodules sometimes provides conclusive evidence that they are benign, e.g. the heavily calcified nodules that are seen following histoplasmosis or chicken pox (varicella) pneumonia. The majority of multiple pulmonary nodules are of soft-tissue density and it may be extremely difficult to judge whether small nodules are of calcific or soft-tissue density

Table 7.1.4 Differential diagnosis of widespread fine nodular shadowing

- Miliary tuberculosis
- Metastatic disease (e.g. melanoma)
- Fungal diseases (e.g. histoplasmosis)
- Sarcoidosis
- Subacute extrinsic allergic alveolitis
- Coal worker's pneumoconiosis
- Idiopathic pulmonary haemorrhage
- Alveolar microlithiasis

because their apparent density depends so critically on the radiographic technique, particularly the voltage used.

Numerous poorly defined, low-density nodules approximately 8 mm in diameter may be seen around areas of pulmonary consolidation. In other areas they may be confluent and so make up a larger, poorly defined opacity. At a pathological level these nodules correspond to individual acini full of, for example, pulmonary oedema, an inflammatory exudate or haemorrhage.

Diffuse lung shadowing

It is important that reproducible terms are used in the description of widespread pulmonary shadowing: vague terms that may convey a pathological meaning (which in fact cannot be inferred from the gross signs of disease on a chest radiograph), e.g. 'inflammatory shadowing', are misleading. Descriptions of the radiographic pattern should ideally be limited to objective terms such as 'reticular' – a fine network, 'nodular' – small dots of a specified size, 'linear' – fine lines that are not vessels, 'ground-glass' – a greying-out of the lungs that makes the vascular markings indistinct (Fig. 7.1.26), and finally 'air-space shadowing' or 'consolidation' – poorly defined areas of opacification in which an air bronchogram may be visible. These descriptors are more reproducible than and preferable to the wide range of imprecise and subjective terms that have been used in the past. Because the morphological detail of interstitial lung diseases are more readily appreciated on cross-sectional imaging, a fuller description of the various types of diffuse lung disease is given in the section on the interpretation of high resolution computed tomography, below.

An analysis of the distribution of the disease on a chest radiograph is often at least as important as a description of the radiographic pattern in reaching a differential diagnosis. This involves an assessment of whether the disease involves all parts of the lung uniformly or whether there is a zonal predominance (upper, mid or lower; central or peripheral). The perihilar, mid- and upper-zone distribution of the reticulonodular pattern in sarcoidosis is quite different from the lower-zone peripheral distribution of cryptogenic fibrosing alveolitis. The differential diagnosis can be further refined by assimilating other radiographic abnormalities, e.g. the presence of pleural disease in the case of asbestosis or enlarged hilar lymph nodes in the case of sarcoidosis or lymphangitis carcinomatosa.

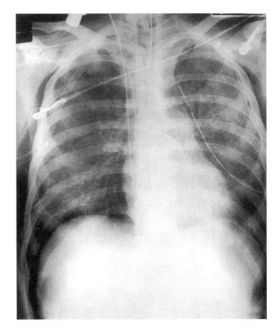

Fig. 7.1.26 Widespread 'ground-glass' pattern obscuring the pulmonary vasculature in a patient with adult respiratory distress syndrome. Note the 'deep-sulcus' sign at both costophrenic angles due to bilateral pneumothoraces in a supine patient.

Increased transradiancy of a hemithorax

There are many causes of increased lucency or transradiancy (darkening) of one hemithorax, ranging from a loss of the soft tissues of the chest wall (e.g. a mastectomy) through to reduced perfusion of one lung due to hypoxic vasoconstriction resulting from underventilation of the lung because of an endobronchial lesion in a main bronchus. It is easy to overlook this important radiographic abnormality when the density difference between the two lungs is slight; a subtle discrepancy in density between the two hemithoraces is more readily appreciated by viewing the radiograph from a distance or through half-closed eyes. The commonest causes of a relatively transradiant hemithorax are shown in Table 7.1.5. Close scrutiny of the chest radiograph will usually indicate which of the categories of causes is responsible for the transradiancy. Specific points to look for are:

- loss of symmetry of the soft tissues of the chest wall
- a discrepancy in the volumes and vascular pattern between the two lungs
- a visceral pleural edge, denoting a pneumothorax.

If there is any clinical suggestion that the cause of the increased transradiancy is an obstructing lesion in a central airway, a chest radiograph taken in full expiration will accentuate the increased transradiancy and will show that the lung fails to empty.

Mediastinum and hilar masses

On a PA chest radiograph the mediastinal structures are superimposed on one another and thus cannot be distinguished individually. The mediastinum is conventionally divided into

Table 7.1.5 Causes of increased transradiancy of one hemithorax

Technical	Rotation of the patient
Chest wall	Loss of soft tissues (radical mastectomy or Poland's syndrome)
Pneumothorax	Particularly in supine patients
Compensatory overinflation	Post lobectomy Overlooked lobar collapse (e.g. left lower lobe) Macleod's syndrome (also caused by reduced perfusion)
Reduced pulmonary perfusion	Hypoxic vasoconstriction due to underventilation caused by an inhaled foreign body or endobronchial tumour Macleod's syndrome Recurrent pulmonary emboli (rarely unilateral)

superior, anterior, middle and posterior compartments; the practical use of these arbitrary divisions is that specific mediastinal pathologies show a definite predilection for individual compartments (e.g. a superior mediastinal mass is most frequently due to intrathoracic extension of the thyroid gland; a middle mediastinal mass is usually due to enlarged lymph nodes). However, it should be borne in mind that the position of a mass within one of these compartments is no guarantee of a specific diagnosis, nor do these boundaries preclude disease from spreading from one compartment to the next.

The density of the cardiac shadow to the left and right of the vertebral column should be identical and any difference signals pulmonary pathology (e.g. consolidation in a lower lobe). A density with a convex lateral border is often seen through the right heart border on a well-penetrated film; this apparent mass is due to the confluence of the pulmonary veins as they enter the left atrium and is of no pathological significance.

The trachea and main bronchi are visible through the upper and middle mediastinum. The trachea is rarely straight and is often to the right of the midline at its midpoint. In elderly patients, the trachea is often dramatically, but inconsequentially, displaced by a dilated aortic arch. The angle of the carina is usually somewhat less than 80°. Splaying of the carina is a sign of gross disease, either in the form of massive subcarinal lymphadenopathy or a markedly enlarged left atrium. A more sensitive, but sometimes subtle, sign of a subcarinal mass is obliteration of the azygo-oesophageal line, which is usually visible on a well-penetrated chest radiograph. The origins of the lobar bronchi, where they are projected over the mediastinal shadow, can usually be made out but the segmental bronchi within the lungs are not generally visible on plain radiography, unless seen end on as ring shadows. The hilar shadows on a chest radiograph are a complex summation of the pulmonary arteries and veins with virtually no contribution from the overlying bronchial walls or normal-sized lymph nodes. The hila are approximately the same size and the left hilum always lies

between 0.5 cm and 1.5 cm above the level of the right hilum. The size and shape of the normal hila show great variation from one individual to another so that subtle abnormalities are difficult to detect. At least as important as an abnormal contour in detecting a mass at the hilum is a discrepancy in density between the two hila: both hilar shadows, at equivalent points, will be of equal density and a mass at the hilum (or an intrapulmonary mass projected over the hilum) will be evident as increased density of that hilum.

Pleural and chest wall disease

Because of the two-dimensional nature of a PA chest radiograph, abnormalities originating in the pleura or chest wall are often difficult to assess. The appearance of a pleural mass on chest radiography depends on whether it is face-on or tangential to the X-ray beam. Generally, a pleural mass will produce a smoothly rounded opacity with a sharp medial border and a less well-defined lateral margin. Although an abnormality of an adjacent rib suggests that an apparent 'pleural' mass is actually of chest-wall origin, the distinction between pleural and chest-wall pathology often cannot be made from a chest radiograph alone.

With extensive pleural pathology it may be difficult to distinguish a pleural effusion, chronic pleural thickening or even a neoplasm of the pleura such as a mesothelioma, and in such cases cross-sectional imaging is invaluable. For example, CT will reveal abnormalities not shown on a plain chest radiograph, such as flecks of calcification within the wall of a chronic empyema (Fig. 7.1.27) or early rib abnormalities in the case of a neoplasm. Furthermore, masses arising from the chest wall that give the appearance of a 'pleural' mass, such as an intercostal lipoma, are readily apparent on CT.

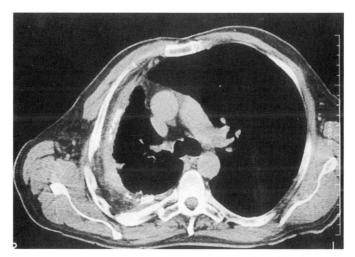

Fig. 7.1.27 Contraction of the right hemithorax secondary to a presumed old tuberculous empyema. The flecks of calcification in the thickened pleura were not visible on an accompanying high-kilovoltage chest radiograph.

Spiral computed tomography for pulmonary embolism

Until the last few years, the traditional diagnostic imaging procedures for the detection of pulmonary embolism were ventilation–perfusion scintigraphy and pulmonary angiography. Recently, pulmonary angiography has progressively been replaced by spiral CT angiography, which allows non-invasive identification of intravascular clots. The CT criteria for acute pulmonary embolism are the equivalent of the classical arteriographic signs of pulmonary embolism, i.e. partial or complete filling defects within an opacified artery (Fig. 7.1.28). It is not generally possible, even with an optimal technique, to detect pulmonary emboli beyond fourth-order vessels (approximately 7 mm in diameter),[160,161] and a negative spiral CT does not exclude small peripheral emboli.

There are many technical factors that may conspire to reduce the diagnostic accuracy of spiral CT for the detection of pulmonary embolism.[162-166] Contrast-enhanced spiral CT should ideally be preceded by an unenhanced scan that covers the entire thorax (a thin section interspaced protocol is usually sufficient). This precontrast scan may reveal secondary features of pulmonary embolism, such as small peripheral infarcts in the costophrenic recesses, pleural effusions or a mosaic perfusion pattern, or an alternative diagnosis to explain the patient's symptoms.[167-170]

When contrast can flow around an embolus, the appearance is of a central or eccentrically placed filling defect within the artery lumen on perpendicular sections, or of a 'railway track' if the artery lies parallel and within the plane of section.[171] If there is complete occlusion of a pulmonary artery by clot, so that there is no surrounding contrast, a pulmonary embolus may be less obvious.

Chronic pulmonary emboli usually appear as crescentic thrombi adhering to the arterial wall; the thrombus may contain calcifications and may show signs of recanalisation.[165,172-174] In patients with severe chronic thromboembolic disease there may be an obvious mosaic perfusion pattern.

Interpretive pitfalls

There are several technical and patient-related causes of misinterpretation of a spiral CT examination. The cause of false-negative results in the segmental, lobar and central pulmonary arteries is almost invariably faulty technique. Lymph nodes immediately adjacent to the central and segmental pulmonary arteries are a common cause of false-positive diagnoses of pulmonary embolism (Fig. 7.1.29).[175,176]

Accuracy of spiral CT in pulmonary embolism

The range of non-diagnostic spiral CT for pulmonary embolism is low (between 2% and 9%).[168,177] This compares favourably with the rate of non-diagnostic $\dot{V}/\dot{Q}$ scans, which is reportedly anywhere between 28% and 87%.[178] In studies including more than 50 patients, the range of sensitivity for spiral CT is 75–96%[170,179] and the range of specificity 76–100%.[177,180] Furthermore, interobserver agreement appears to be good for spiral CT, compared with ventilation–perfusion scanning.[180] In a multicenter European study, observer agreement for spiral CT ($\kappa = 0.72$) was superior to pulmonary angiography ($\kappa = 0.46$) which was in turn superior to ventilation–perfusion scanning ($\kappa = 0.39$).[181]

The spiral CT protocols used in most centres are not designed to detect emboli at the subsegmental pulmonary artery level. Although detection of small subsegmental emboli is possible with pulmonary arteriography, observer agreement at this anatomical level is low (45–66% of cases).[182,183] Questions about

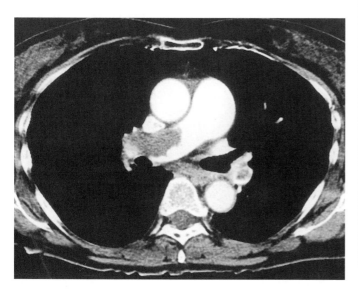

Fig. 7.1.28 Contrast-enhanced spiral CT scan showing filling defects representing emboli in the right and left pulmonary arteries.

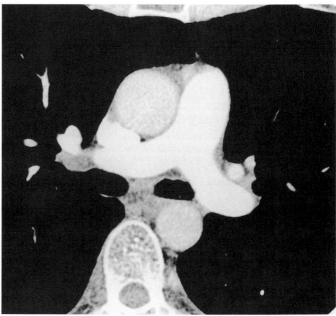

Fig. 7.1.29 Spiral CT for suspected pulmonary embolism. The apparent (low-density) filling defect in the right pulmonary artery is a fibro-fatty lymph node, not an embolus.

the prevalence of emboli confined to the subsegmental pulmonary arteries (anywhere between 2% and 36%[109,184,185]) and their significance remain. The effects of a small subsegmental embolus will be negligible in normal individuals but may be serious in patients with severe cardiopulmonary disease.

There are numerous prescriptive guidelines about which imaging test should be used in patients with suspected pulmonary embolism but the availability of various tests, rather than considerations of diagnostic accuracy, often dictate the sequence of investigations. One approach that has much to recommend it relies on the high specificity of a normal perfusion scintigram and the stratification of patients into outpatients (typically patients with a low pretest probability of pulmonary embolism and no pulmonary disease apparent on chest radiography) and inpatients (patients with a higher probability of pulmonary embolism and often with pre-existing cardiopulmonary disease). For patients with symptoms of deep venous thrombosis and pulmonary embolism, ultrasound of the lower limbs is the first test. A discussion about the potential role of spiral CT in the detection of acute pulmonary embolism can be found in a debate between experts.[186]

In terms of the cost-effectiveness of various strategies used in the investigation of suspected pulmonary embolism, an analysis of 15 combinations of six diagnostic tests (spiral CT, lower limb ultrasonography, $\dot{V}/\dot{Q}$ scanning, pulmonary arteriography and D-dimer plasma levels) has shown that the five most effective strategies (least mortality at 3 months and lowest associated costs per life saved) all include spiral CT, usually in combination with lower limb ultrasonography.[187] A novel approach is the combination of lower limb CT venography and CT pulmonary angiography in a single examination.[188]

Interpretation of high-resolution computed tomography of the lungs

Normal anatomy

Accurate interpretation of HRCT of the lung requires an appreciation of the normal appearances of the bronchi, blood vessels and secondary pulmonary lobules. Throughout the lung the bronchi and pulmonary arteries run and branch together. Both taper slightly as they travel radially; this is most obvious in bronchi running within and parallel to the plane of section. At any given level, the diameter of the bronchus is the same or marginally less than its accompanying artery. The bronchovascular bundle is surrounded by a connective tissue sheath from its origin at the hilum to the respiratory bronchioles in the lung periphery. The concept of separate, but connected, components making up the lung interstitium, propounded by Weibel,[189] is important to the understanding of HRCT findings in interstitial lung disease: the 'peripheral' interstitium surrounds the surface of the lung beneath the visceral pleura and penetrates the lung to surround the secondary pulmonary lobules. Within the lobules, a finer network of 'septal' connective tissue fibres support the alveoli. The 'axial' fibres form a sheath around the bronchovascular bundles extending from the pulmonary hila to

the lung periphery, as far out as the alveolar ducts and sacs. The important point is that the connective tissue stroma of these three separate components are in continuity and thus form a fibrous skeleton for the lungs.

The interface between the bronchovascular bundle and surrounding lung is normally very sharp on HRCT. Any thickening of the connective tissue interstitium will result in apparent bronchial wall thickening and blurring of this interface. The size of the smallest subsegmental bronchi visible on HRCT is determined by the thickness of the bronchial wall rather than the diameter of the bronchus. In general, bronchi with a diameter of less than 3 mm and walls less than 300 μm thick are not identifiable on HRCT.[190-192] Airways reach this size about 3 cm from the surface of the pleura.

The secondary pulmonary lobule is the smallest anatomical unit of the lung surrounded by a connective tissue septum. Within the septa are lymphatic channels and venules. Thickening of the septa between the lobules are responsible for the Kerley B lines seen on the chest radiograph. The lobule contains a variable number of acini, which each measure approximately 6–10 mm in diameter. Each lobule is approximately 2 cm in diameter and has a polyhedral shape, sometimes resembling a misshapen or truncated cone.[193,194] In the lung periphery the base of the cone-shaped lobules lies on a visceral pleural surface and the centrilobular bronchiole and pulmonary artery, each approximately 1 mm in diameter, enter through the apex of the lobule (Fig. 7.1.30).

The connective tissue interlobular septa are well-developed in the subpleural regions, particularly on the diaphragmatic surfaces and anterolateral regions of the lungs. In normal individuals, these interlobular septa measure approximately 100 μm in thickness. Because the lower limit of effective resolution of HRCT in vivo is approximately 300 μm, these structures are usually invisible on HRCT. The few interlobular septa that are visible in normal individuals are usually inconspicuous and are seen as straight lines 1–2 cm in length terminating at a visceral pleural surface (Fig. 7.1.30). Sometimes, several septa joining end to end are seen as a non-branching linear structure measuring up to 4 cm;[192] these are most frequent at the lung bases just above the diaphragmatic surface. Deep within the lung, where the septa are less well developed, these interlobular septa are only recognisable when they are pathologically thickened.

Distribution and patterns of disease on high-resolution computed tomography

A frontal chest radiograph provides valuable information about the distribution of diffuse lung disease: for example, a central or lower zonal predominance may help to narrow the differential diagnosis. Nevertheless, the radiographic pattern of distribution of diffuse lung disease may sometimes be more apparent than real. Some diseases that macroscopically have a truly uniform distribution throughout the lung parenchyma appear to have a mid- and lower-zone predominance on a frontal chest radiograph. In extrinsic allergic alveolitis in the subacute phase, the poorly defined nodular or ground-glass pattern on a chest radiograph appears to be most pronounced in the mid and lower zones.[191] By

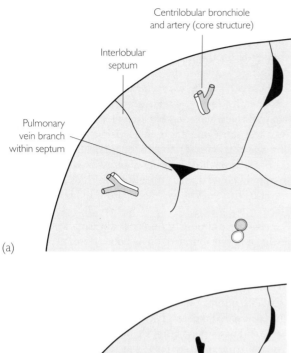

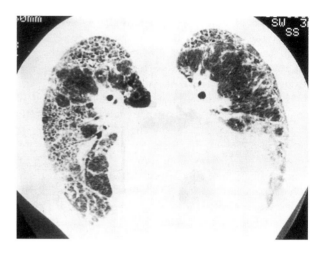

Fig. 7.1.31 A patient with usual interstitial pneumonitis showing the typical subpleural honeycomb pattern (patient scanned in the prone position).

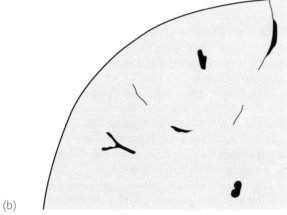

Fig. 7.1.30 (a) Schema of the anatomy of the secondary pulmonary lobule. (b) Structures visible on a corresponding HRCT section; note that the lumina of the bronchioles are not resolved.

contrast the distribution of the nodular or ground-glass pattern on CT in patients with subacute extrinsic allergic alveolitis is seen as uniform, with no zonal predominance.[195] The impression of a concentration of disease in the lower zones on chest radiography can be explained by the greater width of lung traversed by the X-ray beam in the lower zones, resulting in summation of innumerable foci of disease and thus greater X-ray attenuation.[196]

The cross-sectional nature of CT gives an accurate estimation of the uniformity of diffuse disease or the zonal distribution, in both transverse and longitudinal axes. In fibrosing alveolitis (usual interstitial pneumonia subtype) a lower zone and subpleural concentration of disease is typical and it is this distribution that is virtually pathognomonic[197] (Fig. 7.1.31). Quite subtle regional variations in the frequency of lesions may be a pointer to the diagnosis. For example, in Langerhans cell histiocytosis, the lower third of the lung is relatively unaffected and the disease rarely extends into the costophrenic recesses or the anteromedial tips of the right middle lobe and lingula.

Not only does CT confirm the general distribution of disease that may be evident on chest radiography, it also gives important

information about the distribution of disease in relation to the bronchovascular bundles, secondary pulmonary lobules and visceral pleura. Peribronchial disease is elegantly shown by HRCT, particularly around bronchovascular bundles that lie along the plane of section. Conditions that show a 'bronchocentric' distribution are typified by sarcoidosis and lymphangitis carcinomatosa (Fig. 7.1.32) and these diseases tend to have a more central distribution because of the confluence of bronchovascular tree towards the hilum. The demonstration of a bronchocentric distribution is of practical clinical use since it predicts that a transbronchial biopsy is likely to obtain diagnostic material.[198]

The close correlation between HRCT appearances and macroscopic pathological abnormalities often allows accurate anatomical terms to be used in describing patterns of diffuse lung disease. Inexact descriptive terms, so often used in the analysis of plain chest radiographs, can be replaced by precise morphological terms derived from an understanding of normal HRCT anatomy. Nevertheless, there are a few non-specific findings on HRCT that do not always have a definite counterpart at

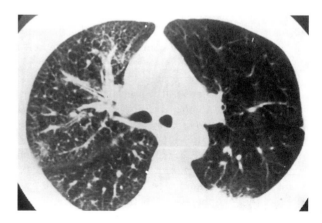

Fig. 7.1.32 Computed tomography scan of a patient with lymphangitis carcinomatosa, showing unilateral thickening of the bronchovascular bundles in the right upper lobe due to infiltration by adenocarcinoma.

a pathological level. Abnormal patterns on HRCT that denote pulmonary disease were initially given many names[66,199,200] but there has been much rationalisation and HRCT abnormalities can be broadly categorised into one of four patterns:

- reticular and short linear opacities
- nodular opacities
- increased lung opacity ('ground-glass')
- cystic air spaces and areas of decreased lung density.

While these HRCT patterns have their corresponding patterns on chest radiography, they are seen with much greater clarity on the cross-sectional images of HRCT and the precise distribution of disease can be more readily appreciated.

Reticular pattern

A reticular pattern recognised on HRCT almost always indicates significant interstitial disease. A reticular pattern due to thickening of interlobular septa is a frequent finding in many different interstitial lung diseases. Numerous interlobular septa that join up to form polygonal outlines indicate an extensive interstitial abnormality (Fig. 7.1.33) caused by infiltration with fibrosis, abnormal cells or fluid (e.g. fibrosing alveolitis, lymphangitis carcinomatosa and alveolar proteinosis, respectively). At a pathological level, interlobular septal thickening due to fibrosis is often associated with bronchovascular thickening, intralobular interstitial thickening (generally beyond the resolution of HRCT) and finally the coarse reticular 'honeycomb' of destroyed lung.

As a consequence of the continuity of the various parts of the lung interstitium,[201] widespread interstitial disease that causes thickening of the interlobular septa also results in bronchovascular interstitial thickening (typified by lymphangitis carcinomatosa). The bronchovascular thickening depicted on HRCT is equivalent to the peribronchial 'cuffing' seen around end-on bronchi on chest radiography. This HRCT finding may be obvious, particularly in regional or unilateral interstitial lung disease, but is sometimes quite subtle when it is minimal and diffuse. The HRCT finding of peribronchovascular thickening in isolation should be interpreted with caution, since it may be a manifestation of reversible airways disease, e.g. asthma.

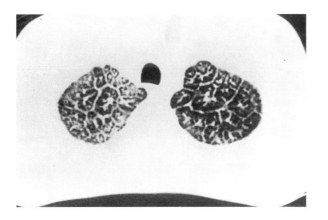

Fig. 7.1.33 The well-defined polygonal outlines at the lung apices represent thickened interlobular septa in a patient with lymphangitis carcinomatosa.

Thickening of the subsegmental and segmental bronchovascular bundles, e.g. due to lymphangitis carcinomatosa, gives the interface between the bronchial wall and surrounding lung an irregular appearance.[190,200,202] At the level of the secondary pulmonary lobule, axial interstitial thickening of the centrilobular artery and bronchiole is seen as a prominent dot or Y-shaped opacity; there is often associated thickening of the interlobular septa. Such thickening is seen in a variety of interstitial lung diseases and is recognised as one of the earliest manifestations of asbestosis.[203,204]

At the other end of the spectrum, extensive pulmonary fibrosis that causes complete destruction of the architecture of the secondary pulmonary lobules results in a characteristic coarse reticular pattern made up of irregular linear opacities. The reticular pattern of end-stage fibrotic or honeycomb lung mirrors the appearances on chest radiography and is characterised by cystic spaces measuring a few millimetres to several centimetres across surrounded by thick irregular walls.[205,206] The distortion of normal lung morphology by extensive fibrosis may result in irregular dilatation of the segmental and subsegmental bronchi; in the lung periphery the dilated bronchi and bronchioles may be indistinguishable from the surrounding cystic air spaces of the honeycomb lung.

Nodular pattern

A nodular pattern, defined in chest radiography as innumerable small discrete opacities ranging in diameter from 2 mm to 10 mm, is a feature of both interstitial and air space disease. The localisation of nodules, as well as other characteristics such as their density, clarity of outline and uniformity of size, may indicate whether the nodules are predominantly within the interstitium or within the air spaces. Since many lung pathologies have both interstitial and air-space components, this distinction is not necessarily helpful in refining the differential diagnosis. The detectability of pulmonary nodules on CT depends upon their size, profusion and density, and on the scanning technique. Narrow-collimation HRCT is superior for the detection of micronodular disease because there is less partial volume effect, which can average out the attenuation of tiny nodules.[150] Many pulmonary diseases, particularly the granulomatous disorders, are characterised by a fine nodular pattern.[207] These include sarcoidosis, pneumoconioses, miliary tuberculosis, Langerhans cell histiocytosis and extrinsic allergic alveolitis. Non-granulomatous diseases responsible for a nodular pattern include miliary metastases and idiopathic pulmonary haemorrhage.

Nodules within the lung interstitium are seen in the interlobular septa, in subpleural regions (particularly in relation to the fissures) and in a peribronchovascular distribution. Nodular thickening of the bronchovascular interstitium results in an irregular interface between the margins of the bronchovascular bundles and the surrounding lung parenchyma. This has been named the 'interface sign'[208] (Fig. 7.1.34). This irregularity may be seen in lymphangitis carcinomatosa[193,202,209] but is at its most obvious in cases of sarcoidosis, when a coalescence of perilymphatic granulomas results in a beaded appearance of the thickened bronchovascular bundles.[59,210] The bronchovascular distribution of nodules, in conjunction with a subpleural nodularity, is highly suggestive of sarcoidosis.

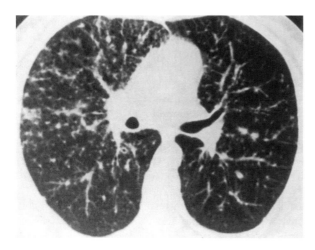

Fig. 7.1.34 Numerous small pulmonary nodules in a patient with sarcoidosis. Many of the nodules surround the bronchovascular bundles, giving a beaded appearance or 'irregular interface' sign.

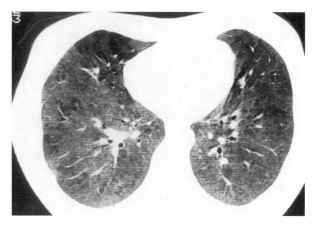

Fig. 7.1.35 A patient with subacute extrinsic allergic alveolitis with widespread ground-glass opacification; note that the abnormal lung is of considerably increased density compared with air within the segmental bronchi.

When the air spaces are filled, or partially filled, with the products of disease, individual acini may become visible on HRCT as low-density poorly defined nodules approximately 8 mm in diameter. Acinar nodules may merge with areas of ground-glass opacification and are often seen around the periphery of areas of dense parenchymal consolidation. Acinar or air-space nodules are usually centrilobular, although this is not invariable and may not be appreciated if these nodules are profuse. Conditions in which this non-specific pattern is seen include organising pneumonia,[211] extrinsic allergic alveolitis,[212] endobronchial spread of tuberculosis,[196] idiopathic pulmonary haemorrhage[192] and pulmonary oedema.[213-215]

Ground glass opacification and increased lung density

A hazy increase in the density of the lung parenchyma on HRCT is usually described as a 'ground-glass' opacification (Fig. 7.1.35). Unlike the analogous abnormality on chest radiography, in which the pulmonary vessels are often indistinct, a ground-glass pattern on HRCT does not obscure the pulmonary vasculature. Although this HRCT abnormality is usually easily recognisable, particularly when it is interspersed with areas of normal lung parenchyma, subtle degrees of increased parenchymal opacification may not be obvious and the conspicuity of this abnormality is susceptible to alterations in window settings. Furthermore, an increase in parenchymal density, mimicking a widespread ground-glass pattern, is seen in healthy individuals breath-holding at near residual volume.

The morphological changes responsible for a ground-glass pattern are complex and include partial filling of the air spaces and thickening of the interstitium or a combination of the two. Thickening of the intralobular interstitium by fluid or a cellular infiltrate is below the limits of resolution of HRCT and volume averaging results in an amorphous increase in lung density. Conditions that are characterised by these pathological changes and result in a ground-glass pattern are shown in Table 7.1.6. In

general, the amorphous ground-glass density seen on HRCT in these conditions represents a potentially reversible phase of the disease. However, mild thickening of the intralobular interstitium by irreversible fibrosis may also produce a ground-glass appearance, but this is usually accompanied by an indirect sign of fibrosis in the form of dilatation and distortion of the bronchi. Furthermore, a ground-glass pattern may be seen in areas of bronchioloalveolar cell carcinoma, usually in conjunction with patches of denser consolidated lung.

A pitfall in identifying a ground-glass pattern on HRCT is encountered in patients with regions of either underperfused or underventilated lung. Regional alterations in pulmonary blood flow may result in striking differences in lung density, e.g. in patients with chronic thromboembolic disease; the density difference between the underperfused lung and the normal lung may give the appearance of a ground-glass density in the normal lung parenchyma. These areas of different density often have

Table 7.1.6 Conditions characterised by predominant ground glass opacification on high-resolution computed tomography

- Subacute extrinsic allergic alveolitis
- Adult respiratory distress syndrome
- Desquamative interstitial pneumonitis
- *Pneumocystis carinii* or cytomegalovirus pneumonia
- Sarcoidosis
- Pulmonary oedema
- Idiopathic pulmonary haemorrhage
- Bronchioloalveolar cell carcinoma
- Eosinophilic pneumonia
- Acute interstitial pneumonitis
- Respiratory bronchiolitis–interstitial lung disease
- Drug toxicity
- Alveolar proteinosis
- Sickle cell disease
- Lymphocytic interstitial pneumonitis

Cystic air spaces as the dominant abnormality are seen in only a few conditions, including lymphangioleiomyomatosis,[217] Langerhans cell histiocytosis,[218] end-stage fibrosing alveolitis[219] and postinfective pneumatoceles. In lymphangioleiomyomatosis the cysts are usually uniformly scattered throughout the lungs with normal intervening lung parenchyma.[205] Paradoxically, as the disease progresses, with coalescence of the larger cystic air spaces, the circumferential well-defined walls of the cysts become disrupted and the HRCT pattern of advanced lymphangioleiomyomatosis, and indeed Langerhans cell histiocytosis, may be difficult to distinguish from severe centrilobular emphysema (Fig. 7.1.37).

Similar confluent cystic air spaces giving a delicate pattern on HRCT are seen in patients with advanced Langerhans cell histiocytosis. However, in the earlier stages of the disease, there is a nodular component and some of the nodules cavitate.[219,220] The constellation of HRCT findings of cavitating nodules, some of which have odd shapes, and cystic air spaces with a predominantly upper-zone distribution is virtually pathognomonic for the diagnosis of Langerhans cell histiocytosis.

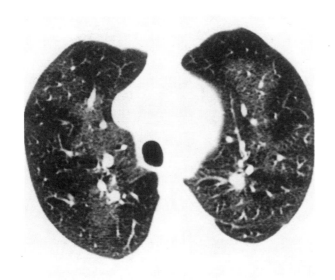

Fig. 7.1.36 Regional inhomogeneity of lung density in a patient with pulmonary hypertension due to chronic thromboembolic disease. The areas of increased density represent regions of lung receiving shunted blood. The proximal pulmonary arteries are dilated.

definable geographical margins and the term mosaic oligaemia has been used to describe this pattern on CT[216] (Fig. 7.1.36). Similarly, in patients with patchy air-trapping due to small-airways disease, e.g. constrictive obliterative bronchiolitis, the relatively transradiant areas of underventilated and underperfused lung may make the normal lung parenchyma appear more than usually dense and thus simulate a ground-glass infiltrate. This mimic can usually be recognised for what it is by the relative paucity of vessels in the underventilated parts of the lungs. By contrast, the vessels in the relatively normal lung of higher density are engorged because of shunting of blood to these regions. If an obliterative bronchiolitis is suspected, additional scans should be performed in full expiration; the regional differences in lung density will then be even more striking.

Cystic air spaces and decreased lung density

The term cystic air space is used to describe a clearly defined air-containing space with a definable, usually thin, wall. Innumerable cystic spaces may not be individually identifiable as such on chest radiography because the superimposition of the thin walls produces a delicate reticular pattern. Several conditions are characterised by profuse cystic air spaces and the size and distribution of these cysts on HRCT is often helpful in refining the differential diagnosis.

The abnormal air spaces of emphysema resulting from destruction of alveolar walls of the distal air spaces produce, on HRCT, areas of low attenuation with, in the case of centrilobular emphysema, a moth-eaten appearance that often appear to merge imperceptibly with normal lung. Although bullae of varying sizes are clearly seen on HRCT in patients with emphysema, there is usually a background of emphysema, which prevents confusion with other conditions in which cystic air spaces are a prominent feature.

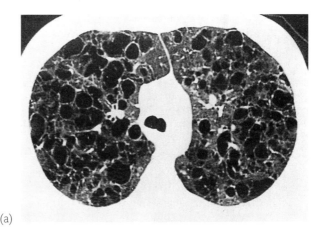
(a)

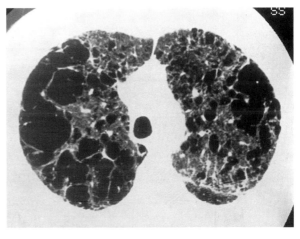
(b)

Fig. 7.1.37 (a) Lymphangioleiomyomatosis at an advanced stage: there is coalescence of the numerous cystic air spaces. (b) Severe centrilobular emphysema. The lung destruction is more permeative than shown in (a); nevertheless, there are similarities between the two patterns.

High-resolution computed tomography of bronchiectasis

The diagnosis of bronchiectasis on chest radiography alone is often uncertain unless the disease is extensive and severe, and HRCT is now the imaging technique of choice for assessing patients with suspected bronchiectasis.

Bronchiectasis is defined as damage to the bronchial wall causing irreversible dilatation of the bronchi, whatever the aetiology. Thus, the cardinal sign of bronchiectasis is dilatation of the bronchi with or without bronchial wall thickening. HRCT criteria for the identification of abnormally dilated bronchi depend on the orientation of the bronchi in relation to the plane of CT section.

Vertically orientated bronchi (in the lower lobes and apical segments of the upper lobes) will be seen in transverse section and reference can then be made to the accompanying pulmonary artery, which in normal individuals is of approximately the same calibre; dilatation of the bronchus will result in the so-called signet-ring sign (Fig. 7.1.38). A false-positive diagnosis of bronchiectasis on HRCT is usually the result of scanning artefacts or another disease that superficially mimics bronchiectasis. Minor degrees of bronchial dilatation (and wall thickening) are a frequent accompaniment of chronic obstructive pulmonary disease and asthma; indeed, bronchiectatic airways by CT criteria may be an incidental finding in such patients and their clinical significance is a source of debate. False negatives are more often due to a technically imperfect examination.

Bronchi that have a more horizontal course on CT, particularly the anterior segmental bronchi of the upper lobes and the segmental bronchi of the lingula and right middle lobe, are demonstrated along their length and abnormal dilatation is seen as non-tapering parallel walls or sometimes distinct flaring of the bronchi as they course distally (Fig. 7.1.39). In more severe cases of bronchiectasis, the bronchi will be obviously dilated and have a concertina or varicose appearance (Fig. 7.1.40). Because

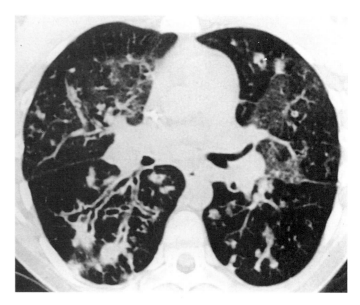

Fig. 7.1.39 Patient with cystic fibrosis showing non-tapering of bronchiectatic airways in the right lower lobe.

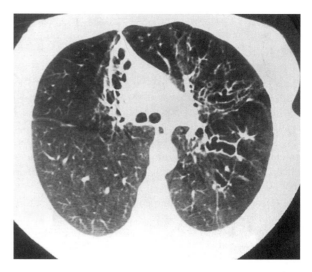

Fig. 7.1.40 Proximal varicose bronchiectasis typical of allergic bronchopulmonary aspergillosis.

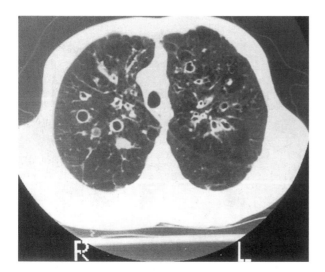

Fig. 7.1.38 Markedly dilated subsegmental bronchi in the upper lobes of a patient with cystic fibrosis. Two of the dilated airways in the right upper lobe are plugged with mucopurulent secretions.

there is usually peribronchial fibrosis, resulting in thickening of the bronchial wall, the small airways can be identified more readily in the periphery of the lung, further than two-thirds of the way out radially from the hilum. Although there is no exact level beyond which visualisation of the bronchi can be regarded as abnormal on HRCT, normal bronchi should not be visible within 3 cm of the pleural surface.[191,192,221]

Supplementary HRCT signs of bronchiectasis are crowding of the affected bronchi with obvious volume loss of the lobe as indicated by position of the fissures. Patients with severe airway involvement by bronchiectasis may show definite regional differences in density of the lung parenchyma (mosaic pattern) because of impaired ventilation that is thought to reflect bronchiolar obstruction. The appearance of elliptical and circular opacities representing mucus- or pus-filled dilated bronchi is a sign of gross bronchiectasis and is almost invariably seen in the presence of other obviously dilated bronchi, some of which may contain air–fluid levels. When there is mucus plugging of the smaller centrilobular airways, minute branching structures or dots in the lung periphery may be identifiable.

High-resolution computed tomography of small-airways disease

There is increasing interest in the ability of HRCT to detect various small-airways diseases.[222-225] Identification of small-airways disease is difficult because of the non-specificity and insensitivity of plain chest radiography and conventional pulmonary function tests. The HRCT signs of constrictive obliterative bronchiolitis are indirect: there are areas of decreased attenuation, which may merge with more normal lung or may have sharply demarcated geographical boundaries (mosaic pattern; see Fig. 7.1.9). By contrast, in the exudative form of bronchiolar disease, HRCT shows thickened and plugged small airways as small irregular branching opacities (Fig. 7.1.41).

Diseases of the small airways have been divided into many histopathologic subtypes. Nevertheless, there are not always obvious clinical or imaging correlates for these various subcategories. A simpler approach is to divide small-airways disease into 'constrictive' and 'exudative' types; this has the advantage that there are recognisable imaging and clinical features in these two subtypes. 'Constrictive' cases show narrowing of the bronchioles by peribronchiolar fibrosis, which has the potential to progress to complete obliteration – the archetypal disease being constrictive obliterative bronchiolitis, which is a non-specific response to injury and is found in association with many diseases. In the 'exudative' type of small-airways disease, typified by diffuse panbronchiolitis, there is inflammatory exudate within and around the affected bronchioles.

The first description of the CT features of adult (constrictive) obliterative bronchiolitis was by Sweatman et al in 1990[226] and subsequent descriptions have confirmed the individual features, listed below:[61,223,224,227-229]

- **Areas of decreased attenuation of the lung parenchyma**. These are regions of reduced density (mosaic pattern), usually with poorly defined margins but sometimes with a well-demarcated geographical outline. The relatively higher density regions represent normal, relatively overperfused lung.
- **Attenuation of the pulmonary vasculature**. In affected areas perfusion is decreased, and vessels within areas of decreased attenuation are of reduced calibre (but are not distorted, as is the case in centrilobular emphysema).

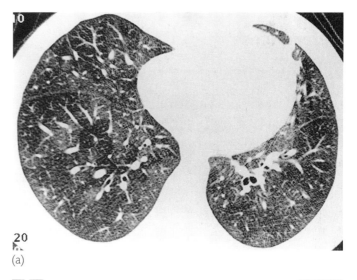

(a)

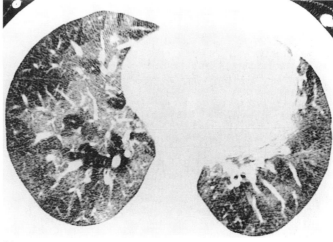

(b)

Fig. 7.1.42 Patient following bone marrow transplant. (a) Subtle inhomogeneity of the density of the lung parenchyma (mosaic pattern) on a standard inspiratory high-resolution computed tomography image. (b) Accentuation of the mosaic pattern on a section obtained at end-expiration.

Fig. 7.1.41 Plugging of small airways in the left lower lobe producing Y-shaped opacities in the lung periphery.

■ **Bronchial abnormalities.** The severity of bronchial dilatation and wall thickening is highly variable but is present in the majority of cases of constrictive obliterative bronchiolitis.[228,230,231]

■ **Air-trapping on expiratory CT.** The regional density differences of the lung are accentuated and small or subtle areas of air-trapping may be revealed on CT performed at end-expiration (Fig. 7.1.42),[222,232,233] and the cross-sectional area of the affected parts of the lung do not decrease in size on the expiratory images.[234,235]

In the exudative form of small-airways disease minute branching structures are identifiable in the lung periphery (see Fig. 7.1.41). The resulting appearance has been termed the 'tree-in-bud' pattern[236,237] and is encountered in many airways diseases, including cystic fibrosis and other causes of bronchiectasis, endobronchial spread of tuberculosis[238] and diffuse panbronchiolitis.[239–241]

References

1. Lodge T. The anatomy of the blood vessels of the human lung as applied to chest radiology. Br J Radiol 1946; 19: 1.
2. Simon M. The pulmonary veins in mitral stenosis. J Faculty Radiol 1958; 9: 25.
3. Kelsey CA, Moseley RD, Mettler FA et al. Comparison of nodule detection with 70-kVp and 120-kVp chest radiographs. Radiology 1982; 143: 609.
4. Peppler WW, Zink F, Naimuddin S et al. Patient-specific beam attenuators. Proceedings of the Chest Imaging Conference, Madison, WI: 1987: 64.
5. Vlasbloem H, Schultze Kool LJ. AMBER: a scanning multiple-beam equalization system for chest radiography. Radiology 1988; 169: 29.
6. Schultze Kool LJ, Busscher DLT, Vlasbloem H et al. Advanced multiple-beam equalization radiography in chest radiology: a simulated nodule detection study. Radiology 1988; 169: 35.
7. Hansell DM, Coleman R, du Bois RM et al. Advanced Multiple Beam Equalisation Radiography (AMBER) in the detection of diffuse lung disease. Clin Radiol 1991; 44: 227–231.
8. Nichols RD, Gurney JW, Jones KK et al. Alveolar consolidation detection: Advanced Multiple Beam Equalization Radiography versus conventional chest radiography. Radiology 1993; 187: 65.
9. Goodman LR, Wilson CR, Foley WD. Digital radiography of the chest: promises and problems. AJR 1988; 150: 1241.
10. Goodman LR, Foley WD, Wilson CR et al. Digital and conventional chest images: observer performance with film digital radiography system. Radiology 1986; 158: 27.
11. MacMahon H, Metz CE, Doi K et al. Digital chest radiography: effect on diagnostic accuracy of hard copy, conventional video, and reversed gray scale video display formats. Radiology 1988; 168: 669.
12. Sonoda M, Takano M, Miyahara J, Kato H. Computed radiography utilizing scanning laser stimulated luminescence. Radiology 1983; 148: 833.
13. Lams PM, Cocklin ML. Spatial resolution requirements for digital chest radiographs: an ROC study of observer performance in selected cases. Radiology 1986; 158: 11.
14. MacMahon H, Vyborny CJ, Metz CE et al. Digital radiography of subtle pulmonary abnormalities; an ROC study of the effect of pixel size on observer performance. Radiology 1986; 158: 21.
15. Fajardo LL, Hillman BJ, Pond GD et al. Detection of pneumothorax: comparison of digital and conventional chest imaging. AJR 1989; 152: 475.
16. Kido S, Ikezoe J, Takeuchi N et al. Interpretation of subtle interstitial lung abnormalities: conventional versus storage phosphor radiography. Radiology 1993; 187: 527.
17. Chotas HG, Dobbins JT, Ravin CE. Principles of digital radiography with large-area electronically readable detectors: a review of the basics. Radiology 1999; 210: 595.
18. Thompson MJ, Kubicka RA, Smith C. Evaluation of cardiopulmonary devices on chest radiographs: digital vs analog radiographs. AJR 1989; 153: 1165.
19. Schaefer CM, Greene R, Hall DA et al. Mediastinal abnormalities: detection with thoracic phosphor digital radiography. Radiology 1991; 178: 169.
20. Gleeson F, Lomas DJ, Flower CDR et al. Powered cutting needle biopsy of the pleura and chest wall. Clin Radiol 1990; 41: 199.
21. Yu CJ, Yang BC, Chang DB et al. Evaluation of ultrasonically guided biopsies of mediastinal masses. Chest 1991; 100: 399.
22. Sawhney S, Jain R, Berry M. Tru-Cut biopsy of mediastinal masses guided by real-time ultrasound. Clin Radiol 1991; 44: 16.
23. Chang DB, Yang PC, Luh KT et al. Ultrasound-guided pleural biopsy with Tru-Cut needle. Chest 1991; 100: 1328.
24. Yang PC, Chang DB, Yu CJ et al. Ultrasound-guided core biopsy of thoracic tumors. Am Rev Respir Dis 1992; 146: 763.
25. Izumi S, Tamaki S, Natori H et al. Ultrasonically guided aspiration needle biopsy in disease of the chest. Am Rev Respir Dis 1982; 125: 460.
26. Yang PC. Ultrasound-guided transthoracic biopsy of peripheral lung, pleural, and chest-wall lesions. J Thorac Imaging 1997; 12: 272.
27. VanSonnenberg E, Nakamoto SK, Mueller PR et al. CT and ultrasound guided catheter drainage of empyemas after chest-tube failure. Radiology 1984; 151: 349.
28. Gleeson FV, Davies RJ. Fibrinolytic treatment of pleural infection. Clin Radiol 1998; 53: 627.
29. Sahn SA. Use of fibrinolytic agents in the management of complicated parapneumonic effusions and empyemas. Thorax 1998; 53(suppl 2): S65.
30. Webb WR, Stern EJ, Kanth N, Gamsu G. Dynamic pulmonary CT: findings in healthy adult men. Radiology 1993; 186: 117.
31. Stern EJ, Graham CM, Webb WR, Gamsu G. Normal trachea during forced expiration: dynamic CT measurements. Radiology 1993; 187: 27.
32. Kalender WA, Seissler W, Klotz E, Vock P. Spiral volumetric CT with single-breath-hold technique, continuous transport, and continuous scanner rotation. Radiology 1990; 176: 181.
33. Vock P, Soucek M, Daepp M, Kalender WA. Lung spiral volumetric CT with single breath-hold technique. Radiology 1990; 176: 864.
34. Remy-Jardin M, Remy J, Giraud F, Marquette CH. Pulmonary nodules: detection with thick-section spiral CT versus conventional CT. Radiology 1993; 187: 513.
35. Remy-Jardin M, Remy J. Spiral CT angiography of the pulmonary circulation. Radiology 1999; 212: 615.
36. Mayo JR, Jackson SA, Müller NL. High-resolution CT of the chest: radiation dose. AJR 1993; 160: 479.
37. Nitta N, Takahashi M, Murata K, Morita R. Ultra low-dose helical CT of the chest: evaluation in clinical cases. Radiat Med 1999; 17: 1.
38. Koehler PR, Anderson RE, Baxter B. The effect of computed tomography viewer controls on anatomical measurements. Radiology 1979; 130: 189.
39. Baxter BS, Sorenson JA. Factors affecting the measurements of size and CT number in computed tomography. Invest Radiol 1981; 16: 337.
40. Harris KM, Adams H, Lloyd DCF, Harvey DJ. The effect on apparent size of simulated pulmonary nodules of using three standard CT window settings. Clin Radiol 1993; 47: 241.
41. Hruban RH, Meziane MA, Zerhouni EA et al. High resolution computed tomography of inflation-fixed lungs. Am Rev Respir Dis 1987; 136: 935.
42. Corcoran HL, Renner WR, Milstein MJ. Review of high-resolution CT of the lung. RadioGraphics 1992; 12: 917.
43. Müller NL, Miller RR. Computed tomography of chronic diffuse infiltrative lung disease (first part). Am Rev Respir Dis 1990; 142: 1206.
44. Müller NL, Miller RR. Computed tomography of chronic diffuse infiltrative lung disease (second part). Am Rev Respir Dis 1990; 142: 1440.
45. Hansell DM. Computed tomography of diffuse infiltrative lung disease: value and limitations. Semin Respir Crit Care Med 1998; 19: 431.
46. Mayo JR, Webb WR, Gould R et al. High-resolution CT of the lungs: an optimal approach. Radiology 1987; 163: 507.
47. Mayo JR. High resolution computed tomography: technical aspects. Radiol Clin North Am 1991; 29: 1043.
48. Murata K, Khan A, Rojas KA, Herman PG. Optimization of computed tomography technique to demonstrate the fine structure of the lung. Invest Radiol 1988; 23: 170.
49. Murata K, Khan A, Herman PG. Pulmonary parenchymal disease: evaluation with high-resolution CT. Radiology 1989; 170: 629.
50. Webb WR, Muller NL, Naidich DP. High-resolution CT technique. In: Anonymous. High-resolution CT of the lung. New York: Raven Press; 1992: 4–13.
51. Kuhns LR, Borlaza G. The 'twinkling star' sign: an aid in differentiating pulmonary vessels from pulmonary nodules on computed tomograms. Radiology 1980; 135: 763.
52. Tarver RD, Conces DJ, Godwin JD. Motion artifacts on CT simulate bronchiectasis. AJR 1988; 151: 1117.
53. Mayo JR, Müller NL, Henkelman RM. The double-fissure sign: a motion artifact on thin-section CT scans. Radiology 1987; 165: 580.

54. Yu CP, Nicolaides P, Soong TT. Effect of random airway sizes on aerosol deposition. Am Ind Hyg Assoc J 1979; 40: 999.

55. Volpe J, Storto ML, Lee K, Webb WR. High-resolution CT of the lung: determination of the usefulness of CT scans obtained with the patient prone based on plain radiographic findings. AJR 1997; 169: 369.

56. Arakawa H, Webb WR, McCowin M et al. Inhomogeneous lung attenuation at thin-section CT: diagnostic value of expiratory scans. Radiology 1998; 206: 89.

57. Evans SH, Cooke DJ, Anderson W. A comparison of radiation doses to the breast in computed tomographic chest examinations for two scanning protocols. Clin Radiol 1989; 40: 45.

58. Zwirewich CV, Mayo JR, Müller NL. Low dose High Resolution CT of lung parenchyma. Radiology 1991; 180: 413.

59. Müller NL, Kullnig P, Miller RR. The CT findings of pulmonary sarcoidosis: analysis of 25 patients. AJR 1989; 152: 1179.

60. Staples CA, Gamsu G, Ray CS, Webb WR. High resolution computed tomography and lung function in asbestos-exposed workers with normal chest radiographs. Am Rev Respir Dis 1989; 139: 1502.

61. Sweatman MC, Millar AB, Strickland B, Turner-Warwick M. Computed tomography in adult obliterative bronchiolitis. Clin Radiol 1990; 41: 116.

62. Schurawitzki H, Stiglbauer R, Graninger W et al. Interstitial lung disease in progressive systemic sclerosis: high resolution CT versus radiography. Radiology 1990; 176: 755.

63. Aberle DR, Gamsu G, Ray CS, Feuerstein IM. Asbestos-related pleural and parenchymal fibrosis: detection with high resolution CT. Radiology 1988; 166: 729.

64. Friedman AC, Fiel SB, Fisher MS et al. Asbestos-related pleural disease and asbestosis: a comparison of CT and chest radiography. AJR 1988; 150: 269.

65. Lenoir S, Grenier P, Brauner MW et al. Pulmonary lymphangiomyomatosis and tuberous sclerosis: comparison of radiographic and thin-section CT findings. Radiology 1990; 175: 329.

66. Mathieson JR, Mayo JR, Staples CA, Müller NL. Chronic diffuse infiltrative lung disease: comparison of diagnostic accuracy of CT and chest radiography. Radiology 1989; 171: 111.

67. Grenier P, Valeyre D, Cluzel P et al. Chronic diffuse interstitial lung disease: diagnostic value of chest radiography and high-resolution CT. Radiology 1991; 179: 123.

68. Padley SPG, Hansell DM, Flower CDR, Jennings P. Comparative accuracy of high resolution computed tomography and chest radiography in the diagnosis of chronic diffuse infiltrative lung disease. Clin Radiol 1991; 44: 227.

69. Nugent KM, Peterson MW, Jolles H et al. Correlation of chest roentgenograms with pulmonary function and bronchoalveolar lavage in interstitial lung disease. Chest 1989; 96: 1224.

70. Harrison NK, Glanville AR, Strickland B et al. Pulmonary involvement in systemic sclerosis: the detection of early changes by thin section CT scan bronchoalveolar lavage and ^{99m}Tc-DTPA clearance. Respir Med 1989; 83: 1.

71. Pantin CF, Valind SO, Sweatman M et al. Measures of the inflammatory response in cryptogenic fibrosing alveolitis. Am Rev Respir Dis 1990; 138: 1234.

72. Panos RJ, Moretensen RL, Niccoli SA, King TE. Clinical deterioration in patients with idiopathic pulmonary fibrosis: causes and assessment. Am J Med 1990; 88: 396.

73. Terriff BA, Kwan SY, Chan-Yeung MM, Müller NL. Fibrosing alveolitis: chest radiography and CT as predictors of clinical and functional impairment at follow-up in 26 patients. Radiology 1992; 184: 445.

74. Wells AU, Hansell DM, Rubens MB et al. The predictive value of thin-section computed tomography in fibrosing alveolitis. Am Rev Respir Dis 1993; 148: 1076.

75. Leung AN, Miller RR, Müller NL. Parenchymal opacification in chronic infiltrative lung diseases: CT-pathologic correlation. Radiology 1993; 188: 209.

76. Bergin CJ, Healy MV, Zincone GE, Castellino RA. MR evaluation of chest wall involvement in malignant lymphoma. J Comput Assist Tomogr 1990; 14: 928.

77. Padovani B, Mouroux J, Seksik L et al. Chest wall invasion by bronchogenic carcinoma: evaluation with MR imaging. Radiology 1993; 187: 33.

78. Webb WR, Gamsu G, Stark DD, Moore EH. Magnetic resonance imaging of the normal and abnormal pulmonary hila. Radiology 1984; 152: 89.

79. Glazer GM, Gross BH, Aisen AM et al. Imaging of the pulmonary hilum: a prospective comparative study in patients with lung cancer. AJR 1985; 145: 245.

80. Link KM, Samuels LJ, Reed JC et al. Magnetic resonance imaging of the mediastinum. J Thorac Imag 1993; 8 (1): 34.

81. Gupta A, Frazer CK, Ferguson JM et al. Acute pulmonary embolism: diagnosis with MR angiography. Radiology 1999; 210: 353.

82. Bergin CJ, Pauly JM, Macovski A. Lung parenchyma: projection reconstruction MR imaging. Radiology 1991; 179: 777.

83. Mayo JR, MacKay A, Müller NL. MR imaging of the lungs: value of short TE spin-echo pulse sequences. AJR 1992; 159: 951.

84. Bergin CJ, Glover GM, Pauly J. Magnetic resonance imaging of the lung parenchyma. J Thorac Imag 1993; 8: 12.

85. McFadden RG, Carr TJ, Wood TE. Proton magnetic resonance imaging to stage activity of interstitial lung disease. Chest 1987; 92: 31.

86. Naidich DP, Weinreb JC, Schinella R. MR imaging of pulmonary parenchyma: comparison with CT in evaluating cadaveric lung specimens. J Comput Assist Tomogr 1990; 14: 595.

87. Mayo JR, MacKay A, Müller NL. T2 relaxation time in MR imaging of normal and abnormal lung parenchyma. Radiology 1990; 177: 313.

88. MacFall JR, Charles HC, Black RD et al. Human lung air spaces: potential for MR imaging with hyperpolarized He-3. Radiology 1996; 200: 553.

89. Pykett IL, Newhouse JH, Buonanno FS et al. Principles of nuclear magnetic resonance imaging. Radiology 1982; 143: 157.

90. Bergin CJ, Glover GH, Pauly JM. Lung parenchyma: magnetic susceptibility in MR imaging. Radiology 1991; 180: 845.

91. Munk PL, Morris DC, Nelems B. Left main bronchial-esophageal fistula: a complication of bronchial artery embolization. Cardiovasc Intervent Radiol 1990; 13: 95.

92. Cho ZH, Ro YM. Reduction of susceptibility artifact in gradient-echo imaging. Magn Reson Med 1992; 23: 193.

93. Edelman RR, Manning W, Burstein D, Paulin S. Coronary arteries: breath-hold MR angiography. Radiology 1991; 181: 641.

94. Shioya S, Haida M, Ono Y et al. Lung cancer: differentiation of tumor, necrosis and atelectasis by means of T1 and T2 values measured in vitro. Radiology 1988; 167: 105.

95. Shioya S, Haida M, Tsuji C et al. T2 of endotoxin lung injury with and without methylprednisolone treatment. Magn Reson Med 1988; 8: 450.

96. Webb WR, Jensen BG, Gamsu G et al. Coronal MRI of the chest: normal and abnormal. Radiology 1984; 153: 729.

97. Naidich DP, Zerhouni EA, Siegelman SS. Principles and techniques of thoracic CT and MR. In: Computed tomography and magnetic resonance of the thorax, 2nd ed. New York: Raven Press; 1991; 1–34.

98. Müller NL, Mayo JR, Zwirewich CV. Value of MR imaging in the evaluation of chronic infiltrative lung diseases: comparison with CT. AJR 1992; 158: 1205.

99. Schmidt HC, Tscholakoff D, Hricak H, Higgins CB. MR image contrast and relaxation times of solid tumours in the chest, abdomen and pelvis. J Comput Assist Tomogr 1985; 9: 738.

100. Swensen SJ, Keller PL, Berquist TH et al. Magnetic resonance imaging of hemorrhage. AJR 1985; 145: 921.

101. Barakos JA, Brown JJ, Brescia RJ, Higgins CB. High signal intensity lesions of the chest in MR imaging. J Comput Assist Tomogr 1989; 13: 797.

102. Webb WR. Magnetic resonance imaging of the hila and mediastinum. Cardiovasc Intervent Radiol 1986; 8: 306.

103. McAdams HP, Hatabu H, Donnelly LF et al. Novel techniques for MR imaging of pulmonary airspaces. Magn Reson Imaging Clin North Am 2000; 8: 205.

104. Bjork L, Ansusinha T. Angiographic diagnosis of acute pulmonary embolism. Acta Radiol 1965; 3: 129.

105. Cheely R, McCartney WH, Perry JR et al. The role of non-invasive tests versus pulmonary angiography in the diagnosis of pulmonary embolism. Am J Med 1981; 70: 17.

106. Cooper TJ, Hayward MW, Hartog M. Survey on the use of pulmonary scintigraphy and angiography for suspected pulmonary thromboembolism in the UK. Clin Radiol 1991; 43: 243.

107. Brown KT, Bach AM. Paucity of angiographic findings despite extensive organized thrombus in chronic thromboembolic pulmonary hypertension. J Vasc Interv Radiol 1992; 3: 99.

108. Auger WR, Fedullo PF, Moser KM et al. Chronic major-vessel thromboembolic pulmonary artery obstruction: appearance at angiography. Radiology 1992; 182: 393.

109. Stein PD, Athanasoulis C, Alavi A et al. Complications and validity of pulmonary angiography in acute pulmonary embolism. Circulation 1992; 85: 462.

110. Mills SR, Jackson DC, Older RA et al. The incidence, etiologies and avoidance of complications of pulmonary angiography in a large series. Radiology 1980; 136: 295.

111. Tajima H, Kumazaki T, Tajima N et al. Effect of iohexol and diatrizoate on pulmonary arterial pressure following pulmonary angiography; a clinical comparison in man. Acta Radiol 1988; 29: 487.

112. Cohen AM, Doershuk CF, Stern RC. Bronchial artery embolization to control hemoptysis in cystic fibrosis. Radiology 1990; 175: 401.

113. Remy J, Arnaud A, Fardou H et al. Treatment of hemoptysis by embolization of bronchial arteries. Radiology 1977; 122: 33.

114. Uflacker R, Kaemmerer A, Neves C, Picon PD. Management of massive hemoptysis by bronchial artery embolization. Radiology 1983; 146: 627.

115. Sweezey NB, Fellows KF. Bronchial artery embolization for severe hemoptysis in cystic fibrosis. Chest 1990; 97: 1322.

116. Garzon AA, Gourin A. Surgical management of massive haemoptysis. Ann Thorac Surg 1978; 187: 267.

117. Tonkin ILD, Hanissian AS, Boulden TF et al. Bronchial arteriography and embolotherapy for hemoptysis in patients with cystic fibrosis. Cardiovasc Interv Radiol 1991; 14: 241.

118. Di Chiro G. Unintentional spinal cord arteriography: a warning. Radiology 1974; 112: 231.

119. Botenga ASJ. Selective bronchial and intercostal arteriography, 1st ed. Baltimore, MD: Williams & Wilkins; 1970.

120. Pump KK. Distribution of bronchial arteries in the human lung. Chest 1972; 62: 447.

121. McPherson S, Routh WD, Nath H, Keller FS. Anomalous origin of bronchial arteries: potential pitfall of embolotherapy for hemoptysis. J Vasc Interv Radiol 1990; 1: 86.

122. Garcarek J, Marciniak R. Application of Spongostan and Mersilene for embolization of bronchial arteries. Eur Radiol 1992; 2: 287.

123. Stoll JF, Bettmann MA. Bronchial artery embolization to control hemoptysis: a review. Cardiovasc Intervent Radiol 1988; 11: 263.

124. Ferris EJ. Pulmonary hemorrhage: vascular evaluation and interventional therapy. Chest 1981; 80: 710.

125. Remy-Jardin M, Wattinne L, Remy J. Transcatheter occlusion of pulmonary arterial circulation and collateral supply: failures, incidents and complications. Radiology 1991; 180: 699.

126. Newton TH, Preger L. Selective bronchial arteriography. Radiology 1965; 84: 1043.

127. Kardjiev V, Symeonov A, Charkov I. Etiology, pathogenesis and prevention of spinal cord lesions in selective angiography of the bronchial and intercostal arteries. Radiology 1974; 112: 81.

128. Ivanick MJ, Thorwarth W, Donohue J et al. Infarction of the left mainstem bronchus: a complication of bronchial artery embolization. AJR 1983; 141: 535.

129. Uflacker R, Kaemmerer A, Picon PD et al. Bronchial artery embolization in the management of hemoptysis: technical aspects and long term results. Radiology 1985; 157: 637.

130. Hayakawa K, Tanaka F, Torizuka T et al. Bronchial artery embolization for hemoptysis: immediate and long-term results. Cardiovasc Intervent Radiol 1992; 15: 154.

131. Rabkin JE, Astafjev VI, Gothman LN, Grigorjev YG. Transcatheter embolization in the management of pulmonary hemorrhage. Radiology 1987; 163: 361.

132. Carrasco CH, Charnsangavej C, Wright KC et al. Use of the Gianturco self-expanding stent in stenoses of the superior and inferior venae cavae. J Vasc Interv Radiol 1992; 3: 409.

133. Solomon N, Holey MH, Jarmolowski CR. Intravascular stents in the management of superior vena cava syndrome. Cathet Cardiovasc Diagn 1991; 23: 245.

134. Watkinson AF, Hansell DM. Expandable Wallstent for the treatment of superior vena cava obstruction. Thorax 1993; 49: 915.

135. Irving JD, Kurdziel JC, Reidy JF et al. Gianturco self expanding stents: clinical experience in the vena cava and large veins. Cardiovasc Intervent Radiol 1992; 15: 328.

136. Ulmer JL, Choplin RH, Reed JC. Image-guided catheter drainage of the infected pleural space. J Thorac Imag 1991; 6: 65.

137. Lee KS, Im JG, Kim YH et al. Treatment of thoracic multiloculated empyemas with intracavitary urokinase: a prospective study. Radiology 1991; 179: 771.

138. Morrison MC, Mueller PR, Lee MJ et al. Sclerotherapy of malignant pleural effusions through sonographically placed small-bore catheters. AJR 1992; 158: 41.

139. Erasmus JJ, Patz EF Jr. Treatment of malignant pleural effusions. Curr Opin Pulm Med 1999; 5: 250.

140. Patz EF Jr, McAdams HP, Erasmus JJ et al. Sclerotherapy for malignant pleural effusions: a prospective randomized trial of bleomycin vs doxycycline with small-bore catheter drainage. Chest 1998; 113: 1305.

141. Patz EF Jr. Malignant pleural effusions: recent advances and ambulatory sclerotherapy. Chest 1998; 113: 74S.

142. Goldberg MA, Mueller PR, Saini S et al. Importance of daily rounds by the radiologist after interventional procedures of the abdomen and chest. Radiology 1991; 180: 767.

143. Hunnam GR, Flower CDR. Radiologically guided percutaneous catheter drainage of empyemas. Clin Radiol 1988; 39: 121.

144. Silverman SG, Mueller PR, Saini S et al. Thoracic empyema: management with image guided catheter drainage. Radiology 1988; 169: 5.

145. Aronberg DJ, Sagel SS, Jost RG et al. Percutaneous drainage of lung abscess. AJR 1979; 132: 282.

146. VanSonnenberg E, D'Agostino HB, Casola G et al. Lung abscess: CT-guided drainage. Radiology 1991; 178: 347.

147. Van Moore A Jr, Zuger JH, Kelley MJ. Lung abscess: an interventional radiology perspective. Semin Intervent Radiol 1991; 8: 36.

148. Westcott JL. Percutaneous catheter drainage of pleural effusion and empyema. AJR 1985; 144: 1189.

149. Wilson AG. The interpretation of shadows on the adult chest radiograph. Br J Hosp Med 1987; 526.

150. Fleischner Society. Glossary of terms for thoracic radiology: recommendations of the nomenclature committee of the Fleischner Society. AJR 1984; 143: 509.

151. Swensen SJ, Silverstein MD, Ilstrup DM et al. The probability of malignancy in solitary pulmonary nodules. Application to small radiologically indeterminate nodules. Arch Intern Med 1997; 157: 849.

152. Swensen SJ, Viggiano RW, Midthun DE et al. Lung nodule enhancement at CT: multicenter study. Radiology 2000; 214: 73.

153. Glazer HS, Kaiser LR, Anderson DJ et al. Indeterminate mediastinal invasion in bronchogenic carcinoma: CT evaluation. Radiology 1989; 173: 37.

154. Seely JM, Mayo JR, Miller RR, Müller NL. T1 lung cancer: prevalence of mediastinal nodal metastases and diagnostic accuracy of CT. Radiology 1993; 186: 129.

155. Primack SL, Lee KS, Logan PM et al. Bronchogenic carcinoma: utility of CT in the evaluation of patients with suspected lesions. Radiology 1994; 193: 795.

156. Goldstraw P. The practice of cardiothoracic surgeons in the perioperative staging of non small cell lung cancer. Thorax 1992; 47: 1.

157. Pearson FG. Staging of the mediastinum. Role of mediastinoscopy and computed tomography. Chest 1993; 103: 346S.

158. Marom EM, McAdams HP, Erasmus JJ et al. Staging non-small cell lung cancer with whole-body PET. Radiology 1999; 212: 803.

159. Erasmus JJ, Patz EF, Jr. Positron emission tomography imaging in the thorax. Clin Chest Med.1999; 20: 715.

160. Geraghty JJ, Stanford W, Landas SK, Galvin JR. Ultrafast computed tomography in experimental pulmonary embolism. Invest Radiol 1992; 27: 60.

161. Remy-Jardin M, Remy J, Wattinne L, Giraud F. Central pulmonary thromboembolism: diagnosis with spiral volumetric CT with the single-breath-hold technique – comparison with pulmonary angiography. Radiology 1992; 185: 381.

162. Brink JA, Woodard PK, Horesh L et al. Depiction of pulmonary emboli with spiral CT: optimization of display window settings in a porcine model. Radiology 1997; 204: 703.

163. Remy-Jardin M, Remy J, Artaud D et al. Peripheral pulmonary arteries: optimization of the spiral CT acquisition protocol. Radiology 1997; 204: 157.

164. Remy-Jardin M, Remy J, Artaud D et al. Spiral CT of pulmonary embolism: technical considerations and interpretive pitfalls. J Thorac Imaging 1997; 12: 103.

165. Kuzo RS, Goodman LR. CT evaluation of pulmonary embolism: technique and interpretation. AJR 1997; 169: 959.

166. Remy-Jardin M, Remy J, Artaud D et al. Spiral CT of pulmonary embolism: diagnostic approach, interpretive pitfalls and current indications. Eur Radiol 1998; 8: 1376.

167. Coche EE, Müller NL, Kim KI et al. Acute pulmonary embolism: ancillary findings at spiral CT. Radiology 1998; 207: 753.

168. Van Rossum AB, Treurniet FE, Kieft GJ et al. Role of spiral volumetric computed tomographic scanning in the assessment of patients with clinical suspicion of pulmonary embolism and an abnormal ventilation/perfusion lung scan. Thorax 1996; 51: 23.

169. Cross JJ, Kemp PM, Walsh CG et al. A randomized trial of spiral CT and ventilation perfusion scintigraphy for the diagnosis of pulmonary embolism. Clin Radiol 1998; 53: 177.

170. Van Rossum AB, Pattynama PM, Mallens WM et al. Can helical CT replace scintigraphy in the diagnostic process in suspected pulmonary embolism? A retrolective-prolective cohort study focusing on total diagnostic yield. Eur Radiol 1998; 8: 90.

171. Greaves SM, Hart EM, Brown K et al. Pulmonary thromboembolism: spectrum of findings on CT. AJR 1995; 165: 1359.

172. Bergin CJ, Sirlin CB, Hauschildt JP et al. Chronic thromboembolism: diagnosis with helical CT and MR imaging with angiographic and surgical correlation. Radiology 1997; 204: 695.

173. Roberts HC, Kauczor HU, Schweden F, Thelen M. Spiral CT of pulmonary hypertension and chronic thromboembolism. J Thorac Imaging 1997; 12: 118.

174. Schwickert HC, Schweden F, Schild HH et al. Pulmonary arteries and lung parenchyma in chronic pulmonary embolism: preoperative and postoperative CT findings. Radiology 1994; 191: 351.

175. Remy-Jardin M, Duyck P, Remy J et al. Hilar lymph nodes: identification with spiral CT and histologic correlation. Radiology 1995; 196: 387.

176. Remy-Jardin M, Remy J. Spiral CT of pulmonary embolism. In: Remy-Jardin M, Remy M, ed. Spiral CT of the chest. Berlin: Springer; 1996: 201–230.

177. Remy-Jardin M, Remy J, Deschildre F et al. Diagnosis of pulmonary embolism with spiral CT: comparison with pulmonary angiography and scintigraphy. Radiology 1996; 200: 699.

178. Van Rossum AB, Pattynama PM, Ton ER et al. Pulmonary embolism: validation of spiral CT angiography in 149 patients. Radiology 1996; 201: 467.

179. Teigen CL, Maus TP, Sheedy PF et al. Pulmonary embolism: diagnosis with contrast-enhanced electron-beam CT and comparison with pulmonary angiography. Radiology 1995; 194: 313.

180. Baghaie F, Remy-Jardin M, Remy J et al. Diagnosis of peripheral acute pulmonary emboli: optimization of the spiral CT acquisition. Radiology 1998; 209: 299.

181. Mayo JR, Remy-Jardin M, Müller NL et al. Pulmonary embolism: prospective comparison of spiral CT with ventilation-perfusion scintigraphy. Radiology 1997; 205: 447.

182. Herold CJ, Remy-Jardin M, Grenier PA et al. Prospective evaluation of pulmonary embolism: initial results of the European multicenter trial (ESTIPEP). Radiology 1998; 123: 334.

183. Diffin DC, Leyendecker JR, Johnson SP et al. Effect of anatomic distribution of pulmonary emboli on interobserver agreement in the interpretation of pulmonary angiography. AJR 1998; 171: 1085.

184. Stein PD, Henry JW. Prevalence of acute pulmonary embolism in central and subsegmental pulmonary arteries and relation to probability interpretation of ventilation/perfusion lung scans. Chest 1997; 111: 1246.

185. Remy-Jardin M, Remy J, Artaud D et al. Opinion response to acute pulmonary embolism: the role of computed tomographic imaging. J Thorac Imaging 1997; 12: 92.

186. Goodman LR, Lipchik RJ, Kuzo RS. Acute pulmonary embolism: the role of computed tomographic imaging. J Thorac Imag 1997; 12: 83.

187. Gefter WB, Palevsky HI. Opinion response to acute pulmonary embolism: the role of computed tomographic imaging. J Thorac Imaging 1997; 12: 97.

188. Van Erkel AR, van Rossum AB, Bloem JL et al. Spiral CT angiography for suspected pulmonary embolism: a cost-effectiveness analysis. Radiology 1996; 201: 29.

189. Loud PA, Grossman ZD, Klippenstein DL, Ray CE. Combined CT venography and pulmonary angiography: a new diagnostic technique for suspected thromboembolic disease. AJR 1998; 170: 951.

190. Weibel ER. Looking into the lung: what can it tell us? AJR 1979; 133: 1021.

191. Webb WR, Stein MG, Finkbeiner WE et al. Normal and diseased isolated lungs: high-resolution CT. Radiology 1988; 166: 81.

192. Murata K, Itoh H, Todo G et al. Centrilobular lesions of the lung: demonstration by high-resolution CT and pathologic correlation. Radiology 1986; 161: 641.

193. Stein MG, Mayo J, Müller N et al. Pulmonary lymphangitic spread of carcinoma: appearance on CT scans. Radiology 1987; 162: 371.

194. Bergin CJ, Roggli V, Coblentz C, Chiles C. The secondary pulmonary lobule: normal and abnormal CT appearances. AJR 1988; 151: 21.

195. Cook PG, Wells IP, McGavin CR. The distribution of pulmonary shadowing in Farmer's Lung. Clin Radiol 1988; 39: 21.

196. Hansell DM, Moskovic E. High-resolution computed tomography in extrinsic allergic alveolitis. Clin Radiol 1991; 43: 8.

197. Mindell HJ. Roentgen findings in Farmer's Lung. Radiology 1970; 97: 341.

198. Tung KT, Wells AU, Rubens MB et al. Accuracy of the typical computed tomographic appearances of fibrosing alveolitis. Thorax 1993; 48: 334.

199. Naidich DP. Pulmonary parenchymal high-resolution CT: to be or not to be. Radiology 1989; 171: 22.

200. Zerhouni EA, Naidich DP, Stitik FP et al. Computed tomography of the pulmonary parenchyma. Part 2: Interstitial disease. J Thorac Imag 1985; 1: 54.

201. Austin JHM, Muller NL, Friedman PJ et al. Glossary of terms for CT of the lungs: recommendations of the nomenclature committee of the Fleischner Society. Radiology 1996; 200: 327.

202. Zerhouni EA. Computed tomography of the pulmonary parenchyma. An overview. Chest 1989; 95: 901.

203. Akira M, Yamamoto S, Yokoyama K et al. Asbestosis: high-resolution CT – pathologic correlation. Radiology 1990; 176: 389.

204. Akira M, Yokoyama K, Yamamoto S et al. Early asbestosis: evaluation with high-resolution CT. Radiology 1991; 178: 409.

205. Müller NL, Miller RR, Webb WR et al. Fibrosing alveolitis: CT pathologic correlation. Radiology 1986; 160: 585.

206. Nishimura K, Kitaichi M, Izumi T et al. Usual interstitial pneumonia: histologic correlation with high-resolution CT. Radiology 1992; 182: 337.

207. Remy-Jardin M, Remy J, Deffontaines C, Duhamel A. Assessment of diffuse infiltrative lung disease: comparison of conventional CT and high-resolution CT. Radiology 1991; 181: 157.

208. Lee KS, Kim TS, Han J et al. Diffuse micronodular lung disease: HRCT and pathologic findings. J Comput Assist Tomogr 1999; 23: 99.

209. Ren H, Hruban RH, Kuhlman JE et al. Computed tomography of inflation-fixed lungs: the beaded septum sign of pulmonary metastases. J Comput Assist Tomogr 1989; 13: 411.

210. Lynch DA, Webb WR, Gamsu G et al. Computed tomography in pulmonary sarcoidosis. J Comput Assist Tomogr 1989; 13: 405.

211. Gruden JF, Webb WR. Identification and evaluation of centrilobular opacities on high-resolution CT. Semin Ultrasound CT MR 1995; 16: 435.

212. Müller NL, Staples CA, Miller RR. Bronchiolitis obliterans organizing pneumonia: CT features in 14 patients. AJR 1990; 5: 983.

213. Cheah FK, Sheppard MN, Hansell DM. Computed tomography of diffuse pulmonary haemorrhage with pathological correlation. Clin Radiol 1993; 48: 89.

214. Murata K, Herman PG, Khan A et al. Intralobular distribution of oleic acid-induced pulmonary edema in the pig. Evaluation by high-resolution CT. Invest Radiol 1989; 24: 647.

215. Stark P, Jasmine J. CT of pulmonary edema. Crit Rev Diagn Imaging 1989; 29: 245.

216. Remy-Jardin M, Remy J, Giraud F et al. Computed tomography (CT) assessment of ground-glass opacity: semiology and significance. J Thorac Imag 1993; 8: 249.

217. Martin KW, Sagel SS, Siegel BA. Mosaic oligemia simulating pulmonary infiltrates on CT. AJR 1986; 147: 670.

218. Aberle DR, Hansell DM, Brown K, Tashkin DP. Lymphangiomyomatosis: CT, chest radiographic and functional correlations. Radiology 1990; 176: 381.

219. Brauner MW, Grenier P, Mouelhi MM et al. Pulmonary histiocytosis X: evaluation with high-resolution CT. Radiology 1989; 172: 255.

220. Templeton PA, McLoud TC, Müller NL et al. Pulmonary lymphangioleiomyomatosis: CT and pathologic findings. J Comput Assist Tomogr 1989; 13: 54.

221. McGuinness G, Naidich DP, Leitman BS, McCauley DI. Bronchiectasis: CT evaluation. AJR 1993; 160: 253.

222. Desai SR, Hansell DM. Small airways disease: expiratory computed tomography comes of age. Clin Radiol 1997; 52: 332.

223. Hwang JH, Kim TS, Lee KS et al. Bronchiolitis in adults: pathology and imaging. J Comput Assist Tomogr 1997; 21: 913.

224. Müller NL, Miller RR. Diseases of the bronchioles: CT and histopathologic findings. Radiology 1995; 196: 3.

225. Wells AU. Computed tomographic imaging of bronchiolar disorders. Curr Opin Pulm Med 1998; 4: 85.

226. Myers JL, Colby TV. Pathologic manifestations of bronchiolitis, constrictive bronchiolitis, cryptogenic organizing pneumonia, and diffuse panbronchiolitis. Clin Chest Med.1993; 14: 611.

227. Hartman TE, Swensen SJ, Müller NL. Bronchiolar diseases: computed tomography. In: Epler GR, ed. Diseases of the bronchioles. New York: Raven Press; 1994: 43–58.

228. Hansell DM, Rubens MB, Padley SPG, Wells AU. Obliterative bronchiolitis: individual CT signs of small airways disease and functional correlation. Radiology 1997; 203: 721.

229. Hansell DM. Small airways diseases: detection and insights with computed tomography. Eur Respir J 2001; 17: 1294–1313.

230. Padley SP, Adler BD, Hansell DM, Müller NL. Bronchiolitis obliterans: high resolution CT findings and correlation with pulmonary function tests. Clin Radiol 1993; 47: 236.

231. Loubeyre P, Revel D, Delignette A et al. Bronchiectasis detected with thin-section CT as a predictor of chronic lung allograft rejection. Radiology 1995; 194: 213.

232. Arakawa H, Webb WR. Air trapping on expiratory high-resolution CT scans in the absence of inspiratory scan abnormalities: correlation with pulmonary function tests and differential diagnosis. AJR 1998; 170: 1349.

233. Lucidarme O, Coche E, Cluzel P et al. Expiratory CT scans for chronic airway disease: correlation with pulmonary function test results. AJR 1998; 170: 301.

234. Marti-Bonmati L, Ruiz Perales F, Catala F et al. CT findings in Swyer–James syndrome. Radiology 1989; 172: 477.

235. Stern EJ, Frank MS. Small-airways disease of the lungs: findings at expiratory CT. AJR 1994; 163: 37.

236. Aquino SL, Webb WR, Zaloudek CJ, Stern EJ. Lung cysts associated with honeycombing: change in size on expiratory CT scans. AJR 1994; 162: 583.

237. Collins J, Blankenbaker D, Stern EJ. CT patterns of bronchiolar disease: what is 'tree-in-bud'? AJR 1998; 171: 365.

238. Lynch DA, Brasch RC, Hardy KA, Webb WR. Pediatric pulmonary disease: assessment with high-resolution ultrafast CT. Radiology 1990; 176: 243.

239. Im JG, Itoh H, Shim YS et al. Pulmonary tuberculosis: CT findings – early active disease and sequential change with antituberculous therapy. Radiology 1993; 186: 653.

240. Akira M, Kitatani F, Yong-Sik L et al. Diffuse panbronchiolitis: evaluation with high-resolution CT. Radiology 1988; 168: 433.

241. Nishimura K, Kitaichi M, Izumi T, Itoh H. Diffuse panbronchiolitis: correlation of high-resolution CT and pathologic findings. Radiology 1992; 184: 779.

7 Imaging

7.2 Scintigraphic imaging

Antonio Palla and Carlo Giuntini

Key points

- Nuclear medicine utilises the emission of radionuclides introduced into the human body.

- Most pulmonary scintigraphies make use of planar large-field-of-view scintillation cameras and technetium-99m (e.g. perfusion and ventilation scintigraphies) or gallium-67 radionuclides.

- Single photon emission computed tomography (SPECT) cameras show advantages over planar ones in that they provide tridimensional imaging of the lung and quantitative measurement of radionuclide uptake in a defined volume.

- Positron emission tomography (PET) cameras allow the construction of several image slices of the organ of interest by utilising the annihilation of two particles, a positron and an electron.

- Positron-emitting tracers (e.g. carbon-11, fluoride-18, nitrogen-13) can label compounds of the physiological human metabolism.

- Cyclotron-produced short-lived positron radiotracers, such as fluoride-18, can tag common organic molecules of the body and thus permit the preparation of molecules specific for a target organ (e.g. the lung) or a target lesion (e.g. a tumour).

Several nuclear techniques can be applied to the diagnosis of pulmonary disease. Perfusion lung scintigraphy is the oldest, but is still widely used, and positron emission tomography (PET) with positron-emitting radiopharmaceuticals is the most recent. The scintigraphic imaging is most helpful in the diagnosis of pulmonary embolism, chronic obstructive lung disease (COPD), inflammatory lung diseases and intrathoracic neoplasms. In the present chapter we review each single technique in relation to the diagnosis of the pulmonary disease taken into consideration.

Diagnosis of pulmonary embolism

Pulmonary embolism is a common medical emergency because the lung arterial tree is often a site of embolism. Thrombi usually form in the deep veins of the lower extremities, break loose via the inferior vena cava through the right heart and fragment under pressure. The fragmented emboli lodge in the pulmonary arterial tree or capillary bed, depending on their size.

Large emboli may lodge in the large branches (trunk, right and left main pulmonary arteries, lobar and segmental arteries) in the initial phase of embolism. These thrombi may break down and move into smaller and more peripheral vessels later. Characteristically, patients with pulmonary embolism complain about acute dyspnoea and chest pain and show arterial hypoxemia, tachycardia and tachypnoea. Clinical diagnosis alone is uncertain: a final diagnosis is needed because the disease is treatable with anticoagulants but such treatment entails some risk.

Perfusion lung scintigraphy

In the diagnosis of pulmonary embolism, perfusion lung scintigraphy plays a role of paramount importance. First introduced by Taplin in the 1960s,[1] it allows a non-invasive, widely available and inexpensive evaluation of the distribution of blood flow in the pulmonary arteries.[2] Either human serum albumin macroaggregates or microspheres labelled with technetium-99m may be used for obtaining perfusion imaging.[3] The particle size range for macroaggregated albumin is 10–90 μ. Once injected intravenously, such particles, because of their size, lodge into the pulmonary arterioles, giving a map of the pulmonary circulation; their distribution is proportional to the amount of pulmonary blood flow and, accordingly, they will be absent where the circulation has stopped because of the presence of emboli.

The recommended number of particles per injection is 60 000–200 000, which occludes transiently 1 in 1500 arterioles in the lung; a dose of 2–4 mCi (74–148 MBq) of ^{99m}Tc pertechnetate is used to label the radiopharmaceutical. The radiopharmaceutical is injected through the antecubital vein; its distribution in the lung is nearly even from apex to base in supine subjects but shows a gradient from base to apex according to gravity in seated or erect subjects (Fig. 7.2.1). This latter position is to be preferred for injection in order to evaluate the preservation of the physiological gravitational distribution of pulmonary blood flow.[4]

Several studies have shown that perfusion lung scintigraphy is a safe procedure even in embolized patients. In over 300 patients with cardiopulmonary diseases, Moser and colleagues did not observe any complications due either to the antigenic effect of injected proteins or to microembolism itself.[5]

A large-field-of-view Anger scintillation camera equipped with a parallel-hole collimator (low-energy, high-resolution) is the most widely used instrument. Such an instrument allows eight pulmonary views to be collected in a reasonable time (around 15 min) – anterior, posterior, right and left lateral, right and left posterior oblique (45°), right and left anterior oblique. While the last two views often are omitted, the posterior oblique views are definitely useful in identifying the posterior and lateral segments of the lower lobes, avoiding the 'shine-through' effect from the opposite lung that is frequent in the lateral views and is responsible for several misdiagnoses that play a part in reducing the specificity of perfusion scintigraphy.[6]

Single photon emission computed tomography (SPECT) offers advantages over planar imaging in that it provides better contrast, edge definition and separation of target from background, thus having the potential for better detection of size, shape and distribution of perfusion.[7] Furthermore, SPECT permits the quantitative measurement of radionuclide uptake in a defined volume of the lung. The technical apparatus includes a large-field-of-view gamma camera with one or two rotating heads, equipped with a low-energy, all-purpose collimator and dedicated computer and software. By achieving a 360° circular orbit around the thorax of the patient, it offers 64 projections in a 64 × 64 matrix in three different planes (transaxial, sagittal, coronal; Fig. 7.2.2).

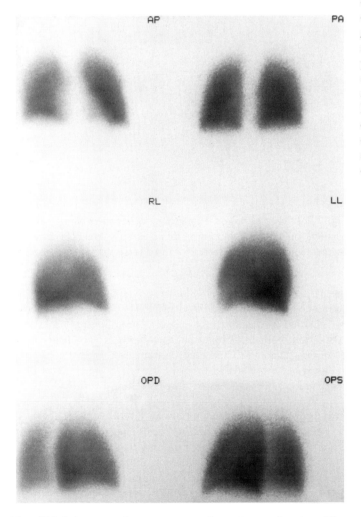

Fig. 7.2.1 Lung perfusion scintigraphy using technetium-99m macroaggregates, showing normal distribution of radionuclide over both lungs. The reported lung views are: anterior (top left), posterior (top right), right lateral (middle left), left lateral (middle right), right posterior oblique (bottom left), left posterior oblique (bottom right).

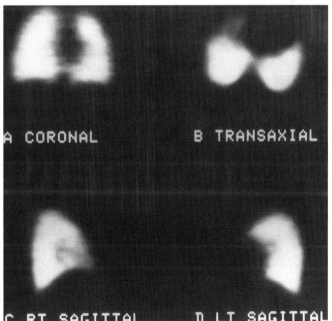

Fig. 7.2.2 Normal single photon emission computed tomography (SPECT) perfusion scintigraphy, illustrating the four views routinely shown. The dark area between the lungs is due to the heart silhouette.

Because of these characteristics, perfusion SPECT has been employed in clinical practice to diagnose pulmonary embolism. The accuracy of SPECT scintigraphy in recognising segmental perfusion defects caused by pulmonary embolism is high but requires a good knowledge of normal segmental pulmonary anatomy as it appears on SPECT scintigraphy,[8] since several normal structures (such as hila) can cause defects that may erroneously be attributed to pulmonary embolism. Therefore, an anatomical lung segment chart on SPECT scintigraphy may be of great help in scintigraphic diagnosis.[9] Moreover, SPECT scintigraphy has been used to evaluate the significance of some controversial scintigraphic findings described on planar imaging, such as the 'stripe sign' whose presence would practically exclude pulmonary embolism; SPECT, however, demonstrated the inconsistency of this sign, which accordingly should not be considered in the future in the diagnosis of pulmonary embolism.[10]

The scintigraphic diagnosis of pulmonary embolism consists of two main criteria:

■ identification of perfusion defects corresponding to one or more segments (segmental defects) or a portion of a segment (subsegmental defects; Fig. 7.2.3)
■ the finding of diversion of pulmonary blood flow from lower and posterior lung regions to upper and anterior ones, with the ensuing development of hyperperfused areas.[4]

Perfusion lung scintigraphy has an extremely high sensitivity in the diagnosis of pulmonary embolism since a normal lung scan virtually excludes the diagnosis. Two prospective studies (and a retrospective one) in patients with clinically suspected pulmonary embolism and a normal lung scan in whom anticoagulants were withheld demonstrated a total event rate (fatal or non-fatal pulmonary embolism) of 0.2% after a follow-up of at least 3 months.[11–13] Therefore, it may be considered a safe practice to withhold anticoagulant therapy in such patients. On the other hand, several authors consider the specificity of perfusion lung scintigraphy to be unsatisfactorily low, because lung pathologies other than pulmonary embolism may cause apparent segmental perfusion defects. However, the ability to recognise perfusion defects as segmental depends greatly on the technical specifications employed and the method used to interpret the results. Pulmonary embolism typically causes multiple, wedge-shaped, bilateral perfusion defects; however, less typical findings may be difficult to interpret. A practical standardisation of the scintigraphic criteria for such a diagnosis has been validated recently in a large clinical trial.[14] Overall, the experience of the person who evaluates the scintigraphy is fundamental; indeed, both inter- and intraobserver disagreement in lung scan reporting are approximately 10–20%, regardless of the classification used.[15] To overcome such disagreement, an anatomical lung segment chart may be of help, since it significantly improves consistency.[16,17] Of course, perfusion lung scanning should be used in conjunction with clinical data according to the quantitative diagnostic approach.[18]

Ventilation lung scintigraphy

Ventilation lung scintigraphy has been introduced as an addition to lung perfusion in the diagnosis of pulmonary embolism on

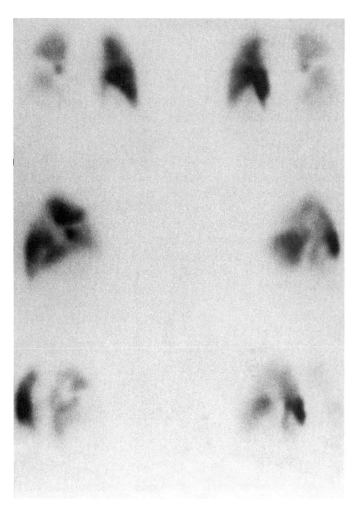

Fig. 7.2.3 Lung perfusion scintigraphy of a patient with massive, bilateral pulmonary embolism, demonstrating multiple bilateral segmental defects characteristic of the disease.

the basis that ventilation should be normal in unperfused areas; consequently, the ventilation/perfusion ($\dot{V}/\dot{Q}$) mismatch should be regarded as diagnostic of pulmonary embolism.[19] To study ventilation, both gases and nebulised aerosols have been used. The gases (xenon-133 and krypton-81m are the most common) demonstrate the distribution of lung volumes, not that of bulk ventilation, since they move into the lung by diffusion; the aerosol tracers (^{99m}Tc-labelled aerosols of homogeneously sized particles) show the distribution of convective ventilation.[20] Accordingly, gaseous tracers have mostly been employed in the diagnosis of pulmonary embolism and labelled aerosols in the study of COPD and in the evaluation of bronchial clearance and the integrity of the bronchial epithelium. A further and more detailed description of the practical performance of the technique is given later in the section on evaluation of COPD in this chapter. Scintillation cameras with low-energy, parallel-hole collimators are generally used to image ventilation. Routinely, the posterior view is chosen; however, if the patient has recently undergone perfusion scintigraphy, ventilation should be imaged using the view that best shows defects in perfusion. By using [81m]Kr or aerosols labelled with ^{99m}Tc all the traditional views may be achieved. Because of its ability to separate target from background activity, SPECT has been employed to image ventilation; however, because the anatomy is not as clear-cut on ventilation as on perfusion, interpretation of the SPECT image is more difficult.

Despite the large number of studies and trials made with $\dot{V}/\dot{Q}$ scintigraphy to diagnose pulmonary embolism, and although there has so far been no large trial comparing the diagnostic efficacy of $\dot{V}/\dot{Q}$ with perfusion alone, the diagnostic strategy based on the simultaneous use of the two techniques has failed. Ventilation does not add specificity to perfusion in most patients and, in addition, it decreases the sensitivity of the former. Indeed, only 13% of patients, those with high-probability $\dot{V}/\dot{Q}$ scan, gain any advantage from this combined strategy,[21] since in this setting specificity rises to 97%. In all other cases the specificity is modest (intermediate or indeterminate probability) or low (low probability) and perhaps worse than with perfusion alone if the patients are correctly assessed clinically before the study. There are several reasons for this, the most important being the actual decrease of ventilation in embolised zones.[22] If we add to this the fact that all methods of performing ventilation suffer from practical limitations we can understand why a realistic diagnostic strategy should not include ventilation routinely, only in selected patients.

To increase the specificity of the diagnosis of pulmonary embolism, the results of perfusion lung scintigraphy should instead be integrated with the clinical judgement of the referring physician, as demonstrated in several studies.[23–25] Indeed, when lung scintigraphic results conflict with clinical judgement (e.g. low clinical probability but high probability on scintigraphy, or vice versa) further diagnostic techniques should be employed.[26] On the basis of the above considerations, a study was designed in the Pisa area, the so called PISA-PED study, that aimed to investigate the diagnostic role of perfusion scintigraphy alone combined with clinical judgement.[18] The authors used a simplified classification of perfusion defects (Table 7.2.1), radiographic signs and clinical findings to express a clinico-scintigraphic probability of pulmonary embolism. Pulmonary angiography

yielded a definitive results in 386 of 607 patients with an abnormal perfusion lung scan. Pulmonary embolism was shown in 236 patients (lung scan positive in 217, sensitivity 92%) while pulmonary embolism was excluded in 154 patients (lung scan normal in 134, specificity 87%). The overall conclusion of this study was that, by considering clinical findings, perfusion lung scan data and follow-up results together, the number of patients with a definitive diagnosis (confirmation or exclusion) of pulmonary embolism could be greatly increased and the number of pulmonary angiographic studies accordingly decreased without the necessity for pulmonary ventilation.

Evaluation of the severity of pulmonary embolism

Perfusion lung scintigraphy is the best technique for evaluating the severity of embolism. This can be achieved by simply counting the number of unperfused lung segments on all six views obtained with the gamma camera,[27] thus obtaining a reliable index of severity of the disease, both acutely and after appropriate therapy. In the acute phase of pulmonary embolism, it has been demonstrated that, in a series of 1000 patients, the mean number of unperfused lung segments was 8.13; this represents an average rate of obstruction of the vascular bed of about 45% (Fig. 7.2.4).[28] Interestingly, the distribution of unperfused segments shows the normal error-frequency curve, the so called gaussian bell; this suggests that pulmonary embolism has a continuous spectrum of severity from cases with minimal perfusion damage to cases with massive embolism.[28] By using SPECT it has become possible to calculate the volume of a reperfused lung region a few minutes after fibrinolytic therapy.[29]

Recovery after therapy

Perfusion lung scanning also enables the evaluation of late recovery of pulmonary perfusion from acute embolism. Once again, the method is based on counting the unperfused lung segments on pulmonary perfusion scintigraphy and shows that perfusion

Table 7.2.1 Perfusion scan categories and interpretation criteria[24]

Normal	No perfusion defects
Near normal	Perfusion defects smaller or equal in size and shape to the following roentgenographic abnormalities:
	Cardiomegaly
	Enlarged aorta, hila and mediastinum
	Elevated diaphragm
	Blunting of the costophrenic angle
	Pleural thickening
	Intrafissural collection of liquid
Abnormal (PE$^+$)	Single or multiple wedge-shaped perfusion defects, with or without matching chest-X-ray abnormalities
	Wedge-shaped areas of overperfusion usually coexist
Abnormal (PE$^-$)	Single or multiple perfusion defects other than wedge-shaped, with or without matching chest-X-ray abnormalities
	Wedge-shaped areas of overperfusion are usually not seen.

PE, pulmonary embolism.

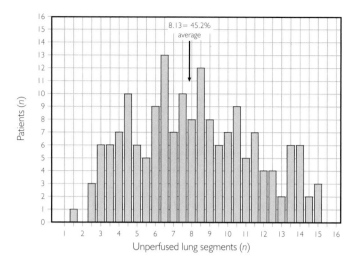

Fig. 7.2.4 Distribution of unperfused lung segments, which takes a 'gaussian' appearance in patients with pulmonary embolism.

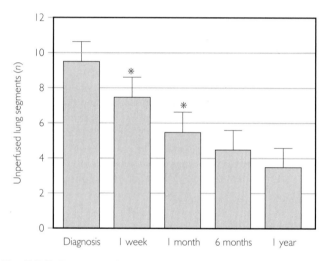

Fig. 7.2.5 Recovery of pulmonary perfusion from acute embolism to 1 year later. Perfusion damage is calculated as the number of unperfused lung segments (*y* axis). Decrease of number of unperfused lung segments is significant ($p^* < 0.05$) 1 week and 1 month after acute embolism.

damage decreases from 50% of the total vascular bed at the beginning to less than 20% 12 months after acute embolism (Fig. 7.2.5).[30] Recovery is greatest during the first month and then proceeds slowly during the successive months of follow-up. Recovery of arterial blood gases parallels that of perfusion in all phases of follow-up.[31,32]

Other scintigraphic modalities

Several scintigraphic techniques have been employed to improve the diagnosis of both deep vein thrombosis and pulmonary embolism. The original method using radio-iodinated fibrinogen, the activity of which may be scanned on the surface over deep vein thrombosis, is very useful in studying the pathophysiology of the thrombosis, since it enables the incorporation of fibrinogen into a forming thrombus to be followed as it occurs in high-risk conditions (e.g. surgery or long-term immobilisation).[33] Unfortunately, the technique is cumbersome and of poor specificity in the proximal veins.

Platelets accumulate at the site of tissue injury during the process of thrombus formation. Therefore, these cells have been labelled in order to image thrombi. To this end, autologous platelets have been labelled with indium-111 and successfully used to detect thrombi.[34] Several disadvantages of this technique have, however, limited its widespread clinical use. First, heparin reduces the adhesion of platelets to the growing thrombus and this decreases the sensitivity of the technique substantially, since heparin is often administered to the patient as soon as the clinical suspicion of pulmonary embolism arises. Second, the isolation of platelets from the individual patient's blood and their labelling must be carried out in rigorously sterile and pyrogen-free conditions, which makes it a complex process only available in specialised laboratories.

The use of radiolabelled antiplatelet monoclonal antibodies seems partly to overcome the above limitations. A monoclonal antibody to the platelet glycoprotein complex GpIIb/IIIa (7E3) was labelled with indium-111 and incubated with whole blood rather than with washed platelets.[35] A more recent idea is based upon the observation that platelets circulate in resting form and become activated at the site of thrombus formation. Thus, the potential exists for more thrombus-specific targeting using antibodies specific to activated platelets. P-selectin (CD62), also known as PADGEM or GMP-140, is a platelet glycoprotein that is translocated from an internal location to the cell membrane upon platelet activation. Therefore, antibodies to P-selectin only bind to activated platelets. A study has been designed on a baboon model with very promising results (thrombus visualisation 10 minutes after the injection, a thrombus:blood-pool ratio of 33:1)[36] that await verification in human studies.

Radiolabelled agents that bind to fibrin have also been used as a target for immunoscintigraphy of the thrombi. The idea is that, upon cleavage of soluble fibrinogen by thrombin, epitopes are exposed on the newly formed fibrin molecules that are not available on the parent molecule. Therefore, monoclonal antibodies that react with fibrin and cross-react only very weakly with circulating fibrinogen have been generated and radiolabelled for thrombus imaging. Although preliminary results seem of great clinical interest, optimal images are available only several hours after injection.[37]

Most recently, interest has been raised by the possibility of using immunoscintigraphy or, even more interestingly, either a terminal peptide of fibrin labelled with technetium-99m[38] or a peptide that binds with high affinity to the glycoprotein IIb/IIIa receptors expressed on activated platelets to image vascular thrombosis;[39] however, once again the results are preliminary and large-scale clinical investigation is lacking.

In conclusion, it is perhaps realistic to state that, so far, the radio-iodinated fibrinogen is the only agent that has produced interesting pathophysiological information and proved to be a helpful diagnostic aid in this field of medicine.

Evaluation of chronic obstructive pulmonary disease

Nuclear medicine may contribute to the evaluation of COPD through pulmonary perfusion scintigraphy and pulmonary ventilation scintigraphy; in addition, the study of bronchial clearance may play a role.

Perfusion lung scintigraphy

Perfusion scintigraphy does not have the paramount role in COPD that it has in pulmonary embolism but it is essential in the evaluation of the disease, mostly in the early phases.

Perfusion lung scintigraphy uses the same technique as was previously described for the diagnosis of pulmonary embolism. Chronic bronchitis causes a patchy, non-segmental decrease of perfusion in the lung parenchyma. Because of the pathogenesis of the disease, defects may be located everywhere in the lungs, although they appear more frequently in the lower regions, especially in exacerbations. Repeated studies after prolonged hospital treatment are useful to show the reversibility of vascular lesions. Pulmonary emphysema causes significant inhomogeneity of distribution of pulmonary blood flow and increase in lung size (Fig. 7.2.6). Since chronic bronchitis and pulmonary emphysema often coexist in the same patient it is not unusual to observe all the above abnormalities in the same scan. In giant bullous emphysema, there is absence of perfusion in the areas of bullous formation (Fig. 7.2.7). The absence of perfusion may correspond quantitatively to the size of the bulla or it may be greater because of compression of relatively normal lung

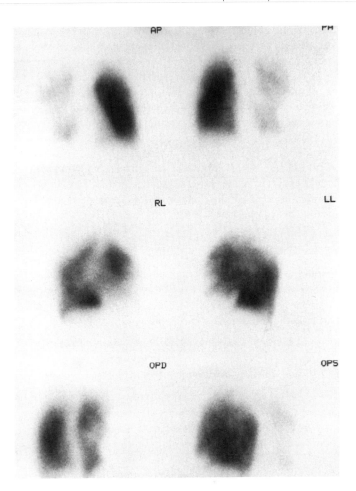

Fig. 7.2.7 Lung perfusion scintigraphy of a patient with giant bullous emphysema. Perfusion in the right lung is almost absent since the lung is entirely occupied by the giant bulla; in the left lung perfusion appears inhomogeneous.

parenchyma around the bulla. This discrepancy is, of course, of interest to the surgeon before the intervention and to the clinician in view of recovery following surgery; indeed, when the lung parenchyma around the bulla is compressed, the patient may benefit from excision[40] and this may allow the compressed healthy tissue to regain its physiological function. Details on this point, unobtainable using pulmonary function tests, might be reliably provided by a perfusion study.[41] Also important is the knowledge of compression of large vessels in the mediastinum and hilum and of the contralateral lung that may accurately be obtained from a perfusion study. The use of SPECT scintigraphy, thanks to three-dimensional imaging and the possibility of imaging only the slice of interest, appears to be indicated for the above purposes.

A quite recent application of perfusion lung scintigraphy is in evaluating the inhomogeneity of pulmonary emphysema when considering surgical intervention to reduce lung volume. Both centriacinar and panacinar emphysema cause alteration of ventilation/perfusion ratio. However, the former affects mainly the superior regions and the latter the inferior regions of the lungs. In both cases, surgery should remove those lung areas that are functionally useless. Therefore, pulmonary perfusion and venti-

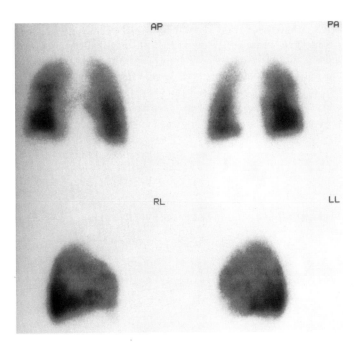

Fig. 7.2.6 Lung perfusion scintigraphy of a patient affected by pulmonary emphysema of moderate degree. Posteroanterior lung diameters are markedly augmented and distribution of radionuclide is inhomogeneous; however, no perfusion defects are present.

lation scintigraphies have been employed to visualise damaged lung areas, investigate the distribution of inhomogeneity of the emphysema and assess whether the residual pulmonary arterial bed is able to accept the whole cardiac output without increasing pulmonary arterial pressure disproportionately. Ingenito and colleagues showed that, among 29 patients with a diffuse, rather homogeneous distribution of pulmonary emphysema (on the basis of ventilation/perfusion scan), significant postsurgical improvement in FEV_1 (> 12% of predicted value) was seen in only 15.[42] In a second study of patients with inhomogeneous emphysema, the same authors demonstrated that the greater the inhomogeneity of distribution of emphysema the greater the improvement in postsurgical FEV_1.[43]

Ventilation lung scintigraphy

Ventilation lung scintigraphy, as previously stated, makes use of both gaseous tracers and nebulised aerosols. In choosing a radiopharmaceutical one should bear in mind that pulmonary ventilation is based on two mechanisms:

- *convection*, the mass movement of air in and out of the airways
- *diffusion*, molecular movement toward lower concentrations inside the airspace.

The former takes place mostly in the convective airways, the latter in the peripheral airspace. Gaseous tracers describe both phenomena, nebulised aerosols describe the distribution of convective ventilation only.[20,44] The most commonly used gas is xenon-133. The patient inhales continuously from a closed circuit to reach equilibrium of the gas in the lungs; the activity over the chest can be recorded with a gamma camera. The rate of equilibration (wash-in) as well as of elimination (wash-out) of activity from the thorax is proportional to the ventilation.[45] Krypton-81m is a gas that, when inhaled continuously, will not reach equilibrium in the airspace on account of its very short half-life (13 s). The patient inhales the gas added to air inspired

through a face mask; each inspiration may be considered as a single dose of the gas, so the images collected by the gamma camera during quiet breathing may be viewed as the sum of the individual breaths (Fig. 7.2.8).[46]

Aerosols are more suitable for evaluating ventilation in COPD. They consist of liquid droplets or solid preformed particles labelled with technetium-99m. To trace ventilation, particles should be deposited in the airways by sedimentation, i.e. they should follow the airflow into the most peripheral airways, avoiding any impact on bronchial walls. To this end, particles of about 1 μm in aerodynamic diameter should be chosen.[20] Images may be collected in all the traditional views. Compared with the distribution of krypton-81m, images in normal subjects do not show differences. In COPD patients, on the other hand, images do differ, particles typically having three patterns of deposition associated with the obstructive type of the disease and gas having less distinctive features.[20] Indeed, peripheral spots of labelled aerosol indicate areas of relative hyperventilation (Fig. 7.2.9) that gaseous tracers fail to visualise because they distribute by diffusion in airspaces ventilated by collateral channels (Fig. 7.2.10). Therefore, in COPD, images of convective ventilation distribution obtained with particles are more closely correlated with functional lung impairment. On the other hand, increased deposition by impaction in the large airways is related to constriction and is characteristically associated with asthma.

Study of bronchial mucociliary clearance

Tracheobronchial clearance may be regarded as an index of bronchial epithelial function, which may be impaired early in several bronchopulmonary pathologies. Therefore, early knowledge of impairment may help with both diagnosis and prognosis of such patients. Aerosols of radiolabelled particles of sufficiently large size have been used to study bronchial clearance,[22] since relatively large particles are deposited along all the bronchi and cleared away by mucociliary transport. Although the rate of removal of particulate material largely depends on the site of

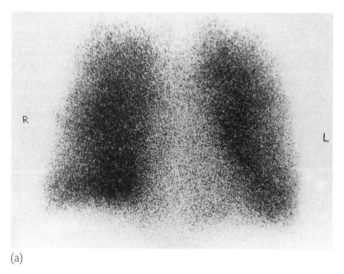

(a)

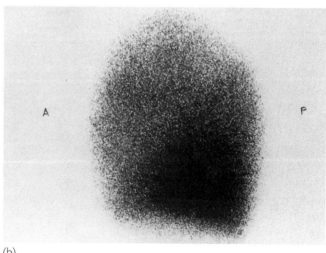

(b)

Fig. 7.2.8 Krypton-81m ventilation obtained in a normal subject. Distribution of gas to both lungs is uniform. Although the same views as on perfusion scintigraphy are obtainable, only anterior (a) and left lateral (b) views are shown for the sake of brevity.

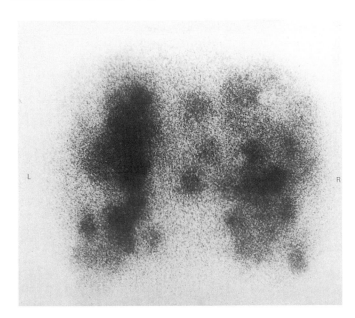

Fig. 7.2.9 Technetium-99m HAMM (human albumin particles) ventilation (posterior view) of a patient affected by severe chronic obstructive pulmonary disease. A typical 'spotty' deposition of particles is appreciable as a result of the significant inhomogeneity of ventilation.

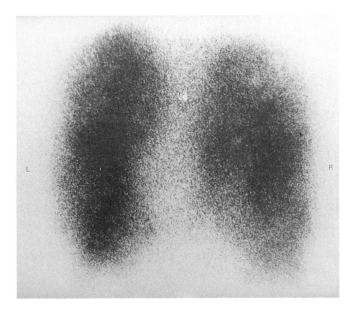

Fig. 7.2.10 Krypton-81m ventilation (anterior view) of the same patient as in Figure 7.2.9. The distribution, although diffusely inhomogeneous, does not show 'spotty' patterns.

deposition, it is also dependent on the presence of airway disease. Particles of about $1\,\mu m$ in aerodynamic diameter should be used, to ensure deposition throughout the bronchial tree and to avoid distribution and diffusion in peripheral airspaces through collateral channels. In particular, monodisperse aerosols of human albumin particles $0.8\,\mu m$ in diameter with a geometric standard deviation of $1.9\,\mu m$, which are easily labelled with technetium-99m (HAMM) have been employed,[22] along with a

planar large-field-of-view gamma camera. Images are taken using a standard view (usually the anterior view) soon after inhalation, 20, 40 and 60 minutes later, thus showing the movement up toward the carina of rounded hot spots caused by lumping of particles. This upward movement may be severely impaired in patients with COPD and bronchiectasis (Fig. 7.2.11). Time–activity curves may also be obtained showing the changing activity (counts) over time (minutes). In this way, the effect of drugs on bronchial clearance may be evaluated.

Diagnosis of inflammatory disease of the lungs

Pathological processes of different types may cause lung inflammation, including bacterial, viral or fungal infections, acute respiratory distress syndrome (ARDS), sarcoidosis and other interstitial lung disease.

In the acute or subacute phase, the diagnosis of pulmonary inflammatory disease is made possible by the use of several radiopharmaceuticals, each exhibiting a quite specific mechanism of accumulation inside the lesion of interest. In particular, radionuclide techniques may be employed to detect the site of intrathoracic infections and in detecting, staging and monitoring pulmonary alveolitis.

In order to detect intrathoracic infections the following techniques may be employed:

- ^{67}Ga-citrate scintigraphy
- autologous white blood cells labelled with ^{111}In oxime
- autologous white blood cells labelled with ^{99m}Tc-hexamethylpropyleneamine oxime (HMPAO)
- ^{99m}Tc-labelled monoclonal antibodies (MAb) specific to human immunoglobulin
- ^{99m}Tc-labelled polyclonal human immunoglobulin
- ^{111}In-labelled chemotactic peptide analogues.

All these tracers have been tested and found to be potentially useful in the detection of pneumonia, abscess, tuberculosis or pulmonary densities in patients with viral, bacterial or mycotic infections.[47] However, most of the above tracers have several disadvantages. These include difficulties in preparing the radiotracer (MAb specific to human immunoglobulin), performing the whole technique (polyclonal human immunoglobulin) or obtaining the radiotracer itself (HMPAO, polyclonal human immunoglobulin). Therefore, these tracers have not been widely adopted in clinical practice. Among them, only ^{67}Ga citrate and, to a lesser extent, autologous white blood cells have been shown to have a practical clinical application.

Gallium-67 scintigraphy

Normally gallium-67 accumulates within liver, bowel, kidneys, bone marrow and spleen. It accumulates inside the cells in lysosomes or lysosome-like granules in normal tissue. However, in inflammatory tissue and in tumours, the mechanism is perhaps different, but not yet thoroughly understood. Gallium-67 (radioactive half-life 3.25 days) is excreted through the kidneys

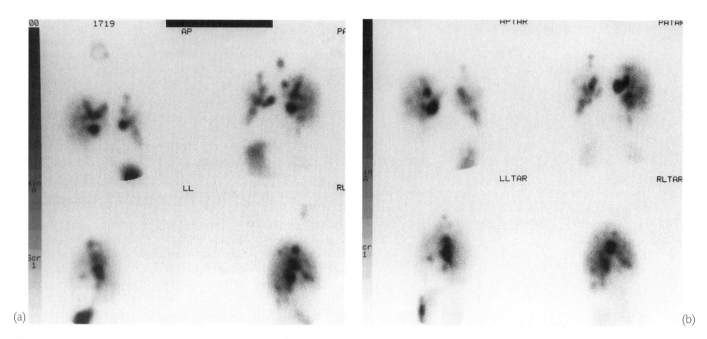

(a)   (b)

Fig. 7.2.11 Study of mucociliary tracheobronchial clearance of a patient with severe chronic bronchitis. A remarkably inhomogeneous deposition of particles is appreciable soon after inhalation in four different views (a). Little modification of particle positioning (black spots) is seen 4 hours later (b), indicating notably reduced clearance.

and, partly, through the bowel after the first 24 hours but even after 72 hours these organs can still be visualised. Once injected intravenously, this radioactive element binds avidly to transferrin, lactoferrin, ferritin and siderophores, low-molecular-weight compounds that normally mediate incorporation of iron into cells and bacteria. In blood, it possesses a half-life of several hours. In general, gallium-67 accumulates where rapid cell growth is present; this characteristic makes it ideal for evaluating the activity of inflammatory processes. It has been calculated that the radiation absorbed dose is 0.90 rad/mCi to the colon, 0.58 to the marrow, 0.53 to the spleen, 0.46 to the liver and 0.26 to the glands. These levels of radiation are quite low in comparison with those of other nuclear medicine techniques used for similar purposes (e.g. [111]In leukocytes); these characteristics, along with wider availability and less complex technique, make gallium-67 scintigraphy the most extensively used scintigraphic technique in both acute and chronic inflammation.

The acquisition of images requires a scintillation gamma camera with a medium-energy collimator for the 184 and 296 KeV emissions of gallium-67; the dose injected ranges between 5 and 10 mCi (185 and 370 MBq). Images should be taken routinely 48 and 72 hours after the injection; in doubtful cases images should also be taken after 120 hours when the background activity has definitely disappeared. An image may be taken 6 hours post-injection if a pulmonary infection is suspected. A whole body planar imaging is routinely performed unless a limited examination is requested; the use of SPECT (with a higher dose of radionuclide) is often necessary for better localisation or identification of a region of abnormal uptake. The amount of gallium-67 uptake may be quantified by a semiquantitative[48] or, ideally, quantitative method, the latter being more accurate than the former.[49,50]

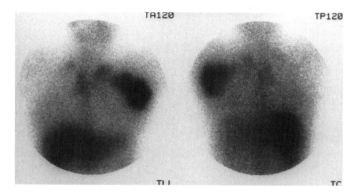

Fig. 7.2.12 Gallium-67 scintigraphy of a patient with acute pulmonary infection of the left lung. The anterior view is shown on the left, the posterior view on the right. A large, intense uptake of gallium is visible in the left upper lobe; mediastinal, paratracheal and supraclavicular lymph nodes also take up the radionuclide avidly. (Courtesy of Dr P. Fazzi, University of Pisa.)

The most important indications for gallium-67 scintigraphy are pulmonary infections, lung involvement in acquired immuno-deficiency syndrome (AIDS), and interstitial lung disease.

In acute pyogenic infections, the abnormal concentration of gallium-67 may be evident early (6 hours after the injection) and better visualised later on (48 hours; Fig. 7.2.12), although it continues to increase for 7–19 days. In chronic abscesses (present for more than 2 weeks) only the edge of the lesion may be visualised as a result of central necrosis and lack of blood supply; in these cases, however, indium-111 leukocyte scintigraphy is often completely negative.

The diagnosis of tuberculosis may be difficult clinically, especially in patients who have already had the disease years earlier; in such patients gallium-67 allows the physician to distinguish pleuroparenchymal fibrosis due to previous infections from recent reinfections with quite a good degree of accuracy. Moreover, scintigraphy is helpful in determining disease activity in sputum-smear-negative patients with tuberculosis.[51] Alternatively, thallium-201 has been proposed for this purpose.[52]

The increase of opportunistic infections in immunodepressed patients and the reappearance, after several years of continuous decline, of tuberculosis has led to increasing clinical use of gallium-67. Indeed, the diagnosis of tuberculosis is even more complicated in AIDS patients, where the classical radiographic manifestations are often lacking while thoracic lymphadenopathies and non-cavitated pulmonary infiltrates in middle and lower lobes are more frequent. In such patients, gallium-67 scintigraphy is often routinely used, although HRCT has been demonstrated to be more helpful in guiding the technique of biopsy and directing the bronchoscopist to the lung segment affected by the disease.[53]

In AIDS patients, *Pneumocystis carinii* pneumonia (PCP) represents a common and life-threatening complication. The gallium-67 scintigraphy shows diffuse increased lung uptake quite characteristic of PCP in the presence of compatible clinical findings; gallium-67 is positive in the lungs in presence of PCP in 100% of patients with AIDS (Fig. 7.2.13), even if the infection is subclinical.[54-55] Gallium-67 scintigraphy is also useful for the diagnosis of Kaposi's sarcoma in such patients. When chest radiography is abnormal and gallium-67 scintigraphy is normal, the diagnosis of Kaposi's sarcoma is likely, since this tumour characteristically does not concentrate gallium-67. A further indication for the use of gallium-67 in patients with AIDS is the differential diagnosis of intracranial masses, to distinguish neoplasms (lymphoma or glioma) from other, non-malignant lesions. For this purpose, both gallium-67 and thallium-201 help to differentiate tumours from infarction or progressive multifocal leukoencephalopathy.[56] Finally, in patients with fever of unknown origin, gallium-67 may be indicated, usually when no immediate significant medical history is present. Since many causes of fever

do not induce a neutrophilic infiltrate, gallium-67 scintigraphy may be preferred to labelled leukocytes.[57]

The use of gallium-67 in interstitial lung disease may help in the evaluation of both disease activity and treatment efficacy[58] In patients with sarcoidosis several studies have shown that gallium-67 scintigraphy has high sensitivity in demonstrating acute alveolitis[59] (Fig. 7.2.14). In particular, the sensitivity is higher than that of chest radiography, serum level of angiotensin-converting enzyme, or levels of T-lymphocyte subpopulations in circulating blood, both in patients with hilar adenopathy only (stage I) and in patients with lung involvement (stage II–III). Furthermore, gallium-67 scintigraphy shows a linear relationship with the number of lymphocytes found in bronchoalveolar lavage in patients with sarcoidosis.[60]

On the other hand, the specificity of gallium-67 scintigraphy is low in these diseases but this is of minor importance since other techniques are available to differentiate among lung disorders. However, when specific patterns can be visualised the specificity rises markedly. This is the case when intense uptake into the salivary and lacrimal glands ('panda sign'; Fig. 7.2.15) or thoracic lymph nodes ('lambda sign'; Fig. 7.2.16) is seen. These patterns may make invasive diagnostic procedures unnecessary.[59] In patients with idiopathic pulmonary fibrosis, gallium-67 scan is abnormal in 70% of cases[61] and the uptake index correlates with the level of neutrophils found in the bronchoalveolar lavage. In patients with hypersensitivity pneumonitis, the uptake of gallium-67 parallels the evolution of the disease.[62]

Because of its low specificity, the routine use of gallium-67 scanning in the initial assessment of sarcoidosis is not recommended. However, gallium-67 scintigraphy is helpful in sarcoidosis when diagnostic difficulties arise, particularly when extrapulmonary involvement (stage IV) is suspected,[63] and then it is advisable to perform a whole-body scan.[64]

Indium-111 leukocyte scintigraphy

White blood cells labelled with ^{111}In oxime are obtained by incubation of a suspension of white blood cells with the ^{111}In oxime. The In^{3+} ion does not pass through the cell membrane, because of its electronic charge, until complexed with the lipophilic agent oxime. Inside the cell, the indium–oxime complex dissociates and

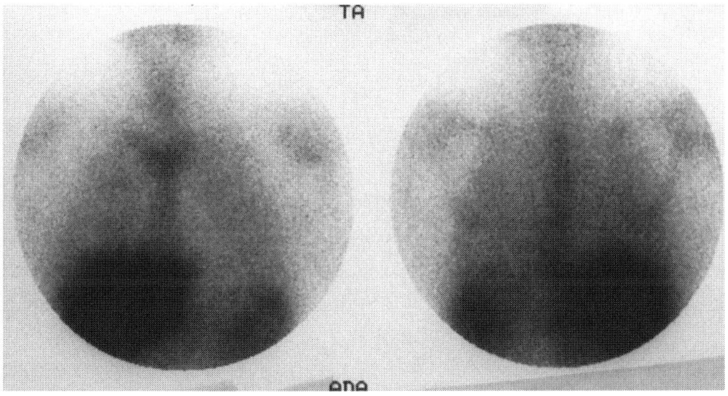

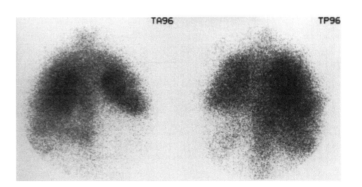

Fig 7.2.13 Gallium-67 scintigraphy of a patient treated for non-Hodgkin's lymphoma who developed *Pneumocystis carinii* pneumonia. A mild, diffuse, homogeneous lung uptake is appreciable bilaterally. (Courtesy of Dr P. Fazzi, University of Pisa.)

Fig 7.2.14 Gallium-67 scintigraphy showing intense, diffuse, homogeneous uptake in a patient with acute alveolitis due to sarcoidosis. (Courtesy of Dr P. Fazzi, University of Pisa.)

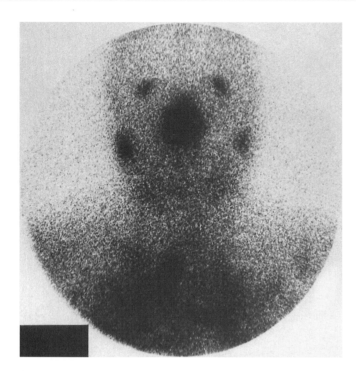

Fig 7.2.15 The typical 'panda' sign of a patient affected by sarcoidosis. The sign is caused by focal gallium uptake in the nose and salivary glands. (Courtesy of Dr P. Fazzi, University of Pisa.)

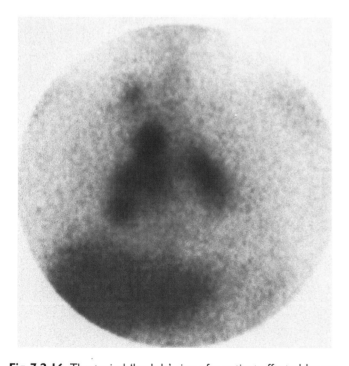

Fig 7.2.16 The typical 'lambda' sign of a patient affected by sarcoidosis. The 'lambda' sign is caused by focal gallium uptake in the hilar and paratracheal lymph nodes. A right supraclavicular lymph node is also visible in this patient. (Courtesy of Dr P. Fazzi, University of Pisa.)

indium-111 binds to intracellular plasma proteins. The process of labelling white blood cells with indium-111 is rather complex and this has perhaps limited its use to specialised centres. About 30–50 ml of venous blood from the patient is necessary for the labelling process. In the sample, white blood cells must be separated from red blood cells. Since the ratio between red blood cells and white blood cells in the blood is 1000:1, it is mandatory that the method employed to remove red blood cells is 100% efficient: even a method that removes 99.9% of red blood cells will result in equal numbers of both types of cell.

Because 60% of normal white blood cells are neutrophils, most of the labelled white blood cells will be neutrophils. Moreover, the method used for labelling white blood cells should not damage the surface sensors responsible for migration of the neutrophils to the site of infection. Finally, the whole procedure must be done in aseptic conditions. About 200–500 μCi of ^{111}In-labelled white blood cells may be injected slowly through a large-bore needle, while injection through plastic tubes should be avoided. After the intravenous injection, an immediate accumulation in the lungs is appreciable; then, unless the lung represents the site of an infection, by 3–4 hours it should be clear of this tracer.[65] Most activity at this time will be present in spleen, liver and bone marrow. Images are usually taken 24 hours after the injection and delay does not increase the accuracy of the examination. The physical half-life of indium-111 is 2.8 days; however, the biological half-life of labelled white blood cells in normal subjects is shorter, about 7 hours, since they are destroyed by the reticuloendothelial system.

In spite of the promising theoretical indications for such a tracer, its clinical applications are limited. First proposed for the diagnosis of bronchiectasis and assessment of their activity and severity,[66] labelled white blood cells did not achieve extensive use for this purpose, because of the valid alternatives represented by endoscopic and radiological techniques, i.e. bronchoalveolar lavage and high-resolution computed tomography (CT). In acute abscesses, labelled white blood cells are still directly indicated, although perhaps replaced by gallium-67 scintigraphy. In lobar pneumonia, leukocyte scintigraphy is usually negative,[67] while it may be positive in diseases showing diffuse and symmetrical accumulation, such as ARDS.[68] However, even in these cases, other techniques seem more suitable on the grounds of efficacy and safety. At present, the usefulness of ^{111}In-leukocyte scintigraphy in patients with fever of unknown origin is under study.

Study of pulmonary clearance

Since most inflammatory lung diseases enhance alveolar–epithelial permeability, measurement of the clearance rate of diethylenetriamine pentaacetic acid (DTPA) from the lung has become a valid tool for evaluating the functional state of the blood–gas barrier. Measurement of the clearance rate of inhaled ^{99m}Tc-labelled DTPA from the lungs using a gamma camera provides an index of the integrity of the pulmonary epithelium.[69] The relatively small size of this molecule allows the tracer to diffuse through the alveolo-capillary membrane and the clearance rate of DTPA predicts the inflammatory activity of pulmonary processes.[70] The technique consists of continuously registering the count over the lung immediately after inhalation of the aerosol; it has been applied to evaluate epithelium integrity in several disorders. A rapid clearance rate has been demonstrated in normal smokers, diffuse interstitial lung disease, ARDS, hyaline membrane disease, bronchopulmonary dysplasia and PCP. In almost all the studies the clearance of DTPA showed consistent parallel changes with clinical status or radiographic appearances. Unfortunately, however, it is sensitive but poorly specific, since the clearance rate in normal smokers and in patients with interstitial lung disease is similar and practically indistinguishable. Moreover, standardisation of the inhalation technique and criteria for assessing the clearance rate is needed to reduce the variability of results and to provide reliable values to identify patients with abnormal clearance rates.

Diagnosis of intrathoracic neoplasms

Two main scintigraphic techniques may be employed in the diagnosis of intrathoracic tumours: gallium-67 scintigraphy and positron emission tomography (PET). Moreover, lung perfusion scintigraphy may play a role in assessment of resectability.

Actually, several other agents have also been employed in the scintigraphic diagnosis of intrathoracic neoplasms but for different reasons none has achieved widespread clinical use. Among these are thallium-201 (^{201}Tl),[71] ^{99m}Tc-labelled hexamethylpropyleneamine oxime (HMPAO)[72] or ^{99m}Tc-labelled methoxyisobutyl isonitrile (MIBI).[73] Of interest in the detection of bronchial carcinoid is ^{111}In-labelled octreotide, a peptide taken up by tumours that express somatostatin receptors.[74] Also rather specific is the detection of phaeochromocytoma by ^{123}I-labelled meta-iodobenzylguanidine (MIBG),[75] a noradrenaline (norepinephrine) analogue taken up into the presynaptic terminals of sympathetic nerves.

Gallium-67 scintigraphy

The technique is described above. In the diagnosis of both non-Hodgkin's and Hodgkin's lymphoma, the use of gallium-67 scintigraphy is a matter of controversy. In fact, it has a sensitivity and specificity close to 100% when high doses (6–10 mCi) of radionuclide and SPECT are employed.[76] The role of gallium-67 scintigraphy in staging lymphoma is limited, however, since radiological imaging techniques such as CT are more effective in showing sites of disease below the diaphragm.[77] According to Tumeh and colleagues[78] gallium-67 SPECT showed foci due to lymphoma that were not clearly demonstrated on planar imaging, and perhaps with greater accuracy than CT.

Most recently, the role of gallium-67 in predicting the outcome of both non-Hodgkin's[79] and Hodgkin's[80] lymphoma has been reassessed, by demonstrating that the early use of such a tracer during chemotherapy is a good indicator of patients who may benefit from a change to a more aggressive treatment. Moreover, gallium-67 scintigraphy is an excellent predictor of residual tumour viability in lymphoma patients

and the persistent positivity of the scan predicts poor outcome.[81] As to the follow-up under therapy, a relevant clinical question is whether a residual mass visible on the chest radiograph after appropriate treatment is due to fibrosis (e.g. resulting from radiotherapy) or to persistent foci of the original neoplasm. Gallium-67 may detect relapse of lymphoma more accurately and much earlier than CT, as well as diagnosing complete remission after treatment.[82] Therefore, gallium-67 scintigraphy either with SPECT or with a planar gamma camera is the technique of choice for monitoring the response of lymphoma to treatment.

The use of gallium-67 scintigraphy to localise lung cancer was first described by Edwards & Hayes in 1969.[83] Since then, the technique has been used for both localisation and staging[84] (Fig. 7.2.17). The sensitivity of gallium-67 scintigraphy in detecting lung cancer is generally moderate. It is low for lesions less than 2 cm in diameter; to overcome this drawback it is possible to increase the amount of the injected dose (from 3 mCi to 10 mCi) since this increases the sensitivity from 43% to 75% in neoplasms of a size between 1.5 cm and 3 cm.[85] Other reasons for false-negative cases, the incidence of which ranges from 9% to 22%, are unfavourable localisation of the neoplasm, necrosis of the lesion and recent therapy with cytostatic drugs. On the other hand, the uptake from the tumour is not dependent on the histological cell type; one exception is bronchioloalveolar carcinoma, which typically takes up gallium-67 strongly.

In staging of lung cancer, the role of gallium-67 scintigraphy is controversial. The capability of gallium-67 in investigating lymph node involvement and the presence of metastases is variable and discrepant in different series. By testing the gallium-67 scintigraphy against mediastinoscopy, the surgical gold standard technique in determining lymph node involvement, Alazraky et al[86] demonstrated that patients with no gallium-67 uptake may undergo surgery without mediastinoscopy while patients with hilar/mediastinal uptake must have mediastinoscopy first, since the gallium-67 sensitivity was 100% but the specificity was only 71%. However, other authors[87] found a lower sensitivity (56%) and a higher specificity (94%) and, accordingly, their conclusion

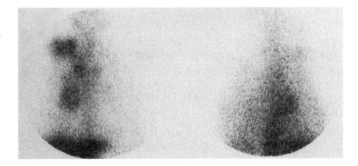

Fig 7.2.17 Gallium-67 scintigraphy of a patient affected by lung cancer. In the anterior view, an intense uptake is visible in the right upper lobe, corresponding to the radiographic density. Moreover, radionuclide uptake is appreciable in correspondence of right hilar and mediastinal lymph nodes. (Courtesy of Dr P. Fazzi, University of Pisa.)

was that mediastinoscopy should be performed only in the absence of gallium-67 uptake.

In searching for extrapulmonary metastases, the probability that extrapulmonary uptake of gallium-67 is due to metastases is about 90% when the scintigraphy shows a positive uptake for lung cancer.[88]

Positron emission tomography (PET) scanning

The use of PET with positron-emitting nuclides has recently been introduced in the diagnosis of neoplastic diseases. The prerequisites were improved instrumentation, the development of computer hardware and software and the development of 'baby' cyclotrons (necessary to generate and make available readily appropriate nuclides). These have made it possible to label compounds of the physiological human metabolism with positron-emitting tracers. PET is unique in its ability to obtain functional images of blood flow and metabolic processes rather than anatomical images such as those supplied by radiography, CT and magnetic resonance imaging (MRI). The production by a cyclotron of short-lived positron radiotracers of basic organic elements such as carbon-11, nitrogen-13, oxygen-15 and fluorine-18 that can be used to tag common organic molecules of the body allows a molecule to be constructed that is specific for the target organ (e.g. the lung) or lesion (e.g. the tumour). The PET camera utilises the annihilation of two particles, a positron and an electron, to generate two photons, each of 511 KeV, with a direction opposite to each other. By reconstructing the planes from which photons originate, the PET camera is able to construct image slices of the organ of interest.

The combination of the PET camera with the glucose analogue ^{18}F-2-fluoro-2 deoxyglucose (FDG) is perhaps the modality most frequently used in the diagnosis, staging and follow-up of patients with bronchogenic carcinoma, pulmonary metastatic disease and Hodgkin's lymphoma. FDG is the ideal tracer for neoplasms since it is a marker of glucose uptake and cancer cells possess an increased glucose metabolism As a consequence, FDG-6-phosphate is trapped within the tumour cells and provides the basis for FDG-PET tumour imaging. Patients must be evaluated in fasting conditions (at least 4 hours) in order to minimise the competitive inhibition of FDG by serum glucose.[89] In patients with diabetes, the FDG should be administered only when their blood sugar is well controlled by therapy; in patients with a history of glucose intolerance a serum glucose level should be obtained and FDG injected only when the value is within an acceptable range.

Positron emission tomographic imaging is presently performed by a tomographic camera that can produce several simultaneous cross-sectional slices with a field of view of at least 14 cm. This operation allows accurate exploration of the region of interest, which is identified on the basis of visual analysis of the CT scan. After the patient has been positioned on the tomographic bed, 10 mCi (370 MBq) of FDG is infused through the antecubital vein, in the arm opposite to the region of interest. Simultaneously, transmission images are acquired. Up to 60 million counts are collected for each scan; such images are sub-

sequently used to generate attenuation correction factors. Then, a 60-minute period is allowed for radiotracer uptake before the acquisition of a static 15-minute image of the region of interest. The correct position should be maintained throughout the whole study, possibly with the help of a light beam and indelible marks on the patient's torso. An anatomical reference point should be identified in each patient in order to ensure reproducibility throughout the studies when these are performed at different times.

The interpretation of FDG-PET studies may be carried out in either a qualitative or a semiquantitative way. In the former case, an abnormal area is compared with background activity. For instance, the interpretation of a lung nodule consists in the comparison of nodule uptake and normal mediastinal/cardiac blood pool intensity. A lesion may be diagnosed as malignant when the nodule uptake is greater than that of the normal blood pool. Conversely, a smaller or similar uptake allows one to consider the lesion to be benign. In the latter case, a semiquantitative index may be derived from glucose metabolism at the level of the region of interest. This is called the standardised uptake ratio[90] and represents the normalisation of the amount of FDG uptake or intensity in a particular area to the total injected dose and the patient's body weight.

It has been demonstrated that, in lung cancer, FDG-PET characterises lesions that are indeterminate on radiological CT;[91] this is because many benign lesions have similar radiological characteristics to malignant ones. This property of FDG-PET is of great clinical importance since half of lesions that are removed are benign and, therefore, the early use of procedures such as video-assisted thoracic surgery may be excessive. The main indication of FDG-PET in pulmonary neoplastic pathology is the evaluation of patients with focal pulmonary opacities on chest radiography[92] (Fig. 7.2.18). Since most malignant pulmonary nodules are adenocarcinomas (now representing the most prevalent type of lung cancer in North America, 40% of the total), the early diagnosis of peripheral lung nodules repre-

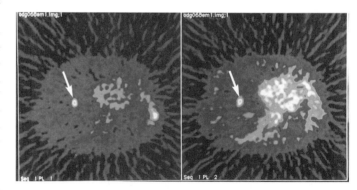

Fig 7.2.18 ^{18}F-2-fluoro-2 deoxyglucose positron emission tomography (FDG-PET) scan of a patient showing a solitary pulmonary nodule in the upper lobe of the right lung on chest radiography. Two consecutive transaxial slices of the region of interest are shown: a focal, intense uptake is visible in the upper lobe of the right lung, corresponding to the radiographic nodule (arrow). Such a finding is highly compatible with the neoplastic nature of the lesion. (Courtesy of Drs G. Mariani and A. Giorgetti, University of Pisa.)

sents a great task for the attending physician. The sensitivity and specificity in differentiating benign from malignant lung lesions are high, sensitivity being around 95–100% and specificity around 80–85% (the latter is lower because inflammatory processes also accumulate FDG avidly). The high negative predictive value of FDG-PET allows all nodules that test negative to be considered benign, thus avoiding the need for biopsies or surgery. It is interesting that no correlation seems to exist between lesion diameter and uptake of FDG; however, lesions less than 0.7 cm in diameter are perhaps below the resolution capability of the scanner.[93] A correlation exists between lesion doubling time and FDG uptake;[94] a correlation was also found between prognosis and amount of FDG uptake in patients with solitary pulmonary nodules subsequently diagnosed as cancer.[95] Of less clinical importance but still useful for the decision making process is the use of FDG-PET in patients with hilar masses.

The second main indication of FDG-PET is the staging of lung cancer. Assessment of lymph node involvement (mostly hilar and mediastinal) in patients with lung cancer is of paramount importance in establishing a management strategy. To this end, the use of FDG-PET is definitely more accurate, sensitive and specific than any radiological technique, including CT and MRI, since radiological staging is only based on a size-dependent criterion (Fig. 7.2.19). Perhaps the combined use of radiological CT and FDG-PET will further improve accuracy.[96] The sensitivity and specificity for N2–N3 mediastinal disease have been shown to be 20% and 90% for CT and 70% and 97% for PET.[97] Only mediastinoscopy is presently superior to FDG-PET in the study of lymph nodes involvement, but it is invasive.[98] Technically, lung-cancer-staging use whole-body imaging. A whole-body study requires four or five different bed positions and acquisition takes about 30–50 minutes.

Lung cancer may metastasise early to various organs and, with whole-body imaging, FDG-PET has been shown to be 100% sensitive and 94% specific in showing distant metastases.[99] It is probable that, in many cases, the management strategy might be changed on the basis of a whole-body study.[91,97] Whole-body PET scintigraphy is also more accurate than bone scintigraphy and brain CT or MRI imaging in staging

bronchogenic carcinoma.[100] FDG-PET has shown promising results in monitoring the response to chemotherapy[101] by showing a decrease in FDG accumulation after therapy. Persistent or recurrent disease may also be detected early,[102] especially in lung regions showing fibrosis following radiotherapy. To differentiate areas of fibrosis from recurrence, the combined use of radiological CT and FDG-PET may be very helpful (Fig. 7.2.20).

Recently, the prognostic value of thoracic FDG-PET imaging after treatment for non-small-cell lung cancer was investigated.[103] The results indicated that FDG-PET strongly correlates with survival rates of patients with treated lung cancer; patients with positive FDG-PET results have a significantly worse prognosis than patients with negative results. Finally, few data exist about the differential diagnosis between benign pleural plaques and lesions due to mesothelioma; FDG-PET may play a role in excluding malignancy when negative.

At present, FDG-PET scintigraphy is not just very promising but essential for the clinical management of lung cancer, especially considering the clinical availability of PET equipment and its relative cost-effectiveness. It reduces the probability that a patient with unresectable disease will undergo an unnecessary intervention.

A great deal of interest was raised by the use of immunoscintigraphy in lung cancer.[104] However, the results of clinical trials must be available before this new promising technique can be accepted into clinical practice.

Perfusion lung scintigraphy

In patients with lung cancer, perfusion lung scintigraphy has a role in the assessment of tumour resectability, by predicting postoperative lung function.

The study of the pulmonary circulation by perfusion scintigraphy in patients with lung cancer provides useful data about the localisation, extension and operability of the tumour. For more details, see Chapter 67.

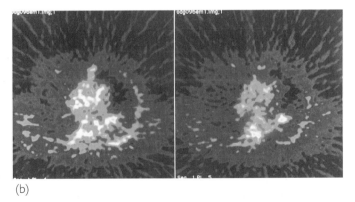

(a) (b)

Fig 7.2.19 (a) Computed tomography (CT) scan (two contiguous slices) of a patient with a squamous cell carcinoma of the main left bronchus. A mass is appreciable around the left hilum, representing perihilar lymph nodes. (b) ^{18}F-2-fluoro-2 deoxyglucose positron emission tomography (FDG-PET) scan of the same patient shows focal, moderate-intensity radionuclide uptake in the perihilar lymph nodes, corresponding to the CT scan, indicating metabolic activity compatible with a metastatic process. (Courtesy of Drs G. Mariani and A. Giorgetti, University of Pisa.)

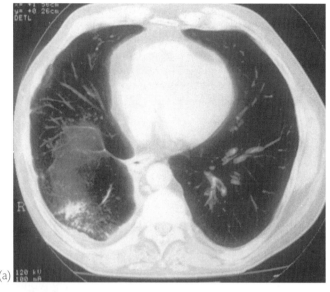

(a)

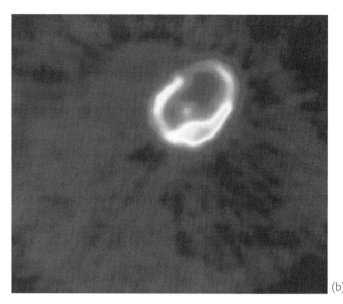

(b)

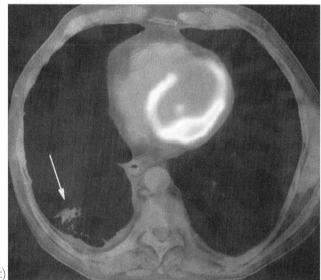

(c)

Fig 7.2.20 (a) Computed tomography (CT) scan showing localised pulmonary fibrosis following radiation therapy for inoperable bronchogenic carcinoma (adenocarcinoma). Differential diagnosis of residual cancer foci is impossible on the basis of the CT. (b) ^{18}F-2-fluoro-2 deoxyglucose positron emission tomography (FDG-PET) scan in the same patient shows no activity corresponding to the radiographic image. (c) An image resulting from the superimposition of the FDG-PET scan on to the corresponding CT slice, the so called 'anatometabolic' method, shows no radionuclide activity in the relevant area (arrow), thus allowing exclusion of cancer recurrence. (Courtesy of Drs G. Mariani and A. Giorgetti, University of Pisa.)

Metabolic functions of the lung

In addition to the function of external gas exchange, the lung also possesses a metabolic function. It is known that the lung activates and deactivates or synthesises many metabolites (peptides, vasoactive amines, etc.). These can be labelled with radioactive tracers and thus studied and potentially used for diagnosis and treatment. For instance, angiotensin-I is converted into angiotensin-II by angiotensin-converting enzyme; other compounds, such as serotonin or bradykinin, are inactivated on coming into contact with the pulmonary endothelium.

Radiolabelled amines have been shown to accumulate in the lung by saturable, receptor-specific mechanisms. Knowledge of the behaviour of such substances in the lung makes it possible to study regional pulmonary metabolism and regional lung function in both health and disease. ^{123}I-labelled *N,N,N'*-trimethyl-*N'*-(2-hydroxy-3methyl-5-iodobenzyl)-1,3-propanediamine (HIPDM) behaves differently in normal smokers and in patients affected by various lung pathologies.[105] This different behaviour may be due to an increased number of cellular binding sites or, alternatively, to unknown processes of HIPDM biotransformation. It is easy to appreciate that an exact knowledge of such mechanisms may reveal interesting fields of study.

Clinical relevance

- Perfusion lung scintigraphy is still the cornerstone of the screening and diagnosis of pulmonary embolism.

- Several nuclear medicine techniques may add relevant physiological information to the radiological diagnosis of chronic obstructive pulmonary disease.

- Gallium scintigraphy may help with the diagnosis, often difficult otherwise, of acute or subacute pulmonary inflammatory disease, such as bacterial, viral or fungal infections, acute respiratory distress syndrome or sarcoidosis.

- The use of PET scintigraphy with positron-emitting nuclides makes it possible to obtain functional images of blood flow and metabolic processes that open new frontiers in the diagnosis, staging and follow-up of thoracic cancer.

- Knowledge of the indications, advantages and limits of each individual nuclear medicine technique is essential for correct clinical use and optimal results.

? Unresolved questions

- Are recently established, effective strategies for the diagnosis of pulmonary embolism applicable to different series of patients?

- Might spiral computed tomography replace pulmonary scintigraphy in the screening and diagnosis of pulmonary embolism?

- Can we find new radiopharmaceuticals able to diagnose pulmonary inflammatory processes earlier and more accurately, especially in immunocompromised patients?

- Will the engineering and biological research progress be able to develop nuclear medicine techniques that can detect intrathoracic cancer in the early, treatable stage?

- Are there potential uses for diagnosis and treatment of pulmonary disease in the knowledge of the metabolic function of the lung?

References

1. Taplin GV, Johnson DE, Dore EK, Kaplan HS. Lung photoscan with macroaggregates of human serum albumin: experimental basis and clinical trials. Health Phys 1964; 10:1219–1227.
2. Palla A, Giuntini C. Is there still a role for radioisotope technique in pulmonary embolism? J Nucl Biol Med 1992; 36: 141–149.
3. Sostman HD, Rapaport S, Gottshalk A, Greenspan RH. Imaging of pulmonary embolism. Invest Radiol 1986; 443–454.
4. Palla A, Petruzzelli S, Donnamaria V et al. Radiographic assessment of perfusion impairment in pulmonary embolism. Eur J Radiol 1985; 5: 252–255.
5. Moser KM, Tisi GM, Rodhes PG et al. Correlation of photoscan with pulmonary angiography in pulmonary embolism. Am J Cardiol 1966; 18: 810–820.
6. Giuntini C. Do radioisotopes techniques fulfil their role in the diagnosis of pulmonary embolism? J Nucl Med Allied Sci 1985; 29: 1–6.
7. Palla A, Tumeh SS, Nagel JS et al. Detection of pulmonary perfusion defects by single photon emission computed tomography (SPECT). J Nucl Med Allied Sci 1988; 32: 27–32.
8. Palla A, Singer SJ, Tumeh SS et al. Segmental pulmonary anatomy in man: a method of study with angiography and single photon emission computed tomography. J Nucl Med Allied Sci 1989; 33: 247–251.
9. Morrell NW, Roberts CM, Jones BE et al. The anatomy of radioisotope lung scanning. J Nucl Med 1992; 33: 676–683.
10. Pace WM, Goris ML. Pulmonary SPECT imaging and the stripe sign. J Nucl Med 1998; 39:721–723.
11. Hull RD, Raskob GE, Coates G, Panju AA. Clinical validity of a normal perfusion lung scan in patients suspected of pulmonary embolism. Chest 1990; 97: 23–26.
12. Van Beek EJR, Kuyer PMM, Shenk BE et al. A normal perfusion lung scan in patients with clinically suspected pulmonary embolism: frequency and clinical validity. Chest 1995; 108: 170–173.
13. Kipper MS, Moser KM, Kortman KE, Ashburn WL Long-term follow-up of patients with suspected pulmonary embolism and a normal lung scan. Chest 1982; 82: 411–415.
14. PISA-PED investigators. Invasive and noninvasive diagnosis of pulmonary embolism. Preliminary results of the prospective investigative study of acute pulmonary embolism diagnosis. Chest 1995; 107: 33S–39S.
15. Hoey JR, Farrer PA, Rosenthal LJ, Spengler RF. Interobserver and intraobserver variability in the lung scan reading in suspected pulmonary embolism. Clin Nucl Med 1980; 5: 509–513.
16. Lensing AWA, van Beek EJR, Demers C et al. Ventilation-perfusion lung scanning and the diagnosis of pulmonary embolism: improvement of observer agreement by the use of a lung segment reference chart. Thrombosis Haemostasis 1992; 68: 245–249.
17. Van Beek EJR, Tiel-van Buul MMC, Hoefnagel CA et al. Reporting of perfusion-ventilation lung scintigraphy with the use of an anatomical lung segment chart: a prospective study. Nucl Med Commun 1994; 15: 746–751.
18. Miniati M, Prediletto R, Formichi B et al. Accuracy of clinical assessment in the diagnosis of pulmonary embolism. Am J Respir Crit Care Med 1999; 159: 864–871.
19. McNeil BJ. A diagnostic strategy using ventilation-perfusion studies in patients suspected of pulmonary embolism. J Nucl Med 1976; 17: 613–616.
20. Santolicandro AM, Ruschi S, Fornai E et al. Imaging of ventilation in chronic obstructive pulmonary disease. J Thorac Imaging 1986; 1: 36–53.
21. Gottshalk A, Sostman HD, Coleman RF et al. Ventilation/perfusion scintigraphy in the PIOPED study. Part II. Evaluation of the scintigraphic criteria and interpretations. J Nucl Med 1993; 34: 1119–1126.
22. Santolicandro AM, Fornai E, Pulerà N et al. Functional aspects of reversible airway obstruction: Respiration 1986: 50: 65–71.
23. PIOPED investigators. Value of the ventilation-perfusion scan in acute pulmonary embolism. JAMA 1990; 263: 2753–2759.
24. PISA-PED investigators. Value of perfusion lung scan in the diagnosis of pulmonary embolism: results of the prospective study of acute pulmonary embolism diagnosis (PISA-PED). Am J Respir Crit Care Med 1996; 154: 1387–1393.

25. Celi A, Palla A, Petruzzelli S et al. Prospective study of a standardized questionnaire to improve clinical estimate of pulmonary embolism. Chest 1989; 95: 332–337.

26. Stein PD, Hull RD, Saltzmann HA, Pineo G. Strategy for diagnosis of patients with suspected acute pulmonary embolism. Chest 1993; 103: 1553–1559.

27. Parker JA, Markis JE, Palla A et al. Pulmonary perfusion after rt-PA therapy for acute embolism: early improvement assessed with segmental perfusion scanning. Radiology 1988; 166: 441–445.

28. Palla A, Giuntini C. Imaging of pulmonary embolism. In: Morpurgo M, ed. Pulmonary embolism. Basel: Marcel Dekker; 1994: 12; 115–151.

29. Palla A, Bellina CR, Marini C et al. A noninvasive, quantitative method to demonstrate the early effect of therapy in acute pulmonary embolism. Eur J Nucl Med 2001; 28: 1605–1609.

30. Palla A, Donnamaria V, Petruzzelli S, Giuntini C. Follow-up of pulmonary perfusion recovery after embolism. J Nucl Med Allied Sci 1986; 30: 23–28.

31. Prediletto R, Paoletti P, Fornai E et al. Natural history of treated pulmonary embolism. Evaluation by perfusion lung scintigraphy, gas exchange, and chest roentgenogram. Chest 1990; 97: 554–561.

32. Marini C, Di Ricco G, Rossi G et al. Fibrinolytic effects of urokinase and heparin in acute pulmonary embolism: a randomized clinical trial. Respiration 1988; 54: 162–173.

33. Kakkar VV. Fibrinogen uptake test for detection of deep vein thrombosis: a review of current practice. Semin Nucl Med 1977; 3: 229–244.

34. McIlmovle G, Davis HH, Welsh MJ et al. Scintigraphic diagnosis of experimental pulmonary embolism with In-111 labeled platelets. J Nucl Med 1977; 18: 910–914.

35. Oster ZH, Srivastava SC, Som P et al. Thrombus radioimmunoscintigraphy: an approach using monoclonal antiplatelet antibody. Proc Natl Acad Sci USA 1985; 82: 3465–3468.

36. Palabrica TM, Furie BC, Konstam MA et al. Thrombus imaging in a primate model with antibodies specific for an external membrane protein of activated platelets. Proc Natl Acad Sci USA 1989; 86: 1036–1040.

37. Wasser MNJM, Koppert PW, Arnolt JW et al. An antifibrin monoclonal antibody useful in immunoscintigraphic detection of thrombi. Blood 1989; 74: 708–714.

38. Thakur ML, Pallela VR, Consigny PM et al. Imaging vascular thrombosis with ^{99m}Tc-labeled fibrin alpha-chain peptide. J Nucl Med 2000; 41: 161–168.

39. Taillefer R, Edell S, Innes G, Lister Jaimes J. Acute thromboscintigraphy with ^{99m}Tc-apcitide: results of the phase 3 multicenter clinical trial comparing ^{99m}Tc-apcitide scintigraphy with contrast venography for imaging acute DVT. Multicenter Trial Investigators. J Nucl Med 2000; 41: 1214–1223.

40. Nakahara K, Nakaoka K, Ohno K et al. Functional modification for bullectomy of giant bulla. Am Thorac Surg 1983; 35: 480–487.

41. Foreman S, Weil H, Duke R et al. Bullous disease of the lung: physiologic improvement after surgery. Ann Intern Med 1968: 69: 757–767.

42. Ingenito EP, Loring SH, Moy M et al. Physiological and radiological criteria identify two distinct groups of patients likely to benefit from lung volume reduction surgery (LVRS). Chest 1998: 114: S350.

43. Ingenito EP, Evans RB, Loring SH et al. Relation between preoperative inspiratory lung resistance and the outcome of lung volume reduction surgery for emphysema. N Engl J Med 1998; 338: 1181–1185.

44. Morrow PE. Aerosol characterization and deposition. Am Rev Respir Dis 1974: 110: 88–89.

45. Coates G, Nahmias C. Xenon-127, a comparison with xenon-133 for ventilation studies. J Nucl Med 1977; 18: 221–225.

46. Fazio F, Jones T. Assessment of regional ventilation by continuous inhalation of radioactive krypton-81m. Br Med J 1975: 3: 673–676.

47. Miller RF, O'Dohorthy MJ. Pulmonary nuclear medicine. Eur J Nucl Med 1992; 19: 335–368.

48. Line BR, Hunninghake GW, Keogh BA et al. Gallium-67 scanning to stage the alveolitis of sarcoidosis: correlation with clinical studies, pulmonary function studies and bronchoalveolar lavage. Am Rev Respir Dis 1981; 123: 440–446.

49. Solfanelli S, Fazzi P, Diviggiano E et al. ^{67}Ga uptake quantification in pulmonary sarcoidosis. An implement to Line's method (abstract). Sarcoidosis 1991; 8: 194.

50. Demeters SL, Cordaseo EM, McIntyre W et al. Quantitation of abnormal Ga-67 uptake in pulmonary interstitial vascular disease. Angiology 1990; 41: 1023–1028.

51. Lai FM, Liam CK, Paramsothy M, George J. The role of ^{67}Gallium scintigraphy and high resolution computed tomography as predictors of disease activity in sputum smear-negative pulmonary tuberculosis. Int J Tuberc Lung Dis 1997; 1: 563–569.

52. Utsunomiya K, Narabayasi I, Nishigaki H et al. Clinical significance of thallium-201 and gallium-67 scintigraphy in pulmonary tuberculosis. Eur J Nucl Med 1997; 24: 252–257.

53. Kirshenbaum KJ, Burke R, Fanapour F et al. Pulmonary high-resolution computed tomography versus gallium scintigraphy: diagnostic utility in the diagnosis of patients with AIDS who have chest symptoms and normal or equivocal chest radiographs. J Thorac Imaging 1998; 13: 52–57.

54. Bitran J, Beckerman C, Weinstein R et al. Patterns of gallium-67 scintigraphy in patients with acquired immune deficiency syndrome. J Nucl Med 1987; 28: 1103–1106.

55. Tuazon CV, Delauly MD, Simon GL et al. Utility of ^{67}Ga-scintigraphy and bronchial washings in the diagnosis and treatment of *Pneumocystis carinii* pneumonia in patients with acquired immune deficiency syndrome. Am Rev Respir Dis 1985; 132: 1087–1092.

56. Lee VW, Antonacci V, Tilak S et al. Intracranial mass lesions: sequential thallium and gallium scintigraphy in patients with AIDS. Radiology 1999; 211: 507–512.

57. Peters AM. The use of nuclear medicine in infections. Br J Radiol 1998; 71: 252–261.

58. Fazzi P, Solfanelli S, Di Pede F et al. Sarcoidosis in Tuscany. A preliminary report. Sarcoidosis 1992; 9: 1–4.

59. Sulavik SB, Spencer RP, Weed DA et al. Recognition of distinctive patterns of Gallium-67 distribution in sarcoidosis. J Nucl Med 1990; 31: 1909–1914.

60. Klech H, Kohn H, Kummor F, Mostbeck A. Assessment of activity in sarcoidosis: sensitivity and specificity of gallium-67 scintigraphy, serum ACE levels, chest roentgenography and blood lymphocyte subpopulations. Chest 1982; 82: 732–738.

61. Line BR, Fulmer JD, Reynolds HY et al. Gallium-67 citrate scanning in the staging of idiopathic pulmonary fibrosis: correlation with physiologic and morphologic features and bronchoalveolar lavage. Am Rev Respir Dis 1978; 118: 355–365.

62. Vanderstappen M, Mornex JF, Lahneche B et al. Gallium-67 scanning in the staging of cryptogenetic fibrosing alveolitis and hypersensitivity pneumonitis. Eur Respir J 1988; 1: 517–522.

63. Sy WM, Seo IS, Homs CJ et al. The evolutional stage changes in sarcoidosis on gallium-67 scintigraphy. Ann Nucl Med 1998; 12: 77–82.

64. Manà J. ^{67}Gallium, ^{201}Thallium, ^{18}F-labeled fluoro-2-deoxy-D-glucose positron emission tomography. Clin Chest Med 1997; 18: 799–811.

65. MacNee W, Selby C. Neutrophil kinetics in the lungs. Clin Sci 1990; 79: 97–107.

66. Currie DC, Saverymuttu SH, Peters AM et al. Indium-111 labeled granulocyte accumulation in the respiratory tract of patients with bronchiectasis. Lancet 1987; i: 1335–1339.

67. Saverymuttu SH, Phillips G, Peters AM, Lavender JP. ^{111}Indium autologous leucocyte scanning in lobar pneumonia and lung abscesses. Thorax 1985; 40: 925–30.

68. Warshawski FJ, Sibbald NJ, Driedger AA, Cheung H. Neutrophil–pulmonary interaction in the adult respiratory distress syndrome. Am Rev Respir Dis 1986; 133: 797–804.

69. O'Brodovich H, Coates G. Pulmonary clearance of ^{99m}Tc-DTPA: a non-invasive assessment of epithelial integrity. Lung 1987; 165: 1–6.

70. Smith RJ, Hydé RW, Waldman DL et al. Effect of pattern of aerosol inhalation of clearance of technetium-99m-labeled diethylenetriamine pentaacetic acid from the lungs of normal humans. Am Rev Respir Dis 1982; 145: 1109–1116.

71. Sehweil AM, McKillop JH, Milroy R et al. Mechanisms of ^{201}Tl uptake in tumours. Eur J Nucl Med 1989; 15: 336–339.

72. Ballinger JR, Duncan J, Hua HA, Ichise M. Accumulation of ^{99m}Tc-HMPAO and ^{99m}Tc-ECD in rodent and human breast tumor cell lines in vitro. Ann Nucl Med 1997; 11: 95–99.

73. Wang H, Murea S, Mainolfi C et al. Tc-99m MIBI scintigraphy in patients with lung cancer. Comparison with CT and fluorine-18 FDG PET imaging. Clin Nucl Med 1997; 22: 243–249.

74. Lamberts SWJ, Bakker WH, Reubi JC, Krenning EP. Somatostatin receptor imaging in the localization of endocrine tumors. N Engl J Med 1990; 323: 1246–1249.

75. Shapiro B. ^{131}I metaiodobenzylguanidine for the locating of suspected pheochromocytoma: experience in 400 cases (441 studies). J Nucl Med 1985; 26: 576–585.

76. Anderson KC, Leonard RCF, Canellos GP et al. High-dose gallium imaging in lymphoma. Am J Med 1983; 75: 327–331.

77. Delcambre C, Reman O, Henry Amar M et al. Clinical relevance of gallium-67 scintigraphy in lymphoma before and after therapy. Eur J Nucl Med 2000; 27: 176–184.

78. Tumeh SS, Rosenthal DS, Kaplan WD et al. Lymphoma: evaluation with Ga-67 SPECT. Radiology 1987; 164: 11–14.

79. Front D, Bar Shalom R, Mor M et al. Aggressive non-Hodgkin lymphoma: early prediction of outcome with ^{67}Ga scintigraphy. Radiology 2000; 214: 253–257.

80. Front D, Bar Shalom R, Mor M et al. Hodgkin disease: prediction of outcome with ^{67}Ga scintigraphy after one cycle of chemotherapy. Radiology 1999; 210: 487–491.

81. Gasparini M, Bombardieri E, Castellani M et al. Gallium-67 scintigraphy evaluation of therapy in non-Hodgkin's lymphoma. J Nucl Med 1998; 39: 1586–1590.

82. Setoain FJ, Pons F, Herranz R et al. [67]Ga scintigraphy for the evaluation of recurrences and residual masses in patients with lymphoma. Nucl Med Commun 1997; 18: 405–411.

83. Edwards CL, Hayes RL. Tumor scanning with 67-Ga citrate. J Nucl Med 1969; 10: 103–105.

84. Bekerman C, Caride VC, Hoffer PB, Boles CA. Noninvasive staging of lung cancer – indications and limitations of gallium-67 citrate imaging. Radiol Clin North Am 1990; 28: 427–510.

85. Waxman AD, Julien PJ, Brachman MB et al. Gallium scintigraphy in bronchogenic carcinoma. The effect of tumor location on sensitivity and specificity. Chest 1984; 86: 178–183.

86. Alazraki NP, Ramsdell JN, Taylor A et al. Reliability of gallium scan chest radiography compared to mediastinoscopy for evaluating mediastinal spread in lung cancer. Am Rev Respir Dis 1978; 117: 415–420.

87. De Meester TR, Golomb HM, Kirchener P et al. The role of gallium-67 scanning in the clinical staging and preoperative evaluation of patients with carcinoma of the lung. Ann Thor Surg 1979; 28: 451–464.

88. Broughton DL, Gibson CJ, Crake T et al. Gallium scanning by conventional imaging and emission computed tomography in the pretreatment evaluation of lung cancer. Thorax 1985; 40: 96–100.

89. Lindholm P, Minn H, Leskinen-Kallio S et al. Influence of the body glucose concentration on FDG uptake in cancer: a PET study. J Nucl Med 1993; 17: 583–589.

90. Lowe VJ, Hoffman JM, De Long DM et al. Semiquantitative and visual analysis of FDG-PET images in pulmonary abnormalities. J Nucl Med 1994; 35: 1771–1776.

91. Graber GM, Gupta NC, Murray GF. Positron emission tomographic imaging with fluorodeoxyglucose is efficacious in evaluating malignant pulmonary disease. J Thorac Cardiovasc Surg 1999; 117: 719–727.

92. Patz EF, Lowe VJ, Hoffman JM et al. Focal pulmonary abnormalities: evaluation with (^{18}F) fluorodeoxyglucose PET scanning. Radiology 1993; 188: 487–490.

93. Coleman RE, Laymon CF, Turkington TG. FDG imaging of lung nodules: a phantom study comparing SPECT, camera-based PET and dedicated PET. Radiology 1999; 210: 823–828.

94. Duhaylongsod F, Lowe VJ, Patz EF et al. Lung tumor growth correlates with glucose metabolism measured by FDG-PET. Ann Thorac Surg 1995; 60: 1348–1352.

95. Ahuia V, Coleman RF, Herndon J, Patz EF. Prognostic significance of FDG-PET imaging in patients with non-small cell lung cancer. Cancer 1998; 83: 918–924.

96. Albes JM, Lietzenmayer R, Schott U et al. Improvement of non-small-cell lung cancer staging by means of positron emission tomography. Thorac Cardiovasc Surg 1999; 47: 42–47.

97. Saunders CA, Dussek JE, O'Doherty MJ, Maisey MN. Evaluation of fluorine-18-fluorodeoxyglucose whole body positron emission tomography imaging in the staging of lung cancer. Ann Thorac Surg 1999; 67: 790–797.

98. Farrell MA, McAdams HP, Herndon JE, Patz EF Jr. Non-small cell lung cancer: FDG-PET for nodal staging in patients with stage I disease. Radiology 2000; 21: 886–890.

99. Bury T, Dowlate A, Corhay JL et al. Whole-body [18]FDG in the staging of non-small cell lung cancer. Eur Respir J 1997; 10: 2529–2534.

100. Marom EM, McAdams HP, Erasmus JJ et al. Staging non-small cell lung cancer with whole body PET. Radiology 1999; 212: 803–809.

101. Vansteenkiste J, Stoobanks S, De Lyn P et al. Prognostic significance of FDG-PET after induction chemotherapy in stage III A-N2 non-small cell lung cancer (N2-NSCLC). Analysis of 13 cases (abstract). Proc Am Soc Clin Oncol 1998; 16: 75.

102. Hebert M, Lowe V, Hoffman J et al. Positron emission tomography in the pre-treatment evaluation and follow-up of non-small cell lung cancer patients treated with radiotherapy. Am J Clin Oncol 1996; 19: 416–421.

103. Patz EF, Connolly J, Herndon J. Prognostic value of thoracic FDG-PET imaging after treatment for non-small cell lung cancer. AJR 2000; 174: 769–774.

104. Dosio F, Magnani P, Paganelli G. Three-step tumor pre-targeting in lung cancer immunoscintigraphy. J Nucl Biol Med 1993; 37: 228–232.

105. Pistolesi M, Miniati M, Petruzzelli S et al. Pulmonary retention of iodobenzylpropanediamine in humans. Effect of cigarette smoking. Am Rev Respir Dis 1988; 138: 1429–1433.

7.3 Ultrasound of the lung and pleura

Angelika Reissig and Claus Kroegel

 Key points

On ultrasound of the lung and pleura:

- **Pneumonia** shows a hypoechoic area with irregular and serrated margins and an inhomogeneous echotexture caused by bronchoaerogram

- **Pulmonary embolism** reveals typical multiple triangular, hypoechoic, pleural-based parenchymal lesions

- **Bronchogenic carcinomas** are mostly echo-poor, rounded or polycyclic areas showing infiltrating growth

- **Lung metastases** are typically weakly echogenic, multiple, rounded or oval, sharply demarcated structures

- **Pleural effusion** presents as an echo-free zone within the pleural space

- **Pneumothorax** shows many hyperechoic reverberations

- **Pulmonary fibrosis** reveals an irregular, thickened, fragmented pleural line and multiple comet tail artefacts.

Ultrasound exploration of the pleura has long been recognised as a useful method for the demonstration of pleural effusion and as a guide to thoracocentesis, pleural biopsy and chest tube placement. However, evaluation of lung parenchyma has not been considered useful. Under normal physiological conditions, the visceral pleura and lung surface will form an echoic line, the so-called 'pleural line' (Fig. 7.3.1). However, the air-containing lung parenchyma interferes with further progression of the ultrasound pulse leading to reverberation artefacts when returning from the lung surface. This may best be visible when under real-time-conditions the lung tissue covers the upper parts of the liver and spleen ('curtain-sign') (Fig. 7.3.2).[1] As a result, the healthy lung parenchyma cannot be penetrated and imaged by sonography, thus limiting the clinical value of the method.

However, under pathophysiological conditions, evacuation of air – either because of pleural fluid collection, malignant cell proliferation within the lung parenchyma or tissue compression – allows ultrasonic waves to penetrate the lung, providing an ultrasound image of the affected section. In recent years, a growing number of reports have suggested that peripheral pulmonary embolism, pneumonia, atelectasis and other condi-tions are all accessible to exploration by ultrasound. Since ultrasonography is a rapid, widely available, non-invasive as well as cost-effective diagnostic technique, this method provides an additional diagnostic tool for the diagnosis of pulmonary disorders (Table 7.3.1).

Technical requirements and technique

Sonographic examination is conducted using a 5 and 3.5 MHz convex scanner, respectively, occasionally supplemented with a 7.5 MHz linear scanner or colour-flow Doppler mode. The exploration is performed with the patients in a seated or prone position, with intercostal application of the scanner to the site of the localised pain followed by a systematic evaluation of the remaining intercostal spaces. Suspicious lesions are assessed along the longitudinal and transversal axes with respect to size, shape, demarcation and echo pattern. If necessary, the inter-costal space can be widened by placing the patients' hands behind the head and elevating the elbows.

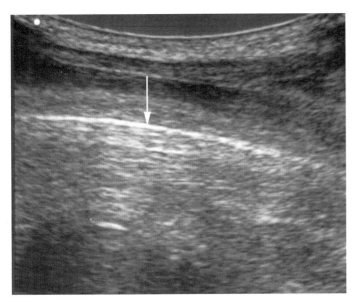

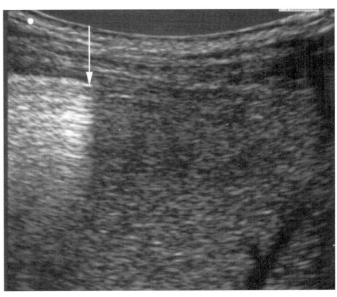

Fig. 7.3.1 Normal sonogram of the pleura. The echogenic 'pleural line' (arrow) is due to the total reflection of the ultrasonic beam at the transition to the normally aerated lung. Thus, normal pulmonary tissue cannot be imaged by sonography.

Fig. 7.3.2 'Curtain-sign'. The breath-dependent movement of the pleural line can easily be assessed in the basal part of the lung. Under real-time-conditions, the pleural line shows a motion reminiscent of a curtain (arrow) covering liver and spleen, respectively.

Table 7.3.1 Differential diagnostic criteria of sonography for distinguishing between pneumonia, pulmonary embolism, bronchogenic carcinoma and compressive atelectasis

	Pneumonia	**Pulmonary embolism**	**Bronchogenic carcinoma**	**Compressive atelectasis**
Echogenicity	Hypoechoic	Hypoechoic	Hypoechoic	Moderately hypoechoic
Echotexture	Non-homogeneous	Homogeneous (early); inhomogeneous (late)	Mostly homogeneous	Mostly non-homogeneous
Shape	Irregular	Triangular > round	Rounded or polycyclic	Concave
Bordering	Serrated margins	Well-demarcated, sharp margins (late)	Infiltrating growth	Sharp and smooth
Bronchoaerogram	A regular feature	None	None	Often
Vascularity	Regularly present; enhanced signal	'Vascular sign'	Irregular neovascularisation	Central vascularity
Characteristic features	Fluid bronchogram may be visible	Occasionally, a single central echo may be present	Tissue necrosis may occur	Associated with large effusion; reduced size following thoracocentesis

Pneumonia

Pneumonia refers to a disease of the peripheral lung tissue and distal bronchioles caused by an overwhelming inflammatory defence reaction of the host directed against pathogenic microorganisms. This reaction is characterised by a flooding of the peripheral airways and alveoli by a neutrophil-rich exudate, leading to air evacuation in the affected tissue and thus providing accessibility to sonographic evaluation. Like any other pulmonary disorders, extension of pulmonary infiltration to the pleura is a prerequisite for the sonographic visualisation of pneumonic lesions.

Sonomorphology of pneumonia

The sonographic appearance of pneumonic lesions can be categorised into parenchymal, pleural and vascular criteria.

Parenchymal criteria

Consolidated lung areas are visible as a small and homogeneous subpleural section without air or fluid bronchograms and are referred to as 'superficial fluid alveolograms' (Fig. 7.3.3).[2] Below the fluid alveologram, a hypoechoic area of varying size and shape with irregular and serrated margins and a non-

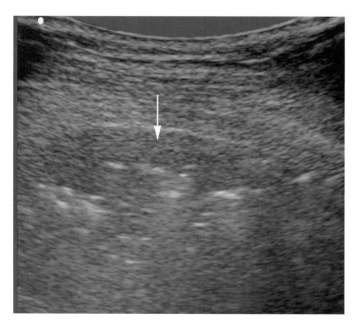

Fig. 7.3.3 Pneumonia. Adjacent to the thin, hypoechoic pleural line, a superficial homogeneous elongated area devoid of air or fluid bronchograms, the so called 'superficial fluid alveolograms' (arrow) is visible. Distal to this sign, a hypoechoic area with irregular and serrated margins and an inhomogeneous echotexture is present. Within this structure, multiple lentil-sized hyperechoic reflexes indicate the presence of air within the lesion (bronchoaerogram).

homogeneous echotexture can be seen.[1] Pneumonia typically reveals a bronchoaerogram, which shows up as multiple lentil-sized air inlets measuring a few millimetres in diameter (Fig. 7.3.3) or as a tree-shaped echogenic structure. These hyperechoic echoes are caused by the residual air within air-conducting airways. Occasionally, the breath-dependent motion of the echoes during real-time investigation can be demonstrated.

Another typical sonographic feature of a pneumonic lesion is the fluid bronchogram. It occurs less frequently than the bronchoaerogram, is characterised by echo-free tubular structures along the airways, which can be differentiated from pulmonary vessels using colour Doppler imaging. The fluid bronchogram reflects exudate-packed conducting airways and may indicate a post-stenotic pneumonia.

Pleural criteria

The corresponding pleural line is mostly fragmented, thinner and hypoechoic as compared to non-pneumonic tissue areas. In addition, pneumonia is frequently accompanied by a pleural effusion adjacent to the pneumonic lung tissue. Excess pleural fluid accumulating in the costophrenic angle is easily detectable by sonography provided the patient is at an upright position.

Vascular criteria

Pneumonia typically shows an enhanced but regular flow signal on colour Doppler imaging.

Course of the disease

Pneumonia can follow different courses. First, it can resolve completely without complications. Second, necrotising pneumonia or a pulmonary abscess may develop, particularly where anaerobic bacteria are the causative pathogen. A lung abscess is characterised by sonography as a hypoechoic area within the pneumonic lesion. Third, irregularities of the pleural line may persist for some weeks or even months because of localised scarring of the lung tissue. Finally, localised pleural thickening may become visible during the course of the disease.

Pulmonary embolism

Detection of thromboembolic lesions of the lung by sonography was first described some 30 years ago.[3,4] Although Mathis and colleagues confirmed the original results recently,[5,6] the diagnostic potential of the technique applied for pulmonary embolism has not been widely appreciated so far.

Complete embolic occlusion of peripheral pulmonary artery results in a rapid breakdown of the surfactant system with consecutive packing of the alveolar lumen by erythrocytes containing exudate.[7,8] These pathophysiologic changes provide the basis for sonographic detection in transthoracic sonography. Again, only consolidations extending to the pleural surface of the lung are accessible to transthoracic sonography.

Sonomorphology of pulmonary embolism

The sonographic findings associated with pulmonary embolism can be classified according to parenchymal, pleural and vascular criteria.[8]

Parenchymal criteria

Typical sonographic findings are multiple, hypoechoic, pleural-based parenchymal lesions, generally well-demarcated from the surrounding tissue.[9] The mostly wedge-shaped lesions are rounded or circular and extend to the pleural surface (Fig. 7.3.4). In addition, a single echo, typically localised at the centre of the lesions (Fig. 7.3.4), may be occasionally detected.[9]

Pleural criteria

Localised and basal effusions are a regular feature of pleural involvement. In addition, the pleura shows a convex outward bulging with a thinned, hypoechoic and fragmented visceral pleural line.

Vascular criteria

Exploration of the lesions by colour Doppler imaging shows a perfusion defect within the hypoechoic parenchymal lesion.[7,10] Occasionally, a congested thromboembolic vessel ('vascular sign') may be visible.[7,11]

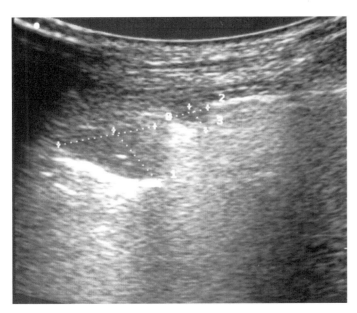

Fig. 7.3.4 Pulmonary embolism. 72-year-old woman with computed-tomography-proven pulmonary embolism. The sonogram reveals two triangular, hypoechoic, pleural-based parenchymal lesions (+). The larger lesion contains a single, centrally located echo.

Course of the disease

Sonography allows monitoring of the course and early detection of complications, such as pneumonia. Sonographic features of end-stage postinfarct pneumonia may be indistinguishable from pneumonia of other aetiology.

Without any complications, pulmonary embolic lesions will decrease in size over time. The margins of the tissue area affected become less distinct and irregular. Eventually, comet-tail artefacts due to local scarring may persist for many years.

Sensitivity and specificity

Sensitivity and specificity of transthoracic sonography for pulmonary embolism are 80%–94% and 87%–92% respectively.[6,9]

Benefits of ultrasound

The basic advantages of transthoracic sonography in diagnosing pulmonary embolism are the identification of very small peripheral events, the opportunity of repeated controls during the treatment period and finally the early detection of possible complications, such as postinfarction pneumonia. Transthoracic sonography is easily accessible at the bedside and requires neither ionising radiation nor contrast medium.

However, a number of 'natural' restrictions to transthoracic sonography may limit the diagnostic potential of the method. In the first instance, embolism-associated lesions can only be detected when they extend up to the lung periphery. Secondly, only about 66% of the peripheral lung areas are accessible to sonographic examination, the remainder being covered by bony structures. Lastly, transthoracic sonography is operator-dependent, relying heavily on the experience of the examiner.

However, inconclusive sonographic images do not exclude pulmonary embolism.

Bronchogenic carcinoma and lung metastases

Lung tumours are detectable by sonography if they extend up to the pleura. Solid tumour tissue may also be visible in the presence of an 'acoustic window', such as pleural effusion or atelectasis, which facilitates penetration of ultrasound waves into the lung parenchyma.

Sonomorphology of bronchogenic carcinoma and lung metastases

Parenchymal criteria

Lung carcinomas (Fig. 7.3.5) characteristically present as echo-poor areas (Fig. 7.3.6) with a polycyclic or oval shape. They are not sharply demarcated and, occasionally, infiltrating growth into the adjacent tissue is visible. In case of carcinoma tissue infiltration into the parietal pleura or the thorax wall, ultrasound fails to show breath-dependent motion of the lesion. In some cases, echo-free zones corresponding with central necrosis are visible within the tumour, whereas hyperechoic lines within the necrotic areas indicate captured air.

Lung metastases are typically less echogenic, round or oval in shape and are sharply demarcated structures (Fig. 7.3.7). Unimpaired breath-dependent motion indicates a strictly intra-pulmonary localisation. Distal to the solid structures, an area of

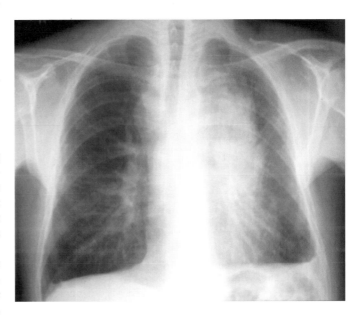

Fig. 7.3.5 Lung carcinoma. The chest radiograph of a 62-year-old man shows left-sided mediastinal consolidation and a small basal effusion. Solids and fluids within the consolidation cannot be differentiated.

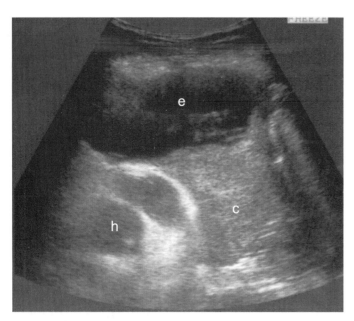

Fig. 7.3.6 Lung carcinoma – corresponding sonogram. By means of ultrasound, effusion (e) and an echo-poor and irregularly demarcated pulmonary consolidation (c) extending up to the heart (h) can be distinguished. Histological examination confirmed the diagnosis of small-cell lung cancer.

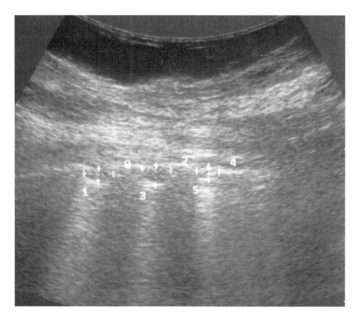

Fig. 7.3.7 Lung metastases in an 82-year-old woman with an adenoid–cystic carcinoma of the lung. The figure demonstrates three hypoechoic, rounded and well demarcated focuses (+) with unrestricted motion during respiration. The sizes of the metastases are 9.8 × 4.6, 9.6 × 6.6 and 7.6 × 4.6 mm. Distal to the solid structures, an area of increased echogenicity with amplification artefacts is present.

increased echogenicity with multiple amplification artefacts is visible.

Pleural criteria

Involvement of the parietal pleura and thorax wall can easily be detected with high sensitivity. Absence of free breath-dependent motion indicates an infiltrating tumour growth. Malignant pleural effusions are frequently seen in sonography. Pleural metastases, which appear as weak, echogenic, rounded or irregular plane structures on the surface of the visceral and parietal pleura, may also be present.

Vascular criteria

Colour Doppler sonography is useful for detecting vascularity in pulmonary masses and may help to differentiate malignant from benign lung tumours. Cancers with detectable flow signals have relatively low-impedance flows or arteriovenous shunting, a lower pulsatility and resistive index, a lower peak systolic velocity and higher end-diastolic velocity than benign lung lesions.[12]

Course of the disease

Estimation of the size and measurement of bronchogenic carcinoma and lung metastases employing sonography can easily be performed and may be a useful parameter for monitoring the size of the tumour in response to therapy.

Pleural effusion

Pleural effusion is defined as a pathologic accumulation of fluid between the parietal and visceral pleura, either caused by a primary pleural disease or due to a condition of the surrounding tissues. Pleural effusions have long been assessed by sonography and remain the most common indication for ultrasound examination. Sonography is the most sensitive technique for the detection of pleural effusions; even small amounts of pleural fluid (about 3–5 ml) are detectable. Effusions yield an 'acoustic window' for ultrasound exploration of adjacent parenchymal alterations such as bronchial carcinoma, pneumonia or pulmonary infarction.

Sonomorphology of pleural effusion

Pleural criteria

Pleural effusion typically presents as an echo-free zone within the pleural space. Typically, the extension and localisation of the pleural effusion is variable, depending on respiration movement and body position,[13] which may be helpful in differentiating effusions from solid pleural mass. The effusion can either be localised or at the bases of the lung. Localised pleural effusion is characterised by a widening of the pleural space by a few millimetres in the section adjacent to a parenchymal lesion. Accumulation of the fluid separates the visceral and the parietal pleura, imposing as distinct hyperechoic lines. Basal effusion can be of varying amount and allows imaging of the diaphragm in a sitting position. Estimation of basal effusion[8] is shown in Figure 7.3.8.

Usually, transudates are echo-free, but under certain conditions echogenic features may be visible.[14] Exudates show an echo-free or echoic pattern, partly with swirling or sedimenting echoes indicating the presence of small particles within the fluid. This is particularly evident when the pleural fluid contains blood (haemothorax). In addition, septa and fibrinous strings are often detected within the exudates, indicating organisation of the effusion. Further, pleural thickening caused by pleural metastases or mesothelioma can be evaluated. However, a distinction between transudates and exudates must be made on the basis of laboratory fluid analysis.

Vascular criteria

Using colour Doppler sonography, the 'fluid colour sign' (Fig. 7.3.9) can be detected. The 'fluid colour sign' refers to a colour signal within fluid accumulation in the pleural cavity during cardiorespiratory cycles that is not visible within stationary solid structures.[15]

Parenchymal criteria

Large effusions will regularly cause atelectases due to mechanical compression of lung tissue (Fig. 7.3.9). These atelectases typically show a breath- and heartbeat-dependent motion within the effusion and will decrease in size after thoracocentesis.

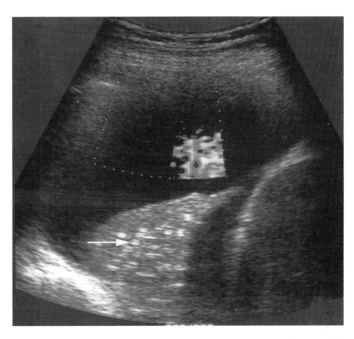

Fig. 7.3.9 'Fluid colour sign' in pleural effusion in an 89-year-old patient suffering from heart failure. Under real-time conditions, a colour signal appears within the fluid, depending on the respiratory and cardiac cycles. Further, the figure shows a sharply demarcated compressive atelectasis (arrow) within the large effusion. During the cardiorespiratory cycles, the atelectasis shows a typical motion, which is sometimes referred as 'flag' or 'waving hand'.

Pneumothorax

Pneumothorax may either develop spontaneously or follow intervention or trauma. Pleural air can be distinguished from normal aerated lung using sonography. However, it is generally necessary to compare the findings with the healthy opposite side of the thorax[8] (Fig. 7.3.10).

Sonomorphology of pneumothorax

Parenchymal criteria

Pulmonary processes previously visible by transthoracic sonography are no longer discernible after a pneumothorax has developed.[16] Further, instead of the typical sonographic lung aspect, multiple hyperechoic reverberations can be seen (Fig. 7.3.10).

Pleural criteria

Normally, the visceral pleural line is hyperechoic and shows a breath-dependent movement that can be assessed during real-time investigation – the so-called 'pleura gliding sign'. In pneumothorax, neither pleural movements nor comet-tail artefacts can be detected. Moreover, the pleural line appears smaller in comparison to the areas not affected. If pneumothorax is accompanied by pleural effusion, some hyperechoic reflexes appear within the fluid, or an 'air–fluid mirror' (Fig. 7.3.11) may be seen.

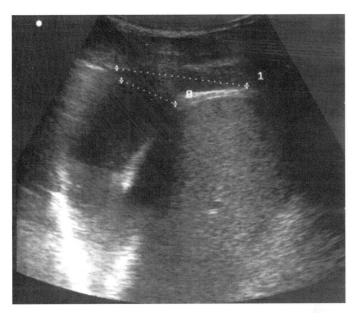

Fig. 7.3.8 Volume estimation of pleural effusion – sonogram in a seated position. The figure shows a pleural effusion in a 59-year-old patient suffering from liver cirrhosis. The relevant distances are as follows: D0, minimal distance between basal lung and diaphragm (cm); D1: maximal lateral length of the effusion (cm). Effusion volume (ml) = (D0 + D1)×k. The constant k = 70 has been estimated empirically.

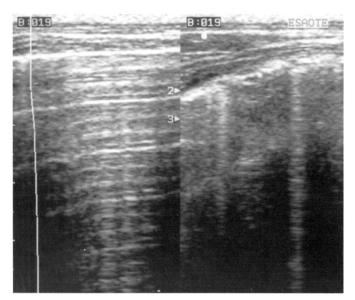

Fig. 7.3.10 Sonogram of a pneumothorax compared to the aerated lung in a 21-year-old patient suffering from a sarcoidosis who developed a spontaneous pneumothorax. On the right, the aerated lung can be seen. Comet-tail artefacts and the thickened pleural line indicates parenchymal involvement. On the left, a typical pleural line cannot be detected. In addition, several hyperechoic reverberations are discernible. During real-time exploration, the 'pleura gliding sign' is absent.

Course of the disease

In emergency situations inaccessible to immediate radiographs, sonography of the lung could facilitate instantaneous decision-making in clinically suspected pneumothorax.[17] However, the extent of the pneumothorax cannot be determined via sonography.

Other pulmonary disorders

Pulmonary fibrosis

Ultrasound imaging in pulmonary fibrosis is non-specific. The basic finding is an irregular, thickened and fragmented visceral pleural line with numerous comet-tail artefacts (Fig. 7.3.12) due to an irregular pleural surface.[8]

Atelectasis

Two different types of atelectasis can be distinguished: atelectasis following compression (compressive atelectasis) and atelectasis following central airway stenosis (resorption atelectasis). *Compressive atelectasis* (Fig. 7.3.9) is more common and regularly associated with a space-occupying pleural effusion. This type of atelectasis usually has sharp and smooth margins and is moderately echoic and of concave shape. It reveals a breath- and heartbeat-dependent motion and decreases in size after thoracocentesis. *Resorption atelectasis* characteristically presents as a homogenous hypoechoic structure with an echogenicity comparable to that of the liver. Its shape remains unchanged during cardiorespiratory cycles and when effusion is drained. This type of atelectasis appears large compared to the extent of effusion. Occasionally, a fluid bronchogram can be detected.

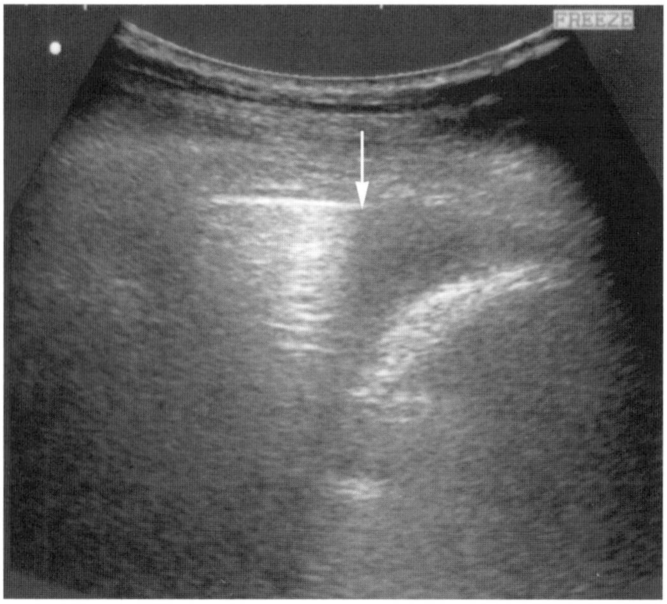

Fig. 7.3.11 Sonogram showing an air–fluid mirror in an 84-year-old patient with seropneumothorax. The sonogram reveals a typical combination of hyperechoic reverberations (arrow) in the upper part and a small pleural effusion above the diaphragm.

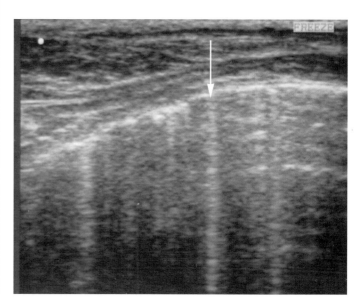

Fig. 7.3.12 Sonogram of a 23-year-old woman suffering from sarcoidosis accompanied by pulmonary fibrosis. Examination with a 7.5 MHz linear scanner reveals multiple comet tail artefacts (arrow) and an irregular, thickened and fragmented pleural line.

Clinical relevance

Ultrasound of the lung and pleura:

- is a useful technique for any physician, especially pneumologists

- is a safe, widely available and cost-effective modality without the need for radiation

- permits localisation and guidance for transthoracic biopsy of peripheral lesions

- allows the immediate detection of complications following transthoracic interventions

- is the most sensitive method for diagnosis of pleural effusion

- allows ultrasound-guided thoracocentesis

- allows the detection and follow-up of peripheral pneumonia

- allows the diagnosis of peripheral pulmonary embolism

- allows the diagnosis of pneumothorax, especially in emergency situations.

? Unresolved questions

- The detection and quantification of vascularity in lung lesions.

- The distinction between benign and malign lung tumours.

- The quantification of pneumonia in comparison to chest radiography.

- Large prospective studies to define the diagnostic role of transthoracic sonography in detecting pulmonary embolism.

References

1. Kroegel C, Reißig A, Hengst U. Diagnosis of parenchymal lung diseases. Diagnostic possibilities and limitations of transthoracic sonography. Dtsch Med Wschr 1999; 124: 765–772.
2. Targhetta R, Chavagneux R, Bourgeois JM et al. Sonographic approach to diagnosing pulmonary consolidations. J Ultrasound Med 1992; 11: 667–672.
3. Joyner C, Miller LD, Dudrick SJ et al. Reflected ultrasound in detection of pulmonary embolism. Trans Assn Am Phys 1966; 79: 262–277.
4. Miller LD, Joyner CR, Dudrick SJ, Eksin DJ. Clinical use of ultrasound in the detection of pulmonary embolism. Trans Assn Am Phys 1966; 166: 381–392.
5. Mathis G, Metzler J, Fußenegger D, Sutterlutti G. Zur Sonomorphologie des Lungeninfarktes. In: Gebhardt et al, eds. Ultraschalldiagnostik. Berlin: Springer; 1990: 388–391.
6. Mathis G, Bitschnau R, Gehmacher O et al. Chest ultrasound in diagnosis of pulmonary embolism in comparison to helical CT. Ultraschall Med 1999; 20: 54–59.
7. Mathis G. Ultrasound diagnosis of pulmonary embolism. Eur J Ultrasound 1996; 3: 153–160.
8. Kroegel C, Reißig A. Transthoracic sonography. Principles and application. An introduction and practical guide with CD-ROM. Stuttgart: Georg Thieme; 2000.
9. Reißig, A, Heyne J-P, Kroegel C. Sonography of lung and plevia in pulmonary embolism: sonomorphologic characterization and comparison with spiral CT scanning. Chest 2001; 120: 1977–1983.
10. Yuan A, Yang PC, Chang CB. Pulmonary infarction: use of color Doppler sonography for diagnosis and assessment of reperfusion of the lung. AJR 1993; 160: 419–420.
11. Mathis G, Dirschmid K. Pulmonary infarction: sonographic appearance with pathologic correlation. Eur J Radiol 1993; 17: 170–174.
12. Yuan A, Chang DR, Y CJ et al. Color Doppler sonography of benign and malignant pulmonary masses. AJR 1994; 163: 545–549.
13. Laing FC, Filly RA. Problems in the application of ultrasonography for the evaluation of pleural opacities. Radiology 1978; 126: 211–214.
14. Yang PC, Luh KT, Chang DR et al. Value of sonography in determining the nature of pleural effusion: analysis of 320 cases. AJR Am J Roentgenol 1992; 159: 29–33.
15. Wu RG, Yang PC, Kuo SH, Luh KT. 'Fluid color' sign: a useful indicator for discrimination between pleural thickening and pleural effusion. J Ultrasound Med 1995; 14: 767–769.
16. Targhetta R, Bourgeois JM, Chavagneux R, Balmes P. Diagnosis of pneumothorax by ultrasound immediately after ultrasonically guided aspiration biopsy. Chest 1992; 101: 855–856.
17. Lichtenstein DA, Menu Y. A bedside ultrasound sign ruling out pneumothorax in critically ill. Chest 1995; 108: 1345–1348.

8 Laboratory methods

8.1 Bacteriology

Roger Freeman

The microbiological diagnosis of pneumonia ideally involves the comprehensive investigation of the exudate within consolidated tissue, entrapped within the parenchyma of the lung. In other respiratory infections (chronic obstructive pulmonary disease – COPD, bronchiectasis) the relevant infected material is secretions inspissated or stagnating within the bronchial tree. Suitable material for examination is usually obtained by one of the following methods:

- expectoration of sputum or suction of inspissated secretions
- invasive sampling, such as bronchoscopic alveolar lavage (BAL), transtracheal aspiration or percutaneous transthoracic aspiration.

In the first method the necessary traversal of the upper respiratory tract and mouth by the sample leads to admixture with saliva and contamination by commensal flora. In the second method the necessary invasive procedures incur varying degrees of risk. Fine judgement is needed in each patient to decide whether the clinical need for accurate microbiological diagnosis justifies the risk of obtaining the necessary samples.

In some patients, e.g. transplantation and other immunosuppressed patients, invasive procedures are justified from the outset. In others, e.g. those with COPD, persistence with non-invasive specimens or trials of empirical chemotherapy may well be reasonable rather than using invasive diagnostic methods.

Some scenarios, e.g. a suspected haematogenous lesion not communicating with the airways, may prompt direct transthoracic sampling. The suspicion of anaerobic infection may also dictate this invasive sampling to show that any upper-respiratory-tract anaerobes isolated have been translocated from their commensal site. Lung abscesses are almost an 'experiment of nature', presenting the investigator with his/her procedure half-completed, since the commonest aetiology is aspiration of upper respiratory tract flora but the subsequent suppuration produces an easily targeted lesion for transthoracic sampling, allowing undoubted incrimination of these 'commensal' bacteria. Long-standing lung abscesses should arouse the suspicion of actinomycosis (as well as of tuberculosis and other causes).

Indirect evidence of the nature of the organisms involved in pneumonia and other chest infections can be obtained by:

- blood cultures, which also give a crude index of severity and prognosis
- serological studies.

These latter, although occasionally the only diagnostic methods available in some settings, tend to delay the diagnosis until therapeutic intervention is either no longer necessary or too late.

In pneumonia complicated by empyema or effusion, the pleural fluid may be a valuable source of microbiological data.

All microbiological specimens are best obtained before the institution of antibiotic therapy and should, without exception, be sent to the laboratory without delay in sterile containers with a screw top. Microbiological samples, especially those obtained by invasive procedures, should always be the first call on the invasively acquired material. Specimen containers used for other pathology tests are often not sterile and may also contain special reagents such as anticoagulants capable of supporting certain bacteria. Syringe squirting can cross-contaminate the microbiology container and lead to 'pseudoisolates' from it. A 'microbiology first; microbiology dry' approach also minimises the risk of the microbiologist receiving the formalin container that was intended for histopathology!

In general, as long as specimens arrive in the laboratory within 24 hours, having been kept at a low temperature (preferably 4°C) meantime, the microbiology cultures will still be meaningful. The common sputum pathogens (even the allegedly fastidious haemophili) are remarkably resilient at refrigerator temperatures.[1] It is also important to remember that anaerobes will not be cultured for in expectorated samples (there being no diagnostic merit in demonstrating their ubiquity in the mouth), so no procedures for their preservation need be taken in such specimens.

Where invasive procedures are used, however, their relative rarity, likely impact on management and, not least, the duty to the patient to gain the maximum benefit from the procedure and so avoid having to repeat it, have suggested the use of additional measures of specimen management in some centres. In fact, the gains achieved by the use of anaerobic atmospheres in the specimen container, and so on, are very modest and probably unjustified in diagnostic settings, given that the difficulties of transport and delay should be avoidable for these patients.

Finally, enrichment techniques at the bedside (commonly, the addition of the specimen to broth) are best avoided since they will destroy forever the relative proportions of different organisms within the sample; data that may be of crucial importance in distinguishing between contaminants and pathogens. If enrichment is required it is best provided in the laboratory after direct procedures have been set up.

Examination of expectorated sputum (and aspirated secretions)

Most laboratories will not examine sputum/secretions unless they are purulent or at least mucopurulent.

Microscopy

Standard microscopy

Gram-stain examination of homogenised sputum (see below) may be helpful. The appearance of numerous Gram-positive lanceolate diplococci (*Streptococcus pneumoniae*), numerous intracellular Gram-negative diplococci (*Moraxella catarrhalis*, previously *Branhamella catarrhalis*) or numerous Gram-positive cocci in grape-like clusters (*Staphylococcus aureus*) can all be diagnostic in the appropriate clinical setting. The overall sensitivity of the Gram stain is not high, however, even in community-acquired pneumococcal pneumonia.[2]

The presence of yeasts is usually easily detected by Gram staining. Other fungi (e.g. *Aspergillus* spp.) must be detected by 'wet microscopy' of unstained samples, special stains (e.g. silver impregnation stains) or both. Very recent, fresh specimens are particularly important when trying to assess the significance of fungal hyphae, particularly in immunodeficient individuals, because these ubiquitous airborne contaminants can multiply during prolonged transit at room temperature.

The microscopic diagnosis of mycobacterial infection is much more secure. Some laboratories perform this on all purulent specimens. In other laboratories such staining must be specifically requested or, at least, the suspicion of mycobacterial disease must be communicated to the microbiologist. Recent assessments of the differing approaches to the microscopical detection of acid-fast bacilli (AFBs) in sputum have shown clearly that auramine staining is significantly more sensitive than Ziehl–Neelsen staining[3] (making nonsense of the common practice of confirming the presence of AFBs detected by the auramine stain by overstaining the slide with the less sensitive Ziehl–Neelsen method!) and that digestion/liquefaction of the sputum (see below) plus some form of concentration (by sedimentation or, preferably, centrifugation) of the specimen also significantly increases the sensitivity.[4] Laboratories continuing to pursue Ziehl–Neelsen staining on untreated sputum are almost

certainly failing to detect significant numbers of mycobacterioses, among them tuberculosis.

In some laboratories differential white-cell stains (e.g. Giemsa) are used. These may be better at detecting intracellular organisms but their main advantage is in demonstrating that purulence may occasionally be caused by eosinophils and not polymorphs.

Additional microscopy

It is possible to detect antigens of certain important bacterial or bacteria-like pathogens in sputum by direct fluorescent antibody tests using high-titre or monoclonal antibodies. Examples include *Legionella pneumophila*, *Pneumocystis carinii* and *Chlamydia pneumoniae*.

In general, such tests are best reserved for the cleaner invasively obtained specimens. In any case, they are now being rivalled by more sensitive methods using DNA-amplification techniques.

Culture

It is remarkably rare to receive sputum that is pure frank pus, although this can occur in pneumococcal lobar pneumonia, when the dense, pure culture of *S. pneumoniae* that results puts the diagnosis beyond doubt. Usually, 'purulent' sputum is a diphasic system containing small globules of pus suspended in a large matrix of mucus. The pus contains high numbers of pathogens ($> 10^8$/ml) and the mucus contains much more modest numbers of commensals ($< 10^5$/ml). As the two phases do not mix naturally, most laboratories homogenise sputum with dithiothreitol or similar chemicals.

Although this dilutes the pathogens to some extent, their very high numbers ensure that they still predominate over the commensals in the resultant homogeneous fluid. However, this will inevitably mean that most cultures of expectorated purulent sputum are a mixture of pathogens and commensals. The experienced microbiologist can usually identify the different organisms by their characteristic colonial appearances, backed up by a few simple and rapid tests (e.g. Optochin sensitivity for *S. pneumoniae*, tributyrin hydrolysis for *M. catarrhalis*, and so on). Commensals comprise those organisms usually found in the healthy upper respiratory tract or mouth, such as α-haemolytic streptococci of several species (formerly '*S. viridans*'), non-pathogenic neisserias (e.g. *Neisseria pharyngis*, *N. sicca*) and staphylococci. Thus, a bacteriological report of 'no pathogens isolated' or 'commensals only' (see later) does not imply no growth, rather that, while organisms have been isolated, they are of those species and in those relative proportions to be expected in a healthy respiratory tract and, therefore, probably not of lower respiratory tract origin and unlikely to be causing disease. However, as discussed earlier, the detection of these very same organisms in invasively acquired samples from the normally sterile lower areas of the respiratory tract, especially lung parenchyma, would imply exactly the opposite conclusion, i.e. a pathogenic role, probably as the result of aspiration. The further detection of anaerobes in the latter situation will confirm this. Thus, the definition of 'commensal' involves a combination of the identity of the organism, the site from which it is isolated, the nature of the other organisms present and the relative numbers of each.

There is a parallel with the well-known adage that a weed (pathogen) is a flower (commensal) growing in the wrong place. Of course, some pathogens, e.g. *Mycobacterium tuberculosis*, are never commensals.

Standard culture

A small range of simple media are usually inoculated. These include blood agar (which may have selective agents such as crystal violet, gentamicin and nalidixic acid incorporated to aid the isolation of pneumococci),[5] heated blood or 'chocolate' agar (which may have diphosphopyridine nucleotide and bacitracin added to aid the growth and isolation of haemophili) and MacConkey's agar (which aids the characterisation of any aerobic Gram-negative bacilli, or 'coliforms', present). Under special circumstances, e.g. with specimens from patients with cystic fibrosis, other, more selective media for certain Gram-negative bacilli may be needed (see below). Both *S. pneumoniae* and *H. influenzae* may grow better with the addition of extra carbon dioxide to the atmosphere. In addition to these organisms, *S. aureus*, *S. pyogenes*, *M. catarrhalis* and *Klebsiella pneumoniae* (Friedländer's bacillus) can be expected to grow well on these media overnight. Although many species can be identified presumptively after overnight incubation for the purposes of choosing antibiotic therapy, full identification often takes a further 24 hours.

The inevitably mixed nature of the overnight culture (even when one organism clearly predominates) does not usually permit concomitant direct sensitivity testing, so that formal sensitivity results cannot reasonably be expected until 48 hours after receipt of the specimen.

The ability to detect the β-lactamase enzyme activity of cultures rapidly, however, allows this information (which implies resistance to agents such as penicillin, amoxicillin and some cephalosporins) to be provided as soon as colonies of the organism are available for testing.[6]

Sabouraud's medium for the isolation of yeasts (most commonly, but not exclusively, *Candida albicans*) is often included in standard cultures, particularly in specimens from hospital inpatients. It is now well-recognised that all yeasts can be pathogens and that non-*albicans Candida* spp. and even non-*Candida* yeasts should be accorded respect. Nor can it any longer be assumed that *C. albicans* isolates are sensitive to fluconazole.

Additional cultures

The most common additional culture is that for mycobacteria, prompted either by a positive AFB stain or by appropriate clinical suspicion. Until recently conventional mycobacterial culture was on Löwenstein–Jensen solid medium (or equivalent). However, mycobacterial culture, especially for the isolation of the members of the *M. tuberculosis* complex, has undergone a revolution with the introduction of continuous automated mycobacterial liquid culture (CAMLiC) techniques[7] (several commercial systems exist). The application of this technology means that *M. tuberculosis* can almost always be grown within 2 weeks and often within less than a week. Similarly, whereas conventional speciation of

mycobacteria requires further subculture and can take several weeks, identification methods based on DNA probes are able securely to identify the CAMLiC isolate as a member of the *M. tuberculosis* complex within a day.[8] These advances, taken together with the use of the same CAMLiC technology for rapid susceptibility tests[9], mean that *M. tuberculosis* can be detected, isolated, identified and assessed for sensitivity/resistance to the usual 'first-line' drugs within 30 days of receipt of a sputum specimen in the vast majority of instances.[10] Gene probes for mycobacteria other than tuberculosis are limited and most of these are identified by slower phenotypic means, although *M. avium–intracellulare* is usually identified by probe.

Culture for *Legionella* spp. is now carried out easily and has the dual advantage of being more sensitive than the direct fluorescent antibody test (see above) and of being able to detect species other than *L. pneumophila*. It takes up to 3 days to complete.

Culture for fungi other than *Candida* spp. has long ceased to be a specialist preserve. In addition to the standard use of Sabouraud's medium for yeasts, more specialised media are now often used for recovery of *Aspergillus* spp., *Cryptococcus* spp. and even saprophytic moulds such as *Penicillium* spp. in heavily immunocompromised patients. Many of these organisms, particularly *Aspergillus* spp., will grow on the usual blood media but specialised media allow early recognition and identification. Non-standard incubation temperatures may be necessary and prior discussion with the microbiologist is essential.

Although it is possible to culture for *Mycoplasma pneumoniae* the technique is insensitive and prone to false-negative results. The isolation of *Chlamydia psittaci* and *C. pneumoniae* requires cell culture methods unsuitable for sputum. Serology (see below) remains the currently preferred method for the diagnosis of these infections, although antigen and/or DNA detection techniques are becoming available. Q fever is almost entirely diagnosed by serology. Attempts to isolate the organism (*Coxiella burnetii*) are strongly discouraged because of the very high risk of laboratory-acquired infection.

Non-cultural methods

In recent years numerous tests have been devised that speed diagnosis by either:

- immunodetection of antigens of microorganisms directly in sputum, invasively acquired bronchial material or, occasionally, urine, or
- molecular biological techniques for detecting the DNA of the organism.

Immunodetection

Pneumococcal capsular polysaccharide antigen (CPS). This is usually performed by reverse passive agglutination of inert particles coated with appropriate antibodies, the detection of the antigen being taken to indicate infection with pneumococci rather than carriage, although this distinction is not reliable. Antigen detection may remain positive when concomitant antibiotic therapy precludes successful culture. However, the diversity of CPS (over 90 serotypes) and the polysaccharide nature of the antigen preclude the use of monoclonal technology so that the sensitivity of this test in routine diagnostic settings is much less than that claimed in research studies.[11] The polyvalent antiserum used (Omniserum®) is also known to cross-react with some commensal (i.e. non-pneumococcal) α-haemolytic streptococci.[12] Antigen can also be detected in serum, urine and pleural exudates, although sensitivity is considerably less than in sputum. Recently, species-specific and highly conserved protein antigens such as pneumolysin have been the target for methods likely to be more specific and sensitive than CPS and early results are encouraging.[13]

Legionella. A soluble antigen from *L. pneumophila* serogroup 1 (by far the commonest infecting variety of this species) is excreted in the urine during the acute phase of the illness. Excretion continues for several days. An enzyme-linked immunosorbent assay (ELISA) method exploits this phenomenon rapidly to diagnose the commonest form of legionellosis (legionnaires' disease).[14] Fluorescent antibody methods for detection in sputum are available for *Legionella* spp. but usually only for some serotypes of *L. pneumophila*, albeit more than just serogroup 1. Hence a negative test by either or both of these methods does not exclude *all* forms of legionellosis.

Pneumocystis carinii is also detected by direct fluorescent antibody test using a monoclonal antibody. This rapid microscopical test works well in most clinical scenarios but it is occasionally found that a very small number of oocysts are detected in lung conditions due to other causes, especially in haematological oncology patients and lung transplant patients.

Molecular biological techniques

DNA probes
Currently these are mainly used for rapid characterisation of *organisms*, especially mycobacteria, rather than for detection of DNA in clinical material. They identify 16S RNA sequences in the organism, this being accepted as the ultimate molecular definition of the microbial species. This approach is too expensive for most routine diagnostic purposes unless it produces a very significant time and/or cost advantage, as in mycobacteria.

DNA amplification by polymerase chain reaction
In simple outline the polymerase chain reaction (PCR) consists of adding specifically synthesised short DNA base sequences (primers) to samples (whether unmodified clinical material or a DNA-rich extract of it) putatively containing the target DNA sequence characteristic of the organism. The primers are made to complement the target DNA sequence. If it is present they will 'lock on' and, in the presence of Taq polymerase and an adequate supply of DNA bases, initiate the PCR and 'grow' more of the target sequence in an exponential fashion until it can be detected by gel electrophoresis (using its molecular weight) or a specific DNA probe.

Even from this barest of descriptions it should be obvious that many things can go wrong with this technique. Substances within the sample that are inimical to Taq polymerase (e.g. haemin, globulin) will prevent DNA synthesis ('inhibitors'). There may be an enormous 'haystack' of unwanted (human) DNA in the sample DNA extract, the 'needle' of the bacterial DNA being lost within it. Detection of target DNA is not necessarily indicative of the live organism – DNA from dead organisms will also be amplified. The method may be too sensitive and thus unhelpfully identify normal carriage as well as true infection. The primers may not be as species- or organism-specific as was intended and related species will also be detected. Cross-contamination with amplified target DNA, giving rise to 'genuine' false positives, can occur in even the best molecular biology laboratories. All these potential problems are in addition to the often-overlooked questions of cost and timeliness.

Despite all this, PCR-based technology has revolutionised some aspects of diagnostic respiratory bacteriology. The present position is one of a measured and judicious use of the technology, seeking to capitalise on its unique attributes but also with a much more sanguine perspective than hitherto. Some important examples now follow.

Mycobacteriology. *M. tuberculosis* can now be detected and identified in sputum by PCR. Most methods target the insertion sequence *IS 6110*,[15] but other targets can be used. Users should be aware that the tuberculosis PCR is reliable in smear-positive samples (i.e. when AFBs have been found), when it can identify the seen AFBs as *M. tuberculosis* (or not), but the PCR will only be positive in a small percentage of the remaining smear-negative but culture-positive specimens. It is, therefore, a valuable adjunct to the AFB smear, not a replacement for it.[16] Culture (and especially CAMLiC culture) remains the most sensitive method for the detection of all common mycobacteria and especially *M. tuberculosis*. PCR-based methods also exist for the direct detection in sputum of some of the mutations leading to rifampicin resistance in *M. tuberculosis*.[17]

The diversity in the numbers of and location of *IS 6110* within populations of *M. tuberculosis* form the basis of several molecular 'strain typing' systems. Other methods are available that utilise other molecular polymorphisms. Thus, *M. tuberculosis* can now be quickly and effectively 'typed'.[18] This is invaluable in outbreaks and possible laboratory cross-contamination incidents.[19] PCR-based methods also exist for other species of mycobacteria and even for some of the individual members of the *M. tuberculosis* complex.[20]

Atypical pneumonia agents. PCR-based tests exist for *Legionella* spp[21] (and not just *L. pneumophila*), *M. pneumoniae*[22] and *C. pneumoniae*.[23] However, whereas in the case of *Legionella* spp. the PCR is diagnostic, since the organism, if present, is clearly an invader, positive results for *M. pneumoniae* (because of asymptomatic carriage) and *C. pneumoniae* (because of latency) will require very cautious interpretation.

Burkholderia cepacia. *B. cepacia* can now rapidly and securely be identified by PCR, whatever the colonial appearances on the selective culture medium and, equally importantly, *B. cepacia* can now be subdivided into several stable 'genomovars', some of which correlate with prognosis.[24]

Pneumocystis carinii. Several PCRs have been described for the detection of this organism, being, in general, significantly more sensitive than the direct fluorescent antibody test described above. The gain in the strength of the signal has meant that *P. carinii* can often be detected by PCR in the saliva/expectorated or induced sputum from patients with autoimmune deficiency syndrome (AIDS), obviating the need for invasive procedures.[25]

Streptococcus pneumoniae. It may seem odd that little mention has been made of PCR-based methods for the commonest of respiratory pathogens – *S. pneumoniae*. However, the sensitivity of PCR on sputum means that carriage will not be distinguished from infection and its cost (in relation to other methods, whether cultural or not) is prohibitive for such common specimens. Nonetheless, *S. pneumoniae* PCRs are of value in epidemiological studies of blood samples from pneumonic patients, when the PCR produces a severalfold increase in diagnoses compared to blood culture, especially in patients on antibiotics at admission.[26] These results better inform empirical therapy, since they reduce considerably the proportion of patients labelled as 'not diagnosed'.

RNA amplification by PCR is also possible, although more difficult, because of the inherent lability of RNA compared to the robustness of DNA. It depends on introducing a reverse transcriptase enzyme at the beginning of the procedure so that the RNA target (if present) is 'converted' into a complementary strand of DNA, the reaction thereafter being as for DNA PCRs. Several different RNAs can be measured (ribosomal, messenger, and so on) and the usefulness of measuring RNA is that it can logically be expected to reflect levels of viability or other important metabolic processes, depending on which RNA target is used. To date, DNA PCR has given invaluable information on the genetics of organisms, but the fact that a microbe *could* produce (i.e. has the gene for) a particular factor (e.g. a toxin) does not necessarily mean that it *does* produce it. RNA PCR can resolve this by showing the gene's activity as well as its mere presence. It is, after all, the phenotype that infects. There are many methodological problems with RNA PCR but it seems likely to increase in importance and value.

Interpretation of sputum examination

Standard examination

The microbiologist will usually look specifically for *S. pneumoniae*, *H. influenzae*, *S. aureus*, *M. catarrhalis*, *K. pneumoniae* and, very rarely, *S. pyogenes*. If none of these is found the usual conclusion is 'no pathogen isolated'.

The presence of *S. pneumoniae* or *H. influenzae* as the predominant organism in material from patients with compatible histories is diagnostic. *H. influenzae* is commonly isolated in small numbers from patients with bronchiectasis between acute exacerbations. The mere isolation of *M. catarrhalis* is not necessarily diagnostic but a heavy growth, supported by typical Gram-stain findings on the sputum specimen, can be taken to be so.

Isolation of *S. aureus* (or *S. pyogenes*) implies contamination from the mouth, nose or throat, but a dense growth of either should prompt a repeat and a review of the patient. In influenza virus epidemics they cause devastating pneumonia.[27]

Yeast isolates almost always represent nasopharyngeal or oral contamination. Genuine *Candida* pneumonia is extremely rare, even in the heavily immunosuppressed.

Isolation of most 'coliforms' implies an altered normal flora consequent on antibiotic use. 'Gram-negative pneumonia' is a much overdiagnosed condition. Invasive sampling may be necessary to support such a diagnosis. Occasionally a devastating and rapidly fatal form of necrotising Gram-negative pneumonia results from contamination of inhalation equipment, typically ventilator humidifiers. Prompt realisation of the source and immediate action to prevent further cases is essential.

Two situations involving the isolation of large numbers of coliform organisms from sputum require very careful interpretation.

Klebsiella spp.

The overwhelming majority are *K. aerogenes* and represent the altered commensal flora induced by antibiotics. A small proportion will be *K. pneumoniae* (Friedländer's bacillus). Distinction need only be made in patients with suggestive features. More rarely, bronchiectatic patients may become chronically colonised with *K. ozaenae*, it being present between exacerbations and more abundant during them.

Pseudomonads

Over 60% of *P. aeruginosa* isolates from patients with cystic fibrosis are of a particular mucoid phenotype and the isolation of such a strain should always raise the suspicion of cystic fibrosis if the diagnosis has not yet been made.

B. cepacia (formerly *Pseudomonas cepacia*) is more difficult to isolate and identify and selective media are required.[28] Identification and 'typing' of this difficult organism has been greatly enhanced by molecular biological techniques (see above). Typing is necessary because of the propensity of *B. cepacia*, infection with some genomovars of which seems to carry an adverse prognosis, to cause person-to-person transmission in cystic fibrosis.

Stenotrophomonas maltophilia (formerly *Pseudomonas maltophilia*) is the most recent pseudomonad to emerge in cystic fibrosis patients. To date, the evidence seems to suggest that it is commonest in the more severely affected patients because it is selected for by the therapy for other organisms, particularly *P. aeruginosa*, rather than because it is itself the cause of any deterioration.[29] There is also good positive evidence that *S. maltophilia* is not spread by person-to-person transmission.[30] There is, therefore, no need for the isolation and cohorting resorted to in *B. cepacia* infection. As with *P. aeruginosa*, the multi-antibiotic resistance of *S. maltophilia* is a problem, but the organism's significance seems more like that of *P. aeruginosa* than *B. cepacia*.

Additional examinations

With the notable exception of tests for pneumococcal antigens and mycobacterial stains and cultures, most of the additional cultural and non-cultural techniques are better employed on specimens obtained by invasive techniques and for those patients with indications to obtain such specimens.

Examination of invasively acquired specimens

All the invasive specimens already outlined should be examined by the most sensitive and rapid methods available, according to the following scheme:

- **Non-immunosuppressed patients.** In addition to standard Gram stain, AFB stain, 'wet microscopy' for fungal hyphae and the standard cultures described above, anaerobic culture and tests for *M. pneumoniae*, mycobacteria, fungi, *Chlamydia* spp. and *Legionella* spp. should be performed.

- **Immunosuppressed patients.** In addition to the above, tests for the presence of *P. carinii* should be included. Invasive specimens from heavily immunosuppressed patients are ideal for PCR techniques, containing little contaminating material to interfere with or inhibit the PCR.

Interpretation of results on invasive samples

In theory these samples will have been obtained from ordinarily sterile sites and therefore any detected microorganism is significant. However, important caveats must be noted.

Extrinsic contamination

It is always possible to introduce small numbers of upper respiratory tract organisms into the sample. This must be borne in mind before concluding that translocated upper respiratory tract organisms are the cause, for instance, of a lung abscess or suppurative pneumonia. In practice the density of growth in the two situations is obviously different and in genuine infection some anaerobes such as *Fusiformis* spp., penicillin-sensitive *Bacteroides* spp. (especially *B. melaninogenicus*) or the microaerophilic varieties of streptococci (especially *S. milleri*) predominate.

Coagulase-negative staphylococci and diphtheroids can contaminate percutaneous samples taken from the lung and extrinsic contamination from water (including *Legionella* spp.) or the air (*Aspergillus* spp.) can occur unless precautions are taken. Extrinsic contamination can also occur within the laboratory and unexpected organisms recovered from enrichment cultures should always prompt a review of their significance.

Inhibition of growth

Inhibition of cultural growth in patients not receiving antibiotics can be due to preservatives in the local anaesthetic used for bronchoscopy or residual antiseptic on inadequately rinsed bronchoscopes.

The contribution of serology to diagnosis

Serology is a means of diagnosing bacterial pneumonias in which isolating the organism is difficult (e.g. *M. pneumoniae*) or hazardous (e.g. *C. burnetii*) and is also useful for retrospective diagnosis and epidemiology.

The two cardinal principles are:

- the detection of specific IgM class antibodies in a single serum specimen, or
- the demonstration that an antibody undergoes a significant (usually fourfold or greater) rise in titre over the course of 10–14 days.

Methods include complement fixation tests (CFTs) for IgG antibodies or, increasingly, ELISAs and immunofluorescence tests that can detect both IgM and IgG.

IgM class antibody detection

Few tests currently use this theoretically attractive option for the diagnosis of bacterial infection but the repertoire is likely to expand in the future. Currently, IgM antibody to *M. pneumoniae* is the best example of an ELISA technique. A micro-immunofluorescence test for IgM to *C. pneumoniae* is being developed. Problems with other serum components, especially rheumatoid factor, occur.[31]

Rising antibody titre testing

This method is widely used for *M. pneumoniae*, *Chlamydia* spp. and *C. burnetii*. It is clearly advantageous to obtain the first, or 'acute', specimen as soon as possible for comparison with the second, or 'convalescent', specimen 10–14 days later. Many laboratories continue to use CFTs in spite of the poor sensitivity and reproducibility of this method compared to ELISA. A major paradox is that testing for antibodies to the uncommon *C. psittaci* is widespread whereas detection of antibodies to *C. pneumoniae*, which may account for about 8% of community-acquired pneumonia, is still rarely performed.

Antibody to *L. pneumophila* is still sought in suspicious cases of atypical pneumonia. Although *Legionella* spp. are now easily cultured from invasive specimens, the detection of *L. pneumophila* serogroup 1 antigen in urine is now a well-accepted test for acute-phase diagnosis of the commonest form of legionellosis, and PCR-based methods on respiratory secretions offer prospects of acute-phase diagnosis of all forms of legionellosis, the antibody test remains valuable as a retrospective test. In low titres it may result from cross-reactions with other bacterial antigens, e.g. campylobacters.[32]

Non-specific serological tests

Acute serum specimens may also contain non-specific IgM-class immunoglobulins, some of which have characteristic associations with certain infections. The most useful example is the detection of IgM-class cold agglutinin antibodies in the acute phase of *M. pneumoniae* infection. Although not always present, cold agglutinins are a very strong pointer to this diagnosis.[33]

Final comments

The foregoing should not be taken to imply that the bacteriological diagnosis of pneumonia is inevitably highly technical, difficult and expensive. This is true of *some* cases but standard examination and culture of expectorated sputum will adequately serve most routine admissions. Indeed, in many cases even these results will often only serve to confirm a clinical diagnosis that has already, justifiably, led to empirical therapy.

Continual dialogue between wards and laboratory at all levels of investigation is an essential prerequisite for providing an optimal service for all patients with respiratory infection. New diagnostic tests require careful evaluation, including proof that they can replace existing tests or that they add something useful to the repertoire, before they are introduced into routine practice (or requested!).

Clinical relevance

Specimens

■ Expectorated sputum is acceptable for common chest infections but its poor quality compromises many investigations

■ Greater certainty is achieved with invasively acquired material (bronchoalveolar lavage, transtracheal aspirate, transthoracic biopsy, and so on)

■ Some diagnoses, especially those involving anaerobes, can only be made on invasively acquired material

■ The 'threshold' for invasive procedures varies with the clinical setting, but discussions with the laboratory are essential to ensure maximum benefit and justification of the risks

Investigations

■ *All* specimens receive standard microscopy and culture (for pneumococcus, *Haemophilus* and *Moraxella*, etc.) and antigen detection may help (for pneumococcus)

■ With specific indications, microscopy and culture for *Mycobacterium tuberculosis* is added

■ Invasive specimens receive standard + mycobacterial + extended detection methods (such as PCR)

■ Correct interpretation of the results, especially of PCR-based tests, is essential

References

1. Gould FK, Freeman R, Hudson S et al. Does storage of sputum specimens adversely affect culture results? J Clin Pathol 1996; 49: 684.

2. British Thoracic Society Research Committee. Community-acquired pneumonia in adults in British hospitals in 1982–83: a survey of aetiology, mortality, prognostic factors and outcome. Q J Med 1987; 62:195.

3. Ba F, Rieder HL. A comparison of fluorescence microscopy with the Ziehl–Neelsen technique in the examination of sputum for acid-fast bacilli. Int J Tuberc Lung Dis 1999; 3: 1101.

4. Peterson FM, Nakasone A, Platon-DeLeon JM et al. Comparison of direct and concentrated acid-fast smears to identify specimens culture positive for *Mycobacterium* spp. J Clin Microbiol 1999; 37: 3564.

5. Nichols T, Freeman R. A new selective medium for *Streptococcus pneumoniae*. J Clin Pathol 1980; 33: 770.

6. O'Callaghan CH, Morris A, Kirby SM, Shingler AH. Novel method for detection of β-lactamases by using a chromogenic cephalosporin substrate. Antimicrob Agents Chemother 1972; 1: 283.

7. Magee JG, Freeman R, Barrett A. Enhanced speed and sensitivity in the cultural diagnosis of pulmonary tuberculosis with a continuous automated mycobacterial liquid culture (CAMLiC) system. J Med Microbiol 1998; 47: 547.

8. Resiner BS, Gatson AM, Woods GL. Use of Gen-Probe AccuProbes to identify *Mycobacterium tuberculosis* complex, *Mycobacterium kansasii* and *Mycobacterium gordonae* directly from BACTEC TB broth cultures. J Clin Microbiol 1994; 32: 2995.

9. Hawkins JE, Wallace RJ, Brown BA. Antibacterial susceptibility tests: mycobacteria. In: Balows A, Hausler WJ, Herrman KL et al, eds. Manual of clinical microbiology, 5th ed. Washington DC: American Society for Microbiology; 1991: 1138.

10. Tenover FC, Crawford JT, Huebner RE et al. The resurgence of tuberculosis: is your laboratory ready? J Clin Microbiol 1993; 31: 767.

11. Farrington M, Rubenstein D. Antigen detection in pneumococcal pneumonia. J Infect Dis 1991; 23: 109.

12. Holmberg H, Danielsson D, Hardie J et al. Cross-reaction between alpha-haemolytic streptococci and Omniserum, a polyvalent pneumococcal serum, demonstrated by direct immunofluorescence, immunoelectroosmophoresis and latex agglutination. J Clin Microbiol 1985; 21: 745.

13. Wheeler J, Freeman R, Steward M et al. Detection of pneumolysin in sputum. J Med Microbiol 1999; 48: 863.

14. Benson RF, Tang PW, Fields BS. Evaluation of the Binax and Biotest urinary antigen kits for detection of Legionnaires' Disease due to multiple serogroups and species of *Legionella*. J Clin Microbiol 2000; 38: 2763.

15. Kearns AM, Freeman R, Steward M et al. A rapid polymerase chain reaction technique for detecting *M. tuberculosis* in a variety of clinical specimens. J Clin Pathol 1998; 51: 922.

16. Afghani B, Stutman HR. Diagnosis of tuberculosis: can the polymerase chain reaction replace acid fast bacillus smear and culture? J Infect Dis 1995; 172: 903.

17. Telenti A, Imboden P, Marchesi F *et al.* Detection of rifampicin-resistance mutations in *Mycobacterium tuberculosis*. Lancet 1993; 341: 647.

18. Kearns AM, Barrett A, Marshall C et al. Epidemiology and molecular typing of an outbreak of tuberculosis in a hostel for homeless men. J Clin Pathol 2000; 53: 122.

19. Bifani P, Moghazeh S, Shopsin B et al. Molecular characterization of *Mycobacterium tuberculosis* H37Rv/Ra variants: distinguishing the mycobacterial laboratory strain. J Clin Microbiol 2000; 38: 3200.

20. Kearns AM, Magee JG, Gennery A et al. Rapid identification of *Mycobacterium bovis* BCG by the detection of the RD1 deletion using a multiplex PCR technique. Int J Tuberc Lung Dis 1999; 3: 635.

21. Cloud JL, Carroll KC, Pixton P et al. Detection of *Legionella* species in respiratory specimens using PCR with sequencing confirmation. J Clin Microbiol 2000; 38: 1709.

22. Honda J, Takafumi Y, Mikako K et al. Clinical use of capillary PCR to diagnose *Mycoplasma pneumoniae* pneumonia. J Clin Microbiol 2000; 38: 1382.

23. Corsaro D, Valassina M, Venditti D et al. Multiplex PCR for rapid and differential diagnosis of *Mycoplasma pneumoniae* and *Chlamydia pneumoniae* in respiratory infections. Diagn Microbiol Infect Dis 1999; 35: 105.

24. Mahenthiralingam E, Bischof J, Byrne SK et al. DNA-based diagnostic approach for identification of *Burkholderia cepacia* complex, *B. vietnamiensis*, *B. mullivorans*, *B. stabilis* and *B. cepacia* genomovars I and III. J Clin Microbiol 2000; 38: 3165.

25. Helweg-Larsen J, Jensen JS, Benfield T et al. Diagnostic use of PCR for detection of *Pneumocystis carinii* in oral wash samples. J Clin Microbiol 1998; 36: 2068.

26. Wheeler JW, Murphy OM, Freeman R et al. PCR can add to detection of pneumococcal disease in pneumonic patients receiving antibiotics at admission. J Clin Microbiol 2000; 38: 3907.

27. Gardner ID. Suppression of antibacterial immunity after infection with influenza virus. J Infect Dis 1981; 144: 225.

28. Nelson JW, Doherty CJ, Brown PH et al. *Pseudomonas cepacia* in inpatients with cystic fibrosis. Lancet 1991; 338: 1525.

29. Talmaciu I, Varlotta L, Mortensen J et al. Risk factors for the emergence of *Stenotrophomonas maltophilia* in cystic fibrosis. Pediatr Pulmonol 2000; 30: 10.

30. Denton M, Todd NJ, Kerr KG et al. Molecular epidemiology of *Stenotrophomonas maltophilia* isolated from clinical specimens from patients with cystic fibrosis and environmental samples. J Clin Microbiol 1998; 36: 1953.

31. Verkooyen RP, Hazenberg MA, van Haaren GH et al. Age-related interference with *Chlamydia pneumoniae* serology due to circulating rheumatoid factor. J Clin Microbiol 1992; 30: 1287.

32. Boswell TCJ, Kudesia G. Seropositivity for *Legionella* in *Campylobacter* infection. Lancet 1992; 339: 191.

33. Sillis M. Modern methods for the diagnosis of *Mycoplasma pneumoniae* pneumonia. Rev Med Microbiol 1993; 4: 24.

8 Laboratory methods

8.2 Detection of respiratory viruses

Paul Taylor and Sebastian L Johnston

Virus infection of the respiratory tract results in a wide spectrum of disease ranging from the trivial common cold to life-threatening pneumonia. The laboratory procedures adopted for viral diagnosis have traditionally been regarded as too prolonged to be of benefit to the individual patient. The advent of specific antiviral agents for respiratory infection, such as ribavirin and the new neuraminidase inhibitors for influenza, has increased the clinical demand to develop and accelerate virus laboratory services. Fortunately, rapid same-day techniques are now available to identify specific viral antigens and nucleic acids in respiratory secretions. Such methods are applicable to diagnosis during the acute stage of disease.

Specimens

Viruses are labile and it is therefore essential that samples should be transported to the virology laboratory without delay. Suitable samples are the following:

- Nose and throat swabs (in viral transport medium)
- Gargle (in saline)
- Nasopharyngeal aspirates
- Endotracheal aspirates
- Sputum
- Bronchoscopic specimens
- Tissue
- Pleural fluid
- Buffy coat (in the immunocompromised patient).

Nose and throat swabs in particular should be placed in a viral transport medium consisting of 2% fetal calf serum in a buffered salt solution, e.g. Hank's. Antibiotics such as penicillin and streptomycin may be added to inhibit bacterial contamination. If transportation to the laboratory is likely to exceed 1 hour samples should be retained in a refrigerator or on ice packs at 4°C. Freezing should be avoided as this destroys the virus and cells necessary for rapid detection methods.

Nose and throat swabs should be carefully taken by a trained individual. The throat (or cough) swab is obtained by swabbing the throat so that the patient gags and coughs on to the swab. Virus isolation is dependent on the presence of an adequate number of infected cells and high-quality samples are imperative. Where throat symptoms are predominant a gargle sample may be appropriate. The patient is requested to gargle with about 10 ml physiological saline, which is then expectorated into a sterile universal container.

In children, aspirates from either the nasopharynx or trachea are ideal for both rapid virus diagnosis and culture. Nasopharyngeal aspirates should be collected from the posterior of the passages using a size 8 sterile feeding tube attached to a sterile plastic mucus extractor and suction applied by a vacuum pump. Tracheal aspirates from intubated patients can be collected into mucus extractors in a similar manner.

In patients with exacerbations of chronic respiratory disease such as asthma, chronic obstructive pulmonary disease (COPD) and cystic fibrosis, sputum may be useful for virus detection. Sputum production may be facilitated by physiotherapy or induced by using aerosols of normal or hypertonic saline delivered by an ultrasonic nebuliser: this non-invasive technique is of particular importance in obtaining secretions from patients with the acquired immune deficiency syndrome (AIDS). Sputum should be expectorated into a sterile universal container and transported immediately to the laboratory.

Suitable samples of various types can be obtained from patients during bronchoscopy. Bronchial secretions can be collected directly or saline may be used to lavage selected lung regions. Such lavages may be obtained from the larger airways (bronchial lavage) or more distally (bronchoalveolar lavage, BAL). Up to 60 ml saline is used in adults and up to 10 ml in children; such specimens produce a high cell yield suitable for both immunofluorescence and culture methods. Bronchial lavage may contain ciliated bronchial epithelial cells, whereas BAL samples are more likely to contain macrophages. The latter cells may give conflicting results by non-specific binding of antibody in immunofluorescence techniques.

Lung tissue samples can be obtained by transbronchial biopsy, percutaneous fine needle aspiration or at thoracotomy. Frozen tissue sections of 20 μm can be processed for immunofluorescence tests although, if sufficient lung material is available, impression smears may be prepared.

Viraemia may be detected in circulating leukocytes obtained from a heparinised blood sample. Ten millilitres of peripheral blood is gently mixed with 500 units of preservative-free heparin and the buffy coat is removed. Lymphocytes are separated by density centrifugation in an iso-osmotic, low-viscosity solution or by allowing the sample to settle for 1 hour at 4°C.

Pleural fluid has been used for viral culture although in the authors' laboratories this has proved unrewarding. This probably reflects low viral yield and the need for sampling to take place during the short period of viraemia.

Laboratory methods

Serology

Serological techniques in general provide a retrospective assessment of a patient's disease. The complement fixation test (CFT) is the method most widely used in virus laboratories to detect specific antibodies to respiratory viruses and other agents that may cause atypical pneumonia, such as *Mycoplasma pneumoniae*, *Chlamydia psittaci* and *Coxiella burnetti*. The CFT, in spite of its flexibility, detects primarily IgG class antibody, requires overnight incubation of the test and is fairly insensitive. For optimum sensitivity, sera collected during the acute and convalescent periods of disease need to be examined. A fourfold or greater rise in titre between these 'paired' sera indicates recent infection with that organism. In some instances a single raised titre above 1:160 may suggest recent infection.

Detection of specific IgM by enzyme immunoassay (EIA) and other systems (radioimmunoassay, fluorescent antibody binding, etc.) may be of greater value than the CFT because the presence of specific IgM indicates recent infection on a single sample collected 10 days or more after onset of symptoms. An EIA is also a more sensitive technique than the CFT.

Patients who are immunodeficient as a result of disease, such as AIDS or immunoglobulin deficiency, treatment with cytotoxic or immunosuppressive drugs or as a result of extremes of age may not respond to viral infection by the production of sufficient detectable antibody. In such instances the specific diagnosis of infection has to depend on the detection of viral antigen or nucleic acid

Virus isolation

The isolation of respiratory viruses requires sensitive cell culture systems.[1] Most virus diagnostic laboratories use three types of cell culture: primary or secondary monkey (e.g. Rhesus) kidney, human embryonic lung (e.g. MRC$_5$) and a continuous cell line such as HEp2. These are capable of supporting the growth of all respiratory viruses except for coronaviruses, which require specialised cell lines such as Clone 16, HRT-18 or organ culture of fetal

trachea. Rhinoviruses grow poorly in these cell cultures and so only a minority of rhinovirus infections are detected by this method.

Once inoculated with clinical material, cell cultures are examined at least twice weekly for the development of cytopathic effects, which develop as a result of viral replication. Some viruses grow rapidly; for example, herpes simplex may produce cytopathic effects within 24 hours. Prolonged incubation may be required for other viruses; for example, cytomegalovirus may require 14 days or more for cytopathic effects to develop. When a typical cytopathic effect has developed it has previously been standard practice to perform neutralisation tests to identify the virus present. This may further delay reporting by a number of days. The introduction of immunofluorescence technology has provided a convenient method for rapidly identifying viruses producing cytopathic effects. Using specific monoclonal antibodies to viral antigens present at an early stage of replication, the immunofluorescence technique can detect virus infection in cell culture before the appearance of recognisable cytopathic effects. Cytomegalovirus, for example, may be detected in infected cell culture 24–36 hours after inoculation.[2] This technique of early cytomegaloviral antigen detection is of particular importance in immunocompromised patients, in whom rapid identification of the virus in the lung may allow prompt and early treatment. Adaptation of this technique to lymphocytes may demonstrate viraemia and the need to consider chemoprophylaxis. Although not yet sufficiently developed for widespread use, it is also possible to use PCR in early cell cultures to detect specific viruses to speed up both detection and identification of the virus type.

Haemadsorption

The replication of influenza and parainfluenza viruses in cell culture promotes antigenic changes at the cell surface, including the production of haemagglutinin. This antigen causes haemadsorption of erythrocytes, which can therefore be used as an indicator of infection caused by these viruses. Immunofluorescence techniques are then used to identify the specific virus.

Immunofluorescence techniques

Viral infection of exfoliated cells in respiratory tract samples may be detected rapidly and specifically using monoclonal antibodies. These vary in sensitivity and each source must be stringently evaluated by the laboratory, particularly if they are to be used for direct detection of viral antigen in clinical material rather than for cell culture confirmation.

Exfoliated cells are isolated by washing and centrifugation until they are free of any mucus. They are then applied to microscope slides, air-dried and fixed in acetone. The supernatant from the first washing step is simultaneously inoculated into cell cultures.

Two major immunofluorescence techniques are in general use: direct and indirect.[3] The direct technique requires the virus-specific monoclonal antibody (MAb) to be labelled with the fluorescent dye fluorescein isothiocyanate (FITC). The indirect technique uses unlabelled mouse MAb and a further step is necessary using an anti-mouse antibody/FITC conjugate. The direct technique is more rapid but is dependent on the availability of conjugated MAbs. Respiratory syncytial virus (RSV), influenza A virus, influenza B virus, adenovirus (group), parainfluenza virus (1, 2 and 3), cytomegalovirus, herpes simplex virus and measles virus are all available as directly conjugated MAbs. Mumps virus and varicella-zoster virus are currently only available unconjugated and therefore require the indirect technique. Cytomegalovirus antigen may be detected directly in peripheral lymphocytes by using an MAb against the 65 kDa lower matrix protein.

Once stained, the preparations are examined microscopically under ultraviolet light, when positive samples exhibit specific immunofluorescence in the cytoplasm or nucleus of infected cells. The immunofluorescence technique is also applicable to other microbes and it may be considered important to test samples from patients with pneumonia for evidence of *Legionella pneumophila* and *Pneumocystis carinii* infection using commercially obtained MAbs.

If an ultraviolet microscope is unavailable, an immunoperoxidase technique can be applied in a similar way to immunofluorescence. The action of peroxidase on its substrate forms a coloured end-product that may be identified with a conventional light microscope

Immunoassays for antigen detection

Viral antigens may be detected by specific antibody conjugated to an enzyme label. When a relevant substrate is added, a coloured end-product is produced, the intensity of which is proportional to the amount of viral antigen present in the sample (EIA). Similar detection methods using thin film optics in optical immunoassays (OIA) also allow detection of viral antigens by specific antibodies bound to silicon wafers. These antibodies capture viral antigens, if present in the clinical sample; addition of a second antibody then changes the thickness of the film, allowing detection by visualisation of colour change.

Commercially available EIAs use immobilised antibody for specific antigenic capture in the form of a 'test pack'. Currently, these are produced for RSV[4] and influenza virus A.[5] OIAs are also commercially available for RSV and influenza, and are being developed for rhinoviruses.[6] These techniques are more rapid and simple than immunofluorescence but at present are less sensitive and should be reserved for urgent acute cases.

An EIA screen for respiratory viruses may be established[7] using a range of antibodies coated on to microtitre plates. This method is most suitable for screening large numbers of samples (over 15 per day) but once established gives reproducible results equal in sensitivity to immunofluorescence. The quality of specimen, which is easy to determine in an immunofluorescence test, is difficult to control in an EIA system, and some form of internal quality control may be required to ensure that cells are present in the sample.

Nucleic acid detection systems

In situ hybridisation (ISH) techniques can be used to detect specific RNA or DNA in paraffin or frozen tissue sections or cytospin preparations. Target viral nucleic acid present in the sample is reacted with complementary labelled nucleic acid.

The hybrid produced can be visualised by a staining reaction directed at the label attached to the probe. Labels include radiolabelled isotopes, fluorochromes and enzymes such as peroxidase. ISH is more sensitive than conventional histological techniques, which depend on detecting inclusion bodies. The technique is rapid, taking about 4 hours to complete; however, it is available only in specialised laboratories and should be regarded as complementing other diagnostic methods.

The polymerase chain reaction (PCR) was first described in 1986 and enables tiny amounts of nucleic acid to be amplified (using specific primers) to detectable levels in a highly specific manner. Since 1989 the technique has been applied to a number of viruses with very encouraging results. It is totally specific and permits detection of viruses with great sensitivity, down to less than 10 copies of viral nucleic acid. It is rapid, results being available within a few hours of arrival of the sample in the laboratory, and can be applied with equal facility to both DNA and RNA viruses. It is particularly suited to two groups of respiratory viruses – rhinoviruses and coronaviruses (which together cause 60–75% of acute respiratory illnesses) – because no other rapid detection methods are available for either agent and standard methods such as cell culture (poor sensitivity) and serology (not available) are inadequate.

Polymerase chain reaction methods have now been developed for all the common respiratory viruses (Table 8.2.1) and in the case of rhinoviruses and coronaviruses are vastly superior to any other method currently available.[8-10] PCR assays for influenza, parainfluenza and RSV also appear to be at least as good as and almost certainly better than standard methods.[11-13]

A further advantage of PCR is the ability to combine primers for several different viruses in the same assay, thus allowing detection of multiple virus types or subtypes in a single test; this is known as multiplex PCR. This method has been used for detection of influenza and RSV together in a single test[14] and even allows detection of up to six virus types in a single test. To date, PCR assays are only used in a research setting and it is likely to be some time before this technique is available as a routine diagnostic method; however, it is used increasingly by PHLS virology laboratories as an adjunct to standard methods[15] and over the coming years it is likely to be even more widely used.

Virus infection in chronic airway disease

Several recent studies suggest that respiratory virus involvement in exacerbations of airway disease is much more frequent than previously believed, rhinoviruses being the predominant pathogens. In a community-based study, 108 asthmatic children were followed up for a year.[16] Virological analysis was extensive, using a combination of standard methodologies, such as culture, immunofluorescence and serology, as well as PCR for rhinoviruses and coronaviruses. Viruses were associated with 80–85% of exacerbations. Rhinoviruses accounted for approximately two-thirds of all identified viruses.

Table 8.2.1 The laboratory diagnosis of respiratory viruses

Respiratory viruses	Number of serotypes	Laboratory techniques			
		Cell culture	MAb IF	PCR	Other
Rhinoviruses	100+	++		+++	
Corona	At least 2	+		+++	o/c
Adenovirus	46		++	+++	+
Respiratory syncytial	1 (2 subtypes)	++	+++	+++	EIA
Influenza A	Multiple, only 1 or 2 in circulation	+	+++	+++	EIA
Influenza B	Only 1 in circulation	+	+++	+++	
Parainfluenza	4		+	+++	+++
Cytomegalovirus	1		+	++	+++
Herpes simplex	2		++	+++	
Human herpes virus 6	1			+	++
Measles	1		+	++	
Enterovirus	22		++	+	+++

o/c, organ culture.

A similarly designed study was performed by Nicholson et al.,[17] in which 138 asthmatic adults were followed up. Virus identification rates were lower, associated with 44% of asthma exacerbations. However, when subjective criteria were used, 80% of asthma exacerbations occurred with symptomatic colds, while 90% of colds were associated with symptoms of asthma. It is possible that the discrepancy between subjective symptomatology and objective virus detection may be attributed to less intensive monitoring and later sampling than was the case in the study in children.

In order to assess whether common colds could also lead to severe asthma requiring hospitalisation, the data obtained from the Southampton paediatric cohort were compared with hospitalisations for asthma in the area during the same time period.[18] Strong correlations were found between the seasonal patterns of upper respiratory infections and hospital admissions for asthma.

Similar studies have been carried out with exacerbations of other airway diseases, including COPD and cystic fibrosis, virus infections again being implicated in a large proportion of exacerbations[19,20]. Further studies such as these using improved diagnosis by PCR should lead to greater awareness of the importance of virus infection in exacerbations of respiratory disease in all age groups. Recent studies have underlined the major contribution of respiratory viral infection to morbidity and mortality in at risk groups such as the young[21,22] and the elderly.[23–25] With the advent of new therapies such as the neuraminidase inhibitors for influenza types A and B and others in development for viruses such as rhinoviruses (Table 8.2.2), the role of respiratory viral infections in respiratory disease is likely to take on increasing clinical as well as research importance.

Virus infections in the immunocompromised host

Knowledge of a patient's immunocompetence enables specific tests for opportunistic viruses such as cytomegalovirus and herpes simplex to be employed. Following organ transplantation, the peak time of viraemia for cytomegalovirus is about 30 days.[26]

Cytomegalovirus can be detected in lymphocytes directly with MAbs or after a short growth cycle in cell culture. A positive result from lymphocytes or specimens obtained at bronchoscopy is of potentially greater clinical relevance than a positive result from urine or throat swabs because cytomegalovirus may persist as a low-grade asymptomatic infection for long periods in the kidney and salivary glands.

In the immunocompromised individual, prolonged viraemia may occur with a number of respiratory viruses; for example, rhinoviruses, parainfluenza viruses and other respiratory viruses can cause fatal pneumonia and systemic infection in transplant recipients.[27] Human herpes virus 6 (HHV-6) has also been shown to cause severe pneumonia in bone marrow transplant recipients.[28] HHV-6 may be detected rapidly by immunofluorescence using a mixture of MAbs on BAL samples and in buffy coat specimens inoculated into cell cultures. Prompt diagnosis of respiratory infections in the immunocompromised patient allows initiation of appropriate antiviral therapy. In view of the inherent toxicity of some important antiviral drugs, such as ganciclovir and foscarnet, it is essential to determine the likely significance of detection of a virus, in terms of the patient's disease, before initiating therapy.

Table 8.2.2 Clinical concepts

Disease type	Virus	Chemotherapy	Vaccine
Upper respiratory tract infection	Rhinovirus	Enviroxime*	No
	Coronavirus		No
Pharyngitis	Adenovirus	Ribavirin	Experimental
Lower respiratory tract infection			
Bronchiolitis	RSV	Ribavirin	No
Croup	Parainfluenza	Ribavirin	No
Influenza like illness	Influenza A+B	ARR	Yes
Pneumonia	Adenovirus	Ribavirin	Experimental
Influenza		ARR	Yes
Chronic airways disease			
Cystic fibrosis	Rhinoviruses	Enviroxime*	No
COPD	Rhinoviruses	Enviroxime*	No
Asthma	Rhinoviruses	Enviroxime	No
Immunocompromised rhinoviruses	Cytomegalovirus	Ganciclovir, foscarnet	No
herpes simplex		Enviroxime*	No
		Acyclovir	No

* In clinical trials.

ARR, Amantadine/rimantadine, Relenza/Tamiflu (neuraminidase inhibitors), ribavirin

Interpretation of results

The viruses associated with infections of the respiratory tract are shown in Table 8.2.2. There is some seasonal variation: most RSV infections, for example, occur between November and February whereas infections caused by parainfluenza virus type 3 generally occur in May and June. In contrast, parainfluenza 1 and 2 viruses and influenza viruses cause well-recognised winter epidemics. Seasonal variation therefore needs to be considered when deciding which MAbs or PCR tests to apply to clinical samples.

Not all MAbs are able to detect the presence of viral antigens in exfoliated cells from the respiratory tract. The high specificity of MAbs to specific viral antigens or epitopes, which may not be present in all cells, may require more than one MAb to be used for a given virus. It is imperative that the quality of all MAbs is carefully monitored with known positive and negative clinical material before being used for diagnostic testing.

Enteroviruses such as Coxsackie B and echoviruses may be detected in respiratory samples from patients with Bornholm disease or pneumonia. In addition to respiratory tract symptoms they usually cause more general disease. Faecal samples or rectal swabs provide the best material for virus isolation but, as excretion may occur for long periods after the initial infection, it is difficult to prove association with active disease. Specific IgM to enteroviruses may also be detected by EIA; PCR can also be used successfully.

With the examination of respiratory samples by both culture and a rapid method such as immunofluorescence and PCR, recognition of dual and even triple infection has become more frequent. In recent studies using PCR, dual infections are found in as many as 10–15% of positive samples and triple infections in up to 5%. The degree of immunofluorescence intensity in a preparation, the strength of a PCR signal and the time to development of cytopathic effects in cell culture may provide a guide to the stage of infection in the individual patient.

It may be possible to detect respiratory viruses in secretions for up to 7 days after the onset of symptoms by culture in cell systems. The duration of detection of viral infection can be extended to 14 days using immunological methods such as immunofluorescence. It is therefore important that the clinician determines the date of onset of infection so that appropriate techniques can be employed and additional methods including specific IgM serology be applied.

? Unresolved questions

- What is the true clinical contribution of acute respiratory virus infections to respiratory disease?

- What is the true clinical contribution of chronic respiratory viral infections in respiratory disease?

- What is the duration of PCR positivity from onset of symptoms in immunocompetent and immunodeficient patients?

- Can rapid diagnostic tests and antiviral therapies be developed to enable treatment of acute respiratory viral illnesses and their complications?

10. Myint S, Johnston S, Sanderson G, Simpson H. Evaluation of nested polymerase chain methods for the detection of human coronaviruses 229E and OC43. Mol Cell Probes 1995; 8: 357–364.
11. Ellis JS, Fleming DM, Zambon MC. Multiplex reverse transcription-PCR for surveillance of influenza A and B viruses in England and Wales in 1995 and 1996. J Clin Microbiol 1997; 35: 2076–2082.
12. Corne J, Green S, Sanderson G, Johnston SL. A multiplex RT-PCR for the detection of parainfluenza viruses 1–3. J Virol Methods 1999; 82: 9–18.
13. Chauhan AJ, Xie P, O'Donnell DR et al. Detection of RS virus by RT-PCR in acute and asymptomatic respiratory samples: a comparison with standard methods. J Virol Methods (submitted).
14. Stockton J, Ellis JS, Saville M et al. Multiplex PCR for typing and subtyping influenza and respiratory syncytial viruses. J Clin Microbiol 1998; 36: 2990–2995.
15. Carman WF, Wallace LA, Walker J et al. Rapid virological surveillance of community influenza infection in general practice. Br Med J 2000; 321: 736–737.
16. Johnston SL, Pattemore PK, Sanderson et al. Community study of role of viral infections in exacerbations of asthma in 9–11-year-old children. Br Med J 1995; 310: 1225–1228.
17. Nicholson KG, Kent J, Ireland DC. Respiratory viruses and exacerbations of asthma in adults. Br Med J 1993; 307: 982–986
18. Johnston SL, Pattemore PK, Sanderson G et al. The relationship between upper respiratory infections and hospital admission for asthma: a time trend analysis. Am J Respir Crit Care Med 1996; 154: 654–660.
19. Seemungal TAR, Donaldson GC, Breuer J et al. Rhinoviruses are associated with exacerbations of COPD. Am J Resp Crit Care Med 1998; 157: A58.
20. Collinson J, Nicholson KG, Cancio E et al. Effects of upper respiratory tract infections in patients with cystic fibrosis. Thorax 1996; 51: 1115–1122.
21. Krilov L, Pierik L, Keller E et al. The association of rhinoviruses with lower respiratory tract disease in hospitalized patients. J Med Virol 1986; 19: 345–352.
22. Chidekel A, Rosen C, Bazzy A. Rhinovirus infection associated with serious lower respiratory illness in patients with bronchopulmonary dysplasia. Pediatr Infect Dis J 1997; 16: 43–47.
23. Nicholson KG, Kent J, Hammersley V, Cancio E. Risk factors for lower respiratory complications of rhinovirus infections in elderly people living in the community: prospective cohort study. Br Med J 1996; 313: 1119–1123.
24. Nicholson KG, Kent J, Hammersley V, Cancio E. Acute viral infections of upper respiratory tract in elderly people living in the community: comparative, prospective, population based study of disease burden. Br Med J 1997; 315: 1060–1064.
25. Wald T, Shult P, Krause P et al. A rhinovirus outbreak among residents of a long-term care facility. Ann Intern Med 1995; 123: 588–593.
26. Guidelines for preventing opportunistic infections among hematopoietic stem cell transplant recipients – recommendations of CDC, the Infectious Disease Society of America, and the American Society of Blood and Marrow Transplantation. MMWR 2000; 49: RR-10.
27. Ghosh S, Champlin R, Couch R, et al. Rhinovirus infections in myelosuppressed adult blood and marrow transplant recipients. Clin Infect Dis 1999; 29: 528–532.
28. Carrigan DR, Drobyski WR, Russler SK et al. Interstitial pneumonitis associated with human herpesvirus-6 infection after marrow transplantation. Lancet 1991; 338: 147.

Clinical relevance

■ A close working relationship needs to be developed between the respiratory physician and the virologist if results relevant to the individual patient are to be obtained.

■ No single diagnostic technique is applicable to all respiratory samples and methods such as immunofluorescence, microscopy and cell culture should be performed simultaneously.

■ As PCR technology becomes more generally available, this too will need to be performed alongside existing methods.

■ Technological advances have led to the recognition that viruses are involved in many more respiratory diseases than was formerly suspected.

References

1. Hsuing GDE. The impact of cell culture sensitivity on rapid viral diagnosis: an historical perspective. Yale J Biol Med 1989; 62: 79.
2. Gleaves CA, Smith TF, Shuster EA et al. Rapid detection of cytomegalovirus in MRC-5 cells inoculated with urine specimens by using low-speed centrifugation and monoclonal antibody to an early antigen. J Clin Microbiol 1984; 19: 917.
3. Gardner PS, McQuillin J. Rapid virus diagnosis: application of immunofluorescence, 2nd ed. London: Butterworths, 1980.
4. Rothbarth PH, Hermus M-C, Schrijnemakers P. Reliability of two new test kits for rapid diagnosis of respiratory syncytial virus infection. J Clin Microbiol 1991; 29: 824–826.
5. Chommel JJ, Remilleux MF, Marchand P, Aymard M. Rapid diagnosis of influenza A. Comparison with ELISA immunocapture and culture. J Virol Methods 1992; 37: 337.
6. Covalciuc KA, Webb KH, Carlson CA. Comparison of four clinical specimen types for detection of influenza A and B viruses by optical immunoassay (FLU OIA Test) and cell culture methods. J Clin Microbiol 1999; 37: 3971–3974.
7. Sarkkinen H. Respiratory viruses. In: Wreghitt TG, Morgan-Capner P, ed. ELISA in the clinical microbiology laboratory. London: Public Health Laboratory Service, 1990: 88.
8. Johnston SL, Sanderson G, Pattemore PK et al. Use of polymerase chain reaction for diagnosis of picornavirus infection in subjects with and without respiratory symptoms. J Clin Microbiol 1993; 31: 111–117.
9. Balfour-Lynn RIM, Valmon HB, Stanway G, Khan M. Use of polymerase chain reaction to detect rhinovirus in wheezy infants. Arch Dis Child 1992; 67: 760.

8.3 Cytopathology

Jennifer A Young

The main clinical application of cytopathology is the investigation of suspected primary or metastatic disease. Cytopathology however, also has a place in the assessment of patients with some benign conditions.

Collection and processing of specimens

A number of specimen collection techniques are available (Table 8.3.1), each appropriate to differing clinical situations and anatomical sites.[1]

Sputum

Three specimens of 'deep cough' sputum, preferably on three consecutive days, should be submitted.

Sputum expectorated following bronchoscopy is a valuable, often overlooked, source of diagnostic material. It is usually highly cellular, especially if brushing or biopsy has been under-

Table 8.3.1 Specimens for pulmonary cytopathology

- Sputum
  - Spontaneous
  - Induced
- Tracheal secretions
- Bronchoscopic specimens
  - Bronchial secretions
  - Bronchial brushings
  - Bronchial washings
  - Transbronchial fine-needle aspiration
  - Bronchoalveolar lavage
- Percutaneous fine-needle aspiration
- Pleural fluid
- Thoracic washings

taken, and is a means of harvesting residual cells from the lumen of the bronchus that would otherwise be lost for diagnostic purposes. Sputum should be collected into clean, dry containers with screw-on lids and transported in biohazard bags.

Induced sputum can be produced by inhalation of the vapours of a warmed (37°C) mixture of 15% sodium chloride and 20% propylene glycol for 20 min.

In the laboratory, the specimen is emptied into a Petri dish and any bloodstained or purulent areas are selectively sampled. A small blob is placed on a slide, squashed down with a second slide, spread out and immediately fixed in 95% ethyl alcohol before staining by the Papanicolaou method. Variations of technique include the Saccomanno system for pooled sputum[2,3] and formalin fixation of centrifuged cell blocks, which are then processed as histological specimens,[4] but neither method has found favour. Homogenisation with dithiothreitol appears, however, to convey some advantages both technically and in enhancement of sensitivity.[5]

Sputum examination is a non-invasive investigation that causes minimal inconvenience to the patient. Definitive evidence of malignancy and tumour typing are both possible, but localisation of the neoplasm is not. Furthermore, it is labour-intensive and many specimens are unsatisfactory as they consist merely of saliva or purulent mucus. Induced sputum is used mainly for the diagnosis of opportunistic infections, particularly *Pneumocystis carinii* pneumonia,[6] and the assessment of eosinophilia.[7] It confers no advantage in the diagnosis of carcinoma.[8] The ready availability of bronchoscopy and associated sampling techniques and the development of percutaneous fine-needle aspiration have reduced the use of sputum cytology.[9] However, it still remains a simple and often effective means of tumour typing in the patient with clinically advanced malignant disease who is unsuitable for surgery. Attempts at screening for detection of early lung cancer still use sputum cytology.[10]

Tracheal secretions

Tracheal secretions obtained by aspiration can be evaluated in neonates to assess the onset of bronchopulmonary dysplasia.[11]

Bronchoscopic techniques

With the exception of bronchoalveolar lavage, bronchoscopic sampling techniques are utilised almost exclusively for the investigation of suspected carcinoma. Guidance for the endoscopist is included in Chapter 10.

Bronchial secretions

Aspiration of secretions sometimes yields only degenerate cellular debris but may provide diagnostic material if brushing is difficult.

Bronchial brushing

This is the method of choice for the investigation of visible endobronchial lesions. More than one brushing is necessary in some cases, as the first specimen may sample only superficial necrotic debris. Each brush should be firmly rolled on to four to six slides and each smear placed immediately in 95% alcohol for rapid fixation.[1]

Bronchial washings

These are useful as a supplement to brushing or can be used to obtain cellular material when an endobronchial abnormality cannot be visualised. From 3–5 ml of fluid is recovered and it is then centrifuged to concentrate the cellular material.

Transbronchial fine-needle aspiration

This technique is suitable for the investigation of submucosal and peribronchial lesions, especially in the upper lobes where biopsy forceps may be difficult to manipulate. An important application is in staging, where transbronchial fine-needle aspiration facilitates investigation of hilar, subcarinal and paratracheal lymph nodes. The device most commonly used is the Wang needle.[12,13] Transbronchial fine-needle aspiration is technically demanding[14,15] and time-consuming but the complication rate is extremely low.[15,16]

Bronchoalveolar lavage

The main applications of bronchoalveolar lavage are the investigation of immunosuppressed patients with respiratory distress[17,18] and the monitoring of interstitial lung disease.[18] Bronchoalveolar lavage can also be used to retrieve diagnostic material from diffuse neoplasia or peripheral lung cancer.[19] The technique of bronchoalveolar lavage is described in Chapter 10.2.

When investigating pulmonary infiltrates in the immunosuppressed an aliquot of the fluid is sent for microbiology (including virology) and the remainder centrifuged and processed with a range of stains including Gram, Ziehl–Neelsen, Perls and Grocott, in addition to the routine cytological methods of Papanicolaou and May–Grünwald–Giemsa. Fluorescence microscopy, immunocytochemistry and polymerase chain reaction (PCR) of DNA may aid the identification of certain infections such as *Pneumocystis carinii*, herpes simplex virus and cytomegalovirus (see Chapter 8.2).[20]

In spite of initial enthusiasm, total cell counts on bronchoalveolar lavage fluid are of relatively little value in the management of interstitial lung disease but differential counts are helpful in diagnosis and in monitoring progress and response to therapy.[18-21] The cells are separated from the fluid by slow centrifugation and resuspended in tissue culture medium to a dilution of 2×10^6 cells/ml. From $100 \mu l$ aliquots of this suspension cytocentrifuge preparations are made, stained with May–Grünwald–Giemsa and 300–500 cells counted by the random field method.

Diagnosis of specific disease is occasionally possible by utilising special stains, for example, oil red O (for lipoid pneumonia), Perls (for past pulmonary haemorrhage and asbestos bodies), diastase–periodic-acid–Schiff (D-PAS; for alveolar proteinosis). If electron microscopy is required (for Langerhans cell histiocytosis, alveolar proteinosis) 25 ml of 5% glutaraldehyde in cacodylate buffer is added as a fixative to 25 ml bronchoalveolar lavage fluid. Additional descriptions of the processing of bronchoalveolar lavage for diagnosis and research are available.[21,22]

Percutaneous fine-needle aspiration

Percutaneous fine-needle aspiration of the lung is valuable for diagnosis and typing of localised primary and secondary tumours, particularly in patients in whom bronchoscopic investigative methods have proved non-diagnostic. The aspirate is obtained under fluoroscopic or computed tomography (CT) guidance[23] and should be collected from the edge rather than the centre of the lesion, which may be necrotic. The technique of percutaneous fine-needle aspiration is dealt with in Chapter 10.3.

Pleural fluid

About 50 ml fluid is required, which is best collected directly into a pot containing heparin/dextran mixture to prevent clotting. The fluid is centrifuged and smears are made from the deposit. Alternatively, fluid can be allowed to clot spontaneously in a dry clean container; the clot can then be removed with forceps and smeared on to slides and the remainder fixed and sectioned. Serial sections of blocks or multiple cytocentrifuge preparations can be used for immunocytochemistry and other special techniques.

Thoracic washings

Washings from the thoracic cavity obtained by instillation of 300 ml saline at the time of resection may give indication of advanced malignancy in patients without pleural effusion.[24]

Interpretation

Lung cancer

Examples of malignant cells are illustrated in Figures 8.3.1–8.3.3. Further guidance on microscopic interpretation can be found in more detailed texts.[25-28]

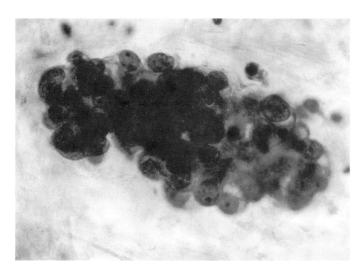

Fig. 8.3.1 Sputum: adenocarcinoma of lung. A large three-dimensional group of malignant cells with pleomorphic, hyperchromatic nuclei containing prominent nucleoli. Papanicolaou stain.

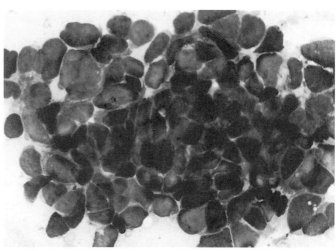

Fig. 8.3.3 Percutaneous fine-needle aspirate: small-cell carcinoma of lung. Small, anaplastic malignant cells with moulded nuclei, diffuse chromatin patterns and inconspicuous nucleoli. May–Grünwald–Giemsa stain.

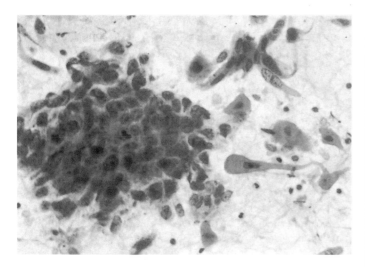

Fig. 8.3.2 Bronchial brushing: squamous-cell carcinoma of lung. Hyperkeratinised, orangeophilic, well-differentiated malignant squamous cells together with a large group of poorly differentiated cells. Papanicolaou stain.

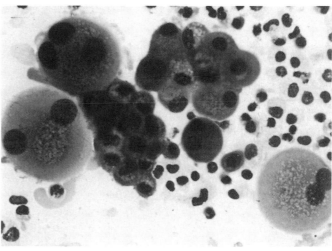

Fig. 8.3.4 Pleural fluid: mesothelioma. Two morula and large, single malignant mesothelial cells. May–Grünwald–Giemsa stain.

Sensitivity and specificity

In a review of *sputum cytology* from 1289 patients with proven lung cancer, sensitivity was 69% and specificity 96%.[29] Similar figures are reported from other large centres[30] but published figures do differ widely. Variation in the number of specimens examined partly contributes to this.[31-34] Bocking[4] gives a good review of results.

At bronchoscopy, maximum diagnostic yield is obtained by a combination of cytological sampling and biopsy.[35-36] The sensitivity of *bronchial brushing* in cases of visible endoscopic abnormality remains in the range 52–90%.[35-43] *Bronchial washings* are more often diagnostic than brushings or biopsy when no endoscopic lesion is visible. The sensitivity of *transbronchial fine-needle aspiration* ranges from 46% to 81%.[44,45] This technique may provide a diagnosis in lesions inaccessible by other sampling methods.[45]

The sensitivity of *percutaneous fine-needle aspiration* in published reports varies from 62% to 96.8%.[46-48] Johnston[49] found it to be the single most sensitive diagnostic technique. CT-guided percutaneous fine-needle aspiration in association with fluoride-18 fluorodeoxyglucose positron-emission tomography can yield a sensitivity of 100%.[50]

Tumour typing

Separation of tumours into small-cell and non-small-cell categories is generally straightforward with all types of cytological material. When more precise classification is considered, typing of well-differentiated keratinising squamous-cell carcinoma and small-cell carcinoma is readily achieved. Distinction between poorly differentiated squamous-cell carcinoma, poorly differentiated adenocarcinoma and large-cell carcinoma is more difficult, particularly on brushings and percutaneous fine-needle aspiration. When compared to post-mortem histological investigations, cytological typing of lung cancer has been reported as being 100% accurate for small-cell carcinoma, 90% for squamous cell carcinoma, 70% for adenocarcinoma and 50% for undifferentiated large-cell carcinoma.[51]

Benign lung disease

Several reviews of cytopathology in benign lung diseases are available.[14,25,26,52,53] Cytology can aid the recognition of specific infections, allergic disorders and industrial exposure.[7,20,54,55] The cytological appearance of many non-neoplastic conditions in percutaneous fine-needle aspiration material is non-specific but conditions such as granulomatous inflammation and hamartoma are sufficiently distinctive to permit an accurate diagnosis and the exclusion of carcinoma.[56,57]

Two major cell patterns, neutrophilic and lymphocytic, are found in bronchoalveolar lavage in interstitial lung disease. The first occurs in cryptogenic fibrosing alveolitis, collagen vascular disease and asbestosis, and the second in granulomatous conditions such as sarcoidosis and extrinsic allergic alveolitis.[21] In sarcoidosis the T-cell helper:suppressor ratio is raised, whereas it is low in extrinsic allergic alveolitis. Figures vary from centre to centre and each laboratory has to establish its own range of normal values (Table 8.3.2).[18]

The role of pulmonary cytopathology in investigating patients with acquired immunodeficiency syndrome (AIDS) is reviewed by Strigle[58] and its role in both AIDS and non-AIDS cases by Young.[17] Cytopathological examination is a very efficient method for diagnosis of *Pneumocystis carinii* pneumonia. The characteristic foamy alveolar casts can be rapidly identified on routine Papanicolaou-processed slides.[59,60] Confirmation by special techniques is possible but does not increase sensitivity,[54] which is 85–98%[54,59] with routine stains. This is superior to induced sputum but the latter is valuable when bronchoscopy is contraindicated.[6] Cytomorphological diagnosis of mycobacteria, certain viral infections (particularly cytomegalovirus) and fungal disease is also possible.[17,20,55] However, pulmonary infiltrates in the immunosuppressed arise from a number of causes and disease is often multifactorial. Problems of interpretation arise when malignancy coexists with infection, drug or radiation damage, graft-versus-host disease or diffuse alveolar damage.[61]

The application of special stains or electron microscopy to bronchoalveolar lavage fluid may be diagnostic in certain conditions. For example, foamy fat-filled macrophages are found in lipoid pneumonia,[62] haemosiderin-laden macrophages in occult pulmonary haemorrhage, periodic-acid–Schiff (PAS)-positive granular material in alveolar proteinosis and excess S100-positive Langerhans cells in Langerhans cell histiocytosis.[21] Electron microscopy shows that the granular material of alveolar proteinosis consists of osmiophilic lamellar bodies and can confirm the presence of Langerhans cells by demonstrating their characteristic Birbeck granules. If the electron microscope is equipped for elemental analysis the nature of any mineral particulates present can be identified.

Pleural effusion

Pleural transudates contain few cells, whereas exudates are usually hypercellular.[63] Neutrophils are most commonly encountered with acute infection, eosinophils with pneumothorax, and lymphocytes in chronic infections such as tuberculosis or immune processes such as rheumatoid disease. Mesothelial cell exfoliation is a common non-specific accompaniment of many pleural diseases. Malignant cells, both primary (mesothelioma) and metastatic (carcinoma, lymphoma), are not uncommon. Identification may be straightforward or require immunocytochemistry.

Unfortunately, there are no cytomorphological features that are both specific for malignant mesothelioma and present in all cases. Nevertheless certain features are diagnostically helpful.[63-66] The malignant cells often form knobbly morula (Fig. 8.3.4) with nuclei bulging from the surface. Single cells tend to be large, often with two or three nuclei, and have plentiful optically dense cytoplasm with occasional sharp-edged vacuoles. The cell borders may be hazy as a result of microvilli and cytoplasmic blebs are sometimes visible. The main diagnostic difficulties are in distinguishing well-differentiated tumours from reactive mesothelial proliferation, and poorly differentiated lesions from metastatic adenocarcinoma. Unequivocal positive staining of malignant cells with D-PAS excludes mesothelioma.

Immunocytochemistry also offers some assistance. Opinions vary as to 'the best panel'.[66,67] Anti-epithelial membrane antigen is the only antibody currently in use that is of any value in distinguishing benign from malignant mesothelial cells.[66,67] Mesothelioma is positive with calretinin, cytokeratin 5/6 and thrombomodulin and negative with Ber-EP4, CEA (monoclonal) and Leu MI.[66,67] However, positive staining may be patchy and,

Table 8.3.2 Bronchoalveolar lavage in interstitial lung diseases

Disease	Proportions of cells in lavage fluid
Cryptogenic fibrosing alveolitis	Neutrophils and eosinophils raised
Sarcoidosis	Lymphocytes and T-cell helper:suppressor ratio both raised
Extrinsic allergic alveolitis	Lymphocytes much raised; helper:suppressor ratio low; mast cells present
Langerhans cell histiocytosis	Langerhans cells raised
Normal values vary between laboratories. At the Brompton Hospital, London, the following normal values have been established: neutrophils ≤ 4%, eosinophils ≤ 3%, lymphocytes ≤ 14%, Langerhans cells ≤ 4% in smokers (generally absent in non-smokers), with macrophages constituting the bulk of the remainder.	

as always, lack of reproducible sensitivity means that interpretation of antibody panels requires a degree of caution.

E-cadherin has also been reported as useful in the detection of carcinoma cells in fluids.[68] Immunophenotyping by means of flow cytometry was investigated by Risberg et al[69] and, while this may enhance the detection of Ber-EP4-positive cells in fluids, the technique was found to be useless in assessing the role of N-cadherin in distinguishing mesothelial cells from adenocarcinoma cells.

With regard to identification of specific metastatic tumours, immunocytochemical staining for prostatic acid phosphatase, prostate-specific antigen, thyroglobulin, CA125 and panels of cytokeratins can all be performed on cytological preparations and first principles applicable to histology should be followed.

Clinical relevance

■ Non-invasive or minimally invasive

■ Low-risk

■ Repeatable

■ Rapid diagnosis and typing of lung tumours

■ Safe investigation of pulmonary infiltrates in the immunosuppressed

■ Management of diffuse lung disease

References

1. Young JA. Techniques in pulmonary cytopathology. ACP Broadsheet 140. J Clin Pathol 1993; 46: 589.
2. Risse EKJ, van't Hof MA, Laurini RN, Vooms PG. Sputum cytology by the Saccomanno method in diagnosing lung malignancy. Diagn Cytopathol 1985; 1: 286.
3. Perlman EJ, Erozan YS, Howdan AH. The role of the Saccomanno technique in sputum cytopathologic diagnosis of lung cancer. Am J Clin Pathol 1989; 91: 57.
4. Bocking A, Bresterfeld S, Chatelain R et al. Diagnosis of bronchial carcinoma on sections of paraffin-embedded sputum: sensitivity and specificity of an alternative to routine cytology. Acta Cytol 1992; 36: 38.
5. Tang C-S, Tang CMC, Lau Y-Y, Kung ITM. Sensitivity of sputum cytology after homogenization with dithiothreitol in lung cancer detection. Acta Cytol 1995; 39: 1137.
6. Carmichael A, Bateman N, Nayagam M. Examination of induced sputum in the diagnosis of Pneumocystis carinii pneumonia. Cytopathology 1991; 2: 61.
7. Wark PA, Gibson PG, Fakes K. Induced sputum eosinophils in the assessment of asthma and chronic cough. Respirology 2000; 5: 51–57.
8. Rogers TK, Lott M, Smith D, Catterall JR. Sputum induction in the cytological diagnosis of bronchogenic carcinoma. Thorax 1992; 47: 881.
9. Fraire AE, McLardy JW, Greenberg SD. Changing utilization of cytopathology versus histopathology in the diagnosis of lung cancer. Diagn Cytopathol 1991; 7: 359.
10. Kennedy TC, Miller Y, Prindiville S. Screening for lung cancer revisited and the role of sputum cytology and fluorescence bronchoscopy in a high-risk group. Chest 2000; 117(suppl 1): 725.
11. Rothberg AD, Miot A, Leman G. Tracheal aspirate cytology and bronchopulmonary dysplasia. Diagn Cytopathol 1986; 2: 212.
12. Wang KP, Marsh BR, Summer WR et al. Transbronchial needle aspiration in the diagnosis of lung cancer. Chest 1981; 80: 458.
13. Wagner ED, Ramzy I, Greenberg SD, Gonzalez JM. Transbronchial fine-needle aspiration. Am J Clin Pathol 1989; 92: 36.
14. Young JA. The lung, pleura and chest wall. In: Young JA, ed. Fine needle aspiration cytophathology. Oxford: Blackwell; 1993: 97.
15. Wang KP, Gupta PK, Haponik EF et al. Flexible transbronchial needle aspiration. Technical considerations. Ann Otol Rhinol Laryngol 1984; 93: 233.
16. Nguyen G-K, York EL, Jones RL, King EG. Transbronchial needle aspiration biopsy via the fiberoptic bronchoscope. Value and limitations in the cytodiagnosis of tumors and tumor-like lesions of the long. Pathol Annu Part 1, 1992; 27: 105.
17. Young JA. Cytological investigation of immune suppressed patients In: Gray W, ed. Diagnostic cytopathology. Edinburgh: Churchill Livingstone; 1995: 543.
18. Stanley MW, Henry MJ, Stanley MJ, Iber C. Bronchoalveolar lavage, cytology and clinical applications. Tokyo: Igahu-Shoin; 1991.
19. DeGracia J, Bravo C, Miravitlles M et al. Diagnostic value of broncho-alveolar lavage in peripheral lung cancer. Am Rev Respir Dis 1993; 147: 649–652.
20. Bewig B, Haacke TC, Tirake A et al. Detection of CMV pneumonitis after lung transplantation using PCR of DNA from bronchoalveolar cells. Respiration 2000; 67: 2, 166.
21. Turner-Warwick M, Haslam PL. Clinical application in bronchoalveolar lavage. Clin Chest Med 1987; 8: 15.
22. Walters EH, Gardiner PV. Bronchoalveolar lavage as a research tool. Thorax 1991; 46: 613.
23. Gouliames A, Giannopoules DH, Panagi GM et al. Computed tomography-guided fine needle aspiration of peripheral lung opacities. Acta Cytol 2000; 44: 344.
24. Vinette-Leduc D, Yazdi H, Valgi A et al;. Pre and post thoracic washings in non-small cell carcinoma of the lung: a cytological study of 44 patients without pleural effusion. Diagn Cytopathol 2000; 22: 218.
25. Young JA. Colour atlas of pulmonary cytology. London: Harvey Miller; 1985.
26. Gray W. Normal respiratory tract and inflammatory conditions. In: Gray W, ed. Diagnostic cytopathology. Edinburgh: Churchill Livingstone; 1995: 13.
27. Sterret G, Frost F, Whitaker D. Tumours of lung and mediastinum. In: Gray W, ed. Diagnostic Cytopathology. Edinburgh: Churchill Livingstone 1995: 69.
28. Young JA. Cytopathology. In: Haselton PS, ed. Spencer's Pathology of lung. New York: McGraw-Hill; 1996: 1221.
29. Kern WH. The diagnostic accuracy of sputum and urine cytology. Acta Cytol 1988; 32: 651.
30. Piletti S, Rilke F, Gribaudi G. Sputum cytology for the diagnosis of carcinoma of the lung. Acta Cytol 1982; 26: 649.
31. Clee MD, Sinclair DJM. Assessment of factors influencing the results of sputum cytology of bronchial carcinoma. Thorax 1981; 36: 143.
32. Jay SJ, Wehr K, Nicholson DP, Smith AL. Diagnostic sensitivity and specificity of pulmonary cytology. Acta Cytol 1980; 24: 304.
33. Frost JK, Ball WC, Levin ML et al. Early lung cancer detection: results of the initial (prevalence) radiologic and cytologic screening in the Johns Hopkins study. Am Rev Respir Dis 1984; 130: 549.
34. Johnston WW. Ten years of respiratory cytopathology at DUMC, I. The cytopathologic diagnosis of lung cancer during the year 1970 to 1974 noting the significance of specimen number and type. Acta Cytol 1981; 25: 103.
35. Mak VHF, Johnston IDA, Heizel MR, Grubb C. Value of washings and brushings at fiberoptic bronchoscopy in the diagnosis of lung cancer. Thorax 1990; 45: 373.
36. Nargshkin S, Daniels J, Young NA. Diagnostic correlation of fiberoptic bronchoscopic biopsy and bronchoscopic cytology performed simultaneously. Diagn Cytopathol 1992; 8: 120.
37. Zavala DC. Diagnostic fiberoptic bronchoscopy: techniques and results of biopsy in 600 patients. Chest 1975; 68: 12.
38. Kvale PA, Bode FR, Kini S. Diagnostic accuracy in lung cancer. Comparison of techniques used in association with flexible fiberoptic bronchoscopy. Chest 1976; 69: 752.
39. Chopra SK, Genovesi MG, Simmons DH, Gothe B. Fiberoptic bronchoscopy in the diagnosis of lung cancer. Comparison of pre- and post-bronchoscopy, sputa, washings, brushings and biopsies. Acta Cytol 1977; 21: 524.
40. Lyall JRW, Summers GD, O'Brien INO et al. Sequential brush biopsy and conventional biopsy: direct comparison of diagnostic sensitivity in lung malignancy. Thorax 1980; 35: 929.
41. Muers MF, Boddington MM, Cole M et al. Cytological sampling at fibreoptic bronchoscopy: comparison of catheter aspirates and brush biopsies. Thorax 1982; 37: 457.
42. Matsuda M, Horai T, Nakamura S et al. Bronchial brushing and bronchial biopsy: comparison of diagnostic accuracy and cell typing in lung cancer. Thorax 1986; 41: 475.
43. Baaklini WA, Reinosa MA, Gorin AB et al. Diagnostic yield of fiberoptic bronchoscopy in evaluating solitary pulmonary nodules. Chest 2000; 117: 1049.
44. Horsley JR, Miller RE, Amy RW, King EC. Bronchial submucosal needle aspiration performed through the fiberoptic bronchoscope. Acta Cytol 1984; 28: 211.
45. Harrow EM, Oldenburg FA, Smith AM. Transbronchial needle aspiration in clinical practice. Thorax 1985; 40: 756.

46. Payne CR, Hadfield JW, Stouin PG et al. Diagnostic accuracy of cytology and biopsy in primary bronchial carcinoma. J Clin Pathol 1981; 34: 773.

47. Yazdi HM, MacDonald LL, Hickey NM. Thoracic fine needle aspiration biopsy versus fine needle cutting biopsy. Acta Cytol 1988; 32: 635.

48. Young CP, Young I, Cowan DF, Blei RL. The reliability of fine needle aspiration biopsy in the diagnosis of deep lesions of the lung and mediastinum: experience with 50 cases using a modified technique. Diagn Cytopathol 1987; 3: 1.

49. Johnston WW. Fine needle aspiration biopsy versus sputum and bronchial material in the diagnosis of lung cancer. Acta Cytol 1988; 32: 641.

50. Collins BT, Lowe VJ, Dunphy FR. Initial evaluation of pulmonary abnormalities : CT-guided fine needle aspiration and fluoride-18 fluorodeoxyglucose position emission tomography correlation. Diagn Cytopathol 2000: 22: 92

51. Di Bonito L, Colauti I, Patriavaca S et al. Cytological typing of primary lung cancer: a study of 100 cases with autopsy confirmation. Diagn Cytopathol 1991; 7: 7.

52. Bedrossian CWM, Acetta PA, Kelly LV. Cytopathology of non-neoplastic pulmonary disease. Lab Med 1983; 14: 86.

53. Rosenthal DL. Cytology in the diagnosis of benign lung diseases. In: Shure D, ed. Clinics in chest medicine. Philadelphia, PA: WB Saunders; 1987: 147.

54. Armbruster C, Pokieser L, Hassl A. Diagnosis of *Pneumocystis carinii* pneumonia by bronchoalveolar lavage in AIDS patients. Acta Cytol 1995; 39: 1089.

55. Lemos LB, Baliga M, Taylor BD et al. Bronchoalveolar lavage for diagnosis of fungal disease. Acta Cytol 1995; 39: 1101.

56. Orell SR, Sterrett GF, Walters M N-I et al. Lung, chest wall and pleura. In: Fine Needle Aspiration Cytology. Edinburgh: Churchill Livingstone; 1999: 202.

57. Dubar F, Leiman G. The aspiration cytology of pulmonary hamartomas. Diagn Cytopathol 1989; 5: 174.

58. Strigle SM, Gal AA. A review of pulmonary cytopathology in the acquired immunodeficiency syndrome. Acta Cytol 1985; 29: 1047.

59. Young JA, Hopkin JM, Cuthbertson WP. Pulmonary infiltrates in immunocompromised patients: diagnosis by cytological examination of bronchoalveolar lavage fluid. J Clin Pathol 1984; 37: 390.

60. Bedrossian CWM, Mason MR, Gupta PK. Rapid cytological diagnosis of *Pneumocystis*: a comparison of effective techniques. Semin Diagn Pathol 1989: 6: 245.

61. Beskow CO, Drachenberg CB, Bourquin PM et al. Diffuse alveolar damage: morphologic features in bronchoalveolar lavage fluid. Acta Cytol 2000; 44: 640.

62. Yang YJ, Steele CT, Anbar RD et al. Quantitation of lipid-laden macrophages in evaluation of lower airway cytology specimens from pediatric patients. Diagn Cytopathol 2001; 24: 98

63. Spriggs AI, Bedding MM. Atlas of serous fluid cytopathology. Dordrecht: Kluwer Academic; 1989.

64. Whitaker D, Shilkin KB. Diagnosis of pleural malignant mesothelioma in life – a practical approach. J Pathol 1984; 143: 147.

65. DiBonito L, Falconieri G, Colault I et al. Cytopathology of malignant mesothelioma: a study of its patterns and histological bases. Diagn Cytopathol 1993; 9: 26.

66. Whitaker D. The cytology of malignant mesothelioma. Cytopathology 2000; 11: 139.

67. Dejmek A. Hjerpe A. Reactivity of six antibodies in effusions of mesothelioma, adenocarcinoma and mesotheliosis: stepwise logistic regression analysis. Cytopathology 2000; 11: 8.

68. Schofield K, D'Aquila T, Rimm DL. E-cadherin expression is a sensitive and specific method for detection of carcinoma cells in fluid specimens. Diagn Cytopathol 2000; 22: 263

69. Risberg B, Davidson B, Dong HP et al. Flow cytometric immunophenotyping of serous effusions and peritoneal washings: comparison with immunocytochemistry and morphological findings. J Clin Pathol 2000; 53: 513–517.

8 Laboratory methods

8.4 Histopathology methods

Richard L Attanoos and Allen R Gibbs

To a large extent the methods used for handling and examination of lung specimens are determined by the type of disease present but in all cases the benefits of close liaison between pathologist, radiologist and clinicians cannot be overemphasised. It is incumbent upon the clinician to inform the pathologist if there is any possibility of the specimen being infectious. Specimens suspected clinically of harbouring infection, particularly tuberculosis, should be submitted unfixed for culture, following which they should be immersed in formaldehyde for 72 hours prior to processing for histopathology. Frozen section should be performed only if deemed absolutely necessary as it poses a risk of infection to laboratory staff. Formaldehyde vapour poses a further health risk to laboratory personnel. The permitted limit of airborne formaldehyde concentration (as outlined by UK government regulations) may be exceeded when copious quantities are used to inflate lung resections. To avoid this, a well-ventilated area, or ideally a dedicated cabinet with extractor fan, should be used. Furthermore, adequate protective clothing, masks and visors are mandatory, in line with the Control of Substances Hazardous to Health (COSHH) and the Reporting of Injuries Diseases and Dangerous Occurrences (RIDDOR) regulations.

Types of specimen

Percutaneous needle and Tru-Cut biopsy specimens

The indication for both these types of biopsy specimen is to identify the nature of suspicious peripheral lung, mediastinal or pleural lesions.[1,2] Less frequently, they are used in the diagnosis of benign neoplasms[3] and non-neoplastic lesions.[4] Macroscopic examination is of limited value. Biopsy size is determined by the biopsy instrument and ranges from 1–2 mm (for needle biopsies) to 10–15 mm tissue cores. At the outset, sections 4–5 μm thick are stained with haematoxylin and eosin, and a number of reserve unstained sections mounted on agar/silane-coated slides should be prepared for possible immunohistochemistry or such other investigations as may be deemed necessary once the initial sections have been evaluated (see Ancillary studies, below).

Bronchial biopsy specimens

The main indication for endobronchial biopsy is the diagnosis of bronchogenic neoplasia[5] but transbronchial biopsy is also usually undertaken as a first-line approach in the investigation of diffuse lung disease and peribronchial infiltrates, the assessment of infection in immunosuppressed patients and, following transplantation, to identify graft rejection.[6–9]

Endobronchial and transbronchial biopsies seldom exceed 3 mm in diameter but diagnostic yield increases with multiple biopsies.[7] In general, the endoscopist should place all specimens for histological examination directly into buffered formalin. If bacterial, mycobacterial, viral or fungal cultures are deemed important, specimens should be sent directly to the corresponding laboratory by the clinician. It is important to document the size and number of fragments sampled so that all are individually examined histologically. Endoscopic biopsies can be sectioned in one of two ways:

- for anticipated neoplastic infiltrates, 4–5 μm sections stained with haematoxylin and eosin are cut at 40 μm intervals, with multiple unstained sections mounted on agar/silane-coated slides suitable for immunohistochemistry
- for post-transplantation transbronchial biopsies, sampling of multiple levels throughout the tissue (complete sampling) is preferred to identify small isolated lesions. Additional stains may he employed according to the initial findings.

Open lung biopsy specimens

Open lung biopsy is the procedure of choice in the diagnosis and assessment of disease activity of diffuse lung disease. In certain patients it also has an important role in the management of solitary peripheral lesions.[10,11]

Biopsy size varies from 2 cm upwards. The tissue to be excised should be handled gently to prevent crushing, haemorrhage and polymorph infiltration. The pathologist should receive the tissue fresh. A frozen-section diagnosis may facilitate both patient management and the prioritisation of additional analyses. For optimal pathological assessment, the metal-stapled line should be excised and the remaining tissue should be gently inflated with formaldehyde using a fine-calibre needle until the pleura is uniformly smooth. The specimen is then left immersed in formaldehyde for 24 hours.[12] This facilitates histological assessment of the distribution of lesions within the lung lobule, which is important in the diagnosis of non-neoplastic pulmonary conditions. Following fixation the biopsy is sectioned into 3–4 mm slices prior to processing. Routine 5 μm sections are cut

and stained with haematoxylin and eosin. Additional stains are commonly performed (Tables 8.4.1 & 8.4.2). In addition, 20 μm unstained sections can be used to assist in the identification of asbestos bodies. Mineral analysis necessitating tissue digestion/incineration can be performed but because of small tissue size it may yield non-representative fibre burden results. This analysis is inappropriate for small biopsies.

Segmental, lobectomy and pneumonectomy specimens

These specimens should be inflated with formaldehyde using a tube or catheter inserted into the lumen of the bronchial resec-

Table 8.4.1   Ancillary techniques in histopathology: histochemistry

Histochemical stain	Indication
Periodic-acid–Schiff (PAS) for glycogen	Fungi, clear cell tumours
PAS with diastase pre-treatment (neutral mucin)	Alveolar lipoproteinosis, adenocarcinoma
Alcian blue pH 2.5 (acid mucin)	Mesothelioma
Combined Alcian blue/diastase PAS (basement membrane/neutral mucin)	Adenoid cystic carcinoma
Grocott	Fungi
Ziehl–Neelsen	*Mycobacteria* spp.
Elastic van Gieson (collagen)	Fibrosis
(elastin)	Vasculature
Reticulin	Architecture/collagen type IV
Toluidine blue/Giemsa	Mast cells
Congo red	Amyloid
Perls Prussian blue (iron)	Pulmonary haemorrhage,
Ferruginous bodies	
Grimelius	Neuroendocrine differentiation

Table 8.4.2   Ancillary techniques in histopathology: immunohistochemistry

Indication	Immunohistochemical marker
Undifferentiated malignancy	
Carcinoma	Cytokeratin (AEI/AE3; CAM 5.2)
Melanoma	S100; HMB-45
Lymphoma	CD45
Sarcoma	Vimentin; actin
Primary bronchogenic carcinoma	Thyroid transcription factor-1 (TTF-1)[*25]
Carcinoma	Carcinoembryonic antigen, Ber EP4, Leu-M1
Neuroendocrine tumours	Chromogranin A, synaptophysin, CD56
Mesothelioma[30,31]	Pancytokeratin, calretinin, cytokeratin 5/6, thrombomodulin

* TTF-1, expressed only by primary bronchogenic and thyroid cancers, is useful in determining whether a thoracic neoplasm is primary pulmonary or metastatic (when used in conjunction with thyroglobulin, which labels thyroid cancers only). TTF-1 is expressed particularly by adenocarcinomas and large and small cell neuroendocrine carcinomas but infrequently by squamous cell carcinomas.

tion margin and connected to a container of fixative at a pressure of 25–30 mmH₂O. The lung should be inflated until the pleura is smooth and then left immersed in formaldehyde for 24 hours. In practice, however, the specimen is often partly dissected before fixation for special procedures and in these circumstances inflation may be difficult. After fixation the whole specimen is sliced sagittally perpendicular to the hilum. For tumours, the bronchi are then opened but in non-neoplastic conditions further parallel sagittal slicing is undertaken at 1–2 cm intervals.

Examination of specimens containing neoplasms[13]

The pathologist has a central role in determining the stage of a lung tumour, and the information required for this largely determines the selection and orientation of tissue blocks. The most widely used staging system for lung tumours is that developed and refined by the American Joint Committee for Cancer Staging.[14,15] This system is based on the size and location of the primary tumour (T), the lymph node state (N) and the presence of metastases (M), and is often referred to as the TNM system.

Accurate TNM staging requires the following information:

- **Tumour size**. The pathologist can accurately assess the size of a tumour in composite tissue sections. For central tumours, the bronchus it arises from or, for peripheral tumours, the segment should be specified. For polypoid tumours the point of attachment of the stalk to the bronchus indicates the origin. At least one block should be taken perpendicular to the bronchial wall to assess the depth of invasion.
- **The distance of the tumour from the carina** should be stated by the surgeon. For central tumours the pathologist should measure the distance from the proximal bronchial resection edge. A transverse block of the proximal bronchial resection edge should be taken to check microscopically for the presence of tumour there. The bronchial mucosa should also be carefully inspected for roughness or loss of the normal bronchial ridges and blocks taken of any suspicious foci, as these may show in-situ malignancy, which is important clinically if it extends near to the proximal bronchial resection edge.
- **Visceral pleural involvement by tumour**. The distance of the tumour from the visceral pleural surface should be measured and if the tumour extends close to the pleura a block should be taken to include both the pleura and the nearest part of the tumour. If there is uncertainty about pleural invasion an elastic van Gieson stain can be useful in demonstrating disruption of the elastic layer.[16]
- **The presence of a malignant pleural effusion** may be known from previous pleural aspirates or determined concurrently with the main resection from fluid obtained by the surgeon at thoracotomy. A cytologically proven malignant effusion results in a T4 tumour designation.
- **Background lung**. At least one section of apparently non-tumorous lung should be examined for occult tumour spread,

the presence and extent of any atelectasis, obstructive pneumonitis, interstitial fibrosis and pneumoconiosis.
- **Lymph node involvement**. The correlation between lymph node size and tumour involvement is poor and therefore formal histological examination, sometimes assisted by immunohistochemistry, is important. Any lymph nodes in the resection specimen such as hilar, lobar, interlobar or segmental (all N1) should be separately identified and blocked.[17] Usually the surgeon will submit separately identified N2 (ipsilateral mediastinal and subcarinal lymph nodes) and N3 (contralateral, mediastinal and hilar lymph nodes and ipsilateral or contralateral scalene or supraclavicular lymph nodes) and the pathologist should examine these separately for neoplastic disease.

Histological typing

Lung tumour classification is based on the World Health Organization (WHO) system.[18] Diagnosis is extensively based on morphological interpretation and identification of specific differentiation patterns. Adjunct studies (see below) such as immunohistochemistry, electron microscopy and molecular genetic analyses (e.g. fluorescent in-situ hybridisation) can assist in pathological diagnosis but as yet some of these techniques are not widely available.

Examination of specimens containing non-neoplastic lesions[13]

The purpose of examining these specimens, whether necropsy or surgical, is to render a diagnosis or assess severity of the disease, or both. The pleura should first be examined for colour, thickness, exudate and any focal lesions such as pleural plaques. The hilar nodes can also be examined at this point and the size, colour, shape and consistency and distribution of such lesions should be recorded. Further sagittal slices of the specimen are then taken at 1–2 cm intervals. Tissue blocks should be taken of abnormal- and normal-looking lung: in some diseases the diagnostic lesions are present in the less severely affected parts of the lung.

Occupational lung disorders

With whole lungs, e.g. post mortem, it is good practice to keep intact one well-inflated whole lung slice for this examination and to take blocks from the other slices. As a *minimum* we recommend that four routine blocks should be taken:

- apex of upper lobe
- apex of lower lobe
- basal segments
- major bronchus to include nodes.

Other blocks should be taken from macroscopically visible lesions. Some of the blocks should include pleura.

Interstitial fibrosis may be recognised if it is severe and the pattern and degree of pulmonary fibrosis can be enhanced by the barium sulphate impregnation technique. The final estimate of severity of pulmonary fibrosis is best done by grading of histological sections taken in a systematic manner, similar to that used for asbestosis.[19]

Several different systems have been developed for quantifying emphysema macroscopically.[20] The method we use, described elsewhere,[21] is quick and convenient and is as accurate as point counting. It can then be used for lungs with or without pneumoconiotic lesions. The average severity in affected lobules is graded on a 0–3 scale, as is the proportion of lobules affected, similar to the assessment of dust lesions.

Frozen-section diagnosis in pulmonary pathology

Frozen sections may be requested for the following purposes:

- assessment of neoplasia
- mediastinal lymph node evaluation in staging
- assessment of lung, bronchial and pleural resection margin clearance
- diagnosis of mesothelial proliferations.

Ancillary studies in histopathology

A wide range of specialised analyses are available that facilitate accurate histopathological diagnosis or, as in the case of industrial disease, causation.

Histochemistry

Histochemistry (see Table 8.4.1) is the most widely available, technically simple and cost-effective ancillary technique in histopathology but in tumour pathology it has been largely replaced by immunohistochemistry.

Immunohistochemistry[22]

Immunohistochemistry (see Table 8.4.2), using either monoclonal or polyclonal antibodies, has application in the following areas:

- tumour differentiation
- prognosis
- identification of infectious agents.

Electron microscopy[23]

Ultrastructural studies are useful in the diagnosis of undifferentiated (anaplastic) neoplasms where tinctorial stains and immunohistochemistry have not been helpful. Identification of various structures such as prekeratin (squamous cell carcinoma), mucin microdroplets, short microvilli with 'fuzzy' glycocalyx (adenocarcinoma), neurosecretory granules (neuroendocrine tumours), melanosomes (melanoma), tight-junctions, long microvilli (mesothelioma), Weibel–Palade bodies (vascular neoplasms) and Birbeck granules (Langerhans cell histiocytosis) may facilitate diagnosis. In infectious diseases, virions, bacteria, fungi and protozoa can be identified by this method. For optimal results appropriate tissue should be cut without delay and without exerting pressure into $1\,mm^3$ fragments and fixed in glutaraldehyde with postfixation in osmium tetroxide.

Electron microscopy is a costly and relatively slow method necessitating access to specialist equipment and interpretive expertise that are not widely available.

Molecular genetic analyses

The techniques in common use are:

- in-situ hybridisation (ISH)
- polymerase chain reaction (PCR)
- interphase cytogenetics
- fluorescent in-situ hybridisation (FISH).

Other techniques, such as comparative genomic hybridisation (CGH) and microarray/'chip' analysis, may prove useful and have diagnostic application in the future.

In-situ hybridisation and PCR are used in the diagnosis of lymphoproliferative disorders. ISH can be used to show light-chain (kappa; lambda) monotypia in B-cell proliferations and PCR can demonstrate clonality in B- and T-cell lymphoid disorders and assist in the designation of lymphoid infiltrates as benign or malignant. Interphase cytogenetics in lung tumours has limited utility in diagnostic application. Fresh tissue needs to be immediately immersed in cytogenetic medium prior to culture. FISH also requires fresh tissue and at present has application only in haematopathology (leukaemia/lymphoma) and soft-tissue tumour pathology.

Mineral analysis[24]

Mineral analysis of lung tissue may detect either fibrous or nonfibrous inorganic materials. Mineral analysis of lung tissue can be used to:

- verify or refute a claimed exposure
- determine the source of the exposure
- correlate mineral content with pathology (e.g. fibrosis, tumour).

A comparison of light microscopic and electron microscopic techniques of mineral analysis is shown in Table 8.4.3.

Table 8.4.3 A comparison of mineral analytical techniques

Method	Advantage	Disadvantage
Light microscopy		
Asbestos body counts on routine (5 µm) or thick (20 µm) slides	Easy, inexpensive Specialised equipment not required Allows confirmation of asbestos exposure and a rough assessment of asbestos load	No reliable quantification of ferruginous bodies or fibres
Phase contrast light microscopy of tissue digests	Fairly easy, inexpensive Specialised equipment not required Data on coated/uncoated fibres Allows for comparisons with normal and asbestos-related diseases	No fibre typing possible Fibres < 0.3 µm diameter not seen
Electron microscopy ± energy-dispersive X-ray spectrometry		
Scanning/transmission electron microscopy	Provides qualitative and quantitative data More accurately quantify fibre burden (SEM < TEM, very thin fibres not detected) Non-fibrous minerals can be determined, e.g. silicates, hard metal constituents	Expensive, time-consuming Atomic weight < 11 undetected
X-ray diffraction	Sensitive and specific Has particular application in the identification of sheet silicates – talc, mica, kaolin	Mixed particles problematic

SEM, scanning electron microscopy; TEM, transmission electron microscopy.

References

1. Harrison BDW, Thorpe RS, Kitchener PG et al. Percutaneous Tru-Cut lung biopsy in the diagnosis of localised pulmonary lesions. Thorax 1984; 39: 493.
2. Tomlinson JR, Sahn SA. Invasive procedures in the diagnosis of pleural disease. Semin Respir Med 1987; 9: 30.
3. Dunbar F, Leiman G. The aspiration cytology of pulmonary hamartomas. Diagn Cytopathol 1989; 5: 174.
4. Wallace JM, Batra P, Gong H Jr et al. Percutaneous needle lung aspiration for diagnosing pneumonitis in the patient with acquired immunodeficiency syndrome (AIDS). Am Rev Respir Dis 1985; 131: 389.
5. Sheppard MN. Bronchial biopsy and its applications. In: Sheppard MN, ed. Practical pulmonary pathology. London: Edward Arnold; 1995: 19.
6. Sheppard MN, Nicholson A. The role of transbronchial and open lung biopsies in non-neoplastic lung disease. In: Kirkham N, Lemoine NR, ed. Progress in pathology 2. Edinburgh: Churchill Livingstone; 1995: 13.
7. Fechner RE, Greenburg SD, Wilson RK. Evaluation of transbronchial biopsy of the lung. Am J Clin Pathol 1977; 68: 17.
8. Haponik EF, Summer WR, Terry PB et al. Clinical decision making with transbronchial biopsy. Am Rev Respir Dis 1981; 123: 280.
9. Wall CP, Gaensler EA, Carrington CP et al. Comparison of transbronchial and open lung biopsies in chronic infiltrative lung disease. Am Rev Respir Dis 1981; 123: 280.
10. Burt ME, Flye W, Webber BL et al. Prospective evaluation of aspiration needle, cutting needle, transbronchial and open lung biopsy in patients with pulmonary infiltrates. Ann Thorac Surg 1981; 32: 146.
11. Sattersfield JR, McLaughlin JS. Open lung biopsy in diagnosing pulmonary infiltrates in immunosuppressed patients. Ann Thorac Surg 1979; 28: 359.
12. Churg A. A procedure for inflation of open lung biopsies. Am J Surg Pathol 1983; 7: 69.
13. Gibbs AR, Attanoos RL. ACP good practice guidelines – examination of lung specimens. J Clin Pathol 2000; 53: 507.
14. Mountain CF. Revisions in the international system for staging lung cancer. Chest 1997; 111: 1710.
15. Sobin LH, Wittekind C, ed. International Union Against Cancer TNM classification of malignant tumours, 5th ed. New York: John Wiley; 1997: 91.
16. Gallagher B, Urbanski SJ. The significance of pleural elastica invasion by lung carcinomas. Hum Pathol 1990; 21: 512.
17. Mountain CF, Dresler CM. Regional lymph node classification for lung cancer staging. Chest 1997; 111: 1718.
18. World Health Organization. Histological typing of lung tumours. In: International histological classification of tumours, 3rd ed, vol 1. Geneva: World Health Organization; 1999.
19. Craighead JE, Abraham IL, Churg A et al. The pathology of asbestos associated diseases of the lungs and pleural cavities: diagnostic criteria and proposed grading scheme. Arch Pathol Lab Med 1982; 106: 542.
20. Thurlbeck WM, Horowitz I, Siemiatycki J et al. Intra- and interobserver variations in the assessment of emphysema. Arch Environ Health 1969; 18: 644.
21. Lyons JP, Ryder RC, Seal RME et al. Emphysema in smoking and non-smoking coal workers with pneumoconiosis. Bull Eur Physiopathol Respir 1981; 17: 75.
22. Attanoos RL, Gibbs AR. Pathology of malignant mesothelioma. Histopathology 1997: 30: 403.
23. Henderson DW, Papadimitriou JM, Coleman M. Ultrastructural appearances of tumours: diagnosis and classification of human neoplasia by electron microscopy, 2nd ed. New York: Churchill Livingstone; 1986.
24. Gibbs AR, Pooley FD. Analysis and interpretation of inorganic mineral particles in 'lung' tissues. Thorax 1996; 51: 327.
25. Bejarono PA, Baughman RP, Biddinger PW et al. Surfactant proteins and thyroid transcription factor-1 in pulmonary and breast carcinoma. Mod Pathol 1996: 9; 445.

9 Non-invasive assessment of inflammation

Andrew M Zurek, Peter J Sterk and Rutko Djukanović

 Key points

- Non-invasive techniques enable assessment of inflammation in a wide range of respiratory diseases by collection of biological samples safely, quickly and repeatedly.

- Inflammation can be measured locally by means of sputum induction and analysis of exhaled gases and breath condensates or systemically by measuring mediators in blood and urine.

- Although there are differences in the methodology used by different groups, a consensus is being reached on standardisation and validation of the various sampling techniques.

- Use of non-invasive methodology has greatly increased the understanding of the pathophysiology of a number of inflammatory conditions, in particular asthma.

- It is hoped that large randomised controlled studies will identify the clinical role of measuring non-invasive inflammatory mediators in respiratory disease.

Historically, the understanding of pathological processes occurring in diseases affecting the respiratory system was largely based on tissue obtained from autopsy. The advent of flexible bronchoscopy, performed without the need of a general anaesthetic, allowed sampling of both the airways and, more recently, the distal portions of the lung. Importantly, this procedure could be performed on both affected patients and normal controls, providing valuable insight into the pathology of airways diseases. However, bronchoscopy is a relatively invasive means of obtaining biological samples. Recognition that inflammation is an important feature in the diagnosis and monitoring of many respiratory diseases has led to the development of less invasive techniques measuring lung inflammation directly or indirectly.

Key features of non-invasive techniques

The ideal non-invasive marker of inflammatory processes should possess the following attributes:

- **safety** – in particular allowing more severe or acutely ill individuals to be studied
- **subject acceptability and tolerability** – fewer individuals should object to non-invasive sampling techniques compared to more invasive ones
- **repeat sampling** – there should be few restrictions on how frequently non-invasive sampling can be performed in any given individual, allowing more detailed measurement of inflammation either during an acute episode or in monitoring a chronic condition over a long time period
- **standardisation and repeatability** – the method should be validated and standardised to allow comparisons between studies and to be valuable in follow up; in addition, the readouts should be repeatable
- **resource issues** – non-invasive sampling should require less expensive equipment, fewer staff, less time and can be performed in the field, enabling larger and more diverse studies to be undertaken.

Utility of non-invasive inflammatory markers

It is envisaged that non-invasive inflammatory markers will:

- aid in confirming or excluding diagnoses in respiratory diseases
- monitor disease activity
- monitor treatment efficacy
- monitor the effects of environmental and occupational pollutants
- provide prospective prognostic information.

Overview of non-invasive techniques studied to date

Non-invasive techniques currently available enable the measurement of inflammatory indices (cells, soluble or secretory compounds and volatile gases) as surrogate markers of inflammatory processes. To date a number of techniques have been developed, although some have been used more widely than others. These can broadly be divided into local measurements (induced sputum and analysis of exhaled air, measuring either gases or condensates containing soluble mediators) and systemic methods, which assess inflammation by studying products spilling over into the blood or measuring mediators or their metabolites excreted into urine. Non-invasive inflammatory markers have been studied most extensively in asthma, followed by other diseases causing airway inflammation. There has been considerably less research into their use in diseases affecting the lung parenchyma.

Validation of non-invasive techniques requires knowledge of marker levels in healthy control subjects, the demonstration of a relationship with disease severity, responsiveness to factors that are associated with disease deterioration, responsiveness to treatment and variation of the marker within individuals over time. Where applicable, non-invasive markers should be compared with similar inflammatory indices obtained by other means, e.g. airway inflammation measured by induced sputum versus bronchoscopy. Standardised methodology should exist in both the sampling technique and subsequent measurement of the inflammatory marker and adequate quality control overseeing these processes should be in place.

Induced sputum

Background

Microscopic examination of spontaneously expectorated sputum has for a long time been an important diagnostic tool in the management of respiratory infections. Several decades ago, it was reported as being able to predict responsiveness to corticosteroids in patients with obstructive airways disease.[1] Sputum induction by means of inhalation of hypertonic saline was developed to overcome the limitations of relying on spontaneously produced sputum. It has been used widely as an alternative to bronchoscopic washings to obtain samples of airway secretions in human immunodeficiency virus (HIV)-infected patients with suspected *Pneumocystis carinii* pneumonia.[2] The recognition that differences exist in the cellular composition of sputum produced by people with asthma or chronic bronchitis compared with controls suggested that examination of sputum could provide additional information about various inflammatory disorders of the airways.[3] By using sputum induction, samples could reliably be obtained in a standardised way, enabling accurate studies to be undertaken.[4,5] The procedure has also been successfully employed in asthmatic children above the age of 7.[6]

Sputum composition

Sputum is composed of cells suspended in mucin, a gelatinous substance secreted by submucosal glands comprising glycoproteins held together by disulphide bonds.[7,8] In normal individuals the most common cell in sputum is the macrophage, accounting for approximately 60% of the cells present. Neutrophils account for most of the remaining cells, with other inflammatory cells (lymphocytes, eosinophils and metachromatic cells) being present in small numbers. Shed ciliated bronchial epithelial cells comprise 1–2% of the total.[9] Squamous cells, originating mainly from the buccal cavity, are also present and give an indication of the degree of salivary contamination in the sputum sample. Within the fluid phase of sputum there are many different types of soluble mediator, including cytokines, proteases, histamine and eicosanoids.[10,11] The extent of interaction with mucins of these mediators is unknown but interaction has been clearly demonstrated for a number of cytokines, such as interleukin (IL)-5[12] and IL-8,[13] resulting in difficulty in detection. The soluble mediators are either secreted by airway inflammatory or structural cells or exude from the circulation. Induced sputum is similar to spontaneous sputum in terms of cellular and soluble mediator composition but has the advantage of producing superior quality samples with greater cell viability.[14]

Methodology

The protocols used thus far by separate investigator groups when performing sputum induction and processing are, broadly speaking, similar. Although minor differences in the methods remain, the relevance of these to many cellular markers of inflammation is not thought to be critical to their correct interpretation. This does not apply to soluble mediators, where detection is greatly dependent on processing and detection methods, including antibodies, used in the assays. The methodology is currently undergoing formal standardisation (European Respiratory Society guidelines are in preparation) and this will allow direct comparison of data from different centres.

Mechanism of sputum induction

Sputum induction is usually performed by inhalation of nebulised hypertonic saline through a mouthpiece. Ultrasonic nebulisers deliver particles of approximately $5\,\mu m$ in size at a high output (greater than 1 ml/min)[15] and achieve a higher success rate than do jet nebulisers. Although there is no difference in cell composition when using isotonic or hypertonic saline, the latter is associated with a higher rate of successful sputum induction.[16,17] The mechanism by which hypertonic saline is thought to induce sputum production is via increased vascular permeability in the bronchial mucosa secondary to the increased osmolarity of the airway lining fluid. In addition, there may be increased mucus production by submucosal glands and increased clearance of airway secretions following inhalation of hypertonic saline. Analysis of the osmolarity or sodium concentration does not show the expectorated sputum samples to be hypertonic.[13]

The concentration of the hypertonic saline used does not appear to influence success rate or sample composition[17] and in general most investigators use concentrations of 3–5%, sometimes increasing the concentration in a stepwise fashion during the induction period. Overall, the success rate of sputum induction is 75–95%.

Duration of sputum induction

Sputum induction is performed for 15–20 min. Sequential analysis of induced sputum indicates that samples expectorated in the first 4 min contain higher percentages of eosinophils and neutrophils and lower percentages of macrophages than do samples collected after 15 min of induction.[18] Mucin is more abundant in the earlier samples whereas surfactant concentrations are higher in the latter samples. This suggests that, as sputum induction progresses, different lung compartments are sampled, with central airway secretions being produced early, followed later by secretions from more peripheral airways, which contain more macrophages and are richer in surfactant.[19] Duration of induction, therefore, has a marked effect on sputum composition and it is important to have a standard induction period for all subjects in a study or in clinical practice.

Safety

Hypertonic saline can cause bronchoconstriction in asthmatics by mechanisms that may include activation of airway mast cells and stimulation of sensory nerve endings. Monitoring of lung function, preferably by measuring forced expiratory volume in 1 second (FEV_1), before and during sputum induction is therefore essential. Pretreatment with the β_2-agonist albuterol (200–400 μg) reduces the fall in FEV_1 seen during inhalation of hypertonic saline, which in most asthmatic individuals is usually less than 10% from baseline and does not effect sputum composition.[20] Premedication with higher doses may limit the effect of additional salbutamol, should induction lead to excessive bronchoconstriction. Overuse of β_2-agonists in the preceding 24 h is associated with increased bronchoconstriction.[21]

Sputum induction should be stopped if excessive broncho-constriction occurs (more than 20% below baseline) or if symptoms, usually cough, dyspnoea or chest tightness, become severe. Conflicting evidence exists regarding the relationship between baseline airway obstruction or bronchial hyperactivity and excessive bronchoconstriction.[22,23] However, less than 20% of severe or uncontrolled asthmatics experience a fall in FEV_1 of greater than 10%, and almost 90% are able to complete sputum induction.[24] Although stronger concentrations of hypertonic saline (up to 5%) and higher nebuliser outputs do impact on subject tolerability of sputum induction, their effect on bronchoconstriction is not known. An approach used by some researchers is to begin induction with isotonic (in patients with severe airway disease) or 3% saline and increase the concentration incrementally if symptoms and lung function do not deteriorate. In high-risk patients (e.g. those with severe asthma) it is advisable to use only isotonic saline and to limit the inhalation period to 8 min. Sputum induction with hypertonic saline is also associated with a small drop in arterial oxygen saturation, in both asthmatics and healthy controls, of approximately 6%

below baseline.[25] However, pulse oximetry is not routinely used to monitor subjects during the procedure.

Use in children

Sputum induction has been performed in a research setting in children above the age of 6.[26] Methodology and safety profile are similar to those used in adults, although the success rate is slightly lower in some studies.[27]

Collection and processing

The collection and processing procedure is summarised in Figure 9.1.

A number of methods have been used during the induction and collection process to optimise the quality of sputum and to ensure that it is representative of lower airways secretions. These include fasting or brushing of teeth prior to induction; the use of nose clips during induction; gargling and rinsing out the mouth with water prior to expectoration and spitting saliva into a separate container before expectorating sputum. The last procedure has been shown to reduce salivary contamination, with decreased numbers of squamous cells and an increased concentration of soluble mediators.[28]

Expectorated sputum should be collected in a Petri dish at 4°C and processed as soon as possible after induction to optimise cell viability and cytospin quality. Some researchers pick out the more viscous, dense portions of the sample using an inverted microscope in order to minimise salivary contamination. Others use the simpler approach of analysing the whole sample.[29] The former method has been suggested to result in fewer salivary cells (squamous cells) although, on balance, the use of either technique does not significantly alter the differential cell count or the ability to distinguish asthmatics from normal subjects.[30] However, concentrations of some soluble mediators are increased in the selected sputum method.[31]

Whichever technique is used, the sample must subsequently be homogenised to allow adequate dispersal of cells and extraction of mediators into the fluid phase. This is achieved by addition of an equal volume of a mucolytic, the most commonly used being dithiothreitol (DTT) at a concentration of 5 mmol/l. The sample is then mixed on a tube rocker or roller mixer for 10–30 min at room temperature before filtration through a 48–70 μm mesh to remove remaining mucous clumps, cell aggregates and debris. The sample is then centrifuged to separate the cell pellet from the fluid phase. The latter is usually frozen at this stage at −70°C for later analysis.

The cell pellet is resuspended and a total cell count is performed manually in a haemocytometer, with cell viability calculated using the trypan blue exclusion method. Cytospins are then prepared and stained with May–Grünwald–Giemsa staining, allowing determination of the differential cell count (Fig. 9.2). If metachromatic cell counts are required, separate staining with toluidine blue is necessary. Manual counting of cytospins has the disadvantage of being relatively slow and requires trained technical staff. Therefore, recently there has been interest in alternative approaches that allow the process to be automated. Quantitative analysis of cell types in induced sputum has been described using laser scanning cytometry.[32] In

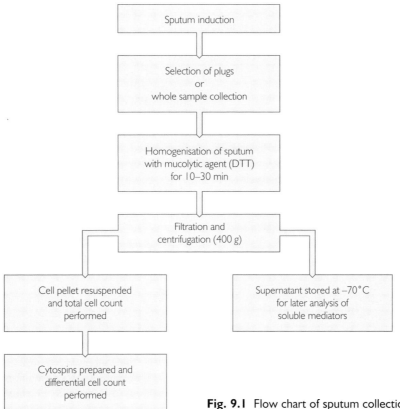

Fig. 9.1 Flow chart of sputum collection and processing.

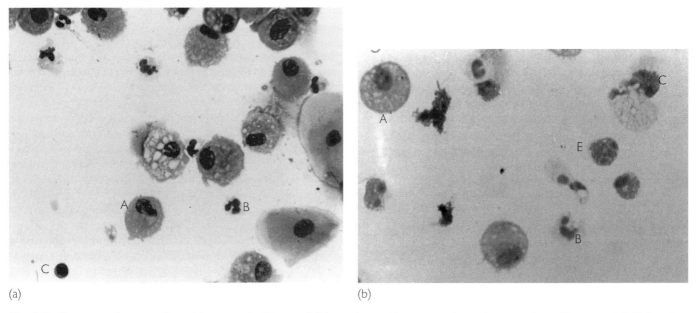

(a)   (b)

Fig. 9.2 Cytospins of sputum from (a) a normal subject and (b) a patient with severe asthma. A, macrophage; B, neutrophil; C, lymphocyte; D, squamous cell; E, eosinophil.

addition, eosinophil cationic protein (ECP) released from lysed sputum cell pellets has been shown to correlate well with the number of eosinophils in the pellet.[33]

The total time required for sputum induction and processing up to the point of producing cytospins is at least 90 min. The need to commence sputum homogenisation shortly after sputum induction currently limits its application to field studies. However, methods involving modified fixation or freezing of freshly expectorated sputum samples are being examined.

It is possible to perform immunocytochemistry and in situ hybridisation on cytospins, although both techniques require high-quality cytospin slides and false-positive staining is common.

Cytokine mRNA can be extracted from cells and measured using the polymerase chain reaction (PCR) technique[34] but the value of the results obtained so far has been limited. Flow cytometry has also been undertaken on the remaining cells after centrifugation[35,36] but is limited by the relatively small numbers of cells obtained in sputum induction compared with peripheral blood, and in addition cell preservation is often poor.

Consequently, most research has concentrated on measuring mediators in the fluid phase. These include cytokines and their receptors, chemokines, adhesion molecules, granulocyte proteins, eicosanoids, proteases and their inhibitors, markers of microvascular leakage and soluble products of nitric oxide. Most assay techniques use specific immunoassays, either radioimmunoassay (RIA) or enzyme-linked immunosorbent assay (ELISA). Bioassays are most commonly used to study chemotaxis. However, it must be remembered that, in general, immunoassays are designed for use in serum or culture fluid and that the environment in processed sputum may affect the results. The mucolytics used for sputum homogenisation can interfere with assay techniques by means of their action of reducing disulphide bonds. This may disrupt the tertiary structure of both the mediator being measured and the capture antibody in the assay. Spiking experiments need to be performed to evaluate the effect of DTT on each particular assay. This has only been done for a small number of mediators. Sputum also contains proteases, binding proteins, autoantibodies and soluble receptors, which may interfere with the assay. Sometimes these problems may be overcome by the addition of protease inhibitors or non-ionic detergents during sputum homogenisation but in other cases different assays will need to be tried.

Reproducibility

The reproducibility of cellular and soluble inflammatory indices derived from sputum induction has been examined in stable asthmatics and healthy controls and found to be of an acceptable level. Interobserver repeatability of sputum differential cell counts is high for eosinophils, macrophages and neutrophils (intraclass correlation coefficient – ICC – greater then 0.8) but is less good for epithelial cells and, in particular, lymphocytes. Interobserver repeatability is dependent on cytospin quality, being lowest when there is low cell viability (less than 50%) or excessive squamous cell contamination (more than 20%).[37] Within-sample reproducibility for differential and total cell counts and ECP concentration, as assessed by analysing different viscous parts from the same sample, is also high.[38]

If sputum induction is repeated after 8 h in the same subjects, there is an increase in the percentage of neutrophils present and a corresponding decrease in the percentage of macrophages. There is no effect on either the total cell count or the populations of other individual inflammatory cell types and epithelial cells. The neutrophilia associated with sputum induction lasts for at least 24 h[39] and has implications for the use of this technique as a means of obtaining repeat samples over a short time period. The behaviour of fluid-phase mediators in this situation has not been investigated. However, within-subject reproducibility of sampling intervals of between 2 days to 2 weeks is acceptable (ICC greater than 0.6) for eosinophils

(in particular), macrophages and neutrophils and a number of soluble mediators, including ECP, major basic protein (MBP), albumin, fibrinogen and IL-8.[38,40,41] Reproducibility over this time interval is poorer for lymphocytes, epithelial cells and the total cell count.

The effect of asthma severity has not been extensively studied but does not appear to significantly affect differential cell count repeatability over this time period. The reproducibility of the majority of fluid-phase mediators still needs to be determined, as does the variation in sputum-derived inflammatory markers over sampling intervals greater than 2 weeks.

Comparison with bronchoscopy

The results of sputum induction in healthy and asthmatic individuals have been compared with data obtained by bronchoscopy from the same subjects. Compared with either bronchial washings or bronchoalveolar lavage (BAL), induced sputum contains a higher concentration of both non-squamous cells and soluble mediators e.g. ECP, albumin, fibrinogen, tryptase and mucin-like glycoprotein. Percentages of neutrophils and possibly eosinophils are higher in sputum than in bronchial washings or BAL but the opposite is true for macrophages and lymphocytes.[42,43] The relative eosinophil counts and ECP levels in sputum correlate with those in bronchial washings and to a lesser extent in BAL, reflecting the part of the airway that each technique samples, i.e. predominately proximal airways in sputum induction and bronchial washings versus predominately distal airways and alveoli in BAL.[44] The relationship between sputum eosinophils and submucosal eosinophils in bronchial biopsies is weak.[45] Correlations also exist for both percentages of neutrophils and CD4[+] T lymphocytes between sputum and BAL.[46] This comparative data helps validate the use of sputum induction as a non-invasive means of studying airway inflammation. However sputum induction should be seen a complementary rather than alternative technique to bronchoscopy.

In both research and clinical practice it is often necessary to measure airway inflammation, sometimes by more than one technique, and airway hyper-reactivity. It is therefore important to ascertain the effect of these various procedures on each other. Current data is very limited but, with regard to airway challenge tests, studies show that methacholine challenge conducted 1 h prior to sputum induction does not significantly alter total or differential cell counts or ECP and albumin concentrations.[47,48] An elegant alternative is to combine measurement of airway hyper-reactivity with sputum induction by measuring the concentration of hypertonic saline required to reduce FEV_1 by 20% (PC_{20}) during induction. Sputum induction performed immediately before bronchoscopy does not lead to significant differences in total or differential cell counts or ECP and albumin levels in bronchial washings or BAL.[44]

Induced sputum in disease

Induced sputum has been extensively used to describe the inflammatory phenotype encountered in respiratory diseases. The majority of studies performed to date have been observational and concentrated on disorders of the airways, especially asthma.

Table 9.1 Induced sputum differential cell counts in normals and in patients with asthma and chronic obstructive pulmonary disease (COPD)

	Macrophages	Neutrophils	Eosinophils
Normals (%)	60–70	30–40	< 2
Asthma	→	→*	↑
COPD	→	↑	→†

* Neutrophils increased in infection, severe/steroid-resistant asthma.
† Eosinophils increased in a subset of COPD patients.

Asthma

Asthma is associated with a sputum eosinophil differential cell count of greater than 2–3% (Fig. 9.2 & Table 9.1). Sputum eosinophils can be increased after exposure to allergens[49] or following reduction in anti-inflammatory treatment.[50] Conversely, initiation of steroid[51-53] (the most potent treatment), theophylline[54,55] or antileukotriene therapy[56] leads to a reduction in sputum eosinophilia and this accompanies improvements in symptoms and lung function. This suggests that the presence or absence of sputum eosinophilia may be useful as an indicator for the need to modify anti-inflammatory therapy. For example, it has been shown that stable asthmatics with higher sputum eosinophil counts are more likely to suffer an exacerbation on reduction of their maintenance inhaled steroid therapy.[57] In the context of poorly controlled asthma, increased eosinophils might indicate inadequate anti-inflammatory treatment or non-compliance. However, if sputum neutrophils predominate in these patients instead of eosinophils, this suggests the presence of viral infection[58] or a subtype of severe disease that is poorly responsive to corticosteroid therapy.[59]

Occupational asthma is also associated with an increase in sputum eosinophils.[60] The degree of eosinophilia relates temporally to exposure to the sensitising agent and thus can be used as a diagnostic aid, with reduced eosinophil percentages observed when the subject is away from work.

In any asthmatic population there will be a wide range of values for sputum eosinophil percentage with a significant proportion of individuals having levels within the normal range (less than 2%). This intersubject variability has a number of causes, the most obvious being level of anti-inflammatory treatment and disease severity. It has been shown that more severe asthma is associated with higher eosinophil counts (Fig. 9.3).[61] However, even when these factors are controlled for there is still a significant degree of heterogeneity. This reflects the fact that asthma is for convenience regarded as a single clinical diagnosis but research into the pathophysiology and underlying genetics of the condition reveals a multitude of different inflammatory pathways and genetic polymorphisms. These will contribute to differing extents to the expression of variable clinical phenotypes in different subjects. Such intersubject heterogeneity is common to all non-invasive inflammatory markers and will have an impact on the sensitivity of these when used as a diagnostic test for asthma. However the presence or absence of elevated levels for a particular marker in asthmatics of similar severity and treatment may

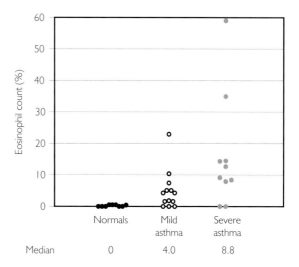

Fig. 9.3 Sputum eosinophilia in normals and asthmatics of varying severity.

identify populations exhibiting different susceptibility to exacerbations or response to a particular treatment.

The relationship between sputum eosinophil percentage and measures of lung function or bronchial hyper-reactivity is complex. Numerous studies report differences in the presence and size of significant correlations between such measures as sputum eosinophilia, FEV_1 and PC_{20} to methacholine.[62-64] This is also the case with other inflammatory indices, such as exhaled nitric oxide (NO).[65,66]

This primarily indicates that variations in single inflammatory pathways do not determine lung function and bronchial hyper-reactivity. Indeed, there would be little additional value in measuring a single parameter of airway inflammation if it only provided similar information to that which could be gained from simpler tests such as the peak flow. Instead, the data from inflammatory markers should be seen as complementary to those obtained from standard tests and may be particularly useful in situations where there is a discrepancy between symptoms and peak flow, FEV_1 and PC_{20}. Symptomatic individuals in whom these values are relatively normal may have significant airway inflammation requiring additional anti-inflammatory treatment, and vice versa. However, prospective studies are required to validate this hypothesis.

A number of studies have identified elevated levels of soluble mediators in asthma patients compared with normal subjects. These include ECP,[67] albumin[5] and cysteinyl leukotrienes.[68] Increased expression of mRNA has been observed in asthmatics for a number of cytokines and chemokines including interleukin (IL)-1, IL-4, IL-5, IL-8 and TNF-α.[69] Several inflammatory mediators, e.g. ECP and albumin, are also related to disease severity.[61,70] Measurement of these inflammatory mediators has helped to identify a number of inflammatory pathways that may be important in the pathogenesis of asthma, although it remains to be seen if they have a role in clinical practice. There has also been considerable interest in airway remodelling processes, which may be particularly important in chronic asthma. It is possible to measure several potential markers of remodelling in sputum, most notably matrix metalloproteinases and their tissue inhibitors.[71]

Chronic obstructive pulmonary disease

In COPD, neutrophils are generally the predominant cell type (Table 9.1)[72] and accompanying this are elevated levels of neutrophil markers such as myeloperoxidase and human neutrophil lipocalin.[73] There is conflicting data on the effect of high-dose inhaled steroids on sputum neutrophilia.[52,74] However, a subgroup of individuals display a sputum eosinophilia similar to that seen in asthma.[75] Such eosinophilic bronchitis has also been observed in some patients with chronic cough[76] and may be a useful indicator of response to treatment with inhaled corticosteroids.[77] Similarly higher levels of IL-6 and IL-8 in stable COPD patients may predict the frequency of exacerbations.[78]

Interstitial lung disease

T-cell subset analysis using flow cytometry has been used to distinguish between sarcoidosis and non-granulomatous interstitial lung disease.[79] Induced sputum can be used to detect hazardous dust particles and has a potential role in the monitoring of workers exposed to silica and hard metals.[80]

Exhaled gases

Interest in the measurement of exhaled gases as non-invasive inflammatory markers was initiated by the discovery of increased levels of NO in the exhaled air of asthmatics.[81,82] Since then, NO and a number of other exhaled gases (e.g. carbon monoxide, ethane, pentane) have been studied in a range of respiratory diseases. Exhaled air can be sampled without the need for unpleasant and potentially hazardous stimulation of the airways as occurs in sputum induction. It tends, therefore, to be more acceptable to patients. However, the equipment needed to analyse these volatile gases is expensive and requires stringent quality control and maintenance. The main advantage over all other non-invasive techniques is that results are available immediately.

Nitric oxide

Nitric oxide is synthesised by the action of nitric oxide synthase (NOS) on L-arginine. NOS exists in several constitutive forms (cNOS), which are activated by an increase in intracellular calcium ion concentration. The amounts of NO produced are small and have local effects, e.g. regulating vasodilatation in vascular endothelial cells or acting as a neurotransmitter in peripheral neurones. An inducible isoform (iNOS) can be expressed by a number of cell types in response to inflammatory stimuli, leading to the production of much larger quantities of NO (nanomolar amounts). Such stimuli include proinflammatory cytokines (e.g. TNF-α, IL-1β) and bacterial lipopolysaccharide. The exact role of increased NO concentrations in these situations, whether beneficial or harmful, is still not known.

Exhaled NO levels in healthy adults are log normally distributed, with a geometric mean of approximately 6–8 parts per billion (ppb).[83] A number of cells can express iNOS, including endothelial cells, smooth muscle cells, macrophages, eosinophils and T lymphocytes. However, the main contribution to exhaled NO comes from bronchial epithelial cells. Epithelial cells in the upper airways, and particularly in the nose, produce much greater levels of NO, with nasal concentrations of 900–1000 ppb.

Methodology[84,85]

Exhaled NO measurement is performed by chemoluminescence. The NO in the sample reacts with ozone to produce oxygen and energised NO_2. The latter returns to its basal energy level by releasing a photon, with the quantity of light emitted corresponding to the concentration of NO in the sample.

There are two main methods of acquiring samples for analysis. The direct or on-line approach involves the subject exhaling from total lung capacity (TLC) into a tube, which is connected to a chemoluminescence analyser. Nitric oxide is measured in real time and, following an initial peak, a plateau concentration is reached after 5–10 s, representing NO produced in the airways (Fig. 9.4). The early peak is caused by higher NO concentrations in the first part of exhaled air secondary to contamination by nasal and ambient NO. The contribution of NO from the nose is reduced by exhaling against resistance, which makes the soft palate shut off the nasopharynx. Alternatively, indirect or off-line techniques usually involve the subject exhaling into a reservoir bag from which samples are subsequently analysed. The bag can be filled either by a single expiratory manoeuvre from TLC, with the first portion exhaled being discarded via a valve, or by tidal breathing. Indirect techniques are useful in situations distant from an analyser such as in field studies or where the subject cannot perform an adequate expiratory manoeuvre, e.g. in young children. All the equipment with which the exhaled air comes into contact must be made of inert materials that will not react with NO in the sample and affect the result. Examples of these include Teflon® and polytetrafluoroethylene (PTFE).

Measured exhaled NO levels are strongly influenced by a number of technical factors, which must be controlled for in order to obtain accurate and reproducible readings. Expiration should be against a resistance of 5–20 cmH$_2$O, to create back pressure in the mouth that closes the soft palate and thus isolates the nasopharynx. This prevents contamination of exhaled air by the much higher amounts of NO produced in the nose. As has already been discussed, the first portion of exhaled air (the dead space) is contaminated by nasal and ambient NO and should not therefore be analysed. Exhaled NO levels are critically dependent on the expiratory flow, with high flow rates producing significantly reduced NO readings, and vice versa with low flow rates. The probable reason for this is the change in the volume of dilution resulting from alterations in the flow rate. In sampling techniques using expiration from TLC, a slow expiratory manoeuvre should be performed with a flow rate of 10–15 l/min. Most on-line analysers include real-time measurement of both expiratory flow and pressure with a visual display providing feedback so that the subject is able to exhale with the optimum force. If tidal breathing sampling techniques are used it is more difficult to exclude nasal contamination and maintain correct flow rates, resulting in higher exhaled NO levels of 14–18 ppb.

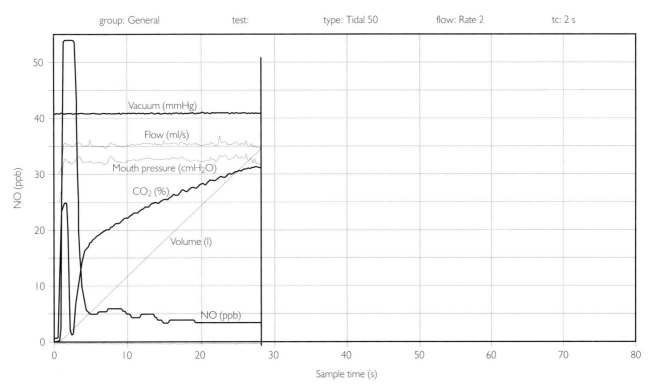

Fig. 9.4 On-line measurement of nitric oxide from a non-asthmatic subject.

Ambient NO levels can vary considerably, from 1 ppb to several hundred. However, inspired NO rapidly combines with haemoglobin and high concentrations fall rapidly during a breath-holding manoeuvre. Therefore, if NO readings are taken from the plateau phase after an exhalation of at least 10 s, the impact of high levels of inspired ambient NO will be very small.[86] This is not necessarily the case in samples obtained by tidal breathing. Cigarette smokers have lower exhaled NO levels than non-smokers and a single cigarette can transiently reduce exhaled NO levels.[87] Forced vital capacity manoeuvres have also been shown to cause a significant fall in exhaled NO readings, with the effect lasting up to 1 h.[88] Therefore, if spirometry is to be performed it should be done after measurement of exhaled NO.

Data on the effect of inhaled β_2-agonist therapy on exhaled NO in asthmatics is conflicting but there is some evidence to suggest that short-acting drugs can increase levels for up to 1 h.[89] Long-acting β_2-agonist use does not appear to have any effect.[90]

The reproducibility of exhaled NO measurement has not been extensively investigated. In normal subjects, duplicate measurements are highly reproducible (ICC 0.98). In stable asthmatics and healthy controls, exhaled NO levels are repeatable over a time interval of approximately 1 week (ICC > 0.8). These data suggest that the reproducibility of exhaled NO measurement is adequate.[91]

Carbon monoxide

Measurement of exhaled carbon monoxide (CO) was first used as a test of tobacco smoke intake. However, CO is also a product of haem oxygenase (HO) activity. Like NOS, this enzyme exists in constitutive (HO-2) and inducible (HO-1) isoforms. HO is part of the body's defence mechanism against oxidative stress from free radicals such as hydrogen peroxide (H_2O_2) and superoxide. These reactive oxygen species are produced in acute and chronic inflammatory conditions and concurrently there is induction of HO-1 by a number of inflammatory mediators, including proinflammatory cytokines, NO, reactive oxygen species and bacterial endotoxin. HO-1 catalyses the initial step in the degradation of haem to bilirubin, an antioxidant, with the release of free iron (also an antioxidant) and CO.

Measurement of exhaled CO could therefore give an indication of oxidative stress in the airways, although to date its use as a non-invasive inflammatory marker has been limited.

Methodology

Exhaled CO is measured by commercially available CO analysers, which can be adapted for direct on-line measurement of CO. The technique is similar to that used in measurement of NO, with the subject exhaling at a slow rate (5 l/min) from TLC for 20–30 s against resistance, at which point exhaled CO is recorded. There is less flow dependence than with measurement of NO and nasal contamination does not occur. However, contamination from environmental CO can influence readings and background levels of CO should be measured prior to each expiratory manoeuvre and subtracted from the recorded exhaled CO. Values in healthy adults are below 5 parts per million (ppm). As would be expected, exhaled CO is markedly increased in smokers, with average values of approximately

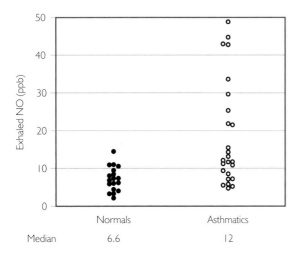

Fig. 9.5 Exhaled nitric oxide (plateau reading) in normals and asthmatic patients.

20 ppm. The majority of exhaled CO is thought to originate from epithelial cells and macrophages.[92]

Exhaled NO and CO in disease

Exhaled NO and CO are elevated in the majority of steroid-naive asthmatics (above 10 ppb and 5 ppm respectively; Fig. 9.5)[81,93] and may be useful tests in the diagnosis of newly presenting patients. In COPD there is conflicting data on whether exhaled NO is elevated in stable disease,[94-96] possibly as a consequence of differing experimental methodology. Levels are high in unstable disease and increase further during exacerbations.[97] In patients with chronic cough, exhaled NO has the potential to identify asthmatics from non-asthmatics.[98]

Both exhaled NO and CO are suppressed with inhaled corticosteroid therapy.[93,99] In the case of NO this only requires relatively low doses, at which sputum eosinophilia is still present. Therefore using only exhaled NO to assess the amount of steroid required may result in persisting airway inflammation. In severe asthmatics NO levels can remain high despite treatment with inhaled or oral steroid therapy, suggesting that these individuals may have a degree of steroid resistance.[100]

In bronchiectasis, exhaled NO is elevated during infective exacerbations but not in clinically stable, steroid-treated patients.[101,102] In contrast, exhaled NO is low in cystic fibrosis patients[103,104] because of increased neutrophilic production of superoxide interacting with NO. However CO is elevated,[105] particularly in unstable disease[106] and may therefore be of value in monitoring inflammation in cystic fibrosis. A similar picture may occur in primary ciliary dyskinesia, with the combination of low NO and high CO in a patient with bronchiectasis providing a diagnostic screening test.

Finally, elevated levels of both exhaled NO and CO are associated with increased disease activity in fibrosing alveolitis.[107]

Ethane and pentane

Ethane and pentane are volatile hydrocarbons produced as a result of the interaction of reactive oxygen species with poly-unsaturated fatty acids in lipid membranes, a process known as lipid peroxidation. They are excreted in exhaled air and have been proposed as indicators of increased oxidative stress. Measurement is by gas chromatography and so far there is only a small body of research describing exhaled ethane or pentane levels in human respiratory diseases. Smokers have been shown to have increased levels of exhaled ethane.[108] Ethane is also elevated in cystic fibrosis patients who are not on steroid therapy.[109] A limitation of their use in monitoring airway inflammation is that they are not specific to disorders of the respiratory tract. Lipid peroxidation occurs in diseases affecting other organ systems (e.g. inflammatory bowel disease and hepatic cirrhosis), resulting in elevated levels in exhaled air.

Breath condensate

Exhaled air contains non-volatile aerosol particles, which originate from the respiratory tract lining fluid. Breath condensate can be collected by freezing exhaled air (e.g. by breathing through tubing passing through ice), with approximately 1 ml of condensate being collected during 5 min of exhalation. This fluid is thought to reflect more closely the composition of alveolar than airway lining fluid because of the greater surface area of the former from which evaporation can occur. It can, therefore, be regarded as a non-invasive, non-cellular equivalent of BAL fluid. Most particles are less than 0.3 μm in diameter and include many protein and lipid inflammatory mediators, nucleic acids and markers of oxidative stress. Hydrogen peroxide, measured spectrofluorometrically, is the most extensively studied component of breath condensate to date. Hydrogen peroxide is increased in asthma,[110,111] COPD,[112] bronchiectasis[113] and adult respiratory distress syndrome[114] and remains elevated in unstable asthmatics despite treatment with steroids.[115] Immunoassays have been used to measure cytokines, leukotrienes and prostaglandins and a variety of other techniques have been used to measure pH, nitrite and amylase. The last is measured to detect significant salivary contamination.

A major advantage of breath condensate analysis over measurement of exhaled gases is that it does not require the subject to perform complex expiratory manoeuvres and is therefore ideally suited for use in young children and even in unconscious, ventilated patients. In addition, the equipment required to collect samples is simple and inexpensive so the technique could easily be performed in the setting of current pulmonary function laboratories.

Blood

Measurement of cells and mediators in blood can provide indirect information of inflammatory processes occurring in the lung. Increased levels of soluble mediators may reflect increased production in a specific tissue or organ spilling over into the circulation. Alternatively, inflammation in the lung may represent a local manifestation of a more systemic inflammatory or immunological condition, which can be studied in the blood.

Blood sampling is a routine and safe procedure that does not require specialised equipment. For many assays little or no processing is necessary post phlebotomy, making it an ideal tool for use in field studies or in primary-care-based clinical practice.

Of the soluble mediators, granulocyte-derived proteins, e.g. ECP, are relatively easy to measure by immunoassay. Chemokines, cytokines and adhesion molecules may present more difficulty. An alternative approach in this case is to extract the mRNA from leukocyte subtypes and measure the signal by semiquantitative PCR. Specific leukocyte and lymphocyte populations, the mRNA they transcribe and the proteins they produce or express can be measured by flow cytometry, in situ hybridisation and immunocytochemistry. In contrast with induced sputum, obtaining adequate cell numbers from blood for such assays is usually not problematic.

Eosinophil cationic protein is the most extensively studied serum inflammatory mediator. Data is conflicting however, with some studies suggesting that it can reliably distinguish asthmatics from normal subjects while others do not.[116,117] As with many other inflammatory markers, serum ECP does appear to be decreased by inhaled steroid therapy.[118] There is some evidence that levels correlate with disease severity.[119]

The ability to measure disease relevant proteins and mRNA is due to be dramatically increased with the development of proteomics and functional genomics. In the former technique, proteins in serum are separated by 3D gel electrophoresis and then identified using mass spectrometry. The mRNA extracted from leukocyte populations can be similarly separated and analysed using rapid sequencing techniques. These methods are quantitative and enable identification of mRNA and proteins that are overexpressed in the disease being studied. In some instances the gene and its product will be novel. It is hoped these techniques could also be applied to induced sputum.

A number of lung-epithelium-specific proteins can diffuse across the alveolar–capillary barrier into the serum. The most studied is Clara cell protein (CC16).[120] Serum CC16 is increased in conditions associated with increased permeability of the alveolar–capillary barrier, e.g. adult respiratory distress syndrome, acute ozone exposure. Because of its lower concentration and shorter half-life in serum, as compared to albumin in airway lining fluid, serum CC16 may be a more sensitive measure of increased alveolar–capillary permeability than albumin in sputum or bronchoalveolar lavage. However, it also has potential as a marker of epithelial damage due to smoking or pollution. Levels may rise if permeability is increased or fall if Clara cell numbers are affected.

Cytokine production by peripheral blood leukocyte populations in culture when exposed to various stimuli, e.g. lipopolysaccharide or allergens, is currently being studied. Cytokine profiles may be dependent on the immunological response of the subject. Therefore, this technique may be able to identify individuals who are at increased risk from potentially hazardous environmental exposures, e.g. cigarette smoke, allergens, organic dusts.

Urine

A number of soluble inflammatory mediators are excreted unaltered or partially degraded in the urine and can be meas-

ured. These include granulocyte proteins (e.g. eosinophil protein X, EPX) and mast-cell-derived methylhistamine. There has been considerable interest in the measurement of urinary EPX in children, where it would appear to have both diagnostic value and be related to symptoms.[121] Cysteinyl leukotrienes are rapidly metabolised in the circulation and difficult to measure in blood. However, after a relatively simple purification method leukotriene $(LT)E_4$ can be measured in urine by ELISA.[122] Levels can be elevated in steroid-naive asthmatics but are normal in individuals on inhaled steroid therapy. Urinary glycosaminoglycans are markers of extracellular matrix turnover. They are increased in acute severe asthma[123] and may be of value in assessing airway remodelling in chronic asthma.

In order to compensate for intersubject variability in urine concentration, mediators in urine are expressed as amount per millimole or microgram of creatinine. Many patients with respiratory disease are treated with inhaled or oral steroids but the effect of these on urinary creatinine excretion is not known.

Clinical applications

Current research has identified certain clinical scenarios where the non-invasive measurement of airway inflammation might provide improvements in patient management. The most promising to date is the identification of patients suffering from chronic cough who have sputum eosinophilia. This subgroup shows an improvement with inhaled steroid therapy[124] not observed in individuals without such eosinophilic bronchitis.[125] The detection of raised eosinophil counts in individuals with COPD also raises the prospect of induced sputum eosinophilia being used to identify patients who should receive inhaled corticosteroids. At present, the value of treatment with inhaled steroids in COPD is questionable[126,127] but it is plausible that a subset of patients with COPD who have sputum eosinophilia may benefit from steroids. Finally, the value of measuring PC_{20}, in addition to symptoms and lung function, as a determinant of level of treatment in asthma has been shown to reduce exacerbations.[128] It is hoped that detection of persistent sputum eosinophilia might, in a similar way, act as a sensitive marker of the need for anti-inflammatory treatment and improve asthma control. In all the situations discussed, large, prospective, randomised controlled trials are now required to determine the size of benefit, practical feasibility and cost-effectiveness.

Conclusion

Techniques for the non-invasive assessment of inflammation are useful tools in the study of diseases affecting the airway and several markers show promise in clinical practice. However before they become accepted as routine investigations, further work is required to standardise and validate the methodology, followed by randomised controlled trials to identify the clinical scenarios to which they can most usefully be applied.

Clinical relevance

Currently the most promising clinical situations where non-invasive techniques may direct management are:

■ asthma diagnosis and treatment (sputum eosinophilia and exhaled NO)

■ occupational lung disease diagnosis (sputum eosinophilia/dust particles)

■ chronic cough diagnosis and treatment (sputum eosinophilia and exhaled NO)

■ bronchiectasis diagnosis (exhaled NO and CO).

? Unresolved questions

■ Large, prospective, randomised, controlled clinical trials are required to determine the place of non-invasive investigations in treatment algorithms.

■ International standardisation of methodology, including safety aspects, needs to be agreed.

References

1. Morrow Brown H. Treatment of chronic asthma with prednisolone. Significance of eosinophils in the sputum. Lancet 1958; 2: 1245–1247.

2. Bigby TD, Margolskee D, Curtis JL et al. The usefulness of induced sputum in the diagnosis of *Pneumocystis carinii* pneumonia in patients with the acquired immunodeficiency syndrome. Am Rev Respir Dis 1986; 133: 515–518.

3. Gibson PG, Girgis-Gabardo A, Morris MM et al. Cellular characteristics of sputum from patients with asthma and chronic bronchitis. Thorax 1989; 44: 693–699.

4. Pin I, Gibson PG, Kolendowicz R et al. Use of induced sputum cell counts to investigate airway inflammation in asthma. Thorax 1992; 47: 25–29.

5. Fahy JV, Liu J, Wong H, Boushey HA. Cellular and biochemical analysis of induced sputum from asthmatic and from healthy subjects. Am Rev Respir Dis 1993; 147: 1126–1131.

6. Gibson PG. Use of induced sputum to examine airway inflammation in childhood asthma. J Allergy Clin Immunol 1998; 102: S100–S101.

7. Chlap Z, Stachura J, Sarnowska K. Investigation of sputum in cases of bronchial asthma. II. Histochemical study of mucous substances in the sputum. Acta Med Pol 1969; 10: 209–217.

8. Keal EE. Biochemistry and rheology of sputum in asthma. Postgrad Med J 1971; 47: 171–177.

9. Belda J, Leigh R, Parameswaran K et al. Induced sputum cell counts in healthy adults. Am J Respir Crit Care Med 2000; 161: 475.

10. Dor PJ, Ackerman SJ, Gleich GJ. Charcot–Leyden crystal protein and eosinophil granule major basic protein in sputum of patients with respiratory diseases. Am Rev Respir Dis 1984; 130: 1072–1077.

11. Frigas E, Loegering DA, Solley GO et al. Elevated levels of the eosinophil granule major basic protein in the sputum of patients with bronchial asthma. Mayo Clin Proc 1981; 56: 345–353.

12. Kelly MM, Leigh R, Horsewood P et al. Induced sputum: validity of fluid-phase IL-5 measurement. J Allergy Clin Immunol 2000; 105: 1162–1168.

13. Louis R, Shute J, Goldring K et al. The effect of processing on inflammatory markers in induced sputum. Eur Respir J 1999; 13: 660–667.

14. Pizzichini MM, Popov TA, Efthimiadis A et al. Spontaneous and induced sputum to measure indices of airway inflammation in asthma. Am J Respir Crit Care Med 1996; 154: 866–869.

15. Goddard RF, Mercer TT, O'Neill PX et al. Output characteristics and clinical efficacy of ultrasonic nebulizers. J Asthma Res 1968; 5: 355–368.

16. Popov TA, Pizzichini MM, Pizzichini E et al. Some technical factors influencing the induction of sputum for cell analysis. Eur Respir J 1995; 8: 559–565.

17. Bacci E, Cianchetti S, Paggiaro PL et al. Comparison between hypertonic and isotonic saline-induced sputum in the evaluation of airway inflammation in subjects with moderate asthma. Clin Exp Allergy 1996; 26: 1395–400.

18. Holz O, Jorres RA, Koschyk S et al. Changes in sputum composition during sputum induction in healthy and asthmatic subjects. Clin Exp Allergy 1998; 28: 284–292.

19. Gershman NH, Liu H, Wong HH et al. Fractional analysis of sequential induced sputum samples during sputum induction: evidence that different lung compartments are sampled at different time points. J Allergy Clin Immunol 1999; 104: 322.

20. Cianchetti S, Bacci E, Ruocco L et al. Salbutamol pretreatment does not change eosinophil percentage and eosinophilic cationic protein concentration in hypertonic saline-induced sputum in asthmatic subjects. Clin Exp Allergy, 1999; 29: 7 12–18.

21. Pizzichini MM, Pizzichini E, Clelland L et al. Sputum in severe exacerbations of asthma: kinetics of inflammatory indices after prednisone treatment. Am J Respir Crit Care Med 1997; 155: 1501–1508.

22. Wong HH, Fahy JV. Safety of one method of sputum induction in asthmatic subjects. Am J Respir Crit Care Med 1997; 156: 299–303.

23. Hunter CJ, Ward R, Woltmann G et al. The safety and success rate of sputum induction using a low output ultrasonic nebuliser. Respir Med 1999; 93: 345–348.

24. De la Fuente PT, Romagnoli M, Godard P et al. Safety of inducing sputum in patients with asthma of varying severity. Am J Respir Crit Care Med 1998; 157: 1127–1130.

25. Castagnaro A, Chetta A, Foresi A et al. Effect of sputum induction on spirometric measurements and arterial oxygen saturation in asthmatic patients, smokers, and healthy subjects. Chest 1999; 116: 941–945.

26. Cai Y, Carty K, Henry RL, Gibson PG. Persistence of sputum eosinophilia in children with controlled asthma when compared with healthy children. Eur Respir J 1998; 11: 848–853.

27. Wilson NM, Bridge P, Spanevello A, Silverman M. Induced sputum in children: feasibility, repeatability, and relation of findings to asthma severity. Thorax 2000; 55: 768–774.

28. Gershman NH, Wong HH, Liu JT et al. Comparison of two methods of collecting induced sputum in asthmatic subjects. Eur Respir J 1996; 9: 2448–2453.

29. Kips JC, Peleman RA, Pauwels RA. Methods of examining induced sputum: do differences matter? Eur Respir J 1998; 11: 529–533.

30. Spanevello A, Beghe B, Bianchi A et al. Comparison of two methods of processing induced sputum: selected versus entire sputum. Am J Respir Crit Care Med 1998; 157: 665–668.

31. Pizzichini E, Pizzichini MM, Efthimiadis A et al. Measurement of inflammatory indices in induced sputum: effects of selection of sputum to minimize salivary contamination. Eur Respir J 1996; 9: 1174–1180.

32. Woltmann G, Ward RJ, Symon FA et al. Objective quantitative analysis of eosinophils and bronchial epithelial cells in induced sputum by laser scanning cytometry. Thorax 1999; 54: 124–130.

33. Gibson PG, Woolley KL, Carty K et al. Induced sputum eosinophil cationic protein (ECP) measurement in asthma and chronic obstructive airway disease (COAD). Clin Exp Allergy 1998; 28: 1081–1088.

34. Gelder CM, Thomas PS, Yates DH et al. Cytokine expression in normal, atopic, and asthmatic subjects using the combination of sputum induction and the polymerase chain reaction. Thorax 1995; 50: 1033–1037.

35. Hansel TT, Braunstein JB, Walker C et al. Sputum eosinophils from asthmatics express ICAM-1 and HLA-DR. Clin Exp Immunol 1991; 86: 271–277.

36. In 't Veen JC, Grootendorst DC, Bel EH et al. CD11β and L-selectin expression on eosinophils and neutrophils in blood and induced sputum of patients with asthma compared with normal subjects. Clin Exp Allergy 1998; 28: 606–615.

37. Ward R, Woltmann G, Wardlaw AJ, Pavord ID. Between-observer repeatability of sputum differential cell counts. Influence of cell viability and squamous cell contamination. Clin Exp Allergy 1999; 29: 248–252.

38. Spanevello A, Migliori GB, Sharara A et al. Induced sputum to assess airway inflammation: a study of reproducibility. Clin Exp Allergy 1997; 27: 1138–1144.

39. Holz O, Richter K, Jorres RA et al. Changes in sputum composition between two inductions performed on consecutive days. Thorax 1998; 53: 83–86.

40. Pizzichini E, Pizzichini MM, Efthimiadis A et al. Indices of airway inflammation in induced sputum: reproducibility and validity of cell and fluid-phase measurements. Am J Respir Crit Care Med 1996; 154: 308–317.

41. in 't Veen JC, de Gouw HW, Smits HH et al. Repeatability of cellular and soluble markers of inflammation in induced sputum from patients with asthma. Eur Respir J 1996; 9: 2441–2447.

42. Keatings VM, Evans DJ, O'Connor BJ, Barnes PJ. Cellular profiles in asthmatic airways: a comparison of induced sputum, bronchial washings, and bronchoalveolar lavage fluid. Thorax 1997; 52: 372–374.

43. Maestrelli P, Saetta M, Di Stefano A et al. Comparison of leukocyte counts in sputum, bronchial biopsies, and bronchoalveolar lavage. Am J Respir Crit Care Med 1995; 152: 1926–1931.

44. Fahy JV, Wong H, Liu J, Boushey HA. Comparison of samples collected by sputum induction and bronchoscopy from asthmatic and healthy subjects. Am J Respir Crit Care Med 1995; 152: 53–58.

45. Grootendorst DC, Sont JK, Willems LN et al. Comparison of inflammatory cell counts in asthma: induced sputum vs bronchoalveolar lavage and bronchial biopsies. Clin Exp Allergy 1997; 27: 769–779.

46. Pizzichini E, Pizzichini MM, Kidney JC et al. Induced sputum, bronchoalveolar lavage and blood from mild asthmatics: inflammatory cells, lymphocyte subsets and soluble markers compared. Eur Respir J 1998; 11: 828–834.

47. Spanevello A, Vignola AM, Bonanno A et al. Effect of methacholine challenge on cellular composition of sputum induction. Thorax 1999; 54: 37–39.

48. Gershman NH, Fahy JV. The effect of methacholine challenge on the cellular composition of induced sputum. J Allergy Clin Immunol 1999; 103: 957–959.

49. Pin I, Freitag AP, O'Byrne PM et al. Changes in the cellular profile of induced sputum after allergen-induced asthmatic responses. Am Rev Respir Dis 1992; 145: 1265–1269.

50. Pizzichini MM, Pizzichini E, Clelland L et al. Prednisone-dependent asthma: inflammatory indices in induced sputum. Eur Respir J 1999; 13: 15–21.

51. Claman DM, Boushey HA, Liu J et al. Analysis of induced sputum to examine the effects of prednisone on airway inflammation in asthmatic subjects. J Allergy Clin Immunol 1994; 94: 861–869.

52. Keatings VM, Jatakanon A, Worsdell YM, Barnes PJ. Effects of inhaled and oral glucocorticoids on inflammatory indices in asthma and COPD. Am J Respir Crit Care Med 1997; 155: 542–548.

53. Jatakanon A, Lim S, Chung KF, Barnes PJ. An inhaled steroid improves markers of airway inflammation in patients with mild asthma. Eur Respir J 1998; 12: 1084–1088.

54. Louis R, Bettiol J, Cataldo D, Radermecker M. Theophylline decreases sputum eosinophilia of asthmatics. Int Arch Allergy Immunol 1999; 118: 343–344.

55. Horiguchi T, Tachikawa S, Kasahara J et al. Suppression of airway inflammation by theophylline in adult bronchial asthma. Respiration 1999; 66: 124–127.

56. Pizzichini E, Leff JA, Reiss TF et al. Montelukast reduces airway eosinophilic inflammation in asthma: a randomized, controlled trial. Eur Respir J 1999; 14: 12–18.

57. Jatakanon A, Lim S, Barnes PJ. Changes in sputum eosinophils predict loss of asthma control. Am J Respir Crit Care Med 2000; 161: 64–72.

58. Pizzichini MM, Pizzichini E, Efthimiadis A et al. Asthma and natural colds. Inflammatory indices in induced sputum: a feasibility study. Am J Respir Crit Care Med 1998; 158: 1178–1184.

59. Cox G. The role of neutrophils in inflammation. Can Respir J 1998; 5(suppl A): 37A–40A.

60. Lemiere C, Pizzichini MM, Balkissoon R et al. Diagnosing occupational asthma: use of induced sputum. Eur Respir J 1999; 13: 482–488.

61. Louis R, Lau LC, Bron AO et al. The relationship between airways inflammation and asthma severity. Am J Respir Crit Care Med 2000; 161: 9–16.

62. Ronchi MC, Piragino C, Rosi E et al. Role of sputum differential cell count in detecting airway inflammation in patients with chronic bronchial asthma or COPD. Thorax 1996; 51: 1000–1004.

63. Crimi E, Spanevello A, Neri M et al. Dissociation between airway inflammation and airway hyperresponsiveness in allergic asthma. Am J Respir Crit Care Med 1998; 157: 4–9.

64. Rosi E, Scano G. Association of sputum parameters with clinical and functional measurements in asthma. Thorax 2000; 55: 235–238.

65. Jatakanon A, Lim S, Kharitonov SA et al. Correlation between exhaled nitric oxide, sputum eosinophils, and methacholine responsiveness in patients with mild asthma. Thorax 1998; 53: 91–95.

66. Lim S, Jatakanon A, Meah S et al. Relationship between exhaled nitric oxide and mucosal eosinophilic inflammation in mild to moderately severe asthma. Thorax 2000; 55: 184–188.

67. Sorva R, Metso T, Turpeinen M et al. Eosinophil cationic protein in induced sputum as a marker of inflammation in asthmatic children. Pediatr Allergy Immunol 1997; 8: 45–50.

68. Pavord ID, Ward R, Woltmann G et al. Induced sputum eicosanoid concentrations in asthma. Am J Respir Crit Care Med 1999; 160: 1905–1909.

69. Konno S, Gonokami Y, Kurokawa M et al. Cytokine concentrations in sputum of asthmatic patients. Int Arch Allergy Immunol 1996; 109: 73–78.

70. Fujimoto K, Kubo K, Matsuzawa Y, Sekiguchi M. Eosinophil cationic protein levels in induced sputum correlate with the severity of bronchial asthma. Chest 1997; 112: 1241–1247.

71. Vignola AM, Riccobono L, Mirabella A et al. Sputum metalloproteinase-9/tissue inhibitor of metalloproteinase-1 ratio correlates with airflow obstruction in asthma and chronic bronchitis. Am J Respir Crit Care Med 1998; 158: 1945–1950.

72. Keatings VM, Collins PD, Scott DM, Barnes PJ. Differences in interleukin-8 and tumor necrosis factor-alpha in induced sputum from patients with chronic obstructive pulmonary disease or asthma. Am J Respir Crit Care Med 1996; 153: 530–534.

73. Keatings VM, Barnes PJ. Granulocyte activation markers in induced sputum: comparison between chronic obstructive pulmonary disease, asthma, and normal subjects. Am J Respir Crit Care Med 1997; 155: 449–453.

74. Confalonieri M, Mainardi E, Della Porta R et al. Inhaled corticosteroids reduce neutrophilic bronchial inflammation in patients with chronic obstructive pulmonary disease. Thorax 1998; 53: 583–585.

75. O'Connell JM, Baird LI, Campbell AH. Sputum eosinophilia in chronic bronchitis and asthma. Respiration 1978; 35: 65–72.

76. Gibson PG, Dolovich J, Denburg J et al. Chronic cough: eosinophilic bronchitis without asthma. Lancet 1989; 1: 1346–1348.

77. Gibson PG, Hargreave FE, Girgis-Gabardo A et al. Chronic cough with eosinophilic bronchitis: examination for variable airflow obstruction and response to corticosteroid. Clin Exp Allergy 1995; 25: 127–132.

78. Peleman RA, Rytila PH, Kips JC et al. The cellular composition of induced sputum in chronic obstructive pulmonary disease. Eur Respir J 1999; 13: 839–843.

79. Fireman E, Topilsky I, Greif J et al. Induced sputum compared to bronchoalveolar lavage for evaluating patients with sarcoidosis and non-granulomatous interstitial lung disease. Respir Med 1999; 93: 827–834.

80. Fireman E, Greif J, Schwarz Y et al. Assessment of hazardous dust exposure by BAL and induced sputum. Chest 1999; 115: 1720–1728.

81. Alving K, Weitzberg E, Lundberg JM. Increased amount of nitric oxide in exhaled air of asthmatics. Eur Respir J 1993; 6: 1368–1370.

82. Kharitonov SA, Yates D, Robbins RA et al. Increased nitric oxide in exhaled air of asthmatic patients. Lancet 1994; 343: 133–135.

83. Salome CM, Roberts AM, Brown NJ et al. Exhaled nitric oxide measurements in a population sample of young adults. Am J Respir Crit Care Med 1999; 159: 911–916.

84. Kharitonov S, Alving K, Barnes PJ. Exhaled and nasal nitric oxide measurements: recommendations. The European Respiratory Society Task Force. Eur Respir J 1997; 10: 1683–1693.

85. American Thoracic Society. Recommendations for standardized procedures for the on-line and off-line measurement of exhaled lower respiratory nitric oxide and nasal nitric oxide in adults and children – 1999. Am J Respir Crit Care Med 1999; 160: 2104-2117.

86. Piacentini GL, Bodini A, Vino L et al. Influence of environmental concentrations of NO on the exhaled NO test. Am J Respir Crit Care Med 1998; 158: 1299–1301.

87. Kharitonov SA, Robbins RA, Yates D et al. Acute and chronic effects of cigarette smoking on exhaled nitric oxide. Am J Respir Crit Care Med 1995; 152: 609–612.

88. Deykin A, Massaro AF, Coulston E et al. Exhaled nitric oxide following repeated spirometry or repeated plethysmography in healthy individuals. Am J Respir Crit Care Med 2000; 161: 1237–1240.

89. Silkoff PE, Wakita S, Chatkin J et al. Exhaled nitric oxide after beta2-agonist inhalation and spirometry in asthma. Am J Respir Crit Care Med 1999; 159: 940–944.

90. Yates DH, Kharitonov SA, Barnes PJ. Effect of short- and long-acting inhaled beta2-agonists on exhaled nitric oxide in asthmatic patients. Eur Respir J 1997; 10: 1483–1488.

91. Purokivi M, Randell J, Hirvonen M-R, Tukiainen H. Reproducibility of measurements of exhaled NO, and cell count and cytokine concentrations in induced sputum. Eur Respir J 2000; 16: 242–246.

92. Horvath I, Donnelly LE, Kiss A et al. Raised levels of exhaled carbon monoxide are associated with an increased expression of heme oxygenase-1 in airway macrophages in asthma: a new marker of oxidative stress. Thorax 1998; 53: 668–672.

93. Zayasu K, Sekizawa K, Okinaga S et al. Increased carbon monoxide in exhaled air of asthmatic patients. Am J Respir Crit Care Med 1997; 156: 1140–1143.

94. Clini E, Bianchi L, Pagani M, Ambrosino N. Endogenous nitric oxide in patients with stable COPD: correlates with severity of disease. Thorax 1998; 53: 881–883.

95. Corradi M, Majori M, Cacciani GC et al. Increased exhaled nitric oxide in patients with stable chronic obstructive pulmonary disease. Thorax 1999; 54: 572–575.

96. Rutgers SR, van der Mark TW, Coers W et al. Markers of nitric oxide metabolism in sputum and exhaled air are not increased in chronic obstructive pulmonary disease. Thorax 1999; 54: 576–580.

97. Agusti AG, Villaverde JM, Togores B, Bosch M. Serial measurements of exhaled nitric oxide during exacerbations of chronic obstructive pulmonary disease. Eur Respir 1999; 14: 523–528.

98. Chatkin JM, Ansarin K, Silkoff PE et al. Exhaled nitric oxide as a noninvasive assessment of chronic cough. Am J Respir Crit Care Med 1999; 159: 1810–1813.

99. Kharitonov SA, Yates DH, Barnes PJ. Inhaled glucocorticoids decrease nitric oxide in exhaled air of asthmatic patients. Am J Respir Crit Care Med 1996; 153: 454–457.

100. Stirling RG, Kharitonov SA, Campbell D et al. Increase in exhaled nitric oxide levels in patients with difficult asthma and correlation with symptoms and disease severity despite treatment with oral and inhaled corticosteroids. Asthma and Allergy Group. Thorax 1998; 53: 1030–1034.

101. Kharitonov SA, Wells AU, O'Connor BJ et al. Elevated levels of exhaled nitric oxide in bronchiectasis. Am J Respir Crit Care Med 1995; 151: 1889–1893.

102. Ho LP, Innes JA, Greening AP. Exhaled nitric oxide is not elevated in the inflammatory airways diseases of cystic fibrosis and bronchiectasis. Eur Respir J 1998; 12: 1290–1294.

103. Grasemann H, Michler E, Wallot M, Ratjen F. Decreased concentration of exhaled nitric oxide (NO) in patients with cystic fibrosis. Pediatr Pulmonol 1997; 24: 173–177.

104. Thomas SR, Kharitonov SA, Scott SF et al. Nasal and exhaled nitric oxide is reduced in adult patients with cystic fibrosis and does not correlate with cystic fibrosis genotype. Chest 2000; 117: 1085–1089.

105. Paredi P, Shah PL, Montuschi P et al. Increased carbon monoxide in exhaled air of patients with cystic fibrosis. Thorax 1999; 54: 917–920.

106. Antuni JD, Kharitonov SA, Hughes D et al. Increase in exhaled carbon monoxide during exacerbations of cystic fibrosis. Thorax 2000; 55: 138–142.

107. Paredi P, Kharitonov SA, Loukides S et al. Exhaled nitric oxide is increased in active fibrosing alveolitis. Chest 1999; 115: 1352–1356.

108. Habib MP, Clements NC, Garewal HS. Cigarette smoking and ethane exhalation in humans. Am J Respir Crit Care Med 1995; 151: 1368–1372.

109. Paredi P, Kharitonov SA, Leak D et al. Exhaled ethane is elevated in cystic fibrosis and correlates with carbon monoxide levels and airway obstruction. Am J Respir Crit Care Med 2000; 161: 1247–1251.

110. Dohlman AW, Black HR, Royall JA. Expired breath hydrogen peroxide is a marker of acute airway inflammation in pediatric patients with asthma. Am Rev Respir Dis 1993; 148: 955–960.

111. Antczak A, Nowak D, Shariati B et al. Increased hydrogen peroxide and thiobarbituric acid-reactive products in expired breath condensate of asthmatic patients. Eur Respir J 1997; 10: 1235–1241.

112. Dekhuijzen PN, Aben KK, Dekker I et al. Increased exhalation of hydrogen peroxide in patients with stable and unstable chronic obstructive pulmonary disease. Am J Respir Crit Care Med 1996; 154: 813–816.

113. Loukides S, Horvath I, Wodehouse T et al. Elevated levels of expired breath hydrogen peroxide in bronchiectasis. Am J Respir Crit Care Med 1998; 158: 991–994.

114. Kietzmann D, Kahl R, Muller M et al. Hydrogen peroxide in expired breath condensate of patients with acute respiratory failure and with ARDS. Intens Care Med 1993; 19: 78–81.

115. Horvath I, Donnelly LE, Kiss A et al. Combined use of exhaled hydrogen peroxide and nitric oxide in monitoring asthma. Am J Respir Crit Care Med 1998; 158: 1042–1046.

116. Bjornsson E, Janson C, Hakansson L et al. Serum eosinophil cationic protein in relation to bronchial asthma in a young Swedish population. Allergy 1994; 49: 730–736.

117. Marks GB, Kjellerby J, Luczynska CM, Burney PG. Serum eosinophil cationic protein: distribution and reproducibility in a randomly selected sample of men living in rural Norfolk, UK. Clin Exp Allergy 1998; 28: 1345–1350.

118. Vatrella A, Ponticiello A, Parrella R et al. Serum eosinophil cationic protein (ECP) as a marker of disease activity and treatment efficacy in seasonal asthma. Allergy 1996; 51: 547–555.

119. Niimi A, Amitani R, Suzuki K et al. Serum eosinophil cationic protein as a marker of eosinophilic inflammation in asthma. Clin Exp Allergy 1998; 28: 233–240.

120. Broeckaert F, Bernard A. Clara cell secretory protein (CC 16): characteristics and perspectives as lung peripheral biomarker. Clin Exp Allergy 2000; 30: 469–475.

121. Lugosi E, Halmerbauer G, Frischer T, Koller DY. Urinary eosinophil protein X in relation to disease activity in childhood asthma. Allergy 1997; 52: 584–588.

122. O'Sullivan S, Roquet A, Dahlen B et al. Urinary excretion of inflammatory mediators during allergen-induced early and late phase asthmatic reactions. Clin Exp Allergy 1998; 28: 1332–133.

123. Shute JK, Parmar J, Holgate ST, Howarth PH. Urinary glycosaminoglycan levels are increased in acute severe asthma – a role for eosinophil-derived gelatinase B? Int Arch Allergy Immunol 1997; 113: 366–367.

124. Brightling CE, Ward R, Goh KL et al. Eosinophilic bronchitis is an important cause of chronic cough. Am J Respir Crit Care Med 1999; 160: 406–410.

125. Pizzichini MM, Pizzichini E, Parameswaran K et al. Nonasthmatic chronic cough: no effect of treatment with an inhaled corticosteroid in patients without sputum eosinophilia. Can Respir J 1999; 6: 323–330.

126. Postma DS, Kerstjens HA. Are inhaled glucocorticosteroids effective in chronic obstructive pulmonary disease? Am J Respir Crit Care Med 1999; 160: 566–571.

127. Burge PS, Calverley PM, Jones PW et al. Randomised, double blind, placebo controlled study of fluticasone propionate in patients with moderate to severe chronic obstructive pulmonary disease: the ISOLDE trial. Br Med J (Clin Res Ed) 2000; 320: 1297–1303.

128. Sont JK, Willems LN, Bel EH et al. Clinical control and histopathologic outcome of asthma when using airway hyperresponsiveness as an additional guide to long-term treatment. The AMPUL Study Group. Am J Respir Crit Care Med 1999; 159: 1043–1051.

10 Invasive techniques

10.1A Diagnostic bronchoscopy

Karl Häussinger, Martin Ja Kohlhäuffl and Chris T Bolliger

Key points

■ The versatility of flexible fibreoptic bronchoscopy performed under local anaesthesia has changed the practice of bronchoscopy enormously.

■ Bronchial washing, brushing, endobronchial and transbronchial biopsies are routinely performed for diagnosis of endobronchial or parenchymal lung diseases and mediastinal processes.

■ The development of new techniques continues to expand the diagnostic armament, e.g. chip technology, endobronchial ultrasound and autofluorescence bronchoscopy.

Historical development

Examination of internal body cavities has been of scientific interest for centuries. Instruments for the inspection of the body cavities such as the mouth, nose, ear, vagina, rectum, urethra and others had been in use for ages before examination of the larynx was first attempted in 1847 by Green. He introduced a technique, passing the larynx and trachea with a gum-elastic catheter into the lower bronchi and introducing silver nitrate solution with a syringe.[1,2] In 1897 G. Killian removed the first foreign body via the translaryngeal route using a Mikulicz–Rosenheim oesophagoscope. During the following years technical improvements included the first glass-fibre bundles for illumination and development of numerous instruments for foreign body extraction.[3-5] In 1904 Chevalier Jackson developed a bronchoscope with a small light at the distal end, in 1930 H. Lamb advocated the application of glass fibres to a flexible gastroscope and in 1940 Edwin N. Broyles developed the optical telescope with forward and angle viewing.

In 1966 the first prototype of a flexible bronchofibrescope was produced by Machida in Japan and was delivered to Shigeto Ikeda, who established standards for the use of it. He introduced and popularised flexible bronchofibrescopy throughout the world. With the rapid progress in electronic devices, Asahi Pentax Corporation developed the first prototype of a videobronchoscope, which was introduced, again by Ikeda, in 1987.[6] This system eliminated the optical fibre bundle and replaced it with a charge-coupled device image sensor on the distal end of the bronchoscope, which made it possible to obtain better image resolution and processing. The television endoscope with a small camera at its tip, the so-called 'videobronchoscope', will probably become the next-generation instrument for visualising the tracheobronchial region.

Indications

Although indication guidelines have been published by the American Thoracic Society[7] (Table 10.1.1), strict guidelines are difficult to establish because of the rapid changes in existing technology as well as the introduction of new advances in

Table 10.1.1 Indications for diagnostic bronchoscopy (Sobolowski et al 1987[7])

Diagnostic uses
- Lung lesions of unknown aetiology that appear on the chest radiograph
- Unexplained haemoptysis
- Unexplained cough
- Localised wheezing
- Stridor
- Unexplained paralysis of vocal cord or hemidiaphragm
- Lung cancer staging
- Airway assessment for patency or injury after trauma
- Diffuse or focal lung disease
- Problems associated with endotracheal tubes
- Unexplained pleural infusion (including chylothorax)
- Suspicious or positive sputum cytology
- Suspected tracheo-oesophageal fistula

clinical practice.[8] Despite the fact that bronchoscopic practice has evolved considerably during the past decade, lung masses and nodules remain the most frequent indication for flexible bronchoscopy, followed by pulmonary infiltrates of suspected infectious aetiology, haemoptysis and interstitial lung disease of unknown origin.[8,9] However, in the USA a recent survey reported that only a minority of bronchoscopists (12%) perform therapeutic bronchoscopy (e.g. laser resection), suggesting a potential move toward development of tertiary care centres of excellence for patients who require advanced therapeutic procedures.[8]

Rigid bronchoscopy

Equipment

Figure 10.1.1 illustrates various types of rigid instruments (Storz) and a Hopkins telescope – which can be equipped with a forward view and a 30° and 90° optic for the lateral view. Different tubes are offered for rigid bronchoscopy. The diameter of the standard tube for investigations of adults should be 8.5 mm – this diameter allows good intraluminal instrumentation – and the length is approximately 40 cm. For smaller openings of the larynx, e.g. in children, smaller tubes are necessary. If children are regularly examined, a bronchoscope with a diameter of 4 mm should be available. The distal one-third of the rigid bronchoscope contains openings that permit ventilation of the opposite lung if the tube is passed deep into the airway on one side (arrows, Fig. 10.1.1).

The operator's end of the bronchoscope may have several parts. The open end can be capped or may allow passage of telescopes or other instruments. A large side port usually comes off at 90° for mechanical ventilation. Newer devices have an angled side port, which can be connected to ventilating equipment for use with Venturi jet ventilation. The tubes have light carriers incorporated into the wall of the scope that provide adequate visualisation for intubation, suctioning or removal of material. Optical telescopes passed through the tube deliver bright light to the airway and provide a magnified, wide-angled view of the lumen. The telescope can be connected to a charge-coupled device chip camera, permitting monitor visualisation. Special instruments include different forceps, scissors, balloon catheters, bougies and suction catheters. Some of the instruments are inserted without the telescope optic. Special forceps are attached to Hopkins telescopes to allow direct visualisation during biopsies.

Patient preparation and anaesthesia

The patient should not have eaten solid foods 8 hours prior to the procedure. Patients who are at risk for perioperative pulmonary aspiration (emergency patients, obese or obstetric patients) can be treated prophylactically with H_2-receptor antagonists or proton-pump inhibitors.[10]

Anaesthesia for rigid bronchoscopy is mostly general anaesthesia produced by short acting intravenous medication. Standard general anaesthesia for rigid bronchoscopy consists of hypnotic agents (e.g. propofol, midazolam, ketamine), analgesia (e.g. remifentanil, alfentanil) and neuromuscular relaxation (e.g. miracurium, atracurium).

Ventilation can be spontaneous, assisted, controlled or manually assisted by hand bag. While a high flow of air-oxygen is applied to the side port of the rigid bronchoscope, the proximal end of the instrument is closed by a glass lens to minimize loss

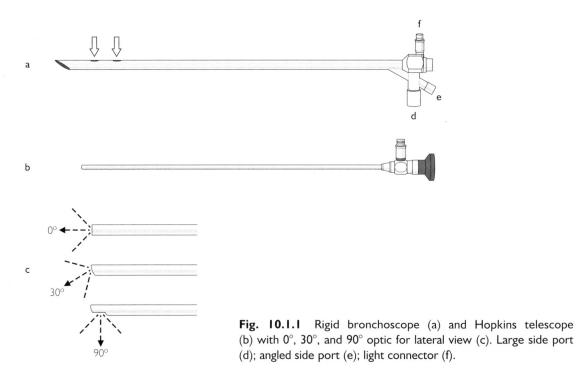

Fig. 10.1.1 Rigid bronchoscope (a) and Hopkins telescope (b) with 0°, 30°, and 90° optic for lateral view (c). Large side port (d); angled side port (e); light connector (f).

of tidal volume. Gas exchange may also be achieved by use of high-frequency jet ventilation via a special Luer-lock connector at the proximal end of the bronchoscope. Most investigators prefer to maintain ventilation by means of a jet ventilator. This allows the proximal end of the bronchoscope to be open, permitting easy introduction of a flexible bronchoscope and additional instruments without influencing ventilation. The jet ventilator achieves ventilation through the Venturi principle.[11]

Monitoring

Adequate monitoring is critical to recognise and prevent respiratory or cardiovascular complications.[12–14] Monitoring should include at least continuous pulsoxymetry, electrocardiography (ECG) and intermittent non-invasive measurement of blood pressure, and optionally capnography and monitoring of neuromuscular relaxation. Transcutaneous measurement of PCO_2 and PO_2[15] are helpful, especially during longer bronchoscopic procedures and when jet ventilation is used.

Techniques of insertion

Once the patient is properly relaxed, the position of the head is adjusted so that the neck is extended, creating a straight line from the oral cavity through the oropharynx to the vocal cords. The rigid bronchoscope is then introduced directly or using a laryngoscope, protecting the lips and teeth with the thumb. Once the uvula is visualised, the proximal portion of the rigid bronchoscope is angled downward. The bronchoscope is then passed under the epiglottis. When approaching the vocal cords the tube is rotated 90° to permit easy passage through the vocal cords. Finally, the teeth and gums are cushioned with gauze or a rubber protector.

Indications

From the beginning of bronchoscopy to the development of flexible bronchoscopy in the early 1970s, the rigid bronchoscope was the sole instrument available for tracheobronchial endoscopy, which was then replaced by flexible bronchoscopy. Since the chip bronchoscope does not allow direct visualization, monitor equipment is necessary. With the development of interventional procedures, rigid bronchoscopy came back into favour, especially in tertiary-care centres. The current main indications for rigid bronchoscopy are predominantly therapeutic procedures, often in emergencies – massive haemoptysis, dilatation of stenosis by bougies, laser resection, cryo- and electrocautery, stent implantation and removal of large foreign bodies. Rare contraindications include patients with unstable cervical spine and laryngeal obstruction.

Flexible bronchoscopy

Equipment

There are only slight differences between the brands of fibreoptic bronchoscope due to recent technological advances. The flexible bronchoscope is a flexible tube containing two or three bundles of tiny glass fibres and can be angulated mechanically when a knob or lever is moved. One bundle serves as the optical bundle and transmits images from the distal objective to the eyepiece. The adjacent bundles transmit light to the distal end of the instrument. The image created is a composite of those formed by the optical bundle, in which each fibre carries one pixel. Newer flexible bronchoscopes contain a tiny camera chip – based on charge-coupled device technology – placed distally on the bronchoscope, thus eliminating the bundle of optic fibres and a suction channel that doubles for insertion of instruments. Flexible fibrescopes are produced in a variety of lengths and diameters, which range from 2.2 mm to about 6.0 mm (Fig. 10.1.2). The diameter of the integrated working channel ranges from 0.5 mm to 3.2 mm. For both sampling of the specimens and therapeutic manoeuvres a variety of instruments have been developed (Fig. 10.1.3). The image that is transmitted through the bronchoscope can be viewed mainly in three different ways:

- observation of the image directly through the eyepiece
- accommodation of a second observer via a side-viewing 'teaching attachment'[3]
- the use of a video camera attached to the eyepiece to follow the progress of the tip of the bronchoscope by watching the monitor.

Patient preparation and anaesthesia

Flexible fibreoptic bronchoscopy is usually performed in sedated, spontaneously breathing patients. Informed written consent should be obtained from all patients. The patients should not have eaten solid foods for several hours before the procedure. In a survey by the American Association for Bronchology, the five most common tests ordered routinely were chest radiograph, platelet count, prothrombin time, complete blood count and electrocardiogram.[8] A chest radiograph has usually been obtained before referral for the procedure. Before and during the procedure, assessment of the level of oxygenation can be carried out by pulse oximetry. Arterial blood gas should be measured if hypercapnia is known or suspected. Routine screening for coagulopathy is no longer recommended, because patients with an increased bleeding tendency can be detected by a focused history. The platelet count should be checked in patients with possible thrombocytopenia (e.g. patients receiving chemotherapy).

Prophylaxis for bacterial endocarditis is not recommended before fibreoptic bronchoscopy with or without biopsy, according to recommendations by the American Heart Association. Prophylaxis is optional for high-risk patients (e.g. patients with prosthetic heart valves, a previous history of endocarditis and complex cyanotic congenital heart disease, or surgically constructed systemic pulmonary shunts or conduits).[16] However, a recent study[17] showed a bacteraemia rate of 6.5%, significantly higher than was previously recognised, in a cohort of 200 consecutive patients undergoing fibreoptic bronchoscopy without either pulmonary infection or an unusually high rate of invasive procedures.

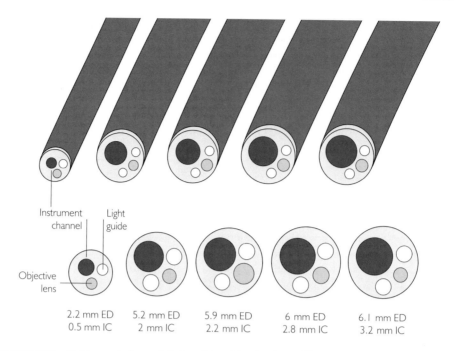

Fig. 10.1.2 Fibreoptic instruments – instrument channel, light guide, objective lens. ED, external diameter; IC, instrument channel.

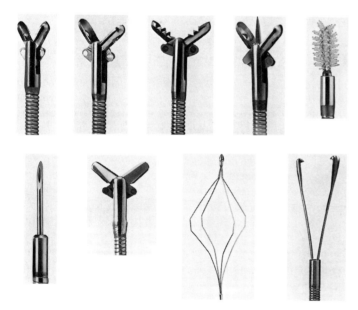

Fig. 10.1.3 Instruments for diagnostic or therapeutic manoeuvres using fibreoptic bronchoscopes.

Although flexible bronchoscopy can be performed without sedation,[18] most involve premedication with sedative agents.[8] The primary objective of conscious sedation during bronchoscopy is to relieve anxiety while maintaining spontaneous respiration and adequate oxygenation. Secondary objectives include amnesia, while maintaining the ability of the patient to cooperate with instructions. The primary objective of systemic and local analgesia during flexible bronchoscopy is to optimise pain control without compromising spontaneous respiration. Secondary objectives include cough suppression and reduction of gag reflex, both of which provide less risk of complication and an increase in patient safety, comfort and cooperation.[19]

Local anaesthesia is routinely induced before bronchoscopy. The posterior pharynx is anaesthetised with spray of 10% lidocaine (lignocaine). Whether topical anaesthetics should be delivered using a hand-held pneumatic atomiser, a nebuliser or directly through the bronchoscope is still a matter of debate. If transnasal passage of the bronchoscope is intended, the nasal mucosa is anaesthetised by topical application of 2% lidocaine gel. When the tracheobronchial tree is entered, additional 1% lidocaine boluses (2–3 ml) are administered through the channel of the bronchoscope into the trachea and into each main bronchus from the level of the carina. Bronchoscopists should be familiar with the potential side effects of excess lidocaine administration (max. total dose 300 mg) and be aware that local anaesthetics applied topically to the posterior pharynx, larynx and tracheobronchial mucosa are rapidly absorbed.[20,21]

At present, midazolam is the most commonly used sedative agent in this procedure – it was used by 87% in a large US survey[8] – because it has a documented rapid onset and a short duration of action. However, intravenous doses of midazolam must be sufficiently spaced to achieve the peak clinical effect before repeat doses are given. The elimination half-time for midazolam is 1–4 hours. Atropin is widely applied by aerosol or parenterally to dry airway secretions and to block vasovagal reactions (e.g. bronchoconstriction, bradykardia).[22] However, several studies have shown that bronchoscopy can be safely carried out without the use of atropine.[18,23,24]

Monitoring

In 1993, guidelines for care during bronchoscopy were published by the British Thoracic Society.[25] Most patients requiring bronchoscopy have lung disease or abnormal lung function and several of the procedures performed during bronchoscopy cause a lowering of arterial oxygenation. For these reasons it is recommended that patients undergoing bronchoscopy are monitored by pulse oximetry during the procedure. This not only allows arterial oxygen saturation to be monitored but also allows detection of dysrhythmias. Supplemental oxygen should be given to maintain the arterial oxygen saturation at or above 90%, since desaturation, defined as a fall in oxygen saturation to less than 90%, occurs in about 50% of the procedures.[26] Patients who become hypoxic and require oxygen during the procedure should continue to receive oxygen during the recovery period, when the lowest oxygen saturation commonly occurs. Standard cardiac and respiratory arrest resuscitation equipment should be available in the bronchoscopy unit. All patients given intravenous sedation should have continuous intravenous access through an indwelling line throughout the procedure. ECG monitoring is not necessary in every patient but would be indicated in patients with known cardiac problems, including dysrhythmias.

Techniques of insertion

The skilled endoscopist should be familiar with all routes for insertion of the fibreoptic bronchoscope. The choice should be based on patient safety, patient comfort, optimal yield in terms of diagnostic and therapeutic goals, and safe care for expensive medical instruments.

There are basically five different routes for insertion of the fibreoptic bronchoscope into the respiratory tract:[27]

- transorally (with or without endotracheal tube)
- transnasally (with or without endotracheal tube)
- through a rigid bronchoscope
- through a tracheostomy tube
- through a tracheostomy.

The transnasal route (without endotracheal tube) was introduced to facilitate introduction and to reduce contamination of the bronchoscope. Over the years, it has replaced the transoral route. It gradually gained popularity because of the smaller diameter of the bronchoscopes and because it eliminates the risk of the patient biting it. Nevertheless, there are certain clinical situations where the oral route has distinct advantages over nasal introductions (Table 10.1.2).

Table 10.1.2 Indications for transoral fibreoptic bronchoscopy (Guntupalli & Siddiqi 1996[27])

- Anatomical obstruction of the nasal passage
- Bleeding diathesis
- Removal of large foreign body from the respiratory tract
- In conjunction with the rigid bronchoscope during special procedures (e.g. laser therapy, airway stent placement)
- In management of a difficult airway requiring oral tracheal intubation
- Checking the position of an orally placed double-lumen endotracheal tube and associated complications

Care of equipment

Bronchoscopy is not a sterile procedure, so there is no need to maintain absolute sterility. Following each use, the instrument has to be cleaned and disinfected or sterilised prior to storage. The instruments used for rigid bronchoscopy can be disinfected or sterilised in the same manner as surgical equipment. The flexible bronchoscope has to be cleaned according to the following schedule.

First, the instrument is wiped off with dry gauze. Then the working channel is cleaned by suctioning sterile water or 70% alcohol. Then a cleaning brush is passed through the channel, followed by irrigation with water. The instrument is then immersed in a cleaning solution. Most units use 2% alkaline glutaraldehyde products[28] with a minimum contact time of 20 minutes.[29,30] Most manufacturers recommend performing a leak test after each use for early detection of damage to the working channel or the outer sheath.[31] Then the instrument is cleaned again with gauze, removed from the cleaning solution and the working channel is again suctioned with cleaning solution, followed by rinsing with sterile water and air-suction drying. For disinfection isopropyl alcohol, glutaraldehyde or phenol can be used. Submersion of the instrument for at least 20 minutes destroys all vegetative pathogens and 99.8% of *Mycobacterium tuberculosis* organisms.

Sterilisation with complete elimination of all viable microorganisms, including spores, can be achieved by submersing the instrument in formaldehyde or ethylene oxide gas. More recently, automatic machines for endoscope disinfection have been used. The Steris system, which is available worldwide, uses 0.2% peracetic acid. However, the system does not include a cleansing stage in the cycle and manual cleaning before the processing is therefore recommended.[32]

Endoscopic view

When inserting the bronchoscope via the nasal passages or the oral route, the bronchoscopist has to be familiar with the anatomy of the upper airway. The bronchoscope is introduced through the nasal vestibule and the posterior choana into the upper oropharynx, passes the epiglottis and is advanced to the vocal cords. The bilateral movement of the vocal cords should be checked during every investigation procedure and signals intact innervation by the vagus nerve. The trachea is entered after passing through the cricoid cartilage and ends at the division into the right and left main-stem bronchus. The shape of the trachea and main bronchi resembles an incomplete circle, formed by the supporting cartilages. A mobile posterior membrane, formed of muscle fibres and long bundles of elastic fibres, completes the tubular structure.

In about 30% of patients there are some anatomical variations, which seem particularly common in the basal segments. These anomalies can be congenital or acquired.[33-35] Many are detected incidentally during bronchoscopic examination and do not cause symptoms or disease.

The colour of the mucosa is usually pale pink but can vary greatly. A distinct reddening of the bronchial mucosa is the most constant sign of inflammatory change. The reddening may consist of simple engorgement of the larger mucosal vessels. Erythema with prominent vascular markings, oedema and increased secretions is most commonly seen in chronic bronchitis but may also be a feature of infection and inflammation from other causes, including neoplasm.

Swelling of the bronchial mucosa is also a common finding in inflammatory conditions. With marked inflammatory swelling there may be appreciable narrowing of small-calibre bronchi and blurring or obliteration of the longitudinal mucosal corrugations. In the elderly, there is often some degree of submucosal atrophy, characterised by a sharper relief of cartilages and carinae.

A very thin surface layer of fluid gives the mucosa its characteristic shine. Normal mucosa produces only sufficient colourless mucus for clearance purposes. The secretions vary widely, from excess of normal clear mucus in simple chronic bronchitis to frank pus in severe infection or purulent bronchitis. In cases of asthma or bronchopulmonary aspergillosis, thick mucoid material can be found, plugging even the smaller bronchi. Rarely, the secretions can be frothy, indicating, for example, pulmonary oedema (when generalised) or bronchioloalveolar carcinoma (especially when localised).

Localised changes raise a number of diagnostic possibilities such as carcinoma, simple pneumonia, localised infections such as lung abscess, bronchiectasis and tuberculosis, or aspiration of foreign secretions or foreign body. Fibrous scarring with obstructive narrowing of the bronchial orifice can occur after local inflammation or ulceration, high-dose radiation and therapeutic endobronchial manipulations (e.g. laser therapy).

The trachea or bronchi may be displaced or distorted in various ways. The most common reason for distortion is local compression by extrabronchial pressure from enlarged lymph nodes. In particular, enlargement of the subcarinal nodes readily produces widening of this area and eventually abolition of the usually keel-sharp edge of the carina.

Information on the condition of the mucous membrane is usually acquired coincidentally during the course of bronchoscopic examination for other reasons. There is a wide normal variation in the posterior membrane of the trachea. During a forced expiratory manoeuvre or cough the posterior membrane prolapses into the lumen of the trachea. This prolapse is more pronounced in the presence of bronchospasm. In patients with chronic obstructive pulmonary diseases the posterior wall may be enlarged and the expiratory manoeuvre may result in subtotal occlusion of the tracheal lumen (Fig. 10.1.4).

Chronic obstructive bronchitis in other cases may cause a U-shaped deformation of the tracheal cartilage. Localised impression of the muscular posterior wall of the trachea can be caused by enlargement of the posterior tracheal nodes.

Abnormal appearances in various diseases

Neoplasms, both primary and metastatic malignancies, can appear in various forms varying from subtle mucosal oedema, erythema and irregularity to exophytic, polypoid tumours, more or less obstructing the lumen of the airway (Fig. 10.1.5).

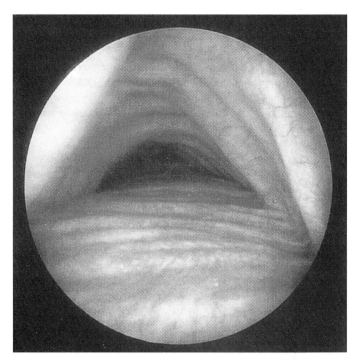

Fig. 10.1.4 Chronic obstructive bronchitis with enlarged posterior wall of the trachea.

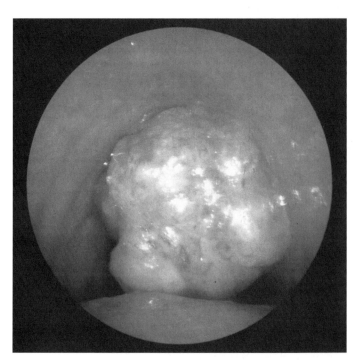

Fig. 10.1.5 Exophytic polypoid malignant tumour, almost completely obstructing the lumen of the trachea.

Tumours located paratracheally or parabronchially, especially enlarged tracheobronchial lymph nodes, can cause extrinsic compression of the tracheobronchial wall, e.g. when located in the tracheobronchial angle or the subcarinal region.

Submucosal mural growth of tumours can cause indirect tumour signs such as elevation, distortion or a break in the longitudinal folds.

Lymphangitic spread often appears with roughening, thickening and vascular irregularity of the mucosal surface (Fig. 10.1.6).

Benign neoplasms, affecting the tracheobronchial tree are rare.

Polypoid tumours, including chondromas, hamartomas and lipomas, most often appear as cherry-like masses, occluding the lumen of a lobar or segmental bronchus and causing more or less purulent retention of secretions.

Similar in appearance is bronchial adenoma, which has a characteristic cherry-red vascular surface and may bleed profusely when biopsied (Fig. 10.1.7).

Papillomatosis is most often located in the upper trachea but can also spread along the wall of the trachea and the main-stem bronchi and appears with polypoid, sometimes yellowish, sometimes transparent smooth masses more or less obstructing the lumen (Fig. 10.1.8).

Amyloidosis is caused by submucosal depositions of amyloid that produce gradual narrowing of the major airways by pseudo-tumour formation. Clinical and radiological examination of the chest often reveal no abnormalities. Bronchoscopically the wall of the trachea or the mainstem bronchi appears abnormally thick. The carina may display an irregular nodular surface and a dark red mass may cause longitudinal stenosis or even complete obstruction of the lumen. Both papillomatosis and amyloidosis tend to bleed when touched by forceps.

Broncholiths are calcified nodules that erode into the wall of a bronchus or enter the tracheobronchial lumen, representing a 'stone' in the wall or lumen of the bronchus. Endoscopically the

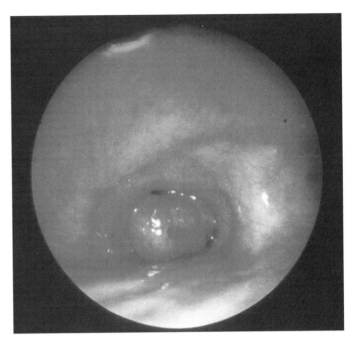

Fig. 10.1.7 Carcinoid tumour partially obstructing the bronchus intermedius. The surface of the tumour is vascular and smooth.

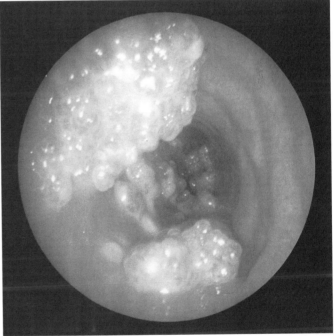

Fig. 10.1.8 Papillomatosis, spreading along the wall of the trachea, appearing as polypoid, yellowish, transparent masses.

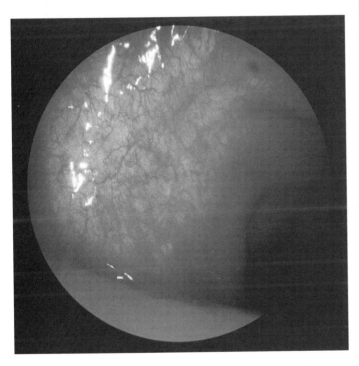

Fig. 10.1.6 Lymphangitic spread in the right wall of the main carina with roughening, thickening and vascular irregularity of the mucosal surface.

feature can vary, appearing as circumscribed inflammation, stenosis or occlusion of the bronchus by granulomatous tissue or a visible, white, calcified mass. Historically the most common aetiologies for broncholithiasis have included tuberculosis and histoplasmosis.

Bronchoscopic findings in *sarcoidosis* may include non-specific reddening and granulomatous involvement, especially in the hilar region and – rarely – yellowish nodules (Fig. 10.1.9). Mucosal biopsy of these nodules show non-caseating granuloma.

Endoscopic signs of *tuberculosis* are often caused by lymphnode enlargement, which may produce distortion and narrowing of the bronchial lumen or even total occlusion, particularly of the middle lobe bronchus. Enlarged tuberculous nodes surrounding the origin of lobar bronchi can result in a thickening and fixation of the spur of the opening mimicking a malignant process. When healing, intrabronchial tuberculosis may encompass fibrotic narrowing of a bronchus with localised stenosis of a single lobar bronchus and bronchiectasis of the lobe or segments distal to the lesion.

Bronchiectasis often appears with purulent secretions caused by severe and chronic bacterial infection (Fig. 10.1.10).

Biopsy techniques

Bronchoscopy should yield as much information as possible. Therefore, the procedures appropriate for each patient should be defined exactly, depending upon the questions to be answered. A high diagnostic yield from bronchoscopy relies on sampling and biopsy of appropriate material from the trachea, bronchi, lung parenchyma and lymph node and its careful preparation and examination. The sampled material can be bronchial secretions or lavage fluid, containing cells or bacteria or tissue from the mucosa, the lung parenchyma or the hilar or mediastinal lymph nodes. The specimens are sampled by

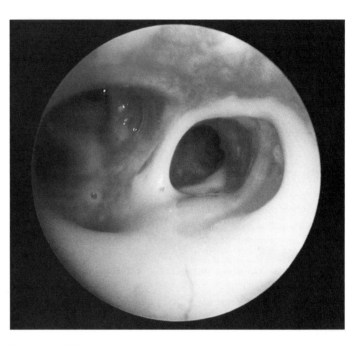

Fig. 10.1.10 Pus, mainly emerging from the right main-stem bronchus, caused by chronic bacterial infection in a patient with severe bronchiectasis.

forceps, brushes, needles, curettes. The material can be collected from the visible region, from paratracheal and parabronchial sites (e.g. mediastinal or hilar lymph nodes) and from the lung parenchyma or the bronchoalveolar region. The samples can be examined microbiologically, cytologically and histologically. Additional diagnostic procedures are immunohistology, special stainings, X-ray spectrometry and electron microscopy.

Cytology samples

The major indication for bronchial brushing is the cytological diagnosis of neoplasms and pulmonary infiltrates of suspected infectious aetiology. The brushes should be initially sterile, disposable and retractable into a plastic sheath. The sheathed brush is passed through the working channel until it just exits the bronchoscope. It is than directed under vision to the desired sampling location, to touch the area. The brush is then briskly withdrawn into the sheath. For peripheral lesions outside the visual range, brushing should be performed under fluoroscopic control in two planes, entering multiple subsegments that pass near the lesion. If the lesion is not visible fluoroscopically, the brush should be directed to the area indicated by the plain chest radiograph. For diagnosis of paratracheal or parabronchial lesions, transbronchial needle biopsy can be performed, which commonly provides cytological samples.

In cases of pulmonary neoplasm the diagnostic yield of bronchial brushing depends on the tumour's location and size and the endobronchial morphology. For bronchoscopically visible tumours, the diagnostic yield is generally reported to be between 62% and 68%.[36] Overall, brushing has been found to have a high diagnostic sensitivity (>80%) when used alone and

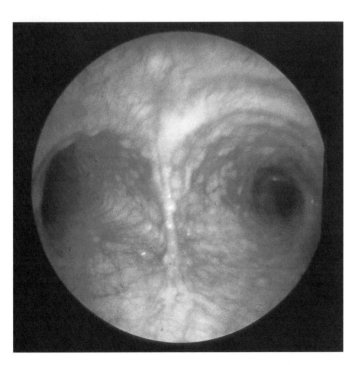

Fig. 10.1.9 Yellowish nodules in the distal trachea and both main stem bronchi in sarcoidosis. Mucosal biopsy reveals non-caseating granuloma.

an enhanced diagnostic sensitivity (up to 97%), when combined with biopsy.[37,38] Further brushing improved the diagnostic yield for lung cancer, which increased to 70.7%[39] and up to 89.6% with five brushings.[40]

For diagnosis of pulmonary infections using protected specimen brushing, sensitivity and specificity was demonstrated to be 82% and specificity 89% respectively compared to post-mortem analysis.[41,42] For patients with human immunodeficiency virus infection, blind bronchial brushing does not add to the diagnostic yield of bronchoalveolar lavage (BAL) alone.[43] Pooling the results of 18 studies evaluating the protected specimen brushing technique in a total of 795 critically ill patients showed the overall accuracy of this technique for diagnosing nosocomial pneumonia to be high, with a sensitivity of 89% and a specificity of 94%.[44]

There are several options for the preparation of diagnostic material after the brushing procedure. For neoplasm, the brush is used to make an immediate smear slide, which is then immersed in 95% alcohol or sprayed with a cytological fixative. After that the brush is rinsed in sterile 0.9% saline. It is helpful to have the pathologist present on site for processing of the specimens.

For non-bacterial microbiological processing, slides are stained in a manner appropriate to the organisms being sought.[45] The brush specimen is rinsed in approximately 5 ml of sterile 0.9% saline. After use the tip can be cut off in an aliquot of sterile 0.9% saline and sent to the laboratory for bacterial culture.

Bronchial biopsies

Forceps biopsy is the most commonly used biopsy method for a central endobronchial tumour. The lesion can be visualised and the location of the bronchial biopsy can be mapped precisely. While biopsies from exophytic tumours or from carinas can be performed easily, biopsies on the lateral wall of the trachea or the main bronchi can be obtained by using special forceps with a central spike to prevent the sample sliding off. However, among forceps with various configurations, no single biopsy forceps was shown to be superior to other types. When the tumour is bronchoscopically visible, the sensitivity of forceps biopsy ranges between 70% and 100%.[36,46,47] When the lesion is not endoscopically visible, the diagnostic sensitivity decreases and depends on location, size and configuration of the findings.

It is generally recommended that multiple biopsy specimens should be taken from endobronchial tumours. The diagnostic yield is directly related to the number of samples obtained: at least five biopsy specimens are required to achieve a probability greater than 90% of obtaining at least one positive sample. Failure to clear overlying blood clots and necrotic tissue can lead to a negative diagnosis.[48–50]

Transbronchial lung biopsies

In 1963 the first bronchoscopic lung biopsy was performed by Howard Andersen, who used rigid bronchoscopes and reported the results of the procedure in 13 patients.[51] Since Andersen's initial description the technique of transbronchial biopsy (TBB) using a flexible bronchoscope has expanded the range of diag-

nostic tools and significantly reduced the rate of open lung biopsies in patients with interstitial lung disease and infiltrates of unknown origin.

Indications for TBB are diffuse or localised interstitial disease with alveolar or fine nodular pattern on chest X-ray or localised densities beyond direct endoscopic vision. TBB offers an attractive alternative to transthoracic needle aspiration or lung biopsy by video-assisted thoracoscopic surgery (VATS). Compared to VATS, TBB provides several biopsy specimens from different areas of one lung. However, the small size of the particles often gives rise to diagnostic problems for the pathologist.

In diffuse lung disease the closed forcep is pushed forward into a small peripheral airway until a slight resistance is felt. Then the forcep is withdrawn about 2–3 cm, opened, pushed forward again, keeping some distance from the pleura, closed and finally withdrawn with a jerk. Using this procedure, biopsies contain small tongues of tissue from between two distal airways (Fig. 10.1.11). If the patient indicates ipsilateral chest pain, the forceps should be withdrawn a few centimetres and repositioned in another subsegment. Special breathing manoeuvres during biopsy procedures have been discussed, but they have not been found to be particularly useful.[52] In diffuse lung diseases, biopsies should routinely be taken from the lower lobe; this seems to reduce the risk of pneumothorax.[53]

The number of biopsies needed for diagnosis is disputed. In clinical practice not all biopsy specimens contain representative lung tissue, so a total of five or six biopsies is reasonable. Additional biopsies add less than 5% to the overall diagnostic yield but significantly increase risk, time and cost.[50,54,55] Floating in formol saline was not found to be helpful in predicting that the specimen contained lung tissue.[56] The need for fluoroscopy during bronchoscopic lung biopsy is also debated.[57,58] TBB for diffuse parenchymal disease do not usually require fluoroscopic guidance.[59] In cases of small, peripheral, localised lesions, however, two-plane fluoroscopy is mandatory to assure proper positioning of the brush, biopsy forceps or needle.[60,61]

Transbronchial lung biopsy offers an attractive alternative to open lung biopsy, but its diagnostic yield varies in different

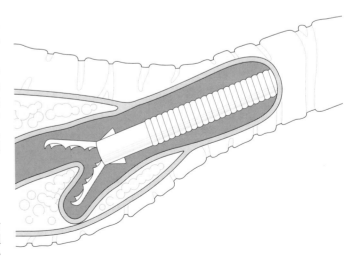

Fig. 10.1.11 Transbronchial biopsy. Forcep positioned beyond visual range – biopsy of lung tissue between two distal airways.

Table 10.1.3 Utility of transbronchial biopsy for selected diagnoses (Villenneuve & Kvale 1995[62])

Histology	Yield (%)
Malignancy	
Peripheral tumours*	21–77
Metastatic lymphangitic carcinoma *	88
Lymphoma	50–57
Alveolar cell carcinoma*	25
Pancoast tumour	36
Interstitial lung disease	
Sarcoidosis (stage I)	56–75
Sarcoidosis (stage II, III)*	83–97
Goodpasture disease	50–100
Wegener's granuloma	50–100
Eosinophilic pneumonia	100[†]
Pneumoconiosis	100[†]
Bronchiolitis obliterans organising pneumonia	50–88
Radiation pneumonitis	50[†]
Infectious lung disease	
Pneumocystis carinii pneumonia*	36–97
Tuberculosis	13–54
Cytomegalovirus pneumonia	11–83
Fungal disease	
Aspergillosis*	20–75[†]
Cryptococcus	75

* Highest specific pathological yield reported for this diagnosis.

† Reported yields for these diagnoses are based on small patient populations, with the highest yields reported in very small samples.

parenchymal lung diseases[62] (Table 10.1.3) and may not be representative of the whole lung because of the small sample size. In pulmonary sarcoidosis and lymphangitis carcinomatosa, a specific diagnosis can readily be obtained in about 80% of patients. In sarcoidosis the diagnostic accuracy correlates with the number of biopsies taken and is influenced by the radiological stage of the disease. The diagnostic yield increased from 46% to 90% in a group of sarcoidosis patients when four biopsies were taken rather than one.[63] Also, the diagnostic yield for this diffuse pulmonary disease was greater for radiological stage II/III disease than for stage I disease (84–83% vs 66%).[64] In contrast, in lymphangitis carcinomatosa there is little difference in diagnostic yield according to different radiographic patterns (diffuse linear interstitial infiltrates versus localised or multiple nodular opacities).[65] The diagnostic accuracy of TBB is lower in solitary pulmonary nodules, alveolitis, histiocytosis X, infectious diseases and cryptogenic organising pneumonia.

Transbronchial lung biopsy for solitary pulmonary nodules combined with brushing has a diagnostic yield of 10% in lesions of less than 2 cm in diameter, and of 40–50% in nodules of 2–4 cm,[66] whereas transthoracic needle aspiration biopsies guided by computed tomography (CT) are more useful in small nodules, with a diagnostic yield of over 60% in malignant nodules less than 2 cm in diameter.[67]

In idiopathic pulmonary fibrosis, TBB is not helpful in making the diagnosis of usual interstitial pneumonia, which is the histopathological pattern that identifies patients with idiopathic pulmonary fibrosis. TBB may, however, exclude usual interstitial pneumonia by identifying an alternative specific diagnosis. Also, because of the small sample size (2–4 mm) TBB should not be used to assess the degree of fibrosis or inflammation.[68]

In patients with suspected extrinsic allergic alveolitis pulmonary histological changes are considered to be only a minor criteria used to substantiate the diagnosis. Although the histopathology of extrinsic allergic alveolitis is distinctive, it is not pathognomonic. In most cases the diagnosis can be established without TBB.[69]

In histiocytosis X the diagnostic yield from TBB specimens is generally reported to be low, perhaps reflecting the focal nature of active lesions. Nevertheless, the diagnosis can be established if sufficient material is obtained and specimens are evaluated using immunohistochemical techniques.[70]

In infectious diseases such as tuberculosis there are two main indications to perform TBB on patients suspected of being infected:

- when sputum smears are negative and a definitive diagnosis is required
- when a coexistent second pulmonary disease, such as carcinoma, is suspected.

However the role of bronchoscopy in the diagnosis of tuberculosis is limited because of the excellent yield of sputum samples. In Acquired immunodeficiency syndrome (AIDS) patients the diagnostic accuracy (90%) of prebronchoscopic sputum samples effectively removes any advantage of diagnosis by TBB.[71]

Where there is a suspicion of *Pneumocystis carinii* pneumonia and a negative sputum examination in AIDS patients, both BAL and TBB guarantee nearly 100% sensitivity and specificity. However, BAL is the initial procedure of choice because of the increased likelihood of haemorrhage or pneumothorax with TBB and the fact that BAL alone clearly has approximately the same diagnostic yield as the combined procedures.[72] TBB has also been useful in the diagnosis of cytomegaly and *Pneumocystis carinii* pneumonia in renal and bone-marrow transplant patients. The diagnostic yield has been reported to be between 58% and 77%.

In order to diagnose cryptogenic organising pneumonia (idiopathic bronchiolitis obliterans with organising pneumonia, BOOP), video-assisted thoracoscopic lung biopsy is currently preferred to TBB as it provides large lung specimens that allow the diagnosis to be made with confidence.[73]

Several studies have demonstrated the safety of TBB in outpatients.[74,75] Relative contraindications are untreated bleeding and severe pulmonary artery hypertension. In patients with diffuse interstitial processes and evidence of mild to moderate pulmonary hypertension, no significant difference in bleeding complication was reported following TBB compared to the control group.[76] Pneumothorax occurs at a rate of 1–2% when the procedure is performed by an experienced bronchoscopist. TBB should only be taken from one lung to avoid the risk of bilateral pneumothoraces. Biopsies taken too peripherally, as well as underlying diseases such as *Pneumocystis carinii* infection, bullous emphysema or shrinking lungs caused by fibrosis, may increase the risk of pneumothorax. Although not mandatory, a routine chest radiograph about two hours after bronchoscopy is recommended to screen for pneumothorax.[75]

A further complication may be significant bleeding, which occurs in about 2% of cases. Biopsies taken from the bronchial wall may increase the risk of bleeding from bronchial arteries. Different techniques to control bleeding rely on saline lavage or wedging the orifice of the segment or subsegment bronchus with the bronchoscope. Usually, bleeding stops spontaneously within a few minutes and can be managed by suction only. The rate of bleeding is especially high in lung-transplant recipients[77] and is not significantly increased in patients with pulmonary hypertension in interstitial lung disease, according to one study.[76]

Transbronchial needle aspiration biopsy

Transbronchial needle aspiration biopsy (TBNA), mostly performed by flexible bronchoscopy, allows tissue to be sampled from paratracheal and parabronchial, i.e. hilar or mediastinal, regions. Applications have been expanded to sampling of submucosal and peripheral lesions.

Initially performed using the rigid bronchoscope and a long metal needle, Oho in 1979[78] and Wang in 1983[79] were the first to use TBNA with the flexible bronchoscope.

Transbronchial needle aspiration biopsy should be based on an exact knowledge of the anatomical structures – i. e. the lymph nodes and major vessels – of the mediastinum. It is essential to select the location for biopsy from a review of the abnormal chest radiograph and computed tomography images and to perform biopsy based on a mapping plan. Indications for TBNA include cytological/histopathological diagnosis of:

- mediastinal/hilar masses
- caused by primary tumour invasion
- caused by lymph node involvement
- submucosal masses
- peripheral tumours or nodules
- drainage of mediastinal structures i.e. bronchogenic cysts or abscesses.

In practice, the most frequent indication is diagnosis and staging of bronchial carcinoma. In these patients, CT may show abnormal mediastinal findings with either direct invasion by tumour or enlarged paratracheal, peribronchial or hilar lymph nodes with or without compression of larger airways or widened carinae. A positive aspirate from a mediastinal node may then prevent the need for mediastinoscopy or even thoracotomy in patients not suitable for surgery.[80,81]

Transbronchial needle aspiration biopsy is also helpful in diagnosing submucosal or peribronchial tumours. Endoscopically the location of biopsy often is signed by infiltration, elevation or compression of tracheal/bronchial walls. Finally, peripheral masses or coin lesions can be diagnosed by TBNA[82–84]

Equipment and technique

Protected transbronchial needles have a diameter of 20–22 gauge for cytological samples and up to 18 gauge for histological samples. Needles can be passed through the channel of flexible bronchoscopes and have a length of at least 10 mm. When the needle is positioned and anchored in the intercartilaginous space under endoscopic vision, the catheter is retracted and the tracheal/bronchial wall is pierced with a quick thrust. For penetration of the wall, different techniques are used and have been described in detail.[85] After insertion, suction with a 60 ml syringe is applied to the proximal end of the sheath, and finally the needle is withdrawn. For cytology, the specimen obtained is blown on to a glass slide (smear technique) and placed immediately in 95% alcohol.[86] Histology is obtained using an 18 or 19 gauge needle, which is inserted by a special technique and increases the risk[86,87] as well as the diagnostic yield.[88] Recently, a study has shown that endoscopic ultrasound-guided transoesophageal biopsy from the mediastinum seems to be superior to blind TBNA.[89] However, in transoesophageal endosonography the pretracheal, right and anterior left hilar structures are out of reach.

Diagnostic yield

Mediastinal disease – staging of bronchial carcinoma
The yield of TBNA in mediastinal disease increases with the presence of endoscopically visible tumour, subcarinal lymph nodes larger than 2 cm, visible tumour masses and widening or erythema of the carina, which indicates tumour involvement. In general, the diagnostic yield from TBNA staging of lung cancer patients in published studies shows a wide range, 43–80%.[79,80,83,90–94] This range is based on different patient selection, different techniques and different methods of training endoscopists. If the carina appears endoscopically normal, the range is only 9–35%. With enlarged lymph nodes, identified by CT scan, TBNA has a total sensitivity of 42%, which decreases to 11% in lymph nodes that appear radiologically normal.

Sarcoidosis
With the development of a flexible histology needle, TBNA was soon used to diagnose sarcoidosis. Wang diagnosed sarcoidosis in 90% of his patients.[95] Morales et al compared TBNA with a 19 gauge needle to transbronchial lung biopsy in 51 patients. Overall he found TBNA to be less sensitive than transbronchial lung biopsy, yielding a diagnosis in 51% and 67% of patients, respectively. However, combining methods, the overall diagnostic yield was 84%.[96] Using the endoscopic ultrasound-guided transoesophageal biopsy technique, Fritscher-Raven and colleagues recently reported a sensitivity of 100% and a specificity of 94% in a small group of sarcoidosis patients.[97]

Peripheral nodules
Transbronchoscopic needle aspiration for the diagnosis of peripheral lesions is performed under fluoroscopic guidance. The success rates vary enormously and depend on the position, size and histology of the tumour as well as on the technique used. The diagnostic yield decreases with peripheral location and small size (smaller than 2 cm yields a diagnostic rate of lower than 30%). For chondromas and tuberculomas, the success rate of TBNA is significantly lower than for malignant lesions. Primary lung cancers have a higher diagnostic yield than metastases.

Table 10.1.4 Yield of biopsy methods in diagnosis of peripheral lung cancer; data are presented as percentages

First author	Washing	Brushing	Biopsy	All methods
Kvale[53,98]	13	26	37	47
McDougall[99]	36	36	49	62
Popovic[53]	–	40	70	75
Mak[100]	38	29	37	56

In most studies, TBNA has a higher diagnostic yield than forceps biopsy alone or a combination of conventional procedures. With reference to the endoscopic techniques used, the diagnostic rate rises with the sequence washing – brushing – biopsy. The highest yield was obtained by combining the three procedures[50,98–100] (Table 10.1.4).

Complications

Transbronchoscopic needle aspiration has a very low incidence of complications.[101,102] Significant bleeding rarely occurs even after vascular puncture, as indicated by blood returning into the suction catheter. Single reports have described pneumothorax, pneumomediastinum and transient bacteraemia.

Contraindications and risks of bronchoscopy

As in all clinical situations, the risk of bronchoscopy and biopsy techniques must be weighed against the potential benefit for the patient. According to the guidelines of the American Thoracic Society for fibreoptic bronchoscopy in adults,[7] the contraindications are as follows:

- absence of consent from the patient or his/her representative
- bronchoscopy by an inexperienced physician without direct supervision
- bronchoscopy without adequate facilities and personnel to care for such emergencies as cardiopulmonary arrest, pneumothorax or bleeding
- inability to adequately oxygenate the patient during the procedure.

The overall morbidity and mortality from fibreoptic bronchoscopy, with or without TBB, is low. Table 10.1.5 summarises the potential complications of fibreoptic bronchoscopy. The danger of serious complications from bronchoscopy is especially high in patients with the following conditions:

- malignant arrhythmia
- profound refractory hypoxaemia
- severe bleeding diathesis that cannot be corrected when biopsy is anticipated.

A review of complications associated with flexible bronchoscopy, soon after the technique was introduced into clinical practice in

Table 10.1.5 Complications of fibreoptic bronchoscopy (Fulkerson 1984[103])

Premedication	Respiratory depression Hypotension or syncope Hyperexcitement
Local anaesthesia	Laryngospasm Bronchospasm Seizures Cardiorespiratory arrest
Bronchoscopy	Bronchospasm Laryngospasm Hypoxaemia Cardiac arrhythmias Fever Pneumonia
Biopsy/brush procedures	Pneumothorax Haemorrhage Pneumonia

the USA, noted that among 24 521 flexible bronchoscopies there was a 0.2% incidence of minor complications, a 0.08% incidence of major complications and a mortality rate of 0.01%.[104] A similar review in 1976 of 48 000 bronchoscopies observed 12 deaths (0.02%) with a 0.3% incidence of major complications.[105] Ten years later a postal survey of bronchoscopic practice by physicians in the UK reported, for a total number of 39 564 bronchoscopies (87% of these being fibreoptic procedures with topical anaesthesia), a similar mortality rate (0.04%) with a lower incidence of major complications (0.12%). TBB carried both an appreciably higher mortality rate (0.12%) and a higher rate of major complications (2.7%).[106] The most common apparent causes of major complications after fibreoptic bronchoscopy alone were biopsy-related haemorrhage ($n = 10$), respiratory depression ($n = 129$), vasovagal episode ($n = 4$), pulmonary oedema ($n = 49$) and arrhythmia ($n = 4$). The leading cause of major complications after fibreoptic bronchoscopy with transbronchial biopsy was pneumothorax ($n = 74$). A recent survey in Germany included a total number of 200 596 bronchoscopies at 681 bronchoscopy units. The mean overall rate of complications was 2.7% with an incidence of 4.6% minor complications and 0.7% major complications. The mortality rate was 0.02%.[107]

Flexible fibreoptic bronchoscopy has also been demonstrated to be safe, even among patients who have recently experienced myocardial infarction or who are in coronary intensive care units.[108,109]

New developments

Endobronchial ultrasound

The endoscopist's view is restricted to the lumen and the inner surface of the airways. Processes within or outside the bronchial wall adjacent to the airways can only be suspected from indirect signs. Radiological imaging procedures, including spiral CT, fail to define structures of the bronchial wall. The predicted sensitivity of CT-scanning in N-staging has a mean value of 60% identified in a recent meta-analysis (range 25–89%).[110] For staging of mediastinal and parabronchial structures, external mediastinal ultrasonography is used in anterior mediastinal or subcarinal lesions but is insufficient for staging of the inferior tracheal or perihilar regions.[111] In transoesophageal endosonography, the pretracheal, right and anterior left hilar structures are out of reach because of the interposition of the airways or lack of anatomical contact.

To improve the accuracy of diagnosis of bronchial, parabronchial and mediastinal structures, the technique of endobronchial ultrasound has been developed. Its clinical use is not yet widely established and evaluation of indications is still continuing.[112,113]

The technique of endobronchial ultrasound is based on the development of flexible introducer catheters for probes equipped with a balloon at the tip. With an outer diameter of 2.6 mm recently developed probes can be introduced through the working channel of a flexible bronchoscope. Once the balloon is filled with water, it completely fills the smaller airways or is brought close to the wall of larger airways. Providing a complete 360° view, endobronchial ultrasound has proved to be useful in high-resolution imaging of the multilayer structures of the bronchial wall and the adjacent mediastinal structures at a distance of up to 4 cm.

The indications for endobronchial ultrasound are listed in Table 10.1.6. Given the increasing detection rate of early central carcinomas by autofluorescence bronchoscopy and the limited depth of penetration of endoscopic treatment modalities, endobronchial ultrasound can be used to analyse local changes in the bronchial wall.[114] In advanced bronchial carcinoma the technique provides valuable information for assessment of tumour invasion of mediastinal organs such as the aorta, vena cava and pulmonary artery. Endobronchial ultrasound may have a significant impact on the sensitivity of transbronchial needle biopsy for histopathological diagnosis of hilar and mediastinal lymph nodes, especially in the N staging of bronchial carcinoma.[115] Further studies are needed to evaluate the role of endobronchial ultrasound in clinical practice.

Fluorescence bronchoscopy

Early malignant changes are difficult to detect by conventional white-light bronchoscopy. For carcinoma-in-situ, this technique has a sensitivity of only 30%.[116] To improve sensitivity for small (pre-)invasive lesions (e.g. moderate to severe dysplasias, carcinoma-in-situ, microinvasive carcinoma), autofluorescence bronchoscopy has been developed. When the bronchial surface is illuminated by blue light, it emits fluorescent light. Malignant and premalignant areas show significantly less intense autofluorescence than normal bronchial tissue.[117] This decrease in autofluorescence in premalignant lesions is caused by epithelial thickening, increase of microvascular density, changes in the tumour matrix and reduced fluorophore concentrations.[118] At the present time several different technical systems have been developed, some of them being in clinical evaluation.[119–122]

As to the number of lesions in a surveyed bronchial system there is no exact information owing to limited sampling. Relative sensitivity is used to quantify the performance of autofluorescence techniques. Relative sensitivity is defined as the ratio of the combined examination mode (i.e. white-light bronchoscopy and autofluorescence bronchoscopy) and white-light bronchoscopy. With the combined investigation, i. e. autofluorescence bronchoscopy + white-light bronchoscopy in one procedure, 1.4–2.7 times more preneoplasias and bronchial cancers were identified than with white-light bronchoscopy alone.[123–126]

The target group for fluorescence bronchoscopy might be patients at greater risk of developing primary, synchronous or metachronous lung cancer:[127]

- patients with lung cancers resected for cure at follow-up
- patients with sputum cytology positive for dysplastic or malignant cells and a normal chest radiograph
- smokers
- persons industrially exposed to carcinogens, e.g. asbestos, radon
- patients admitted to bronchoscopy because of respiratory or radiographic suspicion of lung cancer.

Table 10.1.6 Indications for endobronchial ultrasound

Early endobronchial carcinoma	Intraluminal extent (area) Depth of penetration
Infiltration of mediastinal structures	Trachea, oesophagus Pulmonary artery Aorta, vena cava
Endobronchial-ultrasound-guided biopsy	Mediastinal tumours N staging of bronchial carcinoma

Virtual bronchoscopy

Bronchoscopy is an invasive procedure. Therefore research efforts, especially in the field of radiology, continue to try to replace it with non-invasive imaging techniques. Virtual bronchoscopy has developed as a convergence of advancing CT and computer graphics technology. Based on actual patient data, usually obtained during CT of the chest, virtual bronchoscopy allows the user to manipulate a computer model of a patient's airway, simulating the perspective achieved during real bronchoscopy. Actual technical issues like data acquisition and image display are described in detail by Gladish[128] and will continue to develop with advances in computer and scanner technology.

Evaluation of indications for virtual endoscopy is matter of debate. In general, actual applications are planning of fibreoptic bronchoscopy and guidance, especially in the field of screening and surgical planning.

Special indications for the use of virtual bronchoscopy have been described as:

- detection, localisation and measurement of cross-sectional area and length of airway stenosis[129,130]
- visualisation of airways distal to primary stenosis that cannot be passed with the endoscope[131]
- planning of endobronchial sampling methods such as brushing, washing or forceps biopsy
- follow up after endobronchial intervention[132]
- aid in the selection of TBNA biopsy sites.[133,134] In the future this may be performed during real-time guidance of TBNA biopsy.

In summary, virtual bronchoscopy is a noninvasive rapidly developing method of virtual reality imaging that promises to improve planning for diagnostic and therapeutic interventional bronchoscopy, such as stent placement, laser resection, cryotherapy and brachytherapy.[135]

The main limitations of virtual bronchoscopy are primarily technical (cardiac and respiratory motion) and high costs. Finally, conventional bronchoscopy is mostly performed to obtain a pathohistological diagnosis which cannot be replaced by virtual bronchoscopy.

Clinical relevance

- Direct examination of the tracheobronchial tree by means of flexible fibreoptic bronchoscopy has greatly facilitated the diagnosis, staging and management of pulmonary neoplasms and diseases of the tracheobronchial tract and parenchyma.

- The most frequent diagnostic indications for bronchoscopy include cough, haemoptysis, radiological changes suggestive of tumour, bronchial obstruction and atelectasis. These conditions may be produced by inflammatory processes, tumour or foreign bodies.

- Bronchoscopy is an essential diagnostic tool for lung cancer.

Unresolved questions

- There is a lack of evidence based guidelines by professional societies regarding the clinical application of flexible and rigid bronchoscopy.
- Will chip bronchoscopy substantially improve macroscopic differentiation of subtle mucosal changes?
- What will be the role of three-dimensional ultrasound bronchoscopy for spatial imaging in clinical practice?
- Will on-site analysis of bronchial biopsies or cytological samples improve the diagnostic yield and reduce the number of biopsies performed?

References

1. Patterson EJ. History of bronchoscopy and esophagoscopy for foreign body. Laryngoscopy 1926; 36: 157–175.
2. Donaldson F. The laryngology of Trousseau and Horace Green. An historical review. Proc Am Laryngol Assoc 1891; 10.
3. Kollofrath O. Entfernung eines Knochenstückes aus dem rechten Bronchus auf naturlichem Wege unter Anwendung der direkten Laryngoskopie. MMW 1897; 38: 1038–1039.
4. Von Eiken C. The clinical application of the method of direct examination of the respiratory passages and the upper alimentary tract. Arch Laryngol Rhinol 1904; 15 November.
5. Killian G. Über die Behandlung von Fremdkörpern unter Bronchialstenosen. Zschr Ohrenheilk 1907; 15: 334–370.
6. Ikeda S. The development and progress of endoscopes in the field of bronchooesophagology. J Jpn Bronchooesophagol Soc 1988; 39: 85–96.
7. Sobolowski JW, Burgher LW, Jones FL. Guidelines for fiberoptic bronchoscopy in adults. Am Rev Respir Dis 1987; 136: 1066.
8. Colt HG, Prakash UBS, Offord KP. Bronchoscopy in North America. J Bronchol 2000; 7: 8–25.
9. Prakash UBS, Kenneth PO, Stubbs SE. Bronchoscopy in North America: the ACCP survey. Chest 1991; 100: 1668–1675.
10. Kallar SK, Everett LL. Potential risks and preventive measures for pulmonary aspiration: new concepts in preoperative testing guidelines. Anesth Analg 1993; 77: 171–182.
11. Sanders RD. Two ventilating attachments for bronchoscopes. Del Med J 1967; 39: 170–192.
12. Cote CJ, Rolf N, Liu LM et al. A single-blind study of combined pulse oximetry and capnography in children. Anesthesiology 1991; 74: 980–987.
13. Rolf N, Cote CJ. Frequency and severity of desaturation events during general anesthesia in children with and without upper respiratory infections. J Clin Anesth 1992; 4: 200–203.
14. Cote CJ. Pulse oximetry during conscious sedation. Council of Scientific Affairs, American Medical Association. JAMA 1994; 270: 1463–1468.
15. Palmisano BW, Severinghaus JW. Transcutaneous PCO2 and PO2: a multicenter study of accuracy. J Clin Monit 1990; 6: 189–195.
16. Dajani AS, Taubert KA, Wilson W et al. Prevention of bacterial endocarditis. JAMA1997; 277: 1794–1801.
17. Yigla M, Oren I, Bentur L et al. Incidence of bacteraemia following fibreoptic bronchoscopy. Eur Respir J 1999; 14: 789–791.
18. Colt HG, Morris JF. Fiberoptic bronchoscopy without premedication. A retrospective study. Chest 1990; 98: 1327–1330.
19. Matot I, Kramer MR. Sedation in outpatient flexible bronchoscopy. J Bronchol 1999; 6: 74–77.
20. Ameer B, Burlingame MB, Harman EM. Rapid mucosal absorption of topical lidocaine during bronchoscopy in the presence of oral candidiasis. Chest 1989; 96: 1438–1439.
21. Perry LB. Topical anesthesia for bronchoscopy. Chest 1978; 73: 691–693.
22. Greig JH, Cooper SM, Kasimbazi HJN et al. Sedation for fibreoptic bronchoscopy. Respir Med 1995; 89: 53–56.

23. Roffe C, Smith MJ, Basran GS. Anticholinergic premedication for fibreoptic bronchoscopy. Monaldi Arch Chest Dis 1994; 49: 101–106.

24. Makker H, Kichen R, O'Driscoll R. Atropine as premedication for bronchoscopy. Lancet 1995; 345: 724–725.

25. Harrison BDW. Guidelines for care during bronchoscopy. Thorax 1993; 48: 584.

26. Stanopoulos IT, Pickering R, Beamis JF, Martinez FJ. Oximetric monitoring during routine, oxygen-supplemented flexible bronchoscopy: what role does it have? J Bronchol 1995; 2: 5–11.

27. Guntupalli KK, Siddiqi AJ. Nasal versus oral insertion of the flexible bronchoscope. J Bronchol 1996; 3: 229–233.

28. Uttley AHC, Simpson RA. Audit of bronchoscope disinfection in a survey of procedures in England and Wales and incidence of mycobacterial contamination. J Hosp Infect 1994; 26: 301–308.

29. Rutala WA. APIC guidelines for selection and use of disinfectants. Am J Infect Control 1990; 18: 99–117.

30. Babb JR, Bradley CR, Barnes AR. Question and answer. J Hosp Infect 1992; 20: 51–54.

31. Olympus Academy. Seminar instructions for endoscopy, 2000

32. Fraise AP. Disinfection in endoscopy. Lancet 1995; 346: 787–788.

33. Landing BH, Dixon LG. Congenital malformations and genetic disorders of the respiratory tract (larynx, trachea, bronchi and lungs). Am Rev Respir Dis 1979; 120: 151–185.

34. Warkany J. The lung. In: Warkany M, ed. Congenital malformations. Chicago: Year Book 1971: 64.

35. Wier JA. Congenital anomalies of the lung. Ann Intern Med 1960; 52: 330–348.

36. Arroliga AC, Matthay RA. The role of bronchoscopy in lung cancer. Clin Chest Med 1993; 14: 87–98.

37. Popp W, Rauscher H, Ritschka L et al. Diagnostic sensitivity of different techniques in the diagnosis of lung tumors with the flexible fiberoptic bronchoscope: comparison of brush biopsy, imprint cytology of forceps biopsy and histology of forceps biopsy. Cancer 1991; 67: 72–75.

38. Solomon DA, Solliday NH, Gracey DR. Cytology in fiberoptic bronchoscopy: comparison of bronchial brushing, washing and postbronchoscopy sputum. Chest 1974; 65: 616–619.

39. Rosell A, Monso E, Lores L et al. Cytology of bronchial biopsy rinse fluid to improve the diagnostic yield for lung cancer. Eur Respir J 1998; 12: 1415–1418.

40. Popp W, Merkle M, Schreiber B et al. How much brushing is enough for the diagnosis of lung tumors? Cancer 1992; 70: 2278–2280.

41. Chastre J, Fagon JY, Bornet-Lecso M et al. Evaluation of bronchoscopic techniques for the diagnosis of nosocomial pneumonia. Am J Respir Crit Care Med 1995; 152: 231–240.

42. Meduri GU, Chastre J, Hance AJ et al. The standardization of bronchoscopic techniques for ventilator-associated pneumonia. Chest 1992; 102 (suppl. 5): 557–564.

43. Metersky ML, Harrell JH II, Moser KM. Lack of utility of bronchial brush biopsy in patients infected with the human immunodeficiency virus. Chest 1992; 101: 680–683.

44. Chastre J, Fagon J-Y. Ventilator-associated pneumonia. Am J Respir Crit Care Med 2002; 165: 867–903.

45. Kovitz KL. Bronchoscopic brushing techniques. J Bronchol 1996; 3: 217–223.

46. Govert JA, Kopita JM, Matchara D et al. Cost effectiveness of collecting routine cytologic specimens during fiberoptic bronchoscopy for endoscopically visible lung tumour. Chest 1996; 109: 451–456.

47. Gasparini S. Bronchoscopic biopsy techniques in the diagnosis and staging of lung cancer. Monaldi Arch Chest Dis 1997; 52: 392–398.

48. Gellert AR, Rudd RM, Sinha G, Geddes DM. Fiberoptic bronchoscopy: effect of multiple bronchial biopsies on diagnostic yield in bronchial carcinoma. Thorax 1982; 37: 684–687.

49. Shure D, Astarita RW. Bronchogenic carcinoma presenting as an endobronchial mass. Chest 1983; 83: 865–867.

50. Popovich J, Kvale PA, Eichenhorn MS et al. Diagnostic accuracy of multiple biopsies from flexible fiberoptic bronchoscopy. Am Rev Respir Dis 1982 ;125: 521–523.

51. Andersen HA, Fontana RS, Harrison EG Jr. Transbronchoscopic lung biopsy in diffuse pulmonary disease. Dis Chest 1965; 48: 187–192.

52. Shure D, Abraham JL, Konopka R. How should transbronchial biopsies be performed and processed? Am Rev Respir Dis 1982; 126: 342–343.

53. Kvale PA. Bronchoscopic lung biopsy. J Bronchol 1994; 1: 321–326.

54. Harber P. The optimal number of trans-bronchoscopic biopsies for diagnosing sarcoidosis. Chest 1981; 79: 124–125.

55. Descombes E, Gardiol D, Leuenberger P. Transbronchial lung biopsy: an analysis of 530 cases with reference to the number of samples. Monaldi Arch Chest Dis 1997; 52: 324–329.

56. Curley FJ, Johol JS, Burke ME, Fraire AE. Transbronchial lung biopsy – can specimen quality be predicted at the time of biopsy? Chest 1998; 113: 1037–1041.

57. Judson MA. Is fluoroscopy needed for bronchoscopic lung biopsy? Pro fluoroscopy. J Bronchol 1994; 1: 332–336.

58. Anders GT. Is fluoroscopy needed for bronchoscopic lung biopsy? Con fluoroscopy. J Bronchol 1994; 1: 332–336.

59. Anders GT, Johnson JE, Bush BA. Transbronchial biopsy without fluoroscopy. Chest 1988; 94: 557–560.

60. Metha AL, Kathawalla SA, Chan CC, Arroliga A. Role of bronchoscopy in evaluation of solitary pulmonary nodule. J Bronchol 1995; 2: 315–322.

61. Shure D. Transbronchial biopsy and needle aspiration. Chest 1989; 95: 1130–1138.

62. Villenneuve MR, Kvale PA. Transbronchial lung biopsy. In: Feinsilver SH, Fein AM, ed. Textbook of bronchoscopy. Baltimore: Williams & Wilkins; 1995, ch 5: 77.

63. Gilman MJ, Wang KP. Transbronchial lung biopsy in sarcoidosis: an approach to determine the optimal number of biopsies. Am Rev Respir Dis 1980; 122: 721–724.

64. Roethe RA, Fuller PB, Byrd RB, Hafemann DR. Transbronchial lung biopsy in sarcoidosis. Chest 1980; 77: 400–402.

65. Chuang MT, Padilla ML, Teirstein AS. Flexible fiberoptic bronchoscopy in metastatic cancer to the lungs. Cancer 1983; 52: 1949–1951.

66. Shure D, Fedullo PF. Transbronchial needle aspiration in the diagnosis of submucosal and peribronchial bronchogenic carcinoma. Chest 1985; 88: 49–51.

67. Ost D, Fein A. Evaluation and management of the solitary pulmonary nodule. Am J Respir Crit Care Med 2000; 162: 782–787.

68. King TE, Costabel U, Cordier J-F et al. Idiopathic pulmonary fibrosis: diagnosis and treatment. Am J Respir Crit Care Med 2000; 161: 646–664.

69. Richerson HB, Bernstein IL, Fink JN et al. Guidelines for the clinical evaluation of hypersensitivity pneumonitis. J Allergy Clin Immunol 1989; 84: 839–844.

70. Tazi A, Soler P, Hance AJ. Adult pulmonary Langerhans' cell histiocytosis. Thorax 2000; 55: 405–416.

71. Chan CHS, Chan RCY, Arnold M et al. Bronchoscopy and tuberculostearic acid assay in the diagnosis of sputum smear negative pulmonary tuberculosis: a prospective study with the addition of transbronchial biopsy. Q J Med 1992; 82: 15–23.

72. Huang L, Hecht FM, Stansell JD. Suspected *Pneumocystis carinii* pneumonia with a negative induced sputum examination. Is early bronchoscopy useful? Am J Respir Crit Care Med 1995; 151: 1866–1871.

73. Cordier J-F. Organising pneumonia. Thorax 2000; 55: 318–328.

74. Blasco CH, Hernandez IMS, Garrido VU et al. Safety of transbronchial biopsy in outpatients. Chest 1991; 99: 562–565.

75. Ahmad M, Livingston DR, Golish JA et al. The safety of outpatient transbronchial biopsy. Chest 1986; 90: 403–405.

76. Morris M, Peacock M, Mego D et al. The risk of hemorrhage from bronchoscopic lung biopsy due to pulmonary hypertension in interstitial lung disease. J Bronchol 1998; 5: 117–121.

77. Diette GB, Wiener CM, White P. The higher risk of bleeding in lung transplant recipients from bronchoscopy is independent of traditional bleeding risks. Chest 1999; 115: 397–402.

78. Oho K, Kato H, Ogawa J et al. A new needle for transfiberoptic bronchoscope use. Chest 1979; 76: 492.

79. Wang KP, Terry PB. Transbronchial needle aspiration in the diagnosis and staging of bronchogenic carcinoma. Am Rev Respir Dis 1983; 127: 344–347.

80. Schenk DA, Bower JH, Biyan CL et al. Transbronchial needle aspiration for staging bronchogenic carcinoma. Am Rev Respir Dis 1986; 134: 146–148.

81. Harrow EM, Oldenburg FA, Smith AM. Transbronchial needle aspiration in clinical practice. Thorax 1985; 40: 756–759.

82. Shure D, Fedullo PF. Transbronchial needle aspiration of peripheral masses. Am Rev Respir Dis 1983; 128: 1090–1092.

83. Wang KP, Haponik EF, Britt EJ. Transbronchial needle aspiration of peripheral pulmonary nodules. Chest 1984; 86: 819–823.

84. Wang KP, Britt EJ. Needle brush in the diagnosis of lung mass of nodule through flexible bronchoscopy. Chest 1991; 100: 1148–1150.

85. Dasgupta A, Metha AC, Wang KP. Transbronchial needle aspiration. Semin Respir Crit Care Med 1997; 18: 571–581.

86. Ndukwu J, Wang KP, Davis D et al. Direct smear for cytological examination of transbronchial needle aspiration specimens (abstract). Chest 1991; 100: 888.

87. Wang KP, Harrow EM. Transbronchial needle aspiration: a decade of experience. In: Feinsilver SH, Fein AM, ed. Textbook of bronchoscopy. Baltimore: Williams & Wilkins; 1995: 85–92.

88. Bilaceroglu S, Gunel O, Cagirici U et al. Comparison of endobronchial needle aspiration with forceps and brush biopsies in the diagnosis of endobronchial lung cancer. Monaldi Arch Chest Dis 1997; 52: 13–17.

89. Roberts SA. Obtaining tissue from the mediastinum: endoscopic ultrasound guided transoesophageal biopsy. Thorax 2000; 55: 983–985.

90. Schenk DA, Strollo PJ, Pickard JS et al. Utility of the Wang 18 gauge transbronchial histology needle in the staging of bronchogenic carcinoma. Chest 1989; 92: 271–274.

91. Vansteenkiste J, Lacquet LM, Demedts M et al. Transcarinal needle aspiration biopsy in the staging of lung cancer. Eur Respir J 1994; 7: 265–268.

92. Bilaceroglu S, Cagirici U, Günel Ö et al. Comparison of rigid and flexible transbronchial needle aspiration in the staging of bronchogenic carcinoma. Respiration 1998; 65: 441–449.

93. Shure D, Fedullo PF. The role of transcarinal needle aspiration in the staging of bronchogenic carcinoma. Chest 1984; 86: 693–696.

94. Utz JP, Patel AM, Edell ES. The role of transcarinal needle aspiration in the staging of bronchogenic carcinoma. Chest 1993; 104: 1012–1016.

95. Wang KP, Fuenning C, Johns CJ, Tery PB. Flexible transbronchial needle aspiration for diagnosis of sarcoidosis Ann Otol Rhinolaryngol 1989; 98: 298–300.

96. Morales CF, Patefield AJK, Strollo PJ, Schenk DA. Flexible transbronchial needle aspiration in the diagnosis of sarcoidosis. Chest 1995; 106: 709–711.

97. Fritzscher-Ravens A, Sriram PVJ, Topidis T et al. Diagnosing sarcoidosis using endosonography-guided fine needle aspiration. Chest 2000; 118: 928–935.

98. Kvale PA, Bode FR, Kini S. Diagnostic accuracy in lung cancer. Chest 1976; 69: 752–757.

99. McDougall JC, Cortese DA. Bronchoscopic biopsy and brushing with fluoroscopic guidance in nodular metastatic lung cancer. Chest 1981; 79: 610–611.

100. Mak VHF, Johnston IDA, Hetzel MR, Grubb C. Value of washings and brushings in fibreoptic bronchoscopy in the diagnosis of lung cancer. Thorax 1990; 45: 373–376.

101. Harrow E, Halber M, Hardy S, Halteman W. Bronchogenic and roentgenographic correlates of a positive transbronchial needle aspiration in the staging of lung cancer. Chest 1991; 100: 1592–1596.

102. Salathe M, Soler M, Bolliger CT et al. Tracheobronchial needle aspiration in routine fiberoptic bronchoscopy. Respiration 1992; 59: 5–8.

103. Fulkerson WJ. Current concepts: fiberoptic bronchoscopy. N Engl J Med 1984; 311: 511–515.

104. Credle WJ Jr, Smiddy JF, Elliott RC. Complications of fiberoptic bronchoscopy. Am Rev Respir Dis 1974; 109: 67–72.

105. Suratt PM, Smiddy JF, Gruper B. Deaths and complications associated with fiberoptic bronchoscopy. Chest 1976; 69: 747–751.

106. Simpson FG, Arnold AG, Purvis A et al. Postal survey of bronchoscopic practice by physicians in the United Kingdom. Thorax 1986; 41: 311–317.

107. Markus A, Häußinger K, Hauck RW, Kohlhäufl M. Bronchoskopie in Deutschland: Querschnittserhebung an 681 Institutionen. Pneumologie 2000; 54: 499–507.

108. Dweik RA, Metha AC, Meeker DP, Arroliga AC. Analysis of the safety of bronchoscopy after recent myocardial infarction. Chest 1996; 110: 825–828.

109. Dunaagan DP, Burke HC, Aquino SL et al. Fiberoptic bronchoscopy in coronary care unit patients: indications, safety and clinical implications. Chest 1998; 114: 1660–1667.

110. Dwamena BA, Sonnad SS, Angobaldo Jo et al. Metastases from non-small cell lung cancer: mediastinal staging in the 1990s – meta-analytic comparison of PET and CT. Radiology 1999; 213: 530–536.

111. Wernecke K, Peters P. Mediastinale Sonographie. Dtsch Ärztebl 1993; 90: 506–514.

112. Becker HD. Endobronchialer ultraschall – eine neue Perspektive in der Bronchologie. Ultraschall Med 1996; 17: 106–112.

113. Becker HD, Herth F. Endobronchial ultrasound of the airways and the mediastinum. In: Bolliger CT, Mathur PN, ed. Interventional bronchoscopy. Basel: S Karger; 2000: 80–93.

114. Ono R, Hirano H, Egawa S, Suemasu K. Bronchoscopic ultrasonography and brachytherapy in roentgenologically occult bronchogenic carcinoma. J Bronchol 1994; 1: 281–287.

115. Shannon JJ, Bude RO, Orens JB et al. Endobronchial ultrasound-guided needle aspiration of mediastinal adenopathy. Am J Respir Crit Care Med 1996; 153: 1424–1430.

116. Sato M, Saito Y, Nagamoto N et al. Diagnostic value of differential brushing of all branches of bronchi in patients with sputum-positive or suspected positive for lung cancer. Acta Cytol 1993; 37: 879–883.

117. Hung J, Lam S, Le Riche JC, Palcic B. Autofluorescence of normal and malignant bronchial tissue. Lasers Surg Med 1991; 11: 99–105.

118. Qu J, MacAulay C, Lam S, Palcic B. Laser-induced fluorescence spectroscopy at endoscopy: tissue optics, Monte Carlo modeling, and in vivo measurements. Optic Eng 1995; 34: 3334–3343.

119. Lam S, MacAulay C, Hung J, LeRiche J. Detection of dysplasia and carcinoma in situ with a lung imaging fluorescence device. J Thorac Cardiovasc Surg 1993; 106: 1035–1040.

120. Leonhard M. New incoherent autofluorescence/fluorescence system for early detection of lung cancer. Diagn Ther Endosc 1999; 5: 71–75.

121. Häußinger K, Pichler J, Stanzel F et al. Autofluorescence bronchoscopy. In: Bolliger CT, Mathur PN, ed. Interventional bronchoscopy. Basel: S Karger; 2000: 243–251.

122. Khanavkar M, Il KK, Okunaka T et al. Early detection of bronchial lesions using system of autofluorescence endoscopy (SAFE 1000). Diagn Ther Endosc 1999; 5: 99–104.

123. Lam S, Kennedy T, Unger M et al. Localization of bronchial intraepithelial neoplastic lesions by fluorescence bronchoscopy. Chest 1998; 113: 696–702.

124. Venmans BJW, van Boxem AJM, Smit EF et al. Results of two years experience with fluorescence bronchoscopy in detection of bronchial neoplasia. Diagn Ther Endosc 1999; 5: 77–84.

125. Horvath T, Horvathova M, Salajka F et al. Detection of bronchial neoplasia in uranium miners by autofluorescence endoscopy (SAFE 1000). Diagn Ther Endosc 1999; 5: 91–98.

126. Häußinger K, Stanzel F, Huber RM et al. Autofluorescence detection of bronchial tumors with the D-Light/AF. Diagn Ther Endosc 1999; 5: 105–115.

127. Khanavkar B. Autofluorescence bronchoscopy. J Bronchol 2000; 7: 60–66.

128. Gladish GW, Haponik EF. Virtual bronchoscopy. In: Bolliger CT, Mathur PN, ed. Interventional bronchoscopy. Basel: S Karger; 2000: 253–266.

129. Lacrosse M, Trigauz JP, Van Beers BE, Weynants P. 3D spiral CT of the tracheobronchial tree. J Comput Assist Tomogr 1995; 19: 341–347.

130. Summers RM, Aggarwal NR, Sneller MC et al. CT virtual bronchoscopy of the central airways in patients with Wegener's granulomatosis. Chest 2002; 121: 242–250.

131. Fleiter T, Merkle EM, Aschoff AJ et al. Comparison of real-time virtual and fiberoptic bronchoscopy in patients with bronchial carcinoma. Opportunities and limitations. AJR 1997; 169: 1591–1595.

132. Lee KS, Yoon JH, Kim TK et al. Evaluation of tracheobronchial disease with helical CT with multiplanar and three-dimensional reconstruction correlation with bronchoscopy. Radiographics 1997; 17: 555–570.

133. Vinning DJ, Ferretti G, Stelts DR et al. Mediastinal lymph node mapping using spiral CT and three-dimensional reconstructions in patients with lung cancer: preliminary observations. J Bronchol 1997; 4: 18–25.

134. McAdams HP, Goodman PC, Kussin P. Virtual bronchoscopy for directing transbronchial needle aspiration of hilar and mediastinal lymph nodes: A pilot study. AJR 1998; 170: 1361–1364.

135. Zwischenberger JB, Wittich GR, van Sonnenberg E et al. Airway simulation to guide stent placement for tracheobronchial obstruction in lung cancer. Ann Thorac Surg 1997; 64: 1619–1625.

10.1B Therapeutic bronchoscopy

Chris T Bolliger and Karl Häussinger

Key points

- The scope of therapeutic bronchoscopy has evolved dramatically over the last two decades.

- Originally it was limited to simple therapeutic lavage and removal of foreign bodies.

- Now it is mainly applied in the treatment of central airway obstruction of malignant and less frequently of benign origin.

- Both the rigid and the flexible bronchoscope are being used successfully for all techniques.

- Endoscopic methods to detect and to treat early central lung cancer are currently being tested.

Since its introduction, rigid bronchoscopy has been used both for therapeutic and increasingly for diagnostic purposes. Over the last four decades the flexible bronchoscope has gradually replaced the rigid instrument in many institutions for all diagnostic procedures. Over the last 15 years, however, more and more therapeutic procedures have been developed that have led to a revival of the rigid instrument. Currently, many different techniques, some competitive, some complementary in nature, are being practised with increasing frequency. It is the purpose of this chapter to discuss old and new therapeutic techniques that use the flexible and/or the rigid instrument.

Indications for therapeutic bronchoscopy

Lavage and aspiration of secretions

Tenacious or copious bronchial secretions may lead to atelectasis and respiratory failure. Bronchoscopic aspiration or bronchial toilet of such secretions is indicated whenever patients are unable to actively expectorate them and attempts at mobilising them through intensive chest physiotherapy have failed. This situation classically arises postoperatively, especially after laparotomy of the upper abdomen or after high spinal injuries leading to paralysis of the intercostal musculature and/or the diaphragm. Patients with advanced chronic obstructive pulmonary disease (COPD) with an ineffective cough mechanism due to bronchial collapse and those with refractory severe asthma can both experience relief of airway obstruction through endoscopic aspiration of impacted mucus. However, the use of bronchoscopy in asthma remains controversial. A flexible instrument with a large working channel (diameter 2.8 mm or more) will be adequate for aspiration of most types of secretions. Only rarely does one have to resort to rigid bronchoscopy, which provides the most efficient suction of the central airways. Bronchoscopic aspiration of large quantities of purulent secretions from pulmonary abscesses or irreversibly damaged bronchi in bronchiectasis facilitates drainage and may prevent damage from persisting contamination of healthy areas of the lung.

A further indication for bronchoscopy is clearing the airway after aspiration of food or gastric contents, which should be performed on an emergency basis to avoid severe pneumonia.[1] Massive haemoptysis is another indication for bronchoscopy, that can be life-saving.[2] The choice of the flexible or the rigid instrument will primarily depend on the experience of the bronchoscopist and the available equipment. When working with the flexible bronchoscope, patients often have to be intubated to guarantee adequate ventilation. If double-lumen endotracheal tubes are chosen, one-lung ventilation can be maintained while the other lung is cleaned and inspected for the origin of the haemoptysis. If the active bleeding site can be identified the corresponding bronchus can be effectively blocked by a balloon.[3] Unfortunately, large-channel flexible bronchoscopes cannot readily be passed down through double-lumen tubes because their inner diameters are too small. In life-threatening circumstances, many endoscopists therefore prefer the rigid bronchoscope, which provides better visibility and allows rapid aspiration of even massive blood clots and better control of active bleeding.

Therapeutic bronchoalveolar lavage

Therapeutic bronchoalveolar lavage (BAL) has been proposed for the removal of any pathological material within the airways or alveoli, ranging from the lipoprotein found in alveolar proteinosis, through viscid mucus in asthma and cystic fibrosis to inhaled radioactive dust.[4,5] Under these circumstances, BAL is best described as whole-lung lavage (WLL). It is performed under general anaesthesia, using a double-lumen endotracheal tube, and employs very large volumes of lavage fluid (in the range of 5–10 litres). WLL is effective in alveolar proteinosis[4,6] but its role in other conditions remains unproven.[4]

As well as WLL, true therapeutic BAL via the fibreoptic bronchoscope has been tried in cystic fibrosis and refractory asthma. The effects in cystic fibrosis are at best modest[7] and there seems little indication for such a procedure in a chronic condition, particularly as other mucolytic therapies are becoming available. Therapeutic BAL in patients with acute severe asthma is potentially detrimental and, in spite of an early vogue,[8] has not become established practice. However, therapeutic BAL may have a limited role in less severely ill patients who are slow to respond to therapy as a result of persistent mucus plugging.[4,9]

Bronchoscopy in the intensive care unit

Fibreoptic bronchoscopy can be performed with relative ease in patients receiving mechanical ventilation for both diagnostic and therapeutic purposes.[10-12] The bronchoscope can be passed through the suction port of the endotracheal tube and special adaptors are available that will provide an airtight seal around the bronchoscope. The F_IO_2 should be increased to 1.0 during the procedure. The presence of the bronchoscope within the endotracheal tube creates a high resistance annulus through which air flow is turbulent. Inflation of the lungs can usually be achieved without difficulty; expiratory flow may, however, be severely limited.[13,14] The additional auto-PEEP (positive end-expiratory pressure) that this creates may lead to increased gas trapping, adversely affecting the patient's gas exchange and circulation, and the higher inflation pressures that are required may lead to pulmonary barotrauma.[12] These effects may be minimised by increasing the expiratory time and accepting temporary hypercapnia, while maintaining oxygenation.

In general, the smallest possible bronchoscope should be passed through the largest endotracheal tube for the shortest possible time. If a small endotracheal tube is in place the cuff should be deflated and the bronchoscope inserted alongside. The cuff is then reinflated with the bronchoscope in place. In paediatric patients, even a bronchoscope with a diameter of less than 4 mm will cause almost total obstruction of the airway and it has been suggested that it should not remain in the endotracheal tube for more than 30–40 seconds.[15]

Lavage and aspiration of bronchial secretions under direct vision with the fibreoptic bronchoscope may be beneficial in the management of critically ill patients but its use for this remains controversial and it has not been shown to be better than chest physiotherapy in re-expanding areas of atelectasis.[16,17] The fibreoptic bronchoscope has also been used to aid difficult intubation of patients in intensive care units, and the various techniques that can be used for this have been reviewed.[18]

Removal of foreign bodies

Successful removal of foreign bodies has been a mainstay of therapeutic bronchoscopy since its inception. The large majority (94%) of patients presenting with inhaled foreign bodies are under 15 years of age. A useful algorithm for the management of suspected foreign bodies for children has recently been published.[19] In adults the choice of the flexible or the rigid instrument depends on the type of foreign body, the preference of the endoscopist and the available infrastructure.[20] As a general rule, airway control and protection of the airway walls is superior with the rigid instrument. Larger foreign bodies, and especially objects with cutting edges and needles, can be removed more easily and less traumatically with the rigid bronchoscope. Even if a foreign body cannot be removed through the scope, one can pull part of it into the tip of the barrel and then remove both instrument and foreign body at the same time, thus protecting the airway walls and vocal cords. Needles are most often aspirated with the head down and the tip is usually lodged in the mucosa after several forceful attempts at coughing them up or unsuccessful endoscopic manipulation. In this situation the needle tip will have to be freed by pushing the needle more into the periphery; then advance the tip of the rigid bronchoscope over it and finally remove scope and needle simultaneously.

In recent years a lot of different devices such as snares, loops, baskets, forceps and balloon catheters have been developed that allow removal of foreign bodies with the flexible scope, where before only the rigid instrument was thought to be successful. However, any patient with a foreign body that cannot be removed easily with an initial attempt by fibreoptic bronchoscopy should be transferred to a specialised centre where both flexible and rigid bronchoscopy are performed routinely.[20]

Palliative treatment of central airway obstruction

The distinction between benign and malignant causes of central airway obstruction is of paramount importance. Benign disorders leading to central airway obstruction are mostly granulomatous lesions or strictures due to inflammatory processes. Classically this occurs after prolonged intubation. On the other hand, foreign bodies, or infectious diseases such as tuberculosis, can lead to the formation of obstructing granulomata. Rarer causes are benign airway tumours, such as hamartomas, lipomas, typical carcinoids and others.[21] Extrinsic benign airway compression is rare and usually due to aberrant vessels or enlarged inflamed mediastinal lymph nodes. Another type is dynamic obstruction of unstable airways in tracheomalacia. This is caused by either postintubation destruction of cartilage or highly collapsible airways in patients with advanced COPD. In many instances, surgery is the correct approach; however, there are a number of situations, such as a web-like tracheal postintubation stenosis,[21,22] or benign lesions in patients who are unable or unwilling to undergo surgery, where endoscopic measures can be just as effective and more elegant than surgery.

The large majority of patients with central airway obstruction, however, suffer from malignant disease and, because of the localisation and type of their malignancy, are not candidates for surgery. Even after curative resection, many patients with bronchogenic carcinoma unfortunately suffer recurrence, a substantial proportion of which occurs locally in the chest. Classically, these patients are offered radio- or chemotherapy or a combination of both. The recent emergence of a variety of therapeutic endoscopic techniques, discussed below, makes obstructing lesions of the central airways amenable to local endoscopic treatment. A high degree of obstruction at bronchial or tracheal level leads to dyspnoea, atelectasis or postobstructive pneumonia of the lung parenchyma distal to the obstruction. These complications are often considered at least partial contraindications for radio- or chemotherapy as they can be aggravated by the side effects of these treatment modalities. It is therefore desirable to establish airway patency first to achieve rapid symptom relief.[23]

There are three main types of malignant central airway obstruction: intraluminal, usually by tumour growth, extraluminal by compression from lymph node tumours, and mixed obstructions, which are a combination of both (Fig. 10.1.12). The latter often exhibit quite a marked degree of intramural tumour growth as well. Depending on the type of obstruction and the available equipment, different endoscopic treatment modalities can be chosen; they are discussed in detail below.

Modalities with immediate effect

Laser resection

Laser resection has become the method most frequently used worldwide to treat malignant and benign endoluminal lesions.[21]

The most widely used type of laser is the neodynium–yttrium–aluminium–garnet (Nd:YAG) laser, which has a wavelength of 1064 nm. This laser can be conducted through a flexible catheter, making it easy to use during both flexible and rigid bronchoscopy. As the beam is in the invisible range, an additional helium pilot laser beam in the red light range is added. The technique of endobronchial resection is to use the laser for coagulation purposes only, which entails the use of low-energy impulses (20 W for 0.8–1.0 s). With this technique the tissue to be resected is devitalised by coagulation of the blood supply. The visible effect is 'blanching' of the tissue. If the energy is too high, tissue is immediately carbonised and turns black, which leads to superficial absorption of subsequent laser impulses and lack of tissue penetration. The devitalised tissue is removed mechanically with a forceps or sheared off with the tip of the rigid bronchoscope. Bleeding after removal of tumour masses is again stopped by laser coagulation.

The main advantage of the laser is its immediate effect, making it feasible for virtually all situations and hence very popular (Table 10.1.7). In experienced hands it has very few complications and can be repeated many times. An important limitations, however, is the danger of endobronchial fires in the presence of oxygen concentrations exceeding 40% (50% represents the uppermost limit).[24] In everyday practice this rarely excludes the method but good cooperation between endoscopic surgeon and anesthetist is of vital importance.[25] Laser resection is often used in combination with other endoscopic treatment modalities such as brachytherapy and stent placement. In highly stenotic lesions, for instance, it is used first to re-establish the lumen, which is necessary for the passage of a brachytherapy catheter or the insertion of a stent.

Electrocautery, argon plasma coagulation

Electrocautery or diathermy can be used for the resection of endobronchial (= endoluminal) lesions (Fig. 10.1.12). The method is time-honoured, simple and cheap.[26] Experienced

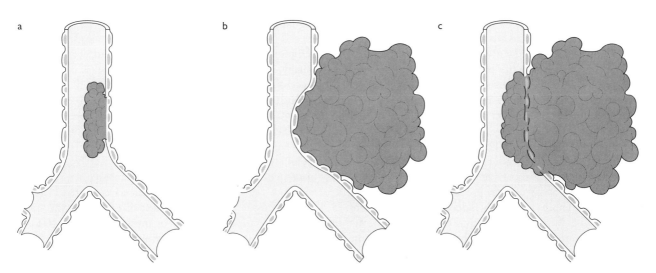

Fig. 10.1.12   Schematic illustration of the three main types of malignant central airway obstruction shown at the tracheal level with identical degrees of narrowing of the lumen. (a) Intraluminal, (b) extraluminal and (c) mixed obstruction.

Table 10.1.7 Indication for endoscopic therapeutic modalities in the three basic types of endobronchial stenosis

Procedure	Endobronchial lesion	Extrinsic lesion	Mixed lesion
Laser	+	−	+
Electrocautery	+	−	+
Cryotherapy	+*	−	+*
Brachytherapy	+*	−	+*
Argon plasma coagulator	+	−	+
Photodynamic therapy	+*	−	+*
Stents	−	+	+†

* Contraindicated in impending respiratory failure. † Indicated if postinterventional airway lumen is less than 50% of normal.

endoscopists using both rigid and flexible probes claim diathermy to be equal to laser resection.[27] The necessary precautions to avoid electrical hazard must be taken. A newer technique is argon plasma coagulation.[28] Successfully used for haemostasis in open surgery, argon plasma coagulation is now available with rigid or flexible probe for gastrointestinal and tracheobronchial use. A high-frequency electric current is transmitted to the tissue via a continuous flow of ionised argon gas (= plasma) blown out of the catheter tip. The electric arch reaches from the tip of the probe to the nearest tissue, which will be coagulated without direct contact. The great advantage of argon plasma coagulation is the limited tissue penetration, 2–3 mm in depth, which prevents perforation of airway walls.[29,30] It clearly presents the best tool for haemostasis as the effect on flowing blood results in immediate coagulation. For this indication it is superior to the Nd:YAG-laser and the equipment is much cheaper. For these reasons, argon plasma coagulation has a promising future in the area of therapeutic endoscopy.

Dilatation

Malignant or benign stenoses of the central airways, defined as reaching from the trachea to the lobar and even segmental bronchi, can be dilated directly with increasing diameters of rigid bronchoscope or more gently with bougies or balloons. The effect is immediate and, at the tracheal level, often life-saving; at the bronchial level, postobstructive atelectasis and/or pneumonia can be treated in this way. Benign tracheal stenoses occurring after prolonged intubation or tracheostemies are often web-like and can be managed by radial laser resection followed by gentle balloon dilatation.[22] This procedure can obviate the need to operate. As a general rule, however, surgery should always be considered for more complex benign obstructions of the central airways, as endoscopic procedures are often second-best. Malignant stenoses are mostly inoperable and are therefore ideally suited to endoscopic treatment. Dilatation is indicated in all cases in which the obstruction of the airway has a significant extraluminal component (Fig. 10.1.12). Unfortunately the effect of pure dilatation rarely lasts for more than a few days, necessitating further endoscopic or tumour-specific treatment (Fig. 10.1.13).

Stents or endoprostheses

Obstructions of the major airways that are primarily of an extraluminal or extrinsic nature (Fig. 10.1.12) and stenoses that are due to collapsible airways resulting from loss of cartilaginous support are not amenable to any of the aforementioned endoscopic treatment modalities. Simple dilatation can be successful in certain benign conditions; however, malignant stenoses, which represent the majority of cases of extraluminal compression, invariably recur a few days after dilatation. Therefore compressed or unstable airways have to be supported with endoprostheses or stents. There has been a tremendous amount of technical development in this area and a variety of different models of stent are commercially available. There are basically two different types: metal and silicone stents. The most widely used stent is the silicone stent designed by Dumon in Marseille. It can be easily inserted and removed, even after years.[31–33] Its disadvantages are the fact that in short, conical or curvilinear stenoses it often migrates and that airways that cannot be dilated to at least 10 mm in diameter are too narrow for the insertion of the delivery device.

For these situations metal stents are ideal as they fit any airway diameter snugly and their application devices generally do not exceed 5 mm in diameters. These stents consist of various types of more or less densely woven wire struts or meshes and are usually inserted under fluoroscopic control. Currently, the most successful metal stent design is the Ultraflex.[34]

Both silicone and metal stents have been shown to lead to dramatic improvement in dyspnoea.[35,36] The most important stent-related complications are migration, retention of secretions and formation of granulomata at their ends. In general, metal stents are more difficult to remove than silicone stents; placement is therefore often permanent.

When the area of the main carina is obstructed, it is very often necessary to stent the most distal part of the trachea and both main bronchi as well. For these situations Y-stents have to be used; the best known types are the Hood stent,[37] the dynamic stent designed by Freitag[38] and the Dumon Y-model.[39] The specific stent to be used will have to meet the individual patient's situation and very often the decision can only be made during therapeutic endoscopy.

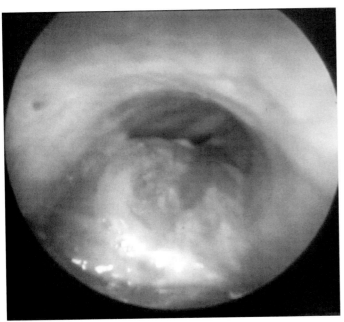
(a)

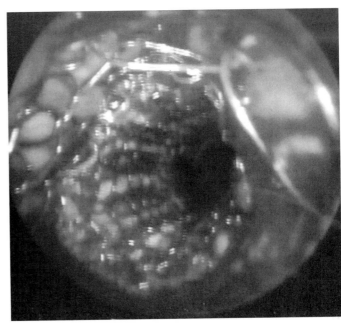
(b)

Fig. 10.1.13   (a) Subtotal occlusion of the trachea by oesophageal tumour pressing on the posterior membrane – patient with life-threatening dyspnoea. (b) Patent tracheal lumen after dilatation with balloon and rigid bronchoscope and subsequent placement of covered Ultraflex stent – disappearance of dyspnoea.

Modalities with delayed effect

Cryotherapy

Cryotherapy is the therapeutic application of extreme cold for local destruction of living tissue. In contrast to laser or electro-cautery, cryodestruction is delayed, occurring from a few hours to a few days under application. Commonly used cryogens are nitrous oxide (N_2O) and liquid nitrogen (N_2).

Cryotherapy exploits the cooling caused by the rapid expansion of liquid gas to freeze the tip of the cryoprobe (Joule–Thompson effect) at a temperature of about −40°C. The cryoprobe is placed on or inserted into the lesion twice or three times to apply repeated cycles of freezing and thawing at the same location before moving to an adjacent site. The effect of freezing/thawing cycles can be monitored either visually or by impedance measurement. The duration of freezing is between 30 and 60 seconds. The thawing time depends upon the type of probe, ranging from a few seconds with a rigid probe to up to 60 seconds with a flexible probe.

A repeat bronchoscopy is usually performed within one week to remove slough tissue and repeat treatment if necessary. Cryotherapy can be safely performed in a high-oxygen environment. It is used mainly for palliation of non-critical endo-bronchial exophytic obstructive lesions and to remove foreign bodies and clots. Other indications may include treatment of low-grade malignant lesions (e.g. adenoid cystic carcinoma) and early cancer (e.g. carcinoma-in-situ).[40–42]

Photodynamic therapy

Photodynamic therapy involves an intravenously administered photosensitiser, which, when exposed to light of the proper wavelength and in the presence of oxygen, causes cell death.[43,44] The method makes use of the fact that certain photosensitisers are preferentially absorbed in tumour tissue when applied intravenously.

Photofrin II (dihaematoporphyrin ester) is the only photosensitiser that has received widespread approval so far for the treatment of lung cancer. The compound is activated by a laser light source of 630 nm wavelength. The treatment fibres used to deliver the light are quartz fibres configured as diffusers for cylindrical or interstitial treatment areas, or as a micro lens for focused surface treatments. A dose of 2–3 mg is injected intravenously 48 hours before therapy. The patient then undergoes bronchoscopy and the area of abnormality is illuminated with light of the appropriate wavelength. The light is delivered in a superficial or interstitial manner (insertion of the probe in the tumour) as needed for homogeneous delivery to target tissue. The effects are not immediate but occur within 48 hours. Therefore, a clean-up bronchoscopy is needed for patients with obstructive lesions. Repeated illumination can be delivered if necessary.

Photodynamic therapy can be used with curative intent for superficial tumours (depth of 5 mm).[45] This makes it an elegant treatment modality for the management of multicentric superficial carcinomas and for patients who are deemed inoperable because of insufficient cardiopulmonary reserves. Another indication for photodynamic therapy is palliation of symptoms caused by central airway obstruction due to late-stage cancer. Like cryotherapy, photodynamic therapy has no immediate effect and it is therefore not feasible as a method for emergency desobstruction of vital airway stenoses.

The major complication of photodynamic therapy is skin photosensitivity, which can occur up to 4–6 weeks after injection. Local airway oedema, tumour necrosis and delayed strictures can cause airway obstruction. Newer photosensitisers such as *m*-tetrahydroxyphenylchlorine (*m*-THPC) or δ-aminolevulinic acid (ALA), which cause less skin sensitisation, are currently being investigated.

Brachytherapy

In contrast to external beam radiation the term 'brachytherapy' is used for radiotherapy whose effect is limited to a very short distance from the source (*brachys* = Greek 'short').[46,47] In the tracheobronchial tree, brachytherapy is performed via an endoscopically placed catheter through which the radioactive probe is advanced. The preferred mode today is high-dose-rate application of iridium-192, which is a very small source of about 1 mm in diameter, allowing its placement through the working channel of a flexible bronchoscope. The distance to be irradiated is measured endoscopically and the radiation dose is calculated by computer. High-dose-rate application has the advantage that one session lasts only a few minutes and can be performed as an outpatient procedure under local anaesthesia. To avoid long term side effects such as haemoptysis and bronchial fistulae, the total dose is usually fractionated and applied in three sessions of 7.5 Gy each measured at 1 cm from the source.[48]

Brachytherapy should be reserved for the treatment of malignancies and is often combined with other endoscopic treatment modalities such as laser resection and stent placement. A major advantage of brachytherapy is its feasibility in patients who have already undergone full-dose external-beam irradiation. Disadvantages are the delayed effect (2–3 weeks), which makes this type of treatment not feasible for emergency intervention; further, the equipment is expensive, which makes this treatment option only feasible for big institutions, preferably with other indications for brachytherapy such as gynaecological or ear, nose and throat cancers.

Gene therapy

The lung is a readily accessible target organ for gene therapy. Viral vectors (e.g. retroviruses, adenoviruses, herpesviruses) and non-viral vectors (e.g. liposomes, 'naked' DNA, protein–DNA complexes) have been used. The two most important areas of pulmonary disease for which in-vivo study results exist are cystic fibrosis and lung cancer. In cystic fibrosis the early results were disappointing but rapid progress in vector technology may lead to a breakthrough for a gene therapy approach for cystic fibrosis in this decade.[49] In lung cancer some encouraging results have been reported by studies using wild-type *p53* gene transfer in patients with advanced disease.[50,51] However, it must be emphasised that, so far, gene therapy for human disease is still in an investigational stage and has not formally proved its efficacy.

Curative treatment of early lung cancer

Endoscopically visible lesions ranging from carcinoma-in-situ to invasive carcinoma not extending beyond the airway wall are usually termed 'early'. If lesions are detected at that stage the chance of cure is up to 95%. Unfortunately such lesions are rarely detected because they hardly ever cause symptoms. They are fortuitous discoveries during bronchoscopy performed for various other reasons or are detected additionally to another lung cancer for which bronchoscopy was performed. There is increasing evidence that endoscopic treatment can be curative for these lesions.[52,53] A precondition for cure by endoscopy is proof, by computed tomography, magnetic resonance imging or endobronchial ultrasound, that the tumour is limited to the airway wall and that there are no lymph-node metastases.

Currently the first-line approach to such lesions is still surgery, with at least a sleeve resection of the involved airway. In patients deemed inoperable because of lack of cardiopulmonary reserves, multiple synchronous lung cancer or simple unwillingness to undergo major thoracic surgery, bronchoscopic treatment with curative intent has been used successfully, using various treatment modalities. To date the place of curative endoscopic treatment of early lung cancer is uncertain as there are no prospective trials comparing cure rates, and thus survival, between surgically and endoscopically treated patients.

Clinical relevance

■ Relieving central airway obstruction invariably results in immediate improvement of respiratory symptoms, provided that the lung parenchyma distal to the obstruction is functional.

■ Treating early lung cancer, defined as carcinoma-in-situ and microinvasive carcinoma not extending beyond the cartilaginous layer of the airway wall, might well become the domain of therapeutic bronchoscopy.

? Unresolved questions

■ There are very few prospective studies comparing various competitive techniques to relieve central airway obstruction (e.g. laser resection versus electrocautery for intraluminal tumours, or brachytherapy versus photodynamic therapy for intramural tumours)

■ What is the long-term compatibility – defined as several years – of metal stents used to relieve extrinsic airway compression?

■ Should endoscopic treatment precede chemo/radiotherapy in untreated malignant central airway obstruction that is not immediately life threatening?

■ Will endoscopic treatment of early lung cancer be equal to surgical resection?

■ Does bronchoscopic gene therapy have a future?

References

1. Lomotan JR, George SS, Brandstetter RD. Aspiration pneumonia. Strategies for early recognition and prevention. Postgrad Med 1997; 102: 225–226.

2. Jean-Baptiste E. Clinical assessment and management of massive hemoptysis. Crit Care Med 2000; 28: 1642–1647.

3. Freitag L, Telkof E, Stamatis G et al. Three years experience with a new balloon catheter for the management of haemoptysis. Eur Respir J 1994; 7: 2033–2037.

4. Danel C, Israel-Biet D, Costabel U, Klech H. Therapeutic applications of bronchoalveolar lavage. Eur Respir J 1992; 5: 1173.

5. Klech H, Hutter C. Clinical guidelines and indications for bronchoalveolar lavage (BAL): report of the European Society of Pneumology Task Group on BAL. Eur Respir J 1990; 3: 937.

6. Du Bois RM, McAllister WAC, Branthwaite MA Alveolar proteinosis: diagnosis and treatment over a ten year period. Thorax 1983; 38: 360.

7. Ewing CW. Role of the fibreoptic bronchoscope in lung lavage of patients with cystic fibrosis. Chest 1978; 5(suppl): 750.

8. Beach FXM, Williams NE. Bronchial lavage in status asthmaticus. A long term review after treatment. Anaesthesia 1970; 25: 378.

9. Lang DM, Simon RA, Mathison DA et al. Safety and possible efficacy of fibreoptic bronchoscopy with lavage in the management of refractory asthma with mucous impaction. Ann Allergy 1991; 67: 324.

10. Olopade CO, Prakash UBS. Bronchoscopy in the critical care unit. Mayo Clin Proc 1989; 64: 1255.

11. Turner JS, Willcox PA, Hayhurst MD, Potgieter PD. Fibreoptic bronchoscopy in the intensive care unit: a prospective study of 147 procedures in 107 patients. Crit Care Med 1993; 22: 259.

12. Jolliet P, Chevrolet JC. Bronchoscopy in the intensive care unit. Intens Care Med 1992; 18: 160.

13. Lindholm CE, Ollman B, Snyder JV et al. Cardiorespiratory effects of flexible fibreoptic bronchoscopy in critically ill patients. Chest 1978; 74: 362.

14. Matsushima Y, Jones RL, King EG et al. Alterations in pulmonary mechanics and gas exchange during routine fibreoptic bronchoscopy. Chest 1984; 86: 184.

15. De Blie J, Scheinmann P. Fibreoptic bronchoscopy in infants. Arch Dis Child 1992; 67: 159.

16. Marini JJ, Pierson DJ, Hudson LD. Acute lobar atelectasis: a prospective comparison of fibreoptic bronchoscopy and respiratory therapy. Am Rev Respir Dis 1979; 119: 971.

17. Luksza AR, Smith P, Coakley J et al. Acute severe asthma treated by mechanical ventilation: 10 years experience from a district general hospital. Thorax 1986; 41: 459.

18. Dellinger RP. Fibreoptic bronchoscopy in adult airway management. Crit Care Med 1987; 18: 88.

19. Martinot A, Closser M, Marquette CH et al. Indications for flexible versus rigid bronchoscopy in children with suspected foreign-body aspiration. Am J Respir Crit Care Med 1997; 155: 1676–79.

20. Marquette CH, Martinot A. Foreign body removal in adults and children. In: Bolliger CT, Mathur PN, ed. Interventional bronchoscopy. Progress in Respiratory Research 30. Basel: S Karger; 2000; 96–107.

21. Cavaliere S, Dumon JF. Laser bronchoscopy. In: Bolliger CT, Mathur PN, ed. Interventional bronchoscopy. Progress in Respiratory Research 30. Basel: S Karger; 2000; 108–119.

22. Mehta AC, Lee FY, Cordasco EM et al. Concentric tracheal and subglottic stenosis. Management using the Nd-YAG laser for mucosal sparing followed by gentle balloon dilatation. Chest 1993; 104: 673–677.

23. Bolliger CT. Multimodality treatment of advanced pulmonary malignancies. In: Bolliger CT, Mathur PN, ed. Interventional bronchoscopy. Progress in Respiratory Research 30. Basel: S Karger; 2000; 187–196.

24. Bolliger CT, Probst R, Tschopp K et al. Silicon-Endoprothesen in der Behandlung von tracheo-bronchialen Stenosen. Schweiz Med Wschr 1991; 121: 1283–1288.

25. Studer W, Bolliger CT, Biro P. Anesthesia for interventional bronchoscopy. n: Bolliger CT, Mathur PN, ed. Interventional bronchoscopy. Progress in Respiratory Research 30. Basel: S Karger; 2000; 44–54.

26. Coulter TD, Mehta AC. The heat is on impact of endobronchial electrosurgery on the need for Nd-YAG laser photoresection. Chest 2000; 118: 516–521.

27. Boxem TV, Muller M, Venmans B et al. Nd-YAG laser vs bronchoscopic electrocautery for palliation of symptomatic airway obstruction: a cost-effectiveness study. Chest 1999; 116: 1108–1112.

28. Sutedja T, Bolliger CT. Endobronchial electrocautery and argon plasma coagulation. In: Bolliger CT, Mathur PN, ed. Interventional bronchoscopy. Progress in Respiratory Research 30. Basel: S Karger; 2000; 120–132.

29. Farin G, Grund KE. Technology of argon-plasma coagulation with particular regard to endoscopic applications: endoscopic surgery and allied technologies. Endosc Surg Allied Technol 1994; 2: 71–77.

30. Storek D, Grund KE, Schutz A et al. Argon-Plasma-Koagulation (APC) in der flexiblen Endoskopie – Kann sie den Laser ersetzen? Endosk Heute 1994; 2: 163–170.

31. Dumon JF. A dedicated tracheobronchial stent. Chest 1990; 97: 328–332.

32. Bolliger CT, Probst R, Tschopp K et al. Silicone stents in the management of inoperable tracheobronchial stenoses: indications, limitations. Chest 1993; 104: 1653–1659.

33. Dumon JF, Cavaliere S, Diaz-Jimenez JP et al. Seven-year experience with the Dumon prosthesis. J Bronchol 1996; 3: 6–109.

34. Miyazawa T, Yamakido M, Ikeda S et al. Implantation of ultraflex nitinol stents in malignant tracheobronchial stenoses. Chest 2000; 118: 959–965.

35. Vergnon JM, Costes F, Bayon MC, Emonot A. Efficacy of tracheal and bronchial stent placement on respiratory functional tests. Chest 1995; 107: 741–746.

36. Bolliger CT, Heitz M, Hauser R et al. An Airway Wallstent of the treatment of tracheobronchial malignancies. Thorax 1996; 51: 1127–1129.

37. Westaby S, Jackson JW, Pearson FG. A bifurcated silicon rubber stent for relief of tracheobronchial obstruction. J Thorax Cardiovasc Surg 1982; 83: 414–417.

38. Freitag L, Eicker R, Linz B, Greschuchna D. Theoretical and experimental basis for the development of a dynamic airway stent. Eur Respir J 1994; 7: 2038–2045.

39. Dumon JF, Dumon MC. Dumon–Novatech Y-stents. A four-year experience with 50 tracheobronchial tumors involving the carina. J Bronchol 2000; 7: 26–32.

40. Homasson JP, Renault P, Angebault M et al. Bronchoscopic cryotherapy for airway strictures caused by tumors. Chest 1986; 90: 159–164.

41. Marasso A, Gallo E, Massaglia GM et al. Cryosurgery in bronchoscopic treatment of tracheobronchial stenosis. Chest 1993; 103: 472–474.

42. Mathur PN, Wolf KM, Busk MF et al. Fiberoptic bronchoscope cryotherapy in the management of tracheobronchial obstruction. Chest 1996; 110: 718–723.

43. Cortese DA, Kinsey JH. Hematoporphyrin derivative phototherapy in the treatment of bronchogenic carcinoma. Chest 1984; 86: 8–13.

44. Marcus SL, Dugan MH. Global status of clinical photodynamic therapy: The registration process for a new therapy. Lasers Surg Med 1992; 12: 318–24.

45. Edell ES, Cortese DA. Bronchoscopic phototherapy with hematoporphyrin derivative for treatment of localized bronchogenic carcinoma: a 5-year experience. Mayo Clin Proc 1987; 62: 8–14.

46. Macha HN, Koch K, Stadler M et al. New technique for treating occlusive and stenosing tumors of the trachea and main bronchi: endobronchial irradiation by high dose iridium-192 combined with laser canalisation. Thorax 1987; 42: 511–515.

47. Mehta M, Shahabi S, Jarjour N et al. Effect of endobronchial radiation therapy on malignant bronchial obstruction. Chest 1990; 97: 662–665.

48. Speisedr BL, Spratling L. Remote afterloading brachytherapy for the local control of endobronchial carcinoma. Int J Radiat Oncol Biol Phys 1993; 25: 579–587.

49. Alton EW, Geddes DM, Gill DR et al. Towards gene therapy for cystic fibrosis. A clinical progress report. Gene Ther 1998; 5: 291–292.

50. Schuler M, Rochlitz CF, Horowitz JA et al. A phase 1 study of adenovirus mediated wild type p53 gene transfer in patients with advanced non-small cell lung cancer. Hum Gene Ther 1998; 9: 2075–2082.

51. Boulay JL, Perruchoud AP, Reuter J et al. P21 gene expression as an indicator for the activity of adenovirus-p53 gene therapy in non-small cell lung cancer patients. Cancer Gene Ther 2000; 7: 1215–1219.

52. Sutedja G, Baris G, van Zandwijk N, Postmus PE. High-dose rate brachytherapy has a curative potential in patients with intraluminal squamous cell lung cancer. Respiration 1993; 61: 167–168.

53. Edell ES. Photodynamic therapy for bronchosgenic carcinoma. Curr Opin Pulm Med 1998; 4: 205–206.

10.2 Bronchoalveolar lavage

Ulrich Costabel and Josune Guzman

 Key points

- Bronchoalveolar lavage (BAL) is a minimally invasive bronchoscopic procedure used to sample material from the terminal airways and the alveolar spaces.

- The technique is not completely standardised but there is general agreement, in adults, that the instillation volume should approximate 100–300 ml saline in 20–25 ml aliquots.

- In diffuse lung disease, the middle or lingular lobe is used as a standard site of BAL..

- In the laboratory, cell differentials, lymphocyte subpopulations, morphological abnormalities and dust particles, including asbestos body counts, can be analysed.

- Bronchoalveolar lavage cell differentials should not be used as an isolated finding but should always be interpreted in the context of disease history and clinical, laboratory and radiological findings.

Bronchoalveolar lavage (BAL) is a minimally invasive bronchoscopic procedure that is used to sample cells, inhaled particles, infectious agents and soluble acellular components from the terminal bronchioli and alveoli of the lung.[1] To achieve this, the fractionated instillation of lavage fluid must be of sufficient volume to ensure a sufficient aspirate. In adults, a minimum of 100 ml instillation should be made, and 300 ml is an acceptable maximum.

Thus this technique serves as a 'window to the lung'. The information gained from BAL is regarded as complementary to histopathology from biopsies but nevertheless has several advantages over biopsy procedures. It is safe and associated with virtually no morbidity. It can therefore be used repeatedly to investigate serial changes. In addition, lavage collects samples from a much larger area of the lungs than can be obtained through the small tissue fragments of transbronchial biopsy or even surgical biopsy specimens, thus giving a more representative picture of inflammatory and immunological changes.

Bronchoalveolar lavage must be clearly differentiated from the following techniques:

- bronchial lavage (or bronchial washing), which requires relatively little instilled fluid (10–30 ml), and is used for bacteriological study and/or tumour cytology; and
- therapeutic lavage which, with small volume as in bronchial lavage, aims to remove sticky bronchial secretions in asthma and cystic fibrosis patients, and which, with very large volumes (10–30 litres) instilled through a double-lumen endotracheal tube during general anaesthesia (whole lung lavage), is used to wash out an entire lung in patients with alveolar proteinosis.

Technical aspects

The technique of BAL is not completely standardised. Details of the different steps of the procedure may vary greatly between institutions and laboratories but attempts have been made to set up a framework that defines the performance of BAL and the laboratory processing and analysis of the recovered constituents. There is general agreement that the instillation volume should approximate 100–300 ml saline in 20–50 ml aliquots and that, in diffuse lung disease, the middle or lingular lobe is used as a standard site. Guidelines and recommendations for a standardised approach have been published.[2–6] The guidelines are based on the principle of the lowest common denominator, hence allowing a number of technical variations in the different steps of the BAL procedure. When the guidelines are followed, however, the results of lavage are sufficiently valid for practical diagnostic purposes. For example, the correct information on cell differentials is important for clinical purposes. In this respect, the total volume of instilled fluid can range from 100–250 ml without affecting the results of cell differentials.[7]

Technical considerations in children

Technical aspects are slightly different in children; for example, different sizes of bronchoscope are used and the instillation volume has to be adapted to the different ages and sizes of children. In this regard, various protocols have been applied. Some investigators used two or four fractions of the same volume (10–20 ml) irrespective of body weight and age. Others adjust BAL volume to bodyweight using 3 ml/kg of normal saline divided into three equal fractions in children weighing less than 20 kg, and 20 ml portions in children weighing more than 20 kg. Also, the normal values for cellular components are slightly different in children, the major difference between children and adults being seen in the CD4+/CD8+ ratio, which has been found to be lower in children in two studies. Detailed recommendations on BAL in children are reported in a recent publication of the European Respiratory Society Task Force on BAL in children.[8] Interestingly, according to a multicentre survey on the diagnostic approach to interstitial lung disease in children, BAL is the most frequently used invasive technique, applied in 63% of the 131 children studied.[9]

Bronchoscopic procedure

Bronchoalveolar lavage is usually performed by fibreoptic bronchoscopy with topical anaesthesia. BAL can also be undertaken under general anaesthesia and in ventilated patients by passing the fibreoptic bronchoscope through either a rigid bronchoscope or an endotracheal tube. To prevent patients from coughing, local anaesthesia must be adequate but superfluous lidocaine (lignocaine), which might otherwise affect cell harvest, viability and function, must be carefully suctioned off before the actual lavage. To avoid lavage contamination by blood, the BAL should always be made before any concomitant procedure, e.g. biopsy or bronchial brushing. If the patient suffers from airway inflammation that is visible at bronchoscopy, the results will be greatly influenced by the contribution of the bronchial spaces and BAL should not be performed until the patient has been treated with antibiotics, because the inflammatory cells from the bronchial spaces will obscure findings at the alveolar level.

Site of bronchoalveolar lavage

The fibreoptic bronchoscope is gently impacted or 'wedged' into a segmental or subsegmental bronchus. In diffuse lung disease, the middle or lingular lobe is used as a standard site of BAL. When the patient is supine, the anatomy favours maximal recovery from these lobes, and over 20% more fluid and cells is recovered from these lobes than from the lower lobes.[2] Several studies have evaluated the interlobar variation of lavage cell differentials, lymphocyte subpopulations and asbestos body counts by performing a bilateral lavage and analysing the right and left sides independently. In general, these studies have shown a good interlobar correlation in patients with non-focal disease on the chest radiograph.[10–12] These observations indicate that, in patients with diffuse lung disease, BAL at one site should yield representative information on the whole lung. Localised shad-

owing naturally requires lavage of the radiographically involved area.

Fluid instillation

Commonly, sterile, unbuffered isotonic saline (0.9% NaCl solution) is used as the instillate, which may be prewarmed to body temperature to decrease coughing and to increase the cellular yield, but many groups continue to use room-temperature saline. The fluid is instilled into the subsegment through the biopsy channel of the bronchoscope, using a standard number of input aliquots (four or five are most commonly recommended), up to a total instillate of 100–300 ml. Smaller instilled volumes (less than 100 ml) increase the likelihood of contamination of lavage fluid by the bronchial spaces, including inflammatory cells derived from the larger airways, which may skew the differential cell count.

Fluid recovery

After each aliquot is instilled, it is immediately recovered by gentle hand suction into the syringe or gentle wall suction into the fluid trap. Suction that is too forceful can cause collapse of the distal airways or trauma of the airway mucosa and so reduce recovery or change the BAL fluid profile. The first aspirated volume is usually smaller than the following ones.

Usually, 40–70% of the instilled volume is recovered. In obstructive airway disease and emphysema the recovery rate is significantly lower and may be less than 30%. Differential evaluation of the 'bronchial' (first aliquot) and 'alveolar' (subsequent aliquots) samples may be useful in airway diseases.

Siliconised glass or plastic vessels should be used for collection and processing of BAL fluid to avoid loss of cells through adhesion to glass surfaces.

Side effects

Bronchoalveolar lavage is generally well tolerated. Side effects are more or less comparable with those of routine fibreoptic bronchoscopy under local anaesthesia. There is practically no mortality and a low complication rate, between 0 and 2.3%, compared to 7% with transbronchial biopsy and 13% with surgical lung biopsy.[13,14]

Side effects include alveolar infiltration, wheezing and bronchospasm, fever in the first 24 hours after BAL and a transient decrease in lung function parameters. These side effects do not last longer than for 24 hours. Patients with severe heart failure can develop pulmonary oedema by stress and hypoxia. The side effects can be reduced by limiting the instilled volume to 100–200 ml. Major or late complications are only seen in patients with severe lung or heart disease. Bleeding is rarely reported even in patients with clotting disorders or thrombocytopenia. Severe complications are extremely rare.[2]

Risk factors for developing adverse effects are extensive pulmonary infiltrates, P_aO_2 below 8.0 kPa (< 60 mmHg), oxygen saturation below 90%, FEV_1 below 1.0 l, prothrombin time below

50%, platelet count below 20 000/ml, significant comorbidity and bronchial hyperreactivity.

Laboratory processing

The total recovered fluid should be transferred to the laboratory as quickly as possible, since the cells are not well preserved in the saline solution. The total volume should be measured. The lavage fluid frequently contains large amounts of mucus, so it is often filtered through gauze. After filtration the fluid is centrifuged for 10 minutes at 500 g. The total cell numbers are counted in a haemocytometer, either of a sample of the pooled native fluid or of a resuspension of the cells after the first centrifugation. Washing procedures result in a loss of total cell numbers but an increase in the viability of the remaining cells. The total cell count is usually expressed as the total number of cells recovered per lavage, and also as the concentration of cells per millilitre of the recovered fluid. Cell viability is assessed by trypan blue exclusion and should range from 80% to 95%.

The differential cell counts are enumerated on slides prepared either by cytocentrifugation or by a cell-smear technique, by counting at least 600 cells after staining with May–Grünwald–Giemsa stain. The Diff-Quick stain should not be used, because it does not stain mast cells. Ciliated or squamous epithelial cells should be noted but not included in the differential cell count. A high percentage of epithelial cells (>5%) is indicative of contamination of the alveolar samples by bronchial cells. Such BAL probes may not be representative for the diagnosis of diffuse parenchymal lung disease. At least three unstained slides should be stored so that special staining with, for example, iron, periodic-acid–Schiff, silver, toluidine blue, fat or Ziehl–Neelsen stains can be performed, if clinically indicated, or indicated by specific observations on the May–Grünwald–Giemsa-stained slides.

If infection is suspected, a complete microbiological assessment, including cultures, can be performed. Quantitative determination of asbestos bodies by the vacuum filtration method can be used to document suspected asbestos exposure. Lymphocyte subpopulations are identified by immunocytochemical methods, immunofluorescence or flow cytometry using monoclonal antibody techniques.

A large number of soluble components have been measured in lavage fluid. Currently, none of them has proved to be useful in clinical settings. Solutes are too non-specific to be of diagnostic value. The prognostic significance of solutes is also uncertain. In general, the quantitative expression of non-cellular lavage constituents is hampered by the lack of satisfactory reference standards to correct for the variable and unpredictable dilutional effects of the epithelial lining fluid during the procedure. A reasonable pragmatic approach was recently taken by the ERS Task Force on measurement of acellular components. It concluded that the results of acellular components should be expressed as amounts per millilitre of recovered BAL fluid, in order to facilitate comparison of data from different workers, until a reliable external marker can be defined.[5]

Interpretation of bronchoalveolar lavage findings

Bronchoalveolar lavage studies should not be limited to counting the cell differentials. At least as important is observation of the morphological appearances of cells and particles. Examples are the different morphology in extrinsic allergic alveolitis (foamy macrophages, heterogeneous macrophage size, presence of plasma cells) versus that of sarcoidosis (more monomorphous appearance of macrophages, less activated lymphocytes), the presence of malignant cells, the characteristic features of alveolar proteinosis, or the detection of dust particles such as asbestos bodies in occupational exposure conditions.[15]

Furthermore, BAL cell differentials should not be used as an isolated finding for making a diagnosis but should always be interpreted in the context of disease history and clinical, laboratory and radiological findings. Combining BAL with high-resolution computed tomography has increased the diagnostic power of both methods (see below).

Bronchoalveolar lavage as an aid to the differential diagnosis of diffuse parenchymal lung disease

Bronchoalveolar lavage has become a widely accepted diagnostic tool in pulmonary medicine. This holds true for both infectious and non-infectious infiltrative and immunological lung diseases. Barriers that restricted its use to research applications and to downplay its clinical value have finally been overcome. In two recently published international statements on the major interstitial lung diseases, BAL was considered helpful in strengthening the diagnosis in patients with sarcoidosis in the absence of biopsy,[16] and BAL and/or transbronchial biopsy were considered requirements for the exclusion of other diseases in a patient with idiopathic pulmonary fibrosis who did not undergo surgical biopsy (one of the four major criteria for making a clinical diagnosis of the disease).[17]

Bronchoalveolar lavage is broadly indicated in every patient with unclear interstitial lung disease or unclear pulmonary shadowing, no matter what cause is suspected. The underlying disorders may be of infectious, non-infectious immunological or malignant aetiology (Table 10.2.1). BAL may also be indicated in patients with normal chest radiographs when clinical and lung function tests are abnormal and point toward a diffuse lung disease.

Changes in the morphological appearance of cells, in the cell yield and in cell differentials have been described in a variety of diffuse lung diseases. BAL findings may, on occasion, be very specific, so that they can directly confirm a particular diagnosis and can then replace lung biopsy. In other selected lung diseases BAL findings are not diagnostic but may help to narrow the differential diagnosis. Sometimes, even a normal lavage may be useful to exclude some disorders with high probability (e.g. extrinsic allergic alveolitis, eosinophilic pneumonia, alveolar haemorrhage) and to focus attention in other directions.

Table 10.2.1 Indications for bronchoalveolar lavage

Interstitial infiltrates
Sarcoidosis
Extrinsic allergic alveolitis
Drug-induced pneumonitis
Idiopathic pulmonary fibrosis
Connective-tissue disorders
Langerhans cell histiocytosis
Pneumoconioses
Lymphangitic carcinomatosis
Alveolar infiltrates
Pneumonia
Alveolar haemorrhage syndromes
Alveolar proteinosis
Eosinophilic pneumonia
Bronchiolitis obliterans/organising pneumonia
Pulmonary infiltrates in the immunocompromised patient
Human immunodeficiency virus infection
Cytostatic treatment, irradiation
Immunosuppressive treatment
Transplant recipients
Occupational dust exposure
Silica
Asbestos
Coal dust

Bronchoalveolar lavage in healthy adults without lung disease

The BAL fluid obtained from healthy, non-smoking adults without lung disease contains only small percentages of lymphocytes, neutrophils and other inflammatory cells.[3,4,15] The alveolar macrophages are the predominant cell population (Fig. 10.2.1a). Cigarette-smoking is a strong confounding factor with significant effects on BAL samples. The alveolar macrophages from smokers show a characteristic appearance: many of them are much larger than those in non-smokers and contain cytoplasmic inclusion bodies (smoker's inclusion bodies) consisting of tar products, lipids, lipofuscin and other substances (Fig. 10.2.1b). The total cell yield is three to five times higher in smokers, due to a three- to fivefold increase in the number of macrophages that leads to a relative decrease in the percentage of lymphocytes. These changes must be known for the interpretation of cell differentials in interstitial lung disease.

Diagnostic bronchoalveolar lavage findings

There are a number of findings that are highly specific for certain disorders. Therefore, if present, such findings obviate the need for biopsy (Table 10.2.2). They include the characteristic findings in pulmonary alveolar proteinosis (Fig. 10.2.2). The gross appearance of the BAL fluid is milky and turbid. Light microscopy reveals (1) acellular oval bodies, (2) few and foamy macrophages, and (3) a dirty background due to the large amounts of amorphous debris. Electron microscopy for confirmation is not necessary in the routine clinical setting. As a non-specific reaction, an increase in lymphocytes with the tendency towards an elevated CD4$^+$/CD8$^+$ ratio can be seen in this disorder.[19]

Diffuse alveolar haemorrhage can be diagnosed by BAL, even if the bleeding is occult, by the demonstration of numerous haemosiderin-laden macrophages and, in patients with fresh bleeding episodes, free red blood cells in the fluid and fragments of red blood cells in the cytoplasm of macrophages (Fig. 10.2.3). Since many syndromes are part of this group of disorders, other clinical and laboratory findings have to establish the cause of the bleeding. On gross examination, the BAL fluid is bloody or pink to orange-brown in colour, depending on the age and the intensity of the bleeding, because of the red blood cells and haemosiderin-laden macrophages in the fluid. In severe haemorrhage, iron stain shows that more than 90% of the macrophages are iron-positive, i.e. haemosiderin-laden. Haemosiderin-laden macrophages do not appear earlier than 48 hours after bleeding. Thus, very early bleeding only shows numerous red blood cells. Endogenous bleeding has to be differentiated from **exogenous iron load** of the lungs, which may be caused by inhalation of iron-rich dust particles in certain occupations, such as metal grinding and welding. Exogenous siderosis does not show the roundish fragments of erythrocytes but instead irregularly shaped dust particles engulfed by the macrophages.

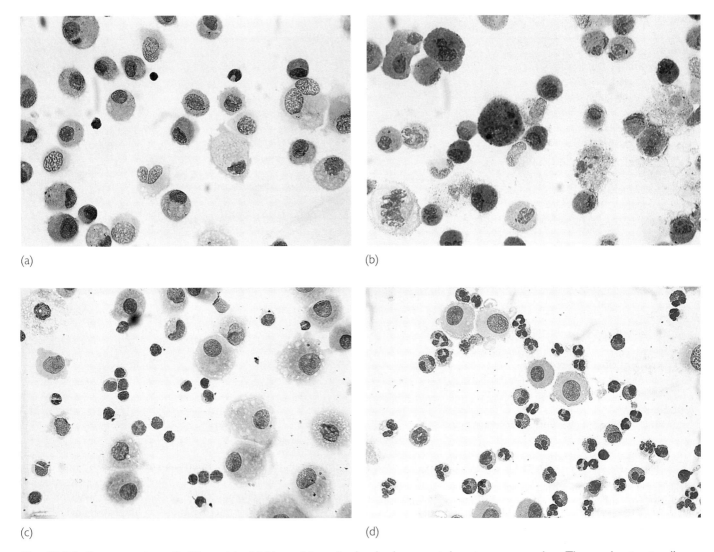

(a)　　　　　　　　　　　　　　　　　　(b)

(c)　　　　　　　　　　　　　　　　　　(d)

Fig. 10.2.1 Representative cell differentials. (a) Normal bronchoalveolar lavage cytology in a non-smoker. The predominant cells are alveolar macrophages; lymphocytes are seen only occasionally. (b) Normal bronchoalveolar lavage cytology in a smoker. The alveolar macrophages are polymorphic, variable in size and display characteristic cytoplasmic smoker's inclusions. (c) Pronounced bronchoalveolar lavage lymphocytosis in extrinsic allergic alveolitis, the alveolar macrophages show foamy cytoplasm. (d) Granulocytic alveolitis in idiopathic pulmonary fibrosis. Predominantly neutrophils, but also many eosinophils. May–Grünwald–Giemsa stain, high-power.

Table 10.2.2 Diagnostic bronchoalveolar lavage findings

Finding	Diagnosis
Pneumocystis carinii, fungi, cytomegalovirus transformed cells	Opportunistic infections
Milky effluent, PAS-positive non-cellular corpuscles, amorphous debris, foamy macrophages	Alveolar proteinosis
Haemosiderin-laden macrophages, intracytoplasmic fragments of red blood cells in macrophages, free red blood cells	Alveolar haemorrhage syndrome
Malignant cells of solid tumours, lymphoma, leukaemia	Malignant infiltrates
Dust particles in macrophages, quantifying asbestos bodies	Dust exposure
Eosinophils greater than 25%	Eosinophilic lung disease
Positive lymphocyte transformation test to beryllium	Chronic beryllium disease
CD1-positive Langerhans cells increased	Langerhans cell histiocytosis

PAS, periodic-acid–Schiff

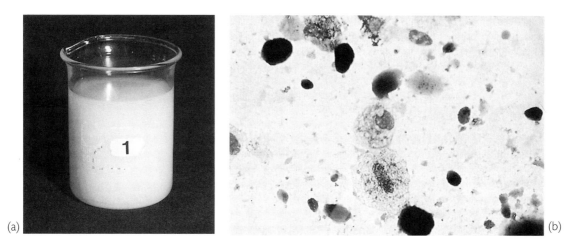

Fig. 10.2.2 Alveolar proteinosis. (a) Milky appearance of bronchoalveolar lavage fluid. (b) Characteristic aspect of bronchoalveolar lavage cytology, showing acellular granules, foamy macrophages and a background of cell debris. May–Grünwald–Giemsa stain. (With permission from Costabel 1994.[18])

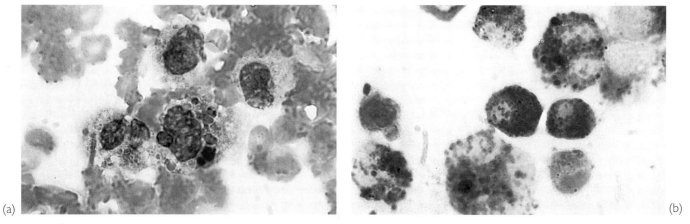

Fig. 10.2.3 Bronchoalveolar lavage cytology in alveolar haemorrhage syndrome: (a) fresh bleeding with numerous red blood cells, both free and phagocytosed within alveolar macrophages, May-Grünwald-Giemsa stain; (b) older bleeding with many haemosiderin-laden macrophages which appear intensely blue with the iron stain. (With permission from Costabel 1994.[18])

Malignant infiltrates, if diffuse, can be reliably diagnosed in 60–90% of cases.[20] The highest yield is seen in widespread malignancies such as primary bronchoalveolar carcinoma or lymphangitic carcinomatosis due to adenocarcinoma. The presence of clusters of type II pneumocytes in the BAL can be misinterpreted as tumour cells. In this regard, even experienced investigators may have difficulty in distinguishing activated type II cells, appearing mainly in diffuse alveolar damage in the BAL fluid, from tumour cells. Even investigations with tumour markers such as some CEA antibodies are not helpful, since they also react with activated type II pneumocytes.

In diffuse lung disease due to **exposure to mineral dust**, BAL can confirm exposure (not disease due to that exposure) by the detection of dust particles such as asbestos bodies.[20,22] Asbestos bodies can also be quantified by a specific filtration technique. The results are given as number of asbestos bodies per millilitre of BAL fluid and there has been shown to be a relatively good correlation with the asbestos body count in lung tissue analysis. An asbestos body count of greater than

1.0/ml indicates an asbestos burden high enough to produce pulmonary asbestosis.

Eosinophilic infiltrates usually show more than 25% eosinophils in the cell differentials if the lavage is performed in the involved segment.[23] In eosinophilic pneumonia, either acute or chronic, the eosinophil count may range from 20% to 90% and is always higher than the neutrophil count (in contrast to Wegener's granulomatosis). In addition, a mild to moderate increase in lymphocytes and a few plasma cells may be present.[3]

In suspected **chronic beryllium disease**, a positive transformation test of BAL lymphocytes in response to beryllium salts may be helpful and confirm the diagnosis.[24]

Increasing numbers of patients who are immunocompromised, either by human immunodeficiency virus (HIV) infection or by receiving immunosuppressive treatment for malignancy or organ transplantation, are prone to develop **pulmonary infections**. In this setting, BAL has probably achieved the greatest practical value in diagnosing such infections and differentiating them from alveolar haemorrhage, pulmonary involvement by the underlying malignancy and drug-induced pneumonitis. The sensitivity of BAL in the diagnosis of bacterial infections ranges from 60% to 90%; in mycobacterial, fungal and most viral infections from 70% to 80%; and in *Pneumocystis carinii* pneumonia 90–95% or higher.[3,25]

Bronchoalveolar lavage as a valuable adjunct to diagnosis

In many types of diffuse parenchymal lung disease, BAL is not specific but can be used as an adjunct to diagnosis. There are many diseases with a lymphocytic, neutrophilic, eosinophilic or mixed cellular pattern (Table 10.2.3). In these settings, BAL may be helpful to narrow the differential diagnosis. In general, the pattern of inflammatory cell populations in the cell differentials will differentiate the fibrosing lung conditions (characterised by neutrophils with or without eosinophils) from the granulomatous or drug-induced lung diseases (characterised by an excess of lymphocytes with or without granulocytes).[26]

Table 10.2.3 Bronchoalveolar lavage cell differentials as an adjunct to diagnosis

Lymphocytic	Sarcoidosis
	Extrinsic allergic alveolitis
	Chronic beryllium disease
	Tuberculosis
	Connective-tissue disorders
	Drug-induced pneumonitis
	Malignant infiltrates
	Silicosis
	Crohn's disease
	Primary biliary cirrhosis
	Human immunodeficiency virus infection
	Viral pneumonia
Neutrophilic (± eosinophilic)	Idiopathic pulmonary fibrosis
	Desquamative interstitial pneumonia (DIP)
	Acute interstitial pneumonia (AIP)
	Acute respiratory distress syndrome
	Bacterial pneumonia
	Connective-tissue disorders
	Asbestosis
	Wegener's granulomatosis
	Diffuse panbronchiolitis
	Transplant bronchiolitis obliterans
	Idiopathic bronchiolitis obliterans
Eosinophilic	Eosinophilic pneumonia
	Churg–Strauss syndrome
	Hypereosinophilic syndrome
	Allergic bronchopulmonary aspergillosis
	Idiopathic pulmonary fibrosis
	Drug-induced reaction
Mixed cellularity	Bronchiolitis obliterans/organising pneumonia
	Connective-tissue disorders
	Non-specific interstitial pneumonia

The CD4+/CD8+ ratio in BAL may also be helpful. Low ratios are commonly observed in the more acute stages of extrinsic allergic alveolitis, certain drug-induced lung diseases, HIV infection and also bronchiolitis obliterans/organising pneumonia (BOOP). A CD4+/CD8+ ratio of more than 3.5 supports the diagnosis of sarcoidosis in the right clinical setting.

Sarcoidosis

Bronchoalveolar lavage shows a lymphocytic alveolitis in 90% of the patients at time of diagnosis. This is a feature common to all stages of sarcoidosis. In late or advanced sarcoidosis, neutrophils may also be increased, as well as the numbers of mast cells.

The value of additional determination of the CD4+/CD8+ ratio has been disputed recently, because of the observed high variability of this ratio in sarcoidosis.[27] Indeed, 15% of patients may even show a decrease to below 1.0 at time of diagnosis, and only about 55% show the characteristic elevated CD4+/CD8+ ratio. Nevertheless, three independent research groups found almost identical values for the sensitivity and specificity of this ratio for diagnosing sarcoidosis.[28–30] Although it is true that the sensitivity is low, reaching only 55%, the specificity is high, at 95%. It was even higher than for transbronchial biopsy in one of these studies.[29] Although an elevated CD4+/CD8+ ratio would obviate biopsy in the appropriate clinical setting, this occurs in only approximately 50% of the patients with sarcoidosis because of the low sensitivity. The CD4+/CD8+ ratio is particularly high in Löfgren's syndrome and other patients with acute disease.[31] In inactive disease, the CD4+/CD8+ ratio is usually in the normal range.

Whether increased numbers of neutrophils in BAL fluid can reliably distinguish patients with sarcoidosis who experience remission from those who will deteriorate, as indicated by Drent et al,[32] has still to be confirmed by other groups.

Extrinsic allergic alveolitis

This disease is characterised by the most striking lymphocytosis in the BAL fluid of all interstitial disease (Fig. 10.2.1c), usually with a relative predominance of CD8+ T cells, resulting in a low CD4+/CD8+ ratio. The CD4+ T cells are also significantly elevated in absolute numbers. In fact, in this disorder, the total cell yield is very high, usually above 20 million from a BAL of 100 ml total instillation. The lymphocyte count is usually more than 50% of total cells (Table 10.2.4). In addition, neutrophils, eosinophils and mast cells may be mildly elevated. Plasma cells and foamy macrophages may be present. The number of activated HLA-DR+ T lymphocytes is high. A normal BAL cytology or an isolated increase in neutrophils or eosinophils effectively excludes extrinsic allergic alveolitis. On the other hand, BAL cannot differentiate between patients with overt disease and healthy exposed subjects who are merely sensitised.[3,33,34]

Acute episodes of extrinsic allergic alveolitis are associated with an influx of neutrophils into the lungs lasting for up to a week. After this period, the cellular profile of the BAL cell differential returns to a significant increase in lymphocytes. In the follow-up, persistent BAL abnormalities indicate that complete avoidance has not been achieved.

Table 10.2.4 Basis data and cell differentials in bronchoalveolar lavage (own data)

	Total cells*	Macrophages (%)	Lymphocytes (%)	Neutrophils (%)	Eosinophils (%)	Mast cells (%)	Plasma cells (%)	Foamy macrophages (%)
Control nonsmokers	7 ± 3	92 ± 4	7 ± 3	1 ± 1	0.1 ± 0.3	0.1 ± 0.1	–	–
Control smokers	23 ± 12	96 ± 3	3 ± 2	1 ± 1	0.4 ± 0.6	0.1 ± 0.3	–	–
Sarcoidosis	16 ± 17	55 ± 21	41 ± 21	3 ± 5	1 ± 1	0.4 ± 0.5	–	–
Extrinsic allergic alveolitis (EAA)	34 ± 22	18 ± 10	78 ± 10	2 ± 2	1 ± 1	0.9 ± 0.9	0.8 ± 0.9	22 ± 17
Idiopathic pulmonary fibrosis (IPF)	14 ± 11	66 ± 23	15 ± 15	14 ± 16	5 ± 5	0.3 ± 0.7	–	14 ± 13
Bronchiolitis obliterans organising pneumonia (BOOP)	14 ± 9	39 ± 19	44 ± 19	10 ± 13	6 ± 8	1.0 ± 0.4	0.1 ± 0.1	25 ± 10
Chronic eosinophilic pneumonia (CEP)	18 ± 22	27 ± 18	22 ± 18	6 ± 6	46 ± 22	1.0 ± 0.9	0.7 ± 0.4	6 ± 11

* × 10^6/100 ml instillation volume; values are mean ± standard deviation

Table 10.2.5 Bronchoalveolar lavage findings in drug-induced interstitial lung disease

Lymphocytosis
- Methotrexate
- Azathioprine
- Cyclophosphamide
- Bleomycin
- Vincristine
- Nitrofurantoin
- Minocycline
- Gold
- Sulfasalazine
- Amiodarone
- Acebutolol
- Atenolol
- Propranolol
- Flecainide
- Diphenylhydantoin
- Nilutamide

Neutrophilia
- Bleomycin
- Busulfan
- Minocycline
- Amiodarone

Eosinophilia
- Bleomycin
- Nitrofurantoin
- Co-trimoxazole
- Penicillin
- Sulfasalazine
- Minocycline
- L-tryptophan

Haemorrhage
- D-penicillamine
- Amphotericin B
- Cytotoxic drugs

Drug-induced pneumonitis

Many drugs can induce an interstitial lung reaction. Any type of alveolitis may be present in BAL (lymphocytic, neutrophilic, eosinophilic or mixed) and also diffuse alveolar haemorrhage[3,15,35] (Table 10.2.5). Most frequently it is a lymphocytic alveolitis, with a predominance of CD8[+] cells, just as in extrinsic allergic alveolitis. In methotrexate-induced pneumonitis, the CD4[+] cells may be preferentially increased, however.[36] Amiodarone causes characteristic changes in the alveolar macrophage population, which shows foamy intracytoplasmic alterations, corresponding to a form of phospholipidosis. This feature is also seen in patients treated with amiodarone but free of clinical lung involvement. If foamy macrophages are not present in BAL, an amiodarone-induced pneumonitis can probably be excluded.

Idiopathic pulmonary fibrosis

The characteristic BAL finding in IPF is an increase in neutrophils, usually to a moderate degree (10–30% of total cells), with or without a parallel increase in eosinophils.[37–39] Usually, the neutrophil level is twice as high as the level of eosinophils (Fig. 10.2.1d). Such an increase in neutrophils is noted in 70–90% of patients, an associated increase in eosinophils in 40–60% of patients and an additional increase in lymphocytes in 10–20% of patients. However, these findings are seen in a wide variety of fibrosing lung conditions other than IPF. A lone and marked increase in lymphocytes is uncommon in IPF (< 10% of patients), so when it is present, another disorder should be excluded (e.g. granulomatous disease, sarcoidosis, extrinsic allergic alveolitis, BOOP, non-specific interstitial pneumonia – NSIP).

Several papers have recently highlighted the prognostic importance of the new histological classification of idiopathic interstitial pneumonia, which limits the definition of IPF to the histopathological pattern of usual interstitial pneumonia (UIP) and discriminates several other subgroups with a better prognosis, including NSIP. The limited data available on BAL cell differentials in NSIP consistently show that this entity is characterised by a predominant lymphocytosis in BAL in addition to a mild increase in neutrophils and eosinophils.[40–42] The BAL pattern seems similar to BOOP and contrasts with the predominant neutrophil and eosinophil increase in UIP or the excessive increase of neutrophils in acute interstitial pneumonia (AIP), thus allowing a certain discrimination between favourable prognostic entities (such as BOOP and NSIP) and the more unfavourable diagnoses (such as UIP or AIP). This is in line with the older observations that a lymphocytic alveolitis in IPF may be associated with a more favourable response to treatment. Today, we can assume that these patients in former studies did not have true IPF/UIP according to the new definition but rather NSIP.

Bronchiolitis obliterans/organising pneumonia

In this disorder, the BAL profile is characterised by a mixed pattern, usually with a predominance of lymphocytes and a more moderate increase in neutrophils, eosinophils and mast cells, as well as the presence of foamy macrophages and, occasionally, plasma cells. Other BAL findings include a decrease in the CD4+/CD8+ ratio and an increase in activated, HLA-DR+ T lymphocytes.[43,44]

Bronchoalveolar lavage may be of value in distinguishing between BOOP and other interstitial lung diseases. In comparison with IPF, patients with BOOP have higher proportions of lymphocytes. A lone increase in neutrophils and/or eosinophils was not seen in any of our patients with BOOP. In chronic eosinophilic pneumonia, BAL eosinophils usually exceed 25% and they are below this threshold in BOOP. In a patient with typical symptoms and signs and with patchy peripheral infiltrates, after infection and malignancy has been excluded by lavage, a BAL cell profile with more than 20% lymphocytes, 2–25% eosinophils and a CD4+/CD8+ ratio less than 1.0 is highly suggestive of idiopathic BOOP and may warrant a therapeutical trial of corticosteroid therapy.

Diagnostic yield of bronchoalveolar lavage in diffuse parenchymal lung disease

As outlined above, there are several rare disorders with specific BAL findings and sufficiently high sensitivity so that biopsy is usually not necessary, including alveolar proteinosis, *P. carinii* pneumonia, alveolar haemorrhage and others (Table 10.2.6).

In many diffuse lung diseases, the cellular BAL profile is abnormal, with either a lymphocytic, neutrophilic, eosinophilic or mixed cellularity. Some of these disorders almost always show an abnormal BAL (high sensitivity), although the specificity is low. In some of them, in combination with clinical and HRCT features, the diagnosis may be possible without biopsy. In this regard, if the CT scan shows the characteristic pattern and distribution of UIP, a simple increase in neutrophils/eosinophils supports the diagnosis of IPF if the major and minor criteria of the recent ATS/ERS statement are fulfilled. Also, if the CT scan shows a patchy ground glass pattern, BAL may be able to reveal that this patient suffers from extrinsic allergic alveolitis (high lymphocyte count), or smoking-related respiratory bronchiolitis/interstitial lung disease (high smoker's macrophage count and normal cell differential), or possibly from alveolar haemorrhage (high count of haemosiderin-laden macrophages). In a patient with predominantly peripheral consolidation plus some ground-glass infiltrates on CT scan, BAL may be suggestive of BOOP (mixed cellular pattern with a relatively low eosinophil count) or chronic eosinophilic pneumonia (major increase in eosinophils).

Role of bronchoalveolar lavage in assessing activity and prognosis

At present it is under debate as to whether or not BAL is useful for assessing the activity of the disease processes with a view to obtaining prognostic information. It is also not proven whether serial BAL has more of a role in monitoring the course of disease and guiding therapy than other indices of change. In sarcoidosis, although differences were observed for several BAL parameters between clinically active and inactive patient groups, the range of overlap between groups is large and none of the investigated findings was able to indicate prognosis reliably enough in a given individual patient. In IPF, a marked increase in neutrophils and/or eosinophils was reported to adversely effect prognosis, whereas elevated lymphocyte counts were found to be more likely to be associated with a good response to corticosteroid treatment.[38,39,45] Today, such patients with increased lymphocyte

Table 10.2.6 Diagnostic yield of bronchoalveolar lavage in diffuse parenchymal lung diseases

Bronchoalveolar lavage without biopsy usually sufficient (high sensitivity and high specificity)	Alveolar proteinosis *Pneumocystis carinii* pneumonia Bronchoalveolar carcinoma Alveolar haemorrhage Eosinophilic pneumonia
Bronchoalveolar lavage in combination with clinical and high-resolution computed tomography (HRCT) features frequently sufficient (high sensitivity, low specificity)	Idiopathic pulmonary fibrosis (neutrophils ± eosinophils) Extrinsic allergic alveolitis (lymphocytes, plasma cells, foamy macrophages) Bronchiolitis obliterans/organising pneumonia (mixed cellularity, CD4+/CD8+ ↓
Bronchoalveolar lavage in only 50% patients typical, biopsy often needed – if CT atypical (moderate sensitivity, high specificity)	Sarcoidosis (CD4+/CD8+ ↑) Langerhans cell histiocytosis (CD1 ↑)
Bronchoalveolar lavage mostly not diagnostic, biopsy required (low sensitivity ± low specificity)	Hodgkin's disease Invasive aspergillosis Lymphangioleiomyomatosis (if CT atypical)

counts most probably have the idiopathic NSIP variant of the idiopathic interstitial pneumonias and not IPF (UIP).

Whether repeated lavage measurements give better information for assessing the evolution of disease activity and the natural history is not clear for the moment. Larger prospective studies are required to clarify this issue before BAL should be routinely used for this purpose. At present, serial BAL cannot be routinely recommended.

Clinical relevance

- Bronchoalveolar lavage (BAL) is broadly indicated in every patient with unclear diffuse lung disease or unclear pulmonary shadowing.

- The information gained from BAL is regarded as complementary to histopathology from biopsies.

- Nevertheless, BAL has several advantages over biopsy procedures: it is safe and associated with virtually no morbidity, and collects samples from a much larger area of the lungs than possible with biopsies, giving a more representative picture of inflammatory and immunological changes.

- In some disorders, specific information may be obtained, e.g. alveolar proteinosis, diffuse alveolar haemorrhage, malignant infiltrates or dust exposure. Here BAL can replace lung biopsy.

- The results of BAL cell differentials with a lymphocytic, neutrophilic, eosinophilic or mixed cellular pattern are not specific but can be used as an adjunct to diagnosis and can be helpful in narrowing the differential diagnosis.

? Unresolved questions

- The technique of induced sputum is even less invasive than bronchoalveolar lavage; what is its diagnostic role in comparison with bronchoalveolar lavage (BAL)?

- What is the diagnostic value of acellular components of BAL?

- Is BAL clinically useful for assessing the activity of disease processes and for providing prognostic information?

- For which patients can serial BAL to monitor the course of disease be recommended?

References

1. Reynolds HY. Use of bronchoalveolar lavage in humans – past necessity and future imperative. Lung 2000; 178: 271–293.
2. Klech H, Pohl W, ed. Technical recommendations and guidelines for bronchoalveolar lavage (BAL). Report of the ERS Task Group. Eur Respir J 1989; 2: 561–585.
3. Klech H, Hutter C, ed. Clinical guidelines and indications for bronchoalveolar lavage (BAL): report of the European Society of Pneumology Task Force on BAL. Eur Respir J 1990; 3: 937–974.
4. American Thoracic Society. Clinical role of bronchoalveolar lavage in adults with pulmonary disease. Am Rev Respir Dis 1990; 142: 481–486.
5. Haslam PL, Baughman RP, ed. Report of European Respiratory Society (ERS) Task Force: guidelines for measurement of acellular components and recommendations for standardization of bronchoalveolar lavage (BAL). Eur Respir Rev 1999; 9: 25–157.
6. Costabel U, Guzman J. Bronchoalveolar lavage in interstitial lung disease. Curr Opin Pulm Med 2001; 7: 255–261.
7. Helmers RA, Dayton CS, Floerchinger C, Hunninghake GW. Bronchoalveolar lavage in interstitial lung disease: effect of volume of fluid infused. J Appl Physiol 1989; 67: 1443–1446.
8. ERS Task Force. Bronchoalveolar lavage in children. Eur Respir J 2000; 15: 217–231.
9. Barbato A, Panizzolo C, Cracco A et al. Interstitial lung disease in children: a multicentre survey on diagnostic approach. Eur Respir J 2000; 16: 509–513.
10. Garcia JGN, Wolven RG, Garcia PL, Keogh BA. Assessment of interlobar variation of bronchoalveolar lavage cellular differentials in interstitial lung diseases. Am Rev Respir Dis 1986; 133: 444–449.
11. Peterson MW, Nugent KM, Jolles H et al. Uniformity of bronchoalveolar lavage in patients with sarcoidosis. Am Rev Respir Dis 1988; 137: 799–784.
12. Teschler H, Konietzko N, Schoenfeld B et al. Distribution of asbestos bodies in the human lung as determined by bronchoalveolar lavage. Am Rev Respir Dis 1993; 147: 1211–1215.
13. Baughman RP. Bronchoalveolar lavage. St Louis, MO: Mosby/Year Book; 1992.
14. Costabel U. CD4/CD8 ratios in bronchoalveolar lavage fluid: of value for diagnosing sarcoidosis? Eur Respir J 1997; 10: 2699–2700.
15. Costabel U. Atlas of bronchoalveolar lavage. London: Chapman & Hall; 1998.
16. Hunninghake GW, Costabel U, Ando M et al. ATS/ERS/WASOG statement on sarcoidosis. Sarcoidosis Vasc Diffuse Lung Dis 1999; 16: 149–173.
17. ATS/ERS Statement. Idiopathic pulmonary fibrosis: diagnosis and treatment. Am J Respir Crit Care Med 2000; 161: 646–664.
18. Costabel U. Atlas der bronchoalveolären Lavage. Stuttgart: Georg Thieme; 1994.
19. Milleron BJ, Costabel U, Teschler H et al. Bronchoalveolar lavage cell data in alveolar proteinosis. Am Rev Respir Dis 1991, 144: 1330–1332.
20. Semenzato G, Poletti V. Bronchoalveolar lavage in lung cancer. Respiration 1992; Suppl 1: 44–46.
21. Costabel U, Donner CF, Haslam PL et al. Clinical role of BAL in occupational lung diseases due to mineral dust exposure. Eur Respir Rev 1992; 2: 89–96.
22. De Vuyst P, Dumortier P, Moulin E et al. Diagnostic value of asbestos bodies in bronchoalveolar lavage fluid. Am Rev Respir Dis 1987; 136: 1219–1224.
23. Allen JN, Bruce Davis W, Pacht ER. Diagnostic significance of increased bronchoalveolar lavage fluid eosinophils. Am Rev Respir Dis 1990; 142: 642–647.
24. Rossmann MD, Kern JA, Elias JA et al. Proliferative response of BAL lymphocytes to beryllium. Ann Intern Med 1988; 108: 687–693.
25. Huaringa J, Leyva FJ, Signes-Costa J et al. Bronchoalveolar lavage in the diagnosis of pulmonary complications of bone marrow transplant patients. Bone Marrow Transplant 2000; 25: 975–979.
26. Drent M, van Nierop MA, Gerritsen FA et al. A computer program using BALF-analysis results as a diagnostic tool in interstitial lung diseases. Am J Respir Crit Care Med 1996; 153: 736–741.
27. Kantrow SP, Meyer KC, Kidd P et al. The CD4/CD8 ratio in BAL fluid is highly variable in sarcoidosis. Eur Respir J 1997; 10: 2716–2721.
28. Costabel U, Zaiss AW, Guzman J. Sensitivity and specificity of BAL findings in sarcoidosis. Sarcoidosis 1992; 9(Suppl. 1): 211–214.
29. Winterbauer RH, Lammert J, Selland M et al. Bronchoalveolar lavage cell populations in the diagnosis of sarcoidosis. Chest 1993; 104: 352–261.
30. Thomeer M, Demedts M. Predictive value of CD4/CD8 ratio in bronchoalveolar lavage in the diagnosis of sarcoidosis (abstract). Sarcoidosis Vasc Diffuse Lung Dis 1997; 14(Suppl. 1): 36.
31. Ward K, O'Connor C, Odlum C, Fitzgerald MX. Prognostic value of bronchoalveolar lavage in sarcoidosis: The critical influence of disease presentation. Thorax 1989; 44: 6–12.
32. Drent M, Jacobs JA, de Vries J et al. Does the cellular bronchoalveolar lavage fluid profile reflect the severity of sarcoidosis? Eur Respir J 1999; 13: 1338–1344.
33. Costabel U. The alveolitis of hypersensitivity pneumonitis. Eur Respir J 1988; 1: 5–9.
34. Haslam PL, Dewar A, Butchers P et al. Mast cells, atypical lymphocytes and neutrophils in bronchoalveolar lavage in extrinsic allergic alveolitis. Am Rev Respir Dis 1987; 135: 35–47.
35. Akoun GM, Cadranel JL, Blanchette G et al. Bronchoalveolar lavage cell data in amiodarone-associated pneumonitis. Chest 1991; 99: 1177–1182.

36. Schnabel A, Richter C, Bauerfeind S, Gross WL. Bronchoalveolar lavage cell profile in methotrexate induced pneumonitis. Thorax 1997; 52: 377–379.

37. Haslam PL, Turton CWG, Heard B et al. Bronchoalveolar lavage in pulmonary fibrosis: comparison of cells obtained with lung biopsy and clinical features. Thorax 1980; 35: 9–18.

38. Haslam PL, Turton CWG, Lukoszek A et al. Bronchoalveolar lavage fluid cell counts in cryptogenic fibrosing alveolitis and their relation to therapy. Thorax 1980; 35: 328–339.

39. Peterson WMW, Monick M, Hunninghake GW. Prognostic role of eosinophils in pulmonary fibrosis. Chest 1987; 92: 51–56.

40. Nagai S, Kitaichi M, Itoh H et al. Idiopathic nonspecific interstitial pneumonia/fibrosis: comparison with idiopathic pulmonary fibrosis and BOOP. Eur Respir J 1998; 12: 1010–1019.

41. Park CS, Chung SW, Ki SY et al. Increased Levels of interleukin-6 are associated with lymphocytosis in bronchoalveolar lavage fluids of idiopathic nonspecific interstitial pneumonia. Am J Respir Crit Care Med 2000; 162: 1162–1168.

42. Suga M, Iyonaga K, Okamoto T et al. Characteristic elevation of matrix metalloproteinase activity in idiopathic interstitial pneumonias. Am J Respir Crit Care Med 2000; 162: 1949–1956.

43. Costabel U, Teschler H, Guzman J. Bronchiolitis obliterans organizing pneumonia (BOOP): the cytological and immunocytological profile of bronchoalveolar lavage. Eur Respir J 1992; 5: 791–797.

44. Cazzato S, Zompatori M, Baruzzi G et al. Bronchiolitis obliterans–organizing pneumonia: an Italian experience. Respir Med 2000; 94: 702–708.

45. Rudd RM, Haslam PL, Turner-Warwick M. Cryptogenic fibrosing alveolitis: relationships of pulmonary physiology and bronchoalveolar lavage to treatment and prognosis. Am Rev Respir Dis 1981; 124, 1–8.

10.3 Lung biopsy

Fergus Gleeson

The first successful percutaneous needle biopsy of the lung was performed by Leyden in 1883[1] but it was almost a century later before this technique became established as an effective procedure in the investigation of suspected pulmonary malignancy.[2] Subsequent improvements in needle design, microbiological and cytohistological techniques, and imaging have resulted in the ever increasing use of percutaneous needle biopsy in the diagnosis of pulmonary disease.[3-4] Recent imaging advances, in particular in computed tomography (CT) scanning has allowed the biopsy of previously inaccessible lesions within the lung, mediastinum and hila.[5-7]

In addition, the development of small-gauge cutting needles has enabled percutaneous biopsy to obtain tissue suitable for histological examination, facilitating the diagnosis of benign lesions and so avoiding more invasive procedures.[8-10] However, percutaneous biopsy is not without risk and should only be performed when it is likely to yield a tissue diagnosis that will affect patient management.[11-12]

Indications and contraindications

Indications

The most common indication for percutaneous needle biopsy is to determine the nature of a solitary pulmonary nodule or mass, and in most patients this is performed for suspected pulmonary malignancy. The value of percutaneous needle biopsy to confirm a diagnosis of bronchogenic carcinoma is unquestioned in patients who are clearly inoperable because of disease extent, poor cardiorespiratory reserve and poor performance status. However the use of needle biopsy in patients that are operable needs to be carefully considered, as the value of a negative biopsy is less certain.[11-12] Confirmation that a solitary pulmonary nodule is benign is less readily achieved by percutaneous needle biopsy and depends on the lesion characteristics, the use of

histological as well as cytological techniques and the pretest probability that the lesion may be benign.[3,4,7-16]

Recently, additional imaging information has aided in the decision on whether to perform bronchoscopy or percutaneous needle biopsy in an attempt to obtain a tissue diagnosis.[17] Computed tomography in particular enables selection of the appropriate investigation, central lesions or those involving a lobar or segmental bronchus being most suitable for bronchoscopic diagnosis and lesions distant from the hilum more suitable for percutaneous needle biopsy.[18]

Percutaneous needle biopsy may be used to confirm a diagnosis of metastatic disease in patients with pulmonary nodules and a known extrathoracic malignancy. Its value in these circumstances depends on the site of the known primary tumour and both the local tumour stage and planned therapy.[19] It may also be used to confirm the presence of a suspected second primary tumour in patients with a diagnosis of extrathoracic malignancy, e.g. head and neck tumours.[20,21] Needle biopsy is less commonly performed to obtain tissue for microbiology but may be of value when sputum cytology and bronchoscopy, including lavage, have been non-diagnostic.[22,23] In these circumstances it has a high success rate, particularly in immunocompromised patients.[24,25]

Contraindications

Although there are no absolute contraindications to percutaneous needle biopsy, there are a number of premorbid conditions that make the likelihood of a complication, or the patient's ability to survive such an event of greater concern.[3] The most frequent is poor respiratory reserve. In each instance the presence of a relative contraindication (Table 10.3.1), warrants considered discussion between the referring physician or surgeon, radiologist and patient. Attempts should be made to minimise the risk by using an experienced operator, correcting coagulopathies and attempting to avoid lung puncture by specialist techniques (see later). In all instances, detailed informed consent from the patient should be obtained.

Table 10.3.1   Relative contraindications to percutaneous needle biopsy

- Contralateral pneumonectomy
- Poor lung function, $FEV_1 < 1.0$ litre
- Intractable cough or uncooperative patient
- Coagulopathy
- Possible arteriovenous malformation or echinococcal cyst
- Pulmonary artery hypertension

Needle selection

Material for cytology, microbiology and histology may be obtained by percutaneous needle biopsy. Biopsy needles are mostly of two types: cutting needles and aspiration needles (Figs 10.3.1 & 10.3.2).

Most aspiration needles range from 19 to 22 gauge and multiple needle types have been designed to increase specimen yield, although there is no evidence to suggest that any one needle is preferable. The use of needles greater than 19 gauge in size has been reported to be associated with a greater incidence of pneumothorax.[26,27]

Cutting needles designed to produce specimens for histological analysis have become increasingly popular. This may be related not only to improvements in design, leading to lighter stiffer needles, but also their ability to provide specimens that enable both a benign diagnosis, and also obviate the need for cytopathologists. The most commonly used cutting needles have

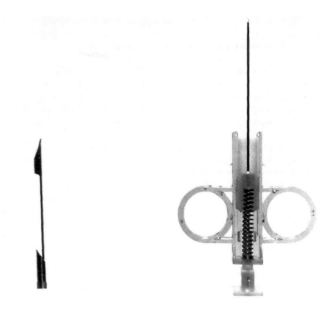

Fig. 10.3.2   Mechanised cutting needle, spring exposed, with insert of needle tip and specimen notch.

a side notch with a throw of up to 2 cm and range from 14 to 20 gauge with 18 gauge being used most frequently.

Initial reports suggested that cutting needle biopsy was associated with a greater incidence of haemorrhage and pneumothorax than aspiration biopsy, but this has recently been challenged.[8-10,28-31]

Both aspiration and cutting needle biopsies may be performed co-axially. The biopsy needle is passed through an outer guiding needle placed in or adjacent to the lesion. This enables multiple passes to be performed without the need for multiple pleural punctures, reducing the risk of a pneumothorax.[32,33] The angle and direction of the outer needle may be altered to allow sampling from different areas of the lesion, and can also be used to inject a small amount of autologous blood along the needle tract – which clots and seals the tract, 'the blood patch technique', at the end of the biopsy further reducing the risk of pneumothorax.[34]

Imaging and biopsy technique

Biopsies may be performed using fluoroscopy, CT or ultrasound. In all instances a prior chest radiograph, preferably posteroanterior and lateral, should be available and if possible a prior chest CT. Factors influencing the choice of imaging modality include the site and size of the lesion, equipment availability and local expertise. Recently, CT has become the preferred imaging technique, enabling the biopsy of smaller, less accessible lesions than previously attempted (Fig. 10.3.3). Fluoroscopy and ultrasound remain valuable imaging modalities for biopsy, being readily available, producing high diagnostic yields and, in particular with ultrasound, a very low complication rate.[35,36] Fluoroscopy is often the imaging technique of choice when the lesion to be biopsied is large and visible on both the posteroanterior and

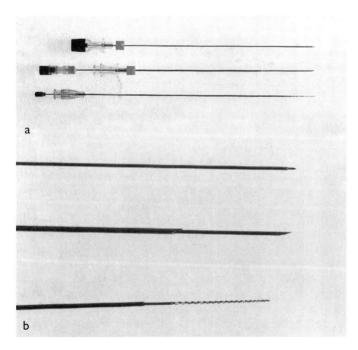

Fig. 10.3.1   Biopsy needles. a. Gauge 22 aspiration needle, coaxial system and screw needle system. b. Close-up of needle tips.

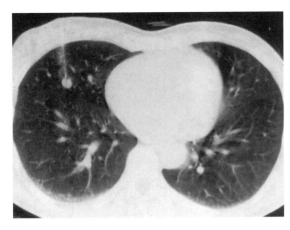

Fig. 10.3.3 Computed-tomography-guided lung biopsy of 7 mm pulmonary nodule poorly seen on fluoroscopy.

lateral radiographs. Ultrasound may only be used when the lesion is in contact with the pleura.

Computed tomography performed prior to biopsy enables assessment of both the lesion and its position, enabling a biopsy route to be planned to avoid bullae and fissures, often avoiding crossing aerated lung, and allowing the shortest pleura-to-lesion distance.[33,37,38] In addition, CT makes it possible to avoid areas of necrosis and to biopsy the wall of a cavitating lesion.

Prior to biopsy, informed consent must be obtained. It is preferable that patient information leaflets are available to the patient at the time of making the appointment for the biopsy, explaining the procedure, its risks and contraindications and the likelihood of a successful outcome considering both the reported literature and the local experience. At the time of consent, any specific risks should be carefully explained. Patients taking anticoagulants and antiplatelet agents should have arrangements made for these to be stopped beforehand. Antiplatelet agents should be stopped at least 5 days before the procedure, and the risks and benefits of this should be discussed with the patient.

Successful percutaneous needle biopsy requires patient cooperation and for this reason most operators do not use sedation. A full blood count, coagulation screen and FEV_1 should be obtained prior to biopsy.

The patient should be positioned supine or prone where possible as maintaining a decubitus position may be difficult. Biopsies should not be performed with the patient seated because of the risk of an air embolus and consequent cerebral catastrophe.[39–41] The requirements of the breathing technique should be explained to the patient and practised before the biopsy. Deep breaths in or out and coughing are to be avoided, and most patients find it more comfortable to hold their breath after a gentle inspiration.

If using fluoroscopy, the best results are usually obtained with a vertical needle insertion. The correct depth of insertion may be measured from a prior CT or lateral chest radiograph, although direct visualisation of needle entry into the lesion using a C-arm unit is preferable. An appropriate needle entry site is readily determined if using ultrasound as the imaging technique,

and the needle is readily visualised entering the lesion. If using CT, a needle entry site avoiding fissures and bullae is chosen if possible. A radio-opaque marker is placed on the skin entry site and a short spiral CT sequence is performed. The distance from skin surface to lesion is measured and marked on the biopsy needle. In all cases the skin should be cleaned and sterilised and infiltrated with local anaesthetic. The needle entry site should be cephalad to a rib to avoid intercostal vessels. Using fluoroscopy or ultrasound, the needle can be advanced continuously into the lesion. If CT is used, and in particular for small or central lesions, the needle alignment may need to be checked and redirected as necessary. In all instances the biopsy needle should only be advanced during suspended respiration. The patient may breathe gently with the needle in place.

For aspiration biopsies, the central stylet is removed and suction is applied with a 10 ml syringe while rotating and moving the needle a short distance to and fro, again during suspended respiration. The appearance of air in the syringe indicates either that there is a poor seal between the syringe and needle or that the needle tip is within lung and not the lesion. If blood appears in the needle hub or syringe, aspiration should cease and the needle should be removed. Prior to needle removal from the patient, aspiration should cease to prevent aspiration of normal lung and soft tissue, i.e. fat and muscle, during removal. If a coaxial technique is being used then the outer sheath remains in place and an inner stylet is placed within it while dealing with the biopsy specimen. The biopsy procedure may be repeatedly performed providing no complication preventing repetition has occurred. For cutting-needle biopsies it is important to ensure, prior to firing the needle, that the tip will either remain within the lesion once fired or stop in a safe place. Histology specimens are placed in formalin and the macroscopic adequacy of the specimen is assessed.

Aspiration biopsy material is expressed on to glass slides. Air-dried slides provide material suitable for Giemsa, Gram and Ziehl–Nielsen staining. Slides fixed in alcohol are stained by the Papanicolaou method and it is imperative that these slides are alcohol-fixed before the cells that they carry can dry. Aspirate may also be put in saline for 'spinning down' and microbiological culture. The essence for all methods is to provide the cytopathologists, histopathologists and microbiologists with the biopsy material in a manner of their choosing as quickly as possible.

Following biopsy the patient is assessed for the presence of complications. A CT section at the site of biopsy readily identifies haemorrhage or a pneumothorax. Fluoroscopy screening only enables identification of larger pneumothoraces and haemorrhage compared to CT. Ultrasound performed following biopsy readily identifies a complicating pneumothorax as the biopsied lesion is no longer against the parietal pleural surface and cannot be identified.

After biopsy the patient is placed puncture-site down where possible and advised to avoid talking, coughing or straining in order to reduce the incidence of pneumothorax and chest-drain insertion. Vital observations are performed immediately following biopsy and thereafter at intervals agreed with the nursing staff caring for the patient. Postbiopsy radiographs performed at 1 and 3 or 4 hours after biopsy are advisable to detect a pneumothorax and assess whether it is enlarging. If there is no or a small non-enlarging pneumothorax the patient may be discharged home with instructions to return immediately if chest pain, shortness of breath or haemoptysis develop.

Complications

Pneumothorax

This is the most common complication. The reported frequency ranges from 0% to 61%,[37–42] with the incidence requiring chest-drain insertion ranging from 0% to 15%.[4,5,37,43,44] The incidence of pneumothorax is lowest if the biopsy is performed under ultrasound and highest using CT.[45,46] It is likely that the incidence reported using CT is high due to its increased sensitivity in detecting pneumothorax compared to fluoroscopy and its use for biopsying technically more difficult lesions.[46,47]

The most important risk factor associated with the development of a pneumothorax is chronic obstructive airways disease. In addition, the need for placement of a chest drain is more likely in these patients.[48–51] Puncture of a superficial bulla is likely to result in a pneumothorax and CT may be used to avoid this. Other factors known to be associated with an increased risk of pneumothorax are mechanical ventilation, intractable coughing, traversing a fissure, deep or small lesions, multiple punctures and operator inexperience.[45,49–51] Needle calibre appears to have little effect on the incidence of pneumothorax until needles larger than 19 gauge are used.[26,27]

A number of techniques have been used in an attempt to reduce the incidence of pneumothorax. If aerated lung is not traversed then a pneumothorax cannot develop and such a biopsy route should be chosen where possible. Traversing a collapsed lobe, the development of an extrapleural window by the injection of saline into the extrapleural space, or decubitus positioning to allow pleural fluid movement have all been used to enable biopsy without crossing aerated lung.[38,52] Multiple pleural punctures may be avoided using a coaxial system enabling multiple biopsies through a single pleural puncture.[32,33] Suspending respiration while removing the biopsy needle has also been reported to reduce the incidence of pneumothorax.

Positioning the patient with the biopsy site dependent may be of benefit and is a practical proposition.[33,52,53] The injection of autologous blood using a coaxial needle technique may or may not be effective.[34] It seems likely that operator skill is one of the most significant factors in the incidence of pneumothorax. Most pneumothoraces occur immediately, a further 9% are detected on a chest radiograph performed at 1 hour and an additional 2% are detected at 4 hours.[54] However, rarely pneumothoraces requiring treatment have been reported up to 24 hours following biopsy.[55] The clinical significance of a pneumothorax depends on its size and the patient's respiratory reserve.

Haemorrhage

This is the second most frequent complication of percutaneous needle biopsy. The reported incidence of biopsy-associated haemorrhage has decreased in recent years, ranging from 0% to 40%, probably as a result of a decrease in needle size.[7–10,30,37,56–58] Significant haemorrhage and fatal haemoptysis are rare.[10,29,57,58] Although there have been a few reports of death after fine-needle aspiration biopsy, almost all deaths from haemorrhage have occurred following the use of cutting needles. The recent development of small-gauge cutting needles has led to an increase in their use, with some series reporting no increase in haemorrhagic complications and others only a slight increase.[58] If haemoptysis occurs the patient should be placed biopsy side down to prevent aspiration into the contralateral lung. In most instances haemoptysis is self-limiting. If it is significant, venous access should be obtained and the patient may require bronchoscopic tamponade or surgery.

Air embolism

This is a rare but potentially fatal complication of needle biopsy.[39–41] It is independent of needle size and appears to occur when the needle lies in a pulmonary vein. This allows air into the vein either from the surrounding lung or via the needle lumen. Suspending respiration while removing the central stylet during aspiration biopsy and attaching the syringe has been suggested to prevent air passage along the needle lumen. In the reported cases, coughing during biopsy occurred and it would seem advisable to remove the needle in this situation. Air embolism may be manifest as a cerebral or cardiac event. Needle-tract seeding is rare and is most likely to occur following biopsy with larger needles and in patients with mesothelioma.[59,60]

Diagnostic accuracy

Percutaneous needle biopsy is extremely accurate for the diagnosis of intrathoracic malignancy, with sensitivities ranging from 70% to 100%.[4–10,29–31,56,58] This range is dependent on needle type, operator experience, the image guidance used and the characteristics of the lesion, its size and site. The ability to make a positive diagnosis of benign disease is less good using aspiration biopsy, with ranges reported from 16% to 68%.[56,61,62] The diagnosis of benign pulmonary disease such as a hamartoma has been significantly improved by the use of cutting needles.[8,9,29,30] The addition of cutting-needle biopsy has improved the ability to diagnose lymphoma, which previously had a low cytological yield.

It is the difficulty in securing a positive diagnosis of benign disease in patients considered to have thoracic malignancy that has led to the value of percutaneous needle biopsy in potentially operable candidates being rightly questioned.[11,12] More recent reports suggest that the use of high-resolution CT and dynamic contrast-enhanced CT can improve the diagnostic accuracy of CT examinations and consequently alter the pretest probability of malignancy in patients referred for percutaneous needle biopsy.[16] The addition of cutting-needle biopsy in more recent reports suggests that the numbers of patients with a false-negative biopsy for malignancy is also significantly reduced.

The differentiation of cell types by percutaneous needle biopsy, although not 100% reliable, is accurate in the important distinction of small-cell from non-small-cell carcinoma.[63–65] A recent study confirmed that the cytological accuracy of small-cell carcinoma was 100%. The accuracy for non-small-cell carcinoma was less good – squamous cell carcinoma 90%, adenocarcinoma 70%, large-cell carcinoma 50%.[66] However, the ability to accurately differentiate among the different cell types of non-small-cell bronchogenic carcinoma is not of practical importance since it does not affect patient management decisions.

The majority of false-negative results are attributable to sampling error rather than judgement error on the part of the cytopathologist. Sampling error may be improved by taking multiple biopsies from different sites. The presence of a cytopathologist on site may also decrease false-negative biopsies and have the added benefit of decreasing the number of passes performed.[67,68] Other false-negative biopsies may result from extensive tumour necrosis and cavitation, or adjacent consolidation or collapse. A non-specific negative result should prompt repetition of the biopsy. Repeat biopsies may provide a true positive result in up to 35–45% cases following an initial negative result.[56] If repeat biopsies are negative then either an alternative means of achieving a tissue diagnosis or following the lesion radiographically with serial chest X-rays or CT examinations should be considered.

The clinical approach to lung biopsy

Centrally placed masses, hilar and paramediastinal masses

Percutaneous needle biopsy has been performed with a high degree of success in hilar and juxtahilar lesions, including patients following a negative bronchoscopy.[69] However it would seem sensible to perform bronchoscopic biopsies for all centrally positioned lesions and in particular those with an endobronchial component.[18] If available, transbronchial needle biopsy may enable a tissue diagnosis to be made in centrally positioned masses with no endobronchial component.[70] Performing a CT

Selection of biopsy technique for peripheral masses

■ There are some instances when the radiographic features or psychological considerations make thoracotomy an inevitable outcome, in which case there is no point in further diagnostic procedures.

■ An endoscopic approach is the choice if:
  – the patient cannot withstand a pneumothorax
  – local operator skills favour this approach.

■ The percutaneous approach is preferred in all other instances:
  – if malignant disease is suspected, needle aspiration is appropriate and highly specific
  – if repeated needle aspiration is negative or a benign diagnosis is suspected, a technique yielding tissue for histological examination, e.g. Tru-Cut® biopsy, is preferred.

Selection of biopsy techniques for centrally positioned masses

■ Bronchoscopy and, if possible, bronchoscopic or transbronchial biopsy should be performed.

■ If bronchoscopy is negative, percutaneous needle aspiration biopsy may be performed.

■ If the operator skills for percutaneous biopsy are not available or it is deemed clinically inappropriate, a surgical approach may be performed.

---

scan may help to identify patients in whom a positive tissue diagnosis is likely to be obtained at bronchoscopy and thereby enable the appropriate biopsy technique to be chosen.[17,18] Percutaneous needle biopsy may be used successfully to obtain a tissue diagnosis in patients with bronchogenic malignancy abutting or invading the mediastinum, either as an alternative to or following a negative bronchoscopy.[71–73]

Allowing for circumstances such as operator skill and considering each patient individually it is possible to suggest a suitable diagnostic pathway for centrally positioned lesions and peripheral lesions.

Diffuse infiltrative lung disease

The advent of high-resolution computed tomography (HRCT), with its ability to define pulmonary interstitial disease not readily diagnosed on chest radiographs, has reduced the need for biopsy in many cases of interstitial lung disease.[74]

However, the need for a tissue diagnosis remains in some cases. Transbronchial biopsy, percutaneous biopsy and open lung biopsy have all been used to provide tissue. Fine needle aspiration, yielding material only suitable for cytological examination, is rarely useful in solving these problems.

Endoscopic techniques

As a relatively safe and simple procedure,[75] transbronchial biopsy via the fibreoptic bronchoscope is likely to be preferred in many units, at least as a first choice. What can be expected from the technique?

The overall yield of positive diagnoses in diffuse lung disease is likely to be around 60% but this depends critically on the type of patient chosen. The chance of producing a positive result is significantly higher in some diagnostic categories than others. This creates a classic dilemma: when the diagnosis is known a biopsy often confirms it; when the diagnosis is in doubt the biopsy is often unhelpful.

Sarcoidosis and lymphangitis carcinomatosa are the two diagnoses most readily made by transbronchial biopsy.[76] Fibrosing alveolitis and the vasculitides are less readily diagnosed.[77,78] It is important to take more than one sample. Even in sarcoidosis one biopsy only gives a 40% positive rate, whereas four or more give a rate of 90% or greater. It is interesting to note that sarcoidosis, lymphangitis carcinomatosa and fibrosing alveolitis are some of the diagnoses most readily made on HRCT.[74]

A positive diagnosis on transbronchial biopsy is unlikely to be wrong but a biopsy that yields normal lung or non-specific histology does not greatly influence clinical management.[79] It must be followed up with other diagnostic tests.

Percutaneous techniques

Cutting-needle biopsy has been performed in the evaluation of diffuse lung disease. However, the increased incidence of haemorrhage and pneumothorax has mostly restricted its use to disease processes with more solid components, e.g. organising pneumonia or sarcoidosis.[10]

Open or thoracoscopic lung biopsy

These approaches cannot fail to give tissue. Even with this advantage the diagnostic yield is not necessarily 100%. In both the important American series of Gaensler & Carrington[80] and the UK series of Venn et al,[81] the figures were close to 92%. Yet others relegate up to 30% of causes to a category labelled 'non-specific'.[82,83] Reviewing the lists of diagnoses in the two former papers, in Gaensler & Carrington up to 13% might be considered not accurately classified, and in the UK series in half of the patients the diagnosis is given as cryptogenic fibrosing alveolitis. Ray et al,[81] by way of comparison, put all their cases that probably had this latter diagnosis (15%) into their 'non-specific' ragbag under the heading 'interstitial pulmonary fibrosis'.

Two observations can help to explain these anomalies. The first is that reporting characteristics, skills and diagnostic criteria differ from one histopathologist to the next. The second is that lung biopsy can only yield a firm diagnosis in those conditions currently defined in anatomical terms. The study of biopsy material seldom gives clues to aetiology. For example, although the alveolitis of extrinsic allergic alveolitis is characteristic and enables a useful diagnosis to be made, the extrinsic cause cannot be identified.

Pleural biopsy

Indications for pleural biopsy may be divided into two groups: to aid in the diagnosis of an unexplained pleural effusion and to help determine the aetiology of focal or diffuse pleural thickening in the absence of an associated effusion.

Pleural biopsy may be performed:

• blind, using a reverse-bevel needle such as a Cope or Abrams needle
• under image guidance, most commonly CT or ultrasound, using an automated cutting needle
• under direct visualisation, using open or thoracoscopic techniques.

Pleural biopsy in the absence of effusion

Biopsy in the absence of pleural fluid is most commonly used to characterise the nature of diffuse or focal pleural thickening detected by chest X-ray or CT (Fig. 10.3.4). Large pleural masses may be biopsied using fluoroscopic or ultrasound guidance,[84] but the majority of image-guided biopsies are performed under CT guidance.[85,86] Using a cutting needle to provide histology specimens, and specialist immunohistochemical techniques, the sensitivity for image-guided biopsy for malignancy is greater than 80% and when combined with the diagnostic CT criteria for malignant pleural thickening[87] it has a specificity of up to 100%.[85] The common desmoplastic pleural response to disease makes aspiration cytology biopsy unhelpful in most cases and specimens for histology should be obtained whenever possible.

Pleural biopsy in the presence of effusion

The diagnostic yield of aspiration cytology for infectious and malignant causes of effusion ranges from 40–80%.[88] The addition of non-image-guided pleural biopsy using a reverse-bevel needle can, when performed by an experienced operator, increase the diagnostic yield for pleural tuberculosis to 80–100%,[89] although this may require up to six biopsies. Inexperienced operators may fail to obtain pleural tissue in up to 60% of patients.[89]

In patients with suspected malignant pleural effusion, the addition of non-image-guided pleural biopsy is of less value than for infectious causes. The yield for the detection of malignant

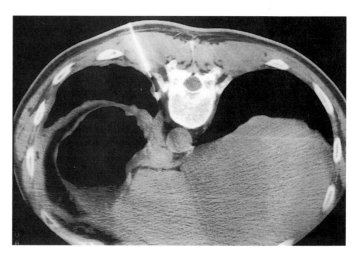

Fig. 10.3.4 Computed-tomography-guided cutting-needle biopsy of irregular pleural thickening providing a histological diagnosis of malignant mesothelioma.

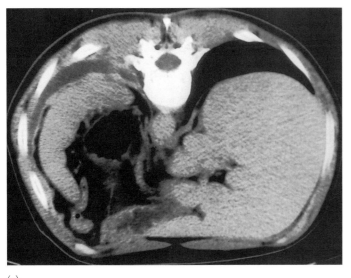
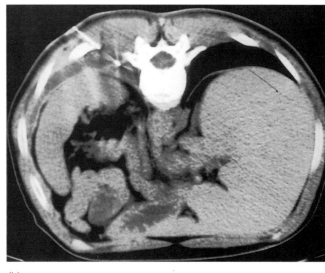

(a)   (b)

Fig. 10.3.5   Contrast-enhanced computed tomography scan demonstrating enhancing irregular pleural thickening (a) and subsequent biopsy providing a histological diagnosis of malignant mesothelioma (b).

mesothelioma is 21–43%[90-92] and for other malignant diseases it is 48–56%.[93-95] In comparison, the use of image guidance has been shown to increase diagnostic yield to more than 90%.[86]

Prior to biopsy a contrast-enhanced CT scan enables pleural thickening to be detected even in the presence of an effusion.[96] Of interest, the impact of the extent of pleural thickening on the success of image-guided biopsy does not appear to be significant. Thickness of as little as 3 mm may be biopsied and produce diagnostic cores of tissue[86] (Fig. 10.3.5). By performing the biopsy along the plane of pleural thickening it is possible to achieve adequate cores for histology in most cases.[86] In reported series, image guidance appears to be a safe technique, with complication rates less than for reverse-bevel needle biopsies.[84-86,97]

Selection of biopsy techniques for biopsy

■ Diffuse or focal pleural thickening detected in the absence of effusion should be biopsied under image guidance using a cutting needle.

■ In the presence of a pleural effusion:
  – non-image-guided reverse-bevel needle biopsy should be performed by an experienced operator in areas with a high incidence of tuberculosis, or if clinical circumstances suggest that this is a likely diagnosis
  – if malignancy is suspected, a cutting-needle image-guided biopsy should be performed, preferably after a contrast-enhanced CT scan has identified the areas of maximal thickness.

■ Thoracoscopic and open pleural biopsy may be performed if prior attempts at diagnosis have been unsuccessful, if the relevant expertise is not available for other biopsy techniques, or in patients with possible malignant effusions requiring pleurodesis.

References

1. Leyden H. Ueber infectiose pneumonia. Dstch Med Wschr 1883; 9: 52.
2. Dahlgren SE, Nordenstrom B. Transthoracic needle biopsy. Chicago: Yearbook Publishers; 1966.
3. Klein JS, Zarka MA. Transthoracic needle biopsy: an overview. J Thor Imaging 1997; 12: 232.
4. Westcott JL. Direct percutaneous needle aspiration of localised pulmonary lesions: results in 422 patients. Radiology 1980; 137: 31.
5. Westcott JL. Percutaneous needle biopsy of hilar and mediastinal masses. Radiology 1981; 141: 323.
6. Gobien RP, Skucas, Paris BS. CT-assisted fluoroscopically guided aspiration biopsy of central hilar and mediastinal masses. Radiology 1981; 141: 443.
7. Westcott JL, Rao N, Colley DP. Transthoracic needle biopsy of small pulmonary nodules. Radiology 1997; 202: 97.
8. Boiselle PM, Shepard JO, Mark, EJ et al. Routine addition of an automated biopsy device to fine-needle aspiration of the lung: a prospective assessment. AJR 1997; 169: 661.
9. Lucidarme O, Howarth N, Finet J-F, Grenier PA. Intrapulmonary lesions: percutaneous automated biopsy with a detachable 18-gauge, coaxial cutting needle. Radiology 1998; 207: 759.
10. Bungay HK, Adams RF, Morris CM et al. Cutting needle biopsy in the diagnosis of clinically suspected non-carcinomatous disease of the lung. B J Radiol 2000; 73: 349.
11. Calhoun P, Feldman PS, Armstrong P et al. The clinical outcome of needle aspirations of the lung when cancer is not diagnosed. Ann Thorac Surg 1976; 41: 592.
12. Charig MJ, Stutley JE, Padley SPG, Hansell DM. The value of negative needle biopsy in suspected operable lung cancer. Clin Radiol 1991; 44: 147.
13. Cummings SR, Lillington GA, Richard RJ. Estimating the probability of malignancy in solitary pulmonary nodules. Am Rev Respir Dis 1986; 134: 449.
14. Gurney JW. Determining the likelihood of malignancy in solitary pulmonary nodules with Bayesian analysis. Radiology 1993; 186: 405.
15. Swensen SJ, Brown LR, Colby TV, Weaver AL. Pulmonary nodules: CT evaluation of enhancement with iodinated contrast material. Radiology 1995; 194: 393.
16. Zhang M, Kono M. Solitary pulmonary nodules: evaluation of blood flow patterns with dynamic CT. Radiology 1997; 205: 471.
17. Laroche C, Fairburn I, Moss H et al. Role of computed tomographic scanning of the thorax prior to bronchoscopy in the investigation of suspected lung cancer. Thorax 2000; 55: 359.
18. Bungay HK, Pal CR, Davies CWH et al. An evaluation of computed tomography as an aid to diagnosis in patients undergoing bronchoscopy for suspected bronchial carcinoma. Clin Radiol 2000; 55: 554.

19. Patz EF Jr, Fidler J, Knelson M et al. Significance of percutaneous needle biopsy in patients with multiple pulmonary nodules and a single known primary malignancy. Chest 1995; 107: 601.

20. Reiner B, Siegal E, Sawyer R et al. The impact of routine CT of the chest on the diagnosis and management of newly diagnosed squamous cell carcinoma of the head and neck. AJR 1997; 169: 667.

21. Quint LE, Park CH, Iannettoni MD. Solitary pulmonary nodules in patients with extrapulmonary neoplasm. Radiology 2000; 217: 257.

22. Castellino RA, Blank N. Etiologic diagnosis of focal pulmonary infection in immunocompromised patients by fluoroscopically guided percutaneous needle aspiration. Radiology 1979; 132: 563.

23. Conces DJ Jr, Clark SA, Tarver RD, Schwenk GR. Transthoracic aspiration needle biopsy: value in the diagnosis of pulmonary infections. AJR 1989; 152: 31.

24. Gruden JF, Klein JS, Webb WR. Percutaneous transthoracic needle biopsy in AIDS: analysis in 32 patients. Radiology 1993; 189: 567.

25. Scott WW Jr, Kuhlman JE. Focal pulmonary lesions in patients with AIDS: percutaneous transthoracic needle biopsy. Radiology 1991; 180: 419.

26. Sinner WN. Complications of percutaneous transthoracic needle aspiration biopsy. Acta Radiol (Diagn) 1976; 17: 813.

27. Berquist TH, Bailey PB, Cortese DA, Miller WE. Transthoracic needle biopsy. Accuracy and complications in relation to location and type of lesion. Mayo Clin Proc 1980; 54: 961.

28. Harrison BDW, Thorpe RS, Kitchener PG et al. Percutaneous Trucut biopsy in the diagnosis of localised pulmonary lesions. Thorax 1884; 39: 493.

29. Hayashi N, Sakai T, Kitagawa M et al. CT-guided biopsy of pulmonary nodules less than 3 cm: usefulness of the spring-operated core biopsy needle and frozen-section pathologic diagnosis. AJR 1998; 170: 329.

30. Laurent F, Latrabe V, Vergier B et al. CT-guided transthoracic needle biopsy of pulmonary nodules smaller than 20 mm: results with an automated 20-gauge coaxial cutting needle. Clin Radiol 2000; 55: 281.

31. Charig MJ, Phillips AJ. CT-guided cutting needle biopsy of lung lesions – safety and efficacy of an out-patient service. Clin Radiol 2000; 55: 964.

32. Greene R. Transthoracic needle aspiration biopsy. In: Athanasoults CA, ed. Interventional radiology. Philadelphia: Pa: WB Saunders; 1982: 587.

33. Moore EH. Technical aspects of needle aspiration lung biopsy: a personal perspective. Radiology 1998; 208: 303.

34. Lang EK, Ghavami R, Schreiner VC et al. Autologous blood clot seal to prevent pneumothorax at CT-guided lung biopsy. Radiology 2000; 216: 93.

35. Yang P-C, Luh K-T, Sheu J-C et al. Peripheral pulmonary lesions: ultrasonography and ultrasonically guided biopsy. Radiology 1985; 155: 451.

36. Pan J-F, Yang P-C, Chang D-B et al. Needle aspiration biopsy of malignant lung masses with necrotic centres: improved sensitivity with ultrasonic guidance. Chest 1993; 103: 1452.

37. Hamarati LB, Austin JHM. Complications after CT-guided needle biopsy of aerated versus nonaerated lung. Radiology 1991; 181: 778.

38. Nashed Z, Klein JS, Zarka MA. Special techniques in CT-guided transthoracic needle biopsy AJR 1998; 171: 1665.

39. Aberle DR, Gamsu G, Golden JA. Fatal systemic arterial air embolism following lung needle aspiration. Radiology 1987; 165: 351.

40. Tolly TL, Feldmeier JE, Czarnecki D. Air embolism complicating percutaneous lung biopsy. AJR 1988; 150: 555.

41. Regge D, Gallo T, Galli J et al. Systemic arterial air embolism and tension pneumothorax: two complications of transthoracic percutaneous thin-needle biopsy in the same patient. Eur Radiol 1997; 7: 173.

42. Fink I, Gamsu G, Harter LP. CT-guided aspiration biopsy of the thorax. J Comput Assist Tomogr 1982; 6: 958.

43. Moore EH, Shepherd JO, McLoud TC et al. Positional precautions in needle aspiration lung biopsy. Radiology 1990; 175: 733.

44. Laurent F, Michel P, Latrabe V et al. Pneumothoraces and chest tube placement after CT-guided transthoracic lung biopsy using a coaxial technique: incidence and risk factors. AJR 1999; 172: 1049.

45. Kazeerooni EA, Lim FT, Mikhail A et al. Risk of pneumothorax in CT-guided transthoracic needle aspiration biopsy of the lung. Radiology 1996; 198: 371.

46. Berger J, Traill Z, Gleeson FV. Incidence of pneumothorax on chest radiographs after CT-guided lung biopsy. Br J Radiol 1998; 71: 84.

47. VanSonnenberg E, Casola G, Ho M et al. Difficult thoracic lesions: CT guided biopsy experience in 150 cases. Radiology 1988; 167: 461.

48. Miller KS, Fish GB, Stanley JH et al. Prediction of pneumothorax rate in percutaneous needle aspiration of the lung. Chest 1988; 93: 742.

49. Cox JE, Chiles C, McManus C et al. Transthoracic needle aspiration biopsy: variables that affect risk of pneumothorax. Radiology 1999; 212: 165.

50. Berquist TH, Bailey PB, Cortese DA, Miller WE. Transthoracic needle biopsy: accuracy and complications in relation to location and type of lesion. Mayo Clin Proc 1980: 55: 475.

51. Fish GD, Stanley JH, Scott Miller K et al. Post biopsy pneumothorax: estimating the risk by chest radiography and pulmonary function tests. AJR 1988; 150: 71.

52. Rozenblit AM, Tuvia J, Rozenblit G, Klink A. CT-guided transthoracic needle biopsy using an ipsilateral dependent position. AJR 2000; 174: 1759.

53. Collings CL, Westcott JL, Banson NL, Lange RC. Pneumothorax and dependent versus nondependent patient position after needle biopsy of the lung. Radiology 1999; 210: 59.

54. Perlmutt LM, Braun SD, Newman GE et al. Timing of chest film follow-up after transthoracic needle aspiration. AJR 1986; 146: 1049.

55. Traill ZC, Gleeson FV. Delayed pneumothorax after CT-guided percutaneous fine needle aspiration lung biopsy. Thorax 1997; 52: 581.

56. Westcott JL. Percutaneous transthoracic needle biopsy. Radiology 1988; 169: 593.

57. Klein JS, Saloman G, Stewart E. Transthoracic needle biopsy with a coaxially placed 20-gauge automated cutting needle: results in 122 patients. Radiology 1996; 198: 715.

58. McLoud T. Should cutting needles replace needle aspiration of lung lesions? Radiology 1998; 208: 569.

59. Sinner WN, Zajieck J. Implantation metastasis after percutaneous transthoracic needle aspiration biopsy. Acta Radiol (Diagn) 1976; 17: 473.

60. Muller NL, Bergin CJ, Miller RR, Ostrow DN. Seeding of malignant cells into the needle tract after lung and pleural biopsy. J Can Assoc Radiol 1986; 37: 192.

61. Khouri NK, Stitik, Erozan YS. Transthoracic needle aspiration biopsy of benign and malignant lung lesions. AJR 1985; 144: 281.

62. Winning AJ, McIvor J, Seed WA et al. Interpretation of negative results in fine needle aspiration of discrete pulmonary lesions. Thorax 1986; 41: 875.

63. Horrigan TP, Bergin KT. Correlation between needle biopsy of lung tumours and histopathologic analysis of resected specimens. Chest 1986; 90: 638.

64. Taft PD, Szyfelbein WM, Green R. A study of variability in cytologic diagnoses based on pulmonary aspiration specimens. Am J Clin Pathol 1980: 73: 36.

65. Thornbury JR, Burke DP, Naylor B. Transthoracic needle aspiration biopsy: accuracy of cytologic typing of malignant neoplasms. AJR 1981; 136: 719.

66. Vielh P. Cytologic typing of primary lung cancer: study of 100 cases with autopsy confirmation. Diagn Cytopathol 1991; 7: 7.

67. Austin JHM, Cohen MB. Value of having a cytopathologist present during percutaneous fine needle aspiration biopsy of lung: report of 55 cancer patients and metanalysis of the literature. AJR 1993; 160: 175.

68. Santambrogio L, Nosotti M, Bellaviti N et al. CT-guided fine-needle aspiration cytology of solitary pulmonary nodules: a prospective randomised study of immediate cytologic evaluation. Chest 1997; 112: 423.

69. Sider I, Davis TM Jr. Hilar masses: evaluation with CT-guided biopsy after negative bronchoscopic examination. Radiology 1987; 164: 107.

70. Harrow EM, Abi-Saleh W, Blum J et al. The utility of transbronchial needle aspiration in the staging of bronchogenic carcinoma. Am J Respir Crit Care Med 2000; 161: 601.

71. Wernecke K, Vassalo P, Peters PE, vonBassewitz DB. Mediastinal tumours: biopsy under ultrasound guidance. Radiology 1999; 172: 473–476.

72. Protopapas Z, Westcott JL. Transthoracic hilar and mediastinal biopsy. J Thorac Imaging 1997; 12: 250–258.

73. Protopapas Z, Westcott JL. Transthoracic biopsy of mediastinal lymph nodes for staging lung and other cancers. Radiology 1996; 199: 489.

74. Webb WR, Muller NL, Naidich DP. High resolution CT of the lung. New York: Raven Press; 1996.

75. Ahmad M, Livingstone DR, Golish JA et al. The safety of outpatient transbronchial biopsy. Chest 1986; 90: 403.

76. Wall CP, Gaensler EA, Carrington CB, Hayes JA. Comparison of transbronchial and open biopsies in chronic infiltrative lung disease. Am Rev Respir Dis 1981; 123: 280.

77. Mitchell DM, Emerson CJ, Collins JV, Stableforth DH. Transbronchial biopsy with the fibreoptic bronchoscope; analysis of results in 433 patients. Br J Dis Chest 1981; 75: 258.

78. Zellweger J-P, Leuenberger PJ. Cytologic and histologic examination of transbronchial lung biopsy. Eur J Respir Dis 1982; 63: 94.

79. Haponik EF, Summer WR, Terry PB, Wang KP. The value of non-specific histological examination. Am Rev Respir Dis 1982; 125: 524.

80. Gaensler EA, Carrington CB. Open biopsy for chronic diffuse infiltrative lung disease: clinical roentgenographic, and physiological correlations in 502 patients. Ann Thorac Surg 1980; 30: 411.

81. Venn GE, Kay PH, Midwood CJ, Goldstraw P. Open biopsy in patients with diffuse pulmonary shadowing. Thorax 1985; 140: 742.

82. Graeve AH, Saul VA, Aki BF. Role of different methods of lung biopsy in the diagnosis of lung lesions. Am J Surg 1980; 140: 742.

83. Ray JF, Lawton BR, Myers WO et al. Open pulmonary biopsy. Chest 1976; 69: 43.

84. Gleeson F, Lomas DJ, Flower CDR et al. Powered cutting needle biopsy of the pleura and chest wall. Clin Radiol 1990; 41: 199.
85. Scott EM, Marshall TJ, Flower CDR. Diffuse pleural thickening: percutaneous CT-guided cutting needle biopsy. Radiology 1995; 194: 867.
86. Adams RF, Gleeson FV. Percutaneous image-guided cutting needle biopsy of the pleura in the presence of a suspected malignant effusion. Radiology 2001; 219: 510.
87. Leung AN, Muller NL, Miller RR. CT in the differential diagnosis of diffuse pleural disease. AJR 1990; 154: 487.
88. Jay SJ. Diagnostic procedures for pleural disease. Clin Chest Med 1985; 6: 33.
89. Kirsch CM, Kroe DM, Azzi RL et al. The optimal number of pleural biopsy specimens for a diagnosis of tuberculous pleurisy. Chest 1997; 112: 702.
90. Ruffie P, Field R, Minkin S et al. Diffuse malignant mesothelioma of the pleura in Ontario and Quebec: a retrospective study of 332 patients. J Clin Oncol 1989; 7: 1157.
91. Boutin C, Rey F. Prevention of malignant seeding after invasive diagnostic procedures in patients with pleural mesothelioma: a randomised trial of local radiotherapy. Chest 1995; 108: 754.
92. Achatzy R, Beba W, Ritschler R et al. The diagnosis, therapy and prognosis of diffuse malignant mesothelioma. Eur J Cadiothorac Surg 1989; 3: 445.
93. Von Hoff DD, Li Volsi V. Diagnostic reliability of needle biopsy of the parietal pleura. A review of 272 biopsies. Am J Clin Pathol 1975; 64: 200–203.
94. Poe RH, Israel RH, Utell JM et al. Sensitivity, specificity and predictive values of closed pleural biopsy. Arch Intern Med 1984; 144: 325.
95. Salyer WR, Eggleston JC, Erozan YS. Efficacy of pleural needle biopsy and pleural fluid cytopathology in the diagnosis of malignant neoplasm involving the pleura. Chest 1975; 67: 536.
96. Traill ZC, Davies RJO, Gleeson FV. Thoracic computed tomography in patients with suspected malignant pleural effusions. Clin Radiol 2001; 56: 193.
97. Screaton NJ, Flower CDR. Percutaneous needle biopsy of the pleura. Radiol Clin North Am 2000; 38: 293.

10.4   Pleural investigations and thoracoscopy

Robert Loddenkemper and Wolfgang Frank

Key points and clinical relevance

■ The requirement for pleural investigation usually arises in the presence of exudative effusions or of pleural thickening of suspected infectious or neoplastic aetiology.

■ Pleural investigations may critically depend on image guidance (fluoroscopy, ultrasound, computed tomography) for safety and targeting reasons.

■ Thoracentesis is the most relevant blind pleural investigation procedure, providing a diagnostic platform for more invasive investigations. Diagnostic patterns describe biochemical, microbiological, molecular and (immuno)cytological features of pleural disease.

■ Closed-needle biopsy has limited sensitivity for diffuse inflammatory and neoplastic disease but is appropriate when contraindications or technical obstacles prevent more invasive procedures.

■ Medical thoracoscopy, classically performed with rigid instruments under local anaesthesia, opens a 'window on the pleural space' providing a diagnostic yield of more than 95% in pleural malignancy and specific infectious disease. It may also significantly improve the management of interstitial lung disease and pneumothorax.

■ Thoracoscopy incorporates highly efficient interventional options, most importantly talc pleurodesis ('poudrage') in malignancy and pneumothorax. Moreover, the management of empyema and tuberculous pleurisy benefits from optimum placement of drains, breaking open of chambers, debridement and fibrinolytic therapy.

■ Thoracoscopy is a remarkably safe procedure with only a few contraindications and significant complications occurring in fewer than 3% of cases, but requires sufficient expertise and continuous practice.

Invasive investigation of pleural disease requires first of all precise localisation and determination of the solid or fluid nature of pleural changes. This is effectively provided by modern imaging techniques, most importantly ultrasonography because of its superior clinical versatility. Invasive techniques are then applied in a stepwise escalating fashion.

Thoracentesis is the basic pleural investigation in all conditions associated with significant pleural effusion. *Blind closed needle biopsy* provides extended diagnostic information in exudative effusion and in solid pleural lesions. *Imaging guidance* is important for all these techniques, to provide optimum results and safety levels. *Endoscopy (thoracoscopy)*, as a 'window on the pleural space', is the gold standard technique and can be used specifically to identify pleurisy with or without effusion and localised lesions alike, but inducible lung detachment from the chest wall (artificial pneumothorax) is an essential prerequisite. The overwhelming majority of invasive diagnostic procedures will require no or only local anaesthesia and may therefore be performed by pulmonologists at the bedside, but are more generally carried out in a standard endoscopic facility.

Thoracentesis

Technique

Thoracentesis is a mandatory diagnostic step if imaging findings show the presence of accessible pleural fluid collections. There are only two exceptions to this general rule: first, if the fluid amount is too small for thoracentesis to be safely performed (< 10 mm fluid film in the lateral decubitus position) and second in apparent 'innocent-bystander'-type pleural involvement, e.g. in congestive heart failure, renal or hepatic disease. Thoracentesis is then only required if an effusion has failed to respond to medical therapy and/or there are clinical signs such as chest pain, fever or clues suggestive of thoracic disease.[1]

Ultrasonic imaging guidance will generally provide optimum safety and efficacy; however, with copious collections bedside percussion-guided thoracentesis is an expedient and safe alternative as well. A 19 gauge needle (to also move viscous aspirates) is adapted to a 20 ml syringe and inserted at the requested costal interspace. The vasculature/nerve-conducting lower edge of the rib is avoided, and penetration should not be too deep. The patient is usually in a sitting or supported position.[1,2] In the severely debilitated patient, e.g. in intensive care, the lateral decubitus position is adequate, with the side of effusion dependent. With skilled technique neither the routine use of local anaesthesia nor a sedative is required. At times, and especially in membranous and trapped collections, it is necessary to perform thoracentesis at various sites to obtain sufficient amounts of fluid and representative samples, since the composition may differ between various compartments. It should also be repeated at other sites in the case of easily recognisable artificial blood contamination.

There is some controversy about the amount of fluid that should be recovered diagnostically. In general a quantity of 20–40 ml will meet all diagnostic demands. Removal of amounts up to 1 litre or even more, as is frequently done, is neither necessary nor desirable, because it may induce pneumothorax and impede subsequent more efficient endoscopic investigations due to the creation of adhesions. Occasionally this may be indicated, however, for palliation of dyspnoea in the case of a massive effusion. Even then a one-step removal of large fluid amounts (> 1.5 litre) should be avoided to prevent hypotensive circulatory effects and re-expansion oedema. When the intention is primarily therapeutic, the use of a kit is advised. These devices consist of a modified needle, often housing a spring-loaded, blunt internal cannula, a three-way stop cock, a 50–100 ml syringe, a safety valve and a 2 litre collection bag, thus avoiding trauma to the lung, infectious contamination and air access to the pleura.

For diagnostic purposes first the general appearance of the fluid is assessed including, colour, viscosity and smell. The effusion may be serous (clear or turbid), suppurative (empyema), sanguinous, chylous or appear as frank blood (haemothorax). In most instances, with the recovery of straw- or amber-coloured, indiscriminate serous fluid, the basic distinction between a transudate or exudate needs next to be established biochemically. For practical purposes, the determination of protein and lactate dehydrogenase is sufficient for this distinction. If there is an exudate, additional investigations as well as cytological analysis may be performed, including a variety of biochemical, haematological, immunological, molecular and microbiological studies, as described in more detail in Chapter 75.[3,4] Importantly, if anaerobic microbiological studies are being requested, the sample should be kept anaerobic and cooled in the original syringe.

The main complication of thoracentesis is pneumothorax, the incidence of which varies in the literature between 3% and 42% depending on the investigator's experience, effusion volume, the use of ultrasound guidance, the type and size of needle used, the quantity of the aspirate and predisposing morbidity (chronic obstructive pulmonary disease, COPD).[1] Chest pain and cough may cause considerable discomfort but rarely amount to a serious problem. Infection should virtually not occur with expert thoracentesis.

Pleural biopsy and endoscopy techniques

When there is clinical suspicion of pleural pathology, but imaging techniques and thoracentesis provide inconclusive or conflicting results, blind pleural biopsy or thoracoscopy may be indicated, but only in the presence of exudates. Prior to proceeding to unnecessary invasive investigations the possibility of a transformed primary transudative effusion (so-called pseudoexudate, see also Chapter 75) should be considered in unexplained exudative effusion or borderline protein or cholesterol values.[5]

Closed needle biopsy

Blind (or closed) needle biopsy is generally indicated in suspected tuberculous or malignant effusion or more generally in lesions expected to reveal specific histological patterns and/or microbiological findings. The hollow-cylinder Tru-Cut® or, more recently, the Radja needle may be preferable to the older but still popular Abrams or Ramel (Cope) needle because of its superior handling, better biopsy quality and for safety reasons.[1,6–8] Needle biopsy is diagnostic in tuberculous pleurisy (combined histology and microbiology) in about 60% of cases.[3–5,7–9] In our series (n = 100), the sensitivity was 63%.[5–11] In neoplastic effusions, the maximum diagnostic yield is in the order of 70%, being usually lower, however, than that of cytology.[12,13] The value of closed-needle biopsy may be defined as augmenting the yield of pleural fluid cytology. In our series, comprising 86 cases of malignant pleurisy, the diagnostic gain was 16% (58%/74%),[14] although in the Mayo Clinic study of 281 patients, pleural biopsy identified only 7% additional malignant effusions when fluid cytology was negative.[15]

Closed-needle biopsy is usually image (ultrasound or fluoroscopy)-guided and may explore pleural changes up to a penetration depth of 15 cm. When the pleural space is obliterated the indication for closed-needle biopsy may be expanded to exploration of deeper structures, including pulmonary lesions adjacent or fused to the pleura.

Safe performance of needle biopsy requires the patient be placed in a stable lateral decubitus position on the side that is not being investigated. Once the specific entry point into the region of interest, and the depth of penetration, has been determined using the preferred imaging technique, local anaesthesia with 1–2% lidocaine (lignocaine) is carefully and generously applied to the relevant intercostal space, with particular attention to the sensitive rib edges. It is even more important than in thoracentesis that too close a proximity to the sulcus at the edge of the lower rib conducting the vasculature/nerve bundle must be strictly avoided to prevent laceration of these structures. It is easier and safer to perform needle biopsy in the thin lateral and anterior regions of the chest wall than in the posterior, and especially the paravertebral, area. However, in the parasternal region the internal mammary artery may be dangerously exposed to

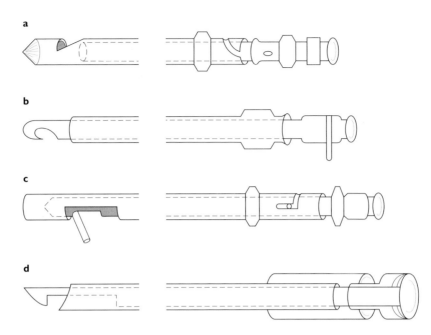

Fig. 10.4.1 The principle of various commonly used closed-biopsy needles. a. The **Abrams needle** consists of a large, blunt outer trocar, an inner cutting cannula and a stylet. After appropriate pleural placement of the needle, removal of the inner stylet and exposure of the notch of the needle by counterclockwise rotation of the inner cannula, fluid can be aspirated and a biopsy obtained. This is achieved by withdrawing the needle until the notch hooks on to the pleura, via back rotation of the cutting cannula. b. The **Cope needle** consists of an outer cannula, a blunt-tipped, hooked biopsy trocar, a bevelled trocar and an obturator or stylet. The whole instrument is introduced to the pleura. A biopsy is obtained by removing the stylet and the bevelled trocar and replacing them with the hooked biopsy trocar. When the hook engages a tissue sample, this can be severed by forward rotation of the outer cannula. c. The **Radja needle** is similar to the Abrams needle but contains a spring-operated, self-opening, stainless-steel biopsy flap. When the needle is withdrawn after insertion and the flap is hooked on to the parietal pleura a biopsy is sheared off by pulling back the outer cannula. d. The **Tru-Cut needle** consists of only two parts, an outer cutting cannula and an inner trocar, carrying the biopsy sampling notch. It does not allow fluid aspiration. When the closed instrument has been placed properly, the outer cutting cannula is withdrawn and then pushed forward again while the trocar is fixed at the distal end by the non-operative hand.

injury. A narrow stab incision of the skin with a scalpel facilitates the introduction of all types of needle.

The principle of the various needles in clinical use is shown in Figure 10.4.1. With the Abrams needle a tissue sample is obtained through a side hole in the outer needle, once the pleura is contacted, by rotation of the cutting inner cylinder. The possibility of first aspirating fluid to confirm a safe position within the pleura is an advantage of this type of needle. The comparatively simple Tru-Cut® (Travenol) needle, which consists only of a hollow external cutting component and an inner tissue sampling trocar, may also be used in the absence of effusion. Because of the pressure that must be exerted with the active hand to penetrate the tissue, protective use of the non-dominant hand is important to prevent sudden excessive penetration of the chest wall. At least three separate biopsies should be obtained, one of which should be saved for sterile bacteriological processing.

Contraindications to needle biopsy are bleeding diathesis and advanced COPD. Needle biopsy has a low complication rate, which varies with the depth of penetration, the site of intervention and the type of needle. Haemorrhage (haemoptysis, haemothorax), pneumothorax, syncope, air embolism, pain and

injury to adjacent organs (liver, spleen) are the most important. Their total incidence has been reported to be 15%; lethal complications occur in 0.09%.[8,15] Therefore, and because the gain in diagnostic yield is limited, the trained clinician will tend to bypass blind pleural biopsy and prefer the higher efficacy of thoracoscopy whenever it is technically feasible. Needle biopsy, however, remains the best alternative if thoracoscopy is not possible or in the presence of technical and clinical obstacles (adhesions, contraindications, non-compliance). In addition, imaging guided closed-needle biopsy is the technique of choice in solid lesions involving deeper structures of the chest wall that may be invisible from the internal pleural surface at thoracoscopy.

Medical thoracoscopy

Medical thoracoscopy was introduced into diagnosis of diseases of the chest by Jacobaeus in Sweden as early as 1910.[16] He also 'invented' minimal invasive surgical thoracoscopy in terms of using the technique for pneumolysis in tuberculosis.[17] Only much later was the diagnostic potential of the technique 'rediscovered' and subsequently developed throughout the second half of the last century, mainly in western Europe.[18-20] Over time the ability, when technically feasible, to biopsy suspicious areas of the pleura under vision control with a remarkable degree of safety has established thoracoscopy worldwide as the gold-standard technique for the diagnosis of pleural disease.[11,21-23] Modern video assisted thoracoscopy is an extended technical application of the original direct vision single entry approach, which has also led to the development of video-assisted thoracic surgery (VATS).[22-26] Unlike traditional thoracoscopy, which can be performed under local anaesthesia and conscious sedation in the endoscopy unit, VATS requires double-lumen intubation and general anaesthesia and is thus less versatile in clinical practice.

Indications

Thoracoscopy allows visualisation of most intrathoracic structures. Therefore, apart from pleural effusion, the classical spectrum of indications also includes interstitial lung disease, pneumothorax and localised disease of the lung, chest wall and diaphragm, as well as mediastinal lesions. The principle of the investigation is illustrated by the CT simulation in Figure 10.4.2.

Pleural effusion is the major classical indication and currently accounts for up to 90% of all investigations.[11,27] With appropriate expertise medical thoracoscopy can clarify the aetiology in 90–95% of pleural effusions. The reported diagnostic yield in malignant effusion is 95% and approaches 98% in tuberculous pleurisy when microscopic, cultural and histological results are combined.[11,19-22] In our prospective series ($n = 101$) the cumulated microbiological/histological yield of thoracentesis (28%), closed-needle biopsy (51%) and thoracoscopy (98%) achieved 100%.[10,11,28] Moreover, in malignant effusion, tissue samples can be used for additional investigations such as immunohistochemistry and hormone receptor staining.[11,23,29]

In the staging of bronchial carcinoma with concomitant effusion, thoracoscopy allows the discrimination between para-malignant effusion and carcinosis, thus avoiding explorative thoracotomy.[11,23] In malignant pleural mesothelioma careful thoracoscopy-based staging is the main determinant of therapeutic decisions (surgical versus non-surgical approaches).[11,20,30-33] Macroscopic findings, such as certain proliferation features ('grapelike' appearance) and the presence of hyaline plaques, may suggest mesothelioma or asbestos exposure respectively.[11,30,31]

The management of pneumothorax benefits considerably from the application of thoracoscopy, visualising cysts, bullae, blebs or pleural leaks to permit rational therapy design.[11,19,34-39] In interstitial lung disease thoracoscopy takes an intermediate position between transbronchial biopsy and surgical techniques (VATS or open lung biopsy) as regards diagnostic yield and invasiveness, with a reported overall sensitivity of 86–93%[19,41] Results are, however, much modified by the distribution, nature and extent of parenchymal changes. Diffuse peripheral location and certain suspected diagnoses such as sarcoidosis or lymphangiosis favour a thoracoscopic approach, especially where anaesthesia is risky.[19,41,42]

The sensitivity of thoracoscopy in focal lesions of the lung and the chest wall is limited. In our series of 151 cases it was only 47.8% in localised lung lesions and 81.3% in various chest wall lesions (fibroma, neurofibroma, lipoma, hamartoma,

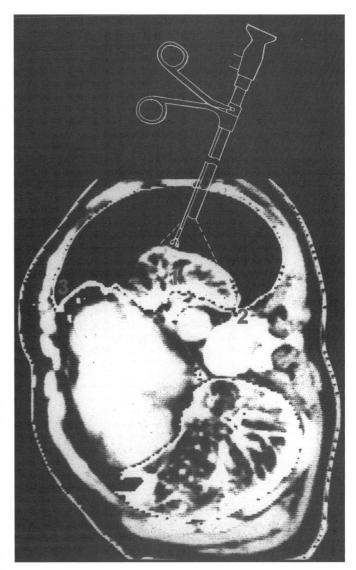

Fig. 10.4.2 Computed tomography simulation of medical thoracoscopy (right thoracic cavity in left lateral position) Visualisation of chest wall pleura, diaphragm, lung, anterior and (partially) posterior mediastinum possible.

chondroma, myoma and others), suggesting the use of thoracoscopy only if surgery is contraindicated, opportunity (pre-existent pneumothorax) or where it is suspected that a lesion is benign.[43]

Thoracoscopy also provides considerable management advantages both in effusion and in pneumothorax because it ensures optimal visual placement of drains. In addition it may be used for therapeutic interventions such as debridement in tuberculosis and empyema, diathermy or laser coagulation in pneumothorax and, most importantly, pleurodesis in malignant effusion and pneumothorax (see Chapter 75).[22,23,44-47]

Technique

Medical thoracoscopy is usually performed under local anaesthesia and conscious sedation (neuroleptanalgesia) in a properly

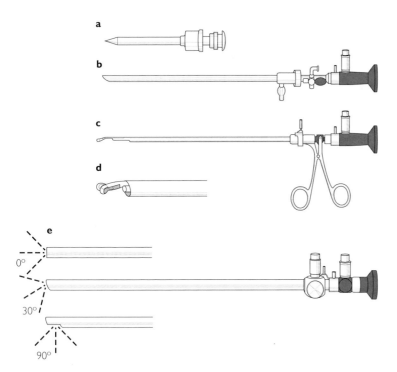

Fig. 10.4.3 Basic instrumental set for medical thoracoscopy. a. Trocar obturator with integrated valve and sharp internal cannula of 7, 9 or 11 mm diameter for single- or two-port technique. b. Single-incision thoracoscope (9 or 11 mm diameter). c. Biopsy forceps with integrated 0° optical system. d. Enlarged view of the optics and forceps in the shaft of the thoracoscope ready for biopsy. e. Various straight- and angled-vision telescopes for the single-entry technique with adapted photographic light shaft

equipped endoscopy suite under sterile conditions (surgical hand-washing, gown and gloves) with the patient lying in the lateral decubitus position on the side that is not to be investigated. Most investigators prefer a single-entry approach, using a 9 mm (sometimes 11 mm) thoracoscope that can provide access for both the scope and accessory instruments. Others prefer a 7 mm port for visualisation and a separate 5 mm instrumentation port.[19] The optimal operating team would include the main investigator, an assistant physician and two specially trained nurses. State-of-the-art thoracoscopy, apart from standard endoscopic equipment, requires the following special components:

- a mobile fluoroscopy and/or ultrasound facility
- needles for induction of pneumothorax (Denneke, Verres)
- pneumothorax apparatus or alternative gas insufflator
- thoracoscopy instruments as shown and specified in Figure 10.4.3 (these are basically rigid and include angled-vision scopes; terminal semiflexible instruments may be sometimes useful but flexible instruments do not confer any advantages and are difficult to sterilise)
- a high-power (> 200 W) cold-light source
- video equipment, including a colour printer
- an optional photographic camera system.

The image-processing components of the system are usually integrated into a mobile rack.

The practice of thoracoscopy requires adequate investigational experience of at least 20 previous supervised examinations and continuous performance of 20 investigations or more per year.[48] Preinvestigation clinical studies should include a chest radiograph (± ultrasonography), arterial or capillary blood gases (optional spirometry), electrolytes and blood coagulation tests. Since thoracoscopy is a demanding procedure in terms of patient compliance, extensive verbal or written patient inform-

ation, supportive counselling and finally informed consent are other important prerequisites.

Thoracoscopy using the more common single-port technique is performed according to the following procedure.[11,18,27]

1. **Induction of premedication 30–45 minutes beforehand**. Most investigators use a combined sedative (midazolam 2–3 mg i.m.) and antitussive medication (hydrocodone 7.5–15 mg i.m.) but various other protocols, including analgesic opiates and neuroleptics, are in use. Dose adjustments may be required in elderly patients and in cardiorespiratory premorbidity. The patient may be allowed a bland meal up to 4 hours prior to the investigation.

2. **Positioning** of the patient, of the monitoring systems (ECG, respiratory rate, pulsoximetry) and of electrodes if cautery is intended; insertion of a venous cannula.

3. **Induction of lung detachment** (artificial pneumothorax) by insufflation of CO_2 as the preferred filling gas. The Denneke or Verres needle (avoiding lung injury) is used in the absence of effusion. Creation of a (sero-)pneumothorax with a regular needle is also a wise precaution in the presence of effusion and will prevent accidental penetration of the trocar into otherwise unrecognised adhesions. A pneumothorax apparatus incorporating a manometer facilitates recognition of the pressure-guided pleural space, and the gas-filling manoeuvre.[11,18] The pleural air (gas) space created should be large enough to allow complete inspection of the pleural cavity. With adhesions an air space of at least 2 cm depth is required to ensure safe introduction of the trocar. The extent of lung detachment needs to be verified by fluoroscopy.

4. **Selection of optimum and safe entry site** using fluoroscopy. The 4th/5th–6th intercostal space in the anterior axillary line has evolved as an almost standard entry point, providing an optimum overview of the pleural cavity and generally allowing bioptic access to all objects of interest. Local adhesions and unusual object locations may modify the entry point.

5. **Implementation of local anaesthesia** using 1% novocaine or 1–2% lidocaine (lignocaine). It is important to carry out an initial trial aspiration of gas from the pleural cavity as the ultimate safeguard against inadequate entry points, followed by withdrawal of the needle and careful and copious infiltration of the pleura, the intercostal space, the rib edges and the skin. Inappropriate anaesthesia may be responsible for severe pain and vagovasal syncope.

6. **A preparatory deep skin incision** about 1.5-cm long. It would appear wise at this step to integrate closed-needle biopsy into the thoracoscopic work-up of pleural effusion, since (1) thoracoscopy may be blinded to the pleural area immediately beneath the point of entry and (2) closed-needle biopsy may provide additional cross-sectional bioptic information about the chest wall, examining deeper structures than are safely accessible by thoracoscopy.

7. **Cautious trocar introduction**, avoiding uncontrolled deep penetration. Forceful trocar handling is a frequent mistake and may lead to haemorrhage and lung injury.

8. **Evacuation of the entire fluid collection**. This ensures complete inspection of the pleural space. It is also necessary for the thoracoscopic approach to pleurodesis (talc *poudrage*). Since rapid removal of massive collections of fluid may provoke circulatory redistribution effects, with systemic hypotension or subsequent re-expansion lung oedema, intravenous isotonic volume replacement and slow post-thoracoscopic lung expansion (over hours) is required as a measure of precaution in profuse effusion (> 3 litres).

9. **Introduction of the telescope and thorough visual examination of the entire pleural cavity**. Basic orientation requires a profound knowledge of the normal anatomy and recognition of landmark structures. The normal pleura presents as a delicate, transparent, light-reflecting surface. Angled telescopes allow inspection of remote or concealed locations such as the paravertebral area, the chest apex, the interlobar space and the mediastinal pleura. Descriptive terms in the evaluation of pleural changes refer to the presence of hyperaemia (hypervascularity), diffuse thickening ('pachypleuritis'), circumscribed thickening (plaques), granulations, lymphangitis, nodules and nodes, large scale tumours, blood-derived exudative deposits (fibrin, septae, membranes, pus, blood) and adhesions or strands. Those for the evaluation of pulmonary changes include: inflation status and colour (hyperinflation, emphysema, atelectasis, anthracosis) and circumscribed changes such as consolidation (focal, segmental, lobar), blebs, bullae, cysts and visible air leaks.

10. **Optional blunt dissection with instruments of impeding adhesions and breaking of septae and membranes**. This procedure is essential to obtain a representative overview and unimpeded bioptic access. A small cavity may be expanded to the full size of the pleural space, as often and typically occurs in tuberculous or rheumatic pleurisy, occasionally also in malignancy. The procedure is also important to ensure full post-thoracoscopic lung expansion. Fibrotic and vascularised adhesions, however, must be spared.

11. **Video and optional photographic documentation**. This is recommended for documentation in the patient files and for teaching purposes.

12. **Biopsy.** Biopsies are generally taken from the parietal pleura. The ribs and intercostal spaces must be clearly identified in order to avoid inadvertent deep forceps penetration at the inferior rib margin. Biopsies certainly cause a short, sharp pain but rarely require additional anaesthesia. Macroscopic visual evaluation alone is remarkably sensitive and specific for a number of aetiologies such as carcinosis, mesothelioma, tuberculosis and rheumatic pleurisy, but may be misleading and should never be relied on. Therefore copious and numerous biopsies even in the normal-appearing situs are recommended. Visceral pleural and lung biopsies should be taken judiciously, considering risks and contraindications (bleeding, pulmonary malexpansion, pulmonary hypertension). Probing of the lung with the forceps helps to define suspect areas. The use of a coagulating forceps with a mean setting of 100 W will minimise or prevent a subsequent air leak. Mediastinal and pericardial biopsies can be obtained but require advanced experience and perfect anatomic knowledge. At times it may be safer, particularly for remote structures and those of uncertain nature such as suspected cysts, to adopt a less aggressive approach using a vision-guided puncture technique. The prior use of a probe stick is recommended for improved assessment of any unclear lesion. A specifically designed angled thoracoscope with a separate optical and interventional port facilitates these procedures. It is also used in interventions such as cautery, laser application and pleurodesis. Bleeding is a regular side-effect of biopsy and rarely requires cautery. Injury to the intercostal artery would appear to be particularly critical. In our experience of more than 6000 cases, haemorrhage has never necessitated surgical intervention.

13. **Assessment of lung expandability**. This is particularly important before induction of pleurodesis. The main causes of impeded lung expansion are membranous inflammatory or malignant parenchymal entrappings ('trapped lung'), large-scale pulmonary consolidation and major air leaks.

14. **Optional induction of pleurodesis** using talc powder (see Chapter 75).

15. **Insertion of tube drainage in the optimum position.** For optimal function and tolerance, the drain should be placed in an apicodorsal direction covering the pulmonary surface as far as possible. Interlobar and mediastinal position of the drainage must be avoided.

16. **Suture fixation of the drain at the penetration site.** Purse string sutures are not needed.

17. **Cautious lung expansion**. The level of suction and the time-setting for complete lung expansion must take into account risks such as re-expansion oedema and well-recognised impediments (trapped/consolidated lung and bronchopleural fistula). Not all investigators use continuing post-thoracoscopic tube drainage after re-expansion when the lung is intact and has not been biopsied. However, an indwelling drain increases safety and facilitates management of effusion in many ways. For correct management of pleurodesis it is indispensable.

18. **Radiographic confirmation of drain position and correct drain function.**

19. **Removal of the drain and clamping/suture of the insertion site** as soon as stable lung expansion and discontinuation of secretions have been confirmed.

Contraindications

Relevant absolute and relative contraindications may be summarised as follows.

Absolute contraindications

- Bleeding disorders (partial thromboplastin time > 40 s, Quick test < 60%, platelets < 40 000)
- Critical cardiac performance, i.e. left ventricular ejection fraction less than 0.35, recent myocardial infarction (< 6 weeks) and cardiac arrhythmias more than Lown IVb despite adequate therapy
- Obliterated pleural space or non-detachment of the lung on pneumothorax induction.

Relative contraindications

- Critical respiratory performance (Po_2 < 50 mmHg, Pco_2 > 50 mmHg), unless caused by pneumothorax or effusion
- Critical small pleural cavity to explore and/or impeded, difficult access
- When lung biopsies are being considered, pulmonary hypertension (pulmonary artery pressure > 35 mmHg), critically decreased compliance as in pulmonary fibrosis (honeycombing), suspicion of vascular malformations.

Safety aspects

Measures and precautions to improve and monitor intrathoracoscopic patient safety include the insertion of an indwelling venous cannula, continuous cardiorespiratory monitoring and establishment of low-flow oxygen insufflation. Prior grounding and placement of electrodes allows rapid implementation of cautery on demand. Verbal contact between the investigating staff and the conscious patient has an important supportive function. The presence of an anaesthetist may be required for modified anaesthetic protocols such as neuroleptanalgesia. Gas exchange during thoracoscopy and its relationship to various procedures has been analysed in a few clinical studies, which have unanimously shown that changes in O_2 saturation do occur subsequent to premedication, positioning manoeuvres, induction of pneumothorax and sometimes during thoracoscopy; however, they virtually never attain critical levels.[49,50] In one study the variability and changes in oxygen saturation measured before, during and after thoracoscopy was 93.5 ± 5%, 91.0 ± 4% and 94.0 ± 3% respectively.[51] In addition, the lateral recumbent position with the 'good' lung dependent – as is typically used in thoracoscopy – represents the optimum in terms of gravity-dependent gas exchange.

Post-thoracoscopic care focuses on cardiocirculatory and respiratory function, maintenance of adequate drainage, monitoring of pleural secretions and lung expansion and finally control of pain and prevention of soft-tissue emphysema (cough control).

Complications

Important complications, especially major bleeding and severe dyspnea, occur in fewer than 3% of cases and lethal complications in fewer than 0.01%.[20,27,52] Infection (empyema) complicates thoracoscopy in fewer than 1%. Mediastinal and soft tissue emphysema are more frequent (< 7%), but rarely represent a significant problem. Air embolism is a serious, but fortunately rare complication (< 0.1%); the preference for CO_2 as the filling gas is already part of a preventive strategy. Persistent air leak (> 7 days) occurs preferentially in pneumothorax and after lung biopsy. Malignant seeding of the chest wall entry port is virtually unique to mesothelioma. Local irradiation post-thoracoscopy has proved to be an effective means of prevention. Re-expansion lung oedema is related to profuse and long-standing effusion and is rarely observed with reasonable preventive strategies (most importantly the use of prolonged low suction levels; < 0.5%). The side effects of pleurodesis are not directly thoracoscopy-related and therefore discussed elsewhere (Chapter 75).

Surgical pleural biopsy

Surgical biopsy is the ultimate investigation for pleural disease if less invasive procedures have failed to clarify the aetiology or in the presence of technical or other obstacles to thoracoscopy. With the diagnostic efficacy of advanced imaging techniques for guiding non-surgical diagnostic interventions, the need for surgical biopsy has become rare.

? Unresolved questions

- How can improved imaging techniques (ultrasound) be employed for optimum targeting?
- What will be the effects of technical progress in biopsy needle design?
- What will be the trends in technical development and preferences in thoracoscopy – single- versus multiple-port technique, semiflexible instruments?
- Medical and surgical (video-assisted thoracic surgery) indication preferences remain to be defined.

References

1. Light RW. Thoracentesis (dagnostic and terapeutic) and pleural biopsy. In: Light RW. Pleural diseases, 3rd ed. Baltimore: Williams & Wilkins; 1995.
2. Collins TR, Sahn SA. Thoracentesis: complications, patients' experience and diagnostic value. Chest 1987; 91: 817–822.
3. Sahn SA. The diagnostic value of pleural fluid analysis. Semin Respir Crit Care Med 1995; 16: 269–278.
4. Light RW. Pleural diseases, 3rd ed. Baltimore: Williams & Wilkins; 1995.
5. Loddenkemper R, Frank W. Pleural effusion, haemothorax, chylothorax. In: Grassi C, ed. Pulmonary diseases. London: McGraw-Hill; 1999: 41; 391–404
6. O'Connor S, Yung T. A comparison of Abrams and Raja pleural biopsy needles Aust NZ J Med 1992; 22: 237.
7. Radja GO, Argaval V, Vizoli LD et al. Comparison of the Raja and the Abrams pleural biopsy needles in patients with pleural effusion. Am Rev Respir Dis 1993; 147:1291–1294.
8. Chretien J, Daniel CJ. Needle pleural biopsy. In: Chretien J, Bignon J, Hirsch A, ed. The pleura in health and disease. New York: Marcel Dekker; 1985: 631–642.

9. Cope C. New pleural biopsy needle – preliminary study. JAMA 1958; 167: 1107–1108.

10. Loddenkemper R, Grosser H, Ma J et al. Diagnostik des tuberkulösen Pleuraergusses: prospektiver Vergleich laborchemischer, bakteriologischer, zytologischer und histologischer Untersuchungsergebnisse. Pneumologie 1983; 37: 1153–1156.

11. Loddenkemper R. Thoracoscopy: state of the art. Eur Respir J 1998 ; 11: 213–221.

12. Canto-Armengod A, Rivas J, Saumench J et al. Points to consider when choosing a biopsy method in cases of pleurisy of unknown origin. Chest 1983; 84:176.

13. Canto-Armengod A. Thoracoscopy: diagnostic results in secondary malignant pleural effusions. Pneumologie 1989; 43: 58–60.

14. Loddenkemper R, Grosser H, Gabler A, Mai J. Prospective evaluation of biopsy methods in the diagnosis of malignant pleural effusions. Intrapatient comparison between pleural fluid cytology, blind needle biopsy and thoracoscopy. Am Rev Respir Dis 1983; 127(suppl. 4): 114

15. Prakash UBS, Reiman HM. Comparison of needle biopsy with cytologic analysis for the evaluation of pleural effusion: analysis of 414 cases. Chest 1983; 84:176.

16. Jacobaeus HC. Über die Möglichkeit, die Zystoskopie bei Untersuchung seröser Höhlen anzuwenden. Münch Med Wschr 1910; 40: 2090–2092.

17. Jacobaeus HC. The cauterization of adhesions in artificial pneumothorax therapy of tuberculosis. Am Rev Tuberc 1922; 6: 871–897.

18. Brandt HJ, Loddenkemper R, Mai J. Atlas of diagnostic thoracoscopy. New York: Thieme; 1985.

19. Boutin C, Viallat JR, Aelony Y. Practical thoracoscopy. Berlin: Springer; 1991.

20. Alcozer G, Dorigoni A. La toracoscopia diagnostica. Florence: Nardini; 1984.

21. Mathur PN, Boutin C, Loddenkemper R. 'Medical' thoracoscopy: technique and indications in pulmonary medicine. J Bronchol 1994; 1: 1153–1156.

22. Colt HG. Thoracoscopy: window to the pleural space. Chest 1999; 116: 1409–1415.

23. Harris RJ, Kavuru MS, Mehta AC et al. The impact of thoracoscopy on the management of pleural disease. Chest 1996; 107: 845–852.

24. Inderbitzi R. Chirurgische Thorakoskopie. Berlin: Springer; 1993.

25. Loddenkemper R, Kaiser D. Thoracoscopy. Stuttgart: Thieme; 2001.

26. Linder A, Friedel G, Toomes H. Prerequisites, indications and techniques of video-assisted thoracoscopic surgery. Thorac Cardiovasc Surg 1993; 41:140–146.

27. Frank W, Herziger D. Medical thoracoscopy in Germany: a current national status report (abstract). Pneumologie 1999; 53: S10.

28. Loddenkemper R. Thoracoscopy: results in non-cancerous and idiopathic pleural effusions. Poumon-Coeur 1981; 37: 261–264.

29. Sahn SA. Pleural diseases related to metastatic malignancies. Eur Respir J 1997; 10: 1907–1913.

30. Boutin C, Frey F, Gouvernet J et al. Thoracoscopy in pleural malignant mesothelioma. A prospective study of 188 consecutive patients. Part 1: Diagnosis; Part 2: Prognosis and staging. Cancer 1993; 72: 389–404.

31. Martensson G, Hagmar B, Zetergren L. Diagnosis and prognosis in malignant pleural mesothelioma: a prospective study. Eur J Respir Dis 1984; 65: 169–178.

32. Rush V. Clinical features and current treatment of diffuse malignant pleural mesothelioma. Lung Cancer 1995; 12(suppl. 2): S127–S146.

33. International Mesothelioma Interest Group. A proposed new international TNM system for malignant mesothelioma. Chest 1995; 108: 1122–1128.

34. Boutin C, Astoul P, Rey F, Mathur PN. Thoracoscopy in the diagnosis of spontaneous pneumothorax. Clin Chest Med 1995; 16: 497–503.

35. Vanderschueren RG. The role of thoracoscopy in the evaluation and management of pneumothorax. Lung Suppl 1990; 1122–1125.

36. Liu HP, Lin PJ, Hsie MJ et al. Thoracoscopic surgery as a routine procedure for spontaneous pneumothorax. Chest 1995; 107: 559–562.

37. Takeno Y. Thoracoscopic treatment of spontaneous pneumothorax. Ann Thorac Surg 1993; 56: 688–690.

38. Inderbitzi RGC, Leiser A, Furrer M, Althaus U. Three years experience in video-assisted thoracic surgery (VATS) for spontaneous pneumothorax. J Thorac Cardiovasc Surg 1994; 107: 1410–1415.

39. Janssen JP, Schramel FMNH, Sutedja TG et al. Videothoracoscopic appearance of first and recurrent pneumothorax. Chest 1995; 108: 330–334.

40. Schaberg T, Raffenberg M. Preussler H, Loddenkemper R. Thoracoscopic lung biopsies in the diagnosis of diffuse and localised lung diseases. Am Rev Respir Dis 1991; 143: A667.

41. Boutin C, Loddenkemper R, Astoul Ph. Diagnostic and therapeutic thoracoscopy: techniques and indications in pulmonary medicine. Tubercle Lung Dis 1993; 74: 225–239.

42. Kadokura M, Colby TV, Pyers JL et al. Pathologic comparison of video-assisted thoracic surgical lung biopsy with traditional open lung biopsy. J Thorac Cardiovasc Surg 1995; 59: 348.

43. Raffenberg M, Schaberg T, Loddenkemper R, Thorakoskopische Diagnostik pleuranaher Herdbefunde. Pneumologie 1992; 46: 298–299.

44. Rodriguez-Panadero F, Antony VB. Pleurodesis: state of the art. Eur Respir J 1997; 10: 1648–1654.

45. Kennedy L, Sahn SA. Talc pleurodesis for the treatment of pneumothorax and pleural effusion. Chest 1994; 106: 1215–1222.

46. Karmy-Jones R, Sorenson V, Horst M et al. Rigid thoracoscopic debridement and continuous pleural irrigation in the management of empyema. Chest 1997; 111: 272–274.

47. Landreneau RJ, Keenan RJ, Hazelrigg SR et al. Thoracoscopy for empyema and haemothorax. Chest 1995; 109: 18–24.

48. Mares DC, Mathur PN. Medical thoracoscopy: the pulmonologist's perspective. Sem Respir Crit Care 1997; 18: 803–816.

49. Faurschou P, Madson F, Viskum K. Thoracoscopy: influence of the procedure on some respiratory and cardiac values. Thorax 1982; 38: 341.

50. Colt HG. Thoracoscopy: a prospective study of safety and outcome. Chest 1995; 108: 324–329.

51. Newhouse M. Pulmonary gas exchange during thoracoscopy. Chest 1989; 96: 246–249.

52. Viskum K, Enk B. Complications of thoracoscopy. Poumon-Coeur 1981; 37: 25–28.

11 Principles of thoracic surgery

Peter Goldstraw

Key points

- The thoracic surgeon has a key role in the curative treatment of many thoracic conditions, both benign and malignant.

- The thoracic surgeon can also assist in obtaining a tissue diagnosis, in assessing treatment options and in the palliation of extensive malignancy.

- A little forethought may allow several minor surgical procedures to be undertaken sequentially, such that a diagnosis is assured and evaluation completed under one anaesthetic.

- The rigid bronchoscope remains a valuable investigative and therapeutic tool.

Over the last 50 years the principles of thoracic surgery have become established, largely as a result of practical experience rather than formal scientific study. A large number of thoracic surgical units developed initially to deal with the needs of tuberculosis; subsequently the management of lung cancer came to dominate practice as the surgical needs of patients with tuberculosis declined. Each of the early units had at its centre an influential and charismatic figure and from each a 'school' of thoracic surgery developed to dominate and populate other surgical units. Major aspects of care therefore became standardised, but many aspects of management have never been subjected to scientific study. For this reason this chapter contains a blend of what is standard practice on the one hand and views derived from personal training and experience on the other.

Diagnostic techniques

There is no clear division between diagnostic and therapeutic surgery and often both aspects are contained within a single pro-

cedure. Discussion between physician and surgeon is important to select the appropriate investigative technique that will provide the maximum amount of information with the least trauma to the patient. An escalating series of minor operations should be avoided, since this can be disheartening and debilitating for the patient. Careful preoperative evaluation should allow a contingency plan to be discussed with the patient such that, if one procedure does not allow complete evaluation, others may be accomplished under a single general anaesthetic. The anaesthetist must be fully aware of the options and will need to choose the muscle relaxant and other drugs accordingly.

Rigid bronchoscopy

During the early years of fibreoptic bronchoscopy, much energy and time was spent in adversarial debate over the superiority of flexible or rigid bronchoscopy. It is now generally agreed that each technique has its advantages and disadvantages and both have a role in patient management.[1] As it is performed under local anaesthetic, fibreoptic bronchoscopy (see Chapter 10.1) is an ideal screening procedure for the investigation of large numbers of patients, a small percentage of whom will require surgical evaluation with the rigid bronchoscope. Rigid bronchoscopy on anaesthetised and paralysed patients allows a still field to make precise evaluation and a wide-bore instrument to permit the instrumentation necessary to restore the patency of an airway or remove a foreign body. Often, the choice of instrument will depend on the facilities available locally and the experience and expertise of the operators.

In current practice the major indications for rigid bronchoscopy are as follows.

Histological diagnosis. Approximately one-quarter of patients referred for pulmonary resection are seen initially by the surgeon without histological diagnosis. In some this is the result of the peripheral location of their tumours, whereas in others bronchial abnormalities have been seen on fibreoptic bronchoscopy but the histological diagnosis has not been established. The bronchial abnormality may be non-specific, merely reflecting compression

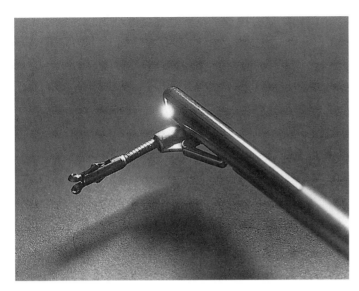

Fig. 11.1 Stortz right-angled biopsy instrument: the biopsy forceps are swung into view by a proximal mechanism then advanced under vision. The biopsies obtained are considerably larger than those of the flexible bronchoscope.

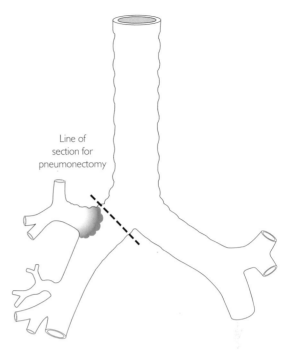

Line of section for pneumonectomy

Fig. 11.2 Tumour extending proximal to the origin of the right upper lobe may be proximal to the carina but still within the main bronchus and resectable by pneumonectomy.

caused by extrabronchial disease, or necrotic slough may cover endobronchial tumours and shallow small biopsies may not show the true underlying pathology. Occasionally, vascular endobronchial tumours may not be biopsied because of the physician's understandable concern regarding bleeding. The large biopsy instrument used with the rigid bronchoscope allows removal of any slough and biopsy of the underlying tumour. Bleeding, even if brisk, can be safely controlled. The improved optics of modern rigid bronchoscopes, coupled with ingenious right-angled biopsy instruments (Fig. 11.1), allows large biopsies under direct vision even from the segments of the upper lobes and the apical segment of the lower lobe.

Assessment of operability. Where tumours are judged to be of borderline resectability, the still field and wide-angled telescopes available to the rigid bronchoscopist allow more precise evaluation. Polypoid tumours may be displaced with the rigid instrument, often demonstrating that their site of origin lies some distance distally within the bronchial tree. The oblique origin of the right main bronchus and its short length may create difficulties in assessing resectability: a tumour at this site may extend along the lateral wall of the right main bronchus so that, even when it appears to be proximal to the carina, it is limited to the main bronchus (Fig. 11.2). The rigid bronchoscope also allows the operator to assess the rigidity of the bronchial wall, which may indicate extrabronchial extension of tumour. For all these reasons it is routine for most surgeons to undertake rigid bronchoscopy at induction of anaesthetic before any pulmonary resection. There may in addition be anatomical considerations that are relevant specifically to the surgeon and to the choice of surgical procedure. Tumours emerging from the right upper lobe bronchus, for example, may be amenable to sleeve resection if bronchial extension proximally and distally is limited. Tumours are often described by the referring physician as 'within the intermediate bronchus' but, if they are sited at the termination of this

bronchus, middle and lower lobectomy is feasible, whereas at its origin pneumonectomy is necessary. Occasionally, anomalies of anatomy will be noted and the surgeon is then forewarned of technical difficulties that may be encountered at thoracotomy.

Endobronchial bleeding. Where endobronchial bleeding is brisk, good views may be difficult or impossible with the flexible bronchoscope. With the rigid instrument, brisk bleeding can be controlled through a large-bore sucker and blood clot lavaged from the bronchial tree. In practice, bleeding, even if massive, frequently stops with the sedative effect of general anaesthesia, and the site of bleeding may have to be inferred from the distribution of blood clot.

It is appropriate in this section to consider also some of the therapeutic applications of rigid bronchoscopy.

Removal of foreign bodies. Although novel techniques are developing to permit foreign-body removal through the fibreoptic bronchoscope, such expertise is not widely available and not applicable to small children, who are the most common group to have endobronchial foreign bodies. The removal of foreign bodies, particularly those of organic nature and particularly in small children, can be fraught with difficulty, and the surgeon would greatly prefer to have the first attempt at their removal. Failure renders subsequent attempts more difficult because of oedema and bruising. The ability to suspend ventilation under general anaesthesia and the wide bore of the rigid bronchoscope gives this technique a high success rate. Successful and complete removal with a single bronchoscopy is possible in 95% of patients. Occasionally, a repeat procedure is necessary to remove residual fragments or check the completeness of removal once oedema has settled. Biplanar imaging and the ingenious instrumentation devised for coronary artery interventions in the catheter laboratory allow one to

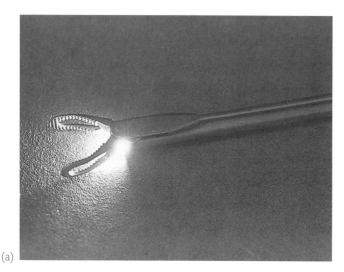

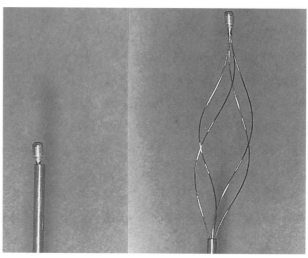

(a)

(b)

Fig. 11.3 Instruments for the removal of foreign bodies. (a) Optical foreign-body forceps permits removal under direct vision and can be accommodated by bronchoscopes larger than 3.0 Stortz – suitable for children around 2 years of age. (b) Foreign-body basket suitable for smaller instruments and younger children but difficult to use in practice because of the limited view obtainable with small bronchoscopes.

retrieve foreign bodies from beyond endoscopic vision. It is rarely necessary to undertake thoracotomy to remove an endobronchial foreign body. The operator should have available a wide range of biopsy forceps and snares as the choice of instrument can only be determined once the situation has been assessed bronchoscopically (Fig. 11.3). It may be helpful to insinuate a Fogarty embolectomy balloon catheter beyond the obstruction. The balloon can then be inflated and the foreign body withdrawn into a more accessible area of the bronchial tree. Once the object has been successfully removed, any damage caused by impaction or attempts at removal should be assessed and both sides of the bronchial tree should be carefully examined for other fragments of foreign body.

Relief of airway obstruction

Obstructing tumours of the trachea are best dealt with by surgical resection, although many prove to be inoperable and suitable only for palliative measures. The bronchoscopic relief of life-threatening obstruction as an initial procedure does, however, allow careful evaluation, and may improve the prospects of subsequent resection. There are many techniques currently available to relieve the intraluminal component of endotracheal and endobronchial obstruction, and it should now rarely be necessary to undertake resection as a matter of urgency. The rigid bronchoscope may be used to core out an adequate airway and large fragments of tumour can be removed with suitably sized biopsy forceps. Prolonged examination is possible, the patient being anaesthetised with incremental doses of intravenous agents and adequately ventilated using the Venturi principle[2] (Fig. 11.4). A diathermy loop (Fig. 11.5) can be used to resect large volumes of tumour from the trachea or main bronchi. Most physicians undertaking laser photoresection have reverted to using a rigid bronchoscope because it allows removal of charred fragments of tumour and frequent cleaning of the laser-carrying cable. Although laser resection is more elegant, it has not been shown to be more effective than the diathermy loop. Once obstruction has been relieved, large

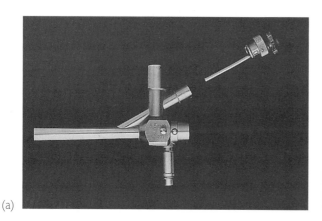

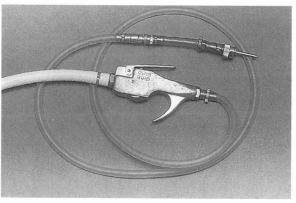

(a)

(b)

Fig. 11.4 The Saunders Venturi equipment for ventilation during rigid bronchoscopy. (a) The Venturi needle attaches to the proximal fitting on the Stortz bronchoscope. (b) The driving gas (oxygen at 410 kPa) is controlled by a trigger mechanism on the pipeline.

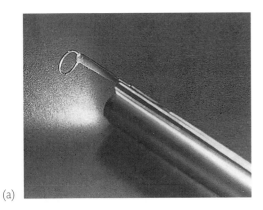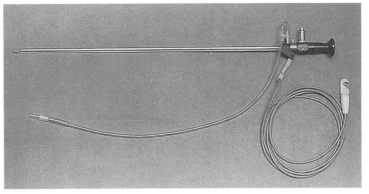

(a)

(b)

Fig. 11.5 Diathermy resectoscope for use with the rigid bronchoscope. (a) The distal diathermy loop attached to the straight telescope. (b) Proximal attachments exhaust smoke and attach to an orthodox diathermy machine. An earth plate is necessary.

amounts of pus may well up from the distal bronchial tree, and the large-bore sucker is an additional advantage of rigid bronchoscopy in this setting.

If the endoscopist judges that endobronchial obstruction will recur rapidly, or if there is a major component due to intramural disease or extramural compression, there is now available a wide range of stents that can be helpful.[3,4] The choice of stent in any situation will depend upon the site and characteristics of the stenosis, its length, calibre and wall consistency (Fig. 11.6). The T-tube or T–Y-tube stents are inserted by a tracheostomy incision but can provide support for the whole trachea, the carina and both main bronchi and can even pass through the larynx. The transverse limb provides vertical stability and allows tracheobronchial suction. This limb should remain spigoted most of the time, thus allowing speech, expectoration and the humidi-

fication of inspired air. Other silicone stents, both tubular and Y-shaped, are inserted through the larynx and manipulated into position using the rigid bronchoscope. Such stents tend to occlude with dried sputum over some weeks and, if needed beyond this period, require renovation. Often, however, they can be removed once chemotherapy or radiotherapy, by external or afterloading techniques, has relieved the underlying obstruction. These types of stent are cheap and impermeable to tumour ingrowth. Expanding wire stents (Fig. 11.7) can be inserted under radiographic control assisted by endoscopic localisation of the upper and lower limits of the stricture, using the rigid or flexible bronchoscope. They should be regarded as permanent implants, although removal is possible if conditions are right.[5] These wire stents are uncovered and subject to tumour ingrowth. They are therefore best suited to relieve obstruction due to extramural compression. Covered wire stents have been

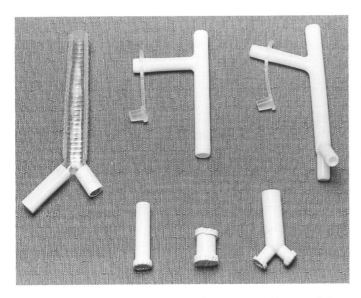

Fig. 11.6 A selection of temporary silicone stents. Top row (left to right): a Freitag Dynamic stent, a T-tube and a T–Y-tube. Bottom row: a selection of 'home-made' stents in tubular and Y configuration. These can be fashioned from silicone T-tubes of varying sizes once the patient's needs are appreciated at bronchoscopy. All but the T-tube and T–Y-tube can be inserted entirely endoscopically.

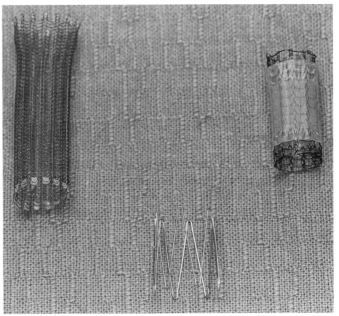

Fig. 11.7 A selection of expanding wire stents, with one example of a covered type.

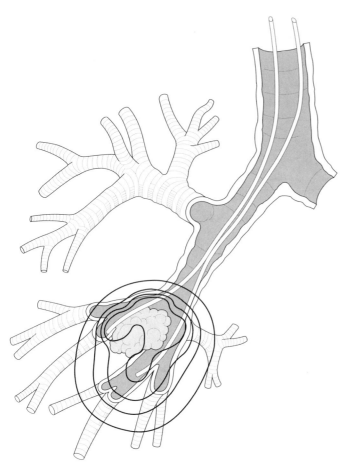

Fig. 11.8 Diagrammatic representation of endobronchial, after-loading radiotherapy using the microSelectron-HDR machine. (Reproduced with permission of Nucletron BV.)

developed but have not been successful because of problems with displacement and chronic colonisation. The use of wire stents in benign disease can be helpful but should only be considered once an experienced endoscopist has decided that conventional surgery is not possible.

Once critical airway obstruction has been relieved, patients will be referred for appropriate oncological advice. One then can remove any temporary stent. If obstruction subsequently recurs, the treatment cycle can be repeated. If tracheal and/or bronchial obstruction recurs following external irradiation, further treatment may be limited by the radiation tolerance of normal tissues. In these circumstances, further treatment is possible using after-loading techniques in which high-activity iridium is introduced via a catheter positioned at fibreoptic bronchoscopy[6] (Fig. 11.8). A temporary stent may have to be inserted to facilitate such therapy.

Mediastinal biopsy

The mediastinum can be approached through various incisions. Mediastinoscopy is an endoscopic examination through a cervical incision used to biopsy tissue adjacent to the anterior or lateral aspects of the trachea. Mediastinotomy is an anterior

approach to the mediastinum usually undertaken through a short transverse incision in the second intercostal space on either side of the sternum. Median sternotomy is a major, vertical midline incision to divide the sternum. It is commonly used to excise anterior mediastinal tumours and has gained great popularity in cardiac surgery.

Mediastinoscopy

Originally introduced by Carlens in 1959,[7] this technique has become valuable in the assessment of mediastinal node involvement by carcinoma of the lung and as a route for biopsy of abnormal lymph nodes visualised radiographically. A short transverse cervical incision is made, and the mediastinoscope is insinuated beneath the pretracheal fascia. As long as the surgeon remains within this plane, damage should not result to other mediastinal structures. The field of view through the mediastinoscope is, however, limited, and all mediastinal structures whether normal or pathological have the same uniform non-pulsatile appearance. Biopsy is therefore hazardous in inexperienced hands. Mediastinoscopy allows the biopsy of nodes within the superior mediastinum, either in the paratracheal chain or at the carina. The superior pole of the right hilum is sometimes accessible but biopsy in this area is hazardous as a result of the proximity of the azygos vein and the upper lobe bronchus and branch of the pulmonary artery. In patients who on radiographic grounds are inoperable, mediastinoscopy may be of value in providing a tissue diagnosis. In potentially operable patients, mediastinoscopy is a valuable staging procedure. Its routine use has been shown to decrease the frequency of 'open and close' thoracotomy, and it identifies those patients with gross mediastinal gland involvement who are incurable,[8] although not excluding those patients with more subtle degrees of involvement who might obtain benefit from resection. Mediastinoscopy is unreliable when used in the diagnosis of patients whose chest radiograph shows only hilar lymphadenopathy and is now not usually undertaken unless mediastinal lymphadenopathy has been demonstrated on computed tomography. In experienced hands, mediastinoscopy may be safely performed in the presence of superior vena caval obstruction,[9] but its diagnostic value is considerably reduced if radiotherapy has been given before mediastinoscopy, when post-irradiation fibrosis may obscure the underlying neoplasm and deeper, more hazardous biopsy may be necessary. The complications of mediastinoscopy are listed in Table 11.1.

Anterior mediastinotomy

This technique was originally introduced by McNeill and Chamberlain in 1966,[13] but has since been modified. A transverse incision is now used and the costal cartilage is no longer resected because its removal does not improve access but results in an ugly sulcus beneath the scar (Fig. 11.9). This technique allows open biopsy of tumours of the anterior mediastinum and may be performed to either side of the sternum. Left anterior mediastinotomy is a valuable adjunct to cervical mediastinoscopy in patients with carcinoma of the bronchus originating within the left upper lobe or those tumours extending to the left main bronchus. In this position, tumours may be unresectable beyond the reach of

Table 11.1 Complications of mediastinoscopy (Adapted with permission from Goldstraw.[10])

No. of cases	2000[10]	4134[11]	3742[11]	11311[12]
Deaths	0	0	3	16
Bleeding requiring thoracotomy*	3	2	4	
Other serious bleeding	2	10	18	19
Vocal cord paresis	5	9	13	47
Pneumothorax	1	7	11	25
Wound infection	3	0	2	37
Mediastinitis	0	2	0	2
Perforation of oesophagus	0	2	1	3
Tumour seedling	1	3	1	0
Total complications	15	39	60	133

* Limited upper sternotomy.

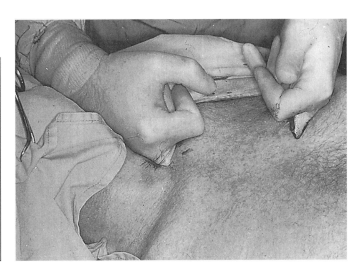

Fig. 11.10 Bidigital examination of the subaortic fossa through cervical (left) and anterior (right) incisions provides a reliable assessment of the subaortic window. In addition, mediastinoscopy will have been performed through the cervical incision.

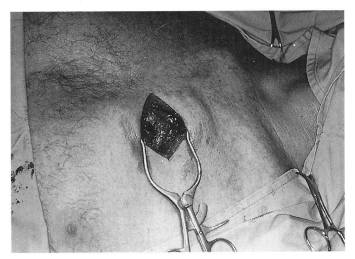

Fig. 11.9 The incision for left anterior mediastinotomy. The pleura is not opened.

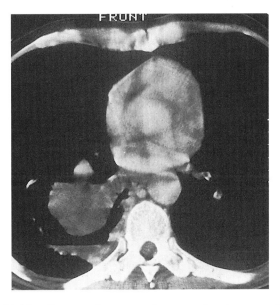

Fig. 11.11 Computed tomography scan showing a cavitating tumour abutting the mediastinum. At thoracotomy tumour was confined within the visceral pleura and resection was feasible.

the mediastinoscope and glands may be involved in the subaortic fossa or anterior mediastinal chain.[14] In the assessment of operability, digital examination provides adequate information in the majority of patients and it is particularly valuable to undertake bidigital examination of the subaortic fossa through the cervical and anterior incisions (Fig. 11.10). The mediastinoscope may be introduced through the anterior mediastinotomy incision if biopsies are necessary but great care is needed when biopsying in the subaortic fossa.

Many studies have evaluated the role of computed tomography (CT) in the preoperative assessment of the mediastinum in patients with carcinoma of the bronchus (see Chapter 70). The consensus opinion suggests that if CT scans of the mediastinum are normal, mediastinal exploration may be omitted before thoracotomy.[15] CT evidence suggesting inoperability should, however, be treated with considerable caution. If tumour abuts the mediastinum (Fig. 11.11) or if glands within the mediastinum are shown to be enlarged, mediastinal explor-

ation should be undertaken because in approximately 50% of such cases the tumour proves to be resectable or the glands are shown to be enlarged by reactive hyperplasia.[16] In patients with lower-lobe tumours the CT scan may show features that suggest inoperability because of invasion or lymph-node involvement beyond the reach of the mediastinoscope. Evaluation of these findings is impossible other than by thoracotomy but one series has shown that resection is still feasible in 65% of such cases.[16]

The role of positron emission tomography (PET) scanning in lung cancer is evolving and increasing. It is a non-invasive method by which one can characterise the nature of peripheral lung lesions that are beyond the reach of the bronchoscope. PET is more accurate than CT in the evaluation of mediastinal nodes[17] and may allow mediastinal exploration to be used more selectively. PET can detect distant metastases missed on CT and characterise any additional abnormalities found on the CT survey for metastatic disease. It is being evaluated for the assessment of response to induction chemotherapy and may better predict those patients who should proceed with second-line surgery. It can detect relapse if this is considered of clinical relevance. PET unfortunately remains expensive, is only available in a few centres and has poor anatomical localisation. It is thus unlikely to succeed CT in standard practice.

Pleural biopsy

The investigation and management of patients with pleural disease is covered in detail in Chapter 75. Patients referred for surgical biopsy of the pleura may have had previous aspirations in attempts at diagnosis or treatment. Thoracoscopy in these circumstances may be contraindicated. Pleural loculi can obscure the underlying pathology and the lung may be adherent in some cases. Thoracoscopy is therefore more hazardous and biopsy can prove falsely reassuring. Open pleural biopsy may be preferable and can be undertaken through a 7–10 cm incision. Either technique may be combined with pleurodesis if this is appropriate for the underlying condition. Pleurodesis can be reliably induced by insufflating talc either through the thoracoscope or at open pleural biopsy, unless fibrin deposits from previous aspirations or attempted pleurodesis prevent talc from impinging uniformly on the naked pleural surface. Such fibrin may be removed at open pleural biopsy. In the author's experience, the most common situation in which pleurodesis fails is where pleural malignancy prevents full expansion of the underlying lung and apposition of the pleural surfaces. In this difficult situation the insertion of a subcutaneous pleuroperitoneal (Denver) shunt (Fig. 11.12) may prove the only palliative measure possible.[18]

Lung biopsy

In patients with diffuse, bilateral lung disease, biopsy may be necessary for diagnosis or assessment of the phase of the disease. Where less invasive procedures have failed, open lung biopsy is safe and reliable, providing accurate diagnosis in as many as 91% of patients in our series.[19] Lung biopsy is now performed using video-assisted thoracoscopic surgery (VATS). This allows one to view a larger area of the lung from which to select the biopsy sites, and is useful where the target area is towards the lung apex. Such technology, however, is costly and does not reduce the morbidity of lung biopsy. Critically ill patients, often already being ventilated, cannot tolerate the single-lung anaesthesia required for VATS. In such a patient population, open techniques are still preferred (Fig. 11.13). With either surgical technique, a high-resolution CT scan of the lungs is essential in choosing the most useful biopsy site.

Exploratory thoracotomy

In some patients with a radiographic abnormality, exploratory thoracotomy may prove to be the only way of confirming a

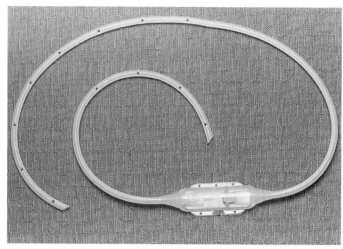

(a)

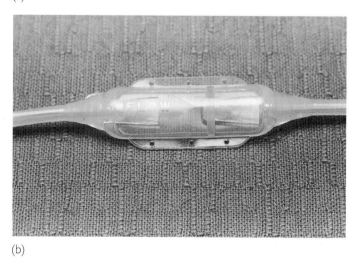

(b)

Fig. 11.12 (a) A Denver pleuroperitoneal shunt for the palliation of malignant effusion in the presence of 'trapped lung'. (b) Detail of the pump chamber.

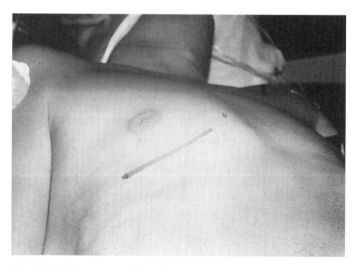

Fig. 11.13 Incision used for right open lung biopsy. A good cosmetic scar will result.

diagnosis. This procedure may, for example, give the only reliable access to hilar abnormalities because overlying vascular structures limit accessibility through short incisions or by VATS. The exploratory nature of this operation should be made clear to the patient and the therapeutic options should be fully discussed. In the author's experience, most patients are able to accept the uncertainty of this approach.

Preoperative evaluation for thoracic surgery

The assessment necessary for 'adequate' preoperative evaluation will vary enormously from patient to patient and from condition to condition. For some patients the assessment may be completed during a single outpatient consultation; for others prolonged investigation as an inpatient may prove necessary. It is helpful to consider the aims of preoperative evaluation as giving the answers to two questions:

- Is the condition suitable for surgical treatment?
- Is the patient suitable for such surgery?

Clearly an affirmative answer is required to both questions if one is to proceed with surgery.

A decision as to whether the condition is suitable for surgery can be made after clinical evaluation supplemented by various investigations. Inadequate preoperative evaluation leads to futile surgery but those tests deemed appropriate vary depending on whether the patient has a benign or malignant condition and whether one is aiming for cure or palliation.

The assessment of patient suitability is essentially one of fitness, and inadequate evaluation in this respect may lead to hazardous surgery. A period of inpatient preparation may prove necessary before it is possible to make a decision and a few days spent improving the patient's condition preoperatively may save weeks postoperatively. Physiotherapy may be of value in dealing with excess sputum production, whether caused by smoking or other conditions such as bronchiectasis, and nebulised bronchodilators are likely to help those with airway obstruction. Cardiac function can be improved by treating hypertension or arrhythmias. Intrapleural sepsis is notoriously difficult to diagnose and particularly debilitating. It is a good rule to undertake drainage of an empyema prior to definitive treatment in all but the fittest of patients. Adequate drainage can improve the patient's general condition and restore stamina, making surgery not only feasible but also less hazardous.

The formal evaluation of fitness for surgery is covered elsewhere but a few comments are appropriate here.

Age. The risk of any surgery increases with age but in this respect 'physiological' age matters more than chronological age and there is no specific age limit above which thoracic operations become prohibitively hazardous or below which risk becomes negligible.

Ischaemic heart disease. Major thoracic surgery is most commonly undertaken in those age groups at risk of myocardial ischaemia, and thoracotomy is frequently necessary for smoking-related illnesses, which are known risk factors for cardiovascular disease. The risk of perioperative reinfarction falls steadily in the months following myocardial infarction and, if possible, surgery should be delayed for at least 3 months and preferably for 6 months.[20] It is usually possible to delay cancer surgery for a short period. If, however, it is necessary to perform surgery within 6 months of an infarct, careful monitoring and control of haemodynamic instability during anaesthesia reduce the perioperative risk.[21] A history of myocardial infarction more than 6 months earlier does not appear to increase the risk of major thoracic surgery if the patient is leading an angina-free active life without drugs. If there is evidence of continuing ischaemia then an exercise test according to the Bruce protocol can be helpful. In the author's experience ischaemic episodes following pulmonary resection are unlikely in patients who can successfully complete stage 2 of the Bruce protocol, provided that their condition is stabilised preoperatively on appropriate therapy.

Respiratory function. Respiratory function testing is important when undertaking any major operation and is of critical importance when considering pulmonary resection (see also Chapter 18). The only tests that have been shown to correlate with the morbidity and mortality of pulmonary resection are the patient's exercise capacity, an elevated arterial carbon dioxide tension and simple spirometric tests such as forced expiratory volume in 1 second and forced vital capacity.[22] A major cause of morbidity and mortality following pulmonary resection is inadequate sputum clearance, and spirometric tests reflect the patient's ability to generate high flows within the bronchial tree, an important component of expectoration. Spirometric measurements are also important as a guide to postoperative function. This depends on the extent of proposed resection and the functional state of the lung tissue to be removed. Isotope scans are occasionally used to predict postoperative spirometry in patients who are being considered for pneumonectomy.[23] The functional consequences are often less than might be anticipated because the lung to be removed is making little contribution preoperatively (Fig. 11.14).

Patient motivation. One should not underestimate the importance of motivation and this should be exploited by the surgeon in the preoperative interviews with patients and their relatives.

The preoperative assessment of patient 'fitness' will never become an exact science. Fitness represents more than the sum function of each individual organ system and is clearly related to the level of daily activity; this is important not only in preoperative evaluation but also when discussing the quality of life following surgery.

Therapeutic surgery may prove damaging and destructive, and the probable benefit must be seen to greatly outweigh the possible risks. Thus, speculative surgery may be reasonable if the operative risks are small, and high-risk surgery may still be reasonable if great benefit is to be expected. In practice the decision is not difficult in most patients, but occasionally it may be finely balanced and critically depend upon the patient's attitude to his/her problem and its treatment options. A full and frank discussion between the patient and the surgeon develops a rapport that greatly eases the management of any postoperative problems. This bond should not

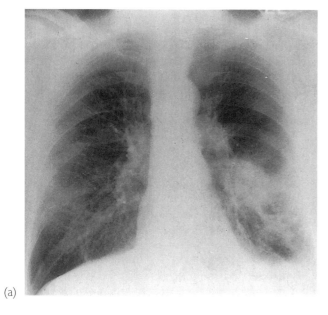

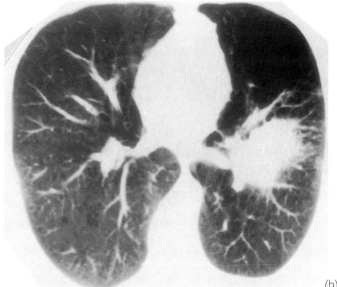

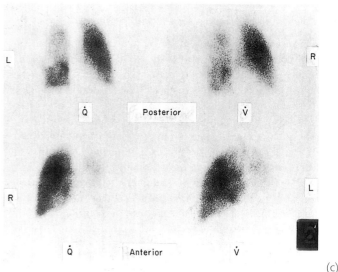

Fig. 11.14 (a) Chest radiograph of a 54-year-old man with gross emphysema and a centrally positioned squamous carcinoma in the left lung. Lung function was extremely poor with FEV_1/FVC of 0.5/2.2. Pneumonectomy was judged necessary. (b) Computed tomography scan showing gross emphysema of the left upper lobe and the central position of the tumour of the lower lobe. (c) Perfusion ($\dot{Q}$) (left) and ventilation ($\dot{V}$) (right) scans, showing the limited contribution made by the left lung. Left pneumonectomy was accomplished without incident.

be underestimated and all patients proceeding to major surgery should be convinced that 'their' surgeon has their best interests at heart.

Intraoperative evaluation

At thoracotomy the first step should be to recheck the preoperative evaluation while avoiding irreversible damage. Even when operating for benign lung disease it is important to examine the whole lung to ensure that the macroscopic extent of disease correlates with radiographic preoperative assessment. Although it is rare to radically change the proposed operation, one occasionally has to resect adjacent segments affected by extension of the disease process. Checking the preoperative evaluation assumes the greatest importance and complexity when operating for a presumed lung cancer. Often, thoracotomy has to be recommended on the basis of a suspicious radiograph or of a broncho-

scopy report, unsupported by histology. The author uses an operative routine that requires thorough and often prolonged dissection to answer four questions before proceeding with resection for a presumed malignant condition.

1. What is the diagnosis?

When no histological diagnosis has been made before surgery, frozen section biopsies at the time of thoracotomy are mandatory and these should be taken from an area that is likely to reflect the true nature of the pathology. It is not uncommon to find inflammatory changes surrounding a tumour, and it is sometimes difficult to dissect into the hilum without risking damage. There will be rare occasions when the surgeon cannot find a safe and reliable site for biopsy and it may then be necessary to proceed on the clinical evidence. Where malignancy is so extensive as to require pneumonectomy, positive biopsy is usually possible at some point around the hilum.

2. With the diagnosis of malignancy confirmed, is complete excision by pneumonectomy feasible?

Dissection around the hilum should be undertaken to show that all hilar structures can be divided at a point clear of macroscopic tumour. Proximal extension of tumour may require intrapericardial assessment but the pericardium should be incised away from the phrenic nerve so as to do least damage if the tumour proves to be inoperable. Where bulky tumours are invading the chest wall, it is sometimes necessary to resect the segment of chest wall before obtaining sufficient access to evaluate the hilum. Occasionally, on the left, it may be necessary to divide the recurrent laryngeal nerve before completely clearing tumour from the aortic adventitia or involved nodes from the subaortic fossa. In these circumstances the surgeon gains considerable reassurance from a preoperative mediastinal exploration that suggests that the tumour is otherwise suitable for resection.

3. If pneumonectomy is feasible, is it desirable?

This question in essence requires a complete review of preoperative staging to ensure that the clinically determined tumour (T) and node (N) categories (see Chapter 70) are not radically altered by intraoperative evidence. Preoperative T stage may be altered by refuting or confirming invasion of important structures or the finding of 'satellite' nodules. Although this is important, it is usually of less importance than the intraoperative reassessment of N stage. A hilar mass may consist of primary tumour or involved hilar lymph nodes. Such nodal disease may affect the extent of resection but not its feasibility or desirability. Mediastinal node involvement is of far greater importance. Surgeons generally do not operate on patients who have been shown on preoperative evaluation by mediastinoscopy to have N2 disease. However in all patients a thorough re-examination of nodal status is recognised as an important component of intrathoracic staging. This evaluation is now termed 'systematic nodal dissection', and comprises two component parts.

The first step involves the removal of all mediastinal nodal stations with the surrounding fat. These are examined macroscopically and, if necessary, by frozen section examination. Each such station is sent to the laboratory labelled according to an internationally agreed nodal chart, such as that devised by Narake[24] (Fig. 11.15). The routine examination of mediastinal nodes, as the first component of systematic nodal dissection, has provided insight into the more subtle degrees of mediastinal node involvement. With increasing experience more and more nodal stations are being examined and surgeons are now applying the same rigorous nodal evaluation to N1 stations. In one study on the value of systematic nodal dissection an average of seven nodal stations, ranging from three to 13 stations, were

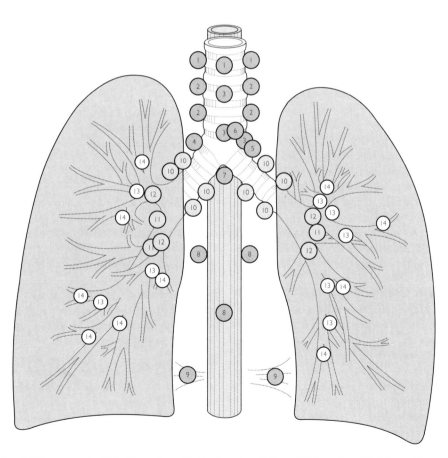

Fig. 11.15 Node 'stations'. The numerical labelling of mediastinal nodes, 1–9, and N1 nodes, 10–14, avoids confusion in terminology.

removed prior to making any decision on the advisability of resection or establishing the extent of resection necessary. This detailed evaluation revealed 'unexpected N2' disease in almost 20% of the patients, despite careful preoperative evaluation using CT in all cases and mediastinal examination selectively, based upon the CT appearances.[25] Although disconcerting, in most cases mediastinal node involvement was limited to a single deposit and it has been shown that such subtle degrees of mediastinal involvement do not preclude a reasonable prospect of cure, and a 5-year survival of around 20%.[26]

The surgeon has at this stage inflicted no permanent damage to lung tissue and can retreat if s/he finds extensive and unexpected mediastinal nodal involvement such that the therapeutic equation has swung against resection. Intraoperative staging is aiding the evaluation of surgical results and may prove of value in the future in deciding adjuvant protocols. In practice, at the present time, it results in few changes in the therapeutic decision to attempt a potentially curative resection.

4. If pneumonectomy is feasible and desirable, is a lesser resection likely to prove successful?

At this point the attention of the surgeon focuses upon the hilum. The prospects for lobectomy, bilobectomy, sleeve resection or segmentectomy depend upon factors such as invasion into the fissures, the involvement of hilar structures supplying adjacent lobes and the presence of fixed N1 nodes. This step is the second phase of systematic nodal dissection, in which N1 nodes are sequentially examined, proceeding centrifugally, until the required extent of resection has been determined. The advantage of approaching the problem in this order is that, while attempting lesser resection, one not infrequently discovers more proximal extension or involvement of small nodes requiring pneumonectomy. If after irreversible damage to hilar structures this is found to be the case, the surgeon is obliged to undertake pneumonectomy, and it is then too late to question whether such an extensive resection is desirable.

There is no therapeutic advantage in making the resection more extensive than is necessary to achieve complete excision, although a randomised, prospective trial has suggested that lobectomy should be considered the minimum resection for patients able to tolerate such surgery.[27] Pneumonectomy carries no survival advantage over lobectomy.[28,29] Bronchoplastic sleeve resection is an excellent operation in patients whose tumours are sufficiently localised to allow this option, carrying a low operative mortality, an excellent long-term prognosis and preservation of lung function.[30] Sleeve resection should be considered preferable to pneumonectomy wherever it is technically possible, even in the presence of N1 disease.[31] Segmentectomy, introduced initially as a resection option for those patients unable to tolerate lobectomy, may remain a valid option in carefully selected cases in which well-localised tumours occur in appropriate segments of the lung.[32]

If, after complete intraoperative evaluation, the surgeon decides not to proceed with resection, a moment should be spared to consider if any further procedure might be helpful. Can further biopsies be taken to completely catalogue the extent of disease? Is it of value to mark tumour deposits with metal clips to aid postoperative radiotherapy? If pleural malignancy has been found, is it reasonable to undertake talc insufflation to prevent subsequent pleural effusion? If hypertrophic pulmonary osteoarthropathy was a troublesome preoperative feature, will division of the vagus nerve provide palliation? In these ways the disastrous impact of an open-and-close thoracotomy may be minimised.

Operative techniques

An extensive description of surgical techniques is given elsewhere.[33]

Pulmonary resection

The extent of resection often depends upon subtle anatomical considerations and is not necessarily related to the size of a tumour. Frequently, small, but involved, glands will be detected at operation, necessitating more extensive resection than was appreciated preoperatively. Small primary tumours may involve hilar structures subtending adjacent lobes, again necessitating more extensive resection. The latter situation not infrequently occurs with tumours within the apical segment of the lower lobe, where small tumours readily extend across fissures, making resection of adjacent lobes necessary. Such tumours may also involve the recurrent branch of the pulmonary artery supplying the posterior segment of the upper lobe, necessitating pneumonectomy. The intraoperative assessment of bronchoalveolar carcinoma may be particularly difficult as a result of the indefinite margins of such tumours and their capacity to stream across alveolar bridges if the fissures separating lobes are incomplete. Removal of the middle lobe with the upper or lower lobe is usually termed 'bilobectomy'. 'Completion pneumonectomy' involves the removal of the remainder of a lung at any time following partial excision.

Bronchoplastic (sleeve) resection

The primary tumour may extend from the lobar bronchus to involve a common bronchus serving other lobes. In these circumstances, lobectomy and resection of a 'sleeve' of the common bronchus may allow anastomosis and preservation of distal lobes. This most commonly occurs with tumours in the right upper lobe, where the interposition of the intermediate bronchus distances the origin of middle and lower lobe bronchi from the site of tumour extension (Fig. 11.16). On the left, the bifurcation of the main bronchus into upper and lower lobe bronchi makes bronchoplastic resection less common. Less malignant tumours such as carcinoid allow closer resection margins and bronchoplastic resection is more common with this type of pathology. Occasionally, tumours confined to a bronchus can be treated by resection of the bronchus alone with preservation of all lung parenchyma. The technical pinnacle of bronchoplastic resection entails resection of the main carina with or without pneumonectomy and reanastomosis of the remaining lung(s).

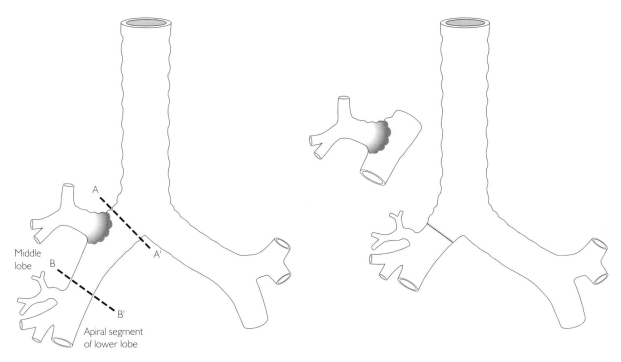

Middle
lobe   B

A'

B'

Apiral segment
of lower lobe

Fig. 11.16 A tumour within the right upper lobe extending into the main bronchus. If this is the only factor preventing lobectomy, then sleeve resection across the main bronchus (A–A') and intermediate bronchus (B–B') will allow conservation and reanastomosis of the middle and lower lobes.

Decortication

When excising an empyema cavity, the parietal cortex is frequently removed along with the parietal pleura, since this has little functional consequence. When resecting the visceral cortex, however, the surgeon hopes to preserve the visceral pleura, so reducing air leak. The success of this operation depends on expansion of the underlying lung and obliteration of the pleural space to prevent further infective problems. Pleurectomy for recurrent pneumothoraces should not be confused with decortication. In the former, the removal of parietal pleura is the strategy used to produce pleurodesis, whereas in the latter the parietal pleura is resected only as a tactical expedient to removal of the parietal cortex.

Pleurectomy

The parietal pleura can be stripped from the lateral chest wall anteriorly as far as the mediastinal reflection, posteriorly to the vertebral bodies, inferiorly to the costodiaphragmatic recess and superiorly over the apex and down the mediastinum as far as the azygos arch on the right and the aortic arch on the left. In other places it is intimately adherent to the diaphragm or mediastinal structures. Removal of the parietal pleura leaves a raw surface and, if the underlying lung is able to expand such that the visceral pleura reaches this raw surface, then obliteration of the pleural space – pleurodesis – can reliably be achieved. By obliterating the pleural space, pleurodesis will prevent the reaccumulation of air or fluid. Equally good results may be achieved by severe abrasion of the pleura at thoracotomy. Chemical pleurodesis, although avoiding thoracotomy, produces less reliable

results and is reserved for those patients unable safely to tolerate an operation.

The majority of these pleural procedures are now accomplished using VATS techniques. This is of enormous advantage when operating upon frail patients or those with advanced disease. However the cosmetic advantages of VATS therapy for patients with primary, spontaneous pneumothorax involves an accepted risk of recurrence in 5% of patients, even in experienced hands. VATS has yet to be shown to be superior in terms of postoperative pain and other morbidity, mortality or length of stay.

Surgery for emphysema

Where large, 'dominant' bullae are a feature of emphysema, surgery has a long-established place. Intracavitary drainage, using a modification of the Monaldi technique, effects collapse of the bullae with a small incision and a short anaesthetic.[34]

The improvement following such surgery has been ascribed to the expansion and recruitment of lung tissue, which, while still emphysematous, is functionally better than the bullous area. The re-emergence of 'bilateral pneumectomy'[35] as a surgical option for patients with more diffuse emphysema has shown the functional benefit of 'volume reduction'. Diaphragmatic function is improved, expiratory collapse of airways is reduced and patients breath more deeply and more comfortably from a lower functional residual capacity.[36] The degree of improvement following volume-reduction surgery is dependent upon the pattern of the emphysema.[37] In patients with diffuse emphysema that is homogeneous, any areas of lung that are resected are as important functionally as the areas that remain, and any improvement must reflect the benefit of volume reduction. If the disease is heterogeneous, then the surgeon will resect the more abnormal parts, adding the benefit attributed to bullectomy to that due to volume reduction. The reported improvement in lung function following emphysema surgery ranges from 10% to 85% of preoperative levels, probably reflecting differences in selection and the patient populations in different studies.

Selection for emphysema surgery must also consider physiological parameters. Patients must be sufficiently disabled to make the risks of surgery justified while remaining sufficiently robust to make these risks acceptable. Selection is based upon spirometry, blood gas determination, degree of air-trapping, gas transfer measurements and walking distance. Rehabilitation is useful in selecting patients who are well-motivated and preparing them for surgery. At least one randomised controlled trial has shown that the improvement in spirometric measurements, exercise capacity and quality of life after volume-reduction surgery are greater and more prolonged that can be achieved by rehabilitation alone.[38]

In experienced units the perioperative mortality of volume reduction can be maintained at around 5% by manipulation of the population accepted for surgery.[39] Adverse prognostic factors include α_1-antitrypsin deficiency, severe hypoxaemia, hypercapnia, concurrent bronchiectasis, ischaemic heart disease and previous surgery. Most departments now perform volume reduction using VATS, and bilateral, concurrent surgery probably provides greater improvement without any greater risk.[40]

Metastasectomy

The excision of pulmonary metastases is an increasingly performed procedure.[41] Preoperative selection demands that certain criteria are fulfilled:

- complete control of the primary site, usually by surgical excision
- exclusion or control of extrathoracic metastases
- accurate documentation of the number and distribution of pulmonary metastases by CT
- patient fitness and respiratory reserve that will withstand the proposed resection.

Since these tumours are of haematogenous origin, conservative resection is undertaken, usually by removing the metastasis with a shallow shell of surrounding lung parenchyma. Occasionally, larger, more proximal deposits may require segmental resection or lobectomy, but pneumonectomy produces poor results. Bilateral deposits may be approached through a median sternotomy but on occasions staged bilateral thoracotomy may be preferred if tumour deposits are large or encroach on the hilum. Oncologists have been critical in the past but are now enthusiastic supporters of this surgical approach. Results are now available on a multinational database of 5206 cases,[42] showing overall actuarial survival of 36% at 5 years, 26% at 10 years and 22% at 15 years following complete resection of pulmonary metastases from a wide range of primary sites and cell types. The results were influenced by the completeness of resection, the disease-free interval, cell-type and number of metastases (Fig. 11.17).

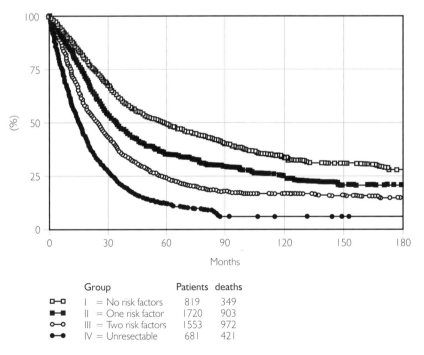

Fig. 11.17 Survival following pulmonary metastasectomy according to prognostic groups. Group I: completely resected cases with disease-free interval of 36 months or greater, and single metastasis. Group II: completely resected cases with *either* disease-free interval less than 36 months *or* more than one metastasis. Group III: completely resectable cases with *both* disease-free interval of less than 36 months *and* more than one metastasis. Group IV: unresectable or incompletely resected cases. (Redrawn with permission from Pastorino et al.[42])

In those selected for repeat surgery for further pulmonary relapse the results were also good, with 44% surviving 5 years. Overall perioperative mortality was 1%.

Tracheal resection

No reliable and safe prosthesis has yet been developed for the trachea and the surgeon is restricted in the length of trachea that can be resected by the need to achieve an end-to-end anastomosis following resection. The principles of such surgery have been well described by Grillo and others.[43] Various techniques have been developed to permit end-to-end anastomosis in the adult following resection of up to 50% of the total tracheal length. The majority of benign strictures follow intubation injury. Nearly all of these can be resected as long as the situation has not been complicated by laser treatment or previous attempts at correction. Few tumours, on the other hand, are sufficiently localised to permit resection but, as surgery usually offers the only prospect of cure, all borderline cases should be assessed by a surgeon with experience in this demanding area. Airway stenting has proved to be a valuable technique in patients with benign or malignant disease assessed as inoperable by an experienced endoscopist.

A cervical approach provides good access to the whole of the trachea, although on occasion exposure may be facilitated by a limited upper sternotomy. If resection of the carina or main bronchus may be required, a right lateral thoracotomy is necessary.

Postoperative management[44]

Most postoperative complications have their origin in the operating room. Clean operations may be contaminated by organisms such as *Staphylococcus aureus* present on the skin of the patient or spread from operating room staff. Prophylactic antibiotics have been shown to reduce the frequency of wound infections if given at induction of anaesthesia.[45]

Pleural infection

Pleural infection may result from air-borne organisms or may arise from the respiratory tract if the bronchus is opened. Although such contamination must be common, it is usually suppressed if expanding lung tissue can obliterate the pleural space. After pneumonectomy, however, such contamination may result in empyema. Following lesser resections, an empyema is associated with persistent air leak, the consequent need for prolonged chest drainage and the presence of a residual space within the chest.

Pulmonary atelectasis

This may be immediately evident on a chest radiograph following thoracotomy. When it occurs on the side of surgery, it may result from handling, retraction or incomplete re-expansion after collapse by a double-lumen endobronchial tube. Contralateral atelectasis can result from a badly positioned double lumen tube that allows spillage into the dependent lung or obstructs a lobar orifice (Figs 11.18 & 11.19). The short right main bronchus

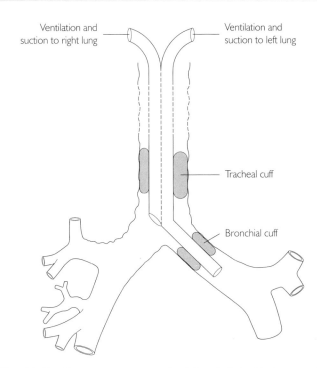

Fig. 11.18 Correct positioning of a left-sided double-lumen tube used when undertaking right-sided resections. Malposition may occur if the tube is down the wrong side, too high – failing to protect the left lung from spillage, or too low – obstructing the left upper lobe orifice.

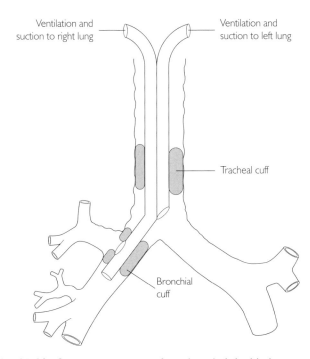

Fig. 11.19 Correct positioning of a right-sided double-lumen tube used when undertaking left-sided resections. The proximal origin of the right upper lobe bronchus complicates the design of these tubes and a side-hole is fashioned within the bronchial cuff. If this hole is not correctly positioned the right upper lobe will become atelectatic. Other options for malposition exist as for the left-sided tube.

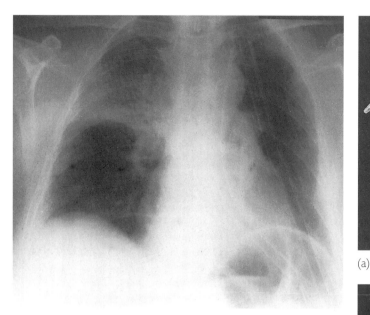

Fig. 11.20 Postoperative chest radiograph. During left upper lobectomy partial collapse of the right upper lobe has occurred, presumably as the result of a malpositioned double-lumen tube.

requires special modification of the double-lumen tube to allow ventilation of the upper lobe through a side hole in the endo-bronchial cuff. If positioned blindly by the anaesthetist, such tubes may not adequately ventilate the right upper lobe, with resultant atelectasis (Fig. 11.20). Increasingly, therefore, such endobronchial tubes are placed under bronchoscopic control.[46] A double-lumen tube cannot be accommodated within the smaller airways of children below 8 or 9 years of age and an endo-bronchial blocker must be used. This may also be preferable to endobronchial intubation when operating for lung sepsis or bronchiectasis in the adult because this device will protect ipsi-lateral lobes as well as the contralateral lung.

Sputum retention

This is particularly common in the smoking patient with chronic sputum production and is aggravated by inhibition of cough as a result of pain and the sedative effect of anaesthesia and analgesia. Other predisposing factors include laryngeal incompetence caused by transection of the recurrent laryngeal nerve and para-doxical motion caused by phrenic nerve damage or resection of the chest wall. Even in such difficult circumstances, however, adequate analgesia and intensive physiotherapy will prevent sputum retention in most cases but great vigilance should be exercised by all contributing to postoperative care. Should sputum retention develop the use of a mini-tracheostomy tube (Fig. 11.21) is of considerable benefit to management. This is inserted under local anaesthesia through the cricothyroid mem-brane. It is kept spigoted to allow speech and expectoration but provides an easy route for endobronchial suction.[47] This tech-nique is not without complications and it is best undertaken by a surgeon experienced in the technique. If sputum retention is not appreciated in spite of maximum treatment, pneumonia will

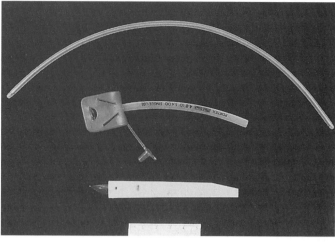

(a)

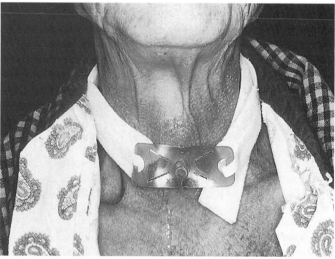

(b)

Fig. 11.21 (a) Mini-tracheostomy set (Portex). At the bottom is the guarded knife used to incise the cricothyroid membrane. The stylet (top) is then inserted into the trachea and the tracheostomy tube (centre) is introduced using a Seldinger technique. (b) The mini-tracheostomy tube in position. It is kept spigoted unless required for suction, hence allowing normal speech and expectoration and minimising crusting. It Is held securely in place with a Velcro strap around the neck.

supervene and formal tracheostomy and artificial ventilation may prove necessary.

Anastomotic dehiscence and bronchopleural fistula

When these occur early in the postoperative period it reflects technical inadequacies during the operation. Early re-explo-ration and repair are necessary. Anastomotic leak and fistula occurring later are associated with empyema and one cannot be sure whether infection has eroded the suture line or small leaks have resulted in infection. Bronchopleural fistula is now rare. The incidence of this previously devastating complication is around 1% in pneumonectomy,[48] the author not having encountered it in the last 14 years. Drainage of the empyema may allow small leaks to close spontaneously but more persistent and larger fistulae require further operation and are often extremely difficult to manage. Chronic empyema in association with a persistent bronchopleural fistula is now managed by complex soft-tissue transfer procedures,[49] thus avoiding the cosmetic and long-term functional problems associated with thoracoplasty.

Supraventricular dysrhythmias

Such complications, principally atrial fibrillation, occur more commonly after thoracotomy in the elderly and in those undergoing extensive resection with intrapericardial dissection, especially if recovery is complicated and prolonged. Prophylactic digoxin may be of value,[50] but this is disputed.[51]

Acute lung injury and adult respiratory distress syndrome

The definitions of adult respiratory distress syndrome and its less severe variant, acute lung injury, have been agreed internationally.[52] Although originally reported after pneumonectomy and attributed to fluid overload[53] (Fig. 11.22), it is known to occur after any injury and all lung operations and recognised to be part of the systemic response to injury. Injury is mediated by neutrophil activation and the release of cytokines, leading to increased permeability of the alveolar–capillary membrane.[54] Progressive hypoxaemia is often overlooked for 2–3 days and pulmonary opacification attributed to lung infection. Undoubtedly in the past many patients suffering from adult respiratory distress syndrome were labelled as dying from other, vague infection leading to organ failure. The incidence and mortality is dependent upon the extent of lung resection. The combined incidence of adult respiratory distress syndrome and acute lung injury in one series was 3.9%, but it ranged from 6.0% after pneumonectomy to 1.0% after only minor resections. Overall, these authors estimated that almost three-quarters of all postoperative deaths could be attributed to acute lung injury or adult respiratory distress syndrome.[55]

Treatment is supportive but survival rates seem to be improving.[56]

Postoperative survival

If the risks of surgery are to be kept low, there must be thorough preoperative evaluation, optimum preoperative preparation, careful surgical technique and attentive postoperative care. Experience from the USA[57] and from the UK[58] suggests that postoperative mortality rate following lobectomy for lung cancer is around 3% and for pneumonectomy 6–8%. Good postoperative care requires experience and attention by the surgical and nursing team supplemented by excellent physiotherapy and support staff.

The management of chest drains

A chest drain inserted at thoracotomy is usually placed as low as possible within the pleural space and directed towards the apex. When inserting a chest drain in the ward, however, the position of the diaphragm can not be ascertained with such certainty. It may be as high as nipple level if the phrenic nerve is paralysed, if there is atelectasis or if an expiratory effort occurs during insertion so that a chest drain should be positioned no lower than the fifth intercostal space; on the left side it should be kept lateral to the nipple to avoid damaging the mediastinal struc-

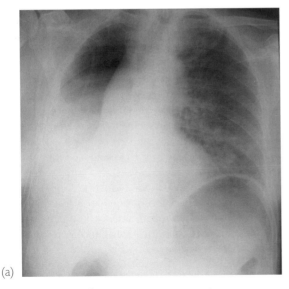
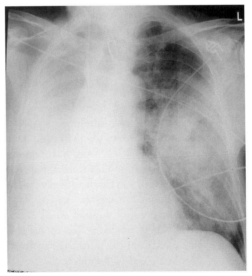

(a)   (b)

Fig. 11.22 (a) Chest radiograph 2 days after right pneumonectomy. There is some contralateral parenchymal shadowing, a mini-tracheostomy tube has been inserted to deal with sputum thought to be responsible for the hypoxaemia and radiographic changes. (b) Chest radiograph at day 8. The patient has had a tracheostomy performed and is dependent on intermittent positive-pressure ventilation for what is clearly now adult respiratory distress syndrome.

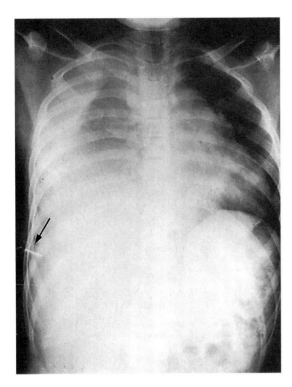

Fig. 11.23 A chest drain inserted to drain a traumatic haemothorax was inserted too low (arrow) and injured the liver. The haemothorax was successfully managed with a further drain in a correct position but laparotomy was necessary to repair the liver.

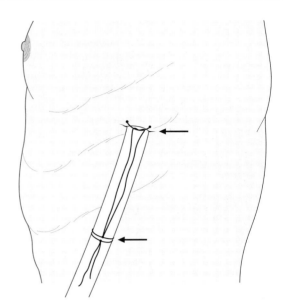

Fig. 11.24 Suture recommended to secure a chest drain. The purse-string component (upper arrow) prevents air entry or fluid drainage around the tube while the retaining component (lower arrow) prevents outward displacement. On removing the chest drain the retaining component is cut distally, leaving two long ends of the suture to secure the purse-string knot

tures (Fig. 11.23). If the drain is positioned anterior to the posterior axillary line the patient may sit or lie comfortably with it in place. The site favoured by some, anteriorly in the midclavicular line through the second interspace, produces an ugly scar.

A drain in the preferred position in the midaxillary line above the fifth intercostal space will reliably remove air and fluid from the pleural space, since with re-expansion of the underlying lung all parts of the pleural space are at an equal pressure when the patient is supine. If a single drain is not rapidly effective, a second tube may be necessary, through a higher interspace or positioned slightly more anteriorly.

Once the site of insertion has been selected, infiltration of local anaesthetic is necessary through the intercostal muscles and adjacent to the parietal pleura. An adequate skin incision should be made to reduce friction against the sides of the drain. A defect is created through the intercostal muscles using a spreading action with strong scissors or a haemostat. This tract should be led to, if not through, the parietal pleura so that the drain can be inserted without force. Once positioned, it may be held in place by a single suture fulfilling the function of a purse string and a retention suture (Fig. 11.24). When removing the drain the retention knot may be cut and the tails of the purse string suture may be then tightened to close the chest-wall defect.

The largest tube that fits comfortably between the ribs should be used. There is little advantage in inserting small chest drains, since they are as uncomfortable but less effective and may easily kink or become obstructed. Intrapleural drains with underwater seal are innately obstructing, requiring that

intrapleural pressure exceed the column of water in the underwater limb of the drainage bottle. Gentle suction is often helpful and on occasion higher suction pressures may be necessary. The suction used should be capable of dealing with high volumes of air leaking from damaged lung tissue, because otherwise functional obstruction may occur intermittently. Suction at −10 to −20 cmH₂O (−1 to −2 kPa) will serve for most situations.

Chest drains cannot function if clamped! The temptation to clamp a tube while moving the patient should be resisted because it may prove dangerous. It is feasible to devise a system of transportation that allows the patient to be moved safely without fear of traction on the drains or tilting or other damage to the chest drain bottle.

The bulky apparatus associated with underwater drainage limits patient mobility, and suction even more so. Since gaining experience with volume reduction surgery, many surgeons are much more relaxed about air leak and the need for suction. Suction undoubtedly exacerbates the air leak, and may cause it to be prolonged. Certainly, the prolonged immobilisation associated with suction demoralises the patient and may increase morbidity. Following volume reduction surgery, the patient with emphysema may have a considerable air leak and, spurred by the need to obtain rapid mobilisation, these patients are converted to a Heimlich bag at an early stage in their recovery (Fig. 11.25). They are often discharged with their drains in place to continue mobilising at home. The success of this policy has led to wider use of such portable systems following all lung operations. This has been shown in one randomised trial to result in a shorter hospital stay.[59]

A chest drain may be removed safely when it no longer functions. It is common surgical practice to leave a tube in situ

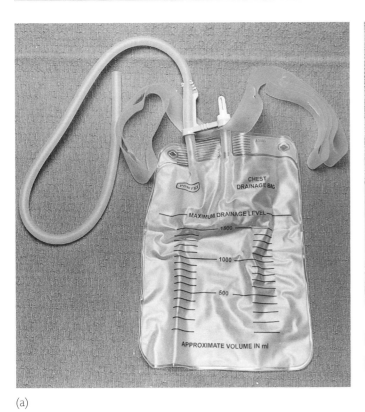

(a)

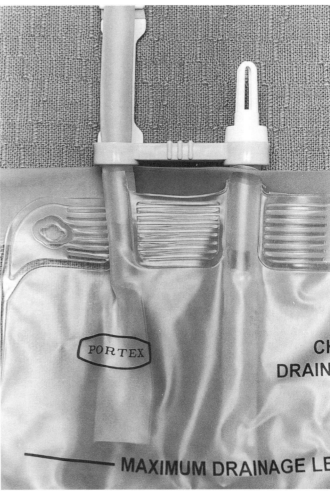

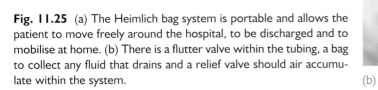

(b)

Fig. 11.25 (a) The Heimlich bag system is portable and allows the patient to move freely around the hospital, to be discharged and to mobilise at home. (b) There is a flutter valve within the tubing, a bag to collect any fluid that drains and a relief valve should air accumulate within the system.

until local obliteration of the pleural space is reflected by dampening of the respiratory swing to 2–3 cmH$_2$O. It is difficult to assess function when a Heimlich bag is being employed, and this is one drawback of this system. The nurse removing the drain must be aware of intrapleural dynamics, removing the tube quickly but smoothly, with the patient maintaining a Valsalva manoeuvre at full inspiration. The associated positive intrapleural pressure prevents air being drawn in to the pleural space from the atmosphere during removal of the tube. Once

the drain has been removed, the purse-string suture should be tied, preventing air from entering the pleural space and fluid from draining from the space, with the consequent risk of empyema.

An open drain inserted into an empyema cavity represents a different situation. Here the rigid walls of the cavity prevent mediastinal shift or collapse of the underlying lung and there is no need for underwater seal drainage. Indeed, such open drains are not truly intrapleural but intracavitary.

Therapeutic principles

- 'Resectability' relates to the prospects for tumour removal. A surgeon should evaluate borderline cases.

- 'Operability' relates to the fitness of the patient to withstand the proposed operation. A surgeon should evaluate borderline cases.

- Age alone is never an absolute contraindication to operation.

Principles of lung cancer surgery

- Careful preoperative staging is necessary prior to thoracotomy.

- All preoperative staging is inaccurate. Detailed intrathoracic staging should be performed after thoracotomy before making the decision to resect.

- Complete resection is necessary for cure.

- There is no survival advantage gained by resection greater than that required to achieve complete resection of the lesion.

- The patient must survive surgery to benefit from cure!

References

1. Collins JV, Dhillon P, Goldstraw P. Practical bronchoscopy, Oxford: Blackwell Scientific; 1987.
2. Gothard JWW, Branthwaite MA. Diagnostic procedures. In: Anaesthesia for thoracic surgery. Oxford: Blackwell Scientific; 1982.
3. Irving JD, Goldstraw P. Tracheobronchial stents. Semin Int Radiol 1991; 8: 295.
4. Petrou M, Goldstraw P. The management of tracheobronchial obstruction: a review of endoscopic techniques. Eur J Cardiothorac Surg 1994; 8: 436.
5. Hind CRK, Donnelly RJ. Expandable metal stents for tracheal obstruction: permanent or temporary? A cautionary tale. Thorax, 1992; 47: 757.
6. Burt PA, O'Driscoll BR, Notley HM et al. Intraluminal irradiation for the palliation of lung cancer with the high dose microSelectron. Thorax, 1990; 45: 765.
7. Carlens E. Mediastinoscopy: a method of inspection and tissue biopsy in the superior mediastinum. Dis Chest 1959; 36: 343.
8. Pearson FG. An evaluation of mediastinoscopy in the management of presumably operable bronchial carcinoma. J Thorac Cardiovasc Surg 1968; 55: 617.
9. Kay PH, Azariades M, Goldstraw P. The role of cervical mediastinoscopy in patients with superior vena caval obstruction. Thorax 1986; 41: 712.
10. Goldstraw P. Mediastinal exploration by mediastinoscopy and mediastinotomy. Br J Dis Chest 1988; 82: 111.
11. Foster ED, Munro PD, Dobell AR. Mediastinoscopy: a review of anatomical relationships and complications. Ann Thorac Surg 1972; 13: 273.
12. Nohl-Oser HC. Mediastinoscopy. Br J Hosp Med 1976; 16: 33.
13. McNeill TM, Chamberlain JM. Diagnostic anterior mediastinotomy. Ann Thorac Surg 1966; 2: 532.
14. Jiao X, Magistrelli P, Goldstraw P. The value of cervical mediastinoscopy combined with anterior mediastinotomy in bronchogenic carcinoma of the left upper lobe. Eur J Cardiothorac Surg 1997; 11: 450.
15. Goldstraw P. CT scanning in the pre-operative assessment of non-small cell lung cancer. In: Hansen HH, ed. Lung cancer: basic and clinical aspects. Boston, MA: Martinus Nijhoff; 1986: 183.
16. Goldstraw P, Kurzer M, Edwards D. Pre-operative staging of lung cancer: accuracy of computed tomography versus mediastinoscopy. Thorax 1983; 38: 10.
17. Vansteenkiste J, Stroobants SG, De Leyn P et al. Lymph node staging in non-small cell lung cancer with FDG-PET scan: a prospective study on 690 lymph node stations from 68 patients. J Clin Oncol 1998; 16: 2142.
18. Petrou M, Kaplan D, Goldstraw P. The management of recurrent malignant pleural effusions: the complementary role of talc pleurodesis and pleuroperitoneal shunting. Cancer 1995; 75: 801.
19. Venn GE, Kay PH, Midwood CJ, Goldstraw P. Open lung biopsy in patients with diffuse pulmonary shadowing. Thorax 1985; 40: 931.
20. Goldman L, Caldera DL, Nussbaum SR et al. Multifactorial index of cardiac risk in noncardiac surgical procedures. N Engl J Med 1977; 297: 845.
21. Rao TLK, Jacobs KH, El Etr AA. Reinfarction following anaesthesia in patients with myocardial infarction. Anesthesiology 1983; 59: 499.
22. Boushy SF, Billig DM, North LB et al. Clinical cause related to pre-operative and post-operative pulmonary function in patients with bronchogenic carcinoma. Chest 1971; 59: 383.
23. Boysen PG, Harris JO, Block AJ et al. Prospective evaluation for pneumonectomy using perfusion scanning. Follow-up beyond one year. Chest 1981; 80: 163
24. Narake T, Suemasu K, Ishikawa S. Lymph node mapping and curability at various levels of metastasis in resected lung cancer. J Thorac Cardiovasc Surg 1978; 76: 832.
25. Graham ANJ, Chan KJM, Pastorino U, Goldstraw P. Systematic nodal dissection in the intrathoracic staging of patients with non-small cell lung cancer. J Thorac Cardiovasc Surg, 1999; 117: 246.
26. Goldstraw P, Mannam GC, Kaplan DK, Michael P. Surgical management of non-small-cell lung cancer with ipsilateral mediastinal node metastasis (N2 disease). J Thorac Cardiovasc Surg 1994; 107: 1.
27. The lung cancer study group, Ginsberg RJ, Rubenstein LV. Randomized trial of lobectomy versus limited resection for T1N0 non-small cell lung cancer. Ann Thorac Surg 1995; 60: 615.
28. Bignall JR, Martin M, Smither DW. Survival in 6086 cases of bronchial carcinoma. Lancet 1967; 1: 1067.
29. Wilkins EW, Scannell JG, Craver JG. Four decades of experience with resection for bronchogenic carcinoma at the Massachusetts General Hospital. J Thorac Cardiovasc Surg 1978; 76: 364.
30. Firmin RK, Azariades M, Lennox SC, Lincoln JCR. Sleeve lobectomy (lobectomy and bronchoplasty) for bronchial carcinoma. Ann Thorac Surg 1983; 35: 442.
31. Mehran RJ, Deslauriers J, Piraux M et al Survival related to nodal status after sleeve resection for lung cancer. J Thorac Cardiovasc Surg 1994; 107: 578.
32. Williams DE, Pairolero PC, Davis CS et al. Survival of patients surgically treated for stage I lung cancer. J Thorac Cardiovasc Surg 1981; 82: 70.
33. Paneth M, Goldstraw P, Hyams B. Fundamental techniques in pulmonary and oesophageal surgery. London: Springer Verlag; 1987.
34. Venn GE, Williams PR, Goldstraw P. Intracavity drainage for bullous emphysematous lung disease; experience with the Brompton technique. Thorax 1988; 43: 998.
35. Cooper JD, Trulock EP, Triantafillou AN et al. Bilateral pneumectomy (volume reduction) for chronic obstructive pulmonary disease. J Thorac Cardiovasc Surg, 1995; 109: 106.
36. Morgan MDL, Denison DM, Strickland B. Value of computed tomography for selecting patients with bullous lung disease for surgery. Thorax 1986; 41: 855.
37. Weder W, Thurnheer R, Stammberger U et al. Radiologic emphysema morphology is associated with outcome after surgical lung volume reduction. Ann Thorac Surg 1997; 64: 313.
38. Geddes D, Davies M, Koyama H et al. Effect of lung-volume-reduction surgery in patients with severe emphysema. N Eng J Med 2000; 343: 239.
39. Cooper JD, Patterson GA, Sundaresan RS et al. Results of 150 consecutive bilateral lung volume reduction procedures in patients with severe emphysema. J Thorac Cardiovasc Surg 1996; 112: 1319.
40. Lowdermilk GA, Keenan RJ, Landreneau RJ et al. Comparison of clinical results for unilateral and bilateral thoracoscopic lung volume reduction. Ann Thorac Surg 200; 69: 1670.
41. Goldstraw P. The surgical management of pulmonary metastases. Baillière's Clin Oncol 1987; 1: 601.
42. Pastorino U, Buyse M, Friedel G et al. Long-term results of lung metastasectomy: prognostic analyses based on 5206 cases. J Thorac Cardiovasc Surg 1997; 113: 37.
43. Grillo HC. Reconstruction of the trachea: experience on 100 consecutive cases. Thorax 1973; 28: 667.
44. Goldstraw P. Postoperative management of the thoracic surgical patient. Clin Anesthesiol 1987; 1: 207.
45. Ilves R, Cooper JD, Todd TRJ, Pearson FG. Prospective, randomised, double-blind study using prophylactic cephalothin for major, elective, general thoracic operations. J Thorac Cardiovasc Surg 1981; 81: 813.
46. Smith G, Hirsch N, Ehrenwerth J. Placement of double-lumen endobronchial tubes: correlation between clinical impressions and bronchoscopic findings. Br J Anaesth 1986; 58: 1317.
47. Matthews HR, Hopkinson RD. Treatment of sputum retention by mini-tracheostomy. Br J Surg 1984; 71: 147.
48. Al-Kattan K, Cattalani L, Goldstraw P. Bronchopleural fistula after pneumonectomy with a hand suture technique. Ann Thorac Surg 1994; 58: 1433.
49. Al-Kattan K, Breach NM, Kaplan DK, Goldstraw P. Soft-tissue reconstruction in thoracic surgery. Ann Thorac Surg 1995; 60: 1372.
50. Burman SO. The prophylactic use of digitalis before thoracotomy. Ann Thorac Surg 1972; 14: 359.
51. Ritchie AJ, Bowe P, Gibbons JRP. Prophylactic digitalization for thoracotomy: assessment. Ann Thorac Surg 1990; 50: 86.
52. Bernard GR, Artigas A, Brigham KL et al. The American-European Consensus Conference on ARDS. Definitions, mechanisms, relevant outcomes and clinical trial coordination. Am J Crit Care Med 1994; 149: 818.
53. Mathru M, Blakeman BP. Don't drown the 'down lung'. Chest, 1993; 103: 1644.
54. Williams E, Quinlan GJ, Goldstraw P et al. Postoperative lung injury and oxidative damage in patients undergoing pulmonary resection. Eur Respir J 1998; 11: 1028.
55. Kutlu CA, Williams EA, Evans TW et al. Acute lung injury and acute respiratory distress syndrome after pulmonary resection. Ann Thorac Surg 2000; 69: 376.
56. Lee J, Turner JS, Morgan CJ et al. Adult respiratory distress syndrome: has there been a change in outcome predictive measures? Thorax 1994; 49: 596.
57. Ginsberg RF, Hill LD, Eagan RT et al. Modern thirty day operative mortality for surgical resections in lung cancer. J Thorac Cardiovasc Surg 1983; 86: 654.
58. Returns of the UK Thoracic Surgery Register 1998/9. London: Society of Cardiothoracic Surgery of Great Britain and Ireland.
59. Graham ANJ, Cosgrove AP, Gibbons JRP, McGuigan JA. Randomised trial of chest drainage systems. Thorax 1992; 47: 461.

12 Lung transplantation

John H Dark and Paul A Corris

 Key points

- Lung and heart–lung transplantation are now established therapeutic options for selected patients with advanced lung disease.

- The majority of patients worldwide undergo either single or bilateral lung transplantation, with heart–lung transplantation kept for patients with severe pulmonary hypertension associated with right ventricular failure or congenital heart disease.

- Despite the development of newer immunosuppressive agents, acute rejection and infection remain common problems.

- Chronic rejection manifest as obliterative bronchiolitis remains the major problem limiting long-term survival and is associated with persistent vascular rejection and lymphocytic bronchiolitis

- Patients free of obliterative bronchiolitis at 5 years enjoy a normal lifestyle and have an excellent chance of surviving more than 10 years.

The modern era of lung transplantation began in 1981 with the introduction of combined transplantation of heart and lungs in patients with end-stage pulmonary vascular disease.[1] The indications for heart–lung transplantation were subsequently widened to include pulmonary parenchymal and airway diseases.[2] Survival rates were good and in marked contrast to the universal failures reported after single-lung transplantation in the preceding 25 years.[3] The success of heart–lung transplantation resulted partly from reliable healing of the tracheal anastomosis compared with the bronchial anastomotic breakdown that frequently followed single-lung transplantation. The better healing reflected a good blood supply to the proximal donor trachea via donor coronary artery/bronchial artery anastomoses. The earlier lack of success with single-lung transplantation was also due to poor selection of potential

recipients, some of whom had sepsis and multiorgan failure, and the apparently insuperable problems at that time of rejection and infection.

With the introduction of successful heart–lung transplantation, however, it was realised that many patients received a new heart unnecessarily. After further research, clinical success in single-lung transplantation for fibrosing lung disease was reported by the Toronto Group in 1986.[4] Factors contributing to success included careful patient selection, introduction of cyclosporin A as the principal immunosuppressant and restoration of a viable blood supply to the bronchial anastomosis by wrapping it with a pedicle of greater omentum. Subsequently this latter practice has largely been abandoned and reliable healing can confidently be achieved without this procedure.

In 1988 double-lung transplantation with a tracheal anastomosis was introduced.[5] This procedure was, however, accompanied by more frequent problems with airway healing than heart–lung transplantation.[6] Furthermore, the operation was more complex than heart–lung transplantation and the extensive mediastinal dissection frequently led to denervation of the native heart. Bleeding was at least as much of a problem as for heart–lung transplantation and by 1989 the procedure as originally described had been abandoned. The solution to the problem of airway healing was to perform two separate bronchial anastomoses,[7] because (as in single-lung transplantation) the donor bronchus is better vascularised initially if the anastomosis is close to the lung parenchyma. This concept was further developed as a bilateral procedure carried out by performing sequential single-lung transplantations.[8] As its name implies, two separate lungs were implanted with separate hilar anastomoses (each of bronchus, pulmonary artery and left atrial cuff). The heart and mediastinum were left largely undisturbed. These improvements in surgical techniques, together with improved prophylaxis for infection and control of rejection, reduced mortality and led to rapid growth in lung transplantation from the late 1980s to mid-1990s. Currently, however, the limited supply of donor lungs has caused the frequency of lung transplantation to plateau at approximately 1500 procedures per year worldwide.

As the number of potential candidates increases, the disparity between the sizes of the donor and candidate pools continues to widen and waiting time for transplantation has lengthened, with the International Society for Heart and Lung Transplantation data base now registering a median of 500 days. This problem has driven the transplant community to consider new ways of increasing the number of available donor organs. Approaches currently under assessment include relaxation on the limits of age and function of the donor lung,[9,10] which has permitted growth in the number of transplants without diminishing early survival. Another approach applicable to paediatric practice is the use of living lobar transplantation whereby a child or small young adult receives two lower lobes from two living donors each implanted using a similar technique to bilateral lung transplantation.[11] The results of more than 100 such procedures to date have proved very satisfactory with no recorded donor deaths. More recent work has demonstrated the feasibility of lung transplantation using non-heart-beating donors and this has the potential for a huge increase the provision of suitable lungs. Finally, work on xenotransplantation continues but this is not a realistic option for those requiring lung transplantation in the immediate future.[12]

Indications and criteria for lung transplantation

A working party of the International Society of Heart and Lung Transplantation has recently published disease specific guidelines on the identification of potential suitable lung transplant candidates.[13] General advice regarding indications and acceptance criteria are discussed below.

Age and underlying condition

The major shortfall in suitable donor organs mentioned above has led the International Society to suggest an upper age limit of 55 years for transplantation of heart and lungs, 60 for both lungs alone and 65 years for single-lung transplantation. The higher age limit reflects the greater availability of suitable single lungs and the relative simplicity of the procedure leading to less surgical trauma than bilateral or heart–lung transplantation. The lower age limit for heart–lung transplantation is influenced by data showing a worse outcome for the procedure as age increases. Patients who develop any end-stage pulmonary or pulmonary vascular disease unresponsive to conventional medical therapy may be considered for transplantation provided they have none of the following established contraindications:

- significant disease of other major organ systems
- active extrapulmonary infection
- current cigarette smoking
- poor rehabilitation potential
- symptomatic osteoporosis
- significant psychosocial problems
- drug abuse or history of medical non-compliance.

Medical conditions leading to ineligibility for lung transplantation

Systemic disease and major organ dysfunction

The presence of uncontrolled systemic disease in patients with respiratory failure precludes lung transplantation. Good renal and hepatic function are essential, particularly in view of the adverse effects of immunosuppression on renal function.[14] A creatinine clearance of more than 50 ml/min prior to transplantation is desirable because both cyclosporin and tacrolimus, the principal immunosuppressive drugs used following lung transplantation, are nephrotoxic. Synthetic function of the liver should be preserved, with no abnormalities of coagulation. A raised hepatic alkaline phosphatase with elevated transaminases requires investigation but does not preclude assessment. This is clearly relevant to patients with α_1-protease inhibitor (antitrypsin) deficiency or cystic fibrosis, who may have coexisting liver disease. Patients with cystic fibrosis who have portal hypertension and varices require individual consideration of suitability for isolated lung transplantation. Diabetes mellitus, if well-controlled and not associated with vascular complications, is not a contraindication.

Patients with collagen vascular disease who are being considered for transplantation for their pulmonary complication may be precluded by the presence of active extrapulmonary disease. Examples would include the lack of mobility as a result of destructive rheumatoid arthritis or evidence of nephritis complicating systemic lupus erythematosus. Patients being considered for transplantation have often been treated with corticosteroids for many years and their intrinsic disease has led to markedly decreased physical activity. These factors, along with age and hormonal deficiencies, frequently result in a substantial loss of bone mineral density, a complication that is accelerated by immunosuppressive agents such as corticosteroids and cyclosporin after transplantation. Accordingly, patients who have severe osteoporosis or those with a history of compression fractures in the pretransplant period are at high risk of fractures postoperatively and symptomatic osteoporosis is regarded as a contraindication for transplant referral until therapy with bisphosphonates improves bone density.[15]

Nutritional state

Many patients with end-stage chronic pulmonary disease suffer from cachexia and malnutrition.[16] All recipients lose weight in the first week following transplantation and severe preoperative nutritional deficiency increases postoperative risk, in particular of infection and poor wound healing. Similarly, obesity predisposes to atelectasis and impairs early postoperative mobility, which is essential for successful lung transplantation. Ideally, recipients should be within 25% of their optimal bodyweight. Many of the early unsuccessful transplant recipients were bedbound and most transplant centres now require that recipients are capable of self-care and able to participate in exercise rehabilitation in attempts to maintain muscle bulk and physical fitness.

Infection

Persistent extrapulmonary sepsis reduces the chances of successful transplantation because it may lead to severe systemic sepsis following immunosuppressive therapy. Patients with recurrent or persistent pulmonary infection are not suitable for single-lung transplantation[17] and require heart–lung or double-lung transplantation. Oral hygiene is important and all patients should have any dental sepsis eradicated preoperatively. Many patients with parenchymal destruction and fibrosis develop chronic pulmonary cavitation, predisposing to development of an aspergilloma or other mycetoma. The presence of an aspergilloma in the periphery of the lung carries a high risk of seeding the pleural space with *Aspergillus* sp., leading to fungal empyema.

Previous surgery

Extensive pleural adhesions are associated with a risk of life-threatening haemorrhage when the natural lungs are removed. Clearly there is a gradation of risk from scarring caused by previous open lung biopsy by limited thoracotomy to previous total pleurectomy. This has important consequences for the management of pneumothorax in potential recipients. Successful transplant surgery can be carried out following talc or tetracycline pleurodesis; however, if pleurectomy is required surgeons should be asked to perform a limited procedure. The use of the antifibrinolytic agent aprotinin during transplant surgery reduces bleeding in patients who have undergone previous thoracotomy[18] and surgeons prefer to carry out bilateral lung transplantation via transverse bilateral thoracotomy, which allows better access to the pleural space than by sternotomy in patients with suspected pleural adhesions.

Systemic corticosteroids

Although early lung transplant programmes insisted on patients being weaned from corticosteroids, this proved very difficult to achieve in practice, particularly in patients with chronic obstructive pulmonary disease (COPD) or idiopathic pulmonary fibrosis. Experience has shown that bronchial anastomoses are at no greater risk in patients receiving up to 20 mg of prednisolone a day than in those taking no prednisolone,[19] providing that there is no evidence of steroid-induced thinning of the skin, osteoporosis or myopathy. Weaning from corticosteroids is therefore no longer essential before referral for transplantation but all patients should reduce the dose to 20 mg per day or less.

Cardiac disease

Patients under consideration for isolated lung transplantation should ideally have sufficient right and left ventricular function to allow single-lung anaesthesia, thereby obviating the need for cardiopulmonary bypass. Patients deemed at risk of haemodynamic instability, however, should be transplanted electively on bypass. Right ventricular function improves considerably after successful surgery and pulmonary vascular resistance falls to normal. Single-lung transplantation has been successful in a patient with a right ventricular ejection fraction of only 12%, although the mean right ventricular ejection fraction in one series was 31% for single- and 38% for double-lung transplantation.[20] Following single-lung transplantation for idiopathic pulmonary fibrosis, pulmonary vascular resistance, pulmonary artery pressure and right ventricular performance return to normal even when markedly abnormal preoperatively.[21]

Clinical evidence of cor pulmonale is not a contraindication to successful isolated lung transplantation. Moreover patients with severe primary pulmonary hypertension have undergone successful isolated lung transplantation with restoration of right ventricular function. Patients being assessed for isolated lung transplantation need to have preserved left ventricular function on echocardiography and those with an ejection fraction of less than 40% require further assessment. Patients at risk of coronary artery disease require full assessment, which may include coronary angiography; the need for this to be performed prior to assessment should be discussed with the individual transplant unit.

Psychological factors

The importance of adequate social support cannot be overemphasised. Despite the treatment advances and experience gained over the past 10 years, recipients still commonly experience life-threatening complications, and emotional stresses associated with transplantation are substantial. Family members or close friends are needed to monitor recipients, assist with their medication, transport them to health-care facilities and provide emotional support. Any potential recipient must be well-motivated, be able to cope and have demonstrated a willingness to comply with medical advice and treatment. Underlying psychiatric illness and abuse of alcohol or drugs, including cigarettes, are contraindications.

Referral population

To be considered for lung transplantation, patients should have advanced pulmonary airway, parenchymal or vascular disease with an estimated life-expectancy of 2 years or less. The most common condition that results in transplantation world wide is emphysema, followed by cystic fibrosis (Fig. 12.1). The guidelines for referral published by the International Society of Heart and Lung Transplantation rely on physiological measurements, which have been shown to predict average survival with a reasonable degree of accuracy, although it is clearly difficult to predict survival precisely in an individual.

Patients with cystic fibrosis whose forced expiratory volume in 1 second (FEV_1) is less than 30% predicted, P_aO_2 below 55 mmHg (7.3 Pa) or P_aCO_2 above 49 mmHg (6.5 kPa) have a 2-year mortality rate of 50%.[22] FEV_1 is the most significant predictor of mortality and recommendations therefore are to consider patients for transplantation when the FEV_1 falls below 30% of the predicted value. The distance a patient walks in 6 minutes is also an important bench mark for lung transplantation. Failure to achieve 180 m has been shown to be associated with an unacceptable postoperative mortality rate and a short preoperative survival.[23]

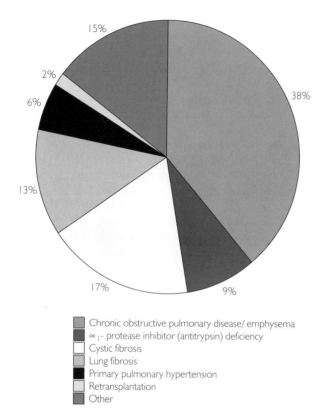

Chronic obstructive pulmonary disease/ emphysema
∝₁- protease inhibitor (antitrypsin) deficiency
Cystic fibrosis
Lung fibrosis
Primary pulmonary hypertension
Retransplantation
Other

Fig. 12.1 Major indications for unilateral or bilateral lung transplantation.

In primary pulmonary hypertension, patients with a poor outcome can be identified on the basis of right heart catheterisation. Recent advances in the medical management of this condition using intravenous, subcutaneous or nebulised prostacyclin and the introduction of atrial septostomy has reduced the need for transplantation in patients with advanced disease.

It can be very difficult to estimate survival in patients with Eisenmenger's syndrome or emphysema. Although patients may survive for several years, they may have an unacceptable quality of life on account of breathlessness and transplantation may be considered in order to improve this alone. Furthermore, it has been shown that patients with emphysema do not show improved life expectancy following lung transplantation, in contrast to those with idiopathic pulmonary fibrosis or cystic fibrosis.

Many patients with cystic fibrosis develop relatively resistant colonising Gram-negative organisms and consequently it is important to monitor antibiotic sensitivities regularly during their pre-operative course. When highly resistant strains are encountered they should be tested for synergy between classes of antibiotics and for high-dose inhibition by aminoglycosides, which can be delivered by aerosol in the postoperative period. Transplantation for patients infected with panresistant strains of *Pseudomonas aeruginosa* or *Burkholderia cepacia* is controversial.[24] The outcome of transplantation is worse in such patients and indeed some transplant units have a policy of not offering transplantation to patients colonised with *B. cepacia*. Molecular techniques have, however, shown that *B. cepacia* is a complex of organisms that can be subdivided into genomovars. Recent work has demonstrated that the adverse outcome in patients undergoing transplantation colonised with *B. cepacia* relates to those colonised with genomovar 3.

Disease-specific guidelines

Chronic obstructive pulmonary disease

■ FEV_1 < 25% of predicted (without reversibility), and/or
■ P_aCO_2 ≥ 55 mmHg (7.3 kPa) and/or
■ Elevated pulmonary artery pressure with progressive deterioration, such as cor pulmonale.

Preference should be given to those patients with elevated P_aCO_2 with progressive deterioration who require long-term oxygen therapy, as they otherwise have the poorest prognosis.[25]

Cystic fibrosis and bronchiectasis

■ FEV_1 ≤ 30% predicted or rapidly progressive respiratory deterioration with FEV_1 >30% predicted. Rapid progressive deterioration may be signalled by, for example an increasing rate of hospitalisation, rapid fall in FEV_1, massive haemoptysis or increasing cachexia, in spite of optimal medical management.
■ Resting arterial blood gases while breathing room air – P_aCO_2 > 50 mmHg (6.7 kPa); P_aO_2 < 55 mmHg (7.3 kPa) – are useful criteria and are associated with less than 50% 2-year survival; however, patients should be considered candidates for transplantation if they meet FEV_1 criteria, even though they may not yet be markedly hypercapnic or hypoxaemic.[22]
■ Young female patients with cystic fibrosis who deteriorate rapidly have a particularly poor prognosis.[26] These patients should be evaluated on an individual basis regardless of functional criteria.

Patients with bronchiectasis from other causes – immunodeficiency syndromes, immotile or dysfunctional cilia syndromes, postinfection or unknown – may also be considered for transplantation. Few data are available on likely survival rates in such patients with advanced disease, which makes formulation of guidelines for selection difficult. In general, in evaluating such patients the lung transplant community has followed the guidelines listed above for cystic fibrosis.

Idiopathic pulmonary fibrosis

■ Symptomatic (including rest or exercise-related oxygen desaturation), progressive disease with failure to improve or maintain lung function while being treated with steroids or other immunosuppressive agents. Clinical assessment at frequent intervals (e.g. every 3 months) is extremely useful in evaluating the progression of disease or failure to improve with drug treatment.[27]
■ Initial evaluation should be considered when pulmonary function deteriorates on treatment, even though the patient may be only mildly symptomatic.
■ Patients are usually symptomatic when the vital capacity falls below 60–70% predicted and the CO transfer coefficient falls below 50–60% predicted.

Systemic disease with pulmonary fibrosis

Pulmonary fibrosis is common in a number of systemic diseases, such as systemic sclerosis, rheumatoid arthritis and sarcoidosis, and following chemotherapy. In patients with these diagnoses, the manifestations of the underlying process are highly variable, and patients should be considered on an individual basis. In general, evidence that the systemic disease is quiescent is required. It is necessary for all patients to meet general selection criteria and to have failed optimal medical therapy to be considered for lung transplantation. The criteria for timing of selection for transplantation listed above should be followed.

Pulmonary hypertension

Potential candidates for lung transplantation with a diagnosis of primary pulmonary hypertension should be assessed by a centre with experience in this condition and all patients should be evaluated for vasodilator therapy and other medical or surgical interventions before considering transplantation. The following criteria should be met to consider a patient within the 'transplant window'.

■ Symptomatic, progressive disease that, despite optimal medical or surgical treatment, is accompanied by New York Heart Association (NYHA) class III or IV disability – where available, prostacyclin should be considered the gold standard for medical vasodilator therapy if there is no objective indication that calcium-channel blockers may be useful.
■ Useful haemodynamic criteria of failure of optimal pretransplant therapy include a cardiac index less than 1 l/min/m², a right atrial pressure above 15 mmHg and a mean pulmonary artery pressure above 55 mmHg.

Pulmonary hypertension secondary to congenital heart disease (Eisenmenger's syndrome)

The prognosis of pulmonary hypertension in patients with congenital heart disease is different from other types of pulmonary hypertension. Haemodynamically, similar pulmonary artery pressures are associated with better cardiac function and lower right atrial pressures and a somewhat better prognosis.[28] Predictors of survival are less reliable. The role of vasodilator therapy in pretransplant management of these patients is not yet clear.

■ Severe progressive symptoms with function at NYHA III or NYHA IV level despite optimal medical management.

Combined pulmonary and other organ failure

Patients presenting with failure of more than one organ have occasionally been considered as candidates for multiorgan transplantation. Advanced liver disease, for example, can be associated with pulmonary hypertension.[29] Selected patients with liver and lung disease may be candidates for liver–lung transplants.[30] Similarly, patients with heart and lung disease or kidney and lung disease or other combined organ failure might occasionally be candidates for a multiorgan transplant. In each case the candidate should meet all the criteria for selection for the individual transplant. Furthermore, because experience in this area is limited and outcomes are not well-studied, only centres with well-established transplant programmes in each of the organ systems involved should consider such procedures.

Paediatric lung transplantation

Cardiopulmonary vascular disease

Lung transplantation in children is evolving.[31] Diseases that are potentially amenable to lung transplantation include primary pulmonary hypertension, pulmonary hypertension associated with structural heart disease, pulmonary vein stenosis, pulmonary hypertension associated with parenchymal lung disease, and congenital abnormalities of lung development or of lung adaptation to extrauterine life. As in adults, maximal medical therapy, including vasodilators and supplemental oxygen, should be instituted before children are considered for transplantation. Because the diagnoses are varied and the disease spectra diverse, prognostic indicators have been difficult to develop. Empirical criteria are the primary means of selecting candidates and include:

■ disease no longer responding to maximum medical and surgical treatment
■ moderately severe or severe functional impairment (NYHA class III or IV)
■ right ventricular failure, severe cyanosis and low cardiac output.

To arrive at appropriate decisions it is necessary to follow these patients with great care in centres that specialise in paediatric work. Careful assessment of all these patients is vital to exclude other correctable cardiac defects contributing to pulmonary hypertension. Pulmonary hypertension with parenchymal lung disease or abnormalities of development or adaptation need to be individually assessed because only single cases of patients receiving transplants have been described. These diseases include congenital diaphragmatic hernia, congenital surfactant protein B deficiency and congenital cystic emphysematous lung disease.

Other diseases

Other diseases presenting in advanced stages in children include, among others, cystic fibrosis, bronchiolitis obliterans, pulmonary fibrosis and bronchopulmonary dysplasia. It is often difficult, because of the limited available data, to make accurate predictions regarding survival. As in the case of the cardiopulmonary diseases, patients may be considered candidates for transplantation when progressive disability occurs (NYHA class III or IV) in spite of optimal medical therapy. With cystic fibrosis, guidelines for adult patients can generally be adapted to the paediatric population.

Choice of procedure

The team listing a patient for lung transplantation has a number of options: the most simple format – single-lung transplantation, paired or double lung transplants with various types of airway anastomosis and combined heart and lung transplantation. Lobar transplants may be isolated but are normally paired and are applicable to smaller recipients and those benefiting from live donation. In most cases the decision will be dependent upon the pretransplant diagnosis but local expertise and also regional differences in organ allocation are important.

Single-lung transplantation

Single-lung transplantation (Figs 12.2 & 12.3) is ideal in the setting of restrictive lung disease as both ventilation and perfusion are directed towards the transplanted lung. However, chronic obstructive pulmonary disease is the most common indication worldwide. Two lungs can be removed from the majority of donors but there will be a number of situations when one donor lung is damaged irretrievably but the other is usable.

Bilateral lung transplantation

Bilateral lung transplantation evolved from en-bloc double-lung transplantation as the option for patients, mainly those with septic disease, who require replacement of both lungs. There was a particular impetus in the USA, where organ allocation rules prevented the widespread application of heart–lung transplantation. After the initial airway problems of en-bloc transplantation,[5] French groups demonstrated better airway healing with bibronchial anastomoses.[7] The current technique, first described by Pasque et al,[8] was the logical continuation, with all the anastomoses at the level of the hilum. The heart remains innervated

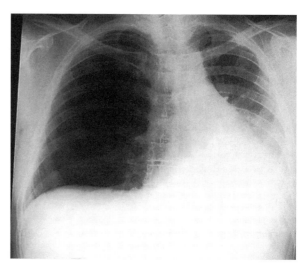

Fig. 12.3 Expiratory chest radiography of patient 2 years after left single-lung transplantation for emphysema, showing mediastinal shift towards transplanted lung.

and the standard transverse thoracosternotomy (clamshell incision) gives excellent access to all areas of the chest. Bleeding from vascular postinflammatory adhesions or from enlarged bronchial arteries buried within inflamed hilar nodes can easily be controlled. The technique can easily be adapted for lobar transplantation and even the use of two lobes from the same lung, as in the elegant split-lung technique of Couteuil.[32]

Heart–lung transplantation

Heart–lung transplantation was the first successful method of pulmonary transplantation, introduced initially for patients with pulmonary vascular disease.[33] It can also be applied to a variety of pulmonary parenchymal conditions, with the potential wastage of a donor heart obviated by use of the 'domino procedure'.[34] There is very reliable healing of the distal trachea because of coronary-to-bronchial collaterals. The transplanted heart is relatively protected from coronary disease,[35] although some late deaths, almost invariably in the setting of obliterative bronchiolitis are clearly cardiac. The heart removed from the pulmonary recipients (domino heart), never having been exposed to the deleterious effects of brain-stem death, functions exceptionally well in cardiac recipients.[36] On the other hand, the pulmonary recipient who then develops obliterative bronchiolitis is rarely a candidate for retransplantation. Isolated lung retransplantation is usually precluded by a degree of concomitant graft coronary disease. Redo heart–lung transplantation is technically very demanding and has such a poor outcome that it has all but been abandoned.[37]

Determinants of choice of procedure

Two main factors decide the procedure for a particular patient. The first is whether the contralateral lung can be left in the recipient (the 'harmless native lung') and only in this setting can single-lung transplantation be performed. Inability to leave the native lung in place, nearly always because of pulmonary sepsis,

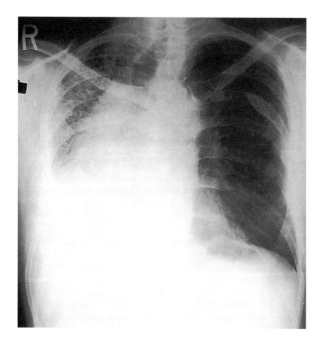

Fig. 12.2 Chest radiograph of patient 2 years after left single-lung transplantation for idiopathic pulmonary fibrosis, showing contraction of natural fibrotic lung with mediastinal shift towards the native lung.

means some form of paired transplant is indicated. The standard choice would be bilateral lung transplantation but heart–lung transplantation with domino donation of the recipient's heart, is used by two experienced UK centres.

For patients with pulmonary vascular disease the reparability or recoverability of cardiac function will decide whether the heart should be replaced (heart–lung transplantation) or retained. Almost any degree of right ventricular failure will recover when pulmonary vascular resistance is normal.[38] This can be achieved most efficiently with a paired lung transplant, although single-lung transplantation has been widely used in pulmonary hypertensive patients. For patients with the Eisenmenger complex there is increasingly good evidence that heart–lung transplantation is a better option than cardiac repair and paired lung transplantation.[39] Left ventricular function is almost always impaired and the resulting elevated left-sided filling pressure exacerbates any post-transplant lung injury and predisposes to a difficult early postoperative course.

Restrictive disease

In the absence of contralateral sepsis, single-lung transplantation is the ideal option. There are several series of lengthy follow-up and functional results are excellent.[40]

Obstructive lung disease

Despite earlier doubts, single-lung transplantation can readily be performed for emphysema[41] and this is now the commonest pre-transplant diagnosis. On occasion, the contralateral lung may be a source of infection, either from pre-existing bronchiectasis or by colonisation of a bulla, often with *Aspergillus* sp. Bilateral lung transplantation is clearly needed in these cases. In addition, there has been a tendency to transplant both lungs in younger patients. It was previously believed that patients with extensive bullae were more at risk of air trapping and overexpansion of the native lung and that they too were candidates for bilateral lung transplantation but it is now clear that this is not the case. It is however undeniable that spirometry is much better after a paired lung transplant, often approaching normal, although functional outcomes such as 6 minute walk distance show little difference between single-lung transplantation and bilateral lung transplantation in patients with COPD.

Some registry data suggest that there is a survival advantage after 3 years for those with paired lung transplants.[42] Presumably obliterative bronchiolitis occurs with a fall in expiratory flow, which is better tolerated when the starting point is higher. In some institutional series there has been a lower early mortality with bilateral lung transplantation.[43] Thus from the point of view of an individual, bilateral lung transplantation is the procedure of choice, with probable longer survival and improved quality of life in the long term and possibly better early function. This finding has to be reconciled with the observation, both in Europe and in North America, that there is no difference in survival after lung transplantation for COPD compared with survival on the waiting list.[44,45] The inference is that, for the majority of patients, transplantation improves quality but not quantity of life. It is difficult to justify performing bilateral lung transplantation in this setting, particularly when these patients compete with others (e.g. with cystic fibrosis) who have a clear improvement in survival after bilateral lung transplantation.

Septic lung disease

These patients will in general suffer either from cystic fibrosis or another type of bronchiectasis. All the infected lung tissue should be removed and in general the procedure of choice is a bilateral lung transplantation. Single-lung transplantation plus contralateral pneumonectomy has been described for cystic fibrosis but is only rarely applicable.[46]

Heart–lung transplantation has been used by two UK centres for this group of patients. In the hands of experts the outcome is equally good. By use of the domino procedure, wastage of donor hearts is minimised but there is a disadvantage to the pulmonary recipient, who receives a denervated organ that will eventually be prone to accelerated graft coronary disease.

Pulmonary vascular disease

Heart–lung transplantation is clearly the procedure of choice if there is irreparable congenital heart disease (e.g. single ventricle or pulmonary atresia), left ventricular dysfunction or significant coronary disease. If the heart can potentially be retained, isolated lung transplantation can be performed. Single-lung transplantation has been championed by some groups but there is probably a higher early mortality and less good functional result. In particular, if obliterative bronchiolitis developed in the transplanted lung, very significant ventilation perfusion mismatching develops.[47] The native lung, almost devoid of perfusion but ventilated because of airway changes in the transplant, comes to represents a very large volume of physiological dead space.

The lung donor

Understanding the pathophysiology of brain-stem death and how its sequelae affect the donor has improved with time. An initial surge in blood pressure, following brief but intense release of noradrenaline (norepinephrine), may result in stress injury to the pulmonary endothelium. There follows a generalised inflammatory state, with activation of a number of cytokine pathways. A degree of lung injury is probably an invariable accompaniment and may predict events in the recipient.[48]

This inflammatory state compounds other causes of lung injury – trauma, aspiration and inadequate bronchial toilet – such that lungs can be removed from only 20% of organ donors.[49] Ideal donor criteria are shown in Table 12.1. P_aO_2, measured during ventilation with an F_1O_2 of 1.0 and positive

Table 12.1   Criteria for ideal donor selection

- Age < 55 years
- < 20 pack-years smoking history
- Lung secretions non-purulent
- ABO compatible
- Clear chest radiograph
- No aspiration
- Gram-stain- and culture-negative
- $P_aO_2 > 300$ mmHg (> 40 kPa) with $F_1O_2 = 1.0$ and positive end-expiratory pressure of 5 cmH$_2$O

end-expiratory pressure (PEEP) of 5 cmH$_2$O, may be the best determinant of lung viability. A single lung may still be usable even if there are radiographic changes in the contralateral lung. Selective measurement of pulmonary vein blood gases when the chest is opened may identify such usable single lungs.[50]

Optimal management of the lung donor includes repeated bronchial toilet and physiotherapy, avoidance of excessive crystalloid infusion, maintenance of normal body temperature and treatment of failing left ventricular function with inotropes. Perhaps because of the cytokine-driven lung injury, relatively modest changes in central venous pressure may result in rapid deterioration of gas exchange.[51] There may be a conflict between maintenance of optimal perfusion of abdominal organs, avoidance of unnecessary catecholamine infusions (from the point of view of the heart) and best management of the lung, avoiding transfusion and keeping left atrial pressure low. High-dose steroids given at an early stage may reduce deterioration in the donor.[52]

Lung retrieval and preservation

Final assessment of the lungs is made by a surgical team after the chest has been opened via sternotomy. As in other organs, ischaemic damage is minimised by cooling. This is achieved by flushing a cold solution through the pulmonary artery, often preceded by a prostaglandin infusion to obtain maximum vasodilatation, together with topical cooling of cold saline solution. Following much laboratory research,[53] a low potassium/dextran solution is gradually replacing the widely used intracellular-type (i.e. high potassium) Euro Collins solutions borrowed from renal transplantation. The lungs are stored inflated and ischaemic times of 6–8 hours are generally tolerated. Longer times are associated with more early dysfunction and possibly an increased frequency of rejection. Registry data show this to be the case particularly for organs from older donors.[42]

Lung implantation

The simplest procedure, single-lung transplantation, is a template for all the others. In general, the side with worse function, as judged from an isotope perfusion scan, is chosen for the transplant. Through a standard lateral thoracotomy, the hilar structures are mobilised. Patients with emphysema can nearly always be maintained on the dependent lung (although air trapping is a potential problem), as can most of those with a restrictive disease, thus avoiding the need for cardiopulmonary bypass. A trial clamping of the pulmonary artery is the final arbiter and, if this is tolerated for 10 minutes, the lung is removed. A cuff of left atrium is prepared around the pulmonary veins of the recipient, after opening the pericardium.

The donor bronchus is trimmed as close as possible to the lung parenchyma, where it is vascularised by pulmonary to bronchial collaterals. With this lung positioned in the chest, the bronchi are anastomosed end to end with apposition of the cut mucosa. This short donor bronchus technique results in very reliable healing, with a complication rate of less than 3%.[54] Dehiscence is now exceedingly rare and the occasional fibrous

stricture can easily be managed with dilatation and endobronchial stenting. Wrapping of the anastomosis, e.g. with omentum or pericardium, is unnecessary. The corresponding atrial cuff on the donor lung is simply sutured to that on the recipient and the implantation is completed with an end-to-end pulmonary artery anastomosis.

Bilateral lung transplantation duplicates all the above for both lungs. The standard 'clamshell' incision gives superb access to all parts of the pleural cavity, invaluable for the control of vascular adhesions, which often accompany long-standing septic lung disease. Sequential removal and implantation of the lung can be performed but this involves very skilful anaesthetic management of one-lung ventilation and there is often a degree of haemodynamic instability. All the pulmonary blood flow has to pass through the first lung while the second is implanted, usually resulting in a degree of pulmonary oedema. An alternative is to use cardiopulmonary bypass for both removal and implantation of both lungs.[55] Airway management is very straightforward, and reperfusion can take place in a controlled manner into both vascular beds. Bypass is essential in smaller recipients, when double-lumen tracheal intubation is impossible, and for lobar transplantation.

The principal disadvantage of the clamshell incision is pain and sometimes sternal instability. If there are no pleural adhesions, e.g. in patients with emphysema, separate anterior thoracotomies (keeping the sternum intact)[56] or a sternotomy[57] can be used for bilateral lung transplantation.

Sternotomy is routine for heart–lung transplantation, which is in some respects a more straightforward procedure. Bypass is obviously essential. The heart and lungs are removed and the new organs are implanted with anastomosis of the trachea, aorta and right atrium and separate caval anastomoses if the heart is used for a cardiac transplant recipient – the domino procedure. The attached heart provides a systemic blood supply through coronary-to-bronchial collaterals to the lungs. As a result the trachea is vascularised from below and airway anastomotic problems are rare after heart–lung transplantation. A sternotomy gives poorer access to pleural adhesions and hilar structures. Bleeding is commoner after heart–lung transplantation, with a re-exploration rate of 20–30% in some series. There is also a risk of phrenic and, more frequently, vagal nerve injury. With less mediastinal dissection and better access, both bleeding and nerve injury are much less common after bilateral lung transplantation.

Postoperative course and management

Reperfusion injury and immediate postoperative management

By the time of implantation, the donor lung has already suffered from the consequences of brain-stem death and cold ischaemic injury. Any damage to the endothelium is exacerbated by interaction with recipient neutrophils and subsequently from free-radical-mediated injury. The end result is frequently a degree of alveolar capillary leak with occasional progression to a full blown acute respiratory distress syndrome (ARDS) picture. Reperfusion injury can be minimised by controlling pulmonary artery pressure during the initial phase and by manoeuvres such as high-dose steroids to reduce neutrophil sequestration within the lung.[58] Rises in pulmonary artery pressure should be avoided and pulmonary venous pressure kept low by avoiding overtransfusion and the use of inotropes if necessary. The tendency for alveolar oedema should be countered by ventilating with PEEP. Inhaled nitric oxide, in concentrations of 20–30 ppm, has proved invaluable in managing established damage and can often completely reverse a picture of pulmonary oedema in 24 hours.[59] The main benefit is probably reduced pulmonary artery pressure but there is a direct effect on neutrophil adhesion. Oxygenation benefits from improved ventilation and perfusion matching. With greater understanding of events during the initial first few minutes of reperfusion and the early addition of nitric oxide, acute lung injury is now rarely fatal.

The patient receiving a single-lung transplant for emphysema who develops primary transplant dysfunction can be particularly difficult to manage. Application of PEEP results in overdistension of the residual native lung and mediastinal shift and impedes expansion of the transplanted lung. Separate lung ventilation for 48 or 72 hours, applying PEEP to the transplanted lung together with inhaled nitric oxide and ventilating the recipient lung to minimise air trapping, may be required to retrieve the situation.[60]

In general, postoperative management follows the routine for any patient undergoing a major thoracotomy. Epidural analgesia is essential for the potentially painful clamshell incision and is preferable for single-lung transplantation via a lateral thoracotomy. If lung function is good, the patient can be extubated early, although supplemental oxygen is frequently required for up to a week. Fluid management has to steer between excessive crystalloid transfusion and the requirement for good renal perfusion in the setting of exposure to nephrotoxic drugs such as cyclosporin.

In non-septic lung disease, only narrow-spectrum, antistaphylococcal prophylaxis is used initially. Secretions from the donor lung are sampled at the time of transplantation and bronchoalveolar lavage (BAL) is performed as a routine before implantation. Antibiotics are altered subsequently if there are significant new organisms in the donor lung. Patients with septic lung disease, particularly those with cystic fibrosis, are often colonised with multiply-resistant organisms and *Aspergillus* spp., and pose a more difficult problem. The main burden is removed with the old lungs. Major efforts are made to avoid contaminating the pleural space during explantation, supplemented by irrigation of the chest with amphotericin solution and the antiseptic tauroline. Antibiotics and antifungals appropriate to the known sensitivities of previous isolates are given systemically over the perioperative period.

Early postoperative management beyond the intensive care unit

After extubation, patients are usually transferred from an intensive care unit to a step-down ward. Central venous and arterial catheters may be removed and oxygen saturation monitored continuously by an oximeter. Chest radiographs are taken twice a day during the first week and monitored for perihilar infiltrates or septal lines, which can suggest acute rejection. The development of a pleural effusion in addition to parenchymal change may indicate acute rejection or empyema. If clinical deterioration occurs, additional chest radiographs are performed. After the first week the frequency of radiographic and other studies can be adjusted according to the patient's clinical status. Chest radiographs have been reported as normal in 26% of cases of acute rejection during the first month and lung function testing is a vital part of graft surveillance.

Spirometry is performed as soon as practicable after surgery. Many transplant units teach patients to monitor their own function using a hand-held battery spirometer. A sustained 5–10% reduction in FEV_1 has been reported as being a sensitive marker of either lung rejection or infection that warrants further investigation, even in the absence of clinical symptoms or chest radiographic abnormalities.

All patients who undergo single-lung transplantation have a perfusion scan within the first week after transplantation. The graft should have immediate preferential perfusion compared with the native lung and any evidence of hypoperfusion of the new lung raises the probability of vascular anastomotic stricture or thrombosis. Vascular anastomotic complications are rare but carry a high mortality. Pulmonary venous obstruction leads to increasing parenchymal infiltrates and both arterial and venous strictures or thromboses lead to persistent hypoxaemia. The diagnosis requires a high index of suspicion and confirmation by transoesophageal echocardiography and pulmonary angiography. Treatment may involve judicious use of thrombolytic agents, where thrombosis is significant, balloon dilatation or surgery.

The principal problem in the early management following lung transplantation is the impossibility of differentiating between opportunist infections of the lung and lung rejection. Both com-

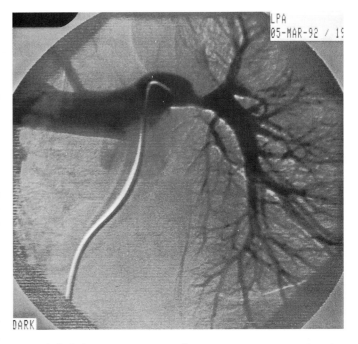

Fig. 12.4 Pulmonary angiogram demonstrating anastomotic stricture of pulmonary artery following single lung transplantation.

plications present with identical respiratory symptoms and physical signs, which include fever, cough, shortness of breath, malaise and crackles on auscultation. Chest radiography is also often unhelpful because pulmonary infiltrates and pleural effusions are common to both and in the early postoperative period may also occur as a result of vascular injury of the donor lung.

Bronchoscopy in the early postoperative period

Fibreoptic bronchoscopy with BAL and transbronchial biopsy have an essential role in the monitoring of a lung allograft in the early postoperative period. Bronchoscopy is carried out in response to the development of respiratory symptoms, a new radiographic infiltrate, a drop in lung function or an unexplained fever. Although transbronchial biopsy may have a 15–28% false-negative rate, it remains the gold standard in practical terms for the diagnosis of acute lung rejection.[61] It is generally believed that four to six biopsies should be taken and that serial sections should be reported by a pathologist familiar with lung transplantation pathology and graded using the guidelines established by the International Society for Heart and Lung Transplantation.[62] A deterioration in clinical condition may also be caused by lung infection and, moreover, a number of studies have shown that infection and rejection may be seen concurrently in the early period following transplantation. For these reasons it is important to perform BAL at the same time as transbronchial biopsy to provide samples for microbiological and cytological examination for bacteria, fungi and viruses.

Immunosuppression

Standard therapy is a three-drug regimen based on either cyclosporin A or tacrolimus. The other components are corticosteroids and either azathioprine or mycophenolate mofetil. Both tacrolimus and cyclosporin A are given orally twice a day, with the concentration in whole blood measured at trough level using a monoclonal assay. Trough levels of 300–350 mg/ml cyclosporin and 10 mg/ml of tacrolimus represent initial targets but these may be adjusted on an individual basis in patients with rejection or infective complications. Oral prednisolone is begun at 1 mg/kg per day and the dose lowered by 0.2 mg/kg per week with a target maintenance dose of 0.2 mg/kg per day at the time of hospital discharge. The initial daily dose of azathioprine is 2–3 mg/kg, the dose being adjusted according to the white cell count. Mycophenolate mofetil is commenced at a dose of 1.5 g twice a day.

Both cyclosporin A and tacrolimus are metabolised by the liver, such that interactions with a number of commonly used drugs may alter the concentrations of both agents. Rapid elevations in levels because of drug interactions cause acute toxicity whereas rapid reductions allow rejection to occur. Table 12.2 summarises drugs that commonly alter the concentrations of cyclosporin and tacrolimus in blood.

Early infection prophylaxis

It is routine for patients to receive prophylactic antibiotics following surgery and it is common to cover staphylococci and

Table 12.2 Drugs that alter the concentration of cyclosporin and tacrolimus in the blood

Raise blood levels	Calcium-channel blockers: diltiazem, verapamil, nicardipine Methylprednisolone Antifungal agents: ketoconazole, itraconazole, fluconazole Macrolide antibiotics: erythromycin, clarithromycin Whole grapefruit and grapefruit juice (tacrolimus only) Other drugs: allopurinol, bromocriptine, danazol, metoclopramide
Decrease blood levels	Anticonvulsants: phenytoin, carbamazepine, phenobarbitone Antibiotics: rifampicin, nafcillin Other drugs: ticlopidine, octreotide

anaerobic organisms until healing of the bronchial anastomosis has been identified. Flucloxacillin, metronidazole and gentamicin are commonly used. Patients who have septic lung conditions are often colonised with *Pseudomonas* species and should receive appropriate antibiotic cover according to pretransplant cultures. Recipients with airways colonised by *Aspergillus* spp. are generally given antifungal treatment to reduce the frequency of disseminated fungal infections as well as infections of the bronchial and anastomotic site. There is no clear consensus and units employ a variety of strategies, including nebulised amphotericin 20 mg twice a day, low-dose intravenous amphotericin or oral itraconazole. Some donor lung lavages show evidence of *Candida* spp. and the prophylactic use of fluconazole is usually employed.

Patients with evidence of lung injury or who have required a prolonged period of mechanical ventilation often continue with nebulised colomycin to help prevent colonisation of lungs with Gram-negative organisms. Patients at high risk of the subsequent development of cytomegalovirus (CMV) disease will often start prophylaxis with oral ganciclovir during this early postoperative period (see below).

Early complications

Acute rejection

Acute rejection is seen in up to 40% of recipients within the first 30 days of transplantation. Episodes that occur in the first 2 weeks typically cause fever, chills, malaise, increasing tightness in the chest, cough and worsening dyspnoea. Physical examination may reveal signs of pleural effusion and crackles. Pulmonary function studies may show deterioration and hypoxaemia. Chest radiographs may demonstrate interstitial infiltrates, with or without pleural effusions.

The principal histopathological change found in acute rejection is a perivascular lymphocytic infiltrate, which may extend into alveolar septa in the later stages of rejection (Fig. 12.5). In

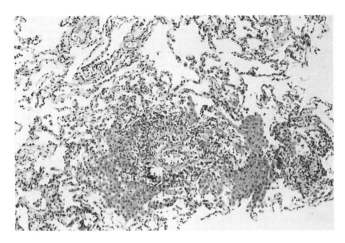

Fig. 12.5 Transbronchial lung biopsy specimen showing acute rejection with lymphocytes surrounding an arteriole and infiltrating the surrounding alveolar walls.

addition, airways may show a lymphocytic infiltrate. It is usual to perform transbronchial biopsy from each lobe from one lung as rejection may be patchy and multiple biopsies from different lobes afford a greater chance of positive diagnosis. Many studies have tried to establish reliable, less invasive methods of diagnosing rejection on blood or BAL cells and fluid. To date, none have proved sufficiently sensitive and specific for routine clinical use, although the Pittsburgh group reported some success using the donor-specific primed lymphocyte response of BAL cells to diagnose lung allograft rejection. The grading of acute pulmonary rejection is based on the intensity of lymphocyte infiltrate, as described in Table 12.3.

Acute rejection is a complex integrated immune response stimulated by the recognition of histocompatability antigens on the surface of donor cells. The most important histocompatability antigens are those of the major histocompatability complex (MHC). T-cell recognition of foreign MHC occurs via complex

Table 12.3 Histological grading for acute rejection

Type of rejection	Description
Acute rejection	
Grade A0 – None	No significant abnormality
Grade A1 – Minimal	Infrequent perivascular infiltrates
Grade A2 – Mild	Frequent perivascular infiltrates surrounding venules and arterioles
Grade A3 – Moderate	Dense perivascular infiltrates extending into alveolar septa and air spaces
Grade A4 – Severe	Diffuse perivascular, interstitial and airspace mononuclear infiltrates with pneumocyte damage, possibly with necrosis infarction or vasculitis
Chronic rejection	
Acute	
Inactive	
Chronic vascular rejection	

interaction between the donor antigens, antigen-presenting cells and the T-cell antigen receptor, together with accessory costimulatory molecules. Adhesion molecules such as vascular cell adhesion molecule (VCAM)-1 and intercellular adhesion molecule (ICAM)-1 facilitate the process. Following interaction, the T cell becomes activated, a term that refers to a cascade of events including signal transduction, gene transcription and release of cytokines. Episodes of acute vascular rejection are usually treated with pulsed methyl prednisolone 10 mg/kg intravenously for 3 days followed by augmented oral prednisolone at 1 mg/kg for a month. Rejection episodes resistant to increased corticosteroids may be treated by T-cell antibody, photophoretic therapy or total lymphoid irradiation. In general, however, the response to methyl prednisolone is brisk, with symptoms improving within 24 hours. Within 1 week of completing therapy, allograft function should have improved dramatically. Failure to achieve this warrants immediate re-evaluation.

Infection

The principal cause of early postoperative death is infection. Bacterial pneumonia is common in the early postoperative period and affects up to 35% of patients.[63] The factors that influence the development of pneumonia include immunosuppression, alteration of the natural defence mechanisms, such as a depressed cough reflex, and reduced clearance, in part because of depressed ciliary beat frequency. The initial approach to determine the cause of pneumonia in a patient who has received a lung allograft is no different from that of any other immunocompromised patient. Transbronchial biopsy, however, is usually carried out at an earlier stage because acute rejection may present with identical clinical features. Sputum should be sent for Gram stain and culture and blood cultures are taken. Fibreoptic bronchoscopy is carried out with lavage and protected brush specimens from the involved segments. The high incidence of pneumonia is caused by Gram-negative rods such as *Pseudomonas* spp. All transplant centres have reported typical pneumonia organisms, such as *Streptococcus pneumoniae*, *Haemophilus influenzae*, *Mycoplasma pneumoniae*, *Legionella pneumophila* and *Staphylococcus aureus*. Although patients with cystic fibrosis do not have a higher frequency of pneumonia, they do have an increased frequency of *Pseudomonas* spp. isolated from sputum and lavage, and such patients benefit from prophylactic nebulised colomycin to prevent the development of pneumonia.

Cytomegalovirus is the most common viral pathogen. A recipient negative for CMV antibody who receives an organ from an antibody-positive donor has the potential for the most severe disease.[64] Antibody-positive patients who receive lungs from either antibody-positive or antibody-negative donors may also develop CMV disease but the risk is not as great as in the former category. Antibody-negative patients who receive lungs from antibody-negative donors have a negligible risk, provided they receive seronegative blood products. CMV disease typically presents with fever, increasing breathlessness and/or abdominal pain and is usually associated with leukopenia.

Much literature has been published concerning the prophylaxis of CMV disease in lung transplant recipients. The high incidence of CMV disease in antibody-negative recipients of lungs from positive donors led to a number of strategies and practice still varies widely. The development of oral ganciclovir taken 1 g three times a day up to 3 months after transplantation has been adopted by many groups. It is virostatic rather than viricidal and so infection typically occurs when prophylaxis is discontinued. The advantage of delaying the onset of CMV disease is that the degree of immunosuppression is usually less and the patient's overall condition more robust at the later date and so the host is more able to deal with the pathogen. A second approach is to use pre-emptive therapy with ganciclovir based on weekly testing for antigenaemia in at risk patients. This is conceptually more scientific but practically challenging as it relies on repeated blood sampling and the availability of a reliable antigenaemia testing service.

Ganciclovir at 5 mg/kg intravenously twice a day for 2–3 weeks is the treatment of choice for established CMV infection. The dose must be adjusted for renal insufficiency and leukopenia. Herpes virus pneumonia was reported as a common problem in early heart and lung transplant recipients and for that reason acyclovir prophylaxis has traditionally been given for up to 6–12 weeks after transplantation.

Pneumocystis carinii is one of the potential opportunist infections following lung transplantation but has been virtually eliminated by the widespread use of prophylaxis. Without prophylaxis, infection was reported in up to 88% of heart–lung transplant recipients. It is rare before 6 months after transplantation but prophylaxis is usually started within the first month. Prophylactic treatment is taken twice daily for 3 days each week using trimethoprim 160 mg and sulfamethoxazole 800 mg in combination (co-trimoxazole).

Infection with *Candida* or *Aspergillus* spp. is a potential problem when these organisms are isolated from the airway of the donor lung at harvest or from the recipient lung following explantation. They may invade the bronchial anastomosis in the early postoperative period and infect not only devitalised tissue at the anastomosis but also ischaemic areas of the bronchus, with the potential to cause life-threatening haemorrhage. Prophylaxis for susceptible patients is as discussed above and frank infection is treated with fluconazole, itraconazole or intravenous amphotericin and flucytosine as indicated previously.

Transition to outpatient management

Most lung transplant recipients remain in hospital for at least 3 weeks after transplantation for surveillance and physiotherapy. Patients also require a good deal of education regarding warning signs of infection or rejection and information relating to their drug therapy. Once recipients have achieved a sufficient level of independence they can be discharged to housing adjacent to the hospital, where they can continue postoperative training and rehabilitation for days or weeks prior to returning home. Highly deconditioned recipients benefit greatly from intensive rehabilitation.

Outpatient management

The number of lung transplant recipients continues to grow and as a consequence respiratory physicians play an increasing role in the management of these patients. They need to be aware, however, of when to refer recipients back to transplant centres for specialist investigation.

The major complications encountered in the first few months following transplantation are similar to those encountered early – rejection and infection. Differences in the presentation of rejection and the causes of infection occur in this stage compared with the early postoperative period In addition, a number of other disorders associated with immune suppression are seen and these require prompt management if the recipient is to realise the maximum potential from transplantation. Although two-thirds of recipients experience at least one episode of acute rejection within the first 2 years, the incidence is greatest in the first 6 months and declines markedly thereafter.[65] After 6 months, chronic rejection, recognised histologically by bronchiolitis obliterans and functionally by the bronchiolitis obliterans syndrome (BOS), begins to emerge.[66]

Bronchiolitis obliterans syndrome

Bronchiolitis obliterans syndrome has become the leading cause of death following lung transplantation and affects up to two-thirds of all long-term survivors.[67,68] Prevention is complicated and remains one of the major challenges facing lung transplantation today.

Histologically, BOS is recognised by obliteration of bronchioles by organising fibrin associated with fibroblasts and mononuclear cells (Fig. 12.6). Immunohistology shows that the walls of the bronchioles are infiltrated by CD8+ lymphocytes.[69] The small bronchioles are left as fibrous bands extending out to the pleura, with associated dilatation and bronchiectasis of proximal airways. Vascular sclerosis affecting both pulmonary arteries and veins may be seen in conjunction with obliterative bronchiolitis.

The leading risk factor for chronic rejection is the severity and persistence of acute rejection. Those recipients affected by recurrent or persistent acute cellular rejection who fail to respond to repeated therapy with corticosteroids are at the highest risk. Other complications that may also increase the risk include infection with CMV, severe lung injury in the early post-transplant period, and mismatch of the HLA-A locus.

The diagnosis of bronchiolitis obliterans syndrome is made on the basis of an irreversible decline in FEV_1 after all other causes of allograft dysfunction have been excluded. It is categorised functionally into four groups, as shown in Table 12.4. Since

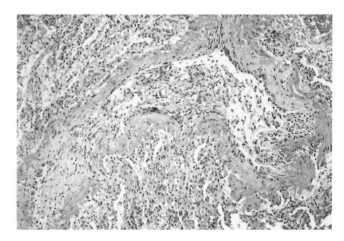

Fig. 12.6 Open lung biopsy showing obliterative bronchiolitis with the bronchiolar lumen obliterated by organising fibrin, fibroblasts and lymphocytes.

Table 12.4 Staging of bronchiolitis obliterans syndrome

Stage 0	$FEV_1 > 90\%$ $FEF_{25-75} > 75\%$
Stage 0-p	FEV_1 81–90% and/or $FEF_{25-75} \leq 75\%$
Stage 1	FEV_1 66–80%
Stage 2	FEV_1 51–65%
Stage 3	$FEV_1 < 50\%$

Percentages refer to baseline value.
FEV_1, forced expiratory volume in 1 second; FEF_{25-75}, forced expiratory flow between 25% and 75% of vital capacity.

biopsy specimens from up to one-third of recipients with chronic rejection do not show bronchiolitis obliterans, histological confirmation via transbronchial biopsy is not necessary. Bronchiolitis obliterans usually results in a progressive loss of function due to airflow obstruction over a period; however, a few patients appear to stabilise, with an attenuation in the loss of FEV_1. The most common clinical manifestations of the condition are dyspnoea on exertion, cough and sputum. Patients with BOS commonly develop proximal bronchiectasis and become colonised with Gram-negative organisms as the disease progresses. Recurrent pulmonary infection is common at this stage.

Effective treatment of BOS remains difficult. The majority of centres begin therapy with a pulse of corticosteroids but this is generally ineffective. Cytolytic therapy may stabilise lung function in some patients and switching patients from cyclosporin-based immunosuppression to tacrolimus appears to stabilise lung function in others. Other approaches include total lymphoid irradiation, cyclophosphamide and rapamycin.

Current research aims to identify those patients at risk prior to functional damage when more targeted immunosuppression may be successful in preventing irreversible bronchiolar obliteration.

Surveillance

Many transplant centres perform surveillance bronchoscopy, which includes transbronchial biopsies at predetermined intervals. Changes in the management take place in up 50% of patients as a result of this practice. Other transplant centres have stopped carrying out biopsies as there is no evidence that the frequency of obliterative bronchiolitis in units carrying out surveillance biopsies is lower than in those centres where bronchoscopy is performed only when required by clinical indication. The development of newer and more specific immunosuppressive drugs however, may necessitate a return to the practice of performing regular surveillance biopsies.

Complications in intermediate and long-term survivors

Infection

Bacterial infection is common in long-term survivors, leading to both lower respiratory tract infections and pneumonia. The usual organisms causing community-acquired pneumonia in a non-transplant population predominate. Although many fungal species have the potential to cause life- threatening infection in lung recipients, *Aspergillus* spp. are by far the most important. Invasive aspergillosis usually occurs in recipients who were previously colonised by *A. fumigatus* and who undergo treatment for rejection. Invasive disease requires treatment with intravenous amphotericin B, usually using a liposomal product. Amphotericin may also be inhaled if there is involvement of the bronchial mucosa. The level of immunosuppression is also lowered. Some centres elect to treat recipients who become colonised by *Aspergillus* with oral itraconazole. It is unclear whether this approach eliminates the possibility of invasive disease. Tuberculosis is a rare cause of infection, probably because of the preoperative prophylaxis of at-risk recipients with isoniazid and careful selection of donors. The few cases reported respond well to therapy. A whole gamut of opportunist infections have been reported in lung transplant recipients, including nocardiasis and, as with other immunocompromised hosts, results of treatment are best with early microbiological confirmation and specific targeted therapy as soon as possible. The use of early bronchoalveolar lavage or fine-needle aspiration of nodules is recommended.

Lymphoproliferative disease

Epstein–Barr virus (EBV) is associated with post-transplant lymphoproliferative disease, which results from immortalisation of B cells that are either monoclonal or polyclonal in origin. Most adult recipients have immunity to EBV but when a seronegative recipient receives an organ from a seropositive donor the risk of primary infection is high and nearly 50% of such infections are associated with lymphoproliferative disease.

Reactivation of latent EBV infection also occurs following intense immunosuppression for rejection. Post-transplant lymphoproliferative disease is usually asymptomatic until the burden of tumour interferes with lung function or leads to symptoms in other sites such as intestinal obstruction. Less commonly, enlargement of peripheral lymph notes occurs.

Recipients at risk of a primary infection may be monitored for EBV antibodies to early antigens or for EBV mRNA in peripheral blood detected by the polymerase chain reaction. Evidence that links a high level of EBV mRNA in the blood with lymphoproliferative disease is emerging and suggests that this approach may identify recipients who have subclinical post-transplant disease.

Many patients who develop post-transplant lymphoproliferative disease respond to a reduction in the level of systemic immunosuppression. Routine chemotherapy carries a high risk of morbidity and subsequent mortality. Newer treatment options include the use of monoclonal antibodies and employing recipients' natural killer cells, obtained by venesection and activated in vitro with interleukin 2 prior to subsequent reinfusion of activated cells.[70] Despite the fact that post-transplant lymphoproliferative disease can be controlled in the majority of instances, it still leads to the premature death of some lung transplant recipients and more research into novel therapeutic approaches is required.

Drug-induced complications

Most transplant recipients have impaired renal function as a result of cyclosporin- or tacrolimus-induced vasoconstriction of the afferent renal arteriole leading to a reduction in glomerular filtration rate. The cause of the vasoconstriction is multifactorial and includes increased production of vasoconstrictors such as endothelin 1 and direct effects of cyclosporin on calcium channels in vascular smooth muscle.[71] Although tubal abnormalities were initially thought to be the cause of cyclosporin-induced renal dysfunction, it is now believed that they occur as a consequence of chronic hypoperfusion. A degree of chronic nephrotoxicity occurs in virtually all patients after lung transplantation but a minority will require renal replacement therapy in the form of haemodialysis or renal transplantation as the result of severe chronic renal failure. The concurrent administration of many drugs can potentiate nephrotoxicity and particular care needs to be taken when coprescribing non-steroidal anti-inflammatory drugs and aminoglycoside antibiotics. Drugs that block calcium channels have been shown to protect at least partly against acute and chronic nephrotoxicity. Systemic hypertension is also a side effect of the calcineurin inhibitors and approximately two-thirds of previously normotensive patients will develop hypertension.

Neuromuscular complications

Approximately 25–30% of lung transplant recipients develop neurological problems, including headache, confusion, seizures, strokes, peripheral neuropathy and myopathy. The majority of complications relate to the neurotoxic affects of cyclosporin and tacrolimus. One important syndrome is posterior leukoencephalopathy, when a patient may present with a constellation of symptoms that include tremor, headache, encephalopathy, seizures, cortical blindness and confusion. Patients become hypertensive and, although the syndrome most commonly appears in the early post-transplant period, it has been recorded much later. The diagnosis is supported by characteristic white-matter changes on T2-weighted magnetic resonance imaging, which reflects microvascular injury. These findings are commonly reversible with initial discontinuation and then a reduction in the level of calcineurin inhibitors. Patients who develop major seizures commonly have co-existent hypomagnesaemia and in general are younger recipients. Control of seizures is best managed with valproate which does not interfere with calcineurin inhibitor levels. Myopathy is a complication of therapy with ciclosporin and corticosteroids. Cyclosporin has been implicated as the causative factor in the development of a proximal myopathy with features of mitochondrial dysfunction. The reduced maximum exercise capacity following successful lung transplantation seems to be caused by reduced peripheral muscle activity as the result of this mitochondrial dysfunction rather than any ventilatory limitation of the lungs themselves.

Osteoporosis

Bone mineral density is reduced in many patients with advanced chronic pulmonary disease and studies have demonstrated a 15% reduction in bone mineral density during the first 6 months after surgery. One study showed that 73% of patients following lung transplantation had spine and femoral bone mineral densities below the fracture threshold. Since the majority of bone loss appears to occur within the first 6 months, prophylactic therapy with bisphosphonates and calcium supplementation should be commenced early.

Gastrointestinal complications

Approximately 20% of patients develop gastrointestinal complications including gastroparesis, gastritis, peptic ulcers, cholelithiasis and colonic perforation. Gastroparesis leads to significant morbidity and occurs as a direct effect of cyclosporin on gastric emptying and also as a result of vagal nerve damage during surgery. Azathioprine, cyclosporin and tacrolimus can be associated with acute pancreatitis.

Non-lymphoproliferative malignancies

Patients after lung transplantation are susceptible to a number of non-lymphatic tumours[72]. Skin tumours are most common, particularly squamous cell carcinoma. As a consequence, lung transplantation recipients must avoid excessive exposure to sunlight. Other tumours seen with greater frequency in the transplant population include sarcomas and carcinomas of the cervix and hepatobiliary system.

Other drug-related complications

Cyclosporin induces gum hypertrophy, hirsuties and diabetes. Tacrolimus causes less gum hypertrophy and hirsuties but is a more potent inducer of diabetes.

Outcome and results

Providing that patients are appropriately selected, the results of heart–lung, single-lung and bilateral lung transplantation are good. Data from the International Society of Heart and Lung Transplantation show an improvement in survival over the last decade, although survival still lags behind that of patients receiving liver, kidney or heart transplantation. Nonetheless, lung transplantation has become an accepted therapy for many end-stage pulmonary or pulmonary vascular diseases. The 1-year survival rate should now be 75–80% with a 5 year survival of 50–55%. Functional results in survivors measured in terms of FEV, and exercise performance are good and recipients of two lungs can expect to attain their normal predicted FEV_1, and vital capacity after 6–12 months in the absence of complications, although the CO transfer factor (diffusing capacity) usually remains reduced. All patients should expect restoration of a normal lifestyle with little or no functional restriction during normal daily activities. Maximum exercise performance is limited by peripheral muscle function rather than cardiac or ventilatory limitation. Successful lung transplant recipients regain a normal 6-minute walking distance by 1 year with no evidence of desaturation on exercise irrespective of the operation. In addition to prolonging life, lung transplantation also improves the quality of life as determined by standardised measures of health status.[73] There are increasing numbers of recipients surviving to 10 years. Patients who have not developed BOS by 5 years and are free of other long-term complications have a good potential for long-term survival.

Disease recurrence

There has been great interest in the study of lungs after successful transplantation to see whether the original lung disease will recur in the allograft. Mature granulomata have been described in the lungs in patients transplanted for sarcoidosis, and alveolar cell carcinoma, lymphangioleiomyomatosis and Langerhans cell granulomatosis[74] have all been demonstrated in the lung allograft following transplantation for these indications. So far there is no evidence that COPD, including emphysema associated with α_1-proteinase inhibitor (antitrypsin) deficiency will recur, presumably because of cessation of smoking. There have been two case reports of recurrent giant-cell interstitial pneumonia in pulmonary allografts after transplantation for this condition[75] but to date there have been no reports of interstitial pulmonary fibrosis of usual type recurring. Nor have there been any reports of recurrence of primary pulmonary hypertension.

Medical management of lung candidates awaiting lung transplantation

Good communication between a potential lung transplant recipient's physician and the transplant centre physician is essential. Transplant centres need to aware of changes in the condition of candidates and all must be aware that candidates may deteriorate to the point where transplantation is no longer feasible. It is important for patients to remain as mobile as possible, emphasising the need for pulmonary rehabilitation, including nutritional support. Some patients who develop cachexia will require parenteral feeding in order to reverse cachexia, and exercise rehabilitation will improve muscle strength.

One area sometimes causing concern relates to the decision as to whether to intubate a young patient awaiting lung transplantation. Clearly this should be considered where there is an acute on chronic deterioration, e.g. due to pneumonia, where control of the acute problem may lead to successful weaning from the ventilator. Patients who develop the need for intubation as a result of progressive deterioration in the natural course of their disease, however, should not be ventilated mechanically since this increases the risk of an adverse outcome of transplantation compared to non-intubated patients. The critical shortage of donor lungs therefore mitigates against intubating patients who develop progressive respiratory failure. Some patients have, however, received chronic ventilatory support by non-invasive ventilation. This does not appear to lead to an adverse outcome and consideration of this form of support should be discussed on an individual basis.

Summary

Lung transplantation is an effective therapy for patients with end-stage lung disease. The major practical problems facing lung transplantation continue to be a shortfall in suitable donor organs compared with the number of potential recipients and the development of obliterative bronchiolitis. Patients with advanced pulmonary airway, parenchymal or vascular disease who receive lung transplantation and remain free of obliterative bronchiolitis enjoy an excellent standard of life, with normal or near-normal restoration of activity and good prospects of prolonged survival.

> **? Unresolved questions**
>
> ■ A major problem facing lung transplantation is the shortfall in donor organs and ways to increase the number of donor organs, including improved management of potential donors and xenotransplantation, remain under intensive research.
>
> ■ The development of newer immunosuppressive agents necessitates clinical trials to determine optimal combinations for lung transplant recipients.
>
> ■ Strategies to both prevent and treat patients developing obliterative bronchiolitis need to be improved.
>
> ■ Newer less invasive strategies to help monitor graft alloreactivity other than fibreoptic bronchoscopy with lung biopsy and lavage continue to be researched.
>
> ■ How best to induce graft tolerance remains important in all types of transplantation.

References

1. Reitz BA, Wallwork J, Hunt SA et al. Heart lung transplantation: a successful therapy for patients with pulmonary vascular disease. N Engl J Med 1982; 306: 557.

2. Penketh A, Higenbottam T, Hakim M, Wallwork J. Heart and lung transplantation in patients with end stage lung disease. Br Med J 1987; 295–331.

3. Wildevuuer CRH, Benfield JR. A review of 23 lung transplantations by 20 surgeons. Ann Thorac Surg 1979; 9: 489.

4. Toronto Lung Transplant Group. Unilateral transplant for pulmonary fibrosis. N Engl J Med 1986; 314: 1140.

5. Patterson GA, Cooper JD, Goldman B et al. Technique of successful clinical double lung transplantation. Ann Thorac Surg 1988; 45: 626.

6. Patterson GA, Todd TR, Cooper JD et al. Airway complications following double lung transplantation. J Thorac Cardiovasc Surg 1990; 99: 14.

7. Noirclerc, Metras D, Vaillant A et al. Bilateral bronchial anastomosis in double lung and heart lung transplantations. Eur J Cardiothorac Surg 1990; 4: 314.

8. Pasque MK, Cooper JD, Kaiser LR et al. Improved technique for bilateral lung transplantations: rationale and initial clinical experience. Ann Thorac Surg 1990; 49: 785.

9. Shumway SJ, Hertz MI, Petty MG, Colman RM III. Liberalization of donor criteria in lung and heart–lung transplantation. Ann Thorac Surg 1994; 57: 92.

10. Fisher AJ, Dark JH, Corris PA. Improving donor lung evaluation – new approach to increase organ supply for lung transplantation. Thorax 1998; 53: 818.

11. Barr ML, Shenkel FA, Cohen RG et al. Living related lobar transplantation. Recipient outcome and early rejection patterns. Transplant Proc 1995; 27: 1995.

12. Cooper DKC, Keogh AM, Brink J et al. Report of the Xenotransplantation Advisory Committee of the International Society of Heart and Lung Transplantation: the present status of xenotransplantation and its potential role in the treatment of end-stage cardiac and pulmonary diseases. J Heart Lung Transplant 2000; 19: 1125.

13. ISHLT International Guidelines for Selection of Lung Transplant Candidates. J Heart Lung Transplant 1998; 17: 703.

14. Bennett WK Pulliam JP. Cyclosporine nephrotoxicity. Ann Intern Med 1983; 99: 851.

15. Aris RM, Neuringer IP, Weiner MA et al. Severe osteoporosis before and after lung transplantation. Chest 1996; 109: 1176.

16. Hunter AMB, Carey MA, Larsh HW. The nutritional status of patients with chronic obstructive pulmonary disease. Am Rev Respir Dis 1981; 124: 376.

17. Colquhoun IW, Gascoigne AD, Gould FK et al. Native pulmonary sepsis following single lung transplantation. Transplantation 1991; 52: 931.

18. Bidstrup BP, Royston D, Supsford RW, Taylor KM. Reduction in blood loss and blood use after cardiopulmonary bypass with high dose aprotinin. J Thorac Cardiovasc Surg 1989; 93: 364.

19. Colquhoun IW, Gasgcoine AD, Dark JH et al. Airway complications following pulmonary transplantation. Ann Thorac Surg 1994; 57: 141.

20. Morrison DI, Maurer JR, Grossman RR Preoperative assessment for lung transplantation. Clin Chest Med 1990; 2: 207.

21. Doig JC, Richens D, Corris PA et al. Resolution of pulmonary hypertension after single lung transplantation. Br Heart J 1991; 66: 431.

22. Kerem E, Reisman J, Corey M et al. Prediction of mortality in patients with cystic fibrosis. N Engl J Med 1992; 326: 1187.

23. Kadikar A, Maurer J, Kesten S. The six minute walk test: a guide to assessment for lung transplantation. J Heart Lung Transplant 1997; 16: 313.

24. Aris RM, Gilligan PH, Neuringer IP et al. The effects of panresistant bacteria in cystic fibrosis patients on lung transplant outcome. Am J Crit Care Med 1997; 155: 1699.

25. Connors H, AF, Dawson NV, Thomas C et al. Outcomes following acute exacerbation of severe chronic obstructive lung disease. Am J Respir Crit Care Med 1996; 154: 959.

26. Dodge JA, Morrison S, Lewis PA et al. Cystic fibrosis in the United Kingdom 1968–1988: incidence, population and survival. Paediatr Perinatal Epidemiol 1993; 7: 157.

27. Turner Warwick M, Burrows B, Johnson A. Cryptogenic fibrosing alveolitis: response to corticosteroid treatment and its effect on survival. Thorax 1980; 35: 593.

28. Hopkins WE, Ochoa LL, Richardson GW et al. Comparison of the haemodynamics and survival of adults with severe primary pulmonary hypertension or Eisenmenger syndrome. J Heart Lung Transplant 1996; 15: 100.

29. Mandell MS, Groves BM. Pulmonary hypertension in chronic liver disease. Clin Chest Med 1996; 16: 17.

30. Wallwork J, Calne RY, Williams R Transplantation of liver, heart and lungs for primary biliary cirrhosis and primary pulmonary hypertension. Lancet 1987; 2: 182.

31. Annitage JM, Kirland G, Michaels, M et al. Critical issues in pediatric lung transplantation. J Thorac Cardiovasc Surg 1995; 109: 60.

32. Couteuil JP, Tolan MP, Loulmet DF et al. Pulmonary bipartitioning and lobar transplantation: a new approach to donor organ shortage. J Thorac Cardiovasc Surg 1997; 113: 529.

33. Reitz BA, Wallwork JL, Hunt SA et al. Heart–lung transplantation: successful therapy for patients with pulmonary vascular disease. N Engl J Med 1982; 306: 557.

34. Yacoub MH, Banner NR, Khaghani A et al. Heart–lung transplantation for cystic fibrosis and subsequent domino heart transplantation. J Heart Transplant 1990; 9: 459.

35. Lim TT, Botas J, Ross H et al. Are heart–lung transplant recipients protected from developing transplant coronary disease? A case-matched intracoronary ultrasound study. Circulation 1996; 94: 1573.

36. Smith JA, Roberts M, McNeil K et al. Excellent outcome of cardiac transplantation using domino donor hearts. Eur J Cardiothorac Surg 1996; 106: 28.

37. Adams DH, Cochrane AD, Khagani A et al. Re-transplantation in heart–lung recipients with obliterative bronchiolitis. J Thorac Cardiovasc Surg 994; 107: 450.

38. Pasque MK, Trulock EP, Kaiser LR, Cooper JD. Single lung transplantation for pulmonary hypertension: three month haemodynamic follow-up. Circulation 1991; 84: 2275.

39. Waddell T et al. Lung or heart–lung transplant for Eisenmenger's syndrome: analysis of the ISHLT/UNOS Joint Thoracic Registry. J Heart Lung Transplant 2000; 19: 57.

40. Chaparro C, Scavuzzo M, Winton T et al. Status of lung transplant recipients surviving beyond five years. J Heart Lung Transplant 1997; 16: 511.

41. Mal H, Andreassian B, Fabrice P et al. Unilateral lung transplantation in end-stage pulmonary emphysema. Am Rev Respir Dis 1989; 140: 797.

42. Hosenpud JD, Bennett LE, Keck BM et al. The registry of the International Society for Heart and Lung Transplantation: sixteenth official report. J Heart Lung Transplant 1999; 18: 611.

43. Bavaria JE, Kodoff R, Palevsky H et al. Bilateral versus single lung transplant for chronic obstructive pulmonary disease. J Thorac Cardiovasc Surg 1997; 113: 520.

44. Geertsma A, van der Bij W de Boer WJ, TenVergert EM. Survival with and without lung transplantation. Transplant Proc 1997; 29: 630.

45. Hosenpud JD, Bednnett LE, Keck BM et al. Effect of diagnosis on survival benefit of lung transplantation for end-stage lung disease. Lancet 1998; 1: 24.

46. Forty J, Hasan A, Gould FK et al. Single lung transplantation with simultaneous contralateral pneumonectomy for cystic fibrosis. J Heart Lung Transplant 1994; 13: 727.

47. Levine SK Jenkinson SG, Bryan CL et al. Ventilation–perfusion irregularities during graft rejection in patients undergoing single lung transplantation for primary pulmonary hypertension. Chest 1992; 101: 401.

48. Fisher AJ, Donnelly SC, Hirani N et al. Levels of interleukin-8 in donor lungs is associated with early graft failure after lung transplantation. Am J Respir Crit Care Med 2001; 163: 259.

49. Egan TM, Boychuk JE, Rosato K, Cooper JD. A study to assess suitability of donor lungs for transplantation. Whence the lung? Transplantation 1992; 53: 420.

50. Aziz T, El-Gamel A, Yonan N. Pulmonary vein gas analysis for assessment of donor lung function. J Heart Lung Transplant 2001; 20: 225.

51. Pennefather SH, Bullock RE, Mantle D, Dark JH Use of low dose arginine vasopressin to support brain-dead organ donors. Transplantation 1995; 59: 58.

52. Follette DM, Rudich SM, Babcock WD. Improved oxygenation and increased lung recovery with high-dose steroid administration after brain death. J Heart Lung Transplant 1998; 17: 423.

53. Kirk AJB, Colquhoun IW, Dark JH. Lung preservation: a review of current practice and future directions. Ann Thorac Surg 1993; 56: 990.

54. Wilson IC, Hasan A, Healy M et al. Healing of the bronchus in pulmonary transplantation. Eur J Cardiothoracic Surg 1996; 1: 521.

55. Rao JN, Forty J, Hasan A et al. Bilateral lung transplant: the procedure of choice for end-stage septic lung disease. Transplant Proc 2001; 33: 1622.

56. Meyers BF, Sundaresan RS, Guthrie T et al. Bilateral sequential lung transplantation without sternal division eliminates post-transplantation sternal complications. J Thorac Cardiovasc Surg 1999; 117: 358.

57. Macchiarini P, Ladurie FL, Cerrina J et al. Clamshell or sternotomy for double lung or heart–lung transplantation? Eur J Cardiothoracic Surgery 1999; 15: 333.

58. Clark SC, Sudarshan C, Khanna R et al. Controlled reperfusion and pentoxifylline modulate reperfusion injury after single lung transplantation. J Thorac Cardiovasc Surg 1998; 115: 1335.

59. Date H, Triantafillou AN, Trulock EP et al: Inhaled nitric oxide reduces human allograft dysfunction. J Thorac Cardiovasc Surg 1996; 111: 913.

60. Smiley RM, Navedo AT, Kirby T et al. Postoperative independent lung ventilation in a single-lung transplant recipient. Anesthesiology 1991; 74: 1144.

61. Gullinger RA, Paradis IC, Dauber JH et al. The importance of bronchoscopy with transbronchial biopsy and bronchoalveolar lavage in the management of lung transplant recipients. Am J Respir Crit Care Med. 1995; 152: 2037.

62. Cooper JD, Billingham M, Egan T et al. A working formulation for the standardization of nomenclature and for clinical staging of chronic dysfunction in lung allografts. J Heart Lung Transplant 1993; 12: 713.

63. Kramer MR, Marshal SE, Stance VA et al. Infectious complications in heart–lung transplantation. Analysis of 200 episodes. Arch Intern Med. 1993; 153: 2010.

64. Wreghitt TG, Hakim M, Gray JJ et al. Cytomegalovirus infections in heart and heart–lung transplant recipients. J Clin Pathol 1988; 41: 660.

65. Bando K, Paradis IL, Komatsu K et al. Analysis of time-dependent risks for infection, rejection and death after pulmonary transplantation. J Thorac Cardiovasc Surg 1995; 109: 49.

66. Bando K, Paradis IL, Konishi H et al. Obliterative bronchiolitis after lung and heart–lung transplantation: an analysis of risk factors and management. J Thorac Cardiovasc Surg 1995; 110: 4.

67. Sundaresan S, Trulock PE, Mohanankumar T et al. Prevalence and outcome of bronchiolitis obliterans syndrome after lung transplantation. Ann Thorac Surg 1995; 60: 1341.

68. Kelly K, Hertz MR Obliterative bronchiolitis. Clin Chest Med 1997; 18: 319.

69. Milne DS, Gascoigne AD, Wilkes et al. The immunological features of obliterative bronchiolitis following lung transplantation. Transplantation 1992; 54: 748.

70. Nalesnik MA, Rao AS, Furukawa H et al. Autologous lymphokine-activated killer cell therapy of Epstein–Barr virus positive and negative lymphoproliferative disorders arising in organ transplant recipients. Transplantation 1997; 63: 1200.

71. Rossi ND, Churchill PC, McDonald FD et al. Mechanism of cyclosporine A-induced renal vasoconstriction in the rat. J Pharmacol Exp Ther 1989; 250: 896.

72. Penn I. Incidence and treatment of neoplasia after transplantation. J Heart Lung Transplant 1993; 12: S328.

73. Gross CR, Savik SK, Bolman RM, Hertz MI. Long-term health status and quality of life outcomes of lung allograft recipients. Chest 1995; 108: 1587.

74. Gabbay E, Derk JH, Ashcroft T et al. Recurrence of Langerhans cell granulomatosis following lung transplantation. Thorax 98: 53: 326.

75. Frost AE, Keller CA, Brown RW et al. Giant cell interstitial pneumonitis: disease recurrence in the transplanted lung. Am Rev Respir Dis 1993; 148: 1401.

13 Principles of oxygen therapy

Jean-Louis Pépin and Patrick Lévy

Key points

- Cellular hypoxia may be hypoxaemic, may result from a reduction in tissue blood flow (local ischaemia) or may be histotoxic.

- Arterial hypoxaemia is due mainly to anatomical right-to-left shunts, ventilation–perfusion mismatching, alveolar hypoventilation or diffusion impairment.

- Chronic hypoxaemia is associated with neuropsychological and autonomic nervous system dysfunction, peripheral neuropathy, pulmonary hypertension, weight loss, skeletal muscle alterations and increased mortality.

- In acute hypoxaemia, additional oxygen is required but oxygen therapy may need to be carefully controlled using a Venturi mask in order to avoid hypercapnic acidaemia.

- Long-term oxygen therapy (LTOT) should be given to chronic obstructive pulmonary disease (COPD) patients with a stable P_aO_2 of less than 7.3 kPa (<55 mmHg) on air. The duration of oxygen therapy should be more than 15 h per day.

- Patients with COPD and a P_aO_2 between 7.3 and 7.8 kPa (55 and 59 mmHg) with polycythaemia, pulmonary hypertension or clinical evidence of cor pulmonale are also candidates for LTOT.

- No controlled studies of LTOT have been performed in cystic fibrosis or in restrictive respiratory diseases such as fibrosing alveolitis or pneumoconiosis.

Oxygen acts as the final acceptor of the electron transfer system in the cellular mitochondria. Aerobic metabolism produces 30 molecules of high-energy adenosine triphosphate (ATP) from each molecule of glucose metabolised in the presence of oxygen, whereas anaerobic glycolysis produces only three molecules of ATP for each glucose molecule, with lactic acid formed as the end-product. Many processes are involved in the movement of oxygen from the atmosphere until it reaches the interior of the body cells, where it is used. The total pathway includes movement through the airway by convection and diffusion, diffusion across the alveolar–capillary membrane, through the plasma and red cell, combination with haemoglobin, movement of blood through the body and finally unloading of oxygen in the tissues and its diffusion through the cells until it reaches the mitochondria (Fig. 13.1). Oxygen therapy, by raising the inspired oxygen concentration, can influence this cascade by increasing alveolar PO_2, and thus the PO_2 of ventilated and perfused alveoli, and thereby the oxygen saturation of haemoglobin in the arterial circulation.

In this chapter, definitions of hypoxia and hypoxaemia are given, together with a description of the mechanisms of hypoxaemia and an examination of its acute and chronic consequences. Oxygen therapy is considered in terms of efficiency, indications, toxicity and monitoring.

Definitions

Cellular hypoxia occurs when the oxygen stores of the cell are insufficient to meet oxygen demand. As oxygen stores are limited, in acute conditions anoxia may rapidly occur, leading to cellular death. In chronic respiratory failure, hypoxia induces several metabolic changes that allow the cell to survive.[2]

Classically, hypoxia can be hypoxaemic (associated with a fall in the oxygen saturation of arterial blood, S_aO_2), anaemic (reduction of haemoglobin concentration which lowers arterial oxygen content, C_aO_2), localised as a result of a reduction of tissue blood flow (local ischaemia) or histotoxic because of an alteration of mitochondrial respiration (Table 13.1).

Hypoxaemia is defined by a fall in S_aO_2. This is almost always associated with a low arterial partial pressure of oxygen (P_aO_2). P_aO_2 can remain normal, however, but S_aO_2 is reduced in the situation where carboxyhaemoglobin (HbCO) or methaemoglobin (MetHb) is elevated, because this reduces the amount of functional haemoglobin. Conversely, a low P_aO_2 can be associated with a normal S_aO_2 when haemoglobin affinity for oxygen is

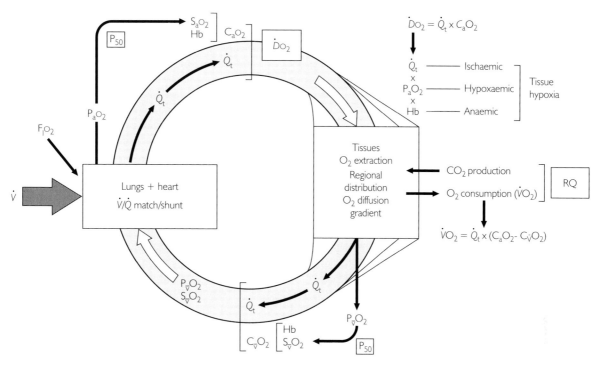

Fig. 13.1 Diagrammatic representation of the different steps in oxygen transport. Oxygen transport can be affected at various levels: failure of ventilation, decrease in cardiac output, reduction in haemoglobin concentration or affinity, altered tissue oxygen extraction, regional distribution of blood flow. This affects tissue oxygenation and may potentially alter lung gas exchange when $P_{\bar{v}}O_2$ is lowered. $\dot{V}$ ventilation; F_IO_2, fractional inspired oxygen concentration; $\dot{Q}$ cardiac output; $P_aO_2/P_{\bar{v}}O_2$, partial pressure of arterial/mixed venous blood; $S_aO_2/S_{\bar{v}}O_2$, percentage saturation of arterial/mixed venous blood; $C_aO_2/C_{\bar{v}}O_2$, oxygen content of arterial/mixed venous blood; Hb, haemoglobin concentration; RQ, respiratory quotient; $\dot{D}O_2$, oxygen delivery. (Modified from Leach & Treacher 1992.[1])

Table 13.1   Mechanisms of hypoxia

Type	Mechanisms	Conditions
Hypoxaemic	Reduction of P_IO_2	Altitude
	Right-to-left shunting	Cyanotic congenital heart disease, pulmonary arteriovenous fistula, acute respiratory distress syndrome, liver cirrhosis
	$\dot{V}_A/\dot{Q}_T$ mismatching	Multiple, e.g. diffuse airway narrowing, pneumonia, pulmonary oedema, fibrosis, etc.
	Hypoventilation	Overall hypoventilation e.g. muscle weakness, scoliosis, etc.
		Alveolar hypoventilation, e.g. above plus chronic obstructive pulmonary disease, etc.
	Impaired diffusion	Pulmonary fibrosis (especially on exercise)
	Low $C_{\bar{v}}O_2$	Pulmonary fibrosis, pulmonary embolism, etc.
Anaemic	Reduction of functional haemoglobin	Anaemia, carbon monoxide poisoning
Ischaemic	Reduction of blood flow	Low cardiac output, local ischaemia
Histotoxic	Tissue poisoning	Cyanide poisoning

increased, as in several variants of normal adult haemoglobin caused by intrinsic changes in the haemoglobin molecule, to an altered response of haemoglobin to 2,3-diphosphoglycerate or to both. Normal values of P_aO_2 fall with age (about 12 kPa or 90 mmHg at 20 years of age versus 8 kPa or 60 mmHg at 80). Both S_aO_2 and P_aO_2 are reduced in normal subjects at altitude as a result of reduction in barometric pressure and inspired PO_2 (P_IO_2).

Mechanisms of arterial hypoxaemia

Reduction of the inspired oxygen partial pressure

At 3000 metres above sea level P_IO_2 is 14.6 kPa or 110 mmHg and the normal P_aO_2 is around 7.3 kPa (55 mmHg). Millions of people live at such altitude and, in contrast to chronic respiratory failure, this chronic hypoxaemia is not associated with increased morbidity. This may be because of adaptive mechanisms occurring in utero, as suggested by recent data in experimental animals on ventilatory and metabolic adaptations during gestation at simulated altitude.[3]

Shunts

If venous blood passes directly to the left side of the circulation without meeting ventilated alveoli, no gas exchange can occur. This results in a reduction in S_aO_2 proportional to the shunted fraction of cardiac output ($\dot{Q}_s/\dot{Q}_t$). Normal subjects have a right-to-left shunt of 2–3% of the cardiac output and this can be greatly increased in lung or cardiac disease. Shunting is the main mechanism of hypoxaemia in cyanotic congenital heart diseases. Shunts in atelectatic regions of lung can contribute to postoperative hypoxaemia and to the severe hypoxaemia that occurs in the acute respiratory distress syndrome (ARDS). In chronic respiratory disease, however, the shunt contribution is generally limited to rare diseases such as pulmonary arteriovenous communications and the hepatopulmonary syndrome complicating progressive liver failure.[4]

Ventilation–perfusion mismatching

Ventilation–perfusion ($\dot{V}_A/\dot{Q}$) mismatching is by far the most common cause of arterial hypoxaemia in lung disease. In normal lungs, the alveolar ventilation–perfusion ratio is on average close to 0.8, with a narrow distribution of values. An active PO_2-dependent increase in pulmonary vascular tone limits inhomogeneity in normal lungs. Hypoxic pulmonary vasoconstriction is, however, only moderately effective in fine adjustment of ($\dot{V}/\dot{Q}$) ratios in healthy or diseased lungs.[5] In lung disease, with pathological changes affecting the bronchi, lung parenchyma and pulmonary vessels, severe ($\dot{V}_A/\dot{Q}$) imbalance can result. Some alveoli receive a reduced ventilation in relation to their perfusion (low ($\dot{V}_A/\dot{Q}$) ratio), resulting in arterial hypoxaemia that cannot be compensated by hyperventilation of normally perfused alveoli (see Chapter 2.5). Oxygen inhalation, even with modest increases in the fractional concentration of inspired oxygen (F_IO_2), can usually correct S_aO_2 in patients whose hypoxaemia results from ($\dot{V}_A/\dot{Q}$) mismatching. ($\dot{V}_A/\dot{Q}$) imbalance is the main determinant of hypoxaemia in common respiratory diseases such as chronic obstructive pulmonary disease (COPD), bronchial asthma, pneumonia, pulmonary oedema and pulmonary fibrosis.[6]

Alveolar hypoventilation

When total ventilation is reduced, the alveoli inevitably receive less inspired gas, and hypoxaemia and hypercapnia result.[7] Hypoxaemia caused by hypoventilation alone, resulting in a normal alveolar–arterial tension gradient (AaPO2), is uncommon. However, if there is no associated ($\dot{V}_A/\dot{Q}$) mismatching the reduction in P_aO_2 and the rise in P_aCO_2 will be proportional to the degree of hypoventilation, as indicated by the alveolar air equation. Effective alveolar ventilation can also be reduced by an increase in the physiological dead space (V_D/V_T). The relationship between P_aCO_2 and V_D/V_T is non-linear, resulting in progressively increasing rises in P_aCO_2 as dead-space volume is elevated. In patients with chronic respiratory failure, V_D/V_T can reach values as large as 0.60, compared to 0.25 in normal subjects. In this situation only a small further increase in V_D/V_T results in a large rise in P_aCO_2. This mechanism may account for at least part of the hypercapnia induced by oxygen inhalation[8,9] in patients with respiratory failure due to COPD.

Diffusion impairment

Hypoxaemia is a common feature of interstitial lung disease such as pulmonary fibrosis, in which it is usually associated with chronic hypocapnia and hyperventilation. This was originally thought to be related to impairment of oxygen diffusion through the thickened alveolar capillary membrane. However, although impaired oxygen diffusion can generate exercise-induced desaturation, it is not the main determinant of hypoxaemia at rest. Arterial hypoxaemia in interstitial disease is the result of low mixed venous PO_2 ($P_{\bar{v}}O_2$), acting together with modest degrees of diffusion limitation and ($\dot{V}_A/\dot{Q}$) mismatching.[6]

Other mechanisms

Anaemia reduces the oxygen content of arterial blood (C_aO_2) and this in turn causes some reduction in mixed venous oxygen content ($C_{\bar{v}}O_2$) and saturation ($S_{\bar{v}}O_2$). The reduction in $S_{\bar{v}}O_2$ is the result of a normal oxygen uptake at tissue level in the face of reduced oxygen transport caused by anaemia. If the relationship between oxygen pressure and saturation is unchanged, $P_{\bar{v}}O_2$ is also lowered. This lowered $P_{\bar{v}}O_2$ is responsible for a secondary reduction in P_aO_2. An increase in cardiac output usually occurs as a compensatory mechanism in severe anaemia and this tends to limit the reduction in P_aO_2.[10]

Polycythaemia is a frequent consequence of chronic hypoxaemia. It also results in a small reduction in P_aO_2 caused by ($\dot{V}_A/\dot{Q}$) mismatching related to polycythaemia per se.[10]

Mechanisms of oxygen sensing and responses to acute and chronic hypoxia

Oxygen sensing[11,12] was previously attributed solely to specialised chemoreceptors such as those of the carotid bodies that regulate cardiovascular and ventilatory rates. It is now appreciated that all nucleated cells in the human body sense O_2 concentration and respond to reduced O_2 availability (hypoxia), whether acute or chronic. However O_2 sensing mechanisms occur in a tissue specific fashion with different time constants and different PO_2 thresholds. Carotid body cells respond to hypoxia promptly by eliciting a ventilatory response whereas chronic changes (e.g. erythropoietin secretion) occur principally as a result of complex alterations in gene expression. At the cellular level, the mitochondrial respiratory chain remains the best identified oxygen sensor but membrane-bound nicotinamide adenine dinucleotide (phosphate) – NAD(P)H – oxidase probably also takes part in the oxygen sensing processes. An exponential increase in response to decreasing PO_2 below 30 mmHg is seen in mitochondria and also in membrane-bound NAD(P)H oxidase. The response involves an increase in calcium ions and shutdown of membrane K^+ and opening of Ca^{2+} channels (Fig. 13.2). Chronic hypoxia works via the same mechanisms but eventually inhibits the proteasome which normally degrades hypoxia-inducible factor (HIF)-1α. HIF-1α then reacts with pre-existing HIF-1β, producing the transcriptional regulator HIF-1. This formation requires time and HIF-1 is then translocated into the nucleus with subsequent activation of a battery of genes (Fig. 13.2). The target genes activated by HIF-1 include those whose protein products are involved in angiogenesis, energy metabolism, erythropoiesis, cell proliferation and viability, vascular remodelling and vasomotor responses.[12]

Consequences of acute and chronic hypoxaemia and effects of oxygen therapy

Central nervous system

Acute hypoxaemia can result in cerebral dysfunction. Clinically, there may be behavioural disturbances, intellectual dysfunction, impairment of consciousness and sometimes coma. Such effects are seen at very low P_aO_2 (around 4 kPa or 30 mmHg), with highly variable individual sensitivity. More subtle changes in

psychomotor function are detectable with acute hypoxaemia when P_aO_2 is around 7.3 kPa (55 mmHg).[13]

A reduction in intellectual ability, a depressive profile and behavioural disturbances are more frequent in COPD patients with chronic hypoxaemia than in controls matched for age, sex, education and socioeconomic status.[14,15] Long-term oxygen therapy (LTOT) improves intelligence quotient and reduces mood disturbances.[16,17] In the Nocturnal Oxygen Therapy Trial (NOTT), there was a greater improvement in neuropsychological function on continuous therapy compared with nocturnal therapy alone over the second 6 months of the study.[17,18] This neuropsychological improvement was mainly in cognitive function and persisted for several hours while the subject was breathing room air.

Sleep quality is generally poor in patients with hypoxaemic COPD with reduced sleep time, increased sleep state changes and increased frequency of arousal.[19-21] Its contribution to impairment of intellectual ability is unknown and the long-term effects of oxygen therapy on sleep quality in COPD are also uncertain.

In COPD, electroencephalographic (EEG) abnormalities have been related to hypoxaemia and hypercapnia. Brezinova et al[22] found a positive correlation between the mean dominant frequency of the EEG and the arterial blood gas tensions, pH and haemoglobin concentration. The changes in EEG activity seen with long-term oxygen therapy suggested a protective effect on the brain.

Peripheral neuropathy

Chronic hypoxaemia is a recognised cause of peripheral neuropathy.[23-25] The peripheral neuropathies seen in hypoxaemic

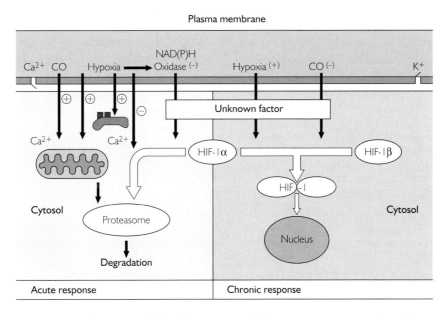

Fig. 13.2 Mode of oxygen sensing and acute and chronic responses. The acute response to hypoxia occurs via mitochondria and membrane-bound NAD(P)H oxidase. It involves an increase in calcium ion concentration with closure of membrane potassium and opening of calcium channels. The chronic effect of hypoxia is mediated via the same mechanisms but involves the formation of hypoxia-inducible factor (HIF)-1, which is then translocated into the nucleus with subsequent activation of a battery of genes.

COPD and diabetes mellitus have both pathological and electrophysiological similarities such as resistance to ischaemic conduction failure, which may result from tissue hypoxia.[25-27] Some of the electrophysiological abnormalities observed in experimental diabetic neuropathy in rats are reversed by oxygen inhalation.[28] No data are available, however, on the effects of long-term oxygen treatment on peripheral neuropathy in humans.

Autonomic nervous system dysfunction

Subclinical autonomic neuropathy is common in hypoxaemic COPD. In a study by Stewart et al,[29] parasympathetic autonomic dysfunction, assessed by heart rate responses to the Valsalva manoeuvre, deep breathing and postural change, was significantly correlated with P_aO_2 whereas tests of sympathetic function were relatively normal. This presumably results from hypoxic damage to autonomic nerves; its significance for prognosis of the underlying disease requires further study. These derangements in the autonomic nervous system may be partially reversed by oxygen administration.[30]

Cardiovascular function

Acute hypoxaemia results in tachycardia, increased cardiac output and hypotension related to peripheral vasodilatation. Conversely, in the pulmonary circulation hypoxia causes vasoconstriction and pulmonary hypertension.[31]

In patients with chronic hypoxaemia, mean pulmonary artery pressure (PAP) is negatively correlated with P_aO_2, although confidence intervals are large.[32] This relationship has been demonstrated in COPD and in fibrosing alveolitis. In COPD, further decreases in P_aO_2 occurring during the long-term course of the disease are also inversely correlated with increases in PAP, suggesting that hypoxaemia determines the progression of pulmonary arterial hypertension.[33] This pulmonary hypertension arises from hypoxic vasoconstriction and structural changes in pulmonary arteries.[34] The mean PAP is related to prognosis in COPD, survival rates being different at 4 and 7 years in a group of 175 patients according to their initial value of PAP.[35]

In some patients, low-flow oxygen therapy leads to lower PAP over 24 h, which indicates the responsiveness of the pulmonary vessels. This response was found to be a reliable indicator of survival with LTOT in one study[36] but this was not confirmed in a more recent study.[37] Conversely, removing oxygen causes an increase in pulmonary vascular resistance, which takes 2–3 h to reach a new steady state.[38]

Long-term oxygen therapy does not completely reverse pulmonary arterial hypertension but produces improvement in some patients and slows its progression.[39-41] As hypoxic vasoconstriction is not the only mechanism of pulmonary arterial hypertension, and structural changes may vary from one patient to another,[42,43] there is a variable haemodynamic response to oxygen. It is also difficult to determine whether a modest improvement in PAP will lead to clinical improvement in right heart failure or a significant reduction in mortality.

Dyspnoea at rest

Some work has suggested that hypoxaemia may cause breathlessness separate from its stimulant effect on ventilation.[44] There are large individual differences in the sensation of dyspnoea for a given level of P_aO_2. Supplemental oxygen reduces breathlessness at rest in hypoxaemic patients with either interstitial lung disease or COPD.[45] The improvement is probably mainly the result of the associated reduction in ventilation. The oxygen cost of breathing is four to 10 times higher in COPD than in normal individuals and is significantly reduced by oxygen inhalation.[46]

Dyspnoea and exercise performance

Exercise ability is reduced in hypoxaemic patients. Although in patients with COPD there is no relationship between oxygen desaturation and walking distance during a 6-minute test,[47] exercise capacity in COPD can be improved by oxygen inhalation.[48] This improvement is limited[49] but not outweighed[50] by the additional work required to carry the supply of gas. Supplemental oxygen improves dyspnoea and exercise tolerance in patients with COPD who have only mild hypoxaemia at rest and the improvement may be considerable even in the absence of exercise-induced desaturation.[51] Administration of supplemental oxygen 10 min before exercise, however, does not improve maximum exercise performance or breathlessness on exertion in COPD patients.[52]

Improvement in exercise tolerance may be achieved by various mechanisms:[53]

- the oxygen delivery to tissues may be increased, allowing the cardiovascular and respiratory systems to work more efficiently (i.e. decrease in heart and respiratory rate)
- the greater availability of oxygen to tissues may shift the anaerobic threshold to a greater work load, reducing the necessity of hyperventilation to compensate for the metabolic acidosis.

Other possible contributory mechanisms include a reduction in ventilatory requirement through the removal of hypoxaemic drive or prevention of diaphragmatic fatigue through reduction in ventilatory demand.

Skeletal muscle function and nutrition

Progressive weight loss is common in COPD and has been shown to carry an independent mortality risk.[54] Although the mechanisms are uncertain, inadequate dietary intake in the face of raised energy requirements (hypermetabolism) may contribute. Disturbances in intermediary metabolism caused by altered anabolic and catabolic mediators such as hormones, cytokines and growth factors have been described.[55,56] Eating-related oxygen desaturation may contribute to the limited dietary intake.[57]

The aerobic capacity of skeletal muscle is impaired in COPD; this may be the result of hypoxaemia[58,59] and can be improved by oxygen inhalation[60] (Fig. 13.3).

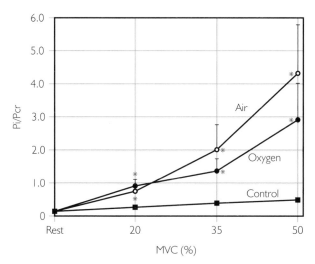

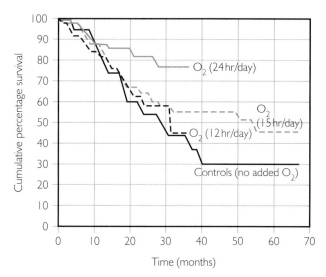

Fig. 13.3 Study of skeletal muscle metabolism using ³¹P magnetic resonance spectroscopy: determination of inorganic phosphate to phosphocreatinine ratio (Pi/PCr) at rest and during the course of exercise at 20, 35 and 50% of maximal voluntary contraction (MVC) of the calf muscle in seven chronic obstructive pulmonary disease (COPD; circles) and seven age-matched control subjects (squares) during air (empty circles) and oxygen (filled circles) administration. Values are mean ± standard error. Asterisks indicate that Pi/PCr values are significantly different ($p < 0.05$) for the COPD group versus the control group (while breathing air or oxygen). Dagger indicates that the Pi/PCr value is significantly different ($p < 0.05$) for air versus oxygen in the COPD group. Pi/PCr increase reflects an impairment of muscular oxidative metabolism that is incompletely corrected during oxygen inhalation (see text). (With permission from Payen et al.[60])

Fig. 13.4 Cumulative percentage survival of patients in the NOTT (dotted line) and MRC (solid line) controlled trials of long-term oxygen therapy for men aged under 70 years. Survival was best in those who received oxygen most of the time.

Quality of life

Neuropsychological disturbances[13,15] dyspnoea,[45] impairment of exercise ability[50] and frequent hospitalisation related to chronic respiratory failure may impair the quality of life in COPD.[14] Oxygen therapy can improve intellectual ability[15,16] and reduce dyspnoea at rest[45] and during exercise.[50,51] The frequency and length of hospitalisation can also be significantly reduced.[18,61] Therefore, the quality of life is improved, albeit not to a large extent. The limited benefit may be the result of marked disability in these patients and restrictions related to equipment for oxygen supply may also be of importance.[62]

Survival

The survival rate is negatively correlated with P_aO_2 or S_aO_2 in hypoxaemic patients whatever the cause.[63] LTOT has been shown to improve survival only in hypoxaemic patients with COPD. This was established in two controlled studies: the Medical Research Council (MRC) trial[40] and the NOTT.[18] The MRC trial clearly indicated that LTOT given for more than 15 h/day improves the survival rate when compared to a group of patients not receiving oxygen. The NOTT showed that the survival rate was better in hypoxaemic COPD patients receiving oxygen for more than 18 h/day when compared to patients

receiving only nocturnal oxygen therapy (Fig. 13.4). In the MRC trial, the improvement in survival was effective only after 500 days of treatment in men, although present from the start of the trial in women. This was not so in the NOTT study, nor has it been confirmed by further studies[64] Cooper et al,[64] in a retrospective study, reported higher survival rates than the previous studies: 62% at 5 years, although only 26% at 10 years. The correction of hypoxaemia, as assessed by the level of P_aO_2 obtained during oxygen inhalation, is also a reliable factor in predicting survival with LTOT.[65] However, although improved survival with oxygen is undoubted in COPD, the exact mechanism is unclear.

Biological and tissue markers of hypoxia

Polycythaemia

Chronic hypoxaemia is associated with polycythaemia. The relation between S_aO_2 and red-cell mass in patients with COPD is, however, highly variable. The differences result partly from variations in carboxyhaemoglobin concentration caused by persistent tobacco consumption.[66]

Long-term oxygen therapy reduces polycythaemia but discrepancies are observed among studies.[18,40,67] These differences may result from variations in the daily duration of oxygen therapy and from persistent smoking by some individuals.[66]

Erythropoietin secretion

Erythropoietin is the primary humoral regulator of erythropoiesis; it acts by stimulation of the proliferation and differentiation of erythroid precursor cells. Its production in the renal cortex is stimulated by local hypoxia, which can be caused by anaemia, hypoxaemia and/or reduced renal blood flow. A circadian rhythm of erythropoietin secretion in human serum has been demonstrated. During acute hypoxaemia, the level of serum erythropoietin increases.[68] Erythropoietin is usually higher than normal in patients with polycythaemia secondary to chronic lung disease, but a single sample does not allow prediction of the occurrence of polycythaemia in COPD.[69] After red-cell mass reduction by erythrophaeresis, serum erythropoietin increases, suggesting that polycythaemia tends to limit endogenous erythropoietin secretion. There is a relationship between the severity of hypoxaemia and the serum level, and this is lowered by oxygen therapy.[70]

Platelets

Platelet size is increased in hypoxaemic COPD patients. After 24 h of oxygen treatment, there is a fall in mean platelet volume.[71] Platelet survival time is shortened in these patients and this is also reversed by oxygen therapy.[72] Platelet aggregation and behaviour are altered in chronic hypoxaemia, factors that may contribute to the pulmonary vascular damage found in these patients.[73]

Electrolytes

Hypoxaemia, in the presence of hypercapnia, may contribute significantly to sodium retention and oedema by adversely affecting glomerular function.[74] The mechanism may possibly involve reduction in renal blood flow, stimulation of the renin–aldosterone system or impairment of renovascular autoregulation.[74,75] An impaired ability to excrete water and a hypertonic saline load has been shown in COPD patients with a history of oedematous exacerbations. Parasympathetic autonomic dysfunction seems to be an important determinant.[76,77] Correction of hypoxaemia improves sodium excretion, supporting the use of oxygen therapy alone as initial conservative management of oedema in hypoxaemic and hypercapnic COPD patient.[75]

Release of ATP degradation products

Cell hypoxia may cause energy depletion, with a resultant decrease in ATP levels, leading to release of a cascade of purine catabolic intermediates (adenosine, inosine, hypoxanthine, xanthine) and ultimately uric acid, which is chemically stable and excreted by the kidney. As a consequence, the urinary uric acid/creatinine ratio is increased overnight in patients with sleep-associated hypoxaemia.[78] Such an effect has yet to be shown in COPD patients.

Oxyhaemoglobin affinity

A shift to the right of the oxyhaemoglobin dissociation curve that improves unloading of oxygen in peripheral tissues is a common compensatory response to conditions of low oxygen delivery, such as anaemia, high-altitude hypoxia or heart failure. The decrease in oxyhaemoglobin affinity is related to an increase in 2,3-diphosphoglycerate (2,3DPG) concentration in erythrocytes. In hypoxaemic COPD patients, however, conflicting results have been found with 2,3DPG levels being either normal or increased. In sleep apnoea syndrome, with repetitive nocturnal hypoxaemic episodes usually without diurnal hypoxaemia, the oxyhaemoglobin dissociation curve is shifted to the right and there is an increase in 2,3DPG.[79]

Hypoxaemia during sleep

Chronic respiratory failure

In patients with COPD, kyphoscoliosis and neuromuscular disorders, exclusive nocturnal desaturation or worsening of diurnal hypoxaemia occur during sleep. Sleep quality is poor in hypoxaemic COPD[19,20] and nocturnal episodes of desaturation are associated with elevations in pulmonary artery pressure.[80] It has been suggested that these intermittent episodes of pulmonary hypertension may, after many years, contribute to the development of chronic pulmonary hypertension.[81] If this hypothesis is valid, nocturnal oxygen therapy might be useful even without significant diurnal hypoxaemia.

The definition of significant nocturnal desaturation is not yet well established. However the most commonly used definitions in the literature are:

- more than 30% of total time in bed spent with oxygen saturation less than 90%
- a drop in oxygen saturation below 90% for longer than 5 min, reaching a nadir of 85% or lower.[82-83]

In a study by Connaughton et al,[84] 97 patients with COPD were followed after sleep studies and there was a significantly higher mortality in patients with the lowest oxygen saturation during sleep. However, similar predictions could be made from the daytime oxygen levels and vital capacity; these were associated with a shorter survival over a mean follow-up period of 70 months, independently of nocturnal S_aO_2. On further analysis, the data from nocturnal polysomnography or oximetry did not influence the prognosis more than either awake S_aO_2 or daytime pulmonary function.

Whether exclusively nocturnal hypoxaemia per se carries a higher mortality risk for COPD patients without daytime hypoxaemia has been much debated. One study[82] showed significantly better survival in subjects without nocturnal desaturation. There was also a trend in this study towards longer survival of patients treated with nocturnal oxygen for exclusively nocturnal desaturations. However, recent data from a European multicentre trial[85] clearly demonstrated that, in patients with daytime P_aO_2 above 60 mmHg and nocturnal desaturation that was much more severe than usually considered (30% of recording time with a $S_aO_2 < 90\%$), there were no significant changes in pulmonary haemodynamics and no difference in terms of haemodynamic changes and survival rate over a 2-year period, when comparing patients with and without oxygen supplementation.

Nocturnal arrhythmias are associated with periods of desaturation[86-88] and can be reduced by oxygen therapy[86,88] but the clinical importance of these findings is uncertain.

In COPD, oxygen desaturation occurring during rapid eye movement (REM) sleep is associated with a myocardial stress similar to that occurring during submaximal exercise. This has been demonstrated by both estimation of coronary blood flow[89] and measurement of left ventricular ejection fraction.[90]

Obstructive sleep apnoea syndrome

The obstructive sleep apnoea syndrome produces intermittent nocturnal hypoxaemia, generally without diurnal hypoxaemia. The neuropsychological consequences are the result of the combination of sleep fragmentation and hypoxaemia. Indices of hypoxaemia, in particular the nadir value of S_aO_2, are good predictors of daytime alertness and sleepiness in these patients. Reductions in general intellectual function, verbal fluency and performance in executive and psychomotor tasks correlate with the severity of nocturnal hypoxaemia.[91]

Hypoxaemia associated with apnoeas also contributes to episodic bradycardia[92] and activation of the sympathetic nervous system.[93] A dose–response relationship between systemic hypertension and obstructive sleep apnoea syndrome, has been demonstrated.[94] This may be related to chronic stimulation of the autonomic nervous system[95] depressed baroreflex sensitivity[96] and increased vasoconstrictor sensitivity.[97] Ventricular ectopy is frequent, especially during the period of maximal heart rate and peak systolic blood pressure immediately after an apnoea[98] and particularly if the S_aO_2 falls below 60%.

Peaks of PAP occur during apnoeas.[99] Sustained pulmonary hypertension, however, is seen only in patients with daytime hypoxaemia and no relationships have been found with the number of apnoeas, the nadir of nocturnal S_aO_2 or the amount of time spent in apnoea.[100] Furthermore, patients with obstructive sleep apnoea usually only develop right heart failure when there is additional daytime hypoxaemia.[101]

Indications for oxygen therapy

Acute hypoxaemia

In acute hypoxaemia additional oxygen is often required urgently because prolonged hypoxaemia leads to tissue hypoxia with potentially irreversible consequences for vital organs. Provided that the circulation is adequate, oxygen will prevent hypoxic tissue damage. In the absence of carbon dioxide retention, oxygen flow rate can be adjusted to that required to maintain adequate oxygenation of tissues.

In the presence of carbon dioxide retention, inspired oxygen concentration needs to be controlled to avoid hypercapnic acidaemia. A recent study showed that aggravating hypercapnia occurred only in a small percentage of patients (13%) when controlled oxygen therapy is given using Venturi masks.[102] Controlled oxygen therapy in COPD patients should proceed as follows: after initial arterial blood gas analysis defines the severity of respiratory failure, oxygen is given by a Venturi mask (e.g. 24.5% or 28%) or by low-flow oxygen (e.g. nasal prongs at 2 l/min). Arterial blood gas analysis should be repeated 30–60 min later. If the P_aO_2 is more than 6.7 kPa (50 mmHg) and

the arterial pH not lower than 7.25, controlled oxygen therapy should continue, along with treatment directed to reverse the cause of the acute exacerbation. If it is impossible to raise P_aO_2 above 6.7 kPa (50 mmHg) in spite of maximal therapy without serious hypercapnic acidosis (pH < 7.25), other measures are likely to be required, e.g. the use of doxapram or intermittent positive pressure ventilation[103] (see Chapter 47.6).

Myocardial infarction

It is usual to give oxygen to patients in the acute phase of a myocardial infarction, because some have moderate hypoxaemia that may be corrected by oxygen. Short-term high inspired oxygen concentrations do lead to a transient reduction of electrocardiographic (ECG) abnormalities during myocardial infarction but a controlled study showed no difference in mortality, incidence of arrhythmias or use of analgesics with or without the use of oxygen at 6 l/min.[104]

Pneumothorax

The rate of resolution of a pneumothorax can be increased threefold by the inhalation of pure oxygen. The mechanism involves generating a pressure gradient between gases in the pleural cavity and the surrounding tissues, which enhances the absorption of nitrogen from the pleural cavity.[105] The efficacy of high concentrations of inhaled oxygen (F_iO_2 60%) to improve resolution of pneumothorax has recently been demonstrated using animal models[106] and such treatment may also be of value in cases of pneumomediastinum.[107]

Hypoxia without hypoxaemia

This occurs in patients who have tissue hypoxia, despite a normal P_aO_2, due to abnormalities in the quantity or type of haemoglobin, impaired release of oxygen from haemoglobin or impaired utilisation of oxygen by tissues.

Anaemia

Although chronic anaemia is usually well-tolerated, this is not the case in acute anaemia ,where the use of high concentration oxygen can be a useful temporary measure in addition to transfusion.

Carbon monoxide poisoning

Accidental or suicidal carbon monoxide inhalation is one of the leading causes of death by poisoning in Western countries. Carbon monoxide combines with haemoglobin to form a stable compound, carboxyhaemoglobin (COHb), reducing the total oxygen-carrying capacity of the blood. The oxyhaemoglobin dissociation curve is also shifted to the left, leading to a concomitant decrease in oxygen delivery. The severity of carbon monoxide poisoning is assessed both by the concentration of COHb and the clinical presentation. The mainstay of management is administration of 100% oxygen through a tight-fitting, non-rebreathing mask at a flow rate of 10 l/min. The use of 100% oxygen can provide one-third of the body's total requirement of oxygen in simple solution in plasma and reduces the half-life of carboxyhaemoglobin from 240 min to approximately 60–80 min. Hyperbaric oxygen can further reduce this half-life to 20–25 min and can provide sufficient oxygen dissolved in plasma to meet the total body oxygen requirements without functioning haemoglobin.[108] In patients with severe carbon monoxide poisoning undergoing mechanical ventilation, hyperbaric oxygen can decrease both the mortality and the frequency of serious neurological deficits.[109]

Methaemoglobinaemia

In acute severe acquired methaemoglobinaemia, inhalation of high concentrations of oxygen is a useful temporary measure until the condition can be reversed.

Oxygen transport deficiency

In patients with oxygen transport deficiency, i.e. inadequate intravascular volume (haemorrhagic shock), inadequate cardiac function or inadequate local oxygen delivery, high concentrations of oxygen may be useful but definitive treatment should be directed at the underlying disease and maintenance of an adequate circulation.

The perioperative state

General anaesthesia, using inhaled agents, commonly causes a decrease in functional residual capacity and an increase in venous admixture. The effects are greatest following abdominal and thoracic surgery, in obese patients and in those with pulmonary disease. In the immediate postoperative period, mild hypoxaemia may result from maldistribution of ventilation. The blood oxygen level should be monitored (e.g. using an oximeter) and oxygen therapy used as appropriate[110] (see Chapter 18). In a recent large study (500 patients), the use of 80% oxygen during the operation and for 2 h afterwards reduced the frequency of surgical wound infections from 11 to 5% when compared with the group of patients receiving only 30% oxygen.[111]

Oxygen to drive nebulisers

Administration of bronchodilators by nebuliser uses the Venturi principle to generate an aerosol. This is widely used in patients with acute attacks of asthma. High flow rates of oxygen (4–8 l/min) are needed. Caution is required in patients with COPD and hypercapnia in whom worsening carbon dioxide retention can occur with such uncontrolled oxygen, but the risk is small when treatment is appropriately supervised.

Hyperbaric oxygenation

Resistant hypoxic cells are found in animal and human solid tumours and are thought to compromise the success of radiotherapy. For this reason hyperbaric oxygen was formerly used in an attempt to overcome the resistance of tumours to radiation. However, two types of hypoxia may coexist in tumours – chronic, or diffusion-limited, and acute, or perfusion-limited hypoxia. Given these two refractory hypoxic cell populations and the technical difficulties of high oxygen administration, other manipulations of oxygen supply are receiving considerable attention, i.e. reduction of haemoglobin affinity for oxygen and

modification of tumour blood flow by vasoactive agents such as calcium antagonists or nicotinamide.[112,113]

Hyperbaric oxygen therapy can also be used to increase oxygen partial pressure and reverse haemoglobin affinity for another gas, as in carbon monoxide poisoning (see above). Treatment of decompression sickness is usually with hyperbaric air without addition of supplementary oxygen (see Chapter 33).

Long-term oxygen therapy

Ideally, LTOT should meet the following objectives:

- correction of hypoxaemia without inducing hypercapnia
- reduction of polycythaemia
- improvement in survival
- improvement in neuropsychological function
- improved quality of sleep
- prevention of right heart failure
- improved quality of life
- reduced costs of health care.

Selection of patients

It is appropriate that each patient should receive optimum therapy before LTOT is prescribed. This includes suitable pharmacological therapy, physical therapy, cessation of smoking, reduced alcohol ingestion and reduction of polycythaemia.

The main criterion for selection of patients[114-116] with COPD who are likely to benefit from oxygen therapy is a low P_aO_2. It has, however, been shown that spontaneous improvement after an acute exacerbation of COPD may take up to 3 months. One-third of patients leaving hospital with low P_aO_2 may improve spontaneously after 3 months to a level no longer qualifying for LTOT.[117] Thus confirmation of hypoxaemia with two measurements of P_aO_2 at least a few weeks apart is recommended before starting LTOT. A recent study has evaluated how often LTOT was re-evaluated 1–3 months after initial prescription in unstable patients.[118] In this study, a significant number of patients remained on LTOT without any re-evaluation and the treatment could potentially have been discontinued in up to 60% of the patient appropriately re-evaluated.[118]

Adequate data on the efficacy of LTOT exist only for COPD but most practitioners and investigators assume that the data in COPD apply to other chronic hypoxaemic lung diseases.[114]

Assessment of oxygen efficiency and tolerance

For optimal treatment oxygen flow should be sufficient to raise P_aO_2 to more than 8.7 kPa (65 mmHg),[115,116] preferably in all diurnal and nocturnal situations. It is difficult to predict oxygen requirements during sleep in patients with COPD. The current recommendations by the American Thoracic Society are to increase the inspired oxygen flow by 1 litre/min during exercise and sleep in those patients who fulfil the requirements for supplemental oxygen.[119] However, it is not clear whether this is adequate and one study suggested that half of COPD patients receiving LTOT need increased oxygen flow during sleep.[120]

Simple exercise tests and nocturnal oximetry without and with oxygen flow are sometimes used to adjust flow rates. The required flow may be different in various situations such as exercise, sleeping or eating and this should be reassessed periodically in each individual.

Nocturnal oxygen does not induce clinically important increases in P_aCO_2 during sleep in most patients with stable obstructive lung disease. Even in moderate to severe hypercapnic COPD, P_aCO_2 changes with sleep are less than 1.33 kPa (10 mmHg), about two-thirds of this change being related to the effect of oxygen per se.[121] Therefore, a single assessment of arterial PCO_2 at the end of a night breathing oxygen is sufficient when starting LTOT.[122]

Indications

Generally accepted indications

After optimising treatment and stopping smoking, LTOT can be given to COPD patients with a stable P_aO_2 of less than 7.3 kPa (<55 mmHg) breathing air. The cut-off point of 7.3 kPa (55 mmHg) was chosen because the shape of the oxygen dissociation curve determines that hypoxaemia rapidly becomes more severe as P_aO_2 falls below 8 kPa (60 mmHg). Oxygen is often prescribed outside the prescription guidelines for patients with a P_aO_2 above 8 kPa. Of 7700 COPD patients prescribed LTOT via the French ANTADIR network, 18.5% had a P_aO_2 of 60 mmHg or more at the start of treatment.[123] On LTOT, there was no difference in the survival rates of patients with a P_aO_2 less than 60 mmHg compared those to with more hypoxaemic COPD. These data suggest that patients with only moderate hypoxaemia may be candidates for LTOT. However, in a randomised study comparing air and LTOT in 135 COPD patients with a stable P_aO_2 between 56 and 65 mmHg, there was no difference in survival rates over at least 3 years between the two groups.[124] On the basis of these data there is no justification for prescribing LTOT in patients with moderate hypoxaemia,[125] although the conclusion might have been different if quality-of-life assessment had been the primary end-point.

Possible indications

Patients with COPD and a P_aO_2 between 7.3 and 7.8 kPa (55–59 mmHg) with polycythaemia, pulmonary hypertension or clinical evidence of cor pulmonale are usually also considered as appropriate candidates for LTOT.[122] In this group of patients, haemodynamic measurements, sleep studies and/or exercise tests may be helpful.

Controversial indications

No controlled studies of LTOT have been performed in cystic fibrosis or in restrictive respiratory diseases such as fibrosing alveolitis or pneumoconiosis.

Long-term oxygen therapy and non-invasive positive pressure ventilation in chronic respiratory failure

In respiratory failure due to kyphoscoliosis, neuromuscular diseases or skeletal disorders related to tuberculosis, oxygen therapy alone is ineffective and may cause marked acceleration of CO_2 retention. In such patients, hypercapnia and hypoxaemia are more appropriately treated by non-invasive ventilation (NIV) without a preliminary trial of LTOT.[126]

In chronic respiratory failure associated with COPD, the use of non-invasive ventilation in combination with LTOT controls nocturnal hypoventilation and improves sleep, quality of life and daytime blood gases in some patients.[126–128] Nasal ventilation is unlikely to produce benefits unless used in association with LTOT. Patients with COPD who show significant daytime hypercapnia (> 50 mmHg) and the greatest reduction in overnight P_aCO_2 with NIV are those patients most likely to benefit from the combination of the two treatments.[126–128]

Palliative use of oxygen

In patients with terminal heart failure, cancer[129] or obstructive or fibrosing lung disease, oxygen may help to reduce dyspnoea and fatigue.

Duration of oxygen therapy

The NOTT study would seem to indicate that, once the decision to use LTOT has been taken, attempts should be made to achieve 24 h compliance or at least 15 h/day. Patients should be encouraged to use their oxygen as much as possible, including situations such as meals, toileting and exercise.[122] They need the appropriate apparatus to make this possible, such as portable systems or extended tubing. There should be insistence on cessation of smoking because cigarette smoking limits the efficacy of LTOT and is potentially dangerous.

In addition to the classic indications for LTOT, there are indications for oxygen therapy for a shorter period each day.

Nocturnal oxygen only

Chronic respiratory failure

Recent data in patients with a daytime P_aO_2 above 8 kPa (> 60 mmHg) and oxygen desaturation during sleep showed that nocturnal oxygen therapy did not modify the evolution of pulmonary haemodynamics during a 2-year follow-up and did not result in any delay in the prescription of continuous oxygen therapy (> 15 h/24 h).[85] Also, there was no effect on survival, although the limited number of deaths precluded any firm conclusion. Consequently, the prescription of nocturnal oxygen alone is probably not justified in COPD and current international guidelines should be reconsidered.[85]

Central sleep apnoea

Congestive heart failure is a common condition and is associated with high morbidity and mortality. Sleep-disordered breathing has been reported as one of the multiple factors that may contribute to its declining course. The published rates of Cheyne–Stokes respiration with central sleep apnoea (CSR–CSA) in patients with congestive heart failure vary from 30% to 100%. Proposed mechanisms for CSR–CSA include:

- increased central controller gain (i.e. raised responses to CO_2 and hypoxia favouring respiratory instability)
- increased circulation time
- hypocapnia
- reduced buffering capacity of arterial blood gases.

A low P_aCO_2 promotes ventilatory instability and the occurrence of central apnoeas is consistent with the physiological notion of apnoea threshold. Thus in one study the positive predictive value of a P_aCO_2 below 35 mmHg for central apnoea in patients with stable cardiac failure was 78%.[130]

A higher mortality has been reported in congestive heart failure patients who show CSR–CSA during sleep. CSR–CSA itself may be sufficient to impair cardiac function by different mechanisms. Changes in pleural pressure with negative swings at the peak of hyperventilation affect both preload and afterload. Sympathoadrenal activation also occurs as a result of arousals, hypoxaemia and hypercapnia. These phenomena may result in an imbalance between oxygen delivery and demand, particularly in the presence of coronary artery disease.

When these patients were treated with nocturnal oxygen a correlation has been found between the improvement in Cheyne–Stokes respiration and the increase in peak oxygen consumption during exercise. Andreas et al suggested that treatment of CSR–CSA by oxygen, with concomitant reduction in arousals and desaturations and a reduction in sympathetic overactivity, is the explanation for the exercise capacity improvement found in congestive heart failure.[131] Sympathetic activation is an important pathophysiological and prognostic factor in heart failure and CSR–CSA per se is a stimulus to sympathetic activation. It can be speculated that treatment of CSR–CSA may reduce sympathetic tone and thus lead to improved survival in such patients. As the use of nasal CPAP remains controversial in patients with congestive heart failure and CSR–CSA, nocturnal oxygen therapy is probably, at the present time, the reference treatment for this type of sleep-disordered breathing.[132–134]

Ambulatory oxygen therapy

Two situations need to be distinguished.[135]

Portable oxygen therapy alone: COPD patients not sufficiently hypoxaemic to merit long-term oxygen therapy but showing exercise desaturation

No data are available on the specific affects of exercise desaturation on survival or pulmonary haemodynamics. Therefore, oxygen is not justified in this situation unless it improves dyspnoea or exercise capacity.[136] When compared to breathing air, use of domiciliary oxygen on exertion did not improve quality of life in mild hypoxaemic COPD patients.[137] In one study supplemental oxygen during pulmonary rehabilitation did little to enhance exercise tolerance although there was a small benefit in terms of dyspnoea.[138] Only patients with severe disabling dyspnoea during training are likely to find symptomatic relief with oxygen.[138] In another study in which patients received either air or oxygen[138] at rest and at the end of standardised stair-climbing, those receiving oxygen clearly felt less breathless.[139] These studies are the first to assess scientifically whether or not oxygen therapy is actually beneficial acutely in the management of COPD patients.[140] Clearly not everyone benefits and there is a need to provide a pragmatic demonstration of benefit from portable oxygen before prescription, ultimately by performing double-blind tests of portable oxygen and compressed air.[141]

Portable oxygen as a means of extending the duration of long-term oxygen therapy

This application of portable oxygen has two aims: to correct effort-related hypoxaemia and to increase the duration of oxygen use over the 24 h.[142]

Who should prescribe oxygen therapy?

It is logical that oxygen should be prescribed by a respiratory physician. In a British study, when LTOT was recommended by a respiratory physician the criteria for prescription were fulfilled in 82% of cases compared with 35% when prescribed by general practitioners or non-specialist physicians.[143]

Contraindications to long-term oxygen therapy

When considering LTOT it is essential that the patient should have stopped smoking and have some understanding of what is required for such demanding therapy. Consideration needs to be given to the practicality of home installation of LTOT and the ability of the family to cope.

Compliance and education

Many studies[144–150] have reported the number of hours of LTOT actually achieved by patients at home. A prospective French multicentre study[151] of a large number of patients ($n = 931$) examined uptake of the medical prescription and compliance with treatment for at least 15 h/day. Only 45% of the patients used oxygen for an average of 15 h or more per day. Previous studies have shown the proportion to be very variable, ranging from 17% to 70% of patients.[142,147,149] The clinical and functional severity of the condition seems to be one of the factors determining compliance. The most compliant patients tend to be those with the most severe blood gas impairment, the most severe spirometric abnormalities and the most frequent hospital admissions.[145–149,151] One study[146] showed further that patients increased their daily consumption of oxygen if their condition deteriorated. Such studies reinforce the need to follow the defined criteria for prescription for LTOT. Initiating this inconvenient and demanding treatment when patients' symptoms and disability are not severe enough to accept the treatment inevitably leads to limited use.

The method of initial advice and prescription of oxygen treatment is crucial for subsequent compliance. One study[151] showed that the likelihood of achieving at least 15 h of oxygen therapy per day was multiplied 4.5-fold when the medical prescription for oxygen therapy stated precisely the required duration as more than 15 h/day. Moreover, it was evident that the patients had received insufficient explanation of how to achieve 15 h of treatment per day, e.g. patients did not understand that oxygen treatment could and should be used during meals, toileting and leisure activities. Obviously, one should verify that smoking has ceased at the time of initial prescription. Last, prescription of ambulatory oxygen therapy whenever required and precise description of the different situations when oxygen could be used increase the likelihood of achieving daily use for 15 h or greater. Compliance is also improved by follow–up education after the initiation of therapy, whether given by a nurse or a physiotherapist.[151] This underlines the importance of technical and medical follow-up to improve education and allow recognition of side effects and intolerance to treatment, which lead to reduced compliance.

Finally, patients tend to become more compliant the longer they are on treatment. This may be the result of deterioration in respiratory function with time but may also be related to the effects of technical and medical education of the patient.[151]

Surveillance and follow-up

There are both technical and medical aspects to the follow-up of patients on LTOT. The function of the equipment needs to be checked regularly.[152,153] The selection of concentrator needs to take into consideration the capacity to deliver the desired concentration at the flow rates chosen. If liquid oxygen systems are used, its delivery needs to be reliable and safe, and the patient needs to understand the equipment.

Medical follow-up includes regular assessment with measurement of blood gases on air and oxygen. Ideally the patient would be best seen at home to assess compliance by examining the counter of the machine. Blood gases measured at home assess both the patient and the efficacy of the machine. Some stable patients show improvement in P_aO_2 over time[154] but whether this indicates that LTOT can then be discontinued is controversial.

Cost and volume of long-term oxygen therapy

The international utilisation of home oxygen therapy is highly variable.[155] For example, the number of LTOT users varies from 20/100 000 in the UK to 241/100 000 in the USA.[155] The total cost of LTOT is estimated at between $1.4 billion and $3 billion annually in the USA. LTOT represents 73% of the total ambulatory cost in a COPD patient at the stage of chronic respiratory failure.[156]

Why is more oxygen prescribed in some countries? The studies are consistent in finding that 25–40% of the patients do not meet the classical criteria for LTOT.[123,156,157] Moreover, unstable patients at the time of initial prescription are generally not adequately re-evaluated.[118] Clearly, large variations exist from one country to another regarding the use of LTOT for oxygen desaturations during sleep and oxygen and exercise in patients with awake resting P_aO_2 over 55 mmHg. Closer adherence to recommendations and guidelines for patient selection, assessment and re-evaluation is desirable.

Devices for oxygen administration

In hospital, oxygen is usually piped to the bedside from a gaseous or liquid source. For domiciliary treatment, three methods of oxygen delivery are available:

- oxygen cylinders
- oxygen concentrators
- liquid oxygen.

The use of oxygen cylinders as the principal source of long-term domiciliary oxygen therapy is now in decline because this mode of delivery is very expensive and cumbersome and requires repeated deliveries. Smaller cylinders of 0.4–1.0 m³, however, remain of value and can be used for travel outside the home.

Oxygen supply by concentrator

An oxygen concentrator (Fig. 13.5) concentrates oxygen from ambient air by absorption of nitrogen. It is compact, easily positioned in the home and avoids the necessity of large stores of gas in the domestic environment. It is relatively cheap to run, easily serviced and transportable outside the home; concentrators weigh around 25 kg and can usually be fitted in the luggage boot of the car. Oxygen concentrators have the disadvantage that portable oxygen therapy has to be provided separately.

Concentrators operate on the molecular sieve principle using a column of synthetic aluminium silicate (Zeolite) to adsorb nitrogen from room air, producing an output gas with a high concentration of oxygen (> 90% at low flow rates). As the flow is increased, a greater volume of gas passes through the molecular sieve and the time spent in contact with the aluminium silicate is less, so that adsorption of nitrogen is less complete and the oxygen concentration delivered falls. Thus, the use of these machines is limited in patients requiring high flow rates. Although recent models can deliver greater (> 90%) oxygen at flow rates of 4 l/min, some patients with severe hypoxaemia require two machines delivering a supply in parallel.

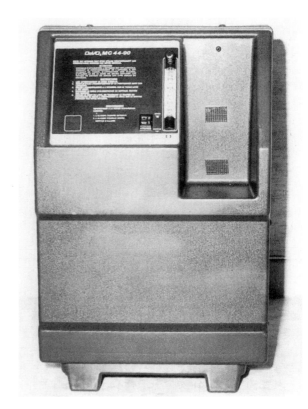

Fig. 13.5 Oxygen concentrator: the most widely used device for long-term oxygen therapy at home.

The machines are reliable and long-lasting, relatively cheap, simple to use and generally well-accepted, although the noise generated by the equipment may be a problem. Finally, standby cylinders are needed in case of power failure, particularly in patients requiring almost continuous oxygen therapy.

Liquid oxygen

This method of oxygen supply (Fig. 13.6) requires the storage of large quantities of liquid oxygen in the home and a frequent delivery service. The supply has to be installed in a space with free air circulation as the refrigeration is maintained by venting continuously a small amount of the liquid source. In most countries the cost of liquid oxygen is two or three times the cost of oxygen provided by a concentrator. The container weighs around 35 kg and contains 20–40 litres of liquid oxygen, 1 litre of liquid oxygen corresponding to 850 litres of gaseous oxygen. Thus, depending on flow rates, the patient may require delivery of oxygen as frequently as twice a week. A small portable oxygen cylinder can be filled from the large reservoir and used for ambulatory oxygen therapy. The capacity of these smaller cylinders allows ambulation of up to 8 h when used at a flow rate of 2 l/min. The main

indications for liquid oxygen are younger patients requiring high flow rates and longer daily duration for oxygen therapy, and also those who are more active.[158] Vergeret et al[142] showed that use of liquid oxygen did not lead to greater use of treatment than a gaseous supply but did improve the quality of life. A recent cost–utility analysis confirmed these findings.[159] The cost of liquid oxygen was three times the cost of concentrator treatment. However, quality of life showed significant differences in favour of liquid oxygen for dimensions of physical function, ambulation, social interaction and global score.[159]

Methods of oxygen delivery

Oxygen is a drug and should be prescribed as such. The concentration to be administered should be clearly stated, as well as the method of supply and the degree of monitoring to be undertaken. This applies to both the acute and chronic situations.[122]

Acute respiratory failure

Face masks

Oxygen masks are designed to fit over the mouth and nose and deliver increased concentrations of oxygen in the inspired gas.

- **High-concentration masks** can increase the inspired oxygen concentration to around 60%, with an inspired oxygen flow exceeding 6 l/min (Fig. 13.7) They allow some rebreathing. This can be overcome by using a valve to separate inspired from expired gas. These masks have two major drawbacks. Patients will not wear them consistently over a long time because they have to be tight-fitting and are thus

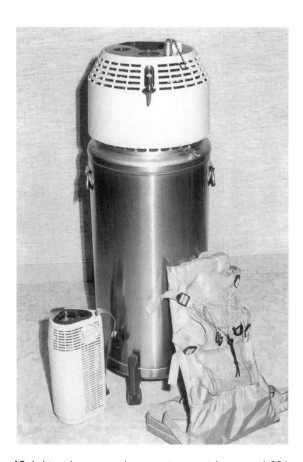

Fig. 13.6 Liquid oxygen: the container weighs around 35 kg and contains 20–40 litres of liquid oxygen, 1 litre of liquid oxygen corresponding to 850 litres of gaseous oxygen. The small portable oxygen cylinder can be filled from the large reservoir and used for ambulatory oxygen therapy. Its capacity allows ambulation of up to 8 h when used at a flow rate of 2 l/min.

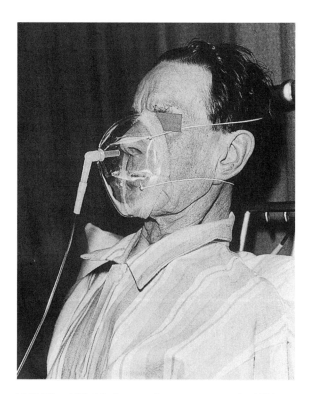

Fig. 13.7 The MC Mask provides approximately 60% inspired oxygen concentration at 6 l/min of oxygen, with some rebreathing.

uncomfortable. Furthermore, if given inadvertently to patients with respiratory failure and carbon dioxide retention, they can lead to increasing hypercapnia, worsening respiratory acidosis and death.

■ **Low concentration masks**[160]

- *Fixed performance masks* deliver a constant predetermined oxygen concentration to the patient's mouth unaffected by tidal volume or pattern of breathing. For example, Ventimasks, which work on the Venturi principle, are colour-coded with their required oxygen flow rate and nominal output concentration (24.5%, 28%, 35%, 40%).

- *Variable performance masks* (e.g. Edinburgh mask, Fig. 13.8) do not deliver a known, fixed oxygen concentration. Oxygen is delivered at a continuous low flow rate, which supplements room air to a limited extent. They allow hypoxaemia to be relieved partially, minimising further carbon dioxide retention.

However, all these masks are uncomfortable for use by patients over long periods. The variability of inspired oxygen concentration delivered with nasal prongs is considerable, similar to that found with uncontrolled masks.[161] Thus, as uncontrolled oxygen therapy may be dangerous during acute hypercapnic exacerbations of COPD, Venturi masks are the safer method.[102,162] If, for reasons of compliance, nasal prongs are used, the clinical status, P_aCO_2 and pH should be carefully monitored.

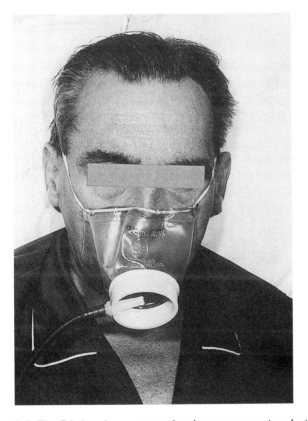

Fig. 13.8 The Edinburgh oxygen mask, a low concentration device that, at a rate of 2 l/min of oxygen provides approximately 25–30% inspired oxygen concentration without significant rise in inspired carbon dioxide concentration.

Nasopharyngeal catheters

These offer an alternative way of maintaining a raised inspired oxygen concentration when nasal prongs or masks have proved inadequate.[163] For maximum efficiency the catheter should be inserted pernasally, so that the tip lies behind and just beneath the soft palate. This distance is similar to that from the nostril to the ear lobe. Firm strapping reduces the risk of the catheter being displaced. They generally need to be changed to the other nostril every 6 h.

Long-term oxygen therapy

Nasal prongs

Nasal prongs overcome the difficulties of face masks and are the most commonly used system for prolonged oxygen delivery. They are simple, cheap, well-tolerated and reliable. Patients can eat, sleep, talk and expectorate without discontinuing therapy.

The oxygen concentration delivered is independent of mouth or nose breathing.[164] Oxygen flow rates up to 3 l/min are well tolerated and do not require humidification. At greater flows humidification may be needed to avoid nasal mucosal drying, irritation and discomfort.

Nasal prongs are visible and this may have cosmetic and psychological effects. Their use is unlikely to cause progressive hypercapnia in patients in the stable state. Displacement of prongs during sleep is difficult to prevent, but is not a major problem in most individuals.

Nasopharyngeal catheters

These are most often used in acute exacerbations as in the home they are poorly tolerated and often badly placed by the patients. They should only be used long-term in patients needing high flow rates and refusing transtracheal catheterisation.

Oxygen-conserving nasal cannulae

Oxygen-conserving cannulae[165,166] consist of nasal prongs with a closely coupled reservoir containing a collapsible membrane, and an oxygen supply line at the distal end of the reservoir on each side. The conserver cannula stores oxygen in the following manner: during early exhalation, the dead space gas pushes the membrane out filling the reservoir. After the reservoir is filled and during the rest of exhalation, oxygen displaces the original dead space gas medially by venting it through the nasal prongs. During early inspiration, the patient inhales the 20 ml bolus of approximately 85% oxygen from the reservoir, thus collapsing its membrane. Thus one can attain a required S_aO_2 level with a flow rate of 0.5–1.0 l/min instead of the usual 2.0 l/min. The efficiency varies between patients, perhaps caused by different breathing patterns. Thus each individual's response has to be assessed. The device is highly visible and may be cosmetically unacceptable to many patients.

Inspired-phase oxygen delivery

Many attempts have been made to conserve oxygen by using intermittent, inspiration-phased oxygen delivery because only oxygen delivered in the early phase of inspiration is used in gas exchange. The usefulness of these devices is in prolonging the time for which a portable device can be used or in reducing the interval between deliveries of liquid oxygen to the home.

Early devices were manual or relied upon chest-wall movement for activation. Most devices activated by temperature or pressure changes require specially modified nasal prongs, which are expensive. Unfortunately rapid breathing, as may occur in breathless patients, causes an almost continuous flow of oxygen and little oxygen conservation.[167] There is little long-term experience with these devices. The effect of mouth breathing on their function is not known and this may be relevant during sleep.

Data on efficacy are few, but in some patients they have been found useful at rest, during exercise and sleep.[168–170] One study on 94 patients showed that overall correction of S_aO_2 was not as good with valved oxygen compared with continuous oxygen at similar flow rates, both by day and by night.[171]

In conclusion, the role of these systems remains marginal and requires individual assessment.

Transtracheal catheter

Transtracheal oxygen delivery involves administration of oxygen percutaneously through a catheter inserted into the suprasternal trachea. There are wide variations in its use among countries and among respiratory units, and its place in treatment remains undefined.[172,173]

Transtracheal oxygen usually improves S_aO_2 at flow rates lower than those used with nasal cannulae, thereby leading to more economical use of oxygen. An additional advantage of transtracheal delivery is the ability to promote continuous oxygen use, an outcome generally associated with a significant reduction in mortality.[18,13] Transtracheal delivery also eliminates problems related to use of nasal cannulae such as nasal crusting and blockage, dry throat, hoarseness and epistaxis.

Transtracheal oxygen delivery is invasive but with little morbidity and no reported mortality related to insertion of the catheter. The most common complications are irritating cough, occasional slight haemoptysis and discomfort at the puncture site. When the cannula track is immature the most frequent problem is the development of mucus ball[174] caused by the drying effect of oxygen, increased sputum production and poor compliance with catheter changing schedules. Daily catheter cleaning prevents these problems. Late complications relate to the tip of the catheter breaking off and being inhaled. There have been reports of accidents in replacing the catheter, with creation of a false track, bacterial cellulitis and subcutaneous emphysema. Problems are obviously greater with inexperience.

Transtracheal oxygen reduces dyspnoea and improves exercise tolerance with a reduction of inspired minute ventilation.[175] Tidal volume is decreased but respiratory rate is unchanged. Improved exercise tolerance[176] may be the result of decreased inspiratory work of breathing. Finally, use of transtracheal catheters has been reported to reduce hospital admissions in patients with COPD.[176]

Humidification

Humidification of inspired oxygen is recommended mainly when delivered directly to the trachea. It is therefore necessary when using transtracheal catheters or tracheostomy. When oxygen is delivered by mask or nasal prongs, the nose usually provides the necessary humidification. Nevertheless, when high flow rates are required, humidification is desirable. For LTOT, bubble-through cold water humidifiers are used almost exclu-

sively. Humidifier attachments on oxygen concentrators are frequently contaminated with potentially pathogenic bacteria. Although in most patients the infection rate is unchanged, microbiological assessment is required at least in patients in whom reduced resistance to colonisation with potential pathogens is suspected.[177] Thus humidification is needed only by the minority of patients who complain of drying of the mucosa.

Conclusions

For LTOT, nasal prongs are generally the most appropriate method of oxygen delivery because of their simplicity, safety and cheapness. Alternative devices need only be used when oxygenation is inadequate with standard nasal prongs and the potential benefit must be weighed against the greater complication rate of other methods of delivery.

Oxygen toxicity

Three categories of hazard have been associated with oxygen therapy. The first includes physical risks such as fire hazard or tank explosions, trauma from catheters or masks and drying of mucous membranes as a result of inadequate humidification. The second category comprises functional effects, including carbon dioxide retention and atelectasis. The third category consists of toxic manifestations of oxygen: increased generation of partially reduced oxygen products, free radicals, is responsible for the cytotoxicity of oxygen.

Pulmonary toxicity

The effects of hyperoxia in normal subjects include substernal discomfort and diminished vital capacity, which develop within several hours. Longer exposures may result in reduced pulmonary compliance and diffusing capacity. Chronic oxygen toxicity results in varying degrees of pulmonary oedema and fibrosis. Chronic oxygen toxicity is not well understood in humans, partly because of the difficulty in separating the effects of oxygen from the manifestations of the underlying disease for which oxygen was administered. This is obviously the case in acute situations such as adult respiratory distress syndrome (see Chapter 28).

Cerebral oxygen toxicity

Hyperbaric oxygenation causes severe cerebral vasoconstriction which can result in epileptic fits. Similarly in neonates, hyperoxia even at atmospheric pressure can lead to retrolental fibroplasia, manifested by damaged retinal blood vessels, and permanent visual impairment.

Limits for safe exposure

Oxygen toxicity develops as a function of the dose and duration of oxygen administered. A precise threshold concentration that is toxic to human lungs has not been established. It can only be extrapolated from animal studies and a limited number of human experiments. Oxygen at a concentration of

100% should be administered for a short period of time for cardiopulmonary resuscitation or instability. Short exposures (2–7 days) to oxygen at F_IO_2 of 50% or less do not lead to clinically significant lung impairment. Although the effects of prolonged exposure at such an F_IO_2 have not been defined, it appears from clinical experience with LTOT that toxicity is limited. However, the goal of oxygen therapy should be to deliver oxygen at the lowest concentration required to achieve adequate tissue oxygenation, thereby minimising the risk oxygen toxicity.

Monitoring oxygen therapy

Techniques available for monitoring oxygen therapy include measurement of arterial blood gases on samples obtained by intermittent puncture or by an intra-arterial line, non-invasive monitoring by oximetry and transcutaneous methods, as well as non-invasive monitoring of inspired or expired air.

Invasive monitoring

The choice of sites for arterial puncture are, in order of preference, the radial, brachial and femoral arteries. The carotid artery should not be used. Complications are uncommon, generally minor and temporary. The presence of an arterial line facilitates monitoring if measurements of blood gases are required at frequent intervals (e.g. more than five per day).

Causes of significant error in arterial blood gas measurements include excessive heparin, failure to keep the sample iced if analysis is not done within 30 min[178] and a high white blood cell count. Dilution of blood with 20% heparin (2 ml blood and 0.5 ml heparin) leads to a mean decrease of 0.03 pH units and 0.96 kPa (7.2 mmHg) in P_aCO_2, whereas P_aO_2 increases by 0.68 kPa (5.1 mmHg) ($n = 14$, personal data). The changes in P_aO_2 are dependent on the initial level of P_aO_2, i.e. the higher the initial P_aO_2 the larger the resulting changes. A leukaemia of 400 000/mm³ can induce a decrease in P_aO_2 of 1.33 kPa (10 mmHg) in 30 s.[179] Finally, technical errors in measurement are probably the most important source of error, especially in calibration of equipment.

Oximetry

Oximetry is now widely used for continuous measurement of S_aO_2. Oximeters are easily used, portable and relatively inexpensive.

Method of oxygen measurement

An oximeter is a spectrophotometric device that measures the differential absorption of light by oxy- and deoxyhaemoglobin. Modern instruments use only two transmitted wavelengths and therefore include in the measurement other forms of haemoglobin such as carboxyhaemoglobin and methaemoglobin. Two sensors are mainly used – ear and finger probes. Studies in normal subjects and patients with respiratory disease have demonstrated that the accuracy of ear oximetry compared to direct arterial blood gas measurement is ± 3–5% saturation, which is adequate

for most clinical situations.[180,181] However, appropriate use of this technique requires a knowledge of its limitations and differences in accuracy in various clinical conditions. Movement artefacts may produce a false fall in saturation.[182] Skin pigmentation may cause inability to obtain a reading or warning messages indicating poor tissue penetration of the signal.[183] Raised concentrations of bilirubin, carboxyhaemoglobin or methaemoglobin may all cause false increases in S_aO_2.[184] Poor perfusion (as in shock) can lead to inadequate S_aO_2 measurement, as also can cardiac arrhythmias. Invasive measurement is then required.

Clinical usefulness

Acutely ill patients
Oximetry is widely used in intensive care and anaesthesia for continuous monitoring of S_aO_2 and to adjust the level of oxygen therapy. This avoids repeated blood gas measurements, provided that hypercapnia is absent. However, it should be noted that many of the conditions that lead to the limitations cited above may be present in critically ill patients.

Monitoring of long-term oxygen therapy
Studies showing the benefit of LTOT were based on oxygenation measured in arterial samples. As oximetry is less accurate, its use could lead to false-negative or false-positive results.[185] The level of carbon dioxide is also of importance in this context and thus oximetry is not sufficient for selection of patients for LTOT.

Assessment of nocturnal S_aO_2 and screening for sleep apnoea syndrome
Oximetry is clinically useful in a variety of settings when intermittent arterial blood gas sampling is impracticable for monitoring of important variations of S_aO_2. This is typically the case in sleep studies. During sleep, oximetry allows identification of nocturnal desaturation as in screening for sleep apnoea.[186-188] It may also be useful for adjusting oxygen flow rate when LTOT is needed.

Exercise testing
Oximetry is of value during exercise to identify patients with exercise desaturation and to adjust the flow rate of oxygen needed during exertion. However, results of ear oximetry during exercise should be interpreted cautiously.[189] Particular care is required in stabilising the sensor because of the movement of the exercising patient. Another problem may be hypoperfusion of the ear. One study of 101 patients showed that the direction of the changes in saturation from rest to exercise is correctly evaluated in most cases but absolute values are not reliable.[190]

Transcutaneous Po2 measurement

Wide application of transcutaneous oxygen ($P_{tc}O_2$) and carbon dioxide ($P_{tc}CO_2$) monitoring[191] has been limited by the high cost of the devices and by technical requirements. The probe must be heated to 43°C and relocation is therefore necessary every 3–4 h, depending on the susceptibility to thermal injury of the individual patient. The technique has received wide acceptance in neonatal and infant monitoring and is of potential value in monitoring paediatric patients undergoing intensive care. In the adult, however, $P_{tc}O_2$ does not consistently correlate with P_aO_2, which limits its use in clinical practice.

Conclusions

Oxygen therapy has several well-established indications in acute conditions and there has been a marked increase in the use of long-term oxygen in the last 15 years. The beneficial effects of LTOT have been assessed in COPD but there is no controlled study on its effects in other patients with chronic respiratory failure. The development of LTOT has stimulated technological improvements in oxygen delivery systems. Documentation of arterial hypoxaemia at rest is the major criterion for selection of patients. Simple estimation of P_aO_2 correlates poorly with the tissue consequences of hypoxaemia, however, and the local cellular and tissue consequences of hypoxia together with the important adaptive mechanisms are active areas of research. The results may contribute to better understanding of respiratory failure and its consequences and may allow development of new criteria for treatment.

? Unresolved questions

- What is the role of nocturnal oxygen treatment in patients with a daytime P_aO_2 > 8 kPa (>60 mmHg) and nocturnal oxygen desaturation? On present evidence it is probably not justified.

- What is the role of portable oxygen therapy alone in chronic obstructive pulmonary disease (COPD) patients not sufficiently hypoxaemic to merit domiciliary LTOT but showing exercise desaturation?

- What is the value of oxygen therapy in patients with congestive heart failure and Cheyne–Stokes respiration with central sleep apnoea?

- In chronic respiratory failure due to COPD, what is the value of non-invasive ventilation together with long-term oxygen therapy?

References

1. Leach RM, Treacher DF. Oxygen transport: the relation between oxygen delivery and consumption. Thorax 1992; 47: 971.
2. Connett RJ, Honig CR, Gayeski TEJ, Brooks GA. Defining hypoxia: a systems view of $\dot{V}O_2$, glycolysis, energetics, and intracellular PO_2. J Appl Physiol 1990; 68: 833.
3. Gleed RD, Mortola JP. Ventilation in newborn rats after gestation at simulated high altitude. J Appl Physiol 1991; 70: 1146.
4. Rodriguez-Roisin R, Agusti AGN, Roca J. The hepatopulmonary syndrome: new name, old complexities. Thorax 1992; 47: 897.
5. Mélot C, Naeije R, Hallemans R et al. Hypoxic pulmonary vasoconstriction and pulmonary gas exchange in normal man. Respir Physiol 1987; 68: 11.
6. Wagner PD, Rodriguez-Roisin R. Clinical advances in pulmonary gas exchange. Am Rev Respir Dis 1991; 143: 883.
7. Weinberger SE, Schwartzstein RM, Weiss W. Hypercapnia. N Engl J Med 1989; 321: 1223.
8. Similowski T, Derenne JPh. Relations entre hypercapnie et hypoxémie des insuffisants respiratoires chroniques obstructifs (IRCO). Rev Mal Respir 1987; 4: 373.
9. Aubier M, Murciano D, Milic-Emili J et al. Effects of administration of O_2 on ventilation and blood gases in patients with chronic obstructive pulmonary disease during acute respiratory failure. Am Rev Respir Dis 1980; 122: 747.
10. Gibson GJ, ed. Blood disorders. In: Clinical tests of respiratory function. New York; Raven Press; 1984: 252.
11. Lahiri S. Historical perspectives of cellular oxygen sensing and responses to hypoxia. J Appl Physiol 2000; 88: 1467
12. Semenza GL. HIF-1: mediator of physiological and pathophysiological responses to hypoxia. J Appl Physiol 2000; 88: 1474
13. Denison DM, Ledwith F, Poulton EC. Complex reaction times at simulated cabin altitudes of 5,000 feet and 8,000 feet. Aerospace Med 1966; 37: 1010.
14. McSweeny AJ, Grant I, Heaton RK et al. Life quality of patients with chronic obstructive pulmonary disease. Arch Intern Med 1982; 142: 473.
15. Grant I, Heaton RK, McSweeny AJ et al. Neuropsychologic findings in hypoxemic chronic obstructive pulmonary disease. Arch Intern Med 1982; 142: 1470.
16. Krop HD, Block AJ, Cohen E. Neuropsychologic effects of continuous oxygen therapy in chronic obstructive pulmonary disease. Chest 1973; 64: 317.
17. Heaton RK, Grant I, McSweeny AJ et al. Psychologic effects of continuous and nocturnal oxygen therapy in hypoxemic chronic obstructive pulmonary disease. Arch Intern Med 1983; 143: 1941.
18. Continuous or nocturnal oxygen therapy in hypoxemic chronic obstructive lung disease. A clinical trial. Nocturnal Oxygen Therapy Trial group (NOTT). Ann Intern Med 1980; 93: 391.
19. Calverley PMA, Brezinova V, Douglas NJ et al. The effects of oxygenation on sleep quality in chronic bronchitis and emphysema. Am Rev Respir Dis 1982; 126: 206.
20. Fleetham J, West P, Mezon B et al. Sleep, arousals, and oxygen desaturation in chronic obstructive pulmonary disease. The effect of oxygen therapy. Am Rev Respir Dis 1982; 126: 429.
21. Douglas NJ. Sleep in patients with chronic obstructive pulmonary, disease. Clin Chest Med 1998; 19: 115
22. Brezinova V, Calverley PMA, Flenley DC, Townsend HRA. The effect of long-term oxygen therapy on the EEG in patients with chronic stable ventilatory failure. Bull Eur Physiopathol Respir 1979; 15: 603.
23. Appenzeller O, Parks RD, MacGee J. Peripheral neuropathy in chronic disease of the respiratory tract. Am J Med 1968; 44: 873.
24. Paramelle B, Vila A, Pollak P et al. Fréquence des polyneuropathies dans les bronchopneumopathies chroniques obstructives. Presse Méd 1986; 15: 563.
25. Malik RA, Masson EA, Sharma AK et al. Hypoxic neuropathy: relevance to human diabetic neuropathy. Diabetologia 1990; 33: 311.
26. Masson EA, Church SE, Woodcock AA et al. Is resistance to ischaemic conduction failure induced by hypoxia? Diabetologia 1988; 31: 762.
27. Hampton KK, Alani SM, Wilson JI, Price DE. Resistance to ischaemic conduction failure in chronic hypoxaemia and diabetes. J Neurol Neurosurg Psychiatry 1989; 52: 1303.
28. Low PA, Tuck RR, Dyck PJ et al. Prevention of some electrophysiologic and biochemical abnormalities with oxygen supplementation in experimental diabetic neuropathy. Proc Natl Acad Sci USA 1984; 81: 6894.
29. Stewart AG, Waterhouse JC, Howard P. Cardiovascular autonomic nerve function in patients with hypoxaemic chronic obstructive pulmonary disease. Eur Respir J 1991; 4: 1207.
30. Scalvini S Porta R Zanelli E et al. Effects of oxygen on autonomic nervous system dysfunction patients with chronic obstructive pulmonary disease. Eur Respir J 1999; 13: 119
31. Weitzenblum E, Schrijen F, Mohan-Kumar T et al. Variability of the pulmonary vascular response to acute hypoxia in chronic bronchitis. Chest 1988; 94: 772.
32. Bishop JM, Cross KW. Use of other physiological variables to predict pulmonary arterial pressure in patients with chronic respiratory disease. Eur Heart J 1981; 2: 509.
33. Weitzenblum E, Sautegeau A, Ehrhart M et al. Long-term course of pulmonary arterial pressure in chronic obstructive pulmonary disease. Am Rev Respir Dis 1984; 130: 993.
34. Reid LM. Structure and function in pulmonary hypertension. Chest 1986; 89: 279.
35. Weitzenblum E, Hirth C, Ducolone A et al. Prognostic value of pulmonary artery pressure in chronic obstructive pulmonary disease. Thorax 1981; 36: 752.
36. Ashutosh K, Dunsky M. Noninvasive tests for responsiveness of pulmonary hypertension to oxygen. Prediction of survival in patients with chronic obstructive lung disease and cor pulmonale. Chest 1987; 92: 393.
37. Sliwinski P, Hawrylkiewicz I, Gorecka D, Zielinski J. Acute effect of oxygen on pulmonary arterial pressure does not predict survival on long-term oxygen therapy in patients with chronic obstructive pulmonary disease. Am Rev Respir Dis 1992; 146: 665.
38. Selinger SR, Kennedy TP, Buescher P et al. Effects of removing oxygen from patients with chronic obstructive pulmonary disease. Am Rev Respir Dis 1987; 136: 85.

39. Weitzenblum E, Sautegeau A, Ehrhart M et al. Long-term oxygen therapy can reverse the progression of pulmonary hypertension in patients with chronic obstructive pulmonary disease. Am Rev Respir Dis 1985; 131: 493.

40. Medical Research Council Working Party (MRC Report). Long term domiciliary oxygen therapy in chronic hypoxic cor pulmonale complicating chronic bronchitis and emphysema. Lancet 1981; 1: 681.

41. Timms RM, Khaja FU, Williams GW and the Nocturnal Oxygen Therapy Trial Group. Hemodynamic response to oxygen therapy in chronic obstructive pulmonary disease. Ann Intern Med 1985; 102: 29.

42. Magee F, Wright JL, Wiggs BR et al. Pulmonary vascular structure and function in chronic obstructive pulmonary disease. Thorax 1988; 43: 183.

43. Andoh Y, Shimura S, Aikawa T et al. Perivascular fibrosis of muscular pulmonary arteries in chronic obstructive pulmonary disease. Chest 1992; 102: 1645.

44. Lane R, Cockcroft A, Adams L, Guz A. Arterial oxygen saturation and breathlessness in patients with chronic obstructive airway disease. Clin Sci 1987; 72: 693.

45. Swinbun CR, Mould H, Stone TN et al. Symptomatic benefit of supplemental oxygen in hypoxemic patients with chronic lung disease. Am Rev Respir Dis 1991; 143: 913.

46. Mannix ET, Manfredi F, Palange P et al. Oxygen may lower the O_2 cost of ventilation in chronic obstructive lung disease. Chest 1992; 101: 910.

47. Mak VHF, Bugler JR, Roberts CM, Spiro SG. Effect of arterial oxygen desaturation on six minute walk distance, perceived effort, and perceived breathlessness in patients with airflow limitation. Thorax 1993; 48: 33.

48. Lilker ES, Karnick A, Lerner L. Portable oxygen in chronic obstructive lung disease with hypoxemia and cor pulmonale. A controlled double-blind crossover study. Chest 1975; 68: 236.

49. Leggett RJE, Flenley DC. Portable oxygen and exercise tolerance in patients with chronic hypoxic cor pulmonale. Br Med J 1977; 2: 84.

50. Leach RM, Davidson AC, Chinn S et al. Portable liquid oxygen and exercise ability in severe respiratory disability. Thorax 1992; 47: 781.

51. Dean NC, Brown JK, Himelman RB et al. Oxygen may improve dyspnea and endurance in patients with chronic obstructive pulmonary disease and only mild hypoxemia. Am Rev Respir Dis 1992; 146: 941.

52. McKeon JL, Murree-Allen K, Saunders NA. Effects of breathing supplemental oxygen before progressive exercise in patients with chronic obstructive lung disease. Thorax 1988; 43: 53.

53. Stein DA, Bradley BL, Miller WC. Mechanisms of oxygen effects on exercise in patients with chronic obstructive pulmonary disease. Chest 1982; 81: 6.

54. Wilson DO, Rogers RM, Wright EC et al. Body weight in chronic obstructive pulmonary disease. Am Rev Respir Dis 1989; 139: 1435.

55. Schols AMWJ, Soeters PB, Mostert R et al. Energy balance in chronic obstructive pulmonary disease. Am Rev Respir Dis 1991; 143: 1248.

56. Schols AM, Wouters EF Nutritional abnormalities and supplementation in chronic obstructive pulmonary disease. Clin Chest Med 2000; 21: 753

57. Schols A, Mostert R, Cobben N et al. Transcutaneous oxygen saturation and carbon dioxide tension during meals in patients with chronic obstructive pulmonary disease. Chest 1991; 100: 1287.

58. Wuyam B, Payen JF, Lévy P et al. Metabolism and aerobic capacity of skeletal muscle in chronic respiratory failure related to chronic obstructive pulmonary disease. Eur Respir J 1992; 5: 157.

59. Skeletal muscle dysfunction in chronic obstructive pulmonary disease. A statement of the American Thoracic Society and European Respiratory Society. Am J Respir Crit Care Med 1999; 159: S1

60. Payen JF, Wuyam B, Lévy P et al. Muscular metabolism during oxygen supplementation in patients with chronic hypoxemia. Am Rev Respir Dis 1993; 147: 592.

61. Petty TL, ed. Long term outpatient oxygen therapy. In: Chronic obstructive pulmonary disease, lung biology in health and disease. New York: Marcel Dekker; 1985: 375.

62. Lahdensuo A, Ojanen M, Ahonen A et al. Psychosocial effects of continuous oxygen therapy in hypoxaemic chronic obstructive pulmonary disease patients. Eur Respir J 1989; 2: 977.

63. Bishop JM, Cross KW. Physiological variables and mortality in patients with various categories of chronic respiratory disease. Bull Eur Physiopathol Respir 1984; 20: 495.

64. Cooper CB, Waterhouse J, Howard P. Twelve year clinical study of patients with hypoxic cor pulmonale given long term domiciliary oxygen therapy. Thorax 1987; 42: 105.

65. Brambilla C, Rigaud D, Kuentz M et al. Oxygénothérapie de longue durée chez les malades hypoxémiques. Facteurs de pronostic. Bull Eur Physiopathol Respir 1982; 18: 253.

66. Calverley PMA, Leggett RJ, McElderry L, Flenley DC. Cigarette smoking and secondary polycythemia in hypoxic cor pulmonale. Am Rev Respir Dis 1982; 125: 507.

67. Levine BE, Bigelow DB, Hamstra RD et al. The role of long-term continuous oxygen administration in patients with chronic airway obstruction with hypoxemia. Ann Intern Med 1967; 66: 639.

68. Eckardt KU, Boutellier U, Kurtz A et al. Rate of erythropoietin formation in humans in response to acute hypobaric hypoxia. J Appl Physiol 1989; 66: 1785.

69. Wedzicha JA, Cotes PM, Empey DW et al Serum immunoreactive erythropoietin in hypoxic lung disease with and without polycythaemia. Clin Sci 1985; 69: 413.

70. Ström K, Odeberg H, Andersson AC et al. Erythropoietin levels decrease in patients with chronic hypoxia starting domiciliary oxygen therapy. Eur Respir J 1991; 4: 820.

71. Wedzicha JA, Cotter FE, Empey DW. Platelet size in patients with chronic airflow obstruction with and without hypoxaemia. Thorax 1988; 43: 61.

72. Johnson TS, Ellis JH Jr, Steele PP. Improvement of platelet survival time with oxygen in patients with chronic obstructive airway disease. Am Rev Respir Dis 1978; 117: 255.

73. Wedzicha JA, Syndercombe-Court D, Tan KC. Increased platelet aggregate formation in patients with chronic airflow obstruction and hypoxaemia. Thorax 1991; 46: 504.

74. Reihman DH, Farber MO, Weinberger MH et al. Effect of hypoxemia on sodium and water excretion in chronic obstructive lung disease. Am J Med 1985; 78: 87.

75. Mannix ET, Dowdeswell I, Carlone S et al. The effect of oxygen on sodium excretion in hypoxemic patients with chronic obstructive lung disease. Chest 1990; 97: 840.

76. Stewart A, Waterhouse J, Billings C, Howard P. Hormonal, renal and neural mechanisms in oedematous COPD (Part 1) ability to excrete a water load. Eur Respir J 1992; 5(Suppl. 15): 49S.

77. Stewart A, Waterhouse J, Billings C, Howard P. Hormonal, renal and neural mechanisms in oedematous COPD (Part 2). Ability to excrete a saline load. Eur Respir J 1992; 5(Suppl. 15): 50S.

78. Hasday JD, Grum CM. Nocturnal increase of urinary uric acid:creatinine ratio. A biochemical correlate of sleep-associated hypoxemia. Am Rev Respir Dis 1987; 135: 534.

79. Maillard D, Fleury B, Housset B et al. Decreased oxyhemoglobin affinity in patients with sleep apnea syndrome. Am Rev Respir Dis 1991; 143: 486.

80. Boysen PG, Block AJ, Wynne JW et al. Nocturnal pulmonary hypertension in patients with chronic obstructive pulmonary disease. Chest 1979; 76: 536.

81. Block AJ, Boysen PG, Wynne JW. The origins of cor pulmonale. A hypothesis. Chest 1979; 75: 109.

82. Fletcher EC, Donner CF, Midgren B et al. Survival in COPD patients with a daytime $P_aO_2 > 60$ mmHg with and without nocturnal oxyhemoglobin desaturation. Chest 1992; 101: 649.

83. Levi Valensi P, Aubry P, Rida Z. Nocturnal hypoxemia and long-term oxygen therapy in chronic obstructive pulmonary disease patients with a daytime P_aO_2 of 60–70 mmHg. Lung 1990; 168: S770.

84. Connaughton JJ, Catterall JR, Elton RA et al. Do sleep studies contribute to the management of patients with severe chronic obstructive pulmonary disease? Am Rev Respir Dis 1988; 138: 341.

85. Chaouat A Weitzenblum E Kessler R, et al. A randomized trial of nocturnal oxygen therapy in chronic obstructive pulmonary disease patients. Eur Respir J 1999; 14: 1002.

86. Flick MR, Block AJ. Nocturnal vs diurnal cardiac arrhythmias in patients with chronic obstructive pulmonary disease. Chest 1979; 75: 8.

87. Shepard JW, Garrison MW, Grither DA et al. Relationship of ventricular ectopy to nocturnal oxygen desaturation in patients with chronic obstructive pulmonary disease. Am J Med 1985; 78: 28.

88. Tirlapur VG, Mir MA. Nocturnal hypoxemia and associated electrocardiographic changes in patients with chronic obstructive airways disease. N Engl J Med 1982; 306: 125.

89. Shepard JW, Schweitzer PK, Keller CA et al. Myocardial stress. Exercise versus sleep in patients with COPD. Chest 1984; 86: 366.

90. Lévy PA, Guilleminault C, Fagret D et al. Changes in left ventricular ejection fraction during REM sleep and exercise in chronic obstructive pulmonary disease and sleep apnoea syndrome. Eur Respir J 1991; 4: 347.

91. Montplaisir J, Bédard MA, Richer F, Rouleau I. Neurobehavioral manifestations in obstructive sleep apnoea syndrome before and after treatment with continuous positive airway pressure. Sleep 1992; 15: S17.

92. Zwillich C, Devlin T, White D et al. Bradycardia during sleep apnoea, characteristics and mechanisms. J Clin Invest 1982; 69: 1286.

93. Narkiewicz K, van de Borne P, Cooley RL et al. Sympathetic activity in obese subjects with and without obstructive sleep apnea. Circulation 1998; 98: 772.

94. Peppard PE, Young T, Palta M, Skatrud J. Prospective study of the association between sleep-disordered breathing and hypertension. N Engl J Med 2000; 342: 1378

95. Veale D, Pépin JL, Lévy PA. Autonomic stress tests in obstructive sleep apnoea syndrome and snoring. Sleep 1992; 15: 505.

96. Carlson JT, Hedner JA, Sellgren J et al. Depressed baroreflex sensitivity in patients with obstructive sleep apnea. Am J Respir Crit Care Med 1996; 154: 1490.

97. Kraiczi H, Hedner J, Peker Y, Carlson J. Increased vasoconstrictor sensitivity in obstructive sleep apnea. J Appl Physiol 2000; 89: 493.

98. Adlakha A Shepard JW. Cardiac arrhythmias during normal sleep and in obstructive sleep apnea syndrome. Sleep Med Rev 1998;2: 45.

99. Coccagna G, Mantovani M, Brignani F et al. Continuous recording of the pulmonary and systemic arterial pressure during sleep in syndromes of hypersomnia with periodic breathing. Bull Eur Physiopathol Respir 1972; 8: 1159.

100. Weitzenblum E, Krieger J, Apprill M et al. Daytime pulmonary hypertension in patients with obstructive sleep apnea syndrome. Am Rev Respir Dis 1988; 138: 341.

101. Whyte KF, Douglas NJ. Peripheral edema in the sleep apnea/hypopnea syndrome. Sleep 1991; 14: 354.

102. Moloney ED, Kiely JL, McNicholas WT. Controlled oxygen therapy and carbon dioxide retention during exacerbations of chronic obstructive pulmonary disease. Lancet 2001; 357: 526.

103. Derenne JPh, Fleury B, Pariente R. Acute respiratory failure of chronic obstructive pulmonary disease. Am Rev Respir Dis 1988; 138: 1006.

104. Rawles JM, Kenmure ACF. Controlled trial of oxygen in uncomplicated myocardial infarction. Br Med J 1976; 1: 1121.

105. Chadha TS, Cohn MA. Noninvasive treatment of pneumothorax with oxygen inhalation. Respiration 1983; 44: 147.

106. Zierold D, Lee SL, Subramanian S, Dubois JJ. Supplemental oxygen improves resolution of injury-induced pneumothorax. J Pediatr Surg 2000; 35: 998.

107. Patel A, Kesler B. Wise RA. Persistent pneumomediastinum in interstitial fibrosis associated with rheumatoid arthritis: treatment with high-concentrations oxygen. Chest 2000; 117: 1809.

108. Ilano AL, Raffin TA. Management of carbon monoxide poisoning. Chest 1990; 97: 165.

109. Hawkins M, Harrison J, Charters P. Severe carbon monoxide poisoning: outcome after hyperbaric oxygen therapy. Br J Anaesth 2000; 84: 584.

110. Fairley BH. Oxygen therapy for surgical patients. Am Rev Respir Dis 1980; 122: S37.

111. Greif R, Akea O, Horn EP et al. Supplemental perioperative oxygen to reduce the incidence of surgical-wound infection. Outcomes research group. N Engl J Med 2000; 342: 161.

112. Horsman MR, Overgaard J. Overcoming tumour radiation resistance resulting from acute hypoxia. Eur J Cancer 1992; 28A: 717.

113. Siemann DW. Tissue oxygen manipulation and tumor blood flow. Int J Radiat Oncol Biol Phys 1992; 22: 393.

114. Zielinski J, Sliwinski P. Indications for and methods of long term oxygen therapy. Eur Respir Rev 1991; 1: 536.

115. Report of a SEP Task group. Recommendations for long term oxygen therapy (LTOT). Eur Respir J 1989; 2: 160.

116. Tarpy SP, Celli BR. Long-term oxygen therapy New Engl J Med 1995; 14: 710.

117. Levi-Valensi P, Weitzenblum E, Pedinielli JL et al. Three months follow-up of arterial blood gas determinations in candidates for long-term oxygen therapy. Am Rev Respir Dis 1986; 133: 547.

118. Oba Y, Salzman GA, Willsie SK. Reevaluation of continuous oxygen therapy after initial prescription in patients with chronic obstructive pulmonary disease. Respir Care 2000; 45: 401.

119. Standards for the diagnosis and care of patients with chronic obstructive pulmonary disease Am J Respir Crit Care Med 1995; 152: S77.

120. Plywaczewski R, Sliwinski P, Nowinski A et al. Incidence of nocturnal desaturation while breathing oxygen in COPD patients undergoing long-term oxygen therapy. Chest 2000; 117: 679.

121. Goldstein RS, Ramcharan V, Bowes G et al. Effect of supplemental nocturnal oxygen on gas exchange in patients with severe obstructive lung disease. N Engl J Med 1984; 310: 425.

122. Conference report. Further recommendations for prescribing and supplying long-term oxygen therapy. Am Rev Respir Dis 1988; 138: 745.

123. Veale D, Chailleux E Taytard A, Cardinaud JP. Characteristics and survival of patients prescribed long-term oxygen therapy outside prescription guidelines. Eur Respir J 1998; 12: 780.

124. Gorecka D, Gorzelak K, Sliwinski P, Tobiasz M, Zielinski J. Effect of long term oxygen therapy on survival in patients with chronic obstructive pulmonary disease with moderate hypoxaemia. Thorax 1997; 52: 674.

125. Zielinski J. Long term oxygen therapy in COPD patients with moderate hypoxaemia: does it add years to life? Eur Respir J 1998; 12: 756.

126. Clinical indications for Noninvasive Positive Pressure Ventilation in Chronic Respiratory Failure Due to Restrictive Lung Disease, COPD, and Nocturnal Hypoventilation-A Consensus conference report. Chest 1999; 116: 521.

127. Wedzicha JA. Long term oxygen therapy vs long-term ventilatory assistance. Respir Care 2000; 45: 178.

128. Meecham Jones DJ, Paul EA. Jones PW, Wedzicha JA. Nasal pressure support ventilation plus oxygen compared with oxygen therapy alone in hypercapnic COPD. Am J Respir Crit Care Med 1995; 152: 538.

129. Bruera E, De Stoutz N, Velasco-Leiva A, Schoeller T, Hanson J. Effects of oxygen on dyspnoea in hypoxaemic terminal-cancer patients. Lancet 1993; 342: 13.

130. Javaheri S, Corbett WS. Association of low P_aCO_2 with central sleep apnea and ventricular arrhythmias in ambulatory patients with stable heart failure. Ann Intern Med 1998; 128: 204–207.

131. Andreas S, Clemens C, Sandholzer Figulla HR Kreuzer H. Improvement of exercise capacity with treatment of Cheyne–Stokes respiration in patients with congestive heart failure. J Am Coll Cardiol 1996; 27: 1486.

132. Quaranta AJ, D'Alonzo GE, Krachman SL Cheyne–Stokes respiration during sleep in congestive heart failure. Chest 1997; 111: 467.

133. Krachman SL, D'Alonzo GE, Berger TJ, Eisen HJ. Comparison of oxygen therapy with nasal continuous positive airway pressure on Cheyne–Stokes respiration during sleep in congestive heart failure. Chest 1999; 116: 1550.

134. Staniforth AD, Kinnear WJ, Starling R et al. Effect of oxygen on sleep quality, cognitive function and sympathetic activity in patients with chronic heart failure and Cheyne–Stokes respiration. Eur Heart J 1998; 19: 922.

135. Donner CF, Braghiroli A, Patessio A. Can long-term oxygen therapy improve exercise capacity and prognosis? Respiration 1992; 59(Suppl. 2): 30.

136. Lock SH, Paul EA, Rudd RM, Wedzicha JA. Portable oxygen therapy: assessment and usage. Respir Med 1991; 85: 407.

137. McDonald CE, Blyth CM, Lazarus MD et al. Exertional oxygen of limited benefit in patients with chronic obstructive pulmonary disease and mild hypoxemia. Am J Respir Crit Care Med 1995; 152: 1616.

138. Garrod R, Paul EA, Wedzicha JA. Supplemental oxygen during pulmonary rehabilitation in patients with COPD with exercise hypoxaemia. Thorax 2000; 55: 539.

139. Killen JWW, Corris PA. A pragmatic assessment of the placement of oxygen when given for exercise induced dyspnoea. Thorax 2000, 55: 544.

140. Calverle PMA. Supplementary oxygen therapy in COPD: is it really useful? Thorax 2000; 55: 537.

141. Working group on oxygen therapy of IUATLD: Howard P, De Haller R. Domiciliary oxygen – by liquid or concentrator? Eur Respir J 1991; 4: 1284.

142. Vergeret J, Brambilla C, Mounier L. Portable oxygen therapy: use and benefit in hypoxaemic COPD patients on long-term oxygen therapy. Eur Respir J 1989; 2: 20.

143. Dilworth JP, Higgs CMB, Jones PA, White RJ. Prescription of oxygen concentrators: adherence to published guidelines. Thorax 1989; 44: 576.

144. Jones MM, Harvey JE, Tattersfield AE. How patients use domiciliary oxygen. Br Med J 1978; 1: 1397.

145. Evans TW, Waterhouse JC, Howard P. Clinical experience with the oxygen concentrator. Br Med J 1983; 287: 459.

146. Vergeret J, Tunon de Lara M, Douvier JJ et al. Compliance of COPD patients with long term oxygen therapy. Eur J Respir Dis 1986; 69: 421.

147. Desrue B, Lecoq C et l'association d'aide aux insuffisants respiratoires de Bretagne. Prescription et observance de l'oxygenotherapie. Rev Mal Respir 1989; 6: 237.

148. Walshaw MJ, Lim R, Evans CC, Hind CRK. Prescription of oxygen concentrators for long term treatment: reassessment in one district. Br Med J 1988; 297: 1030.

149. Walshaw MJ, Lim R, Evans CC, Hind CRK. Factors influencing the compliance of patients using oxygen concentrators for long-term home oxygen therapy. Respir Med 1990; 84: 331.

150. Howard P, Waterhouse JC, Billings CG. Compliance with longterm oxygen therapy by concentrator. Eur Respir J 1992; 5: 128.

151. Pépin JL, Barjhoux CE, Deschaux C, Brambilla C. Long-term oxygen therapy at home. Compliance with medical prescription and effective use of therapy. Chest 1996; 109: 1144.

152. Bongard JP, Pahud C, De Haller R. Insufficient oxygen concentration obtained at domiciliary controls of eighteen concentrators. Eur Respir J 1989; 2: 280.

153. Sous-Commission Technique ANTADIR. Home controls of a sample of 2,414 oxygen concentrators. Eur Respir J 1991; 4: 227.

154. O'Donohue WJ. Effect of oxygen therapy on increasing arterial oxygen tension in hypoxemic patients with stable chronic obstructive pulmonary disease while breathing ambient air. Chest 1991; 100: 968.

155. O'Donohue WJ Plummer AL. Magnitude of usage and costs of home oxygen therapy in the United States. Chest 1995; 107: 301.

156. Pelletier-Fleury N, Lanoe JL, Fleury B, Fardeau M. The cost of treating COPD patients with long-term oxygen therapy in a French population. Chest 1996 110: 411.

157. Guyatt GH, McKim DA, Austin P, et al. Appropriateness of domiciliary oxygen delivery. Chest 2000; 118: 1303.

158. Schaannin J, Strom K, Boe J. Do patients using long-term liquid oxygen differ from those traditional treatment with oxygen concentrators and/or common gas cylinders ? A comparison of two national registers. Respir Med 1998; 92: 84.

159. Andersson A, Strom K, Brodin H, et al. Domiciliary liquid oxygen versus concentrator treatment in hypoxaemia: a cost-utility analysis. Eur Respir J 1998; 12: 1284.

160. Stewart AG, Howard P. Devices for low flow O_2 administration. Eur Respir J 1990; 3: 812.

161. Bazuaye EA, Stone TN, Corris PA, Gibson GJ. Variability of inspired oxygen concentration with nasal cannulas. Thorax 1992; 47: 609.

162. Davies RJO, Hopkin JM. Nasal oxygen in exacerbations of ventilatory failure: an underappreciated risk. Br Med J 1989; 299: 43.

163. Collard Ph, Wautelet F, Delwiche JP et al. Improvement of oxygen delivery in severe hypoxaemia by a reservoir cannula. Eur Respir J 1989; 2: 778.

164. Gould GA, Forsyth IS, Flenley DC. Comparison of two oxygen conserving nasal prong systems and the effects of nose and mouth breathing. Thorax 1986; 41: 808.

165. Tiep BL, Nicotra B, Carter R et al. Evaluation of a low-flow oxygen-conserving nasal cannula. Am Rev Respir Dis 1984; 130: 500.

166. Moore-Gillon JC, George RDJ, Geddes DM. An oxygen conserving nasal cannula. Thorax 1985; 40: 817.

167. Gould GA, Hayhurst MD, Scott W, Flenley DC. Clinical assessment of oxygen conserving devices in chronic bronchitis and emphysema. Thorax 1985; 40: 820.

168. Bower JS, Brook CJ, Zimmer K, Davis D. Performance of a demand oxygen saver system during rest, exercise, and sleep in hypoxemic patients. Chest 1988; 94: 77.

169. Senn S, Wanger J, Fernandez E, Cherniack RM. Efficacy of a pulsed oxygen delivery device during exercise in patients with chronic respiratory disease. Chest 1989; 96: 467.

170. Cuvelier A, Muir JF, Czernichow P, et al. Nocturnal efficiency and tolerance of a demand oxygen delivery system in COPD patients with nocturnal hypoxemia. Chest 1999; 116: 22.

171. Commission médico-technique ANTADIR: Segard B, Muir JF, Bedicam JM, Defouilloy C, Sautegeau A. Qualité de l'oxygénothérapie délivrée avec les valves économiseuses d'oxygéne. Une étude multicentrique. Rev Mal Respir 1992; 9: 197.

172. Hoffman LA, Johnson JT, Wesmiller SW et al. Transtracheal delivery of oxygen: efficacy and safety for long-term continuous therapy. Ann Otol Rhinol Laryngol 1991; 100: 108.

173. Orvidas LJ, Kasperbauer JL, Staats BA, Olsen KD. Long-term clinical experience with transtracheal oxygen catheter. Mayo Clin Proc 1998; 73: 739.

174. Harrow EM, Oldenburg FA, Ligenfelter MS, Leonard J. Respiratory failure and cor pulmonale associated with tracheal mucoid accumulation from a SCOOP transtracheal oxygen catheter. Chest 1992; 101: 580.

175. Couser JI, Make BJ. Transtracheal oxygen decreases inspired minute ventilation. Am Rev Respir Dis 1989; 139: 627.

176. Hoffman LA, Wesmiller SW, Sciurba FC et al. Nasal cannula and transtracheal oxygen delivery. Am Rev Respir Dis 1992; 145: 827.

177. Pendleton N, Cheesbrough JS, Walshaw MJ, Hind CRK. Bacterial colonisation of humidifier attachments on oxygen concentrators prescribed for long term oxygen therapy: a district review. Thorax 1992; 46: 257.

178. Liss HP, Payne CP. Stability of blood gases in ice and at room temperature. Chest 1993; 103: 1120.

179. Hess C, Nichols A, Hunt W, Suratt P. Pseudohypoxemia secondary to leukemia and thrombocytosis. N Engl J Med 1979; 301: 361.

180. Nickerson BG, Sarkisian C, Tremper K. Bias and precision of pulse oximeters and arterial oximeters. Chest 1988; 93: 515.

181. Hannhart B, Michalski H, Delorme N et al. Reliability of six pulse oximeters in chronic obstructive pulmonary disease. Chest 1991; 99: 842.

182. Warley ARH, Mitchell JH, Stradling JR. Evaluation of the Ohmeda 3700 pulse oximeter. Thorax 1987; 42: 892.

183. Ries AL, Prewitt LM, Johnson JJ. Skin color and ear oximetry. Chest 1989; 96: 287.

184. Govaert P, Vanhaesebrouk P, De Praeter C, De Baets F. Pulse oximetry and methaemoglobinaemia. Lancet 1988; 1: 517.

185. Carlin BW, Clausen JL, Ries AL. The use of cutaneous oximetry in the prescription of long-term oxygen therapy. Chest 1988; 94: 239.

186. Williams A, Santiago S, Stein M. Screening for sleep apnea? Chest 1989; 96: 451.

187. George CF, Millar TW, Kryger MH. Identification and quantification of apneas by computer-based analysis of oxygen saturation. Am Rev Respir Dis 1988; 137: 1238.

188. Levy P, Pepin JL, Deschaux-Blanc C et al. Accuracy of oximetry for detection of respiratory disturbances in sleep apnea syndrome. Chest, 1996; 109: 395–9.

189. Hansen JE, Casaburi R. Validity of ear oximetry in clinical exercise testing. Chest 1987; 91: 333.

190. Escourrou PJL, Delaperche MF, Visseaux A. Reliability of pulse oximetry during exercise in pulmonary patients. Chest 1990; 97: 635.

191. Clark JS, Votteri B, Ariagno RL et al. Non invasive assessment of blood gases. Am Rev Respir Dis 1992; 145: 220.

14 Respiratory intensive care

Spyros G Zakynthinos and Charis S Roussos

Key points

- As well as the two classical types of respiratory failure (type I, acute hypoxaemic, and type II, ventilatory failure), two further variants have been described: type III (perioperative, due to atelectasis) and type IV (circulatory, as in shock).

- In type I respiratory failure (e.g. acute respiratory distress syndrome) the aim of ventilatory management is to improve oxygenation and avoid ventilator-associated injury by limiting positive end-expiratory pressure (PEEP) and tidal volume within bounds set by the pressure–volume curve of the respiratory system ('open-lung ventilation'), even at the cost of hypercapnia ('permissive hypercapnia').

- If, in acute-on-chronic respiratory failure, invasive ventilation becomes unavoidable, it should approximate the natural pattern of breathing of such patients in order to avoid overventilation and dangerous alkalaemia.

- In acute severe asthma ventilatory support requires high pressures, with a risk of barotrauma, and excessive ventilation may worsen hyperinflation.

- Weaning from ventilatory support requires a systematic approach to reverse the factors that led to the need for ventilation.

Respiratory intensive care is relevant to the management and the overall care of patients with acute or acute-on-chronic respiratory failure. Respiratory failure is defined conventionally as the condition in which the arterial P_{O_2} (P_aO_2) is less than 60 mmHg (8 kPa), the arterial P_{CO_2} (P_aCO_2) is higher than 45 mmHg (6 kPa), or both. However, as these cut-off values are not rigid, serving rather as a guide in combination with the history and clinical assessment of the patient, respiratory failure could be defined generally as the condition in which the patient loses the ability to provide sufficient oxygen to the blood and systemic organs and/or to ventilate

adequately. Resuscitation of the patient with acute respiratory failure requires urgent airway control, ventilator management and stabilisation of the circulation; on-going care necessitates a differential diagnosis and therapeutic plan derived from an informed clinical and laboratory examination supplemented by the results of special intensive care unit (ICU) interventions, such as right heart catheterisation.[1]

The purpose of this chapter is to review the pathophysiology and the basis for diagnosis and management of acute respiratory failure requiring intensive care, together with the principles of ventilator management and respiratory system monitoring during invasive mechanical ventilation.

Respiratory failure

Types of respiratory failure

According to Wood,[2] four types of respiratory failure with different patterns of pathophysiology can be diagnosed in patients requiring mechanical ventilation for respiratory failure. Each has a predominant mechanism, i.e. increased intrapulmonary shunt $\dot{Q}_S/\dot{Q}_T$ in type I (*acute hypoxaemic*) respiratory failure, decreased alveolar ventilation ($\dot{V}_A$) in type II (*ventilatory*) respiratory failure, atelectasis in type III (*perioperative*) respiratory failure and hypoperfusion in type IV (*shock*) respiratory failure.

Hypoxaemic versus ventilatory failure

These two are the classical and most common types of respiratory failure. In acute hypoxaemic (type I) respiratory failure (AHRF), increased $\dot{Q}_S/\dot{Q}_T$ due to lung air space flooding or collapse causes hypoxaemia refractory to oxygen therapy despite hyperventilation and reduced P_aCO_2. In hypoventilatory respiratory failure, also called ventilatory failure, primary failure of alveolar ventilation caused by decreased respiratory drive, mechanical defect of the respiratory system or respiratory muscle fatigue,[3] leads to CO_2

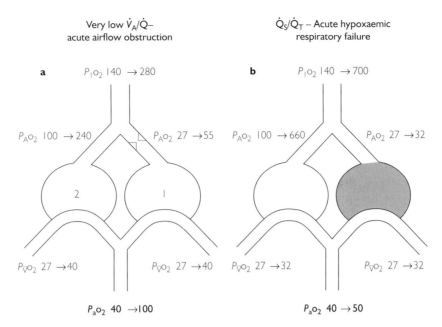

Fig. 14.1 Contrasting effects of oxygen therapy on arterial P_{O_2}: (a) acute airflow obstruction and (b) air-space 'flooding' as in acute hypoxaemic respiratory failure. Each panel depicts a two-compartment lung with perfusing mixed venous P_{O_2} ($P_{\bar{v}O_2}$) of 27 mmHg breathing room air. (a) Because the air space distal to the obstruction is so poorly ventilated, all its inspired oxygen is absorbed and its alveolar P_{O_2} ($P_{A}O_2$) approaches $P_{\bar{v}O_2}$ (27 mmHg). When blood from the well-ventilated alveolus (which is fully saturated) mixes with an equal amount of blood from the obstructed unit (S_{O_2} = 50%), the resulting arterial blood ($S_{a}O_2$ = 75%) has a very low P_{O_2} (40 mmHg). Raising $F_{I}O_2$ to 0.4 (i.e. $P_{I}O_2$ = 280 mmHg) increases the $P_{A}O_2$ of the obstructed unit to 55 mmHg (approximately 90% saturated). Mixture of blood from the two units now produces $S_{a}O_2$ approaching 100% and $P_{a}O_2$ approaching 100 mmHg. Note that mixed venous P_{O_2} has also increased (27→40 mmHg). (b) During room air breathing, conditions are similar to (a). Raising $F_{I}O_2$ to 1.0 increases the dissolved oxygen in the blood from the well-ventilated alveolus by about 2 ml/dl but oxygen is still not absorbed from the flooded air space. Accordingly, $P_{a}O_2$ (from 40 to 50 mmHg) and $P_{\bar{v}O_2}$ (from 27 to 32 mmHg) increase only slightly. (Redrawn with permission from Wood[2].) [7.5 mmHg = 1 kPa]

retention and arterial hypercapnia associated with reduced $P_{a}O_2$; this hypoxaemia is easily corrected with oxygen therapy.

Causes and pulmonary gas exchange abnormalities

The causes of AHRF include cardiogenic or permeability pulmonary oedema, pneumonia or lung haemorrhage. In these diseases, even an inspired oxygen fraction ($F_{I}O_2$) of 1.0 cannot correct the hypoxaemia (Fig. 14.1); this refractory hypoxaemia is often associated with increased total ($\dot{V}_{E}$) and alveolar ventilation and, therefore, decreased $P_{a}CO_2$.[2,4] However, as the underlying condition persists or progresses, fatigue of the respiratory muscles may develop, leading to decrease in $\dot{V}_{A}$ and increase in $P_{a}CO_2$. Respiratory muscle fatigue results from the increased load imposed on the respiratory muscles during spontaneous breathing, combined with tachypnoea, hypoxaemia and acidosis.

When there is either central nervous system (CNS) depression of the drive to breathe or a mechanical defect of the respiratory system (e.g. flail chest, Guillain–Barré syndrome, myopathies), $\dot{V}_{E}$ and $\dot{V}_{A}$ decrease, raising the alveolar and arterial P_{CO_2}. (Since $P_{a}CO_2 = k \times \dot{V}_{CO_2}/\dot{V}_{A}$, where $\dot{V}_{CO_2}$ is the rate of CO_2 production, and k is a constant of proportionality.) Mild alveolar hypoxia develops as the required oxygen uptake ($\dot{V}_{O_2}$) is absorbed from the reduced $\dot{V}_{A}$, so the consequent arterial hypoxaemia can be corrected with small increases in $F_{I}O_2$. In asthma or restrictive lung diseases, the ratio of physiological dead space to tidal volume

(V_{D}/V_{T}) is increased because large numbers of poorly perfused alveoli are ventilated excessively (high $\dot{V}_{A}/\dot{Q}$ units). Accordingly, the patient would have a decreased $\dot{V}_{A}$ were $\dot{V}_{E}$ to remain normal. However, $\dot{V}_{E}$ usually increases in these patients, resulting in increased $\dot{V}_{A}$ and low $P_{a}CO_2$. Alveolar hypoventilation and increase in $P_{a}CO_2$ may develop when the inspiratory muscles become unable to sustain the increased $\dot{V}_{E}$ because of fatigue. Hypoxaemia develops when other alveoli are poorly ventilated in relation to their perfusion (low $\dot{V}_{A}/\dot{Q}$ units), and the hypoxaemia is made worse by low mixed venous oxygen content;[4,5] again, modest increments in $F_{I}O_2$ correct this hypoxaemia (Fig. 14.1).

Treatment goals

The goals of supportive therapy for types I and II respiratory failure are quite different. Therapy for patients with type I failure has four objectives:[6]

- stabilisation of the patient on the ventilator with minimal respiratory work
- ventilation with the least tidal volume providing adequate CO_2 elimination[7]
- addition of the least amount of positive end-expiratory pressure (PEEP) to prevent expiratory collapse of recruited alveoli while attaining oxygen saturation ($S_{a}O_2$) of over 90% with an adequate circulating haemoglobin and a non-toxic $F_{I}O_2$[8,9]

- cardiovascular management to reduce air space oedema by seeking the lowest pulmonary vascular pressures compatible with an adequate cardiac output and oxygen transport to the peripheral tissues[10] (see below and Chapter 28).

Each of these management goals with type I failure differs from those with type II (ventilatory) failure: patients with depressed CNS drive or a mechanically deranged respiratory system require adequate ventilation and minimal oxygen with careful attention to preventing atelectasis and correcting hypoperfusion until the abnormal condition resolves; patients who require ventilation for airflow obstruction are supported with bronchodilator therapy and ventilator settings that minimise intrinsic PEEP (PEEPi) until the airway resistance is reduced sufficiently for the respiratory muscles to achieve adequate spontaneous ventilation off the ventilator (see below).

Perioperative respiratory failure

In the perioperative period many patients develop type III or perioperative respiratory failure with atelectasis as the primary causative mechanism.[11] In general, abnormal abdominal mechanics reduce the end-expired lung volume (FRC) below the increased closing volume in these patients, which leads to progressive collapse of dependent lung units.[11] The end result frequently is type I AHRF.

The identification of atelectasis as a distinct mechanism leading to this type of respiratory failure draws attention to the need to prevent lung collapse by reducing the adverse effects of common clinical circumstances promoting reduction in FRC and of the conditions that promote abnormal airway closure at increased lung volume. Because many of these mechanisms also occur in patients with type I or type II respiratory failure, implementation of approaches to minimise atelectasis should be a part of the management of all patients with respiratory failure.[6] The relevant principles are:[6]

- turning the patient from supine to the lateral decubitus position every 1–2 h, accompanied by vigorous chest physiotherapy and endotracheal suction
- the 30–45° upright position helps by reducing the load imposed by the abdomen
- the addition of sighs, continuous positive airway pressure (CPAP) or PEEP returns the end-expired lung volume to a position above the patient's closing volume
- special attention should also be given to treating incisional or abdominal pain (e.g. epidural anaesthesia), and to minimising intra-abdominal pressure (e.g. from ascites or tight bandages).

Hypoperfusion states causing type IV respiratory failure

Several mechanically ventilated patients do not fit the categories of type I, II or III respiratory failure,[6] in particular those who have been intubated and stabilised with ventilatory support during a hypoperfusion state. Thus, type IV respiratory failure is most commonly due to cardiogenic, hypovolaemic or septic shock without associated pulmonary problems.[12] The rationale for ventilator therapy in these patients, who are frequently tachypnoeic, is to stabilise gas exchange and minimise the 'steal' of limited cardiac output by the working respiratory muscles until the mechanism for the hypoperfusion state is identified and corrected.[3,12] Weaning from the ventilator of the patient with type IV respiratory failure is simple: when shock is corrected, the patient resumes spontaneous breathing and is extubated. Furthermore, when patients with type I, II or III respiratory failure suffer a concurrent hypoperfusion state, the causes of reduced blood flow must be identified and corrected as part of the weaning process.[6]

Acute hypoxaemic respiratory failure

Type 1 or acute hypoxaemic respiratory failure arises from diseases causing collapse or filling of alveoli (or both), with the result that a substantial fraction of mixed venous blood traverses non-ventilated air spaces, completing a right-to-left intrapulmonary shunt[13] (Fig. 14.1). In addition to the adverse consequences on gas exchange, interstitial and alveolar fluid accumulation causes an increase in lung stiffness, imposing a mechanical inspiratory load and increased work of breathing.[14] Uncorrected, the gas exchange and lung mechanical abnormalities may eventually cause tissue hypoxia, respiratory arrest and death.

The disorders causing AHRF may be divided into diffuse conditions, such as pulmonary oedema, and focal lung lesions, such as lobar pneumonia (Table 14.1). As discussed elsewhere (Chapter 2.6), lung liquid flux is determined by the conductance of the pulmonary microcirculation and the accompanying driving pressure. Accordingly, excessive lung liquid accumulation may arise from hydrostatic pressure increases, leading to cardiogenic or increased-pressure oedema (see Chapter 77.1), or from lung injury that causes an increase in conductance and a failure of the microcirculation to maintain an oncotic pressure gradient between the intravascular and interstitial spaces, which causes increased-permeability oedema or the acute (formerly adult) respiratory distress syndrome (ARDS; see Chapter 28).

The general management of the relevant conditions is covered elsewhere and the focus here is on the principles of management of these diseases in the ICU.

Management of cardiogenic pulmonary oedema

The management of cardiogenic pulmonary oedema overlaps considerably with management of left ventricular systolic and diastolic dysfunction. Most patients respond dramatically to pharmacological interventions, and mechanical ventilatory support typically is not required. Nevertheless, on presentation hypoxaemia may be severe and, as with other causes of AHRF, is minimally responsive to oxygen therapy. As many as one-third of patients with cardiogenic pulmonary oedema have modest elevations of P_aCO_2 despite obvious increased respiratory drive and before receiving narcotic drugs.[15] These patients need increased pressure and energy to ventilate the respiratory system because of stiff lungs and excessive dead space ventilation; energy demands are further increased by 'cardiac asthma', which is associated with airway obstruction, gas

Table 14.1 Causes of acute hypoxaemic respiratory failure

Homogenous lung lesions

Cardiogenic or increased-pressure pulmonary oedema
- Left-ventricular (LV) failure
- Acute LV ischaemia
- Accelerated or malignant hypertension
- Mitral regurgitation
- Mitral stenosis
- Ball-valve thrombus
- Volume overload, particularly with coexisting renal and cardiac disease

Increased permeability or low-pressure pulmonary oedema (acute respiratory distress syndrome)
- More common
  - Sepsis and sepsis syndrome
  - Acid aspiration
  - Multiple transfusions for hypovolaemic shock
- Less common
  - Near-drowning
  - Pancreatitis
  - Air or fat emboli
  - Cardiopulmonary bypass
  - Pneumonia
  - Drug reaction or overdose
  - Leukoagglutination
  - Inhalation injury

Pulmonary oedema of unclear or 'mixed' origin
- Reexpansion
- Neurogenic

Diffuse alveolar haemorrhage
- Microscopic angiitis
- Collagen vascular diseases
- Goodpasture's syndrome
- Severe coagulopathy

Focal lung lesions

Lobar pneumonia

Lung contusion

trapping and dynamic hyperinflation. Coexisting hypoxaemia and inadequate cardiac output may diminish the energy supply to the respiratory muscles. This imbalance between the energy supplies and demands of the respiratory muscles may lead to fatigue, alveolar hypoventilation and hypercapnia.

Pharmacological therapy

The primary goal of pharmacological therapy is to reduce the left atrial and pulmonary vascular pressures that are responsible for the pulmonary oedema; this ultimately improves oxygenation and reduces the work of breathing. Reduction in left ventricular preload is achieved with drugs that either translocate central blood volume to a peripheral compartment (morphine, nitrates) or achieve net diuresis (furosemide/frusemide) or both. Because ventricular systolic function is often impaired, inotropic support (dobutamine) and afterload reduction (lowering of systemic blood pressure by treating anxiety, e.g. with morphine, or by specific antihypertensive therapy) are usually required as well.[16]

Positive-pressure ventilation

Most patients respond rapidly to pharmacological agents and do not need mechanical ventilatory support. If improvement is noted but the patient remains in significant respiratory distress with or without hypoxaemia, early consideration should be given to non-invasive positive-pressure ventilation (see Chapter 15), which improves gas exchange, reduces the work of breathing, relieves dyspnoea, reduces ventricular afterload and improves outcome in patients with ventricular dysfunction and cardiogenic pulmonary oedema.[17,18] It is likely that its benefits derive from avoidance of endotracheal intubation and its associated complications. Non-invasive ventilation should begin at low levels of inspiratory and expiratory pressures (e.g. 5 cmH$_2$O). Some systems provide CPAP throughout the respiratory cycle whereas others permit selection of independent inspiratory and expiratory pressure levels. Increasing expiratory pressure benefits gas exchange primarily, whereas increasing inspiratory pressure increases the tidal volume delivered for a given patient effort, thus reducing the work of breathing.

Patients who present with shock, who develop significant hypotension during the course of therapy or who fail to tolerate non-invasive ventilation should be considered for endotracheal intubation and mechanical ventilation.[13] Invasive mechanical ventilation (i.e. institution of mechanical ventilation via an endotracheal tube) offers similar benefits (e.g. reduced work of breathing, diminished oxygen consumption, reduction of left ventricular afterload) but has the risks of intubation. PEEP should be applied and titrated against arterial saturation to permit a reduction in the F_1O_2 to 0.6 or less. PEEP has fewer adverse effects on venous return when the circulatory volume is increased, as in cardiogenic oedema, and it tends to reduce both left ventricular preload and afterload.[19]

Management of acute respiratory distress syndrome

Pharmacological therapy

Supportive management of ARDS is inadequate unless accompanied by diagnosis and aggressive treatment of the predisposing condition or conditions (Table 14.1). Some causes of ARDS tend to have a generally benign course. These include pulmonary oedema associated with opiates or air emboli, which often responds to supplemental oxygen and diuresis alone. When mechanical ventilation is required, it is usually for a brief period. As the sequence of cellular and biochemical events resulting in acute lung injury has been described in increasing detail, a number of pharmacological interventions to interrupt these pathways (corticosteroids, eicosanoids, ketoconazole, surfactant) have been proposed.[20] Unfortunately, none has proved beneficial.[21]

Supportive therapy: circulatory management

The management of ARDS relies on supportive therapy while underlying diseases are diagnosed and treated. Most patients with ARDS do not die during the early phase of disease as a consequence of severe hypoxaemia, but rather days to weeks later, frequently with evidence of hypermetabolism, nosocomial infection and multiple organ failure.[20] The best strategy to minimise oedema production and lessen its adverse effects is by aggressive reduction in ventricular preload without decreasing cardiac output. Reduction of circulating volume can improve lung function but hypoperfusion and other organ failure may occur, since it is difficult to balance low pulmonary vascular pressure against an adequate cardiac output and oxygen delivery. Right heart catheterisation and measurement of the pulmonary capillary wedge pressure (PCWP) are helpful and should be accompanied by close monitoring of organ function, as in all critically ill patients (e.g. mental status, urine output, circulatory adequacy, metabolic evidence of anaerobic metabolism).

Supportive therapy: ventilatory management

Ventilatory management of patients with ARDS has recently been considered following experimental and clinical studies. Early observation showed that mechanical ventilation using large tidal volumes and high inflation pressures could cause fatal lung injury in animals with otherwise normal lungs.[22] The term *ventilator-induced lung injury* has been applied to acute lung injury induced directly by mechanical ventilation in animal models. This condition is indistinguishable morphologically, physiologically and radiologically from diffuse alveolar damage resulting from other causes of acute lung injury. *Ventilator-associated lung injury* is defined as lung injury resembling ARDS that occurs in patients receiving mechanical ventilation. It is associated with pre-existing lung pathology such as ARDS.

Animal experiments exploring the precise mechanisms of ventilation-induced lung injury demonstrated that it appears to be related to the distending volume to which the lung is subjected rather than to the distending pressure.[23] Such observations have created the term *volutrauma*, which differs from the older term *barotrauma* applied to the grosser forms of extra-alveolar air collection that are observed on routine radiographs in patients undergoing mechanical ventilation. In addition to the detrimental effects of overdistension, many investigations have suggested a protective effect of PEEP against ventilator-induced lung injury.[23] This effect may be related to the ability of PEEP to maintain recruitment of collapsed and flooded alveoli, thereby avoiding cyclical recruitment–derecruitment with each breath delivered, a mechanical event thought to lead to shear injuries to terminal airways and alveoli.[23]

The events of alveolar recruitment and alveolar overdistension have been related to the pressure–volume relationships of the respiratory system during inflation (Fig. 14.2). Both in animal models of lung injury and in patients with early ARDS, the respiratory system inflation pressure–volume curve has a sigmoid shape, with both lower and upper inflection points[24] (Fig. 14.2). The lower inflection (about 13 cmH$_2$O) seems to represent the point where massive alveolar recruitment occurs during inflation, while the upper point (about 30 cmH$_2$O) is taken to represent alveolar overdistension with its attendant risks of alveolar injury. These mechanical events – cyclical alveolar recruitment–derecruitment and overdistension – not only have the potential for direct lung injury but also may initiate a series of inflammatory events with widespread consequences. Several studies have shown that the serum and bronchoalveolar lavage profile of cytokines and other mediators of inflammation may be altered by ventilator strategies that result in alveolar overdistension or recruitment–derecruitment. The clinical sig-

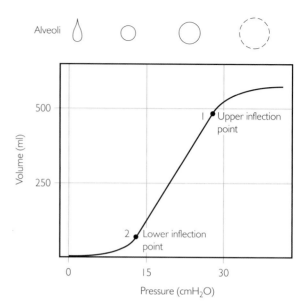

Fig. 14.2 Schematic sigmoid pressure–volume curve of the respiratory system in a patient with acute respiratory distress syndrome, with (top) the relative degree of alveolar inflation. At airway pressures greater than the upper inflection point, 1 (c. 30 cmH$_2$O), the curve flattens as the limits of lung compliance are reached. Airway pressures below the lower inflection point, 2 (c. 13 cmH$_2$O) are also associated with lower compliance and result in alveolar collapse.

nificance of such biochemical markers of inflammation remains to be determined but the linkage of mechanical events during ventilatory support to inflammation could provide an explanation for the evolution of the multisystem organ failure so commonly observed in patients with ARDS.[25,26]

On the basis of the accumulating information from animal and, recently, clinical studies of ventilator-associated lung injury,[7,26] recommendations have been made to select levels of PEEP and tidal volume that maintain the respiratory system between the pressure–volume inflection points, i.e. PEEP level about 2 cmH$_2$O above the lower point and tidal volume sufficiently low (6 ml/kg of predicted body weight) to maintain inflation below the upper point at the end of each inspiration. This strategy has been termed *open-lung ventilation* and it has been recommended that these end-points of ventilation should be used even at the cost of resulting hypercapnia (permissive hypercapnia).

Additional innovative therapies for ARDS include prone positioning, tracheal gas insufflation, high-frequency ventilation, inverse ratio ventilation, extracorporeal gas exchange, partial liquid ventilation, and inhaled nitric oxide (see Chapter 28).

Management of focal lung conditions producing type I respiratory failure

Lobar pneumonia

Pneumonias, even those involving only a modest fraction of the lung volume, can produce significant shunting of blood because of the increase in pulmonary blood flow and aerobic metabolism of the consolidated region.[27] Accordingly, supplemental oxygen often has only a minor effect in resolving the associated hypoxaemia but it may correct arterial desaturation caused by hypoventilation of lung regions mechanically interdependent with the pneumonic consolidation.[13]

The guidelines for ventilator management are similar to those for patients with ARDS. However, PEEP therapy should be added cautiously and should be guided by pulse oximetry. This is particularly true in these patients with focal disease because PEEP may not recruit the consolidated lung but rather hyper-inflate normal lung, redistributing blood flow to the area of con-solidation and worsening intrapulmonary shunt. Nevertheless, a trial of PEEP is warranted in most patients because varying degrees of lung oedema may be present in regions distant from the radiographically apparent pneumonia. If the patient cannot be adequately oxygenated using PEEP, positioning with the healthier lung downward may help. This manoeuvre increases blood flow to normally ventilated lung regions and improves gas exchange. In those patients with substantial airway secretions, such positioning carries the risk of infecting the normal lung; hence airway toilet is of paramount importance.

Lung contusion

Blunt chest trauma, particularly when sufficient to cause rib frac-tures, often contuses the underlying lung. The contusion essen-tially stops blood flow to the consolidated hemorrhagic region, probably by mechanical distortion or obliteration of the vessels. As a result, the shunt in pulmonary contusion is very small but the hypoxia can be quite profound because of the mechanical interdependence of the contused regions with the surrounding lung units, which consequently have low $\dot{V}_A/\dot{Q}$ ratios. This situa-tion is relevant to oxygen therapy, because hypoxaemic patients with large lung contusions often become well-oxygenated with modest amounts of supplemental oxygen delivered via nasal prongs or mask.[13] The not uncommon concurrence of flail chest with lung contusion has little impact on the already small shunt but adds to the hypoventilation of associated regions with very low $\dot{V}_A/\dot{Q}$, leading to severe hypoxaemia. Measures that increase ventilation, such as adequate pain control, often allow simple oxygen supplementation to correct the hypoxaemia and spare the patient intubation and positive-pressure ventilation.

Ventilatory failure

In healthy subjects, P_aCO_2 is maintained within a narrow range (36–44 mmHg, 4.8–5.9 kPa) as $\dot{V}_A$ is adjusted to match the fluc-tuating $\dot{V}CO_2$. Primary failure of $\dot{V}_A$ leads to a rising P_aCO_2, termed *ventilatory failure* or *type II respiratory failure*. From a pathophysiological standpoint, acute ventilatory failure may develop whenever there is:

- a decrease in neuromuscular competence resulting from depressed CNS respiratory drive or a mechanical defect in any part of the respiratory system (chest wall, e.g. flail chest; nerves and neuromuscular transmission, e.g. myasthenia gravis; respiratory muscles, e.g. weakness)
- an increase in the energy demands of the respiratory muscles, mainly due to excessive respiratory system load, and
- a decrease in the energy available to the respiratory muscles.

Increased energy demands and decreased energy available to the respiratory muscles will lead to ventilatory failure through the development of inspiratory muscle fatigue. Of the conditions in which acute ventilatory failure may develop, two account for a substantial proportion of admissions to ICU: acute deterioration of chronic obstructive pulmonary disease (COPD), so-called acute-on-chronic respiratory failure, and acute severe asthma.

Pathophysiology of type II respiratory failure

The ventilatory pump consists of the chest wall and the respir-atory muscles attached to it and its activity is controlled by the respiratory centres in the CNS, together with their connections to the muscles through the spinal cord and the corresponding nerves.[12] Before addressing the issue of how this pump may fail, we shall first consider the conditions that should be met before the ventilatory pump works properly.

In a spontaneous breath, the inspiratory muscles must gener-ate sufficient force to overcome the elastance of the lungs and chest wall (lung and chest-wall elastic loads) as well as the airway and tissue resistance (resistive load). This requires an adequate output of the centres controlling the muscles, anatom-ical and functional integrity of the relevant nerves, unimpaired neuromuscular transmission, an intact chest wall and adequate muscle strength. This can be represented schematically by con-sidering the ability to take a breath as a balance between inspir-atory load and neuromuscular competence[28] (Fig. 14.3). Under normal conditions this system is weighted in favour of neuro-muscular competence, i.e. the available reserves permit consid-erable increases in load. However, to breathe spontaneously the inspiratory muscles need to sustain the load over time and also to adjust the minute ventilation in such a way that there is ade-quate gas exchange. The ability of the respiratory muscles to sustain this load, without the appearance of fatigue, is called 'endurance', and is determined by the balance between energy supply and demand[12] (Fig. 14.3).

Energy supplies depend on:

- the blood flow to the inspiratory muscles
- the blood substrate (fuel) concentration
- the arterial oxygen content
- the ability of the muscles to extract and utilise energy sources and their energy stores.[12,28]

Under normal circumstances, energy supplies are adequate to meet the demands and a large recruitable reserve exists. Energy demands increase proportionally with the mean tidal pressure developed by the inspiratory muscles (P_I) expressed as a fraction of maximum (P_I/P_{Imax}), the overall ventilation, the inspiratory duty cycle (ratio of inspiratory time to duration of total breath-ing cycle, T_I/T_{TOT}) and the mean inspiratory flow rate (tidal volume/inspiratory time, V_T/T_I), and are inversely related to the efficiency of the muscles[12,28] (Fig. 14.3). 'Fatigue' develops when the mean rate of energy demand exceeds the mean rate of energy supply.[28]

But what determines the ratio P_I/P_{Imax}? The numerator, the mean tidal inspiratory pressure, is determined by the elastic and resistive loads imposed on the inspiratory muscles. The denom-inator, the maximum inspiratory pressure, is determined by

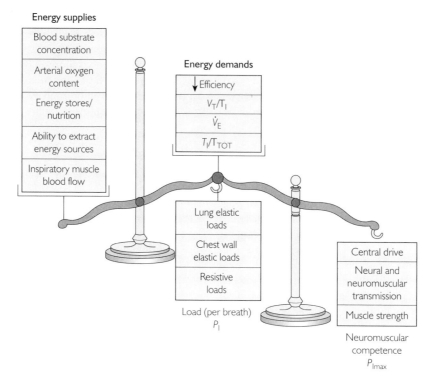

Fig. 14.3 Two balances representing the determinants of load, neuromuscular competence, energy supplies and demands. The ability to take a spontaneous breath is determined by the balance between the load imposed upon the respiratory system (P_I) and the neuromuscular competence of the ventilatory pump (maximal inspiratory pressure, P_{Imax}; right balance). Respiratory muscle endurance is determined by the balance between energy supplies and demands (left balance). Normally, the supplies meet the demands and a large reserve exists. Whenever this balance tips in favour of demand, the respiratory muscles ultimately become fatigued, leading to inability to sustain spontaneous breathing. In this model, P_I/P_{Imax} (one of the determinants of energy demands) is replaced by the balance between load and neuromuscular competence (see text for explanation). T_I/T_{TOT}, duty cycle, i.e. fraction of inspiration to duration of total respiratory cycle; V_T/T_I, mean inspiratory flow; $\dot{V}_E$ = minute ventilation.

neuromuscular competence, i.e. the maximum inspiratory muscle activation that can be achieved. It follows, then, that the value of P_I/P_{Imax} is determined by the balance between load and competence. But P_I/P_{Imax} is also one of the determinants of energy demands; therefore, the two balances, i.e. between load and competence and energy supply and demand, are in essence linked, creating a system. Schematically, when the central hinge of the system moves upwards, or is at least horizontal, an appropriate relationship between ventilatory needs and neurorespiratory capacity exists and spontaneous ventilation can be sustained indefinitely[28] (Fig. 14.3).

It can easily be seen that the ability of a subject to breathe spontaneously depends on the fine interplay of many different factors. Normally this interplay moves the central hinge far upwards and creates a great ventilatory reserve for the healthy individual[28] (Fig. 14.3). When the central hinge of the system, for whatever reason, moves downward, an inappropriate relationship of ventilatory needs to neurorespiratory capacity develops and spontaneous ventilation cannot be sustained. Consequently, ventilatory failure will develop whenever the relationship between ventilatory needs and neurorespiratory capacity becomes inappropriate. This can happen if there is:[12,28]

- an increase in the energy demands
- a decrease in the energy available

- a decrease in neuromuscular competence
- a combination of the above factors – ventilatory failure is usually multifactorial, with each factor contributing its own proportion.

Weaning from mechanical ventilation for patients with type II respiratory failure can be viewed as the mirror image of the cause of ventilatory failure. It therefore requires a systematic approach to reverse the sequence in order to restore an appropriate relationship between ventilatory needs and neurorespiratory capacity. The same approach to weaning is also applicable in patients with other types of respiratory failure. Table 14.2 summarises all possible factors that, by their fine interplay, can lead to ventilatory failure.

Two mechanisms, dynamic hyperinflation and cardiorespiratory interaction, are of particular relevance to the course of ventilatory failure.

Dynamic hyperinflation

Acute dynamic hyperinflation is a highly illustrative example of how the fine interplay of many different factors may drive the central hinge of the mechanical model shown in Figure 14.3 downwards, leading to imbalance between ventilatory needs and neurorespiratory capability, and thus to ventilatory

Table 14.2 Factors contributing to an inappropriate relationship between ventilatory needs and neurorespiratory capacity

↓ Energy supplies	↑ Energy demands			↓ Neuromuscular competence		
	Efficiency ↓	**↑ Load**		**↓ Drive**	**Impaired nerve/ neuromuscular transmission**	**Muscle weakness**

↓ Energy stores
 • Poor nutrition
 • Catabolic states
 • Prolonged submaximal breathing
 ↓ Blood fuel
 • Extreme inanition
 Inability to utilise energy
 • Sepsis
 • Cyanide poisoning
 ↓ Arterial O_2 content
 • Hypoxaemia
 • Anaemia
 ↓ Respiratory muscle blood flow
 • ↓ Cardiac output (shock, left ventricular failure)
 • ↑ Force of contraction
 • ↑ T_I/T_{TOT}
	↑ Minute ventilation loads
	 • ↑ VCO_2
	   – Fever
	   – Sepsis
	   – Shivering
	   – Tetanus
	   – Pain/agitation
	   – Trauma/severe burns
	   – Excess carbohydrate intake
	 • ↑ V_D/V_T
	   – Pulmonary embolism
	   – Emphysema
	   – ARDS
	   – Hypovolaemia
	 ↑ V_T/T_I
	 ↑ T_I/T_{TOT}
		↑ Resistive loads
		 • Broncho-constriction
		 • Airway oedema, secretions
		 • Upper airway obstruction
		 • Obstructive sleep apnoea
		 • Endotracheal tube kinking and secretion encrustation
		 • Ventilatory circuit resistance
			↑ Lung elastic loads
			 • Hyperinflation (PEEPi)
			 • Alveolar oedema
			 • Infection
			 • Atelectasis
			 • Interstitial inflammation and/or oedema
			 • Lung tumour
			
			 ↑ Chest-wall elastic loads
			 • Pleural effusion
			 • Pneumothorax
			 • Flail chest
			 • Tumour
			 • Obesity
			 • Ascites
			 • Abdominal distension
				• Drug overdose
				 • Brainstem lesion
				 • Sleep deprivation
				 • Hypothyroidism
				 • Starvation/ malnutrition
				 • Metabolic alkalosis
				 • Toxic metabolic encephalopathy
				 • Bulbar poliomyelitis
				 • Sleep-induced hypoventilation
					• Phrenic nerve injury
					 • Spinal cord lesion
					 • Neuromuscular blockers
					 • Myasthenia gravis
					 • Aminoglycosides
					 • Guillain–Barré syndrome
					 • Botulism
					 • Critical illness polyneuropathy
					 • Poliomyelitis
						• Electrolyte derangement
						 • Malnutrition
						 • Myopathy/ dystrophy, etc.
						 • Hyperinflation
						 • Drugs – corticosteroids
						 • Disuse atrophy
						 • Sepsis

failure.[29] In patients with acute hyperinflation (usually due to COPD or asthma), the load on the inspiratory muscles is increased for a variety of reasons. First, airway obstruction and/or decreased elastic recoil lead to prolongation of expiration, which cannot be completed before the ensuing inspiration. Expiration therefore ends before the respiratory system reaches elastic equilibrium at FRC, and thus a positive elastic recoil pressure, called intrinsic positive end-expiratory pressure (PEEPi), remains. During the next inspiration, the inspiratory muscles have to develop a pressure equal to this before airflow begins or before assisted breaths are triggered during mechanical ventilation (Fig. 14.4). Therefore, PEEPi represents an inspiratory threshold load. Second, because of hyperinflation, tidal breathing occurs over a less compliant portion of the pressure–volume curve of the lung, further increasing the load. Third, as FRC increases, tidal breathing may take place over that portion of the chest wall static pressure–volume curve where either it has a positive recoil, i.e. the chest wall tends to move inwards, or its expanding tendency is less than when tidal breathing begins from normal FRC. Furthermore, with severe hyperinflation the marked flattening of the diaphragm causes its costal and crural fibres to be arranged in series and perpendicularly to the chest wall. Contraction of these perpendicularly oriented fibres results in paradoxical inward movement of the lower rib cage (Hoover's sign). This distortion of the chest wall during inspiration further increases the elastic load. Finally, the resistive load to breathing is also increased, because of airway narrowing, copious secretions, mucous plugging, etc.

At the same time, neuromuscular competence is decreased because of respiratory muscle weakness associated with impaired geometry, hypercapnia, acidosis, malnutrition and steroid use. Hyperinflation decreases the length of the inspiratory muscles, forcing them to operate in a disadvantageous portion of their force–length relationship. In addition, a flattened diaphragm generates less transmural pressure for a given tension than when normally curved.

Obviously, the energy demands are significantly increased. Concurrently, the available energy is diminished because of a combination of hypoxaemia and insufficient muscle blood flow caused by the increased P_I/P_{Imax}. Thus, many different factors come into play in the hyperinflated patient, which interact and lead to ventilatory failure.[29]

Interactions between respiration and circulation in ventilatory failure

The ventilatory pump is not only linked functionally to the cardiac pump and the vascular conduit for O_2 and CO_2 transport, but also mechanically because of their close apposition within the semirigid thorax. Therefore, the two systems must work in concert for a patient to sustain spontaneous breathing. This means that the cardiovascular system has to provide sufficient blood to the lungs and the working respiratory muscles and, at the same time, the ventilatory pump should not pose any impediment to the heart and blood flow that could either provoke cardiac dysfunction or 'steal' oxygen and blood from other tissues in favour of the respiratory muscles.[29]

Patients with left ventricular dysfunction may develop an increase in pulmonary venous pressure and sometimes, ultimately, a decrease in cardiac output when inspiratory load increases because of bronchoconstriction, pneumonia, airway secretions or upper airway obstruction. This phenomenon has been demonstrated in COPD patients with ventricular dysfunction upon removal from positive-pressure mechanical ventilation.[31] Several factors may be responsible (e.g. increased venous return due to decreased pleural pressure and sympathetic discharge, reduced left ventricular compliance due to ischaemia or right ventricular enlargement/ventricular interdependence, reduced ventricular contractility due to ischaemia and/or hypoxaemia).[31]

The mechanism leading to ventilatory failure in these patients might be considered as follows.[29] During bronchoconstriction or other reason, the increase in respiratory muscle workload as well as anxiety and sympathetic discharge result in an abrupt increase in oxygen and cardiac demands. The failing left ventricle then is unable to respond normally and left ventricular end-diastolic pressure rises, causing interstitial, peribronchiolar and alveolar oedema. This reduces lung compliance, increases airway resistance and worsens $\dot{V}_A/\dot{Q}$ mismatching, leading to hypoxaemia. The energy demands of the respiratory muscles are increased, while energy supplies are either diminished or not sufficiently increased (inadequate cardiac output, hypoxaemia). This eventually leads to the inability to sustain

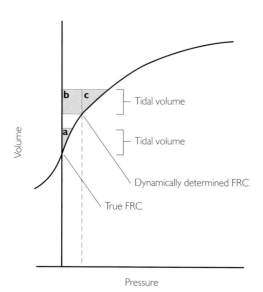

Fig. 14.4 Pressure–volume curve of the respiratory system, illustrating the impact of intrinsic PEEP on work of breathing. Without intrinsic PEEP inspiration begins from 'true' functional residual capacity (FRC), and the external work (pressure × volume) required to produce a tidal volume is area a. With intrinsic PEEP, inspiration begins from the higher, dynamically determined volume and the external work to produce the same tidal volume is shown by areas b and c. The work represented by area b must be performed simply to initiate gas flow (e.g. to trigger a ventilator). Adding continuous positive airway pressure in an amount equal to intrinsic PEEP (shown as the dashed line) reduces the work of each breath to area c. (Redrawn with permission from Schmidt et al[30].)

spontaneous ventilation at a level adequate to achieve normo-capnia, and P_aCO_2 rises. The abnormal blood gases depress cardiac contractility and, at the same time, respiratory muscle function. This further worsens blood gases and creates a vicious circle that may culminate in ventilatory failure.

The pivotal role played by the respiratory muscles in the development of left ventricular dysfunction is mediated through the effects of muscle activation on pleural and abdominal pressures.[29,31] Normally, spontaneous inspiration increases abdominal pressure at the same time as it decreases pleural pressure, through diaphragmatic contraction and descent. The importance of the decreased pleural pressure for augmentation of venous return is easily understood. Furthermore, the negative intra-thoracic pressure increases the afterload of both ventricles and this, combined with the increased venous return, may lead to right ventricular distension. Because the two ventricles are con-strained by a common pericardial sac and share the interven-tricular septum, changes in the volume of one ventricle may affect the function of the other; thus, right ventricular disten-sion impedes the filling of the left ventricle.[31] This occurs both through a generalised increase in pericardial pressure and also because of a shift of the interventricular septum toward the left. Left ventricular filling impediment increases the diastolic stiff-ness of the left ventricle at the same time as afterload is elevated because of the decreased pleural pressure. This combined effect leads to the elevation of left ventricular end-diastolic pressure, with the above-mentioned sequence of events culminating in ventilatory failure.

On the other hand, the role of abdominal pressure is not usually considered significant, yet abdominal pressure surrounds the abdominal venous system through which two-thirds of the venous return passes. Therefore, an increase in abdominal pressure could theoretically compress the abdominal veins and increase the amount of blood returning to the heart.[29,31]

The increased left ventricular preload and afterload resulting from the increased load imposed on the respiratory muscles during an insult (e.g. bronchospasm) may also lead to altered myocardial perfusion and ischaemia, and thus to ventilatory failure. This phenomenon has also been described during weaning failure.[32] Haemodynamic and ventilatory changes asso-ciated with the increased inspiratory load seem to be sufficient to increase myocardial oxygen demands (as evidenced by the increased heart rate and arterial blood pressure) to such an extent that it cannot be met by the available coronary oxygen supply, probably because of coronary atherosclerosis or spasm, thus leading to ischaemia.

In normal subjects breathing quietly, the oxygen cost of breathing ($\dot{V}O_{2,resp}$) is a small proportion (about 2%) of the total oxygen requirement ($\dot{V}O_{2,tot}$). However, in the patient with increased respiratory load because of an insult, $\dot{V}O_{2,resp}$ may be significantly elevated (about 25% of $\dot{V}O_{2,tot}$) at the same time that the energy available may be decreased. This may be the case for the patient with ventricular dysfunction who develops ventilatory failure. In such cases $\dot{V}O_{2,resp}$ may increase to such an extent that the working respiratory muscles may 'steal' oxygen and blood from other tissues. Animal studies provide strong support for this theory. When dogs with cardiogenic or septic shock were mechanically ventilated, only 3% of their cardiac output was directed to their respiratory muscles but when they were allowed to breathe spontaneously their respiratory muscles received up to 20% of the cardiac output, stealing blood from other organs such as the brain, liver and other muscles.[29]

Acute severe asthma

Acute severe asthma (status asthmaticus) can result in ventila-tory failure and death. The general principles of management are discussed in Chapter 48.11. Here we focus on the pharma-cological and ventilator management of the intubated patient treated with mechanical ventilation.

Pharmacological management

Humidified oxygen should be given to achieve full arterial saturation. Resolution of hypoxaemia improves oxygen delivery to the respiratory muscles, relieves any component of hypoxia-induced pulmonary hypertension and protects against any paradoxical worsening of gas exchange with bronchodilator therapy.

Beta-agonists should be administered by inhalation. Inhaled beta-agonists can be delivered equally well by a metered-dose inhaler with a spacer adopted on the inspiratory limb of the ven-tilator or by a hand-held nebulizer.[33] When an metered-dose inhaler is used, tidal volume should be increased above 500 ml, inspiratory flow rate should be lowered to 40 l/min, actuation of the inhaler should be timed to coincide with inspiration, and the breath should be followed by a brief (3 s) pause. The effect on airway resistance should be monitored by using the peak-to-pause pressure gradient of airway pressure at a constant inspir-atory flow. Intravenous infusion of beta-agonists is not recommended. The subcutaneous route can be considered in patients younger than 40 years, without known cardiac disease, who are not responding adequately to several hours of inhaled beta-agonists.[34] Adrenaline (epinephrine) 0.3 ml 1:1000 or terbutaline 0.25 mg every 20 min can be used.

Corticosteroids are given in the usual way. One approach is to give 60–125 mg methylprednisolone intravenously every 6 h during the initial 24 h of treatment. Ipratropium bromide may be of benefit in some patients when administered either by a metered-dose inhaler with a spacer (e.g. 6–10 puffs every 20 min) or by a nebuliser (e.g. 0.5 mg) mixed with a beta-agonist every 20 min, in the acute setting. Theophylline may also be useful, particularly when patients fail to respond initially to beta-agonists and corticosteroids. Especially in patients already taking theophylline, monitoring of serum concentration is required.

Ventilator management

Mechanical ventilation in acute severe asthma is particularly challenging because airway pressures are typically high and interventions to achieve normocapnia often result in more dynamic hyperinflation and greater risk of barotrauma. The goals of therapy are to achieve adequate alveolar ventilation, low levels of PEEPi, minimal circulatory compromise and low risk of barotrauma.

Lung hyperinflation is directly proportional to $\dot{V}_E$[35] and to the degree of airflow obstruction. In the postintubation period, dan-gerous levels of hyperinflation develop when patients are ventilated excessively. The positive intrathoracic pressure associated with positive-pressure ventilation and rising PEEPi act to increase right atrial pressure. This decreases venous return to the right heart, resulting in systemic hypotension and tachycardia. These effects can be demonstrated by hypoventilating the patient (2–3 breaths/min) to prolong expiratory time and allow lung deflation. Restoration of blood pressure generally occurs within 60 s of initiating this manoeuvre. Tension pneumothorax, which may occur bilaterally, should be considered in patients who remain hypotensive despite a trial of hypoventilation.[30]

After intubation, patients should be sedated deeply and sometimes need to be paralysed. These interventions minimise airway pressures, allow determination of PEEPi, P_{peak} and P_{plat} (see below), and lower $\dot{V}CO_2$. In principle, the aim would be to ventilate the patient to a normal P_aCO_2 level while keeping the P_{peak} and PEEPi low enough to avoid barotrauma. When patients with severe asthma are ventilated to eucapnia, however, severe dynamic hyperinflation usually occurs. End-inspired volume can be as large as 3–4 l above apnoeic FRC, a condition that risks barotrauma and cardiovascular compromise. Various combinations of V_T and respiratory frequently at a constant overall ventilation show that at higher rates and smaller tidal volume, P_{peak} and P_{plat} fall, owing to the lower end-inspired lung volume, whereas there is a small increase in end-expired volume and corresponding PEEPi owing to slightly greater air trapping caused by the reduced time for expiration.[35] Moreover, increasing inspiratory flow ($\dot{V}_I$) from 40 l/min to 100 l/min while maintaining V_T and respiratory rate reduces end-expired lung volume and P_{plat} by allowing more time for expiration.[35]

To avoid significant lung hyperinflation, the ventilator should be set to allow sufficient exhalation time. The most important means of achieving this is to reduce the ventilation, mainly by decreasing the respiratory rate; increasing inspiratory flow may also be useful. A strategy aimed at reducing inspiratory time by increasing inspiratory flow in order to lengthen the exhalation time carries a cost of higher P_{peak}. Recent data fail to show a relationship, however, between P_{peak} and complications of mechanical ventilation.[36] The reasons may be that P_{peak} does not predict alveolar pressure or the degree of overdistension of alveolar structures and that the high pressures are encountered largely by narrow proximal airways. In general, therefore, high peak pressures are acceptable for the advantage of reducing PEEPi. Clinical studies demonstrate that an initial ventilation between 8 and 10 l/min (achieved by a tidal volume between 8 and 10 ml/kg and a frequency between 11 and 14 breaths/min), combined with an inspiratory flow of 80–100 l/min, is unlikely to result in dangerous hyperinflation. Surrogate measures of lung hyperinflation are P_{plat} and PEEPi measured with the patient relaxed. Complications are rare when P_{plat} is less than 30 cmH$_2$O and PEEPi is less than 15 cmH$_2$O.[36]

The current approach to mechanical ventilation in the patient with severe asthma is to use low ventilation and high inspiratory flow to minimise dynamic hyperinflation. Initial ventilator settings such as those above will usually lead to a P_aCO_2 level well above the normal range, an approach that trades the risks of barotrauma for the presumably lower risks of hypercapnia (permissive hypercapnia). Several series of asthmatic patients have been treated successfully with this approach.[30] Hypercapnic acidosis causes cerebral vasodilatation, decreased myocardial contractility, peripheral vasodilatation with a hyperdynamic circulation, and pulmonary vasoconstriction.[37] Accordingly, permissive hypercapnia should be avoided in patients with raised intracranial pressure (as might occur with anoxic brain injury from cardiopulmonary arrest) and in patients with severe myocardial dysfunction. Another disadvantage of permissive hypercapnia is that, in addition to full sedation, patients generally need therapeutic paralysis. There are increasing reports of severe muscular weakness due to myopathy following mechanical ventilation for asthma. Most patients were treated with high-dose corticosteroids, alone or combined with paralytic agents.[38,39]

Weaning from mechanical ventilation
Although some patients respond to therapy within hours, more typically 24–48 h of aggressive bronchodilator and anti-inflammatory therapy is required until airway pressures fall. Once this occurs and P_aCO_2 normalises, paralytic agents and sedatives should be withheld and the patient should be allowed to breathe. A quick return to spontaneous breathing and extubation is preferable, without prolonged trials of spontaneous or partially assisted breathing, because the endotracheal tube itself may perpetuate bronchospasm.

Acute-on-chronic respiratory failure

In COPD with severe, stable, chronic respiratory failure, the energy demands are increased as a result of increased load per breath and of decreased efficiency, mainly as a result of hyperinflation. At all times, these increased energy demands are marginally balanced by diminished and barely adequate neuromuscular competence (see Fig. 14.3). Minor additional decrements in strength or increments in load are sufficient to precipitate acute ventilatory failure. Exacerbations of COPD account for a substantial portion of bed days because these patients often require prolonged ventilatory support. In addition, COPD is an important problem in surgical ICUs because it is one of the more common reasons for prolonged postoperative recovery. Clinical presentation, treatment and the use of non-invasive ventilation are described in Chapters 15 and 47. In the present chapter the three phases of management – before intubation, following intubation and during weaning from the ventilator – are discussed.

Management before intubation
The goals of management in the patient not yet intubated are to avoid intubation and invasive mechanical ventilation wherever possible, and to recognise progressive respiratory failure when it is not. Avoiding intubation and invasive mechanical ventilation nearly always depends on detecting the cause of respiratory failure and reversing it. Thus, while non-invasive ventilation is initiated, potentially reversible precipitating factors of acute deterioration of COPD should be diagnosed and treated (see Chapter 47).

Management following intubation
This phase consists of the immediate peri-intubation management and the first few days of mechanical ventilation. In general, treatment begun in the preintubation phase (bronchodilators, antibiotics, etc.) is continued. Care comprises stabilis-

ing the patient on the ventilator, ensuring rest of the patient and respiratory muscles, improving neuromuscular competence, reducing load and giving prophylaxis against complications. Optimal treatment at this time is likely to facilitate eventual weaning from mechanical ventilation.

Peri-intubation risks

There are two common pitfalls in the postintubation period – life-threatening alkalosis and hypotension, both related to overzealous ventilation and avoidable by considering the patient's own ventilatory pattern preceding intubation.[30] Most patients with acute-on-chronic respiratory failure have a ventilation of 10 l/min or less and breathe with a tidal volume of about 300 ml. Physicians commonly choose ventilator settings with higher V_T and $\dot{V}_E$, particularly during the first few minutes of manual-assisted ventilation. In addition, as the work of breathing is assumed by the ventilator, $\dot{V}CO_2$ drops by as much as 20%. All of these factors considerably lower the patient's P_aCO_2 once assisted ventilation begins. Because pre-existing compensatory metabolic alkalosis is the rule, life-threatening alkalaemia (pH > 7.7) can be produced easily. This complication can be avoided by simply applying a ventilation approximating the patient's own pattern of breathing. Hypotension is a consequence of increasing intrathoracic pressure due to escalating PEEPi following intubation and conversion from spontaneous to positive-pressure ventilation. The effect of sedative drugs and sympathetic lysis also contributes to hypotension. The degree of dynamic hyperinflation is proportional to the ventilation; PEEPi has the same deleterious consequences on venous return as externally applied PEEP and can cause serious hypoperfusion. Again, the key to avoiding the pitfall is to prevent excessive ventilation. When hypotension occurs, the circulation can usually be promptly restored by simply ceasing ventilation for 30 s and then reinstituting it along with measures to reduce PEEPi and restore circulating volume.[30]

Ventilator settings

The assist–control mode (see below) is used initially because one of the goals in this phase is to ensure respiratory muscle rest. Tidal volumes of about 5–7 ml/kg are used (about 350–500 ml) with a respiratory rate of 20–24 breaths/min. As previously discussed, PEEPi presents an inspiratory threshold load to these patients. Patients must generate sufficient force to counterbalance PEEPi before their efforts result in any inspiratory flow and before they can trigger the ventilator. This difficulty cannot be overcome by lowering the trigger sensitivity on the ventilator or by using flow triggering. Applying external PEEP roughly equal to the PEEPi reduces the work of breathing (and triggering) by significant amounts,[40] as shown in Figure 14.4. In some patients, externally applied PEEP causes additional hyperinflation with detrimental haemodynamic effects and potentially increased risk of barotrauma. However, most patients have expiratory flow limitation so that external PEEP (in amounts up to about 85% of the PEEPi) has no significant impact on the expiratory flow–volume relationship, hyperinflation or haemodynamics.[41]

Respiratory muscle rest and recovery. The respiratory muscles require 48–72 h for full recovery, so resumption of breathing efforts before that is useless and is likely to lead to

recurrence of respiratory muscle fatigue.[30] Rest can be achieved with any mode of ventilation as long as settings are chosen that minimise patient effort. It is important to emphasise that having the patient connected to a ventilator is no guarantee that s/he is relieved of the work of breathing.[30] Even when the ventilator is set at a very sensitive trigger, the presence of PEEPi causes the patient to have to make a substantial inspiratory effort to get a breath, even on assist–control mode. For example, with a triggered sensitivity of –2 cmH_2O and a PEEPi of 12 cmH_2O, the patient must lower the airway pressure by 14 cmH_2O to trigger a breath. It is important to ensure that the patient is, in fact, rested.

Increasing neuromuscular competence

Each of the factors shown in Figure 14.3 and Table 14.2 that contribute to depressed neuromuscular competence should be reviewed daily in the ventilated patient. In this phase, the importance of nutrition must be recognised. Malnutrition is a common feature of advanced COPD and contributes to respiratory muscle dysfunction as well as immune depression. With refeeding, hypophosphataemia commonly develops while the patient is in the ICU, and serum phosphate content should be monitored.

Decreasing load

Efforts to decrease respiratory load should continue. Once the patient is ventilated, it becomes possible to divide the load into resistive and elastic components (see below). These determinations may provide insight into the precipitants of respiratory failure and serve to guide therapy. It is important to continue treatment with bronchodilators. Both metered-dose inhalers and nebulisers can be used as discussed above in relation to asthma.

Weaning from the ventilator

The principle guiding the management in this phase is that successful weaning from the ventilator requires that the premorbid compensated relationship between ventilatory needs and neuro-respiratory capacity must be re-established. Therefore, a strategy for successfully discontinuing mechanical ventilation emphasises increasing the neuromuscular competence, mainly by increasing the strength, decreasing the energy demands by decreasing the load, and increasing the energy supply by improving circulation and hypoxaemia (Fig. 14.3 & Table 14.2) In either case, when the above-mentioned relationship is re-established the patient will be able to breathe free of assistance. On the other hand, if this relationship cannot be restored, attempts at spontaneous breathing will fail.

Mechanical ventilation

Mechanical ventilation refers to any method of breathing in which a mechanical apparatus is used to augment or satisfy entirely the bulk flow requirements of a patient's breathing; it can be given by negative or positive pressure. Although negative-pressure ventilation obviates the need to intubate the patient, problems mainly in providing routine nursing care have led to its virtual replacement in ICUs by positive-pressure ventilation

(PPV). In PPV, the ventilator creates a superatmospheric pressure at the upper airway during inspiration, thus resulting in a pressure gradient that 'pushes' gases into the alveoli. Expiration is passive. The following sections present some of the principles of invasive (i.e. requiring tracheal intubation) PPV used in ICUs.

Positive-pressure ventilation

Categories of positive-pressure ventilators

Pressure-preset ventilators (and pressure-preset modes)
Ventilators are either pressure-preset or volume-preset (Fig. 14.5). In pressure-preset machines (or modes), the physician sets a pressure by means of a button on the ventilator. When inspiration begins, the ventilator develops the preset pressure and volume enters the lung. Inspiration ceases and the expiratory phase begins either when the preset pressure is reached in the system (old pressure-type ventilators, i.e. Bird Mk VII, Bennett PR-2) or the preset inspiratory time is over (pressure-control modes incorporated in current ventilators). If respiratory compliance should decrease and/or airway resistance increase, volume delivery would fall proportionally, as the preset pressure remains constant. Thus, *pressure* is the independent variable and *volume* is the dependent variable. Clearly, therefore, these ventilators or modes are not well suited for ventilation of patients with changing respiratory mechanics;

otherwise, if they are used, the patient must be monitored closely to avoid inadvertent hypoventilation.

Volume-preset ventilators
These ventilators deliver a volume that is set by the physician on the machine's control panel and, within limits, deliver that volume irrespective of the pressure generated within the system. A reduction in compliance and/or an increase in airway resistance would result in a proportionate increase in pressure. Therefore, *volume* is the independent variable, and *pressure* the dependent one. These ventilators are the machines of choice for ventilation of severely ill patients, and are those currently used in ICUs.

Modes of positive-pressure ventilation

Assist–control mode
The ventilator in this mode is sensitised to respond to the patient's inspiratory effort, if such efforts are preset (Assist), but the machine will cycle automatically in the absence of such efforts (Control). This is the mode most commonly used in the initial phase of full ventilatory support.

Synchronised intermittent mandatory ventilation (SIMV)
This mode can be considered a combination of spontaneous ventilation and assisted ventilation. At intervals determined by the SIMV frequency setting, the machine becomes 'sensitised' to the

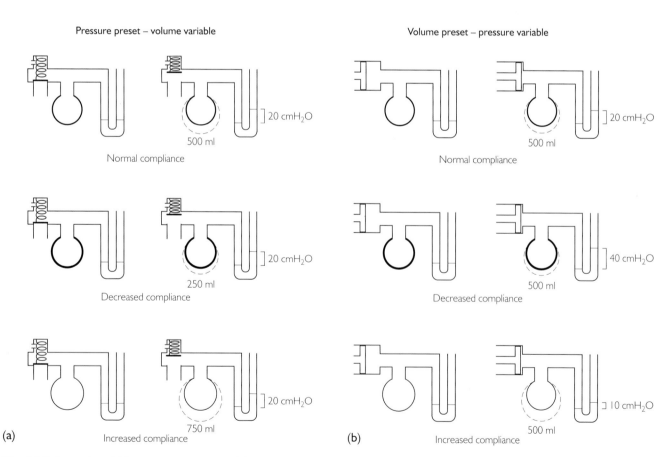

Fig. 14.5 Principles of (a) pressure-preset and (b) volume-preset ventilators. (a) Volume delivery is variable, depending on the compliance (or resistance) of the respiratory system. The ventilator is represented by the spring. (b) Inflation pressure is variable, depending on the compliance (or resistance) of the respiratory system. The ventilator is represented by the piston.

patient's inspiratory effort and responds to that effort by delivering a mechanical 'assisted' breath. Between these assisted cycles, the patient breathes spontaneously at a rate and depth of his/her own choice.

Pressure support ventilation (PSV)

This belongs to the category of partial ventilatory support modes, in which part of the breathing pattern is controlled by the patient. During inspiration, the airway pressure is raised to a preset level – the pressure support level. Each breath is supported, and is triggered and terminated by the patient. SIMV, PSV or their combination are used to aid the transition from full ventilatory support to spontaneous breathing.

Positive end-expiratory pressure and continuous positive airway pressure

PEEP refers to positive end-expiratory pressure applied during mechanical ventilation, including mask ventilatory assistance; thus, airway pressure (P_{AW}) is equal to the level of PEEP at the end of expiration and is higher during inspiration. CPAP signifies the application of positive pressure during spontaneous breathing, in the presence or absence of an endotracheal tube; therefore, airway pressure is equal to the set level of pressure during both inspiration and expiration.

The major aims of PEEP in acute respiratory failure are to improve oxygenation in patients with type I failure and to unload the inspiratory muscles in COPD patients with acute exacerbation. Both indications for PEEP have been discussed above.

Most of the effects of CPAP on the cardiorespiratory system are similar to those of PEEP. A major difference is that spontaneous ventilation during CPAP results in a much lower mean intrathoracic pressure compared with PEEP and mechanical ventilation. Consequently, depression of cardiac output is significantly less with CPAP than at similar levels of PEEP.

Assessment of the need for intubation and mechanical ventilation in respiratory failure

The decision to intubate requires clinical judgement and should be assessed by a physician present at the bedside.[30] Assessment of respiratory failure based solely on results of arterial blood-gas measurements is inappropriate. Certainly, an increasing P_aCO_2 in a patient with progressively worsening symptoms and signs of distress should be interpreted as a sign of impending respiratory arrest. In addition, a P_aO_2 that remains below 50 mmHg (6.7 kPa) despite O_2 therapy and non-invasive ventilation suggests that intubation is probably inevitable. However, the absolute level of P_aCO_2 in isolation from other clinical data may be less useful. Indeed, even with P_aCO_2 higher than 120 mmHg (16 kPa), in COPD patients who are alert and conversing, intubation may not become necessary. On the other hand, many patients with acute severe asthma or hypoxaemic respiratory failure progress to respiratory arrest long before progressive hypercapnia is clearly developed.

In general, in appropriate patients, non-invasive ventilation should be tried first. If this fails to stabilise the patient, the goal at this stage of management is to intubate the patient once invasive mechanical ventilation becomes unavoidable. Useful bedside predictors of impending respiratory arrest include:

- a respiratory rate that remains above 35 breaths/min or rises despite therapy and non-invasive ventilation
- deterioration in mental status
- a rapid and shallow pattern of breathing
- continued use of all accessory respiratory muscles
- the patient's subjective sense of exhaustion.

Concomitant haemodynamic instability or inability to protect the airway may also make intubation essential.

Weaning from mechanical ventilation

In the vast majority of mechanically ventilated patients, resumption of spontaneous ventilation is obtained easily.[42–45] These include those requiring routine postoperative ventilatory support, those with overdoses of sedatives and those with other self-limited causes of ventilatory failure. However, in a substantial number of mechanically ventilated patients, weaning is difficult and likely to fail.[42–45] These patients usually suffer from chronic obstructive or restrictive pulmonary diseases, cardiac failure, central nervous system dysfunction or peripheral neuromuscular disorders.

The aetiology and pathophysiology of weaning failure is usually the same as that discussed for ventilatory failure, i.e. weaning failure is caused by an inappropriate relationship between ventilatory needs and neurorespiratory capacity; thus, weaning is a systematic approach to reverse these factors in order to make this relationship appropriate. Possible factors that, by their fine interplay, can lead to weaning failure are summarised in Table 14.2. Less often, weaning failure is due to hypoxaemia or cardiovascular dysfunction. The mechanism is again the same as that discussed in the ventilatory failure section above.

Reduction of the duration of mechanical ventilation

Although physicians recognise that some of the risks associated with mechanical ventilation (such as nosocomial pneumonia) increase with the duration of ventilatory support, a significant number of patients are kept on machine support for longer than necessary. This is clear from the outcome of patients who have unplanned (i.e. self or accidental) extubation. The reintubation rate in such patients varies from 31% to 78%[46] which means that between 22% and 69% of patients had remained intubated without needing ventilatory support (since they did not require reintubation). This finding probably reflects the fact that even excellent physicians do not accurately judge on clinical grounds when a patient is able to wean. However, recent randomised controlled trials have shown that the total duration of mechanical ventilation[45,47] as well as the time spent on weaning[42,43,48] can be reduced by the adoption of specific stategies. These include, first, the systematic daily screening of respiratory function followed (when appropriate) by trials of spontaneous breathing to identify as early as possible when a patient is able to wean[45] and, second, the implementation of ventilatory protocols in difficult-to-wean patients instead of relying on physicians' personal preferences.[42,43,47,48]

When is a patient able to wean? Indices predicting weaning outcome

Before weaning is considered, the underlying disease process responsible for the acute respiratory failure and mechanical ventilation should have improved. The patient must be haemodynamically stable (absence of myocardial ischaemia or shock as judged by need for vasopressors or recent onset of arrhythmia), adequately oxygenated ($P_aO_2 > 60$ mmHg (8 kPa) with $F_IO_2 < 0.4$ and PEEP < 5 cmH$_2$O), with no agitation, sepsis or overt CNS depression.[49] However, many patients satisfying these preconditions actually fail to wean. It is therefore highly desirable to have objective measurements – indices that can help in making the decision to wean a patient from the ventilator.

Several measured parameters and calculated variables have, over the years, been proposed as indices that can be used to predict the weaning outcome.[49] The most important and relevant are those that:

- record and analyse the pattern of spontaneous breathing in terms of tidal volume (V_T), respiratory rate (f) or f/V_T (a measure of rapid shallow breathing)
- are intended to assess respiratory muscle strength, such as maximal inspiratory pressure (P_{Imax})
- assess simple ventilatory parameters, such as vital capacity (VC) and minute ventilation ($\dot{V}_E$)
- are aimed to assess central respiratory drive, such as the airway pressure developed 100 ms after the beginning of inspiration against an occluded airway ($P_{0.1}$).

However, over the years no index has proved to be ideal, i.e. to be highly predictive of weanability, and it seems that the best approach is to use weaning indices for systematic daily screening of respiratory function in order to proceed or not to a trial of spontaneous breathing. This will make possible the early identification of those patients who are potentially capable of breathing spontaneously and thus more likely to wean successfully,[45] and will certainly lead to a reduction in the duration of mechanical ventilation, since the frequent unnecessary prolongation of ventilator support will be avoided.

The initial trial of spontaneous breathing

Recent multicentre studies using spontaneous breathing trials before extubation have reported that nearly 25% of patients who meet usual weaning criteria fail to complete these trials;[42-44] thus, it seems more prudent to conduct these trials before extubation. This strategy would prevent unnecessary reintubation and the associated risks (such as pneumonia), since patients failing to complete the spontaneous breathing trial would most likely also fail to sustain spontaneous breathing once extubated.

Weaning is considered to have begun with the onset of the spontaneous breathing trial, whose duration is usually 2 h,[42-45] although it has been reported that even 30 min may be sufficient. When the patient remains clinically stable with no sign of poor tolerance (defined below) until the end of this period, it is considered that s/he has been successfully weaned and the patient is extubated. If during this trial the patient develops signs of poor tolerance, weaning has failed and mechanical ven-

tilation is reinstituted. Although not universally agreed, the following are considered signs of poor tolerance:[42-45]

- an increase in respiratory rate above 35 breaths/min
- an increase or decrease in blood pressure by more than 20%, or to above 180 or below 90 mmHg
- an increase or decrease in heart rate of more than 20 beats/min
- an S_aO_2 below 90% or a P_aO_2 below 60 mmHg (8 kPa)
- an increase in P_aCO_2 of more than 5 mmHg (0.7 kPa) and/or a decrease in pH to less than 7.3
- the development of cardiac arrhythmias
- the appearance of sweating and of signs of increased work of breathing, signalling impeding respiratory muscle fatigue (accessory muscle use, markedly paradoxical or asynchronous rib-cage–abdominal breathing movements, intercostal retractions, nasal flaring)
- the development of complaints of dyspnoea or anxiety not relieved by reassurance.

The spontaneous breathing trial can be applied in one of two ways:[44]

- via a T-piece circuit, with supplemental O$_2$ and humidification of gas
- via the ventilator circuit with PSV of 7–8 cmH$_2$O to counterbalance the extra work imposed by breathing through the ventilator circuit.[44,45]

In either case the F_IO_2 should be set at the same level as that used during mechanical ventilation.

The approach of conducting spontaneous breathing trials once a patient meets the weaning criteria and directly extubating the patient upon successful completion of the trial is different from the traditional approach to weaning. In fact, implicit in the concept of the term 'weaning' is the assumption that patients become dependent on the ventilator and that such dependence should be gradually decreased. However, this is not the case for the majority of mechanically ventilated patients. As a general approximation, about 60%[42,43] of patients requiring mechanical ventilation for more than 24 h successfully complete the 2 h spontaneous breathing trial and are extubated without requiring reintubation. Consequently, these patients do not need a gradual withdrawal of ventilatory support, which would only unnecessarily lengthen the duration of mechanical ventilation, with the attendant increases in risk and costs.

In summary, systematic daily screening of respiratory function (by means of weaning indices) followed (when appropriate) by trials of spontaneous breathing reduces the duration of mechanical ventilation[45,47] and has been suggested as a useful strategy for every ICU to adopt.

Strategies and techniques for difficult weaning

About 40% of mechanically ventilated patients either fail the initial spontaneous breathing trial (about 20%) or are extubated and require reintubation (about 20%).[42,43] The cause and pathophysiology of the ventilator dependency in these patients are complex[29,50] but should be thoroughly sought to allow for the application of aetiologically based therapeutic strategies. Specific ventilatory techniques should be applied to wean these patients from mechanical ventilation.[42,43] Furthermore, recent trials have shown that these ventilatory techniques should preferably be applied in a protocol-directed manner, since this approach may shorten the duration of weaning[48] and thus the total duration of mechanical ventilation.[47,48]

Therapeutic strategies

Since the ability to sustain spontaneous breathing depends on the fine interplay of so many different factors, every attempt should be made to correct all the reversible derangements listed in Table 14.2; furthermore, hypoxaemia and cardiovascular dysfunction should be sought and treated. Finally, psychological support should be provided for the patient.

Several therapeutic interventions and the benefits from them have already been discussed (e.g. the use of PEEP or CPAP to counterbalance PEEPi until the underlying pathophysiological mechanisms producing it are reversed).

Ventilatory techniques

There are generally two different ventilatory techniques for the difficult to wean patient: T-piece weaning and partial-support weaning (SIMV, PSV, SIMV+PSV).

Using the T-piece technique, weaning is accomplished by alternating periods of full ventilator support with increasing periods of independent breathing through a T-piece circuit or a CPAP system.[42–44] With this method, periods of spontaneous breathing are progressively lengthened according to tolerance. Judgement of the latter is based on the same criteria used in the initial spontaneous breathing trial. If the patient tolerates the trial for 2 h, extubation follows.

During partial support weaning with SIMV, the patient is allowed to breathe spontaneously and the ventilator delivers a number of breaths with predetermined frequency and tidal volume. During weaning the number of ventilator-delivered breaths (SIMV rate) interspersed between spontaneous efforts is initially set at half the frequency previously used during assist–control mechanical ventilation, keeping V_T and $\dot{V}_I$ constant.[42,43] The SIMV rate is then reduced in a stepwise fashion by 2–4 breaths/min twice or more daily, as tolerated by the patient. The SIMV rate is increased again if the patient develops signs of poor tolerance (listed in the previous section). The cause of weaning difficulty is sought and treated before rate reduction is resumed. Generally, it is useful to allow the patient's respiratory muscles to rest at night by increasing the SIMV rate. In the two large recent multicentre trials that have compared different modes of weaning, the SIMV rate was reduced to 4–5 breaths/min and if the patient could tolerate it for 2 h[43] or 24 h,[42] weaning was considered complete and the patient was extubated.

During partial support weaning with PSV, the airway pressure is initially titrated at a level sufficient to achieve a respiratory rate of 20–30 breaths/min.[42,43] At least twice daily the pressure support level is decreased by 2–4 cmH$_2$O.[42,43] If the patient develops signs of poor tolerance, the support level is increased again and the cause of the deterioration is investigated and whenever possible reversed. Weaning is complete when the patient is able to breathe spontaneously with a low pressure support level (5–8 cmH$_2$O) to account for the resistance of the endotracheal tube and ventilator circuit.[42,43]

Partial-support weaning with SIMV plus PSV theoretically offers a more gradual transition from full ventilatory support to spontaneous breathing, which might be beneficial for 'difficult to wean' patients. However, the time required for weaning is longer with this modality.[51] Furthermore, no study has shown it to be superior to other techniques and consequently it cannot be recommended on a regular basis.

Recently, two randomised clinical trials comparing three ventilatory techniques of weaning (T-piece, SIMV and PSV) concluded that the outcome of difficult weaning was influenced by the ventilatory strategy chosen.[42,43] PSV had a significant benefit over the other methods in terms of failures, reducing the probability of remaining on mechanical ventilation in one study.[42] On the other hand, in the other study[43] T-piece weaning clearly proved superior. SIMV was the least effective ventilatory technique in both studies.[42,43]

Respiratory system monitoring and measurements

As most patients are ventilated, at least initially, with a volume-preset mode (i.e. assist–control or SIMV), and monitoring of respiratory system mechanics in most ICUs is practicable only during volume-preset ventilation, the following discussion is limited largely to this setting. Determination of respiratory system mechanics is an integral part of ventilator management and is a routine part of the examination of the critically ill patient.

Inspiratory airway pressure and PEEPi measurement

When, after muscle relaxation, a patient is ventilated mechanically the inspiratory airway pressure (P_{AW}) consists of three components: one to drive gas across the inspiratory resistance, the second to expand the alveoli against the elastic recoil of the lungs and chest wall, and the third equal to the alveolar pressure present before inspiratory flow begins:

$$P_{AW} = P_{resist} + P_{stat} + PEEPtot$$
$$P_{AW} = \dot{V}I \times R_{AW} + V_T \times E_{RS} + PEEPtot$$

where E_{RS} is elastance of the respiratory system, PEEPtot = PEEP + PEEPi, P_{resist} is the resistive pressure component, P_{stat} is the static elastic pressure term, $\dot{V}_I$ is inspiratory flow, which is constant (square wave), R_{AW} is inspiratory resistance, and V_T is the tidal volume . Diagnostic and therapeutic information can be obtained by separating the individual components of P_{AW}, as follows. First, PEEPi is measured by the end-expiratory port occlusion method (Fig. 14.6). Several ventilators facilitate its determination by providing an expiratory pause switch. This method does not provide accurate estimation of PEEPi if there is a leak in the tubing or around the endotracheal tube cuff, if there is gas flow into the circuit during expiration (as during continuous nebulisation of bronchodilators), or if the patient is

a

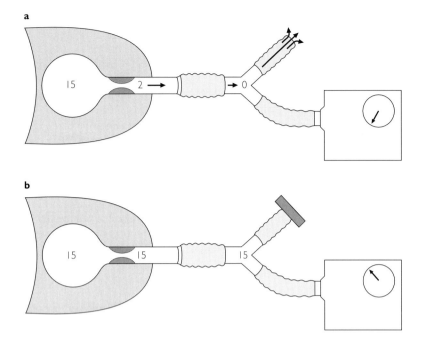

Fig. 14.6 Auto-PEEP measured by the end-expiratory port occlusion manoeuvre. (a) Just before the next inflation, alveolar pressure is markedly positive (15 cmH$_2$O) as flow continues through critically narrowed airways. (b) The manometer approximates auto-PEEP only when pressures equilibrate following occlusion of the expiratory port at end exhalation. (Redrawn with permission from Pepe PE, Marini JJ. Occult positive end-expiratory pressure in mechanically ventilated patients with airflow obstruction: the auto-PEEP effect. Am Rev Respir Dis 1982; 126: 166 Official Journal of the American Thoracic Society, American Lung Association.)

b

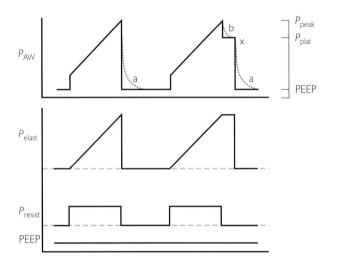

Fig. 14.7 Components of the inspiratory airway pressure (P_{AW}) during mechanical ventilation in volume-preset mode (assist–control or synchronised intermittent mandatory ventilation). The tracings from below up show: PEEP (applied PEEP or intrinsic PEEP); the pressure required to drive flow across the inspiratory resistance (P_{resist}); the static elastic recoil pressure of the respiratory system (P_{elast}); and pressure at the airway opening (P_{AW}). This last during inspiration equals the sum of the three lower tracings. The contribution of PEEP, P_{resist}, and P_{elast} to P_{AW} can be determined in a passive patient by: (1) noting the PEEP (or measuring intrinsic PEEP); (2) stopping flow briefly at end inspiration, during which P_{AW} falls to a lower plateau (x); (3) subtracting the plateau pressure (P_{plat}) from the peak pressure (P_{peak}) to give P_{resist}; and (4) subtracting the PEEP (or intrinsic PEEP) from P_{plat} to give P_{elast}. During expiration P_{AW} does not fall immediately (a) to the PEEP level because of finite resistance in the expiratory limb of the ventilator. Similarly, the P_{peak} does not fall immediately (b) to P_{plat} because of time required for redistribution of gas and viscoelastic properties of the respiratory system. (Redrawn with permission from Schmidt et al[30].)

not completely passive during the manoeuvre. PEEP is set by the ventilator. The remainder of the P_{AW} ($\Delta P = P_{peak} - \text{PEEPtot}$) can be apportioned between its two components, P_{resist} and P_{stat}, by stopping flow at end-inspiration and allowing the P_{AW} to drop to a plateau level (P_{plat}; Fig. 14.7). Then:

$$P_{resist} = P_{peak} - P_{plat}$$

$$P_{stat} = P_{plat} - \text{PEEPtot}.$$

With an inspiratory flow in the range of 1 l/s, P_{resist} is typically between 4 cmH$_2$O and 10 cmH$_2$O. Elevated P_{resist} is found with high $\dot{V}_I$ or increased R_{AW}. When $\dot{V}_I$ remains unchanged, a rise in P_{resist} may indicate, for example, increased bronchospasm or endotracheal tube obstruction. Conversely, falling P_{resist} may correspond to a response to bronchodilators. Because $P_{stat} = V_T \times E_{RS}$, elevated P_{stat} indicates excessive V_T or increased elastic recoil of the lungs or chest wall, as in pulmonary fibrosis, acute lung injury or abdominal distension. Respiratory system static compliance (C_{RS}) is the inverse of E_{RS} and is normally about 70 ml/cmH$_2$O.

Often the cause of ventilatory failure has not been determined by the time of endotracheal intubation. If the P_{peak} is not abnormally high in a passive, ventilated patient, the physician should suspect impaired drive, neuromuscular weakness or a transient, now resolved, problem (e.g. upper airway obstruction bypassed by the endotracheal tube) as the cause for ventilatory failure. When the P_{peak} is high, partitioning its components into the P_{resist}, the P_{stat}, and PEEPi can help to narrow the differential diagnosis and to adapt therapy specifically to the cause of ventilatory failure.

Effect of patient effort on airway pressure

Patients usually perform inspiratory work during assist–control breaths.[52] This may not be obvious despite careful examination of the patient unless intrathoracic pressure (oesophageal pressure, central venous pressure) is measured. Clues to patient effort are often available from the P_{AW} tracing, such as concavity of the rise in P_{AW}, variability of P_{peak}, and a dip in P_{AW} before inspiration, indicating a triggering effort.

Measurement of respiratory muscle strength

The *maximal inspiratory pressure* generated on a voluntary (or involuntary) inspiratory effort from FRC is commonly used to test respiratory muscle strength. Measurement of the voluntary P_{Imax} requires patient effort and coordination and is difficult to perform reproducibly in many intubated critically ill patients. Accordingly, in clinical practice, the measured pressure is not necessarily maximal 'P_{Imax}' has low predictive value for weaning and cannot therefore be used by itself reliably to predict weaning outcome. However, it can help to identify patients with potentially treatable respiratory muscle weakness and to monitor its improvement or deterioration.

The *vital capacity* is also used to assess respiratory muscle strength. A value greater than 10 ml/kg has been suggested to predict weaning success but, again, its predictive value is low. Measurement of VC can help to monitor the respiratory muscle strength of patients with relatively normal lungs and respiratory muscle weakness, as in myasthenia gravis or Guillain–Barré syndrome.

> ## ? Unresolved questions
>
> ■ What is the role of respiratory muscle fatigue in the pathogenesis of respiratory failure?
>
> ■ To what extent does open-lung ventilation improve the prognosis of acute respiratory distress syndrome?
>
> ■ Are there useful pharmacological interventions in the management of acute respiratory distress syndrome?
>
> ■ What are the most appropriate indications for non-invasive positive-pressure ventilation in acute respiratory failure?

References

1. Hall JB, Schmidt GA, Wood LDH. An approach to critical care. In: Hall JB, Schmidt GA, Wood LDH, ed. Principles of critical care. New York: McGraw-Hill; 1998: 3–9.
2. Wood LDH. The pathophysiology and differential diagnosis of acute respiratory failure. In: Hall JB, Schmidt GA, Wood LDH, ed. Principles of critical care. New York: McGraw-Hill; 1998: 499–508.
3. Roussos C. Respiratory muscle fatigue and ventilatory failure. In: Hall JB, Schmidt GA, Wood LDH, ed. Principles of critical care. New York: McGraw-Hill; 1992: 1701–1709.
4. Dantzker RM. Gas exchange in the adult respiratory distress syndrome. Clin Chest Med 1982; 3: 57–67.
5. Wagner P, Dantzker D, Dueck D et al. Ventilation–perfusion inequality in chronic obstructive pulmonary disease. J Clin Invest 1977; 59: 203–216.
6. Wood LDH, Schmidt GA, Hall JB. Principles of critical care of respiratory failure. In: Murray JF, Nadel JA, ed. Textbook of respiratory medicine. Philadelphia, PA: WB Saunders; 2000: 2377–2411.
7. Hickling KG, Walsh J, Handerson S et al. Low mortality rate in adult respiratory distress syndrome using low volume, pressure limited ventilation with permissive hypercapnia: a prospective study. Crit Care Med 1994; 22: 1568–1578.
8. Amato MRP, Barbases N, Medeiros DM et al. Effect of a protective-ventilation strategy on mortality in the acute respiratory distress syndrome. N Engl J Med 1998; 338: 347–354.
9. Sznajder JI, Nahum A, Hansen DE et al. Volume recruitment and oxygenation in pulmonary edema. J Crit Care 1998; 13: 126–135.
10. Mitchel JR Schuiler D, Callandrino FS et al. Improved outcome based on fluid management in critically ill patients requiring pulmonary artery catheterization. Am J Respir Crit Care Med 1992; 145: 990–998.
11. Hedenstierna G. Mechanisms of postoperative pulmonary dysfunction. Acta Chir Scand Suppl 198; 550: 152–158.
12. Walley KR, Wood LDH. Shock. In: Hall JB, Schmidt GA, Wood LDH, ed. Principles of critical care. New York: McGraw-Hill; 1998: 277–301.
13. Hall JB, Schmidt GA, Wood LDH. Acute hypoxemic respiratory failure. In: Murray JF, Nadel JA, ed. Textbook of respiratory medicine. Philadelphia, PA: WB Saunders; 2000: 2413–2442.
14. Polese U, Rossi A, Appendini L et al. Partitioning of respiratory mechanics in mechanically ventilated patients. J Appl Physiol 1991; 71: 2433–2435
15. Aberman A, Fulop M. The metabolic and respiratory acidosis of acute pulmonary edema. Ann Intern Med 1972; 76: 173–184.
16. Goldberg IF, Cohn JN. New inotropic drugs for heart failure. JAMA 1987; 258: 493.
17. Bersten AD, Huh AW, Vedig AE et al. Treatment of severe cardiogenic pulmonary edema with continuous positive airway pressure delivered by face mask. N Engl J Med 1991; 325: 1825–1830.
18. Abou-Shala N, Mcduri U. Noninvasive ventilation in patients with acute respiratory failure. Crit Care Med 1996; 24: 705–715.
19. Calvein JE, Driedger AA, Sibbald WJ. Positive end-expiratory pressure (PEEP) does not depress left ventricular function in patients with pulmonary edema. Am Rev Respir Dis 1981; 124: 121–128.
20. Artigas A, Bernard GR, Carlet I et al. The American–European Consensus Conference on ARDS, part 2: Ventilatory, pharmacologic, supportive therapy, study design strategies, and issues related to recovery and remodeling. Am J Respir Crit Care Med 1998; 157: 1332–1347.
21. Ware LB, Matthay MA. The acute respiratory distress syndrome. N Engl J Med 2000; 342: 1334–1349.
22. Dreyfuss D, Basset U, Soler R et al. Intermittent positive pressure hyperventilation with high inflation pressures produces pulmonary microvascular injury in rats. Am J Respir Crit Care Med 1985; 132: 880–884.
23. Dreyfuss D, Saumon U. Ventilator-induced lung injury: lessons from experimental studies. Am J Respir Crit Care Med 1998; 157: 294–323.
24. Marini JJ. Lung mechanics in the adult respiratory distress syndrome: recent conceptual advances and implications for management. Chest 1990; 11: 673–679.
25. Slutsky AR, Tremblay LN. Multiple system organ failure: is mechanical ventilation a contributing factor? Am J Respir Crit Care Med 1998; 157: 1721–1725.
26. Ranieri VM, Suter PM, Tontorella C et al. Effect of mechanical ventilation on inflammatory mediators in patients with acute respiratory distress syndrome. JAMA 1999; 282: 54–61.
27. Light RB, Mink 5, Wood LDH. Pathophysiology of gas exchange and pulmonary perfusion in pneumococcal lobar pneumonia in dogs. J Appl Physiol 1981; 50: 524–530.
28. Vassilakopoulos T, Zakynthinos S, Roussos C. Respiratory muscles and ventilatory failure. Monaldi Arch Chest Med 1996; 51: 489–498.
29. Vassilakopoulos T, Zakynthinos S, Roussos C. Respiratory muscles and weaning failure. Eur Respir J 199; 9: 2383–2400.
30. Schmidt GA, Hall JB, Wood LDH. Ventilatory failure. In: Murray JF, Nadel JA, ed. Textbook of respiratory medicine. Philadelphia, PA: WB Saunders; 2000: 2443–2470.
31. Lemaire F, Teboul JL, Cinotti L et al. Acute left ventricular dysfunction during unsuccessful weaning from mechanical ventilation. Anesthesiology 1988; 69: 171–179.
32. Hurford WE, Lynch KE, Strauss WH et al. Myocardial perfusion as assessed by thallium 201 scintigraphy during the discontinuation of mechanical ventilation in ventilator dependent patients. Anesthesiology 1991; 74: 1007–1016.
33. Dhand R, Tobin MJ. Inhaled bronchodilator therapy in mechanically ventilated patients. Am J Respir Crit Care Med 1997; 156: 3–10.
34. Appel D, Karpel JP, Sherman M. Epinephrine improves expiratory airflow rates in patients with asthma who do not respond to inhaled metaproterenol sulfate. J Allergy Clin Immunol 1989; 84: 90–98.
35. Tuxen DV, Lane S. The effects of ventilatory pattern on hyperinflation, airway pressures, and circulation in mechanical ventilation of patients with severe air-flow obstruction. Am Rev Respir Dis 1987; 136: 872–879.
36. Williams TJ, Tuxen DV, Scheinkestel CD et al. Risk factors for morbidity in mechanically ventilated patients with acute severe asthma. Am Rev Respir Dis 1992;146: 607–615.
37. Tuxen DV. Permissive hypercapnic ventilation. Am J Respir Crit Care Med 1994; 150: 870–874.

38. Bachmann P, Gaussorgues P, Piperno D et al. Hydrocortisone and pancuronium bromide: acute myopathy during status asthmaticus. Crit Care Med 1988; 16: 731–733.

39. Knox AJ, Mascie-Taylor BH, Muers M. Acute hydrocortisone myopathy in acute severe asthma. Thorax 1986; 41: 411–412.

40. Appendini L, Purro A, Patessio A et al. Partitioning of inspiratory muscle workload and pressure assistance in ventilator-dependent COPD patients. Am J Respir Crit Care Med 1996; 154: 1301–1309.

41. Ranieni VM, Giuliani R, Cinnella G et al. Physiologic effects of positive end-expiratory pressure in patients with chronic obstructive pulmonary disease during acute ventilatory failure and controlled mechanical ventilation. Am Rev Respir Dis 1993; 147: 5–13.

42. Brochard L, Rauss A, Benito S et al. Comparison of three methods of gradual withdrawal from ventilatory support during weaning from mechanical ventilation. Am J Respir Crit Care Med 1994; 150: 896–903.

43. Esteban A, Frutos F, Tobin MJ et al, for the Spanish Lung Failure Collaborative Group. A comparison of four methods of weaning patients from mechanical ventilation. N Engl J Med 1995; 332: 345–350.

44. Esteban A, Alia I, Gordo F et al, for the Spanish Lung Failure Collaborative Group. Extubation outcome after spontaneous breathing trials with T-tube or pressure support ventilation. Am J Respir Crit Care Med 1997; 156: 459–465.

45. Ely EW, Baker AM, Dunagan DP et al. Effect on the duration of mechanical ventilation of identifying patients capable of breathing spontaneously. N Engl J Med 1996; 335: 1864–1869.

46. Boulain T and the Association des Reanimateurs du Centre-Ouest. Unplanned extubations in the Adult Intensive Care Unit. A prospective multicenter study. Am J Respir Crit Care Med 1998; 157: 1131–1137.

47. Saura P, Blanch L, Mestre J et al. Clinical consequences of the implementation of a weaning protocol. Intensive Care Med 1996; 22: 1052–1056.

48. Kollef MH, Shapiro SD, Silver P et al. A randomized, controlled trial of protocol-directed versus physician directed weaning from mechanical ventilation. Crit Care Med 1997; 25: 567–574.

49. Vassilakopoulos T, Roussos C, Zakynthinos S. Weaning from mechanical ventilation. J Crit Care 1999; 14: 38–62.

50. Vassilakopoulos T, Zakynthinos S, Roussos C. The tension-time index and the frequency/tidal volume ratio are the major pathophysiologic determinants of weaning failure and success. Am J Respir Crit Care Med 1998; 158: 1–8.

51. Esteban A, Alia A, Ibanez J et al. Modes of ventilation and weaning. A national survey of Spanish hospitals. The Spanish Lung Failure Collaborative Group. Chest 1994; 106: 1188–1193.

52. Marini JJ, Rodriguez RM, Lamb V. The inspiratory workload of patient-initiated mechanical ventilation. Am Rev Respir Dis 1986.; 134: 902–909.

15 Principles of non-invasive ventilatory support

Mark W Elliott

 Key points

■ There should be a high index of suspicion for patients at risk of nocturnal hypoventilation.

■ The use of non-invasive ventilation is well established in patients with neuromuscular disease and chest-wall deformity.

■ Currently, non-invasive ventilation has a limited role in chronic ventilatory failure due to COPD.

■ Non-invasive ventilation is indicated in patients with mild acidosis due to acute exacerbations of COPD.

■ Non-invasive ventilation is useful in *selected* patients with hypoxaemic respiratory failure due to a variety of different conditions, in postextubation respiratory failure and for weaning.

Until the Copenhagen polio epidemic in the 1950s non-invasive ventilation, using external negative-pressure devices, had been the modality of ventilatory support of choice. During the epidemic, because of the numbers of patients needing ventilatory support and the lack of sufficient negative-pressure equipment, patients were ventilated, via an endotracheal tube, manually by teams working round the clock. Thereafter positive-pressure ventilation via an endotracheal tube became the method of choice, with negative-pressure ventilation confined to a small number of specialist centres and limited to patients with severe chronic ventilatory failure. However in recent years, with the development of interfaces and ventilators suitable for delivering positive-pressure ventilation non-invasively, there has been a resurgence of interest in non-invasive ventilation (NIV) initially for a wider range of patients with chronic ventilatory failure and subsequently for those with acute respiratory failure.

Modes of non-invasive ventilation

Negative-pressure devices

These have largely been superseded by positive-pressure devices but there is still a role in selected patients, primarily those who are unable to tolerate positive-pressure ventilation. The iron lung is the most efficient and modern machines can be triggered in response to patient effort. Although very good results have been reported, even in patients with severe ventilatory failure,[1,2] use of this method is confined to a few specialist centres. Negative-pressure ventilation may also have a role following paediatric cardiac surgery.[3,4] Although portable iron lungs are available, their size and expense precludes widespread domiciliary use and negative-pressure ventilation at home is usually delivered using either a cuirass or poncho wrap ventilator. Apart from the difficulty of achieving an acceptable seal in some patients, the discomfort associated with their use and their cumbersome nature, the major problem is that these devices worsen or precipitate upper airway obstruction during sleep.[5,6] Comparative trials are under way comparing negative-pressure ventilation with NIV by positive pressure in acute exacerbations of COPD and it is quite possible that negative-pressure ventilation may experience a resurgence in the future.

Positive-pressure ventilation

Ventilators usually used for NIV are either volume- or pressure-targeted. Volume-preset ventilators deliver a constant flow of gas and the pressure generated by the machine is that required to achieve a predetermined tidal volume. Pressure-preset ventilators deliver a constant pressure and the resulting tidal volume depends upon lung and chest wall mechanics. The timing of the inspiratory and expiratory phases can be adjusted and positive pressure can be administered during expiration (positive end-expiratory positive pressure – PEEP). Ventilation may be provided totally by the machine or the patient can initiate some or all breaths (triggering), which facilitates in part the transition from fully supported ventilation to spontaneous breathing. There are theoretical advantages to each mode, but broadly speaking they are comparable in efficacy. Volume targeted ventilators have been shown to produce more complete offloading of the respiratory muscles, but at the expense of comfort.[7] In intubated patients, however, assist pressure-controlled ventilation has been shown to be more effective than assist volume-controlled ventilation in reducing various parameters of respiratory muscle effort, although this difference is only seen at moderate tidal volumes and low flow rates.[8] In stable patients little difference in gas exchange is seen with different types of ventilator.[9,10] In terms of outcome, Vitacca et al[11] found that there was no difference whether volume-targeted or pressure-targeted machines were used in acute respiratory failure, but pressure-targeted machines were better tolerated by patients. During domiciliary ventilation a switch from pressure to volume ventilators has been shown to improve the control of nocturnal hypoventilation in some patients,[12] but the contrary has also been shown in others.[13]

A new mode of proportional assist ventilation improves gas exchange and dyspnoea in stable chronic obstructive pulmonary disease (COPD)[14] and has been used successfully in the treatment of acute respiratory failure of various aetiologies.[15] Proportional assist ventilation delivers ventilation according to patient demand, which should theoretically be more comfortable but makes the assumption that the patient with respiratory failure knows best what s/he needs in terms of ventilatory support. Proportional assist ventilation using flow assistance and PEEP achieved the greatest improvement in minute ventilation, dyspnoea and reduction in pressure time product per breath of the respiratory muscles and diaphragm in patients with COPD and acute respiratory failure.[16] It has been shown to decrease patient effort, work of breathing and neuromuscular drive ($P_{0.1}$) in patients with COPD being weaned from invasive mechanical ventilation.[17,18] Further data are needed comparing proportional assist ventilation with conventional modes of ventilation, particularly the effect upon outcome.

Pressure-cycled machines are usually cheaper than volume-cycled flow generators and this, together with their usually better tolerability, makes them the machines of first choice. In addition, because they increase flow to achieve the target pressure, they compensate better for leaks. However, if the impedance to inflation is very high or changes suddenly, tidal volume will fall and in this situation a volume-cycled ventilator is preferable.

Continuous positive airway pressure (CPAP) can be considered as a mode of non-invasive ventilation. In patients with restrictive lung disease it improves oxygenation and reduces the work of breathing by recruiting atelectatic lung, improving ventilation/perfusion relationships and increasing functional residual capacity. In patients with COPD it counterbalances intrinsic PEEP, thereby reducing the work of breathing,[19] but the benefit seen is not as great as when PEEP is added to pressure support ventilation.[10,20] CPAP may also be useful in splinting the upper airway during sleep when there is upper airway obstruction, which in the acute setting may further compromise effective ventilation. It has been shown to reduce inspiratory muscle effort during sleep in chronic stable patients with COPD but without any beneficial effects upon gas exchange or daytime symptoms.[21] CPAP requires a spontaneously breathing patient and is ineffective if the patient makes no or little respiratory effort. PEEP can be added during NIV and has beneficial effects, offloading the respiratory muscles, probably by counterbalancing the inspiratory threshold load imposed by intrinsic PEEP,[22] and lavaging carbon dioxide from the mask.[23]

The advantages and disadvantages of these different modes are summarised in Table 15.1.

Interfaces

The interface is crucial to successful NIV. These can be factory-manufactured or customised. Driven largely by the explosion in the diagnosis and treatment of obstructive sleep apnoea, there are now a wide variety of different factory-made masks of different designs, shapes, sizes and materials. It is usually possible to find something that suits most individuals and there is seldom a need for an individually made interface. Broadly speaking, there are four different types of interface: full face masks (enclosing mouth and nose), nasal masks, nasal pillows or plugs (inserted directly into the nostrils), and mouthpieces. New devices, akin to a diver's helmet, have recently been reported and may prove to be very effective for acute NIV. A review of published studies showed that in acute NIV facial masks predominate (63%), followed by nasal masks (31%) and nasal pillows (6%). In contrast, for chronic NIV nasal masks (73%) are the most commonly used, followed by nasal pillows (11%), facial masks (6%) and mouthpieces (5%).

Non-invasive ventilation in chronic ventilatory failure

The causes of chronic ventilatory failure potentially treatable by non-invasive ventilation are summarised in Table 15.2.

Neuromuscular disease and chest-wall deformity

Several uncontrolled studies have demonstrated benefit from nocturnal NIV in terms of improvement in daytime arterial blood gases, relief of the symptoms of nocturnal hypoventilation and improved survival compared to that which would be expected without treatment[25-29] in patients with neuromuscular and chest wall diseases.

Although there are no large prospective randomised controlled trials, a number of case series have reported excellent results in patients with severely deranged blood gas tensions, who would have been expected to have a very poor prognosis. Simonds & Elliott[30] reported a 5-year actuarial survival for patients with previous polo of 100%, sequelae of tuberculosis 95%, neuromuscular disease 81% and early-onset scoliosis 79%. Health status amongst those ventilated compared favourably with UK population norms and with patients in the USA with chronic disorders. Leger et al reported similar results in 276 patients from a number of centres in France[31] and showed a reduction in hospital charges once NIV was instituted.

Table 15.1 Modes of positive-pressure ventilation used for non-invasive ventilation

Mode	Description	Advantages	Disadvantages
Continuous positive airway pressure (CPAP)	Continuous positive pressure, which is the same throughout inspiration and expiration. Requires spontaneously breathing patient	Simple Cheap	Little evidence to support its use in acute or chronic respiratory failure, except when due to cardiogenic pulmonary oedema or obstructive sleep apnoea
Pressure ventilation (PV)	A predetermined pressure is set – delivered tidal volume will depend upon patient effort and impedance to inflation. Can be used in assist mode only (pressure support), timed mode (pressure controlled) or a combination	Widely used Better evidence base for effectiveness than V V Greater patient comfort than V V Leak compensation Easy to add EPAP/PEEP Machines generally cheaper and smaller than V V	Will fail to ventilate patient if impedance to inflation is high or changing
Volume ventilation (V V)	A predetermined volume is set and the machine generates the pressure necessary to deliver this. Used in assist or control mode or, more usually, combination	Effective when impedance to inflation is high More effective unloading of respiratory muscles (?)	No leak compensation Less well tolerated than pressure ventilators ($\pm$) Machines tend to be more expensive
Proportional assist ventilation (PAV)	Ventilation in response to patient effort	Closer to natural breathing Greater patient comfort than other modes More unloading of respiratory muscles than pressure support	Ineffective if poor patient effort No outcome data to show more effective than existing modes

EPAP, expiratory positive airway pressure; PEEP; positive end-expiratory pressure.

Table 15.2 Causes of chronic ventilatory failure potentially treatable by non-invasive ventilation[24]

Chest-wall deformity
- Early-onset scoliosis
- Thoracoplasty/sequelae of tuberculosis

Non- or slowly progressing neurological conditions
- Central hypoventilation syndrome
- Ondine's curse
- Spinal cord injury – tetraplegia
- Poliomyelitis
- Diaphragmatic paralysis
- Metabolic myopathies
- Spinal muscular atrophy
- Congenital myopathies

Rapidly progressive neuromuscular disorders
- Duchenne muscular dystrophy
- Motor neurone disease

Lung disease
- Chronic obstructive pulmonary disease
- Cystic fibrosis
- Bronchiectasis

However retrospective or uncontrolled studies may bias the literature for a number of reasons. First, negative results are often not published and the literature therefore reflects the experience of a few enthusiastic units, usually tertiary referral centres, limiting the generalisability of the results. Second, the point at which NIV is initiated may affect length of survival. The earlier NIV is started, the longer survival is likely to be; the apparently improved survival may therefore be deceptive. Thirdly, for ease of analysis and presentation, patients with a variety of different disorders are often grouped and good results in one disorder may mask a lack of benefit in another when all are analysed together. Caution should therefore be exercised in the interpretation of survival data from uncontrolled studies.

Often, non-invasive ventilation is started to improve symptoms. In some cases the improvement is dramatic and symptoms return consistently when NIV is withdrawn, but in others it is less clear-cut. There are few data objectively assessing the effect of NIV on quality of life using appropriate scales or objectively confirming end-points that are important to patients, such as exercise capacity. NIV during sleep is often regarded as unpleasant and the fact that patients use it is considered evidence of benefit, in that they would not continue if they did not perceive that the advantages were greater than the disadvantages. The same was also previously thought to be true for CPAP in the treatment of obstructive sleep apnoea. However a recent double-blind randomised controlled trial comparing active with sham CPAP showed a significant placebo effect on symptoms, particularly energy and vitality, although the improvements were substantially and significantly less than those seen in the actively treated group.[32] The placebo effect of a 'breathing machine' on individuals who have problems with breathing and have been told that they have potentially life-threatening ventilatory failure should not be underestimated. Observational studies are, however, valid[33] and the place of NIV in these patient groups is now so well established that most would consider it unethical to perform a prospective randomised controlled trial with survival, or even quality of life, as end-points. Questions remain, however, regarding the appropriate timing of intervention, and further data are needed.

Rapidly progressive neuromuscular disease

In more rapidly progressive neuromuscular disease, e.g. Duchenne muscular dystrophy or motor neurone disease, death from ventilatory failure is common. Assisted ventilation may be instituted when the patient is *in extremis*, sometimes before a firm diagnosis has been made, when there is little doubt from short-term trials of spontaneous breathing that the patient can not sustain sufficient ventilation to support life.

A number of studies have shown symptomatic benefits in patients at an earlier stage in the natural history of their disease.[34-38] In a non-randomised controlled trial, Pinto et al[37] compared the outcome of 10 patients with motor neurone disease treated with NIV to 10 control patients who had refused NIV. Although the forced vital capacity (FVC) of the NIV-treated group was lower, suggesting more severe respiratory muscle weakness, 50% were alive at 2 years, whereas all the control patients had died within 8 months. On the other hand, Raphael et al[39] randomised patients with Duchenne muscular dystrophy to NIV or conventional therapy and found that there was a trend towards increased mortality with NIV. However this study should be interpreted with caution: the patients studied might not be expected to benefit from NIV as they had no evidence of hypoventilation either by day (P_aCO_2 normal) or at night (not measured, but unlikely given normal daytime P_aCO_2). Uncontrolled studies[31,40] have shown excellent results in hypercapnic patients with Duchenne muscular dystrophy in terms of survival, with one reporting a 73% 5-year survival in 24 patients.[40]

In patients with rapidly progressive neuromuscular disease there are a number of potential problems related to extending life by mechanical ventilation. These include life of marginal quality, disruption to the lives of other family members and difficulty in stopping high-technology life-sustaining care once it has been started.[35] For most patients and their carers it is not just a question of survival at any cost. There are a few data on quality of life in patients with motor neurone disease receiving home mechanical ventilation, but when it has been recorded most report significant symptomatic improvement without distressing prolongation of life.[34,41] In a study of ventilator users with Duchenne muscular dystrophy,[42] health-care professionals significantly underestimated the patient's scores in the life satisfaction and general affect instruments and significantly overestimated the relative hardship associated with ventilator dependence, confirming that the patient is in the best position to determine what is, and what is not, an acceptable quality of life.

Patients with neuromuscular disease often have a weak cough and the issue of clearance of secretions often needs to be addressed before NIV becomes necessary. Once the FVC falls below 2 litres, techniques to maximise secretion clearance should be taught.[43] These include abdominal thrust manoeuvres, breath stacking and the use of cough machines.[44] A comprehensive approach targeted at improving secretion clearance has been shown to reduce the need for hospitalisation in such patients.[43,45]

Clinical implications

In general, hypercapnic ventilatory failure worsens during sleep because of a normal physiological reduction of respiratory drive. Initially, patients develop ventilatory failure only at night, managing to maintain a normal carbon dioxide tension during the day; an otherwise unexplained elevation in base excess may be a clue to the presence of nocturnal hypoventilation. As the disease progresses, abnormal blood gas tensions develop by day. Symptoms are non-specific and may be mistaken for a 'normal' effect of the underlying disease; they include lethargy, sleepiness, morning headache, neuropsychiatric symptoms, dyspnoea and ankle oedema.

These patients are at risk of sudden life-threatening deterioration, e.g. with a trivial chest infection. Unfortunately, patients with severe chest-wall or neuromuscular diseases not infrequently present as an emergency, sometimes requiring intubation and mechanical ventilation, with a history typical of nocturnal hypoventilation going back over many months. Because symptoms are so non-specific, it is important to have a high index of suspicion in 'at risk' individuals (Table 15.2) and a low threshold for further investigation. Those at risk of developing nocturnal hypoventilation should be evaluated at an early stage because the need for NIV can often be anticipated by observing trends in physiological measurements. Patients should be warned of the symptoms of nocturnal hypoventilation and those with a weak cough can be taught how to maximise secretion clearance. Suggested investigations are shown in Table 15.3.

Table 15.3 Investigation of a patient at risk for nocturnal hypoventilation

Minimum
- Spirometry (lying and sitting if neuromuscular disease)
- Maximum respiratory pressures (if neuromuscular disease)
- Arterial blood gas tensions
- Overnight monitoring of oxygen saturation ± transcutaneous CO_2

Additional
- More detailed pulmonary function tests
- Sniff nasal inspiratory pressure[47]
- Measurement of transdiaphragmatic pressure during a sniff and following electrical or magnetic stimulation of the phrenic nerves
- Detailed sleep monitoring if obstructive sleep apnoea is suspected

Non-invasive ventilation and chronic ventilatory failure secondary to lung disease

That artificial ventilation should be effective in patients with an abnormality of their own 'ventilator' due to neuromuscular disease or chest wall deformity is not surprising. However, NIV is increasingly offered to patients with ventilatory failure due to chronic lung disease in whom the primary abnormality is in the lungs themselves. A number of studies have shown that domiciliary nocturnal NIV is feasible in patients with COPD[26,30,31,46,48–50] and bronchiectasis[51] and that abnormal physiology can be corrected using NIV; gas exchange during sleep can be improved,[46] excessive respiratory muscle activation reduced[52,53] and exercise capacity and diurnal arterial blood gas tensions can be improved.[46,49] Use of health-care resources is also reduced.[50]

However, there have been few controlled trials and most of these had small numbers of patients followed over a short period of time.[54–57] The studies have generally been characterised by no significant advantage from NIV,[54–56] poor tolerance[54] and worse sleep efficiency.[56] However, Meecham Jones et al[55] showed improvements in daytime arterial blood gas tensions, sleep quality and quality of life during the pressure support limb of a crossover study comparing pressure-support ventilation and oxygen with oxygen alone. This was the only study in which the overnight control of nocturnal hypoventilation was confirmed and the improvement in daytime P_aCO_2 correlated with a reduction in overnight transcutaneous CO_2.

Other possible explanations for the failure of NIV include: patients not hypercapnic, insufficient inflation pressures to achieve adequate ventilation, and inadequate patient acclimatisation to the technique. Larger case series of patients with COPD[30,31] suggest survival comparable to that seen in the patients treated with long-term oxygen in the Medical Research Council and Nocturnal Oxygen Therapy Trial studies.[58–60] The patients included were often those who had 'failed' (not rigorously defined) on oxygen therapy and were usually hypercapnic.

The exact place of NIV in chronic ventilatory failure secondary to COPD remains unclear and needs to be evaluated by further large randomised controlled trials with clearly defined end-points. Long-term oxygen therapy is one of only two interventions that have been shown to prolong life in patients with COPD and remains the gold standard for the treatment of ventilatory failure in this condition. Preliminary results from two multicentre European trials comparing NIV with long-term oxygen therapy in COPD suggest that NIV does not improve survival but may reduce the need for hospitalisation.[61,62]

Until further data are available a trial of NIV can only at present be justified in patients who have symptoms of nocturnal hypoventilation (morning headaches, daytime sleepiness, etc.) despite maximal bronchodilator therapy or who cannot tolerate long-term oxygen therapy. Most studies suggest that it is the patients with more severe hypercapnia who are likely to benefit and there is no place for nocturnal NIV in those without sustained daytime hypercapnia. Adequate control of nocturnal hypoventilation should be confirmed, as this has been a feature of the studies in which benefit has been seen.[46,55]

Effects of non-invasive ventilation

An understanding of how NIV has an effect on unsupported breathing is important in determining the appropriate goal of therapy. Effective ventilation is achieved when the respiratory muscle pump has sufficient capacity to deal with the load imposed upon it and the system receives the necessary drive. It has been suggested that NIV 'works' by resting chronically fatigued respiratory muscles.[63] However, research in this area has been hampered by the absence of good tests of respiratory muscle fatigue and gives conflicting results. Small increases in maximum respiratory pressures have been cited as evidence of improved capacity, although in the absence of a control group these may have been due to learning effects and better motivation.

Other studies[64,65] have reported improved daytime arterial blood gas tensions in the absence of changes in the indices of respiratory muscle strength. In randomised controlled trial, Shapiro et al[66] studied 184 patients with COPD randomised to active or sham domiciliary negative-pressure ventilation using a poncho wrap ventilator. They showed no significant difference between the two groups but compliance with treatment was much less than anticipated. They concluded that respiratory muscle fatigue (measured by a 6 min walking test) was not present and that little was to be gained by resting the respiratory muscles. However, 6 min walking distance is an unconventional measure of respiratory muscle fatigue. It is difficult to draw any meaningful conclusions from this study except that the poor compliance suggests that any symptomatic benefit was outweighed by the disadvantages associated with negative-pressure ventilation. Further carefully designed studies in stable patients, controlling for the effects of motivation and learning upon test performance and using newer techniques to assess respiratory muscle function,[67] are needed.

There are few data about the effect of NIV upon load. Simonds et al[68] showed no change in 'accessible lung volume' in patients using a device delivering large tidal volumes used for 10–15 min per day. However, there was a sustained improvement in vital capacity and maximum voluntary ventilation and it was suggested that this may have been due to changes in chest-wall compliance. In eight patients with COPD, Elliott et al[64] showed a small reduction in gas trapping and increase in dynamic compliance and hypothesised that this was due to a reduction in lung water.

Some data support the hypothesis that restoration of central respiratory drive is important. Berthon Jones et al[69] showed a leftward shift of the ventilatory response curve to progressive hypercapnia in patients with severe obstructive sleep apnoea after 90 days treatment with CPAP. Annane et al[70] found that an improvement in diurnal P_aCO_2 correlated with the improvement in the slope of the ventilatory response to CO_2 in patients with neuromuscular disease and chest-wall deformity. In eight patients with severe COPD ventilated non-invasively during sleep for 6 months, Elliott et al[64] showed a reduction in bicarbonate and base excess and a resetting of the ventilatory response to CO_2 at a lower level. However, Appendini et al[20] recorded a high $P_{0.1}$ (an index of central drive) in eight ventilator-dependent patients with COPD, suggesting that, in these patients, an abnormality of respiratory centre output was unlikely. Schonhofer et al[71] found no change in $P_{0.1}$ after a period of non-invasive ventilation in patients with extra-pulmonary restrictive disorders.

Patients receiving domiciliary ventilation often report an improved sense of well-being and better-quality sleep and this may be accompanied by only small changes in arterial blood gas tensions. Severe sleep disruption occurs in patients with COPD[72] and neuromuscular/chest-wall deformity[73] and is improved during NIV.[46,55,65,70] Masa et al,[74] in a 2-week comparison of NIV with overnight supplemental oxygen, showed that, although oxygen therapy resulted in a greater improvement in overnight oxygen saturation, it did not ameliorate symptoms of morning headache, lethargy or dyspnoea. NIV, by contrast, was effective in improving symptoms and diurnal blood gas tensions. Of the 21 patients studied, 19 opted to continue NIV, one to continue oxygen and one declined both therapies.

Further evidence that sleep quality may be important comes from studies in which NIV was withdrawn for short periods. Hill et al[75] found a return of symptoms of daytime sleepiness, morning headache and dyspnoea and worsening nocturnal oxygen saturation, but no change in diurnal arterial blood gas tensions or maximum pressures when NIV was withdrawn for 1 week in six patients with restrictive chest-wall disease. Jiminez et al[76] also showed a deterioration in sleep quality, accompanied by severe derangements in oxygen saturation, when NIV was stopped for 15 days in five patients who had been using NIV for at least 2 months.

However NIV does not necessarily have to be administered during sleep to improve physiological variables and sleep quality. Schonhofer et al[71] allocated patients to receive NIV either during sleep or while awake during the day for 1 month. Improved diurnal blood gas tensions, increased respiratory

muscle strength and a slight reduction in occlusion pressure $P_{0.1}$ were seen in both groups with no differences between them. At the end of the study, overnight oxygen saturation, transcutaneous CO_2 tension and sleep quality also improved in both groups during spontaneous breathing overnight. The finding of a reduction in $P_{0.1}$ and an improvement in respiratory muscle strength suggests that improvement in muscle function, rather than restoration of central drive, was the important mechanism. Daytime NIV is an option in patients unable to sleep with a ventilator.

In summary, there are conflicting data about mechanisms of benefit from NIV. Further studies are needed in the different patient groups, using more sophisticated tests, particularly of respiratory muscle function. On the basis of current knowledge, NIV should be targeted to improve arterial blood gas tensions, reduce respiratory muscle activity and improve sleep quality. The indications for starting NIV in chronic ventilatory failure are summarised in Table 15.4.

Use of non-invasive ventilation in acute respiratory failure

In contrast to chronic respiratory failure there are now a number of prospective randomised controlled trials of NIV in acute respiratory failure (Table 15.5). It has been shown to be an effective treatment for ventilatory failure, particularly resulting from acute exacerbations of COPD but also hypoxaemic respiratory failure, community-acquired pneumonia, cardiogenic pulmonary oedema and following solid organ transplants in 12 randomised controlled trials. There have also been two randomised controlled trials of NIV in weaning. NIV has been used in a variety of different settings, with different ventilator modes and interfaces and in differing degrees of severity.

The earliest studies were performed mainly in the setting of the Intensive Care Unit (ICU) and the most striking finding was a reduction in the need for intubation and mechanical ventilation, which in the largest study translated into improved survival and reduced complication rates and length of both ICU and hospital stay.[78] However these studies were performed in units committed to the non-invasive approach and with particular expertise and this factor, more than location, may have been important in determining the outcome. Furthermore there are questions over the generalisability of these results to everyday clinical practice; results achieved in enthusiastic units as part of a clinical trial may not be achievable in other units lacking the same skill levels or commitment to making NIV work.

What these studies do show is that successful NIV is possible and that the prevention of intubation is advantageous. A reduction in the incidence of nosocomial infection is a consistent and important advantage of NIV compared with invasive ventilation.[92,93] In intubated patients there is a 1% risk per day of developing nosocomial pneumonia.[94] This complication of invasive ventilation is associated with a longer ICU stay, increased costs and a worse outcome.[95] The reduction in nosocomial infections is probably the most important advantage of avoiding intubation by using NIV.

Table 15.4 Indications for starting non-invasive ventilation in chronic respiratory failure

Chest wall deformity and slowly progressive neuromuscular disease[24]
■ Symptoms and nocturnal desaturation (S_aO_2 <88% for >5 consecutive minutes)
Rapidly progressive neuromuscular disease[24]
■ Timing less critical since tempo of disease will mean that ventilatory support will soon be required anyway
■ Consider when P_{imax} <60 cmH$_2$O
■ Consider when forced vital capacity <50% predicted
■ Hypercapnia
■ Symptoms of nocturnal hypoventilation
■ Severe orthopnoea with sleep disturbance but without evidence of nocturnal hypoventilation
Chronic obstructive pulmonary disease and lung diseases
■ Hypercapnia
■ Failure of long-term oxygen therapy (first ensure optimal bronchodilator therapy and careful titration of oxygen therapy)
■ Intractable cor pulmonale

Table 15.5 Summary of prospective randomised controlled trials of non-invasive ventilation in patients with lung disease. Figures in bold are statistically significant results ($p < 0.05$).

	Disease (n)	Setting	Baseline data (pH or P_a/F_iO_2)*	ETI or 'surrogate'	Mortality	Mode plus settings (cmH$_2$O) and use on day 1 – when stated
Bott et al[77]	COPD (60)	Ward	7.35	0/30 vs 5/30	3/30 vs 9/30	Volume-cycled ventilators. Use 7.63 h on day 1
Brochard et al[78]	COPD (85)	ICU	7.28 vs 7.27	**11/43 vs 31/42**	**4/43 vs 12/42**	PSV 20. Use at least 6 h per day
Kramer et al[79]	Mixed COPD (23)	ICU	7.28 vs 7.27 7.29 vs 7.27	**31% vs 73%** **9% vs 67%**	1/16 vs 2/15	IPAP 11.3 EPAP 2.6. Use 20.1 h on day 1
Barbe et al[80]	COPD (24)	ER and ward	7.33	0/12 vs 0/12	0/12 vs 0.12	IPAP 14.8 EPAP 5. Use 2×3 h sessions per day
Angus et al[81]	COPD (17)	Ward	7.31 vs 7.30	0.9 vs 5/8	0/9 vs 3/8	IPAP 14–18 cmH$_2$O
Wood et al[82]	Mixed (27) COPD (6)	ER	7.35 vs 7.34	7/16 vs 5/11	4/16 vs 0/11	
Celikel et al[83]	COPD (30)	ICU	7.27 vs 7.28	**1/16 vs 6/15**	0/15 vs 1/15	PSV 15.4 for mean of 26.7 h
Bardi et al[84]	COPD (30)	Ward	7.36 vs 7.39	1/15 vs 2/15	0/15 vs 1/15	IPAP 13 EPAP 3
Martin et al[85]	COPD (23) Non-COPD (38)	ICU	7.27 vs 7.28 103 vs 110*	**6.4 vs 21.3/100** ICU days	2.4 vs 4.27/100 ICU days	IPAP 11 EPAP 5.7
Plant et al[86]	COPD (236)	Ward	7.32 vs 7.31	**15% vs 27%**	**10% vs 20%**	IPAP 10–20 EPAP 5 h. Use median 8 h on day 1
Antonelli et al[87]	Hypoxic ARF (64)	ICU	116 vs 124*	10 vs 32	28% vs 47%	PSV – continuous for first 24 h
Antonelli et al[88]	Post-transplant ARF (40)	ICU	129 vs 129*	**20% vs 70%**	35% vs 55%	PSV 14–20 PEEP up to 10
Confalonieri et al[89]	Pneumonia (56) COPD (23)	ICU	183 vs 167*	**21% vs 61%**	7/28 vs 6/28	PSV 14.8 PEEP 4.9
Delclaux et al[90]	Hypoxic ARF	ICU	140 vs 148*	21% vs 24%	19% vs 18%	CPAP
Hilbert et al[91]	Immunocompromised (52)	ICU	141 vs 136*	46% vs 77%	38% vs 69%	PSV at least 45 min every 3 h

* P_a/F_iO_2: P_aO_2 (mmHg) ÷ fractional inspired oxygen concentration.
ARF, acute respiratory failure; COPD, chronic obstructive airways disease; ER, Emergency Room; ETI, endotracheal intubation; ICU, Intensive Care Unit; IPAP/EPAP/CPAP, inspiratory/expiratory/constant positive airway pressure; PEEP, positive end-expiratory pressure; PSV, pressure support ventilation

The use of NIV opens up new opportunities in the management of patients with ventilatory failure, particularly with regard to location and the timing of intervention. With NIV, paralysis and sedation are not needed and ventilation outside the ICU is an option; given the considerable pressure on ICU beds in some countries, the high costs and the distressing experience of admission to ICU for some patients,[96] this is an attractive option. It also means that ventilatory support can be instituted at an earlier stage in the course of the condition before assisted ventilation would normally be considered necessary.

A number of studies have suggested that NIV is less likely to be successful in more severely affected patients.[78,87,97] There have been eight prospective randomised controlled studies of NIV outside the ICU, either on general wards[77–82,84,86] or in the Accident and Emergency Department.[80,82] NIV was instituted at a higher arterial pH than in the ICU studies and most failed to show any significant advantage of NIV when analysed on an intention to treat basis. However, in one study,[77] when those unable to tolerate NIV were excluded, a significant survival benefit was seen (9/30 vs 1/26, $p = 0.014$).

There are a number of possible reasons for the difference between the ICU studies and those performed in the ward or Accident and Emergency Department. Most of the studies were small and may have lacked the power to show any difference in need for intubation and mortality, given that most patients with a mild exacerbation of COPD (defined by the degree of acidosis) would not be expected to need intubation and ventilation.[98] ICUs benefit from high nurse-, therapist- and doctor-to-patient ratios and staff with responsibility for a larger number of patients may not have had time to devote to instituting NIV, which certainly initially requires an investment of time to make it work.[79,99] Furthermore, non-ICU staff are likely to be relatively inexperienced in assisted ventilation and there are less facilities for patient monitoring. Finally, patients are usually admitted to ICU when other therapists have failed, whereas most of those presenting to the Emergency Room or general ward have not received any treatment. A proportion will improve after initiation of standard medical therapy. In a 1-year period prevalence study[100] of acute exacerbations of COPD, of 954 patients admitted through the Emergency Departments in

Leeds, 20% were acidotic on arrival in the Department and of these 25% had completely corrected their pH by the time of arrival on the ward. There was a weak relationship between the $PaCO_2$ on arrival at hospital and the presence of acidosis, suggesting that, in at least some patients, respiratory acidosis had been precipitated by high-flow oxygen therapy administered in the ambulance on the way to hospital.

A multicentre randomised controlled trial of NIV in acute exacerbations of COPD in general respiratory wards in 13 centres ($n = 236$) has recently been reported.[86] NIV was applied by the usual ward staff, most of whom had had little or no previous experience of NIV, using a bilevel device in spontaneous mode, according to a simple protocol. 'Treatment failure', a surrogate for the need for intubation defined by a priori criteria, was reduced from 27% to 15% by NIV ($p < 0.05$). In-hospital mortality was also reduced from 20% to 10% ($p < 0.05$). Subgroup analysis suggested that the outcome in patients with an arterial pH below 7.3 after initial treatment was inferior to that in the studies performed in the ICU. This study suggests that, with adequate staff training, NIV can be applied with benefit outside the ICU by the usual ward staff and that the early introduction of NIV on a general ward results in a better outcome than providing no ventilatory support for acidotic patients outside the ICU. The results in the more severely affected patients (pH < 7.3 after initial management) suggested that this simple approach is not appropriate in these patients and that they are best managed in a higher-dependency setting with a more sophisticated ventilator individually adjusted to their requirements. This study does, however, confirm that early intervention is advantageous.

All the studies have excluded patients who required immediate intubation and ventilation and inevitably a proportion of patients will require intubation after a failed trial of NIV. The role of NIV has been evaluated in weaning[101,102] and for the treatment of postextubation respiratory failure[103] and, although further studies are needed, the results suggest that NIV is useful in selected patients.

Indications for starting NIV in acute exacerbations of COPD are summarised in Table 15.6.

Non-invasive continuous positive airway pressure

Respiratory failure due to lung disease

There is little randomised controlled trial evidence to support the use of non-invasive CPAP, most studies being case

Table 15.6 Indications for starting non-invasive ventilation in acute respiratory failure due to chronic obstructive pulmonary disease

- Consider when pH <7.35 and respiratory rate >23/min
- Unless contraindicated, when pH <7.3
- When patient has been intubated and there is difficulty weaning, or postextubation respiratory failure

series.[104-112] In one recent randomised controlled trial,[90] non-invasive CPAP plus oxygen was compared with oxygen alone in 123 patients, of whom 102 had acute lung injury. After 1 h of treatment, a greater subjective response to treatment and improved oxygenation were seen with CPAP but no further differences in respiratory indices were observed between the groups. There was no difference in endotracheal intubation rate, hospital mortality or length of stay in the ICU. A higher number of adverse events occurred with CPAP treatment. Although it is widely used, therefore, the only available randomised controlled trial showed that, despite early physiological improvement, CPAP neither reduced the need for intubation nor improved outcomes in patients with acute hypoxaemic, non-hypercapnic respiratory insufficiency, primarily due to acute lung injury.

Cardiogenic pulmonary oedema

There is now a significant literature about the use of CPAP in patients with acute cardiogenic pulmonary oedema. Three randomised controlled trials have been performed comparing standard medical treatment plus CPAP with standard medical treatment alone.[113-115] All showed more rapid physiological improvement with CPAP and the pooled results[116] show a risk reduction for intubation of 26% (95% CI 14 to 38%) with CPAP, indicating that four patients with pulmonary oedema need to be treated with CPAP to prevent one intubation. They also suggest a trend towards reduced hospital mortality, with a risk difference of 6.6% between the two treatment groups, but the confidence intervals were wide (95% CI –16% to 3%) and thus do not allow the exclusion of harm with CPAP treatment.

Only one study to date has compared bilevel positive airway pressure (BiPAP) and CPAP in the treatment of acute pulmonary oedema.[117] Performed in the Emergency Department setting, this study of 27 patients showed that BiPAP improved ventilation and vital signs more rapidly than CPAP but there was no difference in intubation rate, mortality rate or ICU or hospital length of stay. There was, however, a trend towards an increased myocardial infarction rate in the BiPAP group, although it was unclear whether this was due to BiPAP ventilation per se, the specific settings used or a higher incidence of chest pain at the outset. Further larger studies are therefore needed comparing NIV and mask CPAP. At present, CPAP should be the mode of ventilatory support of first choice in patients with acute cardiogenic pulmonary oedema.

Monitoring progress

For safety it is recommended that all patients receiving NIV for acute ventilatory failure should have continuous monitoring of oxygen saturation by pulse oximetry and regular assessment of arterial blood gas tensions, since there is no accurate and reliable non-invasive measure of CO_2 tension or, more importantly, pH and recording of respiratory rate. The oxygen saturation should be maintained at around 92%[118] to avoid the twin dangers of dangerous hypoxia and the risk of worsening hypercapnia due to altering the dead space to tidal volume ratio.[119] Arterial blood gases should be checked at baseline and after 1–4 h because a number of studies have shown that an improvement in arterial blood gas tensions, and particularly pH, after a short period of NIV predicts a successful outcome.[77,78,97,120–122] Arterial blood gas tensions should be checked within 1 h of any change in ventilator settings or F_IO_2.

Finally, continuous or intermittent recording of respiratory rate may be useful in determining the likely outcome with NIV. Patients who have been intubated and are likely to fail a weaning attempt adopt a pattern of rapid, shallow breathing when disconnected from the ventilator,[123] indicating that they are breathing against an unsustainable load. A reduction in respiratory rate with NIV has been variably shown in a number of studies, with larger falls generally being associated with a successful outcome from NIV,[78,120,121] although this is not always seen.[124]

However, patients failing NIV do not exclusively fail at the beginning of treatment. Late failure (after 48 h of successful NIV) is recognised, with rates reported at 0–20%, and has been associated with poor outcomes. In one study,[125] 23% of patients with COPD initially successfully treated with NIV subsequently deteriorated after 48 h. Whether the patients were subsequently intubated or NIV was continued, the outcome was poor, with a mortality of more than 50%. Using logistic regression analysis a low pH, a low activities of daily living score and the presence of associated complications at admission were more likely in patients who failed after 48 h or more of NIV. Patients who fail after initial successful NIV have a poor prognosis.[126]

Contraindications to non-invasive ventilation

A number of contraindications to NIV have been suggested. Some of these are self-evident, such as severe facial deformity or trauma, which would prevent effective mask application. Others are primarily theoretical and are suggested because patients with these features have been excluded from previous studies rather than because there is evidence that invasive ventilation is superior in these situations. They include coma or confusion, upper gastrointestinal bleeding, high risk of aspiration, excessive secretions, haemodynamic instability or uncontrolled arrhythmia.[127] Whether patients should receive a trial of NIV in these circumstances very much depends upon the individual situation; for instance, if intubation has been refused or is considered inappropriate there is little to be lost by a trial of NIV.

Implications for staffing and training

Non-invasive ventilation has been reported to be a time-consuming procedure[128] but, as with any new technique, there is a learning curve and the same group have subsequently published more encouraging results.[129] ICU-based studies have shown no increase in workload compared with standard therapy but, certainly initially, a significant amount of time is required to establish the

patient on NIV.[79,99] On general wards Plant et al[86] found that NIV resulted in a modest increase in nursing workload in the first 8 h of the admission, equating to an average 26 m, but no difference was identified thereafter. There are, however, no data on the effect NIV has on the care that other patients on the ward received, nor whether the outcome would have been better if the nurses had spent more time with the patients receiving NIV. Since NIV in the more severely ill patient may require as much input as an invasively ventilated patient,[99] there should usually be one nurse responsible for no more than three or four patients, although clearly this will depend upon the care needs of the other patients. In the less severely affected patient, NIV can be successful with a lower level of staffing.[86] Staff training and experience is more important than location, and adequate numbers of staff skilled in NIV must be available throughout the 24-hour period. Because of the demands of looking after these acutely ill patients, and to aid training and skill retention, NIV is usually best carried out in one single-sex location, with one nurse responsible for no more than three to four patients in total.

Practical implications of providing an acute non-invasive ventilation service

Whether NIV should be performed in an ICU, a High-Dependency Unit or a general ward depends upon individual circumstances. There have been no direct comparisons between outcomes from NIV in the ICU and a general ward and it is unlikely that there ever will be such a trial. It should be appreciated that, while there is some overlap, the skills needed for non-invasive ventilation are different from those required for invasive ventilation and the outcome from NIV is likely to be better in a general ward where the staff have a lot of experience of NIV than in an ICU with high staff-to-patient ratios and a high level of monitoring but little experience of NIV. Other factors to be considered include whether or not intubation is felt to be appropriate should NIV fail, the presence of other system failure, co-morbidity, the severity of the respiratory failure and the likelihood of success with NIV.

Because many patients, particularly those with COPD, breathe via the mouth when dyspnoeic, a full face mask is usually required acutely; occasionally, a mouth piece may be helpful. Once NIV is tolerated, a change can be made to a nasal mask. Having established an adequate mask fit, it is essential to achieve and maintain adequate ventilation and good synchrony between the ventilator and the patient as soon as possible, as failure will often result in non-compliance with NIV. As the clinical situation changes, ventilator settings may need to be adjusted.

Humidification

Non-invasive ventilation can cause excess loss of water vapour, leading to thickened and tenacious secretions as well as the discomfort associated with a dry nose or mouth. In addition, increased nasal resistance has been described with CPAP, leading to increased mouth leak, and this is likely also to be a problem with NIV, particularly when pressure-cycled systems with high inspiratory flow rates are used.[130] Humidification of the inspired gas must be considered for some patients. It can be achieved using a heat and moisture exchange filter but, as the filter becomes saturated with water and secretions, the resistance to gas flow increases. Regular nebulised saline may sometimes be sufficient to prevent secretions becoming dried but will not have any effect on nasal resistance. A water bath humidifier with a heated wire circuit is ideal, but expensive.

Nebulised drugs

These can be administered during NIV by adding the nebuliser into the circuit. This can be done using a T-piece positioned as close to the patient as possible, ideally between the exhale valve and the patient to prevent fall out and loss of the drug, although this does increase the dead space. Most nebulisers will work, but a nebuliser that is able to work at varying angles is useful as the ventilator circuit is often unsupported, leaving the nebuliser to function on its side. In addition, aerosols can be administered into the ventilator circuit using metered dose inhalers and spacer devices[131,132] but peripheral lung deposition of aerosol during mechanical ventilation may not be as good as during spontaneous ventilation and use during NIV has not been evaluated. However, a recent study[133] has suggested that, although peripheral deposition is significantly reduced during mask CPAP, the bronchodilator effect is not compromised, at least in stable patients. Whenever possible patients should receive their inhaled drugs off the ventilator but this is obviously not possible if the patient is ventilator-dependent, in which case nebulisation during NIV is possible.

Physiotherapy

Physiotherapy can be performed during NIV and indeed is sometimes more effective because the patient is less breathless and better able to cooperate.[134] However, physiotherapists require specific training.

Conclusion

Non-invasive ventilation is widely considered to be a very effective treatment in patients with chronic ventilatory failure due to chest-wall deformity and neuromuscular disease. In contrast, NIV cannot at present be recommended for most patients with chronic hypercapnia due to COPD but there is sufficient evidence to warrant treatment in highly selected patients when all other avenues have been exhausted. In acute ventilatory failure due to COPD, there is now considerable randomised controlled trial evidence to support the use of NIV in both mild (pH 7.30–7.35) and moderate (pH < 7.30) exacerbations. In acute hypoxaemic respiratory failure, NIV reduces the intubation rate and complications, with the greatest benefit being seen in milder disease. In cardiogenic pulmonary oedema, non-invasive CPAP results in more rapid physiological improvement and a reduction in the need for intubation. The precise role of NIV in weaning and postextubation respiratory failure needs to be evaluated further, but it has a role in selected patients. Overall, NIV should be seen as complementary to invasive ventilation rather than as a direct alternative. When successful, it has been shown to reduce important complications, particularly nosoco-

mial pneumonia and length of stay in the ICU. There is little to be lost, therefore, and much to be gained, from a trial of NIV in patients with acute respiratory failure of whatever aetiology, unless it is contraindicated or there is a low likelihood of success. There is accumulating evidence that NIV is more likely to be successful when started earlier and assisted ventilation should now be considered earlier in patients with respiratory failure than has been the case hitherto.

?   Unresolved questions

- What is the place of non-invasive ventilation in chronic ventilatory failure due to COPD?

- What is the place of non-invasive ventilation in acute hypoxaemic respiratory failure and weaning?

- What is the best timing for starting non-invasive ventilation in slowly progressive neuromuscular disease and chest wall deformity?

- What is the mechanism by which non-invasive ventilation during sleep improves daytime function?

References

1. Corrado A, Bruscoli G, De Paola E et al. Respiratory muscle insufficiency in acute respiratory failure of subjects with severe COPD: treatment with intermittent negative pressure ventilation. Eur Respir J 1990; 3: 644–648.
2. Corrado A, De Paola E, Gorini M et al. Intermittent negative pressure ventilation in the treatment of hypoxic hypercapnic coma in chronic respiratory insufficiency. Thorax 1996; 51: 1077–1082.
3. Shekerdemian LS, Shore DF, Lincoln C et al. Negative-pressure ventilation improves cardiac output after right heart surgery. Circulation 1996; 94(9 Suppl): II49–II55.
4. Grunstein RR, Stewart DA, Lloyd H et al. Acute withdrawal of nasal CPAP in obstructive sleep apnea does not cause a rise in stress hormones. Sleep 1996; 19: 774–782.
5. Sanna A, Veriter C, Stanescu D. Upper airway obstruction induced by negative-pressure ventilation in awake healthy subjects. J Appl Physiol 1993; 75: 546–552.
6. Levy RD, Cosio MG, Gibbons L et al. Induction of sleep apnoea with negative pressure ventilation in patients with chronic obstructive lung disease. Thorax 1992; 47: 612–615.
7. Girault C, Richard JC, Chevron V et al. Comparative physiologic effects of noninvasive assist–control and pressure support ventilation in acute hypercapnic respiratory failure. Chest 1998; 111: 1639–1648.
8. Cinnella G, Conti G, Lofaso F et al. Effects of assisted ventilation on the work of breathing: volume-controlled versus pressure-controlled ventilation. Am J Respir Crit Care Med 1996; 153: 1025–1033.
9. Meecham Jones DJ, Wedzicha JA. Comparison of pressure and volume preset nasal ventilator systems in stable chronic respiratory failure. Eur Respir J 1993; 6: 1060–1064.
10. Elliott MW, Aquilina R, Green M et al. A comparison of different modes of noninvasive ventilatory support: effects on ventilation and inspiratory muscle effort. Anaesthesia 1994; 49: 279–283.
11. Vitacca M, Rubini F, Foglio K et al. Non-invasive modalities of positive pressure ventilation improve the outcome of acute exacerbations in COLD patients. Intens Care Med 1993; 19: 450–455.
12. Schonhofer B, Sonnerborn M, Haidl P et al. Comparison of two different modes for noninvasive mechanical ventilation in chronic respiratory failure: volume versus pressure controlled device. Eur Respir J 1997; 10: 184–191.
13. Smith IE, Shneerson JM. Secondary failure of nasal intermittent positive pressure ventilation using the Monnal D: effects of changing ventilator. Thorax 1997; 52: 89–91.

14. Ambrosino N, Vitacca M, Polese G et al. Short-term effects of nasal proportional assist ventilation in patients with chronic hypercapnic respiratory insufficiency. Eur Respir J 1997; 10: 2829–2834.

15. Patrick W, Webster K, Ludwig L et al. Non-invasive positive-pressure ventilation in acute respiratory distress without prior respiratory failure. Am J Respir Crit Care Med 1996; 153: 1005–1011.

16. Ranieri VM, Grasso S, Mascia L et al. Effects of proportional assist ventilation on inspiratory muscle effort in patients with chronic obstructive pulmonary disease and acute respiratory failure. Anaesthesiology 1997; 86: 79–91.

17. Wrigge H, Golisch W, Zinserling J et al. Proportional assist versus pressure support ventilation: effects on breathing pattern and respiratory work of patients with chronic obstructive pulmonary disease. Intens Care Med 1999; 25: 790–798.

18. Appendini L, Purro A, Gudjonsdottir M et al. Physiological response of ventilator-dependent patients with chronic obstructive pulmonary disease to proportional assist ventilation and continuous positive airway pressure. Am J Respir Crit Care Med 1999; 159: 1510–1517.

19. Goldberg P, Reissmann H, Maltais F et al. Efficacy of noninvasive CPAP in COPD with acute respiratory failure. Eur Respir J 1995; 8: 1894–1900.

20. Appendini L, Purro A, Patessio A et al. Partitioning of inspiratory muscle workload and pressure assistance in ventilator-dependent COPD patients. Am J Respir Crit Care Med 1996; 154: 1301–1309.

21. Petrof BJ, Kimoff RJ, Levy RD et al. Nasal continuous positive airway pressure facilitates respiratory muscle function during sleep in severe chronic obstructive pulmonary disease. Am Rev Respir Dis 1991; 143: 928–935.

22. Appendini L, Patessio A, Zanaboni S et al. Physiological effects of positive end-expiratory pressure and mask pressure support during exacerbations of chronic obstructive pulmonary disease. Am J Respir Crit Care Med 1994; 149: 1069–1076.

23. Ferguson GT, Gilmarin M. CO_2 rebreathing during BiPAP ventilatory assistance. Am J Respir Crit Care Med 1995; 151: 1126–1135.

24. Leger P, Muir J-F. Selection of patients for long-term nasal intermittent positive pressure ventilation: practical aspects. Eur Respir Mon 1998; 85: 328–347.

25. Bach JR, Alba AS. Management of chronic alveolar hypoventilation by nasal ventilation. Chest 1990; 97: 52–57.

26. Carroll N, Branthwaite MA. Control of nocturnal hypoventilation by nasal intermittent positive pressure ventilation. Thorax 1988; 43: 349–353.

27. Leger P, Jennequin J, Gerard M, Robert D. Home positive pressure ventilation via nasal mask for patients with neuromuscular weakness or restrictive lung or chest-wall disease. Respir Care 1989; 34: 73–77.

28. Ellis ER, Bye PTB, Bruderer JW, Sullivan CE. Treatment of respiratory failure during sleep in patients with neuromuscular disease. Am Rev Respir Dis 1987; 135: 148–152.

29. Polkey MI, Harris ML, Hughes PD et al. The contractile properties of the elderly human diaphragm. Am J Respir Crit Care Med 1997; 155: 1560–1564.

30. Simonds AK, Elliott MW. Outcome of domiciliary nasal intermittent positive pressure ventilation in restrictive and obstructive disorders. Thorax 1995; 50: 604–609.

31. Leger P, Bedicam JM, Cornette A et al. Nasal intermittent positive pressure ventilation. Long-term follow-up in patients with severe chronic respiratory insufficiency. Chest 1994; 105: 100–105.

32. Jenkinson C, Davies RJ, Mullins R, Stradling JR. Comparison of therapeutic and subtherapeutic nasal continuous positive airway pressure for obstructive sleep apnoea: a randomised prospective parallel trial. Lancet 1999; 354: 2100–2105.

33. Black N. Why we need observational studies to evaluate the effectiveness of health care. Br Med J 1996; 312: 1215–1218.

34. Howard RS, Wiles CM, Loh L. Respiratory complications and their management in motor neuron disease. Brain 1989; 112: 1155–1170.

35. Oppenheimer EA. Decision-making in the respiratory care of amyotrophic lateral sclerosis: should home mechanical ventilation be used? Palliative Med 1993; 7: 49–64.

36. Cazzolli PA, Oppenheimer EA. Home mechanical ventilation for amyotrophic lateral sclerosis: nasal compared to tracheostomy-intermittent positive pressure ventilation. J Neurol Sci 1996; 139(suppl): 123–128.

37. Pinto AC, Evangelista T, Carvalho M et al. Respiratory assistance with a non-invasive ventilator (BiPAP) in MND/ALS patients: survival rates in a controlled trial. J Neurol Sci 1995; 129: 19–26.

38. Moxham J. Respiratory muscle testing. Monald Arch Chest Dis 1996; 51: 483–488.

39. Raphael JC, Chevret S, Chastang C, Bouvet F. Randomised trial of preventive nasal ventilation in Duchenne muscular dystrophy. French Multicentre Cooperative Group on Home Mechanical Ventilation Assistance in Duchenne de Boulogne Muscular Dystrophy. Lancet 1994; 343: 1600–1604.

40. Simonds AK, Muntoni F, Heather S, Fielding S. Impact of nasal ventilation on survival in hypercapnic Duchenne muscular dystrophy. Thorax 1998; 53: 949–952.

41. Moss AH, Casey P, Stocking CB et al. Home ventilation for amyotrophic lateral sclerosis patients: outcomes, costs, and patient, family, and physician attitudes. Neurology 1993; 43: 438–443.

42. Bach JR, Campagnolo DI, Hoeman S. Life satisfaction of individuals with Duchenne muscular dystrophy using long-term mechanical ventilatory support. Am J Phys Med Rehab 1991; 70: 129–135.

43. Tzeng AC, Bach JR. Prevention of pulmonary morbidity for patients with neuromuscular disease. Chest 2000; 118: 1390–1396.

44. Bach JR. Mechanical insufflation-exsufflation. Comparison of peak expiratory flows with manually assisted and unassisted coughing techniques. Chest 1993; 104: 1553–1562.

45. Bach JR, Ishikawa Y, Kim H. Prevention of pulmonary morbidity for patients with Duchenne muscular dystrophy. Chest 1997; 112: 1024–1028.

46. Elliott MW, Simonds AK, Carroll MP et al. Domiciliary nocturnal nasal intermittent positive pressure ventilation in hypercapnic respiratory failure due to chronic obstructive lung disease: effects on sleep and quality of life. Thorax 1992; 47: 342–348.

47. Hughes PD, Polkey MI, Kyroussis D et al. Measurement of sniff nasal and diaphragm twitch mouth pressure in patients. Thorax 1998; 53: 96–100.

48. Marino W. Intermittent volume cycled mechanical ventilation via nasal mask in patients with respiratory failure due to COPD. Chest 1991; 99: 681–684.

49. Sivasothy P, Smith IE, Shneerson JM. Mask intermittent positive pressure ventilation in chronic hypercapnic respiratory failure due to chronic obstructive pulmonary disease. Eur Respir J 1998; 11: 34–40.

50. Jones SE, Packham S, Hebden M, Smith AP. Domiciliary nocturnal intermittent positive pressure ventilation in patients with respiratory failure due to severe COPD; long term follow up and effect on survival. Thorax 1998; 53: 495–498.

51. Benhamou D, Muir JF, Raspaud C et al. Long-term efficiency of home nasal mask ventilation in patients with diffuse bronchiectasis and severe chronic respiratory failure: a case-control study. Chest 1997; 112: 1259–1266.

52. Carrey Z, Gottfried SB, Levy RD. Ventilatory muscle support in respiratory failure with nasal positive pressure ventilation. Chest 1990; 97: 150–158.

53. Elliott MW, Mulvey DA, Moxham J et al. Inspiratory muscle effort during nasal intermittent positive pressure ventilation in patients with chronic obstructive airways disease. Anaesthesia 1993; 48: 8–13.

54. Strumpf DA, Millman RP, Carlisle CC et al. Nocturnal positive-pressure ventilation via nasal mask in patients with severe chronic obstructive pulmonary disease. Am Rev Respir Dis 1991; 144: 1234–1239.

55. Meecham Jones DJ, Paul EA, Jones PW, Wedzicha JA. Nasal pressure support ventilation plus oxygen compared with oxygen therapy alone in hypercapnic COPD. Am J Respir Crit Care Med 1995; 152: 538–544.

56. Lin CC. Comparison between nocturnal nasal positive pressure ventilation combined with oxygen therapy and oxygen monotherapy in patients with severe COPD. Am J Respir Crit Care Med 1996; 154: 353–358.

57. Gay PC, Hubmayr RD, Stroetz RW. Efficacy of nocturnal nasal ventilation in stable, severe chronic obstructive pulmonary disease during a 3-month controlled trial. Mayo Clin Proc 1996; 71: 533–542.

58. Medical Research Council Working Party Report. Long term domiciliary oxygen therapy in chronic hypoxic cor pulmonale complicating chronic bronchitis and emphysema. Lancet 1981; 1: 681–685.

59. Nocturnal oxygen therapy trial group. Continuous or nocturnal oxygen therapy in hypoxaemic chronic obstructive lung disease, a clinical trial. Ann Intern Med 1980; 93: 391–398.

60. Hamnegard CH, Wragg SD, Mills GH et al. Clinical assessment of diaphragm strength by cervical magnetic stimulation of the phrenic nerves. Thorax 1996; 51: 1239–1242.

61. Muir JF, de la Salmoniere P, Cuvelier A et al, on behalf of the NIPPV Study Group. Survival of severe hypercapnic COPD under long term home mechanical ventilation with NIPPV + oxygen versus oxygen therapy alone: preliminary results of a European multicentre study. Am J Respir Crit Care Med 1999; 159: A295.

62. Clini E, Sturani C, on behalf of AIPO. The Italian multicentric study: non-invasive nocturnal pressure support ventilation (NPSV) in COPD patients. Am J Respir Crit Care Med 1999; 159: A295.

63. Macklem PT. The clinical relevance of respiratory muscle research: J Burns Amberson Lecture. Am Rev Respir Dis 1986; 134: 812–815.

64. Elliott MW, Mulvey DA, Moxham J et al. Domiciliary nocturnal nasal intermittent positive pressure ventilation in COPD: mechanisms underlying changes in arterial blood gas tensions. Eur Respir J 1991; 4: 1044–1052.

65. Barbe F, Quera-Salva MA, de Lattre J et al. Long-term effects of nasal intermittent positive pressure ventilation on pulmonary function and sleep architecture in patients with neuromuscular diseases. Chest 1996; 110: 1179–1183.

66. Shapiro SH, Ernst P, Gray-Donald K et al. Effect of negative pressure ventilation in severe chronic obstructive pulmonary disease. Lancet 1992; 340: 1425–1429.

67. Mills GH, Kyroussis D, Hamnegard CH et al. Bilateral magnetic stimulation of the phrenic nerves from an anterolateral approach. Am J Respir Crit Care Med 1996; 154: 1099–1105.

68. Simonds AK, Parker RA, Branthwaite MA. The effect of intermittent positive-pressure hyperinflation in restrictive chest wall disease. Respiration 1989; 55: 136–143.

69. Berthon-Jones M, Sullivan CE. Time course of change in ventilatory response to CO_2 with long-term CPAP therapy for obstructive sleep apnea. Am Rev Respir Dis 1987; 135: 144–147.

70. Annane D, Quera-Salva MA, Lofaso F et al. Mechanisms underlying effects of nocturnal ventilation on daytime blood gases in neuromuscular diseases. Eur Respir J 1999; 13: 157–162.

71. Schonhofer B, Geibel M, Sonnerborn M, Kohler D. Daytime mechanical ventilation in chronic respiratory insufficiency. Eur Respir J 1997; 10: 2840–2846.

72. Calverley PMA, Brezinova V, Douglas NJ et al. The effect of oxygenation on sleep quality in chronic bronchitis and emphysema. Am Rev Respir Dis 1982; 126: 206–210.

73. Sawicka EH, Branthwaite MA. Respiration during sleep in kyphoscoliosis. Thorax 1987; 42: 801–808.

74. Masa JF, Celli BR, Riesco JA et al. Noninvasive positive pressure ventilation and not oxygen may prevent overt ventilatory failure in patients with chest wall diseases. Chest 1997; 112: 207–213.

75. Hill NS, Eveloff SE, Carlisle CC, Goff SG. Efficacy of nocturnal nasal ventilation in patients with restrictive thoracic disease. Am Rev Respir Dis 1992; 145: 365–371.

76. Jiminez JFM, Sanchez de Cos Escuin J, Vicente CD et al. Nasal intermittent positive pressure ventilation: analysis of its withdrawal. Chest 1995; 107: 382–388.

77. Bott J, Carroll MP, Conway JH et al. Randomised controlled trial of nasal ventilation in acute ventilatory failure due to chronic obstructive airways disease. Lancet 1993; 341: 1555–1557.

78. Brochard L, Mancebo J, Wysocki M et al. Noninvasive ventilation for acute exacerbations of chronic obstructive pulmonary disease. N Engl J Med 1995; 333: 817–822.

79. Kramer N, Meyer TJ, Meharg J et al. Randomised, prospective trial of noninvasive positive pressure ventilation in acute respiratory failure. Am J Respir Crit Care Med 1995; 151: 1799–1806.

80. Barbe F, Togores B, Rubi M et al. Noninvasive ventilatory support does not facilitate recovery from acute respiratory failure in chronic obstructive pulmonary disease. Eur Respir J 1996; 9: 1240–1245.

81. Angus RM, Ahmed AA, Fenwick LJ, Peacock AJ. Comparison of the acute effects on gas exchange of nasal ventilation and doxapram in exacerbations of chronic obstructive pulmonary disease. Thorax 1996; 51: 1048–1050.

82. Wood KA, Lewis L, Von Harz B, Kollef MH. The use of noninvasive positive pressure ventilation in the Emergency Department. Chest 1998; 113: 1339–1346.

83. Celikel T, Sungur M, Ceyhan B, Karakurt S. Comparison of noninvasive positive pressure ventilation with standard medical therapy in hypercapnic acute respiratory failure. Chest 1998; 114: 1636–1642.

84. Bardi G, Pierotello R, Desideri M et al. Nasal ventilation in COPD exacerbations: early and late results of a prospective, controlled study. Eur Respir J 2000; 15: 98–104.

85. Martin TJ, Hovis JD, Costantino JP et al. A randomized, prospective evaluation of noninvasive ventilation for acute respiratory failure. Am J Respir Crit Care Med 2000; 161: 807–813.

86. Plant PK, Owen JL, Elliott MW. Early use of non-invasive ventilation for acute exacerbations of chronic obstructive pulmonary disease on general respiratory wards: a multicentre randomised controlled trial. Lancet 2000; 355: 1931–1935.

87. Antonelli M, Conti G, Rocco M et al. A comparison of noninvasive positive-pressure ventilation and conventional mechanical ventilation in patients with acute respiratory failure. N Engl J Med 1998; 339: 429–435.

88. Antonelli M, Conti G, Bufi M et al. Noninvasive ventilation for treatment of acute respiratory failure in patients undergoing solid organ transplantation: a randomized trial. JAMA 2000; 282: 235–241.

89. Confalonieri M, Potena A, Carbone G et al. Acute respiratory failure in patients with severe community-acquired pneumonia. A prospective randomized evaluation of noninvasive ventilation. Am J Respir Crit Care Med 1999; 160: 1585–1591.

90. Delclaux C, L'Her E, Alberti C et al. Treatment of acute hypoxemic nonhypercapnic respiratory insufficiency with continuous positive airway pressure delivered by a face mask: a randomized controlled trial. JAMA 2000; 284: 2352–2360.

91. Hilbert G, Gruson D, Vargas F et al. Noninvasive ventilation in immunosuppressed patients with pulmonary infiltrates, fever, and acute respiratory failure. N Engl J Med 2001; 344: 481–487.

92. Nourdine K, Combes P, Carton M-J et al. Does noninvasive ventilation reduce the ICU nosocomial infection risk? A prospective clinical survey. Intens Care Med 1999; 25: 567–573.

93. Girou E, Schortgen F, Delclaux C et al. Association of noninvasive ventilation with nosocomial infections and survival in critically ill patients. JAMA 2000; 284: 2361–2367.

94. Fagon JY, Chastre J, Hance A et al. Nosocomial pneumonia in ventilated patients: a cohort study evaluating attributable mortality and hospital stay. Am J Med 1993; 94: 281–287.

95. Torres A, Aznar R, Gatell JM. Incidence, risk and prognosis factors of nosocomial pneumonia in mechanically ventilated patients. Am Rev Respir Dis 1990; 142: 523–528.

96. Easton C, MacKenzie F. Sensory-perceptual alterations: delirium in the intensive care unit. Heart Lung 1988; 17: 229–237.

97. Ambrosino N, Foglio K, Rubini F et al. Non-invasive mechanical ventilation in acute respiratory failure due to chronic obstructive airways disease: correlates for success. Thorax 1995; 50: 755–757.

98. Jeffrey AA, Warren PM, Flenley DC. Acute hypercapnic respiratory failure in patients with chronic obstructive lung disease: risk factors and use of guidelines for management. Thorax 1992; 47: 34–40.

99. Nava S, Evangelisti I, Rampulla C et al. Human and financial costs of noninvasive mechanical ventilation in patients affected by COPD and acute respiratory failure. Chest 1997; 111: 1631–1638.

100. Plant PK, Owen J, Elliott MW. One year period prevalence study of respiratory acidosis in acute exacerbation of COPD; implications for the provision of non-invasive ventilation and oxygen administration. Thorax 2000; 55: 550–554.

101. Nava S, Ambrosino N, Clini E et al. Noninvasive mechanical ventilation in the weaning of patients with respiratory failure due to chronic obstructive pulmonary disease. A randomized, controlled trial. Ann Intern Med 1998; 128: 721–728.

102. Girault C, Daudenthun I, Chevron V et al. Noninvasive ventilation as a systematic extubation and weaning technique in acute-on-chronic respiratory failure. A prospective, randomized controlled study. Am J Respir Crit Care Med 1999; 160: 86–92.

103. Hilbert G, Gruson D, Porel L et al. Noninvasive pressure support ventilation in COPD patients with post extubation hypercapnic respiratory insufficiency. Eur Respir J 1998; 11: 1349–1353.

104. De Lucas P, Tarancon C, Puente L et al. Nasal continuous positive airway pressure in patients with COPD in acute respiratory failure: a study of the immediate effects. Chest 1993; 104: 1694–1697.

105. Brett A, Sinclair DG. Use of continuous positive airway pressure in the management of community acquired pneumonia. Thorax 1993; 48: 1280–1281.

106. Covelli HD, Weled BJ, Beekman JF. Efficacy of continuous positive airway pressure administered by face mask. Chest 1982; 81: 147–150.

107. Gachot B, Clair B, Wolff M et al. Continuous positive airway pressure by face mask or mechanical ventilation in patients with human immunodeficiency virus infection and severe *Pneumocystis carinii* pneumonia. Intens Care Med 1992; 18: 155–159.

108. Suter PM, Kobel N. Treatment of acute pulmonary failure by CPAP via face mask: when can intubation be avoided? Klin Wochenschr 1981; 59: 613–616.

109. Petrof BJ, Legare M, Goldberg P et al. Continuous positive airway pressure reduces work of breathing and dyspnea during weaning from mechanical ventilation in severe chronic obstructive pulmonary disease. Am Rev Respir Dis 1990; 141: 281–289.

110. DeHaven CB, Hurst JM, Branson RD. Post extubation hypoxaemia treated with continuous positive airways pressure mask. Crit Care Med 1985; 13: 46–48.

111. Putensen C, Hormann, Baum M, Lingnau W. Comparison of mask and nasal continuous positive airway pressure after extubation and mechanical ventilation. Crit Care Med 1993; 21: 357–362.

112. Kilger E, Briegel J, Haller M et al. Effects of noninvasive positive pressure ventilatory support in non-COPD patients with acute respiratory insufficiency after early extubation. Intens Care Med 1999; 25: 1374–1380.

113. Rasanen J, Heikkila J, Downs J et al. Continuous positive airway pressure by face mask in acute cardiogenic pulmonary edema. Am J Cardiol 1985; 55: 296–300.

114. Bersten AD, Holt AW, Vedig AE et al. Treatment of severe cardiogenic pulmonary edema with continuous positive airway pressure delivered by face mask. N Engl J Med 1991; 325: 1825–1830.

115. Lin M, Yang YF, Chiang HT et al. Reappraisal of continuous positive airway pressure therapy in acute cardiogenic pulmonary edema. Short-term results and long-term follow-up. Chest 1995; 107: 1379–1386.

116. Pang D, Keenan SP, Cook DJ, Sibbald WJ. The effect of positive pressure airway support on mortality and the need for intubation in cardiogenic pulmonary edema: a systematic review. Chest 1998; 114: 1185–1192.

117. Mehta S, Jay GD, Woolard RH et al. Randomized prospective trial of bilevel versus continuous positive airway pressure in acute pulmonary oedema. Crit Care Med 1997; 25: 620–628.

118. Jubran A, Tobin MJ. Reliability of pulse oximetry in titrating supplemental oxygen therapy in ventilator-dependent patients. Chest 1990; 97: 1420–1425.

119. Stradling JR. Hypercapnia during oxygen therapy in airways obstruction: a reappraisal. Thorax 1986; 41: 897–902.

120. Meduri GU, Abou-Shala N, Fox RC et al. Noninvasive face mask mechanical ventilation in patients with acute hypercapneic respiratory failure. Chest 1991; 100: 445–454.

121. Soo Hoo GW, Santiago S, Williams AJ. Nasal mechanical ventilation for hypercapnic respiratory failure in chronic obstructive pulmonary disease: determinants of success and failure. Crit Care Med 1994; 22: 1253–1261.

122. Meduri GU, Turner RE, Abou-Shala N et al. Noninvasive positive pressure ventilation via face mask – first line intervention in patients with acute hypercapnic and hypoxemic respiratory failure. Chest 1996; 109: 179–193.

123. Yang KL, Tobin MJ. A prospective study of indexes predicting the outcome of trials of weaning from mechanical ventilation. N Engl J Med 1991; 324: 1445–1450.

124. Anton A, Guell R, Gomez J et al. Predicting the result of noninvasive ventilation in severe acute exacerbations of patients with chronic airflow limitation. Chest 2000; 117: 828–833.

125. Moretti M, Cilione C, Tampieri A et al. Incidence and causes of non-invasive mechanical ventilation failure after initial success. Thorax 2000; 55: 819–825.

126. Lightowler JV, Elliott MW. Predicting the outcome from NIV for acute exacerbations of COPD. Thorax 2000; 55: 815–816.

127. Ambrosino N. Noninvasive mechanical ventilation in acute respiratory failure. Eur Respir J 1996; 9: 795–807.

128. Chevrolet JC, Jolliet P, Abajo B et al. Nasal positive pressure ventilation in patients with acute respiratory failure. Chest 1991; 100: 775–782.

129. Chevrolet JC, Jolliet P. Workload on non-invasive ventilation in acute respiratory failure. In: Vincent JL, ed. Year book of intensive and emergency medicine. Berlin: Springer; 1997: 505–513.

130. Richards GN, Cistulli PA, Ungar RG et al. Mouth leak with nasal continuous positive airway pressure increases nasal airway resistance. Am J Respir Crit Care Med 1996; 154: 182–186.

131. Dhand R, Tobin MJ. Bronchodilator delivery with metered-dose inhalers in mechanically-ventilated patients. Eur Respir J 1996; 9: 585–595.

132. Dhand R, Duarte AG, Jubran A et al. Dose-response to bronchodilator delivered by metered-dose inhaler in ventilator-supported patients. Am J Respir Crit Care Med 1996; 154: 388–393.

133. Parkes SN, Bersten AD. Aerosol kinetics and bronchodilator efficacy during continuous positive airway pressured delivered by face mask. Thorax 1997; 52: 171–175.

134. Bott J, Moran F. Physiotherapy and nasal intermittent positive pressure ventilation. In: Simonds AK, ed. Non-invasive respiratory support. London: Chapman & Hall; 1995: 133–142.

16 Principles of physiotherapy

Rik Gosselink

Key points

- Respiratory physiotherapy enhances airway clearance in lung disease associated with hypersecretion.

- Forced expiratory techniques are the most important treatment modalities to improve short-term airway clearance.

- Respiratory muscle training enhances strength, endurance and symptoms in various conditions associated with respiratory muscle weakness.

- Exercise training and peripheral muscle training are effective components of the rehabilitation of patients with pulmonary disease.

Respiratory physiotherapy is relevant to the treatment not only of patients with acute and chronic lung disease, but also of those with advanced neuromuscular disorders. Physiotherapy contributes to the treatment of various aspects of respiratory disorders such as airflow obstruction, alterations in ventilatory pump function and impaired exercise performance. In addition, physiotherapy aims to improve quality of life. In patients with chronic lung disease, more particularly in chronic obstructive pulmonary disease (COPD), bronchiectasis and cystic fibrosis, physiotherapy includes treatment modalities that improve dyspnoea, airway clearance and exercise performance. In patients with neuromuscular disorders and acute lung disease, physiotherapy aims to improve airway clearance, lung and chest-wall compliance and respiratory muscle function, with the aim of improving pulmonary function or preventing pulmonary deterioration.

Since lack of compliance with treatment is a well-known problem with the prescription of techniques for airway clearance and the maintenance of the effects of exercise training after rehabilitation, physiotherapy also includes patient education. Treatment as well as assessment of the above-mentioned areas is covered by physiotherapists. In this chapter, airway clearance techniques, breathing exercises, exercise training and peripheral and respiratory muscle training in conditions affecting the respiratory system will be discussed.

Techniques for airway clearance and lung inflation

Hypersecretion and impaired mucociliary transport are important pathophysiological features of obstructive lung diseases such as cystic fibrosis and chronic bronchitis, as well as being seen in patients with acute lung disease, i.e. atelectasis and pneumonia. Hypersecretion is associated with an increased rate of decline of pulmonary function and excess mortality in patients with COPD.[1] In patients with more advanced neuromuscular disease, mucus retention and pulmonary complications significantly contribute to morbidity and mortality.[2] Although a cause–effect relationship has not been proved in these conditions, improvement of airway clearance is considered to be an important aim of treatment of such patients.

Mucus retention results from excessive mucus production or abnormal rheological properties on the one hand or impaired mucociliary function or cough clearance on the other. Pharmaceutical interventions and physiotherapy are effective to enhance mucus transport by improving the rheological properties of the mucus layer, stimulating ciliary action or utilising compensatory physical mechanisms such as gravity, airflow–mucus interaction, vibration, oscillation or airway squeezing. In a recent meta-analysis in patients with cystic fibrosis,[3] it was concluded that the combined standard treatment of postural drainage, percussion and vibration resulted in significantly greater sputum expectoration than no treatment. No differences were observed between standard treatment and other treatment modalities. In patients with COPD and bronchiectasis it was concluded in a recent Cochrane library review[4] that the combination of postural drainage, percussion and forced expiration improved airway clearance, but not pulmonary function. There is certainly need for further research to support or refute the use of physiotherapy aimed at improving bronchial hygiene.

Forced expiration

The concept of therapeutic forced expiratory manoeuvres is to enhance mucus transport with high airflow velocities. A higher airflow velocity makes mucus move to the central airways because of the interaction and energy transfer between the air stream and the mucus layer (two-phase gas–liquid interaction). The effectiveness of this transmission and hence of mucus transport depends on the thickness of the mucus layer and airflow velocity. A thicker mucus layer is easier to move as more kinetic energy is transmitted to it.[5] High expiratory flow and dynamic airway compression during forced expiratory manoeuvres accelerate the air stream considerably.

Forced expiratory manoeuvres, huffing and coughing, are considered to be the cornerstone of airway clearance techniques and are an essential part of almost every combination of treatment modalities. Huffing and coughing consist of a deep inspiration followed by a forced expiration, without and with glottis closure, respectively. Lower pleural pressures and peak flow rates are generated during huffing compared to coughing. Huffing and coughing, and to a lesser extent also breathing at rest or during exercise, promote higher airflow velocity and stimulate mucus transport significantly. Both techniques have been shown to

increase mucus clearance from central and intermediate lung zones[6,7] (Fig. 16.1). The forced expiration technique combines huffing, coughing and diaphragmatic breathing. The technique was recently expanded to include deep-breathing exercises to open up collapsed or hypoventilated areas in the lung and renamed the active cycle of breathing technique. Autogenic drainage aims to enhance mucus transport in peripheral airways by forced expirations at low lung volumes. Expiratory force is significantly less in autogenic drainage compared to the other forced expiratory techniques with the aim of preventing airway collapse, but neither technique has been shown to be superior.[8] Airway collapse is a major risk during forced expiration in patients with airway instability and results in significant reduction of mucus transport.[6] Therefore, forced expiratory manoeuvres should be carefully adapted to altered pulmonary mechanics in patients with more severe airflow obstruction. The lack of association between tracheobronchial clearance and peak flow achieved during cough and forced expiration implies that excessive attempts to achieve the highest flow rates are not necessary. Forced expirations also contribute to alterations in viscoelastic properties of the mucus layer. Repetitive strain on the mucus by repeated huffing or coughing reduces viscosity and promotes mucus transport.[9]

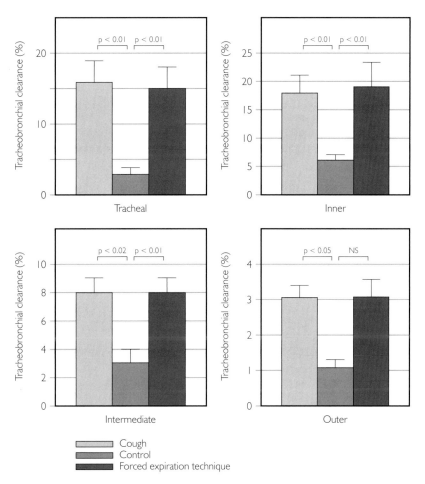

Fig. 16.1 Tracheobronchial clearance of radioaerosol tracer (mean ± SD) in four regions of the lung (tracheal, inner, intermediate, outer) during control conditions (middle bar) and after applying the forced expiration technique (right bar) and coughing (left bar). (Redrawn with permission from Hasani et al.[7])

In neuromuscular disease the reduced expiratory muscle strength limits effective huffing and coughing. Mechanical insufflation and exsufflation and manually assisted coughing are effective and safe methods of facilitating clearance of airway secretions.[10] In addition, deep lung insufflation increases maximum insufflation capacity and peak cough flow in patients with progressive neuromuscular disease.[11] Glossopharyngeal breathing is also used to improve the efficacy of coughing in patients with neuromuscular disease and intact upper airway function. It has been shown that this technique increases vital capacity and thereby improves expiratory flow rates.

Chest expansion and lung inflation

Mechanically ventilated patients are unable to perform forced expiratory manoeuvres effectively. Hyperinflation combined with chest-wall compression during expiration ('bag squeezing') is frequently applied in clinical practice. However, controversy exists regarding the safety and effectiveness of the approach.[12] In particular, the detrimental cardiovascular effects must be taken into consideration when applying manual lung hyperinflation.[13]

Postoperative pulmonary complications after thoracic and abdominal surgery remain a major cause of morbidity and mortality. Prolonged hospitalisation and stay in intensive care may result. Evidence for the effectiveness of physiotherapy in preventing postoperative pulmonary complications after abdominal surgery is provided in randomised controlled trials.[14-16] A meta-analysis confirmed the beneficial effect of physiotherapy on the prevention of complications after abdominal surgery,[17] but it remains unclear which treatment modalities are most effective. In addition to deep-breathing exercises, coughing and early mobilisation, simple devices such as positive expiratory pressure mask breathing and incentive spirometry are provided to patients with the aim of reducing pulmonary complications. Although incentive spirometry is widely used in clinical practice, it has not been shown to be of additional value after major abdominal, lung and cardiac surgery.[18] After abdominal surgery, Hall et al.[19,20] concluded that incentive spirometry was as effective as chest physiotherapy in both low- and high-risk patients. However, in low-risk patients after cholecystectomy no benefit of incentive spirometry was found compared to a control group not receiving any specialised respiratory care. Celli et al.[15] were also unable to detect differences in pulmonary complications (22% on average) between patients using deep-breathing exercises, incentive spirometry and intermittent positive pressure breathing, but the patients in the incentive spirometry group had a significantly shorter hospital stay. In thoracic surgery for lung or oesophageal resection, incentive spirometry had no additional effect on recovery of pulmonary function, pulmonary complications or hospital stay.[21]

Exercise

During exercise, increased ventilation and release of mediators in the airways may be effective in enhancing mucus transport. Indeed, increased mucus transport has been observed during exercise in healthy subjects and patients with chronic bronchitis,[22] but it was less effective than conventional physiotherapy in patients with cystic fibrosis.[23] During exercise combined with physiotherapy, significantly more sputum was expectorated than during physiotherapy alone.[24]

Postural drainage

During postural drainage the major bronchi are positioned in a more vertical position to allow gravitational forces to promote mucus transport to the central airways. Postural drainage is usually combined with other treatment modalities. Studies investigating the efficacy of postural drainage using radioaerosol tracers showed no additional improvement in mucus transport after postural drainage but, in patients with bronchiectasis and excessive mucus production, postural drainage alone enhanced mucus transport and expectoration.[25]

Body position has also been shown to affect oxygenation. This effect has not always been acknowledged in clinical care. In patients with unilateral lung disease, the lateral decubitus position with the unaffected side down in general improves oxygenation.[26] In patients with acute respiratory distress syndrome, the prone position increased arterial P_{O_2}. Alterations in ventilation–perfusion inequality have been suggested as the main reason for improved oxygenation in these body positions.

Percussion and vibration

Manual or mechanical percussion and vibration are based on the assumption of transmission of oscillatory forces to the bronchi. Although such oscillations are observed in the central airways, it is believed that absorption of the forces by air and lung parenchyma prevents transmission to smaller and intermediate airways. This probably explains the lack of additional effects on mucus transport of additive chest percussion and vibration to breathing exercises, postural drainage and coughing.[27] Another explanation might be the frequency dependence of the effects of vibration and oscillation. The optimal frequency enhancing mucus transport appears to be around 12–17 Hz[28] (Fig. 16.2). It seems that manual percussion frequency is too low ($\sim$ 3–5 Hz) and mechanical percussion frequency too high ($\sim$ 40 Hz). However, clinical trials have not shown greater efficacy of high-frequency oscillation with a more optimal oscillation frequency compared to standard physiotherapy in patients with chronic bronchitis or cystic fibrosis.[29]

Positive expiratory pressure mask breathing and flutter breathing

In the early 1980s, positive-expiratory-pressure mask breathing was introduced to further improve physiotherapy treatment modalities that aim to increase mucus transport. Expiration against a resistance may prevent airway collapse and improve collateral ventilation. Indeed, Falk et al.[30] showed that the addition of this technique to forced expiration or postural drainage increased mucus expectoration in cystic fibrosis. Other investigators were unable to show additional short-term effects on mucus transport in cystic fibrosis[31] or chronic bronchitis.[32] However, recently it was demonstrated that positive-expiratory-pressure therapy was superior to standard treatment in preserving pulmonary function in the long term.[33]

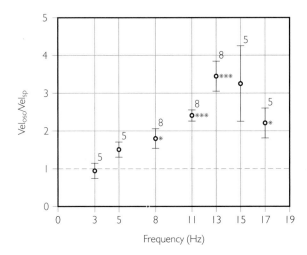

Fig. 16.2 Ratio of velocity of tracheal marker particles during high-frequency chest-wall oscillation (Vel_{osc}) to velocity during spontaneous breathing (Vel_{sp}) as a function of the applied frequency. Numbers beside each symbol indicate number of trials (* $p < 0.05$, ** $p < 0.01$, *** $p < 0.001$ compared to control conditions). Abd., abdominal. (Redrawn with permission from King et al.[28])

Flutter breathing is the addition of a variable, oscillating expiratory pressure and airflow at the mouth to facilitate clearance of mucus. Although in patients with cystic fibrosis Konstan and colleagues[34] observed a fivefold increase in expectorated mucus compared to cough or postural drainage, others were unable to find differences in expectoration.[35] Sputum rheology was significantly altered during flutter breathing, but this did not result in an increased sputum volume.[35]

Breathing exercises and body positions

'Breathing exercises' is an all-embracing term for a range of exercises such as active expiration, pursed-lips breathing, relaxation therapy, specific body positions, inspiratory muscle training and diaphragmatic breathing. The aims of these exercises vary considerably and include the improvement of (regional) ventilation and gas exchange, amelioration of debilitating effects on the ventilatory pump, improvement of respiratory muscle function, decreasing dyspnoea and improvement of exercise tolerance and quality of life. In patients with COPD and asthma, breathing exercises are aimed to:

- reduce hyperinflation of the rib cage
- increase the strength and endurance of the respiratory muscles
- optimise the pattern of thoracoabdominal motion.

Breathing exercises to reduce hyperinflation of the rib cage

The idea of decreasing hyperinflation of the rib cage is based on the assumption that this intervention will result in the inspiratory muscles working over a more advantageous part of their length–tension relationship. Moreover, it is expected to decrease the elastic work of breathing, because the chest wall moves over a more favourable part of its pressure–volume curve. In this way, the work load on the inspiratory muscles should diminish, along with the sensation of dyspnoea. The decrease of hyperinflation implies that the patient is able to breathe at a lower functional reserve capacity, resulting, if tidal volume remains constant, in an increase in alveolar gas 'refreshment'. Several treatment strategies aim to reduce the hyperinflated chest wall.

Relaxation exercises
The rationale for relaxation exercises arises from the idea that, at least in patients with asthma during an exacerbation of the disease, eccentric activity of the inspiratory muscles during expiration increases. This increased activity may continue even after recovery from an acute episode of airway obstruction and hence contributes to hyperinflation. Second, relaxation also aims to reduce the respiratory rate and increase tidal volume and thus to improve breathing efficiency. Relaxation exercises have hardly been studied in patients with lung disease, but a positive trend towards a reduction of symptoms is clearly apparent.

Pursed-lips breathing
Pursed-lips breathing aims to improve expiration both by its prolongation and by preventing airway collapse. The subject performs a moderately active expiration through the half-opened lips inducing expiratory mouth pressures of about 5 cmH_2O. Gandevia[36] observed in patients with severe lung emphysema and tracheobronchial collapse that the expired volume during a relaxed expiration increased, on average, by 20% in comparison to a forced expiration. This suggests that relaxed expiration causes less 'air-trapping', which results in a relatively lower level of hyperinflation. Pursed-lips breathing reduces respiratory rate and dyspnoea and improves tidal volume and oxygen saturation in resting conditions[37] However, its application during treadmill exercise did not change blood gases. Some patients use the technique instinctively. It appears that patients with loss of lung elastic recoil pressure benefit most, while in these patients slowing expiration improves tidal volume and decreases airway compression. Similar adaptations in breathing pattern and oxygen saturation have been observed in patients with myotonic muscular dystrophy.[38] Breslin[37] observed during pursed-lips breathing an increase in rib-cage and accessory muscle recruitment during the entire breathing cycle, while transdiaphragmatic pressure remained unchanged. In addition, the inspiratory duty cycle fell and resulted in a significant decrease of the tension–time index of the diaphragmatic contraction.

Rib cage mobilisation techniques
Specific mobilisation of rib-cage joints appears a specific aim for physiotherapy as the rib-cage mobility seems to be reduced in obstructive lung disease. Uncontrolled studies in patients with cystic fibrosis suggested some improvement in rib-cage mobility and pulmonary function after manipulative therapy of the rib cage and thoracic spine. The potential importance of mobility exercises in these patients is in line with the observed persistent hyperinflation after heart–lung transplantation in cystic fibrosis patients. No studies have been reported in patients with COPD but the basis for such treatment seems weak, as altered chest-wall mechanics are related primarily to loss of elastic recoil and

airway obstruction. In addition, after lung transplantation significant reduction of hyperinflation is observed.

Rib cage mobilisation might be effective in younger patients with cystic fibrosis during growth, whereas in older patients with COPD with altered pulmonary mechanics these techniques will not be of help.

Breathing exercises to improve respiratory muscle function

Reduced endurance and strength of the inspiratory muscles are frequently observed in chronic lung disease and neuromuscular disorders and contribute to dyspnoea, exercise limitation and probably to respiratory failure. Improvement of respiratory muscle function is aimed at reducing the relative load on the muscles (the fraction of the actual pressure and the maximal pressure; PI/PI_{max}) and hence may contribute to reducing dyspnoea and increasing the maximal sustained ventilatory capacity. This might also imply an improvement of exercise capacity in patients with ventilatory limitation during exercise. Breathing exercises and body positions aim to improve the length–tension relationship or geometry of the respiratory muscles (in particular of the diaphragm) or to increase the strength and endurance of the inspiratory muscles. According to the length–tension relationship, the output of the muscle increases when operating at a greater length, for the same neural input. At the same time, the efficacy of the contraction in moving the rib cage improves. Also, the piston-like movement of the diaphragm increases and enhances lung volume changes. The diaphragm can be lengthened by increasing abdominal pressure during active expiration or by adopting body positions such as forward leaning.

Specific training of the respiratory muscles might enhance their strength and/or endurance.

Contraction of the abdominal muscles during expiration
Contraction of the abdominal muscles during expiration is encouraged to support the functioning of the diaphragm. As a result of the increased abdominal pressure during active expiration, the diaphragm is assumed to be lengthened, allowing it to operate closer to its optimal length. In addition, active expiration will increase elastic recoil pressure of the diaphragm and the rib cage. The release of this pressure after relaxation of the expiratory muscles will assist the next inspiration. In healthy subjects, this mechanism is brought into play only with increased ventilation. However, in patients with severe COPD, contraction of abdominal muscles invariably occurs during resting breathing.[39] Active expiration increases transdiaphragmatic pressure (P_{di}) and PI_{max}. The additional effects of active expiration and exercise training in patients with severe COPD were studied by Casciari and colleagues.[40] They observed a significant increase in maximum oxygen uptake during a bicycle ergometer test after a period of additional breathing exercises during a training programme on a treadmill compared to the treadmill programme without breathing exercises.

Although active expiration seems to improve inspiratory muscle function and is commonly observed in resting breathing and during exercise in COPD patients, the significance of abdominal muscle activity remains poorly understood. Indeed, if

expiratory flow limitation is present then abdominal muscle contraction will not enhance expiratory flow and its relaxation will not contribute to inspiratory flow. This means that abdominal muscle contraction will not contribute to the mechanical work of breathing, which is still all performed by the inspiratory muscles. Nevertheless, abdominal muscle recruitment may optimise diaphragm length and geometry. The mechanism is, however, unclear, as Ninane and colleagues[39] observed that there was no overlap between the onset of diaphragm contraction and abdominal muscle contraction. Contraction of the diaphragm started just after the onset of relaxation of the abdominal muscles.

Body position
Relief of dyspnoea is often experienced by patients in different body positions. Forward leaning has been shown to be very effective in COPD[41] and is probably the body position most often adopted by patients with lung disease. The effect of this position seems not to be related to the severity of airway obstruction, changes in minute ventilation or improved oxygenation.[41] Hyperinflation and paradoxical abdominal movement, however, were related to relief of dyspnoea in the forward leaning position.[41] Alternatively, forward leaning is associated with a significant reduction in electromyographic activity of the scalenes and sternomastoid muscles, increase in transdiaphragmatic pressure and a significant improvement in thoracoabdominal movements[41] (Fig. 16.3). From these studies it was concluded that the subjective improvement of dyspnoea in patients with COPD was the result of the more favourable position of the diaphragm on its length–tension curve. In addition, forward leaning with arm support allows accessory muscles (pectoralis minor and major) to contribute significantly to rib-cage elevation. The same holds for the forward leaning position with head support, which allows the accessory neck muscles to assist inspiration.

Abdominal belt
The 'abdominal belt' was developed as an aid to support diaphragmatic function. Early studies in patients with emphysema reported an increase in the excursion of the diaphragm and a reduction of the activity of accessory muscles during application of the abdominal belt. However, its application in patients with severe COPD significantly shortened endurance time on a bicycle ergometer.[42]

The abdominal belt is also used in patients with spinal cord injury, in whom it improves vital capacity.[43] However, increases in expiratory flow and expiratory pressures during abdominal strapping were not consistently observed in these patients.[44]

Respiratory muscle training
Recent studies in patients with COPD have shown natural adaptations of the diaphragm at cellular (increased proportion of type I fibres) and subcellular (shortening of the sarcomeres and increased concentration of mitochondria) levels, contributing to greater resistance to fatigue and to better functional muscle behaviour.[45,46] These spontaneous adaptations may be further enhanced by inspiratory muscle training. In patients with COPD, respiratory muscle training improves inspiratory muscle function, provided that the training intensity exceeds 30% PI_{max}

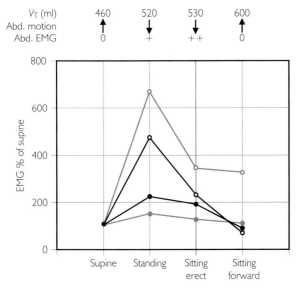

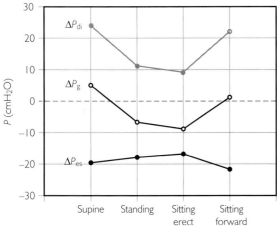

Fig. 16.3 Changes in electromyographic (EMG) activity of the respiratory muscles and pressure (P_{di}, transdiaphragmatic; P_g, gastric; P_{es}, oesophageal) in different body positions. (Redrawn with permission from Sharp et al.[41])

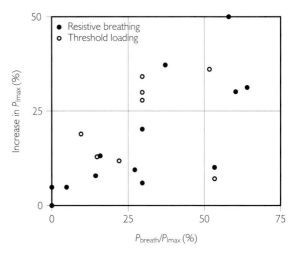

Fig. 16.4 Plot of the relationship between the load during inspiratory muscle training (P_{breath}/PI_{max}) and the improvement in maximal inspiratory pressure in 19 studies in patients with chronic obstructive pulmonary disease. (Modified from Pardy & Rochester.[47])

(Fig. 16.4). The required duration of training is 20–30 minutes a day, aiming to improve endurance capacity. Inspiratory muscle training in addition to exercise training has been shown to result in greater improvements in exercise capacity in patients with a ventilatory limitation to exercise.[48] Improved inspiratory muscle function has been shown to alleviate dyspnoea,[49] reduce nocturnal desaturation[50] and improve quality of life.

No data are available on which method of respiratory muscle training should be practised: resistive loading, threshold loading, maximal inspiratory (Müller) manoeuvres or a combination of all these. Resistive breathing (breathing through a small hole) has the disadvantage that the inspiratory pressure developed is flow-dependent. Threshold loading has the advantage of being independent of inspiratory flow. However, it requires build-up

of negative pressure before flow occurs and hence is inertial in nature. Similar workloads are obtained during resistive loading and threshold loading. Threshold loading enhances the velocity of inspiratory muscle contraction. This might be an important additional effect as it shortens inspiratory time and increases the time for exhalation and relaxation. Since inspiratory muscles are at risk of developing fatigue in these patients, increased relaxation time may prevent the development of fatigue. Whether resistive loading or inertial loading produces different training effects remains to be studied.

In tetraplegic patients, respiratory muscle training has been shown to enhance inspiratory muscle function, dyspnoea and exercise performance.[51,52] In patients with neuromuscular disease, respiratory muscle dysfunction is more complex and is dependent on the precise disease and its stage. It seems that patients with respiratory muscle function greater than 25% of the predicted value are still trainable.[53,54] Although inspiratory muscle function is commonly affected in these diseases, expiratory muscle function is often more impaired, e.g. in tetraplegia and multiple sclerosis. Respiratory muscle training has also been shown to be beneficial in the latter condition.[55] In the long term, the progressive nature of most neuromuscular diseases, affecting the primary function of the muscle, probably impedes the beneficial effects of training.[54,55]

Breathing exercises to optimise thoracoabdominal movements

Alterations of chest wall motion are common in patients with asthma and COPD. Several studies have described an increase in rib-cage contribution to chest-wall motion and/or asynchrony between rib-cage and abdominal motion in these patients. The mechanisms underlying these alterations are not fully elucidated but appear to be related to the degree of airflow obstruction, hyperinflation of the rib cage, changes in diaphragmatic function and an increased contribution of the accessory inspiratory muscles to chest-wall motion. Increased activity of accessory muscles is believed to enhance the sensation of dyspnoea. Consequently, diaphragmatic breathing, or slow and deep breathing, are commonly applied in physiotherapy practice, attempting to correct abnormal chest-wall motion, decrease the work of breathing and dyspnoea, increase the efficiency of breathing and improve the distribution of ventilation.

Diaphragmatic breathing

During diaphragmatic breathing the patient is told to move the abdominal wall exclusively during inspiration and to reduce upper rib-cage motion. This aims to improve chest-wall motion and the distribution of ventilation, to decrease the energy cost of breathing, the contribution of rib cage muscles and dyspnoea, and to improve exercise performance. All studies show that COPD patients are able voluntarily to change their breathing pattern to more abdominal movement and less thoracic excursion.[56] However, diaphragmatic breathing is accompanied by increased asynchronous and paradoxical breathing movements, while no permanent changes of the breathing pattern are observed.[56] Although abdominal and thoracic movement clearly change, no changes in ventilation distribution have been observed.[57] In several studies an increased work of breathing, enhanced oxygen cost of breathing and reduced mechanical efficiency of breathing have been found[56] (Fig. 16.5).

In conclusion, therefore, there is no evidence from controlled studies to support the use of diaphragmatic breathing in COPD patients.

Slow and deep breathing

Since, for a given minute ventilation, alveolar ventilation improves when breathing takes place at a slower rate and higher tidal volume, this type of breathing is encouraged for patients with impaired alveolar ventilation. Several authors have reported a significant reduction of respiratory frequency, and significant rises of tidal volume and P_aO_2 during imposed low-frequency breathing at rest in patients with COPD.[38] Slow and deep breathing exercises as part of pulmonary rehabilitation during exercise

training may add to more efficient breathing during exercise and hence reduce ventilatory demand and dyspnoea.[58]

Unfortunately, these effects are counterbalanced by increased work of breathing. In addition, Bellemare & Grassino[59] demonstrated that, for a given minute ventilation, fatigue of the diaphragm developed earlier during slow and deep breathing. This breathing pattern resulted in a significant increase in the relative force of contraction of the diaphragm (P_{di}/P_{dimax}), pushing it into the critical zone of muscle fatigue.

In summary, slow and deep breathing improves breathing efficiency and oxygen saturation at rest. A similar tendency has been observed during exercise, but needs further research. However, this type of breathing is associated with a breathing pattern prone to induce respiratory muscle fatigue.

Exercise training and peripheral muscle training

Impaired exercise tolerance is a common finding in patients with COPD. Several pieces of evidence point to the fact that this feature is not a simple consequence of loss of pulmonary function. Reduced exercise capacity shows only a weak relationship to impairment of lung function. Other factors, such as peripheral and respiratory muscle weakness and deconditioning, are now recognised as important contributors to reduced exercise tolerance.[60] These are important observations, since peripheral and respiratory muscle training might thus be able to improve physical performance symptoms, quality of life and, perhaps, survival in these patients. Recent randomised controlled studies on the efficacy of pulmonary rehabilitation reported significant improvements in maximal exercise capacity, walking distance and endurance capacity after pulmonary rehabilitation.[61] In addition, improved quality of life and reduced symptoms were observed. Mortality rate tended to decrease after rehabilitation.

Although these programmes are comprehensive, most authors consider exercise training to be a mandatory part of the programme. Training of peripheral muscles can be performed to improve either endurance or strength. Endurance training involves a larger muscle mass working at moderate intensity for a longer period of time. This is discussed in Chapter 17. Strength training, on the other hand, involves a smaller muscle mass working at high intensity for a shorter period. This has the advantage of being less demanding for the ventilatory system and thus creating less dyspnoea. Both types of training might improve exercise performance, symptoms and quality of life.

During peripheral muscle strength training, additional weights are applied to lower and upper limb movement. By varying the additional load or the number of repetitions, the muscle adaptation in strength or endurance can be modified. Strength training performed 3 times a week as three sets of eight repetitions, each at 80% of the one-repetition maximum, increased strength and muscle mass in healthy subjects after 12 weeks.[62] No change was seen in the distribution of muscle fibres, but the number of capillaries per fibre and oxidative enzymes increased significantly.[62] In addition, improvements in maximal oxygen uptake were observed in healthy elderly men.[62] Intensive strength training in elderly subjects is feasible and improves physical performance significantly.[63]

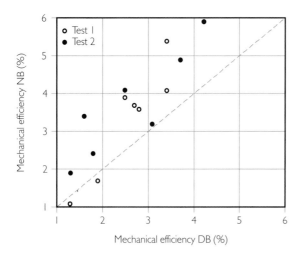

Fig. 16.5 Identity plot of the mechanical efficiency of breathing during natural breathing (NB) and diaphragmatic breathing (DB) in patients with chronic obstructive pulmonary disease. (Redrawn with permission from Gosselink et al.[55])

Peripheral muscle training has the advantage that the ventilatory demand is less than that of general exercise (walking, cycling). Hence, the sensation of dyspnoea will be less during muscle training, allowing training at higher intensities. Simpson et al,[64] in a randomised controlled trial, found that weightlifting, with loads ranging from 50% to 85% of the one-repetition maximum load, resulted in a significantly greater increase in peripheral muscle performance than in the control group. In addition, improvements in endurance exercise capacity and quality of life, but not in maximal exercise capacity, were found. Along the same lines, Clark et al.[65] performed a randomised controlled study to investigate the effects of a low-intensity (no additional loads) leg and arm muscle conditioning programme. As might be expected, significant improvements in muscle endurance, but not in muscle strength, were observed. The endurance walk test and physiological adaptations at submaximal exercise (reduced ventilatory equivalents for oxygen and carbon dioxide) improved significantly in comparison to the control group. As in the study of Simpson et al,[64] no changes in maximal exercise performance were seen.

It remains unclear whether either endurance muscle training, strength training or a combination of both is to be preferred. In COPD patients, the addition of strength training to endurance training enhanced muscle strength and muscle mass significantly more than endurance exercise training but failed to show additional effects on exercise performance and quality of life.[66] However, it is not clear from this study whether these patients had significant muscle weakness. In another study,[47] the combination of strength and endurance training improved peripheral muscle strength, exercise performance and quality of life in COPD patients with muscle weakness compared to a control group. In addition, the improvements in peripheral muscle strength and exercise performance were well-correlated (Fig. 16.6). This finding further substantiates the causal relationship between peripheral muscle function and exercise capacity.

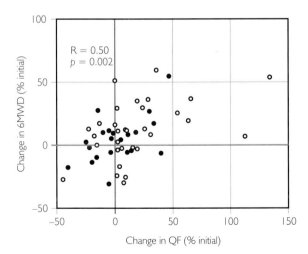

Fig. 16.6 Relation between changes in quadriceps strength (QF) and 6-minute walking distance (6MWD) in patients with chronic obstructive pulmonary disease after exercise training (open circles) or after a control period with no exercise (closed circles). (Modified from Troosters et al.[67])

References

1. Vestbo J, Prescott E, Lange P and the Copenhagen City Heart Study Group. Association of chronic mucus hypersecretion with FEV_1 decline and chronic obstructive pulmonary disease morbidity. Am J Respir Crit Care Med 1996; 153: 1530–1535.

2. Lieberman SL, Shefner JM, Young RR. Neurological disorders affecting respiration. In C. Roussos, ed. The thorax. Part C: Disease, 2nd ed. New York: Marcel Dekker; 1995: 2135–2175.

3. Thomas J, Cook DJ, Brooks D. Chest physical therapy management of patients with cystic fibrosis. A meta-analysis. Am J Respir Crit Care Med 1995; 151: 846–850.

4. Jones AP, Rowe BH. Bronchopulmonary hygiene physical therapy for chronic obstructive pulmonary disease and bronchiectasis. The Cochrane Library 2000; 3: 1–12.

5. Clarke SW, Jones JG, Oliver DR. Resistance to two-phase gas–liquid flow in airways. J Appl Physiol 1970; 29: 464–471.

6. Van der Schans CP, Piers DA, Beekhuis H et al. Effect of forced expirations on mucus clearance in patients with chronic airflow obstruction; effect of lung recoil pressure. Thorax 1990; 45: 623–627.

7. Hasani A, Pavia D, Agnew JE, Clarke SW. Regional lung clearance during cough and forced expiration technique (FET): effects of flow and viscoelasticity. Thorax 1994; 49: 557–561.

8. Miller S, Hall DO, Clayton CB, Nelson R. Chest physiotherapy in cystic fibrosis: a comparative study of autogenic drainage and the active cycle of breathing techniques with postural drainage. Thorax 1995; 50: 165–169.

9. Zahm JM, King M, Duvivier C et al. Role of simulated repetitive coughing in mucus clearance. Eur Respir J 1991; 4: 311–315.

10. Bach JR. Mechanical insufflation–exsufflation. Comparison with peak expiratory flows with manually assisted and unassisted coughing techniques. Chest 1993; 104: 1553–1562.

11. Kang S-W, Bach JR. Maximum insufflation capacity. Chest 2000; 11: 861–865.

12. Denehy L. The use of manual hyperinflation. Eur Respir J 1999; 14: 958–965.

13. Singer M, Vermaat J, Hall G et al. Hemodynamic effects of manual hyperinflation in critically ill mechanically ventilated patients. Chest 1994; 106: 1182–1187.

14. Roukema JA, Carol EJ, Prins JG. The prevention of pulmonary complications after upper abdominal surgery in patients with noncompromised pulmonary status. Arch Surg 1988; 123: 30–34.

15. Celli BR, Rodriguez KS, Snider GL. A controlled trial of intermittent positive pressure breathing, incentive spirometry, and deep breathing exercises in preventing pulmonary complications after abdominal surgery. Am Rev Respir Dis 1984; 130: 12–15.

16. Fagevik Olsen M, Hahn I et al. Randomized controlled trial of prophylactic chest physiotherapy in major abdominal surgery. Br J Surg 1997; 84: 1535–1538.

17. Thomas JA, McIntosh JM. Are incentive spirometry, intermittent positive pressure breathing and deep breathing exercises effective in the prevention of postoperative pulmonary complications after abdominal surgery? A systematic overview and meta-analysis. Phys Ther 1994; 74: 3–10.

18. Crowe JM, Bradley CA. The effectiveness of incentive spirometry with physical therapy for high-risk patients after coronary artery bypass surgery. Phys Ther 1997; 77: 260–268.
19. Hall JC, Tarala R, Harris J et al. Incentive spirometry versus routine chest physiotherapy for prevention of pulmonary complications after abdominal surgery. Lancet 1991; 337: 953–956.
20. Hall JC, Tarala R, Tapper J, Hall JL. Prevention of respiratory complications after abdominal surgery: a randomised clinical trial. Br Med J 1996; 312: 148–153.
21. Gosselink R, Schrever K, De Leyn P et al. Recovery after thoracic surgery is not accelerated with incentive spirometry. Crit Care Med 2000; 28: 679–683.
22. Oldenburg FA, Dolovich MB, Montgomery JM, Newhouse MT. Effects of postural drainage, exercise and cough on mucus clearance in chronic bronchitis. Am Rev Respir Dis 1979; 120: 739–745.
23. Salh W, Bilton D, Dodd M, Webb AK. Effect of exercise and physiotherapy in aiding sputum expectoration in adults with cystic fibrosis. Thorax 1989; 44: 1006–1008.
24. Baldwin DR, Hill AL, Peckham DG, Knox AJ. Effect of addition of exercise to chest physiotherapy on sputum expectoration and lung function in adults with cystic fibrosis. Respir Med 1994; 88: 49–53.
25. Mazzocco MC, Owens GR, Kiriloff LH, Rogers RM. Chest percussion and postural drainage in patients with bronchiectasis. Chest 1985; 88: 360–363.
26. Gillespie DJ, Rehder K. Body position and ventilation–perfusion relationships in unilateral pulmonary disease. Chest 1987; 91: 75–79.
27. Van der Schans CP, Piers DA, Postma DS. Effect of manual percussion on tracheobronchial clearance in patients with chronic airflow obstruction and excessive tracheobronchial secretion. Thorax 1986; 41: 448–452.
28. King M, Philips DM, Gross D et al. Enhanced tracheal mucus clearance with high frequency chest wall compression. Am Rev Respir Dis 1983; 128: 511–515.
29. Arens R, Gozal D, Omlin KJ et al. Comparison of high frequency chest compression and conventional chest physiotherapy in hospitalized patients with cystic fibrosis. Am J Respir Crit Care Med 1994; 150: 1154–1157.
30. Falk M, Kelstrup M, Andersen JB et al. Improving the ketchup bottle method with positive exiratory pressure (PEP), in cystic fibrosis. Eur J Respir Dis 1984; 65: 423–432.
31. Lannefors L, Wollmer P. Mucus clearance with three chest physiotherapy regimes in cystic fibrosis: a comparison between postural drainage, PEP and physical exercise. Eur Respir J 1992; 5: 748–753.
32. Van Hengstum M, Festen J, Beurskens C et al. Effect of positive expiratory pressure mask physiotherapy (PEP) versus forced expiration technique (FET/PD) on regional lung clearance in chronic bronchitics. Eur Respir J 1991; 4: 651–654.
33. McIlwaine PM, Wong LT, Peacock D, Davidson AGF. Long-term comparative trial of conventional postural drainage and percussion versus positive expiratory pressure therapy in the treatment of cystic fibrosis. J Pediatr 1997; 131: 570–574.
34. Konstan MW, Stern RC, Doershuk CF. Efficacy of the Flutter device for airway mucus clearance in patients with cystic fibrosis. J Pediatr 1994; 124: 689–693.
35. App EM, Kieselmann R, Reinhardt D et al. Sputum rheology changes in cystic fibrosis lung disease following two different types of physiotherapy: flutter vs autogenic drainage. Chest 1998; 114: 171–177.
36. Gandevia B. The spirogram of gross expiratory tracheobronchial collapse in emphysema. Q J Med 1963; 32: 23–31.
37. Breslin EH. The pattern of respiratory muscle recruitment during pursed-lips breathing in COPD. Chest 1992; 101: 75–78.
38. Ugalde V, Breslin EH, Walsh SA et al. Pursed lips breathing improves ventilation in myotonic muscular dystrophy. Arch Phys Med Rehabil 2000; 81: 472–478.
39. Ninane V, Rypens F, Yernault JC, De Troyer A. Abdominal muscle use during breathing in patients with chronic airflow obstruction. Am Rev Respir Dis 1992; 146: 16–21.
40. Casciari RJ, Fairshter RD, Harrison A et al. Effects of breathing retraining in patients with chronic obstructive pulmonary disease. Chest 1981; 79: 393–398.
41. Sharp JT, Druz WS, Moisan T et al. Postural relief of dyspnea in severe chronic obstructive pulmonary disease. Am Rev Respir Dis 1980; 122: 201–211.
42. Dodd DS, Brancatisano TP, Engel LA. Effect of abdominal strapping on chest wall mechanics during exercise in patients with severe chronic obstructive pulmonary disease. Am Rev Respir Dis 1985; 131: 816–821.
43. Goldman JM, Rose LS, Williams SJ et al. Effect of abdominal binders on breathing in tetraplegic patients. Thorax 1986; 41: 940–945.
44. Estenne M, Van Muylem A, Gorini M et al. Effects of abdominal strapping on forced expiration in tetraplegic patients. Am J Respir Crit Care Med 1998; 15: 795–798.
45. Levine S, Kaiser L, Leferovich J, Tikunov B. Cellular adaptations in the diaphragm in chronic obstructive pulmonary disease. N Engl J Med 1997; 337: 1799–806.
46. Orozco-Levi M, Gea J, Lloreta JL et al. Subcellular adaptation of the human diaphragm in chronic obstructive pulmonary disease. Eur Respir J 1999; 13: 371–378.
47. Pardy RL, Rochester DL. Respiratory muscle training. Semin Respir Med 1992; 13: 53–62.
48. Wanke T, Formanek D, Lahrmann H et al. The effects of combined inspiratory muscle and cycle ergometer training on exercise performance in patients with COPD. Eur Respir J 1994; 7: 2205–2211.
49. Harver A, Mahler DA, Daubenspeck JA. Targeted inspiratory muscle training improves respiratory muscle function and reduces dyspnea in patients with chronic obstructive pulmonary disease. Ann Intern Med 1989; 111: 117–124.
50. Heijdra YF, Dekhuijzen PNR, van Herwaarden CLA, Folgering HTM. Nocturnal saturation improves by target-flow inspiratory muscle training in patients with COPD. Am J Respir Crit Care Med 1996; 153: 260–265.
51. Uijl SG, Houtman S, Folgering HT, Hopman MT. Training of the respiratory muscles in individuals with tetraplegia. Paraplegia 1999; 37: 575–579.
52. Liauw MY, Lin MC, Cheng PT et al. Resistive inspiratory muscle training: its effectiveness in patients with acute complete cervical cord injury. Arch Phys Med Rehab 2000; 81: 752–756.
53. Wanke T, Toifl K, Merkle M et al. Inspiratory muscle training in patients with Duchenne muscular dystrophy. Chest 1994; 105: 475–482.
54. Gozal D, Thiriet P. Respiratory muscle training in neuromuscular disease: long-term effects on strength and load perception. Med Sci Sports Exerc 1999; 311: 522–527.
55. Gosselink R, Kovacs L, Ketelaer P et al. Respiratory muscle weakness and respiratory muscle training in severely disabled multiple sclerosis patients. Arch Phys Med Rehab 2000; 81: 747–751.
56. Gosselink R, Wagenaar RC, Sargeant AJ et al. Diaphragmatic breathing reduces efficiency of breathing in chronic obstructive pulmonary disease. Am J Respir Crit Care Med 1995; 151: 1136–1142.
57. Grimby G, Oxhoj H, Bake B. Effects of abdominal breathing on distribution of ventilation in obstructive lung disease. Clin Sci Molec Med 1975; 48: 193–199.
58. Casaburi R, Porszasz J, Burns MR et al. Physiologic benefits of exercise training in rehabilitation of patients with severe chronic obstructive pulmonary disease. Am J Respir Crit Care Med 1997; 155: 1541–1551.
59. Bellemare F, Grassino A. Force reserve of the diaphragm in patients with chronic obstructive pulmonary disease. J Appl Physiol 1983; 55: 8–15.
60. Gosselink R, Troosters T, Decramer M. Peripheral muscle weakness contributes to exercise limitation in COPD. Am J Respir Crit Care Med 1996; 153: 976–980.
61. Lacasse Y, Wong E, Guyatt GH et al. Meta-analysis of respiratory rehabilitation in chronic obstructive pulmonary disease. Lancet 1996; 348: 1115–1119.
62. Frontera WR, Meredith CN, O'Reilly KP, Evans WJ. Strength training and determinants of VO$_2$max in older men. J Appl Physiol 1990; 68: 329–333.
63. Fiatarone MA, O'Neill EF, Doyle Ryan N et al. Exercise training and nutritional supplementation for physical frailty in very elderly people. N Engl J Med 1994; 330: 1769–1775.
64. Simpson K, Killian KJ, McCartney N et al. Randomised controlled trial of weightlifting exercise in patients with chronic airflow limitation. Thorax 1992; 47: 70–75.
65. Clark CJ, Cochrane JE, Mackay E. Low intensity peripheral muscle conditioning improves exercise tolerance and breathlessness in COPD. Eur Respir J 1996; 9: 2590–2596.
66. Bernard S, Whittom F, Leblanc P et al. Aerobic and strength training in patients with chronic obstructive pulmonary disease. Am J Respir Crit Care Med 1999; 159: 896–901.
67. Troosters T, Gosselink R, Decramer M. Short and long-term effects of outpatient pulmonary rehabilitation in COPD patients, a randomized controlled trial. Am J Med 2000; 109: 207–212.

17 Pulmonary rehabilitation

Nicolino Ambrosino

Key points

- Pulmonary rehabilitation is a multidisciplinary intervention directed to patients and families with the aim of achieving and maintaining the individual's maximum level of independence and functioning in the community.

- Pulmonary rehabilitation programmes can reduce dyspnoea, increase exercise tolerance and improve health-related quality of life in patients with chronic obstructive pulmonary disease and other respiratory diseases

- The appropriate selection of patients plays a key role in the success.

- Proper measurement of outcomes of rehabilitation is mandatory.

- Pulmonary rehabilitation may be successfully implemented in hospital-based and outpatient programmes, and also at home.

- The key to success is the individual tailoring of the different components of a programme.

Aims of pulmonary rehabilitation

Of various therapeutic interventions only long-term oxygen therapy and smoking cessation have been shown to improve survival in patients with chronic obstructive pulmonary disease (COPD).[1,2] Although the primary pathological changes are confined to the lungs, the consequent physical deconditioning and emotional responses contribute importantly to morbidity. Breathlessness leads to inactivity and consequent peripheral muscle deconditioning, resulting in a vicious cycle leading to further inactivity, social isolation, fear of dyspnoea and depression. Patients with severe COPD become less mobile and reduce their activities of daily living. In a survey of patients with severe COPD treated with long-term oxygen therapy, 50% did not leave the house (Medical Research Council, MRC dyspnoea grade 5) and 78% were breathless walking around at home and performing daily activities.[3] Pulmonary rehabilitation programmes may offer a way to break this downward cycle.[4] Furthermore, it has been shown that the use of health-care services by COPD patients is related more to respiratory and peripheral muscle force than to airway obstruction[5] and, in patients hospitalised with an acute exacerbation of severe COPD, 1-year survival was reported to be independently related, among other factors, to body mass index (BMI) and prior functional status.[6] Peripheral and respiratory muscle function, nutrition and activities of daily living are all factors that can be positively influenced by multidisciplinary rehabilitation.

Once recognised as 'an art of medical practice',[7] pulmonary rehabilitation has been defined as 'a multidimensional continuum of services directed to persons with pulmonary disease and their families, usually by an interdisciplinary team of specialists, with the goal of achieving and maintaining the individual's maximum level of independence and functioning in the community'.[8] Pulmonary rehabilitation reduces symptoms, increases functional ability, and improves health-related quality of life in individuals with chronic respiratory diseases, even in the face of irreversible abnormalities of lung architecture. These benefits are possible since often much of the *disability* (the inability to perform an activity within the normally expected range because of lung disease) and *handicap* (the disadvantage resulting from an impairment or disability within the context of the patient's ability to perform in society or fill expected roles) result, not from the functional respiratory disorder (the *impairment*) per se, but from secondary morbidity that is often treatable once recognised. For example, although the degree of airway obstruction or hyperinflation in COPD does not change appreciably with rehabilitation, it results in reversal of muscle deconditioning and better pacing, enabling these patients to walk further with less breathlessness.[9]

Selection of patients

The appropriate selection of patients plays a key role in the success of pulmonary rehabilitation.[10] Pulmonary rehabilitation programmes are designed to manage patients at all stages of disease, from the onset of symptoms until the final stages.[11]

Age. Until a few years ago, elderly patients were excluded from pulmonary rehabilitation but nowadays age is not considered a limiting factor. Recent literature has highlighted the beneficial effects of regular participation in comprehensive rehabilitation, including education, lower and upper extremity training, breathing retraining and chest physiotherapy, in COPD patients older than 75.[12]

Nutritional status. Factors related to nutritional status have an independent influence on the natural history of COPD.[13] A compromised nutritional state may contribute to reduced exercise performance and a positive association between nutritional state and maximal exercise performance has been found in some studies. Patients with different characteristics of body composition and severity of nutritional depletion may be eligible for pulmonary rehabilitation.[14]

Respiratory impairment. The severity of respiratory impairment as assessed by lung function is often an important factor influencing both patient motivation and compliance with the programme. In one study[15] of a comprehensive programme, however, all patients with COPD of varying severity showed benefit from participation in exercise training. The gains made by participants at different stages of disease did not differ significantly. The authors therefore concluded that all patients with COPD, regardless of their disease severity, should be referred for exercise rehabilitation or be encouraged to begin exercise training on their own.[15]

Level of disability. The level of disability, as assessed by severity of dyspnoea, is more important. Wedzicha et al[16] showed that the effects of training in COPD patients may depend on the initial level of dyspnoea. Patients with moderate dyspnoea (MRC grade 3/4), who were regularly mobile outside the home, showed quite large improvements in exercise capacity after physical training. In contrast, patients with severe disability (MRC grade 5), who were largely housebound owing to dyspnoea, showed no improvement in exercise performance following individualised physical training. The recent development of new therapeutic approaches such as lung transplantation,[17] lung volume reduction surgery[18] or long-term treatment of difficult-to-wean patients[19] means that patients with most severe COPD, and even with chronic respiratory failure, are potential candidates for rehabilitation programmes.

Compliance with therapy. Data on adherence to rehabilitation programmes are generally lacking. It is also noteworthy that in the prospective controlled study of pulmonary rehabilitation by Goldstein et al,[20] as many as 29% of the 126 eligible COPD patients refused to participate.

Other conditions than COPD. Smaller numbers of patients with conditions other than COPD have been included in studies dealing with pulmonary rehabilitation.[21] Rehabilitation programmes are commonly being applied in patients with bronchial asthma, neuromuscular diseases, and cystic fibrosis, as well as in

Table 17.1 Factors influencing the outcome of pulmonary rehabilitation

- Appropriate selection of patients
- Age
- Nutritional status
- Severity of respiratory impairment
- Compliance with therapy

preparation for and during recovery after abdominal and thoracic surgery and lung transplantation.[17,18] Nevertheless large studies devoted specifically to diseases other than COPD are lacking.

Contraindications. Although the only absolute contraindication appears to be lack of compliance or unwillingness to participate, studies on pulmonary rehabilitation usually have some exclusion criteria. In the study by Goldstein et al,[20] subjects regarded as ineligible included those with coexisting diseases (41%) and those who were still smoking (7%), lived too far away from hospital (16%) or had language barriers, cognitive impairment, adverse social circumstances or very severe disability (31%). Whether these conditions should be considered as general criteria for exclusion from routine therapeutic rehabilitation is still a matter of debate, particularly for smoking and severe disability. In a particular patient, potential contraindications should be judged in relation to his/her disease and to the specific therapeutic programme chosen.

Appropriate patients for pulmonary rehabilitation are those who recognise that their symptoms result from lung disease and who are motivated to be active participants in their own care to improve their health status. The benefits of pulmonary rehabilitation programmes in patients with COPD have been extensively documented.[15–29] The only absolute limitation to rehabilitation appears to be unwillingness to participate or poor compliance. Nevertheless, many factors may influence outcome (Table 17.1).

Evaluation of rehabilitation

Proper evaluation of candidates is the keystone of a successful rehabilitation programme.[30] Optimisation depends on the correct evaluation of somatic and physiological issues by the rehabilitation team, taking account of, quantifying and monitoring the variables that are important determinants of a patient's quality of life.

Confirming the diagnosis, characterising the severity of the main symptoms and identifying the impact of the disease on the patient's lifestyle are major aims of clinical assessment for respiratory rehabilitation.[31]

Lung function. Although rehabilitation does not improve pulmonary function, and baseline lung function cannot predict its benefit,[21,32] lung function tests are important for characterisation and quantification of impairment resulting from the patient's lung disease.

Muscle function. Assessment of respiratory muscle function is useful for prescribing and evaluating the results of a rehabilitation programme in conditions such as COPD, pre- and postoperatively and in neuromuscular disease.

Pulmonary rehabilitation programmes may be better planned if peripheral muscle function is also evaluated. Specific quantitative measurement (e.g. by dynamometer, or isokinetic strength) or at least simple clinical assessment may be employed. Chronic inactivity, psychological factors, steroid myopathy and other drug effects may impair skeletal muscle function in patients with COPD. Peripheral muscle force has been reported to be an important determinant of exercise capacity in COPD patients, in whom the utilisation of health-care services is related to ventilatory and peripheral muscle force.[5,33]

Exercise tolerance. An exercise test is necessary to assess the patient's exercise tolerance and to evaluate possible blood gas changes, which cannot be predicted from baseline lung function tests. The exercise test is also used to establish a safe and appropriate prescription for subsequent training. Assessment of exercise is best made using the type of exercise that will be employed in training (e.g. treadmill testing for a walking exercise training programme); however, results from one type of exercise test can be translated to similar forms of exercise.

Laboratory tests are the gold standard measurements. However 'field tests' can provide a useful assessment of task performance when laboratory facilities are unavailable. Timed walking tests can be used to measure exercise capacity indirectly following rehabilitation, particularly when limited resources are available. Measuring the distance covered during a walking test is considered a simple and reproducible way to determine exercise tolerance in patients with chronic lung disease. The main advantages of walking tests are simplicity, minimal resource requirements (i.e. a corridor and a supervisor) and general applicability. The main disadvantages of these tests are problems with patient and supervisor motivation, their non-standardised nature and their dependence on the single quantitative measurement of distance covered. Although walking tests can meet stringent test–retest criteria, the plethora of circumstances in which testing takes place limits comparison of results from different centres.[33] The shuttle walk test is an increasingly used standardised incremental field walking test.[34]

Measurement of dyspnoea. There is evidence that improvement in dyspnoea is the main benefit of pulmonary rehabilitation.[21] The severity of dyspnoea is only weakly related to lung function[35] and they describe different aspects of COPD. There is therefore a need to specifically measure this symptom in order to evaluate the clinical effects of rehabilitation. Several methods are available to measure dyspnoea, including clinical scales, visual analogue and open scales (see Chapter 5.3).[35] All these methods provide useful information when sequential measurements are performed within a single patient but they are unhelpful for comparing dyspnoea between individual patients or groups of patients.

Quality of life. Most patients with chronic respiratory disease seek medical evaluation when difficulty in breathing interferes with their ability to perform various activities of daily living and/or adversely affects their health-related quality of life, i.e. quality of life as it is affected by health status. Health-related quality of life measures are able to provide adequate and often excellent reproducibility; however, physiological indices such as pulmonary function and exercise tolerance do not correlate strongly with these measures.[36]

Psychological evaluation. In patients with COPD, in addition to progressive physical disability, high levels of depression and anxiety as well as impaired performance in tests of memory and concentration have been found. The clinical syndromes of depression and anxiety may further reinforce the patient's social isolation and physical inactivity.

Settings for rehabilitation

Most reported studies of pulmonary rehabilitation have relied on hospital-based[20] and outpatient programmes,[16,22–24,26–28] although recent European trials have confirmed that programmes can also be successfully implemented at home.[16,22,24,25] Goldstein et al[20] performed their programme on an inpatient basis for 2 months and thereafter for another 4 months on an outpatient basis. Similar improvements were observed in that study compared to programmes that were entirely outpatient-based. In a study by Cambach et al[26] in COPD patients and asthmatics, similar improvements were observed in community-based as in outpatient hospital-based programmes. The best location for rehabilitation probably depends on the severity of disease, availability of resources, ability to travel and need for supervision. In the study by Wijkstra et al,[22] patients referred for home rehabilitation performed their exercise unsupervised at home and visited a physiotherapist twice weekly for training, with similar protocols to outpatient rehabilitation programmes. Both short- and long-term benefits can be obtained with a day-hospital-based outpatient programme.[37] Although few data exist directly comparing patient outcomes in different settings, it is probably the structure and components of the programme rather than the setting itself that determine its effectiveness.[9,24]

Components of rehabilitation programmes

Although any patient with symptomatic COPD or other chronic respiratory disease should be considered for pulmonary rehabilitation, the key to success is the individual tailoring of the programme. The improvement attributable to individual elements of a programme is difficult to assess because of the multidisciplinary nature of pulmonary rehabilitation and the wide range of therapeutic modalities (Table 17.2).

An example of this multidisciplinary approach is the study by Foglio et al,[37] in which a team comprising respiratory physicians, nurses, physiotherapists, dietitian and psychologist offered care. The programme included optimisation of the pharmacological treatment, together with three 3-hour sessions per week for 8–10 weeks, including:

- supervised incremental exercise until achieving 30-minute continuous cycling at 50–70% of the maximal workload determined during an initial incremental cycloergometer exercise test
- abdominal, upper and lower limb muscle exercises including lifting progressively increasing light weights, shoulder and full arm circling and other exercises

Table 17.2 Components of pulmonary rehabilitation programmes

- Optimisation of pharmacological therapy
- Smoking cessation
- Education
- Chest physiotherapy
- Exercise training
- Respiratory muscle training
- Peripheral muscle training
- Occupational therapy
- Long-term oxygen therapy
- Respiratory muscle rest (mechanical ventilation)
- Psychosocial support
- Nutrition

- patient and family education
- nutritional programmes and psychosocial counselling.

This introduces the problem of evaluation of individual components of a pulmonary rehabilitation programme. The components still under discussion and the rationale for selection of each modality are reviewed below. Well-accepted adjuncts to rehabilitation already shown to prolong life (smoking cessation and long-term oxygen therapy) are covered elsewhere (Chapters 24 and 13 respectively).

Breathing control techniques

The technique of coordinating the breathing process was previously widely used in rehabilitation but now receives less emphasis. When the term 'breathing retraining' is used, it usually refers to these techniques, including pursed-lips and diaphragmatic breathing (see Chapter 16). Pursed-lips breathing is often used unconsciously by patients with COPD to enhance exercise tolerance during dyspnoea and increased ventilatory demand. Pursed-lips breathing results in slower and deeper breaths with significant increase in oxygenation and in a shift in ventilatory muscle recruitment from the diaphragm to the accessory muscles of ventilation. During exercise, the shift to pursed-lips breathing results in decreased dyspnoea.[38] Studies of diaphragmatic breathing[39,40] have failed to show benefit.

Lower extremity exercise training

Marked functional limitation often occurs in patients with respiratory disease.[3] Dyspnoea, responsible for a vicious cycle of negative feedback, is the main deconditioning stimulus. Progressive decrease of physical activity is in fact the patient's natural response to such an unpleasant symptom. Less exertion leads to reduced muscle mass, which in turn results in more dyspnoea at increasingly lower levels of exertion. Thus, a main goal of exercise training is to break this debilitating pattern. Improvements in exercise tolerance may be achieved through both physiological and psychological interventions.[29]

Although exercise training programmes by cycling and/or treadmill walking, stair climbing etc., have been widely used in different respiratory diseases, in the COPD patient they should not be considered until optimal medical control of the disease has been achieved. It is safe to state that any patient capable of undergoing training will benefit from a programme that includes leg exercise.[21] However the optimal exercise intensity, modality, need for supervision, duration and maintenance programme remain to be determined.[41]

Exercise training is based on general principles of exercise physiology: intensity, specificity and reversibility. Until recently it was commonly held that patients with advanced lung disease had a ventilatory limitation to exercise that precludes the aerobic training levels necessary for beneficial physiological adaptations. However, recent studies have demonstrated that anaerobic metabolism and early onset of lactic acidosis are observed during exercise training of COPD patients.[41] Greater improvements in maximal and submaximal exercise responses can be obtained after exercise at high exercise levels (e.g. 60% of maximal work rate – above the anaerobic threshold).[41] Training respiratory patients at 60–75% of maximal work rate results in substantial increases in maximal exercise capacity with reduction in ventilation and lactate levels at a given work rate. Most rehabilitation programmes include endurance training with periods of sustained exercise for about 20–30 min two to five times a week. In patients who cannot tolerate high-intensity exercise, interval training consisting of 2–3 min of high-intensity training alternating with equal periods of rest, is considered an alternative.

Although in COPD patients with chronic hypoxaemia peripheral muscle function has been shown to deteriorate, the effects of supplemental oxygen during rehabilitation are still debated. In a controlled study, pulmonary rehabilitation improved exercise performance and health-related quality of life in COPD patients with hypoxaemia at peak exercise irrespective of whether they breathed air or supplemental oxygen during the training.[42]

Although the exact underlying physiopathological mechanism is still unclear, there is laboratory evidence that continuous positive airway pressure and different modalities of mechanical ventilation (delivered either by mouthpiece or by facial/nasal mask) may reduce breathlessness and increase exercise tolerance in these patients, allowing them to reach a higher exercise intensity. Respiratory muscle unloading and reduction in intrinsic positive end-expiratory pressure have been considered among mechanisms underlying these effects in COPD patients. Nevertheless the role of mechanical ventilation during rehabilitation (if any) is still to be defined.[43]

Respiratory muscle training

Conditions such as neuromuscular disease, malnutrition, restrictive lung disease and pulmonary hyperinflation may severely affect the respiratory muscles. Respiratory muscle training results in increased strength and endurance. However there are conflicting results about the benefits of respiratory muscle training on both exercise and the activities of daily living in COPD patients. A meta-analysis reported little evidence of clinically important benefits in patients with COPD.[44] The likeliest indications for respiratory muscle training are:

- high spinal cord lesions without diaphragmatic involvement
- preparation for and following abdominal or thoracic surgery
- weaning from ventilatory support.

More research is needed before final recommendations can be made regarding which patients, if any, are likely to benefit from these therapeutic modalities. Although specific physiological effects have been reported with respiratory muscle training, this modality should not be used in patients with damaged or adapted respiratory muscle fibres.[38]

Training of upper extremity muscle groups

Many exercise programmes focus on lower-extremity training. Unfortunately, many daily activities, such as bathing, dressing and grooming, require use of the upper limbs. For a given workload, upper-limb work demands more energy than lower-limb work and a higher ventilatory demand is made. Particularly for elderly patients, the increased energy and ventilatory demands of simple self-care activities may result in marked functional limitation.

Because exercise training must be specific to the muscles involved in the relevant task, it is important that upper limb exercises tailored to the patient's needs are included in the programme. A critical review of the literature suggests that exercise conditioning including leg and arm training improves exercise performance, inducing physiological adaptations rather than simple reduced perception of dyspnoea.[21] COPD patients, moreover, show greater improvements in dyspnoea and health-related quality of life if arm exercise is included in their training in addition to general exercise programmes.[45]

Suitable candidates for such programmes are either COPD patients with dyspnoea associated with the use of upper extremities or patients with long-term deconditioning. Training can be performed using supported arm exercise with ergometry or unsupported arm exercises by lifting weights and dowels, and stretching elastic bands. Both methods can effectively improve arm endurance.

Occupational therapy

Chronic pulmonary diseases are the most common cause of disability and loss of time from work. The goal of occupational therapy is restoration of the patient to occupational or recreational activities with less energy expenditure and fewer symptoms.

Education

Education in the present context may be defined as a learning process that improves patients' ability to cope and to make informed decisions regarding their own care. In this regard, all patients with COPD need to be educated. Education aims to improve the compliance of patients with medication, oxygen therapy, smoking cessation, nutrition, exercise and health preservation. Educational programmes are directed both to the patients and their families. A number of standard topics are addressed in the educational sessions (Table 17.3). There has been particular enthusiasm for educational programmes for

Table 17.3 Common topics for education in rehabilitation programmes

- Lung anatomy and physiology
- Patient-specific lung disease
- Adverse effects of inactivity
- Bronchodilatation and airway clearing
- Breathing training
- Energy conservation techniques
- Drug therapy
- Comprehensive self-management of disease
- Benefits of rehabilitation
- Safety guidelines
- Oxygen therapy
- Non-invasive ventilation
- Environmental hygiene
- Symptom management and control
- Psychological factors/coping strategies (anxiety, panic control)
- Stress management
- Relaxation techniques
- End-of-life planning
- Smoking cessation
- Travel/leisure/sexuality
- Nutrition

patients with bronchial asthma, cystic fibrosis and COPD. Nevertheless, education alone is of little benefit, as demonstrated by studies in which education alone was used as a control intervention and the results were compared to treatment with exercise.[23] Therefore, although more research is needed to assess its value, education should not be considered as an alternative to exercise training in rehabilitation programmes.[21]

Psychosocial support

Anxiety, depression and lack of self-esteem often coexist in patients with chronic pulmonary disease. Indeed, anxiety and depression are the two most commonly reported emotional consequences of asthma. Male COPD patients show both psychophysiological disturbances and depression. Anxiety and depression are also commonly reported in patients with respiratory insufficiency. Psychological problems may result in decreased participation in social activities and are commonly reflected in the sexual sphere. These problems are likely to improve as the patient becomes involved in rehabilitation, resulting in desensitisation of dyspnoea, loss of fear and regaining of self-control.

The effect of rehabilitation on psychological outcomes has not been clearly defined. One controlled, randomised study of outpatient pulmonary rehabilitation showed no significant change in depression.[23] Significant reductions in depression and anxiety have, however, been reported after a rehabilitation programme in one uncontrolled study, in which group psychological counselling and stress management sessions were added to exercise training and educational topics.[46] Nevertheless, rehabilitation sessions including education, exercise breathing techniques and relaxation techniques have been shown to be more effective in reducing anxiety than a similar number of psycho-therapy sessions.

Nutritional programmes

Reduced body weight is a risk factor in COPD independent of the deterioration of airflow.[13] Malnutrition, obesity and weight loss are all associated with respiratory disease and may lead to respiratory muscle dysfunction, effects on the control of ventilation, increased frequency of respiratory infections and alterations in lung parenchymal structure. On the other hand, nutritional supplementation may also result in increased CO_2 production and consequent increased respiratory drive. Nutritional supplementation and/or correction is indicated in COPD patients with either malnutrition or obesity, in cystic fibrosis and bronchiectasis, before and after lung transplantation, in interstitial lung disease and to reduce obesity in obstructive sleep apnoea syndrome.

Results of rehabilitation

The benefits of pulmonary rehabilitation include improved exercise tolerance and symptoms and decreased health care expenditure, in particular, reduced use of expensive medical resources. Published results provide a sound scientific basis for the overall intervention as well as for specific components of it.[19,20,23,27,29] After rehabilitation, patients report improved quality of life with a reduction in respiratory symptoms, increase in exercise tolerance and ability to perform daily activities, more independence and improvement in psychological function, with less anxiety and depression and increased feelings of hope, control and self-esteem.[21] Studies that have examined individual components of rehabilitation have shown that even patients with severe disease can learn to understand their disease better, increase their activity levels and improve their exercise tolerance as a result of training.[17-19] Pulmonary rehabilitation for patients with COPD does not result in significant changes in lung function.[21] Studies of survival have shown variable results. Vocational benefits may be difficult to achieve in the presence of severe, disabling disease. However, patients with less severe disease may return to work and increase vocational and recreational activities considerably (Table 17.4).

Table 17.4 Results of pulmonary rehabilitation

Outcome	Expected improvements
Dyspnoea	+++
Exercise tolerance	++
Health-related quality of life	++
Health resources consumption	+
Respiratory muscle function	++
Survival	?
Lung function	−

Duration of benefit

Several reports[23,27,28,37] confirm that a rehabilitation programme for COPD patients, including lower and upper limb exercise training and education, can achieve benefits in health-related quality of life and hospital admissions that persist for a period of 2 years. In particular, two recent randomised controlled studies[27,28] showed long-term benefits. Griffiths et al,[27] in a randomised controlled study versus standard medical management, evaluated the effect of outpatient rehabilitation on use of health care and patients' wellbeing over 1 year. Compared with the control group, the rehabilitation group showed greater improvements in walking ability and in general and disease-specific health status.[27] In a second randomised controlled study versus standard care, Guell et al[28] examined the short- and long-term effects of an outpatient rehabilitation programme for COPD patients These authors found significant differences between groups in dyspnoea, walking test results and day-to-day dyspnoea, fatigue and emotional function measured by the Chronic Respiratory Disease Questionnaire. The improvements were evident at the third month and continued with somewhat diminished magnitude in the second year of follow-up. These authors[28] found that the rehabilitation group had a significant reduction in exacerbations but not in the number of hospitalisations.

There are relatively few data on the appropriate strategies to maintain the short-term benefits of an initial programme.

Health economics

Most of the observational studies support a positive cost–benefit ratio (the ratio between resources used and saved or created). Although most of these studies are uncontrolled, they usually report long-term follow-up. After rehabilitation some studies show that patients need less frequent hospitalisation.[27,37]

Few studies have carried out cost–utility analysis (the ratio between resources used and quality of life produced). One study showed that rehabilitation might produce 1 QALY (quality-adjusted life year) at a cost at the time of US $23 000. This was better than many other care programmes: for instance, at the time of that study, screening mammography had a cost of US $175 000 to produce 1 QALY. However, other cost–utility studies did not report similar results.[47]

Studies of cost–efficacy (the ratio between resources used and clinical effects) are far more complex. Recently, it has been estimated that the number of patients required to be treated to improve symptoms of a single patient is 4.1 for dyspnoea, 4.4 for fatigue, 3.3 for emotion and 2.5 for mastery (items of the Chronic Respiratory Questionnaire).[48]

Future studies

Despite the progress made in understanding pulmonary rehabilitation, more information is needed to ensure appropriate treatment for the increasing number of patients with chronic respiratory diseases.

There is still confusion in the terminology used in pulmonary rehabilitation for patient outcomes. It has been suggested that the World Health Organization's international classification of impairment, disability and handicap be adopted.[9]

We need more information on the impact on health-care costs and survival. Much of the current evidence is based on retrospective studies. In one study evaluating whether questionnaire-related functional status was predictive of survival, Bowen et al[49] found that variables associated with increased 3-year survival following pulmonary rehabilitation included, among others, a higher postrehabilitation functional activities score, a longer postrehabilitation walking test and referral for outpatient pulmonary rehabilitation.

Although the benefits of exercise training are well-established,[21,29] little is known about the additional benefits of education, breathing retraining strategies, psychosocial support and group therapy. Knowledge of the effectiveness of individual components would be beneficial for patients who are unable to exercise, e.g. those receiving ventilatory support or those who have a severe systemic illness.

Furthermore, we need further information on the intensity, duration and optimum form of exercise training to be tailored to the individual patient. Does the reported effectiveness of high-intensity training[41] result in long-term improved quality of life? Might this negatively influence long-term adherence to exercise? The best modality of upper-extremity training is unknown, as is the best application of ventilatory muscle training.

What is the role (if any) of respiratory muscle rest by non-invasive positive-pressure ventilation (NIV)? Recently Garrod et al[50] randomised severe COPD patients to receive NIV plus exercise training or exercise training alone and found a significantly greater improvement in exercise tolerance and health-related quality of life in the NIV group compared with those undergoing training alone. They concluded that domiciliary ventilatory support could be used successfully to augment the benefits of rehabilitation in severe COPD.

Studies evaluating the long-term effectiveness of pulmonary rehabilitation have generally shown a gradual decrease in improvements in disability and handicap over time. Although the decline may reflect progression of the underlying disease or comorbidity, can this progression be slowed with maintenance exercise programmes?

Although anecdotal information supports its use, little scientific evidence is available on the effectiveness of pulmonary rehabilitation in diseases other than COPD and asthma, and little experience is available in paediatric patients.

Patients with COPD who continue to smoke cigarettes are often most in need of pulmonary rehabilitation but there is no consensus on whether or not they should be included in programmes. Is their inability or unwillingness to quit smoking a predictor of failure in rehabilitation or is it simply another aspect of comorbidity that must be addressed?

In conclusion, there is evidence that pulmonary rehabilitation programmes may reduce dyspnoea, increase exercise tolerance and improve health-related quality of life in patients with COPD and other respiratory diseases. Pulmonary rehabilitation is a costly process and patients should be carefully selected in order to save resources and obtain the maximum benefit. Although several questions remain unresolved, pulmonary rehabilitation programmes should be included in the comprehensive treatment of patients with COPD and other respiratory diseases.

? Unresolved questions

- Who are the patients most likely to benefit from pulmonary rehabilitation programmes?

- What are the benefits of rehabilitation in diseases other than chronic obstructive pulmonary disease?

- What is the most effective form of rehabilitation in patients with severe disability?

- What are the relative indications for, and effectiveness of, single components of rehabilitation?

- What is the best schedule to maintain the benefits?

- What are the effects on survival?

- What are the economic implications?

References

1. Report of British Research Medical Council Working Party. Long-term domiciliary oxygen therapy in chronic hypoxic cor pulmonale complication in chronic bronchitis and emphysema. Lancet 1981; 1: 681–686.
2. Anthonisen NR, Connett JE, Kiley JP et al. Effects of smoking intervention and the use of an inhaled anticholinergic bronchodilator on the rate of decline of FEV1. JAMA 1994; 272: 1497–1505.
3. Restrick LJ, Paul EA, Braid GM et al. Assessment and follow up of patients prescribed long term oxygen therapy. Thorax 1993; 48: 708–713.
4. Donner CF, Decramer M. Pulmonary rehabilitation. Eur Respir Monog 2000; 5: 1–199.
5. Decramer M, Gosselink R, Trooster T et al. Muscle weakness is related to utilization of health care resources in COPD patients. Eur Respir J 1997; 10: 417–423.
6. Connors AF Jr, Dawson NV, Thomas C et al. Outcomes following acute exacerbation of severe chronic obstructive lung disease. Am J Respir Crit Care Med 1996; 154: 959–967.
7. Donner CF, Howard P. Pulmonary rehabilitation in chronic obstructive pulmonary disease (COPD) with recommendations for its use. Eur Respir J 1992; 5: 266–275.
8. NIH Workshop Summary: Pulmonary rehabilitation research. Am J Respir Crit Care Med 1994; 149: 825–833.
9. American Thoracic Society. Pulmonary rehabilitation 1999. Am J Respir Crit Care Med 1999; 159: 1666–168
10. Donner CF, Muir JF. ERS task force position paper. Selection criteria and programmes for pulmonary rehabilitation in COPD patients. Eur Respir J 1997; 10: 744–757.
11. Ambrosino N, Foglio K. Selection criteria for pulmonary rehabilitation. Respir Med 1996; 90: 317–322.
12. Couser JI, Guthmann R, Hamadeh MA, Kane CS. Pulmonary rehabilitation improves exercise capacity in older elderly patients with COPD. Chest 1995; 107: 730–734
13. Schols MWJ, Slangen J, Volovics L, Wouters EFM. Weight loss is a reversible factor in the prognosis of chronic obstructive pulmonary disease. Am J Respir Crit Care Med 1998; 157: 1791–1797.
14. Schols AMWJ, Soeters PB, Dingemans AMC et al. Prevalence and characteristics of nutritional depletion in patients with stable COPD eligible for pulmonary rehabilitation. Am Rev Respir Dis 1993; 147: 1151–1156.
15. Berry MJ, Rejeski WJ, Adair NE, Zaccaro D. Exercise rehabilitation and chronic obstructive pulmonary disease stage. Am J Respir Crit Care Med 1999; 160: 1248–1253.
16. Wedzicha JA, Bestall JC, Garrod R et al. Randomized controlled trial of pulmonary rehabilitation in severe chronic obstructive pulmonary disease patients, stratified with the MRC dyspnoea scale. Eur Respir J 1998; 12: 363–369.
17. Stiebellehner L, Quittan M, End A et al. Aerobic endurance training programme improves exercise performance in lung transplant recipients. Chest 1998; 113: 906–912.
18. Criner GJ, Cordova FC, Furukawa S et al. Prospective randomized trial comparing bilateral lung volume reduction surgery to pulmonary rehabilitation in severe chronic obstructive pulmonary disease. Am J Respir Crit Care Med 1999; 160: 2018–2027.

19. Nava S. Rehabilitation of patients admitted to a respiratory intensive care unit. Arch Phys Med Rehabil 1998; 79: 849–854.

20. Goldstein RS, Gort EH, Stubbing D et al. Randomised controlled trial of respiratory rehabilitation. Lancet 1994; 344: 1394–1397.

21. ACCP/AACVPR. Pulmonary rehabilitation. Joint ACCP/AACVPR evidence-based guidelines. Chest 1997; 112: 1363–1396.

22. Wijkstra PJ, Van Altena R, Kraan J et al. Quality of life in patients with chronic obstructive pulmonary disease improves after rehabilitation at home. Eur Respir J 1994; 7: 269–273

23. Ries AI, Kaplan RM, Limberg TM, Prewitt LM. Effects of pulmonary rehabilitation on physiologic and psychosocial outcomes in patients with chronic obstructive pulmonary disease. Ann Intern Med 1995; 122: 823–832.

24. Strijbos JH, Postma DS, Van Altena R et al. A comparison between an outpatient hospital-based pulmonary rehabilitation programme and a home-care pulmonary rehabilitation programme in patients with COPD: a follow-up of 18 months. Chest 1996; 109: 366–372.

25. Elias MT, Rubio TM, Ortega F et al. Results of a home-based training programme for patients with COPD. Chest 2000; 118: 106–114.

26. Cambach W, Chadwick-Straver RVM, Wagenaar RC et al. The effects of a community-based pulmonary rehabilitation programme on exercise tolerance and quality of life: a randomized controlled trial. Eur Respir J 1997; 10: 104–113.

27. Griffiths TL, Burr ML, Campbell IA et al. Results at 1 year of outpatient multidisciplinary pulmonary rehabilitation: a randomized controlled trial. Lancet 2000; 355: 362–368.

28. Guell R, Casan P, Belda J et al. Long-term effects of outpatient rehabilitation of COPD. A randomized trial. Chest 2000; 117: 976–983.

29. Lacasse Y, Wong E, Guyatt GH et al. Meta-analysis of respiratory rehabilitation in chronic obstructive pulmonary disease. Lancet 1996; 348: 1115–1119.

30. Ambrosino N, Clini E. Evaluation in pulmonary rehabilitation. Respir Med 1996; 90: 395–400.

31. Goldstein RS, Avendano MA. Candidate evaluation. In: Casaburi R, Petty TL, ed. Principles and practice of pulmonary rehabilitation. Philadelphia, PA: WB Saunders; 1993: 317–321.

32. Niederman MS, Clemente PH, Fein AM et al. Benefits of a multidisciplinary pulmonary rehabilitation programme. Improvements are independent of lung function. Chest 1991; 99: 798–804.

33. ERS task force. Clinical exercise testing with reference to lung diseases: indications, standardization and interpretation strategies. Eur Respir J 1997; 10: 2662–2689.

34. Singh SJ, Morgan MDL, Scott S et al. Development of a shuttle walking test of disability in patients with chronic airflow obstruction. Thorax 1992; 47: 1019–1024.

35. Mahler D, Guyatt GH, Jones PW. Clinical measurement of dyspnea. In: Mahler D. Dyspnea. New York: Marcel Dekker; 1998: 149–198.

36. Jones PW, Quirk FH, Baveystock CM, Littlejohns P. A self-complete measure of health status for chronic airflow limitation. Am Rev Respir Dis 1992; 145: 1321–1327.

37. Foglio K, Bianchi L, Bruletti G et al. Long-term effectiveness of pulmonary rehabilitation in patients with chronic airway obstruction (CAO). Eur Respir J 1999; 11: 125–132.

38. Gosselink R, Foglio K, Ambrosino N. Breathing exercises. In: Ambrosino N, Donner CF, Rampulla C. Topics in pulmonary rehabilitation. Pavia, Italy: Maugeri Foundations; 1999: 209–228.

39. Gosselink RAAM, Wagenaar RC, Rijswijk H et al. Diaphragmatic breathing reduces efficiency of breathing in patients with chronic obstructive pulmonary disease. Am J Respir Crit Care Med 1995; 151: 1136–1142.

40. Vitacca M, Clini E, Bianchi L, Ambrosino N. Acute effects of deep diaphragmatic breathing in COPD patients with chronic respiratory insufficiency. Eur Respir J 1998; 11, 408–415.

41. Casaburi R, Patessio A, Ioli F et al. Reductions in exercise lactic acidosis and ventilation as a result of exercise training in patients with obstructive lung disease. Am Rev Respir Dis 1991; 143: 9–18.

42. Garrod R, Paul EA, Wedzicha JA. Supplemental oxygen during pulmonary rehabilitation in patients with COPD with exercise hypoxaemia. Thorax 2000; 55: 539–543.

43. Ambrosino N. Exercise and noninvasive ventilatory support. Monaldi Arch Chest Dis 2000; 55; 242–246.

44. Smith K, Cook D, Guyatt GH et al. Respiratory muscle training in chronic airflow limitation: a meta-analysis. Am Rev Respir Dis 1992; 145: 533–539.

45. Clark CJ, Cochrane L, Mackay E. Low intensity peripheral muscle conditioning improves exercise tolerance and breathlessness in COPD. Eur Respir J 1996; 9: 2590–2596.

46. Emery C, Leatherman NE, Burker EJ, MacIntyre NR. Psychological outcomes of a pulmonary rehabilitation programme. Chest 1991; 100: 613–617.

47. Kaplan RM, Ries AL. Cost-effectiveness of pulmonary rehabilitation. In: Fishman AP. Pulmonary rehabilitation. New York: Marcel Dekker; 1996: 379–398.

48. Goldstein RS, Gort EH, Guyatt GH, Feeny D. Economic analysis of respiratory rehabilitation. Chest 1997; 112: 370–379.

49. Bowen JB, Votto JJ, Thrall RS et al. Functional status and survival following pulmonary rehabilitation. Chest 2000; 118: 697–703.

50. Garrod R, Mikelsons C, Paul EA, Wedzicha JA. Randomized controlled trial of domiciliary noninvasive positive pressure ventilation and physical training in severe chronic obstructive pulmonary disease. Am J Respir Crit Care Med 2000; 162; 1335–1341.

18 Assessment for anaesthesia with respiratory disease

Brian F Keogh and Caroline J Bateman

 Key points

■ Assessment involves medical optimisation and assessment of risk.

■ Rejection as a candidate for anaesthesia on the basis of pulmonary disease is rare.

■ Individual likely postoperative requirements should be matched to available resources by effective scheduling processes.

■ No single test accurately predicts perioperative risk or the likelihood of postoperative pulmonary complications.

■ Reasonable risk stratification for patients with pulmonary disease exists for thoracic surgery but is poorly defined for other disciplines.

■ Advances in surgical techniques, anaesthesia, recovery facilities and pain-control techniques mandate that the limits of operability are continually redefined.

Patients with respiratory disease who require anaesthesia present with a diverse range of pulmonary pathology and associated comorbidity. The preoperative assessment of these patients is of great importance since it will help identify those at risk of developing perioperative complications and aid in the appropriate allocation of resources for postoperative care. Optimisation of the patient's preoperative state, addressing both pulmonary and comorbid conditions, is a key element of anaesthetic management, should invoke a multidisciplinary approach and can favourably influence the postoperative course. Postoperative pulmonary complications may prolong hospital stay by an average of between 1 and 2 weeks and this has obvious implications for both the patient and hospital resources.[1]

The definition of a postoperative pulmonary complication varies considerably and ranges from a fever with a cough to the requirement for prolonged ventilatory support. As a result, com-parison of studies addressing the incidence of pulmonary complications is difficult, and a further confounding factor is the impact of the type and duration of surgery. In patients undergoing thoracic surgery, recent data suggests that major respiratory complications such as atelectasis, pneumonia and respiratory failure occur in 15–20% of patients and account for most of the expected 3–4% mortality.[2] Data available on the incidence of pulmonary complications in abdominal and peripheral surgery is generally much less current and may not adequately reflect advances in perioperative medicine nor the recent trend towards acceptance for surgery of patients with more severe comorbid disease.

Recent advances in anaesthesia, surgery and postoperative care now result in very few patients being rejected as operative candidates by the anaesthetist on the basis of preoperative pulmonary disease. The risk of undertaking the procedure must obviously be balanced against the risk of not doing so and, with the current emphasis on risk evaluation and informed consent,[3] it should become increasingly possible to provide each patient with a reasonable risk/benefit assessment. The degree to which this assessment in patients with respiratory disease is currently evidence-based varies. In a review of literature available on preoperative assessment of pulmonary risk, Ferguson concluded in 1999 that appropriate assessment of risk was well-defined for thoracic surgery but was less so for general surgical and cardiovascular procedures.[4]

Risk assessment in anaesthesia

The risk of anaesthesia as the sole cause of death is gratifyingly low. An early UK estimate in 1982 suggested an incidence of death due primarily to anaesthesia of 1:10 000.[5] More recent studies have suggested an incidence of death directly attributable to anaesthesia perhaps 20 times lower,[6,7] although the number of deaths classified as anaesthesia-associated has correspondingly risen. Much data has been derived from risk studies, not the least being from the series of National Confidential

Enquiry into Perioperative Deaths (NCEPOD) reports from the UK, which have in general stressed the multifactorial nature of perioperative deaths. Analysis of data from NCEPOD confirms, in both anaesthesia and surgical assessments, that patients whose deaths were considered as part of the 2000 report were more likely to be older, require urgent operation and be less well in terms of comorbidity than patients who died in 1990.[8]

The risk of anaesthesia is inextricably linked to the overall risk of the procedure and is greatly influenced by comorbidity. There are many risk stratification systems but two are commonly applied. An almost routine assessment is the American Society of Anesthesiologists (ASA) Physical Status classification, in existence since the 1940s but modified to its current structure (Table 18.1) by Dripps and colleagues in 1961.[9] This has been shown to be strongly predictive of postoperative pulmonary complications in patients with pulmonary disease.[10] The Goldman cardiac-risk index, a more elaborate combination of patient history, examination and laboratory data, is also commonly used and predicts both cardiac and pulmonary complications.[1]

Postoperative pulmonary complications and general risk issues

No consensus exists as to what constitutes a postoperative pulmonary complication.[11] Those most commonly cited in the literature include pneumonia, fever with cough, radiographic infiltrates or atelectasis, bronchospasm, need for prolonged ventilation and respiratory failure. Retrospective studies of the incidence of complications are inherently flawed by the lack of a standard definition and reliance on the quality and discriminatory value of past medical records. Length of stay in the intensive care unit or postoperative length of stay in hospital have been suggested as relatively objective but indirect measures of postoperative pulmonary complications.

A review of the medical literature reveals that, with a few notable exceptions, there is relatively little recent information on the incidence of postoperative pulmonary complications in non-cardiothoracic patients and much of the data available is more than 20 years old. Patients undergoing emergency surgery are at greater risk of complications generally, and specifically of postoperative pulmonary complications, than those undergoing elective procedures and this holds true for patients with pre-existing pulmonary disease.[10] Abdominal surgery carries a particular risk of pulmonary complications and the incidence is much higher than for peripheral procedures.[12] The duration of anaesthesia (or total procedure time) has also been shown to be an independent predictor of postoperative pulmonary complications in general elective surgery[13] and in patients with chronic obstructive pulmonary disease.[10] Operations lasting more than 4 hours, regardless of operative site, are associated with an increased risk of pneumonia.[14] A recent report of 89 patients undergoing lung volume reduction surgery similarly found a poor outcome associated with anaesthetic time more than 3.5 hours.[15]

Effects of anaesthesia on the respiratory system

Anaesthesia in the supine position is associated with changes in pulmonary mechanics that may particularly adversely affect patients with already compromised pulmonary function. The diaphragm moves in a cephalad direction, resulting in a reduction in thoracic volume and regional atelectasis. Functional residual capacity (FRC) falls and, as it approaches closing volume, airways resistance increases, particularly in obese patients. FRC may actually impinge upon the closing capacity, especially in the obese and the elderly. Dependent lung atelectasis can be demonstrated on computed tomography (CT) scan, usually in the posterobasal segments, and may persist for several days postoperatively. Atelectasis results in increased intrapulmonary shunt and patients with existing pulmonary disease are particularly at risk of substantial increases in resultant intrapulmonary shunt levels. Physiological dead space is also increased and can adversely impact on patients with pre-existing lung disease, especially those with chronic obstructive pulmonary disease.

Postoperative hypoxaemia to quite profound levels (e.g. P_aO_2 6 kPa or 44 mmHg) is common in patients with pre-existing lung disease. This is usually multifactorial, combining existing $\dot{V}/\dot{Q}$ disturbance with postoperative atelectasis and possibly exacerbated by diaphragm dysfunction and/or chest wall splinting due to discomfort or the effects of surgery. In addition, sedative drugs may compound the situation by contributing to upper airway obstruction and shallow respiration in patients with existing atelectasis. Accordingly, P_aCO_2 values encountered in the recovery room (7–9 kPa, 50–65 mmHg) are often higher than might be ordinarily accepted. These levels should not necessarily cause alarm in an appropriately monitored and observed patients and may be expected in a postoperative patient with pre-existing respiratory disease given adequate analgesia. The recovery room phase is a key element of the perioperative care of such patients and will be considered later in the chapter.

Table 18.1 American Society of Anesthesiologists Physical Status classification.[9]

Class	Physical status
I	Normal, healthy
II	Mild systemic disease
III	Severe systemic disease that limits activity but is not incapacitating
IV	Incapacitating systemic disease that is a constant threat to life
V	Moribund. Not expected to survive 24 hours with or without operation

Emergency procedures are indicated by the prefix: E

Preoperative anaesthetic assessment of the patient with pulmonary disease

Preliminary assessment

In addition to the general medical history, problems with previous anaesthesia, especially the requirement for postoperative ventilation, should be specifically elicited from the history. Current medications should be detailed, the degree of compliance with medication should be ascertained if respiratory symptoms are unstable and any recent history of corticosteroid therapy should be established. Any history of allergy, upper airway problems, difficulty with mouth opening, precarious dentition or limitation of neck flexibility should be documented.

Indicators of cardiopulmonary reserve and ASA status should be determined. Patients who are ASA I or II with no limitation of activity or exercise capacity do not need further cardiorespiratory screening before surgery.[2] The majority of patients with pre-existing parenchymal pulmonary disease are ASA III and require further investigation. Patients who are receiving domiciliary oxygen clearly require both investigation and preoperative optimisation. Pulmonary function testing, plus or minus exercise testing and/or $\dot{V}/\dot{Q}$ scanning, should be arranged as indicated in each individual patient. The patient's current status in relation to their best personal baseline symptoms should be determined and recent exacerbation of pulmonary infection or sputum production should be excluded. Any new symptoms such as increasing dyspnoea, cough, increasing effort intolerance or chest pain should be verified and investigated.

Clinical examination should specifically elicit signs of respiratory obstruction or use of accessory muscles. Cyanosis, dyspnoea or a 'barrel' chest represent anaesthetic alerts. The high incidence of cardiac comorbidity should be recognised and any evidence of cardiac insufficiency identified. Electrocardiography should be performed and patients with advanced pulmonary disease should undergo echocardiography to document the degree of pulmonary hypertension and to assess right ventricular function. Routine blood investigations should include assessments of hepatorenal function and arterial blood gases should be measured in patients who are ASA III or higher, in order to determine baseline gas exchange and identify patients with resting elevated P_aCO_2 levels. A recent chest radiograph should be available and, in patients with severe, non-homogenous pulmonary pathology, a CT scan may prove useful in directing anaesthetic conduct.

General patient-related issues

Smoking

It is commonly held that patients should cease cigarette smoking as long as possible before a planned surgical procedure. It is difficult to predict who will be successful in achieving this goal and what tangible benefit it will provide. In addition, the smoker often feels the need to admit to smoking a cigarette on the morning of surgery and may do so just prior to, or during the early phase of, induction of anaesthesia. While this admission may help to resolve the anxieties of the patient, it places the anaesthetist in a difficult position, particularly if the patient is already thought to be at high risk of postoperative complications.

Carboxyhaemoglobin represents 2% of circulating haemoglobin (up to 4% in city dwellers) and may rise to 15% in cigarette chain smokers. Heavy smokers may therefore undergo general anaesthesia with a significant reduction in their functional oxygen-carrying capacity.[16] The half-life of carboxyhaemoglobin is approximately 6 hours and levels fall substantially if smoking is stopped more than 12 hours before surgery. Current smokers are at risk of tissue hypoxia and it is recognised that wound tissue oxygen tension correlates with wound healing and resistance to infection.[17]

The major cardiovascular effects of nicotine include increase in heart rate, myocardial contractility and systemic vascular resistance and these combine to increase myocardial oxygen consumption. At the same time, nicotine has a direct vasoconstrictor effect on the coronary arteries and, in patients with pre-existing coronary artery disease, results in an unfavourable effect on myocardial oxygen supply–demand ratio.[18] Nicotine has a half-life of 30–60 min and should be almost completely cleared after 5 hours. Its primary metabolite, cotinine, has a much more benign cardiovascular profile and is thought to result in a mild vasodilation of vascular beds. There is therefore a strong suggestion of theoretical benefit from a brief (6–12 hours) cessation of smoking preoperatively on the grounds of nicotine pharmacokinetics alone. A recent study of the effect of acute smoking and general anaesthesia showed that patients older than 65 years who had smoked shortly before surgery had more episodes of rate-pressure-product-related ST segment depression than non-smokers, ex-smokers or chronic smokers who had not smoked before surgery.[19]

The incidence of pulmonary complications is lower in thoracic surgical patients who are not smoking as opposed to those who smoke until surgery. In one study of 117 thoracotomy patients, current smoking was associated with a more than doubling of both the risk of all complications and that of pulmonary complications.[20] In a prospective study of 200 smokers who underwent coronary surgery, a lower risk of pulmonary complications (14.5%) was found in ex-smokers who had not smoked for 2 months when compared to current smokers (33%).[21] Conversely, patients who had stopped smoking within 2 months had a pulmonary complication rate (57%) almost twice that of current smokers. Along similar lines, a recent study showed that, while the incidence of postoperative pulmonary complications in smokers was more than four times that of never-smokers (22% versus 4.9%), current smokers who reported a reduction in cigarette consumption but failed to stop were nearly seven times more likely to suffer postoperative pulmonary complications than those who did not alter their smoking habits.[22] Differences in complication rates were admittedly only noted in the 'minor' categories, which included increased aerosol use and atelectasis.

Several explanations have been proposed to explain these counterintuitive findings of apparently increased risk of postoperative complications for those in the early stages of changes in smoking habit. These include an increase in sputum production, a reduction in bronchial irritation, which precedes any reduction in bronchial hypersecretion and therefore may result in sputum retention and bronchial obstruction, and possible selection bias in that the sickest cigarette-dependent patients are more likely to cut down than those who are relatively symptom free.

Smoking is also directly relevant to anaesthesia. The tracheo-bronchial tree in smokers is hyper-responsive, resulting in coughing, laryngospasm, bronchospasm, requirement for deeper and longer anaesthesia and in some cases unacceptable hypoxia. In addition, the combination of excessive sputum production and reduced mucociliary clearance may lead not only to ventilation–perfusion mismatching but, in association with repetitive and often poorly effective coughing, may secondarily impact on pain control requirements and wound healing in thoracoabdominal procedures.

Patients are being increasingly empowered to influence the treatment they receive and it may prove difficult to deny treatment to smokers even if this approach is thought to be based on solid medical grounds. If the patient who smokes is to be reviewed at an anaesthesia preassessment clinic, these smoking-related matters should be addressed but if not, the surgeon and referring physician should raise them with the patient during the preoperative preparation, as long as possible before the planned intervention. A list of procedure-related issues that should be discussed with smokers is listed in Table 18.2.

In summary, current evidence suggests that smoking cessation for a period of at least 2 months is associated with a lower incidence of postoperative complications and that, after that period, the longer the period of abstinence the better.

Table 18.2 Preanaesthetic counselling for smokers

Pulmonary
- Increased airway irritability
- Increased, but less effective cough
- Difficulty in expectorating effectively
- Risk of atelectasis and hypoxia
- Difficulty in controlling pain associated with coughing

Cardiovascular
- Nicotine mediated coronary vasoconstriction
- Imbalance of myocardial supply and demand
- Increased risk of coronary ischaemia
- Increased risk of arrhythmia in older patients

Oxygen carriage
- Inefficient O_2 carriage in blood (COHb levels)
- Decreased O_2 availability to tissues and risk of delayed healing

Immunity
- Increased risk of pulmonary infections (2–6×non-smokers)
- Decreased immunity leading to risk of other infections

Issues listed are those that might be discussed with a smoking patient in a preoperative counselling session. At the very least a 12-hour cigarette fast should be encouraged.

Refractory smokers, to whom the possibilities of postoperative complications should be explained in detail, or smokers who are first seen shortly before surgery, should be advised to undergo a smoking fast of 12 or preferably 24 hours, especially if there is a risk of coronary artery disease. Consideration should be given to the problems of nicotine withdrawal. An overnight fast is reported to be tolerable and associated with less anxiety than several days of abstinence.[23] Pharmacological assistance has been recommended to increase the number of successful quitters.[24] Residual questions remain about the best advice for patients who are unable to cease smoking completely for 8 weeks preoperatively or in whom the scheduling of surgery precludes this. Although these patients should be advised to at least achieve a 24-hour smoking fast preoperatively, it is not clear whether beyond this they should be advised to alter or to maintain their baseline smoking patterns.[24]

Obesity

Obesity is defined as body mass index (BMI) more than 30 and morbid obesity as BMI more than 40. Obese patients have an increased risk of postoperative atelectasis.[25] Early evidence suggested that moderate weight loss prior to surgery decreased the risk of pulmonary complications[26] but this was not confirmed by a more recent evaluation.[27] In addition, a review of 10 series of morbidly obese patients undergoing gastric bypass surgery found an incidence of postoperative pneumonia and atelectasis of only 3.9%, comparable to non-obese patients. Current evidence suggests that obesity alone is not a significant risk factor for pulmonary complications.[28] Despite this, a recent study comparing pulmonary mechanics in normal versus morbidly obese patients undergoing abdominal surgery has highlighted the marked reduction in total, lung and chest-wall static compliance, increased total respiratory resistance and reduction in functional residual capacity (to 40% of non-obese values) in the morbidly obese (Fig. 18.1).[29] These findings have considerable implications for anaesthetic techniques but also may influence the risk assessment in patients with combined morbid obesity and pulmonary disease.

The combination of obesity and coexisting respiratory disease was associated in one study with a 38% incidence of postoperative pulmonary complications as compared to 12% in obese patients without respiratory disease.[30] Although postoperative ventilation is rarely required for obesity per se, it is much more likely in the presence of coexisting cardiac or pulmonary disease.[31] A programme of gradual weight reduction prior to surgery is therefore desirable. Obese patients with respiratory diseases are likely to require at least a high-dependency bed and possibly an intensive-care bed and preoperative assessment should allow appropriate resource allocation.

Specific additional preoperative assessment issues in obese patients include careful assessment of the upper airway, vascular and epidural access, and evaluation of the risk of acid aspiration and of commonly associated conditions such as diabetes. Patients should be introduced to physiotherapy exercises preoperatively and the importance of these and of early mobilisation in the obese patient should be stressed.

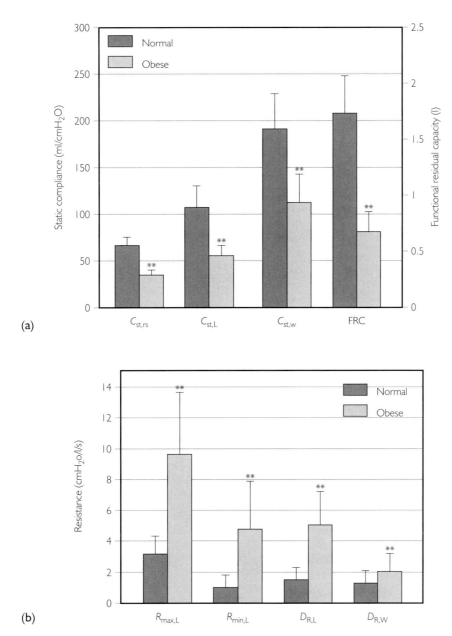

Fig. 18.1 Impact of morbid obesity on static compliance, functional residual capacity (FRC) and resistance characteristics in anaesthetised patients. a. In sedated and paralysed patients, a substantial reduction in total respiratory ($C_{st,rs}$), lung ($C_{st,L}$) and chest wall ($C_{st,w}$) static compliance, and particularly in FRC values, was observed in obese compared to normal patients. b. Similarly, the maximum resistance of the respiratory system ($R_{max,rs}$) was significantly increased in the obese, due mainly to an increase in maximum lung resistance ($R_{max,L}$), the result of increased airway resistance ($R_{min,L}$) and 'additional' lung resistance ($D_{R,L}$). A slight increase in chest wall resistance ($D_{R,w}$) did not account for the overall marked change in $R_{max,rs}$. These unfavourable alterations in pulmonary mechanics are particularly relevant to obese patients with pre-existing pulmonary disease. Modified with permission from Pelosi et al 1996.[29]

Age

There are conflicting data on the impact of age on the risk of postoperative pulmonary complications. In patients older than 80 years undergoing thoracic surgery, Osaki reported a remarkably low mortality of 3%. The rate of respiratory and cardiac complications were both reported at 40%, representing twice and three times the expected incidence of younger patients

respectively.[32] In another series, a high mortality of 22% was reported for pneumonectomy in patients over 70 years.[33] This high mortality, particularly for right pneumonectomy, has been attributed to the cardiac sequelae of the resected pulmonary vascular bed.[2]

In non-thoracic surgery, age does not seem to be an independent predictor of outcome or of pulmonary complications.[34] The 30-day mortality in 500 patients older than 80 years undergoing anaesthesia and surgery was 6.2% for all ASA classes, with most deaths due to cardiac complications or infection.[35] Age was also not found to predict postoperative pulmonary complications in two studies of patients with severe chronic obstructive pulmonary disease.[10,36] In a recent review of preoperative pulmonary evaluation, Smetana concluded that current evidence indicated that pulmonary complications were more strongly related to coexisting conditions than to chronological age, and that advanced age alone was not therefore a reason to withhold surgery.[28]

Physiological changes in the respiratory system associated with ageing may nevertheless influence the conduct of anaesthesia and surgery. These include chest-wall rigidity and an increase in the proportion of the total elastic work of breathing expended on chest-wall movement (70% in a 70-year-old male versus 40% in a 20-year-old), a reduction in respiratory muscle strength and endurance and an increase in closing volume to approximately 30% of total lung capacity at age 70. In addition there is a diminished response to hypoxia and hypercapnia and a higher incidence of respiratory depression in response to opiates or sedatives.[37]

Respiratory tract infection

The majority of studies assessing the implications of respiratory tract infection have been in children with upper respiratory tract infections. A review in 1997 recommended that children with moderate to severe respiratory tract infection should have elective surgery postponed for 6 weeks.[38] Less conservative approaches are generally recommended for mild infections, and a 2-week delay following infection is commonly advised. In a prospective study of more than 2000 children, these same authors found that a 'cold' on the day of surgery, nasal congestion or a productive cough were associated with an increased risk of adverse anaesthetic events (cough, breath-holding, desaturation or airway obstruction among others) but that neither a history of respiratory tract infection nor previous cancellation of surgery due to respiratory tract infection within the previous 6 weeks predicted an increase in anaesthetic adverse events.[39]

There is very limited information on respiratory tract infection in adults scheduled for anaesthesia or the impact of pre-existing lower respiratory tract infection on outcome. Upper respiratory tract infection has been shown to increase upper airway irritability in adults for up to 15 days.[40] Airway irritability correlated well with symptoms, implying that a 2-week delay and resolution of symptoms might be advisable in adults before undergoing elective surgery. Surprisingly, a study of patients with asthma found no increase in postoperative pulmonary complications in patients who had had symptoms of an upper respiratory tract infection within the previous month.[41]

Current respiratory tract infection in a patient with pre-existing pulmonary disease should be treated prior to elective surgery. This would be perceived by the anaesthetist as an integral part of preoperative preparation, and ideally such patients should be treated by a pulmonary physician. There is limited recent data but infected sputum has long been considered to warrant antibiotic therapy.[42] In chronic obstructive pulmonary disease, a course of antibiotics in patients with increased cough or sputum production may be of benefit in reducing postoperative complica-

tions.[43] There are no studies that have evaluated the impact of mild, presumably viral, upper respiratory tract infection in high-risk patients undergoing major surgery. Although this may cause inconvenience for the patient and disrupt surgical planning, it is appropriate to delay truly elective procedures until symptoms have settled. In urgent or emergency procedures, the pressing need for surgery is likely to override these concerns.

Cardiac disease

Heart and lung disease often occur together and cardiac complications are second to pulmonary in thoracic surgical patients although, in the general surgical population, these rankings are reversed. In a broad classification of surgery-specific cardiac risk, thoracic surgical procedures were stratified as intermediate, below emergency and major vascular procedures.[44]

Major clinical predictors of increased perioperative cardiovascular risk are:[44]

- unstable coronary syndromes (recent myocardial infarction with evidence of ischaemia, unstable or severe angina)
- decompensated congestive cardiac failure
- severe valvular disease
- significant arrhythmia (high-grade atrioventricular block, supraventricular arrhythmias with uncontrolled ventricular rate and symptomatic arrhythmias with underlying heart disease).

Intermediate risk predictors include:

- mild angina
- previous myocardial infarction
- compensated or previous congestive cardiac failure
- diabetes.

Minor predictors of risk include:

- advanced age
- abnormal electrocardiogram (ECG)
- cardiac rhythm other than sinus
- history of stroke
- uncontrolled systemic hypertension.

Ischaemic heart disease

Patients with respiratory disease commonly present with several risk factors for coronary artery disease. In one study of 598 thoracic surgical procedures the incidence of perioperative myocardial ischaemia was 5% and that of myocardial infarction was 1.2%.[45]

There has been considerable debate about the value of routine invasive screening for patients prior to major thoracic surgical procedures. It is generally accepted that standard history, physical examination, assessment of functional status and ECG should identify the majority of patients at high risk and that specialised cardiac screening is not cost-effective.[2,46] This view is also currently held in relation to non-thoracic surgical procedures.[44,47] Patients should undergo further non-invasive investigation and/or angiography in the presence of major or intermediate risk predictors as listed above.

Some refinements of this broad statement have been suggested, particularly on cost-effectiveness grounds, in the ACC/AHA Task Force Guidelines.[44] This report has proposed an algorithm for preoperative assessment of coronary risk, suggesting that patients with intermediate risk factors (above) and moderate or excellent functional capacity can undergo intermediate-risk procedures (includes thoracic and non-vascular and non-emergency surgery) without further cardiac investigation. A reasonable sequence of testing in patients thought to require further investigation would be exercise ECG, thallium scan and angiography if findings are positive. Patients thought at high risk of significant coronary artery disease on the basis of history or ECG may proceed directly to angiography, especially if pulmonary disease limits exercise capability. Additional investigations include ambulatory ECG, radionuclide scanning and exercise echocardiography. The value and/or cost effectiveness of these investigations, and indeed of thallium scanning, is the subject of ongoing debate.[47]

Patients with significant coronary artery disease may undergo optimisation of medical therapy, angioplasty with or without stenting or coronary artery surgery. Although it is an attractive approach, the impact on outcome of angioplasty/coronary stenting preoperatively in surgical patients with or without pulmonary disease is not yet known. Combined procedures for coronary grafting and pulmonary resections have been reported[48] but for more major resections, pulmonary resection is often delayed for 4–6 weeks after cardiac surgery until the patient has regained weight and muscle mass. Patients who have suffered a myocardial infarction present particular difficulties. Although current practice is to delay elective procedures for up to 6 months following infarction, pulmonary resection is often an urgent procedure and may be performed with acceptable risk in optimised patients within 4–6 weeks.[2]

Cardiac valve disease

Severe valvular heart disease is recognised to be a high-risk predictor of cardiovascular adverse events. The exact nature and extent of valve lesions should be determined by echocardiography, as should ventricular performance. A low threshold for investigation of coronary artery status is appropriate. Functional status is a useful indicator of disease severity and of perioperative risk. There are no substantial data on postoperative outcome in patients with combined pulmonary disease and cardiac valve disease. In patients requiring major surgery, including pulmonary resections, the issue of surgical priority in the presence of a newly diagnosed valve lesion may arise.

Valve surgery should be advised on standard cardiological criteria, should not be specifically influenced by the need for other surgery and, if indicated, should in most cases precede a planned other procedure. Although risk is increased, the presence of severe valve disease should not be prohibitive in the decision-making process. A report of 48 patients with severe aortic stenosis, 75% of whom had congestive cardiac failure, angina or syncope, who underwent surgical procedures either with general anaesthesia or sedation combined with local anaesthesia, suggested a low risk and reported no intraoperative deaths.[49]

Renal insufficiency

Screening blood tests are abnormal in 2–5% of patients[50] and these usually relate to elevated blood glucose and/or serum urea/creatinine levels. In a study of more than 7000 patients undergoing abdominal and peripheral, non-vascular surgery, renal disease was significantly predictive of increased risk.[51] In the same study, the development of renal failure postoperatively was associated with a 1–2% mortality rate after elective surgery in patients older than 50 years and a 2% mortality for emergency procedures in patients aged 50–70 years, rising to 9% in those over 70 years old. Perioperative management of patients with renal insufficiency relies on maintenance of intravascular volume, haemodynamic support and avoidance of nephrotoxins. A variety of pharmacological agents are recommended including mannitol, loop diuretics, dopamine, dopexamine and more recently fenoldopam, but none have definitively been shown to be renal-protective.

Difficulties in preservation of renal function are compounded in patients with pulmonary disease, particularly those undergoing pulmonary resection. In general surgery, patients with renal insufficiency are maintained at high intravascular filling pressures while in thoracic surgery, intravenous fluids, while not necessarily being restricted, should be administered judiciously and patients should be kept on the 'dry' side in order to prevent pulmonary microvascular leakage. A balance is even more difficult to achieve in patients with cardiac insufficiency and elevated pulmonary venous pressure. In a study of 130 patients undergoing major thoracic procedures, 24% developed renal impairment and, while there were no deaths in the patients without renal impairment, 6/31 (19%) of those who developed renal impairment died.[52] Postoperative renal impairment was associated with preoperative renal impairment or diuretic intake, pneumonectomy, postoperative infection and blood loss.

Respiratory disease specific issues

Chronic obstructive pulmonary disease

Patients with chronic obstructive pulmonary disease (COPD) commonly present for anaesthesia and surgery; in thoracic surgery patients, COPD is the commonest comorbid condition encountered. Disease control may be suboptimal, because of variable patient compliance or recent exacerbation, and referral to a pulmonary physician for medical optimisation is often required.

Patients with COPD have an increased risk of postoperative pulmonary complications. The incidence depends on the definition of a complication and the severity of pulmonary disease (Table 18.3).[28] Most studies suggest that patients with COPD are between two and five times more likely to suffer postoperative pulmonary complications. In addition, a recent study of 105 patients with severe COPD ($FEV_1 < 1.2$ l and $FEV_1/FVC < 75\%$) who underwent non-cardiothoracic surgery reported 6.6% in-hospital mortality but disappointing long-term survival (Fig. 18.2).[10] The observed survival rates (e.g. 53% at 2 years, 30% at 4 years) were lower than those observed in other longitudinal studies of COPD patients without surgery.

Although the data demonstrating increased risk of postoperative complications in COPD patients is considerable, there is

Table 18.3 Patient-related risk factors for postoperative pulmonary complications. Modified from Smetana 1999.[28]

| Risk factor | Type of surgery | Incidence of pulmonary complications (%) | | Unadjusted relative risk associated with factor |
		Factor present	Factor absent	
Smoking	Coronary bypass	39	11	3.4
	Abdominal	15–46	6–21	1.4–4.3
ASA	Unselected	26	16	1.7
Class >II	Thoracic or abdominal	26–44	13–18	1.5–3.2
Age > 70	Unselected	9–17	4–9	1.9–2.4
	Thoracic or abdominal	17–22	12–21	0.9–1.9
Obesity	Unselected	11	9	1.3
	Thoracic or abdominal	19–36	17–27	0.8–1.7
Chronic obstructive	Unselected	6–26	2–8	2.7–3.6
pulmonary disease	Thoracic or abdominal	18	4	4.7

Range of reported values from selected key publications.

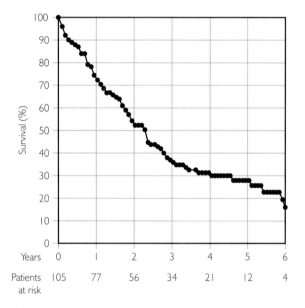

Fig. 18.2 Long-term survival of patients with severe chronic obstructive pulmonary disease following non-cardiothoracic surgery. Observed survival rates in 105 patients (53 general, 52 regional or local anaesthesia) following surgery. In-hospital mortality was 6.6%. The mortality rate of 47% at 2 years is higher than other longitudinal studies. The added mortality was thought to be due either to the effect of surgery and anaesthesia or to the underlying disease for which surgery was required. Redrawn with permission from Wong et al 1995.[10]

little recent information about the preoperative benefit of specific therapies in COPD. Aggressive therapy for patients who do not have optimal treatment of symptoms or airflow obstruction or who are not at their best baseline exercise capacity is recommended[28] and surgery should be deferred until treatment is optimised. Combinations of bronchodilators, physiotherapy, antibiotics, smoking cessation and corticosteroids were shown

to reduce the risk of postoperative pulmonary complications more than 25 years ago[42,53] but there is limited recent data and it is generally lacking in relation to individual therapeutic agents. The combination of inhaled ipratropium bromide and inhaled beta-agonists is recommended[54] and steroids preoperatively will improve the reversible component of ongoing bronchospasm.[55] In another study, the incidence of postoperative pneumonia in patients with COPD was reduced by the combination of bronchodilators and steroids.[43] Although most COPD patients do not respond to steroids, a preoperative course of systemic steroids may be valuable in patients who do not achieve their best personal baseline level despite bronchodilator therapy.[28,56] Their use in an individual patient must be balanced against the potential disadvantages of administering steroids preoperatively.

Chronic obstructive pulmonary disease and physiotherapy
Patients with COPD are reported to have fewer postoperative pulmonary complications if they undergo intensive preoperative chest physiotherapy.[42] There is no definite evidence of superiority for any particular form of physiotherapy and the important variable is the amount of time devoted to physiotherapy.[2] Incentive spirometry is resource-efficient but since it is self-administered it depends on patient motivation. Exercise tolerance can be improved in the most severe COPD patients,[57] suggesting that it should be considered in all high-risk patients. In practice, the time from diagnosis to surgery for malignant disease means that substantial benefit will not be possible in this group. Patients with COPD who produce considerable amounts of sputum benefit most from physiotherapy.[58]

Pulmonary rehabilitation programmes, including physiotherapy, physical exercise, nutritional support and education, in addition to medical therapy have been shown to improve exercise tolerance and functional capacity in COPD patients.[59] This process takes several months and is extremely relevant to preparation for lung volume reduction surgery, although less so for surgery for malignant disease. Nutritional status, which is often poor in COPD patients, should be assessed and short-term benefits may be achieved with preoperative supplements. Whitaker and colleagues demonstrated that 16 days of enteral feeding supplemented to 1000 kcal above normal intake resulted in weight gain and improved muscle strength.[60]

Asthma

Patients with asthma present commonly for anaesthetic procedures and are at increased risk of perioperative complications, particularly exacerbation of bronchospasm. From the anaesthetic perspective, the known asthmatic is less of a problem than a previously unrecognised asthmatic who develops acute severe asthma in the perioperative period, either as a response to airway instrumentation or as an adverse reaction to drug therapy. The latter group may present immediate diagnostic difficulties and inevitably encounter a stormy intraoperative course as a succession of bronchodilators, anti-inflammatory and adrenergic agents may be administered in quick succession. High-dependency or intensive care may be required to stabilise and monitor such patients postoperatively. Cheney and colleagues reported 40 cases of bronchospasm, of which 33 had sustained neurological damage or died, from the American Society of Anesthesiologists Closed Claims Project.[61] Approximately 50% gave no history of asthma or COPD, confirming that bronchospasm can occur under anaesthesia in patients with no history of reactive airways disease and with dire consequences.[61]

The true incidence of perioperative respiratory complications in asthmatic patients is not clear. Although older studies have reported incidences of approximately 20%,[62] the most recent large study of 706 asthmatic patients reported bronchospasm in only 12 (1.7%).[41] This retrospective study probably underestimates the true incidence and smaller studies suggest exacerbation of asthma in 5–10% of patients[63] and a higher incidence of mild wheezing (0–45%), depending on anaesthesia technique.[64]

Preoperative assessment in asthma clearly includes optimisation of therapy. Patients should be free of wheezing and guidelines have been published that suggest that peak flow should be greater than 80% of predicted or personal best value.[65] In patients who are unstable or in whom compliance with therapy is questionable, a period of preoperative admission for supervised therapy with nebulised agents may be advisable. The use of short courses of corticosteroids to optimise asthmatic patients preoperatively does not appear to be associated with an increase in complications, particularly wound infections.[63,66]

Cystic fibrosis

The increased longevity of patients with cystic fibrosis renders it likely that sufferers will increasingly present for anaesthesia for a variety of indications, most commonly related to the disease (nasal polyps, pneumothoraces, vascular access or enteral feeding procedures) but also for unrelated conditions.

The information available on anaesthesia in cystic fibrosis is limited. There have been few studies published and these are limited to retrospective analyses of cases performed over long intervals, during which both anaesthetic and therapeutic options have evolved considerably. A series of 144 patients reflecting practice in the 1960s reported a perioperative mortality of 4%,[67] although subsequent reviews have suggested more favourable outcomes. In a series published in 1985, there was no perioperative mortality from 126 anaesthetics administered over a 3-year period, although postoperative pulmonary complications were noted in 9% of cases.[68] A more recent review published in 1995, but spanning 16 years, reported a perioperative mortality of less than 1%.[69]

Although there is a tendency to prefer alternatives to general anaesthesia in cystic fibrosis if possible, there is, in fact, little evidence to suggest that general anaesthesia per se causes a deterioration in pulmonary function. A retrospective review of pulmonary function tests showed no evidence that anaesthesia had long-term detrimental effects.[67] One small study showed deterioration in pulmonary function tests at 48 hours following injection sclerotherapy for varices[70] but no longer-term follow-up was performed and these patients may represent an at-risk subgroup for immediate postoperative pulmonary dysfunction. Although procedures under local or regional techniques may be preferred, it is possible that some patients might benefit from a short period of very aggressive physiotherapy, bronchial toilet and possibly even bronchoscopy, which could be afforded as adjunctive procedures under general anaesthesia.

Patients with cystic fibrosis presenting for truly elective surgery should be at their optimum level of pulmonary function and any infective exacerbation should be treated beforehand. The incidence of gastro-oesophageal reflux is higher than the general population and antiacid prophylaxis should be considered. Intensive pre- and postoperative physiotherapy is essential and the procedure should be scheduled appropriately to ensure these facilities are available. Perioperative antibiotic cover is routine and is usually administered intravenously. Adequate analgesia must be ensured in order that postprocedural pain does not adversely impact on the ability to perform effective physiotherapy.

In clinical practice, it is much more common for patients with cystic fibrosis to present for procedures that are not truly elective. Vascular access procedures, particularly in younger patients, may be required during an acute infective exacerbation, thoracic complications require urgent intervention and even procedures for enteral feeding access may be required when patients are not at their baseline best function. Such procedures, which may be surgically minor, require considerable resources, particularly in the postoperative period. Patients should undergo immediate preoperative physiotherapy and be receiving appropriate antibiotic and bronchodilator therapy. Anaesthesia care should involve regular intraoperative bronchial toilet and provision of effective postoperative pain relief. Patients should receive postoperative physiotherapy in the recovery room. It is the authors' practice to maintain the patient on a short-acting anaesthetic infusion (propofol) for a variable period in the recovery room, during which time aggressive physiotherapy is conducted by nurses and the cystic fibrosis physiotherapy team while access to the airway is still available. When secretions have been effectively cleared, or no further benefit is thought likely, the sedative infusion is ceased and the patient is rapidly extubated, and then undergoes further physiotherapy before discharge to the ward. Many such patients require a period of postoperative monitoring in a high-dependency unit and a small percentage will require intensive-care unit facilities.

At the extreme end of the spectrum, patients with cystic fibrosis who are being bridged to transplantation with non-invasive ventilation (NIV) may present for surgical procedures during the terminal phase of their respiratory condition. Pulmonary function is so deranged that such patients would ordinarily not be considered for anaesthesia but the possibility of transplantation and the extreme motivation of these patients often dictates that surgery should proceed. An additional consideration is that intubation and continued invasive ventilation in such patients may predispose to bacteraemia, endotoxin release, systemic inflammatory syndrome and multiorgan damage,[71,72] so that the aim is to return such patients to NIV as soon as possible after the procedure, following recovery-room physiotherapy as outlined above.

Interstitial lung disease

There is very little information in the literature about anaesthesia for patients with interstitial lung disease and data on risk assessment is non-existent.[73] In the authors' experience, elevated pulmonary vascular resistance places a patient with cryptogenic fibrosing alveolitis at high risk of complications and a poor outcome from intensive care.[74]

Chest wall abnormalities

Patients presenting for correction of scoliosis may have restrictive lung disease, and in more severe cases, pulmonary hypertension. Vital capacity (VC) reduction occurs in direct proportion to the severity of the thoracic distortion. Respiratory reserve is said to be adequate if VC is more than 70% of the predicted value, whereas postoperative ventilation is required if it is less than 50%.[75] Preoperative cardiac assessment in at-risk cases should include echocardiography, although the echo window may be poor, and possibly right-heart catheterisation. An increased risk of malignant hyperthermia is recognised in these patients.

Patients with kyphoscoliosis requiring anaesthesia for other elective and emergency procedures often need a period of postoperative ventilation and a prolonged weaning programme, sometimes with NIV. Severe cases, particularly with upper thoracic and cervical-spine abnormalities, represent a technically very challenging group for the anaesthetist and airway management, central vascular access and regional analgesic techniques may prove difficult. Cardiopulmonary reserve may be limited and circulatory management includes preventing a mismatch of demand and perfusion in the pulmonary hypertensive right ventricle. Airway assessment and access is a key issue and thoracic or ear-nose-and-throat surgical assistance may be required. Elective tracheostomy may be appropriate and, in extreme cases, although technically difficult and uncomfortable for the patient, this can be performed under local anaesthesia.

Respiratory muscle weakness

This group encompasses a range of conditions, many of which previously caused death in childhood but now demonstrate enhanced survival well into adult life. Anaesthetic difficulties

relate to associated cardiomyopathy, for which these patients should be thoroughly assessed preoperatively, potassium metabolism and adverse reactions to depolarising neuromuscular blockade, technical and logistic difficulties and an association with malignant hyperthermia. A recent study of 219 general anaesthetic procedures reported an 8.2% incidence of complications, mainly pulmonary, and that the risk of pulmonary complications was significantly higher after upper abdominal surgery or in patients with severe muscular disability, as assessed by the presence of proximal limb weakness.[76]

Chronically ventilated patients

A study in 1990 of 139 mainly ventilator-dependent patients with restrictive disease or muscle weakness who required surgical procedures found a perioperative mortality of only 2%.[77] The authors concluded that aggressive surgery was not inappropriate in severely disabled, ventilator-dependent patients. Such patients may provide few logistic difficulties for the anaesthetist as their recovery phase does not involve weaning or extubation. Preoperative assessment of cardiac performance is highly desirable but it may prove difficult to achieve meaningful stress testing and optimal views may not be possible on transthoracic echocardiography.

Procedure-specific issues

Thoracic surgery

Preoperative assessment and the estimate of risk are perhaps most advanced in this area. Postoperative major respiratory complications (atelectasis, pneumonia and respiratory failure) occur in 15–20% of thoracic surgical patients and this group accounts for the majority of the 3–4% mortality rate observed.[78] Cardiac complications, the leading cause of postoperative morbidity and mortality in other areas of surgery, are seen in 10–15% of thoracic surgical patients.[79] The risk of anaesthesia per se is difficult to tease out in these patients and is inextricably linked to the risks of the overall procedure.

Assessment of respiratory function

A very useful assessment of respiratory function is the patient's quality of life. An ASA Class I or II patient, with full exercise capacity, does not need cardiorespiratory screening prior to surgical procedures.[2]

Attempts to find a single respiratory function test with sufficient sensitivity and specificity to predict outcome for pulmonary resection have not been successful. Slinger has proposed a 'three-legged-stool' approach, outlined in Table 18.4, combining assessments of respiratory mechanics, gas exchange and cardiopulmonary interaction.[2]

Respiratory mechanics

Various tests have shown correlation with postoperative outcome including forced expiratory volume in 1 second (FEV_1), forced vital capacity (FVC), maximal voluntary ventila-

Table 18.4 'Three-legged stool' of prethoracotomy respiratory assessment. Modified from Slinger & Johnston 2000.[2]

Respiratory mechanics	Cardiopulmonary reserve	Lung parenchymal function
FEV_1 ppo > 40%	$\dot{V}_{O_2 max}$ > 15 ml/kg/min	D_LCO ppo > 40%
MVV, RV/TLC, FVC	Stair climb > 2 flights	P_aO_2 > 8.3 kPa (60 mmHg)
	6-minute walk test.	
	Exercise SpO_2 fall < 4%	P_aCO_2 < 6.3 kPa (45 mmHg)

D_LCO, diffusing capacity for carbon monoxide; FEV_1, forced expiratory volume in 1 second; FVC, forced vital capacity; MVV, maximal voluntary ventilation; ppo, predicted postoperative; RV, residual volume; SpO_2, peripheral oxygen saturated ion from pulse oximetry; TLC, total lung capacity; $\dot{V}_{O_2 max}$, maximum oxygen consumption.

tion (MVV) and residual volume to total lung capacity ratio (RV/TLC) as expressed as a percentage of predicted volumes. The most valid single test is predicted postoperative (ppo) FEV_1 percentage. This is calculated as:

$$ppo\ FEV_1\% = preoperative\ FEV_1\% \times (1 - \%functional\ lung\ tissue\ removed/100).$$

The percentage of functional lung tissue remaining can be calculated on the basis of the number of functioning subsegments of lung removed (*b*) but subtracting from that number any subsegments obstructed by tumour (n)[80] (Fig. 18.3):

$$\%\ functional\ lung\ tissue\ removed = (b - n/42 - n)/100.$$

In one series from Nakahara and colleagues of 156 patients, all 10 patients with ppo $FEV_1\%$ less than 30% required postoperative ventilation, and six died.[78] Thus ppo $FEV_1\%$ values of less than 30% predict an extremely high risk of postoperative morbidity and values between 30% and 40% an intermediate risk. These data reflect practice in the early 1980s and more recent data from Cerfolio and colleagues, possibly reflecting in part the impact of epidural anaesthesia, have suggested lower com-

plication rates in the high-risk groups.[81] These workers identified a correlation of ppo $FEV_1\%$ below 43% with the need for supplemental home oxygen. Markos and colleagues reported no postoperative complications in 47 patients with ppo $FEV_1\%$ above 40% but mortality of 50% in 6 patients with values below 40%.[82]

Kearney and colleagues did not standardise FEV_1 values and identified a low ppo FEV_1 (but not preoperative FEV_1) as the only significant correlate of complications when the effects of other potential risk factors were controlled for in multivariate analysis.[79] In a series of 331 patients undergoing pulmonary resections, with a low overall mortality of less than 1% and an all-complications rate of 17%, they found that, although a ppo FEV_1 below 1 litre was the best predictor of complications, it was not prohibitive (of 47 patients with ppo FEV_1 less than 1 litre, 45 survived and 66% had an uncomplicated postoperative course). Their findings also suggested that the magnitude of change from pre- to postoperative FEV_1 values may predict complications, an observation supported by the higher rate of complications observed in pneumonectomy.

Gas exchange

Arterial blood-gas data should be measured preoperatively in the majority of patients with pulmonary disease. Traditional alert values of P_aO_2 less than 60 mmHg (8.3 kPa) and P_aCO_2 more than 45 mmHg (6.3 kPa) may be of use but do not strongly predict postoperative pulmonary complications. Although these or similar values are commonly cited as risk factors, there are no large studies or prospective evaluations correlating arterial blood gases with outcome.[83] Additionally, although most authorities would agree that elevated P_aCO_2 places patients at high risk, no stratification is available and it is unclear if, or at what level, the risk is prohibitive.[83]

The most useful test of gas-exchanging capacity is the diffusing capacity for carbon monoxide (D_LCO) as a percentage of the predicted value. A similar equation to that used above for FEV_1 can be applied to give a predicted postoperative corrected value:

$$ppo\ D_LCO\% = preoperative\ D_LCO\% \times (1 - \%functional\ lung\ tissue\ removed/100).$$

A ppo $D_LCO\%$ value of less than 40% correlates with increased risk of respiratory and cardiac complications[2,82] and values above 40% indicate patients at low risk (Table 18.5)[4,82]

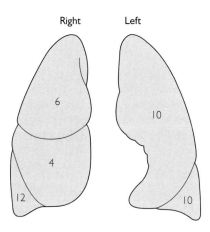

Fig. 18.3 Calculation of predicted postoperative (ppo) pulmonary function. The number of subsegments of each lobe for calculation of ppo values is shown. Non-functioning or obstructed subsegments are subtracted from both numerator and denominator when calculating percentage of functional lung tissue removed. With permission from Slinger & Johnston 2000.[2]

Table 18.5 Preoperative tests for assessing pulmonary risk prior to major lung resection. Modified from Ferguson 1999.[4]

Test	Value range for low-risk patients
FEV_1%	> 60%
D_LCO%	> 60%
ppo FEV_1	> 800 ml
ppo FEV_1%	> 40%
ppo D_LCO%	> 40%
$\dot{V}O_{2\,max}$ during exercise	> 15 ml/kg/min

Cardiopulmonary interactions

Stair-climbing in ambulatory patients has been used to assess cardiopulmonary reserve. This is usually described as the number of flights achieved without stopping, although there is no standard definition of what constitutes a flight of stairs. The ability to climb three or more flights is associated with decreased mortality. Inability to complete two flights suggests increased risk.[2] In a recent study of ventilatory reserve by stair-climbing in COPD patients, Pollock and colleagues advocated a symptom-limited, maximal stair-climbing assessment rather than confirming the ability to complete a certain number of flights.[84] In this study, the ability to climb 83 standardised steps correlated with a maximum oxygen consumption ($\dot{V}O_{2\,max}$) of 20 ml/kg/min, a level that would generally be thought acceptable for major pulmonary resection.[85] Stair-climbing is a simple test that provides a broad indication of cardiopulmonary reserve but requires standardisation before it can be used as a reliable predictive tool.[85]

Formal exercise testing is the gold standard for assessment of pulmonary function and maximal oxygen consumption ($\dot{V}O_{2\,max}$) has been advocated by several groups as the most useful assessment of cardiopulmonary reserve. In a small cohort of 22 patients undergoing pulmonary resection, the group with no cardiopulmonary complications (11 patients) had mean preoperative $\dot{V}O_{2\,max}$ values of 22.4 versus 14.9 ml/kg/min for those with complications.[86] In another study of 50 patients, the only deaths (2) and 3/7 cases of morbidity occurred in patients with $\dot{V}O_{2\,max}$ less than 10 ml/kg/min.[87] No patients with $\dot{V}O_{2\,max}$ over 20 ml/kg/min suffered complications. In a high-risk group (mean preoperative FEV_1 41% predicted), Walsh reported no mortality and a 40% complication rate in 20 patients with $\dot{V}O_{2\,max}$ above 15 ml/kg/min.[88] In another study of 80 patients, $\dot{V}O_{2\,max}$% below 60% predicted suggested a high risk of morbidity and mortality.[89] In a more recent paper, these workers again found that $\dot{V}O_{2\,max}$% was the best independent predictor of postoperative complications and that a $\dot{V}O_{2\,max}$% below 60% predicted indicated postoperative complications with 99% specificity and a positive predictive value of 86%.[90]

Formal laboratory assessment and exercise testing are expensive and labour-intensive and less expensive alternatives have been considered. The 6-minute walk test has been shown to correlate well with $\dot{V}O_{2\,max}$ values in patients with end-stage lung disease undergoing pretransplant assessment.[91] The test is used increasingly in the assessment for lung volume reduction surgery and inability to walk 200 m correlates with poor outcome in this group.[92] Exercise oximetry has also been pro-

posed as an alternative, easily performed assessment tool. A recent prospective study in 46 patients undergoing pneumonectomy suggested that resting peripheral oxygen saturation below 90% or a reduction of 4% or more during exercise was highly predictive of major morbidity and prolonged intensive-care stay after pneumonectomy.[93]

Summary of the anaesthetic perspective

The three-legged-stool approach has been advocated by Slinger as a reasonably simple, standard approach to the anaesthetic assessment of patients for thoracic surgery.[2] Of the parameters listed, ppo FEV_1% above 40%, ppo D_LCO% above 40% and $\dot{V}O_{2\,max}$ above 15 ml/kg/min are thresholds below which patients face increased risk. As Slinger emphasises in his recent review, anaesthetists are rarely required to determine the suitability of a patient as an operative candidate; rather they use the preoperative assessment to identify patients at high risk and to outline, in concert with medical and surgical colleagues, the degree of perceived risk to the patient as part of the informed consent process.[2] In the authors' experience it is now extraordinarily rare for patients to be refused surgical intervention in a thoracic surgical facility on anaesthetic grounds alone.

Other preoperative assessments of pulmonary function

Ventilation–perfusion lung scanning
Although not necessarily regarded as a first-line assessment tool, ventilation–perfusion scanning can further refine assessments of predicted postoperative pulmonary function.[82] Clearly spirometry, D_LCO values and exercise capacity take no account of differential function in lung regions. Postoperative predictions can be altered on the basis of $\dot{V}/\dot{Q}$ scan demonstration of areas of non-functioning lung and may confer operability on patients who would otherwise be considered borderline or inoperable. $\dot{V}/\dot{Q}$ scanning also provides useful information for the anaesthetist in relation to the conduct of one-lung anaesthesia and is routine in many centres for patients undergoing major pulmonary resections.

Flow–volume loops
These may identify a variable intrathoracic airway obstruction in the presence of a tumour mass that may impact on anaesthetic management. Flow–volume loops are not thought to be required routinely from the anaesthetic perspective in patients who do not describe a supine exacerbation of dyspnoea or cough.[2]

Assessment of cardiopulmonary reserve – algorithms for lung resection candidates

It is clear that no single investigation correlates with the risk of postoperative complications or outcome. Similarly, there are no threshold low values that convincingly confer lack of operability, and the whole issue of conferring inoperable status on a patient has been challenged in the light of improved outcomes in high-risk patients, developments in video-assisted techniques, lung-sparing surgery, volume-reduction surgery and even long-term ventilatory support.[94]

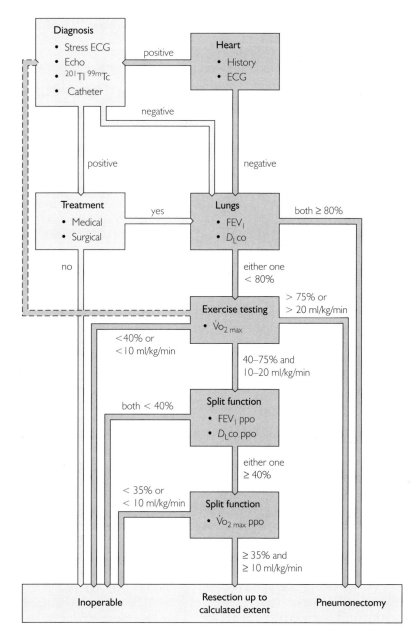

Fig. 18.4 Algorithm for preoperative assessment of functional operability for lung resection. This is the current version, modified to exclude patients with absolute $\dot{V}O_{2\,max}$ ppo values under 10 ml/kg/min, following prospective evaluation of the original version. While the algorithm is not presented as a gold standard, it does address key information of anaesthetic relevance. (Modified from Wyser et al[95] with permission.)

Wyser and colleagues have proposed an algorithm for preoperative assessment incorporating:

- cardiac history and ECG
- FEV_1, D_LCO and $\dot{V}O_{2\,max}$ and their respective ppo values based on radionuclide perfusion scanning.[95]

The algorithm is outlined in Figure 18.4. They reported prospective evaluation of this algorithm in 137 patients. Five patients were deemed functionally inoperable and 132 passed the algorithm, including 38 pneumonectomies. All were extubated within 24 hours, mean ICU stay was 1.4 days, overall complication rate was 11%, with two deaths (1.5%). They concluded that adherence to this algorithm resulted in a 50% reduction in complications, despite the percentage of inoperable patients remaining similar.

Tracheal surgery

The principles of assessment of patients for tracheal surgery are as for other forms of thoracic surgery. Patients may present with extreme degrees of obstruction in malignant disease and even benign strictures may require urgent intervention. Patients who have previously received ventilatory support are at risk of airway strictures and, although signs and symptoms may suggest adult-onset asthma, they should be presumed to have an organic airway lesion until proven otherwise.[96]

Flow–volume loops may localise the site of obstruction to the intra- or extrathoracic airway. Linear tomography is probably the investigation of choice for characterising the nature and extent of the obstruction, while computed tomography will evaluate extraluminal and mediastinal involvement.[97] In addition to general issues, anaesthetic assessment includes assessment of neck mobility, particularly the possible degree of extreme flexion and extension, and the ability to tolerate the supine position.

Oesophageal surgery

The risk of postoperative pulmonary complications following oesophageal surgery ranges from 25% to 50%.[4,98] Risk factors include the type of surgical approach, intraoperative factors such as blood loss, and patient factors such as age, history of smoking, spirometry and diffusing capacity values and performance, and nutritional status. Patients with COPD are at increased risk after oesophagectomy, as are patients in whom early extubation is not possible. The development of pulmonary complications increases the mortality risk sevenfold, and accounts for 40–60% of the operative mortality.[4]

Abdominal surgery

Abdominal surgery is a recognised risk factor for the development of postoperative respiratory complications. The incidence reported in the literature varies from 10–70%, with recent data suggesting 15–30%,[99–101] and this compares to 0–4% for peripheral surgery. Upper abdominal procedures result in diaphragm dysfunction, irrespective of the effectiveness of pain control, and the incidence of pulmonary complications in several studies has exceeded twice that of lower abdominal procedures.[28] The impact of minimally invasive procedures is still being assessed but favourable pulmonary complication rates for laparoscopic (< 1%) versus open (13–33%) cholecystectomy have been reported.[28] The presence of, or need for, a nasogastric tube is also associated with increased risk of postoperative pulmonary complications.

Despite the high incidence of complications, preoperative risk indices are considerably less developed than those for thoracic procedures and many of the studies available have been retrospective. Hall and colleagues, in a prospective study of 1000 patients undergoing abdominal surgery, reported ASA Class more than II as the most powerful indicator of risk and, when combined with age more than 59 years, these two groups accounted for 88% of patients with pulmonary complications following surgery.[101] In patients with pre-existing pulmonary disease, various parameters have been assessed as predictive of postoperative complications. In one recent study, pulmonary hyperinflation, as evidenced by an increased residual volume, preoperative FEV_1 and D_LCO were found to be highly predictive of postoperative complications.[102] Another study found FEV_1 below 61% predicted and P_aO_2 below 9.33 kPa to be the main predictors of pulmonary complications (overall incidence 18%) in 480 patients undergoing abdominal surgery.[99] Other recent studies have not shown spirometric values to be useful in predicting risk.[28,103]

Uncommon situations in perioperative respiratory care

Non-invasive ventilation

The proliferation of non-invasive ventilation (NIV) as a ventilatory support mode in a range of conditions renders it inevitable that anaesthetists will increasingly encounter patients presenting for surgical procedures who are receiving NIV. The most likely patient groups include those with slowly progressive neuromuscular disease, restrictive chest-wall disease or obstructive sleep apnoea but, as the debate about the role of NIV in COPD evolves, increasing numbers of patients with COPD may also present having been established on NIV. Important anaesthetic issues include the indication for NIV, associated cardiac pathophysiology, particularly pulmonary hypertension, and the possibility of a difficult intubation, which might be encountered.[104]

The need for NIV in a patient with relatively stable chronic pulmonary disease should not represent a contraindication to anaesthesia or surgery. The impact of the type of surgery needs to be considered: thoracic or abdominal procedures may carry increased risk and may require a period of formal postoperative ventilation in the ICU prior to return to NIV. More peripheral surgical procedures can usually be performed smoothly in such patients and they can be managed postoperatively in the recovery room or high-dependency area. The patient's home ventilator should always be available in the recovery room and staff dealing with the patient should be familiar with its use.[104] There are clear resource issues that must be satisfied and such procedures should therefore only be undertaken in centres with established NIV units that have the appropriate expertise in nursing, physiotherapy or respiratory therapy to support patients on NIV during the recovery phase.

In practice, while most anaesthetists would favour securing a more reliable airway in patients dependent on NIV, minor or very short procedures can be performed using the NIV apparatus. More usually, a more secure airway is established and the patient is transferred back to NIV early in the re-emergence phase. Clearance of oropharyngeal secretions and effective analgesia are key to the smooth transition back to NIV.

In the recent literature there has been interest in the use of NIV following solid organ transplantation. Concern about immunosuppression and the desire to avoid the increased risk of nosocomial infection associated with endotracheal intubation[105] has led to examination of the role of NIV immediately postoperatively in such patients. Antonelli and colleagues randomised 40 patients who developed respiratory insufficiency following solid organ transplants to receive either NIV or standard oxygen therapy via face mask. The use of NIV was associated with a significant reduction in the rate of endotracheal intubation (20% NIV versus 70% conventional therapy) and reduction in ICU stay (5.5 versus 9 days), although overall hospital mortality did not differ.[106] A similarly low reintubation rate (2/15) was found in another study of NIV in early postoperative respiratory failure in which the majority (11/15) of patients had undergone transplantation.[107]

Patients already ventilated in the intensive care unit

Patients requiring ventilatory support for acute severe pulmonary failure occasionally require surgical intervention during the acute phase of illness and, although minor procedures may be performed in the intensive care unit, surgical preference and logistics usually dictate that patients are transferred to the operating room for more major procedures. Trauma patients in the acute phase of acute respiratory distress syndrome (ARDS) may require fixation of fractures. In addition, a minority of patients with ARDS or pneumonia may require an exploratory laparotomy or other emergency procedure during the course of their illness.

Surgical procedures can be safely undertaken in patients requiring high levels of ventilatory support. Many intensive-care ventilators have integral power sources and the most severely affected patients should not necessarily require disconnection, resulting in alveolar derecruitment, during transfer. Similarly, nitric oxide administration, if employed, can be maintained throughout transfer and intraoperatively with current delivery systems. Lung-protective ventilation (low tidal volume, high positive end-expiratory pressure) should be maintained and this is best achieved by using an intensive-care-type ventilator and providing intravenous anaesthesia for the procedure. Particular attention should be paid to maintaining lung volume and preventing derecruitment of unstable alveoli. In practice, ventilatory support can usually be satisfactorily maintained and management problems are much more likely to relate to the presence of associated cardiovascular instability.

Patients with extreme derangement of pulmonary function

Patients with extreme pulmonary dysfunction who require constant oxygen supplementation, have minimal exercise tolerance and may be receiving intermittent or continuous ventilatory support may be proposed as surgical candidates. This is most likely to occur if lung-volume reduction surgery is thought likely to be of benefit or in lung cancer surgery combined with lung-volume reduction in a patient who might not meet standard criteria for surgery. Urgent or emergency procedures might also be indicated in such patients in whom the risk–benefit analysis suggests that surgery should proceed.

A possible approach to this difficult dilemma is to plan preoperatively for prolonged postoperative rehabilitation in the intensive care unit. Preoptimisation should be achieved as much as is possible, surgery performed and the patient transferred to the intensive care unit for full ventilatory and multiorgan support. An early tracheostomy would be appropriate, and analgesia/sedation should be continued until the patient is pain-free at the surgical site. An epidural may be employed in the early phase but is not necessarily integral to this prolonged postoperative rehabilitation approach. The patient should receive full ventilatory support during this period (incorporating but fully supporting patient-initiated breaths if present) and effective postoperative enteral nutrition should be established early. The patient is thus fully awake, cooperative, pain-free and able to interact positively with pulmonary physiotherapy before weaning from ventilation is attempted. Gradual weaning from ventilation is then instituted and can be expected to take many days or even weeks. Transfer to intermittent non-invasive ventilation should be considered in the latter phase of the weaning programme.

Although this approach is labour-intensive and requires substantial resources, the resource issues may be balanced by the resulting discharge home of a patient who would be otherwise be ventilator-bound in hospital. Recent reports of combined lung cancer and lung-volume reduction surgery in patients with severe emphysema who were poor candidates for traditional surgical approaches have suggested encouraging outcomes.[108,109] Our own experience using the above preplanned but extended postoperative support programme in a ventilator-dependent patient undergoing lung-volume reduction surgery has also been encouraging (Fig. 18.5).[110]

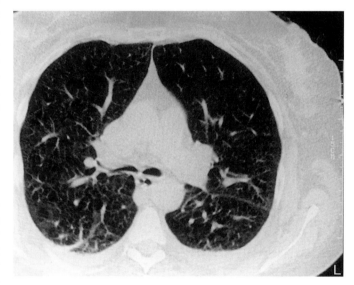

Fig. 18.5 Extreme derangement of pulmonary function. Preoperative computed tomography (CT) scan of a 48-year-old patient with severe chronic obstructive pulmonary disease in whom weaning from ventilation proved impossible at 6 weeks following acute exacerbation. Pulmonary function tests 8 months previously revealed FEV_1 0.43 litres, FEV_1/FVC 0.26 and RV 3.2 litres. Although the indication for lung volume reduction surgery was not classical, CT scan revealed a paucity of vessels anteriorly, consistent with emphysema. The patient refused transplantation and underwent lung-volume reduction surgery. Despite very unfavourable pulmonary function, weaning from ventilation as described proved successful after 14 days and the patient was discharged, independently mobile and with nocturnal non-invasive ventilation, on day 30. Weaning was not attempted until the patient was fully cooperative and pain-free.

Organisational issues and anaesthesia for respiratory disease

As with other medical specialties, the nature and provision of anaesthetic services are constantly evolving and subject to ever-increasing scrutiny, not only in terms of the quality of medical care delivered but also in terms of patient satisfaction and the economics of health-care provision. Several aspects of recent service evolution have particular relevance to patients with respiratory disease.

Preoperative anaesthesia clinics

The establishment of preoperative anaesthesia clinics, often conducted in parallel with surgical clinics, has been a feature of the 1990s in many health-care systems. This approach has many advantages, including facilitation of a well-structured, multi-disciplinary assessment and optimisation programme and identification of high-risk surgical candidates in advance, thereby allowing efficient anaesthesia and postoperative care resource allocation. A potential disadvantage is that patients are often assessed and counselled in the clinic by an anaesthetist who may not actually be involved in their perioperative care.

The provision of information and the opportunity to discuss concerns reasonably in advance of the procedure, and hence allowing time for reflection and clarification of often difficult issues, is almost universally well-received by patients in an era of increasing expectation. Patients with pulmonary disease represent a subgroup most likely to benefit from this approach, not only because of the high incidence of comorbidity encountered but also because of the potential opportunities provided. Specifically in relation to anaesthesia, these opportunities might include preoperative education in, and implementation of, physiotherapy programmes, smoking cessation, judicious weight reduction in the obese and nutritional support in cachectic patients. In a recent appraisal of the scheduling efficiency of anaesthesia clinics,[111] mean consultation times were found to be long (28 min ± ≈ 20 min) in two USA centres, inferring benefit from both assessment and patient perspectives. Patients with respiratory disease, particularly those with advanced disease, should ideally be offered this facility and should be encouraged by the referring physician to attend. Although there is limited data about the influence of such clinics on outcome, there is a potential, and commonly realised, benefit in terms of patient comprehension, satisfaction and morale.

Acute pain services

One of the current and ongoing controversies in anaesthesia concerns the optimum approach to postoperative pain control. Epidural anaesthesia has an established place in providing postoperative pain relief, particularly in the high-risk patient.[112] A current controversy, relevant to patients with pulmonary disease, concerns the appropriate application of thoracic epidural anaesthesia in thoracic surgical practice.[113,114] Simple techniques such as local infiltration, nerve blocks and postoper-

ative local anaesthetic delivery to surgical sites via indwelling catheters should also be considered.

Although the details of postoperative analgesic techniques are beyond the scope of this chapter, the delivery of effective pain relief is vital to successful postoperative care, and the prevention of pulmonary complications, in the majority of patients with respiratory disease. This need has been recognised in the last 15 years and many institutions have now established formal acute pain services. The service must be proactive rather than reactive and be capable of prompt and effective troubleshooting when problems arise. Preoperative identification of patients at particular risk of severe postoperative pain or those with limited pulmonary reserve should result in referral to the service for assessment of options and patient education.

Recovery-room facilities

The scope of recovery-room activities and the acuity of care provided has consistently increased during the last decade. Recovery rooms now commonly provide ventilatory facilities, allowing planned, but reasonably short-term ventilatory support and stabilisation in the postoperative period. The quality of care during the recovery process depends largely on the expertise and commitment of the recovery nursing team. Close liaison, or even shared organisational structure and exchange of personnel, with the intensive-care unit is advantageous, particularly in a unit with a high volume of high-risk and thoracic surgical patients. The ability to manage unexpected complications and provide a flexible, dual facility approach to postoperative care, in concert with the intensive care unit, enhances not only the safety and quality of care but also the efficiency of resource utilisation.

In addition to the standard recovery-room monitoring and resuscitation facilities, units receiving a significant volume of high-risk pulmonary disease or thoracic surgical patients should provide a range of respiratory support technology, including traditional ventilation, continuous positive airway pressure systems and facilities for, and expertise in, non-invasive ventilation. Related facilities include near-patient testing of basic blood profile and arterial blood gases, rapidly responsive mobile radiology, bronchoscopy equipment and a high-profile physiotherapy service. Invasive monitoring, including pulmonary artery catheterisation, should be routinely available, and non-invasive techniques for cardiac output measurement, such as oesophageal Doppler transducers, will be increasingly used in the future. Relative hypothermia is common, particularly after thoracic surgery, and shivering is undesirable in patients with borderline gas exchange or limited cardiopulmonary reserve. Facilities for active rewarming should therefore be available and, in very high-risk patients, rewarming should be achieved prior to attempted extubation.

References

1. Lawrence VA, Hilsenbeck SG, Mulrow CD et al. Incidence and hospital stay for cardiac and pulmonary complications after abdominal surgery. J Gen Intern Med 1995; 10: 671–678.
2. Slinger PD, Johnston MR. Preoperative assessment for pulmonary resection. J Cardiothorac Vasc Anaesth 2000; 14: 202–211.

3. Department of Health. Reference guide to consent for examination or treatment. London: Department of Health; March 2001: www.doh.gov.uk/consent.

4. Ferguson MK. Preoperative assessment of pulmonary risk. Chest 1999; 115: 58S–63S.

5. Lunn JN, Mushin WW. Mortality associated with anaesthesia. London: Nuffield Provincial Hospitals Trust; 1982.

6. Buck N, Devlin HB, Lunn JN. Report on the confidential enquiry into post-operative deaths. London: Nuffield Provincial Hospitals Trust/Kings Fund; 1987.

7. Eichorn JH. Prevention of intraoperative anaesthesia accidents and related severe injury through safety monitoring. Anesthesiology 1989; 70: 572–577.

8. National Confidential Enquiry into Perioperative Deaths. Then and now: 1990–2000. The 2000 Report of the National Confidential Enquiry into Perioperative Deaths. London: NCEPOD; 2000.

9. Dripps RD, Lamont A, Eckenhoff JE. The role of anesthesia in surgical mortality. JAMA 1961; 178: 261.

10. Wong D, Weber EC, Schell MJ et al Factors associated with postoperative pulmonary complications in patients with severe chronic obstructive pulmonary disease. Anesth Analg 1995; 80: 276–284.

11. Zibrak JD, O'Donnell CR, Marton K. Indications for pulmonary function testing. Ann Intern Med 1990; 763–771.

12. Wightman JA. A prospective survey of the incidence of postoperative pulmonary complications. Br J Surg 1968; 55: 85–91.

13. Mitchell CK, Smoger SH, Pfeifer MP et al. Multivariate analysis of factors associated with pulmonary complications following general elective surgery. Arch Surg 1998; 133: 194–198.

14. Garibaldi RA, Britt MR, Coleman ML et al. Risk factors for post-operative pneumonia. Am J Med 1981; 70: 677–680.

15. Glaspole IN, Gabbay E, Smith JA et al. Predictors of perioperative morbidity and mortality in lung volume reduction surgery. Ann Thorac Surg 2000; 69: 1711–1716.

16. Howells TH, Pettit JE. Haematological disorders. In: Vickers MD ed. Medicine for anaesthetists, 2nd ed. Oxford: Blackwell Scientific; 1982: 334–384.

17. Jonsson K, Hunt TK, Mathes SJ. Oxygen as an isolated variable influences resistance to infection. Ann Surg 1988; 208: 783–787.

18. Akrawi W, Benumof JL. A pathophysiological basis for informed preoperative smoking cessation counselling. J Cardiothorac Vasc Anesth 1997; 11: 629–640.

19. Woehlck HJ, Connolly LA, Cinquegrani MP et al. Acute smoking increases ST depression in humans during general anesthesia. Anesth Analg 1999; 89: 856–860.

20. Dales RE, Dionne G, Leech JA et al. Preoperative prediction of pulmonary complications following thoracic surgery. Chest 1993; 104: 155–159.

21. Warner MA, Offord KP, Warner ME et al. Role of preoperative cessation of smoking and other factors in postoperative pulmonary complications: a blinded prospective study of coronary artery bypass patients. Mayo Clin Proc 1989; 64: 609–616.

22. Bluman LG, Mosca L, Newman N, Simon DG. Preoperative smoking habits and postoperative pulmonary complications. Chest 1998; 113: 883–889.

23. Gritz E, Carr CR, Marcus AC. The tobacco withdrawal syndrome in unaided quitters. Br J Addiction 1991; 86: 57–69.

24. Lillington GA, Sachs DPL. Preoperative smoking reduction. All or nothing at all. Chest 1998; 113: 856–858.

25. Latimer RG, Dickman M, Day WC et al. Ventilatory patterns and pulmonary complications after upper abdominal surgery determined by preoperative and postoperative computerized spirometry and blood gas analysis. Am J Surg 1971; 122: 622–632.

26. Gould A. Effect of obesity on respiratory complications following general anesthesia. Anesth Analg 1962; 41: 448–452.

27. Shenkman Z, Shir Y, Brodsky JB. Perioperative management of the obese patient. Br J Anaesth. 1993; 70: 349–359.

28. Smetana GW. Preoperative pulmonary evaluation. N Engl J Med 1999; 340: 937–944.

29. Pelosi P, Croci M, Ravagnan I et al. Total respiratory system, lung and chest wall mechanics in sedated–paralysed postoperative morbidly obese patients. Chest 1996; 109: 144–151.

30. Buckley FP, Robinson NB, Simonowitz DA, Dellinger EP. Anaesthesia in the morbidly obese. A comparison of anaesthetic and analgesic regimens for upper abdominal surgery. Anaesthesia 1983; 38: 840–851.

31. Cooper JR, Brodsky JB. Anesthetic management of the morbidly obese patient. Semin Anesth 1987; 6: 260–270.

32. Osaki T, Shirakusa T, Kodate M et al. Surgical treatment of lung cancer in the octogenarian. Ann Thorac Surg 1994; 57: 183–193.

33. Van Mieghem W, Demedts M. Cardiopulmonary function after lobectomy or pneumonectomy for pulmonary neoplasm. Respir Med 1989; 83: 199–206.

34. Marx GF, Mateo CV, Orkin LR. Computer analysis of postanesthetic deaths. Anesthesiology 1973; 39: 54–58.

35. Djokovic JL, Hedley-Whyte J. Prediction of outcome of surgery and anesthesia in patients over 80. JAMA 1979; 242: 2301–2306.

36. Kroenke K, Lawrence VA, Theroux JF, Tuley MR. Operative risk in patients with severe obstructive pulmonary disease. Arch Intern Med 1992; 152: 967–971.

37. Oskvig K. Special problems in the elderly. Chest 1999; 115: 158S–164S.

38. Van der Walt J. Anaesthesia in children with viral respiratory tract infections. Paediatr Anaesth 1997; 7: 353–354.

39. Parnis SJ, Barker DS, van der Walt JH. Clinical predictors of anaesthetic complications in children with respiratory tract infections. Paediatr Anaesth 2001; 11: 29–40.

40. Nandwani N, Raphael JH, Langton JA. Effect of an upper respiratory tract infection on upper airway reactivity. Brit J Anaesth 1997; 78: 352–355.

41. Warner DO, Warner MA, Barnes RD et al. Perioperative respiratory complications in patients with asthma. Anesthesiology 1996; 85: 460–467.

42. Stein M, Cassara EL. Preoperative pulmonary evaluation and therapy for surgical patients. JAMA 1970; 211; 787–790.

43. Garibaldi RA, Britt MR, Coleman ML et al. Risk factors for post-operative pneumonia. Am J Med 1981; 70: 677–680.

44. ACC/AHA Task Force Report: guidelines for perioperative cardiovascular evaluation for noncardiac surgery. Circulation 1996; 93: 1278–1317.

45. Von Knorring J, Lepantalo M, Lindgren L, Lindfors O. Cardiac arrhythmias and myocardial ischaemia after thoracotomy for lung cancer. Ann Thorac Surg 1992; 53: 642–647.

46. Ghent WS, Olsen GN, Hornung CA, et al. Routinely performed multigated blood pool imaging (MUGA) as a predictor of postoperative complication of lung resection. Chest 1994; 105: 1454–1457.

47. Mangano DT. Assessment of the patient with cardiac disease. Anesthesiology 1999; 91: 1521–1526.

48. Rao V, Todd TRJ, Weisel RD et al. Results of combined pulmonary resection and cardiac operation. Ann Thor Surg 1996; 62: 342–347.

49. O'Keefe JH Jr, Shub C, Rettke SR. Risk of noncardiac surgical procedures in patients with aortic stenosis. Mayo Clin Proc 1989; 64: 400–405.

50. Roizen MF. Preoperative evaluation. In Miller RD (ed), Anesthesia, 4th ed. New York: Churchill Livingstone; 1994: 827–882.

51. Pedersen T, Eliasen K, Henriksen E. A prospective study of mortality associated with anaesthesia and surgery: risk indicators of mortality in hospital. Acta Anaesthesiol Scand 1990; 34; 176–182.

52. Golledge J, Goldstraw P. Renal impairment after thoracotomy: incidence, risk factors and significance. Ann Thorac Surg 1994; 58: 524–528.

53. Tarhan S, Moffitt EA, Sessler AD et al. Risk of anesthesia and surgery in patients with chronic bronchitis and chronic obstructive pulmonary disease. Surgery 1973; 74: 720–726.

54. The COMBIVENT Inhalation Aerosol Study Group. In chronic obstructive pulmonary disease, a combination of ipratropium and albuterol is more effective than either agent alone: an 85-day multicenter trial. Chest 1994; 105: 1411–1419.

55. Celli B. Perioperative respiratory care of the patient undergoing upper abdominal surgery. Clin Chest Med 1993; 14: 253–261.

56. Mendella LA, Manfreda J, Warren CP, Anthonisen SR. Steroid response in stable chronic obstructive pulmonary disease. Ann Intern Med 1982; 96: 17–21.

57. Niederman MS, Clemente P, Fein AM et al. Benefits of a multidisciplinary pulmonary rehabilitation program. Chest 1991; 99: 798–804.

58. Selsby D, Jones JG. Some physiological and clinical aspects of chest physiotherapy. Br J Anaesth 1990; 64: 621–631.

59. Kesten S. Pulmonary rehabilitation and surgery for end-stage lung disease. Clin Chest Med 1997; 18: 174–181.

60. Whittaker JS, Ryan CF, Buckley PA, Road JD. The effect of refeeding on peripheral and respiratory muscle function in malnourished chronic obstructive pulmonary disease patients. Am Rev Respir Dis 1990; 142: 283–288.

61. Cheney FW, Posner KL, Caplan RA. Adverse respiratory events infrequently leading to malpractice suits. A closed claims analysis. Anesthesiology 1991; 75: 932–939.

62. Gold MI, Helrich M. A study of complications related to anesthesia in asthmatic patients. Anesth Analg 1963; 42: 238–293.

63. Kabalin CS, Yarnold PR, Grammer LC. Low complication rate of corticosteroid-treated asthmatics undergoing surgical procedures. Arch Intern Med 1995; 155: 1379–1384.

64. Pizov R, Brown RH, Weiss YS et al. Wheezing during induction of anaesthesia in patients with and without asthma. Anesthesiology 1995; 82: 1111–1116.

65. Guidelines for the diagnosis and management of asthma. National Heart, Lung and Blood Institute, National Asthma Education Program, expert panel report. X. Special considerations. J Allergy Clin Immunol 1991; 88(suppl.): 523–534.

66. Pien LC, Grammer LC, Patterson R. Minimal complications in a surgical population with severe asthma receiving prophylactic corticosteroids. J Allergy Clin Immunol 1988; 82: 696–700.

67. Doershuk CF, Reyes AL, Regan AG, Matthews LW. Anesthesia and surgery in cystic fibrosis. Anesth Analg 1972; 51: 413–421.
68. Lamberty JM, Rubin BK. The management of anaesthesia for patients with cystic fibrosis. Anaesthesia 1985; 40: 448–459.
69. Weeks AM, Buckland MR. Anaesthesia for adults with cystic fibrosis. Anaesth Intens Care 1995; 23: 332–338.
70. Richardson VF, Robertson CF, Mowat AP et al. Deterioration in lung function after general anaesthesia in patients with cystic fibrosis. Acta Paediatr Scand 1984; 73: 75–79.
71. Hodson ME, Madden BP, Steven MH et al. Non-invasive mechanical ventilation for cystic fibrosis patients – a potential bridge to transplantation. Eur Respir J 1991; 4: 524–527.
72. Swami A, Evans TW, Morgan CJ et al. Conventional ventilation as a bridge to heart–lung transplantation in cystic fibrosis. Eur Respir J. 1991; 4(suppl. 14): 188s.
73. Kheradmand F, Wiener-Kronish JP, Corry DB. Assessment of operative risk for patients with advanced lung disease. Clin Chest Med 1997; 18: 483–494.
74. Lewis NL, Guest CK, Morgan CJ et al. Ventilation in cryptogenic fibrosing alveolitis – prognosis and critical care implications. Eur Respir J 1998; 12(suppl. 28): 51s.
75. Winkler M, Marker E, Hetz H. The peri-operative management of major orthopaedic procedures. Anaesthesia 1998; 53(suppl. 2): 37–41.
76. Mathieu J, Allard P, Gobeil G et al. Anesthetic and surgical complications in 219 cases of myotonic dystrophy. Neurology 1997; 49: 1646–1650.
77. Patrick JA, Meyer-Witting M, Reynolds F, Spencer GT. Peri-operative care in restrictive pulmonary disease. Anaesthesia 1990; 45: 390–395.
78. Nakahara K, Ohno K, Hashimoto J et al. Prediction of postoperative respiratory failure in patients undergoing lung resection for lung cancer. Ann Thorac Surg 1988; 46: 549–552.
79. Kearney DJ, Lee TH, Reilly JJ et al. Assessment of operative risk in patients undergoing lung resection. Chest 1994; 105: 753–759.
80. Nakahara K, Monden Y, Ohno K et al. A method for predicting postoperative lung function and its relation to postoperative complications in patients with lung cancer. Ann Thorac Surg 1985; 39; 260–265.
81. Cerfolio RJ, Allen MS, Trastek VF et al. Lung resection in patients with compromised pulmonary function. Ann Thorac Surg 1996; 62: 348–351.
82. Markos J, Mullan BP, Hillman DR et al. Preoperative assessment as a predictor of mortality and morbidity after lung resection. Am Rev Respir Dis 1989; 139: 902–910.
83. Reilly JJ, Mentzer SJ, Sugarbaker DJ. Preoperative assessment of patients undergoing pulmonary resection. Chest 1993; 103: 342S–345S.
84. Tanoue LT. Preoperative evaluation of the high-risk surgical patient for lung cancer resection. Semin Respir Crit Care Med 2000; 21: 421–432.
85. Pollock M, Roa J, Benditt J, Celli B. Estimation of ventilatory reserve by stair climbing. A study in patients with chronic airflow obstruction. Chest 1993: 104: 1378–1383.
86. Smith TP, Kinasewitz GT, Tucker WY et al. Exercise capacity as a predictor of post-thoracotomy morbidity. Am Rev Respir Dis 1984; 129: 730–734.
87. Bechard D, Wetstein L. Assessment of oxygen consumption as preoperative criterion for lung resection. Ann Thorac Surg 1987; 44: 344–349.
88. Walsh GL, Morice RC, Putnam JB Jr et al. Resection of lung cancer is justified in high risk patients selected by exercise oxygen consumption. Ann Thorac Surg 1994; 58: 704–710.
89. Bolliger CT, Jordan P, Soler M et al. Exercise capacity as a predictor of postoperative complications in lung resection candidates. Am J Respir Crit Care Med 1995; 151: 1472–1480.
90. Brutsche MH, Spiliopoulos A, Bolliger CT et al. Exercise capacity and extent of resection as predictors of surgical risk in lung cancer. Eur Respir J 2000; 15: 828–832.
91. Cahalin L, Pappagianopoulos P, Prevost S et al. The relationship of the 6-min walk test to maximal oxygen consumption in transplant candidates with end-stage lung disease. Chest 1995: 108; 452–459.
92. Szekely LA, Oelberg DA, Wright C, et al. Preoperative predictors of operative morbidity and mortality in COPD patients undergoing bilateral lung volume reduction surgery. Chest 1997; 111; 550–558.
93. Ninan M, Sommers KE, Landreneau RJ et al. Standardized exercise oximetry predicts postpneumonectomy outcome. Ann Thorac Surg 1997; 64: 328–332.
94. Olsen GN. Lung cancer resection. Who's inoperable? Chest 1995: 108: 298–299.
95. Wyser C, Stulz P, Soler M et al. Prospective evaluation of an algorithm for the functional assessment of lung resection candidates. Am J Respir Crit Care Med 1999; 159: 1450–1456.
96. Grillo HC, Donahue DM. Post intubation tracheal stenosis. Semin Thorac Cardiovasc Surg 1996; 8: 370–380.
97. Pinsonneault C, Fortier J, Donati F. Tracheal resection and reconstruction. Can J Anesth 1999; 46: 439–455.
98. Law SY, Fok M, Wong J. Risk analysis in resection of squamous cell carcinoma of the oesophagus. World J Surg 1994; 18: 339–346.
99. Fuso L, Cisternino L, Di Napoli A, et al. Role of spirometric and arterial gas data in predicting pulmonary complications after abdominal surgery. Respir Med 2000; 94: 1171–1176.
100. Brooks-Brunn JA. Validation of a predictive model for postoperative pulmonary complications. Heart Lung 1998; 27: 151–158.
101. Hall JC, Tarala RA, Hall JL, Mander J. A multivariate analysis of the risk of pulmonary complications after laparotomy. Chest 1991; 99: 923–927.
102. Barisione G, Rovida S, Gazzaniga, Fontana L. Upper abdominal surgery: does a lung function test exist to predict early severe postoperative pulmonary complications? Eur Respir J 1997; 10: 1301–1308.
103. Lawrence VA, Dhanda R, Hilsenbeck SG, Page CP. Risk of pulmonary complications after elective abdominal surgery. Chest 1996; 110: 744–750.
104. Dinner L, Goldstone JC. Non-invasive ventilation in the intensive care unit and operating theatre. Br J Hosp Med 1997; 57: 91–94.
105. Meduri GU. Noninvasive ventilation. In: Marini JJ, Slutsky AS, ed. Physiological basis of ventilatory support: a series on lung biology in health and disease. New York: Marcel Dekker; 1998: 921–998.
106. Antonelli M, Conti G, Bufi et al. Noninvasive ventilation for treatment of acute respiratory failure in patients undergoing solid organ transplantation. JAMA 2000; 283: 235–241.
107. Kilger E, Briegel J, Haller M, et al. Effects of non-invasive positive pressure ventilatory support in non-COPD patients with acute respiratory insufficiency after early extubation. Intens Care Med 1999; 25; 1374–1379.
108. De Meester SR, Patterson GA, Sundareson RS, Cooper JD. Lobectomy combined with volume reduction for patients with lung cancer and advanced emphysema. J Thorac Cardiovasc Surg 1998; 115: 681–685.
109. McKenna RJ Jr, Fischel RJ, Brenner M, Gelb AF. Combined operations for lung volume reduction and lung cancer. Chest 1996; 110: 885–888.
110. Murtuza B, Keogh BF, Simonds AK, Pepper JR. Lung volume reduction surgery in a ventilated patient with severe pulmonary emphysema. Ann Thorac Surg 2001; 71: 1037–1038.
111. Dexter F. Design of appointment systems for preanesthesia evaluation clinics to minimize patient waiting times: a review of computer simulation and patient survey studies. Anesth Analg 1999; 89: 925–931.
112. Yeager MP, Glass DD, Neff RK, Brink-Johnsen T. Epidural anesthesia and analgesia in high-risk surgical patients. Anesthesiology 1987; 729–736.
113. Slinger PD. Every postthoracotomy patient deserves thoracic epidural analgesia. J Cardiothorac Vasc Anesth 1999; 13: 350–354.
114. Grant RP. Every postthoracotomy patient does not deserve thoracic epidural analgesia. J Cardiothorac Vasc Anesth 1999; 13: 355–357.

19 Principles of inhaled therapy

Eric Derom

Key points

- Each formulation is a unique combination of a drug and a device.

- Inhaled drugs with negligible bioavailability from the gastrointestinal tract may exert systemic effects.

- Large drug particles are deposited in the oropharynx and the trachea, small drug particles in the small airways.

- The use of a nebuliser should be restricted to specific categories of patients.

- A formulation generating a monodisperse aerosol allows prescribing lower doses.

- Nebulisers and pressurised metered-dose inhalers are effective in delivering aerosolised drugs to ventilated patients.

- Systemic effects may develop with inhaled drugs that have a prolonged plasma elimination half-life.

- Extrapulmonary deposition may contribute to the development of systemic effects for inhaled corticosteroids with high gastrointestinal bioavailability.

- Many patients are unable to use pressurised metered-dose inhalers correctly.

- Spacer–pressurised metered-dose inhaler combinations should be considered as individual entities.

- Pressurised metered-dose inhalers should be used at an inhalation flow as low as possible, and dry-powder inhalers at a high inhalation flow

- The clinical significance of preference and acceptance studies is difficult to assess.

- The L/T ratio is only useful in comparing different formulations of the same drug.

The primary aim of a treatment with inhaled drugs is to reach symptomatic and functional improvement by delivering the drug in the form of respirable particles to the airways. The categories of device currently used to generate aerosolised drugs in medicine are pressurised metered-dose inhalers (pMDIs), dry-powder inhalers (DPIs) and nebulisers. Each formulation is a unique combination of a drug and a device. That combination, rather than the drug itself, causes one portion of the emitted dose to be deposited in the airways, another portion to impact on the tongue or back of the pharynx, while small portions of drug are retained in the inhaler or exhaled.

Pulmonary deposition of a drug delivered from a given formulation is generally expressed as a fraction of a reference dose, which is generally the metered dose (Table 19.1). The nominal dose can be based on either the metered or the delivered dose. For example, budesonide delivered via a pMDI attached to a spacer device has a lung deposition of 34% with reference to the normal metered dose but of 76% with reference to the dose delivered from the spacer, as a substantial part of the drug delivered by the pMDI is retained in the spacer.[1] In this chapter, nominal dose will be used as the dose reference, unless otherwise mentioned.

The amount of drug deposited in the airways is responsible for the clinical effects. The portion that is deposited on the pharynx will be swallowed down (unless the patient rinses his/her mouth) and may contribute to local side effects. Systemic bioavailability is the rate and extent of a drug's appearance in the systemic circulation where it exerts its biological effects. Drug that is absorbed via the lung membrane or gut and escapes first-pass metabolism in the gut wall and liver becomes systemically available. Thus, systemic bioavailability after inhalation has two components: drug absorbed via the gastroin-

Table 19.1 Dose definitions

Expression	Definition
Nominal dose	Dose written on the package label; also called labelled dose
Metered dose	Amount of drug leaving or contained in the metering unit
Delivered dose	Amount of drug leaving the device
Fine particle dose	Amount of drug contained in particles less than 0.5 μm
Retained amount	Amount of drug retained in the device
Inhaled dose	Amount of drug entering the subject through inhalation
Exhaled amount	Amount exhaled
Recovered amount	Amount recovered from, for example, wiping the face and the hands with a tissue
Dose to subject	Inhaled dose minus the amount of drug leaving the subject through exhalation and mouth rinsing
Lung dose	Amount of drug deposited in the lungs

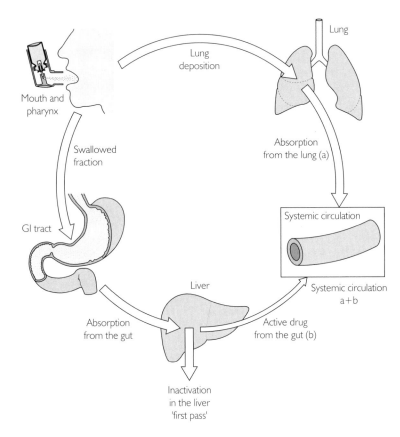

Fig. 19.1 The fate of an inhaled drug. The amount of drug reaching the systemic circulation is the sum of the pulmonarily (a) and orally (b) available fractions. The fraction deposited in the airways is almost completely absorbed. Systemic absorption of the fraction deposited in the oropharynx will depend on the degree of absorption from the gastrointestinal tract and of first-pass metabolism.

testinal *and* the pulmonary route. Systemic side effects are related to the total systemic bioavailability (Fig. 19.1).

Health-care providers involved in aerosol therapy should be informed about the differences between the available inhalers and the pharmacokinetic and pharmacodynamic properties of the drugs they contain, in order to make appropriate comparisons and intelligent choices for their patients. Moreover, they should inform their patients about the aims of the treatment, potential side effects, handling of the device and in which circumstances the drugs should be inhaled.

Basic principles of aerosol behaviour in the lungs

Physical and chemical properties

An aerosol is a two-phase system consisting of a gaseous continuous phase (usually air) and a discontinuous phase made up of fine, individual particles, with a range of sizes between 0.01 μm and 100 μm. A mist is an aerosol of liquid particles, whereas dust (caused by dispersion) and smoke (caused by condensation) are aerosols of solid particles. Liquid particles are spherically shaped because of surface tension. Some solid particles are also spherical; others will crystallise to form a regular solid.

A therapeutic aerosol consists of particles whose sizes are expressed by their aerodynamic diameter. The aerodynamic diameter attributed to a particle is the diameter of a spherical particle of unit density that has the same settling velocity in air as the particle in question. Thus, a very dense particle of drug will have a different aerodynamic behaviour to an equivalently sized but less dense particle.

Most therapeutic aerosols and the particles it contains exhibit an approximately log normal distribution, which can be described by giving the mass median aerodynamic diameter (MMAD) and the geometric standard deviation (GSD). Lung deposition characteristics and efficacy depend largely on particle or droplet size. The MMAD is the diameter around which the mass of particles of a given aerosol is equally distributed. A MMAD of $5 \mu m$ means that 50% of total aerosol mass is to be found in droplets or particles with aerodynamic diameters above 5 μm and 50% below. Particle mass distribution is more meaningful than particle size distribution, since the therapeutic effects of aerosols depend on the mass of drug that these particles represent and not on the number of particles that will eventually reach the airways. In terms of mass, one single particle of $10 \mu m$ diameter equals as many as 1000 drug particles of $1 \mu m$ diameter.

Aerosols used for medical purposes are invariably poly- (or hetero-) disperse and the geometric standard deviation gives an indication of the scatter of particle size. A histogram in which nearly all particles fall into one range is said to be monodisperse (GSD < 1.22), whereas heterodisperse aerosols (GSD > 1.22) are made of particles of different sizes.

Deposition of aerosols within the respiratory tract

Deposition is the process that determines what fraction of inspired particles will eventually be caught in the respiratory tract. All particles that touch a surface are likely to be deposited, the site of deposition being the site of initial contact. Aerosol therapy is in essence a problem of aerosol deposition, since drugs must be targeted to their receptor sites, wherever they may be, in order to be effective. It is thought that drugs with site-specific actions on mucous glands or smooth muscle should be deposited in proximal airways, drugs affecting airway inflammation should be deposited throughout the tracheo-bronchial tree, and drugs affecting alveolar function should be deposited in the alveoli.

Inertial impaction is the principal mechanism of deposition in the large airways for particles greater than a few millimetres in diameter, and may be of importance for any particle larger than $1 \mu m$. Large particles or particles travelling at high velocities in more proximal airways may be unable to follow the airstream when it changes direction in the throat or at bifurcations between successive generations of airways. Indeed, when the airstream passes round a corner of angle θ, the probability of impaction is proportional to $u \cdot d^2 \cdot \sin\theta/r$, where u is airstream

velocity, d particle aerodynamic diameter and r airway radius. Inertial impaction tends to occur in central airways (trachea and larger bronchi) and in partially obstructed airways, where the total cross-sectional area is small, the air flow high and turbulence may develop.

Gravity causes all particles with a density (δ_{part}) greater than that of air (δ_{air}) to experience a downward force. The magnitude of this gravitational force (F_{grav}) equals $V_{part} \times (\delta_{part} - \delta_{air}) \times g$, where V_{part} is the volume of the particle and g is gravitational acceleration. Gravitational sedimentation is time-dependent and occurs at low airflow. Small particles are more likely to settle down in more distal airways by gravity, as the increase in overall cross-sectional area of the airways ensures a low flow of air. Slow inhalation and breath-holding are believed to promote sedimentation and deposition for the same reason.[2,3]

Brownian motion is the continuous and irregular movement of particles of less than $0.5 \mu m$ diameter caused by impaction of surrounding molecules. It plays little part in deposition of therapeutically used aerosols, since their MMADs are generally much larger than $0.5 \mu m$. Electrical forces, thermophoresis and simple contact with airway walls are less important mechanisms of deposition.

Larger particles (MMAD > $10 \mu m$) or particles inhaled at high flow have a greater chance to be deposited in the oropharynx and the central airways (Fig. 19.2). Particles ranging between 5 and $10 \mu m$ are deposited in the larger intrapulmonary airways, from the trachea down to the larger bronchi. Particles with an aerodynamic diameter of less than $5 \mu m$ are deposited more frequently in the lower airways and are therefore considered to be in the respirable range.[4] Very fine particles (MMAD < $0.5 \mu m$) are too small to settle down and will leave the lung during expiration.[4] As deposition within the tracheobronchial tree is highly dependent on particle size, drug targeting may be improved by using monodisperse aerosols, which may allow the use of lower drug doses.[5]

Other factors, however, such as inhalation technique, airway diameter and alteration in particle size (evaporation, hygroscopic growth and particle agglomeration), also affect airway

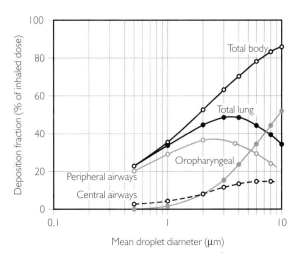

Fig. 19.2 Deposition profiles predicted from an empirical model for an inhaled aerosol cloud produced by nebulisation with a geometric standard deviation of 2.2. Redrawn from Rudolph et al.[4]

deposition. For example, a more proximal deposition has been reported in patients with airways obstruction[4,6] compared to healthy subjects.

Lung residence time

The functional effect of an inhaled drug results from its interaction with cellular receptors. Slow absorption from the lung prolongs exposure to airway receptors and may enhance the functional effect. For example, β_2-agonists have been characterised as:

- those that directly activate the receptor and appear rapidly in the systemic circulation (salbutamol)
- those that directly activate the receptor and are taken up into a membrane depot (formoterol)
- those that are taken up in a membrane depot before interacting with the receptor (salmeterol).

These differences in residence time are reflected in the kinetics of airway smooth muscle relaxation in vitro[7] and in the time course of the bronchodilatation in asthmatic patients.[8] For salmeterol, the enhanced retention in lung tissue appears to be at the expense of the onset of action in patients with asthma, which is slower than salbutamol[9] and formoterol.[8,10]

Retention in lung tissue of inhaled glucocorticosteroids has not been studied extensively. Slow absorption from the lung and prolonged exposure of inhaled corticosteroids to the airways may enhance the anti-inflammatory effect without a concomitant increase in systemic glucocorticosteroid activity. The prolonged pharmacodynamic response of budesonide[11,12] has been attributed to its association with intracellular formation of long-chain fatty acid esters.[13] Preliminary data indicate that liposome encapsulation of drugs also offers prolonged retention and drug action in the lower airways.[14,15]

Pulmonary clearance

Particles deposited between the larynx and the terminal bronchioles may be cleared via two different mechanisms. Insoluble substances or large particles deposited on the mucociliary escalator are cleared within less than 24 h. Mucociliary transport may, however, be somewhat slower in patients with pulmonary disease.[16] Pulmonary absorption is the primary, most effective mechanism by which inhaled drugs are cleared[17,18] Maximum serum concentrations of inhaled drug generally occur within the hour of inhalation, even when gastrointestinal absorption is blocked. Soluble particles deposited in the alveoli are eliminated by alveolar absorption, which is even more rapid than bronchial absorption.[19] Insoluble particles deposited in the alveoli are cleared via alveolar macrophages, the interstitial space, and lymphatics. Any particle remaining in the lungs after 24 h is deemed to be alveolar in site, with a half-life which may range between weeks and months.

Systemic elimination

Drug that is absorbed via the lung membrane or gut and escapes the first-pass metabolism becomes systemically available. Once in the systemic circulation, this drug behaves like an intravenous dose and is eliminated by hepatic and renal clearance. Clearance and volume of distribution determine elimination half-life. Systemic accumulation of an inhaled substance will occur if the dosing interval is shorter than the time required for its elimination.[20] Accumulation of inhaled bronchodilators does not occur, as they are cleared rapidly. Differences between corticosteroids have, however, been reported. For example, the elimination half time of fluticasone exceeds 7 h[20,21] whereas that of triamcinolone, flunisolide and budesonide is less than 3 h.[20,22] Suppression of cortisol secretion in patients treated with inhaled fluticasone and budesonide in both healthy volunteers and in asthmatic patients has been attributed to this difference in half-life.[23,24]

Aerosol generation and inhalation devices

To reach the airways, the drug must be aerosolised and subsequently inhaled. The process of aerosolisation can be divided into two fundamental types:

- condensation from the vapour or gaseous phase
- communitation (= break-up) from the macroscopic solid or liquid phase.

Condensation is not used to generate medicinal aerosols.

The inhalation process consists of three steps:

1. dose delivery from the inhaler
2. pulmonary deposition of part of the delivered dose
3. functional response to the deposited dose.

The third step, the functional response, is dependent on different factors, such as potency of the drug, potential for inhaler-induced bronchoconstriction and site of aerosol deposition within the tracheobronchial tree. The first two steps include factors such as preparation, priming and handling of the inhaler, inhalation technique and physiological variables, such as airway narrowing, airway closure and mucous plugging. As aerosol system design has a considerable impact on aerosol generation and inhalation process, formulation-dependent effects on dose delivery, pulmonary deposition and functional response may be expected.

Nebulisers

Aerosol generation and jet nebulisers

The most prevalent method of liquid aerosol formation is the shearing of liquid by relative motion of liquid and gas. This can be accomplished by either causing liquid to flow at a high velocity into relatively calm air (hydraulic atomisation) or by causing gas to flow at high velocity with respect to liquid (pneumatic atomisation). The latter technique is used in medicine, as only pneumatic atomisation allows the generation of aerosols containing small enough particles.

The driving gas, usually compressed air, passes through a very narrow hole from a high-pressure system over a liquid feed tube (Fig. 19.3). Because of the fall in pressure and the increase in gas velocity, the Bernoulli effect draws liquid to the surface. The liquid is propelled forward as a thin sheet, then breaks up into droplets by shear-induced instability. This typically produces droplets ranging between 15 and 500 μm. Most large particles are removed by impacting on a baffle in front of the jet. Smaller droplets may leave the nebuliser, unless they land on the internal walls of the nebuliser for renebulisation. Constant-output nebulisers produce aerosols at a constant rate, but are highly inefficient, because the aerosol is diluted during inspiration by air entrainment via the T-piece. In addition, more than 50% of the delivered aerosol is wasted during exhalation, as the nebuliser nebulises during both inspiration and expiration.[25]

New types of nebuliser were designed some years ago to reduce these inefficiencies.[26] First, the open vent nebuliser, in which an extra vent is incorporated, causes more small particles to be inspired in a given time. Second, the breath-enhanced nebuliser contains a valve on top of the device (Fig. 19.4), which allows extra air to be drawn through the nebuliser during inspiration. This increases aerosol production during inspiration and decreases it during expiration, such that up to 70% of the generated aerosol is delivered to the patient and nebulisation time may be reduced. Third, the dosimetric nebuliser releases electronically controlled doses of aerosols only during inspiration

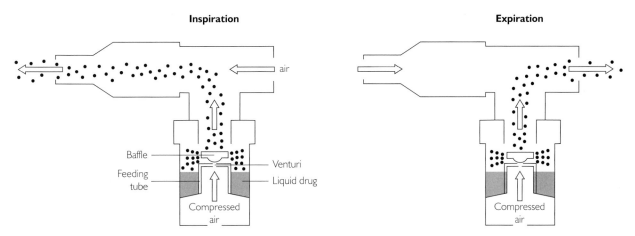

Fig. 19.3 Conventional nebuliser design. Air from the compressor passes through a small hole, called Venturi. Larger particles impact on baffles and on the walls of the chamber, and are returned for nebulisation. Small particles leave the nebuliser continuously. The aerosol generated during expiration is wasted.

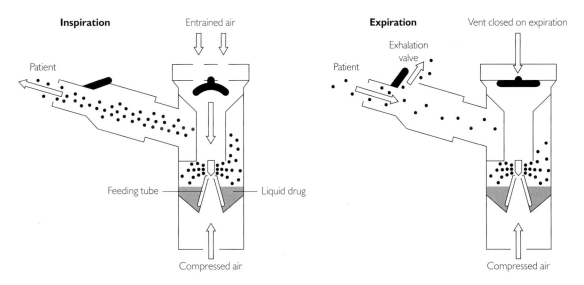

Fig. 19.4 A breath-assisted, open vent nebuliser. On inspiration, the valve on top of the chamber opens, pulling more aerosol from the nebuliser and increasing the dose to the patient. On expiration, the vent closes and aerosol exits via a one-way valve near the mouthpiece.

(Fig. 19.5) or a portion thereof, and may theoretically improve delivery up to 100% of the generated aerosol.

Aerosol generation and ultrasonic nebulisers

In the ultrasonic nebuliser, ultrasonic waves from an oscillating piezoelectric crystal are focused on the surface of the drug solution to form unstable microwaves, which break up to produce airborne droplets. As some of the energy from the crystal is converted into heat, the aerosol is warmer and the concentrating effect less than for the jet nebuliser. The process of nebulisation in ultrasonic nebulisers does not require airflow. Mean particle size is inversely proportional to the frequency of the ultrasonic vibrations of the crystal. As with jet nebulisers, baffles within the nebulisers remove larger droplets and much of the aerosol produced impacts on these, falling back into the drug reservoir.

Jet nebulisers are by far the most common type of nebuliser used worldwide. Ultrasonic nebulisers do not appear to nebulise drug suspensions as efficiently as jet nebulisers,[27] and should be avoided for this task until technical progress has allowed newer models to be developed. Some patients prefer ultrasonic nebulisers for routine bronchodilator treatment because they are smaller and quieter.

Nebuliser performance and pulmonary deposition

Drug output is obviously determined by the volume of drug solution initially put in the nebuliser (fill volume), the residual volume (the volume of solution left in a nebuliser once nebulisation has ceased) and the rate of nebulisation, which is determined by nebuliser design. Nebulisers with a low residual volume are preferable in order to reduce the amount of wasted drug. Increasing driving gas flow through jet nebulisers will increase drug output, reduce particle size and decrease nebuli-

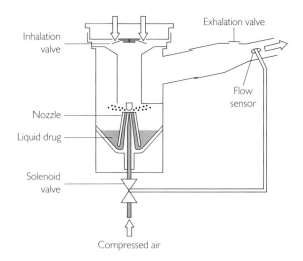

Fig. 19.5 A dosimetric nebuliser releases electronically controlled doses of aerosol only during inspiration. The solenoid valve is opened by generation of an inspiratory flow. During expiration, no compressed air is allowed to enter the nebuliser chamber, and no aerosol is produced.

sation time. Highly viscous solutions nebulise slowly and require powerful compressors. Other factors affecting drug output are the gradual evaporation of solvent during nebulisation (responsible for a gradual increase in the concentration of the drug in the solution) and solution temperature. Factors such as environmental conditions, nebuliser ageing and static charge are not thought to be of clinical relevance.[25] Nebuliser design has also a significant impact on the properties of the aerosol produced and hence on pulmonary deposition.[28,29] Differences in drug delivery exist, even between nebulisers of the same class, and not all nebulisers produce enough aerosol particles of adequate size. According to a recent survey, manufacturers' information on particle size was unavailable for more than 30% of the jet nebulisers, while virtually no information on ultrasonic nebulisers has been published recently.[30] Current recommendations for jet nebulisers are a fill volume of 2.0–2.5 ml and a residual volume of less than 1.0 ml. Moreover, 50% of the particles should have a MMAD under 5 μm and at least 50% of the solution should be nebulised within 5 min. Nebuliser chamber and compressor should be matched. Ultrasonic nebulisers are less recommendable because of their less efficient nebulisation of drug suspensions and the potential for breakdown of complex molecules.[25]

Lung deposition from nebulisers is generally below 10% of the fill dose and devices delivering more than 15% of the fill dose to the lungs are relatively rare.[29] Recently introduced nebulisers that use vents to augment aerosol delivery produce slightly higher deposition rates, even when used with relatively weak compressors and flow rates.

Inhalation technique and pulmonary deposition

It is generally recommended that aerosols generated by nebulisers should be inhaled during quiet breathing. Fast inspiration promotes inertial impaction in the upper airways and proximal deposition, whereas slow controlled inhalation promotes pulmonary deposition and reduces upper airway deposition.[31] Nose breathing reduces lung deposition of aerosols approximately by half. Nevertheless, the use of a mask has been shown to be an effective method of drug delivery to children who are too young to use a mouthpiece. However, if the mask is not well-sealed to the face, some of the drug may land on the face or in the eyes. It remains uncertain whether systematic use of a mouthpiece enhances pulmonary deposition of nebulised drugs in patients capable of using a facemask correctly.

Advantages and disadvantages

The main advantage of a nebuliser (Table 19.2) is that the aerosol can be inhaled during tidal breathing. Nebulisers are, however, expensive, time-consuming, bulky and inefficient. Moreover, they should be cleaned after use, as inappropriate maintenance leads to bacterial contamination of the wet parts.[32] Nebulisers should therefore be primarily reserved for:

- patients unable or too ill to use hand-held devices, which are more difficult to handle
- when medications are not formulated in hand-held devices (e.g. rhDNase, surfactant, antimicrobial drugs, gene therapy)
- when large doses are needed.

Table 19.2 Inhalation devices: advantages and disadvantages

	Nebuliser	**pMDI**	**pMDI + spacer**	**DPI**
Time consumption	Extensive	Minimal	Minimal	Minimal
Portability	Bulky	Portable	Bulky	Portable
Power supply	Yes	No	No	No
Cost	Much more expensive than pMDI	Cheap	Somewhat more expensive than pMDI alone	More expensive than pMDI
Maintenance	Complex	Unnecessary	Somewhat complex	Unnecessary
Preparation	Complex	Simple	Moderately simple	Simple
Handling/loading	Easy	Complex	Less complex than pMDI	Easy
Inhalation	Tidal breathing	Slow inhalation after actuation	Co-ordination less critical than pMDI	Forceful inhalation
Dose delivered	Variable time dependent	Reproducible	Time-dependent	Effort-dependent
Environmentally friendly	Yes	If CFC-free	If CFC-free	Yes
Pulmonary deposition	Low	Medium	High	Medium to high
Oropharyngeal deposition	Low	High	Low	Moderate to high

Attention should be paid to the combination of nebuliser and compressor. Medium- to high-power compressors and high-output nebulisers are needed to nebulise highly viscous solutions of glucocorticosteroids, pentamidine, deoxyribonuclease (rhDNase), tobramycin, colistin and gentamicin.[30]

Portable nebulisers

A novel multidose, hand-held nebuliser, Respimat®, delivers metered doses of aerosolised drug solution. The mechanical power of a spring, rather than volatile gas propellants, is used to generate the aerosol. The active substance is gently released over more than 1 s as a soft mist, which is eventually inhaled by the patient.[33] Preliminary comparisons between Respimat® and pMDI indicated that lung deposition was higher with Respimat® (39% versus 11–15%) and oropharyngeal deposition lower (37–39% versus 72%).[34,35]

Pressurised metered-dose inhalers

Aerosol generation

Introduced in 1956, pMDIs remain the most widely used aerosol systems for inhaled drugs. A pMDI consists of a sealed canister at pressures up to 400 kPa containing one or two drugs that are either dissolved or suspended as a fine powder in a propellant (Fig. 19.6). To that propellant, a low dose of surfactant has been added as a lubricant to improve the physical stability of the drug suspension and to prevent aggregation of particles. Chlorofluorocarbons (CFCs or freons) have been used as propellants for years. Replacement of CFC propellants by more environmentally friendly hydrofluoroalkane (HFA) propellants

is scheduled for the coming years, in accordance with the Montreal Agreement.

At actuation (Fig. 19.6), a metered volume of the content (between 25 and 100 μl, depending on the design of the canister) is released through the valve stem, and the liquid phase is broken up into a stream of rapidly moving droplets. Nozzle design and pressure inside the canister determine particle size, particle speed and plume geometry.

Most pMDIs deliver aerosol particles at a high velocity (30–100 m/s) with an initial MMAD of about 30 μm. The velocity of the aerosol particles decreases within a few centimetres of the actuator orifice and the MMAD falls because of rapid evaporation of propellant and deposition by impaction of larger droplets. The final MMAD of aerosols released by the currently used pMDIs has been estimated to range between 2.8 and 5.5 μm, although larger diameters have been reported. Particle velocities and sizes generated by the newly developed HFA pMDIs are slower and smaller.[36]

Inhalation technique and pulmonary deposition

Using an optimal inhalation technique (Table 19.3), pulmonary deposition of drugs administered via most pMDIs ranges between 8% and 12%.[37] A recently developed pMDI, containing an HFA solution formulation of beclometasone dipropionate, exhibits a pulmonary deposition of about 50% of the nominal dose[38] but this feature has not been observed with the HFA suspension formulation of salbutamol or fenoterol.[39,40] Omission of priming and shaking reduces the total and fine-particle dose delivered by a CFC-containing pMDI by 25% and 36% respectively[41] but does not affect the function of HFA solution formulations. As actuations separated by less than 1 s decrease

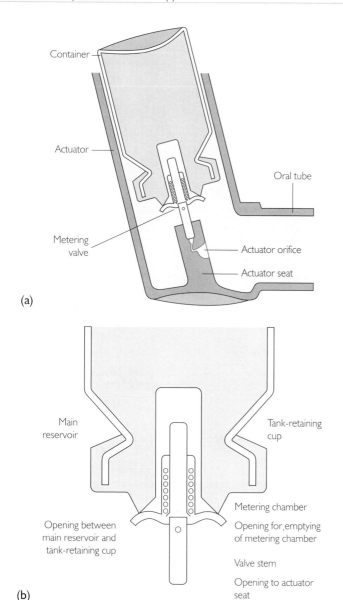

Fig. 19.6 A schematic section through a typical pressurised metered dose inhaler (a) and its metering valve (b). The container contains a mixture of drugs, surfactants and propellants. The metering chamber contains the next dose. In the resting state, it communicates with the contents of the larger tank-retaining cup. Compressing the valve stem activates the valve and closes the communication between the metering chamber and the tank-retaining cup, causing the metering chamber to empty through the opening in the valve stem.

Table 19.3 Correct use of a pressurised metered-dose inhaler

1. Remove the protective cap
2. Shake the canister thoroughly
3. Place the mouthpiece between the lips
4. Breathe out quietly
5. Fire the inhaler while taking a slow, deep inhalation
6. Hold the breath at full inspiration while counting up to 10
7. Restart the procedure from point 2 if a second inhalation is required

fine-particle dose by 16%, it is currently recommended that actuations are separated by at least 3 s to allow the valve to refill. The use of a longer breath-holding time (10 s versus 4 s), a low inhalation flow (30 l/min versus 80 l/min), and actuating at the beginning of inspiration improves pulmonary deposition markedly.[2,3]

Coordination between actuation and inhalation is required, since the aerosol cloud leaves the canister immediately after actuation. Breath-actuated pMDIs offer the advantage that the dose is released upon actuation. The use of breath-actuated pMDIs increases pulmonary deposition in 'bad coordinators', but not in 'good co-ordinators'.

Advantages and disadvantages

Portability, low cost and reproducibility of dose released are obvious advantages of pMDIs. The complexity of handling of pMDIs is the main disadvantage (Table 19.2). Although many patients are unable to use pMDIs without mistakes, an education programme may lead to a correct inhalation technique in 80% of patients.[42] High oropharyngeal deposition of inhaled corticosteroids may give rise to local side effects. The 'cold freon effect', which may stop or halt inhalation, can be circumvented by prescribing a nebuliser or DPI containing the same drug. Adverse reactions, such as bronchoconstriction, are rare.[43]

Spacers

For a number of patients using a pMDI, coordination of actuation and inhalation is difficult to achieve. Large and small spacers, holding chambers, tube extensions and other add-on devices have been developed in an attempt to overcome this problem. In daily practice, the term 'spacer' is used to denote these different inhalation aids.

Fate of an aerosol in a spacer

At actuation, the aerosol particles released by a pMDI enter the spacer, where they decelerate and decrease in size, because of the evaporation of the propellant enveloping the particles. Some of the aerosol will stick to the wall of the spacer between actuation and the start of the patient's inhalation. The dose available for inhalation equals the dose delivered by the pMDI minus the dose lost in the spacer.[44]

Three different mechanisms contribute to aerosol loss in a spacer. *Impaction*, which depends on the relationship between the volume of the spacer and the speed of the jet, accounts for the instantaneous removal of the largest droplets. A greater amount of drug will remain airborne in longer and larger spacers,[45] or if the pMDI releases the aerosol jet at a lower speed. For example, the HFA pMDI formulation of salbutamol delivers a higher output from a spacer than the original CFC formulation, despite the fact that the HFA formulation releases less drug as fine particles.[36] Spacer length is also critical for both the fine-particle dose and the ratio of fine to coarse particles.[46]

Sedimentation shortens the time available for inhalation after actuation and causes drug delivery from a spacer to be time-dependent. Sedimentation is responsible for the more pronounced loss of aerosol in small-volume tubes.[46]

Electrostatic attraction also reduces aerosol half-life by attraction of aerosol particles on to plastic surfaces. New plastic spacers with a high electrostatic charge delivered in vitro 23% less salbutamol particles of less than 6.8 μm than used ones, whereas washing them with an anionic or cationic detergent increased small-particle dose from 55% to 70% compared to delivery from new spacers.[47] Electrostatic charges may be circumvented by using a metal spacer[44] or antistatic paint,[48] by immersion in household ionic detergents without rinsing or drying with a cloth,[49] by rinsing with benzalkonium chloride[50] or priming by firing the actuator several times in the spacer.[50] Abolishing static charge increased aerosol half-life from 10 s to 30 s for a given spacer[44,47,50] and improved the amount of salbutamol deposited in the lung.[48,51] It thus appears that every spacer–pMDI combination should be considered as an individual entity.[52]

Inhalation technique and pulmonary deposition

Spacers improve drug targeting to the lungs and reduce oropharyngeal deposition. Indeed, with a pMDI attached to a large-volume spacer, the aerosol is presented as a standing cloud of particles, which contains a smaller amount of larger particles and has no inherent flow. This explains why oropharyngeal deposition ranges from 30% to 80% without and 10% to 20% with a spacer,[1,53] and why lung deposition with a pMDI connected to intermediate- and large-volume spacers ranges between 20% and 38%, which is more than that of a pMDI alone.[1,53,54] Doses should be given separately.[55] A slow inspiratory flow should be used, since impaction of particles is proportional to flow rate. The spacer should be emptied in one or two inhalations for adults and older children, five breaths in toddlers and 10 breaths in infants.[46] In young children up to 4 years of age, it is generally recommended to connect a facemask to the spacer.

Advantages and disadvantages

The use of a spacer improves the predictability of drug delivery from a pMDI in patients with potential coordination difficulty. Spacers are the devices of choice in children until they are sufficiently mature to use a DPI or a breath-actuated pMDI. Spacers are as effective as nebulisers in patients with an acute asthma attack.[56] Spacers reduce oropharyngeal deposition of inhaled drugs, decrease the likelihood of developing local side effects[57] and improve the therapeutic index and safety of the treatment with drugs with high oral bioavailability.[58] Improving drug targeting to the lungs may also lead to reductions in prescribed dose and in cost of treatment.

Dry powder inhalers

Aerosol generation

All DPIs contain relatively large 'secondary' particles, which are deaggregated into small 'primary' particles during inhalation. The drug is contained within the 'primary' particles. The 'secondary' particles are manufactured by aggregation of primary particles or by partially covering a carrier (e.g. lactose) with drug particles, because small primary particles are very difficult to

handle during pharmaceutical production. The final formulation is generated when the patient inhales through the inhaler. DPIs do not contain freons and surfactants.

Dry powder inhalers are breath-actuated. Single-dose inhalers such as the Spinhaler®, Rotahaler® or Cyclohaler® require the introduction of a capsule in the inhaler. The capsule needs to be pierced or opened before inhalation. Multidose capsule or blister DPIs, such as the Diskhaler®, the Diskus® and the Spiros® contain a number of doses, which are metered during the production process and made available for inhalation by piercing or opening the capsule or the blister. For multidose powder reservoir DPIs such as the Turbuhaler®, Pulvinal® and Easyhaler®, the patient has to meter the dose just before the inhalation.

Inhalation technique and pulmonary deposition

The inhalation effort critically determines the intrinsic properties of the aerosol[59] and has to be sufficiently high to produce an aerosol containing a sufficient amount of fine particles.[59,60] The intrinsic resistance of the inhaler and the negative pressure generated by the patient[59] determines the inhalation flow.

With an optimal inhalation technique, lung deposition ranged between 6.2% and 9.2% after inhaling via a Rotahaler®,[37] and averaged 11.6% for salbutamol Diskhaler®.[37] Although mean peripheral deposition with Diskhaler® was lower in patients with airway narrowing than in healthy subjects, total pulmonary deposition was similar in both groups. Studies with Turbuhaler® containing budesonide, terbutaline and formoterol yielded depositions ranging between 16.8% in a first and between 20 and 32% in later studies.[18,37,60,61] Lung deposition of 32% has been reported with still another multidose DPI.[62]

For Rotahaler®, the use of a low and high inhalation flow resulted in a pulmonary deposition of 3.6% and 7.0% respectively.[63] For Turbuhaler®, lung deposition was similarly reduced by half at low inhalation flow,[60] whereas for another inhaler, deposition decreased by 30% if inhalation flow fell from 99 l/min to 54 l/min.[62]

Advantages and disadvantages

Dry powder inhalers are breath-actuated, are easier to handle than nebulisers or pMDIs and exhibit pulmonary depositions that at least equal and sometimes exceed pMDIs and nebulisers, which are three considerable advantages (Table 19.2). DPIs are, however, more expensive. Some formulations are moisture-sensitive.[64,65] Inhalation-flow-related delivery and deposition of the drug is another disadvantage. Indeed, children below 5 years of age and disabled patients may be unable to use some devices, in particular these with a high intrinsic resistance, as their respiratory muscles are unable to generate sufficient negative pressure.

Aerosol therapy in ventilated patients

In mechanically ventilated patients, drug delivery by inhalation is a common route of administration of bronchodilators, antibiotics and surfactant, and is particularly useful as an alternate route for drug administration. In these patients, however, efficiency of aerosol delivery to the lower respiratory tract is altered by a number of factors that are not a concern in ambulatory patients. In particular, deposition of aerosol in the endotracheal tube and ventilator circuits causes a significant reduction in the fraction of aerosol reaching the lower respiratory tract. Moreover, the characteristics of the ventilator-delivered breath are quite different from a spontaneous breath. Nevertheless, nebulisers and pMDIs are considered to be effective in delivering aerosols when careful attention is given to the technique of administration, and both devices can be adapted for use in ventilator circuits.

Deposition of nebulised aerosols ranges between 1% and 15%.[66,67] This variation has been attributed to differences in the radiolabel used, types of nebuliser, treatment time and humidity in the circuit. In vivo data indicate that approximately 6% of the dose from a pMDI is deposited in the lungs.[66]

In vitro studies have allowed a number of factors to be elucidated that may affect pulmonary deposition of aerosols in mechanically ventilated patients. Nebulisers producing aerosol with MMADs between $1\,\mu m$ and $3\,\mu m$ are likely to achieve greater deposition, as larger particles impact on the ventilator circuit and the endotracheal tube.[68] Heat and humidification reduce aerosol deposition,[68,69] whereas placing a nebuliser at a distance of 30 cm from the endotracheal tube is more efficient than placing it between the patient Y and the endotracheal tube.[68] For pMDIs, it appears that a combination with a chamber device results in a four- to sixfold greater delivery of aerosol than pMDI actuation into a connector attached directly to the endotracheal tube.[66,69,70] In-vitro studies further indicate that synchronisation of aerosol generation with inspiratory airflow, a tidal volume greater than 500 ml and a longer duty cycle are associated with greater aerosol delivery to the lower respiratory tract.[68,69]

The use of nebulisers in mechanically ventilated patients

When using a nebuliser to administer a drug to mechanically ventilated patients, the methods should be close to the optimal operating characteristics of the device in terms of fill volume and gas flow rate.[68] Nebulisers operating only during inspiration are more efficient. During nebuliser use, appropriate ventilator adjustments in minute volume and alarm systems should be made. The ventilation strategy should not compromise the patient's respiratory mechanics. For example, increasing the duty cycle may enhance lung deposition but worsen dynamic hyperinflation. Whether the humidifier should be bypassed during nebulisation remains a matter of debate.[67,68,71] General recommendations for using nebulisers in ventilated patients, proposed by Dhand & Tobin,[71] are summarised in Table 19.4.

The use of pressurised metered-dose inhalers in mechanically ventilated patients

In the past, pMDIs were considered to be ineffective for delivering bronchodilator therapy to mechanically ventilated patients. Recent studies, however, have clearly established their efficacy, if appropriate methods are used. The use of specially designed spacers[66,69,70] reduces the aerosol impaction on the tubing observed with elbow and in-line adapters, and is therefore strongly recommended.[71] Aerosol delivery should be in synchrony with a sponta-

Table 19.4 Technique for using nebulisers and pressurised metered-dose inhalers in mechanically ventilated patients. Slightly modified with permission from Dhand & Tobin.[71]

Nebulisers
- Place drug solution in nebuliser, employing a fill volume (2–6 ml) that ensures greatest aerosol-generating efficacy
- Place nebuliser in inspiratory line at least 30 cm from the patient Y
- Ensure airflow of 6–8 l/min through the nebuliser
- Ensure adequate tidal volume (> 500 ml in adults); attempt to use duty cycle > 0.3 if possible
- Adjust minute volume to compensate for additional airflow through the nebuliser, if required
- Turn off flow-by or continuous flow mode on ventilator
- Observe nebuliser for adequate aerosol generation throughout use
- Disconnect nebuliser when all medication is nebulised or when no more aerosol is being produced
- Reconnect ventilator circuit and return to original ventilator settings

Pressurised metered-dose inhalers
- Ensure V_T > 500 ml (in adults) during assisted ventilation
- Aim for an inspiratory time (excluding the inspiratory pause) >0.3 of total breath duration
- Ensure that the ventilator breath is synchronised with the patient's inspiration
- Shake the inhaler vigorously
- Place canister in actuator of a cylindrical spacer situated in inspiratory limb of ventilator circuit
- Actuate inhaler to synchronise with precise onset of inspiration by the ventilator
- Allow a breath-hold at end-inspiration for 3–5 s
- Allow passive exhalation
- Repeat actuations after 20–30 s until total dose is delivered

neous breath and given with assisted modes of ventilation. The influence of breath-holding manoeuvres, proposed by some investigators,[72] on bronchodilator response has not been evaluated. Bypassing the humidifier has been suggested but not universally accepted. General recommendations for the use of pMDIs in ventilated patients are summarised in Table 19.4.[71]

Aerosolised drugs

Aerosolised drugs are frequently used in the treatment of pulmonary disorders. Topical administration of a drug allows high local concentrations to be achieved in the airways, the site of the disease, while avoiding high systemic concentrations. A further advantage is that the onset of action of drugs such as bronchodilators is more rapid than if they had been administered orally. In this section, the clinical effects, indications and adverse effects of the currently prescribed inhaled drugs will be briefly discussed. A more detailed discussion of the exact place of these drugs in the prevention and treatment of pulmonary disorders will be found in other chapters of this book.

Aerosolised drugs in pulmonary medicine

Bronchodilating drugs

Inhaled β_2-agonists and anticholinergics may increase airflow and protect against a variety of bronchoconstrictive stimuli. Most β_2-agonists and anticholinergics exhibit a duration of action of 4–6 hours. However, the effects of the long-acting β_2-agonists salmeterol and formoterol last for 12 hours[8,10,73] and those of the anticholinergic tiotropium for at least 24 hours.[74,75]

Despite topical administration, systemic side effects such as tachycardia, prolongation of the Q–Tc interval, skeletal muscle tremor, headache, decreases in serum potassium and arterial P_{O_2}, and increases in lactic acid and serum glucose may develop with higher than conventional doses of inhaled β_2-agonists.[76–78] The clinical relevance of these biochemical changes is unclear. Full agonists, such as fenoterol, are more likely to elicit cardiovascular effects[76] or pronounced reductions in plasma potassium[79] than the partial agonists salbutamol and terbutaline.

A bitter metallic taste, drying of the mouth and blurred vision if sprayed in the eyes are the most frequent side effects of inhaled anticholinergics.

Anti-inflammatory drugs

Cromolyn sodium and nedocromil inhibit the early and late asthmatic response to allergen challenge and exercise-induced bronchoconstriction. These drugs are scarcely absorbed from the gut and are only active when inhaled. An unpleasant taste is the only reported side effect of nedocromil.

Corticosteroids are the most potent and effective anti-inflammatory medications currently available. Oral candidiasis, dysphonia, reflex cough and bronchospasm are the most common local adverse effects of inhaled corticosteroids, but can generally be prevented by mouth-rinsing, the systematic use of a spacer or a holding chamber, pretreatment with a β_2-agonist or

the use of another formulation. High doses of inhaled corticosteroids may promote skin bruising and dermal thinning,[80] reduce 24-hour cortisol secretion[24] and alter some metabolic markers of bone synthesis and resorption.[80] It remains unclear whether the presence of measurable systemic effects is predictive of long-term adverse events such as reduced linear growth, osteoporosis, cataract or glaucoma.

Antimicrobial drugs

Nebulised pentamidine, which is sometimes used in the prophylaxis and treatment of pulmonary infections with *Pneumocystis carinii*, produces adverse reactions if it is deposited in the upper airways, including nausea, cough, dyspnoea and bronchoconstriction.[81] Systemic effects of inhaled pentamidine have not been reported. Nebulisation of pentamidine should be carried out in a room separate from other patients. The health-care worker should leave the room immediately after starting the compressor, until nebulisation is complete.

Aerosolised colistin, gentamicin and tobramycin are sometimes prescribed to treat or prevent pulmonary infections with *Pseudomonas aeruginosa*, without demonstrable adverse effects. In hospital, a nebuliser should be fitted with a high-efficiency breathing filter on the expiratory port to prevent environmental contamination. At home, patients should nebulise their antibiotics in a separate room. Case reports indicate that the role of nebulised liposomal amphotericin B in pulmonary infections with *Aspergillus* spp. merits further assessment.[82] Conversely, the effects of aerosolised ribavirin on the course of bronchiolitis caused by respiratory syncytial virus remain controversial.[83]

Deoxyribonuclease and mucolytic agents

Although it is frequently prescribed to patients with cystic fibrosis, it remains unclear whether inhaled deoxyribonuclease (rhDNase) reduces mortality or the number of exacerbations.[84] High-power nebuliser systems are generally recommended for generating rhDNase-containing aerosols, while ultrasonic nebulisers should be avoided.[30]

Mucolytic agents such as *N*-acetylcysteine are generally prescribed to thin viscous sputum. Although widely used, few studies show objective benefit. Bronchoconstriction after inhalation of *N*-acetylcysteine has been reported.

Saline and water

Inhalation of an aerosol of hypertonic (3–5%) saline is sometimes used to induce sputum production in the context of the non-invasive diagnosis of respiratory infections in immunosuppressed patients. Hypertonic saline draws fluid from the lung interstitium into the alveoli where inflammatory casts and debris are loosened and can move via the mucociliary escalator to the central airways. Occasional adverse effects are retching and nausea, as well as dyspnoea, bronchoconstriction and hypoxaemia.[85]

Water inhaled as cooling steam from a boiling kettle has a traditional role in the treatment of childhood croup. However, being hypotonic, it may cause bronchoconstriction.

Other agents

Current research is directed towards the aerosolised surfactant or nebulisation for administration of genes to the lungs.

Aerosolised drugs in the systemic treatment of other diseases

As substances delivered into the deep lung are rapidly absorbed, current research focuses on the lungs as a route for systemic administration of drugs. For example, the bioavailability of aerosolised morphine appears to be close to 100% while with peptides and proteins a bioavailability exceeding 50% has been reported.[86] From a clinical point of view, the pulmonary route of administration of molecules such as insulin offers the potential for pulsatile delivery, while liposome encapsulation delivered to the alveolar space could be used for controlled release of drugs such as morphine. Preliminary studies have shown that insulin inhaled by healthy volunteers reached the systemic circulation even more rapidly than after subcutaneous administration.[87] Other potential applications of these new technologies are the use of dry-powder inhalers for the administration of vaccines.[88]

Methodologies to predict or assess pulmonary deposition of aerosols

In-vitro methods are sometimes used to predict pulmonary deposition of a given formulation, but in-vivo measurements are always needed to obtain a correct estimation of lung deposition of inhaled particles.

In-vitro characterisation of devices

Impactors allow estimating particle mass, mass distribution and MMAD of aerosols. Twin impactors make an arbitrary division between small 'respirable' particles and larger 'non-respirable' particles. More sophisticated samplers, such as the Andersen impactor or laser-beam devices, allow aerosol properties to be described in detail.

In-vitro measurements are primarily developed to monitor the quality of a manufactured aerosol during its production process. In addition, in-vitro techniques can be used to compare generic formulations to the original when trying to bridge one formulation to another.[15] Although a good description of the particle size properties of an aerosolised drug may give some predictive information about its gross behaviour within the tracheobronchial tree, fine-particle dose is not the only variable influencing pulmonary deposition. Particle inertia and intrinsic velocity (high, from a pMDI; low, from a nebuliser, effort-dependent in the case of a DPI), the negative pressure and inhalation flow generated by the patient, breathing pattern and alterations in flows within the respiratory tract caused by disease-related changes in local geometry of the airways, will inevitably modify aerodynamic behaviour and pulmonary deposition of aerosolised drugs.

The use of simulated breathing patterns and/or actual patient breathing patterns may increase somewhat the reliability of the obtained information. Nevertheless, determinations of equivalence of different formulations should not rely on in-vitro measurements alone and pulmonary deposition studies remain necessary to bridge between in-vitro measurements and the clinical effect.

Direct assay of drug in lung deposition

Interspecies differences in airway architecture and patterns of respiration limit the relevance of studies of lung deposition in animals. Drug concentrations in lung tissue of patients undergoing lung surgery can, however, be assayed and compared with the concentration in blood taken at the same time-point, if inhaled preoperatively.[89]

Lung imaging

Measurements of dose deposited in the lung and distribution of this dose within the lung can be made using scintigraphic techniques including planar two-dimensional gamma imaging[90] and three-dimensional scintigraphic methods such as single photon emission computed tomography (SPECT) and positron emission tomography (PET). Both planar gamma scintigraphy and SPECT use low energy gamma emitters, mainly technetium-99m. The use of PET has the advantages that the tracers are isotopes of the basic biological molecules carbon, oxygen, fluorine and nitrogen, which can be incorporated directly into the drug molecule. This allows functional imaging as well as deposition measurements. The use of SPECT and PET for the study of drug-deposition patterns needs further validation.[15] Unless a radiolabel is directly incorporated into the drug molecule, the quality of the labelling procedure must be confirmed before use. This requires in-vitro measurements of emitted dose and the aerosol size distribution of both radioactivity and drug, to ensure that the radiolabel follows the drug in the radiolabelled product and that the drug is not altered by the labelling procedure. Visualisation of the topical distribution of the aerosol within the lung and of extrathoracic deposition of the drug represents a major advantage of scintigraphic investigations. Its two-dimensional nature does not, however, permit differentiation of deposition in small bronchioles from alveolar deposition as the planar image can only be divided into 'regions of interest'.[6]

Pharmacokinetic studies

Pharmacokinetic methods are based on the assumption that systemic bioavailability of the drug equals pulmonary deposition, if the drug is not metabolised in the lung or absorbed from the gastrointestinal tract. For drugs absorbed from the gastrointestinal tract, activated charcoal can be used to block gastrointestinal absorption.[18] Intravenous administration of a known amount of drug labelled with an isotope as an internal standard allows an absolute estimation of the pulmonary deposition of the drug from the appearance of the labelled and unlabelled compound in serum and urine.[91] As the doses delivered are generally small and the resulting plasma levels correspondingly low, sensitive assay systems should be used. Major advantages of this method over scintigraphic methods are that inadvertent changes in formulation at labelling and repeated exposition to radiation are avoided.

Pharmacokinetic methods sometimes yield lower lung deposition data than scintigraphic methods. Some part of the drug deposited in central airways may be detected by scintigraphy but removed by rapid mucociliary transport, whereas pharmacokinetic methods measure only the drug absorbed across the lung epithelium.[17,18]

The early appearance of a drug in plasma or urine after inhalation yields indices that are in some way related to lung deposition but do not permit the expression of lung deposition in absolute terms.

Practical considerations

Until a decade ago, most health-care providers believed that successful implementation of a treatment with inhaled drugs depended on the efficacy and side effects of the drug and the formulation-dependent inhalation technique. In recent years, factors such as cost, patient preference, in-vitro data, therapeutic index and pulmonary and extrathoracic deposition have been increasingly used to convince health-care providers of the superiority of one formulation over another. This section represents an attempt to put into perspective the various factors and data that should, could or might be taken into account before making a final choice.

Data on the in-vitro performance of the formulation

The particle size of the aerosol, as measured in vitro, should definitely be taken into account when choosing a nebuliser, as substantial differences appear to exist even between nebulisers of apparently the same class.[92] A generally accepted recommendation is that at least 50% of particle mass generated by a nebuliser should be within the respirable range (MMAD $< 5 \mu m$) at an appropriate airflow. As pointed out above, nebuliser output, rate of nebulisation and residual volume should also be taken into consideration as they all affect nebulisation time.

Conversely, in-vitro studies dealing with emitted dose, particle size or fine-particle dose are less helpful in the selection of a pMDI or a DPI. In-vitro measurements do not predict the in-vivo behaviour of aerosolised drugs in a reliable way. For example, several generic pMDIs with fine-particle fractions comparable to the original formulation (as measured in vitro) behaved differently once attached to a large volume spacer,[36,93] a discrepancy that has been attributed to differences in plume geometry.

Extrapolation of in-vitro data to the in-vivo situation should always be done with caution. For example, it has been demonstrated that variability in lung deposition of terbutaline inhaled via Turbuhaler® is lower than with the corresponding pMDI in healthy volunteers and in patients with asthma,[94] despite the fact that the in vitro dose variability is greater with Turbuhaler® than with the pMDI formulation.[95]

Studies on acceptability, preference and compliance

Studies on acceptability, preference and compliance rarely exceed 7 weeks, are usually sponsored by the pharmaceutical industry and often tend to have a biased questionnaire. Patients and physicians often express spontaneous preferences for new devices over old one. Although preference for one or another device may affect patient compliance, the clinical significance of this phenomenon is difficult to value.

Compliance with nebulisers is poor, averaging 50% in two studies[96,97] and 70% in a third.[98] Predictors of good compliance are age, better education, more pronounced pulmonary symptoms and reduced forced expiratory volume in 1 s (FEV_1). Reasons not to comply are lack of time, insufficient insight into the aim of the treatment and duration of nebulisation exceeding 5–10 min.

Although pMDIs are more practical than nebulisers, self-reported compliance and canister weight tend to overestimate adherence to treatment and might explain why the overall compliance of 70%, reported over a 2-year follow-up period in the Lung Health Study,[99] might represent a overestimate. Other studies have indicated that up to 40% of the patients tend to underuse[100] and about 20% to overuse medication formulated in a pMDI, despite adequate study supervision.[101] A retrospective comparison between DPIs and pMDIs from New Zealand indicated that the mean daily inhaled dose of inhaled glucocorticosteroids was significantly higher for DPIs.[102] Regular teaching and education improve patient compliance.[103]

As there is current evidence that addition of long-acting β_2-agonists to inhaled corticosteroids in patients with persistent asthma provides greater clinical benefit than doubling the dosage of inhaled corticosteroids, fixed combinations of the two drugs have been formulated into one device. Combination treatment with salmeterol $50 \mu g$ and fluticasone $250 \mu g$ given twice daily provided better asthma control and greater improvement in pulmonary function than did the individual agents.[104] This confirms earlier studies,[12,105] which showed that a reduction in the number of inhalations improved compliance. Interestingly, combination treatment not only simplified the management of asthma in patients who needed both classes of drugs for optimal control of their disease, but appeared to be cost-effective.[106]

Treatment efficacy measured as the total number of exacerbations, days with exacerbations and hospitalisations, and healthcare utilisation assessed over at least 1 year in a sufficient number of patients is far more informative than studies in which only one aspect of the treatment, be it preference, acceptance or compliance, is assessed. In such studies, cost of treatment, as well as direct and indirect costs related to the disease, should be included. However, differences between countries in cost and patient preference (often related to cultural background) make it difficult to extrapolate data obtained in one specific country[107,108] to other parts of the world.

Data on pharmacodynamic and pharmacokinetic properties of inhaled drugs

Each drug is characterised by pharmacodynamic and pharmacokinetic properties such as receptor-binding affinity, retention in lung tissue, distribution volume and clearance. Differences in pharmacokinetic properties within one specific drug class may have important clinical consequences. For example, it has been claimed that the degree of β_2-selectivity and the presence of a partial antagonistic activity are the reasons why salbutamol and terbutaline are less associated with worsening control of asthma symptoms than fenoterol.

A greater potency for a drug within a given drug category may represent an advantage if a greater maximum effect can be obtained. If, however, potency is used in the context of comparison of effects on a weight-for-weight basis, a lower receptor-binding affinity can generally be compensated by the use of a formulation with a high pulmonary deposition or by prescribing a higher dose.

Prolonged pulmonary residence time represents an obvious advantage, as is now clear from studies with long-acting β_2-agonists. For inhaled glucocorticosteroids, clinical studies have pointed out that budesonide once daily is as effective as half the dose given twice daily,[12] a feature that is not shared by other inhaled glucocorticosteroids. Conversely, prolonged plasma elimination half-life is a disadvantage, as this may cause accumulation of the drug in the systemic circulation.[20,21]

Handling and maintenance of the inhaler

Inappropriate use or mistakes in inhalation technique reduce the dose delivered and compromise the efficacy of the treatment. For example, it was demonstrated that the increase in FEV_1 was 80% of maximum achievable after inhalation from the unprimed pMDI, compared to 92% after inhalation from the primed one.[109] In a study with plastic spacers, priming the spacer by actuating the pMDI a few times increased pulmonary deposition of glucocorticosteroids in asthmatic patients by 40–50%[110] whereas, in another study, pulmonary deposition of salbutamol was doubled if the spacer was coated with benzalkonium chloride.[48] The use of an inappropriate inhalation flow is of relevance for a DPI[59] and may eventually affect the clinical response. Incorrect handling of nebulisers includes the use of an incorrect flow setting or of a wrong dilution of drug in the solvent.

Maintenance is not required for DPIs and pMDIs. As reported previously, however, poor maintenance of nebulisers may lead to contamination of its wet parts[32] and cause bacterial respiratory tract infections. For spacers and add-on devices, the amount of electrostatic charge present may depend on how much the device has been used and on washing procedures.[49]

Handling and maintenance of devices by patients should be taught, practised and checked regularly. Nevertheless, inappropriate use of inhalers and mistakes in the inhalation technique occur frequently. As patients unable to use one device sometimes do better with another, physicians should develop a rational inhaler strategy, taking various factors, such as age, ability to learn correct use and patient preference, into account.

Data on pulmonary deposition

The move towards generic inhaler products and the banning of chlorofluorocarbons has increased the need to demonstrate the effectiveness of new formulated drugs and to determine their equivalence with established formulations. As the design of the aerosol system can have significant impact on the amount and characteristics of the delivered aerosol, the clinical response of each new inhaler product has to be measured directly. Measures of clinical response are, however, relatively insensitive for comparing different inhalation devices. For bronchodilators, changes in FEV_1 are often used to assess their therapeutic response. Pulmonary function measurements may, however, fail to detect important differences in lung deposition between two formulations of the same drug, since the plateau or level of maximal response is easily reached with normal treatment doses. A well-designed comparative study with bronchodilators should thus include at least two dose levels for at least one of the formulations, and it is necessary to demonstrate a difference in response between the two dose levels to draw conclusions.[37] Comparative studies with inhaled corticosteroids are even more difficult to conduct,[80] as no rapid response occurs and clinical effect is based on relatively imprecise clinical end-points such as diary recordings of peak expiratory flow, symptom scores and use of bronchodilator medication, measured over longer periods of time. As pointed out above, the predictive value of in-vitro studies for pulmonary deposition and clinical effect is low.

Evidence is accumulating that lung-deposition data may act as a parameter for the clinical response to inhaled drugs in asthma patients. Indeed, correlations between pulmonary deposition and clinical effects have been investigated in a restricted number of studies and found to be excellent.[2,3,54,61,111–113] In one of these studies,[61] lung deposition of terbutaline, measured with the charcoal block method, was 21.5% of the nominal dose after DPI (Turbuhaler®)and 8.2% after pMDI. The 0.25 mg terbutaline dose given by DPI resulted in a significantly higher FEV_1 response than 0.25 mg inhaled via pMDI. The increase in FEV_1 after the 0.5 mg dose given via pMDI and the 0.25 mg dose inhaled via DPI was similar, indicating that the amount of drug reaching the lungs, not the nominal dose, determined the clinical effect. The difference in clinical effect between 0.25 mg and 0.5 mg given by DPI did not reach statistical significance, because 0.25 mg terbutaline administered via DPI already resulted in a close-to-maximum effect. In a subsequent study from the same research group, the bronchoprotective effects of terbutaline were more related to the amount of drug deposited in the lungs than to the nominal dose or the dose delivered from the inhaler.[113]

The correlation between pulmonary deposition and clinical response observed in these and other studies has three important consequences. First, formulations leading to high pulmonary deposition may represent an advantage for the clinician, as substitution of 'device A' with low pulmonary deposition for 'device B' with high pulmonary deposition might lead to better control of symptoms. Secondly, an attempt should always be made to reduce the prescribed dose if the disease is well under control, especially if a device with a high pulmonary deposition is used, in order to avoid unnecessary systemic exposure and spare medication. Finally, as the aforementioned studies provide convincing evidence that lung-deposition data are predictive of the clinical response to inhaled asthma drugs, lung-deposition studies might, in certain circumstances, supplement or substitute clinical response and bioequivalence studies.

Data on extrathoracic deposition, local side effects, and systemic effects

The fraction of the drug delivered by the inhaler that deposits on the oropharynx (Fig. 19.1) may contribute to local side effects and to systemic effects, at least if the patient does not rinse his/her mouth and if the part of the drug absorbed in the gastrointestinal tract is not completely inactivated by the first-pass metabolism.

Local side effects such as candidiasis occur in 5% of the patients on inhaled corticosteroids. The use of large-volume spacers[57] or inhalation via Turbuhaler® followed by mouth-rinsing[114] not only reduces oropharyngeal deposition but decreases the incidence of candidiasis significantly. Thus, in patients prone to corticosteroid-induced local side effects, mouth-rinsing and the use of formulations characterised by a high pulmonary and a low pharyngeal deposition are recommended. Conversely, extrapulmonary deposition does not represent a clinically relevant issue for inhaled β_2-agonists and anticholinergics.

Extrathoracic deposition of drugs with negligible oral bioavailability, such as fluticasone, does not contribute to the development of systemic effects.[20] If these develop, they are caused by the pulmonary bioavailability of the drug (Fig. 19.1). Conversely, about 20% of the extrapulmonary fraction of beclometasone reaches the systemic circulation[115] through gastrointestinal absorption. This explains why reduced extrapulmonary deposition with a large-volume spacer reduces the systemic effects of beclometasone inhaled via a pMDI.[58]

Lung versus total bioavailability ratio

It is possible to evaluate the balance between pulmonary bioavailability and systemic bioavailability if the following data are known:

- the degree of retention of the drug in the inhaler
- the percentage of pulmonary and oropharyngeal deposition of the drug
- the degree of gastrointestinal absorption
- the degree of inactivation by the first-pass metabolism.

From these data the L/T ratio (L = local bioavailability, T= systemic bioavailability) can be derived.

Calculations have shown that, for terbutaline, the L/T ratio averages 0.55 for a pMDI and 0.81 for Turbuhaler®.[116] For salbutamol, the L/T ratio averages 0.35 for a pMDI, 0.15 for Rotahaler®, 0.24 for Diskhaler® and 0.45 for Turbuhaler®.[116] The differences in value between salbutamol and terbutaline are a reflection of inherent differences in gastrointestinal absorption and first-pass metabolism between these drugs. For budesonide, similar calculations have yielded 0.59 for pMDI, 0.84 for Turbuhaler® and 0.95 for pMDI with Nebuhaler®.[117]

A higher L/T ratio will always indicate a more favourable ratio with respect to the balance between desired and undesired effect, resulting from a good targeting ability of the combination of substance and device, or from a low contribution of the gastrointestinal tract.

The clinical relevance of the L/T ratio, a theoretical concept, is, however, less clear. Indeed, the L/T ratio is only useful in comparisons of different formulations of the same drug. A high L/T ratio always implies that it is the pulmonary bioavailability that determines the systemic activity. Comparisons between drugs, however, should not be made, as different substances may differ in terms of relative activity in the lungs and the systemic circulation. Moreover, the L/T ratio should always be verified clinically. One example of this is that inhaled fluticasone has been shown to exert systemic effects[24] despite its minimal gastrointestinal bioavailability, and its very high L/T ratio. Another example is that vast differences appear to exists between healthy volunteers and asthmatic patients in terms of 24-hour cortisol suppression after inhalation of high doses of inhaled glucocorticosteroids,[23,24] a difference that may be attributed to a difference in systemic bioavailability of glucocorticosteroids between healthy subjects and patients with asthma.[118]

> ### ? Unresolved questions
>
> It remains to be investigated whether:
>
> - The systematic use of a mouthpiece enhances lung deposition of nebulised drugs in patients capable of using a facemask correctly
> - Lung deposition may substitute for or supplement clinical response data when comparing different inhalation devices or drugs formulations
> - In- vitro determination of fine-particle dose predicts pulmonary deposition of a formulation
> - Improved drug targeting by using monodisperse aerosols is cost-saving, since the reduction in drug consumption may mean using a more expensive inhalation device
> - Cost-effectiveness studies with inhaled drugs performed in one country may not be extrapolated to other parts of the world.

References

1. Thorsson L, Edsbäcker S. Lung deposition of budesonide from a pressurized metered-dose inhaler attached to a spacer. Eur Respir J 1998; 12: 1340–1345.
2. Newman S, Pavia D, Garland N, Clarke SW. Effects of various inhalation modes on the deposition of radioactive pressurized aerosols. Eur J Respir Dis 1982; 63(suppl. 119): 57–65.
3. Newman S, Pavia D, Clarke S. Simple instructions for using pressurized aerosol bronchodilators. J R Soc Med 1980; 73: 776–779.
4. Rudolph G, Kobrich R, Stahlhofen W. Modelling and algebraic formulation of regional aerosol deposition in man. J Aerosol Med 1990; 21(suppl 1): S306–S406.
5. Zanen P, Go LT, Lammers JW. The efficacy of a low-dose, monodisperse parasympatholytic aerosol compared with a standard aerosol from a metered-dose inhaler. Eur J Clin Pharmacol 1998; 54: 27–30.
6. Newman SP, Hirst PH, Pitcairn GR. Understanding regional lung deposition data in gamma scintigraphy. In: Dalby RN, Byron PR, Farr SJ, ed. Respiratory drug delivery VI. Buffalo Grove, IL: Interpharm Press; 1998: 9–16.
7. Linden A, Rabe KF, Lofdahl CG. Pharmacological basis for duration of effect: formoterol and salmeterol versus short-acting beta 2-adrenoceptor agonists. Lung 1996; 174: 1–22.
8. Derom EY, Pauwels RA. Time course of bronchodilating effect of inhaled formoterol, a potent and long acting sympathomimetic. Thorax 1992; 47: 30–33.
9. Ullman A, Svedmyr N. Salmeterol, a new long acting inhaled beta₂ adrenoceptor agonist: comparison with salbutamol in adult asthmatic patients. Thorax 1988; 43: 674–678.

10. Palmqvist M, Persson G, Lazer L et al. Inhaled dry-powder formoterol and salmeterol in asthmatic patients: onset of action, duration of effect and potency. Eur Respir J 1997; 10: 2484–2489.

11. McFadden ER, Casale TB, Edwards TB et al. Administration of budesonide once daily by means of Turbuhaler to subjects with stable asthma. J Allergy Clin Immunol 1999; 104: 46–52.

12. Campbell LM. Once-daily inhaled corticosteroids in mild to moderate asthma: improving acceptance of treatment. Drugs 1999; 58(suppl. 4): 25–33.

13. Miller-Larsson A, Mattsson H, Hjertberg E et al. Reversible fatty acid conjugation of budesonide. Novel mechanism for prolonged retention of topically applied steroid in airway tissue. Drug Metab Dispos 1998; 26: 623–630.

14. Saari M, Vidgren MT, Koskinen MO et al. Pulmonary distribution and clearance of two beclomethasone liposome formulations in healthy volunteers. Int J Pharm 1999; 181: 1–9.

15. Snell NJ, Ganderton D. Assessing lung deposition of inhaled medications. Consensus statement from a workshop of the British Association for Lung Research, held at the Institute of Biology, London, UK on 17 April 1998. Respir Med 1999; 93: 123–133.

16. Currie DC, Pavia D, Agnew JE et al. Impaired tracheobronchial clearance in bronchiectasis. Thorax 1987; 42: 126–130.

17. Newman S, Steed K, Hooper G et al. Comparison of gamma scintigraphy and a pharmacokinetic technique for assessing pulmonary deposition of terbutaline sulphate delivered by pressurized metered dose inhaler. Pharmacol Res 1995; 12: 231–236.

18. Borgström L, Newman S, Weisz A, Morén F. Pulmonary deposition of inhaled terbutaline: comparison of scanning gamma camera and urinary excretion methods. J Pharmacol Sci 1992; 81: 753–755.

19. Bennett WD, Ilowite JS. Dual pathway clearance of ^{99m}Tc-DTPA from the bronchial mucosa. Am Rev Respir Dis 1989; 139: 1132–1138.

20. Hochhaus G, Mollmann H, Derendorf H, Gonzalez-Rothi RJ. Pharmacokinetic/pharmacodynamic aspects of aerosol therapy using glucocorticoids as a model. J Clin Pharmacol 1997; 37: 881–892.

21. Thorsson L, Dahlstrom K, Edsbäcker S et al. Pharmacokinetics and systemic effects of inhaled fluticasone propionate in healthy subjects. Br J Clin Pharmacol 1997; 43: 155–161.

22. Ryrfeldt Å, Andersson P, Edsbäcker S et al. Pharmacokinetics and metabolism of budesonide, a selective glucocorticoid. Eur J Respir Dis Suppl 119 1982; 122: 86–95.

23. Lönnebo A, Grahnén A, Jansson B et al. An assessment of the systemic effects of single and repeated doses of inhaled fluticasone propionate and inhaled budesonide in healthy volunteers. Eur J Clin Pharmacol 1996; 49: 459–463.

24. Derom E, Van Schoor J, Verhaeghe W et al. Systemic effects of inhaled fluticasone propionate and budesonide in adult patients with asthma. Am J Respir Crit Care Med 1999; 160: 157–161.

25. O'Callaghan C, Barry PW. The science of nebulised drug delivery. Thorax 1997; 52 Suppl 2: S31–S44.

26. Knoch M, Sommer E. Jet nebulizer design and function. Eur Respir Rev 2000; 10: 183–186.

27. Thomas SH, O'Doherty MJ, Graham A et al. Pulmonary deposition of nebulised amiloride in cystic fibrosis: comparison of two nebulisers. Thorax 1991; 46: 717–721.

28. Clark AR. The use of laser defraction for the evaluation of the aerosol clouds generated by medical nebulisers. Int J Pharm 1995; 115: 69–78.

29. Newman S. Lung deposition from nebulizers. Eur Respir Rev 2000; 10: 224–227.

30. Kendrick AH, Smith EC, Wilson RS. Selecting and using nebuliser equipment. Thorax 1997; 52(suppl. 2): S92–S101.

31. Hakkinen AM, Uusi-Heikkila H, Jarvinen M et al. The effect of breathing frequency on deposition of drug aerosol using an inhalation-synchronized dosimeter in healthy adults. Clin Physiol 1999; 19: 269–274.

32. Barnes KL, Clifford R, Holgate ST et al. Bacterial contamination of home nebuliser. Br Med J (Clin Res Ed) 1987; 295: 812.

33. Zierenberg B, Eicher J, Dunne S, Freund B. Boehringer Ingelheim Nebulizer Bineb, a new approach to inhalation therapy. In: Dalby RN, Byron PR, Farr SJ, ed. Respiratory Drug delivery V. Buffalo Grove, IL: Interpharm Press; 1996: 187–94.

34. Newman SP, Steed KP, Reader SJ et al. Efficient delivery to the lungs of flunisolide aerosol from a new portable hand-held multidose nebulizer. J Pharm Sci 1996; 85: 960–964.

35. Newman SP, Brown J, Steed KP et al. Lung deposition of fenoterol and flunisolide delivered using a novel device for inhaled medicines: comparison of RESPIMAT with conventional metered-dose inhalers with and without spacer devices. Chest 1998; 113: 957–963.

36. Barry PW, O'Callaghan C. In vitro comparison of the amount of salbutamol available for inhalation from different formulations used with different spacer devices. Eur Respir J 1997; 10: 1345–1348.

37. Pauwels R, Newman S, Borgström L. Airway deposition and airway effects of antiasthma drugs delivered from metered-dose inhalers. Eur Respir J 1997; 10: 2127–2138.

38. Leach C. Effect of formulation parameters on hydrofluoroalkane-beclomethasone dipropionate drug deposition in humans. J Allergy Clin Immunol 1999; 104: S250–S252.

39. Newman S, Pitcairn G, Steed K et al. Deposition of fenoterol from pressurized metered dose inhalers containing hydrofluoroalkanes. J Allergy Clin Immunol 1999; 104: S253–S257.

40. Ramsdell JW, Colice GL, Ekholm BP, Klinger NM. Cumulative dose response study comparing HFA-134a albuterol sulfate and conventional CFC albuterol in patients with asthma. Ann Allergy Asthma Immunol 1998; 81: 593–599.

41. Everard ML, Devadason SG, Summers QA, LeSoüef PN. Factors affecting total and 'respirable' dose delivered by a salbutamol metered dose inhaler. Thorax 1995; 50: 746–749.

42. Van der Palen J, Klein JJ, Kerkhoff AH et al. Inhalation technique of 166 adult asthmatics prior to and following a self-management program. J Asthma 1999; 36: 441–447.

43. Snell NJ. Adverse reactions to inhaled drugs (editorial). Respir Med 1990; 84: 345–348.

44. Bisgaard H, Anhøj J, Klug B, Berg E. A non-electrostatic spacer for aerosol delivery. Arch Dis Child 1995; 73: 226–230.

45. Zak M, Madsen J, Berg E et al. A mathematical model of aerosol holding chambers. J Aerosol Med 1999; 12: 187–196.

46. Bisgaard H, Anhøj J, Wildhaber JH. Spacer devices. In: Bisgaard H, O'Callaghan C, Smaldone GC, ed. Drug delivery to the lung: clinical aspects. New York: Marcel Dekker; 2001

47. Wildhaber JH, Devadason SG, Hayden MJ et al. Electrostatic charge on a plastic spacer device influences the delivery of salbutamol. Eur Respir J 1996; 9: 1943–1946.

48. Anhøj J, Bisgaard H, Lipworth BJ. Effect of electrostatic charge in plastic spacers on the lung delivery of HFA-salbutamol in children. Br J Clin Pharmacol 1999; 47: 333–336.

49. Piérart F, Wildhaber JH, Vrancken I et al. Washing plastic spacers in household detergent reduces electrostatic charge and greatly improves delivery. Eur Respir J 1999; 13: 673–678.

50. Berg E, Madsen J, Bisgaard H. In vitro performance of three combinations of spacers and pressurized metered dose inhalers for treatment in children. Eur Respir J 1998; 12: 472–476.

51. Clark DJ, Lipworth BJ. Effect of multiple actuations, delayed inhalation and antistatic treatment on the lung bioavailability of salbutamol via a spacer device. Thorax 1996; 51: 981–984.

52. Barry PW, O'Callaghan C. A comparative analysis of the particle size output of beclomethasone diproprionate, salmeterol xinafoate and fluticasone propionate metered dose inhalers used with the Babyhaler, Volumatic and Aerochamber spacer devices. Br J Clin Pharmacol 1999; 47: 357–360.

53. Thorsson L, Kenyon C, Newman S, Borgström L. Lung deposition of budesonide in asthmatics: a comparison of different formulations. Int J Pharm 1998; 168: 119–127.

54. Newman S. The correct use of inhalers. In: Clark T, editor. Steroids in asthma. Auckland: Adis Press; 1982: 210–216.

55. Barry PW, O'Callaghan C. The effect of delay, multiple actuations and spacer static charge on the in vitro delivery of budesonide from the Nebuhaler. Br J Clin Pharmacol 1995; 40: 76–78.

56. Dewar AL, Stewart A, Cogswell JJ, Connett GJ. A randomised controlled trial to assess the relative benefits of large volume spacers and nebulisers to treat acute asthma in hospital. Arch Dis Child 1999; 80: 421–423.

57. Salzman GA, Pyszczynski DR. Oropharyngeal candidiasis in patients treated with beclomethasone dipropionate delivered by metered-dose inhaler alone and with Aerochamber. J Allergy Clin Immunol 1988; 81: 424–428.

58. Brown PH, Blundell G, Greening AP, Crompton GK. Do large volume spacer devices reduce the systemic effects of high dose inhaled corticosteroids? Thorax 1990; 45: 736–739.

59. Olsson B, Asking L. Critical aspects of the function of inspiratory flow driven inhalers. J Aerosol Med 1994; 7: S43–S47.

60. Newman S, Morén F, Trofast E et al Terbutaline sulphate terbutaline: effect of inhaled flow rate on drug deposition and efficacy. Int J Pharm 1991; 74: 209–213.

61. Borgström L, Derom E, Ståhl E et al. The inhalation device influences lung deposition and bronchodilating effect of terbutaline. Am J Respir Crit Care Med 1996; 153: 1636–1640.

62. Newman SP, Pitcairn GR, Hirst PH et al. Scintigraphic comparison of budesonide deposition from two dry powder inhalers. Eur Respir J 2000; 16: 178–183.

63. Olsson B, Borgström L, Asking L, Bondesson E. Effect of inlet throat on the correlation between fine particle dose and lung deposition. In: Dalby RN, Byron PR, Farr SJ, ed. Respiratory drug delivery V. Buffalo Grove, IL: Interpharm Press; 1996: 273–81.

64. Maggi L, Bruni R, Conte U. Influence of the moisture on the performance of a new dry powder inhaler. Int J Pharm 1999; 177: 83–91.

65. Meakin BJ, Cainey J, Woodcock PM. Effect of exposure to humidity on terbutaline delivery from Turbuhaler dry power inhalation devices. Eur Respir J 1993; 6: 760–761.

66. Fuller HD, Dolovich MB, Turpie FH, Newhouse MT. Efficiency of bronchodilator aerosol delivery to the lungs from the metered dose inhaler in mechanically ventilated patients. A study comparing four different actuator devices. Chest 1994; 105: 214–218.

67. O'Riordan TG, Palmer LB, Smaldone GC. Aerosol deposition in mechanically ventilated patients. Optimizing nebulizer delivery. Am J Respir Crit Care Med 1994; 149: 214–219.

68. O'Riordan TG, Greco MJ, Perry RJ, Smaldone GC. Nebulizer function during mechanical ventilation. Am Rev Respir Dis 1992; 145: 1117–1122.

69. Diot P, Morra L, Smaldone GC. Albuterol delivery in a model of mechanical ventilation. Comparison of metered-dose inhaler and nebulizer efficiency. Am J Respir Crit Care Med 1995; 152: 1391–1394.

70. Rau JL, Harwood RJ, Groff JL. Evaluation of a reservoir device for metered-dose bronchodilator delivery to intubated adults. An in vitro study. Chest 1992; 102: 924–930.

71. Dhand R, Tobin MJ. Inhaled bronchodilator therapy in mechanically ventilated patients. Am J Respir Crit Care Med 1997156: 3–10.

72. Fernandez A, Lazaro A, Garcia A et al. Bronchodilators in patients with chronic obstructive pulmonary disease on mechanical ventilation. Utilization of metered-dose inhalers. Am Rev Respir Dis 1990; 141: 164–168.

73. Derom E, Pauwels R, Van der Straeten ME. The effect of inhaled salmeterol on methacholine responsiveness in subjects with asthma up to 12 hours. J Allergy Clin Immunol 1992; 89: 811–815.

74. Maesen FP, Smeets JJ, Sledsens TJ et al. Tiotropium bromide, a new long-acting antimuscarinic bronchodilator: a pharmacodynamic study in patients with chronic obstructive pulmonary disease (COPD). Dutch Study Group. Eur Respir J 1995; 8: 1506–1513.

75. O'Connor BJ, Towse U, Barnes PJ. Prolonged effect of tiotropium bromide on methacholine-induced bronchoconstriction in asthma. Am J Respir Crit Care Med 1996; 154: 876–880.

76. Wong CS, Pavord ID, Williams J et al. Bronchodilator, cardiovascular, and hypokalaemic effects of fenoterol, salbutamol, and terbutaline in asthma. Lancet 1990; 336: 1396–1399.

77. Bondesson E, Friberg K, Soliman S, Lofdahl CG. Safety and efficacy of a high cumulative dose of salbutamol inhaled via Turbuhaler or via a pressurised metered-dose inhaler in patients with asthma. Respir Med 1998; 92: 325–330.

78. Lecaillon JB, Kaiser G, Palmisano M et al. Pharmacokinetics and tolerability of formoterol in healthy volunteers after a single high dose of Foradil dry powder inhalation via Aerolizer. Eur J Clin Pharmacol 1999; 55: 131–138.

79. Burgess C, Beasley R, Crane J, Pearce N. Adverse effects of beta2-agonists. In: Pauwels R, O'Byrne PO, ed. Asthma treatment. New York: Marcel Dekker; 1997: 257–282.

80. Barnes PJ, Pedersen S, Busse WW. Efficacy and safety of inhaled corticosteroids. New developments. Am J Respir Crit Care Med 1998; 157: S1–S53.

81. Leigh TR, Wiggins J, Gazzard B, Collins JV. A comparison of several agents with two delivery systems for the prevention of airway narrowing induced by nebulised pentamidine isethionate. Respir Med 1991; 85: 527–531.

82. Purcell IF, Corris PA. Use of nebulised liposomal amphotericin B in the treatment of *Aspergillus fumigatus* empyema. Thorax 1995; 50: 1321–1323.

83. Guerguerian AM, Gauthier M, Lebel MH et al. Ribavirin in ventilated respiratory syncytial virus bronchiolitis. A randomized, placebo-controlled trial. Am J Respir Crit Care Med 1999; 160: 829–834.

84. Kearney CE, Wallis CE. Deoxyribonuclease for cystic fibrosis. Cochrane Database Syst Rev 2000: CD001127.

85. Miller RF, Buckland J, Semple SJ. Arterial desaturation in HIV positive patients undergoing sputum induction. Thorax 1991; 46: 449–451.

86. Davis SS. Peptide delivery-advantages and disadvantages of alternative mucosal routes of administration. In: Dalby RN, Byron PR, Farr SJ, ed. Respiratory drug delivery VI. Buffalo Grove, IL: Interpharm Press; 1998: 1–8.

87. Farr SJ, Gonda I, Licko V. Physicochemical physiological factors influencing the effectiveness of inhaled insulin. In: Dalby RN, Byron PR, Farr SJ, ed. Respiratory drug delivery VI. Buffalo Grove, IL: Interpharm Press; 1998: 25–33.

88. LiCalsi C, Christensen T, Bennett JV et al. Dry powder inhalation as a potential delivery method for vaccines. Vaccine 1999; 17: 1796–1803.

89. Esmailpour N, Hogger P, Rabe KF et al. Distribution of inhaled fluticasone propionate between human lung tissue and serum in vivo. Eur Respir J 1997; 10: 1496–1499.

90. Newman S. Scintigraphic assessment of pulmonary delivery systems. Pharm Tech 1998; 22: 78–94.

91. Borgström L, Nilsson M. A method for determination of the absolute pulmonary bioavailability of inhaled drugs: terbutaline. Pharm Res 1990; 7: 1068–1070.

92. Barry PW, O'Callaghan C. An in vitro analysis of the output of budesonide from different nebulizers. J Allergy Clin Immunol 1999; 104: 1168–73.

93. Derom E, Pauwels R. Bioequivalence of inhaled drugs. Eur Respir J 1995; 8: 1634–1636.

94. Borgström L, Bengtsson T, Derom E, Pauwels R. Variability in lung deposition of inhaled drug, within and between asthmatic patients, with a pMDI and a dry powder inhaler, Turbuhaler®. Int J Pharm, 2000; 193: 227–230.

95. Borgström L, Asking L, Beckman O et al. Discrepancy between in vitro and in vivo dose variability for a pressurized metered dose inhaler and a dry powder. J Aerosol Med 1998; 11: S59–S64.

96. Schöni MH, Horak E, Nikolaizik WH. Compliance with therapy in children with respiratory diseases. Eur J Pediatr 1995; 154: S77–S81.

97. Turner J, Wright E, Mendella L, Anthonisen N. Predictors of patient adherence to long-term home nebulizer therapy for COPD. The IPPB Study Group. Intermittent Positive Pressure Breathing. Chest 1995; 108: 394–400.

98. Cochrane GM. Compliance with nebulized therapy. Eur Respir Rev 1997; 7: 383–384.

99. Rand CS, Nides M, Cowles MK et al. Long-term metered-dose inhaler adherence in a clinical trial. The Lung Health Study Research Group. Am J Respir Crit Care Med 1995; 152: 580–588.

100. Milgrom H, Bender B, Ackerson L et al. Noncompliance and treatment failure in children with asthma. J Allergy Clin Immunol 1996; 98: 1051–1057.

101. Mawhinney H, Spector SL, Kinsman RA et al. Compliance in clinical trials of two nonbronchodilator, antiasthma medications. Ann Allergy 1991; 66: 294–299.

102. Frost GD, Penrose A, Hall J, MacKenzie DI. Asthma-related prescribing patterns with four different corticosteroid inhaler devices. Respir Med 1998; 92: 1352–1358.

103. Cochrane GM. Compliance and outcomes in patients with asthma. Drugs 1996; 52(suppl) 6: 12–19.

104. Shapiro G, Lumry W, Wolfe J et al. Combined salmeterol 50 microg and fluticasone propionate 250 microg in the Diskus device for the treatment of asthma. Am J Respir Crit Care Med 2000; 161: 527–534.

105. Mann M, Eliasson O, Patel K, ZuWallack RL. A comparison of the effects of bid and qid dosing on compliance with inhaled flunisolide. Chest 1992; 101 : 496–499.

106. Lundback B, Jenkins C, Price MJ, Thwaites RM. Cost-effectiveness of salmeterol/fluticasone propionate combination product 50/250 microg twice daily and budesonide 800 microg twice daily in the treatment of adults and adolescents with asthma. International Study Group. Respir Med 2000; 94: 724–732.

107. Liljas B, Sta[o]hl E, Pauwels RA. Cost-effectiveness analysis of a dry powder inhaler (Turbuhaler) versus a pressurised metered dose inhaler in patients with asthma. Pharmacoeconomics 1997; 12: 267–277.

108. Rutten-van Molken MP, van Doorslaer EK, Till MD. Cost-effectiveness analysis of formoterol versus salmeterol in patients with asthma. Pharmacoeconomics 1998; 14: 671–684.

109. Blake KV, Harman E, Hendeles L. Evaluation of a generic albuterol metered-dose inhaler: importance of priming the MDI. Ann Allergy 1992; 68: 169–174.

110. Kenyon CJ, Thorsson L, Borgström L, Newman SP. The effects of static charge in spacer devices on glucocorticosteroid aerosol deposition in asthmatic patients. Eur Respir J 1998; 11: 606–610.

111. Zainudin BM, Biddiscombe M, Tolfree SE et al. Comparison of bronchodilator responses and deposition patterns of salbutamol inhaled from a pressurised metered dose inhaler, as a dry powder, and as a nebulised solution. Thorax 1990; 45: 469–473.

112. Laube BL, Edwards AM, Dalby RN et al. The efficacy of slow versus faster inhalation of cromolyn sodium in protecting against allergen challenge in patients with asthma. J Allergy Clin Immunol 1998; 101: 475–483.

113. Derom E , Van Schoor J, Borgström L et al. Lung deposition and clinical effect of terbutaline delivered from pMDI and Turbuhaler on airway responsiveness in patients with asthma. Am J Respir Crit Care Med 2001; 164: 1398–1402.

114. Selroos O, Backman R, Forsen KO et al. Local side-effects during 4-year treatment with inhaled corticosteroids: a comparison between pressurized metered-dose inhalers and Turbuhaler. Allergy 1994; 49: 888–890.

115. Lipworth BJ. New perspectives on inhaled drug delivery and systemic bioactivity. Thorax 1995; 50: 105–110.

116. Borgström L. Local versus total systemic bioavailability as a means to compare different inhaled formulations of the same substance. J Aerosol Med 1998; 11: 55–63.

117. Thorsson L. Studies on the deposition, bioavailability and systemic activity of glucocorticoids in man. Thesis/Dissertation, Lund University, Lund, Sweden; 1998.

118. Brutsche MH, Brutsche IC, Munawar M et al. Comparison of pharmacokinetics and systemic effects of inhaled fluticasone propionate in patients with asthma and healthy volunteers: a randomised crossover study. Lancet 2000; 356: 556–561.

20 Genetics and gene therapy

Duncan M Geddes

 Key points

■ Most respiratory diseases have genetic linkages.

■ These linkages inform pathogenesis.

■ Genetic linkage may lead to screening, early diagnosis and new treatment.

■ Drug treatment may be individualised by genetic information.

■ Many proposed linkages are not confirmed in further studies.

In 1865 Mendel published his findings on the inheritance of peas. His concept of pairs of genes, one inherited from each parent, was politely ignored for 35 years until in 1900 three biologists independently came up with the same conclusions and acknowledged Mendel's foresight. For the next 50 years genetics developed slowly; progress then accelerated and there has been an explosion of knowledge over the past 10 years. DNA was discovered in 1953, the first complete genome sequence (for yeast) in 1996 and the first genome of a multicellular organism (a roundworm) in 1998. The year 2000 saw the first draft of the human genome.

A recent part of this explosion has been the linking of diseases to specific genes. First, for monogenic disorders such as cystic fibrosis and α_1-antitrypsin deficiency and then for more complex disorders with multiple genetic and environmental causes such as asthma and chronic obstructive pulmonary disease (COPD). The single-gene defects are relatively easy to study but the diseases they cause are all, because of natural selection, rare. In contrast, the polygenic disorders are common but difficult to study because of the variable interactions of the different genes with each other and with the environment. Recently, the study of genetic linkages has been simplified by a number of advances in analytical technique. As the map of the human genome becomes more complete, many more markers are available and so linkage becomes more precise. Micro-array

DNA and RNA chip technology allow many thousands of analyses in a single step.[1] The breeding of transgenic animals helps to define the function of genes, as does the developing discipline of proteomics.[2]

The potential of this genetic information is enormous and many have predicted a new chapter in the screening, prevention and treatment of human disease.[3] Others, however, have been more cautious, pointing out that simple concepts that can be applied to monogenic disease will be impossible to use for the benefit of complex common ones.[4] There have also been warnings about the ethical and societal conflicts that new genetic information will bring.[5] Whichever way the future evolves, doctors will need to digest and use this new genetic information for the benefit of their patients. This chapter summarises these recent advances as applied to respiratory medicine, together with their implications for the clinician. More details of the genetics of the individual conditions will be found in the relevant disease chapters.

Methodology

There are three basic steps in analysing the genetic components of a disease.[6] First, a linkage is established between the disease phenotype and a location on a human chromosome. Second, the gene responsible for this association is identified and third, the way in which mutations in the gene give rise to the disease is explored.

Linkage studies

These explore the way in which the expression of some trait (a phenotype) can be linked to some markers on human chromosomes, and were originally relatively crude because of the paucity of these markers. An early example was linking haemophilia to the X chromosome and at first cytogenetic differences were the only markers that could be used. Subsequently, as the human genome has become progressively better characterised, so more and more markers have become available and linkage studies have become simpler, quicker and more precise. Now using 80 000 single-nucleotide polymorphisms, diseases can be linked to relatively small stretches of DNA. Such linkage studies work best with well-defined phenotypes such as occur in monogenic diseases; for example, the presence or absence of cystic fibrosis within family members is very clear-cut. Linkage studies can screen the whole genome but are relatively insensitive and need large numbers of families unless the linkage is very strong. Furthermore, since many comparisons are made, statistical power is reduced. An alternative is to do an association study in which a possible association between a disease and a single genetic marker is explored usually in a case-control study. This is much more sensitive and uses conventional statistical significance but a candidate site needs to be identified first. Also there can be major difficulties with the precise definition of the disease phenotype as a result of incomplete expression or differences in ethnic background or environmental exposure.

The second step of moving from a linkage or association to a single gene used to involve cloning of fragments of DNA in order to establish more precise genetic linkage and to characterise the genes in that fragment of DNA. This so-called positional cloning has become much simpler as more genes have been identified together with their associated markers. It is therefore frequently possible to identify a likely gene close to an established linkage and to do further association studies to test its relevance (*positional candidate cloning*). For all these linkage and association studies an alternative is to use a so-called intermediate phenotype rather than the disease itself to establish the association. For example, the serum level of α_1-antitrypsin and IgE are intermediate phenotypes for inherited emphysema and asthma respectively.

Gene sequencing

The final step involves sequencing the gene itself and establishing some form of association between the disease phenotype (or intermediate phenotype) and a mutation. While originally this seemed to be a relatively clear-cut exercise, experience from monogenic diseases shows how complicated it can be. There are, for example, over 1000 separate disease-associated mutations on the cystic fibrosis gene alone. The situation for complex polygenic disorders in which multiple genes are involved may make a full analysis of the genetic components impossibly complex. With the technological advances of whole-genome mapping, together with DNA chips, the task of identifying disease-associated genes for the monogenic disorders has become relatively simple. In contrast, accurate case definition, the selection of appropriate controls and the range and diversity of genetic and environmental interactions are major challenges for the study of the polygenic disorders.

Monogenic diseases

Cystic fibrosis[7]

Cystic fibrosis is one of the commonest monogenic recessive diseases, affecting 1 in 2500 births in northern European popu-

lations. Carriers are healthy, although associations with asthma or increased fertility have been claimed. The CF gene was one of the first to be identified by chromosomal linkage followed by positional cloning and sequencing. The gene is on the long arm of chromosome 7 and its 27 exons express a 1480-residue transmembrane protein that functions as an epithelial cell chloride channel. Most of the disease-associated mutations occur in the nucleotide-binding domains of the protein, suggesting that these sites are critical for normal function. The discovery of the gene has led to an impressive increase in the understanding of the pathophysiology of the disease as well as the development of transgenic mice for further study of pathogenesis and new treatments. Mutational analysis has allowed a detailed study of the relationship between mutations (genotype) and the disease severity (phenotype). As a result, the clinical spectrum of cystic fibrosis disease now extends from congenital absence of the vas deferens, causing infertility in otherwise healthy males, through sinusitis and recurrent pancreatitis without lung disease to the full classical clinical disorder of lung infection with pancreatic insufficiency. The definition of this spectrum has made the clinical diagnosis more difficult and has raised wider societal issues such as the possible effect of the diagnostic label of cystic fibrosis on the insurance or mortgage prospects of somebody with the mildest form of the disease. Conversely, the ability to screen carriers and provide prenatal diagnosis is of undoubted benefit to couples at risk and could have major implications for the future prevalence of the condition. More controversially, genetic analysis allows neonatal screening for cystic fibrosis, but the value of this is still debated and such screening has not yet become routine. In spite of much promise and research activity, the identification of the gene has not yet led to any new genetic or small-molecule drug treatment.

Alpha-1-antitrypsin deficiency[8]

This recessively inherited deficiency of a serum antiprotease affects 1 in 10 000 of the population and is responsible for about 1% of cases of emphysema. The association of lung and liver disease with low circulating levels of the protein was well established before the discovery of the gene, and the two important disease-associated mutations (S and Z) were characterised by protein electrophoresis. Heterozygotes for the common M phenotype are healthy. Genetic analysis has led to characterisation of the mutations at codon 264 (S phenotype) and 342 (Z phenotype) and elucidation of the protein structure and structure–function relationships, but no new drugs have yet been developed because of this knowledge. The finding of an association between emphysema and polymorphisms in the untranslated region of the gene emphasises the complexity of genetic studies and their mechanisms. Population or neonatal screening for low levels of serum α_1-antitrypsin has not been thought worthwhile.

Immotile cilia syndrome[9]

This disorder of ciliary function is responsible for a variable combination of infertility, sinusitis, bronchiectasis and situs inversus and results from an abnormality of the dynein protein involved in ciliary movement. The disorder is recessively inherited, with a population frequency of about 1 in 34 000. Approximately 10 candidate genes encoding dynein heavy arms have been identified but the relevant gene for human disease is not yet known. Benefits from the discovery of the genetic basis of the disorder may include early diagnosis and treatment, an understanding of the pathophysiology and new drug targets. However, the disease is so rare that new treatments will not necessarily be developed.

Polygenic disorders

A genetic predisposition to common disorders may be suspected from clinical experience and confirmed by twin studies and more detailed epidemiology. Genetic analysis is much more complex than for monogenic disorders because of the influence of other genes and the environment. For example, it can be argued that genetic factors are important in COPD since only 16% of smokers develop the disorder. Alternatively, since there would be little COPD without smoking, genetic factors are arguably irrelevant. Nevertheless, there is great interest and activity in the study of the genetics of the common polygenic diseases with a view to prevention, early diagnosis and particularly the development of new treatments.

Asthma[10]

Epidemiological and twin studies have established that asthma runs in families and IgE levels have shown up to 70% inheritance. Genetic studies have therefore concentrated both on the clinical diagnosis of asthma within families and also on intermediate phenotypes such as IgE levels, bronchial hyper-responsiveness, eosinophil counts and atopy. So far, genome screens using techniques with relatively low sensitivity have identified around 10 candidate regions of interest with possible functional linkages (Table 20.1). Although not all these associations have been confirmed, there is a developing consensus, largely from epidemiological studies, that genes responsible for IgE and atopy are (not surprisingly) linked to asthma. Because of the complexity of the genetic associations and the fact that they may operate differently in different ethnic groups, it is difficult to see any immediate clinical applications and in particular no added value to diagnosis. While it is conceivable that screening

methods could identify high-risk families or individuals, such screening would need to be more sensitive than simpler measures such as atopy, family history or IgE levels.

The most immediate application is likely to be in drug discovery and drug prescribing. The best example so far is the β_2-adrenoreceptor. Homozygotes for a variant with glycine at position 16 (35% of Caucasians) have reduced responses to chronic beta-agonist treatment and this could help define ideal treatment (see below).

Chronic obstructive pulmonary disease[11]

Family and twin studies show a threefold variation in risk of developing COPD among European smokers due to inheritance. Conversely, Chinese and Japanese smokers appear to be less susceptible to COPD. There are many biologically plausible candidates for genetic linkage including proteases, antiproteases, inflammatory mediators, oxidants and antioxidants. Many linkages have been proposed (Table 20.2) but most have not been confirmed on retesting in other populations. So far, only α_1-antitrypsin deficiency is fully established as an inherited form of COPD.

Venous thrombosis and pulmonary embolism[12]

The blood-clotting cascade is well characterised and many genetic linkages have been confirmed (Table 20.3). Factor V Leiden (FVL) has a frequency of up to 20% of European populations, while deficiency of protein C or S is relatively rare

Table 20.2 Proposed genetic linkages and associations with chronic obstructive pulmonary disease

Category	Candidate
Antiproteases	α_1-antitrypsin, α_1-chymotrypsin
Blood group	Group A, B, Lewis non-secretor
Major histocompatibility complex	HLA-B7
Enzymes	Glutathione-S-transferase, microsomal epoxide hydrolase, cytochrome P450
Other	Vitamin D binding protein, TNF-α

Table 20.1 Genes and functions proposed as influencing the development of severity of asthma

Phenotype	Candidate
IgE, bronchial hyper-responsiveness	IL-4, IL-5, IL-9, IL-13
Eosinophils	MHC, TNF-α
Atopy, asthma	FcϵRIβ, CC16, TCR-α
Asthma	IFN-γ, IL-4α
Asthma severity	β-adrenergic receptor

Table 20.3 Genetic linkages and associations for thrombophilia

- Anti-thrombin
- Protein C
- Protein S
- Factor V Leiden
- Prothrombin
- Thrombomodulin
- Homocystinuria and homocystinaemia

(1 in 300). About 10% of first thrombotic episodes are associated with deficiency of protein S, C or antithrombin, rising to 50% when FVL is added. It is likely that interactions between thrombophilia genes and between genetic and other risk factors are much more important than any single genetic risk by itself. For example, the presence of FVL alone does not increase the risk of recurrence of thrombosis among those who have had a single previous episode, whereas the combination of FVL and a prothrombin mutation more than doubles the risk. Also, the genotype may affect the pattern of disease, FVL being more closely linked with deep-vein thrombosis than with pulmonary embolism.

A known thrombophilia risk alters future medical and surgical management, but neither the clinical value nor the cost-effectiveness of routine testing of people at risk of thrombosis (e.g. pregnancy, oral contraceptive use) has yet been established.

Lung cancer[13]

Unlike cancers of the breast or colon, no clear-cut inherited component of lung cancer has been found. This may be because of the overwhelming influence of cigarette smoking, with uncontrolled variables such as quantity smoked, brand and smoking technique. Nonetheless, genes are always involved in cancer and it has been estimated that the build-up of six to seven mutations in a single cell is responsible for malignant change. Such mutations are induced by chemical carcinogens in cigarette smoke, which can interact directly with oncogenes and with DNA repair. Oncogenes implicated in small-cell carcinoma and non-small-cell carcinoma of the lung are listed in Table 20.4.

Genetic study of lung cancer may benefit patients in three ways. First, genetic assays may be a sensitive screening tool for early diagnosis. The polymerase chain reaction assay on sputum stored from previous screening studies was more sensitive than cytology. Second, the genetic make-up of a tumour may predict prognosis. Third, prediction of chemotherapy response or the development of novel drugs (e.g. antibodies directed at oncogene products) may help treatment.

Table 20.4 Genetic linkages and associations for lung cancer

Gene	Oncogene/ suppressor	% frequency in SCCL	NSCCL
Fragile histidine triad	Suppressor	100	60
MYC	Oncogene	30	
P16	Suppressor	80	50
k-Ras	Oncogene		30
Rb	Suppressor	90	
Bcl2	Oncogene	25	10
p53	Suppressor	75	50
c-erb, B-2/neu	Oncogene		30

NSCCL, non-small-cell carcinoma of the lung; SCCL, small-cell carcinoma of the lung.

Table 20.5 Candidate genes for susceptibility to tuberculosis

Human leukocyte antigen	Vitamin D receptor
NRAMP1	Complement receptor 1
Tumour necrosis factor	Fucosyltransferase 2
Mannose-binding protein	INOS
Interferon-γ receptor	Chemokine receptors
Interleukin-1α, -1β, -4, -6, -10, RA	TH2 cluster

Tuberculosis[14]

Clinical experience suggests that genetic factors are important in tuberculosis. For example, susceptibility alters rapidly after a naive population is first exposed to the disease. This was observed in 1890 in an American Indian reservation, where the initial mortality of 10% dropped to 0.2%, presumably from selection of the genetically better protected. Similarly, monozygotic twins share susceptibility to tuberculosis. Genetic susceptibility has been studied in mice and rabbits as well as man and a number of genetic linkages have been discovered (Table 20.5). Interestingly, the susceptibility gene NRAMP appears to protect against sarcoidosis.

While population benefits have yet to be shown, screening for risk could provide better targeted vaccination and surveillance programmes.

Others

A range of genetic linkages to other pulmonary diseases as well as to normal lung function has been reported. These include sarcoidosis (NRAMP), obstructive sleep apnoea (many candidates), alveolar proteinosis and infant respiratory distress (surfactant proteins). This list is inevitably out of date as there are new additions almost every month. Indeed, it has been claimed that all human disease, with the possible exception of trauma, has a genetic component. There is much more to come.

Genetics and microbiology

The genomes of many viruses, bacterial and fungi have been mapped and others will follow. This information will inevitably inform the study of microbial virulence, pathogenicity and susceptibility to antibiotics as well as defining new targets for drug discovery. For example, drug resistance in tuberculosis is largely due to mutation of the bacterial genes encoding the targets used by these drugs. Although beyond the scope of this chapter, the possibilities of improvements in antibiotic treatment are exciting and imminent.

Genetics and pharmacology[15]

Pharmaceutical companies are investing in genetics in the belief that genetic information will revolutionise prescribing. There may be the following changes:

- **Drug discovery**. Any gene shown to be important in a disease may reveal a new pathogenetic mechanism as well as providing the protein structure involved. This predicts a new generation of drugs precisely aimed at individual molecules. The possibility of genetic therapies aimed at or comprising the genes themselves will be discussed below.
- **Disease variation**. Genetic analysis will help to define subgroups of common diseases. For example, there may well be quite different profiles of mediators among different asthmatics identifiable by genetic screening. Treatment could then be tailored accordingly.
- **Patient variation**. The response to a drug depends on many genetically controlled factors such as absorption, distribution, metabolism and elimination. Again, genetic screening could provide a pharmacological response profile to improve efficacy and reduce the risk of side effects. The acetylator status, which determines the metabolic speed and therefore risk of neuropathy from isoniazid, provides one simple example, while for asthma, genetic variation in the β_2-adrenoreceptor and polymorphism in the 5-lipoxygenase promoter region in relation to leukotriene therapy[16] may prove important. Nevertheless, this variant is rare in African and Japanese populations, emphasising how any genetic approach to prescribing will need to be individualised. In the future, clinical subsets of patients (steroid-resistant, aspirin-sensitive, etc.) may be identified by genetic testing, thus allowing more appropriate and safer prescribing.
- **Clinical trials and surveillance**. By defining the appropriate subjects for a new drug undergoing trial the numbers needed to show benefit would be reduced. More new drugs might therefore reach the market at lower cost. Furthermore, post marketing surveillance of rare side effects might be linked to a certain genotype, defining the at-risk population and limiting the damage done.

A single nucleotide polymorphism markers (a *Snip chip*) could be used to define an individual's drug response profile and so tell the prescriber what to do.

Genetics, ethics and society[5]

The chief areas of concern involve individuals' privacy and the possible misuse of genetic information, particularly in insurance, banking, employment and medical research. In particular, there are both personal and wider societal concerns about the prediction of future disease in a healthy person. As a result, many countries have already laid down far-sighted rules to protect the individual. In particular, laws are now in place to prevent genetic discrimination in insurance and employment, but such laws are new, have seldom been tested and may need to be amended in the light of experience and future changes. Research ethics committees now require statements about the confidentiality of any genetic tests done in the course of research and the requirement to ask for further consent for any additional tests to be performed on retained specimens. The situation with tests performed for clinical reasons is less clear.

Unfortunately, the word 'genetic' has acquired negative connotations in connection with genetic engineering, genetically modified foods and the debate about human cloning. There is, therefore, a danger that valuable medical advances may be impeded by over-restrictive legislation. The pharmaceutical industry has argued cogently that disease-susceptibility testing is very different from the genetic profile of drug response and that the concept of 'genetic testing' should not be applied to both.

Gene therapy

Genes ultimately control the structure and function of all cells in the body. It is therefore logical to attempt to modify disease by altering genetic control. Indeed, many drug treatments already act in this way: corticosteroids, for example, interact with the promoter regions of genes that control inflammation. Gene-therapy strategies differ according to the disorder and its pathogenesis. These strategies range from over-riding a mutant gene with the normal version in inherited diseases such as cystic fibrosis, through the introduction of a new gene or antisense oligonucleotide to modify function in an acquired disease such as cancer, to the more visionary concept of gene repair by homologous recombination. All these strategies require that genetic material reaches the right part of the cell and works when it gets there. The technological difficulties are formidable and although, during the 1990s, many experiments showed that the concepts underlying gene therapy were sound, by the year 2002 no such treatment had been developed for clinical use.

Delivering the gene to the cell

Molecules enter cells more easily when they are small and lipid-soluble than when they are large and carry an electric charge. Since the molecular weight of even the smallest gene is thousands of times larger than that of conventional drugs and all DNA is negatively charged, the problems of cell entry are considerable. Furthermore any DNA that enters a cell is likely to be broken down in the endosome or by nucleases in the cytoplasm, so very little reaches the nucleus. The two main ways round these problems are to load the DNA on to a virus that has evolved techniques of nuclear delivery or to link plasmid DNA to a liposome. Many viruses can deliver therapeutic genes but none is perfect for the job. Retroviruses are efficient but they are too small to accommodate large genes and only infect dividing cells. In contrast, the less efficient adenovirus can carry larger genes[17] and infect non-dividing cells but provokes an immune response. All viruses have to be inactivated to prevent replication and none as yet has a blameless safety record. In contrast, liposomes[18] are inherently safer but, so far, somewhat less efficient than viruses at gene transfer. Furthermore, plasmid DNA is grown in bacteria and so differs from mammalian DNA, resulting in a tendency to cause inflammation.[19]

Complete cDNA is likely to be necessary for replacement gene therapy for inherited disorders. In contrast, smaller fragments of nucleotides are much easier to deliver to cells and may have greater potential for human gene therapy for acquired diseases. Such oligonucleotides may be antisense to bind to and inactivate a gene or specially designed to bind to genomic DNA and induce single-nucleotide switching to repair mutant genes.

Delivering the gene to the lungs

Nebulisers, which deliver drugs to the airways, are also likely to be suitable for gene therapy. There are, however, some important problems to be overcome. First, DNA is relatively fragile and easily denatured, requiring a trade-off between nebuliser power and efficiency on the one hand and DNA stability on the other. Second, the effect of particle size, an important variable for nebulised drug delivery, on gene transfer efficiency is not known. Third, aerosols are preferentially delivered to healthy parts of the lung. This means that gene therapy for destructive lung diseases such as cystic fibrosis needs to be administered early and before the airways are damaged. Various vascular routes of delivery to the airways have been proposed, such as peripheral venous or bronchial arterial injection with subsequent passage of the gene through the vessel wall and then into the cells. This route avoids airway mucosal defences such as mucus and cilia but introduces other barriers.

Delivery to the pulmonary vessels and alveoli poses different but possibly less daunting challenges. Both viral and non-viral systems can be formulated to survive in the circulation and, since the pulmonary vascular bed is the first encountered after an intravenous injection, relative high levels of lung uptake are achievable. However, systemic administration inevitably reaches all other organs, including ovaries and testes, with the risk of unwanted effects and in particular germ-line gene transfer.

Gene therapy – which respiratory diseases?

Inherited disorders such as cystic fibrosis and α_1-antitrypsin deficiency are both suitable candidates and have attracted considerable research interest. Early clinical trials in cystic fibrosis have shown gene transfer to the airway epithelium and measurable change in chloride transport.[20-23] The challenge is to improve the efficiency of airway gene transfer. Similarly, early studies have shown expression of normal α_1-antitrypsin after gene transfer to the lungs but circulating levels are low and much more efficient gene transfer is needed.[24] It is much more likely that protein replacement therapy will be used for this indication.

All acquired respiratory diseases are potential candidates for gene therapy but few have yet reached the stage of human studies. Speculation has included anti-inflammatory gene therapy for airway inflammation in asthma, COPD or acute respiratory distress syndrome, lung water clearance in pulmonary oedema using genes for sodium transport, and a variety of gene-based approaches for lung cancer. There will be much more to come but, in view of the technical difficulties involved, it is unlikely that gene therapy for acquired diseases will be available before 2010.

? Unresolved questions

- Will multiple genetic linkages be too complex to apply to patient care?
- When will gene therapy be available?
- Will a personal gene chip be useful and, if so, when?
- How will society handle the ethics of genetic information?

References

1. Robinson BWS, Erle DJ, Jones DA et al. Recent advances in molecular biological techniques and their relevance to pulmonary research Thorax 2000; 55: 329–339.
2. Banks RE, Dunn MJ, Hochstrasser DF et al. Proteomics: new perspectives, new biomedical opportunities Lancet 2000; 356: 1749–1756.
3. Bell J. The new genetics in clinical practice. Br Med J 1998; 316: 618–620.
4. Holtzman NA, Marteau TM. Will genetics revolutionise medicine? N Engl J Med 2000; 343: 141–144.
5. Collins FS. Medical and societal consequences of the human genome project. N Engl J Med 1999; 341: 28–37.
6. Kaprio J. Genetic epidemiology. Br Med J 2000; 320: 1257–1259.
7. Davidson DJ, Porteous DJ. Genetics and pulmonary medicine – 1: The genetics of cystic fibrosis lung disease. Thorax 1998; 53: 389–397.
8. Mahadeva R, Lomas DA. Genetics and pulmonary medicine – 2: Alpha-1 antitrypsin deficiency, cirrhosis and emphysema. Thorax 1998; 53: 501–505.
9. Afzelius BA. Genetics and pulmonary medicine – 6: Immotile cilia syndrome: past, present and prospects for the future. Thorax 1998; 53: 894–897.
10. Hall IP. Genetics and pulmonary medicine – 8: Asthma. Thorax 1999; 54: 65–69.
11. Barnes PJ. Genetics and pulmonary medicine – 9: Molecular genetics of chronic obstructive pulmonary disease. Thorax 1999; 54: 245–252.
12. Laffan M. Genetics and pulmonary medicine – 4: Pulmonary embolism. Thorax 1998; 53: 698–702.
13. Roland M, Rudd RM. Genetics and pulmonary medicine – 7: Somatic mutations in the development of lung cancer. Thorax 1998; 53: 979–983.
14. Bellamy R. Genetics and pulmonary medicine – 3: Genetic susceptibility to tuberculosis in human populations. Thorax 1998; 53: 588–593.
15. Roses AD. Pharmacogenetics and future drug development and delivery. Lancet 2000; 355: 1358–1361.
16. Drazen J, Yandava CN, Dube I et al. Pharmacogenetic association between ALOX5 promoter genotype and the response to anti-asthma treatment. Nat Genet 1999; 22: 168–170.
17. Rosenfeld MA, Siegfried W, Yoshimura K. Adenovirus-mediated transfer of a recombinant alpha-1-antitrypsin gene to the lung epithelium. Science 1991; 252: 431–434.
18. Gao X, Huang L. A novel cationic liposome for efficient transfection of mammalian cells. Biochem Biophys Res Commun 1991; 179: 280–285.
19. Schwartz DA, Quinn TJ, Thorne PS. CpG motifs in bacterial DNA cause inflammation in the lower respiratory tract. J Clin Invest 1997; 100: 68–73.
20. Zabner J, Couture LA, Gregory RJ et al. Adenovirus-mediated gene transfer transiently corrects the chloride transport defect in nasal epithelia of patients with CF. Cell 1993; 75: 207–216.
21. Crystal RG, McElvaney NG, Rosenfeld MA et al. Administration of an adenovirus containing the human CFTR cDNA to the respiratory tract of individuals with cystic fibrosis. Nat Genet 1994; 8: 42–51.
22. Caplen NJ, Alton EWFW, Middleton PG et al. Liposome-mediated CFTR gene transfer to the nasal epithelium of patients with cystic fibrosis. Nat Med 1995; 1: 39–46.
21. Alton EFW, Stem M, Farley R et al. Cationic lipid mediated CFTR gene transfer to the lungs and nose of patients with cystic fibrosis: a double blind placebo controlled trial. Lancet 1999; 353: 947–954.
23. Wagner JA, Reynolds T, Moran ML et al. Efficient and persistent gene transfer of AAV-CFTR in maxillary sinus. Lancet 1998; 352: 1702–1703.
24. Canonico AE, Conary JT, Meyrick BO, Brigham KL. Aerosol and intravenous administration of human alpha 1 antitrypsin gene to the lungs of rabbits Am J Respir Cell Mol Biol 1994; 10: 24–29.

DEVELOPMENTAL ABNORMALITIES

21 Malformations

Andrew Bush

Key points

- Congenital lung malformations should be described clinically and pathologically using everyday language, without recourse to embryological speculation.

- The six pulmonary trees should be investigated systematically if a congenital malformation is suspected.

- Other areas that may impact on the respiratory system should be considered for potential malformations (heart and great vessels, chest wall, abdomen).

- The possibility of multisystem disease must be remembered.

- These principles will allow a clear description of the problem and facilitate the planning of appropriate treatment.

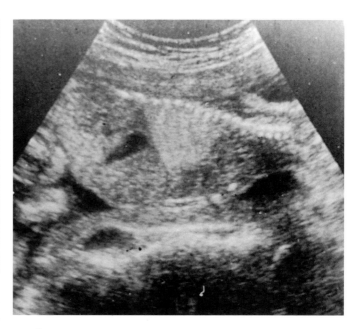

Fig. 21.1 Antenatal ultrasound showing a large, brightly echogenic congenital thoracic malformation (CTM) abutting the fetal spine.

Increasing skill in antenatal ultrasound has brought new problems. Virtually every fetus has been scanned by the second trimester, and abnormalities that would in the past have escaped detection are now being discovered. It is often unclear what advice should be offered to the parents to be. In the field of paediatric urology, harm was caused in the past by precipitate action. Dilated upper urinary tracts were drained in utero without it being appreciated that they were not obstructed and could have resolved without any treatment. Similarly, it has become clear that many large lung malformations seen at the routine 20 weeks gestation scan have largely disappeared by term (Fig. 21.1).

Furthermore, it is uncertain how these malformations should be described. The nomenclature of congenital lung disease was never very clear, with terms such as 'sequestrated segment', 'cystic adenomatoid malformation', 'hypoplastic lung' and 'malinosculation' being used to describe abnormalities that often overlap. Now, however, they are used inconsistently before and after birth. For example, 'congenital cystic adenomatoid malformation' is used by perinatologists to describe a lesion that may well disappear before birth[1] but is used postnatally to describe an abnormality that may require lobectomy. Congenital cystic adenomatoid malformation may have a pulmonary arterial supply or be supplied like a sequestration from systemic arteries, and histological features of these lesions may overlap.[2] New imaging modalities such as magnetic resonance imaging (MRI) and new treatment options such as embolisation of supplying vessels have become available. A complete reappraisal of the diagnosis, investigation and management of congenital lung disease is thus timely. This chapter will first describe a new approach to the nomenclature of congenital lung disease and then use this framework to describe in a logical manner the various abnormalities encountered in clinical practice.

Principles of classification of congenital lung disease

It is suggested that the following principles should be followed:

- What is *actually seen* should be described, without indulgence in embryological speculation, which may later be proved wrong.
- The description should be in everyday language, discarding Latin.
- The lung and associated organs should be approached in a systematic manner, because abnormalities are often multiple and associated lesions will be missed unless carefully sought.
- Clinical descriptions should not include pathological assumptions as the same clinical appearance (e.g. a multicystic mass) may have different pathological phenotypes.

Describe what is actually seen

This recommendation should be followed both before and after birth. In principle, antenatal ultrasound abnormalities should be described using such terms as 'increased echogenicity' or 'multiple cysts' rather than 'congenital cystic adenomatoid malformation'. In the postnatal period, a radiographic abnormality should be described as solid or cystic. If cystic, the cysts are either single or multiple, and the uniformity and thickness of the walls should be described. The cysts may be filled with air, or partially or completely with fluid; and their size should be recorded. Postnatally an air–fluid level implies that the abnormality is ventilated, albeit with a long time constant. If the lesion has been excised, the pathologist should describe the tissues found (epithelial, mesenchymal) and the contents of any cysts that may be present, thus giving a simple description of what is seen down the microscope. Any classification system that is to be robust cannot be based on embryological speculation.

Use everyday language

Many current medical terms are ambiguous and are best avoided. For example 'hypoplastic lung' could be taken as meaning a lung that is small but otherwise normal, or small because the underlying structure is abnormal; the term 'congenital small lung' (which for convenience can be shortened to CSL) avoids such ambiguity. The use of the term 'emphysema' in congenital lobar emphysema is another source of confusion as it implies lung destruction whereas in at least some variants (polyalveolar lobe) there may be too many, not too few alveoli.[3] What is actually seen is a congenital large hyperlucent lobe (which can be shortened to CLHL), which term should be used in clinical practice. Throughout this chapter, unwarranted established terms will be given in brackets after the proposed new term; for the convenience of the reader, the new terms will be spelled out in full, in addition to the abbreviated form being given. A summary comparison of old and new nomenclature is given in Table 21.1.

Use a systematic approach

The lung can be considered to be formed from six 'trees': bronchial, arterial (systemic and pulmonary), venous (systemic and pulmonary) and lymphatic. This chapter describes these trees in turn, followed by three other areas where malformations may impact on the respiratory system and which should thus also be assessed. These are the heart and great vessels, the chest wall including the respiratory neuromuscular apparatus, and the abdomen. Finally, the possibility of multisystem disease, for example tuberous sclerosis, should be considered. Each patient suspected of having a congenital lung malformation should be systematically evaluated along these lines, if important coexisting abnormalities are not to be missed.

Keep clinical descriptions and pathological diagnoses separate

This is an extension of the principle of describing what is seen. Black and white images on a scan are unlikely to be pathogno-

Table 21.1 Comparison of new and old terms

New nomenclature	Old terms superseded
Congenital large hyperlucent lobe (CLHL)	Congenital lobar emphysema Polyalveolar lobe
Congenital thoracic malformation (CTM; can also be numbered if that is shown to be helpful)	Cystic adenomatoid malformation (type 0–4) Sequestration (intra- and extrapulmonary) Bronchogenic cyst Reduplication cyst Foregut cyst
Congenital small lung (CSL)	Pulmonary hypoplasia
Absent lung, absent trachea	Agenesis of lung, tracheal aplasia
Absent bronchus	Bronchial atresia

monic of a single histological entity. It is more logical to describe the clinical appearances and construct a pathological differential diagnosis.

Classification of congenital lung disease

Abnormalities of the bronchial tree

Laryngeal and subglottic area

Abnormalities of the larynx and subglottic region usually present as a baby with severe respiratory distress or as stridor, which may or may not be associated with breathing difficulty. Severe abnormalities may result in endotracheal intubation being difficult or impossible. Absent larynx (laryngeal atresia) is usually due to cartilaginous overgrowth just below the vocal cords leaving only an inadequate channel. Viewed from above the larynx appears normal but attempts at intubation are unsuccessful and tracheostomy is required. The lungs are normal or large (congenital large lung – CLL, hyperplastic).[4] The commonest cause of stridor, characteristically starting shortly after but not at birth, is laryngomalacia, in which an abnormally long epiglottis partially occludes the laryngeal inlet during inspiration. This may be associated with variable amounts of pharyngo- and tracheomalacia. Congenital laryngeal cysts and webs are other causes of congenital stridor. With total or partial absence of the trachea (tracheal aplasia), the main bronchi either communicate only with each other or with the oesophagus.[5] In Down's syndrome, the trachea may be smaller than normal in both the sagittal and coronal planes.[6] Congenital intrinsic tracheal narrowing (stenosis) may take the form of a gradual tapering, an isolated segmental narrowing or a membranous web, or be due to a nodule of ectopic oesophageal tissue. Congenital extrinsic compression may be due to a vascular ring or pulmonary artery sling (left pulmonary artery arising from the right and looping behind the trachea, see below). This sling syndrome may form part of a ring–sling complex, in which the tracheal cartilages form complete rings, the left bronchus is short and the right is long (bronchial pseudoisomerism).[7] The abnormally long trachea is narrowed and usually funnel-shaped. This abnormality is difficult to correct surgically and the prognosis is poor. The trachea normally has 22 cartilages, with more in the ring–sling complex and fewer in infants with a congenitally short neck.

Bronchial arrangements and connections

Variations of the usual arrangement (situs solitus) are usually asymptomatic; these are mirror image arrangement (situs inversus), right isomerism, left isomerism, indeterminate, crossover segment and absence of one lung with contralateral usual bronchial arrangement. Abnormal connections that are often symptomatic may be to the oesophagus, a mediastinal cyst or a pulmonary parenchymal abnormality. Presentation may be with recurrent infection or (with H-type tracheo-oesophageal fistula) choking on feeding. Such abnormalities are best visualised by using bronchoscopy, a pressure injection of barium into the oesophagus (tube oesophagram) for tracheo-oesophageal fistula, or oesophagoscopy.

Abnormal arrangements require consideration of what makes, for example, a right lung. It is *not* being in the right hemithorax. In clinical practice, the two most useful determinants of right lung morphology are the presence of three, not two lobes and a very short main bronchus prior to the take-off of the upper lobe bronchus. A third criterion is the presence of an eparterial bronchus. Mirror-image arrangement must be distinguished from the superficially similar congenitally small (hypoplastic) right lung (Fig. 21.2) with right-sided heart (dextroposition) by determining bronchial morphology. This is important because each has a different implication and requires different investigation. Mirror image arrangement may be a feature of primary ciliary dyskinesia (discussed in Chapter 49, whereas a congenital small lung needs to have its vascular supply delineated (see below).

The term 'isomerism' is so entrenched that it is probably not feasible to replace it with, for example, bilateral right lung (BRL), which would be more logical. Nearly 80% of children with right isomerism (BRL) lack a spleen, leading to a risk of overwhelming pneumococcal sepsis. A similar proportion with left isomerism (bilateral left lung, BLL) have multiple small spleens.[8,9] The Ivemark syndrome consists of right isomerism (BRL), asplenia, a midline liver, malrotation of the gut and a variety of cardiac abnormalities including a common ventricle, totally anomalous pulmonary venous drainage and bilateral superior caval veins and right atria.[8] Left isomerism (BLL) is associated with multiple small spleens (polysplenia), a midline liver,

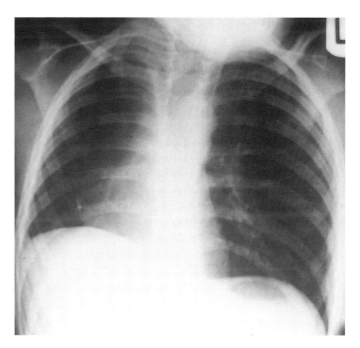

Fig. 21.2 Chest radiograph showing a right-sided congenital small lung (CSL), with the heart displaced into the right hemithorax. This is be distinguished from the superficially similar mirror-image organ arrangement.

malrotation of the gut, partially anomalous pulmonary venous drainage and cardiac septal defects.[9] Although non-familial, Ivemark's syndrome is confined to males whereas the other isomerism syndromes may affect either sex. Recently a syndrome of left bronchial isomerism, normal atrial arrangement, and severe tracheobronchomalacia has been described, extending the spectrum of left isomerism (BLL).[10]

Occasionally, a congenitally small lung may be so abnormal that its morphology can only be described as indeterminate. The contralateral lung morphology is, however, usually obvious. Quite commonly, minor deviations from the normal bronchial branching pattern may be seen, which may be associated with spontaneous pneumothorax.[11] A tracheal origin of one or more of the right upper lobe bronchi is usually of no clinical significance but may be a cause of recurrent right upper lobe collapse in an intubated patient if the endotracheal tube is low.

Abnormal bronchial branching and pulmonary lobation form a spectrum of abnormalities. Main bronchi may be displaced so that one or both whole lungs arise from the alimentary tract rather than the trachea.[5] This often accompanies absent trachea and probably represents a variety of tracheo-oesophageal fistula, but a bronchobiliary fistula (connecting the biliary and tracheobronchial trees, usually near the carina) may be part of a duplication of the upper alimentary tract from the level of the fistula to the ampulla of Vater.[12] Bile causes intense inflammation of the bronchial tree and in infancy the combination of cough with bile-stained sputum is typical of the condition. Bronchial diverticulosis possibly represents abnormal bronchial branching.[13] Other abnormalities of the bronchi include a double upper lobe bronchus and an accessory cardiac lobe bronchus arising from the intermediate bronchus. A 'bridging bronchus' crossing the mediastinum from left to right represents origin of the right lower lobe bronchus from the left bronchial tree.[14] Abnormalities of segmental bronchi include double bronchi to the apical segment of either upper lobe, either displaced or supernumerary, an absent right upper lobe apical segmental bronchus and separate origin of the apical segmental bronchus of the left lower lobe from the main bronchus.

A crossover lung segment is one with bronchial and arterial connections from the other side.[15] The crossover is usually from right to left, the right lung is small and the venous drainage anomalous, a variant of the 'scimitar' syndrome (see below). These are features that crossover lung segment shares with the equally rare condition 'horseshoe' lung, where there is fusion of the lungs behind the heart and in front of the oesophagus.[16] However, unlike 'horseshoe' lung, there is no fusion of the lungs; the pleural cavities are separate and the crossover segment lies in a pleural recess behind the heart that communicates with the pleural cavity on the side from which the segment derives.

Abnormal lobation of the lungs does not imply an abnormal pattern of bronchial branching: lack or incomplete development of one or more interlobar fissures is common despite the presence of five lobar bronchi. Extra fissures separating off lung segments as extra lobes are also common, particularly the lingula and the medial basal and apical segments of the lower lobes.[17] Fissures accommodating blood vessels may also be found, so that an azygos lobe may be formed by the parasagittal separation of the medial part of the right or left upper lobes by the azygos

and hemiazygos veins respectively. Absence of a lobe (and its bronchus) is rare.

Specific disorders of the bronchial tree

Absent lung

Absent lung (aplasia) is not uncommon but absence of a lobe (which must be distinguished from left isomerism) or of both lungs is rare. There may be a rudimentary bronchial stump, an important point in unilateral absence as secretions tend to pool in the stump, become infected and spill over to infect the contralateral lung.[18] With bilateral absence of the lungs the trachea ends blindly and the pulmonary artery arises from the aorta. Absent lung is often associated with other malformations and in unilateral absence these are often on the same side of the body.[19] In unilateral absence (Fig. 21.3) the surviving lung is enlarged and the number of alveoli is doubled but the bronchi are normal.[20] Nevertheless, there is a significant reduction in vital capacity and exercise tolerance may be reduced. The congenital bronchial branching pattern abnormalities and their appearances on computed tomography (CT) have recently been reviewed.[21]

Small lungs

Small lungs (hypoplasia) may be normal or abnormal in form. Alveoli are reduced in number or size. Normal right and left lung weights at term are 21 g and 18 g respectively and the lung/body weight ratio exceeds 0.012.[22] The reduction in alveoli may be associated with fewer airway generations, the degree of loss depending upon how early lung development was impaired. Development of airways down to the terminal bronchioles is complete by 16 weeks and the whole gas conductive system is complete by birth, unlike the alveoli and alveolar ducts, which continue to grow postnatally.[23] It follows that correction after birth of such causes of small lung as diaphragmatic hernia may permit at least some growth of alveoli, but not airways.[24]

Small lungs are seldom an isolated finding and are usually associated with a variety of other malformations.[25] These include diaphragmatic defects, renal anomalies, extralobar pulmonary parenchymal malformations and severe neuromuscular and musculoskeletal disorders. Most of these associations have a causal relationship (see below) but some, such as that with Down's syndrome,[26] are unexplained. Lung growth before birth is dependent upon blood supply, availability of space, respiratory movements taking place in utero and fluid filling the airways. The causes of small lungs therefore include the following (Tables 21.2 & 21.3):

- **Congenital abnormalities of blood vessels supplying the lungs**, e.g. isolated pulmonary stenosis and Tetralogy of Fallot. Even subtle disturbances of pulmonary haemodynamics have been shown to perturb lung development.
- **Compression of the lungs by intrathoracic masses**, e.g. congenital diaphragmatic hernia.
- **Compression of the lungs by chest-wall deformity**, e.g. Jeune's asphyxiating thoracic dystrophy. The lungs continue to grow after birth, so infantile scoliosis may cause postnatal hypoplasia.[27]

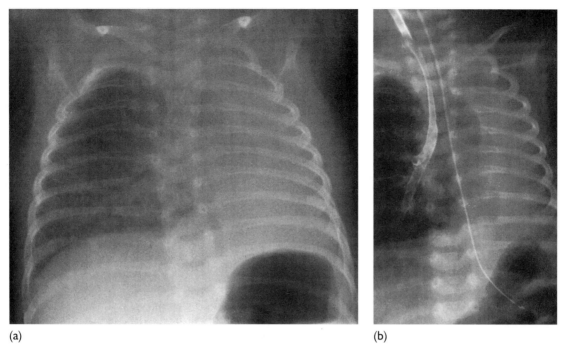

(a) (b)

Fig. 21.3 Left lung agenesis. a. Chest X-ray shows an opaque left hemithorax that is small and has narrowed intercostal spaces. The right lung is herniating across the midline. b. Bronchogram shows absent left bronchus and a segment of complete cartilage rings in the trachea.

Table 21.2 Causes of bilateral congenital small lungs

System fault	Example
Lack of space	Abnormal thoracic, abdominal or amniotic cavity contents (Table 21.3)
Abnormal vascular supply	Pulmonary valve or artery stenosis, tetralogy of Fallot
Neuromuscular disease	Central nervous system, anterior horn cell, peripheral nerve or muscle disease reducing fetal breathing movements

Table 21.3 Congenital small lungs due to extrapulmonary mechanical factors

Abnormal thoracic contents	Diaphragmatic hernia Pleural effusion Large congenital thoracic malformation
Thoracic compression from below	Abdominal tumours Ascites
Thoracic compression from the sides	Amniotic bands Oligohydramnios Asphyxiating dystrophy/scoliosis

■ **Lack of respiratory movements in utero** because of neuromuscular disease. Any interruption of the pathway from the brainstem to the muscle fibres will have this effect, e.g. antenatal onset of spinal muscular atrophy and myotonic

dystrophy inherited from the mother, who may herself be undiagnosed until after the birth of the affected baby.
■ **Oligohydramnios**, caused by either chronic leakage or deficient production of amniotic fluid. The mechanism whereby oligohydramnios causes small lungs could again be compressive but manometry shows that amniotic pressure is reduced rather than raised in oligohydramnios.[28] Loss of lung liquid is probably more important; experimental tracheal ligation prevents the adverse pulmonary effects of oligohydramnios[29] and human fetuses with renal agenesis and an absent larynx have large lungs.[4,15] Fetal urine contributes to amniotic fluid and renal agenesis and posterior urethral valves are important causes of oligohydramnios. Potter's syndrome consists of an abnormal facial appearance, small lungs and absent kidneys. Although oligohydramnios is commonly thought to be the cause of the pulmonary abnormality,[30] a lack of renal metabolites has also been proposed.[31]

Disorders of the bronchial walls

Abnormalities in bronchial wall calibre may result in all or part of the bronchial tree being too large or too small. They may present with recurrent infections, steroid unresponsive wheeze or stridor. Congenital tracheobronchomegaly (Mounier-Kuhn's syndrome) is characterised by tracheomalacia and bronchiectasis. The major airways are greatly dilated; in the normal adult the maximum transverse diameters of the trachea and main bronchi are 20 mm and 14.5 mm respectively.[32] There are saccular bulges between the cartilages. Bronchial clearance is impaired, resulting in recurrent respiratory infection.[33]

This syndrome generally presents between the ages of 30 and 50 years and is more common in males.[34] An autosomal recessive connective-tissue defect has been postulated.[35] This is supported by the occasional association of Mounier-Kuhn's syndrome with Ehlers–Danlos syndrome,[36] cutis laxa[37] or Kenny–Caffey syndrome.[38]

A rare cause of congenital tracheobronchomalacia is the presence of oesophageal remnants in the wall of the trachea, which is generally seen in association with oesophageal atresia and tracheo-oesophageal fistula.[39]

Localised narrowing, and in particular obstruction due to an absent bronchus, often results in cystic degeneration of the lobe distal to the obstruction before birth, as fetal lung liquid continues to be secreted and cannot drain into the amniotic cavity. Absent bronchus may be detected radiographically in an asymptomatic individual (Fig. 21.4) and presentation may be late, on average at age 17 years.[40,41] The radiological appearances are virtually diagnostic, consisting of an ovoid hilar opacity, most commonly in the left upper lobe, with branches radiating out into a distal area of hyperlucency. The opacity represents a distended, mucus-filled bronchus that is continuous with the distal airways but has no proximal connection. Infection may result in inflammation and fibrosis. The interruption to the airway may take the form of a membrane, a fibrous cord or a gap. The distal hyperlucency is due to collateral ventilation and air-trapping. Failure to identify the congenital nature of the problem may lead to a misdiagnosis of mucus plugging. Unlike in absent bronchus, there is no focal opacity in CLHL (congenital lobar emphysema). The continuity of the cyst with the distal airways and the hyperinflation of the distal lung distinguish absent bronchus from bronchogenic cyst (the nomenclature of which is

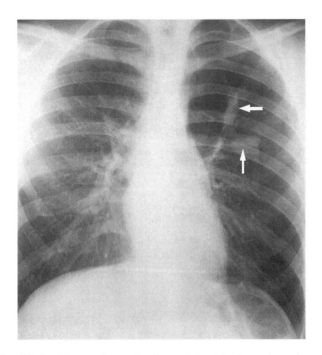

Fig. 21.4 Chest radiograph of an adult with absent bronchus: a branching density radiates into the hyperlucent left upper lobe (arrows).

discussed later) but the two conditions are occasionally associated.[42] True congenital bronchiectasis is much rarer than was previously thought.

Congenital bronchomalacia may be isolated, often with a good prognosis, at least in the short term,[43] or associated with other congenital abnormalities, including connective tissue disorders and Larsen's and Fryn's syndromes.[44–46] Williams & Campbell described a syndrome of diffuse bronchomalacia affecting the second to the seventh generations of bronchi.[47] Its occurrence in siblings[48] and the very early onset of symptoms suggests a congenital aetiology. Bronchomalacia may also be secondary to other congenital abnormalities such as vascular rings. Fixed bronchial narrowing may be due to defects in the wall (e.g. complete cartilage rings) or extrinsic compression by an abnormal vessel or cyst.

Abnormal airway connections

The separation of those parts of the primitive foregut destined to form the lower respiratory tract normally proceeds in a cephalad direction and if this is incomplete the two may communicate in a tracheo-oesophageal fistula (Fig. 21.5). The proximal part of the oesophagus usually ends in a blind sac and the distal part takes origin from the lower trachea, but the anatomy varies. Presentation is in the newborn period if the oesophagus is blind-ended. A direct connection between an otherwise normal oesophagus and trachea (H-type fistula) may present late, with recurrent infection and even lung abscess.[49] Symptoms may include bouts of coughing after drinking. Treatment is surgical and the prognosis is good. Histological examination shows that abnormalities in the wall of the trachea extend beyond the fistula: there is often widespread loss of cartilage and squamous metaplasia.[39,50] Communication between the trachea and a congenital cyst is also recorded.[51] Late presentations of such abnormal connections have been described.[52]

Alveolar disorders

Counting numbers of alveoli requires an open lung biopsy and is usually only of theoretical importance. CLHL (congenital lobar emphysema) is an example of an alveolar disorder. In some cases it is due to partial obstruction of the lobar bronchus leading to air-trapping. The obstruction may be caused by external compression by a cyst or abnormal blood vessel or by intrinsic abnormalities such as mucosal flaps, mucous plugs or twisting of the lobe on its pedicle.[53] A deficiency of bronchial cartilage is diagnosed by exclusion; in practice the cause of CLHL is frequently not identified. Some patients also have congenital cardiac anomalies.

Congenital large hyperlucent lobe affects the left upper lobe in about half of cases and the right middle and right upper lobes in most of the remainder; the lower lobes are affected in less than 10% of cases. It may cause severe respiratory distress in the neonatal period but may also be a chance finding in an adult.[54] Curiously, it almost never becomes infected; if CLHL is the seat of recurrent infection, suspect that the appearances are secondary to bronchial stenosis. Males are affected more than females but the condition is usually not familial. Some patients require early surgical excision because of respiratory embarrassment

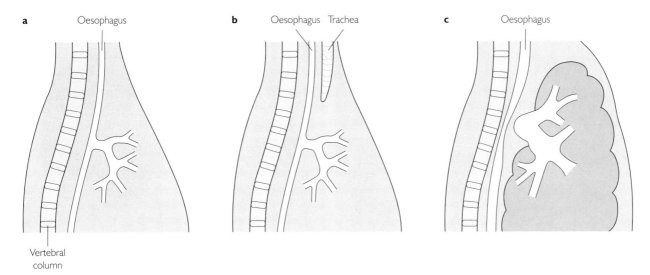

a Oesophagus   b Oesophagus Trachea   c Oesophagus

Vertebral
column

Fig. 21.5 Abnormal tracheal development and abnormal connections between trachea and oesophagus. a. Absent trachea, bronchi arise from oesophagus. b. Blind-ended proximal trachea, distal segment arises from oesophagus. c. Absent trachea, no proximal bronchial connection, lungs distended with fluid.

but, if there are no clinical problems, observation suffices and the long-term outlook is good (Fig. 21.6).

Another cause of CLHL is a polyalveolar lobe, which can only be diagnosed pathologically. A polyalveolar lobe has a normal number of conductive airways but an increased number of alveoli in each acinus.[3] The affected lobe is large and hyperlucent but individual alveoli are not increased in size. The number of alveoli in an acinus is best assessed by counting the intercepts made by alveolar walls on a line from the terminal bronchiole to the interlobular septum.[55] The number of alveoli depends on the age of the child but, in general, the radial count is 2–5 in fetuses, 5–10 in infants and 10–12 in children a few years old. These figures are greatly exceeded in a polyalveolar lobe.

Solid and cystic lesions: clinical approach

Clinical presentation varies with age (Table 21.4). Antenatally the lesions present as an abnormality on ultrasound, rarely associated with a pleural effusion or fetal hydrops. In the newborn period, they may be asymptomatic or present with respiratory distress. Infection is rare under 1 year of age.[56] In later childhood or adulthood, they may be a chance finding, cause recurrent unifocal infection, haemoptysis[57] or haemothorax,[58] or undergo malignant change.[59] Unusual infections such as tuberculosis and aspergillosis[60] have been described. Other presentations include bronchiectasis, bronchopleural fistula and airway obstruction mimicking asthma.[61]

When assessing patients with a suspected congenital lung malformation, it is more logical to describe cystic abnormalities by their appearance, whether on images or pathologically. The use of terms like 'reduplication cyst' and 'bronchogenic cyst' in clinical practice, prior to the resection of the abnormality, implies embryological and/or pathological information and is to be discouraged. A better clinical term, which makes no assumptions, is congenital thoracic malformation (CTM), some forms

Table 21.4 Presentation by age of congenital thoracic malformation

Age	Presenting feature
Antenatal	Intrathoracic mass Pleural effusion Fetal hydrops
Newborn period	Respiratory distress Stridor Cardiac failure Chance finding
Later childhood/adulthood	Recurrent infection (including tuberculosis, aspergillosis) Haemoptysis, haemothorax Bronchiectasis, bronchopleural fistula Steroid-resistant airway obstruction Cardiac failure Chance finding Malignant transformation

of which have been described as a congenital cystic adenomatoid malformation, CCAM, or congenital pulmonary airway malformation, CPAM. CTM encompasses a spectrum of conditions, clinically described as either cystic, intermediate or solid.[62] It will be seen that the clinical definition of CTM includes what the pathologist may subsequently describe as a CCAM, a bronchogenic or reduplication cyst, or other more specific term (Fig. 21.7). CTMs may be calcified.[63] Critical to the clinical approach is the definition of the other pulmonary trees (see above); even a 'simple' cyst may be rather more complex than first thought after more detailed investigation.

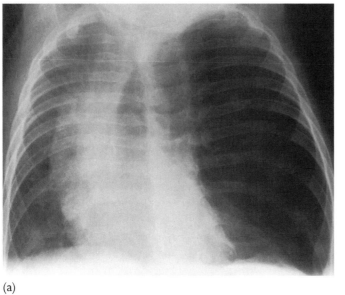

(a)

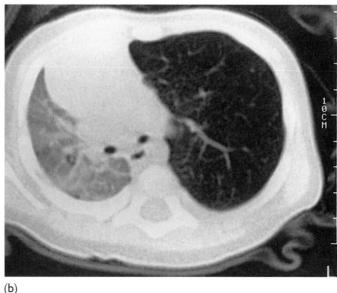

(b)

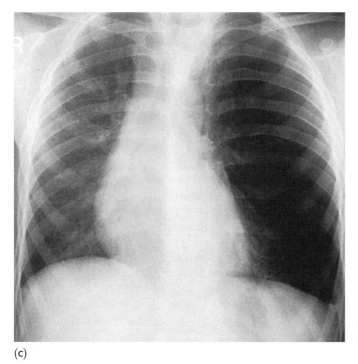

(c)

Fig. 21.6 Natural history of congenital large hyperlucent lobe (CLHL) (congenital lobar emphysema). a. The chest radiograph shows a hugely distended left upper lobe with marked mediastinal displacement and collapse of the left lower lobe in an infant aged 6 months. b. The corresponding computed tomography appearances. The infant was asymptomatic despite these dramatic appearances. c. Chest radiograph 2 years later. Although the changes of CLHL are still present, they are much less dramatic. The child has remained well without treatment.

Solid and cystic lesions: pathological approach

The same constraints of clarity outlined above should apply to the pathologist as to the clinician. The term congenital thoracic malformation is preferred in pathological descriptions, attaching the qualifier cystic, intermediate or solid, as above, and describing the nature of the cellular components in terms of what is seen down the microscope, without speculating about what tissue they may have been derived from and how the journey was accomplished.

'Bronchogenic and other foregut cysts' are one type of CTM recognisable by cartilage and glands in their wall and a lining of respiratory epithelium. They are usually situated in the mediastinum close to the carina (51%) but may be found in the right paratracheal region (19%), alongside the oesophagus (14%), at the hilum of the lung (9%) or in a variety of other locations (7%), including the substance of the lungs and even beneath the diaphragm.[64] Some cysts are lined by respiratory epithelium but lack cartilage in their walls. Congenital lung cysts are often not discovered until adult life, either as an incidental radiographic finding or because of complications, which include infection, haemorrhage and, in rare instances, neoplastic transformation.[65] Cysts may also have a gastric, intestinal or squamous epithelial lining, a muscle coat and an absence of

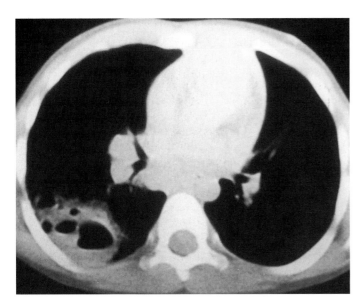

Fig. 21.7 Computed tomography showing a chronically infected, multicystic congenital thoracic malformation (CTM) that presented as recurrent chest infections. Lobectomy was undertaken, with a good result.

cartilage. This type is usually situated in the posterior mediastinum or, as they may be associated with vertebral malformations, even within the spine.[66] They may also be associated with abdominal cysts.

Pathologically, five patterns of CPAM have been recognised. Clinically, they may also be mimicked by other conditions such as pulmonary hamartoma or ectopic tissue (below), which are readily distinguished pathologically. If the preferred CTM nomenclature is used, these five types are seen as part of an extended pathological spectrum incorporating other cystic lesions as above. The nomenclature of the five types may be retained and, if thought useful, numbers may be allocated to the various pathological types of cyst. Whether such an extended pathological classification is useful or practical is beyond the scope of this chapter. Type 0, previously described as acinar dysplasia[67] or congenital acinar aplasia,[68] is composed of tissue looking like primitive bronchi whereas type 4 is of alveolar appearance in structure. As with any CTM, the blood supply may be from either or both the pulmonary artery and the aorta.

Some workers incorporate sequestration into what was previously described as the CPAM spectrum.[69] The fact that extralobar sequestrations may contain tissue identical to CTM underscores the logic of combining rather than separating these two conditions[2,70] and dropping the terms sequestration, CPAM and CCAM in favour of a single, catch-all term such as CTM. The five pathological types formerly described as CPAM, now replaced by the extended spectrum of CTM, will be described in turn. These types are not separate entities; overlap has been described.

Type 0 CTM (acinar dysplasia) is incompatible with life, being seen in term or premature babies who are cyanosed at birth and survive only a few hours. It is usually associated with cardiovascular anomalies and dermal hypoplasia. The lungs are small and firm throughout. Microscopically, bronchial-type

airways that have cartilage, smooth muscle and glands are separated by abundant mesenchymal tissue.

Type 1 CTM (cystic CCAM) is the commonest type and is usually readily resectable. The boundary between the lesion and the adjacent normal lobe is sharply delineated but there is no capsule. Presentation is usually with neonatal respiratory distress but the condition is increasingly detected in utero by ultrasonography.[71] Alternatively, recurrent infections in older children or even in young adults may first prompt investigation.[72] Radiographically, air-filled cysts, usually limited to one lobe, compress the rest of the lung, depress the diaphragm and cause mediastinal shift. The cysts range in size from 1 cm to 10 cm. They are lined by pseudostratified ciliated columnar epithelium interspersed with rows of mucous cells of pyloric type. The latter cells may be the site of malignant change (see below).[65,73] The relevant bronchus is often absent,[74] yet the cysts are usually radiolucent, presumably as a result of collateral ventilation.

Type 2 CTM (intermediate-type CCAM) is the second most frequent type. It is seen in the first month of life and is usually associated with other anomalies that adversely affect the prognosis – renal agenesis, cardiovascular defects, diaphragmatic hernia and syringomyelia. This variety is sponge-like, consisting of multiple small cysts as well as solid, pale, tumour-like tissue. Microscopically the cysts are seen to be dilated bronchioles separated by normal alveoli. Occasional examples contain striated muscle. This type of lesion may be also identified within extralobar sequestrations.[70,75]

Type 3 CTM (solid-type CCAM) is uncommon and occurs almost exclusively in male babies, often causing hydramnios.[71] It is a large, bulky lesion that typically involves and expands a whole lobe, the others being compressed and the mediastinum displaced. The remaining pulmonary tissue is underdeveloped. The prognosis is dependent upon the amount of unaffected lung. Microscopically, an excess of bronchiole-like structures are separated by small air spaces that have a cuboidal lining. Unlike the preceding types there is no cystic change.

Type 4 CTM is relatively uncommon (10–15%) and presents as infantile respiratory distress or repeated childhood pneumonia. Radiographically, there are large air-filled cysts with compression of the other thoracic structures; pneumothorax occasionally complicates this condition. The cysts are peripheral and thin-walled. They have a simple lining composed of type I alveolar epithelial cells resting upon loose mesenchymal tissue.

So-called mesenchymal cystic hamartoma is classified as a further type of CTM. This lesion was first described in 1986,[76] since when only a few more cases have been reported.[77] The condition may cause no symptoms until adult life, when it may present with haemoptysis, pneumothorax, haemothorax or pleuritic pain. Chest radiograph shows one or more cystic nodules, sometimes with air–fluid levels, generally bilateral. Sarcomatous transformation has been described.[77,78] Mesenchymal cystic hamartoma may represent a late-presenting, low-grade pleuropulmonary blastoma but its predilection for adults and common bilaterality is against this. The lesions may be supplied by bronchial, intercostal or phrenic arteries, underscoring the similarity with the CTM spectrum. Pathological examination shows them to consist of multilocular, thin-walled cysts lined by primitive mesenchymal cells that support a ciliated cuboidal epithelium. In places the epithelium is continuous with that lining adjacent bronchioles. The mesenchymal cells have dark, oval nuclei and inconspicuous cytoplasm and show only rare mitoses. They do not stain for smooth-muscle actin, a reaction that is usually positive in both myometrial stromal sarcoma and lymphangioleiomyomatosis, from which these lesions have to be distinguished.

Muscular hamartomas, which are small focal proliferations of smooth muscle, are occasionally observed incidentally in the lung. They are generally stellate in outline and almost always the muscle is intermingled with fibrous tissue. They are often considered to be hamartomatous but it is possible that they represent old scars in which there is prominent reactive smooth muscle hyperplasia. A case reported as 'diffuse fibro-leiomyomatous hamartomatosis'[79] is possibly just a further example; while some 'multiple pulmonary leiomyomatous hamartomas' possibly represent the condition of so-called benign metastasising leiomyomas. Despite these cautions, apparently genuine examples of smooth muscle hamartomas are occasionally reported in the lung, sometimes associated with similar lesions in the bowel and liver.[80]

'The sequestration spectrum' has been used to indicate that a portion of lung exists without appropriate bronchial and vascular connections. Classically, no airway connects the lesion to the tracheobronchial tree and the blood supply is systemic, but in some cases there is a normal airway.[81] Alternatively, an airway may connect the sequestration to the oesophagus or stomach in a complex bronchopulmonary–foregut malformation,[82] or ectopic pancreatic tissue may be present within the sequestration.[83] Occasionally, sequestration is associated with duplication of the oesophagus, stomach or pancreas.[83]

There is therefore a spectrum of abnormalities associated with pulmonary sequestration.[69,84] Conventionally, two forms are recognised, extralobar, which has its own covering of visceral pleura, and intralobar, which is embedded in otherwise normal lung. Both are probably part of the CTM spectrum. Extralobar sequestration is generally detected in infancy because of associated malformations and affects males four times more frequently than females. In contrast, intralobar sequestration is often an isolated anomaly and therefore unrecognised until adult life. It has a male-to-female ratio of 3:2.[85] About two thirds of all sequestrations are found on the left.[85] Intralobar sequestrations are typically located in the posterior basal segment of the left lower lobe and extralobar sequestrations beneath the left lower lobe. There is often a defect in the diaphragm and about 15% of extralobar sequestrations are abdominal. The veins leaving an extralobar sequestration generally join the azygos or other systemic veins whereas an intralobar sequestration usually has normal pulmonary venous connections, but as with all CTMs, any combination of arterial supply and venous drainage is possible.

Some workers believe that the intralobar variety is an acquired condition in which the aberrant artery is a dilated systemic collateral to a focus of infection, basing this on the relative sparsity of other malformations associated with this type of sequestration and its rarity in perinatal autopsies.[86] However, although the incidence of associated anomalies is lower than with extralobar sequestrations (50–70%), it is still appreciable

(6-12%)[87] and the rarity of the condition in neonates may be because it is easily overlooked until there is cystic degeneration or infection.

The lung tissue in a sequestration is often poorly developed and cystically dilated. The cysts are lined by columnar or cuboidal epithelium, or the sequestered lung may be entirely composed of structures resembling alveolar ducts. Mucus distends the multiple intercommunicating spaces and the lesion appears solid radiographically, unless air enters through a bronchial connection or, in the case of intralobar sequestration, by collateral ventilation, when fluid levels are often seen. In the absence of associated anomalies, detection is unlikely unless a chest radiograph is requested for some other reason or infection ensues.

Abnormally placed pulmonary tissue ('pulmonary ectopia') and abnormal intrapleural tissue

Two categories of ectopia need to be considered – ectopia of nonpulmonary tissues in the thorax and ectopia of lung tissue outside the thoracic cavity.

Abnormal intrapleural adrenocortical tissue,[88] thyroid (lacking C-cells)[89] and liver[90] have all been described in the lung and pancreatic tissue has been noted within so-called intralobar sequestrations with gastrointestinal connections.[74,83] Ectopic striated muscle is recorded in sequestered or small lungs[91] and occasionally as an isolated pulmonary abnormality,[92] sometimes tumour-like.[93] Rarely, a whole kidney may be found above the diaphragm but outside the lung.[94] There may be ectopic lung tissue in the neck, the abdomen or the chest wall, often associated with skeletal or diaphragmatic abnormalities. Some examples of abdominal pulmonary ectopia have been considered to represent extralobar sequestration as well as ectopia.[95]

Abnormalities of the arterial tree

When surgery is contemplated for any CTM, it is important that any abnormal vasculature is identified in advance. Inadvertent severance of anomalous systemic arteries has led to fatal haemorrhage, while ligation of anomalous veins from adjacent non-sequestered lung has led to infarction of normal tissue. The pulmonary and systemic arterial trees need to be considered separately. Systemic arterial abnormalities of the great vessels of the mediastinum can be separated from those of the bronchial circulation (normally 1–2% of the left ventricular output) and other pathological collaterals. The pulmonary capillary bed may be bypassed, leading to direct arteriovenous communication; or absent, resulting in minimal pulmonary arteriovenous connections.

Pulmonary arterial abnormalities

In general, pulmonary arterial and venous arrangement mirrors bronchial arrangement. Exceptions to this include congenital origin of the left pulmonary artery from the right (pulmonary artery sling, see above; Fig. 21.8). There may also be a crossover arterial segment, with the right upper lobe supplied by a branch from the left pulmonary artery, so preoperative pulmonary

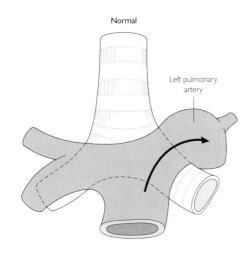

Normal

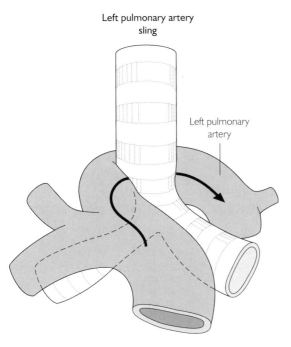

Left pulmonary artery
sling

Fig. 21.8 Left pulmonary artery sling syndrome. a. The normal arrangement; the arrow indicates the course of the left pulmonary artery. b. In the left pulmonary artery sling syndrome the left pulmonary artery passes to the right and then backwards over the origin of the right main bronchus before crossing to the left side behind the trachea at its bifurcation and in front of the oesophagus

angiography is essential. Surgical repair of a sling with a crossover may result in infarction of the right upper lobe if the abnormal vessel has not been discovered. Isolated crossover pulmonary artery branches in the absence of bronchial crossover are occasionally seen. They cross the mediastinum to supply lung segments that often are abnormal in other ways.

Pulmonary stenosis may affect lobar and segmental vessels as well as the main pulmonary arteries and the narrowings may be multiple. Unilateral absence of a pulmonary artery leads to

the lung on that side receiving only systemic blood, through either anomalous systemic arteries or enlarged bronchial arteries.[96] The two sides are affected equally frequently and the defect may be isolated or associated with other cardiovascular anomalies, typically tetralogy of Fallot with absent left pulmonary artery and patent arterial duct when the right pulmonary artery is missing.[96] Patients with isolated unilateral absence may lead a normal life or symptoms may not arise until adult life; one third remain completely asymptomatic.[97] Symptoms include pulmonary infection or bleeding from bronchopulmonary anastomoses.[98] Ipsilateral lung tumour has been reported.[99] Pulmonary hypertension may also develop.[100] Clinically, the condition may be difficult to distinguish from embolic occlusion and obliterative bronchiolitis. The presence of other congenital defects would militate against these, and the absence of mosaic attenuation on computed tomography would point away from obliterative bronchiolitis. Only a short segment of the artery may be lacking and surgical correction may be possible.[101] In other cases, pulmonary arteries may be difficult to identify histologically and they tend to be overshadowed by hypertrophied bronchial arteries. Pulmonary hypertension develops in 18% of patients with an isolated defect and more often when there are other vascular anomalies: surgical ligation of one artery has little effect on the contralateral vasculature in adults but the high fetal pulmonary vascular resistance persists if ligation is perinatal.[96]

Anomalous systemic arteries supplying the lung may be associated with any CTM or even be an isolated finding.[102] They are also found if the pulmonary artery is absent and may also be part of complex arteriovenous malformations. They may also be an isolated finding. One or both pulmonary arteries may take origin from the aorta.[103] Bilateral origin from the aorta is part of the spectrum of common arterial trunk, and usually presents to the paediatric or fetal cardiologist. Unilateral origin of a pulmonary artery from the aorta may be an isolated abnormality, sometimes presenting with persistent tachypnoea.

Congenitally small unilateral pulmonary artery is usually seen in association with an ipsilateral small lung. Normal pulmonary blood flow is needed for normal lung development. Bilateral small or absent pulmonary arteries are usually part of the spectrum of pulmonary valve atresia/tetralogy of Fallot, presenting to the paediatric cardiologist with cyanosis in the newborn period.

Abnormalities of the systemic arteries

Two groups of abnormalities are relevant to the lung. The first includes those producing a vascular ring, such as double aortic arch or right-sided arch with aberrant origin of the left subclavian from a diverticulum of Kommerell with left duct/ligament. The second group includes collateral vessels arising from the aorta and supplying all or part of one or both lungs, or a CTM. These vessels may be hypertrophied bronchial arteries or abnormal non-bronchial arteries; there may be multiple collaterals.[104] This last group may be seen in association with direct pulmonary arteriovenous connections (pulmonary arteriovenous malformations). Aneurysm of aortopulmonary collateral vessels has been described.[99]

Abnormalities of the venous tree

Disorders of the systemic (bronchial) venous tree

The bronchial venous system drains into the systemic venous network and thence into the right atrium. No disorders of the systemic (bronchial venous) tree have been described.

Disorders of the pulmonary venous tree

Anomalous pulmonary veins result in blood from the lungs returning to the right side of the heart rather than entering the left atrium. The anomalous veins may join the inferior caval vein or hepatic, portal or splenic veins below the diaphragm, or above the diaphragm they may drain into the superior caval vein or its tributaries, the coronary sinus or the right atrium. The anomaly may be total or partial, unilateral or bilateral, and isolated or associated with other cardiopulmonary developmental defects. These include bronchial isomerism, mirror image arrangement, asplenia, pulmonary stenosis, patent arterial duct and a small interatrial communication.[105] The type of isomerism gives a good indication as to whether the anomaly is total or partial, right-sided isomerism suggesting totally anomalous veins and left-sided isomerism suggesting a partial anomaly.[106] Occasionally the anomalous vein runs much of its course buried within the lung substance.[107] Anomalous pulmonary venous connections are often narrow and this may cause relatively mild pulmonary hypertension.[108]

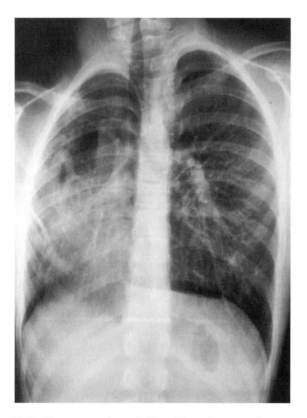

Fig. 21.9 'Scimitar syndrome'. Chest X-ray showing right congenital small lung with hemianomalous venous drainage.

The 'scimitar' syndrome is a particular clinical problem characterised by a small right lung, resulting in the heart moving to the right (cardiac dextroposition) and an abnormal band shadow representing the abnormal venous drainage to the systemic veins (Fig. 21.9), fancifully compared to a scimitar (a sign that is in fact often absent[109]). Infants with this condition presenting in heart failure have a worse prognosis,[109] often because of associated abnormalities, among which may be malformations in the left side of the heart.[110] Aortopulmonary collaterals should be sought and occluded.[111] More invasive treatment options include reimplantation of the vein and pneumonectomy.[112] Severe pulmonary hypertension is an adverse prognostic feature.[110] An association with horseshoe lung has been described; this usually causes early death but occasional long term survival has been reported.[113]

Absence of the pulmonary veins[114] or narrowing of their ostia into the left atrium results in pulmonary venous obstruction. Partial anomalous pulmonary venous drainage may be obstructed or unobstructed. Unilateral anomalous venous drainage may be part of complex lung malformations; it may also be seen in association with what appears to be a simple lung cyst. This underscores the need for accurate delineation of all abnormalities even in straightforward-appearing cases. Minor abnormalities of venous connection, such as a segment draining directly into the azygos system, are not uncommon and usually not of practical significance.

Abnormalities of the connections between the pulmonary arterial and venous trees

Pulmonary arteriovenous malformations

An important group of abnormalities, which potentially involves systemic and pulmonary arterial and venous trees, includes the various forms of 'pulmonary arteriovenous fistula'. These are discussed in detail elsewhere (see Chapter 66). In summary, they range from the diffuse, microscopic to the single or multiple large abnormality. The large connections may have both a systemic and a pulmonary arterial supply (see above). It is important to know if there is a systemic component, since this may cause high-output cardiac failure. Furthermore, whereas embolisation of an abnormal pulmonary arteriovenous connection via the feeding pulmonary artery may be curative, more extensive procedures may be needed to deal with systemic arterial components.

Congenital alveolar capillary dysplasia (misalignment of lung vessels)[115]

This malformation represents a failure of capillaries to extend into the alveolar tissue of the lung and is an unusual cause of congenital pulmonary hypertension, persistent fetal circulation and respiratory distress in the newborn. Cases reported to date have all been rapidly fatal. Many have associated gastrointestinal or genitourinary malformations. Occasionally, siblings are affected. Histology shows increased septal connective tissue and pulmonary veins accompanying small pulmonary arteries in the centres of the acini rather than occupying their normal position in the interlobular septa (misalignment of lung vessels). The pulmonary arteries are decreased in number and show increased muscularisation. Pulmonary lobules are small and radial alveolar counts may be decreased. Alveoli are decreased in complexity, their walls contain few capillaries and there is poor contact of capillaries with alveolar epithelium. The primary fault is poorly understood. The relationship of congenital alveolar capillary dysplasia to a condition previously described as congenital alveolar dysplasia[116] is unclear; the latter does not show the paucity of capillaries or arteriovenous misalignment described in the former but some regard one as a variant of the other while others believe the two conditions to be distinct.

Abnormalities of the lymphatic tree

This tree is the hardest to delineate and in most malformations it is not relevant. Lymphatic tree disorders usually require histological confirmation. Lymphatic hypoplasia of varied distribution underlies the yellow nail syndrome in which lymphoedema is accompanied by discoloration of the nails and pleural effusions.[117] Although inherited it is not usually manifest until adult life. The Klippel–Trenaunay syndrome, usually characterised by varicosities of systemic veins, cutaneous haemangiomas and soft-tissue hypertrophy, is another congenital disorder in which pleuropulmonary abnormalities are described, including pulmonary lymphatic hyperplasia, pleural effusions, pulmonary thromboembolism and pulmonary vein varicosities.[118]

Congenital pulmonary lymphangiectasia

This may be secondary to obstruction of pulmonary lymphatic or venous drainage, or primary, the latter either limited to the lung or part of generalised lymphangiectasia. There is a high degree of association of primary pulmonary lymphangiectasia with other congenital abnormalities, particularly asplenia[119] and cardiac anomalies. It causes severe respiratory distress and is generally fatal in the neonatal period but presentation may be delayed until adult life.[120] The lungs are heavy, with widened interlobular septa, and on the visceral pleural surface there is a pronounced reticular pattern of small cysts which accentuates the lobular architecture of the lungs. The cysts measure up to 5 mm in diameter and are situated in the interlobular septa and about the bronchovascular bundles. Near the hila of the lungs the cysts are elongated.[121] Microscopy confirms that the cysts are located in connective tissue under the pleura, in the interlobular septa and about the bronchioles and arteries. Serial sections show that they are part of an intricate network of intercommunicating channels, which vary greatly in width and are devoid of valves.[121] The cysts are lined by an attenuated simple endothelium. The absence of multinucleate foreign-body giant-cell reaction distinguishes this condition from interstitial emphysema. The clinical history is also usually quite different: interstitial emphysema is usually a complication of positive pressure ventilation in a very preterm baby.

Congenital chylothorax

Congenital chylothorax may be part of congenital lymphatic dilatation, an isolated abnormality or associated with congenital abnormality of the main lymphatic duct or pulmonary lymphatics.[122] Associations with Noonan's, Ullrich–Turner and Down's syndromes,[122,123] fetal thyrotoxicosis,[124] H-type tracheo-oesophageal fistula[125] and mediastinal neuroblastoma[126] have been described; familial cases have also been reported.[122,127] If there is a large antenatal chylothorax, antenatal drainage may be necessary.[128] Postnatally, treatment is with a medium-chain triglyceride diet, with paracentesis as necessary, in the first instance, and total parenteral nutrition if this fails.[129] Surgical options include pleurodesis, ligation of the thoracic duct[130] and pleuroperitoneal shunting.[128,131]

Other relevant abnormalities

Cardiac abnormalities

Cardiac malformations may be coincidental to, or a fundamental part of a pulmonary malformation. They are sufficiently common that echocardiography should be a routine part of the work-up of congenital lung disease. Coincidental malformations are seen with, for example, CLHL (congenital lobar emphysema). Around 10% have an atrial or ventricular septal defect. Lung abnormalities in which heart disease is fundamental include those with the pulmonary atresia spectrum (see above). By definition, lung blood supply is abnormal. However, these cases usually present to paediatric cardiologists.

Abnormalities of the chest wall, including the diaphragm

Diaphragmatic anomalies

The posterolateral diaphragm contains the foramen of Bochdalek, through which herniation of abdominal viscera is prone to occur, particularly on the left resulting in mediastinal shift to the right. Hernias of this type are among the commonest congenital defects. They occur in about 1 in 2000 fetuses but many have other major anomalies and are aborted after diagnostic antenatal ultrasound or are stillborn. If the infant is suitable for surgical correction, respiratory insufficiency and persistent fetal circulation are frequent postoperative problems. The foramina are normally sealed at about 8 weeks gestation so that hernias forming after this time tend to be enclosed in a serosal sac. Anterior Morgagni hernia is usually a chance finding in an asymptomatic child (Fig. 21.10).

The diaphragmatic muscle is formed between the pleural and peritoneal membranes and if it is deficient the whole diaphragm, or more usually one side, is elevated, a process known as eventration of the diaphragm. Posterolateral herniation and eventration are both commoner on the left and affect boys twice as often as girls. Unilateral eventration usually requires no treatment (Fig. 21.11); bilateral lesions may require

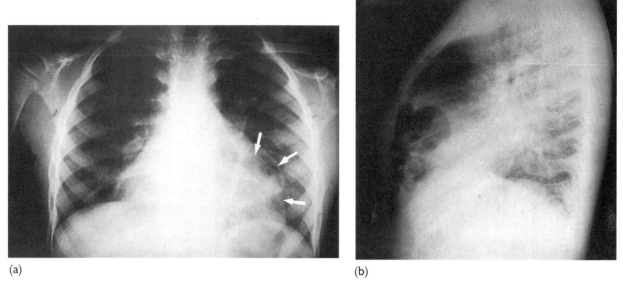

(a)   (b)

Fig. 21.10 Anterior (Morgagni) diaphragmatic hernia. a. Chest radiograph from a 5-year-old asymptomatic boy. There is a segmented gas shadow superimposed on the cardiac opacity (arrows). b. Lateral chest radiograph revealing the anterior hernia containing large intestine.

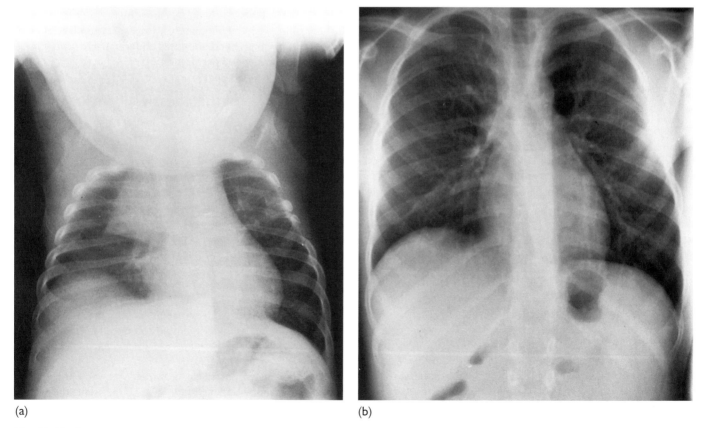

(a)   (b)

Fig. 21.11 Chest radiographs demonstrating the natural history of eventration. a. Right-sided eventration in an infant, with apparent compression of the right lung. Note the prominent thymic shadow ('sail sign'). b. The same child 10 years later, having had no treatment. The eventration is barely discernible.

surgery if there is respiratory distress in the newborn period. Anterior and paraoesophageal hernias each account for only 5% of the total, while total absence of half or the whole diaphragm is very unusual.[132] Duplication of the diaphragm results in a fibromuscular septum subdividing a pleural cavity, usually between the right upper and middle lobes. Associated anomalies of the heart and lungs are frequently found.

Pectus carinatum (pigeon breast)

In this condition, the sternum protrudes anteriorly, and may lie obliquely if the excessive growth of the ribs is asymmetrical. It may be present at birth but usually becomes prominent during adolescence. Respiratory function is normal as there is no loss of lung volume and little interference with rib movement.

Pectus excavatum (funnel chest)

This condition appears soon after birth and is occasionally associated with kyphosis, scoliosis or mitral valve prolapse. It may be familial or associated with Marfan's or Ehlers–Danlos syndrome, or isolated hyperflexibility of the joints. It may also be acquired in infancy secondary to obstructive sleep apnoea. Initially the condition is reversible but it may become permanent. There is no evidence that surgical correction is other than cosmetic. It has been suggested that a thoracoscopic correction could be less risky to growing bone, and should be used in young children, but there is no evidence that this new procedure offers any advantage over conventional surgery.

Asphyxiating thoracic dystrophy (Jeune's syndrome)

This is a rare disorder of the costal cartilages in which the ribs are shortened and the rib cage narrowed so that lung development is retarded and the lungs are small. Less severe degrees are compatible with life but respiratory movements are entirely abdominal and respiratory failure often develops in infancy or childhood. Surgical enlargement of the chest cavity has been undertaken but is controversial.

Scoliosis

Scoliosis (lateral curvature of the spine) is generally accompanied by rotation of the spine. If the condition is present at birth there is often a recognisable congenital abnormality of the spine, such as hemivertebra, and other congenital skeletal abnormalities such as absent or fused ribs may also be present. Most cases are idiopathic, and some present in infancy. They tend to progress to respiratory failure in later life.[27] However, it is commoner for idiopathic scoliosis to appear during adolescence and not progress in this way. Scoliosis may also be secondary to neuromuscular disorders, both hereditary and acquired; these conditions are discussed elsewhere (see Chapter 73).

Abdominal abnormalities

Any large abdominal mass or fluid may compress the lungs, thus impairing development. Congenital absence of the kidneys causes oligohydramnios and small lungs (above). Rare CTMs may connect with the stomach[133] and be associated with abdominal visceral malrotation.[134]

Multisystem abnormalities

Most congenital lung abnormalities are isolated but a few are part of a more generalised disorder. Complex abnormalities of lung development may be associated with chromosomal abnormalities.[135]

Tuberous sclerosis may affect the lungs as well as kidneys, heart and brain, resulting in pulmonary lymphangioleiomyomatosis (see Chapter 60) or micronodular type II pneumocyte hyperplasia.[136] The latter is a multifocal microscopic lesion that usually has no clinical significance. The hyperplastic cells show no atypia and appear to be devoid of any malignant potential. Micronodular type II pneumocyte hyperplasia may be seen in otherwise normal lungs or in association with pulmonary lymphangioleiomyomatosis. Unlike lymphangioleiomyomatosis, it affects tuberous sclerosis patients of either sex and the hyperplastic type II cells fail to stain for HMB-45.[136]

Investigation of congenital lung disease

Antenatal investigation

A detailed account of the technicalities of antenatal ultrasound is beyond the scope of this chapter. The role this investigation has played in setting new management problems has been discussed above. The same general principles of describing what is actually seen should be applied. It is difficult to see much role for biopsy of the fetal lung but, if it is deemed essential, caution in interpreting the histology is advisable.[1]

Postnatal investigation

There is currently no consensus as to how best (if at all) to investigate a well, thriving infant with a small lung malformation. If treatment is being contemplated, which is usually because of symptoms or the presence of a large malformation, then investigation should aim systematically to delineate all possible relevant aspects of the malformation, as emphasised above. The next sections outline the possible roles of the different available tests.

Chest radiography

All infants in whom any suggestion of a lung malformation has been made antenatally require a chest radiograph prior to discharge. In many it will be normal, but more detailed imaging may reveal tiny malformations. Specific points in the chest radiograph in the context of congenital lung disease include the determination of bronchial arrangement; and the side of the aortic arch (Fig. 21.12). Although in some cases the chest radio-

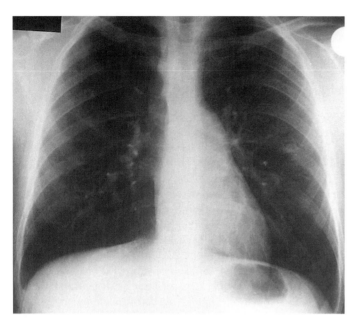

Fig. 21.12 Chest radiograph in a child with steroid-resistant wheeze. There is a right aortic arch, a clue to the fact that this child has a vascular ring.

graph will be clearly abnormal (e.g. CLHL) (congenital lobar emphysema), in most, further imaging will be required.

$\dot{V}/\dot{Q}$ scanning

This technique gives functional information. Unilateral absent perfusion and ventilation is seen in complete absence of one lung. Unilateral absence of perfusion, which may be combined with secondary abnormalities in ventilation, is seen in unilateral absence of the pulmonary artery, unilateral origin of pulmonary artery from aorta and unilateral absence of pulmonary veins. Bilateral absent perfusion is seen in common arterial trunk (truncus arteriosus); the pattern of ventilation is normal. Focal defects are seen with large CTMs. Increased uptake of technetium-99m microspheres given by peripheral vein injection is seen in the brain and kidneys as a feature of pulmonary arteriovenous fistulae (as well as in congenital heart disease with right to left shunt) and has been used to quantitate shunt. Split lung function may be useful in determining whether operation on a unilateral bronchial or pulmonary artery stenosis is advisable. In cases of doubt, $\dot{V}/\dot{Q}$ scanning can differentiate CLHL from hyperinflation of a normal lobe secondary to contralateral congenital small lung or lobar atelectasis; in this case, the lucent area is functional, whereas CLHL causes a filling defect.

Ultrasound scanning (including echocardiography)

Cardiac abnormality is so bound up in the consideration of congenital lung malformations that virtually all infants need an echocardiogram. Indeed, antenatal ultrasound will have already detected many cardiac abnormalities. Echocardiography detects relevant abnormalities of the systemic arteries in the mediastinum, such as double aortic arch and aberrant origin of sub-

clavian artery. The pulmonary arteries and veins should be imaged and unilateral abnormal (hemianomalous) venous drainage excluded. Injection of saline into a peripheral vein allows detection of a right-to-left shunt; in such cases, bubbles appear in the left atrium. Pulmonary artery pressure may be estimated from the Bernoulli equation if there is physiological tricuspid or pulmonary regurgitation. It may be possible to image abnormal collateral arteries arising from the abdominal aorta. In small, sick infants, in whom angiography may carry an unacceptably high morbidity, it is necessary to rely solely on ultrasound to delineate the vascular anatomy of the lungs and malformation. Parenchymal ultrasound imaging is generally less helpful. Defects in the diaphragm may be identified and pleural disease confirmed. Ultrasound is useful in differentiating thymic abnormalities from mediastinal cysts.

Computed tomography (CT)

This technique gives the best images of parenchymal abnormalities, and is probably the first investigation of choice in an adult with suspected CTM.[137] Modern fast-acquisition-time scanners do not require general anaesthesia. Many abnormalities that are not visible on the chest radiograph are delineated by computed tomography (CT), at a cost of a higher radiation dosage. Whether the detection of tiny abnormalities is worthwhile can only be solved by prospective studies. However, cystic CTMs large enough to have the potential to be infected may be invisible on chest radiographs, so CT is recommended for all infants in whom an antenatal diagnosis of a lung malformation has been made, even if the chest radiograph after birth appears normal. Scanning after contrast injection, possibly using modern reconstruction techniques, may delineate abnormal aortopulmonary collaterals, obviating the need for angiography.[138]

Magnetic resonance imaging (MRI)

At present this technique is limited by the need for general anaesthesia, at least in small children but if image acquisition times can be shortened the lack of radiation exposure will make this an attractive technique. Currently, MRI can delineate some parenchymal abnormalities but probably with less spatial resolution than CT. MRI is the best way of detecting extension of a neurogenic tumour into the spinal canal. MRI is also used to outline the systemic and pulmonary circulations, and to image any airway compression and its cause. The images may also alert the clinician to the presence of an aortic blood supply to a CTM.

Barium swallow

This investigation is most used to diagnose a vascular ring (Fig. 21.13). If the appearances are those of an anomalous subclavian artery, which may be a variant of no consequence, airway compression may be confirmed by bronchoscopy. A barium swallow cannot rule out fistulae from the oesophagus.

Oesophageal tube injection

Abnormal connections between oesophagus and the trachea or a CTM are best delineated by a tube oesophagram. The pressure

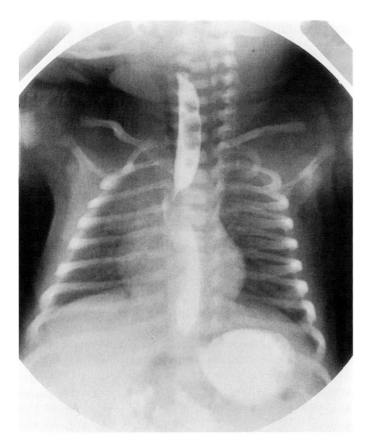

Fig. 21.13 Barium swallow demonstrating a vascular ring, due in this case to a double aortic arch.

injection of barium will reveal a connection that a simple barium swallow will miss. This investigation is only needed in selected cases in which either the malformation is close to the bronchial tree or severe infection (particularly anaerobic) is a feature.

Angiography

In complex cases, angiography will be needed to plan surgery. A rare exception may be the sick, acidotic infant. In these cases, ultrasound techniques have to be relied upon. The operator must completely delineate the anatomy of the pulmonary and systemic trees, including establishing whether there are any arterial collaterals (above). It should be remembered that a CTM may be supplied from the coronary,[139] internal mammary,[140] intercostal[141] or subclavian arteries.[142] At the same time, any embolisation that might be indicated can be performed, including occlusion of pulmonary arteriovenous malformations and systemic arterial collaterals. This may be the only treatment required (see below).

Bronchoscopy and bronchography

The most clear-cut use of bronchoscopy is in the investigation of stridor. In all but typical cases of laryngomalacia, this investigation should be performed at an early stage. Multiple causes of stridor are not uncommon and all the accessible respiratory tract should be examined. Bronchoscopy should not be delayed by

performing a series of non-diagnostic imaging studies. A rigid bronchoscope may be best for excluding laryngeal cleft and tracheo-oesophageal fistula. In other contexts, bronchoscopy is probably best combined with other procedures requiring a general anaesthetic, such as angiography (above); rarely can an anaesthetic be justified solely for bronchoscopy. Ideally the procedure should be performed via a laryngeal mask, so that the whole of the lower airway can be inspected.

First, bronchial arrangement can be verified. Second, abnormalities of the bronchial wall such as complete cartilage rings or compression by a vascular ring can be ascertained. Airway malacia can be visualised directly, and further documented by performing a limited bronchogram with a soluble contrast medium. Unlike the bronchograms carried out prior to the advent of CT scanning, the purpose is to delineate the major airways, not to achieve alveolar filling, and only very small volumes of water-soluble contrast are required. Finally, the presence of blind-ending bronchial stumps can be determined; these may act as a sump for infection. Another role for bronchoscopy is the assessment of airway narrowing in the case of aberrant origin of left subclavian artery. This may be a harmless normal variant or cause significant airway narrowing if a left arterial ligament completes a vascular ring. In doubtful cases, bronchoscopic inspection of the airway is indicated.

Reasons for treating congenital lung malformations

Intervention should serve a purpose. Possible reasons for therapeutic intervention in congenital lung disease might include risk of infection, of interference with lung growth, of high-output heart failure and of malignant change. Each of these risks and the appropriate response will now be considered in turn. Treatment advice is relatively straightforward if an established complication has developed. The major difficulty is in giving advice about prophylactic treatment; it is difficult to calculate risks as it is not known how many undiagnosed malformations never cause any trouble, because we have no good prevalence data.

Risk of infection

Cystic CTMs may present as a severe pneumonia responding poorly to treatment, or a lung abscess, usually after 1 year of age.[56] Initial treatment is with intravenous antibiotics. Surgery is usually advisable to prevent recurrent infection, which is probably inevitable. The differential diagnosis of a residual single cyst after severe pneumonia is a post-staphylococcal pneumatocele, which should be managed conservatively and frequently resolves completely, unlike a congenital malformation. It may be difficult to distinguish the two conditions; a previous chest radiograph if one exists, is often a useful pointer.

It is more difficult to advise on a cystic lesion that has been discovered by chance as it is impossible to calculate the risk of subsequent infection. We advise elective removal of all but the smallest lesions because surgery after or in the throes of an infection may be difficult and mean that more normal lung has to be sacrificed. Nevertheless, some families may prefer to postpone surgery.

Risk of interference with lung growth

Alveoli are mainly formed in the first 18–24 months of life.[143] A CLHL (congenital lobar emphysema) may cause impressive mediastinal shift and compression of normal lung and it might be thought that this could impair lung growth. However, if the baby is asymptomatic, the lesion can safely be left alone. In the long term, regression is usual and good lung function can be anticipated. Indeed, CLHL may be a chance finding in an asymptomatic adult. It would seem that there is little risk of interference with lung growth in an asymptomatic child with this condition, and by extrapolation, probably not to other asymptomatic lesions.

Risk of high-output heart failure

A CTM with a systemic arterial supply is the equivalent in haemodynamic terms of a systemic arteriovenous fistula, and as such may cause high-output heart failure.[144] Prophylactic treatment for this indication is probably not indicated but, if heart failure is thought to be impending, excision of the malformation or embolic occlusion of the abnormal vessel (below) is recommended.

Risk of malignant change

There are isolated case reports of malignant tumours in children with a CTM. The risk attributable to the malformation is not known. Metaplasia or preneoplastic change is not a feature of excised CTMs.[145] Furthermore, malignant disease may develop in sites distant from the original malformation, implying that the malformation is merely a marker of increased malignant potential throughout the lungs, in which case removing the malformation would not deal with the underlying problem. Some advocate removal of even the tiniest malformations, while others are more conservative.

Treatment options

Do nothing

Before birth, careful observation is the best option for all but a tiny minority.[146] After birth, no action may be needed for tiny malformations, or asymptomatic cases of CLHL (congenital lobar emphysema). Some advocate the removal of even a tiny CTM to prevent the development of malignancy but the evidence that this is worthwhile and actually does prevent malignancy is poor.

Antenatal options

Where there is a large fetal pleural effusion, with or without hydrops, fetal thoraco- or abdominal paracentesis, or antenatal placement of a pleuroamniotic shunt, may allow the pregnancy to continue.[146] Careful deliberation is required before recommending intervention, because of the good prognosis untreated of many antenatally diagnosed CTMs.[1,2,146]

Surgical resection

This is the definitive treatment. Proper delineation of all components of the malformation preoperatively is essential. Excision of CTM is usually straightforward and long-term prognosis excellent if nothing more extensive than a lobectomy is required;[56,61,145,147] rare cases of re-expansion pulmonary oedema[56] and death from congenital small lungs[147] have been described after extensive resection. Pneumonectomy is a major procedure, particularly in a prepubertal child, and should be avoided if at all possible. If this operation is carried out, there is a high risk of major scoliosis, worsening particularly during puberty. Consideration should be given to trying to prevent this by replacing the excised lung with a saline bag, which can be inflated from the outside to variable volumes after implantation. More recently, thoracoscopic excision of CTMs has been described.[104,148]

Another surgical option that may be considered if an otherwise normal lung has an abnormal arterial supply or venous drainage is reimplantation of the abnormal vein.[102] However, if this is to be undertaken, it is important to be sure that the lung is capable of gas exchange, by performing a pre-operative CT or $\dot{V}/\dot{Q}$ scan. Surgical correction of scimitar syndrome does not usually restore a normal pulmonary blood flow.[149] Ligation of the feeding artery is rarely needed nowadays, coil embolisation generally being preferred.

Tracheal stenosis has been treated by surgical procedures to widen the narrowed segment and in complex cases tracheal transplantation has been used; the indications for, details of and complexities involved in this surgery are beyond the scope of this chapter.

Options at cardiac catheterisation

Therapeutic embolisation

This is the treatment of choice for pulmonary arteriovenous fistula and may be all that is needed in CTM with a systemic arterial supply. The procedure is usually performed under anaesthetic at the same time as diagnostic angiography (Fig. 21.14). Occlusion of the collateral supply may result in total obliteration of the abnormality (Fig. 21.15); however, even if it does not, subsequent surgery is arguably easier.

Balloon dilatation and stenting

Localised vascular narrowing can be treated in this way.[110] However, if dilatation of a vessel to a small lung is contemplated, it is important to be sure that there is functional tissue that would benefit from an increase in blood supply. If the lung is small, with a balanced reduction in blood flow, it is unlikely that dilatation will be beneficial.

Bronchoscopic options

Balloon dilatation of complete cartilage rings has been advocated but must still be considered experimental. Airway stenting for non-malignant disease has been reported, but the interaction between growth and the stent may pose problems.

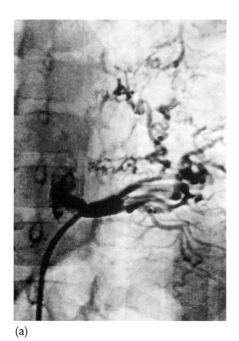
(a)

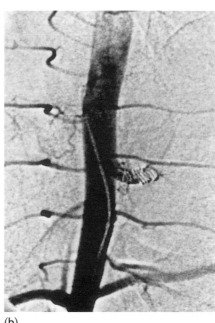
(b)

Fig. 21.14 a. A large aortopulmonary collateral, shown at angiography, which supplied a left lower lobe congenital thoracic malformation. b. Appearances after coil occlusion (digital subtraction technique in both cases).

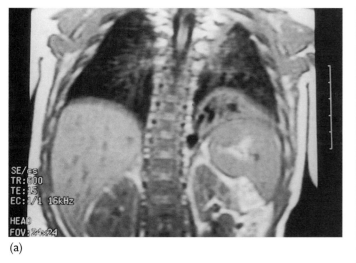
(a)

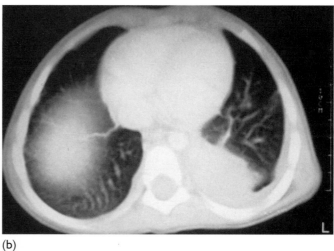
(b)

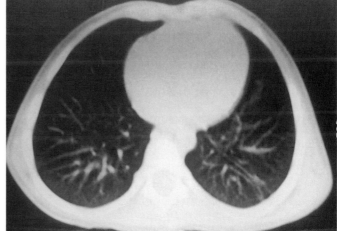
(c)

Fig. 21.15 Treatment of a congenital thoracic malformation by occlusion of feeding vessel. a. Magnetic resonance imaging of the malformation, which abuts the diaphragm and contains a large feeding vessel. b. Computed tomography appearances after coil occlusion: there is a pleural effusion and parenchymal shadowing on the left. c. Follow-up computed tomography. The malformation has completely disappeared. No other treatment was undertaken.

Future directions

There are many areas of uncertainty as to the natural history of antenatally detected congenital lung malformations. These can only be remedied by carefully structured prospective observations. There are clear reasons for discarding past nomenclature before commencing this process. The first is that many terms are irretrievably tarnished with embryological speculation, most of which is probably incorrect. The second is that many of them merely describe extremes of a spectrum rather than discrete entities. The third is the risk that the search for the right name obscures the real clinical need for a systematic approach to the lungs. Finally and most compellingly, terms like cystic adenomatoid malformation have come to mean different things pre- and postnatally and thus any use they once had has now gone.

If the descriptive approach set out above is applied both antenatally and postnatally, it can be the basis of standardised protocols for follow-up. There is a clear need for a national register of these abnormalities. If a standardised approach can be applied both before and after birth, many uncertainties will be resolved. If the current ad hoc basis is maintained, then it will be difficult to give sensible advice to patients and their parents.

? Unresolved questions

- What is the natural history of antenatally diagnosed congenital thoracic malformations, in particular with regard to the likelihood of infection and malignant change?

- What imaging should be performed in a baby with an antenatally diagnosed congenital thoracic malformation who has a normal chest X-ray at birth?

- What is the best option for, and timing of, treatment for a congenital thoracic malformation?

- How frequently and with what investigations should a baby with a known congenital thoracic malformation be followed up, and how does surgical excision modify those recommendations?

References

1. Khakkoo GA, Jawad MH, Bush A et al. Conservative management of fetal lung lesions. Early Hum Dev 1993; 35: 55–62.
2. Samuel M, Burge DM. Management of antenatally diagnosed pulmonary sequestration associated with congenital cystic adenomatoid malformation. Thorax 1999; 54: 701–706.
3. Hislop A, Reid L. New pathological findings in emphysema in childhood: 1. Polyalveolar lobe with emphysema. Thorax 1970; 25: 682–690.
4. Wigglesworth JS, Hislop A, Desai R. Fetal lung growth in congenital laryngeal atresia. Pediatr Pathol 1987; 7: 515–525.
5. Hopkinson JM. Congenital absence of the trachea. J Pathol 1972; 107: 63–67.
6. Aboussouan LS, Odonovan PB, Moodie DS et al. Hypoplastic trachea in Down's syndrome. Am Rev Respir Dis 1993; 147: 72–75.
7. Berdon WE, Baker DH, Wung J-T et al. Complete cartilage-ring tracheal stenosis associated with anomalous left pulmonary artery: the ring-sling complex. J Radiol 1984; 152: 57–64.
8. Landing BH, Lawrence TK, Payne CV, Wells TR. Bronchial anatomy in syndromes with abnormal visceral situs, abnormal spleen and congenital heart disease. Am J Cardiol 1971; 28: 456–462.
9. McArtney FJ, Zuberbuhler JR, Anderson RH. Morphological considerations pertaining to recognition of atrial isomerism. Consequences for chamber localisation. Br Heart J 1980; 44: 657–667.
10. Bush A. Left bronchial isomerism, normal atrial arrangement and bronchomalacia mimicking asthma: a new syndrome? Eur Respir J 1999; 14: 475–477.
11. Bense L, Eklund G, Wiman LG. Bilateral bronchial anomaly; a pathogenetic factor in spontaneous pneumothorax. Am Rev Respir Dis 1992; 146: 513–516.
12. De Carvalho CRR, Barbas CSV, Guarnieri RDdG et al. Congenital bronchobiliary fistula: first case in an adult. Thorax 1988; 43: 792–793.
13. Barbato A, Novello A, Zanolin D et al. Diverticulosis of the main bronchi – a rare cause of recurrent bronchopneumonia in a child. Thorax 1993; 48: 187–188.
14. Gonzalez-Crussi F, Padilla L, Miller JK, Grosfeld JL. 'Bridging bronchus', a previously undescribed airway anomaly. Am J Dis Child 1976; 130: 1015–1018.
15. Clements BS, Warner JO. The crossover lung segment: congenital malformation associated with a variant of scimitar syndrome. Thorax 1987; 42: 417–419.
16. Frank JL, Poole CA, Rosas G. Horseshoe lung: clinical, pathologic, and radiologic features and a new plain film finding. AJR 1986; 146: 217–226.
17. Langlois SL, Henderson DW. Variant pulmonary lobation. Australas Radiol 1980; 24: 255–261.
18. Borja AR, Ransdell HT, Villa S. Congenital developmental arrest of the lung. Ann Thorac Surg 1970; 10: 317–326.
19. Cunningham ML, Mann N. Pulmonary agenesis: a predictor of ipsilateral malformations. Am J Med Genet 1997; 70: 391–398.
20. Ryland D, Reid L. Pulmonary aplasia – a quantitative analysis of the development of the single lung. Thorax 1971; 26: 602–609.
21. Beigelman C, Howarth NR, Chartrand-Lefebvre C, Grenier P. Congenital anomalies of tracheobronchial branching patterns: spiral CT aspects in adults. Eur Radiol 1998; 8: 79–85.
22. Reale FR, Esterly JR. Pulmonary hypoplasia: a morphometric study of the lungs of infants with diaphragmatic hernia, anencephaly, and renal malformations. Pediatrics 1972; 51: 91–96.
23. Reid L. Lung growth in health and disease. Br J Dis Chest 1984; 78: 113–134.
24. Hislop A, Reid L. Persistent hypoplasia of the lung after repair of congenital diaphragmatic hernia. Thorax 1976; 31: 450–455.
25. Page DV, Stocker JT. Anomalies associated with pulmonary hypoplasia. Am Rev Respir Dis 1982; 125: 216–221.
26. Cooney TP, Thurlbeck WM. Pulmonary hypoplasia in Down's syndrome. N Engl J Med 1982; 307: 1170–1173.
27. Boffa P, Stovin P, Shneerson J. Lung developmental abnormalities in severe scoliosis. Thorax 1984; 39: 681–682.
28. Nicolini U, Fisk NM, Rodeck CH et al. Low amniotic pressure in oligohydramnios – is this the cause of pulmonary hypoplasia? Am J Obstet Gynecol 1989; 161: 1098–1101.
29. Adzick NS, Harrison MR, Glick PL et al. Experimental pulmonary hypoplasia and oligohydramnios: relative contributions of lung fluid and fetal breathing movements. J Pediatr Surg 1984; 19: 658–665.
30. Thomas IT, Smith DW. Oligohydramnios, cause of the non-renal features of Potter's syndrome, including pulmonary hypoplasia. J Pediatr 1974; 84: 811–814.
31. Hislop A, Hey E, Reid L. The lungs in congenital bilateral renal agenesis and dysplasia. Arch Dis Child 1979; 54: 32–38.
32. Katz I, Levine M, Herman P. Tracheobronchiomegaly: the Mounier–Kuhn syndrome. AJR 1962; 88: 1084–1093.
33. Schwartz M, Rossoff L. Tracheobronchomegaly. Chest 1994; 106: 1589–1590.
34. Vidal C, Pena F, Mosquera MR, Quintela AG. Tracheobronchomegaly associated with interstitial pulmonary fibrosis. Respiration 1991; 58: 207–210.
35. Johnston RF, Green RA. Tracheobronchiomegaly: Report of five cases and demonstration of familial occurrence. Am Rev Respir Dis 1965; 91: 35–50.
36. Aaby GV, Blake HA. Tracheobronchiomegaly. Ann Thorac Surg 1966; 2: 64–70.
37. Wanderer AA, Ellis EF, Goltz RW, Cotton EK. Tracheobronchiomegaly and acquired cutis laxa in a child. Pediatrics 1969; 44: 709–715.
38. Sane AC, Effmann EL, Brown SD. Tracheobronchiomegaly – the Mounier–Kuhn syndrome in a patient with the Kenny–Caffey syndrome. Chest 1992; 102: 618–619.
39. Wailoo MP, Emery JL. The trachea in children with tracheo-oesophageal fistula. Histopathology 1979; 3: 329–338.
40. Jederlinic PJ, Sicilian LS, Baigelman W, Gaensler EA. Congenital bronchial atresia. A report of 4 cases and a review of the literature. Medicine (Baltimore) 1986; 65: 73–83.
41. Rossoff LJ, Steinberg H. Bronchial atresia and mucocele: a report of two cases. Respir Med 1994; 88: 789–791.
42. Williams AJ, Schuster SR. Bronchial atresia associated with a bronchogenic cyst. Evidence of early appearance of atretic segments. Chest 1985; 87: 396–398.

43. Finder JD. Primary bronchomalacia of infants and children. J Pediatr 1997; 130: 59–66.
44. Godfrey S. Association between pectus excavatum and segmental bronchomalacia. J Pediatr 1980; 96: 649–52.
45. Rock MJ, Green CG, Pauli RM, Peters ME. Tracheomalacia and bronchomalacia associated with Larsen syndrome. Pediatr Pulmonol 1988; 5: 55–9.
46. Strattion RF, Young RS, Heiman HS, Carter JM. Fryn's syndrome. Am J Med Genet 1993; 45: 562–4.
47. Williams H, Campbell P. Generalised bronchiectasis associated with deficiency of cartilage in the bronchial tree. Arch Dis Child 1960; 35: 182–191.
48. Wayne KS, Taussig LM. Probable familial congenital bronchiectasis due to cartilage deficiency (Williams Campbell syndrome). Am Rev Respir Dis 1976; 114: 15–22.
49. Danton MH, McMahon J, McGuigan J, Gibbons JR. Congenital oesophageal respiratory tract fistula presenting in adult life. Eur Respir J 1993; 6: 1412–1414.
50. Emery JL, Haddadin AJ. Squamous epithelium in the respiratory tract of children with tracheo-oesophageal fistula. Arch Dis Child 1971; 46: 236–242.
51. Tanaka H, Igarashi T, Teramoto S et al. Lymphoepithelial cysts in the mediastinum with an opening to the trachea. Respiration 1995; 62: 110–113.
52. Evers WB, Vissers R, van Noord JA. Pulmonary sequestration with congenital broncho-oesophageal fistula. Eur Respir J 1990; 3: 1067–1069.
53. Hislop A, Reid L. New pathological findings in emphysema in childhood: 2. Overinflation of a normal lobe. Thorax 1971; 26: 190–194.
54. Critchley PS, Forrester-Wood CP, Ridley PD. Adult congenital lobar emphysema in pregnancy. Thorax 1995; 50: 909–910.
55. Emery JL, Mithal A. The number of alveoli in the terminal respiratory unit of man during late intrauterine life and childhood. Arch Dis Child 1960; 35: 544–547.
56. Takeda S, Miyoshi S, Inoue M et al. Clinical spectrum of congenital cystic disease of the lung in children. Eur J Cardiothorac Surg 1999; 15: 11–17.
57. Hayakawa K, Soga T, Hamamoto K et al. Massive hemoptysis from a pulmonary sequestration controlled by embolization of aberrant pulmonary arteries: case report. Cardiovasc Intervent Radiol 1991; 14: 345–348.
58. Zapatero J, Baamonde C, Bellan JM et al. Hemothorax as a rare presentation of intralobar pulmonary sequestration. Scand J Thorac Cardiovasc Surg 1983; 17: 177–179.
59. Bell-Thomson J, Missier P, Sommers SC. Lung carcinoma arising in bronchopulmonary sequestration. Cancer 1979; 44: 334–339.
60. Freixinet J, de Cos J, Rodriguez de Castro F et al. Colonisation with Aspergillus of an intralobar pulmonary sequestration. Thorax 1995; 50: 810–811.
61. Al-Bassam A, Al-Rabeeah A, Al-Nassur S et al. Congenital cystic disease of the lung in infants and children (experience with 57 cases). Eur J Pediatr Surg 1999; 9: 364–368.
62. Stocker JT, Madewell JE, Drake RM. Congenital cystic adenomatoid malformation of the lung. Hum Pathol 1977; 8: 155–171.
63. Van Dyke JA, Sagel SS. Calcified pulmonary sequestration: CT demonstration. J Comput Assist Tomography 1985; 9: 372–374.
64. Aktogu S, Yuncu G, Halilcolar H et al. Bronchogenic cysts: clinicopathological presentation and treatment. Eur Respir J 1996; 9: 2017–2021.
65. Sheffield EA, Addis BJ, Corrin B, McCabe MM. Epithelial hyperplasia and malignant change in congenital lung cysts. J Clin Pathol 1987; 40: 612–614.
66. Fallon M, Gordon ARG, Lendrum AC. Mediastinal cysts of foregut origin associated with vertebral anomalies. Br J Surg 1954; 41: 520–533.
67. Rutledge JC, Jensen P. Acinar dysplasia: a new form of pulmonary maldevelopment. Hum Pathol 1986; 17: 1290–1293.
68. Chambers HM. Congenital acinar aplasia – an extreme form of pulmonary maldevelopment. Pathology 1991; 23: 69–71.
69. Heithoff KB, Sane SM, Williams HJ et al. Bronchopulmonary foregut malformations. A unifying etiological concept. AJR 1976; 126: 46–55.
70. Aulicino MR, Reis ED, Dolgin SE et al. Intra-abdominal pulmonary sequestration exhibiting congenital cystic adenomatoid malformation – report of a case and review of the literature. Arch Pathol Lab Med 1994; 118: 1034–1037.
71. Mendoza A, Wolf P, Edwards DK et al. Prenatal ultrasonographic diagnosis of congenital adenomatoid malformation of the lung. Arch Pathol Lab Med 1986; 110: 402–404.
72. Avitabile AM, Hulnick DH, Greco MA, Feiner HD. Congenital cystic adenomatoid malformation of the lung in adults. Am J Surg Pathol 1984; 8: 193–202.
73. Ribet ME, Copin MC, Soots JG, Gosselin BH. Bronchioloalveolar carcinoma and congenital cystic adenomatoid malformation. Ann Thorac Surg 1995; 60: 1126–1128.
74. Miller RK, Sieber WK, Yunis EJ. Congenital adenomatoid malformation of the lung. A report of 17 cases and review of the literature. In: Sommers SC, Rosen PP, ed. Pathology annual, vol 15, part 1. New York: Appleton-Century-Crofts; 1980: 387–406.
75. Samuel M, Burge DM. Management of antenatally diagnosed pulmonary sequestration associated with congenital cystic adenomatoid malformation. Thorax 1999; 54: 701–706.
76. Mark EJ. Mesenchymal cystic hamartoma of the lung. N Engl J Med 1986; 315: 1255–1259.
77. Hedlund GL, Bisset GSI, Bove KE. Malignant neoplasms arising in cystic hamartomas of the lung in childhood. Radiology 1989; 173: 77–79.
78. Ueda K, Gruppo R, Unger F et al. Rhabdomyosarcoma of lung arising in congenital cystic adenomatoid malformation. Cancer 1977; 40: 383–388.
79. Cruickshank DB, Harrison GK. Diffuse fibro-leiomyomatous hamartomatosis of the lung. Thorax 1953; 8: 316–318.
80. Rosenmann E, Maayan C, Lernau O. Leiomyomatous hamartosis with congenital jejunoileal atresia. Israel J Med Sci 1980; 16: 775–779.
81. Gustafson RA, Murray GF, Wardon HE et al. Intralobar sequestration. A missed diagnosis. Ann Thorac Surg 1989; 47: 841–847.
82. Gerle RD, Jaretzkia A, Ashley CA, Berne AS. Congenital bronchopulmonary-foregut malformation: pulmonary sequestration communicating with the gastrointestinal tract. N Engl J Med 1968; 278: 1413–1419.
83. Corrin B, Danel C, Allaway A et al. Intralobar pulmonary sequestration of ectopic pancreatic tissue with gastro-pancreatic duplication. Thorax 1985; 40: 637–638.
84. Sade RM, Clouse M, Ellis FH Jr. The spectrum of pulmonary sequestration. Ann Thorac Surg 1974; 18: 644–655.
85. Carter R. Pulmonary sequestration. Ann Thorac Surg 1969; 7: 68–85.
86. Stocker JT, Malczak HT. A study of pulmonary ligament arteries. Relationship to intralobar sequestration. Chest 1984; 86: 611–615.
87. Stocker JT. Sequestration of the lung. Semin Diagn Pathol 1986; 3: 106–121.
88. Armin A, Castelli M. Congenital adrenal tissue in the lung with adrenal cytomegaly. Case report and review of the literature. Am J Clin Pathol 1984; 82: 225–228.
89. Bando T, Genka K, Ishikawa K et al. Ectopic intrapulmonary thyroid. Chest 1993; 103: 1278–1279.
90. Mendoza A, Voland J, Wolf P, Benirschke K. Supradiaphragmatic liver in the lung. Arch Pathol Lab Med 1986; 110: 1085–1086.
91. Remberger K, Hubner G. Rhabdomyomatous dysplasia of the lung. Virchows Arch A Pathol Anat Histopathol 1974; 363: 363–369.
92. Hardisson D, Garcia Jimenez JA, Jimenez Heffernan JA, Nistal M. Rhabdomyomatosis of the newborn lung unassociated with other malformations. Histopathology 1997; 31: 474–479.
93. Ramaswamy A, Weyers I, Duda V et al. A tumorous type of pulmonary rhabdomyomatous dysplasia. Pathol Res Pract 1998; 194: 639–642.
94. Burke EC, Wenzl JE, Utz DC. The intrathoracic kidney. Report of a case. Am J Dis Child 1967; 113: 487–490.
95. Lager DJ, Kuper KA, Haake GK. Subdiaphragmatic extralobar pulmonary sequestration. Arch Pathol Lab Med 1991; 115: 536–538.
96. Pool PE, Vogel JHK, Blount SG. Congenital unilateral absence of a pulmonary artery. Am J Cardiol 1962; 10: 706–732.
97. Bahler RC, Carson P, Traks E et al. Absent pulmonary artery: problems in diagnosis and management. Am J Med 1969; 46: 64–71.
98. Ko T, Gatz MG, Reisz GR. Congenital unilateral absence of a pulmonary artery: report of two adult cases. Am Rev Respir Dis 1990; 141: 795–798.
99. Roman J, Jones S. Congenital absence of the pulmonary artery accompanied by ipsilateral emphysema and adenocarcinoma. Am J Med Sci 1995; 309: 188–190.
100. Wang TZ, Lin YM, Hwang JJ. Unilateral pulmonary artery agenesis in adulthood – not always a benign disease. Chest 1997; 111: 832–833.
101. Presbitero P, Bull C, Haworth SG, de Laval MR. Absent or occult pulmonary artery. Br Heart J 1984; 52: 178–185.
102. Yamanaka A, Hirai T, Fujimoto T et al. Anomalous systemic supply to normal basal segments of the left lower lobe. Annals Thorac Surg 1999; 68: 332–338.
103. Nashef SAM, Jamieson MPG, Pollock JCS, Houston AB. Aortic origin of right pulmonary artery: successful surgical correction in three consecutive patients. Ann Thorac Surg 1987; 44: 536–538.
104. Nakamura H, Makihara K, Taniguchi Y et al. Thoracoscopic surgery for intralobar pulmonary sequestration. Ann Thoracic Cardiovasc Surg 1999; 5: 405–407.
105. Petersen RC, Edwards WD. Pulmonary vascular disease in 57 necropsy cases of total anomalous pulmonary venous connection. Histopathology 1983; 7: 487–496.
106. Bloor CM, Liebow AA, Sonnenblick E, Parmley WW, ed. The pulmonary and bronchial circulations in congenital heart disease. New York: Plenum Press; 1980.
107. Wang JK, Chiu IS, How SW et al. Anomalous pulmonary venous pathway traversing pulmonary parenchyma: diagnosis and implication. Chest 1996; 110: 1363–1366.
108. Haworth SG, Reid L. Structural study of pulmonary circulation and of heart in total anomalous pulmonary venous return in early infancy. Br Heart J 1977; 39: 80–92.
109. Huddleston CB, Exil V, Canter CE, Mendelhoff EN. Scimitar syndrome presenting in infancy. Ann Thorac Surg 1999; 67: 154–159.

110. Gao YA, Burrows PE, Benson LN et al. Scimitar syndrome in infancy. J Am Coll Cardiol 1993; 22: 873–882.

111. Dupuis C, Charaf LA, Breviere GM, Abou P. 'Infantile' form of the scimitar syndrome with pulmonary hypertension. Am J Cardiol 1993; 71: 1326–1330.

112. Honey M. Anomalous pulmonary venous drainage of right lung to inferior vena cava ('Scimitar Syndrome'): clinical spectrum in older patients and role of surgery. Q J Med 1977; 184: 463–483.

113. Dupuis C, Remy J, Remy-Jardin M et al. The 'horseshoe' lung: six new cases. Pediatr Pulmonol 1994; 17: 124–130.

114. Sun CC, Doyle T, Ringel RE. Pulmonary vein stenosis. Hum Pathol 1995; 26: 880–886.

115. Vassal HB, Malone M, Petros AJ, Winter RM. Familial persistent pulmonary hypertension of the newborn resulting from misalignment of the pulmonary vessels (congenital alveolar capillary dysplasia). J Med Genet 1998; 35: 58–60.

116. MacMahon HE. Congenital alveolar dysplasia of the lungs. Am J Pathol 1948; 24: 919–931.

117. Beer DJ, Pereira W, Snider GL. Pleural effusion associated with primary lymphedema: a perspective on the yellow nail syndrome. Am Rev Respir Dis 1978; 117: 595–599.

118. Gianlupi A, Harper RW, Dwyre DM, Marelich GP. Recurrent pulmonary embolism associated with Klippel–Trenaunay–Weber syndrome. Chest 1999; 115: 1199–1201.

119. Esterly JR, Oppenheimer EH. Lymphangiectasis and other pulmonary lesions in the asplenia syndrome. Arch Pathol 1970; 90: 553–560.

120. White JES, Veale D, Fishwick D et al. Generalised lymphangiectasia: pulmonary presentation in an adult. Thorax 1996; 51: 767–768.

121. Laurence KM. Congenital pulmonary lymphangiectasis. J Clin Pathol 1959; 12: 62–69.

122. Moermans P, Vandenberghe K, Devlieger H et al. Congenital pulmonary lymphangiectasis with chylothorax: a heterogeneous lymphatic vessel abnormality. Am J Med Genet 1993; 47: 54–58.

123. Yammamoto T, Koeda T, Tamura A et al. Congenital chylothorax in a patient with 21 trisomy syndrome. Acta Paediatr Jpn 1996; 38: 689–691.

124. Ibrahim H, Asamoah A, Krouskop RW et al. Congenital chylothorax in neonatal thyrotoxicosis. J Perinatol 1999; 19: 68–71.

125. Harvey JG, Houlsby W, Sherman K, Gough MH. Congenital chylothorax: report of a unique case associated with 'H'-type tracheo-oesophageal fistula. Br J Surg 1979; 66: 485–487.

126. Easa D, Balaraman V, Ash K et al. Congenital chylothorax and mediastinal neuroblastoma. J Pediatr Surg 1991; 26: 96–98.

127. Fox GF, Challis D, O'Brien KK et al. Congenital chylothorax in syndromes. Acta Paediatr 1998; 87: 1010–1012.

128. Mussat P, Dommergues M, Parat S et al. Congenital chylothorax with hydrops: postnatal care and outcome following antenatal diagnosis. Acta Paediatr 1995; 84: 749–755.

129. Fernandez Alvarez JR, Kalache KD, Grauel EL. Management of spontaneous congenital chylothorax: oral medium-chain triglycerides versus total parenteral nutrition. Am J Perinatol 1999; 16: 415–420.

130. Andersen EA, Hertel J, Pedersen SA, Sorensen HR. Congenital chylothorax: management by ligature of the thoracic duct. Scand J Thorac Cardiovasc Surg 1984; 18: 193–194.

131. Hartman H, Samuels MP, Noyes JP et al. A case of congenital chylothorax treated by pleuroperitoneal drainage. J Perinatol 1994; 14: 313–315.

132. Sheehan JJ, Kearns SR, McNamara DA et al. Adult presentation of agenesis of the hemidiaphragm. Chest 2000; 117: 901–902.

133. Stanley P, Vachon L, Gilsanz V. Pulmonary sequestration with congenital gastroesophageal communication. Report of two cases. Pediatr Radiol 1985; 15: 343–345.

134. Weitzmann JJ, Brennan LP. Bronchogastric fistula, pulmonary sequestration, malrotation of the intestine, and Meckel's diverticulum – a new association. J Pediatr Surg 1998; 33: 1655–1657.

135. Davies J, Jaffe A, Bush A. Distal 10q trisomy syndrome with unusual cardiac and pulmonary abnormalities. J Med Genet 1998; 35: 72–74.

136. Muir TE, Leslie KO, Popper H et al. Micronodular pneumocyte hyperplasia. Am J Surg Pathol 1998; 22: 465–472.

137. Rappaport DC, Herman SJ, Weisbrod GL. Congenital bronchopulmonary diseases in adults: CT findings. AJR 1994; 162: 1295–1299.

138. Franco J, Aliaga R, Domingo ML, Plaza P. Diagnosis of pulmonary sequestration by spiral CT angiography. Thorax 1998; 53: 1089–1092.

139. Bertsch G, Market T, Hahn D et al. Intralobar lung sequestration with systemic coronary arterial supply. Eur Radiol 1999; 9: 1324–1326.

140. Yiu MWC, Ooi GC, Chan JKF, Tsang KWT. Hypolucent lung in a woman with recurrent haemoptysis. Respiration 2000; 67: 341–345.

141. Werber J, Ramilo JL, London R, Harris VJ. Unilateral absence of a pulmonary artery. Chest 1983; 84: 729–733.

142. Gamillscheg A, Beitzke A, Smolle-Juttner FM et al. Extralobar sequestration with unusual arterial supply and venous drainage. Pediatr Cardiol 1996; 17: 57–59.

143. McDonald JA, ed. Lung biology in health and disease. Lung growth and development, vol 100. New York: Marcel Dekker; 1997.

144. Levine MM, Nudel DB, Gootman N et al. Pulmonary sequestration causing congestive heart failure in infancy: a report of two cases and review of the literature. Ann Thorac Surg 1982; 34: 581–585.

145. Halkic N, Cuenoud PF, Corthesy ME et al. Pulmonary sequestration: a review of 26 cases. Eur J Cardiothorac Surg 1998; 14: 127–133.

146. Becmeur F, Horta-Geraud P, Donato L, Sauvage P. Pulmonary sequestrations: prenatal ultrasound diagnosis, treatment, and outcome. J Pediatr Surg 1998; 33: 492–496.

147. Coran AG, Drongowski R. Congenital cystic disease of the tracheobronchial tree in infants and children. Experience with 44 consecutive cases. Arch Surg 1994; 129: 521–527.

148. Mezzeti M, Dell'Agnola CA, Bedoni M et al. Video-assisted thoracoscopic resection of pulmonary sequestration in an infant. Ann Thorac Surg 1996; 61: 1836–1837.

149. Najm HK, Williams WG, Coles JG et al. Scimitar syndrome: twenty years' experience and results of repair. J Thorac Cardiovasc Surg 1996; 112: 1161–1168.

22 Bronchopulmonary dysplasia

Anne Greenough

 Key points

- Bronchopulmonary dysplasia, prolonged oxygen dependency after birth in association with an abnormal chest radiograph appearance, is increasing.

- Bronchopulmonary dysplasia has a multifactorial aetiology but improved survival of very immature infants is primarily responsible for the growing numbers with the condition.

- Bronchopulmonary dysplasia children require frequent readmissions to hospital in the first 2 years, particularly for lower respiratory tract infection.

- Lung function abnormalities (airways obstruction) are detected in adolescents and young adults who had bronchopulmonary dysplasia.

Definition

Bronchopulmonary dysplasia (BPD) was first described by Northway in 1967.[1] Infants with BPD developed chronic pulmonary morbidity following acute respiratory failure; there were four stages based on distinctive chest radiograph appearances. Those abnormalities, particularly the severe cystic lesions characterising stage 4 BPD, are now uncommon. As a consequence, BPD is usually diagnosed if an infant has prolonged dependency on supplementary oxygen. Infants will usually have been ventilated in the perinatal period and have at least interstitial abnormalities on their 28-day chest radiograph.[2] Many, however, would describe such infants as suffering from chronic lung disease and reserve the diagnosis of BPD for those who have the classical chest radiograph changes described by Northway.[1] Unfortunately, there is no consensus in the literature and the terms chronic lung disease and BPD are used interchangeably. There is also controversy as to the exact duration of oxygen dependency that best defines chronic

lung disease/BPD. In an early study,[3] oxygen dependency beyond 36 weeks postconceptional age rather than 28 days correlated more closely with continuing morbidity after discharge. In infants usually exposed to antenatal steroids and postnatal surfactant, however, oxygen dependency beyond 28 days, particularly if associated with an abnormal chest radiograph appearance, performed better with regard to prediction of ongoing respiratory morbidity, even throughout the preschool years.[4] In this chapter, BPD will be used to describe infants who remained dependent on supplementary oxygen beyond 28 days.

Epidemiology

Infants born at very early gestations are most likely to develop BPD. The incidence of BPD in very-low-birthweight infants has increased over the last two decades from approximately 10% to 30%, most of the extra cases explained by improved survival of very immature infants. A further factor contributing to increased susceptibility is an inability to secrete adequate amounts of cortisol in settings of increased stress.[5] Whether a family history of asthma increases the likelihood of developing BPD is controversial, but it is associated with a slower resolution of BPD.[6]

Aetiology

The aetiology of BPD is summarised in Figure 22.1.

Antenatal infection

Infants exposed to chorioamnionitis are at increased risk of BPD.[7] Meta-analysis of 17 reports, including term and preterm infants showed that the relative risk for BPD development in infants colonised with *Ureaplasma urealyticum* was 1.72 (95% confidence intervals (CI) 1.5 to 1. 96).[8] The pooled relative risk for high risk infants (<1500 g and/or <31 weeks gestational

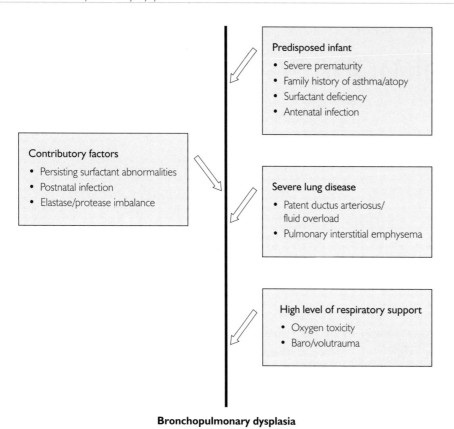

Fig. 22.1 Aetiology of bronchopulmonary dysplasia.

Bronchopulmonary dysplasia

age) was 5.21 (95% CI 0.9 to 47.7). Colonisation is significantly associated with younger maternal age, premature labour and prolonged rupture of the membranes.

Patent ductus arteriosus

Infants who develop a patent ductus arteriosus are at increased risk of BPD. Infection, particularly if temporally related, potentiates the effect of a patent ductus arteriosus on the risk of BPD.[9] Fluid overload may explain the association of patent ductus arteriosus and BPD. A retrospective review[10] demonstrated that BPD infants had received greater quantities of fluid and generally gained weight in the first four days in contrast to the weight loss seen in non-BPD infants.

Pulmonary interstitial emphysema

This condition has been associated with a high incidence of BPD.[11] In pulmonary interstitial emphysema, respiratory function is compromised by air dissection into false air spaces compressing lung tissue.

Oxygen toxicity

Northway[1] originally ascribed BPD to oxygen toxicity, as the chronic phase was invariably seen in infants in high oxygen concentrations for more than 150 hours. Oxygen toxicity is still felt to be a contributory factor. Prolonged exposure to high oxygen concentrations has complex biochemical, microscopic and gross anatomical effects on lung tissues.

Positive pressure support

Initially BPD was only described in infants exposed to a concentration of supplementary oxygen of 100%. Later it became apparent that BPD also occurred in infants who received oxygen concentrations of less than 60%, if this was used with continuous positive airways pressure (CPAP) or mechanical ventilation. The longer infants are ventilated the more likely they are to develop BPD, particularly if very high peak inflating pressures are used. An inverse relationship has been demonstrated between hypocapnia and subsequent BPD development,[12] further incriminating baro- or volutrauma. At follow up, airways resistance was higher in infants who had been ventilated compared to those who had required supplementary oxygen or no form of respiratory support.[13]

Surfactant abnormalities

Prolonged exposure to high inspired oxygen concentrations results in alterations in type 2 pneumocyte function and impaired surfactant biosynthesis via oxidant-induced injury. In infants with BPD, the lecithin/sphingomyelin ratio increases slowly and even at term BPD infants have low levels of phosphatidylinositol. There may also be inadequate levels of surfactant proteins, deficiency of surfactant protein A (SP-A) mRNA expression was present at term in a model of chronic lung injury.[14] In addition, oxygen free radicals degrade SP-A. Infants with BPD are further disadvantaged as they have surfactant inhibitors, e.g. glycolipids and proteins, present in their airways.

Disturbance of elastase/protease system

The granulocytes present in the tracheal aspirates of BPD infants release elastase, collagenase and phospholipase A2, which destroy lung parenchyma and break down surfactant. In BPD patients there is a significantly less favourable protease antiprotease balance, with a higher elastase activity than similarly aged non-BPD infants.[15]

Pathophysiology

Respiratory distress syndrome is associated with a pulmonary inflammatory reaction, as indicated by an excess of neutrophils and alveolar macrophages in the lung effluent. This is associated with a loss of endothelial, basement membrane and interstitial sulphated glycosaminoglycans.[16] Barotrauma and oxygen toxicity further contribute to the inflammatory reaction, which persists in those infants who develop BPD; thus the majority still have neutrophils in their aspirates at 11–15 days. The activated neutrophils mediate endothelial cytotoxicity and inhibit phosphatidyl choline synthesis. C5a and interleukin (IL)-8, important chemoattractants for human neutrophils, are detected in the bronchoalveolar lavage (BAL) fluid and may contribute to the abnormal lung permeability of early BPD.[17] Proinflammatory cytokines IL-1β and IL-6, which may have a role in initiating the inflammatory response, are also increased in the BAL fluid from infants who develop BPD. In addition, the β-chemokine macrophage inflammatory protein (MIP)-1α is increased from birth and is associated with the later development of fibrosis.[18] Tumour necrosis factor (TNF)-α increases at a later stage and may contribute to the chronic inflammation. TNF-α, IL-6 and IL-8 concentrations in tracheal aspirates collected on days 2 and 3 are significantly related to gestational age and the duration of supplemental oxygen.[19] BAL-derived macrophages from preterm newborns with respiratory distress syndrome may not contain IL-10 during the early stages of lung inflammation.[20] IL-10 inhibits the production of proinflammatory cytokines by monocytes and macrophages; thus the macrophages in preterm lungs may not control the inflammatory process as effectively as more mature hosts.

Leukotriene B4 is detected in the BAL fluid of BPD infants. Urinary leukotriene levels are also high at 28 days and even at 6 months in BPD infants.[21] Leukotrienes cause bronchoconstriction, vasoconstriction, oedema, neutrophil chemotaxis and mucus production in the lung. Eicosanoids and platelet-activating factor, other potent lipid mediators with injurious effects on the lung, are also found in large quantities in the tracheobronchial effluent of infants in whom BPD subsequently develops.

Pathology

There is an early reparative stage in weeks 1–2 and then a subacute fibroproliferative stage in weeks 2–4. These stages represent a continuum from acute lung injury. There is severe bronchial and bronchiolar injury with a loss of respiratory epithelium and a fibroblastic proliferative response. In the respiratory units, there is interstitial fibrosis, smooth muscle proliferation and type II pneumocyte metaplasia. After approximately 1 month of age there is a chronic proliferative phase.[22] Airway injury is marked by smooth muscle hypertrophy, squamous metaplasia of the respiratory epithelium and glandular hyperplasia.[23] In the respiratory units there may be areas of severe fibrosis alternating with areas of emphysema. Such changes are, however, unusual except in infants who had the classical chest radiograph appearance of Northway stage 4 BPD. Hypertrophy of the pulmonary arterial smooth muscle in the media and adventitial fibrous tissue may be present;[24] hence pulmonary hypertension can complicate the progress of BPD infants.

Clinical presentation

The majority of infants are born very prematurely and remain dyspnoeic despite oxygen supplementation. Chronic hypoxia can lead to the development of cor pulmonale; thus infants are usually nursed in sufficient supplementary oxygen to maintain their oxygen saturation level at least above 92% (see Management, below). Nevertheless, some infants suffer episodes of spontaneous desaturation (BPD spells). BPD infants have frequent respiratory relapses, usually due to bacterial or viral infections. In infants who remain chronically ventilator-dependent, endotracheal secretions are common; there may be chronic carbon dioxide retention, persistent atelectasis, lobar hyperinflation, tracheo- and/or bronchomalacia.[25] A minority, with severe BPD, are oedematous and have obvious signs of right heart failure, but infants with milder disease are often intolerant of standard maintenance fluid volumes. Feeding difficulties and aspiration occur frequently, as does growth failure and osteopenia with resultant fractures (Fig. 22.2). The increased risk of aspiration in BPD infants is related to their predisposition to gastro-oesophageal reflux.

Investigations

Imaging

Northway et al[1] described four distinct radiographic appearances. The first stage was radiographically indistinguishable from severe respiratory distress syndrome and was usually seen between 1 and 3 days. In stage 2 there was marked radioopacity of the lungs occurring between 4 and 10 days and in stage 3 clearing of the radio opacity occurred but a cystic, bubbly pattern developed at 10–20 days (Fig. 22.3). Stage 4 was characterised by hyperexpansion, streaks of abnormal density and areas of emphysema with variable cardiomegaly, which was seen from 1 month of age (Fig. 22.4).

The chest radiograph appearances of BPD infants at 28 days have more recently been divided into two types.[11] Type I BPD was characterised by homogeneous or patchy ill-defined opacification in the lungs without coarse reticulation and type II

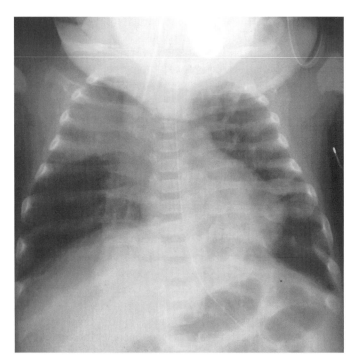

Fig. 22.2 Chest radiograph of a 24-week gestation infant with Northway stage 4 bronchopulmonary dysplasia. There are healing rib fractures (callus) on the left side of the chest and right upper lobe consolidation.

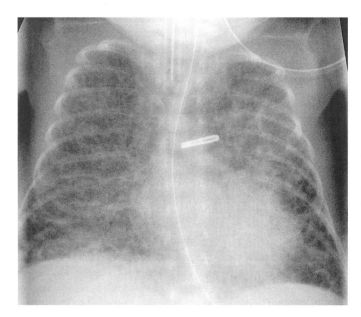

Fig. 22.3 Chest radiograph of a 25-week gestation infant with Northway stage 4 bronchopulmonary dysplasia. There are fibrotic changes and a cystic, bubbly pattern. The infant has undergone ligation of a patent ductus arteriosus.

disease by coarse reticulation and streaky densities interspersed with small cystic translucencies. Type I BPD resolved and was the more common appearance; type II BPD followed pulmonary interstitial emphysema and had a poorer prognosis. Chest radio-

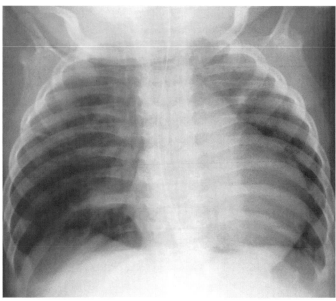

Fig. 22.4 Chest radiograph of a 26-week gestation infant with Northway stage 4 bronchopulmonary dysplasia. There is marked hyperexpansion, with areas of emphysema and bullae.

graph scoring systems have been developed to quantify disease severity and/or predict prognosis. At follow-up, lesions in BPD infants with chronic pulmonary dysfunction are better visualised on a computerised tomography (CT) scan than a chest radiograph. Findings include multifocal areas of hyperaeration and linear and triangular subpleural opacities.[26]

Lung function abnormalities

In the first months after birth, BPD infants may have a low functional residual capacity (FRC), compliance and specific compliance but high airways resistance. There is also evidence of impaired gas mixing. Supplementary oxygen is required to maintain adequate oxygen saturations and a compensated respiratory acidosis is frequently present. A low FRC and impaired gas mixture are seen in all infants with BPD but changes in lung mechanics are usually restricted to those with more severe disease.

Differential diagnosis

A number of infants become chronically oxygen-dependent despite initially having no or only mild respiratory distress syndrome and without a requirement for ventilatory support. This can occur in very immature infants, usually of birthweight less than 1000 g. Some have used the term chronic pulmonary insufficiency[27] of prematurity to describe affected infants, particularly if they present at between 4 and 7 days with respiratory distress, frequent apnoea and a requirement for supplemental oxygen, the abnormalities persisting for several weeks. The infants have small-volume lungs with hazy lung fields. Continuous positive airways pressure (CPAP) is useful to treat worsening hypoxaemia and apnoea; the prognosis is good. Infants who develop Wilson–Mikity syndrome also have no respiratory problems in the first week but progressive respiratory failure develops during the second week. The diagnosis is supported by diffuse, small, bilateral cystic translucencies on the chest radiograph. The condition occurs in infants of less than 32 completed weeks of gestation. Elevated plasma IgM levels in the first day of life and a high incidence of chorioamnionitis in mothers of infants with Wilson–Mikity syndrome, associated with a raised cord-blood IgM, suggests that intrauterine infection[28] is a contributory factor. Symptoms may persist for many months. Abnormal lung function, suggesting persistent small-airway damage, has been found in survivors even at 8–10 years of age but the usual tendency is for the pulmonary disease to resolve.

Prophylaxis

Antenatal therapy

Neither antenatal steroid nor thyrotropin-releasing hormone treatment favourably impacts on the incidence of BPD.[29,30]

Surfactant

Exogenous surfactant replacement therapy does not reduce the incidence of BPD.[31] Inositol supplementation (80 mg/kg) during the first 5 days of life, however, improved survival without chronic lung disease from 55% to 71%.[32]

Steroids

Dexamethasone given to ventilated infants reduces the pulmonary inflammatory response, microvascular permeability and release of inflammatory mediators and neutrophil influx into the airways. There have now been at least 10 trials assessing the impact of early systemic administration of corticosteroids on the incidence of BPD. Meta-analysis of those trials[33] demonstrated that steroid administration, if started within the first 2 weeks, was associated with a significant reduction in the incidence of BPD and, if given between 7 and 14 days, a reduction in mortality. The size of dose and duration of treatment varied between the trials; therefore, a sensitivity analysis was undertaken. It demonstrated that dexamethasone had similar effects when given at a dosage of 0.5 mg/kg per day for 7–14 days compared to when given at a higher dose for longer.[33] Shorter courses, i.e. 3 days or less, even if followed by inhaled therapy, have usually not been associated with a significant reduction in chronic lung disease. Repeating the short course or starting it within the first 48 hours after birth may be more effective but early administration has been associated with an increased risk of intestinal perforations.

Numerous other side effects of systemically administered corticosteroids have been reported. These include pneumothorax, sepsis, necrotising enterocolitis, hyperglycaemia, hypertension, periventricular densities and leukomalacia, diabetic ketoacidosis,

hypertrophic cardiomyopathy and weight loss. Some infants develop hypertensive encephalopathy and dexamethasone can cause secondary adrenal suppression at the hypothalamic–pituitary level. More important, however, is the considerable concern that systemically administered corticosteroids may have long-term adverse effects. Corticosteroids have significant negative effects on cell multiplication in the central nervous system and lung. Follow-up of infants from randomised trials has demonstrated a significant excess of infants with adverse neurodevelopmental outcome following steroid treatment.[34]

Studies in animal models have also suggested that dexamethasone treatment has an adverse effect on the lung. Given at a critical period of between 4 and 14 days after birth, corticosteroids resulted in rats of normal body size but with increased lung volumes and enlarged air spaces, decreased alveolar surface area and reduced total DNA content. The outgrowth of new alveolar septa was partly suppressed[35] and after drug withdrawal, although the trend towards precocious maturation of the lung was reversed, the lungs remained emphysematous, with larger and fewer airspaces. These worrying data urge caution when contemplating systemic administration of corticosteroids.

To avoid the side-effects of systemically administered steroids, this therapy has been given by inhalation. Although the only adverse effect seen was tongue hypertrophy, which resolved after cessation of treatment, randomised trials suggest that the benefits associated with this mode of administration are also less. Inhaled steroids only facilitate extubation and reduce the need for later 'rescue' systemic steroids but do not influence the occurrence of BPD.[36] Two randomised trials[37,38] comparing the effect of inhaled and systemically administered steroids have confirmed that the former route is less effective. The impact on lung function was of a lower magnitude and slower onset[37] and there was less impact on inflammatory mediators.[38]

Antioxidants

Although preterm infants are deficient in antioxidants, supplementation has had variable success. Randomised trials demonstrated that, although BPD was not significantly reduced by administration of vitamin E,[39] it was favourably affected by superoxide dismutase supplementation from 24 hours of age in infants with severe respiratory distress.[40] Toxicity of superoxide dismutase has not been reported but antioxidants affect the bactericidal activity of polymorphonuclear cells. Allopurinol, a synthetic competitive inhibitor of xanthine oxidase and a free radical scavenger, also failed in a randomised placebo-controlled trial to significantly reduce the incidence of BPD.[41] Administration of recombinant human erythropoietin reduces the transfusion rate in preterm infants, decreasing the iron infusion, which may exacerbate free radical damage, leading to BPD. In a randomised trial, however, erythropoietin only significantly reduced the number of days in oxygen[42] but the sample size was relatively small.

Vitamin A

Premature infants are deprived of transplacental acquisition of vitamin A and, as parenteral administration of vitamin A is inefficient, it is not surprising that BPD infants have low vitamin A levels. Meta-analysis of randomised trials demonstrated a trend towards a reduction in death or BPD associated with vitamin A supplementation.[43] Differing conclusions from individual studies may reflect the relatively small numbers of patients included in each trial and/or the differences in dosage and patient populations.[43]

Ventilatory mode

Avoidance of 'aggressive' respiratory support may reduce BPD. Continuous positive airways pressure employed soon after birth in preference to ventilation has been associated with a low incidence of BPD.[44,45] Those results, however, were not generated from randomised trials and the low incidence of BPD could have other explanations, including avoidance of hyperventilation and muscle relaxants and use of permissive hypercapnia.[44]

Synchronised ventilation, which can be achieved by using either high frequency positive-pressure ventilation (HFPPV) or patient-triggered ventilation (PTV), has been associated with improved blood gases and a lower work of breathing. Meta-analysis of randomised trials comparing high frequency positive-pressure ventilation or patient-triggered ventilation to conventional ventilation, however, demonstrated that neither method of respiratory support reduces BPD.[46]

During high-frequency oscillation, small tidal volumes are delivered at very fast frequencies, usually 10–15 times per second. Initial trials failed to demonstrate that high-frequency oscillation (HFO) compared to conventional ventilation reduced BPD. Subsequent studies, however, demonstrated that, if a high-volume strategy was used – i.e. the mean airway pressure was elevated to optimise lung volume[47] – high-frequency oscillation was associated with a lower BPD incidence. Unfortunately, it remains controversial whether the reduction in BPD is at the expense of an increase in intracranial pathology, particularly in very immature infants.[47]

Nitric oxide

Nitric oxide can improve oxygenation in prematurely born infants. Thus it was postulated that NO administration might reduce the incidence of BPD by lowering the exposure to high inspired oxygen concentrations. Randomised trials, however, have failed to demonstrate that early administration of NO impacted favourably on BPD development. The only benefits seen have been a reduction in ventilator days[48] and a lower requirement for bronchodilators or systemically administered corticosteroids.[49]

Fluid balance

Fluid overload compromises respiratory function but promotion of an early diuresis with diuretics or albumin infusion does not significantly improve respiratory status. In addition, randomised trials have highlighted that, although fluid restriction is associated with a lower incidence of necrotising enterocolitis and patent ductus arteriosus, it does not reduce BPD.[50] Providing sodium supplementation is controlled, preterm infants can adapt to differing amounts of fluid input by altering their urine output and osmolality. Withholding early sodium supplementation may reduce BPD.[51] Colloid infusion has a detrimental effect on lung function and oxygen dependency in preterm infants.[50]

Erythromycin

Colonisation with *Ureaplasma urealyticum* may increase the incidence of BPD but to date administration of erythromycin has not impacted favourably on BPD. However, in one trial only 13% of the population was positive for *U. urealyticum*.[52]

Management

To prevent further lung damage, peak inspiratory pressures and inspired oxygen concentrations should be reduced to the minimum compatible with acceptable blood gases and every attempt should be made to wean the infant from the ventilator. Oxygen supplementation should be used to achieve oxygen saturation levels of at least 92%. However, maintaining the level at more than 95%, rather than at a lower saturation, may improve weight gain and reduce hospital readmission rates.[53] Monitoring of oxygen saturation rather than transcutaneous oxygen is more reliable in BPD infants. Carbon dioxide tension can be allowed to rise when the risk of periventricular haemorrhage is reduced, providing that this does not result in a respiratory acidosis. Sedation should be kept to a minimum but may be necessary to achieve adequate mechanical ventilation in certain BPD infants; some even require neuromuscular blocking agents.

Both nitric oxide and surfactant can improve oxygenation in infants with BPD; whether such therapies improve the long-term outcome require to be assessed in randomised trials. Many BPD infants require prolonged ventilation and chronic use of either an oral or nasal endotracheal tube can result in cosmetic defects. Tracheostomy avoids those problems but can be difficult to close.

Bronchopulmonary dysplasia infants are often intolerant of standard maintenance volumes of fluid. Diuretics (see later) should be considered for those who are gaining weight in excess of 20 g/kg per day on such a regimen, as this may indicate fluid retention. Energy requirements above 150 kcal/kg are rare and may be associated with malabsorption.[54] BPD infants benefit from use of a premature formula until they reach approximately 3.0 kg. If the infant is receiving human milk, a fortifier should be used. Addition of modular components such as carbohydrate or fat, or both, can be used to concentrate a formula to 30 kcal/oz, but fat should not provide more than 60% of the total calories to avoid the risk of ketosis and slowing gastric emptying. Infants with BPD may have limited fat absorption and suffer from gastro-oesophageal reflux. If feed thickeners are used and the infant is on a concentrated feed, the osmolality should be checked.

Infants should be considered for home oxygen therapy if they are feeding by mouth and gaining weight but have a supplementary oxygen concentration requirement of more than 25%.

Some infants require years of home oxygen. Only a very small number of BPD infants have been discharged on home ventilation; they must have a tracheostomy. Home ventilation requires an enormous investment in equipment, community services and education for parents.[55]

Drug therapy

Corticosteroids

Systemic administration of corticosteroids to infants with established BPD on the neonatal intensive care unit results in only short-term benefits: reduction in respiratory rate, peak inspiration pressure, fractional inspired oxygen concentration and alveolar oxygen gradient and an improved rate of weaning. Meta-analysis of randomised trials have demonstrated that administration of dexamethasone after the first 3 weeks only facilitates extubation from ventilatory support[56] and there are considerable concerns regarding the long-term adverse effects of corticosteroids (see Prophylaxis, above). Thus, this therapy should be used with extreme caution. Research is urgently required to identify the smallest dose with a positive risk/benefit ratio.

Diuretics

Diuretics improve lung function, resulting in transient improvements in blood gases in both ventilated and non-ventilated babies. Randomised trials, however, have not demonstrated that prolonged diuretic therapy improves long-term outcome.[57] Inhaled furosemide (frusemide) appears to be ineffective in ventilated infants,[58] apart from resulting in transient improvement of lung function in infants with mild disease.

Diuretics, particularly furosemide, have many side-effects, including hypochloraemia, hyponatraemia, hypokalaemia, hypocalcaemia and metabolic alkalosis. Other complications include secondary hyperparathyroidism, rickets and ototoxicity. The ototoxicity of furosemide is a synergistic effect with aminoglycosides. Chronic diuretic therapy may cause hypercalcuria, renal calcification and nephrocalcinosis, leading to haematuria and urinary tract infections. The risk of nephrocalcinosis is increased in infants with a positive family history, or who are receiving parenteral nutrition or concurrent treatment with methylxanthines. Even at 4–5 years of age, renal calcification may persist and be associated with abnormal glomerular filtrate rate. Diuretic therapy, then, should be restricted to intermittent courses for those intolerant of standard fluid volumes.

Anti-asthma medication

Bronchopulmonary dysplasia infants have peribronchiolar smooth muscle hypertrophy and can have a positive response to inhaled bronchodilators even while on the neonatal intensive care unit. Salbutamol causes a dose-related improvement in lung mechanics in ventilator-dependent infants but the beneficial effects of $200\,\mu g$ of salbutamol lasted only 3 hours.[59] Synergism occurs between ipratropium bromide and salbutamol but the effect is seen for only up to 1–2 hours after administration. After discharge, therapy with inhaled ipratropium bromide or terbutaline, using a coffee-cup spacer device, improves lung function and reduces symptoms in wheezy, very-low-birthweight survivors.[60] In non-symptomatic infants, however, nebulised bronchodilator may cause a deterioration in lung function, as evidenced by an increase in airways resistance.[61] This paradoxical effect can be avoided by administering the bronchodilator by inhaler and spacer device rather than by means of a nebuliser. At follow-up, both inhaled sodium cromoglycate and corticosteroids reduce troublesome respiratory symptoms and bronchodilator usage in very-low-birthweight infants.[62,63]

Respiratory syncytial virus prophylaxis

Bronchopulmonary dysplasia infants suffer severe consequences of respiratory syncytial virus (RSV) infection, as evidenced by their high hospitalisation and admission rate to the paediatric intensive care unit. Currently there are no safe and effective vaccines against RSV. Immunoprophylaxis, however, has been shown to reduce the hospitalisation rate of BPD infants. Administration of RSV immunoglobulin (RSV-IgIV), which contains high levels of RSV-neutralising antibodies, was associated with a 40% reduction in hospitalisation rate from RSV infection.[64] RSV-IgIV was given as a 15 ml/kg infusion and 13% of infants with BPD required diuretics at the time of treatment – this may have been caused by fluid overload.

Palivizumab, a humanised immunoglobulin monoclonal antibody, has also been found to reduce the hospitalisation rate in BPD infants.[65] It has a major advantage over RSV-IgIV as it is given by intramuscular injection and is therefore cheaper to administer. Nevertheless, there are concerns that, except in BPD infants receiving home oxygen, administration of palivizumab may not be cost-effective. Studies to date, however, have only assessed the potential savings related to the initial hospitalisation episode. BPD infants, as healthy infants born at term, are likely to suffer ongoing respiratory morbidity following RSV infection; this should also be taken into account as an outcome in any future study.

Prognosis

The mortality of stage 4 BPD is 40%. Infants usually die at about 3 months of age and between 67% and 80% of deaths occur during the initial hospitalisation. Death is due to intercurrent infection, cor pulmonale or respiratory failure. Predictors of death in hospital include male gender and length of time on ventilatory support and supplementary oxygen.[66]

The average weight and height at term of infants with BPD is frequently at or below the third centile. Growth retardation is associated with severe and prolonged respiratory dysfunction.[67] Growth accelerates as pulmonary status improves and, at school age, children who had BPD had similar growth to controls.[68] In the first 2 years, developmental delay is common. At 12 and 18 months, BPD infants performed significantly less well at cognitive, sensorimotor and language tests than infants who had had respiratory distress syndrome.[67]

Poor developmental outcome correlated with prolonged hospitalisation and requirement for oxygen,[67] as well as prolonged ventilation. Neurodevelopmental problems are less common in older children. At 3 years of age, 29% of those who had stage 4 BPD had minor abnormalities and only 34% significant handicap (cerebral palsy, mental retardation, deafness or blindness). The degree of handicap was not dissimilar to that found in preterm infants who had had severe respiratory distress syndrome but, although ventilated for longer than 24 hours, did not develop BPD.[67] In school-age BPD children, low height and intelligence scores[69] appear to relate to prematurity, perinatal events, central nervous system injury and social adversity rather than pulmonary disease.[70]

Rehospitalisation is required in up to 50% of infants in the first year and between 20% and 37% in the second year.[71] Infants with BPD are readmitted an average of five times during the first 2 years. The primary reason for readmission is lower respiratory tract viral infections, particularly RSV. Risk factors for acquisition of RSV infection in BPD infants include large family size, passive smoking and requirement for home oxygen therapy. RSV infection in BPD patients has severe consequences even in the second year of life.

Pulmonary function abnormalities have been frequently documented at follow-up of BPD children (Table 22.1). In the first year, these include a high airways resistance, increased gas trapping, low dynamic pulmonary compliance, reduced FRC, abnormal gas exchange (hypercapnia, low oxygen saturation), elevated minute volume and lower mixing index. The most consistent finding is an elevated pulmonary or airway resistance.[72] Lung function usually improves with age[73] but severe lower airway obstruction persists,[74] particularly in those who have recurrent respiratory symptoms. Pulmonary function tests may still be abnormal in school-age children, with airways obstruction and hyperinflation and reduced exercise tolerance.[75] BPD children at school age are also more likely to have a positive methacholine challenge test and response to bronchodilator therapy.[76] Although lung function abnormalities are also seen in children born prematurely who did not develop BPD, at 8–11 years BPD children had poorer respiratory function, as indicated by a lower forced expiratory volume in 1 second (FEV$_1$) and higher residual volume/total lung capacity.[77]

Airflow obstruction may still be present in 15-year-old children[78] and even in young adults who had BPD – not all the airways obstruction is reversible.[79] The longer-term outlook for affected individuals remains speculative and whether subsequent generations routinely exposed to antenatal steroids and postnatal surfactant will fare better as adults is also uncertain.

Table 22.1 Lung function abnormalities in BPD survivors

First year	High airways resistance and gas trapping Low pulmonary compliance and functional residual capacity
3 years	Certain lung function abnormalities resolve Still evidence of airways obstruction and bronchial hyper-responsiveness
School age	Reduced exercise tolerance Bronchial hyper-responsiveness and airways obstruction
Young adults	Airways obstruction

? Unresolved questions

- How can we achieve accurate detection of high-risk infants to ensure appropriate targeting of interventions at an early stage?
- What are the most effective and safe prophylactic strategies, including the optimum ventilatory mode, particularly for very immature infants?
- What will be the long-term consequences of bronchopulmonary dysplasia and its treatment in children who were routinely exposed to antenatal steroids and postnatal surfactant?

Therapeutic principles

Drug	Effect	Target population
On the NICU		
Diuretics	Short term improvements in lung function	Incipient right heart failure
Bronchodilators	Short term improvements in lung function	Wheezy infants
Corticosteroids	Facilitates extubation	Severe BPD (>3 weeks of age)
After discharge		
Bronchodilators	Improves lung function and relieves symptoms	Infants with troublesome wheeze/cough
Inhaled steroids	Improves lung function Reduces bronchodilator usage	Wheezy BPD infants requiring regular bronchodilators
RSV immunoprophylaxis	Reduces hospitalisation	BPD infants requiring home oxygen

BPD, bronchopulmonary dysplasia; NICU, neonatal intensive care unit; RSV, respiratory syncytial virus

References

1. Northway WHJ, Rosan RC, Porter DY. Pulmonary disease following respiratory therapy of hyaline membrane disease: bronchopulmonary dysplasia. N Engl J Med 1967; 276: 357–368.

2. Greenough A, Kavvadia K, Johnson AH et al. A simple chest radiograph score to predict chronic lung disease in prematurely born infants. Br J Radiol 1999; 72: 530–533.

3. Shennan AT, Dunn MS, Ohlsson A et al. Abnormal pulmonary outcomes in premature infants: prediction from oxygen requirement in the neonatal period. Pediatrics 1988; 82: 527–532.

4. Kinali M, Greenough A, Dimitriou G, Yuksel B. Chronic respiratory morbidity following premature delivery – prediction of prolonged respiratory support requirement. Eur J Pediatr 1999; 158: 493–496.

5. Watterberg KL, Scott SM. Evidence of early adrenal insufficiency in babies who develop bronchopulmonary dysplasia. Pediatrics 1995; 95: 120–125.

6. Hagan R, Minutillo C, French N et al. Neonatal chronic lung disease, oxygen dependency and a family history of asthma. Pediatr Pulmonol 1995; 20: 277–283.

7. Watterberg KL, Demers LM, Scott SM, Murphy S. Chorioamnionitis and early lung inflammation in infants in whom bronchopulmonary dysplasia develops. Pediatrics 1996; 97: 210–215.

8. Wang EE, Ohlsson A, Kellner JD. Association of *Ureaplasma urealyticum* colonization with chronic lung disease of prematurity: result of meta-analysis. J Pediatr 1995; 127: 640–644.

9. Gonzalez A, Sosenko IRS, Chandar J et al. Influence of infection on patent ductus arteriosus and chronic lung disease in premature infants weighing 1000 g or less. J Pediatr 1996; 128: 470–478.

10. Van Marter LJ, Leviton A, Allred EN et al. Hydration during the first days of life and the risk of bronchopulmonary dysplasia in low birth weight infants. J Pediatr 1990; 116(6): 942–949.

11. Hyde I, English ER, Williams JA. The changing pattern of chronic lung disease of prematurity. Arch Dis Child 1989;64: 448–451.

12. Garland JS, Buck RK, Allred EN, Leviton A. Hypocarbia before surfactant therapy appears to increase bronchopulmonary dysplasia risk in infants with respiratory distress syndrome. Arch Pediatr Adolesc Med 1995; 149: 617–622.

13. Yüksel B, Greenough A. Neonatal respiratory support and lung function abnormalities at follow-up. Respir Med 1992; 86: 97–100.

14. Coalson JJ, Winter V, deLemos RA. Decreased alveolarization in baboon survivors with bronchopulmonary dysplasia. Am J Respir Crit Care Med 1995;152:640–646.

15. Watterberg KL, Carmichael DF, Gerdes JS et al. Secretory leukocyte protease inhibitor and lung inflammation in developing bronchopulmonary dysplasia. J Pediatr 1994; 125: 264–269.

16. Murch SH, Costeloe K, Klein NJ et al. Mucosal tumour necrosis factor-α production and extensive disruption of sulfated glycosaminoglycans begin within hours of birth in neonatal respiratory distress syndrome. Pediatr Res 1996; 40: 484–489.

17. Groneck P, Speer CP. Inflammatory mediators and bronchopulmonary dysplasia. Arch Dis Child 1995; 73: F1–F3.

18. Murch SH, Costeloe K, Klein NJ, McDonald TT. Early production of macrophage of inflammatory protein-1α occurs in respiratory distress syndrome and is associated with poor outcome. Pediatr Res 1996; 40: 490–497.

19. Jonsson B, Tullus K, Brauner A et al. Early increase of TNFalpha and IL-6 in tracheobronchial aspirate fluid indicator of subsequent chronic lung disease in preterm infants. Arch Dis Child 1997; 77: F198–F201.

20. Jones CA, Cayabyab RG, Kwong KYC et al. Undetectable interleukin (IL)-10 and persistent IL-8 expression early in hyaline membrane disease: a possible developmental basis for the predisposition to chronic lung inflammation in preterm newborns. Pediatr Res 1996; 39(6): 966–975.

21. Cook AJ, Yuksel B, Sampson AP et al. Cysteinyl leukotriene involvement in chronic lung disease in premature infants. Eur Respir J 1996; 9: 1907–1912.

22 Askin F. Respiratory tract disorders in the fetus and neonate. In: Wigglesworth JS, Singer DB, ed. Textbook of fetal and perinatal pathology, Oxford: Blackwell Scientific; 1991: 643–688.

23. Margraf LR, Tomashefski JF, Bruce MC, Dahms BB. Morphometric analysis of the lung in bronchopulmonary dysplasia. Am Rev Respir Dis 1991; 143: 391–400.

24. Hislop AA, Wharton J, Allen KM et al. Immunohistochemical localization of peptide-containing nerves in human airways: age-related changes. Am J Respir Cell Mol Biol 1990; 3: 191–198.

25. Miller RW, Woo P, Kellman RK, Slagle TS. Tracheobronchial abnormalities in infants with bronchopulmonary dysplasia. J Pediatr 1987; 111: 779–782.

26. Oppenheim C, Marmou-Mani T, Sayegh N et al. Bronchopulmonary dysplasia: value of CT in identifying pulmonary sequelae. AJR 1994; 163: 169–172.

27. Krauss AN, Klain DB, Auld PAM. Chronic pulmonary insufficiency of prematurity (CPIP). Pediatrics 1975; 55: 55–58.

28. Fujimura M, Takeuchi T, Kitajima H, Nakayama M. Chorioamnionitis and serum IgM in Wilson–Mikity syndrome. Arch Dis Child 1989; 64: 1379–1383.

29. Crowley P. Prophylactic corticosteroids for preterm birth (Cochrane Review). In: The Cochrane Library, Issue 4. Oxford: Update Software; 1999.

30. Crowther CA, Alfirevic Z, Haslam RR. Prenatal thyrotropin-releasing hormone for preterm birth (Cochrane review). In: The Cochrane Library, Issue 4. Oxford: Update Software; 1999.

31. Soll RF. Natural surfactant extract versus synthetic surfactant for neonatal respiratory distress syndrome (Cochrane Review). In: The Cochrane Library, Issue 3. Oxford: Update Software; 1999.

32. Hallman M, Bry K, Hoppu K et al. Inositol supplementation in premature infants with respiratory distress syndrome. N Engl J Med 1992; 326: 1233–1239.

33. Bhuta T, Ohlsson A. Systematic review and meta-analysis of early postnatal dexamethasone for prevention of chronic lung disease. Arch Dis Child Fetal Neonatal Ed 1998; 79: F26–F33.

34. Yeh TF, Lin YJ, Huang CC et al. Early dexamethasone therapy in preterm infants: a follow-up study. Pediatrics 1998; 101: e7.

35. Tschanz SA, Damke BM, Burri PH. Influence of postnatally administered glucocorticoids on rat lung growth. Biol Neonate 1995; 68: 229–245.

36. Greenough A. Chronic lung disease of prematurity – prevention by inhaled corticosteroids. Lancet 1999; 354: 266–267.

37. Dimitriou G, Greenough A, Giffin FJ, Kavvadia V. Inhaled versus systemic steroids in chronic oxygen dependency in preterm infants. Eur J Pediatr 1997; 156: 51–55.

38. Groneck P, Goetze-Speer B, Speer CP. Effects of inhaled beclomethasone compared to systemic dexamethasone on lung inflammation in preterm infants at risk of chronic lung disease. Pediatr Pulmonol 1999; 27: 383–387.

39. Saldanha RL, Cepeda EE, Poland RL. The effect of vitamin E prophylaxis on the incidence and severity of bronchopulmonary dysplasia. J Pediatr 1982; 101: 89–93.

40. Rosenfeld W, Evans H, Concepcion L et al. Prevention of bronchopulmonary dysplasia by administration of bovine superoxide dismutase in preterm infants with respiratory distress syndrome. J Pediatr 1984; 105: 781–785.

41. Russell GAB, Cooke RWI. Randomised controlled trial of allopurinol prophylaxis in very preterm infants. Arch Dis Child 1995; 73: F27–F31.

42. Griffiths G, Lall R, Chatfield S et al. Randomised controlled double blind study of role of recombinant erythropoietin in the prevention of chronic lung disease. Arch Dis Child 1997; 76: F190–F192.

43. Kennedy KA, Stoll BJ, Ehrenkranz RA et al. Vitamin A to prevent bronchopulmonary dysplasia in very low birth weight infants: has the dose been too low? Early Hum Dev 1997; 49: 19–31.

44. Avery ME, Tooley WH, Keller JB et al. Is chronic lung disease in low birthweight infants preventable? A survey of 8 centres. Pediatrics 1987; 79: 26–30.

45. Poets CF, Sens B. Changes in intubation rates and outcome of very low birth weight infants: a population-based study. Pediatrics 1996; 98: 24–27.

46. Greenough A, Milner AD, Dimitriou G. Synchronized ventilation (Cochrane review). In: The Cochrane Library, Issue 1. Oxford: Update Software; 2000.

47. Henderson-Smart DJ, Bhuta T, Cools F, Offringa M. Elective high frequency oscillatory ventilation versus conventional ventilation for acute pulmonary dysfunction in preterm infants. (Cochrane review). In: The Cochrane Library, issue 4. Oxford: Update Software; 1999.

48. Kinsella JP, Walsh WF, Bose CL et al. Inhaled nitric oxide in premature neonates with severe hypoxaemic respiratory failure: a randomised controlled trial. Lancet 1999; 354: 1061–1065.

49. The Franco-Belgium Collaborative NO Trial Group. Early compared with delayed inhaled nitric oxide in moderately hypoxaemic neonates with respiratory failure: a randomised controlled trial. Lancet 1999; 354: 1066–1071.

50. Kavvadia V, Greenough A, Dimitriou G, Hooper R. Randomized trial of fluid restriction in ventilated very low birthweight infants. Arch Dis Child 2000; 83: F91–F96.

51. Hartnoll G, Betremieux P, Modi N. Randomised controlled trial of postnatal sodium supplementation on oxygen dependency and body weight in 25–30 week gestational age infants. Arch Dis Child Fetal Neonatal Ed 2000; 82: F19–F23.

52. Lyon AJ, McColm J, Middlemist L et al. Randomised trial of erythromycin on the development of chronic lung disease in preterm infants. Arch Dis Child Fetal Neonatal Ed 1998; 78: F10–F14.

53. Garg M, Kurzner SI, Bautista DB, Keens TG. Clinically unsuspected hypoxia during sleep and feeding in infants with bronchopulmonary dysplasia. Pediatrics 1988; 81: 635–642.

54. Reimers KJ, Carlson SJ, Lombard KA. Nutritional management of infants with bronchopulmonary dysplasia. Nutr Clin Pract 1992; 7: 127–132.

55. Panitch HB, Downes JJ, Kennedy JS et al. Guidelines for home care of children with chronic respiratory insufficiency. Pediatr Pulmonol 1996; 21: 52–56.

56. Halliday HL, Ehrenkranz RA. Delayed (>3 weeks) postnatal corticosteroids for chronic lung disease in preterm infants (Cochrane Review). In: The Cochrane Library, Issue 1. Oxford: Update Software; 2000.

57. Kao LC, Durand DJ, McCrea RC et al. Randomized trial of long-term diuretic therapy for infants with oxygen-dependent bronchopulmonary dysplasia. J Pediatr 1994; 124: 772–781.
58. Kugelman A, Durand M, Garg M. Pulmonary effect of inhaled furosemide in ventilated infants with severe bronchopulmonary dysplasia. Pediatrics 1997; 99: 71–75.
59. Denjean A, Gulmaraes H, Migdal M et al. Dose-related bronchodilator response to aerosolized salbutamol (albuterol) in ventilator-dependent premature infants. J Pediatr 1992; 120: 974–979.
60. Yüksel B, Greenough A, Maconochie I. Effective bronchodilator therapy by a simple spacer device for wheezy premature infants in the first two years of life. Arch Dis Child 1990; 65: 782–785.
61. Yüksel B, Greenough A, Green S. Paradoxical response to nebulized ipratropium bromide in preterm infants asymptomatic at follow-up. Respir Med 1991; 85: 189–194.
62. Yüksel B, Greenough A. Inhaled sodium cromoglycate for preterm children with respiratory symptoms at follow-up. Respir Med 1992; 86: 131–134.
63. Yüksel B, Greenough A. Randomized trial of inhaled steroids in preterm infants symptomatic at follow-up. Thorax 1992; 47: 910–913.
64. The PREVENT study group. Reduction of respiratory syncytial virus hospitalization among premature infants and infants with bronchopulmonary dysplasia using respiratory syncytial virus immune globulin prophylaxis. Pediatrics 1997; 99: 93–99.
65. Anonymous. Palivizumab, a humanized respiratory syncytial virus monoclonal antibody, reduces hospitalization from respiratory syncytial virus infection in high-risk infants. The IMpact-RSV Study Group. Pediatrics 1998; 102: 531–537.
66. Shaw NJ, Ruggins N, Cooke RWI. Infants with chronic lung disease: predictors of mortality at Day 28. J Perinatol 1993; 13: 464–467.
67. Markestad T, Fitzhardinge PM. Growth and development in children recovering from bronchopulmonary dysplasia. J Pediatr 1981; 98: 597–602.
68. Vrlenich LA, Bozynski MEA, Shyr Y et al. The effect of bronchopulmonary dysplasia on growth at school age. Pediatrics 1995; 95: 855–859.
69. Hughes CA, O'Gorman LA, Shyr Y et al. Cognitive performance at school age of very low birth weight infants with bronchopulmonary dysplasia. Dev Behav Pediatr 1999; 20(1): 1–8.
70. Giacoia GP, Venkataraman PS, West-Wilson KI, Faulkner MJ. Follow-up of school age children with bronchopulmonary dysplasia. J Pediatr 1997; 130: 400–408.
71. Furman L, Baley J, Borawski-Clark E et al. Hospitalization as a measure of morbidity among very low birth weight infants with chronic lung disease. J Pediatr 1996; 128: 447–452.
72. Yüksel B, Greenough A. Relationship of symptoms to lung function abnormalities in preterm infants at follow-up. Pediatr Pulmonol 1991; 11: 202–206.
73. Gerhardt T, Hehre D, Feller R et al. Pulmonary mechanics in normal infants and young children during first 5 years of life. Pediatr Pulmonol 1987; 3: 309–316.
74. Mallory GB, Chaney M, Mutich RL, Motoyama RL. Longitudinal changes in lung function during the first three years of premature infants with moderate to severe bronchopulmonary dysplasia. Pediatr Pulmonol 1991; 11: 8–14.
75. McLeod A, Ross P, Mitchell S et al. Respiratory health in a total very low birthweight cohort and their classroom controls. Arch Dis Child 1996; 74: 188–194.
76. Gross SJ, Iannuzzi DM, Kveselis DA, Anbar RD. Effect of preterm birth on pulmonary function at school age: a prospective controlled study. J Pediatr 1999; 133: 188–192.
77. Doyle LW, Ford GW, Olinsky A et al. Bronchopulmonary dysplasia and very low birthweight: lung function at 11 years of age. J Pediatr Child Health 1996; 32: 339–343.
78. Koumbourlis AC, Motoyama EK, Mutich RL et al. Longitudinal follow-up of lung function from childhood to adolescence in prematurely born patients with neonatal chronic lung disease. Pediatr Pulmonol 1996; 21: 28–34.
79. Northway WH, Moss RB, Carlisle KB et al. Late pulmonary sequelae of bronchopulmonary dysplasia. N Engl J Med 1990; 323: 1793–1799.

ENVIRONMENTAL PROBLEMS AND LUNG INJURY

23 Air pollution

Thomas Sandström, Anders Blomberg and Ragnberth Helleday

Key points

- Air pollutants are associated with adverse health effects.

- There are clear associations between NO_2, O_3 and particulate matter pollution and deterioration in lung function, increased symptoms, days off work, hospitalisation, accident and emergency admissions and even mortality.

- The associations appear strongest for particulate pollution.

- Air pollution causes aggravation of symptoms and diseases in individuals and results in substantial health-care and work absence costs.

Air pollution has been an issue of increasing concern for respiratory health during the last decades. Exposure to a variety of pollutants, their sources and their ambient air levels are core information for the understanding of trends in environmentally related health outcomes. Consequently, in this chapter such information is given. This may serve as a basis for a better appreciation of population-based and experimental exposure studies that show how air pollution interferes with living in today's society.

Pollutants, sources and levels

The major combustion-generated air pollutants with adverse health effects are nitric oxides (nitric oxide, NO and nitrogen dioxide, NO_2), ozone (O_3), sulphur dioxide (SO_2), particulate matter and nitric and sulphuric acids. Other combustion- or traffic-related pollutants are hydrocarbons, aldehydes and carbon monoxide. In certain environments organic and inorganic dusts may play a role, and road dust – including particles from tyres, brake discs, etc. – may be of importance, although it has not yet received much attention.

Ozone

Ozone is a secondary photochemical oxidant produced in the atmosphere by photochemical reactions in the presence of nitric oxides, hydrocarbons and ultraviolet radiation. It is poorly soluble in water and is an extremely powerful oxidant, causing oxidative damage when it encounters the epithelial lining fluid and biomolecules in the airways.[1] The toxicity of O_3 appears further to be mediated through a cascade of secondary and tertiary oxidation and free radical derived products, inducing adverse cellular events. Deposition occurs all through the airways, but the main effects are seen in the terminal bronchioles at ambient exposure levels.[2]

European levels are usually less than 15 parts per billion (ppb) but can be as high as 60 ppb. During hot summers with stagnant air, ground levels have been reported to occasionally exceed 200 ppb in central Europe.

Nitrogen dioxide

Nitrogen dioxide is a common air pollutant in ambient air. The major source of NO_2 in the atmosphere is the combustion of fossil fuels for heating and power generation, as well as from motor vehicles. Urban levels of NO_2 vary according to the time of day, season, meteorological condition and human activities. The NO_2 concentration in urban air is characterised by two daily peaks during the morning and afternoon rush-hour traffic. Annual average concentrations in urban areas are mainly below 0.03 ppm but during peaks hourly averages may exceed 0.2 ppm. Indoor concentrations may be considerably higher than outdoors, especially in certain industries and in homes using gas cookers. Here, 24-hour averages may reach 0.5 ppm and peak concentrations may occasionally exceed 1–2 ppm.[3]

Nitrogen dioxide is a highly reactive free radical and oxidant and is poorly water-soluble. It is therefore deposited far more peripherally in the air spaces compared to highly water-soluble gases like SO_2. Absorption of NO_2 still occurs all through the respiratory tract but the major target is the terminal bronchiole, as with O_3. NO_2, being a potent oxidant as well as a free radical itself, may cause lipid peroxidation in cell membranes and oxidative damage to various structural and functional molecules, and also react with the antioxidant defences in the epithelial lining fluid.[1]

Sulphur dioxide

Sulphur dioxide has previously been of more concern to the public with regard to pollution effects. The use of lower-sulphur fuels for petrol and diesel engines and heating has reduced ambient levels greatly. However, in many less-developed countries in the world, liquid fuels and coal containing quite high levels of sulphur are still in use. SO_2 exists as a water-soluble gas, and sulphuric acid may be produced, together with sulphites and sulphates, through reactions with water droplets.[1] The mechanisms of action are not completely understood.

Since SO_2 is highly water-soluble, it is not believed to enter the lungs in major amounts during normal breathing but mainly to be deposited in the upper airways. It has been suggested that neural reflex mechanisms may be involved in the development of bronchoconstriction and airway inflammation.

Particulate matter

Air pollution in Europe emanates mainly from five sources: vehicles, wood and oil combustion, certain industries and long-range transport. Particulate matter pollution is to a large extent produced by vehicles. Due to the associated health effects particulate matter pollution is high on the list for research and further regulation within the European Union as well as the USA and other regions.

Particles can be divided into different size ranges. Fine (<0.1–$2.5\,\mu$m) and ultrafine ($< 0.1\,\mu$m) particles are mainly formed during combustion processes, while coarse particles ($> 2.5\,\mu$m) are often formed mechanically. The most commonly used size-specific indicator is PM_{10} (particulate matter, all particles $< 10\,\mu$m) but this does not discriminate between the three size fractions mentioned above. The number of ultrafine particles per unit volume can be very high in the proximity of combustion processes. It is notable that the number of ultrafine particles has to be enormous to make up a certain particle mass, which may equal just a few very large particles. Current toxicological theories suggest that these fine and ultrafine particles may be more biologically active than larger ones.[4] This could be related to their size and interaction with cell membranes as well as to their intracellular effects. The enormously large surface area of very high numbers of small particles may add to their reactivity. Chemical characteristics on the surface of particles may also be critical. Current theories suggest that transition metals are of some importance.[5-7] Hydrocarbons, aldehydes, and nitric and sulphuric components may also be bioactive and be responsible for toxic effects.

Air-pollution levels in Western countries have shown a trend towards a decrease. In particular, compounds of sulphur and nitrogen have been reduced. This is also true for O_3 in many, if not all, areas. As regards particulate matter pollution, the situation is not so clear-cut. PM_{10} and black smoke levels may often

have decreased but the smaller fractions, which are more harmful, have often not been measured, so that it is unknown whether substantial reductions have really occurred in the levels of fine and ultrafine particles.

The contribution of diesel exhaust particulates to ambient particulate matter is important and varies from 10% to 87% in different reports. Most studies suggest that diesel exhaust particles are a major component of particulate matter.[8] The variability partly results from differences in the way estimations have been made and also whether PM_{10}, $PM_{2.5}$ or particle number has been of concern. Some new diesel engines may emit higher numbers of smaller particles than older ones,[9] and this has also been demonstrated for certain petrol engines. American investigators have reported that diesel exhaust particles are a major component in Los Angeles air, despite the fact that the majority of the car fleet is petrol-powered.[10] As there is still some debate as regards the actual contributions of various sources, we expect to see more detailed descriptions and characteristics, mainly on the hydrocarbon components, reflecting combustion sources for individual particles from different areas.

In the world's ten Megacities (population in excess of 10 million), the United Nations environmental programme and the World Health Organization (WHO) have reported particulate matter to be the most serious global air pollution problem. Among these cities over half have very serious particulate-matter pollution problems, exceeding the WHO guidelines by a factor of more than 2. The majority have concentrations of particulate matter in the range of 200–600 μg/m³ with peaks over 1000 μg/m³. Five megacities had moderate to serious levels, with only three megacities having particulate-matter levels within the WHO guidelines. In Beijing the WHO PM_{10} 24-hour average (air quality standard of 70 μg/m³) was exceeded on every single day of the year, with the highest measurements being above 1000 μg/m³. Similar levels have been reported from Mexico City, Bangkok, Manila, Sao Paolo, Bombay, Karachi and Calcutta. This can be compared with the concentration during the notorious London smog episode of 1952, when the particulate matter was estimated to have reached 1400 μg/m³, in association with high SO_2 levels, which added to the harmful effects.

The annual mean PM_{10} concentrations in UK generally lie between 10 and 45 μg/m³, with peak daily averages of 70–150 μg/m³. Hourly means may exceed 300–400 μg/m³ with peaks over 600 μg/m³. With some variations, metropolitan areas over Europe fall into a similar concentration range.

Health effects

Pollution in ambient air has been recognised as a nuisance to people for many centuries. Indeed, the records from Roman courts report regulations and cases for the handling of burning of fuels to avoid symptoms and discomfort to citizens, who were then mainly affected by the development of early industries. As the Chinese were pioneers in the burning of coal, it is likely that they had already experienced a certain degree of discomfort from this combustion millennia ago. In Europe, chronicles from the 14th century report that English citizens and courts were irritated and increasingly observant of the discomfort associated with coal smoke.

The amounts of combustion increased very significantly during the Industrial Revolution, when heavy industries were developed and workers migrated to the growing population centres. London smog became famous for being so thick that it both reduced visibility and caused airway discomfort, well documented in, for example, Sir Arthur Conan Doyle's classic Sherlock Holmes stories. In parallel with this development workers in highly air-polluted workplaces were apparently exposed to very high concentrations of gases and particles from combustion, greatly exceeding what could ever be reached in outdoors air. Many workers undoubtedly suffered from the consequences of these high levels of exposure but the attention given to this was perhaps modest compared with the attention attracted by outbreaks of ambient air pollution affecting larger numbers of citizens. The events in the Meuse Valley in 1930, in Donora, Pennsylvania in 1948[11] and the London smog episode of 1952[12] made the public aware of the health issues associated with ambient air pollution, with consequences for government legislation. Bronchitis symptoms were already common in London and had been associated with the smog for some time but the excessive death rates induced by the smog of 1952 provided definite proof that air pollution had more serious endpoints than previously assumed. In 1965, Holland & Reid demonstrated in an elegant study that postal workers in London had reduced lung function in comparison with colleagues living in regions with less pronounced air pollution.[13]

Population-based studies

Following the demonstrated excess mortality in London in 1952, and the earlier outbreaks, epidemiological studies demonstrated adverse health effects associated with exposure to particulate matter, O_3, NO_2, SO_2 and acid compounds.

The epidemiological studies can be divided into acute exposure studies and studies of chronic exposure. Both types of study were often population-based, to evaluate mortality, emergency admissions and hospitalisation. Additionally selected cohorts have been studied for symptoms and changes in lung function, normally measured as peak expiratory flow (PEF).[14]

The chronic exposure studies are usually large-scale investigations comparing differences in air pollution between different population centres or urban areas in relation to health-effect parameters. Often the studies covered periods of several years. The acute studies evaluate the temporal relationship between variability in air pollutants and changes in symptoms and physiological parameters, often in association with lag times for effects of 1–3 days.[15,16]

For obvious reasons, results cannot be stronger than the links of the chain. Consequently, exposure measurements are extremely crucial for the evaluation of the relationship between air pollutants and health-effect outcomes. Quite early on, adequate techniques for measuring sulphur and nitrogen compounds were developed. However, estimates of particulate air pollution were for a long time relatively rough, often in terms of the degree of black staining on filters (black smoke, BS). As mentioned earlier, a transition to a particulate matter measure-

ment of PM_{10}, nowadays often also $PM_{2.5}$ and ultrafine particles, or even numbers of particles of different sizes, has improved the description of particulate-matter pollution.[17]

When it comes to health effects, at present the major attention is focused on particulate matter effects. Still, the effects of gaseous pollutants such as NO_2 and O_3 are also important. In some regions, where high-sulphur fuels are in use, SO_2 and sulphuric acid are still a problem.[15]

As far back as the 1970s, a correlation between cardiopulmonary disease events and very high concentrations of particulates and SO_2 had been established. Gradually, sulphur-based air pollution decreased and with sharper epidemiological tools scientists were able to demonstrate that particulate matter causes air-pollution effects on health not only at high levels but also at common ambient levels.

The Six Cities Study is one of the key studies in air pollution science and deserves specific attention. It demonstrated that PM_{10} is associated with an increase in respiratory illness in children as well as an increased risk of cardiopulmonary mortality[18,19] (Table 23.1).

In this much cited large prospective study in six US cities, chosen to represent a wide range of levels of particulate-matter pollution, 8000 individuals were followed over 15 years, various health-outcome parameters being monitored together with measurements of ambient levels of air pollutants. After controlling for confounding factors such as weather, smoking, body weight and socioeconomic status, there was a strong relationship between excess mortality and the concentration of PM_{10} in the atmosphere. For every increase of $100\,\mu g/m^3$ in PM_{10}, mortality increased by 17%. Interestingly, particulate matter was linked with deaths not only from respiratory diseases but also from cardiovascular events.[20] A much larger second study of over half a million citizens in more than 150 US cities confirmed the results from the Six Cities Study, after adjusting for a variety of confounding variables.[21]

Additional studies in the US demonstrated that particulate-matter pollution is associated with an increase in symptoms, lung function deterioration, hospitalisation because of respiratory illness and days off school, in addition to confirming correlations with mortality.[21-25] These findings resulted in extensive research in many continents and it is now fairly well established that cardiorespiratory mortality, morbidity, lung function, symptoms, lung growth in children and school absences correlate with particulate-matter pollution (Tables 23.1 & 23.2). In some studies, correlations are indeed stronger for nitric oxides or O_3, but the general trend is towards stronger associations with particulate-matter pollution. This support usually becomes stronger when $PM_{2.5}$, representing more of the smaller particles, is considered. These smaller particles ($< 5\,\mu m$) are able to enter the lung, which larger particles cannot do.

Apart from the physical features, chemical and toxicological characteristics also point strongly towards adverse biomedical effects related to health outcome. Data are now available from Europe, North and South America, Australia and Asia, all with similar trends.[26-28] It is notable that the effects are not limited to adults or older children. Neonatal and infant death rates have also been associated with variability in particulate-matter pollution.[29-33]

Table 23.1 Long-term respiratory effects of air pollution on adults. Data from Ackerman-Liebrich U. Outdoor air pollution. Eur Respir Monogr 2000; 5: 400–411.

Health outcome	Study type	Population studied	Pollutants	Author
Cardiopulmonary mortality	Cohort	8000 US Americans, 6 cities, 15-year follow-up 5 520 000 US Americans, 50 cities, 8-year follow-up	PM_{10}, $PM_{2.5}$, sulphates $PM_{2.5}$, sulphates	Dockery et al 1993[19] Pope 1995[21]
Lung cancer mortality	Cohort	552 000 US Americans, 50 cities, 8-year follow-up 8000 US Americans, 50 cities, 8-year follow-up	Sulphates $PM_{2.5}$	Pope 1995[21] Dockery et al 1993[19]
Lung function	Cross-sectional Cohort	France USA Switzerland	SO_2, NO_2 Sulphates, PM_{10} PM_{10}, NO_2, SO_2	PAARC 1982 Abbey 1998 Ackermann-Liebrich 1997
Chronic bronchitis, asthma symptoms	Cohort	USA	TSP, PM_{10}, $PM_{2.5}$	Abbey 1995
Phlegm, wheezing, asthma symptoms	Birth cohort	UK, 23-year follow-up	Black smoke	Scarlett 1995
Cough, respiratory symptoms	Cross-sectional	Sweden	NO_2, SO_2	Forsberg 1997
Respiratory symptoms		France	SO_2, NO_2	PAARC 1982
Lower respiratory symptoms		Switzerland	PM_{10}, NO_2, SO_2	Zemp 1999

PM_{10}, $PM_{2.5}$, particles with a 50% cut-off aerodynamic diameter of 10/2.5 µg; PAARC; Pollution Atmospherique Affections Respiratoires Chroniques; TSP: total suspended particular.

The WHO estimates that particulate-matter pollution is responsible for half a million excess deaths every year. For the UK the estimates are around 11 000 per year. Adverse effects have been observed at all concentrations, even at levels far below the WHO safety guidelines. Currently there seems to be no threshold that can be considered safe for human health. Concentrations as low as 20 µg/m³ or lower have been associated with adverse health effects.[34]

Nitrogen dioxide and particulate matter are both produced during combustion and correlate highly, often making it difficult to evaluate which, if not both, is actually responsible for the health outcome. Likewise, O_3 also often correlates well with NO_2 and particulate matter levels, which makes evaluation even more difficult. NO_2 and O_3 independently act as potent agents in air pollution, but in real life effects are almost always mixed in exposed individuals, distorting the evaluation models. Both these pollutants are associated with similar health effects as described for particulate matter. Only if we could substantially reduce one or more of these major components in ambient air pollution could the contribution of each individual agent be estimated. Until then the estimates of attributed health effects are only reasonably good and not optimal.

Air pollution and asthma

In asthmatics, epidemiological studies have generally demonstrated more prominent increases in hospitalisation and related health-care visits, symptoms and effects on lung function than in the general population. Up to the present, a large number of asthma studies have demonstrated strong associations between respiratory symptoms, from the upper respiratory tract as well as lower respiratory symptoms (including wheezing, dry cough, phlegm, shortness of breath and chest discomfort or pain).[14,15,35,36] Associations occur with NO_2, PM_{10} and O_3. A more prominent role for particulate matter has been suggested, partly because there was a stronger association when fine particulates, $PM_{2.5}$, were evaluated. Commonly there is a lag effect of up to several days until the strongest associations between symptoms and decline in lung function are evident.

In experimental chamber or mouthpiece inhalation studies, the effects of air pollutants on bronchoconstriction and bronchial hyperresponsiveness have been studied. They showed that asthmatics responded with more bronchoconstriction and at lower concentrations than healthy individuals after exposure to NO_2 and SO_2.[1,15,35,36,41] While healthy individuals normally respond with bronchoconstriction to high levels of NO_2, such as 2–5 ppm, asthmatics may respond to 0.5 ppm or far less. The same applies to bronchial hyper-responsiveness, which in asthmatics may be elicited after exposure to concentrations as low as 0.1 ppm and in healthy individuals only after high concentrations.

The situation is very different for O_3. It appears that approximately 20% of the general population are 'bronchoconstriction responders', demonstrated as a fall of more than 10% in forced

Table 23.2 Short-term effects of air pollutants on the respiratory health of adults. Data from Ackerman-Liebrich U. Outdoor air pollution. Eur Respir Monogr 2000; 5: 400–411.

Health outcome	Population studied	Pollutants	Author
Panel studies			
Lung function	Cyclists, Netherlands	O_3	Brunekreef 1994
	Jogging, adults, USA	O_3	Spektor 1988
	Farmers, Canada	O_3	Brauer 1996
	Smokers, USA	PM_{10}	Pope 1993
	Hikers, USA	O_3, $PM_{2.5}$, acid aerosols	Korrick 1998
	Asthmatics, USA	NO_2, SO_2, black smoke	Taggart 1996
Asthmatic symptoms	Asthmatics, Netherlands	O_3, PM_{10}	Hiltermann 1998
Time-series studies			
Respiratory mortality	Paris	PM_{13}	Dab 1996
	Milan	TSP, SO_2	Vigotti 1996
	Philadelphia, London	TSP	Schwartz 1994
	London	O_3	Anderson 1996
	Mexico City	TSP	Borja-Aburto 1997
COPD mortality	Birmingham	PM_{10}	Wordley 1997
	6 US cities	PM_{10}, PM2.5, sulphates	Schwartz 1997
Respiratory hospital admissions	Paris	Black smoke, PM_{13}, SO_2	Dab 1996
	London	O_3	Ponce de Leon 1996
	Milan	TSP, SO_2	Vigoutti 1996
	5 European cities	O_3	Spix 1998
COPD hospital admissions	Paris	SO_2, NO_2	Dab 1996
	6 European cities	SO_2, black smoke, NO_2, TSP, O_3	Anderson 1997
Asthma admissions	Helsinki, adults + children	SO_2, O_3	Pönkä 1996
	Atlanta children	O_3, PM_{10}	White 1994
	4 European cities	NO_2, SO_2	Sunyer 19979

PM_{10}, PM_{13}, $PM_{2.5}$, particles with a 50% cut-off aerodynamic diameter of 10, 13 or 2.5 μm; COPD, chronic obstructive pulmonary disease; TSP: total suspended particulates

expiratory volume in 1 second (FEV_1) after exposure to O_3 in the order of 0.2–0.4 ppm. This is true equally of healthy individuals, asthmatics and elderly subjects. Some authors suggested that the effects are stronger in females. Increased bronchial hyperresponsiveness is a prominent feature associated with O_3 exposure. Exposure to as little as 80 ppb seems to elicit increased bronchial hyper-responsiveness in asthmatics and healthy people alike but the lowest threshold for response has not been identified with certainty.[1] These laboratory findings are not absolutely supported by many epidemiological studies, which have found associations between O_3 and bronchoconstriction to be stronger in asthmatics than in healthy people.

Of major concern have been data showing that asthmatics develop bronchoconstriction or hyper-responsiveness when exposed to O_3, NO_2 or SO_2 prior to allergen challenge. This suggests that air pollutants are able to enhance sensitivity to allergens and enhance T-helper cell type 2 (Th2) response. Molfino and coworkers were the first to demonstrate such an effect after O_3 and were soon followed by several other groups of investigators.[37–40]

In experimental studies only few investigators have evaluated airway inflammation following O_3 inhalation in asthmatics compared with healthy subjects. In an American collaborative study the investigators reported a slightly more pronounced neutrophilic airway inflammatory response in a group of asthmatic individuals compared to healthy subjects.[41] This confirms data from a small bronchoalveolar lavage study.[42] In a more recent study the authors demonstrated enhanced eosinophilic inflammation in asthmatics after O_3 exposure, which still remains to be confirmed.[43]

In diesel exhaust the main effects have been attributed to the particulate-matter component. So far only two studies have been presented evaluating the response to diesel engine exhaust exposure in healthy and asthmatic subjects. Both showed that asthmatics are more responsive than healthy individuals. Nordenhäll et al showed that diesel-engine exhaust with a PM_{10} of 300 μg/m^3 caused almost a doubling of bronchial responsiveness to methacholine in 14 asthmatic individuals being treated with inhaled corticosteroids 800–1200 μg BDP.[44] The effect was determined 1 day after exposure, which ties in well with data from epidemiological studies. It should be noted that the increase in bronchial responsiveness was much more evident than the bronchoconstrictive response, which was of similar magnitude as in healthy individuals. Possibly, measurements of bronchial hyper-responsiveness in epidemiological studies too could have added stronger associations with particulate-matter pollution than the probably less sensitive measurement of PEF.

Recent data suggest that the bronchial airway mucosa in asthmatics responds quite differently from that of healthy individuals when exposed to diesel-engine exhaust with PM_{10} 100 $\mu g/m^3$. While healthy individuals decrease their bronchial epithelial cytokine expression of interleukin (IL)-10 by half, there is almost a threefold increase in expression in asthmatics. This may result in an increased Th2 response on subsequent days, which, at least partly, may be necessary for restitution of integrity.[45]

Air pollution and healthy individuals

Even in individuals who have been defined as healthy in epidemiological studies, there are significant associations between air pollution and symptoms. Associations are usually found between particulate pollution and respiratory symptoms, restricted activity and days off work. Restriction due to respiratory morbidity has been especially associated with particulate-matter pollution.[15,46,47] An increased susceptibility to virus infections has been suggested as at least partly mediated by binding of the virus surface to the adhesion molecule ICAM-1 in the nose and airways. ICAM-1 has been shown to be commonly upregulated by exposure to air pollutants. Secondary pneumonia may account for a proportion of the health-care visits or hospitalisation in epidemiological studies. Obviously, individuals with pre-existing respiratory diseases like asthma, chronic obstructive pulmonary disease and possibly other diseases such as pulmonary fibrosis may be even more affected.[48]

Experimental studies using controlled-chamber exposure in humans have demonstrated O_3 and NO_2 but also diesel-engine particulates to be particularly active in producing oxidative stress and free-radical activity in the airways. This has been shown by consumption and subsequent repletion of antioxidants such as ascorbic acid, uric acid and glutathione in the nose and intrapulmonary airways, as reflected in nasal lavage, bronchial washes and bronchoalveolar lavage.[49–51] When the first-line antioxidant defence in the epithelial lining fluid, consisting of ascorbic acid, uric acid and glutathione, is overwhelmed, this leads to oxidation and structural changes in molecules, resulting in secondary and tertiary reactive products of mainly protein and lipid origin. α-tocopherol is an important substance that is involved in second-line defence by scavenging peroxyl radicals and limiting free-radical reactions. Extracellular superoxide dismutase scavenges superoxide anions in order to limit the adverse reactions of these highly reactive species. The inflammatory events that occur subsequent to oxidative challenge from gases and particulates have been suggested to be mediated via oxidative-stress-sensitive transcription factors, such as activation protein (AP)-1 and nuclear factor (NF)-κB, which regulate key chemokine and cytokine transcriptions.[52]

Exposure to 2 ppm of NO_2 has been demonstrated to cause neutrophilic airway inflammation in the bronchi, mediated by release of cytokines such as IL-8, regulating cell migration. The infiltration of activated neutrophils has been accompanied by effects on mast cells and lymphocytes. Studies of time kinetics have described in detail the consumption of antioxidants such as ascorbate and uric acid at 1.5 h after exposure, returning to normal at 6 and 24 h respectively. In contrast, secretions of glutathione into the epithelial lining fluid occurred at 1.5 and 6 h, thereafter returning to normal levels.[53] Repeated exposure on sequential days did not allow the defence systems to recuperate and resulted in an enhanced neutrophilic inflammation in the airways, despite complete attenuation of lung function response.[54]

Even more prominent cascade phenomena occur in the airways following exposure to O_3. Ambiently occurring levels have been demonstrated to cause airway inflammation. In a series of papers, Koren & Devlin described neutrophilic cell influx into the airways following exposures in the range of 80–400 ppb.[55,56] Prominent secretion of cytokines and other proinflammatory substances occurred, with an increase in bronchoalveolar lavage fluid levels of tissue factor, albumin, lactate dehydrogenase, IL-6, IL-8 and prostaglandin E_2. Subsequently, it was shown that repeated exposures limited some of the O_3-induced effects such as bronchoconstriction in these healthy individuals, but the tissue damage, expressed as release of lactate dehydrogenase into lavage fluids, still remained. The inflammation has been further characterised by bronchial mucosal biopsies, which also showed that mast cells were prominent mediators of inflammation even in healthy individuals and that the neutrophilic inflammation followed enhanced expression of vascular adhesion molecules in the superficial blood vessels in the bronchial submucosa close to the basal membrane. Enhanced expression of the adhesion molecule P-selectin and ICAM-1 in the superficial venules in the bronchial mucosa preceded the cell migration (Fig. 23.1). These mechanisms allowed for a prominent migration of inflammatory cells from the blood stream 6 h after exposure, probably via their LFA-1 ligands. Lymphocyte migration and activation was also demonstrated.

An important aspect, which has been more extensively explored during recent years, is whether early lung function decrements would predict subsequent airway inflammation.

Despite some early studies suggesting an association, it is now evident that this is not the case.[57,58] This is an important issue, which has to be taken into consideration for population-based studies.

Healthy individuals also demonstrated prominent airway inflammation following a controlled-chamber exposure to diesel-engine exhaust at levels of particulate matter that occur in busy streets.[51] Figures 23.2 & 23.3 describe current understanding of the interaction of diesel particulate matter with the epithelial lining fluid, the bronchial epithelium, signalling via cytokine release, increase in adhesion molecule expression and inflammatory cell migration into the airway wall and air spaces, based on a series of studies.[50,51,59] Diesel engine particles at a concentration of 300 $\mu g/m^3$ from a running engine for 1 h caused antioxidant changes in airways, prominent recruitment of neutrophils into air spaces and bronchial mucosa, and migration of $CD4^+$ and $CD8^+$ lymphocytes to the airways. The major neutrophil chemotactic factors were identified as IL-8 and GRO-α, which were found to be produced in enhanced amounts in the bronchial epithelium (Fig. 23.4). Even in perfectly healthy indi-

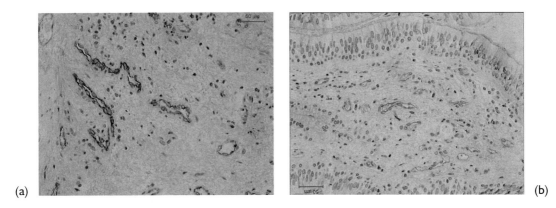

Fig. 23.1 Enhanced vascular adhesion molecule expression after ozone exposure, assisting in inflammatory cell migration from blood stream to bronchial wall and air spaces. (a) P-selectin. (b) ICAM-1. Arrows indicate vessels positively stained using monoclonal antibodies and immunohistochemistry. Bar represents 50 μm.

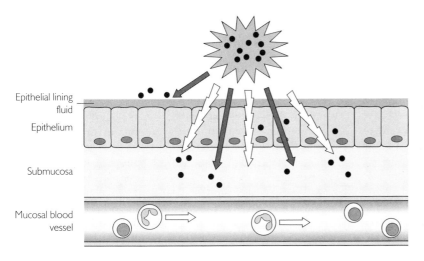

Fig. 23.2 Exhaust particles interact with airway lining fluid, epithelial and submucosal cells, resulting in cytokine and chemokine signals.

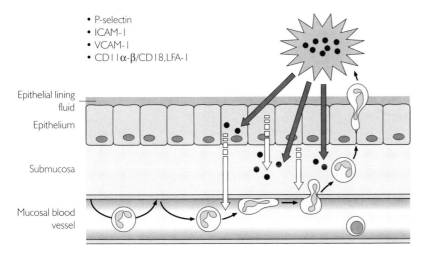

Fig. 23.3 Inflammatory cell recruitment to bronchial wall and air spaces, assisted by enhanced expression of vascular adhesion molecules, resulted in enhanced adhesion rolling, firm adhesion and migration.

viduals, mast cells were recruited and activated to secrete histamine into the air spaces. Furthermore, thrombocytosis was demonstrated in peripheral blood at 6 h after exposure, suggesting that there might be a link with the epidemiological studies and experimental lung models proposing that cardiovascular coagulation disturbances are at least partly responsible for the increase in cardiovascular events. Impaired alveolar macrophage phagocytosis has also been demonstrated to be a physiological token of adverse particulate-matter effects.[59] Subsequently. an even lower concentration of diesel engine particles (100 μg/m³)

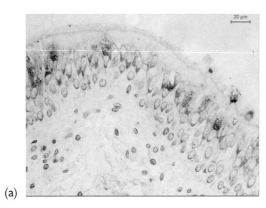 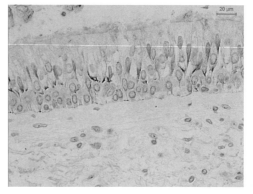

Fig. 23.4 Increased production of neutrophil chemotactic cytokines in the bronchial epithelium following diesel engine particle exposure. (a) GRO-α seen as dark granular staining. (b) IL-8 seen as thin, dark, subnuclear basal staining in epithelial cells using monoclonal antibodies and immunohistochemistry. Bar represents 20 μm.

was demonstrated to cause similar, although less prominent effects, which may be partly due to a slower onset of inflammation following a lower exposure dose.

Air pollution and allergy

Air pollution experiments in cell cultures and animals have demonstrated that sensitisation to allergens and development of an allergic response may be enhanced by NO_2, O_3, SO_2 and most prominently by diesel-engine exhaust particles.[60,61] Epidemiological studies are not supportive of a prominent role for air pollution in allergy development, which seems to be more associated with lifestyle factors. The widely cited allergy studies by Diaz-Sanchez and co-workers with local diesel-exhaust-particle installation in the nose clearly suggest the possibility that particulate-matter pollutants may play some role.[62-65] It is difficult to be entirely sure whether this is related to certain phenotypes or genotypes of atopy or whether other factors are strong enough to make associations that are relatively weak in epidemiological studies. Currently this is a controversial issue.

An interesting observation is that in one study nasal steroid treatment caused an enhanced rather than a diminished ragweed allergen response when diesel exhaust particles were present.[66] This needs confirmation by other studies, however.

Air pollution and the elderly

Epidemiological studies suggest that individuals with pre-existing severe cardiorespiratory disease, including chronic obstructive pulmonary disease, asthma and cardiovascular disease, are more prone to respond adversely to air pollution.[15,16,26,48] The majority of severe, life-threatening or mortal events in this population seem to be most strongly associated with particulate-matter pollution. A controversial issue was whether the air pollutants were just responsible for 'preharvesting', i.e. whether extremely ill individuals might simply be dying some

days earlier than would have been the case without exposure. Recent analyses suggest this not to be the case.[67] Today over 40 studies from different continents have shown the same relationship of enhanced morbidity and mortality with air pollution. With prospective designs, more detailed information on susceptible cohorts may yield further insights into the pathophysiological events responsible for major physical disturbances, hospitalisation or death. A number of theories are currently being investigated in epidemiological, human experimental, animal experimental and cell culture studies.

At present we are not totally confident as to how to protect sensitive individuals from the adverse effects of air pollution. In certain countries, alerts are given for high levels of NO_2, O_3 or PM_{10}. Probably, staying indoors adds some level of protection. Whether cardiovascular, anti-inflammatory, antioxidant or other medication would be protective is yet to be determined.

Therapeutic principles

- Reduction of air pollution (similarly to smoking) is the primary action to prevent the adverse events.

- Trials with pharmaceutical interventions are scarce and there are no evidence-based data to suggest effective treatments.

- Bronchoconstriction by air pollutants is common in individuals with obstructive lung diseases, and bronchodilators are expected to be efficient counteracting agents.

- Inhaled corticosteroids have not been evaluated in air-pollution research. Such studies are presently ongoing.

- There is some limited information suggesting that antioxidant supplementation can reduce the bronchoconstriction and hyperresponsiveness induced by oxidative air pollutants.

References

1. Sandström T. Respiratory effects of air pollutants. Experimental studies in humans. Eur Respir J 1995; 8: 976–995.
2. Mudway IS, Kelly FJ. Ozone and the lung: a sensitive issue. Mol Aspects Med 2000; 21: 1–48.
3. Samet JM, Marbury MC, Spengler JD. Health effects and sources of indoor air pollution. Part I. Am Rev Respir Dis 1987; 136: 1486–1508.
4. Donaldson K, Li XY, MacNee W. Ultrafine (nanometer) particle mediated lung injury. J Aerosol Sci 1998; 29: 553–560.
5. Ghio AJ, Stonehuerner J, Dailey LA, Carter JD. Metals associated with both the water-soluble and insoluble fractions of an ambient air pollution particle catalyze an oxidative stress. Inhal Toxicol 1999; 11: 37–49.
6. Samet JM, Graves LM, Quay J et al. Activation of MAPKs in human bronchial epithelial cells exposed to metals. Am J Physiol 1998; 275: L551–L558.
7. Frampton MW, Ghio AJ, Samet JM et al. Effects of aqueous extracts of PM(10) filters from the Utah valley on human airway epithelial cells. Am J Physiol 1999; 277: L960–L967.
8. Quality of Urban Air Review Group. Airborne particulate matter in the United Kingdom. Boston Spa Report. UK: Quality of Urban Air Review Group; 1996.
9. Airborne Particles Expert Group. Source apportionment of airborne particulate matter in the United Kingdom. London: Airborne Particles Expert Group; 1999.
10. Cass GR, Gray HA. Regional emissions and atmospheric concentrations of diesel engine particulate matter: Los Angeles as a case study. In: Diesel exhaust: A critical analysis of emissions, exposure, and health effects. Cambridge, MA: Health Effects Institute; 1995: 125–137.
11. Ciocco A, Thompson DJ. A follow-up of Donora ten years after: methodology and findings. Am J Publ Health 1961; 51: 155–164.
12. Logan WPD. Mortality in the London fog incident, 1952. Lancet 1953; 1: 336–338.
13. Holland WW, Reid DD. The urban factor in chronic bronchitis. Lancet 1965;1: 445–448.
14. Lebowits MD. Epidemiological studies of the respiratory effects of air pollution. Eur Respir J 1996; 9: 1029.
15. State of the art. Health effects of outdoor air pollution. Am J Respir Crit Care Med 1996; 153: 3–50.
16. Pope CA III, Bates BV, Riazene ME. Health effects of particulate air pollution: Time for measurement. Environ Health Perspect 1995; 103: 472–480.
17. Karg E, Beck-Speier I, Ferron GA et al. Characterization of ambient particles. Third Colloquium on Particulate Air Pollution and Human Health, Durham, NC, 1999.
18. Dockery DW, Speizer FE, Stram DO et al. Effects of inhalable particles on respiratory health of children. Am Rev Respir Dis 1989; 139: 587–594.
19. Dockery DW, Pope CA III, Xu X et al. An association between air pollution and mortality in six US cities. N Engl J Med 1993; 329: 1753–1759.
20. Schwartz J, Dockery DW. Particulate matter air pollution and daily mortality in Steubenville. Am J Epidemiol 1992; 135: 12–19.
21. Pope CA III, Thun MJ, Namboodiri MM et al. Particulate air pollution as a predictor of mortality in a prospective study of US adults. Am J Respir Crit Care Med 1995; 151: 669–674.
22. Pope CA III, Schwartz J, Ranson MR. Daily mortality and PM$_{10}$ pollution in Utah valley. Arch Environ Health 1992; 47: 211–217.
23. Pope CA. Respiratory disease associated with community air pollution and a steel mill in Utah Valley. Am J Public Health 1989; 79: 623–628.
24. Pope CA. Respiratory hospital admissions associated with PM$_{10}$ pollution in Utah, Salt Lake, and Cache Valleys. Arch Environ Health 1991; 46: 90–97.
25. Pope CA, Dockery DW. Acute health effects of PM$_{10}$ pollution on symptomatic and asymptomatic children. Am Rev Respir Dis 1992; 145: 1123–1128.
26. Anderson HR, Ponce de Leon A, Bland JM et al. Air pollution and daily mortality in London 1987–1992. Br Med J 1996; 312: 665–669.
27. Anderson HR, Spix C, Medina S et al. Air pollution and daily admissions for chronic obstructive pulmonary disease on six European cities; results from the APHEA project. Eur Respir J 1997; 10: 1071.
28. Brunekreef B, Hoek G, Breugelmans O, Leentvaar M. Respiratory effects of low-level photochemical air pollution in amateur cyclists. Am J Respir Crit Care Med 1994; 150: 962–966.
29. Brunekreef B, Janssen NAH, Hartog J et al. Air pollution from truck traffic and lung function in children living near motorways. Epidemiology 1997; 8: 298–303.
30. Romieu I, Meneses F, Sienra-Monge JJ et al. Effects of urban air pollutants on emergency visits for childhood asthma in Mexico City. Am J Epidemiol 1995; 141: 546–553.
31. Romieu I, Meneses F, Ruiz S et al. Effects of intermittent ozone exposure on peak expiratory flow and respiratory symptoms among asthmatic children in Mexico City. Arch Environ Health 1997; 52: 368–376.
32. Van Vliet P, Knape M, de Hartog J et al. Motor vehicle exhaust and chronic respiratory symptoms in children living near freeways. Environ Res 1997; 74: 122–132.
33. Smith KR, Samet JM, Romieu I, Bruce N. Indoor air pollution in developing countries and acute lower respiratory infections in children. Thorax 2000; 55: 518–532.
34. Air pollution of the worlds megacities. A report from the UN Environment Programme and WHO. Environment 1994; 36: 5–37.
35. Yu O, Sheppard L, Lumley T et al. Effects of ambient air pollution on symptoms of asthma in Seattle-area children enrolled in the CAMP study. Environ Health Perspect 2000; 108: 1209–1214
36. Roemer W, Hoek G, Brunekreef B. Pollution effects on asthmatic children in Europe, the PEACE study. Clin Exp Allergy 2000; 30: 1067–1075.
37. Molfino NA, Wright SC, Katz I et al. Effect of low concentrations of ozone on inhaled allergen responses in asthmatic subjects. Lancet 1991; 338: 199–203.
38. Jorres R, Nowak D, Magnussen H. The effect of ozone exposure on allergen responsiveness in subjects with asthma or rhinitis. Am J Respir Crit Care Med 1996; 153: 56–64.
39. Tunnicliffe WS, Burge PS, Ayres JG. Effect of domestic concentrations of nitrogen dioxide on airway responses to inhaled allergen in asthmatic patients. Lancet 1994; 344: 1733–1736.
40. Devalia JL, Rusznak C, Herdman MJ et al. Effect of nitrogen dioxide and sulphur dioxide on airway response of mild asthmatic patients to allergen inhalation. Lancet 1994; 344: 1668–1671.
41. Frampton MW, Balmes JR, Cox C et al. Effects of ozone on normal and potentially sensitive human subjects. Part III: Mediators of inflammation in bronchoalveolar lavage fluid from non-smokers, smokers, and asthmatic subjects exposed to ozone: a collaborative study. Res Respir Health Eff Inst 1997; 78: 73–79.
42. Scannell C, Chen L, Aris RM et al. Greater ozone-induced inflammatory responses in subjects with asthma. Am J Respir Crit Care Med 1996; 154: 24–29.
43. Peden DB, Boehlecke B, Horstman D, Devlin R. Prolonged acute exposure to 0.16 ppm ozone induces eosinophilic airway inflammation in asthmatic subjects with allergies. J Allergy Clin Immunol 1997; 100: 802–808.
44. Nordenhäll C, Pourazar J, Ledin M-C et al. Diesel exhaust enhances airway responsiveness in asthmatic subjects. Eur Respir J 2001; 17: 909–15.
45 Stenfors N, Nordenhäll C, Salvi S et al. Different airway inflammatory responses in asthmatic and normal humans exposed to diesel exhaust. Submitted
46. Forsberg B, Stjernberg N, Wall S. People can detect poor air quality well below guideline concentrations: a prevalence study of annoyance reactions and air pollution from traffic. Occup Environ Med 1997; 54: 44–48.
47. Ostro BD, Rothschild S. Air pollution and acute respiratory morbidity: an observational study of multiple pollutants. Environ Res.1989; 50: 238–247.

48. Pope CA III, Dockery DW. In: Holgate ST, Samet JM, Koren HS, Maynard RL, ed. Air pollution and health. San Diego, CA: Academic Press; 1999: 73–706.
49. Kelly FJ, Blomberg A, Frew A et al. Antioxidant kinetics in lung lavage fluid following exposure of humans to nitrogen dioxide. Am J Respir Crit Care Med 1996; 1: 1700–1705.
50. Mudway IS, Blomberg A, Frew AJ et al. Antioxidant consumption and repletion kinetics in nasal lavage fluid following exposure of healthy human volunteers to ozone. Eur Respir J 1999; 13: 1429–1438.
51. Salvi S, Blomberg A, Rudell B et al. Acute inflammatory responses in the airways and peripheral blood following term exposure to diesel exhaust in healthy human volunteers. Am J Respir Crit Care Med 1999; 159: 702–709.
52. MacNee W, Donaldson K. Particulate air pollution: injurious and protective mechanisms in the lungs. In: Holgate ST, Samet JM, Koren HS, Maynard RL, ed. Air pollution and health. San Diego, CA: Academic Press; 1999: 653–672.
53. Blomberg A, Krishna MT, Bocchino V et al. The inflammatory effects of 2 ppm NO_2 on the airways of healthy subjects. Am J Respir Crit Care Med 1997; 156: 418–424.
54. Blomberg A, Krishna MT, Helleday R et al. Persistent airway inflammation but accommodated antioxidant responses and lung function after repeated daily exposure to nitrogen dioxide. Am J Respir Crit Care Med 1999; 159: 536–543.
55. Koren HS, Devlin RB, Graham DE et al. Ozone-induced inflammation in the lower airways of human subjects. Am Rev Respir Dis 1989; 139: 407–415.
56. Devlin RB, McDonnell WF, Becker S et al. Time-dependent changes of inflammatory mediators in the lungs of humans exposed to 0.4 ppm ozone for 2 hr: a comparison of mediators found in bronchoalveolar lavage fluid 1 and 18 hr after exposure. Toxicol App Pharmacol 1996; 138: 176–185.
57. Balmes JR, Chen LL, Scannell C et al. Ozone-induced decrements in FEV_1 and FVC do not correlate with measures of inflammation. Am J Respir Crit Care Med 1996; 153: 904–909.
58. Blomberg A, Mudway I, Nordenhäll C et al. Ozone-induced lung function decrements do not correlate with early airway inflammatory or antioxidant responses. Eur Respir J 1999; 19: 1418–1428.
59. Rudell B, Wass U, Östberg Y et al. Efficacy of filters to reduce acute health effects of diesel exhaust in humans. Occup Environ Health 1999; 56: 222–231.
60. Sandström T, Blomberg A, Helleday R, Rudell B. Air pollution effects on allergen responses – experiences from animal studies. Eur Respir Rev 1998; 53:168–174.
61. Sandström T, Blomberg A, Helleday R, Rudell B. Allergy and automobile pollution: experiments in animals. Rev Fr Allergol 2000; 40: 47–51.
62. Diaz-Sanchez D, Dotson AR, Takenaka H, Saxon A. Diesel exhaust particles induce local IgE production in vivo and alter the pattern of IgE mRNA isoform. J Clin Invest 1994; 94: 1417–1425.
63. Diaz-Sanchez D, Tsien A, Cacillas A et al. Enhanced nasal cytokine production in human beings after in vivo challenge with diesel exhaust particles. J Allergy Clin Immunol 1996; 98: 114–123.
64. Diaz-Sanchez D, Tsien A, Fleming J, Saxon A. Combined diesel exhaust particulate and ragweed allergen challenge markedly enhances human in-vivo nasal ragweed specific IgE and skews cytokine production to a Th2 type phenotype. J Immunol 1997; 158: 2406–2413.
65. Diaz-Sanchez D. The role of diesel exhaust particles and their associated PAHs in the induction of allergic airway disease. Allergy 1997; 52: 52–56.
66. Diaz-Sanchez D, Tsien A, Fleming J, Saxon A. Effect of topical fluticasone propionate on the mucosal allergic response induced by ragweed allergen and diesel exhaust particle challenge. Clin Immunol 1999; 90: 313–322.
67. Zeger SL, Dominici F, Samet J. Harvesting-resistant estimates of air pollution effects on mortality. Epidemiology 1999; 10: 171–175.

24 Smoking

John F Golding

Key points

- Smoking is the greatest preventable cause of death in the developed world.

- The decline in prevalence of smoking in developed countries has been greater in men than in women, such that in many countries the prevalence in women is now close to that of men.

- The prevalence continues to increase in many less developed countries.

- The main health hazards of cigarette smoke are tars (cancer), carbon monoxide, and/or nicotine (cardiovascular diseases) with both gas and particulates implicated in COPD.

- Recent smoking can be assessed by measurements of blood carboxyhaemoglobin, or expired carbon monoxide concentration; urinary or salivary cotinine has a much longer half-life.

- Environmental tobacco smoke (passive smoking) is associated in childhood with respiratory infections, sudden infant death, and asthma and in adults with cancer and cardiovascular disease.

- Prevention of starting smoking is more effective than attempts at giving up.

History

The nicotine molecule was produced over 60 million years ago by the ancestral tobacco plant to punish insect herbivores. Today tobacco smoking punishes the bodies of the most highly evolved species on this planet.

The earliest European explorers of the Americas observed the practices of smoking, snuffing and chewing of leaves from *Nicotiana tabacum*, its relative *N. rustica*, together with *Lobelia* spp., which produces the related molecule lobeline. These prac-

tices were geographically widespread in the Americas for ritual, social and medicinal purposes. This diverse geographical and functional usage implies that tobacco had been used by Indians of the American continent for a long time. However, the earliest hard evidence for the antiquity of smoking comes from a stone bas-relief depicting a Mayan priest in the act of smoking (Fig. 24.1). The adjacent Mayan date glyphs give an equivalent date of AD 692.[1]

The date of introduction of tobacco to Europe can be taken as 1492 when Christopher Columbus sailed to America. In the following century, tobacco cultivation was spread around the world by Spanish and Portuguese sailors to West Africa, India, Ceylon, Indonesia, China and Japan, as well as southern Europe. Tobacco was introduced to England somewhat later, most probably by Sir John Hawkins (1565) – although Sir Walter Raleigh later became associated with the 'weed' – and its use only became common in England about 1600. The popularity of what was at first an extremely expensive import, available only to the rich or to sailors who had access to it, was increased by its widely touted medicinal virtues and supposed aphrodisiac qualities. Jean Nicot (hence 'nicotine') wrote (1573): 'Nicotaine: a herb of marvelous virtue against all wounds, ulcers... '

The rapid increase in the popularity of tobacco was opposed from the outset. For example, the Pope outlawed smoking in the Vatican (1590). King James I issued a pamphlet, *A Counterblaste to Tobacco*, in 1604, rapidly backed by an import duty (cultivation in England was subsequently suppressed). His feelings towards the 'weed' were summarised in the following extract:[2] 'A custome lothsome to the eye, hatefull to the Nose, harmefull to the braine, dangerous to the Lungs, and in the blacke stinking fume thereof, neerest resembling the horrible Stigian smoke of the pit that is bottomless'.

Other countries, such as Russia and Turkey, took stronger anti-tobacco measures.[3]

By the 17th century tobacco had passed what may be termed its stage of persecution. Increasing popularity, together with expanding economic and revenue importance, warmed govern-

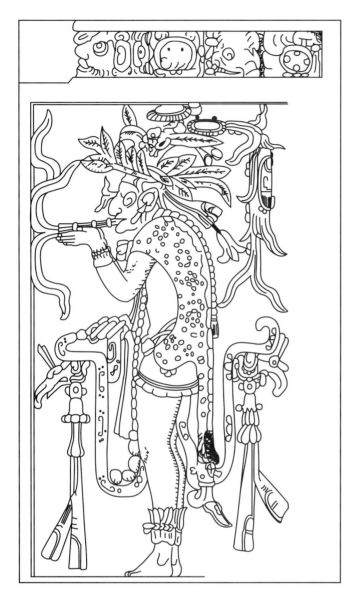

Fig. 24.1 Mayan figure of an individual in the act of smoking. Stone bas-relief in the Temple of the Foliated Cross, Palenque, Chiapas, Mexico. Middle Classic Period (AD 642–783). Temple dedication date glyphs give a Mayan date equivalent to AD 692. (After Mangan & Golding 1984.[1])

ment opinions towards it. The subsequent history of tobacco up to the early 20th century mainly concerns the mode of usage and its increasing commercial importance. Pipe smoking and snuff taking were dominant in the 17th and 18th centuries. Snuff achieved its height of popularity in the 18th century, when the elegant snuff box became the hallmark of social distinction. Since then it has declined to near-negligible levels today. A later but similar growth and decline occurred with chewing tobacco, although some present-day revival can be detected in the growth of smokeless or 'wet tobacco' use, and in the transmuted guise of nicotine chewing gum. The cigar had always been popular with the Spanish, but gained more general popularity in the 19th century. The precursors of cigarettes may

be traced to the Aztecs, who smoked long, tobacco-filled reeds. The Spaniards added the refinement of using paper tubes (*papeletes*) but until the mid- to late 19th century the cigarette was never more than an oddity by comparison with the cigar. From the 1870s hand-rolled cigarettes were gradually replaced by machine-made cigarettes. By the beginning of the 20th century the combination of newly developed flue-cured with air-cured tobacco resulted in an eminently inhalable mild cigarette smoke. The pleasure of inhalation-style smoking, allied with the efficiency of modern manufacturing and sales techniques, led to the cigarette becoming the dominant mode of tobacco usage during the First World War. The period from the First World War to shortly after the Second World War might be termed the 'golden age for the golden leaf'. Production was increasing and women were joining the ranks of smokers in increasing numbers. However, by the 1950s medical statisticians had begun to note a later and more sinister harvest.

Multinational companies now dominate tobacco production and the manufacture and distribution of cigarettes, the dominant mode of usage. These multinationals have diversified into related activities (e.g. paper-making) as well as a host of seemingly unrelated ventures. Although tobacco consumption has levelled off and is now declining in industrialised nations, a new wave of growth is occurring in the expanding populations and economies of developing countries in Africa, South America and parts of Asia.

Prevalence and trends

A wind of change is blowing in social attitudes toward smoking. From being a majority (among males at least), smokers have become a minority group (about 30%) in many countries.[4] The decline in prevalence of smoking has been dramatic; for example, in the UK 70% of men were smokers in the 1950s but by 1998 this had dropped towards 28%.[5–7] An example of recent trends in smoking prevalence is given in Figure 24.2a. The reduction in female smoking has been less dramatic and the prevalence of female smoking was increasing slightly until relatively recently. In many countries women smokers are approaching the prevalence rates seen in men. Women in particular have become heavier smokers. For example, over a 20-year period in the USA, the percentage of women smoking more than 25 cigarettes per day almost doubled from 13% in 1965 to 23% in 1985. Moreover, women are starting to smoke earlier. In some countries, including the UK, the frequency of smoking in girls now exceeds that in boys.[4,7]

On a more positive note, men in particular are giving up smoking in increasing numbers, and fewer men and women are starting to smoke. As most smokers start in their teens (Fig. 24.2b), it may be expected that the growing number of those who have never smoked will remain 'never-smokers' in the years to come. Socioeconomic gradients in smoking became apparent over 20 years ago; the prevalence of smoking has fallen in the professional/white-collar groups but less so for the manual and unskilled (Fig. 24.2c). This difference between socioeconomic groups has widened in recent years, with smoking prevalence remaining unchanged in the most socially deprived groups.[7]

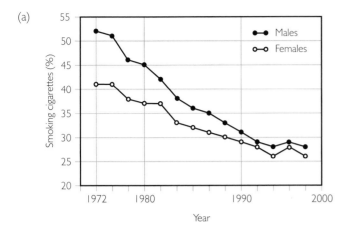

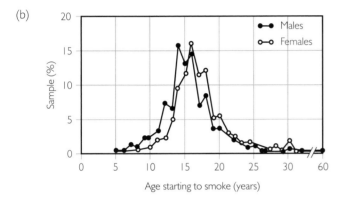

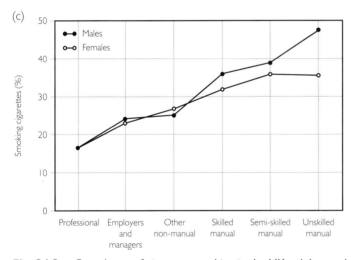

Fig. 24.2 a. Prevalence of cigarette smoking in the UK, adults aged 16 years plus. (Redrawn from General Household Survey 1997.[6]) b. Distribution of age of starting to smoke cigarettes in current regular cigarette smokers in the UK.[5] c. Cigarette smoking by socioeconomic group in the UK. (Redrawn from General Household Survey 1997.[6])

In less developed countries the picture is different; the prevalence of cigarette smoking is increasing, as are the numbers of cigarettes consumed per smoker, although some developing countries have apparently reversed this trend.[8]

The nature of tobacco smoke

Burning tobacco generates a complex mixture of compounds (over 4000 have been identified), which are conventionally divided into gas- and particulate-phase components (Table 24.1). Apart from nitrogen, oxygen and carbon dioxide, gas-phase components include carbon monoxide in significant concentration (about 4% by volume) and smaller but significantly undesirable quantities of nitrogen oxides, ammonia, nitrosamines, hydrogen cyanide, nitriles, volatile hydrocarbons, acetaldehydes, formaldehyde and acrolein. The particulate phase consists of an aerosol of tar/nicotine particles (diameter range $0.1-1.0\,\mu m$, mean $0.2\,\mu m$, approximate concentration 10^{10} particles/ml of mainstream smoke from the cigarette mouthpiece).[4] Tar is the sticky brown residual substance left after removal of nicotine and moisture from the particulate phase. Tar consists of a complex mixture of

Table 24.1 Distribution of selected toxic compounds in cigarette mainstream smoke (MS) and sidestream smoke (SS) of non-filter cigarettes[9]

Compound	MS	SS/MS
Gas phase		
Carbon monoxide	10–23 mg	2.5–4.7
Carbon dioxide	20–60 mg	8–11
Formaldehyde	70–100 µg	0.1–≈50
Acrolein	60–100 µg	8–15
Acetone	100–250 µg	2–5
Pyridine	20–40 µg	10–20
3-vinylpyridine	15–30 µg	20–40
Hydrogen cyanide	400–500 µg	0.1–0.25
Nitrogen oxides	100–600 µg	4–10
Ammonia	50–130 µg	40–130
N-nitrosodimethylamine	10–40 ng	20–100
N-nitrosopyrrolidine	6–30 ng	6–30
Particulate phase		
Particulate matter	15–40 mg	1.3–1.9
Nicotine	1–2.3 mg	2.6–3.3
Phenol	60–120 µg	2.0–3.0
Catechol	100–280 µg	0.6–0.9
Aniline	360 ng	30
2-toluidine	160 ng	19
2-naphthylamine	1.7 ng	30
Benz[a]anthracene	2.0–7.0 ng	2–4
Benzo[a]pyrene	20–40 ng	2.5–3.5
Quinoline	500–2000 ng	8–11
N-nitrosonornicotine	200–3000 µg	0.5–3
N-nitrosodiethanolamine	20–70 ng	1.2
Nickel	20–80 ng	13–30
Polonium-210	0.03–0.5 pCi	?

'Tar' is conventionally taken to consist of the particulate phase minus nicotine and water. The delivery of smoke compounds is varied by both the characteristics of the cigarette, such as the type of tobacco and the addition of a filter tip, and by the vigour with which an individual smokes a cigarette.

polynuclear aromatic hydrocarbons including such carcinogens as non-volatile nitrosamines, aromatic amines and benzopyrene. The use of some flavour additives in cigarettes may also represent a hazard.[4,9-11]

Broadly speaking, the major components representing health hazards are tar (for lung cancer), carbon monoxide and/or nicotine (for cardiovascular disease). Both gas- and particulate-phase components are implicated in the development of chronic obstructive pulmonary disease (COPD). With regard to muco-ciliary function, toxic effects have been demonstrated experimentally by smoke components including acrolein, acetaldehyde, formaldehyde, hydrogen cyanide and phenol. The role of nicotine is somewhat confused by its biphasic action on cilia, acting as a stimulant at low concentration and a depressant at higher concentrations.[11]

The tobacco industry has made attempts to reduce the yields of these various toxic components by each cigarette while preserving taste and flavour.[4] For example, for cigarettes manufactured in the UK between 1934 and 1979, the average tar yield decreased by 49%, nicotine by 31% and carbon monoxide by 11%.[12] This has been achieved by changes in the genetic strains of tobacco plants, fertiliser use, the time and manner of harvesting, leaf storage and curing, and processing techniques such as tobacco sheet reconstruction. However it has been suggested that the toxicity of tar itself may have varied, further complicating interpretation of effects over and above estimates of yields and variations in the manner in which the cigarette is smoked.[7] The design of cigarettes has also changed in terms of packing density, length, paper porosity, side ventilation and filtration efficiency of the butt. Lowered tar and nicotine yields have been achieved mainly by reducing levels in the tobacco itself and the addition of filter tips. Reductions of carbon monoxide have proved more difficult because it cannot be reduced by analogous reductions in preburnt tobacco levels nor, being a small molecule, can it be trapped in the filter tip. Carbon monoxide is produced in the burning cone and the immediately proximal high-temperature tobacco pyrolysis region. Methods have concentrated on cigarette construction to alter the burning rate and the temperature of the tobacco and to encourage side-diffusion from the tobacco rod through the paper and via filter ventilation holes. The latter also provides smoke dilution and reduction of other toxic smoke components.[10]

However, the way in which a cigarette is smoked critically affects tar, nicotine and carbon monoxide delivery. At the simplest level, the tobacco rod acts as a fractionation column, concentrating compounds towards the butt. Particulate matter is produced at much higher concentrations (up to twice as high) towards finishing a cigarette, hence the advice to leave longer stubs.[11] The following section details the effects of smoking style and compensatory behaviour in the face of low-delivery cigarettes.

Smoke intake

Methods of assessing smoke exposure include manner of tobacco use (cigarette, pipes, cigars), years of smoking, numbers smoked daily, machine smoked yields (of tar, nicotine, carbon monoxide), residual butt length, butt filter nicotine, smoking behaviour (number of puffs, puff pressure profile, puff volume, depth and duration of inhalation), blood carboxyhaemoglobin, exhaled carbon monoxide, blood and urinary levels of nicotine and its metabolites such as cotinine, and thiocyanates in saliva, urine or blood.[1,7,10] The measures employed vary tremendously in accuracy, complexity, invasiveness and cost, and consequently in their areas of research application.

Intake

For large-scale epidemiological work, self-report of type and amount of tobacco consumption has formed the basis of the well-known relations of dose-response (e.g. 'pack-years') and mode of usage (e.g. cigarette/cigar/pipe) with mortality and morbidity. However, cigarette yields vary considerably and may change the degree of hazard to some extent. For example, low-tar cigarettes may produce limited reductions in lung cancer. 'Standardised' yields are produced by machine smoking.

Unfortunately, the standard cigarette yields do not take into account actual individual variation in the manner of smoking a cigarette. To take the example of low-tar, ventilated, filter cigarettes: the blocking of the filter perforations by fingers or lips, which is observed in 32–69% of low-tar smokers, increases the yield of toxic products by 59–293%.[11] Standard machine-smoked yields do not take this into account. Another example is the observation that the nominal nicotine yields of various strengths of cigarette accounted for only 25% of the individual differences in rise in blood nicotine levels following a cigarette, whereas 50–60% of the variation was accounted for by individual differences in smoking behaviour.[13]

Residual stub length is a very crude indicator of smoking vigour, which is confounded by the fact that unpuffed and puffed burnt tobacco rod both contribute, i.e. the implied side-stream and mainstream smoke production is not distinguished. Butt-filter nicotine is a better method (which is also non-invasive) of assessing the amount of nicotine (and correlated tar) presented to the smoker. However, butt-filtration efficiencies are based on standard machine smoking and differences between studies indicate that butt-filtration efficiency values themselves change to some extent as a function of individual smoking behaviour. More sophisticated smoking simulators allow a recorded pattern of an individual's smoking behaviour (puff number, interval, duration, pressure profile) to be applied to the cigarette. Consequently a more realistic estimate can be made of the amount of tar, nicotine and carbon monoxide presented to the smoker. Measures of smoking behaviour can be obtained using a flowmeter in a short cigarette holder; other methods include remote infrared sensing of the burning tobacco cone as well as cheek inductive plethysmography.[1,11] Together with measurements of inhalation depth and duration (e.g. chest-wall movement, impedance plethysmography, tracer gases), these methods can provide some estimate of smoke intake.

Deposition

Most of the available information on the actual deposition of cigarette smoke particulates is based on theoretical or physical models of the lungs and measurements of differences in the concentration of aerosol between inhaled and exhaled air. Models predict that with inhalation 30–40% of tar/nicotine particles are deposited in the alveolar region and 5–10% in the tracheobronchial region. Holding smoke in the mouth for 2 seconds can remove 16% of particulate matter. The upper airways absorb 60% of the water-soluble components of the gas phase. Understanding of the dynamics of the process is complicated by the fact that particle size changes within the respiratory tract – increasing with coagulating collisions between particles, decreasing with evaporation of volatile substances and increasing with hygroscopicity.

Physical models of human lungs using double-casting techniques of postmortem material indicate preferential deposition patterns. For example, deposition occurs preferentially at airway bifurcations, which may be the reason for these being common sites of bronchogenic carcinomas in humans. Patterns of inspiration will affect deposition: large tidal volumes favour alveolar deposition. The collection efficiency (the difference between the quantity of smoke component inhaled versus exhaled) for the particulate phase has been demonstrated to be slightly higher for male (57% mean collection efficiency) compared with female (40%) smokers. Collection efficiency appears to be much lower in non-smokers (10%). This probably reflects differences in non-smokers' inhalational patterns. Thus intentional breath-holding following smoke inspiration occurs in smokers and this increases retention.[11]

Carbon monoxide and carboxyhaemoglobin measurements

Blood carboxyhaemoglobin level is a good index of the extent of recent inhalation-style smoking (it has a half-life of less than 4 hours). Exhaled carbon monoxide concentration relates linearly to blood carboxyhaemoglobin. Exhaled carbon monoxide levels greater than 8 parts per million (ppm) are strongly suggestive of smoking and typical levels in an average smoker are around 20–30 ppm, depending on the number and time since smoking. An extremely heavy cigarette smoker may attain up to 80 ppm of carbon monoxide at the end of a day's indulgence in the habit (approximately equivalent to a blood carboxyhaemoglobin of 14%). Measurement of exhaled carbon monoxide has the advantage of being quick and non-invasive, and inexpensive portable carbon monoxide gas analysers are now available. Basal carbon monoxide levels correlate well with venous trough nicotine levels within cigarettes of the same brand.[14] By contrast, the rise in blood nicotine following smoking a single cigarette correlates poorly with the rise in carbon monoxide. This probably reflects the differential lung distribution for gas (carbon monoxide) versus particle (nicotine–tar), quite apart from the fact that the ratio of carbon monoxide to nicotine delivered in a given volume of smoke is determined to some extent by the exact shape of the pressure profile produced by individual smokers. When carbon monoxide is used as an index of smoking, the possibility of its absorption from other sources (e.g. stoves, gas fires, automobiles) should be borne in mind.

Measurement of nicotine and cotinine

Levels of nicotine and its metabolites in biological fluids have the advantage of being the most tobacco-specific of all measurements. Moreover, for cigarette smoking they indicate the extent of particulate phase intake to the lungs because nicotine from cigarette smoke is not well absorbed in the mouth whereas nicotine from pipe/cigar smoke can be absorbed by this route (see Pharmacology of nicotine, below). Nicotine itself has a fairly short half-life (about 2 h from venous trough levels) and so is best used as an index of recent smoking. Its main metabolite, cotinine, with a longer half-life of 19 h, is a better index of chronic smoking and urinary or salivary cotinine sampling has the advantage of being less invasive.[9,15]

Measurement of other substances

Thiocyanates from hydrogen cyanide in tobacco smoke may be measured in blood, urine or saliva. They have an even longer half-life (about 14 days) than cotinine but have the disadvantage of being less tobacco-specific. Other sources include diet (cassava root, cabbage, broccoli, etc.) and less frequently industrial sources (e.g. electroplating works). The differences for regular smoking are large; for example, typical blood levels of thiocyanate are 18 μmol/l in non-smokers, 25 μmol/l in vegetarian non-smokers and 80–100 μmol/l in regular smokers.[16] Less frequently used measures of smoke intake include radioactively labelled 'nicotine-spiked' cigarettes, radiolabelled tracer gases incorporated into the mainstream tobacco smoke and radiolabelled polystyrene latex beads of diameters equivalent to nicotine-tar particles.[11]

Active smoking and ill health

Tobacco smoking is the largest preventable cause of death in the developed world. Epidemiological studies in many countries have consistently pointed to a strong association between smoking and serious disease.[17] For example, for all male smokers the overall mortality ratio is around 1.7 compared to non-smokers. Heavy smokers of two packs a day show a higher mortality ratio of 2.0.[10] The excess mortality can also be expressed in terms of 'lost years'. By this approach, a 35-year-old male cigarette smoker who continues to smoke can expect to die, on average, more than 7 years earlier than a man who has never smoked, the equivalent for the female smoker being 6 lost years.[7] The excess mortality for smokers reaches a peak in middle age, with some decline towards old age. This does not imply a decreasing effect of smoking on health with old age but rather reflects a lower risk in the survivors as a result of a process of selection in which the more susceptible smokers have already died.[10]

Various lines of evidence indicate that the smoking–mortality link is causal. First, the toxic nature of the constituents of tobacco smoke has been demonstrated in laboratory animals. Second, the likelihood of serious disease is related to the degree of exposure, e.g. as expressed in 'pack-years' or cigarettes per day, and it is higher in inhalers than non-inhalers.

Similarly, cigar and pipe smokers show less excess mortality than cigarette smokers, which is related to the lesser inhalation of cigar/pipe smoke, a pattern of exposure to the toxic constituents of tobacco smoke that is consistent with their lesser incidence of cancer of the lung as opposed to cancer of the oral cavity. Third, the risk of serious tobacco-related disease declines as a function of number of years elapsed since giving up smoking, reaching near-equivalence with never-smokers after 15 years off tobacco (the decline in risk is more rapid for cardiovascular disease). Fourth, the increase in smoking prevalence among women smokers during the 20th century has been followed, with a predictable time lag, by an increase in smoking-related diseases such as lung cancer and coronary heart disease in women. A similar predictable rise is beginning to occur in the less developed countries. Finally, epidemiological studies of smoking and non-smoking monozygotic and dizygotic twins have allowed control of genetic and psychosocial factors. This leaves little doubt that the link is causal as regards lung cancer and other lung disease, although the same studies suggest that the link is more complicated with regard to cardiovascular disease, perhaps because smoking is only one of the major risk factors.[1,9,10]

The catalogue of tobacco-related disease is extensive. An example of a classic study of smoking-related mortality is given in Table 24.2.[18] The more important diseases are cardiovascular (including coronary artery disease, cerebrovascular disease, peripheral vascular disease), neoplastic (including cancer of the lung, larynx, oral cavity, oesophagus, bladder, pancreas) and COPD (chronic bronchitis, emphysema). In addition, maternal smoking would appear to produce deleterious effects on the fetus (perhaps by fetal hypoxia), because birth weights are lower and gestation and birth complications greater, even when such relevant factors as social class and maternal weight are taken into account.[10] Exposure in utero to maternal smoking also appears to be a contributor to increased asthma in children (see Associations between ill health and passive smoking, below). Although smoking-related mortality ratios are highest for lung cancer and COPD, in terms of actual number of deaths the major contributor to cause-specific mortality among smokers is cardiovascular disease (Table 24.2).

For cardiovascular disease the smoke components of major interest are carbon monoxide (and related hypoxaemia) and the effects of nicotine on cardiac rhythm, free fatty acids in plasma, lipoproteins, coronary vasoconstriction and the coagulability of blood. Smoking-related neoplastic diseases (e.g. lung cancer) doubtless result from one or more of the known carcinogens and co-carcinogens in tobacco smoke rather than from nicotine or carbon monoxide. COPD is probably caused by the effects of substances in both the gas and particulate phases of smoke on proteolytic enzymes (increased elastase, reduced amounts of its inhibitor, α_1-antiprotease), interference with immune mechanisms and inhibition of mucociliary clearance mechanisms. The latter ciliotoxic effects of tobacco smoke may contribute to carcinogenicity of tobacco smoke, potentiate the effects of other environmental carcinogens, such as asbestos, and increase the risk of respiratory infections. Reliable differences in indices of expiratory airflow exist between smokers and non-smokers after age 25 years. The observation of marked individual differences

Table 24.2 An example of an epidemiological study of mortality related to tobacco smoking: observed deaths (O), expected deaths (E) and mortality ratios (O/E) for pure cigarette smokers, pure cigar smokers and pure pipe smokers for selected causes of death. Adapted from Rogot & Murray.[18]

Cause of death*	Pure cigarette smokers			Pure cigar smokers			Pure pipe smokers		
	Observed deaths	Expected deaths	O/E†	Observed deaths	Expected deaths	O/E†	Observed deaths	Expected deaths	O/E†
All causes	15091	8112	1.86	2653	2302	1.15	1545	1432	1.08
Cardiovascular diseases	8920	5257	1.70	1681	1522	1.10	984	948	1.04
Cancers, all sites	3138	1401	2.24	510	386	1.32	307	237	1.29
Coronary heart disease	5740	3414	1.68	1077	965	1.12	606	596	1.02
Stroke	1172	796	1.47	267	249	1.07	157	159	0.99
Influenza and pneumonia	200	96	2.08	28	34	0.82	22	23	0.97
Aortic aneurysm	359	68	5.28	38	19	2.04	24	12	2.07
Respiratory diseases	879	185	4.75	51	61	0.84	57	39	1.44
Bronchitis and emphysema	568	43	13.13	10	14	‡	22	9	2.53
Lung cancer	1095	91	12.06	41	25	1.66	32	15	2.14

* 'All causes' refers to all deaths observed, most but not all of which can be classified under the general categories of 'Cardiovascular diseases', 'Cancers, all sites' and 'Respiratory diseases'. In addition, a number of more specific categories of major interest are also given, which can be subsumed under the above; for example, the category 'Lung cancer' is one of the categories subsumed under 'Cancers, all sites'. † Based on expected number to 2 decimal places. ‡ Ratio not shown for observed values of less than 20.

in smoking-induced decline in such measures as forced expiratory volume in 1 second (FEV$_1$) has led to the suggestion that those with a particularly rapid decline early in life may represent a group particularly susceptible to later development of COPD.[4,9-11]

Finally, the negative association between smoking and Parkinson's and Alzheimer's disease (perhaps caused by nicotine) may be noted, although these possible protective effects are trivial by comparison with the health risks of smoking.[19] It has been estimated that smoking causes 85 times more deaths than it prevents.[7]

Passive smoking and ill health

Passive (involuntary) smoking refers to the exposure to tobacco combustion products from the smoking of others, often referred to as environmental tobacco smoke (ETS) exposure. Most interest concerns the passive smoking effects on non-smokers because the major tobacco-smoke exposure for smokers comes directly from their own smoking, rather than involuntary smoke intake from the smoking activity of others.

Assessment of exposure

Tobacco smoke in the environment derives from mainstream and sidestream smoke. Mainstream smoke is first filtered by the cigarette and, in the case of the inhaling smoker, by the lungs before emerging into the environment. Sidestream smoke emerges directly into the environment. Many potentially toxic constituents are present in higher concentrations in sidestream than in mainstream smoke. Moreover, sidestream smoke contributes nearly 85% of the total smoke in a room. Quantification of the exposure of a passive smoker is difficult because it is dependent on a number of factors, including type and number of cigarettes burned, size of room and ventilation rate. Elevated levels of indoor by-products of tobacco smoke (acrolein, aromatic hydrocarbons, carbon monoxide, nicotine, oxides of nitrogen, nitrosamines and particulate matter) under realistic conditions, e.g. in cafés, bars, restaurants, trains, cars, hospitals, etc., have been measured in a number of studies. Typical ranges of respirable particulates in smoking areas are 100–700 $\mu g/m^3$, which is up to 25 times the levels found in non-smoking areas.[11]

Indices of passive smoke exposure include those validated in smokers themselves – carbon monoxide, nicotine, metabolites such as cotinine and thiocyanate. None of these is perfect. For example, carboxyhaemoglobin (or exhaled carbon monoxide) has a relatively short half-life of less than 4 h, which allows measurement of acute but not chronic exposure and, at the relatively low levels under consideration, significant non-tobacco sources of carbon monoxide, including (indoor) stoves and (outdoor) combustion engines, may represent frequent sources of error. Although nicotine is the most tobacco-specific index, it settles out of the air with the particulate matter, making it a poor indicator of gas-phase constituents. Moreover, nicotine may subse-

quently evaporate into the environment from surfaces on which it has been deposited.[11] Direct absorption through the skin from deposited nicotine cannot be excluded as an unwanted artefact at the low nicotine levels under consideration. Dietary intake of nicotine in non-smokers can be of importance in the interpretation of low nicotine levels because many common vegetables contain low concentrations of nicotine. For example, it has been suggested that 10 g of aubergine may provide nicotine equivalent to 3 h in a mildly smoky room.[20] Although no single index of exposure has been accepted as yet, one estimate of the exposure in non-smokers to one of the most toxic constituents, tar, has been an 'average population exposure' of 1.43 mg tar/day. Another estimate for a non-smoker breathing 500 $\mu g/m^3$ tobacco smoke for an 8-hour day is that 0.55 mg of particulates would deposit in his or her lungs. For comparison, a two-pack-a-day smoker of average rated 20 mg tar cigarettes would deposit approximately 400 mg of tar in his or her lungs per day. Such calculations make allowance for retention coefficients of 11% and 70% for passive and active smokers respectively.[11]

Associations between ill health and passive smoking

The most frequent symptom of the non-smoker's reaction to passive smoke exposure is eye irritation in approximately 70% of people, a symptom that has been objectively related to smoke exposure using eye blink rates. Headache, nasal irritation and cough are also commonly reported. Small but statistically significant acute decreases in pulmonary function (forced vital capacity – FVC, FEV$_1$, maximum expiratory flow at 50% and 25% FVC) have been demonstrated in non-smokers under experimental chamber conditions of moderate-to-high smoke exposure levels. However, general irritant responses occur below the levels of smoke exposure that produce these acute pulmonary effects.

Half the world's children may be exposed to environmental tobacco smoke. Involuntary smoking among children causes respiratory tract infections, middle-ear disease, sudden infant death syndrome and asthma. The exact mechanisms are still unclear, as are the relative contributions of prenatal versus postnatal exposure.[21] Although direct postnatal environmental tobacco exposure is the most obvious mechanism, recent research indicates that exposure to maternal smoking in utero, with or without subsequent exposure to environmental tobacco smoke, increases the risk of asthma in children. It has been suggested that exposure in utero may increase the occurrence of asthma by altering critical developmental pathways, leading to poorer lung function. In children, many studies have shown a positive relation between parental smoking and respiratory symptoms such as chronic cough, chronic sputum production, persistent wheezing and respiratory infections. Some increased symptoms may be confounded by increased reporting of children's symptoms by parents who smoke and have similar symptoms, by the child's own smoking habits or by other related factors that may have a bearing on the child's health such as socioeconomic group and family size. However, these confounding factors have been controlled in some studies and a relationship remains.

It is possible that young children represent a more susceptible population for the adverse effects of passive smoking than older children or adults. Especially important are the increases in severe respiratory illnesses in children less than 2 years of age.[11] By contrast, objective measurements of pulmonary function in the general population of children, unselected for the minority with severe symptoms, demonstrate differences between children of smoking versus non-smoking parents of small magnitude (a few per cent, e.g. for FEV$_1$). It is not known what implication such small early differences may have for the later development of lung disease.

Objective markers of passive smoke exposure such as salivary or urinary cotinine enable more quantitative relationships with reduced respiratory function in children to be established.[22] As the degree of passive smoke exposure is variable among smoking households and as exposure can occur outside the home in children of non-smoking parents, the use of objective markers for exposure to environmental tobacco smoke may reveal small effects that would otherwise be obscured. Studies of passive smoking and symptoms in patients with known pulmonary disease (e.g. asthmatic patients) have produced some variation in results of objective pulmonary measurements, although subjective symptoms such as chest tightness are related consistently to passive smoke exposure.[4,10] On an optimistic note, evidence from cotinine concentrations in non-smoking children in the UK demonstrates that smoke exposure has almost halved in the last decade, probably by reduction in parental smoking in the home and perhaps by reductions in exposure outside the home.[23]

The evidence that passive smoking is associated with serious health hazards, principally lung cancer, comes from epidemiological studies. Most of these studies have compared the frequency of lung cancer in various groups of non-smokers living with smoking as opposed to non-smoking spouses. A number of artefacts may distort studies of this nature. Thus, smokers tend to congregate and socialise together and this extends to living together. The extent to which smokers preferentially live with other smokers rather than with non-smokers may be termed an 'aggregation factor'. As ex-smokers can in practice be misclassified as 'never-smokers', and as they will be over-represented among non-smokers living with current smokers, the still significant elevated risk from lung cancer in ex-smokers distorts (increases) 'passive smoking' effects. Estimated allowances can be made for ex-smokers among the non-smokers 'boosting' mortality ratios.

A major review of case-control and prospective studies indicated that the mean relative risk for lung cancer in non-smokers living with smoking spouses was 1.35 (1.0 = no difference; less than 1.0 = opposite effect) with a range of 0.5–3.25.[24] Other reviews of the relative risk from smoking spouses have produced somewhat lower values for excess risk of lung cancer, in the range 1.05–1.10.[25] It has been claimed that such results are consistent with risk estimates based on biochemical markers of passive smoke exposure such as cotinine.

Estimates of the relative risk of cardiovascular disease in non-smokers exposed to environmental tobacco smoke have been around 1.2–1.3. Since the total smoke dose experienced by the non-smoker has recently been estimated as some 100–300 times less than that for a typical 20-cigarettes-per-day active smoker

(relative risk of cardiovascular disease around 1.8), non-linear dose–response relationships have been invoked to account for such large effects of passive smoking and the question of the extent of the contribution of epidemiological biases and confounders remains unresolved.[26]

The objective measurement of degree of passive smoke exposure, and relating this to elevated morbidity and mortality, are both qualitatively and quantitatively more difficult than the analogous measurements of smoke exposure and ill health in active smokers. The trend of the evidence indicates that, apart from the well-known irritant effects, passive smoke exposure is associated with increases in respiratory symptoms and infections in the young children of smokers and with small but statistically significant reductions in pulmonary function. For adult non-smokers living with smoking spouses some elevation of lung cancer risk has been observed, which varies between studies, and it remains difficult to estimate the true size of the effect. However, if there is no level below which carcinogens cease to have an effect, it is likely that an elevation of risk for lung cancer from passive smoke exposure does occur.

Importance of nicotine

Evidence for nicotine being the primary motivator for smoking includes the following:

- Nicotine is absorbed from tobacco smoke in sufficient quantities to produce clear-cut pharmacological effects in the brain.
- The most popular form of nicotine self-administration, inhalation of cigarette smoke, is the most rate- and concentration-efficient method for delivering nicotine to the brain.
- Nicotine is the only pharmacologically active constituent obtained in common from the various forms of tobacco use: inhalation of cigarette smoke, non-inhalation of pipe/cigar smoke, tobacco snuffing and tobacco chewing.
- Nicotine replacement therapy (nicotine gum, nicotine transdermal patch) is an effective aid to smoking cessation.
- In experimental conditions, animals will voluntarily self-administer nicotine.
- Self-administration of nicotine can be altered in both animals and humans by central (but not peripheral) nicotinic cholinergic receptor antagonists.
- Smokers downregulate and upregulate nicotine intake in response to variations in tobacco nicotine delivery.
- Smoking or snuffing behaviour in humans is not practised in the absence of the known pharmacological rewards obtained from drugs such as opiates, cannabis, cocaine, organic solvents or nicotine.[1,27]

To stress the importance of nicotine is not to deny the contributions of other factors in determining smoking behaviour. Non-pharmacological sources of reward can be significant and the possibility of the presence of other psychoactive substances in tobacco apart from nicotine cannot be excluded.[7] Other, mostly learned or associated, cues add to smoking satisfaction. Tar components provide taste and smell and are responsible for the 'scratch' of inhaled smoke at the back of the throat; these may become pleasurable by a process of classic conditioned association as predictors of the arrival of nicotine in the brain. Practised smokers may use them as cues for estimating the nicotine strength of the cigarette. Manipulations of the cigarette, pipe or rolling tobacco, lighting-up routines, situational and social pressures all play a part, but these lose their motivational power without the reinforcing effect of nicotine. Thus a knowledge of the properties of nicotine is necessary to understand the motivation in smoking and cessation.

Pharmacology of nicotine

The alkaloid nicotine is a colourless volatile base ($pK_a = 8.5$) that turns brown and acquires the odour of tobacco on exposure to air. At atmospheric pressure it boils at 246°C, volatilising in the cone of burning tobacco at 800°C. It is readily soluble in water, alcohol and ether, and forms water-soluble salts. At blood pH it is in a mainly ionised form, which is the pharmacologically active form.[15,28]

Nicotine in cigarette smoke is suspended on minute droplets of tar and is quickly absorbed from the lung, almost with the efficiency of intravenous injection. It reaches the brain within 10–19 s of inhalation. Using ^{14}C-labelled nicotine cigarettes it has been demonstrated that some inhaling smokers absorb up to 90% of the nicotine from the smoke taken in.[29] The speed, efficiency and controllability of self-dosing with nicotine afforded by cigarette smoking (the so-called 'puff by puff fingertip control') partly explain its popularity over other modes of tobacco use.

The absorption of nicotine is to some extent pH-dependent. Thus nicotine in cigarette smoke, which is somewhat acidic, is not well absorbed from the mouth and is usually inhaled. By contrast, pipe and cigar smoke is more alkaline and thus better absorbed in the mouth. Nicotine chewing gum is formulated with a slightly alkaline buffer to promote nicotine absorption in the mouth. However, the massive absorption area provided by the lungs is the predominant controlling factor in cigarette smoking. Plasma nicotine levels in non-inhaling pipe and cigar smokers are still low (and achieved more slowly) by comparison with inhaling cigarette smokers. A rank order of absorption efficiency is: inhalation > snuffing > buccal absorption (corresponding to cigarettes versus snuff versus chewing tobacco, nicotine gum, non-inhaled pipe/cigar smoke, respectively). Although absorption of nicotine through the skin (transdermal nicotine patch) is efficient with a bioavailability of approximately 80%, it is slow; an initial delay of 0.25–4 h may be observed before detection of nicotine in the plasma. Reasonably steady plasma levels of nicotine may be achieved by 8 h or so, and can be maintained at plasma levels approximately equivalent to those achieved by repeated chewing of nicotine gum, or approximately half of the plasma levels achieved after a day's cigarette smoking. Depending on the formulation, a single application of a nicotine patch will sustain nicotine release for up to 24 h or more.[30]

Pharmacokinetics of nicotine in smoking

Peak plasma nicotine concentrations after inhalation-style cigarette smoking are typically 20–30 ng/ml (100–200 nmol/l). Example time courses and distribution of concentration levels are shown in Figures 24.3[31,32] & 24.4. Pipe/cigar smoking curves (not shown) vary between the curves (Fig. 24.3a) shown for inhaling cigarette smoking versus nicotine gum, as a function of degree of inhalation. Plasma nicotine levels from inhalation smoking probably represent an underestimate of the pharmacological impact on the brain. This is the result of the nicotine 'bolus' effect in arterial blood pumped from the lungs, with each inhaled puff.[28] Arterial blood concentrations of nicotine 1 min following cigarette smoking are approximately two to six times those of venous blood concentrations but equilibrate rapidly, the arterial–venous differences equalising within 5 min.[33] The arterial–venous nicotine concentration difference would be much greater (more than fourfold) if an arterial blood sample was drawn from a passing nicotine 'bolus' during smoking. The occurrence of high but transient levels of nicotine reaching the brain helps explain the perniciousness of the addiction that develops to cigarette smoke and, by analogy, to smoked forms of cocaine (e.g. 'crack'). The concentration and half-life of nicotine in the human brain is not known for certain. Animal experiments indicate that nicotine from the (arterial) blood is rapidly sequestered in the brain but that it washes out again quickly.[1] In the case of slow transdermal (nicotine patch) or buccal absorption (pipe/cigar/nicotine chewing gum), steadier, albeit lower, concentrations of nicotine in the brain might be expected than with inhalation-style smoking. Following a single cigarette, plasma nicotine concentrations decline rapidly over 5–10 min, reflecting redistribution among body tissues. The subsequent elimination half-life of 'trough' plasma nicotine levels is approximately 2 h. In spite of this rapid elimination, the trough plasma nicotine level of a typical smoker will gradually rise over the course of a day's regular smoking.

Metabolism of nicotine

The principal metabolite of nicotine is cotinine (half-life about 19 h). Smaller amounts of nicotine N-oxide are produced and other less important metabolites are nornicotine and the isomethylnicotinium ion. Only nornicotine has any pharmacological potency and no metabolite is thought to exert significant pharmacological actions at the concentrations observed.[15,28] Metabolism and pH account for why ingestion is an inefficient and slow route and thus not used as a mode of tobacco use.

Conversion of nicotine to cotinine occurs in the liver, to a lesser extent in the kidney and lung but not in the brain. Metabolic conversion of nicotine is higher in smokers than in non-smokers, reflecting enzyme induction. Indeed, smokers metabolise a wide variety of drugs more rapidly. Upon tobacco abstinence, over a period of weeks to months, this smoking-induced acceleration wanes and drug degradation approaches the norm for non-smokers. Only a small amount of unmetabolised nicotine is normally excreted in the urine but acidification of urine can increase the proportion of active nicotine excreted (by decreasing renal tubular reuptake and subsequent recirculation and metabolism). This has little effect on blood nicotine levels.[1,15]

(a)

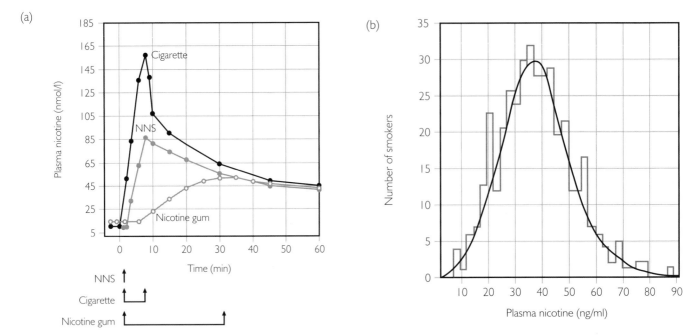

(b)

Fig. 24.3 a. Average plasma nicotine concentrations of three subjects after smoking a cigarette, taking nasal nicotine solution (NNS) and chewing nicotine gum. Doses of nicotine were 2 mg for NNS and nicotine gum and averaged 1.97 mg for the cigarette (1 nmol/l is equivalent to 0.16 ng/ml). (With permission from Russell et al 1981.[31]) b. Distribution of peak plasma nicotine concentrations in a sample of 393 heavy smokers (250 women, 143 men) with a mean cigarette consumption of 30 per day. Blood was taken 2 min after completing a cigarette during the afternoon of a day of usual smoking. The average plasma nicotine concentration was 35.8 ng/ml (SD 13.7) and was not significantly different between men and women. (With permission from Russell & Jarvis 1985.[32])

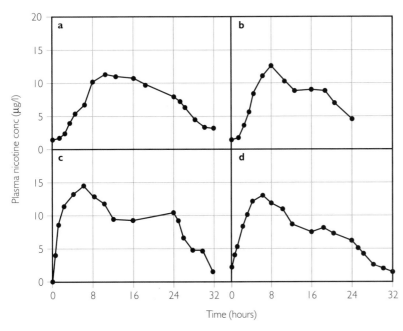

Fig. 24.4 Plasma nicotine levels after application of transdermal nicotine patches of various types: a. Habitrol (n = 11); b. Nicotrol (n = 11); c. Nicoderm (n = 13); d. Prostep (n = 11). All patches were worn for 24 hours apart from the Nicotrol patch, which was worn for 16 hours. Nicotine is absorbed more slowly by the transdermal method than by smoking or chewing. Nicotine levels are sustained for much longer and with less variability with the patch. (Modified from Benowitz 1992.[34])

Actions of nicotine

Nicotine exerts its pharmacological action at cholinergic receptors of the nicotinic type (hence the name) but not those of the muscarinic type. Initial combination with the receptor stimulates a response but persistent occupation blocks further responses.[15]

Briefly, the nicotinic receptor can exist in three interchangeable states, resting (ion channels closed), active (channels open) and desensitised (channels closed). Binding of the natural ligand (acetylcholine) or nicotine converts the resting to the active state for a very short period of time, which is then followed by a longer duration of the desensitised state (refractory and unresponsive) before change to the resting state again. However, low doses of an agonist such as nicotine can maintain cholinergic receptors in the desensitised state without activating them. Receptors are heterogeneous and vary in their binding affinities to nicotine; consequently, it is possible that a smoker's average plasma level of nicotine sustained throughout the day may be sufficient to desensitise a proportion of the cholinergic receptor population, whereas the higher levels of the nicotine bolus will affect other less sensitive receptors to varying extents.[7] In general, small doses of nicotine produce predominantly stimulant effects and larger doses mainly depressant effects. The complexity of nicotine action in smoking is not only the result of its biphasic dose-related stimulant versus depressant properties at the nicotinic receptor. Nicotine may stimulate inhibitory systems and inhibit stimulatory systems by virtue of the secondary release of other transmitters. Thus, in the central nervous system, nicotine-induced release of acetylcholine, dopamine, noradrenaline (norepinephrine), 5-hydroxytryptamine (5-HT), vasopressin and opioid peptides has been demonstrated.

In addition, tolerance to nicotine occurs, both metabolic through enzyme induction and pharmacodynamic. Both acute and chronic types of pharmacodynamic tolerance have been identified, which are unlikely to be explained by metabolic tolerance. Acute tolerance or 'tachyphylaxis' develops and subsides within minute or hours of a single nicotine injection or single cigarette, probably reflecting reversible receptor desensitisation. An example is the increase in autonomic and subjective effects pro-duced by the first (but not subsequent) cigarettes smoked after a period of abstinence which is commonly observed by smokers. Chronic tolerance is only gradually lost, lasting days or weeks. This may reflect up- and downregulation in receptor numbers. In animals, chronic nicotine exposure results in an increased number of nicotine receptors in the brain and the change over time in the number of nicotine receptors parallels change in tolerance. At postmortem examination, the number of nicotine receptors is greater in the brains of smokers than non-smokers.[34]

Nicotine in doses absorbed by the typical smoker causes a wide variety of effects on various systems (Table 24.3).[35-37] The mechanism may involve both peripheral and central actions of nicotine; for example, a rise in heart rate, which is initially caused by direct actions of nicotine on the heart and central nervous system, is sustained by the release of catecholamines from the adrenal medulla.[35]

Nicotine has central effects involving both reward and arousal systems. Although nicotine overdose can cause nausea and vomiting, this is avoided by the smoker through control of self-administration. Subjectively, nicotine in doses obtained from smoking is rewarding and intravenous injection of nicotine is also perceived as rewarding.[38] Self-administration experiments in animals suggest that it is a less powerful reinforcer than amphetamine or cocaine and is maintained under a narrower range of conditions.

The effects of nicotine, in doses equivalent to smoking, on electrocortical activity in animals have been demonstrated to be

Table 24.3 Selected acute physiological effects of nicotine in doses absorbed by the typical smoker

Physiological system or variable	Typical acute effect of nicotine in 'smoking doses'	References
EEG	Shift towards higher frequencies when individual is relaxed	36
Evoked potentials	Inconsistent amplitude changes, which may be related to nicotine dose and the nature of the eliciting stimulus	36,37
Sensory receptors	Stimulated: receptors in the skin, tongue, lung, mechanoreceptors, chemoreceptor of carotid body (skin/tongue/lung receptors also stimulated by other smoke components)	15
Electrodermal	Rise in skin conductance level; reduction in skin conductance responses and spontaneous fluctuations	1
Cardiovascular	Increased pulse rate, peripheral vasoconstriction, small rise in blood pressure, coronary vasoconstriction	15,35
Circulatory hormones	Release of: catecholamines, vasopressin, cortisol and growth hormone	15, 35
Respiratory	Minimal effects on respiration rate or depth (increased airway resistance – uncertain relative role of nicotine versus other smoke components)	1,11,15
Skeletal muscle	Muscle reflexes depressed somewhat, slight decrease in muscle tone, increased finger tremor	1
Gut	Increased tone and motor activity of the bowel	1, 15
Body weight (non-acute: long-term effect)	May be slightly reduced in some smokers by increased metabolic rate, less efficient absorption of food from the gut and decreased appetite	1,15

The intensity and sometimes even direction of the effect is dependent on nicotine dose, which is under the smoker's control; acute nicotine tolerance (tachyphylaxis) from prior smoking will also moderate many of these effects, especially on the cardiovascular system.

dose- and rate-dependent, small doses producing electrocortical arousal, higher doses producing depressant effects. In humans, the most common effect of smoking by a relaxed individual on electrocortical activity is a shift towards higher frequencies, which is consistent with its alerting effects. By contrast, under experimentally stressful conditions, smoking has been observed to produce signs of electrocortical de-arousal that may reflect subjectively experienced 'relaxing' effects. The effects of smoking on evoked potentials is variable and may be dose-related, as in animal experiments.[36,37]

Subjectively, smoking has been reported to relieve feelings of anxiety and stress, and to offset loss of concentration or fatigue. These latter subjective performance enhancements have also been demonstrated using objective indices of information processing, attention, vigilance and memory.[1,39] Nicotine has also been shown to improve mental performance in non-smokers. Equivalent (as far as is possible) tests on animals using nicotine injections in appropriate doses have demonstrated similar effects, although high doses can reverse this.

It can be argued that some or all of these 'beneficial' effects on mood and cognitive performance can be explained from the reverse point of view. In other words, what appear at first sight to be improvements in mood and alertness merely reflect the reversal of a nicotine withdrawal syndrome (see below).

Smoking motivation and models

Smoking is a complex pattern of behaviour, with nicotine acquisition overlaid by social and psychological factors. A variety of theories and models are available that emphasise these factors to differing degrees to explain the motivation to smoke. These theories range from 'psychoanalytical' (including 'oral fixation'), 'social learning', 'smoking typologies', to those placing more emphasis on particular actions of nicotine such as 'arousal modulation' (and similar variants such as 'psychological tool', 'stimulus filter') and 'nicotine addiction' (including more advanced variants such as 'opponent process'), as well as 'genetic predisposition' theories.[1,10] None of these theories or models is sufficient individually, but abstraction of important elements from them enables some (admittedly incomplete) understanding to be achieved. For convenience, smoking is seen in three stages: initiation, maintenance and cessation (the latter is discussed mainly under Prevention and cessation, below).

The initiation stage usually occurs in the early teens (Fig. 24.2c) and begins with experimentation with cigarettes. Social approval or disapproval would appear to be of overriding importance. This is the explanation for the dramatic rise in prevalence of smoking among women over the 20th century, which has paralleled emancipation in other spheres. The highly significant association between adolescent smoking and smoking by adolescent peer group, siblings or parents, indicates that social forces are exerted at an immediate level through these agencies. However, this is not to deny that other individuals such as schoolteachers, high-status individuals in the media and, more mundanely, the degree of enforcement of any legal sanctions against the sale of cigarettes to minors, also have a role.

Within these external limiting factors there is evidence that adolescents of a more rebellious, risk-taking, outgoing nature are more likely to take up smoking, as are individuals with more neurotic personalities. Moreover, a few studies indicate that these personality traits appear to be predictors of future smoking even before experimentation with cigarettes occur. Some degree of genetic predisposition to smoke has been shown, which is probably not specific for nicotine per se but for subsequent greater use of psychoactive drugs in general (including alcohol, caffeine, etc., consumption of which has been shown to be correlated with smoking). Such genetic predisposition may be exerting its effects through genetically linked aspects of personality. Thus it is possible that the personality characteristics of many smokers reflect some 'innate' deficit in central control systems for mood and arousal.

Maintenance of smoking continues through a variety of direct and indirect rewards (see also Pharmacology of nicotine, above). Direct pharmacological reward from nicotine occurs, perhaps through central release of dopamine, noradrenaline (norepinephrine) and opioid peptides. Smoking may also serve as a coping strategy in the face of stress. The mechanism for the tranquillising action of nicotine is still incompletely understood. It is possible that cigarette smokers may obtain stimulant or depressant/tranquillising actions by varying their nicotine intake, by virtue of the biphasic dose- and rate-related stimulant versus depressant nature of nicotine action. Such effects may also explain why smoking can increase mental performance in a variety of tasks.

However, a price, quite apart from physical health hazards, has to be paid by the smoker for these benefits. 'Dependence' on smoking develops in both an obvious and a less obvious fashion. The most obvious is that of physical addiction to nicotine. A definite withdrawal syndrome is experienced by most smokers for days to weeks following cessation. To some extent, continued smoking in long-term heavy users is reinforced by the avoidance of nicotine withdrawal symptoms. Indeed, this is one of the criteria used by the American Psychiatric Association in classifying tobacco smoking, together with use of other drugs such as heroin, under the same diagnosis of 'psychoactive substance dependence'.[34] Weight increase following cessation of smoking may also act as a disincentive for some individuals. However, a more subtle dependence is that many smokers will have learned to use smoking as a coping strategy for dealing with stress, fatigue and boredom. Indeed the personality characteristics of smokers indicate that a disproportionate number are inherently more susceptible to such mood and arousal perturbations. By default, it seems that alternative non-pharmacological coping mechanisms fail to develop or are allowed to 'atrophy' over the years in which the long-term smoker has come to use smoking as a 'psychological tool'.

Given the short latency of puffing, inhalation and nicotine reward in the central nervous system, and given the large number (thousands) of such pairings, the various sensory aspects of smoking (motor movements, lip contact, taste, 'scratch', inhalation) acquire secondary reinforcing properties by a process of conditioning. Similarly, smoking becomes inextricably linked with a wide variety of situations, both work and social.

The involvement of a host of reinforcing factors in smoking explains why it is such a difficult habit to give up for many smokers.[27] Overcoming the initial nicotine withdrawal symptoms would appear to be insufficient to ensure continued success in many ex-smokers (see Prevention and cessation, below). However, humans are rational animals able to look beyond immediate rewards and punishments to the future health risks, which may have seemed remote to the adolescent smoker. Millions of successful ex-smokers testify to the ability of humans both to overcome initial withdrawal symptoms and to devise alternative sources of reward and methods of mood control.

Changing use of tobacco and nicotine

Changing use of tobacco implies different (safer) methods of enjoyment of nicotine by the smoker. It also implies an endpoint, which is reduction of risk rather than total elimination of nicotine use. Nicotine in the high rate concentrations achieved with cigarette smoking (but not with the transdermal patch or gum), irrespective of the other toxic smoke compounds, tar, carbon monoxide, etc., itself carries some cardiovascular risk,[9] although nicotine with the lower rate concentrations via the transdermal patch or gum is regarded as relatively 'safe'.[7] It has been argued, with some force, that changing use is a misconceived goal and clouds the issue, because by offering a 'safer' (but not safe) use of tobacco, it can reduce the motivation to give up all uses of tobacco. Nevertheless smoking is not going to disappear overnight and it is actually increasing in some developing countries and in some subpopulations, e.g. female teenagers, in some developed countries.

For those who will not give up in the immediate future, and for those yet to start, some damage limitation may be possible. Three main approaches are: first, production of a 'safer' cigarette; second, transfer to pipe/cigar smoking, 'smokeless' tobacco use, e.g. chewing tobacco, snuff; and third, change to other formulations of nicotine (nicotine gum, nasal solutions, transdermal patches, inhalable aerosols). From the alternative perspective of cessation, the last of these three approaches is often denoted nicotine replacement therapy (NRT).

With regard to the 'safer' cigarette it can be said with some certainty that no cigarette can be safe, for the simple reason that burning complex hydrocarbons will always produce toxic products that cannot be eliminated without also removing the desired nicotine. The unpopularity of ultra-low-yield cigarettes testifies to this unpalatable truth. Even the more limited goal of producing a medium-nicotine (1.0 mg yield), low tar, low-carbon-monoxide cigarette with acceptable taste has encountered difficulties, although some progress has been made. It is possible that for some smokers reduction of nicotine delivery to low yields simply produces more vigorous compensatory puffing to maintain nicotine intake. The impact of such changes in cigarette design on mortality/morbidity is uncertain. For example, although some studies have indicated risk reduction due to lower tar delivery cigarettes for lung cancer and other tobacco-related cancers,[4] more recent studies in the USA and the UK have cast doubts on whether the trends are attributable to reductions in cigarette tar yields.[7]

Transfer to pipe/cigar smoking could represent a real reduction in hazard for the lungs and cardiovascular system, although not for the upper aerodigestive tract. Unfortunately, the smoker who has migrated from cigarettes often continues smoke inhalational habits with cigar or pipe smoke. Carboxyhaemoglobin measurements indicate that many ex-cigarette smokers who transfer to cigar/pipe smoking continue to inhale in spite of the 'harshness' of this type of tobacco smoke.[10]

Smokeless tobacco use has enjoyed some revival. It is certainly safer than smoking, but the habitual use of wet tobacco sachets poses the hazard of oral diseases, including cancer.[4] Concern has also been expressed that, marketed as a 'safe' form of tobacco use, adolescent users may be introduced to nicotine and then progress to the more dangerous use of cigarettes. Dry tobacco snuff has historically been popular (see above) and would seem to offer some nicotine satisfaction, as well as being relatively safe by comparison with cigarettes.

A more efficient mode of nicotine use is the nasal nicotine spray (see Pharmacology of nicotine, above). Absorption of nicotine is far more rapid than with nicotine gum, and blood nicotine levels are closer to those achieved with cigarette smoking. A variety of transdermal delivery systems using self-adhesive patches have now been developed. However, the lack of sufficient sensory stimulus and sensorimotor ritual, and slow rate of nicotine absorption, limit their use to the alleviation of some nicotine withdrawal symptoms.

Inhalable nicotine aerosols are potentially the most attractive solution to the problem of replacing inhalation-style cigarette smoking. So far, the available aerosol devices have been too clumsy and the nicotine aerosol too irritating. Smoke-free cigarettes have undergone trials but problems with the draw characteristics and the resultant nicotine vapour/aerosol, presumably reflecting a failure to mimic tobacco-smoke aerosol particle size, seem to have limited delivery of sufficient dose to the large absorption area of the lung. Moreover, olfactory and taste satisfaction may be problematical in achieving acceptance with smokers as a replacement for their habitual cigarettes.

Prevention and cessation

Most smokers say that they would like to give up and also report one or more serious attempts to do so. Although it has been difficult to distinguish and demonstrate a direct effect of any particular anti-smoking public health education or media campaign, there is no reason to doubt the source and nature of the self-reported motivation of ex-smokers. This is the wish to avoid future ill health and in some cases actual ill health at the time of giving up. For many pregnant women smokers (and some smoking spouses) concern for the health of the unborn child is the motivator and opportunity to give up smoking.[5] Social pressures to quit smoking can be exerted by the immediate family and peer group. Concern over passive smoking now also works as an additional pressure. Bans or restrictions on smoking in the workplace, on public transport and in various other public places have made smoking more difficult and tend to marginalise the smoker.[4,40] The price of cigarettes, which may be varied by tax, is certainly a factor limiting cigarette consumption (and perhaps smoking prevalence).[41] Socioeconometric models suggest that for, every 1% increase in price, consumption drops by approximately 0.5%.[4] The effects of price increases appear greatest for those with small incomes. Smuggling of cigarettes and tobacco has become extensive in response to the large taxation-driven price differentials between adjacent countries, and this may reduce the impact of 'official' price increases on consumption. Other factors affecting smoking are more difficult to quantify. Probably important are the presence or absence of cigarette advertising and the perceived status of smoking in terms of images and associations in films, television, computer games, sport sponsorship, etc.[1,42]

The proportion of individuals continuing successful abstinence follows a roughly exponential decline after giving up smoking. It approaches an asymptote at 6 months to 1 year, with around 10–30% successful abstinence (varying between studies and type of smoker at entry, see below). This type of decline may also be observed with other drug dependencies, with relapse to alcoholism, opiate or other drug use. Individual factors indicating greater long-term successful smoking cessation include former low daily cigarette consumption or delayed first cigarette of the day, lower consumption rates of alcohol and coffee, higher socioeconomic group, non-smoking spouses or partners and less neurotic or depressive personality. There is some slight evidence that women find it harder to give up smoking.[1] Of importance seems to be the degree of self-confidence from the outset that the goal will be achieved and the absence of stressful episodes that precipitate the desire for a cigarette.[43]

Aids to smoking cessation

Most smokers give up through their own efforts. For those who cannot manage this, a variety of specific methods have been proposed. Various counselling methods have produced some success, especially when combined with social support from friends, family and workplace,[44] although the evidence that more intensive counselling (so-called 'talking therapies') further improves success rates is disputed.[45] With many other methods initial success has been claimed but little or no extra benefit in long-term successful smoking cessation has been shown. Such ineffective methods are many, including progressive reduction of consumption, desensitisation, hypnotic suggestion, acupuncture and aversion therapy, whether by electric shocks associated with smoking, rapid smoking to nicotine nausea or oral silver acetate producing an unpleasant taste when smoking cigarettes. The major failing in these types of method lies not so much in the initial stage of cessation but in their failure reliably to improve long-term abstinence by comparison with unaided quitting.[1] Indeed, it may be important for most successful ex-smokers to experience self-confidence that they have succeeded through their own efforts. For many novice ex-smokers, major difficulties emerge after the initial 'euphoria' of successfully having overcome the first week(s) of withdrawal symptoms. The more complex task then begins of finding alternative sources of enjoyment, different coping strategies in the face of stress and other ways of maintaining concentration during sustained tasks. If, as has been suggested earlier (see Smoking motivation and models), many smokers have inherently poor central control systems for arousal, reward and punishment, then possible alternative strategies may involve physical sports, mental relaxation, assertiveness techniques and different scheduling of work activities if appropriate or possible.

Drugs used to aid smoking cessation may be divided into nicotinic agonists (nicotine and lobeline), nicotinic antagonists (mecamylamine) and a variety of other drugs that may mimic some of the actions of nicotine and/or counteract unpleasant aspects of nicotine withdrawal, which include mixed symptoms of hyper- and hypoarousal (amphetamine, tranquillisers such as benzodiazepines, adrenocorticotrophic hormone, vasopressin, clonidine (an α_2-adrenergic agonist), various antidepressants including fluoxetine (a 5-HT reuptake inhibitor), bupropion (a dopamine uptake inhibitor), and opioid antagonists such as naloxone.[7,34]

To date, the only preparations with demonstrated practical usefulness are nicotine (but not lobeline) via chewing gum, transdermal patch, nasal spray or inhaler, and the antidepressant bupropion (sustained-release Zyban®).[46] These medications appear equally effective and relatively safe, i.e. they all double quit rates and are associated with less than 5% dropout rate due to adverse events caused by the medication itself.[47] Combinations of the above have also been trialled. For example, combining nicotine gum, spray or inhaler with the patch has been proposed to be superior to single treatments alone, perhaps because the combination allows 'nicotine boosts' to be superimposed upon the steadier levels provided by the patch, avoiding to some extent a build-up of central nervous system tolerance as a result of steady levels of nicotine. However, the evidence that such combinations produce added effectiveness is not yet conclusive.[7] There are a few reports that mecamylamine, a nicotinic-receptor antagonist, may assist in cessation but more evidence is required as to its efficacy and long-term practical usefulness. Combining counselling therapy with medication may also further boost quit rates but again this has not been demonstrated conclusively.[44]

The powerful effect of hospital physicians' advice to a smoker who has suffered some serious smoking-related illness has been noted. For example, survivors of myocardial infarction have success rates for giving up smoking of 50%. However, success rates of physician advice for unselected patients in general practice are much lower, around 5% (as judged by long-term validation smoking cessation, e.g. carbon monoxide validation at 1 year follow-up).[11] Nevertheless, given the large number of patients in the latter situation and the minimal cost of such interventions this approach is of potential large-scale use.[48] Other settings for channelling advice are dental, family-planning and prenatal clinics (pregnancy is cited frequently as a reason for having given up smoking.)[5,11] The incorporation of face-to-face advice on smoking cessation from physicians and other health professionals has formed one element of community-based programmes for prevention of chronic disease, which involve other agencies such as schools and workplaces. Although there are methodological limitations to nearly all community studies, positive results have been obtained and it appears that person-to-person communication is a necessary part of such broad-based programmes.[11]

Prevention

Although much attention has been devoted to smoking cessation, it is a truism that prevention is better than cessation and offers the slower but more certain long-term hope of elimination of cigarette smoking. Progress is being made. Fewer young people are taking up the habit, although this trend seems to have levelled off or even reversed recently in some countries (see Prevalence and trends, above). Much remains to be done. Laws restricting the sale of cigarettes to adolescents require enforcement. Of great importance is the role of the image of smoking through associations in the media, including the Internet, marketing – such as free branded gifts, clothing or competitions – and advertising.[49] The reduction of smoking's image as 'something exciting and sophisticated' is required, because this would lower motivation to experiment with cigarettes. Various specific school programmes involving 'peer teaching' and demonstration of immediate effects of smoking to offset what to the adolescent seem distant and personally irrelevant health risks have been tried, in addition to more direct health education messages. As in the case of adult-directed media campaigns it is often difficult to demonstrate specific results.[1,50] However, the message is taking effect gradually and, as adult smokers become a minority, the 'role model' of smoking as an adult activity to emulate will be diminished.

? Unresolved questions

- How best to target preventative and cessation policies?
- How to limit the progressively rising smoking rates in less developed countries?
- Can more effective and safe aids to smoking cessation be developed?

References

1. Mangan GL, Golding JF. The psychopharmacology of smoking. Cambridge: Cambridge University Press; 1984.
2. James I. A counter-blaste to tobacco. (Published under pseudonym 'R.B.' with royal coat of arms). London: R.B. (Bodleian Library copy, Oxford); 1604.
3. Corti C. A history of smoking. London: George G. Harrap; 1931.
4. US Department of Health and Human Services. Reducing the health consequences of smoking: 25 years of progress. A report of the Surgeon General. Washington DC: US Government Printing Office; 1989.
5. Golding JF. Smoking. In: Cox B, ed. The health and lifestyle survey. London: Health Promotion Research Trust; 1987: 97.
6. General Household Survey. Office for National Statistics. London: HMSO; 1997.
7. Royal College of Physicians. Nicotine addiction in Britain. London: Royal College of Physicians of London; 2000.
8. Cox HS, Williams JW, de Courten MP et al. Decreasing prevalence of cigarette smoking in the middle income country of Mauritius: questionnaire survey. Br Med J 2000; 321: 345–349.
9. US Department of Health and Human Services. The health consequences of smoking: cardiovascular disease. A report of the Surgeon General. Washington DC: US Government Printing Office; 1983.
10. US Department of Health and Human Services. Smoking and health. A report of the Surgeon General. Washington DC: US Government Printing Office; 1979.
11. US Department of Health and Human Services. The health consequences of smoking: chronic obstructive lung disease. A report of the Surgeon General. Washington DC: US Government Printing Office; 1984.
12. Wald N, Doll R, Copeland G. Trends in tar, nicotine, and carbon monoxide yields of UK cigarettes manufactured since 1934. Br Med J 1981; 282: 763.
13. Herning RI, Jones RT, Benowitz NL, Mines AH. How a cigarette is smoked determines blood nicotine levels. Clin Pharmacol Ther 1983; 33: 84.
14. Ashton CH, Stepney R, Thompson JW. Should intake of carbon monoxide be used as a guide to intake of other smoke constituents? Br Med J 1981; 282: 10.
15. Goodman Gilman A, Rall RW, Nies AS, Taylor P, eds. The pharmacological basis of therapeutics, 8th ed. New York: Pergamon Press; 1990.
16. Vogt T, Selvin S, Widdowson G, Hulley S. Expired air, carbon monoxide and serum thiocyanate as objective measures of cigarette exposure. Am J Publ Health 1977; 67: 545.
17. Peto R, Darby S, Deo H et al. Smoking, smoking cessation, and lung cancer in the UK since 1950: combination of national statistics with two case-control studies. Br Med J 2000; 321: 323–329.
18. Rogot E, Murray JL. Smoking and causes of death among US veterans: 16 years of observation. Public Health Rep 1980; 95: 213.
19. Van Duijn CM, Hofman A. Relation between nicotine intake and Alzheimer's disease. Br Med J 1991; 302: 1491.
20. Domino EF, Hornback E, Demana T. The nicotine content of common vegetables. N Engl J Med 1993; 329: 437.
21. Wahlgren DR, Hovell MF, Meltzer EO, Meltzer SB. Involuntary smoking and asthma. Curr Opin Pulmon Med 2000; 6: 31–6.
22. Cook DG, Strachan DP. Health effects of passive smoking – 10: summary of effects of parental smoking on respiratory health of children and implications for research. Thorax 1999; 54: 357–366.
23. Jarvis MJ, Goddard E, Higgins V et al. Children's exposure to passive smoking in England since the 1980s: cotinine evidence from population surveys. Br Med J 2000; 321: 343–345.
24. Wald NJ, Nanchahal K, Thompson SG, Cuckle HS. Does breathing other people's tobacco smoke cause lung cancer? Br Med J 1986; 293: 1217.
25. Tweedie RL, Mengerson KL. Lung cancer and passive smoking: reconciling the biochemical and epidemiological approaches. Br J Cancer 1992; 66: 700.
26. Smith CJ, Fischer TH, Sears SB. Environmental tobacco smoke, cardiovascular disease, and the nonlinear dose-response hypothesis. Toxicol Sci 2000; 54: 462–472.
27. Ashton CH, Golding JF. Smoking: motivation and models. In: Ney T, Gale A, ed. Smoking behaviour. Chichester: John Wiley, 1989: 21.
28. Russell MAH, Feyerabend C. Cigarette smoking: a dependence on high-nicotine boli. Drug Metab Rev 1978; 8: 29.
29. Armitage AK, Dollery CT, George CF et al. Absorption and metabolism of nicotine from cigarettes. Br Med J 1975; 4: 313.
30. Benowitz NL. Nicotine replacement therapy. Drugs 1993; 45: 157.
31. Russell MAH, Jarvis MJ, Devitt G, Feyerabend C. Nicotine intake by snuff users. Br Med J 1981; 283: 814.
32. Russell MAH, Jarvis MJ. Theoretical background and clinical use of nicotine chewing gum. In: Hall SM, ed. Pharmacological adjuncts in smoking cessation. Department of Health and Human Services, NIDA Monograph 53. DHHS Pub No (ADM) 85–1333. Washington DC: Public Health Office; 1985: 110.
33. Gourlay SG, Benowitz NL. Arteriovenous differences in plasma concentration of nicotine and catecholamines and related cardiovascular effects after smoking, nicotine nasal spray, and intravenous nicotine. Clin Pharmacol Ther 1997; 62: 453–463.
34. Benowitz NL. Cigarette smoking and nicotine addiction. Med Clin North Am 1992; 76: 415.
35. Cryer PE, Haymond MW, Santiago JV, Shah SD. Norepinephrine and epinephrine release and adrenergic mediation of smoking-associated hemodynamic and metabolic events. N Engl J Med 1976; 295: 573.
36. Golding JF. The effects of cigarette smoking on resting EEG, evoked potentials and photic driving. Pharmacol Biochem Behav 1988; 29: 23.
37. Ashton CH, Marsh VR, Millman JE et al. Biphasic dose-related responses of the CNV (contingent negative variation) to i.v. nicotine in man. Br J Clin Pharmacol 1980; 10: 579.
38. Henningfield JE. How tobacco produces drug dependence. In: Ockene JK, ed. The pharmacologic treatment of tobacco dependence. Cambridge, MA: Institute for Study of Smoking Behavior and Policy, Harvard University; 1986: 19.
39. Warburton DM. Psychopharmacological aspects of nicotine. In: Wonnacott S, Russell MAH, Stolerman IP, ed. Nicotine psychopharmacology: molecular, cellular, and behavioural aspects. Oxford: Oxford University Press; 1990: 77.
40. Woodruff TJ, Rosbrook B, Pierce J, Glantz SA. Lower levels of cigarette consumption found in smoke-free workplaces in California. Arch Intern Med 1993; 153: 1485.

41. Wasserman J. How effective are excise increases in reducing cigarette smoking? Am J Publ Health 1992; 82: 19.

42. Laugesen M, Meads C. Tobacco advertising restrictions, price, consumption in OECD countries, 1960–1986. Br J Addiction 1991; 86: 1343.

43. Shiffman S. Psychosocial factors in smoking and quitting: health beliefs, self-efficacy and stress. In: Ockene JK, ed. The pharmacologic treatment of tobacco dependence. Cambridge, MA: Institute for Study of Smoking Behavior and Policy, Harvard University; 1986: 48.

44. A clinical practice guideline for treating tobacco use and dependence: a US Public Health Service report. Tobacco Use and Dependence Clinical Practice Guideline Panel, Staff Consortium Representatives. JAMA 2000; 283: 3244–3254.

45. Lancaster T, Stead LF. Individual behavioural counselling for smoking cessation. Cochrane database Syst Rev 2000; 2: CD001292.

46. Holm KJ, Spencer CM. Bupropion: a review of its use in the management of smoking cessation. Drugs 2000; 59: 1007–1024.

47. Hughes JR. New treatments for smoking cessation. CA Cancer J Clin 2000; 50: 143–151.

48. Chapman S. The role of doctors in promoting smoking cessation. Br Med J 1993; 307: 518.

49. Macfadyen L, Hastings G, MacKintosh AM. Cross sectional study of young people's awareness of and involvement with tobacco marketing. Br Med J 2001; 322: 513–517.

50. Nutbeam D, Macaskill P, Smith C et al. Evaluation of two school smoking education programmes under normal classroom conditions. Br Med J 1993; 306: 102.

25 Pneumoconioses

Maurits Demedts, Benoît Nemery and Peter Elmes

 Key points

■ High dust exposure conditions are no longer socially or legally acceptable in countries with high standards of living.

■ Nevertheless pneumoconioses may still become manifest as a consequence of exposures far in the past to dusts that are retained in the lung.

■ In addition, unexpected new exposure risks still emerge.

■ Therefore, in compatible clinical settings, especially of interstitial lung diseases of unknown origin, one should always take a very detailed history of past and present occupational and environmental exposure.

General aspects

Definition

Pneumoconiosis is a lung disease that results from dust deposition in the lung and the subsequent host response.[1] In its broadest sense it could, therefore, relate to a variety of disease entities, even including occupational airway disease such as asthma (Chapter 48.13), chronic bronchitis and chronic obstructive pulmonary disease (COPD) with emphysema, hypersensitivity pneumonitis or extrinsic allergic alveolitis (Chapter 55) and cancer (Table 25.1).

Parkes[2] defined pneumoconiosis in a more restricted sense, as a non-neoplastic reaction of the lung to mineral or organic dusts and the resultant alteration in the pulmonary structure, excluding asthma, bronchitis and emphysema.

In this chapter the term pneumoconiosis is used in an even more restricted sense, i.e. diffuse alveolar and parenchymal lung disease due to mineral dust exposure. Pneumoconiosis is classified as 'simple' when the changes produced by the retention of dust are discrete. The collections of dust are separated from each other by normal lung tissue and the disturbance of function is often minor. Serial measurements of spirometric indices such as forced expiratory volume in 1 second (FEV_1) and forced vital capacity (FVC) are usually the most sensitive methods for detecting an abnormal decline in lung function in workers exposed to dust. Coalescent lesions due to relatively non-fibrogenic mineral dust (e.g. kaolin) may cavitate and bleed and become secondarily infected by opportunistic microorganisms; however, these lesions generally appear against a background of simple pneumoconiosis without marked distortion or emphysema, and lung function may remain relatively well preserved.

Progression of the disease is characterised by confluence of the dust foci, increased scarring and distortion of the lung structure. This is described as 'complicated pneumonoconiosis' and the disturbance of function is usually marked, causing breathlessness at exercise and later on even at rest. Such progressive massive fibrosis may even aggravate further after exposure has been stopped, e.g. in silicosis or in coal-worker's pneumoconiosis. In progressive massive fibrosis due to silicosis the other parts of the lung show emphysematous destruction.

Table 25.2 shows a schematic overview of the mineral and metal dust pneumoconioses. Respiratory diseases in coal miners are covered in Chapter 26, and asbestos-related diseases in Chapter 27. This chapter, therefore, deals with general aspects of pneumoconiosis and with the diseases other than coal-worker's pneumoconiosis and asbestos-related diseases. It briefly describes, first, the general mechanisms of lung defences and of the pathogenesis of inorganic dust diseases and the diagnosis of these diseases. Then, different types of diseases related to non-fibrous mineral dust, to fibrous mineral dust and to metal dusts and fumes are described.

History

Before the Industrial Revolution, the amount of respirable dust created with hand tools was small, so that only the most dangerous dusts, such as quartz, were inhaled in sufficient quantity to cause disease.

Table 25.1 Types of pulmonary disease caused by mineral dust and metals

Disease	Cause
Pulmonary fibrosis	Asbestos Crystalline silica (stone cutting, drilling and tunnelling) Kaolin (in china, ceramics and pharmaceuticals) Talc (in paint, ceramics, leather, fabric and paper industries) Cobalt (with or without tungsten carbide)
Alveolar proteinosis	Fine crystalline silica (in silica flour, produced by sand-blasting)
Granulomatous disease	Beryllium (aerospace industry, beryllium copper alloy machining)
Chronic obstructive pulmonary disease	Coal dust Crystalline silica Cadmium (in electronics, metal plating and batteries)
Bronchitis	Rock and mineral dust (road construction, digging of foundations) Cement dust
Asthma	Cobalt
Lung cancer	Asbestos (e.g. boiler and pipe insulation) Cadmium Chromium Nickel
Nasal ulceration and perforation of septum	Arsenic Copper Chromates

Table 25.2 Schematic classification of pneumoconioses due to mineral dusts and metals

Non-fibrous mineral dusts	Quartz and related dust: silicosis Coal dust: coal-worker's pneumoconiosis Mixed dust containing quartz: 'silicatoses', e.g. slate-worker's pneumoconiosis, kaolin pneumoconiosis, talcosis, mica and vermicule pneumoconiosis, diatomite pneumoconiosis, pneumoconioses due to other non-fibrous clays
Fibrous mineral dusts	Asbestos minerals: asbestosis Other natural fibres or synthetic mineral fibres
Metal dusts and fumes	Siderosis, aluminium lung, beryllium lung, hard-metal lung disease (or cobalt lung)

Many pneumoconioses have taken their highest human toll during the industrial age; yet, despite innovations in industrial techniques and more stringent occupational health and safety controls, and although these diseases can be prevented, they have not disappeared in our time and even new entities continue to emerge.

In the second half of the 20th century the majority of pneumoconioses listed on death certificates were coal-worker's pneumoconiosis, silicosis and asbestosis. The rate of death from coal-worker's pneumoconiosis is declining but silicosis remains prevalent in many regions and industries, and shows new exposure risks. Also, other dusts such as talc, kaolin, etc. are of concern as causes of new cases of disease.

In countries with high standard of living, high dust exposure conditions are no longer socially or legally acceptable, yet in many developing countries dusty situations are allowed to persist.

The lung's defences[3]

Most inhaled dust is filtered out by the upper airways or cleared by the ciliated epithelium of large airways. The key sites of deposition of both compact particles and fibres[4,5] are the regions of the terminal bronchioli and the proximal alveoli, including the ridges of the alveolar duct bifurcations. If the defences are overwhelmed by fine dust of less than $10\,\mu m$ in diameter, however, the lung reacts with mainly alveolar and interstitial inflammation that may culminate in disease, or fine dust may have a direct toxic effect.

Defence levels

Schematically, the following defence levels may be considered:

- The upper airway filter, consisting of the hairs and the mucosa folds over the turbinates of the nose, retains most particles over 15 μm diameter, which are carried in the mucus to the pharynx and swallowed.
- The lower airway filter, consisting of the mucociliary epithelium (with mucus secretion both by the goblet cells and by the submucosal seromucous glands) removes nearly all of the particles down to about 5 μm and a proportion of the smaller ones. These particles are carried back to the larynx and swallowed.
- Macrophages clear small particles, partly via the airways. The smaller particles (below 5 μm), which are also termed the respirable or alveolar fraction of inhaled dust, fall on to the lining of the alveolar ducts and alveoli, which are coated with surfactant. Clearance of the deposited particles depends on effective phagocytosis by the alveolar macrophages. Macrophages move out from the walls and engulf the particles. Many dust particles are dissolved by lysosomal enzymes and most of these are carried with the macrophages by the mucus to the larynx and are swallowed.
- Macrophages clear particles partly via the lymphatics. If there is a combination of dust overload and cell damage, macrophages may carry the particles to the hilar lymph nodes, where pneumoconiotic dust may be sequestered. Dust-laden cells can be cleared slowly from the hilar lymph nodes, either along the lymph node chains (up into the neck or down into the abdomen) or via the thoracic duct into the blood stream and so to the related cell systems in the liver and spleen. Drainage towards the pleura is also a possibility.
- When the overload is very heavy, then the type II and even the type I alveolar lining cells may take on a phagocytic role.

Defence systems

Cell defence against oxidative attack has attracted particular interest in biochemical research related to fibrogenesis.[6] Various enzymatic and non-enzymatic defence systems exist to protect cells and tissues against oxidants.[7-10] The enzymes involved in this cellular defence against toxic oxygen species include the superoxide dismutases, catalase and glutathione peroxidase, and the glutathione system. The changes that occur in the pulmonary antioxidant system upon oxidative stress have been outlined in several studies but are not yet fully understood or defined. Both the inflammatory response and fibrosis due to particles (e.g. quartz), fibres (e.g. asbestos) and also ambient air particles (particulate matter < 10 μm, PM_{10}), could be reduced in animal models by the concomitant administration of antioxidant enzymes, such as polyethylene-glycol-associated catalase.[7] Several studies show abnormal values of several antioxidant enzymes in macrophages, red blood cells or serum from patients with coal-worker's pneumoconiosis, with or without progressive massive fibrosis,[8] and especially an upregulation of glutathione-dependent enzymes in red blood cells in the later stages of the disease.

The mechanisms of defence related to immunological sensitisation are still poorly understood. They do not seem to play a major role in pneumoconiosis in general but are of obvious relevance to chronic beryllium disease (see Chapter 48.13),

hypersensitivity pneumonitis (see Chapter 55) and some drug-induced lung diseases (see Chapter 29).

Mechanisms of pneumoconiosis[8,11,12]

Characteristics of inhaled particles

There is without doubt some particle specificity in the response of the lung. The severity and pattern of disease resulting from dust inhalation depend mainly on the concentration of dust and the size distribution of the particles, but also on the shape and surface characteristics of the particles. Even materials that in the form of larger particles are not toxic to the lung may, as ultrafine particles, have biological activity and be toxic, probably because these gain access to the interstitium.[13] However, pneumoconiotic particles are not generally considered to be ultrafine. Especially long fibres, leading to incomplete phagocytosis by macrophages, can cause more inflammation than short fibres.[14] The surface characteristics of the particles, e.g. their electric charge, are a current topic of interest. The surface characteristics also play a part in the ability of particles to cause pneumoconiosis, probably through free radicals at the surface.

This surface chemistry may activate multiple signalling pathways in cells and some transcription factors that are involved in immune responses and proliferation. In particular, the importance of iron on the surface of asbestos fibres has been demonstrated[15] and this is related to the fact that iron, as a transition metal, has the ability to generate free radicals via Fenton chemistry.

Variations in individual clearance systems and susceptibility to fibrogenesis

Genetic and acquired characteristics of the subject, as far as clearance and other defence reactions are concerned, play a role in susceptibility to pneumoconiosis.[8] Indeed, the difference in 'cell-damaging capability' among various dusts also depends on the duration of their persistence in the lung.

Individuals may vary in the way particles or fibres penetrate into and are cleared from the respiratory tract. It is, for instance, established that exercise enhances the pollutant dose delivered to the lung because it increases minute ventilation and because it leads to a switch from nasal to oronasal breathing.[16]

In smokers the response to dust is different from that in non-smokers: smokers usually show more disease than non-smokers at a given exposure level. Cigarette smoke adds to the particulate burden and delays mucociliary clearance by interfering with ciliary action and by causing excessive mucus secretion.

Some diseases such as chronic bronchitis and COPD cause an increased deposition of inhaled particles in experimental animals as well as in patients[17-19] and the deposition rate appears to be proportional to the degree of airways obstruction. In addition, the clearance of particles in the small airways has been shown to be reduced in patients with chronic bronchitis. The deleterious role of increased deposition (and persistence) of inhaled fibrogenic fibres has been studied most in the area of asbestosis. In men with established asbestosis, mineral analyses of bronchoalveolar lavage (BAL) fluid or lung tissue have consistently shown higher burdens of asbestos fibres or asbestos bodies than in exposed men with no apparent disease or disease limited to the airways or pleura.[20-22]

The development or resolution of inflammation and fibrogenesis also depends on genetic or acquired individual variations in susceptibility.[8] The degree to which dust particles such as silica or asbestos lead to fibrosis has been shown to be under genetic control, probably via the response of cytokine networks and growth factors, which determine the cumulative lung load by attenuating clearance and which also regulate the cascade of events leading to fibrogenesis. Thus experimental animals have varying susceptibility to silica depending on species (e.g. the rat is more sensitive than the mouse or hamster) and, within the same species, significant differences of susceptibility to the development of silicosis have been noted among different mouse strains. Various studies, e.g. using knock-out mice, indicate that variations in cytokines or their receptors are critical for inducing fibroproliferative responses in the lung.

Activation of target cells and fibrogenesis

Substantial research has been performed over the past decade in the field of molecular mechanisms of particle-induced lung damage.[23-25] The key mechanism is the direct or indirect activation of inflammatory target cells with subsequent release of mediators. There are probably two major pathways:[25] first, the production of reactive oxygen species in relation to the antioxidant protection and second, the expression and release of cytokines, growth factors and related factors such as eicosanoids and cytokine receptors.

Oxidative stress
Oxidants are mainly leukocyte-derived and particle-surface-mediated.

These reactive oxygen species damage lung tissue, either directly by cellular damage, with loss of epithelial integrity and disruption of the extracellular matrix, or indirectly via induction of inflammation. The most common pathogenic free radical is the hydroxyl radical, which is highly toxic.

Inflammatory mediators
The mediators most probably involved in the pathogenesis of pneumoconiosis are tumour necrosis factor (TNF)-α,[26] interleukin (IL)-6 and IL-8, platelet-derived growth factor and transforming growth factor (TGF)-β (which is most important for fibrogenesis).[23-32]

The early lesions of pneumoconiosis in humans arise highly focussed in the respiratory bronchioles and proximal alveoli, at which level there are a variety of the potential target cell types intervening in the pathogenesis of pneumoconiosis.[33] However, before making contact with cells, deposited particles interact with lung lining fluid, which is largely made up of the secretions of the type II epithelial cells and products from plasma, such as phospholipids and proteins of various types, including immunoglobulin (Ig)G. Coating of particles with IgG has been shown to enhance the ability of macrophages to release cytokine and oxidant in response to asbestos and to generate an oxidative burst in response to quartz.[34]

Target cells
Research has mainly been focussed on alveolar macrophages, which form the principal defensive cells and, furthermore, on type I and II epithelial cells and to a lesser degree on fibroblasts. The other cells include especially ciliated cells, mucus-secreting cells and Clara cells, but the mucociliary clearance system is much less effective in this region than in the upper airways. In addition, the interstitial macrophages should be mentioned as target cells because their response is probably central to the pathogenic events, although few experimental data are available on this.

There is overwhelming evidence from BAL data that the inhalation of pneumoconiotic particles causes neutrophilic inflammation in occupationally exposed humans and in experimentally exposed animals.[21,22] However, it appears that the principal events in the pneumoconiotic lung occur independently of neutrophils[35,36] but are related to activation of macrophages, epithelial cells and fibroblasts, with accumulation of connective tissue cells and their products. For macrophages the role of the Fc receptor and the scavenger receptor[37] has been demonstrated but virtually nothing is known of the specific receptors that are involved in the binding of pneumoconiotic particles to epithelial cells or fibroblasts.

Depending on the toxicity of the dust and the level of exposure, macrophages may die in the alveoli, but they especially die in aggregations around the centrilobular bronchioles or along the lymphatics leading to the hilar lymph nodes. This pathological process may halt after exposure ends but often continues to progress thereafter, because of the continuing reaction to the retained dust.[39,40]

Fibrogenesis
With time there is more diffuse pulmonary involvement, characterised by loss of alveolar type I and II cells and by an increase in the number of alveolar and interstitial macrophages, neutrophils, lymphocytes and eosinophils, and ultimately fibroblast proliferation and collagen accumulation resulting in lung fibrosis. The increased proteolytic activity of the inflammatory leukocytes recruited to the sites of dust deposition is, furthermore, likely to be accompanied by proteolysis of structural proteins in the lung parenchyma, leading to focal emphysema and the dramatic remodelling that characterises pneumoconosis.[38]

With coal dusts and other relatively low-toxicity dusts, there is typically some nodular fibrosis around the terminal bronchiole with some surrounding centrilobular emphysema, which, however, may progress to massive fibrosis and severe emphysema with heavy exposure. Silica, which is more toxic, causes a more severe nodular fibrosis, with adjacent foci of scarring, and blood vessel walls may become involved, leading to thrombosis and patchy necrosis. Asbestos more typically leads to a more diffuse fibrosis with the characteristics of a usual interstitial pneumonia.

The paradigm that lung fibrosis is always preceded by and dependent on the severity of inflammation is valid in many situations but it has been argued more recently, mainly on the basis of pathological observations, that fibrogenesis, i.e. excessive deposition of extracellular matrix and cell proliferation, may represent a more 'independent' disease process.

Finally, radicals can react with and damage a variety of cellular macromolecules and may disrupt DNA to give rise to malignancy.

Diagnosis

The diagnosis of pneumoconiosis is in general a clinical one. There are three major criteria for the diagnosis.[1] The first is a sufficient exposure to a mineral dust known to cause pneumoconiosis, with an appropriate latency period. In order to make any conclusions concerning this point a detailed knowledge of the dust levels in the work environment, the risks and duration of exposure and the use of respiratory protective devices is essential. Sometimes this requires examination of the work place and collecting and counting dust samples. In general, symptoms of persistent productive cough and/or breathlessness on exertion may exist for years before radiographic changes, which may not develop until 10–20 years after exposure started and which may progress long after exposure has ceased.

The second criterion is the recognition of a characteristic disease pattern and especially chest radiographic abnormalities that meet recognised standards for this type of pneumoconiosis. Although respiratory signs and symptoms, as well as lung function abnormalities, are commonly found in patients with pneumoconiosis, neither is a requisite for the diagnosis.

The third criterion is absence of a disease that might mimic pneumoconiosis. Pneumoconiosis may be confused with diffuse interstitial lung diseases of unknown aetiology, such as sarcoidosis, idiopathic pulmonary fibrosis or interstitial lung disease associated with collagen vascular disease.[12]

The chest radiograph is of particular value not only for epidemiological purposes but especially in the diagnosis of the individual case. Yet many occupational lung diseases have non-specific radiographic features and the degree of radiographic abnormality is poorly related to the pathological severity of disease for many dusts. Some dusts produce dramatic radiographic shadows with little or no loss of lung function or blood gas abnormalities, and vice versa.

In the International Labour Office (ILO) in Geneva a classification of the pattern and severity of the radiographic changes in groups of pneumoconiotic workers has been developed that is intended for epidemiological purposes and for use in occupational medicine.[41] It is not intended as a method of diagnosis or for estimating the severity in an individual case, although it may also be very useful here to describe the abnormalities using a standardised, semiquantitative scale. The method of reading is to compare each film with a set of standard films supplied by the ILO in Geneva. The results are recorded on a special form, the content of which is summarised in Table 25.3. The 'small parenchymal opacities' in this table correspond with simple pneumoconiosis (Fig. 25.1) and the 'large coalescent opacities' with progressive massive fibrosis (Fig. 25.2).

Computed tomography (CT) scanning is not part of the official classification of pneumoconiosis. Yet scoring systems for CT scans (especially high-resolution CT scan) similar to the ILO classification of chest radiographs have been described.[42] CT

Table 25.3 Schematic summary of content of the ILO-form for reading chest radiographs

1. **Film number:** date of radiograph; reader; date of reading

2. **Film quality:** grade: 1 good, 2 acceptable, 3 poor, 4 unacceptable

3. **Small (parenchymal) opacities**
   Profusion (or concentration) indicated by a 12-point scale (of two symbols) going from particularly obvious absence of opacities (0/–) to extremely marked profusion (3/+): 0/–, 0/0, 0/1; 1/0, 1/1, 1/2; 2/1, 2/2, 2/3; 3/2, 3/3, 3/+.
   Extent: the lungs are divided into six zones: upper, middle, lower; and right, left
   Shape and size: indicated by two letters, e.g. p/p, q/r, s/s, t/u, q/t, p/u, etc. Rounded opacities are denoted by: p = diameter ≤ 1.5 mm, q = 1.5–3 mm, r = 3–10 mm; irregular opacities are denoted by: s = width ≤ 1.5 mm, t = 1.5–3 mm, u = 3–10 mm

4. **Large opacities,** i.e. greater than 10 mm in diameter: four categories: none, A, B, C.
   A = one or more opacities with diameters between 10 and 50 mm, and sum of diameters ≤ 50 mm
   B = one or more large opacities with sum of diameters > 50 mm and combined area ≤ the equivalent of the right upper lobe
   C = one or more large opacities with combined diameters > the equivalent of right upper lobe

5. **Pleural thickening**
   Chest wall: type: circumscribed (plaques), and/or diffuse
           site: right/left chest wall
           width: a < 5 mm; b 5–10 mm, c > 10 mm
           extent: 1 = length ≤ 1/4 lateral chest wall, 2 = 1/4–1/2, 3 => 1/2
   Diaphragm: none/right/left
   Costophrenic angle obliteration: none/right/left

6. **Pleural calcification**
   Site: wall, diaphragm, other (mediastinal and pericardial pleura)
   Extent: 1 = (sum of) diameter(s) ≤ 20 mm, 2 = 20–100 mm, 3 => 100 mm

7. **Symbols for additional radiographic features of importance**
   ax = coalescence of small opacities, bu = bulla(e), ca = cancer of lung or pleura, cn = calcification in small opacities, co = abnormalities of cardiac size or shape; cp = cor pulmonale, cv = cavity, di = marked distortion of intrathoracic organs, ef = effusion, em = definite emphysema, es = eggshell calcification of lymph nodes, fr = fractured rib(s), hi = enlarged lymph nodes, ho = honeycomb lung, id = ill-defined diaphragm, ih = ill-defined heart outline, kl = septal (Kerley) lines, px = pneumothorax, tb = tuberculosis, etc.

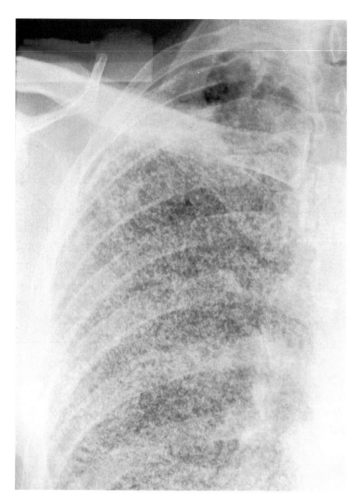

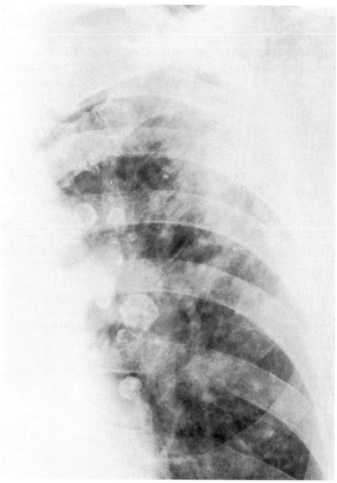

Fig. 25.1 Detail of chest radiograph showing small rounded opacities (ILO 3/+pp) in a symptom-free 45-year old man. He had for 29 years ground small samples of tin ore by hand for analysis. The clear apical region may be due to bullae or a small pneumothorax. (Courtesy of the MRC Pneumoconiosis Unit Collection of standard films, kept at the Univ. Dept. of Respiratory Medicine, Llandough Hospital, Penarth and photographed by Mr R. Harris.)

Fig. 25.2 Detail of chest radiograph showing massive fibrosis with eggshell calcification of hilar nodes (ILO 3/2 rr es) in a retired slate worker. Note the irregular indistinct outline of the subpleural massive shadow due to coalescence of 'r' shadows. (Courtesy of the MRC Pneumoconiosis Unit Collection of standard films, kept at the Univ. Dept. of Respiratory Medicine, Llandough Hospital, Penarth and photographed by Mr R. Harris.)

scanning may be very useful in individual patients to estimate the severity of interstitial fibrosis, to delineate necrosis or abscess formation in confluent opacities, to gauge the extent of emphysema or pleural changes, etc.

Lung function tests may be used for two purposes in inorganic dust exposure: first to study exposed populations of workers, in which case spirometry is a suitable measure; second to diagnose individual patients with occupational lung disease, in which case a battery of tests, including lung volumes and diffusing capacity (transfer factor), is useful. Severity of the functional deficit is estimated by comparison with appropriate age-, height- and sex-matched predicted values derived from large series of normal individuals.[3] In this respect several semiquantitative scoring systems of functional impairment have been published and in most of them the severity of the functional impairment is derived from the abnormalities in some lung function tests expressed as a percentage of the predicted values. An example of such a table, proposed by a working group of the

Belgian Society for Pneumology,[43] is presented in Table 25.4. Such tables are useful as an overall estimate of the severity of impairment in a group of patients but one should be aware that these are an arbitrary and schematic oversimplification when used in an individual patient.

In some cases, examination of the sputum and/or BAL may confirm the diagnosis by showing dust-loaded macrophages and the nature of the dust may be identified under the electron microscope. Asbestos bodies can be detected with the light microscope and their profusion is a useful indication of the asbestos burden.[3] Only in an unusual situation is an open or thoracoscopic lung biopsy with dust analysis indicated to make the diagnosis. However, 'crystals' or 'fibres' may be found in lung biopsies obtained for diagnosing interstitial lung disease without occupational exposure and it may then be difficult to assign a causal or incidental role to these materials.

Post-mortem examination of the lungs removed en bloc, fixed in inflation, cut in 0.1–1.0 cm thick slices and examined in

Table 25.4 Estimation of physical impairment based on lung function (from the `Officiële Belgische Schaal' 1990[43])

Lung function	Physical impairment (%)[†]				
	≤ 20 Minor	21–40 Moderate	41–60 Severe	61–80 Very severe	> 81 Extreme
FEV$_1$ (% predicted)*	84–70	69–55	54–45	44–35	< 35
VC (% predicted)*	84–70	69–60	59–50	49–40	< 40
D_LCO (% predicted)*	79–65	64–55	54–45	44–35	< 35
P_aO$_2$ (mmHg)	74–68	67–60	59–55	54–50	< 50
$\dot{V}$O$_{2\,max}$ (ml/min/kg)	24–20	19–15	14–11	10–8	< 8

* Predicted values of ECSC (Bull Eur Physiopathol Respir 1983; 19(suppl.5): 1–95). † The degree of impairment is derived mainly from the most abnormal lung function test.

detail has been a major source of information about the nature of occupational lung diseases in the last 100 years. In individual cases who have died and in whom a pneumoconiosis is suspected it may still be useful for the granting of a widow's pension to perform a histological examination of autopsy material and to analyse the dust extracted from the lung.

Treatment

There is no effective treatment for pneumoconiosis that is able to induce regression of the disorder or even to stop progression. Prevention is, therefore, of utmost importance. Work regulations and measures to control exposure were set up many decades ago, especially in industrialised countries, and continue to be improved. If, notwithstanding, pneumoconiosis is 'detected', adequate safety measures for the patient and also for coworkers are indicated, with cessation of exposure if warranted.

In subacute forms of pneumoconiosis with much inflammation, corticosteroids are sometimes applied but generally they have no clear long-lasting effect if the offending agent remains in the lung, thus causing a continuing burden.

General health measures are, furthermore, indicated: smoking cessation should be strongly advised, adequate treatment of an associated COPD is mandatory, infection prevention with appropriate vaccines should be advocated.

Association between pneumoconiosis and other abnormalities

Rheumatoid pneumoconiosis

This abnormality was first identified by Caplan in coal miners in south Wales,[44] although sporadic cases have been described in many other dusty occupations. It consists of rounded shadows in the periphery of the midzones of both lungs in individuals with serum-positive rheumatoid arthritis but these lung lesions often precede the joint manifestations. The lung lesions show the histological features of active rheumatoid disease – palisading of chronic inflammatory cells, active arteritis or arteriolitis and the laying down of collagen. The lesions are often about 1 cm in diameter when they are first detected and usually there is a category 1 or 2 simple pneumoconiosis. The lesions may enlarge, perhaps in association with episodes of active joint disease, and they may cavitate, which can lead to serious haemoptysis.

Tuberculosis and pneumoconiosis

The risk of tuberculosis is greatly increased in workers exposed to quartz dust and may also be raised in those exposed to mixed dust containing silica, in which case the risk appears to be proportionate to the extent of silicotic changes.

Patients with silicosis have an about 20-fold increased risk of developing tuberculosis;[45] the mechanisms could be related to the fact that macrophages in the presence of quartz dust in vitro appear to be less able to engulf and kill tuberde bacilli, and that the lymphatic drainage of the lung is damaged, which is important for the control of tuberculous infection. The diagnosis of silicotuberculosis is often difficult, since the organisms may be hard to find: examination of the sputum and even bronchial lavage fluid may be negative in the presence of low-grade active tuberculosis. It is often necessary to treat such cases on suspicion, without microbiological confirmation of the diagnosis, because of haemoptysis and cavitation of lung masses. There is evidence that antituberculous treatment should be more prolonged than in the absence of silicosis and there is a grossly elevated mortality from tuberculosis among silicotics.[46] There is also an increased risk for infections with non-tuberculous mycobacteria.

Other dusts, even the fibrous minerals, do not seem to increase the risk for tuberculosis.

Cancer and pneumoconiosis

Radioactive dusts, such as those encountered by miners of uranium or pitchblende (radium), cause cancer. The greatly increased risk of lung cancer in asbestosis patients, especially smokers, is also well known.

In haematite miners and in other metal miners, radon daughters in the ground water have been shown to be the main risk factor.[47,48] In addition, hard-rock miners have an increased risk of lung cancer that has been attributed to quartz or to the metal ores themselves. The risk of lung cancer is now considered to be increased in the presence of silicosis; yet uncertainty remains as to whether this is related to the level of silica exposure itself or to the silicosis and the related fibrogenic reactions.[49,50]

Another occupation causing silicosis and an increased risk of lung cancer is iron foundry work: many potential carcinogens resulting from the effect of heat on fossil fuels may play a part but no agent has definitely been identified.

Specific disorders

A schematic overview of the pneumoconioses due to dust from non-fibrous minerals, fibrous mineral dust or metal dusts and fumes is given in Table 25.2.

Lung disorders caused by non-fibrous minerals

The lung disorders caused by non-fibrous mineral dusts are generally labelled silicosis, silicate dust pneumoconiosis (or 'silicatosis') and coal worker's pneumoconiosis. This pathology is well-known and a review in 1988 by an international panel of pathologists is still largely relevant.[51]

Although the pulmonary risks of inhalation of non-fibrous mineral dusts are well controlled by government regulation, these pneumoconioses still occur, sometimes also in serious outbreaks. In a number of developing countries especially, where many workers are exposed to dangerous levels of dust in industry and particularly in mining, quarrying and civil engineering, non-fibrous mineral dusts may still be an important cause of fatal lung disease. If these dusts are inhaled for long enough at levels above lung clearance capacity they will cause pneumoconiosis.

Quartz dust is among the most toxic of the non-fibrous dusts and can cause fatal disease after exposure for only a few months to concentrations not perceptible to the naked eye. Indeed, 1–5 g of respired quartz dust can cause fatal silicosis, whereas serious disability in British coal miners seldom occurred unless the lung dust burden was over 100 g. But even quartz dust is relatively inert compared with durable mineral fibres (such as asbestos), which can cause fatal lung fibrosis at 50–100 mg, lung cancer at about 1.2 mg, and mesothelioma at less than 0.01 mg.

It should be kept in mind that, in pneumoconioses due to unusual exposures, the latter probably often remain undetected and the disorders are wrongly labelled idiopathic interstitial lung disease. Wrong diagnoses of sarcoidosis have been made in the granulomatous forms and of idiopathic pulmonary fibrosis in the more fibrotic forms.[52] A careful and detailed history of present and previous home conditions, hobbies and especially occupations is mandatory. Although most information on these unusual exposures comes from descriptive case reports, these may sometimes help to unravel mechanisms and to delineate disease patterns.

Silicosis

Silicosis results from the inhalation of one of the three crystalline forms of silicon dioxide: quartz, cristobalite and tridymite. It is a recognised occupational risk of sand-blasters, stone-cutters, grinders and workers in stone quarries, in factories making glass and sandpaper, in the ceramic industry, in tunnelling, etc. It may present as an acute or chronic pneumoconiosis. The pathogenesis of silicosis is a complex inflammatory process (see above), in which especially the role of macrophages, fibroblasts and epithelial and endothelial cells have been examined. These cell types contribute to the production of a variety of cytokines, among which TNF-α plays an important role. Furthermore, TGF-β and especially oxidative stress reactions interfere in the process of cell damage and fibrosis. A characteristic feature of silicosis is the continuing clinical, functional and radiological progression of the disease for many years after cessation of exposure.[51]

Acute silicosis

This disease is also known as 'silicotic alveolar proteinosis' or 'silicotic alveolar lipoproteinosis'. It has especially been reported after high uncontrolled silica exposure in tunnelling,[53] in sand-blasting metal parts or in making silica flour.

This acute alveolitis may be present within weeks after high-level exposure; for example, it occurs when the respirable levels of dust containing 50% or more crystalline quartz exceed 2–5 mg/m³ and when exposure lasts for more than 1–2 h per day. Such high exposure causes immediate damage in the alveolus. with death of the type I and II pneumocytes as well as the macrophages. Protein fluid, followed by inflammatory cells, leaks from the capillaries into the alveoli, mingling with the surfactant, and the alveoli become obliterated with fibrous tissue. However, the symptoms mostly start within a few months to a year after exposure and consist of gradually worsening dry cough, chest breathlessness, and cyanosis. Fine crackles are generally heard over the lower lung zones. The radiograph shows patchy ground-glass infiltrates suggestive of alveolar filling or pulmonary oedema, with especially dense shadows in the central lung zones. Lung function tests show a restrictive defect with very low diffusing capacity and severe hypoxia.

There is no effective medical treatment and the disease is often fatal, sometimes within a few months. In some cases alveolar proteinosis may be a dominant feature and in some of these therapeutic whole lung washings have been performed, with variable results. The first successful lung transplantation, with 10 months survival, was performed three decades ago in a patient with acute silicosis.[54] In Western countries the main sources of dust capable of causing this pattern of disease have been recognised and subjected to statutory control for many years. The following should still be subjected to close control in all countries: hard-rock mining and tunnelling; the working of granite for building purposes or crushing for aggregate; the preparation of silica flour for industrial purposes and its use especially in the ceramics industry; the use of sand in metal casting; the use of sand in grinding wheels, etc.

Preventive measures consist of working wet and using ventilation systems.

Chronic silicosis

Generally, symptoms are a late manifestation, occurring 10–30 years after the start of the exposure, and mainly consist of a dry cough and progressive dyspnoea on exercise. Clubbing is not a feature. A restrictive lung function is found with decreased diffusing capacity and eventually hypoxia and cyanosis, first at exercise, later at rest. Silicosis in smokers mostly presents with a mixed restrictive and obstructive pattern and complaints are those of COPD.

The first radiographic shadows to appear are medium (1–3 mm) to large (3–10 mm) small rounded opacities (q or r on the ILO scale, see Table 25.3), and these tend to be more frequent in the upper zones. Hilar node enlargement is common. Fibrous bands link the nodules and contract, while the nodules become more profuse and tend to coalesce to form irregular masses (Fig. 25.3). In smokers a combination of coalescent nodules and emphysematous lung zones, especially in the lung bases, is found.

After 20–30 years the nodules may become inactive and calcify from the periphery inwards, which gives rise to the appearance of eggshell calcification in the hilar nodes. Calcification is considered an indication that a silicotic lesion is no longer active.

The histology of the lesions in the lung is diagnostic: the nodules are made of concentric layers of macrophages, fibroblasts and lymphocytes around a dense collagen tissue with a core containing birefringent quartz particles. The nodules are first formed in the centrilobular area near the respiratory bronchiolus and then extend along the lymphatics both to the hilar nodes and to the pleura while linear fibrous tissue is formed linking them together. These nodules conglomerate to form larger masses.

Patients with silicosis have a markedly increased risk for developing lung tuberculosis and also for infections with non-tuberculous mycobacteria. There is probably also an increased risk for lung cancer.

Depending possibly on the presence of amorphous silica in the dust, severe silicosis may be associated with liver and renal damage by silica. An increased incidence of autoimmune diseases such as scleroderma has also been described.[55]

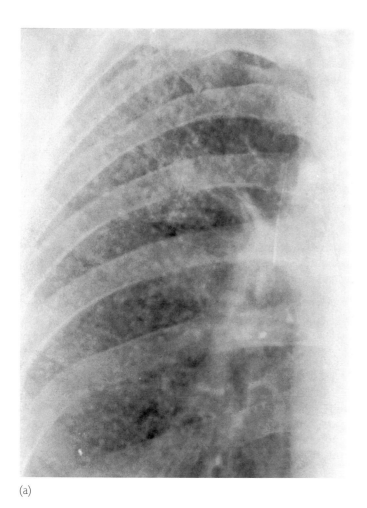

(a)

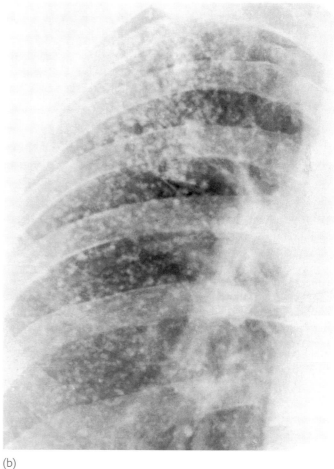

(b)

Fig. 25.3 Details of chest radiographs showing progression in silicosis. This man had been employed in hard-rock mining for 15 years at the time of film (a) and for 24 years at the time of film (b), when he became too disabled to do heavy work: the small rounded opacities (mainly 'q' and 'r') increase in profusion and density with calcifications and coalescence; hilar lymph nodes become slightly enlarged and calcified. Tests for tuberculosis had always been negative. (Courtesy of the MRC Pneumoconiosis Unit collection of standard films, kept at Llandough Hospital, the University Department of Respiratory Medicine, Penarth, and photographed by Mr R. Harris.)

Death in silicotic patients is usually due to cor pulmonale and often occurs 30–50 years after the start of the exposure. In the first half of the last century, a more accelerated form of silicosis was sometimes encountered, with symptoms already experienced within a year of the start of exposure and potential death within 5 years.

Coal-worker's pneumoconiosis

Workers in the coal mining-industry are exposed to a variety of mineral dusts besides coal. The shafts and roadways must be driven through other strata than coal, which may contain hard rock with 75% or more of quartz. The coal seams also contain rock: the proportions of quartz and other mineral dust, however, vary greatly. Therefore, lesions of accelerated or chronic silicosis have been seen in coal miners who have been exposed to quartz while working on shafts and drifts or with rock-contaminated coal.

Otherwise, coal-workers may present the more typical lesions of simple or complicated coal-worker's pneumoconiosis. These diseases are described in detail in Chapter 26.

Pneumoconiosis due to mixed dust containing quartz

Mixed dusts containing silicon dioxide and oxides of aluminium, calcium, magnesium, etc. are also called silicates, and the pneumoconioses attributed to such exposures may be labelled 'silicatoses' (see Table 25.2).

When there is heavy admixture of inert dust containing only a very small proportion of quartz, a simple pneumoconiosis with small opacities (p or q) may be found, with no clear tendency for progression, no symptoms and normal lung function tests.

Slate-workers' pneumoconiosis

Slate is formed by the sedimentation of a mixture of finely divided mineral particles on to a flat surface, and contains variable amounts of mica, feldspar and crystalline quartz (10–70%). Slate-workers' pneumoconiosis was recognised over 100 years ago, especially in north Wales, where the slate quarries and mines supplied large quantities of slate for roofing. The pneumoconiosis was mainly attributed to dry sawing of slates and dry engraving of tombstones, and the problem is believed to have been solved by the introduction of wet working.

The chest radiograph showed small, rounded opacities, especially in the upper zones, which sometimes calcified and coalesced to irregular shadows. There were, generally, massive bilateral hilar gland enlargements with eggshell calcifications (see Fig. 25.2). Pathological examination showed mixed lesions with some silicotic nodules and confluent masses, and also lesions similar to those found in coal workers (centrilobular dust collection and emphysema) and even masses full of slate dust.[56]

Kaolin pneumoconiosis

Kaolinite is a (hydrated) multilayered particle made of alternating plates of aluminium hydroxide and silicon oxide. It is a powerful absorbent. It was in the past mainly used for making china but is nowadays more used as a filler for paper and also as a thickener for paints and an ingredient of special plasters. Kaolin or china clay may be contaminated by silica, sand, mica, feldspar and undegraded granite. Hazards from kaolin may thus be swamped by the effect of silica contamination.

It has been shown, especially by epidemiological surveys in Cornwall, that at relatively high cumulative exposure levels kaolin workers develop an exposure-related simple pneumoconiosis with only minor lung-function changes.[57,58] Radiological progressive massive fibrosis, calcifications and hilar gland changes are rare and probably attributable to silica contamination. Therefore, kaolin itself is considered almost as a nuisance dust.

Talc pneumoconiosis

Talc consists of magnesium silicate that has crystallised into thin plates, which readily split and slide over each other.

The quarrying and mining of talc and its subsequent milling to a powder were known to be especially risky occupations. Powdered talc is the traditional coating for rubber tubing, balloons, gloves, etc. to prevent these from sticking together; it is further used as a lubricant, as a filler and for powdering, especially babies after bathing. Disease (i.e. talcosis) has been described after heavy dust exposure in several of these applications. Examples are talc pneumoconiosis in a magician whose favourite act involved inflating as many balloons as he could as fast as possible[59] (Fig. 25.4) or in an elderly woman whose job three decades before had been to fill rubber hoses with talc[60].

The presumed abnormality in pure talc pneumoconiosis is that of a simple non-disabling pneumoconiosis, without significant loss of lung function, and irregular as well as rounded, small opacities on chest X-ray. The histology of talc pneumoconiosis initially shows a diffuse granulomatous lesion with the in latter stages interstitial fibrosis and few if any silicotic nodules. Diagnosis is confirmed by showing birefringent 'talc bodies' on BAL or lung biopsy.

Talc is often contaminated with other minerals, especially quartz, explaining the occurrence of disabling progressive massive lung fibrosis in some people, and asbestos fibres such as tremolite, actinolite or anthophyllite, explaining disabling pleural changes, mesothelioma and lung cancer in others.[61] Since the early 1960s cosmetic talc and talc for medical use has been monitored to exclude contamination with fibre. Industrial talcs may still contain fibres.

Mica pneumoconiosis

Mica consists of aluminium and potassium silicates with varying amounts of other elements that have crystallised into thin sheets. The traditional mineral of commercial value was muscovite, which can be split into translucent sheets several inches across and was used in the windows of furnaces or as an electrical insulator. In both these uses it has been superseded by synthetic materials. Powdered or ground mica can be produced as a by-product in the separation of sheets during quarrying of other minerals such as feldspar, kaolin and lithium ores – quartz is a frequent component of these mixtures also. Ground mica is used in paints, plasters, ceramics and as a filler in plastics. Radiographic changes are not specific (Fig. 25.5).

A benign simple pneumoconiosis has been reported in people mining and milling mica (mostly in India and South America). More serious cases are probably due to contaminating minerals.[62]

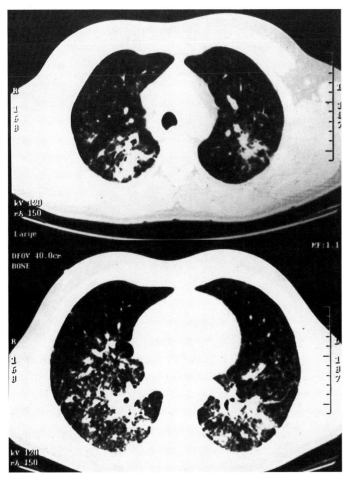

Fig. 25.4 Computed tomography scan of the lungs showing dense coalescences, especially in the best-ventilated dorsobasal lung zones, due to talc. This patient was a magician with minor complaints of dyspnoea whose favourite act for the past 13 years had been blowing up talc-containing figure-balloons as fast as possible (up to 200 balloons in 1 hour) (With permission from Thomeer et al 1999.[59]).

Vermiculite is a poorly compacted form of mica that exfoliates to occupy more than 10 times its original volume when heated. Like the other micas, pure vermiculite does not appear to be a significant risk. However, all commercial deposits of vermiculite should be monitored for contamination by fibrous tremolite, which has been shown to induce a high incidence of mesothelioma in the Montana deposit workers.[63]

Diatomite (Kieselgühr) pneumoconiosis
Diatomite is a soft rock or clay consisting of the skeletons of dead diatoms or plankton and is made up of amorphous non-crystalline silica with some calcium, magnesium and aluminium silicates.

Diatomite is milled into a fine powder, which is used generally as a replacement for asbestos for filtering and clearing liquids, for polishing, as a filler for cosmetic products, and in special plasters and cements. Diatomite pneumoconiosis is rather rare but may be found in a variety of occupations, e.g.

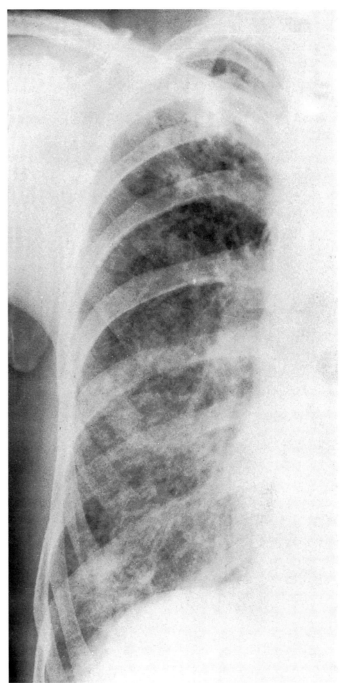

Fig. 25.5 Mica pneumoconiosis. Chest radiograph showing ill-defined nodular and irregular opacities (ILO 2/3 qt) with coalescence at the apex and the base attributed to mica. This 44-year-old man with complaints of slight dyspnoea had spent 18 years grinding mica to a fine powder and 10 years weighing and inspecting the dry powder under dusty conditions. Without a lung dust analysis it is impossible to conclude whether this pneumoconiosis is due to mica or to contaminating quartz or other minerals. (Courtesy of the MRC Pneumoconiosis Unit collection of standard films, kept at the Univ. Dept. of Respiratory Medicine, Llandough Hospital, Penarth and photographed by Mr R. Harris.)

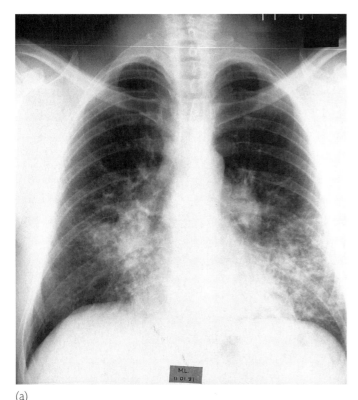

(a)

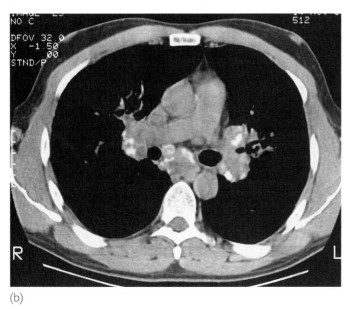

(b)

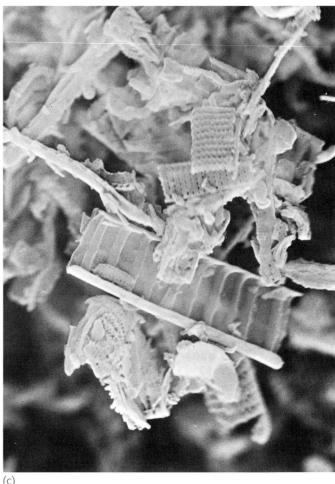

(c)

Fig. 25.6 (a) Chest radiograph showing non-symmetrical lower-zone reticulomicronodular coalescent infiltrates diagnosed as diatomite pneumoconiosis. This 37-year-old non-smoker had worked for the previous 17 years in a brewery, emptying 25–30 bags of diatom earth (Kieselgühr) daily into the filters. (b) Mediastinal computed tomography scan of the same patient shows large, partly calcified lymph nodes. (c) Electron micrograph of diatom earth.

workers in breweries who handle large quantities of diatomite used for filtering the beer[64] (Fig. 25.6). The extraction process for diatomite may include a stage of calcining at high temperature that converts the amorphous silica to cristobalite, which is very fibrogenic.

Exposure to raw diatomite rock or clay or to the extract that is kiln-dried and milled at low temperature only causes a simple pneumoconiosis with a cellular reaction similar to that found with talc. Yet, exposure to the calcined product containing cristobalite may lead to serious progressive pneumoconiosis even with fatal outcome.[65]

Pneumoconiosis due to fibrous mineral dusts

Long, thin respirable fibres, especially if more than 10 times longer than they are thick, are very much more dangerous than other particles. A high proportion of inhaled fibres are caught in the lung and very few are cleared again. These fibres are not only fibrogenic but also carcinogenic if retained for a prolonged period. The most important are the asbestos fibres.

Asbestosis

Asbestos fibres are compound crystallised metallic silicates and include chrysotile (white) and the amphiboles such as crocidolite (blue), amosite (brown) and anthophyllite. The fibres penetrate the wall of the distal airspaces and migrate into the interstitium, causing a low-grade inflammatory response followed by fibrosis first in the centrilobular zone and later in the interstitium. Asbestos bodies, comprising an asbestos fibre coated with an amber layer of a ferritin-like substance containing iron, are found in the alveoli (and BAL fluid) and in the interstitium, and are the sign of exposure.

The radiographic changes in asbestosis are seen on CT scan earlier than on plain chest X-ray and consist of lower-zone bilateral irregular opacities that later become coarse, more profuse and extend further up the lung, with the appearance of honeycombing. The clinical features are late inspiratory crepitations, very gradually increasing breathlessness, and chest tightness, but unless the patient is a smoker he/she will have no cough or sputum until the disease is very far advanced.

The characteristics of asbestosis and other asbestos-related diseases are discussed in detail in Chapter 27.

Other natural fibres

Zeolites are hydrated aluminium silicates with other metal ions, which are formed by recrystallisation from water that has percolated through deposits of volcanic ash. Many of the deposits are of cubic crystals. They are used commercially and form nuisance dusts. However, some forms (e.g. erionite), are fibrous. Coarse, fibrous deposits such as those at the southern end of the Rocky Mountains are too coarse to be dangerous, but the finer deposits, as in Montana, the North Island of New Zealand and especially in Cappadocia (Turkey), are within the respirable range and very dangerous. Virtually 100% mortality due to mesothelioma was recorded in the adult population of one village in Cappadocia. In animal studies this erionite is the most potent cause of mesothelioma in low-dose inhalation studies. Deposits of erionite should never be worked commercially.

Clays and soft rocks with very fine fibre crystals consist mainly of aluminium silicates (e.g. sepiolite, meerschaum), but may also contain some calcium silicate (wollastonite). Laboratory examinations have shown that longer-fibre samples show a potential for both lung fibrosis and cancer in cell culture tests.[66] Yet after inhalation the fibres may not survive long enough in the tissues to present a serious risk in humans.[67] Because of the demand for asbestos substitutes, ore bodies that produce longer (and potentially more dangerous) crystalline fibres of wollastonite have been selected. Yet exposed workers show at the most simple pneumoconiosis, with irregular and rounded opacities and a slight exposure-related loss of lung function. There is no evidence of an increased risk of lung cancer or mesothelioma.[68]

Synthetic man-made mineral fibres

The most common synthetic man-made mineral fibres are the vitreous fibres, which comprise glass fibres, mineral wool (i.e. rock wool and slag wool) and refractory ceramic fibres. Various materials are used as additives and the fibres are often held together with binders (i.e. resins). Exposure to man-made vitreous fibres is well known to cause acute skin, eye and upper airway irritation; however, lower respiratory diseases have not been demonstrated, except for a possible relationship between refractory ceramic fibres and pleural plaques.[69] However, there are still insufficient data on the effects of these latter type of fibres.

Following exposure to synthetic man-made mineral fibres other than vitreous fibres, no human health effects have been reported except for the possibility of pneumoconiosis due to silicon carbide fibres and for an outbreak of chronic interstitial lung disease due to nylon microfibres (labelled 'flock worker's lung').[70]

Lung diseases induced by metal dusts and fumes

Metal-induced lung diseases can be quite diverse: they range from airway diseases to parenchymal disorders and from acute inhalation injury to more chronic pneumoconiosis and even to lung cancer.[71] Usually, metals and their alloys are subdivided into ferrous metals (iron and various types of steel) and nonferrous metals. The latter especially can cause a number of respiratory complications. These may include acute toxic effects such as metal fume fever and acute inhalation injury (which may lead to acute respiratory distress syndrome) or chronic disorders such as COPD or interstitial lung diseases. These may have various pathological presentations; usual interstitial pneumonitis, granulomatous lung disease, giant cell interstitial pneumonitis, etc.

These interstitial lung diseases may in some instances be due to the toxic accumulation of these metals in the lung, causing a cumulative dose-dependent pneumoconiosis of which siderosis is an example. In other instances, as in berylliosis and hard-metal lung disease, the individual predisposition or allergic sensitisation may be the determining factor for developing disease. It should also be noted that subjects with idiopathic pulmonary fibrosis are more likely than controls to have been occupationally exposed to metals, and also to wood.[72,73]

Siderosis

This is the most frequent metallic pneumoconiosis since exposure to iron is extremely widespread. Siderosis is mainly a radiological finding of small, very radiodense opacities with uniform distribution throughout the lung without respiratory symptoms or functional impairment, e.g. welder's pneumoconiosis. With cessation of exposure the radiographic opacities may gradually disappear. However, jobs that involve exposure to iron often also have risks for exposure to silica (siderosilicosis) or to asbestos (sideroasbestosis) with their associated morbidity as a consequence.

Aluminium lung

In view of the extensive industrial use of aluminium, pneumoconiosis caused by exposure to this metal appears to be uncommon. Nevertheless, the risk is not absent.

There are reports of cases of granulomatous lung disease, fibrosis and alveolar proteinosis in aluminium welders or polishers.[74]

Other 'benign' metal pneumoconioses

These include the 'benign' pneumoconioses caused by tin (stannosis), barium (baritosis), antimony (antimoniosis), etc.

Beryllium lung

Modern exposures are mainly associated with chronic beryllium disease.[75] This disease shows a striking histological and clinical resemblance to sarcoidosis because of the presence of non-caseating epithelioid granulomas in the lung interstitium, the bronchial submucosa, the subpleural region and the intrathoracic lymph nodes. The pathology may also suggest extrinsic allergic alveolitis, or finally may present as endstage lung fibrosis with honeycombing.

International exposure limits for air born beryllium are very low (1–2 μg/m³). Cases of chronic beryllium disease still occur in industrial settings, such as the extractions, ceramics, metallurgic and nuclear undustries, as well as among metal workers, and dental workers.

The development of disease is not directly dose-related, and the latency between exposure and disease is unpredictable, may vary from less than one month to more than 10 years. The progression of the disease is also variable, the disease can develop rapidly or progress more slowly over many years. The reported mortality rates vary between 18 and 60%.

The diagnosis is based on the clinical and radiological presentation, including the demonstration of non-caseating epithelioid granulomas in the tissue, very similar to sarcoidosis. The diagnosis requires a positive history of exposure to beryllium, and the proof of sensitisation to beryllium. Patch testing with beryllium has been used previously, but has rarely been applied since the demonstration that healthy exposed individuals may become sensitised through the skin test.

The lymphocyte proliferation test is specific to beryllium salts and reaches sensitivities in the range of 80 to 100% for the blood lymphocytes, and even higher for bronchoalveolar lavage lymphocytes. Thus, this test is now recommended as the standard diagnostic test for berylliosis, discriminating sufficiently unexposed subjects and beryllium-exposed normal subjects without disease.

In chronic progressive disease, the patients are treated by long-term administration of prednisone, in doses and regimen similar to those used in sarcoidosis.

Hard-metal lung disease or 'cobalt lung'

This specific form of interstitial lung disease occurs as a result of exposure to cobalt-containing dusts during the manufacture or use of hard metal or diamond tools.[76,77] While the role of cobalt in the causation of interstitial lung disease is undisputed, exposure to cobalt appears not to lead to parenchymal disease and fibrosis unless it is sintered to microdiamond or hard-metal carbides.[78,79] Hard metal is composed mainly of a carbide (especially tungsten, but also some tantalum, titanium and niobium) and cobalt (5–25%), which functions as a binder. Microdiamond cobalt composite tools are mainly used for drilling, sawing, cutting, grinding or polishing various materials, all of which may give rise to significant exposure especially in factories without efficient exhaust ventilation.[77,80]

Hard-metal or cobalt lung disease may present as a subacute alveolitis with fever and other systemic reactions such as asthenia and weight loss, and it may even evolve to an acute respiratory distress syndrome (Fig. 25.7). It may also progress more insidiously, leading to lung fibrosis (Fig. 25.8). In some patients the interstitial lung disease may coexist with occupational asthma,[81] or the bronchial asthma may be the dominant feature.[82] Overt disease only occurs in a minority of exposed workers, suggesting a specific, perhaps immunological, susceptibility.[78] The known dermal and respiratory sensitising properties of cobalt and some of the clinical features of the disease favour immunological sensitisation as a possible mechanism. However, several pathological features argue against an underlying delayed-type hypersensitivity: in most biopsies no epithelioid cell granulomas and lymphocytic infiltration as in hypersensitivity pneumonitis have been found.[78,83,84]

The combination of both early and late asthmatic responses, development of airway hyper-responsiveness, neutrophilic infiltration after challenge and interstitial lung disease in chronic exposure may also be mediated by non-immunological inflammatory mechanisms in which activated macrophages

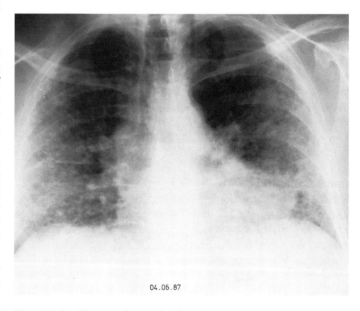

04.06.87

Fig. 25.7 Chest radiograph of a diamond polisher, showing a 'cobalt lung'. There is a diffuse interstitial lung fibrosis, especially in the peripheral zones, with increased heart size, evolving to an acute respiratory distress syndrome. (With permission from Nemery et al 1990.[85]

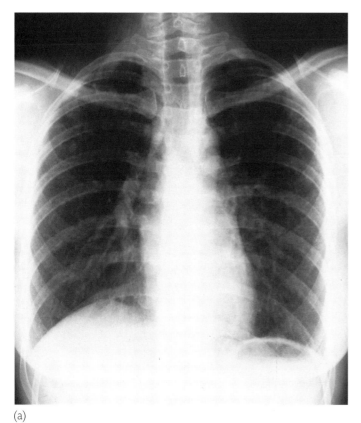
(a)

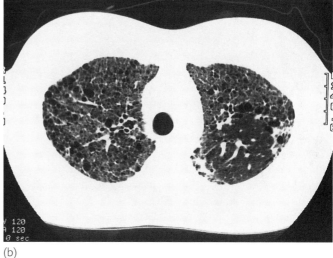
(b)

Fig. 25.8 Chest radiograph (a) and computed tomography scan (b) showing diffuse interstitial lung fibrosis with honeycombing in a 24-year-old female diamond polisher. She had worked with diamond-cobalt disks for 6 years and complained of severe dyspnoea (TLC 45% and $D_L$co 27% predicted), cough, weight loss and nasal congestion. Bronchoalveolar lavage showed 3% lymphocytes, 9% neutrophils, 4% eosinophils and multinucleated giant cells.

release a variety of mediators.[78] Also, oxidative stress may be involved, at least in some cases.[85]

The most characteristic, but not obligatory, pathological finding is a giant cell interstitial pneumonitis with so-called 'bizarre' or 'cannibalistic' multinucleated giant cells, which are also found in the BAL fluid[77,86] (Fig. 25.9).

The evolution is variable but cessation of exposure, sometimes in combination with administration of corticosteroids, usually results in clinical improvement and good recovery in subacute disease.

Lung diseases induced by other fumes, mists and gases

Exposure to industrial airborne agents, including chlorine, phosgene, nitrogen oxides, sulphur dioxide, ammonia and hydrogen sulphide, can lead to a variety of acute respiratory problems from chest discomfort to pulmonary oedema. While in most instances no long-term sequelae are observed following intoxication, occasionally lung fibrosis or bronchiolitis obliterans organising pneumonia[87] may ensue, besides reactive airway dysfunction syndrome, bronchiectasis, emphysema, etc.[88-90]

Typical examples of novel occupational or environmental lung diseases include the exposure to acramin-containing paint aerosols in textile workers, causing bronchiolitis obliterans organising pneumonia (also labelled the ardystil syndrome),[91,92] the toxic oil syndrome[93] and the bronchiolitis obliterans caused by fumes of stoves.[94]

These outbreaks clearly point to the need to improve the protection of workers exposed to mists of uncertain toxicity or unproven innocuity.[87] They also guarantee that novel respiratory diseases, and causes for them, may emerge at any time.

Accordingly, a careful medical observation and follow-up of workers exposed to new or modified working procedures and conditions is of the utmost importance to prevent the occurrence of pneumoconioses and other occupational or environmental respiratory illnesses.

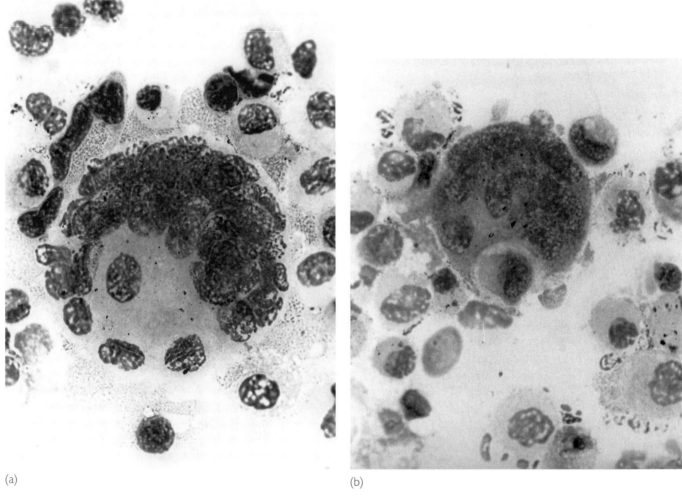

(a)

(b)

Fig. 25.9   (a & b) 'Cannibalistic' multinucleated giant cells. These cells were found in the bronchoalveolar lavage fluid of two diamond polishers with 'cobalt lung'.

Therapeutic principles

- As long as the offending agent remains caught in the lung, the noxious burden continues.

- Therefore, most pneumoconioses cannot be treated successfully and some even progress further after exposure ceases.

- Preventive measures are therefore of key importance.

- Corticosteroids may alleviate symptoms in subacute disorders but often have no long-lasting favourable effect.

- General health measures are still indicated in pneumoconiosis: smoking cessation, treatment of associated chronic obstructive pulmonary disease, prevention and adequate anti-infectious treatment.

? Unresolved questions

- Many aspects in the pathogenesis of pneumoconiosis are only beginning to be unravelled; the interaction of the different processes of direct toxicity and indirect inflammatory burden remains largely unknown.

- The variations in susceptibility between exposed subjects appear to be genetic as well as acquired but the exact underlying mechanism for these variations is still largely unknown.

References

1. Wilt JL, Parker JE, Banks DE. The diagnosis of pneumoconiosis and novel therapies. In: Banks DE, Parker JE, ed. Occupational lung disease, an international perspective. London: Chapman & Hall; 1998: 119–138.

2. Parkes WR. Occupational lung disorders, 3th ed. Oxford: Butterworth-Heinemann; 1994: 35.

3. Elmes P, Cockcroft A, Nemery B. Inorganic dusts. In: Baxter PJ, Adams PH, Aw TC et al, ed. Hunter's diseases of occupation, 9th ed. London: Edward Arnold; 2000: 663–708.

4. Brody AR, Roe MW. Deposition pattern of inorganic particles at the alveolar level in the lungs of rats and mice. Am Rev Respir Dis 1983; 128: 724–729.

5. Brody AR, Hill LH, Adkins B, O'Connor RW. Chrysotile asbestos inhalation in rats: deposition pattern and reaction of alveolar epithelium and pulmonary macrophages. Am Rev Respir Dis 1981; 123: 670–679.

6. Poli G, Parola M. Oxidative damage and fibrogenesis. Free Radicals Biol Med 1997; 22: 287–305.

7. Mossman BT, Marsh JP, Sesko A et al. Inhibition of lung injury, inflammation and interstitial pulmonary fibrosis by polyethylene glycol-conjugated catalase in a rapid inhalation model of asbestosis. Am Rev Respir Dis 1990; 141: 1266–1271.

8. Nemery B, Bast A, Behr J et al. Interstitial lung disease induced by exogenous agents: factors governing susceptibility. In: Demedts M, du Bois RM, Nemery B, Verleden G, ed. Interstitial lung diseases: a clinical update. Eur Respir J 2001; 18 (Suppl 32): 30S–42S.

9. Janssen YMW, Marsh JP, Absher MP et al. Expression of antioxidant enzymes in rat lung after inhalation of asbestos or silica. J Biol Chem 1992; 267: 625–630.

10. Lombard-Gillooly K, Hubbard AK. Modulation of silica-induced lung injury by reducing lung non-protein sulfhydryls with buthionine sulfoximine. Toxicol Lett 1993; 66: 305–315.

11. Donaldson K. Mechanisms of pneumoconiosis. In: Banks DE, Parker JE, ed. Occupational lung disease, an international perspective. London: Chapman & Hall; 1998: 139–160.

12. Wilt JL, Banks DE. Reactions of inorganic dust. In: Walters EH, du Bois RM, ed. Immunology and management of interstitial lung disease. London, Chapman & Hall; 1995: 199–222.

13. Ferin J, Oberdorster G, Penney DP. Pulmonary retention of ultrafine and fine particles in rats. Am J Respir Cell Mol Biol 1992; 6: 535–542.

14. Hill I, Beswick PH, Donaldson K. Differential release of superoxide anion by macrophages treated with long and short fibre amosite asbestos is a consequence of differential affinity for opsonin. Occup Environ Med 1995; 52: 92–96.

15. Simenova PP, Luster MI. Iron and reactive oxygen species in the asbestos-induced tumor necrosis factor-alpha response from alveolar macrophages. Am J Respir Cell Mol Biol 1995; 12: 676–683.

16. Frampton MW, Utell MJ, Clinical studies of airborne pollutants. In: Gardner DE, Crapo JD, McClellan RO, ed. Toxicology of the lung, 3rd ed. Philadelphia: Taylor & Francis; 1999: 455–481.

17. Sweeney TD, Shornik WA, Brain JD et al. Chronic bronchitis alters the pattern of aerosol deposition in to lung. Am J Respir Crit Care Med 1995; 151: 482–488.

18. Bennett WD, Zeman KL, Kim C, Mascarella J. Enhanced deposition of fine particles in COPD patients spontaneously breathing at rest. Inhal Toxicol 1997; 9: 1–14.

19. Svartengren K, Ericsson CH, Svartengren M et al. Deposition and clearance in large and small airways in chronic bronchitis. Exp Lung Res 1996; 22: 555–576.

20. De Vuyst P, Karjalainen A, Dumortier P et al. Guidelines for mineral fibre analyses in biological samples: report of the ERS Working group. Eur Respir J 1998; 11: 1416–1426.

21. Begin R. Assessment of disease activity by gallium-67 scan and lung lavage in the pneumoconioses. Semin Respir Dis 1986; 7: 275–280.

22. Donaldson K, Brown GM, Brown DM et al. Contrasting bronchoalveolar leukocyte responses in rats inhaling coalmine dust, quartz or titanium dioxide: effects, coalrank, airborne mass concentration, and cessation of exposure. Environ Res 1990; 52: 62–76.

23. Mossman BT, Churl A. Mechanisms in the pathogenesis of asbestosis and silicosis. Am J Respir Crit Care Med 1998; 157: 1666–1680.

24. Vanhee D, Gosset P, Boitelle A et al. Cytokines and cytokine network in silicosis and coal workers' pneumoconiosis. Eur Respir J 1995; 8: 834–842.

25. Schins RPF, Borm PJA. Mechanisms and mediators in coal dust induced toxicity, a review. Ann Occup Hyg 1999; 43: 7–33.

26. Driscoll KE. The role of interleukin-1 and tumor necrosis factor alpha in the lung's response to silica. In: Costanova S, Vallyathan V, Wallace WE, ed. Silica and silica-induced disease. Boca Raton, FL: CRC Press; 1996: 163–184.

27. Schins RP, Borm PJ. Epidemiological evaluation of release of monocyte TNF-alpha as an exposure and effect marker in pneumoconiosis: a five-year follow-up study of coal workers. Occup Environ Med 1995; 52: 441–450.

28. Van Hee D, Gosset P, Wallaert B et al. Mechanisms of fibrosis in coal worker's pneumoconiosis. Increased production of platelet-derived growth factor, insulin-like growth factor type I, and transforming growth factor beta and relationship to disease severity. Am J Respir Crit Care Med 1994; 150: 1049–1055.

29. Zhai R, Jetten M, Schins RP et al. Polymorphisms in the promotor of the tumor necrosis factor-alpha gene in coal miners. Am J Ind Med 1998; 34: 318–324.

30. Van Hee D, Gosset P, Marquette CH et al. Secretion and mRNA expression of TNF-alpha and IL-6 in the lungs of pneumoconiosis patients. Am J Respir Crit Care Med 1995; 152: 298–306.

31. Huaux F, Lardot C, Arras M et al. Lung fibrosis induced by silica particles in NMRI mice is associated with an upregulation of the p40 subunit of interleukin-12 and Th-2 manifestations. Am J Respir Cell Mol Biol 1999; 20: 561–572.

32. Huaux F, Arras M, Vink A et al. Soluble tumour necrosis factor (TNF) receptors p55 and p75 and interleukin-10 downregulate TNF-alpha activity during the lung response to silica particles in NMRI mice. Am J Respir Cell Mol Biol 1999; 21: 137–145.

33. Gibbs AR, Seal RME, Wagner JC. Pathological reactions of the lung to dust. In: Morgan WKC, Seaton A, ed. Occupational lung disease, 2nd ed. Philadelphia, PA: WB Saunders; 1984: 129–162.

34. Nyberg P, Klockars M. Effect of immunoglobulins on mineral dust-induced production of reactive oxygen metabolites by human macrophages. Inflammation 1990; 14: 621–629.

35. Henderson RF, Harkema JR, Hotchkiss JA, Boehme DS. Effect of blood leukocyte depletion on the inflammatory response of the lung to quartz. Toxicol Appl Pharmacol 1991; 109: 127–136.

36. Chang LY, Overby LH, Brody AR, Crapo JD. Progressive lung cell reactions and extracellular matrix production after a brief exposure to asbestos. Am J Pathol 1988; 131: 156–161.

37. Resnick D, Freedman NJ, Krieger M. Secreted extracellular domains of macrophage scavenger receptors from elongated trimers which specifically bind crocidolite asbestos. J Biol Chem 1993; 268: 3538–3545.

38. Brown GM, Donaldson K. Inflammatory responses in lungs of rats inhaling coalmine dust: enhanced proteolysis of fibronectin by bronchoalveolar leukocytes. Br J Ind Med 1990; 46: 866–872.

39. Rom WN. Relationship of inflammatory cell cytokines to disease severity in individuals with occupational inorganic dust exposure. Am J Ind Med 1991; 19: 15–27.

40. Li XY, Donaldson K, Brown D, MacNee W. The role of neutrophils, tumour necrosis factor and glutathione in increasing airspace epithelial permeability in acute lung inflammation Am J Respir Cell Mol Biol 1995; 13: 185–189.

41. International Labour Office. Guidelines for the use of ILO international classification of radiographs of pneumoconiosis. Occupational Safety and Health series 22. Geneva: International Labour Office; 1980.

42. Al Jarad N, Wilkinson P, Pearson MC, Rudd RM. A new high resolution computed tomography scoring system for pulmonary fibrosis, pleural disease, and emphysema in patients with asbestos related disease. Br J Ind Med 1992; 49: 73–84.

43. Officiële Belgische Schaal ter bepaling van de graad van invaliditeit. Deel IV: Ademhalingsstelsel. Brussels: Belgische Vereniging voor Pneumologie; 1990: 5–8.

44. Caplan A. Certain unusual radiological appearances in the chest of miners suffering from rheumatoid arthritis. Thorax 1953; 8: 29–37.

45. Westerholm P, Ahlmark A, Maasing R, Segelberg JJ. Silicosis and risk of lung cancer or lung tuberculosis in a cohort study. Environ Res 1986; 41: 339–350.

46. Goldsmith DF, Beaumont JJ, Morrin LA, Schenker MB. Respiratory cancer and other chronic disease mortality among silicotics in California. Am J Ind Med 1995; 28:459–467.

47. International Agency for Research in Cancer. Monographs on the evaluation of the carcinogenic risk of chemicals to humans. Suppl. 7. Lyon: IARC; 1987: 216–219.

48. International Agency for Research in Cancer. Monographs on the evaluation of the carcinogenic risk of chemicals to humans: silica and some silicates. Suppl. 4.2. Lyon: IARC; 1987: 9–143.

49. International Agency for Research on Cancer. Monographs on the evaluation of carcinogenic risks to humans. 68: Quartz. Lyon: IARC; 1997.

50. Finkelstein MM. Radiographic silicosis and lung cancer risk among workers in Ontario. Am J Ind Med 1998; 94: 244–251.

51. Craighead JE, Kleinerman J. Silicosis and silicate committee, NIOSH. Diseases associated with exposure to silica and non-fibrous silica minerals. Arch Pathol Lab Med 1988; 112: 673–720.

52. Demedts M, Thomeer M. Rare diffuse lung diseases and mimics of diffuse lung diseases. In: Olivieri D, du Bois RM, ed. Interstitial lung diseases. Eur Respir Mon 2000; 14: 267–288.

53. Cherniack M. The hawk's nest incident: America's worst industrial disaster. New Haven, CT: Yale University Press; 1986.

54. Derom F, Barbier F, Ringoir S et al. Ten month survival after lung homotransplantation in man. J. Thorac Cardiovasc Surg 1971; 61: 835–846.

55. Sluis-Cremer GK, Hessel PA, Nizdo EH et al. Silica, silicosis and progressive systemic sclerosis. Br J Ind Med 1985; 42: 838–843.

56. Craighead JE, Emerson RJ, Stanley DE. Slateworker's pneumoconiosis. Hum Pathol 1992; 23: 1098–1105.

57. Rundle EM, Sugar ET, Ogle CJ. Analyses of the 1990 chest health care survey of China clay workers. Br J Ind Med 1993; 50: 913–919.

58. Smeers G. The china clay industry lessons for the future of occupational health. Respir Med 1989; 83: 173–175.

59. Thomeer M, Van Bleyenbergh P, Nemery B, Demedts M. A breathless accountant who blew up balloons. Lancet 1999; 354: 124.

60. Gysbrechts C, Michiels E, Verbeken E et al. Interstitial lung disease more than 40 years after a 5 year occupational exposure to talc. Eur Respir J 1998; 11: 1412–1415.

61. Gamble J, Griefe A, Hancock J. An epidemiological industrial hygiene study of talc workers. Ann Occup Hyg 1982; 26: 841–859.

62. Skulberg KR, Gylseth B, Skaug V, Hanoa R. Mica pneumoconiosis: a literature review. Scand J Work Environ Health 1985; 11: 65–74.

63. Amandus HE, Wheeler R, Armstrong B et al. Mortality of vermiculite workers exposed to tremolite. Sixth BOHS International Conference of Inhaled Particles, Cambridge, 1986. Ann Occup Hyg 1988; 32(suppl. 1): 459.

64. Nemery B, Van Kerckhoven W, Verbeken EK et al. An unexpected risk of pneumoconiosis in breweries. Proceedings of the Eight International Conference on Occupational Lung Diseases, Prague, 1992: 658–663.

65. Clark WC, Crally LJ. Pneumoconiosis in diatomite mining and processing. Publication 601. US Department of Health, Education and Welfare. Washington, DC: Public Health Service; 1958.

66. Pott F, Roller M, Zeim U et al. Carcinogenicity studies on natural and manmade fibres with the intraperitoneal test in rats. IARC 1989; 8: 173.

67. McConnochie K, Bevan C, Newcombe RG et al. A study of Spanish sepiolite workers. Thorax 1993; 48: 370–374.

68. Huuskonen MS, Tossavainen A, Koskinen H et al. Wollastonite exposure and lung fibrosis. Environ Res 1983; 30: 291–304.

69. Lockey J, Lemasters G, Rice C et al. Refractory ceramic fiber exposure and pleural plaques. Am J Respir Crit Care Med 1996; 154: 1405–1410.

70. Kern DG, Crausman RS, Durand KTH et al. Flock worker's lung: chronic interstitial lung disease in the nylon flocking industry. Ann Intern Med 1998; 129: 261–272.

71. Nemery B. Lung disease from metal exposure. In: Banks DE, Parker JE, ed. Occupational lung disease, an international perspective. London: Chapman & Hall; 1998: 279–306.

72. Hubbard R, Lewis S, Richards K et al. Occupational exposure to metals or wood dust and aetiology of cryptogenic fibrosing alveolitis. Lancet 1996; 347: 284–289.

73. Demedts M, du Bois RM, Nemery B, Verleden G. Interstitial lung disease: a clinical update. Eur Respir J 2001; 18(suppl. 32): 1S–133S.

74. Jederlinic PJ, Abraham JC, Churg A et al. Pulmonary fibrosis in aluminium oxide workers. Investigation of nine workers with pathologic examination and microanalysis in three of them. Am Rev Respir Dis 1990; 143: 1179–1184.

75. Newman LS, Maier LA, Nemery B. Interstitial lung disorders due to beryllium and cobalt. In: Schwartz MI, King TE, ed. Interstitial lung disease, 3rd ed. St Louis, MO: Mosby; 1998: 367–392.

76. Cugell DW, Morgan WKC, Perkins DG, Rubin A. The respiratory effects of cobalt. Arch Intern Med 1990; 150: 177–183.

77. Demedts M, Gheysens B, Nagels J et al. Cobalt lung in diamond polishers. Am Rev Respir Dis 1984; 130: 130–135.

78. Demedts M, Ceuppens J. Respiratory diseases from hard metal or cobalt exposure. Solving the enigma. Chest 1989; 95: 2–3.

79. Lison D, Lauwerys S, Demedts M, Nemery B. Experimental research into the pathogenesis of cobalt/hard metal lung disease. Eur Respir J 1996; 9: 1024–1028.

80. Figuera S, Gerstenhaber B, Welch L et al. Hard metal interstitial pulmonary disease associated with a form of welding in a metal part coating plant. Am J Ind Med 1992; 21: 313–373.

81. Van Cutsem EJ, Ceuppens JL, Lacquet LM, Demedts M. Combined asthma and alveolitis induced by cobalt in a diamond polisher. Eur J Respir Dis 1987; 70: 54–61.

82. Gheysens B, Auwerx J, van den Eeckhout A, Demedts M. Cobalt induced asthma in diamond polishers. Chest 1985; 88: 740–744.

83. Davison AG, Haslam PL, Corin II et al. Interstitial lung disease and asthma in hard metal workers: bronchoalveolar lavage, ultrastructural and analytical findings and results of bronchial provocation tests. Thorax 1983; 38: 119–128.

84. Anttiula S, Sutinen S, Paanan M et al. Hard metal lung disease: a clinical, histological, ultrastructural and X-ray micro-analytical study. Eur J Respir Dis 1986; 69: 83–94.

85. Nemery B, Nagels J, Verbeken E et al. Rapidly fatal progression of cobalt lung in a diamond polisher. Am Rev Respir Dis 1990;141:1373–1378.

86. Ohori NP, Sciurba FC, Owens GR et al. Giant cell interstitial pneumonia and hard metal pneumoconiosis. A clinicopathological study of four cases and review of the literature. Am J Surg Pathol 1989;13: 581–587.

87. Camus P, Nemery B. A novel cause of bronchiolitis obliterans organizing pneumonia: exposure to paint aerosols in textile workshops. Eur Respir J 1998; 11: 259–262.

88. White CS, Templeton PA. Chemical pneumonitis. Radiol Clin North Am 1992; 30: 1231–1243.

89. Schwartz DA. Acute inhalation injury. State Art Rev Occup Med 1987; 2: 297–318.

90. Nemery B. Late consequences and accidental exposure to inhaled irritants: RADS and the Bhopal disaster. Eur Respir J 1996; 9: 1973–1976.

91. Moya C, Anto JM, Newman-Taylor AJ et al. Outbreak of organizing pneumonia in textile printing sprayers. Lancet 1994; 344: 498–502.

92. Romero S, Hernandez L, Gil J et al. Organizing pneumonia in textile printing workers. A clinical description. Eur Respir J 1998; 11: 265–271.

93. Alonso-Ruiz A, Calabozo M, Perez-Ruiz F, Mancebo L. Toxic oil syndrome. A long-term follow-up of a cohort of 322 patients. Medicine (Baltimore) 1973; 72: 285–295.

94. Janigan DT, Hilp T, Michael R, McCleane JJ. Bronchiolitis obliterans in a man who used his wood-burning stove to burn synthetic construction materials. Can Med Assoc J 1997; 156: 1171–1173.

26 Respiratory disease in coal miners

Benoît Wallaert
Based on a chapter by WKC Morgan

 Key points

- Coal-worker's pneumoconiosis is usually recognised by identification of diffuse, small rounded opacities (simple pneumoconiosis) and/or large opacities exceeding 10 mm (progressive massive fibrosis) on chest radiograph or computed tomography scan.

- Emphysema may be present.

- Abnormalities of lung function usually occur in the presence of progressive massive fibrosis and/or emphysema.

Coal is mined in many countries and still features prominently as a source of energy. Initially it was removed from surface out-croppings but, as the demand for it increased, both open-cast and underground mines were opened. Coal mining remains an important industry in the USA, Germany, South Africa, Australia, Russia, Poland, India and China. In France and the UK, the demand for coal as a source of energy has declined greatly.

Background

Coal is not a mineral of uniform composition. Its nature and its potential to cause pneumoconiosis vary widely from mine to mine and from coalfield to coalfield. It is graded by rank, which reflects its carbon content and thus combustibility. It may contain hazardous impurities, especially silica. The rank of coal has an influence on the risk of pneumoconiosis: the higher the rank, the greater the risk.[1] Anthracite is coal of the highest rank, with a carbon content around 98%. Lower-ranked coals, bituminous and sub-bituminous (i.e. softer coals), have carbon contents of 90–95%. There is a gradual transition from the higher-ranked bituminous coals, such as steam coal, to the

youngest and softest, known as lignite or brown coal. The latter contains the most volatile matter but generates the least heat per gram of coal.

Coal consists mainly of carbon, coal-tar derivatives and coal gas. The last consists of a mixture of methane and carbon monoxide. Coal, depending on its rank and geological formation, also contains a number of other minerals, including some free silica and, for the most part, the higher the rank of the coal the lower the percentage of quartz. Mica and kaolinite are also present and may be detected in the lungs of coal miners when examined post-mortem.[2,3] In addition, the lungs of deceased miners contain a number of iron-containing minerals, along with various other trace metals including beryllium, cobalt and copper.[4-6] The presence of these trace elements seems to have no clinical significance.

Coal was formed from ancient forests that were present on the earth's surface 200–300 million years ago. The organic material was initially covered and then compressed by movements of the earth's crust, and in doing so formed seams varying in thickness from a few centimetres to 30 m.

The workforce in coal mining can be divided into those who work underground and those who work on the surface. Face workers have the most dusty jobs. Behind them are those who work on transportation and removal of the coal from the face to the pit shaft. Their job is still dusty but less so than that of the face workers. They are responsible for loading coal on to either small diesel trains or the conveyer belt. Next, there is a small group of workers who maintain and repair the machinery and who, for the most part, are exposed to little in the way of dust. Finally, there are the surface workers, who similarly, are exposed to little dust. Open-cast coal mining is not a dusty job but there are a few people, who drill holes to place the charges, who may be exposed to high concentrations of free silica. The underground miner, especially the face worker, roof bolter, or tunnel driller, encounters the most obvious risk of inhaling hazardous amounts of dust, depending on how effective is the mine's ventilation and its method of dust suppression. A less obvious risk comes from the use of sand on rail tracks in some mines to increase friction and wheel holding. This may be crushed to produce respirable silica, and silica may have contaminated the dusts that are used in some mines to suppress the risk of fire/explosion.

Over the last 50 years in the UK, Germany, the USA, South Africa and Australia there has been a gradual decline in coal-dust levels in underground mines. This has been effected mainly by improved ventilation but, in addition, a number of measures have been adopted to lessen the formation of dust. These include infiltrating seams with water under high pressure and spraying water on to the cutting and boring surfaces of the equipment used in rapping and cutting coal from the seams. In open-cast coal mines, dust levels rarely approach those in the confined environments of underground mines. However, drill operators and labourers who are not protected by working in enclosed machine cabins may nevertheless be exposed to high levels of dust. In previous generations 'coal trimmers' in ships faced similar risks. They worked in the confined environment of the hold to distribute coal so that the ship was properly balanced and fit to set sail.

Once coal has been burned in power stations, the residual dust (known as fly ash) has a variable composition depending on the combustion process, the coal source and the fly ash precipitation technique. Experimental studies suggest that fly ash has much lower toxicity with respect to inflammatory potential and fibrogenicity that coal-mine dust or silica.[7]

Silica contamination increases the pneumoconiosis risk considerably and, if this is in the form of quartz at a concentration of 15% or more, there is a high risk of rapidly progressive pneumoconiosis simulating silicosis itself. Local geographical variation consequently exerts considerable influence and the risk of pneumoconiosis is particularly increased when coal seams are thin and separated by silica-containing rock.[8] Pneumoconiosis in some coal miners may consequently represent a mixed picture of coal-worker's pneumoconiosis (CWP) and silicosis.

Overall, coal rank and the degree of silica contamination are probably the principal factors accounting for the observed variability in risk between one coal mine and another. Pneumoconiosis does, nevertheless, occur when coal dust exposure is encountered without any silica contamination, and it is clear that coal dust itself poses a significant hazard.

Respiratory effects of coal dust exposure

The prolonged inhalation of coal-mine dust may result in the development of three conditions:

- coal-worker's pneumoconiosis
- silicosis,
- industrial chronic bronchitis and emphysema, either singly or in various combinations.

Coal-worker's pneumoconiosis is the term generally applied to interstitial disease of the lung resulting from chronic exposure to coal dust, its inhalation and deposition, and the tissue reaction of the host to its presence. Silicosis is related to inhalation of dust containing crystalline silicon dioxide (silica), mostly in occupational settings. However silicosis in coal miners is rarely an isolated form of pneumoconiosis and is usually found in conjunction with simple CWP. The pneumoconiosis differs in a number of ways from the acute allergic and toxic interstitial diseases that are associated with exposure to organic dusts, principally because of the long latency periods (usually 10–20 years or more) between exposure onset and disease recognition.

Coal-worker's pneumoconiosis and silicosis

Coal-worker's pneumoconiosis was first recognised in Scottish miners in 1830.[9] For many years it was believed that the lung disease that developed in coal miners with long exposure to coal-mine dust was silicosis but it is now widely considered that CWP is distinct from silicosis. Hart & Aslett reported that it could arise in coal miners exposed only to washed coal that was free of silica.[10] Later, it was demonstrated that the prevalence of radiographic abnormalities in coal miners bore little or no relation to the silica content of the coal-mine dust to which the miners were exposed.[11,12] In contrast, the extent of the radiographic abnormality correlated excellently with the coal-dust content of the lungs.[3,4,11] The proof came when workers exposed to pure carbon were shown to develop a condition that was radiologically indistinguishable from coal-worker's pneumoconiosis and silicosis[13,14] but the macroscopic and microscopic pathological appearances of which differed from those of classical silicosis.[14] Although, in general, quartz has little or no effect in producing the radiographic changes exhibited in coal miners, there may be a few exceptions to this rule: Seaton and colleagues noted that a minority of coal miners at a Scottish colliery showed rapid radiographic progression in spite of relatively low exposures to dust.[15]

Epidemiology

The association between decreased life expectancy and coal mining has been noted repeatedly in the statistics compiled by the Registrar General. In 1936, the British Medical Research Council recognised the seriousness of CWP and established its Pneumoconiosis Unit. The Unit began an extensive epidemiological programme in 1950 with the British National Coal Board, which is known as its Pneumoconiosis Field Research.[16] In parallel, considerable attention was given to coal-miners' respiratory diseases in the USA, beginning with a pilot prevalence study of CWP conducted from 1962–63.[17] These and other studies led to important advances in measuring personal levels of exposure to respirable dust and in understanding the principles of dust control, and these in turn helped to clarify the nature of CWP.

In recent decades the incidence of CWP has been declining in industrial countries because of improved dust controls, and current dust conditions are leading to a considerably lower prevalence of CWP than were seen in the past. During the period 1950–80, the annual UK rate for the recognition of CWP in current and retired miners for state compensation decreased from about 7% to 1–2%. The overall prevalence of CWP, which reflects more distant exposure and earlier incidence, declined from about 13% to 5%, but there were substantial regional differences. Similar regional differences and similar declines have been noted in the USA and other countries. A prevalence study conducted from 1969–71 showed that 46% of American coal miners in eastern states had simple CWP and 14% progressive massive fibrosis (PMF).[18] By contrast, in western miners, who worked a lower-rank coal, often from surface mines, 4.6% of miners had simple CWP and none had PMF. By the late 1970s, the risk varied from 14% to 1.4% for CWP and PMF, respectively, for low–medium-rank coal. Clearly, miners in high-rank coal areas appear to be at greater risk than those mining medium- and low-rank coals.[19]

Pathology

The macroscopic and microscopic pathological appearances of CWP differ considerably from those of classical silicosis.[13,14,20] The histopathological hallmark of CWP is the coal macule, and of silicosis the silicotic nodule.

The lesions of CWP are focal. Simple CWP is associated with the macular and nodular lesions whereas complicated CWP is associated with PMF and the lesions of rheumatoid pneumoconiosis (Caplan's syndrome).[21–25]

On gross examination the pleural surfaces of a coal-worker's lung show an irregular pattern of bluish-black pigmentation outlining the junction sites of septal-lymphatic vessels and the pleura. The pleura is not appreciably thickened unless subpleural nodules or PMF are present. Peribronchial, hilar and paratracheal lymph nodes are enlarged, black and firm.

In simple CWP the cut sections of the lung show black pigmentation in the centres of the lobules, often associated with mild emphysema. These lesions constitute the coal macule with associated focal emphysema. In theory, coal macules are nonfibrotic and not palpable but in practice they may be quite fibrotic. Microscopically, the macule is composed of macrophages laden with coal dust within the walls of the respiratory bronchioles and adjacent alveoli (Fig. 26.1). The focal emphysema resembles a mild form of cigarette-smoke-induced centrilobular emphysema. Another feature of simple CWP are

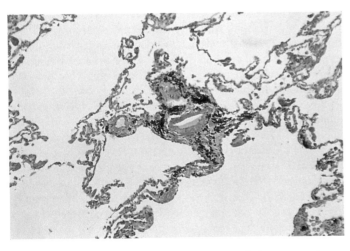

Fig. 26.1 Coal macules composed of dust-laden macrophages within the walls of respiratory bronchioles and adjacent alveoli.

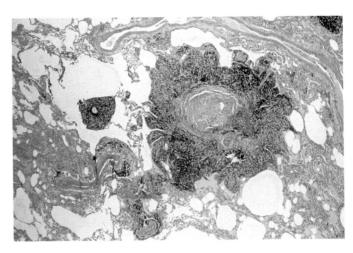

Fig. 26.2 Larger coal nodule showing coal dust, dust-laden macrophages, reticulin fibres and collagenous fibrosis.

the coal nodules. These are rounded lesions with collagenous centres and a rim of dust and macrophages (Fig. 26.2). They represent a form of mixed-dust fibrosis (i.e. coal dust plus silica exposure). Nodules are usually found in association with macules, and in some instances may develop from pre-existing macules. The lymph nodes show large numbers of pigmented histiocytes and variable degree of fibrosis.

Progressive massive fibrosis is defined as an opacity or fibrotic pneumoconiotic lesion of 1 cm in diameter or greater. PMF almost invariably occurs against a background of severe simple CWP (usually of nodular type) and is usually bilateral. PMF lesions appear as black fibrotic masses that may be round oval or irregular in shape; they are well demarcated from the surrounding lung but are not encapsulated. Satellite nodules are usually found in the adjacent lung. The lung and bronchovascular rays become markedly distorted – a characteristic feature of PMF is the tendency of the lesion to transgress normal anatomical boundaries, with fissures, bronchi and vessels becoming obliterated as the lesion progresses. Microscopically, the lesions are composed of bundles of haphazardly arranged hyalinised collagen fibres and/or reticulin fibres and coal dust. Dust particles near the periphery of the lesion are mainly found within macrophages, whereas, in the centre, the dust tends to lie free in clefts and cavities. Necrosis of PMF lesions is common and may be manifested clinically by the sudden coughing up of thick, black material. A giant-cell reaction may be seen in association with the necrotic collagen.

Caplan nodules differ morphologically from ordinary PMF lesions: they are typically rounded, may be multiple and histologically show a necrotic centre with a peripheral palisade of histiocytes and giant cells. They are not distinguishable pathologically from necrobiotic nodules of rheumatoid disease unassociated with coal-dust exposure, and may be difficult to separate morphologically from tuberculous granulomas. Miners with PMF have more severe emphysema than do those with less severe categories of CWP; all types of emphysema may be observed.

In silicosis,[26] the initial lesion is the silicotic nodule, which is less than 1 cm in diameter in simple silicosis, whereas in conglomerate silicosis the nodules become confluent. The silicotic nodule characteristically arises in the region of the respiratory bronchiole, around the pulmonary arterioles and in paraseptal and subpleural tissues. The nodules are well-demarcated, round and firm. Microscopically, the nodule can be divided into three zones: a central zone composed of whorls of dense, hyalinised fibrous tissue, a middle zone made up of concentrically arranged collagen fibres (onion skinning), and a peripheral zone of more randomly oriented collagen fibres, mixed with dust-laden macrophages and lymphoid cells (Fig. 26.3). 'Old' inactive nodules are often relatively acellular. Particles of silica may be demonstrated in the nodules as birefringent particles under polarised light. In silicosis, the pleural surface of the lungs often reveals focal fibrosis associated with silicotic nodules; occasionally, the lesions become confluent to form an arborised network of plaquelike lesions; these lesions form on the visceral pleural surface of the lung. In PMF, nodules are confluent and emphysematous bullae often surround the areas of massive fibrosis. Focal interstitial fibrosis can be observed in the lungs of workers exposed to dust containing a combination of silica and silicates, with sometimes sufficiently advanced lesions to result in honeycomb changes. Silicotic nodules are often found in proximity to areas of interstitial fibrosis. In severe silicosis, there may be structural alterations of the pulmonary vasculature resulting from the accumulation of dust in the adventitia of large vessels and involvement of the smaller blood vessels by silicotic nodules. Hilar and mediastinal lymph nodes exhibit isolated or confluent silicotic nodules.

The pathology of acute silicosis is quite different from the chronic form: the lungs are firm and oedematous, the pleural cavities may contain fibrinous adhesions. There is infiltration of the alveolar walls with plasma cells, lymphocytes and fibroblasts, with some collagenisation. The alveoli are filled with an eosinophilic coagulum. Electron microscopy shows widening of alveolar walls with some collagen and clusters of type II cells; the alveolar spaces contain degenerating cells that are probably type II alveolar cells and macrophages. Silica particles may be demonstrated in the lungs and lymph nodes; silicotic nodules are few or absent.

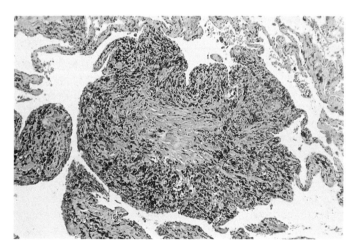

Fig. 26.3 Classic silicotic nodule: onion-skin appearance, with dust-laden macrophages and fibrotic stroma composed of collagen and reticulin.

Pathophysiology

There are three factors that are known to influence the character and severity of lung-tissue reaction to mineral dust. The risk of pneumoconiosis is related to the intensity and years of exposure. However, among a group of workers exposed to the same dust, only a fraction develops pneumoconiosis because of individual susceptibility. The nature and properties of each specific dust constitute the third factor under consideration; for each mineral, geometric and aerodynamic properties, chemistry and surface properties have to be considered.[27] The particles that can cause pneumoconiosis are those aerodynamically and geometrically small enough to reach the respiratory bronchioles and be deposited there; this generally means spherical particles between 0.5 and 5 μm.

The pathogenesis of pneumoconiosis is similar to that of all interstitial lung diseases, with a chronic inflammatory status (alveolitis) in which inflammatory cells are activated and damage the pulmonary architecture, which forms the basis of the fibrotic scar. The following mechanisms have been proposed:[28]

- a direct cytotoxicity due to chemical features of dust that directly damage cells and induce the release of intracellular enzymes causing tissue damage
- activation of oxidant production by alveolar macrophages
- stimulation of the secretion of inflammatory cytokines and chemokines by alveolar macrophages and epithelial cells
- stimulation of secretion of fibroblast growth factors by alveolar macrophages and epithelial cells.

Macrophages are activated after phagocytosis and release inflammatory mediators such as cytokines[29] and arachidonic acid metabolites.[30] These mediators induce recruitment of inflammatory cells in the alveolar wall and on the alveolar epithelial surface. The alveolitis is dominated by alveolar macrophages.[31] Toxic oxygen derivatives and proteolytic enzymes are released by inflammatory cells, which cause cellular damage and disruption of the extracellular matrix.[32] Matrix metalloproteinases and elastase are proteolytic enzymes directed against extracellular matrix components and are secreted by inflammatory cells such as activated alveolar macrophages and neutrophils.[33]

The inflammatory phase is followed by a reparative phase in which growth factors stimulate the recruitment and proliferation of mesenchymal cells and regulate neovascularisation and re-epithelialisation of injured tissues. During this phase, abnormal or uncontrolled reparative mechanisms may result in the development of fibrosis.[34]

Fibrogenic particles activate proinflammatory cytokine production within the respiratory tract. Normal human and/or rat alveolar macrophages exposed in vitro to silica or coal-mine dust release tumour necrosis factor (TNF)-α, interleukin (IL)-1 and IL-6[35] (Fig. 26.4). In-vivo studies show that alveolar macrophages from animals exposed to silica also overproduce TNF-α and IL1 early after treatment.[36] Pro-inflammatory cytokines such as chemokines are also expressed after exposure to fibrogenic dusts. For example, expression of macrophage inflammatory protein (MIP)-1α and MIP-2 mRNA and protein expressions are increased in rats exposed to silica, and the upregulation of these chemokines precedes the influx of

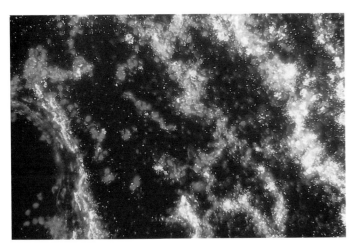

Fig. 26.4 Expression of TNF-α in alveolar macrophages by in-situ hybridisation on lung sections from a patient with coal-worker's pneumoconiosis.

inflammatory cells into the respiratory airways.[37-39] Inert dusts are less effective in stimulating a proinflammatory cytokine production.[35,40] They do not induce in the rat similar increased release of TNF-α or IL-1 by alveolar macrophages. TNF-α seems to play a key role in the recruitment of inflammatory cells induced by toxic dusts.[41]

- In silica-exposed rats, there is a significant correlation between in-vivo activation of macrophages, TNF-α release and the recruitment of neutrophils in the lung.
- Pre-treatment of rats with a monoclonal antibody against TNF-α significantly attenuates the pulmonary recruitment of neutrophils and decreased lung MIP-2 expression in response to silica.
- TNF-α release facilitates the attachment of leukocytes to the endothelium of blood vessels by stimulating the expression of adhesion molecules such as intercellular adhesion molecule (ICAM)-1 on vascular endothelium cells in humans or mice exposed to coal mine or silica dust.[42,43]

In addition, neutrophils recruited in the area of inflammation can also contribute to amplify alveolitis by secreting TNF-α or IL-1.[44] Respiratory and endothelial cells may also play a role in the alveolitis induced by inhaled particles, by releasing inflammatory mediators such as MIP-2, IL-8 and ICAM-1.[38,45]

Several studies demonstrate a key role for transforming growth factor (TGF)-β in the pathogenesis of lung fibrosis. TGF-β directly stimulates fibroblast proliferation[46] and expression of extracellular matrix proteins such as collagen[47] and fibronectin, and causes inactivation of proteases.[48] In humans, elevated TGF-β expression has been observed in silicosis[49] and CWP.[50] TGF-α has mitogenic activity for epithelial and mesenchymal cells and is also upregulated in the fibrotic lungs of rats exposed to silica particles. TGF-α may be critical in directing the proliferation of type II pneumocytes that is associated with pneumoconiosis. TNF-α and IL-1 can have a fibrogenic effect in inducing the accumulation of collagen and fibronectin in lung fibroblast cultures[51] and in stimulating fibroblast proliferation.[52] Thus, increased levels of TNF-α and IL-1 have been

observed in both human and animal lungs under conditions of developing fibrosis such as silicosis[53] and CWP.[54,55] Monocyte chemotactic peptide(MCP)-1 can also stimulate fibroblast collagen expression via specific receptors and endogenous upregulation of TGF-β.

Several human studies have shown that alveolar macrophages of individuals with silicosis and CWP spontaneously release significant amounts of growth factors such as platelet-derived growth factor (PDGF),[50] insulin-like growth factor (IGF) and fibroblast growth factor (FGF).[56] In the same conditions, inert particles had no effect on growth-factor production.[57] These mediators are involved in the proliferative response of type II epithelial cells occurring in progressive massive fibrosis.

Others cytokines, such as interferon (IFN)-γ [58] or granulocyte–macrophage-colony-stimulating factor (GM-CSF),[59] may be involved in the pathogenesis of pneumoconiosis but their role in the fibrotic disease is unclear.

Clinical assessment

Coal-worker's pneumoconiosis is generally first recognised from the plain chest radiograph, which is critical also in evaluating disease progression. The radiographic appearances are usefully described by the coding system devised for standard films of pneumoconiosis under the auspices of the International Labour Office (ILO). In clinical practice, simple CWP is characterised by small rounded opacities (nodules) rather than small irregular opacities, although the latter may be seen in much less profusion. In some coal-mining communities, particularly in past generations, large opacities occurred, characterising PMF.

Clinical features

Simple CWP and category A complicated CWP are not associated with respiratory symptoms. Coal miners with milder forms of CWP usually have no symptoms. As in most populations engaged in manual work, breathlessness and cough in coal miners are usually a consequence of cigarette-smoking. Coal miners, however, typically smoke less than other manual workers yet show a greater prevalence of chronic productive cough irrespective of pneumoconiosis, and it has become clear that coal-mine dust may itself cause chronic bronchitis.

By contrast, complicated pneumoconiosis (PMF) in categories B and C may present with undue breathlessness and productive cough, the sputum being mucoid, mucopurulent, or discoloured as if mixed with black ink (melanoptysis). This is the result of necrosis within the conglomerate, coal-containing lesions that characterise PMF. Progressive undue exertional dyspnoea is usually the dominant symptom but there may rarely be breathlessness at rest.

There are no specific abnormal physical signs in CWP but when complicated CWP is very advanced the signs of emphysema or fibrotic lobar shrinkage may be detected. Finger clubbing and fine inspiratory crackles are not features of the disease and, if these are present, another explanation should be sought. Only in a small proportion of severe cases of complicated disease does CWP evolve to produce chronic respiratory failure and pulmonary heart disease (cor pulmonale). When this does occur, extensive and multifocal conglomerate lesions are to be expected, generally with emphysema and concomitant disabling chronic airways obstruction. Bronchopneumonia commonly follows.

Associated disorders

Irrespective of PMF, there are a number of other disorders with which CWP may be associated – most notably the autoimmune disorders rheumatoid disease and progressive systemic sclerosis. The latter, however, is more clearly associated with silicosis and it is not clear whether it occurs with a greater incidence than expected when there is occupational exposure to coal alone.

The association of *rheumatoid disease* with CWP is known as Caplan's syndrome.[60] The diagnosis is suggested by the association of coal-dust exposure, rheumatoid arthritis and multiple, well-defined, large rounded opacities (nodules with diameter >10 mm) on the chest radiograph. Caplan showed that most subjects with these features have rheumatoid factor in the serum. Radiographically, the nodules may appear calcified or cavitary, and the differential diagnosis from tuberculosis can be difficult. The nodules are typically circular, 0.5–5 cm in diameter and smooth in outline, although rarely completely homogenous. Spontaneous disappearance is common, with or without initial cavitation, and new nodules commonly emerge in different locations. If the nodules become superimposed, suggesting conglomerate masses, PMF may be simulated, but often the radiological appearances of simple CWP are absent and there is a need to consider the possibility of primary lung tumour.

In some cases, the appearances of simple CWP or PMF have been present for years when additional changes develop in relation to the development of rheumatoid arthritis. There is no evident relationship between the severity of the rheumatoid disease and the extent of Caplan's syndrome. It is difficult to assess its prevalence because it is rare and there are difficulties in recognising it.

Pathologically, the Caplan (or rheumatoid) nodule is generally bigger than the nodule of complicated CWP, smoother in outline and distributed at random within the lung fields. Large opacities of complicated CWP more characteristically affect the upper zones. The Caplan nodule is also more likely to cavitate, thus producing a concentric ring pattern, and so is also known as a necrobiotic nodule, indistinguishable from rheumatoid nodules in non-miners. Central necrosis is rare in pneumoconiotic nodules of CWP, although it may occur in conglomerate lesions. When it does, the affected subject may expectorate coal-discoloured sputum, so that 'melanoptysis' is produced.

Coal-worker's pneumoconiosis has also been linked with a number of specific infections, the most prominent of which historically has been *tuberculosis*. A prospective study of 53 753 coal miners in Spain during the period 1971–85 showed an incidence of about 150 cases per 100 000 miners per year of bacterially confirmed pulmonary tuberculosis. The risk was three times greater than that for the general population of the same area.[61] Une and colleagues similarly founded a high annual incidence of tuberculosis (81.6 per 100 000/year) in a health district of Japan. The incidence was 58.1 in the surrounding region and 46 throughout Japan.[62] In contrast to silicosis, however, CWP does not increase significantly the risk for infection with *Mycobacterium tuberculosis*. The association observed with coal mining (and hence CWP) in some countries appears to have been a consequence only of close contact during long hours of work in the confined mine environment.

Non-tuberculous mycobacteria, on the other hand, may infect lungs damaged by CWP and other types of pneumoconiosis with greater than usual frequency, and so CWP does appear to increase the risk for infection with opportunistic organisms. *Mycobacterium avium* is probably the most important of these and is poorly sensitive to antibiotic agents. *Mycobacterium kansasii* and *M. malmoense* may also be pathogenic in this setting, although they are more readily eradicated with antimycobacterial agents. The development of mycobacterial infection in a patient with CWP may be symptomless, at least in its early course, and it may be difficult or impossible to distinguish radiographic evidence of it from PMF lesions, since both characteristically begin in the apices. It may similarly be difficult to attribute change in the radiographic appearances to advancing infection or progressive PMF. Experimental studies additionally suggest that mycobacterial infection is a factor that helps explain the progression from simple to complicated peumoconiosis.[63,64]

Other opportunistic infections reported in association with CWP have included nocardiosis, sporotrichosis, and cryptococcosis, and *Aspergillus* species have been noted to colonise cavities in conglomerate lesions of complicated CWP.[65]

A further association with complicated CWP, if manifested by bullous emphysema, is *spontaneous pneumothorax*, although this is not likely to occur with excess incidence in simple pneumoconiosis. There is no evidence of a causal relationship between CWP and carcinoma of the lung, although there is strengthening evidence linking silica exposure with lung cancer.[66,67] In practice, coal miners smoke less heavily than other manual workers, as noted above, and lung cancer rates are diminished as a result. However one cannot exclude the possibility that silica acts as a cocarcinogen. The advanced stages of complicated CWP are additionally associated with recurrent episodes of acute and subacute bronchitis, as well as a regular productive cough.

Investigations

Radiology

The appearances of the standard high-voltage posteroanterior and lateral chest radiograph are described by reference to the ILO standard films,[68] the classification of which is shown in Table 25.3 (see Chapter 25).

In simple pneumoconiosis, the radiograph typically shows small opacities, which appear first in the upper zones. The opacities involve middle and lower zones as the number of opacities increases. The size of opacities is noted p, q, r for regular opacities and s, t, u for irregular ones. The profusion of opacities is scored in four major categories (0–3), each major category being divided into three minor categories and providing a full range of 12 categories. The grouping of opacities or confluence is classified as a coalescence when the confluence is smaller than 10 mm in diameter or as a large opacity when the confluence is greater than 10 mm. The rounded shadows increase in profusion with increasing dust exposure; a change in profusion after dust exposure has ceased is very unusual.[1]

Complicated pneumoconiosis is defined as a lesion of 1 cm or greater in longest diameter. Complicated pneumoconiosis

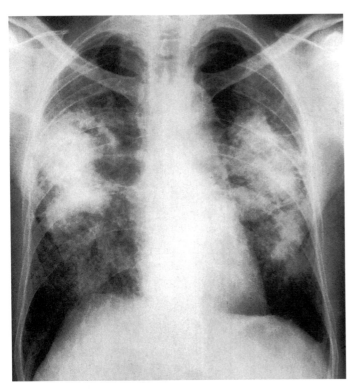

Fig. 26.5 Complicated pneumoconiosis (progressive massive fibrosis): opacities greater than 1 cm in diameter are present and there is the background appearance of simple coal-worker's pneumoconiosis elsewhere. The film was classed as stage C as opacities occupy more than one-third of one lung field.

(PMF) is divided in categories A, B and C, based on the size of the large opacities. The large opacities are usually predominant in the upper lobes and may be unilateral or bilateral, symmetrically or asymmetrically distributed (Fig. 26.5). The pattern of change in size is variable and unpredictable. Most PMF occurs on a background of simple pneumoconiosis and may occur after dust exposure has ceased. A cavity can develop within a PMF lesion. An occasional feature of PMF is a dense peripheral arc or rim at its lower pole, which represents calcification.[69] Dense calcification with the lesion is also sometimes seen. PMF is often associated with bullous emphysema, distortion of the lung and shift of the trachea and mediastinum to the affected side, caused by fibrotic scarring. Irregular, mainly basal, opacities may also be seen on standard radiographs. Cockroft and colleagues[70,71] reported that they were associated pathologically with emphysema and to a lesser degree with diffuse interstitial fibrosis, often in combination.

Progressive massive fibrosis can pose diagnostic difficulties. Nodular opacities can be rheumatoid nodules in Caplan's syndrome. Differential diagnosis with a lung cancer must be kept in mind. A finding pathognomonic of silicosis is the presence of eggshell calcifications in intrapulmonary, hilar or mediastinal lymph nodes.

Pleural effusion is uncommon in CWP. Its presence may be related to an associated infection or an interaction with a systemic collagen vascular disease such as rheumatoid arthritis or progressive systemic sclerosis.

It is natural to wonder whether computed tomography (CT) would demonstrate radiographic changes of pneumoconiosis earlier or with better definition.[72,73] There is a lack of consensus concerning the size of lesions: micronodules are lesions up to 7 mm of diameter; nodules are lesions larger than 7 mm and up to 20 mm; micronodules and nodules define simple pneumoconiosis. Masses of PMF are identified as lesions larger than 20 mm in diameter.

In simple CWP, CT shows parenchymal lesions that can be detected even in exposed workers with normal chest radiographs. There is a posterior and right-sided predominance in the upper zones (Fig. 26.6); in patients with more severe involvement, micronodules are diffusely distributed through the lungs. Detection is dramatically influenced by CT technique: a 10 mm collimation is considered as the best technique. Micronodules can be detected in the subpleural areas; they are detected in 87% of coal miners with radiographic evidence of CWP. Confluence of subpleural micronodules is referred to as pseudoplaques. However, isolated subpleural micronodules cannot be considered as an early sign of CWP because they may be observed among smokers and ex-smokers.

Nodules are usually observed against a background of parenchymal micronodules and generally associated with subpleural micronodules.[74] Two categories of lesion can be observed in PMF: lesions with irregular borders associated with disruption of the pulmonary parenchyma, leading to typical scar emphysema, and lesions with regular borders and absence of scar emphysema. When the lesions are larger than 4 cm in diameter, irregular areas of aseptic necrosis can be observed, with or without cavitation (Fig. 26.7).

Other disorders can be associated with CWP lesions: all types of emphysematous lesion have been observed in the lungs of coal miners. *Focal lung emphysema* indicates distension of the bronchioles with macules and is considered an integral part of the lesions of CWP. Two major forms of emphysema occurring in coal workers can be detected on CT: bullous changes around PMF lesions are referred to as *paracicatricial* or *scar emphysema*

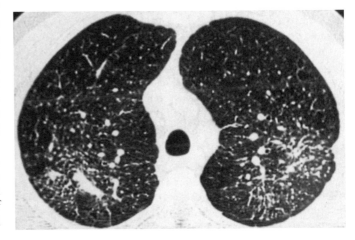

Fig. 26.6 High-resolution computed tomography scan at the level of the upper lobes, showing bilateral parenchymal micronodules and coalescence in the right upper lobe. Note the additional presence of subpleural micronodules and pseudoplaques.

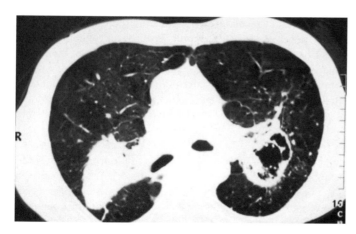

Fig. 26.7 Computed tomography scan showing bilateral masses with necrosis of the left mass. Note features of retraction demonstrated by the right main bronchus orientation and bilateral emphysema.

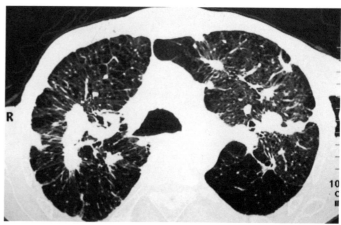

Fig. 26.8 High-resolution computed tomography scan showing bilateral masses consistent with progressive massive fibrosis. There is a background of nodules associated with bullous changes around progressive massive fibrosis lesions referred to as paracicatricial emphysema.

(Fig. 26.8); non-bullous emphysematous lesions are defined as *irregular emphysema* (Fig. 26.9).

Lesions of diffuse pulmonary fibrosis can be detected on high-resolution CT as honeycombing or areas of ground-glass attenuation. Two specific aetiologies of fibrosis of coal miners should be considered: exposure to coal dust or silica particles, both known to predispose to lung fibrosis, or association with scleroderma. It is impossible to distinguish lung fibrosis resulting from occupational exposure from fibrosis of non-occupational origin on the basis of CT appearances alone.[75]

Eggshell calcification of hilar and mediastinal lymph nodes may be present in CWP. Punctuate or massive calcification of nodes may be also observed. Lymph node enlargement can occur in all mediastinal sites.[74]

High-resolution CT images demonstrate radiographic abnormalities in coal miners more frequently than standard radiography interpreted by ILO criteria.[76] CT appears to detect simple pneumoconiosis in its early stages better than standard radiography but is equivalent to radiography for complicated pneumoconiosis (except in the identification of necrosis in PMF lesions).[72]

In silicosis, Bégin et al[77] report that chest radiograph and CT yield similar average scores for detection of opacities. Chest radiograph and CT results are similar in patients with complicated silicosis. CT identifies significantly more coalescence and large opacities in patients with simple silicosis, and does detect earlier changes of coalescence in workers exposed to silica.

Lung function

In studies of lung function in pneumoconiotic patients, a number of different and confounding influences should be considered. The effects of smoking are of major importance. It can be stated that simple CWP has no important effect on spirometric measures, when prior dust exposure is taken into account and when smoking habits are also considered.[78,79] Several studies have shown more subtle changes in lung function, with a lower diffusing capacity in the category of pneumoconiosis with p shadows than with q or r shadows.[80] Arterial oxygen pressure

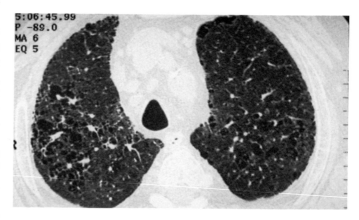

Fig. 26.9 High-resolution computed tomography scan showing small bullae and low attenuation, without progressive massive fibrosis lesions, defined as centrilobular (non-paracicatricial) emphysema.

may be slightly reduced at rest in simple pneumoconiosis, especially in category p cases, although this tends to normalise on effort. The changes are minimal in miners who do not smoke.[80] In PMF, lung function depends on the extent of the lesions and of associated emphysema. Studies of lung function in the more advanced stages of PMF have shown an obstructive and restrictive pattern;[81] the diffusing capacity is usually reduced. Compliance is usually somewhat decreased.[79] Ultimately, hypoxaemic respiratory failure may occur.

Simple silicosis has no appreciable effect on lung function. In more advanced disease, slight reduction in volume, compliance and gas transfer can be present; there is a predominantly restrictive pattern. Slight reduction in arterial oxygen tension on effort may be observed in advanced disease. Oxygen desaturation is not present at rest or on moderate effort in the non-conglomerate stages of disease. As in the case of radiographic progression, the changes in pulmonary function are more likely to occur in workers who have had intense exposure to dust. In addition, it must be pointed out that miners who did not have CWP on chest radiography exhibited lower forced expiratory ventilation in 1 minute (FEV_1) than controls, suggesting the frequent presence of coal-dust-induced chronic obstructive pulmonary disease.[82]

Serological and immunological features

There are no specific biological features of pneumoconiosis. However, immunological abnormalities are now well described. Lippman et al.[83] report 34% of positive circulating antinuclear antibodies among miners with radiographic opacities of pneumoconiosis, with a higher prevalence in the anthracite miners and. a lower one in bituminous miners. Soutar et al.[84] report 17% of positive antinuclear antibodies, with a lower prevalence in simple CWP (9%) than in PMF (27%). Rheumatoid factor is observed in 4–10% of miners with radiographic opacities of pneumoconiosis.[83,84] Serum immunoglobulins IgA and IgG levels are significantly raised in miners with pneumoconiosis compared to non-miners.[85,86] In workers heavily exposed to quartz, such as sand-blasters, rheumatoid factor, antinuclear antibodies and increased immunoglobulin levels are noted in 20–40% of cases.[87] Finally, increased serum angiotensin-converting enzyme levels are observed in 45% of pneumoconiotic coal miners, whatever the radiological classification of pneumoconiosis.[88] Constitutional differences may explain the variations in response to inhaled dust.

Bronchoalveolar lavage

Bronchoalveolar lavage (BAL) studies in CWP are controversial. Two studies have demonstrated similar total and differential cell counts in miners compared with control subjects, and similar oxygen radical release, while a third has shown a significant increase in cell number.[31,89,90] The latter was marked in miners with PMF and was evident after making allowances for smoking habits. There was no change in differential cell count, in contrast to a number of other interstitial disorders of the lung (e.g. sarcoidosis, chronic idiopathic interstitial pneumonia, hypersensitivity pneumonitis) in which an abnormal percentage of lymphocytes and/or neutrophils is usually present.[91] Alveolar inflammatory cells from patients with simple CWP released spontaneously more superoxide anion than did those from control subjects.[90] Superoxide release by alveolar inflammatory cells from patients with PMF was dramatically increased when compared with both control subjects and miners with simple CWP, and among the non-smokers those with PMF demonstrated significantly lower values for lung volumes and diffusing capacity than did those with simple pneumoconiosis. However, no correlation was found between the cellular characteristics of BAL and pulmonary function abnormalities.

In silicosis, there is an increased cellularity with an increased number of macrophages,[92] and a trend towards an increase in lymphocytes and neutrophils. However BAL is not different amongst silica-exposed workers with different severity of disease.

Prognosis

Although mortality statistics for coal miners during the first half of the 20th century suggested a greater risk of premature death in coal miners than in non-miners, much of this was a consequence of accidents and less privileged living standards. Studies over the second half of the century indicated no difference in mortality from the general population, though moderate differences remain between white-collar and blue-collar workers. Since standardised mortality ratios for lung cancer and heart disease tend to be lower for coal miners than the populations from which they arise because of slightly lower consumption of tobacco (they are not allowed to smoke while in the mine), there may still be a minor occupational survival disadvantage resulting from non-malignant respiratory disease. This cannot be attributed to simple pneumoconiosis; it appears to be chiefly a consequence of airway disease, although complicated pneumoconiosis of advanced degree (now very rare) plays some role, since a higher standardised mortality ratio for this has been a consistent observation. Even so, mean life expectancy for coal miners with complicated pneumoconiosis extends into the eighth decade. Simple CWP is not associated with premature mortality but approximately 4% of deaths in coal miners are directly due to complicated pneumoconiosis.[1,93] Among 346 south Wales miners and ex-miners with category B or C complicated CWP, death was attributed to the pneumoconiosis in about one-third of cases.[94] In categories 1, 2, and 3 of simple CWP and category A of complicated CWP, life expectancy is the same as that among the general population without pneumoconiosis.[95] The rate of progression to PMF appears to be influenced chiefly by the age at which the miner begins to show radiographic changes of CWP – the earlier the diagnosis, the more likely is there to be progression.[96] This in turn is likely to reflect individual susceptibility and the level of cumulative exposure.

Industrial bronchitis and emphysema

As in the general population, cigarette smoking is the major cause of cough and sputum production; however, it is clear that non-smoking miners may also develop bronchitis and the longer and greater the dust exposure, the more likely are cough and sputum to be present.

Industrial bronchitis

Industrial bronchitis is a response to the inhalation of a variety of agents including inert dusts, various gases and vapours, and is characterised by cough and sputum.[97] Although often associated, bronchitis and airway obstruction should be considered as separate responses to the same injury.[98]

In 1971 Rae et al reported for the first time an increased prevalence of bronchitis among British coal miners as their cumulative dust exposures increased.[99] Several studies then demonstrated a higher prevalence of chronic bronchitis in coal-face workers than in surface workers.[100,101] Industrial bronchitis is also associated with some minor degree of ventilatory impairment. Increasing severity of bronchitic symptoms is associated with a loss of FEV_1 greater than expected from the effects of measured dust exposure, smoking, age and anthropometry.[102] However, Soutar & Hurley demonstrated a similar effect of dust exposure on FEV_1 in coal miners with or without chronic bronchitis.[103] Airflow obstruction may occur in the absence of symptoms of chronic bronchitis. A relationship between airflow obstruction (and decline in ventilatory capacity) and dust exposure has been suggested in several studies, including longitudinal epidemiological surveys.[1,104-106] Rogan et al reported a loss of FEV_1 of 150 ml at a cumulative dust exposure of 240 gh/m³;[102] Marine & Guar[101] found between 90 and 100 ml decrements in FEV_1 for every 100 gh/m³ exposure to coal dust.

Clearly, bronchitis is not systematically associated with pneumoconiosis. The lack of relationship between pneumoconiosis and bronchitis might be explained by the fact that the particle size required to produce bronchitis is different. Coal and other particles that induce bronchitis are probably between 3 and 10 μm in size, and somewhat larger than the respirable fraction reaching the alveolar space that is responsible for the development of pneumoconiosis. Such larger particles are removed by the mucociliary escalator; they are not associated with radiological evidence of pneumoconiosis.

Emphysema

The occurrence of emphysema in coal miners has been reported by Osler[107] and Cummings.[108] However the causal relationship between respirable dust and emphysema is still a matter of debate.

A series of papers from south Wales has put forward the thesis that coal miners have a higher prevalence of emphysema than do non-miners and that the reduced ventilatory capacity observed in coal miners is a consequence of emphysema.[109,110] These studies have attempted to relate emphysema demonstrated post-mortem to measurements of lung function and radiological category made during life. It was claimed that a relationship existed between the presence of simple and complicated CWP and decreased lung function during life, as diagnosed by a reduction in FEV_1. It was also suggested that the p type of opacity of simple CWP was associated more often with emphysema than the larger q and r types of opacities. Ryder and colleagues[109] showed that the radiographic category of pneumoconiosis was related to emphysema, although they made no distinction between subjects with simple and those with complicated disease. It was also apparent that there was a lack of relationship between FEV_1 and increasing category of simple pneumoconiosis.

There is no doubt that simple CWP is frequently accompanied by focal emphysema[70] and that in the higher categories of simple CWP more focal emphysema is present in the lungs. The proportion of subjects with any emphysema was 47% in 92 men with no palpable dust lesions, 65% in 183 with simple pneumoconiotic lesions and 83% in 175 miners with PMF.[111] The occurrence of centriacinar emphysema was associated with increasing amounts of dust retained in the lungs and dust-related fibrosis, suggesting that the extent and nature of fibrosis may be a crucial factor in determining the presence of emphysema. Usually more than 15–20% of the lung has to be involved before obstruction occurs. Centrilobular (or centriacinar) emphysema is located in the smaller airways (second division of respiratory bronchioles) and is the commonest type of emphysema in both smoking and non-smoking miners but is seldom associated with significant airway obstruction. If focal emphysema were a cause of the airway obstruction that is noted in coal miners, then with increasing category of simple CWP there would be a concomitant increase in the amount of emphysema, and a reduction of FEV_1 would also be expected. This does not occur.

Likewise, the presence of emphysema detected post-mortem is by no means invariably associated with the presence of ante-mortem airway obstruction.[112] Focal emphysema seen in non-smoking miners with simple CWP is seldom that extensive, is not associated with significant airway obstruction nor with loss of diffusing capacity. Nevertheless, the increasing emphysema is reflected in an increased residual volume and is associated with some minor loss of elastic recoil[81,113] and minor ventilation perfusion inequalities.

An editorial entitled 'Coal mining, emphysema and compensation' puts forward the view that coal-induced emphysema is responsible for significant disablement in, British coal miners.[114] Much of the evidence used to support this thesis is based on a report that showed that the relationship between dust and emphysema was evident only in those miners who showed a fibrotic response to inhaled dust, i.e. those with CWP.[115] Moreover, although dust is associated with the development of centriacinar emphysema, no relationship was found between dust and panacinar emphysema. The authors of the report add that the results suggest that non-smokers with the highest lifetime exposures have a lower risk of developing centriacinar emphysema than a smoker with minimal exposure. The report provides no support for the hypothesis that disabling emphysema occurs in non-smoking coal miners, and indeed provides evidence to the contrary.

Another argument against emphysema being responsible for the decrement in ventilatory capacity is the fact that the greatest annual decrement in FEV_1, at least until after the age of 50 years, occurs in the first 3–4 years after starting to work as a coal miner.[116] The FEV_1, after the initial decrement, remains almost constant or declines very little for the next 12–13 years, before staring to decline again, but at a rate that does not match the rapid decline of the early years. The rapid initial decrease described above is unlikely to be the result of emphysema, which appears slowly and progresses inexorably unless the inciting cause is no longer operative.

Management and prevention

No specific treatment affects the course of CWP, although treatment options are available for complications such as tuberculosis and chronic hypoxaemia. Early pneumoconiosis is easily detected by chest radiography. When a miner is found to have CWP, further dust exposure should be prevented. Simple pneumoconiosis does not necessarily require complete exclusion from mining, especially in elderly subjects, whereas when PMF is detected all further dusty work should be avoided. Additional information is obtained from pulmonary function tests, since the development of an obstructive ventilatory defect (due to dust exposure) may occur in the absence of CWP. In all smoking patients advice and support in smoking cessation should be given. If a physician concludes that there is disablement from CWP, he/she should be able to direct the patient towards whatever mechanism for compensation exists.

The prevention of pneumoconiosis depends on controlling concentrations of ambient dust to levels known to be associated with minimal and acceptable risk. Dust control is effected primarily by ventilation, although water sprayed at points of dust generation is a useful measure for dust suppression. When each process is limited by practical constraints in unusual situations (e.g. during development or in emergencies), individual miners can be provided with respiratory protection equipment or their duration of exposure can be limited.

The effectiveness of such measures should be monitored by regular measurement of dust concentrations and by regular clinical and radiological surveillance of the workforce. Static samplers are commonly used at the coal face and other potential sites of exposure to monitor exposure levels, relevant respirable particles of $1–7\,\mu m$ diameter being collected by size-selective, gravimetric elutriators. In other mining situations, personal samplers worn by individual miners can be used. Surveillance allows early recognition of workers with simple pneumoconiosis, who are likely to be those with greatest susceptibility, so that ongoing exposure can be restricted (perhaps by transfer to jobs with lower exposure) and the risk of future disablement from PMF reduced.[1,117,118]

Permissible levels of respirable dust inevitably differ in different countries, although they are often based on the same epidemiological studies. The following standards are active at present:[119] USA: $1\,mg/m^3$; UK: $3.8\,mg/m^3$; Australia: $3\,mg/m^3$; Germany: $4\,mg/m^3$.

Variability of individual susceptibility is likely to be an important determinant for CWP, as it is for most occupational disorders, and a number of predictive factors may be useful in identifying miners with higher than average risk. Indeed marked interindividual differences have been reported in populations of miners exposed to equal dust types and concentrations. Case-control studies have investigated the differences in relation to physical exercise, nasal versus mouth breathing, nutritional factors, co-exposures and constitutional factors such as blood types and histocompatibility.[120] In addition, it is now clear that cytokines and growth factors play a crucial role in particle-induced respiratory disorders.[121] Since gene screening for polymorphisms is now easily performed, an alternative approach for the future might involve genetic screening. TNF-α is known to be important in the development of fibrosis due to silica exposure and is probably relevant to the development of PMF in coal miners. Crucial animal experiments were reported by Piguet et al,[122] demonstrating that silica-induced fibrosis could be ameliorated using a specific anti-TNF antibody and that the infusion of soluble TNF receptors that complex free TNF could prevent and reduce existing fibrosis.[123] A recent study showed a polymorphism in the promoter of the *TNFα* gene in coal miners, with a predominance of the genotype A308 in miners with PMF compared to simple pneumoconiosis,[124] and a further study has

shown an increased plasma level of soluble TNF-α receptors in coal miners with pneumoconiosis.[125] Other genes that are related to CWP pathogenesis (such as IL-1, IL-1 RA, TGF-β, MCP-1, IL-10, IL-6, RANTES and others) should be further screened for. All these findings may provide markers of undue susceptibility.

In any event, control of exposure levels alone is likely to prevent most cases of disabling PMF, and it has been predicted that an exposure concentration over 35 working years that does not exceed an average of $4.3\,mg/m^3$ is associated with a probability for the development of category 2 or more CWP of no more than 3.4%.[126] This represents a dramatic reduction in risk over the last 50 years.

Therapeutic principles

- No specific treatment is available for the management of patients with coal-worker's pneumoconiosis.

- Non-specific treatment should be given for complications such as pneumothorax, hypoxaemia or infectious complications such as tuberculosis.

- Prevention is mainly achieved through the suppression of massive dust exposure (water spraying, ventilation) and regular monitoring of respirable exposure levels.

? Unresolved questions

- Does the extent of exposure play a major role in the development of coal-worker's pneumoconiosis and/or emphysema?

- What is the role of oxidant burden and/or inflammatory processes in the progression to progressive massive fibrosis?

- What are the mechanisms responsible for the development of emphysema in a subgroup of patients?

- What is the true incidence of lung cancer related to coal-dust exposure?

References

1. Seaton A. Coal workers' pneumoconiosis. In: Morgan WK, Seaton A, ed. Occupational lung diseases, 3rd ed. London: WB Saunders; 1995: 374–406.
2. Bergman I, Casswell C. Lung dust and lung iron contents of coal workers in different coalfields in Great Britain. Br J Ind Med 1972; 29: 160.
3. Rossiter CE. Relation of lung dust content to radiological changes in coal workers. Ann NY Acad Sci 1972; 200: 465.
4. Rivers D, Wise ME, King EJ, Nagelschmidt G. Dust content, radiology, and pathology in simple pneumoconiosis of coal workers. Br J Ind Med 1960; 17: 87.
5. Crable JV, Keenan RG, Wolowicz FR et al. The mineral content of bituminous coal miners' lung. Am Ind Hyg Assoc J 1967; 28: 8.
6. Crable JV, Keenan RG, Kinser RE et al. Metal and mineral concentrations in lungs of bituminous coal miners. Am Ind Hyg Assoc J 1968; 29: 106.

7. Borm PJ. Toxicity and occupational health hazards of coal fly ash (CFA). A review of data and comparison to coal mine dust. Ann Occup Hyg 1997; 41: 659–676.
8. Green FHY, Laqueur WA. Coal worker's pneumoconiosis. Pathol Annu 1980 15: 333–341.
9. Gregory JC. Case of peculiar black infiltration of the whole lungs, resembling melanosis. Edin Med Surg J 1831; 36: 389.
10. Hart Pd'A, Aslett EA. Medical Research Council, Special Report Series No. 243. London: His Majesty's Stationery Office; 1942.
11. Nagelschmidt G. The study of lung dust in pneumoconiosis. Am Ind Hyg Assoc J 1965; 26: 1.
12. Casswell C, Bergman I, Rossiter CE. The relation of radiological appearance in simple pneumoconiosis of coal workers to the content and composition of the lung. In: Walton WH, ed. Inhaled particles III, vol. 2. London: Unwin Brothers; 1970: 713.
13. Watson AJ, Black J, Doig AT, Nagelschmidt G. Pneumoconiosis in carbon electrode makers. Br J Ind Med 1959; 16: 274.
14. Gaensler EA, Cadigan JB, Sasahara AA et al. Graphite pneumoconiosis of electrotypers. Am J Med 1966; 41: 864.
15. Seaton A, Dick JA, Dodgson J, Jacobsen M. Quartz and pneumoconiosis in coal miners. Lancet 1981; 2: 1272.
16. Fay JWJ. The National Coal Board's pneumoconiosis field research. Nature 1957; 180: 309.
17. Lainhart WS, Doyle HM Enterline PE et al. Pneumoconiosis in Appalachian bituminous coal miners. US Department of Health, Education and Welfare, Washington DC: US Government Printing Office; 1969.
18. Morgan WKC, Lapp NL. Respiratory disease in coal miners. State of the art. Am Rev Respir Dis 1976; 113: 531.
19. Attfield MD, Seixas NS. Prevalence of pneumoconiosis and its relationship to dust exposure in a cohort of US Bituminous coal miners and ex-miners. Am J Ind Med 1995; 27: 137–151.
20. Ruttner JR, Bovet P, Aufdermaur M. Graphit, Carborund, Staublunge. Dtsch Med Wschr 1952; 77: 1413.
21. Green FHY, Laqueur WA. Coal worker's pneumoconiosis. Pathol Annu 1980; 15: 333–341.
22. Green FHY. Coal workers' pneumoconiosis and pneumoconiosis due to other carbonaceous dusts. In: Pathology of occupational lung disease, 2nd ed. Baltimore, MD: Williams & Wilkins 1998: 129–208.
23. Kleinerman J, Green FHY, Harley R et al. Pathology standards for coal workers' pneumoconiosis: report of the Pneumoconiosis Committee of the College of American Pathologists to the National institute for Occupational Safety and Health. Arch Pathol Lab Med 1979; 103: 375–431.
24. Heppleston AG. The essential lesion of pneumoconiosis in Welsh coal workers. J Pathol Bacteriol 1947; 59: 453.
25. Heppleston AG. The pathogenesis of simple pneumoconiosis in coal workers. J Pathol Bacteriol 1954; 67: 51.
26. Silicosis and Silicate Diseases Committee. Diseases associated with exposure to silica and non fibrous silicate materials. Arch Pathol Lab Med 1988; 112: 673–720.
27. Bégin R, Cantin A, Massé S. Recent advances in the pathogenesis and clinical assessment of mineral dust pneumoconiosis. asbestosis, silicosis and coal pneumoconiosis. Eur Respir J 1989; 2: 988–1001.
28. Castranova V, Vallyathan V. 2000 Silicosis and coal workers' pneumoconiosis. Environ Health Perspect 108 (suppl 4) 675–684
29. Vanhée D, Gosset P, Boitelle A et al. Cytokines and cytokine network in silicosis and coal workers, pneumoconiosis. Eur Respir J 1995; 8: 1–9.
30. Demers LM, Kuhn DC. Influence of mineral dusts on metabolism of arachidonic acid by alveolar macrophage. Environ Health Perspect 1994; 102(suppl. 10): 97–100.
31. Rom WN, Bitterman PB, Rennard SI et al. Characterization of the lower respiratory tract inflammation of nonsmoking individuals with interstitial lung disease associated with chronic inhalation of inorganic dust. Am Rev Respir Dis 1987; 136: 1429–1434.
32. Weiss SJ. Tissue destruction by neutrophils. N Engl J Med 1989; 320: 365–376.
33. Ferry G, Lonchampt M, Pennel L et al. Activation of MMP-9 by neutrophil elastase in an in vivo model of acute lung injury. FEBS Lett 1997; 402: 111–115.
34. Limper AH, Roman J. Fibronectin. A versatile matrix protein with roles in thoracic development, repair and infection. Chest 1992; 101: 1663–1673.
35. Gosset P, Lassalle P, Vanhée D et al. Production of tumor necrosis factor-alpha and interleukin-6 by human alveolar macrophages exposed in vitro to coal mine dust. Am J Respir Cell Mol Biol 1991; 5: 431–436.
36. Oghiso Y, Kubota Y. Enhanced interleukin 1 production by alveolar macrophages and increase in Ia-positive lung cells in silica-exposed rats. Microbiol Immunol 1986; 30: 1189–1198.
37. Driscoll KE, Hassenbein DG, Carter J et al. Macrophage inflammatory proteins 1 and 2: expression by rat alveolar macrophages, fibroblasts, and epithelial cells and in rat lung after mineral dust exposure. Am J Respir Cell Mol Biol 1993; 8: 311–318.
38. Driscoll KE, Howard BW, Carter JM et al. Alpha-quartz-induced chemokine expression by rat lung epithelial cells: effects of in vivo and in vitro particle exposure. Am J Pathol 1996; 149: 1627–1637.
39. Yuen IS, Hartsky MA, Snajdr SI, Warheit DB. Time course of chemotactic factor generation and neutrophil recruitment in the lungs of dust-exposed rats. Respir Cell Mol Biol 1996; 15: 268–274.
40. Driscoll KE, Higgins JM, Leytart MJ, Crosby L. Differential effects of mineral dusts on the in vitro activation of alveolar macrophages eicosanoid and cytokine release. Toxic in Vitro 1990 ; 4: 284–288.
41. Driscoll KE. Macrophage inflammatory proteins: biology and role in pulmonary inflammation. Exp Lung Res 1994; 20: 473–490.
42. Vanhée D, Molet S, Gosset P et al. Expression of leucocyte-endothelial adhesion molecules is limited to intercellular adhesion molecule-1 (ICAM-1) in the lung of pneumoconiotic patients role of tumor necrosis factor-alpha (TNF-alpha). Clin Exp Immunol 1996; 106: 541–548.
43. Nario RC, Hubbard AK. Silica exposure increases expression of intercellular adhesion molecule-1 (ICAM-1) in C57B1/6 mice. J Toxicol Environ Health 1996; 49: 599–617.
44. Kusaka Y, Cullen RT, Donaldson K. Immunomodulation in mineral dust-exposed lungs: stimulatory effect and interleukin-1 release by neutrophils from quartz-elicited alveolitis. Clin Exp Immunol 1990; 80: 293–298.
45. Stringer B, Imrich A, Kobzik L. Lung epithelial cell (A549) interaction with unopsonised environmental particles: quantitation of particle-specific binding and IL-8 production. Exp Lung Res 1996; 22: 495–508.
46. Border WA, Noble NA. Transforming growth factor beta in tissue fibrosis. N Engl J Med 1994; 331: 1286–1292.
47. Roberts CJ, Birkenmeier TM, McQuillan JJ et al. Transforming growth factor beta stimulates the expression of fibronectin and of both subunits of the human fibronectin receptor by cultured human lung fibroblasts. J Biol Chem 1988; 263: 4586–4592.
48. Roberts AB, Sporn MB. Regulation of endothelial cell growth, architecture and matrix synthesis by TGF-beta. Am Rev Respir Dis 1989; 140: 1126–1128.
49. Jagirdar J, Begin R, Dufresne A et al. Transforming growth factor beta (TGF-beta) in silicosis. Am J Respir Crit Care Med 1996; 154: 1076–1081.
50. Vanhée D, Gosset P, Wallaert B et al. Mechanisms of fibrosis in coal workers' pneumoconiosis. Increased production of platelet-derived growth factor, insuline-like growth factor type I, and transforming growth factor beta and relationship to disease severity. Am J Respir Crit Care Med 1994; 150: 1049–1055.
51. Zhang Y, Lee TC, Guillemin B et al. Enhanced IL-1 beta and tumor necrosis factor-alpha release and messenger RNA expression in macrophages from idiopathic pulmonary fibrosis or after asbestos exposure. J Immunol 1993; 150: 4188–4196.
52. Battegay EJ, Raines EW, Seifert RA et al. TGF-beta induces bimodal proliferation of connective tissue cells via complex control of an autocrine PDGF loop. Cell 1990; 63: 515–524.
53. Struhar DJ, Harbeck RT, Gegen N et al. Increased expression of class II antigens of the major histocompatibility complex on alveolar macrophages and alveolar type II cells and interleukin-1 (IL-1) secretion from alveolar macrophages in an animal model of silicosis. Clin Exp Immunol 1989; 77: 281–284.
54. Lassalle P, Gosset P, Aerts C et al. Abnormal secretion of interleukin-1 and tumor necrosis factor alpha by alveolar macrophages in coal workers' pneumoconiosis: comparison between simple pneumoconiosis and progressive massive fibrosis. Exp Lung Res 1990; 16: 73–80.
55. Vanhée D, Gosset P, Marquette CH et al. Secretion and mRNA expression of TNFα and IL-6 in the lungs of pneumoconiosis patients. Am J Respir Crit Care Med 1995; 152: 298–306.
56. Lesur O, Melloni B, Cantin AM, Begin R. Silica-exposed lung fluids have a proliferative activity for type II epithelial cells: a study on man and sheep alveolar fluids. Exp Lung Res 1992; 18: 633–654.
57. Melloni B, Lesur O, Cantin A, Begin R. Silica-exposed macrophages release a growth-promoting activity for type II pneumocytes. J Leukocyte Biol 1993; 53: 327–335.
58. Lesur OJ, Mancini NM, Humbert JC et al. Interleukin-6, interferon-gamma, and phospholipid levels in the alveolar lining fluid of human lungs. Profiles in coal workers' pneumoconiosis and idiopathic pulmonary fibrosis. Chest 1994; 106: 407–413.
59. Xing Z, Tremblay GM, Sime PJ, Gauldie J. Overexpression of granulocyte-macrophage colony-stimulating factor induces pulmonary granulation tissue

formation and fibrosis by induction of transforming growth factor-beta 1 and myofibroblast accumulation. J Leukocyte Biol 1996; 97: 1102–1110.

60. Caplan A, Payne RB, Withey JL. A broader concept of Caplan's syndrome related to rheumatoid factors. Thorax 1962; 17: 205.

61. Mosquera JA, Rodrogo L, Gonzalvez F. The evolution of pulmonary tuberculosis in coal miners in Asturia, northern Spain. An attempt to reduce the rate over a 15-year period 1971–1985. Eur J Epidemiol 1994; 10: 291–297.

62. Une H, Esaki H. An epidemiological study of tuberculosis in the former coal-mining area of Chikuho. An analysis of newly registered tuberculosis patients in Iizuka Health Center District. Nippon Eiseigaku Zasshi 1993; 47: 994–1000.

63. James WRL. The relationship of tuberculosis to the development of massive pneumoconiosis in coal workers. Br J Tuberc 1954; 48: 89–101.

64. Gernez-Rieux C, Tacquet A, Devulder B et al. Experimental studies of interactions between pneumoconiosis and mycobacterial infection. Ann NY Acad Sci 1972; 200: 106–126.

65. Nomoto Y, Kuwano K, Hagimoto N et al. *Aspergillus fumigatus* Asp-f-l DNA is prevalent in sputum from patients with coal workers pneumoconiosis. Respiration 1997l 64: 291–295.

66. International Agency for Research on Cancer. Silica, some silicates, coal dust and para-aramid fibers. Lyon: IARC; 1996.

67. Honma K, Chiyotani K, Kimura K. Silicosis, mixed dust pneumoconiosis and lung cancer. Am J Ind Med 1997; 32: 595–599.

68. International Labour Office. Guidelines for the use of ILO international classification of radiographs of pneumoconiosis, rev ed. International Labour Office Occupational Safety and Health Series No 22 (Rev 80). Geneva: International Labour Office; 1980.

69. Parkes WR. Pneumoconiosis associated with coal and other carbonaceous materials. In: Parkes WR, ed. Occupational lung disorders, 3rd ed. Oxford: Butterworth-Heinemann ; 1994: 366–368.

70. Cockcroft A, Seal RME, Wagner JC et al. Post mortem study of emphysema in coal workers and non-coal workers. Lancet 1982; 2: 600–603.

71. Cockroft AE, Wagner JC, Seal EME, Lyons JP, Campbell MJ. 1982. Irregular opacities in coal workers' pneumoconiosis – correlation with pulmonary function and pathology. Ann Occup Hyg 26: 767–787.

72. Rémy-Jardin M, Degreef JM, Beuscart R et al. Coal worker's pneumoconiosis: CT assessment in exposed workers and correlation with radiographic findings. Radiology 1990; 177: 363–371.

73. Bégin R, Ostiguy G, Fillion R, Colman N. Computed tomography scan in the early detection of silicosis. Am Rev Respir Dis 1991; 144: 697–705.

74. Rémy-Jardin M, Remy J, Farre I, Marquette CH. Computed tomography evaluation of silicosis and coal worker's pneumoconiosis. Radiol Clin North Am 1992; 30: 1155–1176

75. Brichet A, Wallaert B, Gosselin B et al. Fibrose interstitielle diffuse 'primitive' du mineur de charbon: une entité nouvelle? Rev Mat Respir 1997; 4: 277–285

76. Collins LC, Willing S, Bretz R et al. High-resolution CT in simple coal workers' pneumoconiosis. Lack of correlation with pulmonary function tests and arterial blood gas values. Chest 1993; 104: 1156–1162.

77. Bégin R, Bergeron D, Samson L et al. CT assessment of silicosis in exposed workers. AJR 1987; 148: 509–514.

78. Cochrane AL, Higgins ITT. Pulmonary ventilatory function of coal miners in various areas in relation to the X-ray category of pneumoconiosis. Br J Prev Soc Med 1961; 15: 1–11.

79. Morgan WKC, Haudelsman L, Kibelstis J et al. Ventilatory capacity and lung volumes of US coal miners. Arch Environ Health 1974; 28: 182–189.

80. Frans A, Veriter C, Brasseur L. Pulmonary diffusing capacity for carbon monoxide in simple CWP. Bull Physiopathol Respir (Nancy) 1975; 11: 479–502.

81. Morgan WKC, Burgess DB, Lapp NL et al. Hyperinflation of the lungs in coal miners. Thorax 1971; 26: 585.

82. Coggon D, Newman Taylor A. Coal mining and chronic obstructive pulmonary disease: a review of the evidence. Thorax 1998; 53: 398–407.

83. Lippmann M, Eckert HL, Hahon N, Morgan WKC. Circulating antinuclear and rheumatoid factor in coal miners. Ann Intern Med 1973; 79: 807–811.

84. Soutar CA, Turner-Warwick M, Parkes WR. Circulating antinuclear antibody and rheumatoid factor in coal miners. Br Med J 1974; 3: 145–147.

85. Hahon N, Morgan WKC, Petersen M. Serum immunoglobulin levels in coal workers' pneumoconiosis. Ann Occup Hyg 1980; 23: 165–174.

86. Robertson MD, Boyd JE, Collins HPR, Davis JMG. Serum immunoglobulin levels and humoral immune competence in coal workers. Am J Ind Med 1984; 6: 387–393.

87. Doll NJ, Stankus J, Hughes J et al. Immune complexes and autoantibodies in silicosis. J Allergy Clin Immunol 1981; 68: 281–285.

88. Wallaert B, Deflandre T, Ramon Ph, Voisin C. Serum angiotensin-converting enzyme in coal worker's pneumoconiosis. Chest 1985; 87: 844–845.

89. Lapp NL, Lewis D, Schwegler-Berry D et al. Bronchoalveolar lavage in asymptomatic underground coal miners. Chest 1990; 98: 67S.

90. Wallaert B, Lasalle P, Fortin F et al. superoxide anion generation by alveolar inflammatory cells in simple pneumoconiosis and in progressive massive fibrosis of non smoking coal workers. Am Rev Respir Dis 1990; 141: 129–133.

91. Voisin B, Gosselin P, Ramon B et al. Le lavage broncho-alvéolaire dans la pneumoconiose des mineurs de charbon. Rev Fr Mal Respir 1983; 11: 455–466.

92. Bégin R, Cantin A, Bolleau R, Bisson G. Spectrum of alveolitis in quartz-exposed human subjects. Chest 1987; 92: 1061–1067.

93. Carpenter GR, Cochrane AL, Clarke WG et al. Death rates of miners and ex-miners with and without CWP in South Wales. Br J Ind Med 1956; 13: 102–109.

94. Sadler RL. Attributability of death to pneumoconiosis in beneficiaries. Thorax 1974; 29: 699–702.

95. Cochrane AL, Haley TJL, Moore F, Hole D. The mortality of men in the Rhonda Fach 1950–1970. Br J Ind Med 1979; 36: 15–22.

96. McLintock JS, Rae S, Jacobsen M. The attack rate of progressive massive fibrosis in British coal miners. In Walton WH, ed. Inhaled particles III. Woking: Unwin Brothers; 1971: 933–950.

97. Morgan WKC. Industrial bronchitis. Br J Ind Med 1978; 35: 285–291.

98. Bates DV. The fate of the chronic bronchitic: a report of the ten-year follow-up in the Canadian Department of Veteran's Affairs coordinated study of chronic bronchitis. Am Rev Respir Dis 1973; 108: 1043.

99. Rae S, Walker DD, Attfield MD. Chronic bronchitis and dust exposure in British coalminers. Inhaled Part 1970; 2: 883–896.

100. Kibelstis JA, Morgan EJ, Reger R et al. Prevalence of bronchitis and airway obstruction in American bituminous coal miners. Am Rev Respir Dis 1973; 108: 886–893.

101. Marine WM, Guar D. Clinically important respiratory effects of dust exposure and smoking in British coal miners. Am Rev Respir Dis 1988; 137: 106–112.

102. Rogan JM, Attfield MD, Jacobsen MD et al. Role of dust in the working environment in development of chronic bronchitis in British coal miners. Br J Ind Med 1973; 34: 217–226.

103. Soutar CA, Hurley JF. Relation between dust exposure and lung function in miners and ex-miners. Br J Ind Med 1986; 43: 307–320.

104. Love RG, Miller BG. Longitudinal study of lung function in coal-miners. Thorax 1982; 37: 193–197.

105. Attfield MD. Longitudinal decline in FEV_1 in United States coalminers. Thorax 1995; 40: 132–137.

106. Wouters EFM, Jorna THJM, Westenend M. Respiratory effects of coal dust exposure: clinical effects and diagnosis. Exp Lung Res 1994; 20: 385–394.

107. Osler W. The principles and practice of medicine, 2nd ed. Edinburgh: Young & Pentland; 1895: 588.

108. Cummins SL. The pneumoconioses in South Wales. J Hyg 1936; 36: 547–548.

109. Ryder RC, Lyons JP, Campbell H, Gough J. Emphysema and coal worker's pneumoconiosis. Br Med J 1970; 3: 481–487.

110. Lyons JP, Ryder RC, Seal RM, Wagner JC. Emphysema in smoking and non-smoking coalworkers with pneumoconiosis. Bull Physiopathol Respir (Nancy) 1981; 17: 75–85.

111. Ruckley VA, Gauld SJ, Chapman JS et al. Emphysema and dust exposure in a group of coal workers. Am Rev Respir Dis 1984; 129: 528–532.

112. Fletcher C. Some observations of the bronchial and emphysematous types of patient with severe generalized airways obstruction. In: Cumming G, Hunt LB, ed. Form and function in the human lung. Baltimore, MD: Williams & Wilkins; 1968: 231.

113. Lapp NL, Seaton A. Lung mechanics in coal workers' pneumoconiosis. Ann NY Acad Sci 1972; 200: 433.

114. Seaton A. Coalmining, emphysema, and compensation. Editorial. Br J Ind Med 1990; 47: 433–435.

115. Ruckley VA, Fernie JM, Campbell SJ, Cowie HA. Causes of disability in coal miners: a clinico-pathological study of emphysema, airways obstruction and massive fibrosis. Institute of occupational Medicine, Report No. TM-89/05. Edinburgh: Institute of Occupational Medicine; 1989.

116. Cochrane AL. Relation between radiographic categories of coalworker's pneumoconiosis and expectation of life. Br Med J 1973; 2: 532–534.

117. LeRoy Lapp N, Parker JE. Coal workers' pneumoconiosis. In: Epler GR, ed. Clinics in chest medicine vol 13 part 2. Occupational lung diseases. London: WB Saunders; 1992: 243–252.

118. Beckett W, Abraham J, Becklake M et al. Adverse effects of crystalline silica exposure (Official Statement of ATS). Am J Respir Crit Care Med 1997; 155: 761–765.

119. National Institute for Occupational Safety and Health. Criteria for a recommended standard: occupational exposure to respirable coal mine dust. Publication 95–106. Cincinnati, OH: National Institute for Occupational Safety and Health; 1995.

120. Rihs HP, Lipps P, May-Taube K et al. Immunogenetic studies on HLA-DR in German coal miners with and without coal workers' pneumoconiosis. Lung 1994; 172: 347–354.

121. Schins RPF, Borm J. Mechanisms and mediators in coal dust induced toxicity: a review. Ann Occup Hyg 1999 43: 7–33.

122. Piguet PF, Collart MA, Grau GE et al. Requirement of tumour necrosis factor for development of silica-induced pulmonary fibrosis. Nature 1990; 344: 245–247.

123. Piguet PF, Vesin C. Treatment by human recombinant soluble TNF receptor of pulmonary fibrosis induced by bleomycin or silica in mice. Eur Respir J 1994; 7: 515–518.

124. Zhai R, Jetten M, Schins RP et al. Polymorphisms in the promoter of the tumor necrosis factor alpha in coal miners. Ann Ind Med 1998; 34: 318–324.

125. Schins RPF, Borm JPA. Plasma level of soluble tumor necrosis factor receptors are increased in coal miners with pneumoconiosis. Eur Respir J1995; 8: 1658–1663.

126. Jacobsen M. Progression of coal workers' pneumoconiosis in Britain in relation to environmental conditions underground. Proceedings of a Conference on Technical Measures of Dust Prevention and suppression in Mines. Luxembourg: Commission of the European Communities; 1973: 77–93.

27 Asbestos-related disease

Robin M Rudd

Key points

- All types of asbestos cause asbestosis, benign pleural disease, mesothelioma and lung cancer.

- Amphiboles are more carcinogenic than chrysotile.

- The risk of development of all asbestos-induced diseases increases with dose.

- Asbestosis requires much higher doses of asbestos than the minimum necessary to cause mesothelioma and benign pleural disease.

- Asbestos-induced disease seldom appears less than 20 years after first exposure.

'Asbestos' is a term used to describe a number of naturally occurring fibrous mineral silicates whose fire-resistant properties have been recognised for thousands of years.

Types of asbestos fibre

In medical literature a particle with a length-to-breadth ratio of 3:1 or more has generally been accepted as a fibre. Asbestos fibres are of two main types: serpentine fibres, which are curly and flexible, and amphibole fibres, which are straight and stiff. The only important example of the serpentine group is chrysotile (white asbestos). The industrially important members of the amphibole group are crocidolite (blue) and amosite (brown or grey). Other amphiboles include tremolite, a common contaminant of chrysotile, and anthophyllite, which has limited commercial value but was a common contaminant of talc in industrial use.

Commercial use of asbestos

In the mid-19th century the discovery of large deposits of asbestos in Canada and South Africa led to its large-scale exploitation. This accelerated with the development of techniques for spinning and weaving the fibres. During the first four decades of the 20th century the uses of asbestos multiplied, mainly for its properties of fire resistance and poor conduction of heat, electricity and sound.

In the UK and other industrial countries, heavy exposure of workers to asbestos occurred in several industries. Dockers unloaded asbestos in sacks that leaked and split. Factories manufactured asbestos textiles, cement and friction materials such as brake and clutch linings. Asbestos was used in many forms to insulate pipes and boilers in ships, power stations, factories and other large buildings. Tradesmen in ship building and repair such as welders, platers, plumbers and electricians sustained 'neighbourhood exposure' to asbestos used by insulators ('laggers') and carpenters frequently cut asbestos sheets. Construction workers frequently had similar neighbourhood exposure and are accounting for an increasing proportion of cases of asbestos disease. In earlier times, masks were seldom available to the workers in any industry and even if they were offered they usually consisted of a simple gauze filter, which provided inadequate protection. In the UK the Asbestos Industry Regulations 1931 was the first legislation to control asbestos exposure at work. Stricter controls were imposed by the Asbestos Industry Regulations 1969 but it was often not until the early to mid-1970s that adequate respirators and precautions, such as exhaust ventilation and vacuum cleaning rather than sweeping to remove waste asbestos, became usual practice.

Exposure to undisturbed asbestos in buildings has been suggested to carry a negligible risk of disease, on the assumptions that chrysotile would be the only fibre involved and that surfaces would be well maintained to prevent shedding of dust.[1] Unfortunately, amphiboles have been used in ceiling and wall coverings that are still in place and removal is costly. In the UK the Control of Asbestos at Work Regulations 1987 require the use of respirators, protective clothing and decontamination procedures at the end of a shift for asbestos removal workers. The Control Limits for exposure averaged over 4 hours are for amosite and crocidolite 0.2 and for chrysotile 0.5 fibres per millilitre of air. These represent a tiny fraction of the levels of hundreds of fibres per millilitre encountered in dusty industries in the past. Nevertheless, they should not be regarded as 'safe' levels but levels calculated to give an 'acceptably' low risk of death.[1]

Annual imports of asbestos into the UK reached a peak in 1973 and declined thereafter, particularly after 1979 when the Advisory Committee on Asbestos recommended its gradual substitution by other materials, a ban on the use of sprayed asbestos and control of the asbestos removal industry.[2] In the UK the Asbestos (Prohibition) Regulations 1985 banned the importation, supply and use of amosite and crocidolite and in 1999 an amendment to the regulations extended them to chrysotile, with certain exceptions in safety specific areas until 1 January 2005, by which date the marketing and use of all asbestos will be illegal throughout the European Union. The use of asbestos has also virtually ceased in North America but its use is still widespread throughout the developing world and in countries of the former Soviet Union.

The fate of inhaled asbestos particles

The maximum diameter of respirable particles lies between $3\,\mu m$ and $3.5\,\mu m$. Shorter, thinner fibres have a greater chance of penetrating to the lung periphery and most fibres found in lung tissue are less than $50\,\mu m$ in length, although fibres up to $200\,\mu m$ can be identified. Chrysotile, because of its curly configuration, has a relatively broad cross-sectional area and penetrates less readily to the periphery than the needle-like amphiboles.

Most fibres are removed by mucociliary clearance or via the lymphatics after being partially or completely engulfed by macrophages and by epithelial cells lining the airways. Chrysotile is cleared more effectively than the other fibre types, perhaps because of its tendency to separate into tiny fibres and to dissolve in weakly acid environments. Of those fibres that remain in the lung, some become coated with the iron-containing protein ferritin to form asbestos bodies, also known as ferruginous bodies (Fig. 27.1). The tendency to become coated varies with fibre type and size, being greatest for larger amphibole fibres and least for chrysotile.[3] It may be that only fibres too large to be engulfed

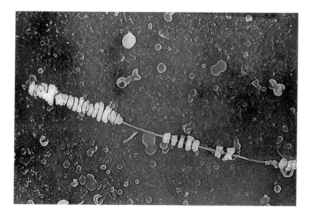

Fig. 27.1 Electron micrograph showing an asbestos body. The coating is gradually built up in segmental fashion.

by a single macrophage become coated, as bodies seldom form on fibres shorter than $10\,\mu m$. Individual subjects vary in their propensity to coat fibres. The coating of the fibre probably renders it less pathogenic.

Asbestosis

Definition

Asbestosis was defined by the Advisory Committee on Asbestos (1979)[4] as 'fibrosis of the lungs caused by asbestos dusts which may or may not be associated with fibrosis of the parietal or pulmonary layer of the pleura'.

Epidemiology

The interval between the onset of exposure to asbestos and the development of symptoms of asbestosis is commonly 20 years or longer, although in earlier years, when continuous extremely heavy exposure occurred, fibrosis occasionally became evident as early as 5 years after the first exposure. New lung and pleural lesions continue to appear more than 40 years after first exposure.[5] Asbestos fibres remain in the lungs for long periods, many permanently, and disease may appear and progress long after exposure has ceased.

Because of the reduction in exposure from the 1970s onwards the incidence in the UK is declining and there are fewer new cases of asbestosis than of mesothelioma.

Dose and response

The long latent period contributes to the difficulty in determining the attack rate among exposed persons and its relation to the dose of asbestos inhaled. Other problems arise from the paucity of studies in which more than a crude estimate of exposure is provided and the fact that many workers were involved with asbestos for relatively short periods, subsequently moving on to other industries.

The frequency and severity of asbestosis increase with increasing dose of asbestos.[6] Dose comprises the product of intensity of exposure in fibres per millilitre and duration of exposure in working years. There is a threshold dose for the development of clinical asbestosis which is probably around 25 fibres/ml · years.[1] The dose of asbestos is not the sole determining factor for the development of asbestosis.[7,8] Immune and non-immune related genes are important in determining susceptibility to experimental interstitial lung disease and may well play a part in determining the response to inhaled asbestos.[9]

Fibre types and dimensions

All types of asbestos fibre are fibrogenic. Animal experiments suggest that chrysotile is at least as fibrogenic as the amphiboles[10,11] but in the human situation the much greater biopersistence of amphiboles than chrysotile probably accounts for the greater tendency to progression of asbestosis caused by amphiboles.

Experimentally, long thin fibres are more fibrogenic than short fibres but human studies have not demonstrated any systematic difference in fibre sizes between subjects with and without asbestosis. This may be partly a consequence of smoking, which interferes with clearance of short more than long fibres, thereby increasing effective dose of short fibres so that they play an increased part in fibrogenesis. Tobacco smoke also increases fibre uptake by pulmonary epithelial cells, resulting in cell damage and cytokine production.[12]

Pathogenesis

In animal models of the disease the deposition of inhaled asbestos particles in respiratory bronchioles and alveoli is followed by accumulation of alveolar macrophages. Incomplete phagocytosis of asbestos fibres by macrophages may result in release of lysosomal enzymes, soluble fibrogenic factors, cytokines and oxygen free radicals. Both inflammation and fibrosis as well as expression of genes linked to cell proliferation and antioxidant defence occur in a dose-related fashion after inhalation of asbestos.[13] Whereas lower intensity exposure evokes reversible inflammatory lesions consisting of focal aggregations of mineral-laden alveolar macrophages without disruption of the normal architecture of the lung, higher exposure causes intense inflammatory changes, cell proliferation in various compartments of the lung, and excessive deposition of collagen and other extracellular matrix components by mesenchymal cells.

Current ideas on the cellular mechanisms underlying the pathogenesis of asbestosis have been reviewed in detail.[12,14] Reactive oxygen species such as hydrogen peroxide, superoxide anion and the hydroxyl radical, and reactive nitrogen species induced by the presence of asbestos are probably important mediators of toxicity.[14] The molecular targets of asbestos and its second messengers, reactive oxygen species and reactive nitrogen species, include critical biological macromolecules such as lipid membranes, DNA and signal transduction proteins. In addition, various cell types of the immune system, including neutrophils, T-lymphocytes and mast cells, accumulate in interstitial regions and are implicated in the development of cell injury, proliferation, apoptosis and fibrosis.[12]

Smoking increases the risk of development of radiographic signs suggesting asbestosis[15] and of progression of asbestosis,[16] and animal studies have provided evidence for a synergistic effect.[17]

Various immunological abnormalities have been reported in asbestosis. Elevation of serum immunoglobulins IgG, IgA and IgM is common and an increased prevalence of circulating autoantibodies has been reported. Antinuclear factor occurred in 25% and rheumatoid factor in 23% of subjects with asbestosis in one series, but each occurred in less than 3% of those with asbestos exposure but not asbestosis.[18] Other studies, many of which were inadequately controlled, have given different results.[19] Whether these antibodies are involved in pathogenesis or whether they are epiphenomena remains uncertain.

Lung structure is probably also important in determining individual susceptibility. A case control study in Quebec showed that cases were shorter than controls, possibly because shorter men have shorter tracheas that are less effective in trapping inhaled fibres, so that more fibres reach alveolar areas.[20] Differences between subjects in retention of asbestos fibres probably contribute to differences in susceptibility to disease.[21]

Pathology

The changes of asbestosis are usually more pronounced in the lower lobes, but often extend to involve the middle lobe and lingula. In advanced cases the upper lobes may be involved and in exceptional cases the upper lobes are most severely involved.[22] In advanced disease there may be honeycombing as in end-stage lung fibrosis of other causes.[23] Visceral pleural thickening is commonly, but by no means always, present and hyaline plaques are present in less than half the cases.

The earliest changes of asbestosis seen microscopically consist of peribronchiolar and alveolar fibrosis. This often occurs in islands preferentially distributed in the subpleural regions. Areas of fibrosis enlarge and coalesce, eventually obliterating the alveolar architecture. Asbestos bodies are usually seen within and adjacent to areas of fibrosis (Fig. 27.2). Occasionally, electron microscopy may demonstrate substantial numbers of uncoated fibres when asbestos bodies are few or absent on light microscopy.[24] This is particularly likely to occur when exposure has been mainly or exclusively to chrysotile fibres, on which asbestos bodies seldom form.

In the UK the severity of fibrosis is often graded according to a five-point scale: none, minimal, slight, moderate and severe.[25] Minimal and slight asbestosis detected microscopically are commonly not detectable by clinical and radiological signs. In the USA a more complex grading scheme has been proposed.[23]

Pathophysiology

As in other interstitial fibrotic lung diseases there is a reduction in pulmonary compliance and disordered gas exchange arising mainly from disturbances of the distribution of ventilation and perfusion (see 'Lung function tests' below).

Clinical features

Presentation

Patients usually present with shortness of breath on exertion of insidious onset. A cough that is dry or productive of scanty mucoid sputum is present in the majority of cases and may become more prominent as the disease advances.

Physical findings

Late inspiratory fine crackles are localised at first to the posterior or posterolateral aspects of the lower zones and gradually become more widespread as the disease progresses. Crackles may be heard before radiographic evidence of asbestosis appears.[26] Occasionally, crackles may be absent despite radiographic evidence of lung disease.

Clubbing of the fingers occurs in a proportion of cases that has been variously reported as from 20% to more than 80%. In one UK series there was clubbing at presentation in 43% of

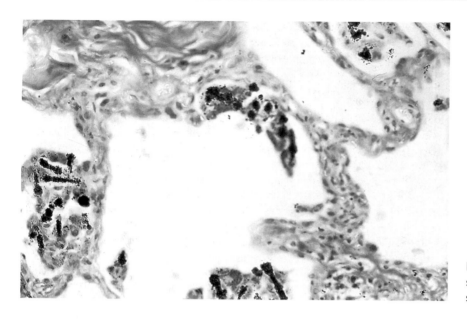

Fig. 27.2 Histological section showing asbestosis. There is fibrous thickening of the alveolar septa associated with asbestos bodies.

cases and it seldom developed subsequently.[27] Cyanosis and cor pulmonale may occur when fibrosis is advanced.

Investigations

Radiography

The most common radiographic features of asbestosis are scattered small opacities, usually irregular and small, between 2 mm and 4 mm in diameter.[28] Smaller rounded opacities occur less frequently. Short horizontal lines are frequently seen above the costophrenic angles and may be the earliest sign of the disease. A diffuse haziness is less commonly seen. A 'shaggy' cardiac outline may occur. Honeycomb or ring shadows also occur in more advanced disease. There is a marked lower zone predominance, although the middle zones are involved also in more than 50% (Fig. 27.3). The upper zones are involved as well in a quarter of cases. The profusion of shadows may be scored using

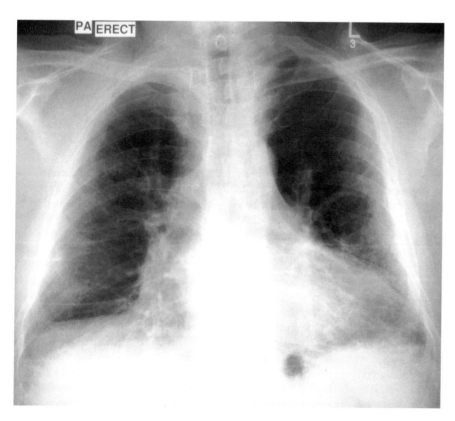

Fig. 27.3 Chest radiograph showing asbestosis. The shadowing is most profuse in the lower zones.

the ILO (International Labour Organization) classification of radiographs, which makes use of a set of standard radiographs illustrating each profusion category[29] (see Chapter 26).

Pleural changes are present in the majority of cases with intrapulmonary shadowing: 75% in one series.[28] The most common features are band-like shadowing along the lateral chest wall and irregularity of the diaphragm, sometimes with calcification. Pleural plaques may be seen along the chest wall and overlying the lung fields. Pleural shadows are often better demonstrated in oblique views which also facilitate assessment of the lung fields when there is overlying pleural disease.

Computed tomography

Computed tomography is more sensitive than conventional radiography in detecting both pleural and parenchymal lung disease[30,31] (Fig. 27.4). High-resolution computed tomography (HRCT) of the thorax, i.e. a scan performed using a thin slice (1–3 mm) technique and a bone algorithm, is more sensitive than routine computed tomography using 10 mm slices with a soft tissue algorithm in detecting asbestosis and pleural disease.[32]

An early feature of asbestosis is a subpleural curvilinear opacity, usually first seen in the posterior parts of the lower lobes.[33] A study that correlated HRCT and histological findings showed that these opacities represent peribronchiolar fibrosis, generally regarded as the earliest histological lesion of asbestosis, while band-shaped opacities represent fibrosis along bronchovascular sheaths or interlobular septa.[34] Minimal asbestosis may be associated with only focal interstitial thickening and in some cases of histologically confirmed asbestosis the HRCT may show normal or near-normal appearances.[35]

Scans in the supine and prone positions allow assessment of the gravity dependence of perfusion. Posterior basal subpleural

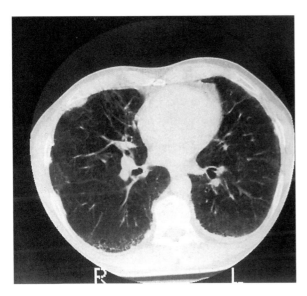

Fig. 27.4 High-resolution computed tomography scan showing posterior basal subpleural reticular opacification with small cysts, particularly in the right lung, indicating mild asbestosis, scattered pleural plaques and posterior pleural thickening, well-marked around the left lung.

curvilinear opacities which are seen in the supine view but which disappear in the prone view are generally regarded as representing gravity-dependent distribution of perfusion rather than evidence of asbestosis. However, the presence of gravity dependent fine 'pencil line' as distinct from ill-defined subpleural lines may be associated with persistent fine inspiratory crackles detected by computerised lung sound analysis, suggesting that these lines may in fact represent very early interstitial fibrosis.[36]

Although an HRCT scan is not essential in the assessment of asbestosis, it is helpful in the detection of early disease and in the assessment of the lungs when there is extensive pleural disease. It is also useful in deciding whether impairment of carbon monoxide transfer should be attributed to emphysema, asbestosis or both in a breathless asbestos worker who has been a smoker.[37] An HRCT scan may also assist in distinguishing asbestosis from cryptogenic fibrosing alveolitis in cases where the occupational history is unclear as to the extent of asbestos exposure. Pleural plaques or thickening can be detected by HRCT in more than 80% of cases of asbestosis and are not found in cryptogenic fibrosing alveolitis. Band-like opacities, often merging with the pleura, are common in asbestosis but uncommon in cryptogenic fibrosing alveolitis while extensive reticulation, ground-glass opacification and upper zone involvement are more common in cryptogenic fibrosing alveolitis than asbestosis.[38] In asbestosis, mediastinal lymph node enlargement can commonly be detected by HRCT,[39] although this feature can also be seen in other interstitial lung diseases.

Lung function tests

Lung function tests show features of interstitial fibrotic lung disease – a restrictive ventilatory defect and impairment of gas transfer. The latter is usually manifested in a reduction in both the carbon monoxide transfer factor (T_LCO) and coefficient (KCO). However, if there is sufficient pleural thickening to contribute to restriction of expansion of the lungs the KCO may be normal or even increased although the T_LCO is reduced. Evidence of airflow limitation is also commonly present.[40] In advanced asbestosis there may not be a typical restrictive pattern, because of an increase in residual volume and consequently in total lung capacity resulting from small airway narrowing.[41]

Lung function impairment correlates well with the extent of pulmonary fibrosis and pleural disease as assessed by plain radiography.[42,43] Asbestosis detectable by HRCT but not by plain radiography is associated with minor reductions in FVC and T_LCO and with a higher dyspnoea score than in subjects without asbestosis.[31] Emphysema, as quantified by HRCT, also frequently contributes to impairment of lung function in asbestos workers, who have usually been smokers.[38]

Exercise testing

Exercise testing on a cycle ergometer or treadmill may be useful in demonstrating physiological disturbances in symptomatic patients with early disease in whom routine lung function test results are within normal limits. There is usually an excessive increase in ventilation in relation to oxygen consumption, reflecting reduced compliance with a consequent increase in the V_D/V_T ratio (proportion of tidal volume ventilating dead space). There is commonly a rise in the $AaPO_2$ (alveolar–arterial PO_2 gradient) on exercise, reflecting disturbed gas exchange. In one study there was a significant although weak correlation between the percentage disability assessed by submaximal exercise test and the assessment of total cardiorespiratory disability by a medical board ($r = 0.51$) but a poor correlation between the exercise test and breathlessness grade.[44] Factors such as mood and attitude play an important part in determining clinical disability.

Sputum examination

The presence of asbestos bodies in sputum indicates occupational exposure but not necessarily the presence of disease. However, sputum examination is an unreliable means of determining whether exposure has occurred and bronchoalveolar lavage is more sensitive.[45]

Bronchoalveolar lavage

There is commonly an increase in total cell counts and a reduced percentage of macrophages, reflecting an increased percentage of one or more of the other cell types. An increase in neutrophils, with or without an increase in eosinophils, occurs in about half of patients while in just under a third increased lymphocyte percentages are seen.[46] The cell profile is different from that seen in subjects with asbestos exposure but without clinical and radiological evidence of asbestosis, who more frequently have increased lymphocytes and less frequently have increased neutrophils.[47]

Asbestos body counts in BAL fluid correlate with asbestos body counts in lung parenchyma,[48] and with the extent of exposure as assessed by occupational history.[49] The number detectable declines after cessation of exposure, probably because of clearance of asbestos from the lungs. Asbestos bodies are rarely found in BAL fluid from patients with interstitial lung diseases other than asbestosis,[50] indicating that exposure to asbestos from ordinary air pollution is seldom sufficient to give rise to asbestos bodies in BAL samples.[48,51]

Lung biopsy

Transbronchial biopsy using larger forceps occasionally provides sufficient material for a diagnosis of asbestosis but a finding of non-specific inflammation or fibrosis may reflect only sampling error and should not be taken as evidence against a diagnosis of asbestosis. Thoracoscopic lung biopsy is less traumatic than open lung biopsy, which is an alternative procedure (see 'Diagnostic strategy' below).

Histological diagnosis

Histological diagnosis may be required in the interpretation of lung biopsy specimens or, more frequently, of postmortem specimens obtained after a death has been reported as possibly due to industrial disease.

There is a lack of uniformity of the minimum histological criteria for the diagnosis of asbestosis. Not uncommonly in the UK

a diagnosis of cryptogenic fibrosing alveolitis is suggested on the grounds that there are too few asbestos bodies present for asbestosis. However, minimum criteria defined in the USA require only discrete foci of fibrosis in the walls of respiratory bronchioles associated with more than one asbestos body.[23] Although asbestos bodies can be found in persons without known exposure because of atmospheric pollution, it can be calculated that an average of 100 sections would have to be examined to find a single asbestos body in a member of the general population.[52] Hence, if even one body is seen in the presence of diffuse interstitial fibrosis, the odds favour a diagnosis of asbestosis.[53]

Light microscopic fibre counts

The fibre burden in the lungs may be assessed by a fibre count performed on digested lung tissue.[54] The results are usually expressed as the number of fibres per gram of dry lung tissue. Fibres are counted by phase-contrast light microscopy, which improves the visibility of uncoated fibres. In control subjects without occupational exposure counts are usually less than 20 000 fibres per gram of dried lung.[55]

In asbestosis, mean total fibre counts have varied greatly in different series, probably reflecting different exposure experiences and interlaboratory variation.[54-56] There is some correlation between severity of fibrosis and fibre counts.

Electron microscopic fibre counts

Electron microscopy can demonstrate the presence of fibres too small to be seen by light microscopy. Estimates of the proportion of fibres demonstrated by electron microscopy that are visible by light microscopy have varied widely, e.g. 12–30%[54] and much less than 1%.[56] The proportion visible by light microscopy would be expected to increase with increasing time since cessation of exposure because of preferential clearance from the lung of shorter, uncoated fibres. The proportion visible by light microscopy is much lower for chrysotile than amphiboles because fewer fibres are coated.

Fibres can be counted in lung tissue by scanning electron microscopy (SEM) and by transmission electron microscopy (TEM). The latter technique gives higher fibre counts because it can detect smaller fibres. The identity of an asbestos fibre can be determined by X-ray energy dispersive microanalysis (XEDS) or less satisfactorily by X-ray diffraction. XEDS determines the elemental composition of the fibre and, by comparison with standard samples of various fibre types, the identity of the fibre can be established.[57] A differential count can be obtained by analysis of a number of fibres.

Electron microscopic fibre counts in subjects with no documented asbestos exposure are generally low, as shown in Table 27.1.[58,59] It is important to note that counts from different parts of the same lung may vary widely[58,60,61] and caution should be exercised in interpretation of a count on a single sample.[62]

Relationships have been demonstrated between histological grades of asbestosis and electron microscopic fibre counts.[56,63,64] Correlations were found between the severity of fibrosis and the number of amphibole fibres but not the number of chrysotile fibres. Within each grade of asbestosis, however, there were considerable variations in the counts. The total counts ranged from less than 10^6 to 10^9 per gram of dry lung in grade 1–2 asbestosis, and from less than 10^7 to 10^{10} in grades 3–4.

Table 27.1 Electron microscopic fibre counts* in subjects not known to have been exposed to asbestos; tissue obtained at post-mortem examination[58,59]

	Cardiff, sex unspecified, n = 55 Geometric mean (range)	Various areas, females, n = 31 Geometric mean (range)
Crocidolite	0.02 (0–1.7)	0.02 (0–0.5)
Amosite	0.02 (0–1.0)	0.02 (0–0.5)
Chrysotile	1.4 (0–11.7)	4.4 (0–20.1)

* $\times 10^6$ fibres per gram of dry lung.

A fibre count by electron microscopy is of diagnostic value in cases of interstitial lung fibrosis in which there is a questionable history of asbestos exposure and asbestos bodies are not seen by light microscopy. The tendency to form asbestos bodies on asbestos fibres varies and in some cases light microscopy may show few or no asbestos bodies whereas substantial numbers of uncoated fibres may be demonstrated by electron microscopy.[24] The demonstration of asbestos fibre counts within the range found in asbestosis in the same laboratory favours a diagnosis of asbestosis but a count well below that range favours an alternative diagnosis.[65,66]

Diagnostic strategy

In many cases the diagnosis is reasonably secure on the basis of a history of exposure, clinical features and radiological signs. If there is doubt additional information may be obtained from HRCT scanning and from BAL. In the unusual case where doubt still remains a lung biopsy may be indicated, mainly to exclude the possibility of other and more easily treatable conditions. If interstitial fibrosis is confirmed on lung biopsy but asbestos bodies are not visible, a fibre count, preferably by electron microscopy, is helpful.

Management

Prevention of further exposure

Prevention of further exposure is obviously advisable but action to achieve this is seldom required. Large quantities of asbestos inhaled in the past remain in the lungs of patients with asbestosis. Levels of exposure currently permitted in Western counties are orders of magnitude lower than those experienced in earlier years and would not cause asbestosis or materially contribute to worsening of pre-existing asbestosis. Thus there is no overriding reason to remove from work an insulation engineer who strips old asbestos lagging while wearing full protective clothing and a positive pressure respirator and who is consequently not exposed to higher than permitted levels. Many sufferers from the disease are, however, understandably very anxious and prefer not to continue in work involving any contact with asbestos, even with full protective equipment. Many employers are reluctant to take on or to continue to employ sufferers from asbestos-induced diseases in work involving any contact with asbestos.

Drug treatment

Because substantial numbers of asbestos fibres remain in the lungs of those affected, and cannot be removed, any treatment must be directed towards suppression of the response to the fibres. Asbestosis is generally regarded as resistant to drug treatment. There are, however, no controlled comparisons of the outcome in those given drug treatment and those left untreated. Because the disease is in many cases only slowly progressive, such a trial would have to be carried out over a very long period and would be a difficult undertaking.

In the uncommon cases with evidence of more rapid than average disease progression, e.g. as manifested by increasing breathlessness and deterioration in lung function over a period of a few months and perhaps with evidence of an active 'alveolitis' on HRCT or BAL, corticosteroids and immunosuppressive drugs such as cyclophosphamide or azathioprine in regimens similar to those employed for cryptogenic fibrosing alveolitis occasionally lead to improvement.

Follow-up

Regular follow-up at intervals of not more than 1 year is advisable for patients with asbestosis. They are at a substantial risk of lung cancer, which may be operable if detected at an early stage. Most patients gain reassurance from regular medical supervision and periodic reassessment of disability is also useful in relation to compensation arrangements.

Prognosis and complications

Asbestosis usually progresses relentlessly, leading to increasing breathlessness and disability. Progression is, however, usually slow and may cease, sometimes to resume after a quiescent interval. Occasionally, progression is more rapid and the disease follows a course similar to that of the more aggressive forms of cryptogenic fibrosing alveolitis.

Several factors are related to the likelihood and rate of progression. Clubbing of the fingers is associated with a greater likelihood of more severe and more rapidly progressive disease.[27] Those with less severe radiological profusion and lesser impairment of lung function at presentation are less likely to show progression in the short to medium term. Smoking accelerates progression of disease.[67] BAL findings relate to rate of deterioration; patients with higher proportions of lymphocytes deteriorate less rapidly than those with increased proportions of neutrophils and eosinophils, as assessed by gas transfer and chest radiograph.[67]

The disease as seen today is on average much less severe than in earlier years when it followed much heavier exposure. Consequently, death from respiratory failure and cor pulmonale has become infrequent and sufferers tend to survive longer, eventually often dying of malignancy.[68] A study from the Factory Inspectorate of England and Wales found that, among men in whom the death certificate recorded the presence of asbestosis, the proportion who also had lung cancer or pleural tumours increased from 19.7% for the period 1931–40 to 54.5% for 1961–63.[69] A study of 665 men with asbestosis diagnosed by the UK Pneumoconiosis Medical Panel between 1952 and 1976 found that, of 283 deaths, 39% were due to lung cancer and 9% were due to mesothelioma.[70] In this study the main factor influencing prognosis was the clinical state at the time of examination. For a man aged 55 years it was estimated that life expectation would be reduced by 3, 5, 8 or 12 years according to whether his disability had been assessed at 10%, 20%, 30–40% or 50% or more respectively. In another study of 59 deaths in asbestosis, 39% were due to lung cancer and 10% were due to mesothelioma.[71] Perhaps because of the relatively small numbers and high mortality from malignant diseases, increasing profusion of small opacities on the chest radiograph did not predict prognosis, a finding in contrast to other studies.[72,73]

Asbestos-induced airway disease

Most asbestos workers are or have been smokers and this undoubtedly contributes to the commonly seen airflow limitation, although smoking is not the whole explanation. Evidence of small-airways dysfunction has been found in asbestos workers who have never smoked, in studies including unexposed non-smoking control subjects.[74,75] Patients with asbestos-related pleural thickening or plaques commonly have evidence of airflow limitation, even when non-smokers, reflecting asbestos airway disease.[76] This is rarely of sufficient degree to cause breathlessness, however. A predominantly obstructive ventilatory defect occurs in some patients with asbestosis, including some who have never smoked.[40] As fibrosis progresses there is not uncommonly a rise in residual volume, suggesting airflow limitation.

On the basis of observations in an animal model it has been suggested that an asbestos-induced inflammatory and fibrotic reaction compresses the small airways.[77] A study of 36 long-term chrysotile miners without asbestosis found evidence of severe diffuse small-airway abnormalities.[78] A further study of 17 lifetime non-smoking asbestos workers, seven of whom had asbestosis, showed evidence of small-airway dysfunction, which was more marked in those with asbestosis than in those without.[79]

Benign pleural disease

Asbestos causes several types of benign pleural disease: pleural plaque, diffuse pleural thickening and pleurisy with or without effusion.

Pleural plaques

Definition

Plaques are circumscribed areas of thickening of the parietal pleura of the chest wall, mediastinum and diaphragm. Occasionally they affect the visceral pleura, including that in the fissures.

Epidemiology

Pleural plaques are strongly associated with a history of asbestos exposure, both occupational and non-occupational, and are the commonest asbestos-induced condition. They can occur after a much lower dose of asbestos than is necessary to cause asbestosis. Plaques are occasionally apparent radiologically in subjects without identifiable asbestos exposure. Plaques have a higher prevalence at autopsy than on radiographic surveys because autopsy is more sensitive for their detection and because autopsy populations involve older subjects. Among an urban population the frequency and extent of plaques at autopsy increases in relation to lung asbestos fibre content.[80] Among occupationally exposed persons the prevalence of plaques increases in relation to the degree of asbestos exposure and in relation to the time elapsed since first exposure.[81] They occur after inhalation of all types of asbestos, although anthophyllite appears to be the most potent. Plaques occur with increased frequency in populations living in areas where the soil is contaminated with asbestiform minerals, for example in areas of Finland, Bulgaria, Czechoslovakia, Turkey and Greece, and in those living in proximity to asbestos mines or factories. Pleural plaques are apparent seldom, and calcified plaques rarely, on plain chest radiographs less than 20 years after first exposure to asbestos.[82]

Aetiology and pathogenesis

The route by which asbestos fibres reach the parietal pleura has not been fully elucidated. Suggestions include retrograde flow in the lymphatic system and direct penetration from the lung across the pleura. Amphibole fibres that have migrated directly through the visceral pleura may be reabsorbed into the parietal pleura through 'black spots' located near lymphatic vessels, at which anthracotic pigment also accumulates in coal miners.[83] The accumulation of amphiboles in such areas may explain the susceptibility of the parietal pleura to plaque formation and mesothelioma. The way in which fibres provoke localised fibrosis of the pleura resulting in formation of a plaque as distinct from diffuse pleural fibrosis is incompletely understood.[84]

Pathology

Plaques appear as grey-white areas, usually on the parietal pleura of the chest wall, the diaphragm, the pericardium and the mediastinum. The lesions are commonly bilateral. They may follow the contour of a rib, be disc-shaped or irregular. The thickness of the plaques may vary from a millimetre or two to a centimetre or more.

Plaques are composed of featureless hyalinised fibrous tissue. Calcification is common. Asbestos bodies can usually be found in the lung tissue and electron microscopy may demonstrate small numbers of uncoated asbestos fibres within the plaques.

Association with asbestosis

The frequency with which plaques are associated with asbestosis is higher in more heavily exposed than in less heavily exposed populations. Histological examination of the lung at post mortem reveals asbestosis in a higher proportion of cases than had been apparent on radiological examination. In a series of 56 cases selected on the basis that pleural plaques were identified at postmortem examination there had been clinical evidence of asbestosis in 16 (29%) and histological evidence of asbestosis was found in a further eight (14%).[85]

Pathophysiology

Pleural plaques do not usually cause symptomatic impairment of lung function. If their extent is great, the plaques may fuse to form sheets, which can interfere with the expansion of the lungs by making the chest wall and diaphragm stiff and resistant to movement. Plaques are frequently associated with evidence of limitation to airflow in the small airways[74,76] and with minor reductions in vital capacity[86,87] but these abnormalities are of insufficient magnitude to be a plausible cause of symptoms.

Clinical features

Usually, pleural plaques are an incidental finding on the chest radiograph, whether this is performed for routine employment health screening or some other purpose. In the unusual case where the plaques are very extensive and fused to form a cuirass-like structure, or where there are adhesions, they may give rise to shortness of breath on exertion. Rarely, pleuritic pain occurs, probably caused by adhesions, and occasionally extensively calcified plaques may give rise to an uncomfortable grating sensation during breathing, which may be audible on auscultation.

Investigations

Radiology

Pleural plaques are commonly seen in profile on the posteroanterior radiograph but are better shown in oblique views. Plaques are usually bilateral but unilateral plaques are not uncommon, constituting 19.3% of definite and 33.9% of probable plaques in one study.[88] Among subjects with unilateral plaques there is an unexplained left sided predominance.[88,89] They appear as ill-defined protrusions along the inner aspect of the rib cage which must be distinguished from normal 'companion shadows' caused by intercostal muscles or fat. Plaques may also be seen face-on as a vague haziness or, if they are calcified, as an irregular 'holly leaf' or 'candle-grease' pattern (Fig. 27.5). Diaphragmatic plaques may be gross or manifested only as an irregularity of the outline or as a sliver of calcification. Postmortem studies show that plaques of minor extent are frequently not detected by radiological examination.[85] Radiological evidence of interstitial

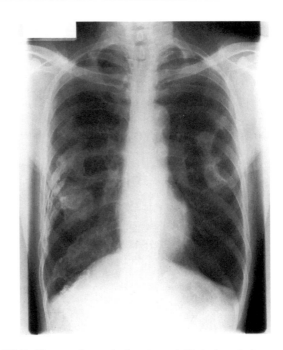

Fig. 27.5 Chest radiograph showing calcified pleural plaques.

lung disease representing asbestosis is present in addition in a minority of cases.

Computed tomography

Computed tomography demonstrates the extent of pleural plaques more accurately than does a plain radiograph. Multiple plaques visually superimposed upon each other may be impossible to distinguish from diffuse pleural thickening on the plain radiograph but the CT scan allows differentiation.[90] It may also reveal evidence of intrapulmonary fibrosis that was not evident on the plain radiograph.

Management, prognosis and complications

There is no treatment for pleural plaques. Pleural plaques are not themselves precursors of malignant change but, in so far as they reflect asbestos exposure, they are associated with an increased risk of asbestos-induced benign and malignant diseases. Among 155 dockyard workers who were re-examined 10 years after detection of benign pleural changes, mostly plaques, 10.3% had small parenchymal opacities and 4.5% had both clinical and radiological signs of asbestosis.[91] The attack rate was substantially higher than among men with no initial pleural abnormality. Of 143 men who initially had plaques, 33 (23%) had diffuse pleural thickening at follow-up 10 years later, or before death, if this occurred within 10 years.

A study of shipyard workers in the UK found a significant excess of deaths from both lung cancer and mesothelioma in those with plaques compared with unexposed controls matched for age and sex,[92] although this study was subject to selection bias. A necropsy-based Italian study found that the odds ratio for mesothelioma increased with the size of plaques, suggesting that larger plaques were associated with higher doses of asbestos.[93] In a Swedish study of 1596 men with plaques followed for 16 369 person years, there were nine mesotheliomas compared with 0.8 expected and 50 bronchial carcinomas compared with 32.1 expected after correcting for smoking habits, indicating a relative risk of 1.4.[94] In a Finnish study, men with benign pleural disease had a raised risk of mesothelioma (standard incidence ratio (SIR) = 5.5, CI = 1.5–14) and a slightly elevated risk of lung cancer (SIR = 1.3, CI = 1.0–1.8).[95] Not all studies have shown patients with plaques to be at increased risk of lung cancer and a recent review suggested that those that have shown a risk are the most subject to selection bias,[96] a suggestion not accepted in an accompanying editorial.[97] Many studies in this area are unsatisfactory in one or more ways: they have concerned populations with unknown or low level asbestos exposure, control for the effect of smoking was unsatisfactory, latency was ignored, follow-up was incomplete, and statistical power to detect small increases in risk was not estimated. It is probable that the extent to which persons with plaques are at risk of cancer depends upon the exposure experienced rather than the presence of the plaques and therefore the risk will vary between different populations with plaques. Unrealistically large population studies would be needed to demonstrate small increases in risk of the order of 1.1 resulting from relatively low levels of environmental asbestos exposure, whereas studies of heavily exposed persons with plaques have demonstrated significantly increased risks of up to two to threefold.[98,99]

Acute asbestos pleurisy and pleural effusion

Definition

Acute pleurisy consists of inflammation of the pleura, often associated with an effusion.

Epidemiology

It has been estimated that 21% of subjects exposed to asbestos will develop the syndrome at some stage.[100] A history of asbestos exposure is significantly more common in subjects with otherwise 'idiopathic' pleural effusion than in control subjects.[101] In a series of 20 cases, effusions occurred a mean of 26 years after first exposure to asbestos but in four cases it was seen after an interval of less than 10 years,[102] indicating that benign effusion may occasionally occur sooner after exposure than other manifestations of asbestos-related disease. The risk of benign effusion increases with the dose of asbestos.[103]

Pathogenesis and pathology

Injection of crocidolite into the pleura of the rabbit induces chemotactic activity resulting in a polymorphonuclear effusion. The process is not dependent on complement activation but is probably a result of a direct effect of the fibres on pleural tissue.[104] The pathology is that of an acute exudative pleurisy.

Clinical features

Symptoms at presentation are variable but often consist of pleuritic pain accompanied by breathlessness if effusions are present. Mild fever and systemic disturbance are common. Episodes are commonly unilateral, although recurrent episodes affecting both sides occur frequently and may be separated by several years. Signs of pleural effusion may be present. Uncommonly, a pleural rub is heard.

Investigations

The chest radiograph shows a pleural effusion of variable size. Converging linear pleural shadows may be seen.[101] Pleural aspiration reveals an exudate, which may be bloodstained, in the absence of malignancy. Investigations for other known causes of pleural effusion are negative. Pleural biopsy shows only nonspecific pleural inflammation and fibrosis. Asbestos bodies or fibres are rarely evident by light microscopy, although fibres may be seen by electron microscopy.

Management

Pleural aspiration relieves breathlessness and anti-inflammatory analgesics relieve pain. Spontaneous resolution of each episode is usual.

Prognosis

The condition may be recurrent and increasing diffuse pleural thickening after each episode is usual.[102] Eventually this may lead to breathlessness and disability. As in other individuals with asbestos exposure, there are risks of mesothelioma and lung cancer, but there is no evidence that the risks are greater than in individuals with similar exposure but without benign pleural disease.

Diffuse pleural thickening

Definition

Diffuse pleural thickening is pleural fibrosis that extends continuously over a variable proportion of the thoracic cavity without well circumscribed margins. It principally involves the visceral pleura, although this is often adherent to the parietal pleura.

Epidemiology

Diffuse pleural thickening is a less common manifestation than pleural plaque formation. It is less clearly dose-related than asbestosis or the malignant diseases[7,8] and its occurrence may be determined partly by other factors. A wide range of fibre counts is observed in association with the condition, but mean counts appear to be somewhat lower than in groups of patients with asbestosis.[105] Amphibole counts were higher than usually seen in non-occupationally-exposed individuals in six of seven cases in this series. In another series, in which fibre counts were comparable to those seen in mild asbestosis, amphiboles were the main fibre type in the lungs although chrysotile was the main fibre type in the pleura.[58] Another study suggested some relation between the incidence of mesothelioma and pleural thickening following asbestos pleurisy lending support to the role of amphiboles in its genesis.[106]

Pathogenesis

Diffuse pleural thickening often follows episodes of acute pleurisy with effusion. In some cases there is no history of such episodes but it is probable that they are frequently subclinical.[107] It is believed to represent the outcome when the resolution of benign pleural effusion involves fibroblast infiltration and a fibrotic healing response. There are features suggestive of an immunological basis for the disease. The erythrocyte sedimentation rate is raised more frequently in patients with diffuse thickening than in those with plaques, and non-specific alterations in serum immunoglobulins occur.[108] Sometimes general malaise, occasionally with febrile episodes, accompanies the pleural disease.

Pathology

There is extensive visceral pleural fibrosis, usually most marked at the bases but often extending to the apex. It is usually, but not always, bilateral. There are commonly adhesions between the pleura and chest wall. Areas of wrinkling and folding of the visceral pleura with deep invaginations into pulmonary tissue, which is compressed and in some cases shows interstitial fibrosis,[109] show as rounded atelectasis on radiographs. This may occur either when diffuse fibrotic changes in the pleura contract, forcing part of the adjacent lung to become atelectatic, or when a pleural effusion causes a segment of lung to become atelectatic so that its components become adherent to each other and remain so after the effusion has been reabsorbed.[109,110] Discrete pleural plaques are often present also. Histological examination shows a basket-weave pattern of pleural fibrosis. Dense, subpleural, lung parenchymal interstitial fibrosis was present in all cases in one series.[105]

Pathophysiology

The dense layer of thickened pleura adherent to the chest wall impedes expansion of the lungs. In advanced cases there may be a progressively shrinking cuirass of thickened pleura squeezing the lung.

Clinical features

The principal symptom is shortness of breath on exertion. There may have been a history of episodes of pleurisy in the past and there may also be pleuritic pain due to adhesions. Occasionally, pain is a persistent feature and may be disabling.[111]

On examination there is usually little to find. There may be reduced chest expansion and quiet breath sounds when the disease is extensive. In some cases inspiratory crackles are present, either because of associated asbestosis or because of the

pleural disease itself, in which case they have a characteristic waveform detectable by computerised lung sound analysis, which differs from that seen in asbestosis.[112] In some cases, crackles may be absent even when asbestosis is present because of masking of their audibility by the thickened pleura.

Investigations
Radiology

The chest radiograph shows pleural thickening along the chest walls. The costophrenic angles are usually obliterated and, when the condition is extensive, the diaphragmatic and cardiac contours may be obscured (Fig. 27.6). Fibrous strands extending from a thickened pleura may have a 'crow's feet' appearance. The appearance of 'shrinking pleuritis with rounded atelectasis', otherwise known as 'folded lung', may be seen. It was first described by Blesovsky in three patients who had been exposed to asbestos.[113] Radiological changes are sometimes unilateral although they may become bilateral later. The pleural changes make assessment of the lung fields difficult and definite radiographic evidence of asbestosis of the lungs is usually not seen.

Occasionally, the pleural thickening involves exclusively or mainly the upper lobes, and there may be fibrosis of the upper lobes of the lungs also.[22,114] The radiological appearances may be difficult to distinguish from those of past tuberculosis. An association between upper lobe asbestos disease and *Aspergillus* infection has been observed and it is suggested that exposure to asbestos leads to changes in the bronchi and the lung parenchyma, i.e. 'scar emphysema', which can facilitate growth of the fungus.[115]

High-resolution computed tomography

High-resolution computed tomography demonstrates the extent of the pleural thickening more clearly than the plain chest radiograph, particularly in the region of the paravertebral gutter, which is very frequently involved and difficult to assess on the plain radiograph. HRCT aids differentiation between multiple discrete plaques and diffuse pleural thickening, which can be impossible on plain radiographs.[90] It is helpful in identifying what may appear to be a mass lesion on the plain radiograph as an area of infolded lung (Fig. 27.7). HRCT may reveal evidence of asbestosis of lung tissue that is not apparent on plain radiograph.

Lung function tests

The characteristic features are a restrictive ventilatory defect, decreased compliance, a reduction in total lung capacity and impairment of gas transfer characterised by a low T_LCO with a normal or increased KCO.[116] The latter is the main difference from asbestosis of the lungs and probably reflects the external constriction of the lung characteristic of pleural disease with a reduction in T_LCO primarily as a result of reduction in lung volume rather than derangement of the alveolar tissue. The KCO correlates directly with the degree of pleural thickening.[117] This is of importance because a normal or raised KCO should not be construed as indicating the absence of coexisting parenchymal asbestosis.

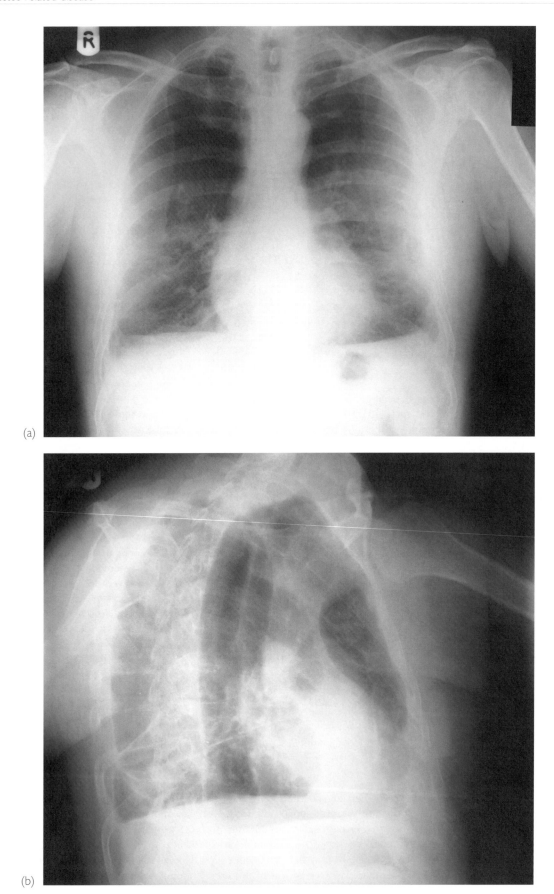

(a)

(b)

Fig. 27.6 *For captions, see opposite.*

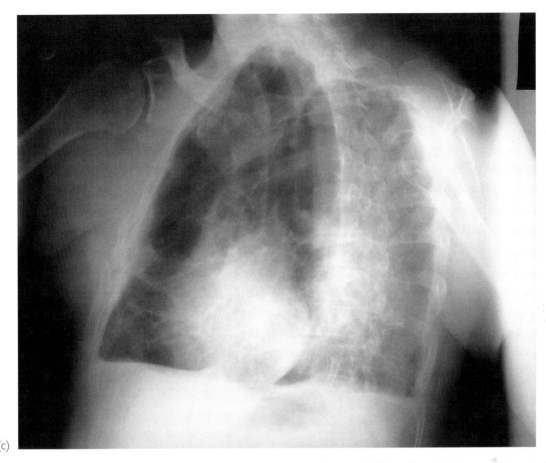

(c)

Fig. 27.6 Postero-anterior and right and left anterior/oblique films showing bilateral diffuse pleural thickening. Posteriorly on the right there is the typical crow's foot appearance of linear opacities splaying out from the thickened pleura.

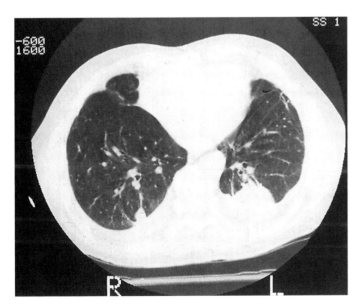

Fig. 27.7 High-resolution computed tomography scan showing bilateral infolded lung, more extensive in the left lung; the characteristic features are the attachment of the mass to the pleura and vessels radiating from the mass towards the hilum.

The severity of breathlessness and disability increase with increasing severity of pleural disease.[90,118–120] The extent of chest-wall pleural thickening and obliteration of the costophrenic angles are the radiological features best associated with degree of disability. The latter feature implies that the parietal pleura over the lower chest wall is stuck to the parietal pleura over the periphery of the diaphragm, preventing the lung from expanding into this potential space. This does not happen with plaques and is possibly an important mechanism by which diffuse pleural thickening usually impairs ventilatory function while plaques usually do not.[121] Unilateral disease may cause disability, although it is generally less severe than that associated with bilateral disease.

Biopsy procedures

Pleural biopsy is usually unnecessary but there is occasionally doubt as to the diagnosis, particularly when the pleural changes are unilateral, suggesting the possibility of mesothelioma. Pleural biopsy by Abrams needle is not satisfactory in the absence of pleural fluid. A CT- or ultrasound-guided cutting needle biopsy may be helpful if there is sufficient pleural thickening for the procedure to be performed safely. Occasionally, sufficient doubt remains after these procedures for thoracotomy to be undertaken, sometimes for the dual purpose of diagnosis and treatment.

Bronchoalveolar lavage

In cases where there is diffuse pleural disease and a doubtful history of asbestos exposure, examination of bronchoalveolar lavage fluid for asbestos bodies or fibres can be helpful.

Management

In most cases no treatment is advisable. If there is severe impairment of lung function and consequent disability, decortication may be attempted. It seldom produces any worthwhile improvement in lung function[122] but may relieve pain.[123]

Prognosis

There is a tendency for the condition to progress. It often begins on one side with effusion followed by pleural thickening, to be followed months or years later by a similar episode on the other side. Once established, pleural thickening tends to progress, mainly in the first 15 years after its onset.[124] Longitudinal lung function data over a mean period of 9 years in 36 subjects showed a significant decrement in FEV_1 and FVC in excess of that predicted from ageing alone.[125] Microscopic examination of subpleural lung tissue usually shows evidence of fibrosis of lung tissue, and clinically overt asbestosis may eventually emerge. Risks of mesothelioma and lung cancer are a function of past asbestos exposure.

Pericarditis

Asbestos exposure occasionally causes benign pericardial effusion, thickening and calcification.[126] These manifestations are analogous to the effects of asbestos on the pleura, by which pericardial changes are usually accompanied. The pericardial thickening may result in constrictive pericarditis with functional consequences of impaired right ventricular filling. This may be suspected in patients with breathlessness disproportionately severe for the apparent degree of respiratory disease. Anatomical and functional aspects of pericardial constriction may be demonstrated by magnetic resonance imaging.[127]

Malignant mesothelioma

Definition

Malignant mesothelioma is a tumour that arises from mesothelial or possibly more primitive submesothelial cells. It occurs most commonly in the pleura but also in the peritoneum and, rarely, can arise in the pericardium or tunica vaginalis testis.

Epidemiology

The existence of primary mesothelial tumours was not generally accepted until the late 1950s although reports of probable cases can be recognised earlier. In 1960 Wagner and colleagues described 33 cases of diffuse pleural mesothelioma and all but one had experienced probable exposure to crocidolite.[128] Much evidence has since accumulated to indicate that asbestos exposure is responsible for the great majority of mesotheliomas. Among subjects with no history of asbestos exposure the annual incidence has been estimated at around 1/1 000 000 population,[129] although this estimate has been questioned in a recent review, which suggested that the true background incidence may be much lower.[130] A few childhood cases, apparently unrelated to exposure to asbestos or other fibrous minerals have occurred.[131]

In 1964 a case-control study was made of patients who had died of mesothelioma at the London Hospital.[132] Evidence of asbestos exposure was found in a majority of cases even though information was often obtainable only from surviving relatives or medical records. Of considerable interest was the observation that some of the patients had not worked with asbestos but had been exposed via dust brought home on the clothes of asbestos workers or from residence in the vicinity of an asbestos factory. Subsequently, further cases of mesothelioma attributable to domestic or residential exposure were identified and this led to the view that even trivial exposure to asbestos could be associated with a substantial risk of mesothelioma. However, situations that might be assumed to be associated with slight exposure, such as domestic contact with contaminated clothing and working in an office with a deteriorating sprayed asbestos ceiling, have been shown to be capable of giving rise to fibre levels in the lung comparable to those found in persons with mild occupational exposure.[133-135] Cases reported after non-occupational exposure have occurred among a very large population at risk, so that the risk associated with such exposure is probably small. A case-control study suggested that exposure derived only from residence in the vicinity of asbestos plants in Yorkshire, UK accounted for only 3% of cases in the area, with the majority of cases occurring in persons who had sustained occupational or para-occupational exposure.[136]

However, there is no clear evidence for a threshold dose of asbestos below which there is no risk of mesothelioma[1,137] A review that suggested that there is a threshold did not address the lack of statistical power of studies to demonstrate a small risk at low levels of exposure.[138] In the UK the criteria for attribution of mesothelioma to asbestos exposure recommended by the Industrial Injuries Advisory Council for the award of state compensation require evidence of asbestos exposure 'above that commonly found in the air in buildings and the general outdoor environment'.[139]

In persons with heavy exposure the risk of mesothelioma is high. Mortality from mesothelioma among employees at an asbestos textile factory before 1964 was estimated at 7.3–10.8% for men and 9.1–12.0% for women.[140] In insulation workers whose exposure began before age 20 the death rate from mesothelioma may be as high as 15%.[141]

The incidence of mesothelioma in the UK (Fig. 27.8) and other industrial countries is still rising and it is likely to continue to do so until around 2020,[142] reflecting the increasing use of asbestos, largely without protection, until about 1970. By 2020 it is expected that there will be between 2700 and 3300 male deaths annually. Female deaths comprised 12% of the total in 1996, although they are increasing less steeply than

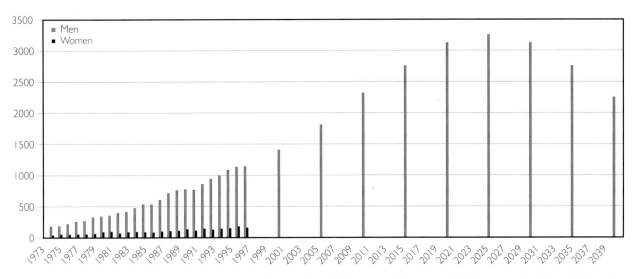

Fig. 27.8 Annual deaths from mesothelioma in England, Scotland and Wales; actual figures to 1996 (source: Health and Safety Executive) and projected for men beyond 2000 (data from Peto et al.[142]).

male deaths, reflecting less frequent occupational exposure to asbestos in women.[142] For the worst affected cohorts, men born in the 1940s, mesothelioma may account for 1% of all deaths and asbestos exposure at work in construction and building maintenance will account for many of these. A similar picture applies to western Europe, where asbestos use remained high until 1980 and where it is expected that mesothelioma deaths will almost double from 5000 in 1998 to 9000 by 2018, and will account for 250 000 deaths over the next 35 years.[143] In the USA, where controls on use of asbestos were introduced earlier and where use of amphiboles was always less than in the UK, the incidence may already have peaked, at around 2300 deaths annually.[144]

Dose–response relation

All the available evidence supports the view that the risk of mesothelioma increases with the dose of asbestos. The dose represents two factors: the concentration of fibres to which exposure occurred and the duration of exposure. It is probable that each brief period of exposure subsequent to the first causes an addition to the total risk that is approximately proportional to the dose of asbestos received.

There are no ideal studies that report the dose-specific mesothelioma risk based on individual exposure estimates but several studies have shown a relation between the risk of mesothelioma and cumulative exposure. For example, among workers at an asbestos factory in east London approximately 8% of deaths were due to mesothelioma.[145] The risk of mesothelioma increased with both the duration of exposure and the estimated intensity of exposure. Similar relationships were reported among crocidolite miners in Western Australia[146] and among gas-mask assemblers.[147] A recent case-control study using a semi-quantitative assessment of exposure showed a clear dose–response relation with a significant excess of mesothelioma at levels of exposure far below limits adopted in most industrial countries during the 1980s.[148] Animal studies confirm the dose–response relationship.[149]

Time since first exposure

The incidence of mesothelioma increases with time elapsed since first exposure to asbestos in proportion to a power function of the time elapsed.[141] This can be explained on the assumption that each brief period of exposure causes an addition to subsequent incidence, which increases approximately as the cube of time since the exposure occurred. For continuous exposure the fourth power of time since first exposure fits the data better.

In two UK series in which 85%[150] and 87%[151] of cases had a history of definite or probable asbestos exposure, mean latent intervals between first exposure and death were 38 (range 3.5–53) years[150] and 41 (15–67) years.[151] Intervals of less than 20 years were uncommon in both series. The case with the shortest latency (3.5 years) was not well documented[150] and there must be doubt as to its validity. The latency between first exposure and appearance of disease is unrelated to the heaviness of exposure.[152]

It is not likely that the tumour actually grows throughout the latent period because this would imply a very long doubling time, which would be reflected in prolonged survival from the onset of clinical manifestations. It is very difficult to obtain direct evidence about the period between the commencement of growth of mesothelioma and death in humans. On the basis of knowledge of the times taken for tumours to double their bulk it has been calculated that the period between commencement of growth of lung cancer and the onset of clinical manifestations probably averages about 10 years.[153] The time between the onset of clinical manifestations and death is approximately similar for mesothelioma and untreated lung cancer, in the range of 12–18 months, and it is reasonable to assume that mesothelioma also starts to grow about 10 years, on average, before clinical manifestations appear. This assumption fits the epidemiological data well.[141]

Fibre type

Fibre types differ in their potential for causing mesothelioma. Assessment of the effects of different types has been difficult because most workers have been exposed to a mixture of the commercial fibre types. The weight of the evidence strongly suggests that amphiboles are more potent than chrysotile in causing mesothelioma and that, among the amphiboles, crocidolite is more potent than amosite.[1,154] However, chrysotile is not without risk. A case control study from Australia demonstrated an increase in risk of mesothelioma with increasing counts of crocidolite, amosite and chrysotile, including cases in which only chrysotile was present.[155] Human cases in which chrysotile was the only type of asbestos in the lungs have been reported from Japan,[156] and animal experiments confirm that chrysotile alone can cause mesothelioma.[149] A recent World Health Organization review of the evidence concluded that chrysotile poses a risk for mesothelioma in a dose-dependent manner with no evidence of a threshold below which there is no risk.[157]

It has been suggested that the mesotheliomas occurring in workers exposed only to chrysotile may have been caused by small quantities, usually less than 1%, of tremolite contaminating the chrysotile. This forms part of the so-called 'amphibole hypothesis' to the effect that most, if not all, asbestos-induced mesotheliomas are caused by amphiboles.[158] The main evidence for this hypothesis has come from Canadian studies. Analysis of lung tissue from chrysotile workers showed higher ratios of counts in mesothelioma cases to those in controls for tremolite than for chrysotile.[159] A further study found substantially higher odds ratios for mesothelioma and lung cancer among workers in central mines, where tremolite contamination was high, than among workers in peripheral mines, where tremolite contamination was lower.[160] In contrast, a study of two chrysotile mining towns in Quebec in which the tremolite content of the air and of lung tissue differed by a factor of 7.5 found no difference in incidence of mesothelioma as a proportion of the workforce.[161] The amphibole hypothesis has been questioned[162] and it has been argued that, even though chrysotile is a less potent cause of mesothelioma than amphiboles, because it accounts for a large majority of asbestos used commercially, it may nevertheless be an important cause of pleural mesothelioma.[163]

Observations of differing incidence of mesothelioma in different areas and industries led to the hypothesis that it is the dimensions of the fibres that relate to the risk of mesothelioma and that the finer fibres appear to be more dangerous. This has been substantiated by analysis of fibre content of lung tissue.[155] Support for this view also comes from animal experiments, in which samples of fibrous glass less than 1.5μ in diameter and longer than 8μ were more potent than other sizes in producing pleural sarcomas.[164] Fortunately, commercially used synthetic mineral fibres are mostly of much larger dimensions and a study of 25 000 workers engaged in their manufacture found only one of 1505 deaths to be due to mesothelioma.[165]

Non-industrial mesothelioma

Endemic pleural mesothelioma in Karain, a remote village in the Cappadocian region of Turkey, was first reported in 1978 by Baris and colleagues.[166] More recent results showed that mesothelioma had caused 50 of 76 deaths among a population averaging approximately 400 adults aged 20 or more over a 9-year period.[167] Exposure to a carcinogenic agent from birth was

suspected. The materials responsible were found to be a fibrous zeolite called erionite and possibly other environmental asbestos minerals, including tremolite, present in the volcanic tuff, which is quarried and used for building. Very recently a kinship study demonstrated that there is a genetic susceptibility to mesothelioma in Cappadocia, perhaps mediating susceptibility to the carcinogenic effect of erionite.[168] Naturally occurring asbestos minerals, including tremolite and perhaps chrysotile, have also been reported to cause mesothelioma in Cyprus,[169] Greece and Turkey.

Site of mesothelioma

Pleural mesothelioma is much more common than the peritoneal form, although the ratio between the sites is variable from entirely pleural to only about 2:1 in favour of pleural in different series.[170] Factors favouring the peritoneal site are longer and heavier exposure, and exposure to amphiboles. Clinical evidence of asbestosis of the lungs is found in association with peritoneal mesothelioma more commonly than with pleural mesothelioma.[170,171]

Smoking and age at first exposure

The risk of mesothelioma is not affected by smoking. The relative risk is not related to age at first exposure, although the absolute risk is greater with earlier exposure because there is more time for mesothelioma to develop.

Aetiology and pathogenesis

As discussed in relation to pleural plaques, fibres that have migrated directly through the visceral pleura may be reabsorbed into the parietal pleura through 'black spots' located near lymphatic vessels.[83] The way in which asbestos fibres reach the peritoneum is a matter of speculation. They may be transported in the lymphatics from the lungs to the abdomen where they have been found in lymph nodes and other abdominal organs.[172] Asbestos is also transported across the mucosa of the intestinal tract after ingestion.[173] Asbestos is a complete carcinogen for mesothelioma.

The mechanism of malignant transformation is incompletely understood. Asbestos is an established genotoxic agent that can induce DNA damage, gene transcription and protein expression important in modulating cell proliferation and cell death.[14] Asbestos, unlike non-fibrogenic particulates, induces apoptosis in mesothelial cells and free radicals. Mesothelioma cell lines are more resistant to apoptosis than non-transformed cells, at least partly because they are more resistant to the cytotoxic effects of an oxidant stress. Asbestos mutagenicity is probably due partly to reactive oxygen and nitrogen species, which cause multiple genotoxic effects including single DNA base substitutions, intrastrand linking, point mutations and large chromosomal deletions.[14] It has also been suggested that asbestos may act as a promoter of mesothelioma.[174] Impairment of lymphatic clearance of asbestos fibres by fibrosis[174] and impairment of non-specific defence mechanisms against malignant disease[175,176] may be relevant.

Recently it has been suggested that simian virus 40 (SV40) may be a co-carcinogen with asbestos for mesothelioma.[177] The virus can transform human cells *in vitro* and induce tumours, including mesothelioma, in laboratory animals, so a causative role for human malignancy is plausible although not proven.[178] The frequency of detection of SV40 in mesothelioma tissue varies from study to study. In the UK a Welsh study found evidence of SV40 in six of nine mesotheliomas[179] while a London study found it in none of 12 cases.[180] A multi-institutional study found SV40 frequently in US mesotheliomas but not in Finnish cases tested in the same laboratory,[181] which suggests that demographic differences are more likely to account for the variation than methodological differences. It has been suggested that the virus infected humans via contaminated parenteral polio vaccine used in the 1950s and early 1960s, most widely in the USA, but SV40 has been identified in persons too young to have received the vaccine, indicating an alternative route of transmission.[178] After more than 30 years of follow-up there is so far no increase in deaths from mesothelioma among the cohort that received contaminated polio vaccine in the USA, although it has not yet reached the age of peak incidence of mesothelioma.[182] Another point that is against SV40 playing an important part in causation of mesothelioma in the UK is the markedly greater increase in deaths in men compared to women; if SV40 were important independent of asbestos, a sex differential effect would not be expected.

Pathology

The right pleura is more commonly involved, perhaps reflecting its greater size,[183] although the contrast with the left-sided predominance of plaques is unexplained. The tumour can arise from either pleural layer. It is often associated with an effusion, particularly in the early stages. As the tumour enlarges, invasion and thickening of the parietal pleura eventually lead to partial or complete encasement of the lung with retraction of the chest wall (Fig. 27.9). Spread by direct extension to the pericardium, contralateral pleura and peritoneum is common, as are blood-borne metastases.

Malignant mesothelioma demonstrates a wide range of histological appearances. The main varieties are the epithelial, sarcomatous and mixed patterns (Fig. 27.10). The epithelial type shows some resemblance to carcinoma, particularly adenocarcinoma, with tubule formation. The sarcomatous type is composed of spindle-shaped cells, often associated with collagen deposition.

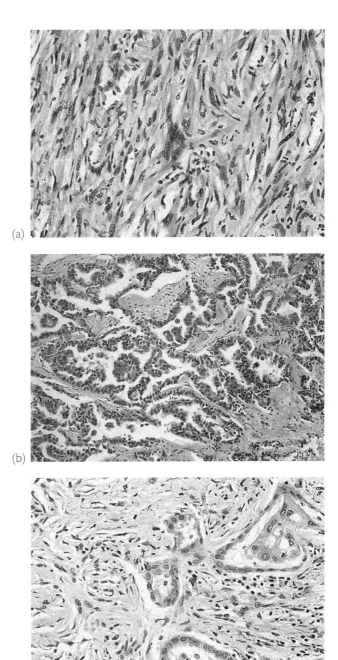

(a)

(b)

(c)

Fig. 27.10 (a) Histological section showing the sarcomatous type of mesothelioma; the spindle cell pattern is evident. (b) Histological section showing the epithelial type of mesothelioma; the tubulo-papillary pattern is evident. (c) Histological section showing the mixed type of mesothelioma; there is sarcomatous stroma surrounding areas of epithelial malignant components.

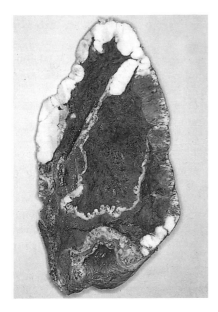

Fig. 27.9 Sagittal section of lung partly encased by a mesothelioma.

Mixed tumours show elements of both of the other types in varying proportions.

Direct extension is more common with epithelial tumours although it occurs commonly with all types. In a series of 115 cases large pleural effusions occurred in over 70% of both epithelial and mixed tumours but in only 16% of the sarcomatous tumours.[184] In 60 of the cases in which autopsies were performed, distant metastases occurred in 37% of epithelial tumours, 33% of mixed tumours and 78% of sarcomatous tumours. Asbestos bodies are usually found in the lung tissue, although not in the tumour tissue.

Pathophysiology

Pleural mesothelioma gradually encases the lung like a cuirass, causing a restrictive ventilatory defect. Peritoneal mesothelioma gradually fills the abdominal cavity and eventually may constrict the intestines, causing obstruction. Pericardial tumour leads to constriction of the heart.

Clinical features

The tumour is more common in males, reflecting the greater frequency with which they have been exposed to asbestos. Mesothelioma is most commonly diagnosed between the ages of 50 and 70 years but may arise at any age.

Pleural mesothelioma commonly presents with dull chest pain of insidious onset, although the pain is sometimes severe and pleuritic. Shortness of breath is common and initially is usually due to pleural effusion. As the tumour progresses tiredness, weight loss and cough commonly develop and profuse sweats may occur. In the later stages severe pain resulting from invasion of thoracic nerve roots may occur.

Peritoneal mesothelioma presents with even vaguer symptoms of tiredness, progressive weakness and loss of appetite. Later abdominal distension due to ascites points to the diagnosis. Ascites is usually recurrent and abdominal distension due to fluid and to tumour mass is frequently gross. Abdominal pain due to subacute intestinal obstruction commonly occurs.

Physical findings

In pleural mesothelioma signs of effusion are common. Later there are signs of gross pleural thickening with reduced or absent respiratory movement and retraction of the chest wall on the affected side. In peritoneal mesothelioma signs may be absent at first. Later, ascites or a doughy abdominal distension becomes apparent. Clubbing of the fingers is uncommon unless there is associated asbestosis of the lungs. Pericardial tumour is often associated with signs of constriction and there may be cardiac arrhythmias due to involvement of conducting tissue. In the late stages, tumour nodules may be found in the skin and these have a predilection for the sites of previous diagnostic or therapeutic intervention.

Investigations

Radiology

The chest radiograph usually shows an effusion initially. Pleural thickening may be visible above the fluid or after aspiration of fluid and, as the tumour progresses, a lobulated outline to the thickening is characteristic (Fig. 27.11) although by no means always present. These features may be demonstrated more clearly by a CT scan (Fig. 27.12a) or MRI. With advanced disease marked contraction of the affected hemithorax becomes apparent. Preservation of a fat line between the thickened pleura and surrounding structures favours a benign process while involvement of the mediastinal pleura or lymph nodes favours a malignant process. However, it may be difficult to distinguish benign from malignant pleural disease. Non-malignant pleural or pulmonary changes attributable to asbestos exposure are also present in the majority of cases.[185]

Staging according to the International Mesothelioma Interest Group (IMIG) TNM-based system[186] may be difficult on the basis of CT and MRI, and thoracoscopic findings are needed for accurate assessment.

Pleural aspiration

Pleural fluid is usually aspirated for therapeutic as well as diagnostic purposes. It is usually bloodstained and shows a high protein content characteristic of an exudate. Cytological examination of pleural fluid has a sensitivity of only 32% in diagnosis of mesothelioma.[187] Immunocytochemistry may assist in distinguishing mesothelioma from adenocarcinoma and from reactive mesothelial cells.

Pleural biopsy

Blind percutaneous needle biopsy, for example by Abrams needle, gives a diagnosis in less than 50% of cases[188] Ultrasound- or CT-guided cutting needle biopsy gives much better results and thoracoscopic biopsy under direct vision will yield a diagnosis in most cases.[189] Open biopsy is occasionally necessary but even then the diagnosis may remain elusive because the tumour often evokes a marked fibrous response and the malignant tissue may not be sampled.

Histological diagnosis

The main problems are the differentiation between mesothelioma and secondary adenocarcinoma of the pleura, usually of pulmonary origin, and the separation of benign from malignant pleural disease.[188] Normal mesothelial cells react to a variety of stimuli by mitotic activity, resulting in the development of rounded cells that float off the normal pavement layer of flattened cells. Papillary or pseudoacinar structures may be formed and it may be impossible to distinguish benign from malignant changes on purely morphological grounds.

Interobserver disagreement in the diagnosis of mesothelioma has diminished in recent years with improvements in histochemical and immunohistochemical techniques. Table 27.2 shows the most useful techniques for differentiation of epithelioid mesothelioma from metastatic adenocarcinoma.[190] If there is mesothelial proliferation suspicious of malignancy but no evidence of invasive activity epithelial membrane antigen (EMA) is often helpful, usually positive if the process is malignant, in both mesothelioma and adenocarcinoma, but not if the process represents mesothelial hyperplasia.

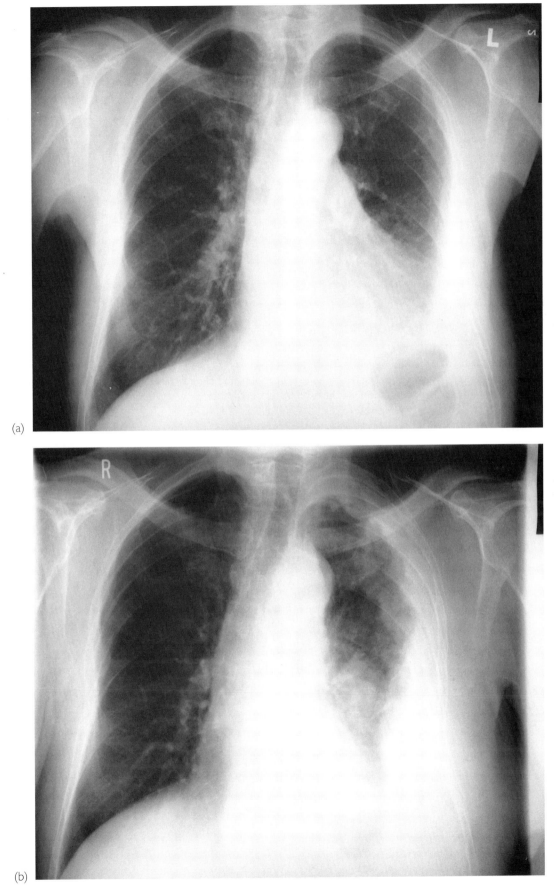

(a)

(b)

Fig. 27.11 Two radiographs from the same patient showing the development of irregular pleural thickening characteristic of mesothelioma.

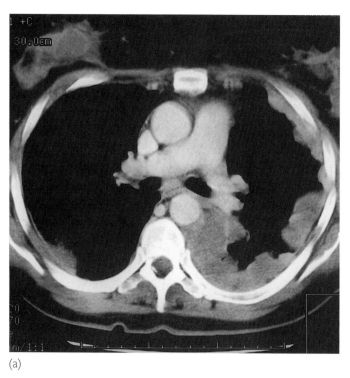
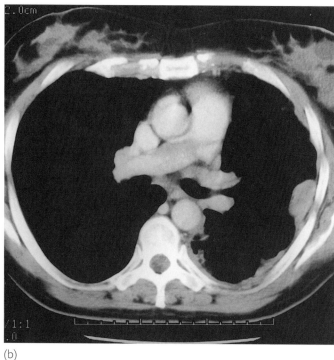

(a)   (b)

Fig. 27.12 (a) Computed tomography scan showing left-sided irregular lobulated pleural thickening characteristic of mesothelioma; the tumour has spread to involve the right posterior chest wall also. (b) After chemotherapy with vinorelbine there has been marked regression of disease on the left and that on the right has resolved.

Table 27.2 Differentiation of mesothelioma from adenocarcinoma. PAS, periodic-acid–Schiff.

Mesothelioma	Adenocarcinoma
Cytoplasm contains glycogen but no diastase-resistant PAS-positive material	Glycogen content is small. May contain diastase-resistant PAS-positive mucin
Alcian-blue-positive hyaluronic acid in glands or on tumour cell surface	No hyaluronic acid within or on tumour cells
CEA, Leu M₁, Ber Ep4 and AUA1 negative	CEA, Leu M₁, Ber Ep4 and AUA1 positive
Calretinin nuclear staining*, cytokeratin 5/6 and thrombomodulin positive	Calretinin nuclear staining*, cytokeratin 5/6 and thrombomodulin negative

* Calretinin stains the cytoplasm of both mesothelioma and adenocarcinoma.

In the sarcomatoid variety, spindle-shaped cells are set in a varying amount of collagenised stroma. If there are few bland spindle cells, differentiation from benign fibrosis may be difficult, while at the other end of the spectrum markedly pleomorphic cellular foci showing mitotic activity are indistinguishable from other forms of undifferentiated sarcoma. Cartilaginous, osseous, muscular or fatty differentiation occasionally occurs in mesothelioma and does not necessarily imply sarcoma.

Immunostains for broad-spectrum cytokeratins are usually positive in mesothelioma and negative in sarcoma.

Karyotype analysis may be used to distinguish benign from malignant epithelial proliferation and electron microscopy also allows identification of cells with an abnormal morphology suggesting malignancy.[191] These methods are, however, of limited availability.

Fibre counts

Fibre counts in the lungs in cases of mesothelioma are, on average, lower than in cases of asbestosis but higher than in control groups without known asbestos exposure.[55] Counts and distribution of fibre types vary according to geographical location of cases.[192] It has been calculated that a count of more than 10^6 amphibole fibres per gram of dry lung confers a risk factor of about 8 for mesothelioma.[152,192]

Caution should be exercised in using the results of fibre counts in an attempt to determine whether a particular mesothelioma was caused by asbestos exposure.[62] There is overlap between the range seen in persons without known exposure and persons with known low-level exposure, and European Respiratory Society guidelines on the interpretation of mineral fibre analysis of lung tissue state that, while a fibre count in the occupational range can support exposure, a count within the background range cannot overrule a clear history of occupational exposure.[193]

A factor that should be taken into account in interpreting fibre counts is elimination of fibres from the lung. Clearance is particularly rapid for chrysotile, with clearance half times of the order of weeks or months,[194] but also occurs with amphiboles with estimated. half times of 20 years for amosite[195] and 7 to 8 years for crocidolite.[196] A count on lung tissue removed at post-mortem examination decades after exposure occurred will be a small fraction of what the count would have been at the time exposure ceased. With increasing time since cessation of exposure, the number of fibres left in the lung diminishes and yet the risk of mesothelioma increases, so the relation between fibre count and mesothelioma risk is complex.

Diagnostic strategy

If the diagnosis is reasonably certain on the basis of typical clinical and radiological features, it is reasonable to accept it without a biopsy, particularly in a frail patient. However, in most cases it is preferable to obtain pathological confirmation and, if the patient is to be included in a clinical trial of therapy, pathological confirmation of the diagnosis is essential. Incorrect diagnosis of mesothelioma may lead to a missed opportunity for treatment of a tumour more responsive to therapy. An incorrect diagnosis of an incurable malignant disease when in fact the patient has benign asbestos-related pleural thickening will cause unnecessary distress and may prompt irreversible decisions, for example about employment, before time disproves the diagnosis. Although pathological confirmation is not essential for a compensation claim to be pursued, in practice lack of confirmation may make this more difficult.

Management

Mesothelioma is generally regarded as incurable although there is renewed interest in radical surgery, from which there are long-term survivors. In a series of 183 patients treated by extrapleural pneumonectomy combined with postoperative chemotherapy and radiotherapy – so-called trimodality therapy – perioperative mortality was 3.8%, no more than would be expected with standard pneumonectomy for lung cancer.[197] Among the remaining 176 patients, 38% survived 2 years and 15% 5 years, with a median of 19 months. Epithelial cell type, extrapleural lymph nodes uninvolved and resection margins clear were favourable prognostic factors and, among 31 patients with all three, 5-year survival was 46% with a median of 51 months. Similar results have been reported by others.[198]

Radiotherapy may provide pain relief but results are often disappointing unless there is a localised area of pain, e.g. due to invasion of a nerve root, rib or vertebra. It may also reduce chest wall masses. Benefits from radiotherapy are usually short-lived.[199] Prophylactic radiotherapy is effective in preventing growth of tumour through biopsy tracks.[200]

Most of the available chemotherapeutic agents have been tried in mesothelioma and agents that have been reported to produce response rates of 10–20% include doxorubicin, epirubicin, mitomycin, cyclophosphamide, ifosfamide, cisplatin, carboplatin and antifolates.[201] Combination chemotherapy regimens have not demonstrated consistently greater response rates than single-agent trials, although several regimes produce response rates around 20%.[202] Symptomatic improvement has been reported following chemotherapy, even in the absence of

demonstrable tumour regression, with regimes employing mitomycin, vinblastine and cisplatin[203], cisplatin and gemcitabine[204] and single agent vinorelbine[205] (Fig. 27.12b). However, there are no randomised studies that demonstrate improved survival or improved quality of life in patients treated with chemotherapy as compared with active supportive care. Such a study, sponsored by the British Thoracic Society, commenced in the UK in 2000.

There is a theoretical basis for immunotherapy[206] and it has been attempted in a number of clinical trials employing various agents including interferons and interleukin-2, of which the latter appears the more promising.[207] Gene therapy is under investigation.[208]

Pleural drainage and chemical pleurodesis with intrapleural tetracycline, talc or other agents are useful for recurrent pleural effusions. For refractory pleural effusions when the lung is bound down so that pleurodesis cannot work, some advocate a pleuroperitoneal shunt (Denver shunt).[209] However, in the author's experience they either become blocked or, if they remain patent, transfer malignancy to the abdomen.

Opiates, often in very large doses, remain the mainstay of treatment in the later stages of the disease and newer agents with improved side-effect profiles, such as transdermal fentanyl, are often helpful. Transcutaneous electrical stimulation of nerves, nerve blocks and cordotomy should be considered for refractory pain.[210]

Prognosis

A recent UK study of 248 patients found a median survival from onset of symptoms of 14 months, with variation according to histological type as follows: 16.2 months for epithelioid, 10.1 months for sarcomatoid and 14.7 months for biphasic tumours.[151] The small minority who survive for more than 3 years are almost exclusively from the epithelioid group [183,184] Various adverse prognostic factors (in addition to histological type other than epithelioid), including more advanced stage of disease,[211] older age, poor performance status, chest pain, weight loss, low haemoglobin, raised white cell count and thrombocytosis, have been identified[212,213] and validated prospectively.[214] Survival from onset of symptoms in peritoneal mesothelioma is even shorter[215], probably because the non-specific nature of symptoms often leads to delayed diagnosis.

Lung cancer

Epidemiology

It had been suspected since the mid-1930s that subjects who had been exposed to asbestos were at an increased risk of developing lung cancer but it was not until the classic paper by Doll in 1955 reporting a substantially increased risk of lung cancer in workers in an asbestos textile factory that the relationship between exposure and disease was conclusively established.[216] In this study, subsequently extended,[217] men exposed to asbestos for 10 years or more before 1933 had a 10-fold increased risk of

Table 27.3 The effect of asbestos exposure and smoking on the risk of lung cancer (after Hammond et al.[218]; the population consisted of insulation workers)

Subjects	Mortality ratio
Non-smokers, not exposed to asbestos	1.00
Non-smokers, exposed to asbestos	5.17
Smokers, not exposed to asbestos	10.85
Smokers, exposed to asbestos	53.24

lung cancer. Many other studies have subsequently confirmed an increased risk in asbestos workers.

The interaction between asbestos exposure and smoking is greater than additive. A study of mortality among insulation workers in the USA demonstrated that the risk of lung cancer was about five times greater in men exposed to asbestos than in men not so exposed, whether or not they also smoked, although the absolute risk was greater in asbestos-exposed smokers than in asbestos-exposed non-smokers[218] (Table 27.3). Saracci reviewed several studies and concluded that the data support the view that the effects of asbestos exposure and smoking on the risk of lung cancer are multiplicative.[219] Since this review several other studies have been published and the conclusions remain broadly similar, although the estimated relative asbestos effect in smokers and non-smokers has varied.[220,221]

Dose–response relation

Most epidemiological studies that have considered the relation between dose of asbestos and the risk of lung cancer have produced results consistent with an approximately linear relation between dose and mortality, with no threshold dose below which there is no increased risk of lung cancer.[1,137,219]

Other factors influencing risk

Age at the time of exposure does not affect the relative risk produced by asbestos exposure.[1] Amphiboles are probably more potent than chrysotile in causing lung cancer in humans but the evidence is less consistent than for mesothelioma[222] and chrysotile is a very potent carcinogen in animal models.[162] The relative risk associated with chrysotile and amphiboles varies between industries. Chrysotile textile workers are at a much higher risk of lung cancer than miners and millers of the same variety of asbestos.[223] It has been hypothesised that the physical characteristics of fibres, depending on the processes to which they have been subjected, may affect the lung cancer risk. However, an electron microscopic study of lung tissue from these two populations indicated that differences in fibre dimensions could not explain the higher risk of lung cancer in asbestos textile workers.[224] The authors suggested that a co-carcinogenic effect of mineral oils used in textile plants to control dust was another possible explanation, but there is no firm evidence for this.

Latent period between exposure and onset of lung cancer

The latent period is variable. Some cases occur between 5 and 9 years after the onset of exposure but the risk rises until at least 30 years after first exposure.[1] A study of USA amosite factory workers suggested that the latent period may be shorter when first exposure occurs at older ages.[225] A study of Quebec chrysotile miners and millers found no evidence for a relation between latency and dose.[226]

Lung cancer and asbestosis

The risk of asbestosis and the risk of lung cancer are both related to the dose of asbestos inhaled, so the conditions frequently occur in the same individual. The association is analogous to that between emphysema and lung cancer in smokers, although no-one suggests that emphysema is a necessary precursor of tobacco-induced lung cancer. The risk of asbestos-induced lung cancer was first identified in persons with asbestosis[216] and, in the context of ideas about 'scar cancers' that were then current but are now anachronistic,[221] the view became prevalent that the lung fibrosis of asbestosis led to the development of cancer. In the mid-1980s, Doll and Peto suggested that, in the light of modern knowledge of carcinogenesis, the idea no longer seemed plausible,[1] but controversy has continued.

Direct support for the hypothesis that the risk of cancer may be confined to those with asbestosis comes mainly from three studies. A pathological study of North American insulation workers reported that histological evidence of asbestosis was present in every case of lung cancer.[227] The diagnostic criteria for asbestosis were idiosyncratic, including cases in which asbestos bodies were absent and in which fibrosis was confined to sub-pleural connective tissue, and histological assessment for the presence of asbestosis was not carried out blind to the presence or absence of cancer.

A post-mortem study of 339 amphibole asbestos miners found that, of 35 cases of cancer, 24 were associated with asbestosis.[228] Standardised proportional mortality ratios indicated no excess of bronchial cancer in 302 exposed men without asbestosis whereas these rates were progressively raised in men with slight or moderate and severe asbestosis. There was selection bias in that the cases studied were those in which compensation claims were pending and the necropsy rate in the population of miners was only 37%.[229] A further analysis of the data showed that dose of asbestos, as represented by years of exposure, could account for most of the variation in lung cancer mortality, although the grade of asbestosis still had a significant effect.[229]

A radiological study of men employed in cement manufacture in New Orleans found that, 20 years or more after hire, no excess of lung cancer was found among workers without radiographically detectable lung fibrosis whereas those with radiographic evidence of fibrosis had a significantly raised risk of lung cancer, with nine observed deaths compared with 2.1 expected.[230] The overall mortality from lung cancer in this study was very low, with an observed to expected ratio of only 1.69 for lung cancer, so that the statistical power to detect a small increase in risk in persons without asbestosis was limited.

In contrast to the latter study, a prospective study of Ontario asbestos cement workers, among whom mortality from lung cancer was much higher, found that the standardised mortality ratio among men without asbestosis at 20 years latency was 5.53 (95% CI: 2.9–9.7). The author concluded that the results demonstrated that lung cancer risk may be elevated in the absence of radiographic asbestosis.[231]

Other studies using different epidemiological methods, have also supported the view that asbestosis is not a necessary precursor of asbestos-induced lung cancer. A hospital-based case control study found an increased odds ratio for lung cancer of around 1.5 in persons whose occupational history indicated a likelihood of asbestos exposure even in the absence of radiological evidence of asbestosis.[232] Criticisms of this study[233–236] were countered by the authors[237] and others.[221] An ecological correlation study of the incidence of lung cancer in Glasgow and the west of Scotland suggested that a considerable proportion of cases of lung cancer were asbestos-related, far more than could be accounted for by an increased risk of cancer in the relatively small number of subjects developing asbestosis.[238]

Proponents of the view that the lung fibrosis of asbestosis is an essential factor in the causation of lung cancer by asbestos exposure[239,240] advance an argument by analogy with cryptogenic fibrosing alveolitis, in which there is also an increased risk of lung cancer.[241,242] However, the cause or causes of cryptogenic fibrosing alveolitis are not established and it is possible that one or more agents concerned may also be carcinogenic. The frequency of death from lung cancer is substantially higher in patients with asbestosis than in those with cryptogenic fibrosing alveolitis[70,71,243], suggesting an additional specific effect of asbestos. The ratio of deaths from lung cancer to those from asbestosis varies considerably in different populations, as does the steepness of the dose–response curve for the risk of lung cancer from asbestos exposure.[224] These observations also suggests that factors other than fibrosis are involved in determining the incidence of asbestos-induced lung cancer.

Pathogenesis

The mechanisms by which asbestos causes lung cancer remain incompletely understood. A recent Consensus Report from the IARC stated that fibre carcinogenesis appears to be a multistage process that may arise from the ability of fibres to cause:

- altered expression or function of key genes arising from genetic or epigenetic alterations;
- altered cell proliferation;
- altered regulation of apoptosis; and
- chronic inflammation.[244]

At a molecular level, interactions between asbestos fibres and target cells may lead to activation of oncogenes or inactivation of tumour suppressor genes that prevent clonal expansion, cell growth and metastasis of cells with altered DNA to allow time for DNA repair or apoptosis after the onset of DNA damage. Increasing evidence suggests that alterations in the function of $p53$, a tumour suppressor gene, are important in asbestos induced lung cancer.[14] Asbestos and asbestos-derived free radicals can also act as tumour promoters to augment cellular pro-

liferation important in the development of a malignant clone of cells.[14] Proponents of the theory that asbestosis is a necessary condition for asbestos-induced cancer suggest that persistence of fibres in numbers sufficient to cause proliferation of airspace epithelial cells, resulting in increased susceptibility to neoplastic transformation, will inevitably lead also to chronic stimulation of interstitial fibroblasts, leading to fibrosis.[239,240]

In vitro studies showed that all types of asbestos fibre caused a dose-related suppression of the ability of natural killer cells to lyse target tumour cells[245] and an *in vivo* study found a reduction in circulating CD16-positive lymphocytes, a subset of natural killer cells, which correlated with the duration of asbestos exposure,[176] and this may be an additional carcinogenic mechanism. Epidemiological evidence suggests that asbestos acts predominantly at one or more of the later stages in carcinogenesis of lung cancer.[141] Synergy between asbestos and tobacco smoke may be mediated by asbestos augmenting the carcinogenic potential of polycyclic aromatic hydrocarbons, which are constituents of cigarette smoke and air pollution. This may occur as a result of adsorption of carcinogens on to the fibres, resulting in their persistence in lung tissue.

A comprehensive review of the evidence concluded that carcinogenicity and fibrogenicity are distinct biological responses to asbestos fibres and that there has been a substantial change in the balance of evidence, supporting the proposition that it is the asbestos fibre load in lung tissue that is the main determinant for carcinogenesis, although not the only factor.[221] The IARC Consensus Report concluded that there are many weaknesses and gaps in current theories and that mechanisms may vary with dose. The evidence in favour of or against any particular theory of carcinogenesis was evaluated as weak.[244]

Pathology

Like lung cancers of other causes (see Chapter 69), those that are caused by asbestos arise principally in the main bronchi and occur in all the common histological forms, including squamous cell, small (oat) cell, adenocarcinoma and large cell.[1] They also occur in the smaller bronchi and in the peripheral parts of the lung. While a lower-lobe preponderance for asbestos-related cancer, increasing with duration of exposure irrespective of the presence of fibrosis, was reported in a Finnish series,[246] a US study found upper lobe predominance in relation to both smoking and asbestos exposure.[247]

Some series have reported an increased frequency of adenocarcinoma in asbestos workers, particularly those with asbestosis,[71] but this may partly reflect the ways in which histological diagnoses were obtained. Adenocarcinoma tends to be peripheral and more frequently beyond the reach of bronchoscopic diagnosis. Hence, postmortem series in which peripheral tumours were identified tend to show an apparent excess of adenocarcinoma compared with bronchoscopic series.[1,248] Many of the studies that have reported an apparent excess of adenocarcinoma in asbestos workers or those with asbestosis were based on autopsy findings, but the higher autopsy rate in asbestos workers than in the general population makes interpretation difficult. A Swedish case-control study that controlled for the source of the histological material as well as year of diagnosis and sex found a significantly increased frequency of adenocarcinoma in asbestos cement workers.[249] However, a US case-control study found no association between asbestos exposure and histological type.[247]

Clinical investigation, management and prognosis

Investigation and treatment proceed along the same lines as for lung cancer of other causes. If asbestosis is present to a substantial degree, poor lung function commonly precludes surgery. The prognosis is otherwise the same as that for lung cancer of other causes.

Attribution of lung cancer to asbestos exposure for compensation purposes

The criteria for attribution of lung cancer to asbestos exposure for compensation purposes remain variable and controversial. An International Consensus Report produced the Helsinki criteria, which suggest that, while asbestosis may contribute some additional risk beyond that conferred by asbestos exposure alone, cumulative exposure should be the main criterion for attribution of lung cancer to asbestos.[66] The criteria further suggest that cumulative exposure of 25 fibres/ml · years, i.e. the threshold level for the development of clinical asbestosis, or a retained fibre burden of 5 000 000 amphibole fibres per gram of dried lung, are associated with a doubling of lung cancer risk. In view of the uncertainty concerning mechanisms of carcinogenesis,[244] reliance on one particular theory of carcinogenesis, i.e. that asbestosis is a necessary precursor of asbestos-related cancer, to determine eligibility for compensation is open to question. Asbestosis is not mandatory for the award of compensation by the state for asbestos-induced lung cancer in Finland, Norway, Sweden, Denmark, Germany or the UK (where diffuse pleural thickening is an alternative criterion).[221] In the UK in 1998 only 26 awards were made for asbestos-related lung cancer, compared with 523 for mesothelioma.[250] Since epidemiological evidence indicates that there are more asbestos-related lung cancers than mesotheliomas[222], present UK prescription rules probably exclude many patients with asbestos-related lung cancer.

Other malignant diseases

There is some evidence that risks of malignant diseases other than lung cancer and mesothelioma are increased in asbestos workers.

Laryngeal cancer

Some inhaled asbestos fibres will inevitably be deposited in the larynx and it is plausible that they should cause cancer at this site. Only one of six case-control studies and one of eight cohort studies considered by Doll and Peto[1] did not show an increased risk of laryngeal cancer in asbestos workers, although the magnitude of the increased risk was approximately twofold or less in

most of the positive studies. They concluded that asbestos should be regarded as one of the causes of laryngeal cancer. The matter remains controversial, however, with three recent reviews reaching conflicting conclusions.[251-3] In the UK the Industrial Injuries Advisory Council declined to recommend that laryngeal cancer should become a prescribed disease in relation to asbestos exposure.[254]

Gastrointestinal cancer

Several published studies have reported an increased risk of cancer at all sites within the gastrointestinal tract, including the oral cavity, in asbestos workers. Many asbestos fibres are swallowed and can therefore reach all parts of the gastrointestinal tract. Asbestos fibres have been found in the wall of the colon in close proximity to colonic cancer tissue.[255] A causal connection between the exposure and the diseases is therefore biologically plausible.[256]

Doll and Peto favoured misdiagnosis of mesothelioma as gastrointestinal cancer as the explanation for the reported excesses of the latter, but did not rule out the possibility that the reported excesses are real.[1] One review concluded that there was no evidence to support a causative association between asbestos exposure and gastrointestinal cancer,[257] but another pointed out that many studies that have not demonstrated an increased risk have not had the statistical power to detect a risk of the size demonstrated in positive studies.[258] A further review that stratified cohorts by dose concluded that the evidence supported an association between asbestos exposure and increased gastrointestinal cancer.[259] However, a more recent review of the evidence relating to colorectal cancer again considered there to be no evidence of a risk.[260] The matter remains controversial but the prevailing view is that a causal link has not been proved.

Cancer at other sites

Increased incidence of several other malignancies has been reported in asbestos workers. These include cancer of the ovary, kidney and prostate, lymphomas and other haematological malignancies.[1] A relationship between these tumours and asbestos exposure is generally regarded as unproven, although the detection of asbestos bodies in many organs other than the lungs[172] suggests that it is not implausible.

Compensation for asbestos-induced diseases

Many industrial countries have arrangements for compensation of affected workers by the state. In the UK the Medical Boarding Centre (Respiratory Diseases), formerly known as the Pneumoconiosis Medical Panel, examines claimants on behalf of the Benefits Agency, which awards Industrial Injuries Disablement Benefit if a prescribed asbestos-related disease is diagnosed. According to the terms of reference, a disease should be diagnosed if, on the balance of probabilities, it is present. In 2000 the conditions for which compensation could be awarded were mesothelioma, asbestosis, diffuse pleural thickening causing disability, and lung cancer if accompanied by either asbestosis or diffuse pleural thickening, intended as markers of substantial asbestos exposure. In the UK, damages may also be obtained by action at common law against employers who can be shown to have negligently failed to provide adequate protection from exposure to asbestos.

? Unresolved questions

- Are all mesotheliomas following chrysotile exposure caused by amphibole contaminants?

- Does simian virus 40 (SV40) play a part in causation of human mesothelioma and if so can SV40 act alone or does it act only as a cofactor with asbestos?

- What value do surgery and chemotherapy have in treatment of mesothelioma and what do new approaches such as gene therapy have to offer?

- Is asbestosis a necessary precursor of asbestos induced lung cancer?

- What are the pathogenetic mechanisms underlying formation of pleural plaques?

References

1. Doll R, Peto J. Asbestos: effects on health of exposure to asbestos. London: HMSO; 1985.
2. Health and Safety Commission. Asbestos: final report of the advisory committee, vol 1. London: HMSO; 1979.
3. Morgan A, Holmes A. Concentrations and dimensions of coated and uncoated asbestos fibres in the human lung. Br J Ind Med 1980; 37: 25–32.
4. Acheson ED, Gardner MJ. The ill effects of asbestos upon health. Asbestos: final report of the advisory committee, vol. 2. London: HMSO; 1979.
5. Lilis R, Miller A, Godbold J et al. Radiographic abnormalities in asbestos insulators: effects of duration from onset of exposure and smoking. Relationships of dyspnea with parenchymal and pleural fibrosis. Am J Ind Med 1991; 20: 1–15.
6. Berry G, Gilson JC, Holmes S et al. Asbestos: a study of dose–response relationships in an asbestos textile factory. Br Ind Med 1979; 36: 98–112.
7. Becklake MR, Case BW. Fiber burden and asbestos-related lung disease: determinants of dose–response relationships. Am J Respir Crit Care Med 1994;150:1488–1492.
8. Finkelstein MM. A study of dose-response relationships for asbestos associated disease. Br J Ind Med 1985; 42: 319–325.
9. Ross GA, Szapiel S, Ferrans VJ, Crystal RG. Susceptibility to experimental interstitial lung disease is modified by immune- and non-immune-related genes. Am Rev Respir Dis 1987; 135: 448–455.
10. Wagner JC, Berry G, Skidmore JW, Timbrell V. The effects of the inhalation of asbestos in rats. Br J Cancer 1974; 29: 252–269.
11. Davis JMG, Beckett ST, Bolton RE et al. Mass and number of fibres in the pathogenesis of asbestos related lung disease in rats. Br J Cancer 1978; 37: 673–688.
12. Mossman BT, Churg A. Mechanisms in the pathogenesis of asbestosis and silicosis. Am J Respir Crit Care Med 1998; 157: 1666–1680.
13. Quinlan TR, Marsh JP, Janssen YMW et al. Dose responsive increases in pulmonary fibrosis after inhalation of asbestos. Am J Respir Crit Care Med 1994; 150: 200–206.
14. Kamp DW, Weitzman SA. The molecular basis of asbestos induced lung injury. Thorax 1999; 54: 638–652.
15. McMillan GHG, Pethybridge RJ, Sheers G. Effect of smoking on attack rates of pulmonary and pleural lesions related to exposure to asbestos dust. Br J Ind Med 1980; 37: 268–272.
16. Samet JM, Epler GR, Gaensler EA, Rosner B. Absence of synergism between exposure to asbestos and cigarette smoking in asbestosis. Am Rev Respir Dis 1979; 120: 75–82.
17. Tron V, Wright JL, Harrison N et al. Cigarette smoke makes airway and early parenchymal asbestos-induced lung disease worse in the guinea-pig. Am Rev Respir Dis 1987; 136: 271–275.
18. Turner-Warwick M, Haslam P. Antibodies in some chronic fibrosing lung diseases. 1. Non-organ specific autoantibodies. Clin Allergy 1971; 1: 83–95.
19. Morris DL, Greenberg SD, Lawrence EC. Immune responses in asbestos-exposed individuals. Chest 1985; 87: 278–280.
20. Becklake MR, Toyota B, Stewart M et al. Lung structure as a risk factor in adverse pulmonary responses to asbestos exposure. Am Rev Respir Dis 1983; 128: 385–8.
21. Begin R, Sebastien P. Excessive accumulation of asbestos fibre in the bronchoalveolar space may be a marker of in individual susceptibility to developing asbestosis: experimental evidence. Br J Ind Med 1989; 46: 853–855.
22. Hillerdal G. Pleural and parenchymal fibrosis mainly affecting the upper lung lobes in persons exposed to asbestos. Respir Med 1990; 84: 129–134.
23. Craighead JE, Abraham JL, Churg A et al. The pathology of asbestos-associated diseases of the lungs and pleural cavities: diagnostic criteria and proposed grading schema. Report of the Pneumoconiosis Committee of the College of American Pathologists and the National Institute for Occupational Safety and Health. Arch Pathol Lab Med 1982; 106: 544–596.
24. Dodson RF, Williams MG, O'Sullivan MF et al. A comparison of the ferruginous body and uncoated fibre content in the lungs of former asbestos workers. Am Rev Respir Dis 1985; 132: 143–147.
25. Hinson KFW, Otto H, Webster I, Rossiter CE. Criteria for the diagnosis and grading of asbestosis. In: Bogovski P et al., ed. Biological effects of asbestos. IARC Scientific Publications No. 8. Lyon: IARC; 1973: 54–57.
26. Shirai F, Kudoh, S, Shibuya A et al. Crackles in asbestos workers: auscultation and lung sound analysis. Br J Dis Chest 1981; 75: 386–396.
27. Coutts I, Gilson JC, Kerr IH et al. Significance of finger clubbing in asbestosis. Thorax 1987; 42: 117–119.
28. Soutar CA, Simon G, Turner-Warwick M. The radiology of asbestos-induced disease of the lungs. Br J Dis Chest 1974; 68: 235–252.
29. International Labour Office. Guidelines for the use of IL international classification of radiographs of pneumoconioses. Occupational Safety and Health Series 22 (Rev 80). Geneva: ILO; 1980.
30. Lozewicz S, Reznek RH, Herdman M et al. Role of computed tomography in evaluation of asbestos related lung disease. Br J Ind Med 1989; 46: 777–781.
31. Staples CA, Gamsu G, Ray CS, Webb WR. High resolution computed tomography and lung function in asbestos-exposed workers with normal chest radiographs. Am Rev Respir Dis 1989; 139: 1502–1508.
32. Aberle DR, Gamsu G, Ray CS, Feuerstein IM. Asbestos-related pleural and parenchymal fibrosis: detection with high-resolution CT. Radiology 1988; 166: 729–734.
33. Yoshimura H, Hatakeyama M, Otsuji H et al. Pulmonary asbestosis: CT study of subpleural curvilinear shadow. Thorac Radiol 1986; 158: 653–658.
34. Akira M, Yamamoto S, Yokoyama K et al. Asbestosis: high resolution CT-pathologic correlation. Radiology 1990; 176: 389–394.
35. Gamsu G, Salmon CJ, Warnock ML, Blanc PD. CT quantification of interstitial fibrosis in patients with asbestosis: a comparison of two methods. AJR 1995; 164: 63–68.
36. Al Jarad N, Strickland B, Bothamley G et al. Diagnosis of asbestosis using a time-expanded wave form analysis, auscultation and high resolution computerised tomography: a comparative study. Thorax 1993; 48: 347–353.
37. Al Jarad N, Wilkinson P, Pearson MC, Rudd RM. A new high resolution computed tomography scoring system for pulmonary fibrosis, pleural disease and emphysma in patients with asbestos related disease. Br J Ind Med 1992; 49: 73–84.
38. Al Jarad N, Strickland B, Pearson MC et al. High resolution computerised tomographic assessment of asbestosis and cryptogenic fibrosing alveolitis: a comparative study. Thorax 1992; 47: 645–650.
39. Sampson C, Hansell DM. The prevalence of enlarged mediastinal lymph nodes in asbestos-exposed individuals: a CT study. Clin Radiol 1992; 45: 340–342.
40. Muldoon BC, Turner-Warwick M. Lung function in asbestos workers. Br J Dis Chest 1972; 66: 121–132.
41. Kilburn KH, Miller A, Warshaw RH. Measuring lung volumes in advanced asbestosis: comparability of plethysmographic and radiographic versus helium rebreathing and single breath methods. Respir Med 1993; 87: 115–120.
42. Cotes JE, King B. Relationship of lung function to radiographic reading (ILO) in patients with asbestos related lung disease. Thorax 1988; 43: 777–783.

43. Miller A, Lilis R, Godbold J et al. Relationship of pulmoanry function to radiographic interstitial fibrosis in 2611 long-term asbestos insulators. Am Rev Respir Dis 1992; 145: 263–270.

44. Cotes JE, Chinn DJ, Reed JW, Hutchinson JEM. Experience of a standardised method for assessing respiratory disability. Eur Respir J 1994; 7: 875–880.

45. Teschler H, Thompson AB, Dollenkamp R et al. Relevance of asbestos bodies in sputum. Eur Respir J 1996; 9: 680–686.

46. Gellert AR, Langford JA, Winter RJD et al. Asbestosis: assessment by broncho-alveolar lavage and measurement of pulmonary epithelial permeability. Thorax 1985; 40: 508–514.

47. Gellert AR, Langford JA, Uthayakumar S, Rudd RM. Bronchoalveolar lavage and clearance of 99-Tc-DTPA in asbestos workers without evidence of asbestosis. Br J Dis Chest 1985; 79: 251–257.

48. Sebastien P, Armstrong B, Monchaux G, Bignon J. Asbestos bodies in bronchoalveolar lavage fluid and in lung parenchyma. Am Rev Respir Dis 1988; 137: 75–78.

49. Karjalainen A, Anttila S, Mantyla T et al. Asbestos bodies in bronchoalveolar lavage fluid in relation to occupational history. Am J Ind Med 1994; 26: 645–654.

50. De Vuyst P, Dumortier P, Moulin E et al. Diagnostic value of asbestos bodies in bronchoalveolar lavage fluid. Am Rev Respir Dis 1987; 136: 1219–1224.

51. Dodson RF, Garcia JGN, O'Sullivan M et al. The usefulness of bronchoalveolar lavage in identifying past occupational exposure to asbestos: a light and electron microscopic study. Am J Ind Med 1991; 19: 619–628.

52. Roggli VL, Pratt PC. Numbers of asbestos bodies on iron-stained tissue sections in relation to asbestos body count in lung tissue digests. Hum Pathol 1983; 14: 355–361.

53. Churg A. The diagnosis of asbestosis. Hum Pathol 1989; 20: 97–99.

54. Ashcroft T, Heppleston AG. The optical and electron microscopic determination of pulmonary asbestos fibre con-centration and its relation to the human pathological reaction. J Clin Pathol 1973; 26: 224–234.

55. Whitwell F, Scott J, Grimshaw M. Relationship between occupations and asbestos-fibre content of the lungs in patients with pleural mesothelioma, lung cancer and other diseases. Thorax 1977; 32: 377–386.

56. Wagner JC, Moncrieff CB, Coles R et al. Correlation between fibre content of the lungs and disease in naval dockyard workers. Br J Ind Med 1986; 43: 391–395.

57. Pooley FD. The identification of asbestos dust with an electron microscope microprobe analyser. Ann Occup Hyg 1975; 18: 181–186.

58. Gibbs AR, Stephens M, Griffiths DM et al. Fibre distribution in the lungs and pleura of subjects with asbestos related diffuse pleural fibrosis. Br J Ind Med 1991; 48: 762–770.

59. Dawson A, Gibbs AR, Pooley FD et al. Malignant mesothelioma in women. Thorax 1993; 48: 269–274.

60. Churg A, Wood P. Observations on the distribution of asbestos fibres in human lungs. Environ Res 1983; 31: 374–380.

61. Churg A. Analysis of lung asbestos content. Br J Ind Med 1991; 48: 649–652.

62. Baker DB. Limitations in drawing etiologic inferences based on measurements of asbestos fibers from lung tissue. Ann NY Acad Sci 1991; 643: 61–70.

63. Wagner JC, Pooley FD, Berry G et al. A pathological and mineralogical study of asbestos-related deaths in the United Kingdom in 1977. Ann Occup Hyg 1982; 26: 423–431.

64. Wagner JC, Newhouse ML, Corrin B et al. Correlation between fibre content of the lung and disease in east London asbestos factory workers. Br J Ind Med 1988; 45: 305–308.

65. Gaensler EA, Jederlinic PJ, Churg A. Idiopathic pulmonary fibrosis in asbestos-exposed workers. Am Rev Respir Dis 1991; 144: 689–696.

66. Anonymous. Asbestos, asbestosis, and cancer: the Helsinki criteria for diagnosis and attribution. Scand J Work Environ Health 1997; 23: 311–316.

67. Al Jarad N, Gellert AR, Rudd RM. Bronchoalveolar lavage and ^{99m}Tc-DTPA clearance as prognostic factors in asbestos workers with and without asbestosis. Respir Med 1993; 87: 365–374.

68. Elmes PC, Simpson MJC. Insulation workers in Belfast. A further study of mortality due to asbestos exposure (1940–75). Br J Ind Med 1977; 34: 174–180.

69. Buchanan WD. Asbestosis and primary intrathoracic neoplasms. Ann NY Acad Sci 1965; 132: 507–518.

70. Berry G. Mortality of workers certified by pneumoconiosis medical panels as having asbestosis. Br J Ind Med 1981; 38: 130–137.

71. Coutts II, Gilson JC, Kerr IH et al. Mortality in cases of asbestosis diagnosed by a pneumoconiosis medical panel. Thorax 1987; 42: 111–116.

72. Cookson WOC, Musk AW, Glancy JJ et al. Compensation, radiographic changes and survival in applicants for asbestosis compensation. Br J Ind Med 1985; 42: 461–468.

73. Liddell FDK, McDonald JC. Radiological findings as predictors of mortality in Quebec asbestos workers. Br J Ind Med 1980; 37: 257–267.

74. Hjortsberg U, Orbaek P, Arborelius M Jr et al. Railroad workers with pleural plaques: II. Small airway dysfunction among asbestos-exposed workers. Am J Ind Med 1988; 14: 643–647.

75. Dossing M, Groth S, Vestbo J, Lyngenbo O. Small airway dysfunction in never smoking asbestos exposed Danish plumbers. Int Arch Environ Health 1990; 62: 209–212.

76. Kilburn KH, Warshaw R. Pulmonary functional impairment associated with pleural asbestos disease: circumscribed and diffuse thickening. Chest 1990; 98: 965–972.

77. Begin R, Masse S, Bureau MA. Morphological features and function of the airways in early asbestosis in the sheep model. Am Rev Respir Dis 1982; 126: 870–876.

78. Wright JL, Churg A. Severe diffuse small airways abnormalities in long term chrysotile asbestos miners. Br J Ind Med 1985; 42: 556–559.

79. Begin R, Cantin A, Berthiaume Y et al. Airway function in lifetime-nonsmoking older asbestos workers. Am J Med 1983; 75: 631–638.

80. Karjalainen A, Karhunen PJ, Lalu K et al. Pleural plaques and exposure to mineral fibres in a male urban necropsy population. Occup Environ Med 1994; 51: 456–460.

81. Harries PG, Mackenzie FA, Sheers G et al. Radiological survey of men exposed to asbestos in naval dockyards. Br J Ind Med 1972; 29: 274–279.

82. Selikoff IJ. The occurrence of pleural calcification among asbestos insulation workers. Ann NY Acad Sci 1965; 132: 351–367.

83. Boutin C, Dumortier P, Rey F et al. Black spots concentrate oncogenic asbestos fibers in the parietal pleura. Thoracoscopic and mineralogic study. Am J Respir Crit Care Med 1996; 153: 444–449.

84. Churg A. The pathogenesis of pleural plaques. Indoor Built Environ 1997; 6: 73–78.

85. Hourihane DO'B, Lessof L, Richardson PC. Hyaline and calcified pleural plaques as an index of exposure to asbestos. A study of radiological and pathological features of 100 cases with a consideration of epidemiology. Br Med J 1966; 1: 1069–1074.

86. Oliver LC, Eisen EA, Greene R, Sprince NL. Asbestos-related pleural plaques and lung function. Am J Ind Med 1988; 14: 649–656.

87. Bourbeau J, Ernst P, Chrome J et al. The relationship between respiratory impairment and asbestos-related pleural abnormality in an active work force. Am Rev Respir Dis 1990; 142: 837–842.

88. Withers BF, Ducatman AM, Yang WN. Roentgenographic evidence for predominant left-sided location of unilateral pleural plaques. Chest 1989; 95: 1262–1264.

89. Hu H, Beckett L, Kelsey K, Christiani D. The left-sided predominance of asbestos-related pleural disease. Am Rev Respir Dis 1993; 148: 981–984.

90. Al Jarad N, Poulakis N, Pearson MC et al. Assessment of asbestos induced pleural disease by computed tomography – correlation with chest radiograph and lung function. Respir Med 1991; 85: 203–208.

91. McMillan GHG, Rossiter CE. Development of radiological and clinical evidence of parenchymal fibrosis in men with non-malignant asbestos-related pleural lesions. Br J Ind Med 1982; 39: 54–59.

92. Edge JR. Incidence of bronchial carcinoma in shipyard workers with pleural plaques. Ann NY Acad Sci 1979; 330: 289–294.

93. Bianchi C, Brollo A, Ramani L, Zuch C. Pleural plaques as risk indicators for malignant pleural mesothelioma: a necropsy-based study. Am J Ind Med 1997; 32: 445–449.

94. Hillerdal G. Pleural plaques and risk for bronchial carcinoma and mesothelioma. A prospective study. Chest 1994; 105: 144–150.

95. Karjalainen A, Pukkala E, Kauppinen T, Partanen T. Incidence of cancer among Finnish patients with asbestos-related pulmonary or pleural fibrosis. Cancer Causes Control 1999; 10: 51–57.

96. Weiss W. Asbestosis: a marker for the increased risk of lung cancer among workers exposed to asbestos. Chest 1999; 115: 536–549.

97. Banks DE, Wang M, Parker JE. Asbestos exposure, asbestosis and lung cancer. Chest 1999; 115: 320–322.

98. Nurminen M, Tossavainen A. Is there an association between pleural plaques and lung cancer without asbestosis? Scand J Work Environ Health 1994; 20: 62–64.

99. Hillerdal G, Henderson DW. Asbestos, asbestosis, pleural plaques and lung cancer. Scand J Work Environ Health 1997; 23: 93–103.

100. Gaensler EA, Kaplan AI. Asbestos pleural effusion. Ann Intern Med 1971; 74: 178–191.

101. Martensson G, Hagberg S, Pettersson K, Thiringer G. Asbestos pleural effusion: a clinical entity. Thorax 1987; 42: 646–651.

102. Lilis R, Lerman Y, Selikoff IJ. Symptomatic benign pleural effusions among asbestos insulation workers: residual radiographic abnormalities. Br J Ind Med 1988; 45: 443–449.

103. Epler GR, McLoud TC, Gaensler EA. Prevalence and incidence of benign asbestos pleural effusion in a working population. JAMA 1982; 247: 617–622.

104. Shore B, Daughaday CC, Spilberg 1. Benign asbestos pleurisy in the rabbit: a model for the study of pathogenesis. Am Rev Respir Dis 1983; 128: 481–485.

105. Stephens M, Gibbs AR, Pooley FD, Wagner JC. Asbestos induced diffuse pleural fibrosis: pathology and mineralogy. Thorax 1987; 42: 583–588.

106. Hillerdal G, Baris YI. Radiological study of pleural changes in relation to mesothelioma in Turkey. Thorax 1983; 38: 443–448.

107. Hillerdal G. Non-malignant asbestos pleural disease. Thorax 1981; 36: 669–675.

108. Hillerdal G. Asbestos related pleuropulmonary lesions and the erythrocyte sedimentation rate. Thorax 1984; 39: 752–758.

109. Menzies R, Fraser R. Round atelectasis. Pathologic and pathogenetic features. Am J Surg Pathol 1987; 11: 674–681.

110. Hillerdal G. Rounded atelectasis. Clinical experience with 74 patients. Chest 1989; 95: 836–841.

111. Miller A. Chronic pleuritic pain in four patients with asbestos induced pleural fibrosis. Br J Ind Med 1990; 47: 147–153.

112. Al Jarad N, Davies SW, Logan-Sinclair R, Rudd RM. Lung crackle characteristics in patients with asbestosis, asbestos-related pleural disease and left ventricular failure using a time-expanded waveform (TEW) analysis. Respir Med 1994; 88: 37–46.

113. Blesovsky A. The folded lung. Br J Dis Chest 1966; 60: 19–22.

114. Oliver RM, Neville E. Progressive apical pleural fibrosis: a 'constrictive' defect. Br J Dis Chest; 1988 82: 439–443.

115. Hillerdal G, Heckscher T. Asbestos exposure and aspergillus infection. Eur J Respir Dis 1982; 63: 420–424.

116. Wright PH, Hanson A, Kreel L, Capel LH. Respiratory function changes after asbestos pleurisy. Thorax 1980; 35: 31–36.

117. Cookson WOC, Musk AW, Glancy JJ. Pleural thickening and gas transfer in asbestosis. Thorax 1983; 38: 657–661.

118. Britton MG. Asbestos pleural disease. Br J Dis Chest 1982; 76: 1–10.

119. McGavin CR, Sheers G. Diffuse pleural thickening in asbestos workers: disability and function. Thorax 1984; 39: 604–607.

120. Lilis R, Miller A, Godbold J et al. Pulmonary function and pleural fibrosis: quantitative relationships with an integrative index of pleural abnormalities. Am J Ind Med 1991; 20: 145–161.

121. Singh B, Eastwood PR, Finucane KE et al. Effect of asbestos-related pleural fibrosis on excursion of the lower chest wall and diaphragm. Am J Respir Crit Care Med 1999; 160: 1507–1515.

122. Dernevik L, Gatzinsky P. Long term results of operation for shrinking pleuritis with atelectasis. Thorax 1985; 40: 448–452.

123. Fielding DI, McKeon JL, Oliver WA et al. Pleurectomy for persistent pain in benign asbestos-related pleural disease. Thorax 1995; 50: 181–183.

124. De Klerk NH, Cookson WOC, Musk AW et al. Natural history of pleural thickening after exposure to crocidolite. Br J Ind Med 1989; 46: 461–467.

125. Yates DH, Browne K, Stidolph PN, Neville E. Asbestos-related bilateral diffuse pleural thickening: natural history of radiographic and lung function abnormalities. Am J Respir Crit Care Med 1996; 153: 301–306.

126. Davies D, Andrews MIJ, Jones JSP. Asbestos induced pericardial effusion and constrictive pericarditis. Thorax 1991; 46: 429–432.

127. Al Jarad N, Underwood SR, Rudd RM. Asbestos-related pericardial thickening detected by magnetic resonance imaging. Respir Med 1993; 87: 309–312.

128. Wagner JC, Sleggs CA, Marchand P. Diffuse pleural mesothelioma and asbestos exposure in the North Western Cape Province. Br J Ind Med 1960; 17; 260–271.

129. McDonald JC. Health implications of environmental exposure to asbestos. Environ Health Perspect 1985; 62; 319–328.

130. Hillerdal G. Mesothelioma: cases associated with non-occupational and low dose exposures. Occup Environ Med 1999; 56: 505–513.

131. Brenner J, Sordillo PP, Magius GB. Malignant mesothelioma in children: report of seven cases and review of the literature. Med Pediatr Oncol 1981; 9: 367–373.

132. Newhouse ML, Thompson H. Mesothelioma of the pleura and peritoneum following exposure to asbestos in the London area. Br J Ind Med 1965; 22: 261–269.

133. Huncharek M, Caotorto JV, Muscat J. Domestic asbestos exposure, lung fibre burden, and pleural mesothelioma in a housewife. Br J Ind Med 1989; 46 354–355.

134. Stein RC, Kitajewska JB, Kirkham N et al. Respir Med 1989; 83: 237–239.

135. Gibbs AR, Griffiths DM, Pooley FD, Jones JSP. Comparison of fibre types and size distributions in lung tissues of paraoccupational and occupational cases of malignant mesothelioma. Br J Ind Med 1990; 47: 621–626.

136. Howel D, Arblaster L, Swinburne L et al. Routes of asbestos exposure and the development of mesothelioma in an English region. Occup Environ Med 1997; 54: 403–409.

137. Report of the Royal Commission on matters of health and safety arising from the use of asbestos in Ontario. Toronto??: Ontario Ministry of the Attorney General; 1984: 281.

138. Ilgren EB, Browne K. Asbestos-related mesothelioma: evidence for a threshold in animals and humans. Regul Toxicol Pharmacol 1991; 13: 116–132.

139. Asbestos related diseases. HMSO; 1996.

140. Newhouse ML, Berry G. Predictions of mortality from mesothelial tumours in asbestos factory workers. Br J Ind Med 1976; 33: 147–151.

141. Peto J, Seidman H, Selikoff IJ. Mesothelioma mortality in asbestos workers: implications for models of carcinogenesis and risk assessment. Br J Cancer 1982; 45: 124–135.

142. Peto J, Hodgson JT, Matthews FE, Jones JR. Continuing increase in mesothelioma mortality in Britain. Lancet 1995; 345: 535–539.

143. Peto J, Decarli A, La Vecchia C et al. The European mesothelioma epidemic. Br J Cancer 1999; 79: 666–672.

144. Price B. Analysis of current trends in United States mesothelioma incidence. Am J Epidemiol 1997; 145: 211–218.

145. Newhouse ML, Berry G, Wagner JC. Mortality of factor workers in East London 1933–1980. Br J Ind Med 1985; 42: 4–11.

146. Hobbs MST, Woodward SD, Murphy B et al. The incidence of pneumoconiosis, mesothelioma and other respiratory cancer in men engaged in mining and milling crocidolite in Western Australia. In: Wagner JC, Davis W, ed. Biological effects of mineral fibres. IARC Scientific Publications No 30. Lyon: IARC; 1980: 615–624.

147. Jones JSP, Smith PG, Pooley FD et al. The consequences of exposure to asbestos dust in a wartime gas-mask factory. In: Wagner JC, Davis W, ed. Biological effects of mineral fibres. IARC Scientific Publications No 30. Lyon: IARC; 1980: 637–653.

148. Iwatsubo Y, Pairon JC, Boutin C et al. Pleural mesothelioma: dose–response relation at low levels of asbestos exposure in a french population-based case-control study. Am J Epidemiol 1998; 148: 133–142.

149. Wagner JC, Berry G, Timbrell V. Mesothelitomata in rats after inoculation with asbestos and other materials. Br J Cancer 1973; 28: 173–185.

150. Greenberg M, Davies TAL. Mesothelioma register 1967–68. Br J Ind Med 1974; 31: 91–104.

151. Yates DH, Corrin B, Stidolph PN, Browne K. Malignant mesothelioma in south east England: clinicopathological experience of 272 cases. Thorax 1997; 52: 507–512 [published erratum appears in Thorax 1997; 52: 1018].

152. Mowe G, Gylseth B, Hartveit F, Skaug V. Occupational asbestos exposure, lung-fiber concentration and latency time in malignant mesothelioma. Scand J Work Environ Health 1984; 10: 293–298.

153. Geddes DM. The natural history of lung cancer: a review based on rates of tumour growth. Br J Dis Chest 1979; 73: 1–17.

154. Gibbs AR. Role of asbestos and other fibres in the development of diffuse malignant mesothelioma. Thorax 1990; 45: 649–654.

155. Rogers AJ, Leigh J, Berry G et al. Relationship between lung asbestos fiber type and concentration and relative risk of mesothelioma; a case control study. Cancer 1991; 67: 1912–1920.

156. Morinaga K, Kohyama N, Yokoyama K et al. Asbestos fibre content of lungs with mesotheliomas in Osaka, Japan: a preliminary report. In: Bignon J, Peto J, Saracci R. Non-occupational exposure to mineral fibres. IARC Scientific Publications No 90. Lyon: IARC; 1989: 438–443.

157. Chrysotile asbestos. Environmental Health Criteria 203. Geneva: World Health Organization; 1998.

158. McDonald JC, McDonald AD. The epidemiology of mesothelioma in historical context. Eur Respir J 1996; 9: 1932–1942.

159. Churg A, Wiggs B, Depaoli L et al. Lung asbestos content in chrysotile workers with mesothelioma. Am Rev Respir Dis 1984; 130: 1042–1045.

160. McDonald JC, McDonald AD. Chrysotile, tremolite and carcinogenicity. Ann Occup Hyg 1997; 41: 699–705.

161. Begin R, Gauthier J-J, Desmeules M. Work-related mesothelioma in Quebec, 1967–1990. Am J Ind Med 1992; 22: 531–542.

162. Stayner LT, Dankovic DA, Lemen RA. Occupational exposure to chrysotile asbestos and cancer risk: a review of the amphibole hypothesis. Am J Public Health 1996; 86: 179–186.

163. Smith AH, Wright CC. Chrysotile asbestos is the main cause of pleural mesothelioma. Am J Ind Med 1996; 30: 252–266.

164. Stanton MF, Lagard M, Tegeris A et al. Carcinogenicity of fibrous glass: pleural response in the rat in relation to fiber dimension. J Natl Cancer Inst 1977; 58: 587–603.

165. Saracci R, Simanto L, Acheson ED et al. Mortality and incidence of cancer in workers in the man made vitreous fibres producing industry: an international investigation at 13 European plants. Br J Ind Med 1984; 41: 425–436.

166. Baris YI, Sahin AA, Ozesmi M et al. An outbreak of pleural mesothelioma and chronic fibrosing pleurisy in the village of Karain/Urgup in Anatolia. Thorax 1978; 33: 181–192.

167. Saracci R, Simonato L, Baris Y et al. The age–mortality curve of endemic pleural mesothelioma in Karain, central Turkey. Br J Cancer 1982; 45: 147–149.

168. Roushdy-Hammady I, Siegel J, Emri S, Testa JR, Carbone M. Genetic susceptibility factor and malignant mesothelioma in the Cappadocian region of Turkey. Lancet 2001; 357: 444–445.

169. McConncohie K, Simonato L, Mavrides P et al. Mesothelioma in Cyprus: the role of tremolite. Thorax 1987; 42: 342–347.

170. Browne K, Smither WJ. Asbestos-related mesothelioma: factors discriminating between pleural and peritoneal sites. Br J Ind Med 1983; 40: 145–152.

171. Elmes PC, Simpson MJC. The clinical aspects of mesothelioma. Q J Med 1976; 179: 427–449.

172. Auerbach C, Conston AS, Garfinkel L et al. Presence of asbestos bodies in organs other than the lung. Chest 1980; 77: 133–137.

173. Bolton RE, Davis LMG, Lamb D. The pathological effects of prolonged asbestos ingestion in rats. Environ Res 1982; 29; 134–150.

174. Browne K. Asbestos-related mesothelioma: epidemiological evidence for asbestos as a promoter. Arch Environ Health 1983; 38: 261–266.

175. Kubota M, Kagamimori S, Yokoyama K, Okada A. Reduced killer cell activity of lymphocytes from patients with asbestosis. Br J Ind Med 1985; 42: 276–280.

176. Al Jarad N, Macey M, Uthayakumar S et al. Lymphocyte subsets in asbestos-exposed subjects: changes in circulating natural killer cells. Br J Ind Med 1992; 49: 811–814.

177. Carbone M, Pass HI, Rizzo P et al. Simian virus 40-like DNA sequences in human pleural mesothelioma. Oncogene 1994; 9: 1781–1790.

178. Butel JS, Lednicky JA. Cell and molecular biology of simian virus 40: implications for human infections and disease. J Natl Cancer Inst 1999; 91: 119–134.

179. Pepper C, Jasani B, Navabi H et al. Simian virus 40 large T antigen (SV40LTAg) primer specific DNA amplification in human pleural mesothelioma tissue. Thorax 1996; 51: 1074–1076.

180. Mulatero C, Surentheran T, Breuer J, Rudd RM. Simian virus 40 and human pleural mesothelioma. Thorax 1999; 54: 60–61.

181. Testa JR, Carbone M, Hirvonen A et al. A multi-institutional study confirms the presence and expression of simian virus 40 in human malignant mesotheliomas. Cancer Res 1998; 58: 4505–4509.

182. Strickler HD, Rosenberg PS, Devesa SS et al. Contamination of poliovirus vaccines with simian virus 40 (1955–1963) and subsequent cancer rates. JAMA 1998; 279: 292–295.

183. Hillerdal G. Malignant mesothelioma 1982: review of 4710 published cases. Br J Dis Chest 1983; 77: 321–343.

184. Law MR, Hodson ME, Heard B. Malignant mesothelioma of the pleura: relation between histological type and clinical behaviour. Thorax 1982; 37: 810–815.

185. Lilis R, Ribak J, Suzuki Y et al. Non-malignant Chest X-ray changes in patients with mesothelioma in a large cohort of asbestos insulation workers. Br J Ind Med 1987; 44: 402–406.

186. Rusch VW. A proposed new international TNM staging system for malignant pleural mesothelioma from the International Mesothelioma Interest Group. Lung Cancer 1996; 14: 1–12.

187. Renshaw AA, Dean BR, Antman KH et al. The role of cytologic evaluation of pleural fluid in the diagnosis of malignant mesothelioma. Chest 1997; 111: 106–109.

188. Whitaker D, Shilkin KB. Diagnosis of pleural mesothelioma in life – a practical approach. J Pathol 1984; 143: 147–175.

189. Boutin C, Rey F. Thoracoscopy in pleural malignant mesothelioma: a prospective study of 188 consecutive patients. Part 1: Diagnosis. Cancer 1993; 72: 389–393.

190. Cury PM, Butcher DN, Fisher C et al. Value of the mesothelium-associated antibodies thrombomodulin, cytokeratin 5/6, calretinin, and cd44h in distinguishing epithelioid pleural mesothelioma from adenocarcinoma metastatic to the pleura. Modern Pathol 2000; 13: 107–112.

191. Warhol MJ. Electron microscopy in the diagnosis of mesothelioma with routine biopsy, needle biopsy, and fluid cytology. In: Antman K, Aisner J, ed. Asbestos-related malignancy. Orlando, FL: Grune & Stratton, 1987: 201–221.

192. Berry G, Rogers AJ, Pooley FD. Mesotheliomas – asbestos exposure and lung burden. In: Bignon J, Peto J, Saracci R, ed. Non-occupational exposure to mineral fibres. IARC Scientific Publications No 90. Lyon: IARC; 1989: 486–496.

193. De Vuyst P, Karjalainen A, Dumortier P et al. Guidelines for mineral fibre analyses in biological samples: report of the ERS working group. Eur Respir J 1998; 11: 1416–1426.

194. Churg A. Deposition and clearance of chrysotile asbestos. Ann Occup Hyg 1994; 38: 625–633.

195. Churg A, Vedal S. Fiber burden and patterns of asbestos-related disease in workers with heavy mixed amosite and chrysotile exposure. Am J Respir Crit Care Med 1994; 150: 663–669.

196. De Klerk NH, Musk AW, Williams V et al. Comparison of measures of exposure to asbestos in former crocidolite workers from Wittenoom gorge, W. Australia. Am J Ind Med 1996; 30: 579–587.

197. Sugarbaker DJ, Flores RM, Jaklitsch MT et al. Resection margins, extrapleural nodal status, and cell type determine postoperative long-term survival in trimodality therapy of malignant pleural mesothelioma: results in 183 patients. J Thorac Cardiovasc Surg 1999; 117: 54–63.

198. Rusch VW, Venkatraman E. The importance of surgical staging in the treatment of malignant pleural mesothelioma. J Thorac Cardiovasc Surg 1996; 111: 815–825.

199. Bissett D, Macbeth FR, Cram I. The role of palliative radiotherapy in malignant mesothelioma. Clin Oncol (R Coll Radiol) 1991; 3: 315–317.

200. Boutin C, Rey F, Viallat JR. Prevention of malignant seeding after invasive diagnostic procedures in patients with pleural mesothelioma. A randomized trial of local radiotherapy. Chest 1995; 108: 754–758.

201. Ong ST, Vogelzang NJ. Chemotherapy in malignant pleural mesothelioma. A review. J Clin Oncol 1996; 14: 1007–1017.

202. Ryan CW, Herndon J, Vogelzang NJ. A review of chemotherapy trials for malignant mesothelioma. Chest 1998; 113: 66S–73S.

203. Middleton GW, Smith IE, O'Brien ME et al. Good symptom relief with palliative MVP (mitomycin-C, vinblastine and cisplatin) chemotherapy in malignant mesothelioma. Ann Oncol 1998; 9: 269–273.

204. Byrne MJ, Davidson JA, Musk AW et al. Cisplatin and gemcitabine treatment for malignant mesothelioma: a phase II study. J Clin Oncol 1999; 17: 25–30.

205. Steele JPC, Shamash J, Evans M et al. Phase II Study of vinorelbine in patients with malignant pleural mesothelioma. J Clin Oncol 2000; 18: 3912–3917.

206. Robinson BWS, Manning LS, Bowman RV et al. The scientific basis for the immunotherapy of human malignant mesothelioma. Eur Respir Rev 1993; 3: 195–198.

207. Astoul P, Picat-Joossen D, Viallat JR, Boutin C. Intrapleural administration of interleukin-2 for the treatment of patients with malignant pleural mesothelioma: a Phase II study. Cancer 1998; 83: 2099–2104.

208. Sterman DH, Treat J, Litzky LA et al. Adenovirus-mediated herpes simplex virus thymidine kinase/ganciclovir gene therapy in patients with localized malignancy: results of a phase I clinical trial in malignant mesothelioma. Hum Gene Ther 1998; 9: 1083–1092.

209. Tsang V, Fernando HC, Goldstraw P. Pleuroperitoneal shunt for recurrent malignant pleural effusions. Thorax 1990; 45: 369–372.

210. Jackson MB, Pounder D, Price C et al. Percutaneous cervical cordotomy for the control of pain in patients with pleural mesothelioma. Thorax 1999; 54: 238–241.

211. Van Gelder T, Damhuis RA, Hoogsteden HC. Prognostic factors and survival in malignant pleural mesothelioma. Eur Respir J 1994; 7: 1035–1038.

212. Curran D, Sahmoud T, Therasse P et al. Prognostic factors in patients with pleural mesothelioma: the European Organisation for Research and Treatment of Cancer experience. J Clin Oncol 1998; 16: 145–152.

213. Herndon JE, Green MR, Chahinian AP et al. Factors predictive of survival among 337 patients with mesothelioma treated between 1984 and 1994 by the Cancer and Leukemia Group B. Chest 1998; 113: 723–731.

214. Edwards JG, Abrams KR, Leverment JN et al. Prognostic factors for malignant mesothelioma in 142 patients: validation of CALGB and EORTC prognostic scoring systems. Thorax 2000; 55: 731–735.

215. Ribak J, Selikoff IJ. Survival of asbestos insulation workers with mesothelioma. Br J Ind Med 1992; 49: 732–735.

216. Doll R. Mortality from lung cancer in asbestos workers. Br J Ind Med 1955; 12: 81–86.

217. Knox JF, Holmes S, Doll R, Hill ID. Mortality from lung cancer and other causes among workers in an asbestos textile factory. Br J Ind Med 1968; 25: 293–303.

218. Hammond EC, Selikoff IJ, Seidman H. Asbestos exposure, cigarette smoking and death rates. Ann NY Acad Sci 1979; 330: 473–490.

219. Saracci R. Asbestos and lung cancer: an analysis of the epidemiological evidence on the asbestos–smoking interaction. Int. J Cancer 1977; 20: 323–331.

220. Berry G, Newhouse ML, Antonis P. Combined effect of asbestos and smoking on mortality from lung cancer and mesothelioma in factory workers. Br J Ind Med 1985; 42: 12–18.

221. Henderson DW, de Klerk NH, Hammar SP et al. Asbestos and lung cancer: is it attributable to asbestosis or to asbestos fiber burden? In: Corrin B, ed. Pathology of lung tumours. New York: Churchill Livingstone;1997: 83–118.

222. McDonald JC, McDonald AD. Epidemiology of asbestos-related lung cancer. In: Antman K, Aisner J. Asbestos-related malignancy. Orlando, FL. Grune & Stratton; 1987: 57–79.

223. McDonald AD, Fry JS, Woolley AJ, McDonald J. Dust exposure and mortality in an American chrysotile textile plant. Br J Ind Med 1983; 40: 361–367.

224. Sebastien P, McDonald JC, McDonald AD et al. Respiratory cancer in chrysotile textile and mining industries: exposure inferences from lung analysis. Br J Ind Med 1989; 46: 180–187.

225. Seidman H, Selikoff IJ, Hammond EC. Short-term asbestos work exposure and long-term observation. Ann NY Acad Sci 1979; 330: 61–89.

226. Liddell FDK. Latent periods in lung cancer mortality in relation to asbestos dose and smoking. In: Wagner JC, Davis W, ed. Biological effects of mineral fibres. IARC Scientific Publications No 30. Lyon: IARC; 1980: 661–665.

227. Kipen HM, Lilis R, Suzuki Y et al. Pulmonary fibrosis in asbestos insulation workers with lung cancer: a radiological and histopathological evaluation. Br J Ind Med 1987; 44: 96–100.

228. Sluis-Cremer GK, Bezuidenhout BN. Relation between asbestosis and bronchial cancer in amphibole asbestos miners. Br J Ind Med 1989; 46: 537–540.

229. Rudd RM. Relation between asbestosis and bronchial cancer in amphibole asbestos miners. Br J Ind Med 1990; 47: 215–216.

230. Hughes JM, Weill H. Asbestosis as a precursor of asbestos related lung cancer: results of a prospective study. Br J Ind Med 1991; 48: 229–233.

231. Finkelstein MM. Radiographic asbestosis is not a prerequisite for asbestos-associated lung cancer in Ontario asbestos-cement workers. Am J Ind Med 1997; 32: 341–348.

232. Wilkinson P, Hansell D, Janssens J et al. Is lung cancer associated with asbestos exposure when there are no small opacities on the chest radiograph? Lancet 1995; 345: 1074–1078.

233. Jones RN, Hughes JM, Weill H. Asbestos exposure, asbestosis, and asbestos-attributable lung cancer. Thorax 1996; 51(Suppl 2): S9–15.

234. Browne K. Asbestos: a risk too far? Lancet 1995; 346: 305–306.

235. Weiss W. Asbestos: a risk too far? Lancet 1995; 346: 305.

236. Weill H, Hughes JM, Jones RN. Asbestos: a risk too far? Lancet 1995; 346: 304.

237. McDonald JC, Newman Taylor AJ. Asbestos: a risk too far? Lancet 1995; 346: 306

238. De Vos Irvine H, Lamont DW, Hole DJ, Gillis CR. Asbestos and lung cancer in Glasgow and the west of Scotland. Br Med J 1993; 306: 1503–1506.

239. Browne K. Is asbestos or asbestosis the cause of the increased risk of lung cancer in asbestos workers? Br J Ind Med 1986; 43: 145–149.

240. Browne K. Asbestos related malignancy and the Cairns hypothesis. Br J Ind Med 1991; 48: 73–76.

241. Turner-Warwick M, Lebowitz M, Burrows B, Johnson A. Cryptogenic fibrosing alveolitis and lung cancer. Thorax 1980; 35: 496–499.

242. Hubbard R, Venn A, Lewis S, Britton J. Lung cancer and cryptogenic fibrosing alveolitis. A population-based cohort study. Am J Respir Crit Care Med 2000; 161; 5–8.

243. Johnston ID, Prescott RJ, Chalmers JC, Rudd RM. British Thoracic Society study of cryptogenic fibrosing alveolitis: current presentation and initial management. Fibrosing alveolitis subcommittee of the research committee of the British Thoracic Society. Thorax 1997; 52: 38–44.

244. Kane AB, Boffetta P, Saracci R, Wilbourn JD. Mechanisms of fibre carcinogenesis. IARC Scientific Publications No 140. Lyon: IARC; 1996.

245. Robinson BWS. Asbestos and cancer: human natural killer cell activity is suppressed by asbestos fibers but can be restored by recombinant interleukins. Am Rev Respir Dis 1989; 139: 897–901.

246. Anttila S, Karjalainen A, Taikina-aho O et al. Lung cancer in the lower lobe is associated with pulmonary asbestos fiber count and fiber size. Environ Health Perspect 1993; 101: 166–170.

247. Lee BW, Wain JC, Kelsey KT et al. Association of cigarette smoking and asbestos exposure with location and histology of lung cancer. Am J Respir Crit Care Med 1998; 157: 748–755.

248. Ives JC, Buffler PA, Greenberg SD. Environmental associations and histopathologic patterns of carcinoma of the lung: the challenge and dilemma in epidemiologic studies. Am Rev Respir Dis 1983; 128: 195–209.

249. Johansson L, Albin M, Jakobsson K, Mikoczy Z. Histological type of lung carcinoma in asbestos cement workers and matched controls. Br J Ind Med 1992; 49: 626–630.

250. UK Social Security statistics. London: HMSO; 1999.

251. Smith AH, Handley MA, Wood R. Epidemiological evidence indicates asbestos causes laryngeal cancer. J Occup Med 1990; 32: 499–507.

252. Liddell FDK. Laryngeal cancer and asbestos. Br J Ind Med 1990; 47: 289–291.

253. Browne K, Gee JB. Asbestos exposure and laryngeal cancer. Ann Occup Hyg 2000: 44; 239–250.

254. Industrial Injuries Advisory Council. Report on cancer of the larynx. London: HMSO; 1989.

255. Ehrlich A, Gordon RE, Dikman SH. Carcinoma of the colon in asbestos-exposed workers: analysis of asbestos content in colon tissue. Am J Ind Med 1991; 19: 629–636.

256. Miller AB. Asbestos fibre dust and gastrointestinal malignancies. Review of the literature with regard to a cause/effect relationship. J Chron Dis 1978; 31: 23–33.

257. Edelman DA. Exposure to asbestos and the risk of gastro-intestinal cancer: a reassessment. Br J Ind Med 1988; 45: 75–82.

258. Davis DL, Mandula B, van Ryzin J. Assessing the power and quality of epidemiologic studies of asbestos-exposed populations. Toxicol Ind Health 1985; 1: 93.

259. Frumkin H, Berlin J. Asbestos exposure and gastrointestinal malignancy: review and meta-analysis. Am J Ind Med 1988; 14: 79–95.

260. Weiss W. The lack of causality between asbestos and colorectal cancer. J Occup Environ Med 1995; 37: 1364–1373.

28 Acute respiratory distress syndrome

Mark J D Griffiths and Timothy W Evans

 Key points – what's the diagnosis?

- Acute lung injury and acute respiratory distress syndrome reflect the lung's response to any severe insult.

- The definitions of these syndromes are easily applicable but identify a relatively inhomogeneous group of patients.

- Investigate and treat the factors precipitating respiratory failure and their effects on other organ systems while supporting the injured lung.

The acute respiratory distress syndrome in adults (ARDS) and its less severe manifestation, acute lung injury (ALI) were defined by an American–European Consensus Conference in 1993 (under review at the time of writing)[1] and are common complications of severe illness. ARDS continues to be associated with significant morbidity and mortality. While defined by its pulmonary manifestations, ARDS is usually accompanied by significant systemic disturbance and death most frequently results from multiple organ failure. ARDS therefore assumes considerable clinical and fiscal significance, which has stimulated many investigators to evaluate the potential of both supportive and therapeutic interventions in the light of advances in the understanding of the pathogenesis of the syndrome. A plan for supportive therapy is presented, based on a combination of current evidence and the authors' practice.

Definition and severity scoring

Definitions of acute respiratory distress syndrome

The first formal description of ARDS is ascribed to Ashbaugh and colleagues in 1967,[2] although army surgeons engaged in the Second World War in Europe reported cases of pulmonary oedema in the absence of cardiac disease in casualties who were managed with 'positive pressure breathing'. The classical defining criteria are refractory hypoxaemia in association with bilateral pulmonary infiltrates with no evidence of elevated left atrial pressure in the presence of a clinical condition known to precipitate ARDS (Table 28.1). The American–European Consensus Conference proposed that ARDS/ALI be defined as a syndrome of inflammation and increased permeability associated with a constellation of radiological and physiological abnormalities that cannot be explained by, but may coexist with left atrial or pulmonary capillary hypertension.[1] Routine measurement of the pulmonary artery occlusion pressure was not recommended, but should be considered if diagnostic doubt persisted after non-invasive (clinical, radiographic and echocardiographic) assessment. The group simultaneously changed the name from the adult respiratory distress syndrome, recognising that, while the pathological appearances are superficially similar to the respiratory distress syndrome of the newborn, the condition occurs in children and is otherwise distinct.

Table 28.1 American–European Consensus Conference (1993) criteria for acute lung injury (ALI) and acute respiratory distress syndrome (ARDS)

	Timing	Oxygenation	Chest radiograph	Pulmonary artery occlusion pressure
ALI	Acute	$P_aO_2/F_IO_2 \leq 300\,mmHg$	Bilateral opacities consistent with pulmonary oedema	< 18 mmHg if measured or no clinical evidence of left atrial hypertension
ARDS		$P_aO_2/F_IO_2 \leq 200\,mmHg$		

P_aO_2/F_IO_2, arterial partial pressure of oxygen/inspired oxygen fraction.

The declared goal of the American–European Consensus Conference was to bring clarity and uniformity to the definition of ARDS. The inclusion of patients with less severe manifestations of lung injury facilitates earlier enrolment of affected patients in clinical trials. However, the assumptions that patients fulfilling the criteria for ALI progress to ARDS and/or have a better prognosis than those with more severely impaired gas exchange remain unproven. Inevitably with a simple definition, the omission of exclusion criteria tends to result in patients with different pathologies being included and 'misclassified' as having ARDS (Table 28.2). For example, factors that influence the outcome, such as the underlying cause (Table 28.3) and whether other organ systems are affected, are not assessed. In addition, the criterion for the presence of bilateral infiltrates on chest radiography consistent with the presence of pulmonary oedema is not sufficiently specific to be applied consistently. Despite these reservations, this definition of ARDS had a sensitivity of 84% and a specificity of 94% in 208 cases of ARDS confirmed at autopsy.[3] However, because there is no practical gold standard for the diagnosis, the only aspect of the definition of lung injury that can be studied is its reliability, i.e. the reproducibility of findings between observers.

Severity scoring

Ideally, two indices of severity are needed: one that would quantify lung injury per se and one that would measure the overall severity of the patient's illness. Most methods of measuring lung injury in ARDS incorporate semiquantitative scores of the

Table 28.2 Conditions that cause acute lung injury and acute respiratory distress syndrome that may have a distinct pathology and specific treatment

Condition			Specific treatment
Pneumonia	Bacterial	Miliary tuberculosis	Yes
		Cytomegalovirus	Yes
	Viral	Herpes simplex	Yes
		Hantavirus	No
	Fungal	Pneumocystis carinii	Yes
	Others	Strongyloidiasis	Yes
Cryptogenic	Acute interstitial pneumonia		Yes
	Cryptogenic organising pneumonia		Yes
	Acute eosinophilic pneumonia		Yes
Malignancy	Bronchoalveolar-cell carcinoma		No
	Lymphangitis		Yes/No
	Acute leukaemia		Yes
	Lymphoma		Yes
Pulmonary vascular disease	Diffuse alveolar haemorrhage		Yes
	Sickle lung		Yes

Table 28.3 Clinical risk factors for acute respiratory distress syndrome

Direct lung injury	Indirect lung injury
Aspiration of gastric contents	Sepsis syndrome
Thoracic trauma/pulmonary contusion	Multiple trauma
	Shock
Diffuse pneumonia	Massive blood transfusion
Ventilator-associated lung injury	Acute pancreatitis
Inhalation injury (smoke, toxin)	Drug overdose/drug reaction
Near drowning	Cardiopulmonary bypass
Pulmonary vasculitis	Pregnancy related (eclampsia, amniotic fluid embolism)
Reperfusion injury (lung transplant)	Fat embolism syndrome
Thoracic irradiation	Tumour lysis syndrome
Following acute upper airway obstruction	Head injury/raised intracranial pressure

extent of pulmonary infiltration on a chest radiograph, the degree of hypoxaemia, the ventilator settings and a measure of respiratory system compliance. Several pulmonary scoring indices have been described and correlated with outcome, although generally not in large groups of patients. There is poor correlation between pulmonary severity of injury scores and outcome, which is related primarily to non-pulmonary factors such as systemic hypotension, chronic liver disease and non-pulmonary organ dysfunction.[4]

In 1988, a four-point lung injury scoring system (Murray Score) was proposed as a means of quantifying the respiratory impairment based on the level of positive end-expiratory pressure (PEEP), the ratio of the partial pressure of arterial oxygen (P_aO_2) to the fraction of inspired oxygen (F_IO_2), the static lung compliance and the degree of radiographic infiltration.[5] Respiratory system compliance can be calculated in intubated patients by dividing the delivered tidal volume by the unlimited plateau airway pressure minus PEEP. Other factors included in the assessment were the inciting clinical disorder and the presence or absence of non-pulmonary organ dysfunction. Although the lung injury scoring system has been widely used in clinical studies, it cannot predict outcome during the first 24–72 hours of ALI/ARDS and thus has limited usefulness.[6] When the scoring system is used 4–7 days after the onset of the syndrome, scores of 2.5 or higher predict a complicated course requiring prolonged mechanical ventilation.[7] Nevertheless, the widespread acceptance of both the American–European Consensus Conference definition and the lung injury scoring system has helped to standardise and quantify lung injury for the purposes of clinical research.

Considerable advances have been made in the application of severity of illness models to describe critically ill patients. These models provide a method of risk stratification for clinical research and for making quality of care comparisons between units with a similar case mix. The new versions of the Mortality Probability Model (MPM II), the Simplified Acute Physiologic Score (SAPS II) and the APACHE III system are based on much larger databases and have used better statistical methods for development, validation and field testing. Lung injury scoring alone was less accurate in its predictive value than was the use of overall physiological derangement represented by the risk of death calculated by Acute Physiology and Chronic Health Evaluation (APACHE III).[8] Similar validation exercises suggest that an accurate estimate of in-hospital mortality in patients with lung injury can be achieved using a general severity score that accounts for both pulmonary and extrapulmonary organ system dysfunction. The independent variables related to mortality were:

- age
- previous disease
- aetiology
- immunosuppression
- the number and type of organ system failures at admission and during the evolution of the disease
- gas exchange after 24 hours of mechanical ventilation
- SAPS.[9]

Recently, the American–European Consensus Conference introduced the gas exchange, organ failure, cause and associated diseases (GOCA) stratification system, which both encompasses an assessment of lung injury and incorporates additional factors that influence prognosis (Table 28.4).

Risk factors

A great number and variety of conditions are associated with ARDS. The risk factors for ARDS can be divided into two groups depending on whether injury to the lung is direct or indirect (Table 28.3). Indirect injury, via blood-borne inflammatory mediators that have escaped their usual controls, is more common. Sepsis (including pneumonia) is the commonest risk factor, as well as being the risk factor most likely to cause ARDS. Diagnosing and treating conditions that mimic or are associated with lung injury is the first principal of successful management of these patients (Table 28.2).

Table 28.4 The GOCA scoring system for acute lung injury and the acute respiratory distress syndrome

Letter	Meaning	Scale	Definition
G	Gas exchange	0	$P_aO_2/F_IO_2 \geq 301$
		1	P_aO_2/F_IO_2 201–300
		2	P_aO_2/F_IO_2 101–200
		3	$P_aO_2/F_IO_2 \geq 100$
	Gas exchange (to be combined with the numeric descriptor)	A	Spontaneous breathing, no PEEP
		B	Assisted, PEEP 0–5 cmH$_2$O
		C	Assisted, PEEP 6–10 cmH$_2$O
		D	Assisted, PEEP = 10 cm H$_2$O
O	Organ failure	0	Lung only
		1	Lung + 1 organ
		2	Lung + 2 organs
		3	Lung + 3 organs
C	Cause	0	Unknown
		1	Direct lung injury
		2	Indirect lung injury
A	Associated diseases	0	No coexisting diseases that will cause death within 5 years
		1	Coexisting disease that will cause death within 5 years but not 6 months
		2	Coexisting disease that will cause death within 6 months

Three studies have prospectively examined the incidence of ARDS associated with the most frequently associated clinical risk factors[10–12] (Fig. 28.1). Secondary factors associated with an increased risk for ARDS include an elevated APACHE III score in patients with sepsis, and increased APACHE III and Injury Severity scores in trauma victims. Mortality was three times

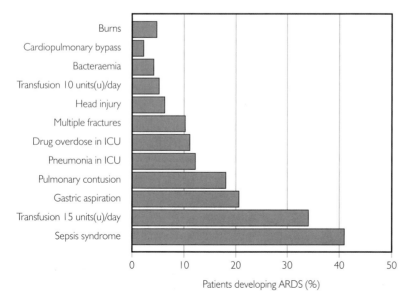

Fig. 28.1 Percentage of patients with single risk factors that develop the acute respiratory distress syndrome (ARDS). 'Transfusion' indicates blood transfusion dose given as units per day. ICU, intensive care unit.

Patients developing ARDS (%)

higher in those succumbing to ARDS (62%) than among patients with clinical risk factors who did not develop ARDS (19%). The difference in mortality if ARDS developed was particularly striking in patients with trauma (56% versus 13%) but less in those with sepsis (69% versus 49%).

Inherited characteristics and chronic comorbidities affect individual susceptibility to and outcome from ARDS. Alcohol abuse is associated with an increased incidence of ARDS and greater mortality,[13] whereas diabetic patients with sepsis have a lower incidence of ARDS than non-diabetic controls.[14] Improvements in molecular technology and mapping of the human genome have increased awareness of the potential to predict those most likely to develop ARDS by screening for genomic polymorphisms. These investigations to date have concentrated on polymorphisms of genes for known modulators of the inflammatory response and for endogenous factors that mediate cytoprotection. This burgeoning field of investigation has not yet produced data that is clinically applicable.[15]

Epidemiology

Incidence

A National Institutes of Health panel estimated in 1972 that there were 150 000 new cases of ARDS per year in the USA, an incidence roughly of 75 cases per 100 000/year. The incidence of ARDS has been difficult to determine accurately because of changing definitions, failure to capture complete data and uncertainty about the true population base or denominator. Several more recent prospective cohort studies have found much lower incidence rates, varying from 1.5–3.5 per 100 000 inhabitants/year in the Canary Islands[16] to a range of 4.8–8.3 cases per 100 000 inhabitants/year in the state of Utah.[17] Other studies found incidences of 4.5 and 3.0 per 100 000 inhabitants/year in the UK[18] and in Berlin[19] respectively. Out of the total 17 440 intensive care unit (ICU) admissions in the APACHE III database, 423 patients (2.4%) had both acute respiratory failure and a hospital diagnosis of ARDS.[8]

Much less information is available on the incidence of ALI. Two recent studies reported that 16–18% of the ventilated ICU population suffer from ARDS and 4–5% from ALI.[20,21] This translates, for example, into a US national incidence of 3600–24 300 adult cases of ARDS per year.

Prognosis

The indicators of a poor outcome in ARDS are age, severity of illness (SAPSII), shock and multiple organ failure.[6,22–24] Of patients over 70 years, 82% do not survive. The mortality rate is directly related to the number of organ-system failures and increases to 83% when three or more are present; patients without other organ failures have a lower mortality rate (38%). The most frequent complications appearing during the course of ARDS are circulatory shock and acute renal failure, associated with a mortality rate of over 90%. The majority of late deaths are related to sepsis syndrome, present in 73% of ARDS patients[25] in whom the predominant site is the lung. Several investigators have indicated that sepsis rather than respiratory failure is the leading cause of death in patients with ARDS.[6,24,26]

Once treatment and patient support has begun, prognostic factors relate to the patient's response to therapy. Although oxygenation (P_aO_2/F_iO_2) is an unreliable prognostic indicator at the onset of ARDS,[6] subsequent changes in P_aO_2 and alveolar–arterial O_2 tension difference ($AaDO_2$) may indicate the evolution of lung injury and provide useful prognostic information. A progressive increase of P_aCO_2 despite increased tidal volume, an increase in the dead space to tidal volume ratio over 70%, an increase of arterial–end-tidal CO_2 difference and a persistently high pulmonary vascular resistance are associated with destruction of the pulmonary circulation and a poor prognosis.[9]

Pathology

The response of the lung to injury is stereotyped; hence, morphological studies can provide few clues to the factors that initiated lung injury. Interpretation of lung biopsies or postmortem specimens is confused by the effects of common events in the clinical course of patients with ARDS, such as nosocomial pneumonia, injury caused by mechanical ventilation and high concentrations of inspired oxygen. There are few indications for lung biopsy in critically ill patients with ARDS; therefore antemortem histopathological data are scarce.

The pathological features of the lung in ARDS result from an evolving process of inflammation, resolution and repair. The appearances termed 'diffuse alveolar damage', particularly in the later stages and in the absence of clinical information, may be confused with cryptogenic organising pneumonia or acute interstitial pneumonia. ARDS can be divided into three overlapping phases that correlate with the clinical evolution of the disease[27] (Fig. 28.2):

1. the *exudative phase* of oedema and haemorrhage
2. the *proliferative phase* of organisation and repair
3. the *fibrotic phase*.

Exudative phase

This phase of diffuse alveolar damage occupies approximately the first week after the onset of respiratory failure. Macroscopically the lungs are rigid, dull red and heavy. Unlike classic pulmonary oedema, the cut surface of the lung does not exude fluid, because the proteinaceous alveolar exudate coagulates.

Eosinophilic hyaline membranes, most prominent in alveolar ducts, are distinctive features of early ARDS. These are composed of plasma proteins and cell debris that leak through the damaged endothelial–epithelial barrier into the alveolar space. Immunohistochemical staining demonstrates immunoglobulin, fibrinogen and, to a lesser extent, complement in hyaline membranes.[28]

There is ultrastructural evidence of endothelial injury but features of severe damage such as cellular necrosis, denudation

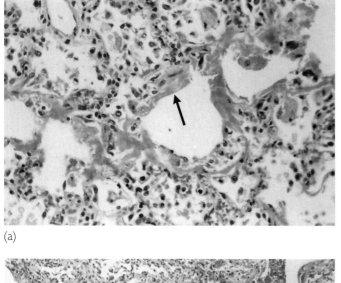

(a)

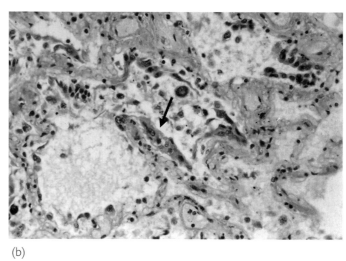

(b)

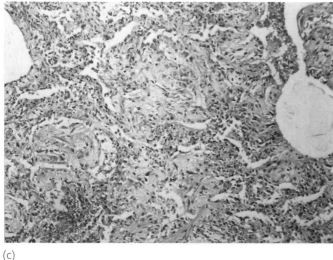

(c)

Fig. 28.2 Pathological features of diffuse alveolar damage associated with acute lung injury and the acute respiratory distress syndrome. a. Exudative phase: extensive hyaline membranes (arrow) line alveoli. Note the large numbers of inflammatory cells in the interstitium. b. Proliferative phase: regenerating type 2 cells (arrow) line alveoli after reabsorption of hyaline membranes. c. Fibrotic phase: extensive fibrosis involves both the alveoli and the interstitium. Haematoxylin & eosin. (Courtesy of Dr MS Shepphard, Department of Lung Pathology, Royal Brompton National Heart and Lung Hospital.)

of the capillary basement membrane and intravascular fibrin accumulation are often absent.[29] Focal intracapillary aggregates of neutrophils are prominent, especially in cases associated with sepsis.[29] However, compact masses of neutrophils in alveolar spaces suggest complicating infection. Alveolar septae are widened by interstitial oedema, fibrin and extravasated red cells, frequently out of proportion to visible endothelial disruption.

By contrast to the irregular and often slight endothelial changes, the alveolar epithelium usually demonstrates extensive necrosis of type I cells. These slough from the alveolar surface to be replaced by hyaline membranes adhering to the denuded basement membrane. Type II cells are more resistant to injury and, in addition to secreting surfactant, provide a population of cells capable of replication and differentiation to replace type I cells.[30] This begins as early as the third day after the onset of ARDS, heralding the beginning of the proliferative phase.

Proliferative phase

The proliferative phase of diffuse alveolar damage is characterised by organisation of intra-alveolar and interstitial exudates.

Typically, between the first and third weeks after injury, the lung parenchymal surface is macroscopically solid, pale grey and glistening, with a slippery texture attributable to newly formed connective tissue.

Epithelial regeneration manifests as rows of cuboidal cells extending along alveolar walls to cover previously denuded basement membrane. Many of these cells stain for surfactant apoprotein indicative of alveolar type II cell differentiation.[28] Within the alveolar wall, fibroblasts and myofibroblasts proliferate and subsequently migrate through defects in the alveolar basement membrane into the fibrinous intra-alveolar exudate. Thus, the exudate is converted to cellular granulation tissue and ultimately into fibrous tissue. Staining for acid mucopolysaccharides is strongly positive in organising granulation tissue. These intra-alveolar materials may act as a sponge, which retains fluid, but they also serve as a framework over which leukocytes and fibroblasts migrate, transforming the exudate into connective tissue, a process termed 'fibrosis by accretion'. Two other mechanisms contribute to remodelling of the lung in ARDS. Fibroblasts within the alveolar wall, stimulated by interstitial oedema, cause alveolar septal fibrosis. The third mechanism, termed 'collapse induration' follows collapse of damaged alveolar walls, which become sealed in apposition by organising fibrin and hyperplastic epithelium. Collapse induration results in fewer but larger alveoli and dilated alveolar ducts and macroscopic 'honeycombing'.

Fibrotic phase

Histologically, fibrosis begins as early as a week after the onset of ARDS. Total lung collagen is measurably increased in ARDS patients surviving more than 14 days and there is a progressive increase in lung collagen with the duration of the disease.[31]

Macroscopically, the pleural surface has a coarse, cobblestone appearance. The cut parenchymal surface is pale and spongy, consisting of areas of microcystic air spaces and irregular scarring. Healed abscesses and chronic interstitial emphysema cause larger cysts in chronic ARDS. However, the appearance of contiguous large air spaces, termed 'adult bronchopulmonary dysplasia', is unusual.

Pulmonary vascular disease in acute respiratory distress syndrome

The pulmonary vascular bed is extensively remodelled in the late proliferative and fibrotic phases of ARDS. Post-mortem specimens from the fibrotic phase reveal tortuous, narrowed arteries with mural fibrous thickening. Pulmonary arteries demonstrate muscularisation of pre- and intra-acinar vessels, which contributes to irreversible pulmonary hypertension in patients with pulmonary fibrosis secondary to ARDS.[32] Increased blood flow, chronic hypoxia and vasoconstriction, and oxygen toxicity may contribute to pulmonary vascular remodelling.

In lungs examined post-mortem, thromboemboli are present in up to 95% of patients. Macrothrombi (in arteries more than 1 mm in diameter) are found in 86% of patients by post-mortem arteriography but are more prevalent in patients dying in the early phase of ARDS. Microthrombi detected by light microscopy are equally common but are evenly distributed through the histopathological phases.[32] Haemorrhagic infarcts are not uncommon, the visceral pleura being particularly susceptible to ischaemic necrosis, probably because of insufficient collateral flow from other pulmonary arteries or the bronchial circulation. These necrotic areas are susceptible to infection and to the development of pneumothorax.

Pathogenesis

Injury to the alveolar–capillary membrane

The microvascular endothelium, the alveolar epithelium and a shared basement membrane constitute the alveolar–capillary membrane. In health, alveolar type II cells occupy only 7% of the alveolar surface despite constituting roughly half of the alveolar epithelium numerically. This structure is ideally suited to gas exchange but type I alveolar epithelial cells in particular are vulnerable to injury that is manifest clinically by leakage of protein-rich oedema fluid into the air spaces. Injury to alveolar type II cells disrupts both epithelial fluid transport, impairing

the removal of oedema fluid from the alveolar space,[33] and the metabolism of surfactant. Compared to healthy individuals, the surfactant obtained by bronchoalveolar lavage (BAL) from patients with ARDS showed increased minimal surface tension and decreased hysteresis of the surface-tension–surface-area relationship, two critical indices of surfactant function in vivo.[34] This impairment of surface activity was equally pronounced in patients with indirect and direct ARDS. Surfactant deficiency and dysfunction, in part caused by plasma proteins in the air space, may contribute to the pathophysiology of ARDS via a number of mechanisms[35] including exacerbation of atelectasis, impairment of gas exchange, increased oedema formation and impairment of local host defence.

Pulmonary inflammation

In the late 1980s it was realised that inflammatory conditions like sepsis, the systemic inflammatory response syndrome and at an organ level ARDS, were caused by an imbalance between pro- and anti-inflammatory mediators.[36] This resulted in uncontrolled and injurious activation of mechanisms that normally protect the host against local microbial invasion and tissue damage. The role of circulating mediators in driving pulmonary inflammation is implied by the observation that more than half of ARDS cases are initiated by a severe systemic condition that lacks a primary pulmonary component. More recently, it has been recognised that elements of the inflammatory response may become primed by a seemingly innocuous insult to later produce an exaggerated reaction to a subsequent stimulus. This mechanism probably underlies the additive effect of clinical risk factors but also suggests that the timing of lesser stimuli is clinically important.

Histological studies of lung tissue obtained early in the course of ARDS show a marked accumulation of neutrophils. Neutrophils predominate in BAL fluid obtained from affected patients[37] and persistent neutrophilia in sequential lavages appears to be a marker of a prolonged requirement for ventilatory support and a poor outlook.[38] While it is probable that neutrophils play an important role in lung injury, as they do in host defence, ARDS may occur in neutropenic patients[39] and not all models of lung injury are neutrophil-dependent. In order to accumulate in tissue, neutrophils adhere to the microvascular endothelium, migrate through the vessel wall and, in the lung, penetrate the alveolar epithelial cell layer to reach the airspace. There are critical differences between the processes governing neutrophil emigration in the pulmonary and systemic microcirculation.[40]

The neutrophil is ideally equipped to be an effector of lung damage associated with parenchymal inflammation. First, analysis of samples from patients at risk of developing ARDS has revealed evidence of both an increased serum concentration of neutrophil elastase[41] and increased alveolar levels of the potent neutrophil chemokine interleukin (IL)-8 in those patients who progress to ARDS.[42] Second, activated neutrophils release cytotoxic reactive oxygen species and potent proteases that kill invading microorganisms or damage local tissues. Finally, the diameter of a neutrophil is greater than that of a pulmonary capillary, which maximises the opportunity for interaction (mutual activation, migration or release of mediators) with the endothelium.

A complex network proinflammatory mediators with considerable overlap and redundancy are produced by resident lung cells (alveolar macrophages and epithelium) and invading leukocytes (Tables 28.5 & 28.6). These initiate and amplify the inflammatory response that characterises lung injury. Individual mediators have been implicated by their detection in the blood and, more tellingly, in the BAL fluid of patients with lung injury and animal models. Certain agents may initiate animal models of ARDS and, conversely, antagonism of individual mediators prevents or attenuates experimental lung injury, although this approach has universally yielded negative results when identical antagonists are used clinically (see below). Several endogenous inhibitors of proinflammatory agents have been described, including IL-1-receptor antagonist, soluble tumour necrosis factor (TNF) receptor, and anti-inflammatory cytokines such as IL-10 and IL-11. The individual mediators (cytokines, proteases and lipid-based molecules), and their interactions, orchestrating parenchymal pulmonary inflammation are too numerous to discuss in detail.

Resolution of inflammation and repair

The first step in resolving lung injury is to remove the initiating cause(s) and to prevent further proinflammatory stimuli that attract leukocytes to the lung and encourage the longevity of distinct populations, e.g. by delaying neutrophil apoptosis.[43] When the balance is tipped in favour of resolution, neutrophil apoptosis followed by macrophage phagocytosis, unlike necrosis, removes the potential for further local tissue damage by preventing the release of proteases and reactive oxygen species. Furthermore, this process induces macrophages to release anti-inflammatory and proapoptotic mediators such as transforming growth factor (TGF)-β and Fas ligand.[44] Macrophages and lymphocytes, rather than undergoing apoptosis, emigrate from the lungs via lymphatics to draining nodes as inflammation resolves.[45]

Following lung injury, functional recovery depends on alveolar type II cell dedifferentiation, migration and proliferation to cover the provisional matrix of the denuded alveolar membrane as the first step towards restoring the type 1 cell population and normal alveolar architecture.[46] Alveolar oedema is resolved by the active transport of sodium and perhaps chloride from the distal air spaces into the lung interstitium.[47] Water follows passively, probably through transcellular water channels, the aquaporins, located primarily on type I cells.[48] In clinical studies, clearance of alveolar fluid can occur very early in the course of lung injury and is associated with a favourable outcome.[49]

Table 28.5 Cellular mediators of acute lung injury and the acute respiratory distress syndrome

	Proinflammatory	Anti-inflammatory	Fibrogenesis
Endothelium	Directs leukocyte migration by chemokine secretion and adhesion molecule expression. Modulates local vascular tone and coagulation mechanisms	Possible role of shedding of soluble adhesion molecules	Secretes proinflammatory and fibrogenic mediators
Epithelium	Expresses ICAM to facilitate leukocyte migration. Secretes chemokines and proinflammatory cytokines. Release of RO/NS	Recovers exposed alveolar basement membrane. Secretes surfactant	Secretion and activation of TGFβ-1. Direct contact with fibroblasts
Macrophage/monocyte	Pivotal mediator of acute and chronic inflammation. Secretes chemokines and proinflammatory cytokines. Release of RO/NS	Removes apoptotic cells by phagocytosis and lymphatic emigration. Release of IL-10	Secretes proinflammatory and fibrogenic mediators
Neutrophil	Effectors of tissue damage and host defence through local release of proteases and RO/NS. Secretes chemokines and proinflammatory cytokines	Removed by apoptosis. Release IL-1ra	Presence in BAL correlates with a poor outlook in fibrotic lung diseases
Platelet	Thrombocytopenia in 50% ARDS patients. Co-factor in coagulation cascades. Potential source of proinflammatory mediators		
Lymphocyte	Potential source of proinflammatory mediators	Source of IL-10. Removed by lymphatic emigration	Source of pro (IL-4) and antifibrotic (IFN-γ) mediators
Myofibroblast			Proliferates and deposits extracellular matrix

ICAM, intercellular adhesion molecule; IFN, Interferon; IL, Interleukin; IL-1ra, Interleukin-1 receptor antagonist; RO/NS, Reactive oxygen/nitrogen species; TGF, transforming growth factor.

Table 28.6 Humoral modulators of inflammation and tissue damage in acute lung injury and the acute respiratory distress syndrome

Action	Class	Mediator(s)	Comment
Proinflammatory	Initiators	Endotoxin, LTA	Gram-negative and -positive cell-wall constituents
		IL-1β, TNF-α	Synergistic and overlapping effects. Induce synthesis of downstream mediators. TNF induces apoptosis
	Chemokines	IL-8, ENA-78, MIP-1α	Neutrophil chemoattractants and activators
	Late mediators and effectors of tissue damage	Lipid derived – PLA_2, COX-2	PAF, prostaglandins, leukotrienes
		Peptide cascades	Coagulation and contact systems, complement, kinins
		Reactive oxygen/nitrogen species – iNOS	Nitric oxide, superoxide, hydrogen peroxide, peroxynitrite
		Proteases	Elastase, metalloproteinases
Anti-inflammatory†	Cytokines	IL-4, -6*, -10, -11, -13, TGF-β	Inhibitors of proinflammatory cytokine production
		IL-1ra	Specific antagonist of the IL-1 receptor
	Soluble receptors	sTNFRI and II, sIL-1RII	Binds and inactivates circulating ligand
	Cytoprotectors	Intracellular	Enzymes (SOD, catalase), heat shock proteins
		Extracellular	Enzymes (antiproteases, TIMP), glutathione

* IL-6 is a typical cytokine in that it has anti- and proinflammatory activities. It inhibits the synthesis of mediators that have predominantly proinflammatory actions without affecting the synthesis of IL-10 and TGF-β. IL-6 promotes the synthesis of corticosteroids and IL-1ra. However, it also induces the acute phase response and is frequently used as a marker for systemic activation of proinflammatory cytokines.

† Concentrations of pro- and anti-inflammatory cytokines are elevated in the bronchoalveolar lavage fluid of patients early in the course of lung injury. Low levels of IL-10 and IL-1ra correlate with mortality while high levels of proinflammatory mediators do not.[54]

COX-2, inducible cyclo-oxygenase; ENA, epithelial-cell-derived neutrophil-activating protein; IL, interleukin; IL-1ra, interleukin-1 receptor antagonist; iNOS, inducible nitric oxide synthase; LTA, lipoteichoic acid; MIP, macrophage inflammatory protein; PAF, platelet activating factor; PLA_2, phospholipase A_2; SOD, superoxide dismutase; sTNFR, soluble tumour necrosis factor receptor; TGF, transforming growth factor; TIMP, tissue inhibitor of metalloproteinase; TNF, tumour necrosis factor.

Soluble protein appears to be removed by diffusion between alveolar epithelial cells. Insoluble protein may be removed by endocytosis and transcytosis by alveolar epithelial cells and by phagocytosis by macrophages.[50]

Lung injury taken in its broadest context may result in a spectrum of parenchymal lung diseases including at each extreme, from the point of view of recovery, ARDS and idiopathic pulmonary fibrosis. Of those patients with ARDS who survive, only a small percentage suffer from a degree of pulmonary dysfunction that interferes with their activities of daily living.[51] An important histological characteristic of fibrosing lung conditions is the persistence of hyperplastic cuboidal type II cells, suggesting that these cells are unable to differentiate. It has been suggested that failure of alveolar epithelial recovery after injury is central to the pathogenesis of fibrosis, although causality has not been proved.

The three-phase pathological model of ARDS and the assertion that fibrosis is an inevitable consequence of unresolved inflammation are gross oversimplifications. Fibrosis is evident histologically as early as a week after the onset of the disorder[52] and procollagen III peptide, a precursor of collagen synthesis, is elevated in the BAL fluid of ARDS patients at the time of endotracheal intubation.[53] Similarly, while several proinflammatory mediators are profibrotic (Table 28.6), it has recently been demonstrated that distinct patterns of gene expression are associated with these processes in the lung.[55] The development of pulmonary fibrosis in a patient with ARDS predicts the requirement for prolonged respiratory support and a poor outcome.[56]

Matrix metalloproteinases (MMP) are enzymes that digest collagens. At least two of these, MMP-2 and MMP-9, are elevated in the lungs in patients with ARDS[57] and it is likely that they facilitate remodelling by removing type III collagen, which is deposited soon after lung injury. Under profibrotic conditions, this matrix is subsequently remodelled so that the thicker and more resistant type I collagen predominates.[58]

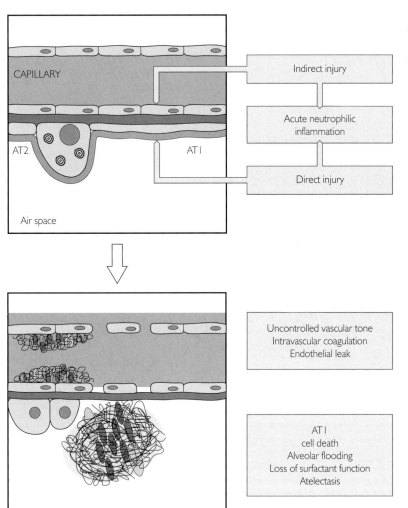

Pathophysiology

The pathophysiology of ARDS reflects the consequences of damage to the alveolar–capillary membrane and acute neutrophilic inflammation. We have divided the strictly pulmonary from the vascular aspects for convenience, although they are co-dependent and overlapping entities (Fig. 28.3).

Pulmonary pathophysiology

Atelectasis, alveolar and interstitial oedema affect the pressure–volume (P/V) relationship of the injured lung (Fig. 28.4). In early ARDS, decreased compliance, marked hysteresis and inflexion points on inflation and deflation are apparent. In mechanically ventilated patients, the initial part of the curve (low lung volume) is flatter, reflecting the relatively large pressures required to open or recruit collapsed peripheral airways and/or alveoli. The lower inflexion point appears when sufficient pressure is generated to open atelectatic lung units. Above the lower inflection point, compliance increases because more lung is available for ventilation. Identifying the lower inflection

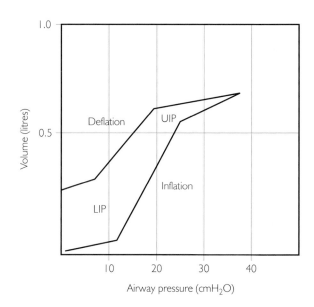

Fig. 28.4 Diagrammatic representation of the pressure–volume curve of a patient with lung injury. LIP, lower inflexion point; UIP, upper inflexion point.

point may be a helpful way to determine in individual patients the amount of PEEP necessary to prevent tidal atelectasis – the 'open lung approach'.[59] Animal experiments suggest that recruitment occurs throughout the entire lung inflation from end-expiratory lung volume to total lung capacity rather than being confined to the region below the lower inflection point.[60] The upper inflection point appears to correspond to the onset of alveolar overinflation. In normal humans, the upper inflection point is seen only after several litres are inspired, corresponding to total lung capacity.[61] In ARDS, the upper inflection point occurs at low volumes, often well below 1 litre and within the range of tidal volume. The clinical value of plotting P/V curves is unknown.

Gas dilution studies have shown that as little as a third to a half of the total lung volume at functional residual capacity (FRC) is gas-filled during the acute phase of lung injury.[62] Only this fraction participates in tidal ventilation, so that it is functionally like a 'baby lung'.[63] Much of the lung, especially in dependent regions, is consolidated and cannot be recruited for gas exchange. By contrast, the remaining, less affected lung must accommodate most of the tidal volume, placing it at risk of overinflation. Depletion of functional surfactant in ARDS promotes the development of widespread atelectasis, which may be exacerbated when low tidal volume strategies are employed. In addition, some areas of the lung appear to collapse cyclically, expanding on inhalation and collapsing on exhalation, a process called 'cyclical or tidal atelectasis.' With each breath, the adjacent lung units that remain open are distended and distorted. Animal models of lung injury suggest that PEEP may protect against ventilator-associated lung injury by preventing cyclical atelectasis.[64]

Pulmonary vascular dysfunction

Changes to the structure and function of the pulmonary vasculature are central to the pathophysiology of ARDS (Table 28.7). Mild pulmonary hypertension is a common observation in both the acute and chronic phases of ARDS,[65] even in the setting of the lowered systemic vascular resistance that characterises the systemic inflammatory response syndrome and septic shock. Associated with these inflammatory conditions there is con-

siderable inhomogeneity between and within different tissue beds in that cutaneous vessels vasodilate while the pulmonary, mesenteric and renal circulations are characterised by vasoconstriction. In health, the endothelium exerts active control over the underlying vascular smooth muscle and tone through the synthesis and release of a wide variety of substances, principally nitric oxide (NO), endothelins (ETs) and cyclo-oxygenase (COX) products. Under inflammatory conditions, the same mediators that propagate widespread inflammation induce expression of enzymes in the endothelium and vascular smooth muscle that produce large amounts of vasoactive agents. Hence the normal mechanisms that control vascular tone are overridden, causing not only local changes in vascular resistance but also a loss of ventilation perfusion matching in the pulmonary circulation and mismatch between oxygen delivery and consumption in systemic tissues.[66] The increase in pulmonary vascular tone associated with ARDS is possibly caused by increased activity of the locally produced vasoconstrictors thromboxane $(TX)A_2$[67] and ET-1,[68] which contribute to the early and late phases of endotoxin-induced pulmonary hypertension.

The loss of hypoxic pulmonary vasoconstriction (HPV) and resulting ventilation–perfusion mismatch in ARDS results in a degree of intrapulmonary shunt, sufficient (> 40% in many cases) to account for the $AaDo_2$ without invoking a decrease in diffusion capacity (Fig. 28.5).[69] This contention is supported by the lack of correlation between pulmonary extravascular water content and hypoxaemia, both in patients[70] and in sheep after endotoxin administration.[71] The increased pulmonary vascular resistance results from both functional (vasoconstriction) and structural (emboli, vascular compression and remodelling) effects of the forces applied by positive pressure ventilation, pulmonary inflammation and damage. Pulmonary hypertension, which is rarely severe, is probably a marker of disease severity and, in the absence of right ventricular dysfunction, of questionable clinical significance. Finally, the association with disseminated intravascular coagulation, histological data and the finding that BAL fluid from ARDS patients has procoagulant activity[72] are consistent with inappropriate activation of coagulation cascades in injured lungs. Injury to the pulmonary microvascular endothelium deprives it of its antiaggregation and

Table 28.7 Pulmonary vascular dysfunction in acute lung injury and the acute respiratory distress syndrome

Target	Mechanism	Effect
Resistance artery	Patchy and dysregulated vasoconstriction/dilation, remodelling in chronic ARDS	Mild pulmonary hypertension Loss of HPV and $\dot{V}/\dot{Q}$ mismatching
Microvasculature	Endothelial inflammation	Increased permeability oedema Leukocyte activation and tissue invasion Intravascular thrombosis
	Extravascular compression	Increased dead space
Postcapillary venule	Vasoconstriction and compression	Mild pulmonary hypertension Increased oedema formation

HPV, hypoxic pulmonary vasoconstriction; $\dot{V}/\dot{Q}$, ventilation/perfusion ratio.

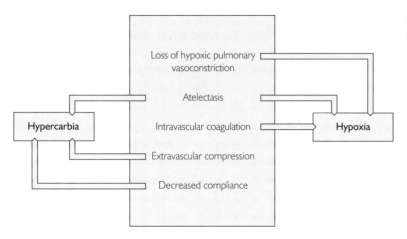

Fig. 28.5 Pathophysiology of gas exchange abnormalities in lung injury.

anticoagulant properties. Apart from causing intravascular thrombosis and embolism, several peptide intermediates in the clotting cascade have potent proinflammatory effects.[73]

Sepsis and multiple organ failure

Definitions are shown in Table 28.8.[36] The coexistence of sepsis, ARDS and other organ failures is to be expected given the common inflammatory mediators and shared pathogenesis of microcirculatory failure and cellular dysfunction. Sepsis is the commonest cause of lung injury accounting for 25–40% of cases.[74] Conversely, 18–38% of patients with systemic infection, defined as bacteraemia or sepsis, develop ARDS. In patients with sepsis, shock and disseminated intravascular coagulation correlate with the incidence of ARDS. Lung injury, shock and renal failure are the earliest and commonest organ failures associated with sepsis.[75] Sepsis is a common and important complication for patients with ARDS; an autopsy study of patients who died with ARDS revealed that 98% had evidence of infection, the commonest site of origin being the lung.[76]

Table 28.8 Definitions of sepsis, septic shock and the systemic inflammatory response syndrome

Sepsis	**The systemic response to infection** Includes two or more of the following: Temperature > 38°C or < 36°C Heart rate > 90/min Respiratory rate > 20/min or P_aCO_2 < 4.3 kPa White cell count > 12 000/mm³ or < 4000/mm³, or > 10% band (immature) forms

Septic shock	**Sepsis with hypotension**
	Sepsis as defined above plus either:
	
	Decrease in systolic blood pressure < 90 mmHg, or a drop of > 40 mmHg for at least 1 h
	in spite of adequate fluid resuscitation
	or
	Perfusion abnormalities, e.g.:
	    Lactic acidosis
	    Oliguria
	    Acutely altered mental status

Systemic inflammatory response syndrome	**Sepsis without infection**
	The response to a variety of severe insults that is indistinguishable from sepsis, but does not have an infectious aetiology. Examples include:
	    Acute pancreatitis
	    Acute infarction
	    Fat embolism syndrome
	    Transfusion reaction
	    Drug hypersensitivity
	    Adrenal insufficiency
	    Over-diuresis

As a risk factor for ARDS, sepsis confers a poor prognosis and is relatively over-represented in patients over 60 years old.[77] Infection and sepsis occurring in the context of ARDS is common because patients are subjected to interventions that impair local host defences, such as endotracheal intubation, central venous catheters and the alteration of normal microbial populations by broad-spectrum antibiotics. Furthermore, the ability of critically ill patients to mount an immune response to infection may be impaired by anti-inflammatory drugs or after a period of systemic inflammation, the so called compensatory anti-inflammatory response syndrome.[78] In the case of a patient with existing ARDS, systemic infection or inflammation may aggravate or rekindle pulmonary inflammation and secondary pneumonia may exacerbate local tissue damage.

Diagnosis and clinical features

At presentation the predisposing condition(s) or complications may dominate the clinical picture so that features of early ARDS are obscured, particularly during recovery from surgery or major trauma when the patient may be mechanically ventilated. Arterial blood gases taken early in the evolution of lung injury usually reveal respiratory alkalosis and hypoxaemia that is often resistant to supplemental oxygen.

Chest radiography and computed tomography

Hypoxaemia often precedes the radiological appearance of pulmonary oedema in ARDS; indeed diffuse bilateral alveolar infiltrates usually appear 4–24 hours after the first abnormal signs. The opacities typical of ARDS tend to be more peripheral and apical than those associated with left ventricular failure.[79] Normal heart size (cardiothoracic ratio < 0.55), vascular pedicle width (< 68–70 mm), absent septal lines, air bronchograms and a peripheral distribution are the most discriminating features associated with non-cardiogenic pulmonary oedema. However, the appearances of ARDS on plain radiography are non-specific. Radiologists can consistently assess the chest radiograph component of the lung injury score but significant variations may be introduced when assessment is performed by other clinicians.[80]

In the later stages of ARDS, consolidation becomes less confluent and an interstitial or ground-glass pattern may appear, with areas of lucency corresponding to pneumatoceles. The appearance of the radiograph can be strongly influenced by the effects of therapy and the radiographic technique. Aggressive administration of fluid may worsen the picture, whereas the use of diuretics reduces oedema formation. Similarly, the technique of mechanical ventilation may affect regional lung density by increasing inflation, giving the radiographic appearance of improvement despite continued severe abnormalities in gas exchange. The authors recommend routine daily radiographs on all patients with ALI/ARDS requiring intensive care. Thoracic ultrasound imaging at the bedside is used to localise and facilitate drainage of pleural effusions.

Despite the involvement of all lung fields on a frontal chest radiograph, computed tomography (CT; Fig. 28.6) often reveals patchy infiltrates interspersed with normal-looking lung, indicating that ARDS is not a global process but a regional disease. The extent of lung involvement on CT correlates with gas exchange and lung compliance[81] and can reveal evidence of ventilator-associated lung injury, localised infection or pleural effusion not evident on plain films. In ARDS a gradient of lung density from ventral to dorsal lung is present: dense parenchymal opacification predominates in the dependent lung and merges with ground-glass opacification and normally aerated lung in the non-dependent regions (Fig. 28.7). In general, ground-glass opacification (increased lung attenuation that does not obscure bronchovascular markings) is the most extensive and common CT pattern seen during the acute illness. It may represent filling of the alveoli and interstitium with oedema fluid, inflammatory debris and red blood cells or, in the later phases, fine intralobular fibrosis. The most frequent and extensive CT abnormality detectable in survivors is a reticular pattern, which was recorded in 23/27 (85%) patients at follow-up.[82] Ground-glass opacification was present but far less extensive. A unique feature of the reticular pattern was its distribution in the axial plane: there was a striking predilection for the non-dependent lung. There was a strong relationship between the duration of mechanical ventilation and the extent of the reticular pattern, suggesting that this chronic abnormality is contributed to by ventilator-associated lung injury, from which the dependent atelectatic lung is protected.

There is evidence from CT that ARDS due to direct and indirect pulmonary injury may be distinct entities (Fig. 28.7). Hence, consolidation was more extensive in patients with pulmonary/direct ARDS and ground-glass opacification was more extensive in the extrapulmonary group.[83] Furthermore, a 'typical' CT appearance (dependent areas of dense parenchymal opacification and non-dependent areas of ground-glass) is more frequent in ARDS due to indirect injury. Importantly, the CT pattern seems to be independently if loosely related to the aetiology of ARDS but not to the delay between endotracheal intubation and CT scanning.

Pulmonary artery catheterisation

Although pulmonary artery catheterisation has been recommended to differentiate cardiogenic from increased-permeability pulmonary oedema, opinions differ about the indications. The American–European Consensus Conference definition of ARDS stipulates that pulmonary artery catheterisation is not required and should be used as indicated by the need to guide haemodynamic management. In the relatively unusual cases in which there is diagnostic doubt, non-invasive techniques such as echocardiography may suffice to exclude cardiac insufficiency. While a high cardiac output and a low pulmonary artery occlusion pressure are characteristic of ARDS, cardiogenic pulmonary oedema may occur with a 'normal' pulmonary artery occlusion pressure in patients whose pressures had been increased during a previous transient episode of left ventricular dysfunction. Conversely, high pressures may be recorded in

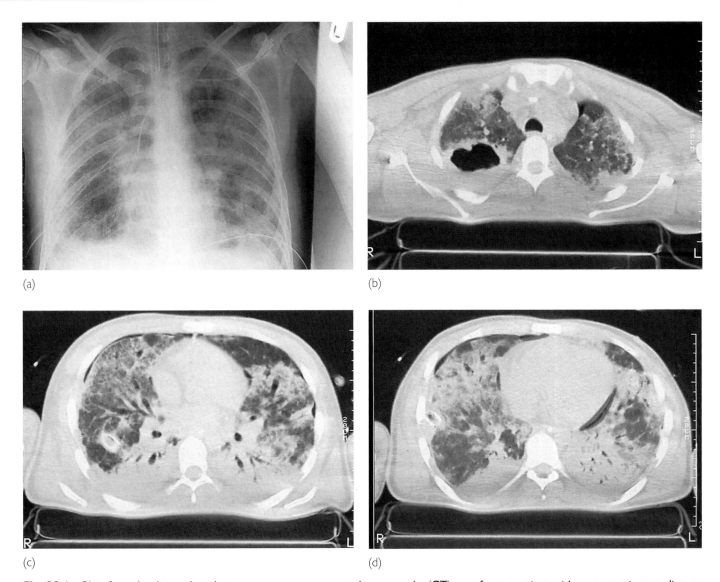

(a)

(b)

(c)

(d)

Fig. 28.6 Plain frontal radiograph and contemporaneous computed tomography (CT) scan from a patient with acute respiratory distress syndrome following chest trauma. The CT scan demonstrates a cavity in the right upper lobe adjacent to a scapula fracture. There is a small right anterior pneumothorax and pneumomediastinum: the right-sided intercostal chest drain is sited in the oblique fissure.

patients with ALI/ARDS who have been resuscitated with large volumes of fluid or in those with increased intrathoracic pressures.

Lung biopsy

Reluctance to undertake lung biopsy in critically ill patients has been tempered by recent advances in minimally invasive surgery. Such techniques are not, however widely available and the risks remain substantial despite reassuring case series.[84] It is rarely necessary to exclude differential diagnoses of diffuse pulmonary shadowing and respiratory failure (Table 28.2). However, microbiological investigation of biopsy specimens may be helpful in diagnosing opportunistic infections associated with ARDS in the immunocompromised host.

Measurements of endothelial and alveolar epithelial barrier function

The integrity of the alveolar–capillary membrane can be evaluated by measuring the protein content of alveolar fluid[85] or the flux of radiolabelled proteins from blood to lung tissue. These procedures are rarely used outside experimental studies. Hydrostatic and high-permeability pulmonary oedema can be distinguished from the ratio of protein concentration in pulmonary oedema fluid to that in plasma. If this ratio is greater than 0.75, an increase in permeability is suggested and if the ratio is between 0.65 and 0.75, the mechanism of oedema formation is indeterminate. Greatest specificity would be expected early after the onset of pulmonary oedema, because alveolar proteins are cleared in a size-dependent

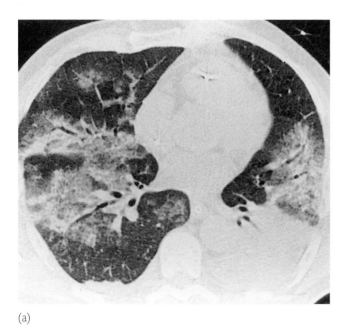
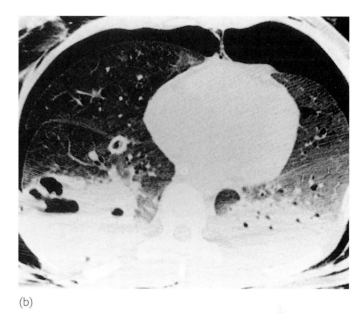

(a)   (b)

Fig. 28.7 Different computed tomographic appearances of lung injury characterise direct and indirect injury. The patterns of direct (a) and indirect (b) lung injury differ. Direct insults to the lung cause inhomogeneous patchy shadowing. Blood-borne injury affects the lung diffusely, the dependent parts becoming more densely consolidated. (Courtesy of Prof. D. Hausell, Radiology Dept., RBH.)

fashion. There is no evidence that a value above 0.75 correlates with the severity of injury to the alveolar–capillary membrane. However, since injury interferes with the size selectivity of the endothelial barrier, analysis of the oedema fluid based on protein size might quantify injury.

Extravascular lung water can be measured at the bedside by the thermal indocyanine green double-indicator dilution method.[86] The amount of extravascular lung water measured in patients with ARDS is about three times the upper limit of normal (500 ml) but may be as much as six to eight times greater. The disadvantages of this technique are that it is invasive and prone to error.

Biological markers

For patients with suspected or confirmed lung injury, having a sensitive and specific marker of disease could have several benefits. First, it might improve the ability to predict which patients with risk factors develop clinically significant ALI, so that potentially protective measures could be assessed and developed. Second, it might help to quantify the severity of disease and to predict complications such as fibrosis and superadded infection. Finally, as understanding of the pathogenesis of ALI/ARDS increases, the use of markers of disease may provide insights into mechanisms giving rise to pathophysiologically based definitions. These novel methods of disease classification may provide more homogenous groups of patients for clinical trials.

Most studies have involved assays on plasma samples or BAL fluid.[37] Unilateral BAL with 60–180 ml of fluid is safe in the majority of patients with ARDS.[87] Analysis may provide information about the cell populations (neutrophil, macrophage, etc.), soluble mediators (TNF-α, IL-1, IL-8, etc.; Table 28.6)

and by-products of inflammation (shed adhesion molecules, elastase, peroxynitrite, etc.) in the distal airways and air spaces.[37] Currently, assay of potential biomarkers is used exclusively in research.

Complications

The complications of the conditions that put patients at risk for developing ARDS and the support that they inevitably require are so intimately associated with the pathogenesis of lung injury that they are considered before the specific management.

Ventilator-associated lung injury

Mechanical ventilation at high volumes (volutrauma) and pressures (barotrauma) can cause a similar histological appearance to other models of lung injury.[88] This is associated with high-permeability pulmonary oedema in the uninjured lung[88] and exacerbated damage in the already injured lung.[89] Alveolar overdistension and the forces generated by repeated opening of recruitable lung units (atelectrauma) are possibly more damaging than the effects of high mean airway pressures and a high inspired oxygen tension. Thus, injurious ventilation of rats is associated with a 50-fold increase in the recovery of proinflammatory cytokines from BAL.[90] Pulmonary production of inflammatory mediators (biotrauma) is likely to exacerbate lung injury and overspill of proinflammatory agents into the systemic circulation of patients may contribute to the development of multiple organ failure and thereby increase mortality.[91] These issues have led to a number of clinical trials of protective ventilatory strategies to reduce alveolar overdistension and increase the recruitment of atelectatic alveoli.[92]

Pneumothorax, subcutaneous emphysema, pneumomedia-stinum, interstitial emphysema and rarely air embolism are manifestations of ventilator-associated lung injury that have traditionally been identified with barotrauma (Fig. 28.8). One study of 100 consecutive patients meeting the criteria for ALI and requiring mechanical ventilation found that 13% of patients

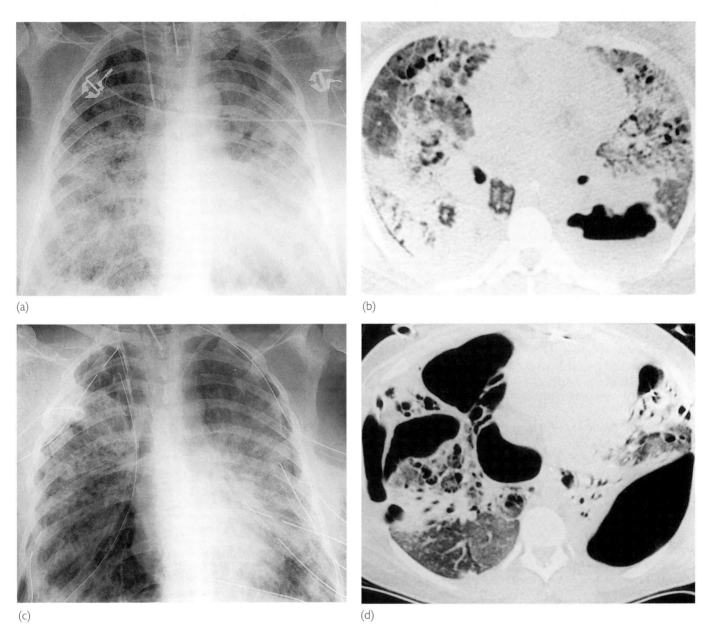

(a)

(b)

(c)

(d)

Fig. 28.8 Severe ventilator-associated lung injury in the recovery phase of acute respiratory distress syndrome. a, b. This 26-year-old patient suffered from ARDS 2 weeks post-partum following left lower lobe pneumonia. The sputum initially grew pneumococcus and sub-sequently methicillin-resistant *Staphylococcus aureus*. Note the abscess in the apical segment of the left lower lobe that is obvious on the CT scan (b) but not on the contemporaneous plain radiograph (a). c, d. After 5 months in intensive care, there were large bilateral multiloculated pneumothoraces, for which several intercostal chest drains had been placed. The CT scan at this stage (d) was useful in locating pneumothoraces and in targeting intercostal drains. Conventional medical treatment and weaning having failed, the patient under-went bilateral open talc pleurodesis and deroofing of the abscess cavity at staged procedures. e. A year later and 6 months after discharge from hospital there are no pneumothoraces and the abscess cavity is largely collapsed. Linear and reticular shadowing, together with trac-tion bronchiectasis, suggest fibrotic scarring. Despite pressure-limited ventilation and prone positioning there is more marked lung damage in the anterior half of the right lung. This observation is consistent with the dependent/posterior portion of the lung being protected against ventilator-induced lung injury by collapse.

Figure 28.8 e, see opposite

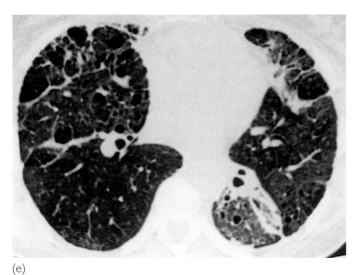

(e)

Fig. 28.8 *Continued.*

experienced air leaks during their illness.[93] Air leaks are rarely a direct cause of death but it is an important cause of morbidity and may contribute to death in patients with other risk factors for poor outcome. Detection can be challenging but worsening hypoxaemia, hypotension or a rapid deterioration in respiratory mechanics should be assumed to have been caused by a pneumothorax. Small pneumothoraces may have profound haemodynamic effects in patients with ARDS because the forces compressing the heart and great veins are transmitted by stiff lung tissue and because the patients are commonly relatively intravascular-fluid-depleted.

Ventilator-associated pneumonia

Nosocomial pneumonia, a complication of prolonged mechanical ventilation, is an important cause of morbidity and probably mortality in patients with ARDS.[94] The frequency of nosocomial pneumonia is not entirely clear owing to diagnostic uncertainty. One study of 243 consecutive mechanically ventilated patients found that patients with ARDS were significantly more likely to develop pneumonia than controls (55% versus 28%), probably because patients with ARDS required longer periods of mechanical ventilation.[95] The symptoms, signs and radiographic appearance of pneumonia are non-specific and easily confused with the underlying disease. Furthermore, because most patients become colonised with potential pathogens within days of intubation, cultures of respiratory secretions can be misleading. One autopsy study of patients with ARDS documented pneumonia in 58% of patients, although the diagnosis was suspected ante-mortem in only 20%.[96] At the same time, 20% of patients thought to have pneumonia on clinical and microbiological grounds did not have histological pneumonia.

It is uncertain whether bronchoscopic techniques such as protected specimen brush or quantitative BAL permit a more accurate diagnosis of ventilator-associated pneumonia compared with tracheal aspiration or blind lavage through a protected catheter. Because no technique is completely sensitive, empirical treatment should not be withheld when clinical suspicion of

pneumonia is high, although it has not been possible to demonstrate that accurate empirical therapy improves outcome. The most common organisms causing ventilator-associated pneumonia are Gram-negative bacteria, particularly *Pseudomonas* spp., although the incidence of Gram-positive infection is increasing and the results of local surveillance should be paramount when establishing an antibiotic policy.

Efforts to prevent ventilator-associated pneumonia have been disappointing. Selective gut decontamination may decrease the risk of pneumonia in selected groups.[97] Unfortunately, evidence supporting this practice is uncertain at best; in addition, the procedure raises the cost of ICU care and may promote the emergence of resistant organisms. Continuous subglottic aspiration may decrease infection by enteric organisms, but not by *Pseudomonas* species.[98]

Miscellaneous complications

Survivors of ARDS are likely to spend weeks or months in intensive care and consequently are exposed to the risk of numerous complications. Optimising mechanical ventilation in patients with severe lung damage often mandates the prolonged use of muscle relaxants and high doses of sedative agents. These agents are associated with failure of enteral feeding, which may be combated by the use of prokinetic agents, aperients and the siting of a nasojejunal feeding tube. Similarly patients with ARDS are at high risk of critical illness neuropathy and myopathy, especially if they have suffered from systemic sepsis and/or have been treated with corticosteroids.[99,100] For similar reasons, corneal and pressure area protection is of paramount importance; these areas are especially vulnerable when patients are placed in the prone position. Finally, immobilised patients require prophylaxis against venous thrombosis; ARDS patients are at greatest risk if their disease is associated with lower-leg trauma and/or sepsis. Our practice is to use low-molecular-weight heparin subcutaneously and compressive stockings.

Respiratory support

Almost all patients with ALI/ARDS require mechanical ventilatory support via an endotracheal tube. A few patients with mild injury may be sustained with continuous positive airways pressure (CPAP) and confidence is growing in using non-invasive ventilation in a closely supervised setting, again in patients with ALI who are haemodynamically stable.[101]

Mechanical ventilation

Currently it is not possible to describe a recipe for optimal ventilation of the ARDS patient. However the recent re-evaluation of ventilator-associated lung injury and results of comparing ventilatory strategies have provided some useful guidelines (Table 28.9). An international survey in the early 1990s found that most patients with ARDS were ventilated with tidal volumes of at least 10 ml/kg.[102] These large tidal volumes (compared with about 7 ml/kg spontaneously breathing at rest) tend to maintain a normal P_aCO_2 and prevent atelectasis in patients with lung injury but are disproportionately harmful when applied to the 'baby lung' of ARDS. Conversely, pressure and volume limitation lead to carbon-dioxide retention with potentially harmful effects.[103] While the pros and cons of hypercapnia are still debated, this approach – 'permissive hypercapnia' – was associated with a low mortality in an unrandomised study in patients with ARDS.[104] In 1993 a consensus conference, while acknowledging the lack of convincing human data, recommended adopting this approach by limiting tidal volume to as low as 5–7 ml/kg and plateau pressure to 35 cmH_2O.[105]

Subsequently, five studies have been published comparing protective with conventional ventilatory strategies; it is debatable whether conventional ventilation groups were ventilated in accordance with best practice because prescribed limits[105] were exceeded. Two of the five studies (Table 28.9) detected a benefit from protective ventilation; however, the data perhaps more convincingly demonstrate the negative effect on outcome of high tidal volumes and pressures.[109] The ARDS Network study provides the most compelling data supporting the hypothesis that low tidal volume ventilation benefits patients with lung injury, because the number of patients recruited (861) was sufficient to show a survival advantage and because the greatest difference in tidal volume was achieved between the two groups (Table 28.9).[110] However, features of the ARDS Network trial protocol were unique and provide less biologically plausible explanations for the survival difference. Despite these caveats we recommend limiting tidal volume and inflation pressures (Table 28.10), and accept that the management of hypercapnia and the definition of the optimal PEEP level remains to be standardised.

Positive end-expiratory ventilation increases FRC, thereby decreasing intrapulmonary shunting of blood through regions with collapsed alveoli. The use of PEEP in established ARDS can help to achieve adequate haemoglobin saturation and a decrease in the requirement for high F_IO_2. Experimental models have suggested that, by preventing atelectrauma, PEEP may impact positively upon the development and course of ARDS, although this has not been demonstrated in patients.[112] PEEP may benefit patients with lung injury by shifting oedema fluid from the airspace into the interstitium. However, positive intrathoracic pressure also has haemodynamic effects that may result in decreased ventricular filling, cardiac output and hence oxygen delivery. These adverse effects are most noticeable in patients who are fluid-depleted. High PEEP levels and permissive hypercapnia are contraindicated in patients who would be harmed by a raised intracranial pressure, most often an issue in patients with multiple trauma. PEEP is set in the 'open lung' approach at 2 cmH_2O above the lower infection point of the pressure–volume curve. If this cannot be determined, a PEEP of 16 cmH_2O is used.[59,109] The driving pressure, defined as plateau pressure minus PEEP, is kept below 20 cmH_2O and peak pressure is limited to 40 cmH_2O. Patients are ventilated using pressure-controlled inverse ratio ventilation or pressure support ventilation; the respiratory rate is kept below 30 breaths per minute. When the patient is disconnected from the ventilator, a 'recruiting manoeuvre' using CPAP of 35 cmH_2O is given for 40 seconds prior to reinstituting the previous level of PEEP. This is because even a single breath without PEEP results in compressive atelectasis and derecruitment.

During inverse ratio ventilation, increased mean airway pressure is achieved by prolonging the inspiratory-to-expiratory ratio. This technique improves oxygenation by recruiting atelectatic alveoli with long time constants. However, whether these effects are preferentially produced by inverse ratio ventilation is controversial.[113] We favour using inverse ration ventilation and levels of PEEP up to 18 cmH_2O, depending on the response of individual patients, but acknowledge that these opinions are not yet supported by adequate clinical studies.

High-frequency ventilation is another strategy that may protect against ventilator-associated lung injury while recruiting atelectatic lung and minimising haemodynamic compromise.[114] There are three techniques: positive pressure, jet and oscillation. Each uses tidal volumes below that of the anatomic dead space at frequencies greater than 60 breaths per minute. Complications include desiccation and inspissation of mucus, airway damage due to high gas velocity, air trapping and high shear forces at interfaces between areas of the lung with different impedances. High-frequency jet ventilation has received most attention. One randomised study of 309 patients found that oxygenation was maintained with lower peak airway pressures and tidal volumes with jet compared with conventional ventilation.[115] However as in other studies, high-frequency jet ventilation did not improve mortality or length of stay.

Prone positioning

Mechanical ventilation in the prone position can recruit collapsed alveolar units and possibly minimise ventilator-associated lung injury[116] early in the course of ARDS. Multiple small prospective studies have confirmed that use of the prone position improves oxygenation in 60–80% of patients to a degree enabling a reduction in F_IO_2.[117] More than 50% of the responders maintained an improvement in oxygenation for at least 1 hour following return to the supine position.

Mechanisms underlying this improvement in oxygenation are complex and incompletely understood.[118] In the supine position, alveolar inflation is greater in the non-dependent lung regions. Lung weight, cardiac mass, cephalic displacement of the abdomen and the regional mechanical properties and shape of the lung and thoracic cage are the main factors that influence transpulmonary pressure and the gravitational distribution of density. In the prone position ventilation redistributes from ventral (over-distended when supine, collapsed in the prone position) to dorsal regions and ventilation is more uniform owing to relief of mechanical factors that contribute to dorsal atelectasis in the supine position. Recruitment manoeuvres, such as high levels of PEEP, are likely to act synergistically with prone positioning and have a more prolonged beneficial effect in prone ARDS patients. Experimental evidence suggests that the distribution of perfusion is also more homogenous in the prone position and $\dot{V}/\dot{Q}$ matching is improved.[119] Other beneficial effects include improved mobilisation of secretions and redistribution of oedema fluid. In addition, more homogeneous ventilation could improve the delivery of aerosolised bronchodilators and inhaled vasodilators.[120]

Table 28.9 Clinical trials of protective versus conventional ventilation strategies in patients with acute lung injury and the acute respiratory distress syndrome

Study	n	Target V_T		Mean V_T (ml/kg)		Target pressure		Mean plateau pressure (cmH_2O)		PEEP (cmH_2O)		Mortality			Comment
		P	C	P	C	P	C	P	C	P	C	P	C	p	
Stewart[106]	120	< 8	10–15	6.8	10.1	≤ 30	50	20	28.6	9.6	8.0	50	47	NS	Mean values for day 7 given. In-hospital mortality
Brower[107]	52	5–8	10–12	7.3	10.2	≤ 30	45–55	24.9	30.6	Not given		50	46	NS	Mean of daily values given
Brochard[108]	116	6–10	10–15	7.4	10.7	≤ 25	≤ 60	24.5	30.5	9.6	8.5	46.6	37.9	NS	Mean values for day 7 given. 60-day mortality
Amato[109]	53	≤ 6	12	387	738	< 20–40	NL	24	37.8	13.2	9.3	38	71	< 0.001	Mean of daily values given. 28-day mortality. PEEP targeted at 2 cmH_2O above LIP on P/V curve vs. optimised for Fio_2 and Do_2. High mortality in C group
*Network[110]	861	6	12	6.5	11.4	≤ 30	≤ 50	26	37	8.1	9.1	31	39.8	0.007	Mean values for day 7 given. In-hospital mortality and breathing without assistance. Significant benefit in ventilator-free days and non-pulmonary organ failures

* A network of 10 centres, 24 hospitals and 75 intensive care units with a special interest in ARDS established recently to organise and run multicentre studies to answer outstanding clinical questions in the field. This institution is supported by the US National Institute of Health (website http://hedwig.mgh.harvard.edu/ardsnet).

C, conventional ventilation strategy; LIP, lower inflection point; NL, no limit; NS, not statistically significant; p, probability value; P, protected ventilation strategy; PEEP positive end-expiratory pressure; P/V, pressure–volume; V_T, tidal volume (ml/kg, except for Amato et al[109], where the figure is in millilitres).

Table 28.10 System-based targets for management of a patient with acute lung injury and the acute respiratory distress syndrome

Respiratory	Arterial oxygen saturation (S_aO_2) 88–92% Arterial blood pH > 7.2 Peak airway pressure < 30 cmH$_2$O Tidal volume 5–7 ml/kg
Cardiovascular	Mean arterial pressure 60–80 mmHg* Cardiac index > 2.2 l/m² Lactate < 1.5 mmol/l Minimal right atrial pressure or pulmonary artery occlusion pressure
Renal	Urine output > 0.5 ml/kg/h
Gut	Enteral feeding established Stress ulceration prevention
Nervous system	Adequate sedation for patient comfort Adequate paralysis for ventilatory management
Musculoskeletal	Early fixation of fractures Contracture prevention
Haematology	Haemoglobin concentration 7–9 g/dl† Thrombosis prevention
Skin	Pressure area and corneal protection
Microbiology	Prompt investigation and treatment of suspected infection
Social	Family and patient fully informed of progress and prognosis

* Target blood pressures vary according to the patient's age, comorbidities and past medical history. † In the absence of ischaemic heart disease.[111]

Predicting a positive response to prone positioning is imprecise. Patients with early diffuse injury characterised by dependent collapse typical of indirect lung injury would be expected to respond best. A brief test is recommended to assess responsiveness.[121] In patients with ARDS, a 10 mmHg increase in P_aO_2 in the first 30 minutes of prone positioning predicted continued improvement over a 2-hour trial, while non-responders at 30 minutes showed no subsequent improvement. Elevated intra-abdominal pressure and anterior chest wall compliance might also predict a positive response. How long to employ the prone position is another question that needs to be answered by prospective studies. We favour periods of 6–12 hours, alternating between the prone and supine positions.

There is no standard method but adequate numbers and teamwork are needed to perform the turn safely without dislodging catheters and tubes. Patients are placed in a modified swimmer's position with one arm extended fully and the head turned toward the extended arm. To allow free abdominal expansion, many practitioners recommend supporting the chest and pelvis. Spinal instability is the major absolute con-

traindication. Haemodynamic instability is a relative cotraindication, since cardiopulmonary resuscitation requires immediate repositioning. One review reported a very low incidence of critical adverse events in 240 patients over 746 prone cycles.[122] Repositioning and soft padding minimise skin breakdown over pressure points, which is the commonest significant complication.

Inhaled vasodilators

Inhaled vasodilators, nitric oxide and prostacyclin (prostaglandin 1$_2$), selectively dilate vessels that perfuse ventilated lung units resulting in improved $\dot{V}/\dot{Q}$ matching, better oxygenation and amelioration of pulmonary hypertension (Fig. 28.9). Because of their short half-lives, both vasodilators lack significant systemic haemodynamic effects when given by inhalation. Nitric oxide at doses between 1.25 and 80 parts per million (ppm) has been investigated extensively for use in ARDS. The majority of responders to nitric oxide do so at 10 ppm, although higher doses may be required to decrease pulmonary artery pressure and it is important to titrate individual responses so that the lowest effective concentration is administered. In the larger studies roughly 60% of patients with lung injury respond to nitric oxide inhalation with a 20% improvement in P_aO_2.[123]

The factors that determine responsiveness to nitric oxide are difficult to identify. One retrospective study found that patients with sepsis or septic shock responded less frequently to nitric oxide than those without (33% versus 64%).[124] A high baseline pulmonary vascular resistance and responsiveness to PEEP predict a positive response.[125] The improvement in $\dot{V}/\dot{Q}$ matching due to nitric oxide may be magnified by concomitant administration of intravenous almitrine, which enhances hypoxic pulmonary vasoconstriction.[126]

The significance of the many other chemical and biological effects of nitric oxide, including anti-inflammatory properties, antiplatelet activity and diminished vascular permeability, are difficult to assess when it is administered clinically.[123] Toxic nitrogen dioxide and methaemoglobin concentrations may increase when high doses of nitric oxide are given, and the concentration of both of these species should be monitored.[127] Most studies show comparable decreases in hypoxia and pulmonary artery pressure with nebulised prostacyclin solution.[128] In contrast to nitric oxide, prostacyclin does not require sophisticated equipment for administration.

While it is clear that many patients develop short-term improvements in oxygenation and pulmonary haemodynamics, it is unclear if these responses are clinically significant. Neither agent has been shown to improve survival in ARDS.

Moreover, the sustained physiological improvement has been modest in many studies. One trial compared increasing concentrations of nitric oxide with placebo in 177 patients and found that the improvement in oxygenation was modest and not sustained and 28-day mortality was not significantly different.[129] At present, inhaled vasodilators may be useful in patients with life-threatening hypoxaemia despite conventional management, but routine application should await further clinical trials.

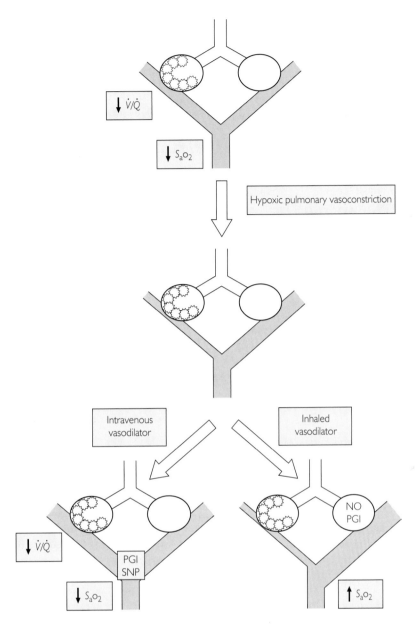

Fig. 28.9 Effect of intravenous and inhaled vasodilators in lung injury. NO, nitric oxide; PGI, prostacyclin; S_aO_2, arterial oxygen saturation; SNP, sodium nitroprusside; $\dot{V}/\dot{Q}$, ventilation/perfusion ratio.

Alternative means of supporting gas exchange

The following techniques are being evaluated as adjuncts to standard respiratory support and are uncommonly used in routine practice.

Surfactant dysfunction may contribute to the pathophysiology and exogenous surfactant has been beneficial in several animal models.[35] Clinical trials have yielded variable results that may reflect important differences in the methods of drug delivery or in the many forms of surfactant available. A high dose and/or repetitive treatment regimen appears to be necessary to overcome inhibitory agents in the alveolar space of ARDS patients and to achieve sustained alveolar recruitment. A study

in 59 patients with ARDS demonstrated significant improvement in oxygenation and a trend towards lower mortality in the bovine surfactant-treated group (19% versus 44%).[130] However, the largest study of surfactant therapy in ARDS involving 725 patients demonstrated no effect on 30-day mortality, length of intensive care unit stay, duration of mechanical ventilation or indices of oxygenation.[131] Future studies of exogenous surfactant should define optimal formulations and delivery systems as well as investigating its effect on pulmonary inflammation, host defence and fibrosis.

Extracorporeal membrane oxygenation is an adaptation of conventional cardiopulmonary bypass technique that involves withdrawing venous blood, passing it through a membrane oxygenator and returning it to the arterial or venous circulation.[132]

Enthusiasm for these techniques in adult practice has waned over the last 10 years because of a high rate of adverse events, especially bleeding. It has recently been suggested that extracorporeal carbon dioxide removal may be a useful adjunct to protective ventilation strategies, especially now that technical advances have improved, allaying some safety concerns. Currently there are no data to support the routine use in adults of these methods, which are confined to rescue therapy in specialist centres.

One of the most exciting treatments proposed for ARDS is partial liquid ventilation during which the lungs are filled to FRC with a perfluorocarbon, most commonly perflubron, a dense, colourless liquid capable of gas transport. Mechanical ventilation continues with the perflubron in place. The main potential benefits include improved oxygenation and decreased ventilator-associated lung injury. Mechanisms of action suggested by animal experiments include reversal of atelectasis, redistribution of pulmonary blood flow, clearance of debris, decrease of total lung water and reduction of inflammation.[133] Experience with partial liquid ventilation in patients with ARDS is limited. In one series of 10 patients with ARDS the shunt fraction fell and static pulmonary compliance improved at 72 hours.[134] No major side effects were noted but subsequent experiences have suggested an increased incidence of pneumothorax and mucus plugging. The impact on survival, mechanical ventilation requirements, length of stay and cost remain unknown.

Non-respiratory support

Haemodynamics and fluid balance

While pulmonary oedema in patients with lung injury is not caused by fluid overload, the high permeability of the pulmonary microvasculature results in leakage of osmotically active molecules into the interstitial space. The formation of oedema, therefore, depends directly on hydrostatic pressure, because osmotic forces are less able to retain fluid in capillaries. As a result, pulmonary oedema is more likely to develop in ARDS for any given pulmonary capillary hydrostatic pressure. Therefore, even in patients who are not volume-overloaded, diuresis may be beneficial by reducing oedema formation[135,136] as long as blood pressure and cardiac output are maintained. The setting of supranormal targets for oxygen delivery (DO_2 – the product of cardiac output and the oxygen content of blood) in unselected ARDS patients to maximise oxygen consumption cannot be recommended.[137,138] Neither optimum haemodynamic targets nor the best technology to monitor relevant parameters has been established for patients with ARDS. Our practice is to maintain intravascular volume at the lowest level compatible with an adequate cardiac output (both measured with a pulmonary artery catheter) and tissue perfusion. The latter is assessed globally using acid–base balance and serial blood lactate estimations, and at an organ-specific level by, for example, measuring hourly urine output. Low-dose diuretic infusions, vasopressors, inotropes and fluid challenges are used to manipulate variables.

Nutrition

Avoiding nutritional depletion while delivering a high-fat, low-carbohydrate diet to reduce CO_2 production and thus ventilatory demand is appropriate for all patients with respiratory failure. Enteral nutrition is preferable, not only because the disadvantages of parenteral feeding, such as catheter-related infection, expense and impaired hypoxic pulmonary vasoconstriction, are avoided. The advantages of enteral feeding include increased blood flow, improved barrier function (decreasing translocation of bacteria and their toxins) and a decreased incidence of stress ulceration.

So-called 'immunonutrition' is designed to influence specifically inflammatory responses and gastrointestinal integrity. A comparison of standard enteral feed with immunonutrition supplemented with antioxidants in patients with ARDS for at least 4 days showed that immunonutrition was associated with reduced pulmonary neutrophil recruitment, improved oxygenation, a shortened duration of mechanical ventilation and fewer new organ failures.[139] However, there was no difference in mortality between the control and treatment groups. A meta-analysis of 12 trials in critically ill patients comparing standard enteral nutrition with immunonutrition suggested reduced rates of infection (including pulmonary) but again no effect on mortality.[140] The data suggested that immunonutrition benefits critically ill surgical and trauma patients, but a large, randomised controlled trial is still required.

Management algorithm

The targets for therapy and a management algorithm as used in the authors' institution are given in Figure 28.10 and Table 28.10. The needs of individual patients modify practice and we would not suggest that this guidance should be applied universally. The indications for adjuncts to ventilatory support such as prone positioning are controversial. Considerable support is required to transfer patients for a CT scan, the threshold for undertaking this investigation depends on local arrangements. Similarly, the decision of when and how to start weaning once stability has been achieved requires judgement and experience. In our experience, patients with severe lung injury require a minimum of 1–2 weeks of ventilatory support, so we proceed relatively slowly with weaning. Adequate PEEP levels are needed to prevent tidal derecruitment; we decrease the I: E ratio and then lower the F_IO_2 to less than 45% before decreasing PEEP levels. Finally, we use high-dose corticosteroid treatment in patients who are failing to progress as judged by their respiratory physiology and chest radiograph.

Pharmacotherapy

Clinical trials and strategy

Why have clinical trials of drugs for the treatment of sepsis and ARDS almost exclusively yielded negative results despite being based on sound theories and promising experimental data? The

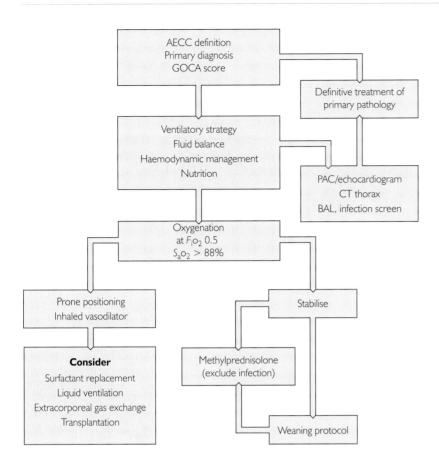

Fig. 28.10 Suggested treatment algorithm for acute lung injury and acute respiratory distress syndrome. AECC, American–European Consensus Conference 1993; BAL, bronchoalveolar lavage; CT, computed tomography; F_iO_2, fractional inspired oxygen concentration; GOCA, lung injury and acute physiology score; PAC, pulmonary artery catheter; S_aO_2, arterial oxygen saturation.

current definition of ARDS identifies a heterogeneous patient population. Incorporation of lung injury and acute physiology scores would obviate this problem but would also necessitate larger and more complex trials. The alternative designs for ARDS studies are therefore either large, multicentre, randomised controlled clinical trials that account for population heterogeneity or small studies of patients with a common aetiology of ARDS that accept the limited application of their findings. Secondly, the 'magic bullet' approach may have to give way to assessing combined techniques that may improve physiology without affecting mortality. Finally, while the early phase of ARDS is not readily treatable, the later phases of the illness involve processes, such as fibrosing alveolitis, neutrophil apoptosis and alveolar epithelial reconstitution, that are susceptible to pharmacotherapy.

The incidence of ALI/ARDS is dependent not only on the nature of the precipitating insult but also on individual susceptibility. Hence, by characterising genomic polymorphisms, advances in identifying risk factors for developing ARDS and the likelihood that a patient will respond to a given intervention may be made. Targeting patients within specific 'at-risk' populations may be a more fruitful approach, because intervening early in the inflammatory process rather than when a cascade with ample redundancy is established is more likely to be effective. Finally, the improved and standardised support of patients with ALI/ARDS will buy more time for drug intervention and facilitate the performance of clinical trials. These considerations raise

the possibility that some agents (see below) discarded on the basis of previous trials should be re-examined.

Corticosteroids

Corticosteroids may modify the course of lung injury by reducing the production and activity of a variety of proinflammatory and fibrogenic mediators.[141] Corticosteroids enhance endothelial integrity in part by the inhibition of inflammatory mediators but also by increasing the number and activity of β-adrenergic receptors and through other membrane-stabilising effects. Finally, dexamethasone upregulated alveolar fluid clearance in an alveolar type II cell line in vitro.[142] However, not all of the effects of corticosteroids are anti-inflammatory, and the anti-inflammatory effects are associated with impaired antimicrobial host defence mechanisms.

The rationale for using high-dose corticosteroids for ARDS was based on small clinical studies showing improvements in cardiac output, pulmonary vascular resistance and oxygen transport. However, trials of short-term, high-dose steroid therapy have failed to demonstrate a mortality advantage in patients at risk of ARDS or with early ARDS due to sepsis, aspiration and trauma.[143,144] Apart from the reasons outlined above accounting for the failure of such studies, later experimental evidence showed that stopping steroid therapy acutely during pulmonary inflammation increased alveolar–capillary membrane permeability and lung fibrosis.[145]

In the 1990s lower-dose, longer-term corticosteroid treatment was assessed, targeting the fibroproliferative phase of the syndrome. A total of 24 patients were randomised to receive either placebo or a 32-day treatment course of methylprednisolone with aggressive surveillance for infection.[146] Corticosteroid-treated patients had a significantly lower mortality (12% versus 62%) and improved P_aO_2/F_iO_2 ratio, lung injury score, multiple organ failure score and extubation rate. Interpretation is complicated by the small number of patients enrolled, the fact that half of the placebo-treated patients crossed over to the methylprednisolone group and the finding that the incidence of infection was nearly twice as high in the steroid-treated group, although this difference was not statistically significant. Despite concerns about the clinical trial data, our practice is to use corticosteroids in patients who are failing to progress after 10 days of mechanical ventilation for ARDS and who demonstrate no evidence of active infection. BAL is performed for microbiological screening prior to steroid administration as follows: methylprednisolone 1 g daily for 3 days followed by 2 mg/kg for at least 2 weeks and up to 4 weeks depending on the patient's response.

Antioxidants

The damage caused by reactive oxygen and nitrogen species to matrix and cellular proteins, lipids and nucleic acids is a central component of the pathogenesis of ARDS. Superoxide ($O_2^{\cdot-}$), hydrogen peroxide (H_2O_2) and nitric oxide ($\cdot NO$) have important physiological roles but their generation and ability to induce a cascade of further radical release are normally carefully controlled. Levels of reactive oxygen species produced by the leukocytes of patients with ARDS are high and increased by the administration of oxygen to levels that overwhelm extra- and intracellular antioxidant defences, resulting in tissue damage.[147] It has therefore been proposed that tissue destruction, counter-productive biological responses and cell death could be prevented by the administration of antioxidants.

The concentration and reducing ability of the endogenous antioxidant glutathione in the BAL fluid of patients with ARDS is depleted.[148] Intracellular glutathione synthesis is stimulated by the cysteine precursors N-acetylcysteine and procysteine (L-2-oxothiazolidine-4-carboxylate). Administration of these precursors increases plasma and BAL fluid levels of glutathione in patients with ARDS, although a complete effect may take 10 days of therapy. After encouraging experimental results, no difference was found between N-acetylcysteine- and placebo-treated groups with established ARDS in the mortality, length of ventilatory support or indices of oxygenation.[149] A large phase III trial of procysteine has been stopped early because of concern over mortality in the treatment arm of the study. Currently, there is little evidence that antioxidant therapy is beneficial to patients with ARDS.

Manipulation of lipid-derived mediators

Lipid mediators such as thromboxanes (TX), leukotrienes (LT), platelet activating factor (PAF) and various prostaglandins (PG) probably contribute to the pathogenesis of ARDS. The monoenoic prostaglandin PGE_1 causes pulmonary and systemic vasodilation and inhibits platelet aggregation and neutrophil adhesion. PGE_1 improved survival in trauma patients with respiratory failure but this benefit could not be reproduced in a subsequent multicentre trial in patients suffering from lung injury precipitated by surgery, trauma or sepsis.[150] The dose of PGE_1 was limited by systemic hypotension and recent trials have used liposome technology to increase drug delivery while mitigating side effects.[151] However, phase II and III trials have shown that patients with ARDS receiving liposomal PGE_1 benefited in terms of P_aO_2/F_iO_2 ratio but not in survival or a reduced requirement for ventilatory support.

Pulmonary hypertension and hypoxaemia in ARDS are in part caused by COX-derived arachidonic acid metabolites such as the vasoconstrictor and platelet aggregator thromboxane. Leukotrienes are derived from arachidonic acid by the enzyme 5-lipoxygenase. In animal models, LTB_4 is a potent neutrophil chemokine while LTC_4 and LTD_4 cause vasoconstriction and pulmonary oedema. BAL fluid from patients with ARDS contains elevated concentrations of LTB_4, LTC_4 and LTD_4, which may be markers for developing ALI.[37] Both thromboxanes and leukotrienes mediate the effects of IL-1 and TNF-α, which are elevated early in ARDS. Two early trials of the selective thromboxane-synthase-inhibitor dazoxiben for the treatment of ARDS showed no mortality benefit.

Ketoconazole is an imidazole antifungal agent that also inhibits thromboxane synthase and 5-lipoxygenase without inhibiting cyclo-oxygenase. Ketoconazole has dual anti-inflammatory actions by inhibiting inflammatory eicosanoid synthesis and directing cyclo-oxygenase products down other less inflammatory metabolic paths, such as those synthesising prostacyclin or PGE_2.[152] Preliminary studies suggested that ketoconazole decreased the incidence of ARDS in at-risk surgical patients. However, an ARDS Network trial in patients with established ARDS of medical and surgical aetiology found no differences in in-hospital mortality, ventilator-free days at day 28, organ-failure-free days or markers of gas exchange between patients given ketoconazole or placebo.[153] The plasma ketoconazole levels achieved were an order of magnitude higher than those obtained previously but there was no demonstrable effect of the drug on the generation of thromboxane.

Pentoxifylline and its more potent metabolite lisofylline are lysophosphatidic acyl transferase inhibitors. These compounds reduce serum free fatty acids in humans, lower cytokine production, neutrophil activation and pulmonary neutrophil sequestration and attenuate lung injury in animal models. A randomised, multicentre, placebo-controlled study of lisofylline in 235 patients with ALI/ARDS was stopped at the first interim analysis because the prespecified level of improvement for the treatment arm of the trial was not achieved.[154]

Future directions

Inhalation of salmeterol prevented high-altitude pulmonary oedema in predisposed subjects,[155] suggesting that β-adrenergic-agonist therapy might hasten the resolution of alveolar oedema and that this method of drug delivery is clinically effective. In addition to β-adrenergic agonists, other treatments should be evaluated, such as stimulation of alveolar fluid clearance by gene therapy and/or stimulation of alveolar type II cell proliferation by growth factors, for example hepatocyte growth factor.[156] Gene therapy may provide a novel approach for treatment of pulmonary oedema because short-term expression may be sufficient for clinical benefit. However, several questions should be addressed before clinical use may be evaluated. The potential for viral vectors to increase inflammation in already damaged lungs may limit its beneficial effects. It is also possible that the time course for viral transfection may prohibit its use in the acute setting.

Preliminary data from pilot studies involving manipulation of clotting cascades in sepsis has been the cause for cautious optimism.[73] A number of agents are undergoing clinical trial and it is hoped that benefit will accrue both for patients with sepsis and those with ARDS, possibly associated with other risk factors.

Outcomes

Published mortality rates for patients with ARDS vary from 10% to 90%. Recent reports from specialist centres suggest that the mortality may have decreased from 66% to around 36%.[157,158] Meta-analysis of data from 3264 patients in 101 studies between 1967 and 1994 gave a mortality rate of $53 \pm 22\%$ with no apparent trend towards a higher survival.[159] The mortality rate in the placebo groups of recent large multicentre ARDS studies ranges between 40% and 48%.[106,108,110,129]

Since the 1993 American European Consensus Conference, most clinical series continue to report mortality rates for patients with ARDS that range from 25% to 70%. This wide variation may be explained by differences in the distribution of prognostic risk factors, exclusion criteria and the definition of mortality (e.g. 28 days versus hospital mortality). One systematic difference between series is the lower mortality reported in clinical trial populations relative to that reported in observational series. This difference is probably due to exclusion criteria in clinical trials that identify a subgroup of patients with ARDS. An obvious implication is that generalising findings from these clinical trials to the larger population of ARDS patients may be inappropriate.

Estimates of the attributable mortality from lung injury are complicated by difficulties in estimating which deaths in critically ill patients with ALI/ARDS are due to lung injury and which are due to other factors. However, it is helpful to compare some simple estimates of cause-specific mortality rates of ALI/ARDS with other diseases. Using the only incidence value available for American–European-Consensus-Conference-defined ALI/ARDS and a mortality of 40% there are 16 350 adult deaths in the USA each year associated with ALI/ARDS. This is similar to the number of deaths associated with emphysema (17 518) and with HIV/AIDS (16 516) and exceeds the number of deaths associated with asthma (5434: CDC National Center for Health Statistics; http: //www.cdc.gov/nchs/fastats/). The results of the ARDS Network trial suggest that 9% of patients with ARDS who are ventilated with 12 ml/kg predicted body weight die because of their ventilator management.[110] If similar treatment benefits were observed in all patients with ARDS in the USA, then approxi-

mately 10 deaths occur every day that could be prevented in ALI/ARDS patients by changes in ventilator management.[160] Therefore, both the number of deaths and the number of preventable deaths in patients with lung injury make it a disease with significant implications for population health.

Quality of life and functional status

Survivors of ARDS are frequently able to return to their prior activities 6–12 months after hospital discharge. Thus, the poor short-term prognosis of ARDS is balanced by the potential for an excellent quality of life in survivors. Nearly all patients have reached their maximum recovery 6 months after endotracheal extubation and this time-point can be used for the evaluation of pulmonary function following ARDS.

Although most patients' pulmonary function markedly improves during recovery, approximately half continue to suffer mild impairment with significant detriment to their quality of life.[161] This is either a mild restriction or more often a small decrease in diffusing capacity and a decrease in expiratory flow rate with airway hyper-reactivity and air-trapping due to small airways disease.[51] Persistent symptoms 1 year after recovery correlate with the duration of mechanical ventilation, the lowest recorded lung compliance and the requirement of an F_1O_2 more than 0.6 for more than 24 hours.[162] Survivors of ARDS also suffer psychological impairments that are typically mild and are not perceived by patients to be related to their pulmonary condition.[161] No link between different ventilatory strategies and long-term outcomes has yet been demonstrated.[161]

Conclusions

Acute lung injury/ARDS results either from direct lung damage that causes acute inflammation or from uncontrolled systemic inflammation that damages the lung. The resulting syndrome cannot as yet be prevented or treated specifically but improvements in supportive care may have improved the survival rates of patients in certain centres. While the mortality of patients with ARDS remains high, most survivors suffer only a mild impairment of respiratory function.

Therapeutic principles

- Mechanical ventilation with large tidal volumes and high pressures is associated with a poor outcome.

- Fluid overload may exacerbate pulmonary oedema while circulatory insufficiency secondary to dehydration may precipitate multiple organ failure.

- Prolonged courses of high-dose corticosteroids may hasten the recovery of patients with chronic acute respiratory distress syndrome in whom active infection can be excluded.

> **?** **Unresolved questions**
>
> - Which patients at risk develop acute respiratory distress syndrome and how can they be prospectively identified?
>
> - How is pulmonary inflammation turned off and what determines the extent and persistence of pulmonary fibrosis?
>
> - What is the optimum management of respiratory acidosis and setting of level of positive end-expiratory pressure?
>
> - What is the role of prone positioning, inhaled vasodilators, surfactant supplementation and extracorporeal gas exchange?
>
> - What are the indications and dosing regimen for corticosteroids?

References

1. Bernard GR, Artigas A, Brigham KL et al. The American–European Consensus Conference on ARDS. Definitions, mechanisms, relevant outcomes, and clinical trial coordination Am J Respir Crit Care Med 1994; 149: 818–824.

2. Ashbaugh DG, Bigelow DB, Petty TL, Levine BE. Acute respiratory distress in adults. Lancet 1967; 2: 319–323.

3. Esteban A, Fdez-Segoviano P, Gordo F et al. Correlation among clinical and post-mortem diagnosis of ARDS. Am J Respir Crit Care Med 1999; 159: A718.

4. Artigas A. Prognostic factors and outcome of ALI. In: Marini JJ, Evans TW, ed. Acute lung injury. Berlin: Springer Verlag; 1998: 16–38.

5. Murray JF, Matthay MA, Luce JM, Flick MR. An expanded definition of the adult respiratory distress syndrome. Am Rev Respir Dis 1988; 138: 720–723.

6. Doyle RL, Szaflarski N, Modin GW et al. Identification of patients with acute lung injury. Predictors of mortality. Am J Respir Crit Care Med 1995; 152: 1818–1824.

7. Heffner JE, Brown LK, Barbieri CA et al. Prospective validation of an acute respiratory distress syndrome predictive score. Am J Respir Crit Care Med 1995; 152: 1518–1526.

8. Knaus WA, Sun X, Hakim RB, Wagner DP. Evaluation of definitions for adult respiratory distress syndrome. Am J Respir Crit Care Med 1994; 150: 311–317.

9. Ferring M, Vincent JL. Is outcome from ARDS related to the severity of respiratory failure? Eur Respir J 1997; 10: 1297–1300.

10. Fowler AA, Hamman RF, Good JT et al. Adult respiratory distress syndrome: risk with common predispositions. Ann Intern Med 1983; 98: 593–597.

11. Montgomery AB, Stager MA, Carrico CJ, Hudson LD. Causes of mortality in patients with the adult respiratory distress syndrome. Am Rev Respir Dis 1985; 132: 485–489.

12. Hudson LD, Milberg JA, Anardi D, Maunder RJ. Clinical risks for development of the acute respiratory distress syndrome. Am J Respir Crit Care Med 1995; 151: 293–301.

13. Moss M, Bucher B, Moore FA et al. The role of chronic alcohol abuse in the development of acute respiratory distress syndrome in adults. JAMA 1996; 275: 50–54.

14. Moss M, Guidot DM, Steinberg KP et al. Diabetic patients have a decreased incidence of acute respiratory distress syndrome. Crit Care Med 2000; 28: 2187–2192.

15. Parsons PE. Mediators and mechanisms of acute lung injury. Clin Chest Med 2000; 21: 467–476.

16. Villar J, Slutsky AS. The incidence of the adult respiratory distress syndrome. Am Rev Respir Dis 1989; 140: 814–816.

17. Thomsen GE, Morris AH. Incidence of the adult respiratory distress syndrome in the state of Utah. Am J Respir Crit Care Med 1995; 152: 965–971.

18. Webster NR, Cohen AT, Nunn JF. Adult respiratory distress syndrome – how many cases in the UK? Anaesthesia 1988; 43: 923–926.

19. Lewandowski K, Metz J, Deutschmann C et al. Incidence, severity, and mortality of acute respiratory failure in Berlin, Germany. Am J Respir Crit Care Med 1995; 151: 1121–1125.

20. Luhr OR, Antonsen K, Karlsson M et al. Incidence and mortality after acute respiratory failure and acute respiratory distress syndrome in Sweden, Denmark, and Iceland. The ARF Study Group. Am J Respir Crit Care Med 1999; 159: 1849–1861.

21. Roupie E, Lepage E, Wysocki M et al. Prevalence, etiologies and outcome of the acute respiratory distress syndrome among hypoxemic ventilated patients. SRLF Collaborative Group on Mechanical Ventilation. Societé de Réanimation de Langue Française. Intensive Care Med 1999; 25: 920–929.

22. Fowler M, Hamman RF, Zerbe GO et al. Adult respiratory distress syndrome. Prognosis after onset. Am Rev Respir Dis 1985; 132: 472–478.

23. Bone RC, Balk R, Slotman G et al Adult respiratory distress syndrome. Sequence and importance of development of multiple organ failure. The Prostaglandin E1 Study Group. Chest 1992; 101: 320–326.

24. Luhr OR, Karlsson M, Thorsteinsson A et al. The impact of respiratory variables on mortality in non-ARDS and ARDS patients requiring mechanical ventilation. Intensive Care Med 2000; 26: 508–517.

25. Bachofen M, Weibel ER. Structural alterations of lung parenchyma in the adult respiratory distress syndrome. Clin Chest Med 1982; 3: 35–56.

26. Fein AM, Lippmann M, Holtzman H et al. The risk factors, incidence, and prognosis of ARDS following septicemia. Chest 1983; 83: 40–42.

27. Tomashefski JF Jr. Pulmonary pathology of acute respiratory distress syndrome. Clin Chest Med 2000; 21: 435–466.

28. Fukuda Y, Ishizaki M, Masuda Y et al. The role of intraalveolar fibrosis in the process of pulmonary structural remodeling in patients with diffuse alveolar damage. Am J Pathol 1987; 126: 171–182.

29. Bachofen M, Weibel ER. Alterations of the gas exchange apparatus in adult respiratory insufficiency associated with septicemia. Am Rev Respir Dis 1977; 116: 589–615.

30. Uhal BD. Cell cycle kinetics in the alveolar epithelium. Am J Physiol 1997; 272: L1031–L1045.

31. Zapol WM, Trelstad RL, Coffey JW et al. Pulmonary fibrosis in severe acute respiratory failure. Am Rev Respir Dis 1979; 119: 547–554.

32. Tomashefski JF Jr, Davies P, Boggis C et al. The pulmonary vascular lesions of the adult respiratory distress syndrome. Am J Pathol 1983; 112: 112–126.

33. Matthay MA, Fukuda N, Frank J et al. Alveolar epithelial barrier. Role in lung fluid balance in clinical lung injury. Clin Chest Med 2000; 21: 477–490.

34. Gunther A, Siebert C, Schmidt R et al. Surfactant alterations in severe pneumonia, acute respiratory distress syndrome, and cardiogenic lung edema. Am J Respir Crit Care Med 1996; 153: 176–184.

35. Günther A, Walmrath D, Grimminger F, Seeger W. Surfactant metabolism and replacement in ARDS. In: Evans TW, Griffiths MJD, Keogh B, ed. European Respiratory Monograph: ARDS. Copenhagen: International Publishers; 2002: (in press).

36. Bone RC, Balk RA, Cerra FB et al. Definitions for sepsis and organ failure and guidelines for the use of innovative therapies in sepsis. The ACCP/SCCM Consensus Conference Committee. American College of Chest Physicians/Society of Critical Care Medicine. Chest 1992; 101: 1644–1655.

37. Pittet JF, Mackersie RC, Martin TR, Matthay MA. Biological markers of acute lung injury: prognostic and pathogenetic significance. Am J Respir Crit Care Med 1997; 155: 1187–1205.

38. Steinberg KP, Milberg JA, Martin TR et al. Evolution of bronchoalveolar cell populations in the adult respiratory distress syndrome. Am J Respir Crit Care Med 1994; 150: 113–122.

39. Laufe MD, Simon RH, Flint A, Keller JB. Adult respiratory distress syndrome in neutropenic patients. Am J Med 1986; 80: 1022–1026.

40. Burke-Gaffney A, Griffiths M. Adhesion molecules in acute lung injury. In: Evans TW, Griffiths MJD, Keogh B, ed. European Respiratory Monograph: ARDS. Copenhagen: International Publishers; 2002: (in press).

41. Donnelly SC, MacGregor I, Zamani A et al Plasma elastase levels and the development of the adult respiratory distress syndrome. Am J Respir Crit Care Med 1995; 151: 1428–1433.

42. Donnelly SC, Strieter RM, Kunkel SL et al. Interleukin-8 and development of adult respiratory distress syndrome in at-risk patient groups. Lancet 1993; 341: 643–647.

43. Lee A, Whyte MK, Haslett C. Inhibition of apoptosis and prolongation of neutrophil functional longevity by inflammatory mediators. J Leukocyte Biol 1993; 54: 283–288.

44. Bellingham G. Resolution of inflammation and repair. In: Evans TW, Griffiths MJD, Keogh B, ed. European Respiratory Monograph: ARDS. Copenhagen: International Publishers; 2002: (in press).

45. Bellingan GJ, Caldwell H, Howie SE et al. In vivo fate of the inflammatory macrophage during the resolution of inflammation: inflammatory macrophages do not die locally, but emigrate to the draining lymph nodes. J Immunol 1996; 157: 2577–2585.

46. Witschi H. Role of the epithelium in lung repair. Chest 1991; 99: 22S–25S.

47. Matthay MA, Folkesson HG, Verkman AS. Salt and water transport across alveolar and distal airway epithelia in the adult lung. Am J Physiol 1996; 270: L487–L503.

48. Dobbs LG, Gonzalez R, Matthay MA et al. Highly water-permeable type I alveolar epithelial cells confer high water permeability between the airspace and vasculature in rat lung. Proc Natl Acad Sci USA 1998; 95: 2991–2996.

49. Ware LB, Matthay M. Maximal alveolar epithelial fluid clearance in clinical acute lung injury: an excellent predictor of survival and the duration of mechanical ventilation. Am J Respir Crit Care Med 1999; 159: A694.

50. Folkesson HG, Matthay MA, Westrom BR et al. Alveolar epithelial clearance of protein. J Appl Physiol 1996; 80: 1431–1445.

51. Ghio AJ, Elliott CG, Crapo RO et al. Impairment after adult respiratory distress syndrome. An evaluation based on American Thoracic Society recommendations. Am Rev Respir Dis 1989; 139: 1158–1162.

52. Pratt PC, Vollmer RT, Shelburne JD, Crapo JD. Pulmonary morphology in a multihospital collaborative extracorporeal membrane oxygenation project. I. Light microscopy. Am J Pathol 1979; 95: 191–214.

53. Chesnutt AN, Matthay MA, Tibayan FA, Clark JG. Early detection of type III procollagen peptide in acute lung injury. Pathogenetic and prognostic significance. Am J Respir Crit Care Med 1997; 156: 840–845.

54. Donnelly SC, Strieter RM, Reid PT et al. The association between mortality rates and decreased concentrations of interleukin-10 and interleukin-1 receptor antagonist in the lung fluids of patients with the adult respiratory distress syndrome. Ann Intern Med 1996; 125: 191–196.

55. Kaminski N, Allard JD, Pittet JF et al. Global analysis of gene expression in pulmonary fibrosis reveals distinct programs regulating lung inflammation and fibrosis. Proc Natl Acad Sci USA 2000; 97: 1778–1783.

56. Martin C, Papazian L, Payan MJ et al. Pulmonary fibrosis correlates with outcome in adult respiratory distress syndrome. A study in mechanically ventilated patients. Chest 1995; 107: 196–200.

57. Torii K, Iida K, Miyazaki Y et al. Higher concentrations of matrix metalloproteinases in bronchoalveolar lavage fluid of patients with adult respiratory distress syndrome. Am J Respir Crit Care Med 1997; 155: 43–46.

58. Raghu G, Striker LJ, Hudson LD Striker GE. Extracellular matrix in normal and fibrotic human lungs. Am Rev Respir Dis 1985; 131: 281–289.

59. Amato MB, Barbas CS, Medeiros DM et al. Beneficial effects of the 'open lung approach' with low distending pressures in acute respiratory distress syndrome. A prospective randomized study on mechanical ventilation. Am J Respir Crit Care Med 1995; 152: 1835–1846.

60. Suki B, Barabasi AL, Hantos Z et al. Avalanches and power-law behaviour in lung inflation. Nature 1994; 368: 615–618.

61. Roupie E, Dambrosio M, Servillo G et al. Titration of tidal volume and induced hypercapnia in acute respiratory distress syndrome. Am J Respir Crit Care Med 1995; 152: 121–128.

62. Suter PM, Schlobohm RM. Determination of functional residual capacity during mechanical ventilation. Anesthesiology 1974; 41: 605–607.

63. Gattinoni L, Pesenti A, Avalli L et al. Pressure–volume curve of total respiratory system in acute respiratory failure. Computed tomographic scan study. Am Rev Respir Dis 1987; 136: 730–736.

64. Muscedere JG, Mullen JB, Gan, K, Slutsky AS. Tidal ventilation at low airway pressures can augment lung injury. Am J Respir Crit Care Med 1994; 149: 1327–1334.

65. Zapol WM, Snider MT. Pulmonary hypertension in severe acute respiratory failure. N Engl J Med 1977; 296: 476–480.

66. Wort SJ, Evans TW. The role of the endothelium in modulating vascular control in sepsis and related conditions. Br Med Bull 1999; 55: 30–48.

67. Winn R, Harlan J, Nadir B et al. Thromboxane A2 mediates lung vasoconstriction but not permeability after endotoxin. J Clin Invest 1983; 72: 911–918.

68. Snapper JR, Thabes JS, Lefferts PL, Lu W. Role of endothelin in endotoxin-induced sustained pulmonary hypertension in sheep. Am J Respir Crit Care Med 1998; 157: 81–88.

69. Dantzker DR, Brook CJ, Dehart P et al. Ventilation–perfusion distributions in the adult respiratory distress syndrome. Am Rev Respir Dis 1979; 120: 1039–1052.

70. Brigham KL, Kariman K, Harris TR et al. Correlation of oxygenation with vascular permeability–surface area but not with lung water in humans with acute respiratory failure and pulmonary edema. J Clin Invest 1983; 72: 339–349.

71. Esbenshade AM, Newman JH, Lams PM et al. Respiratory failure after endotoxin infusion in sheep: lung mechanics and lung fluid balance. J Appl Physiol 1982; 53: 967–976.

72. Idell S, Gonzalez K, Bradford H et al. Procoagulant activity in bronchoalveolar lavage in the adult respiratory distress syndrome. Contribution of tissue factor associated with factor VII. Am Rev Respir Dis 1987; 136: 1466–1474.

73. Abraham E. Coagulation abnormalities in acute lung injury and sepsis. Am J Respir Cell Mol Biol 2000; 22: 401–404.

74. Fein AM, Calalang-Colucci MG. Acute lung injury and acute respiratory distress syndrome in sepsis and septic shock. Crit Care Clin 2000; 16: 289–317.

75. Bernard GR, Wheeler AP, Russell JA et al. The effects of ibuprofen on the physiology and survival of patients with sepsis. The Ibuprofen in Sepsis Study Group. N Engl J Med 1997; 336: 912–918.

76. Bell RC, Coalson JJ, Smith JD, Johanson WG Jr. Multiple organ system failure and infection in adult respiratory distress syndrome. Ann Intern Med 1983; 99: 293–298.

77. Hyers TM. Prediction of survival and mortality in patients with adult respiratory distress syndrome. New Horiz 1993; 1: 466–470.

78. Kox WJ et al. Interferon gamma-1b in the treatment of compensatory anti-inflammatory response syndrome. A new approach: proof of principle. Arch Intern Med 1997; 157: 389–393.

79. Milne EN, Pistolesi M, Miniati M, Giuntini C. The radiologic distinction of cardiogenic and noncardiogenic edema. AJR 1985; 144: 879–894.

80. Meade MO, Cook RJ, Guyatt GH et al. Interobserver variation in interpreting chest radiographs for the diagnosis of acute respiratory distress syndrome. Am J Respir Crit Care Med 2000; 161: 85–90.

81. Gattinoni L, Pesenti A, Bombino M et al. Relationships between lung computed tomographic density, gas exchange, and PEEP in acute respiratory failure. Anesthesiology 1988; 69: 824–832.

82. Desai SR, Wells AU, Rubens MB et al. Acute respiratory distress syndrome: CT abnormalities at long-term follow-up. Radiology 1999; 210: 29–35.

83. Goodman LR, Fumagalli R, Tagliabue Pet al. Adult respiratory distress syndrome due to pulmonary and extrapulmonary causes: CT, clinical, and functional correlations. Radiology 1999; 213: 545–552.

84. Papazian L, Thomas P, Bregeon F et al. Open-lung biopsy in patients with acute respiratory distress syndrome. Anesthesiology 1998; 88: 935–944.

85. Fein A, Grossman RF, Jones JG et al. The value of edema fluid protein measurement in patients with pulmonary edema. Am J Med 1979; 67: 32–38.

86. Schuster D. Quantifying lung injury in ARDS. In: Marini JJ, Evans TW, ed. Acute lung injury. Berlin: Springer Verlag; 1996: 181–196.

87. Steinberg KP, Mitchell DR, Maunder RJ et al. Safety of bronchoalveolar lavage in patients with adult respiratory distress syndrome. Am Rev Respir Dis 1993; 148: 556–561.

88. Dreyfuss D, Basset G, Soler P, Saumon G. Intermittent positive-pressure hyperventilation with high inflation pressures produces pulmonary microvascular injury in rats. Am Rev Respir Dis 1985; 132: 880–884.

89. Corbridge TC, Wood LD, Crawford GP et al. Adverse effects of large tidal volume and low PEEP in canine acid aspiration. Am Rev Respir Dis 1990; 142: 311–315.

90. Tremblay L, Valenza F, Ribeiro SP et al. Injurious ventilatory strategies increase cytokines and c-fos m-RNA expression in an isolated rat lung model. J Clin Invest 1997; 99: 944–952.

91. Ranieri VM, Suter PM, Tortorella C et al. Effect of mechanical ventilation on inflammatory mediators in patients with acute respiratory distress syndrome: a randomized controlled trial. JAMA 1999; 282: 54–61.

92. Slutsky AS, Tremblay LN. Multiple system organ failure. Is mechanical ventilation a contributing factor? Am J Respir Crit Care Med 1998; 157: 1721–1725.

93. Schnapp LM, Chin DP, Szaflarski N, Matthay MA. Frequency and importance of barotrauma in 100 patients with acute lung injury. Crit Care Med 1995; 23: 272–278.

94. Fagon JY, Chastre J, Vuagnat A et al. Nosocomial pneumonia and mortality among patients in intensive care units. JAMA 1996; 275: 866–869.

95. Chastre J, Trouillet JL, Vuagnat A et al. Nosocomial pneumonia in patients with acute respiratory distress syndrome. Am J Respir Crit Care Med 1998; 157: 1165–1172.

96. Andrews CP, Coalson JJ, Smith JD, Johanson WG Jr. Diagnosis of nosocomial bacterial pneumonia in acute, diffuse lung injury. Chest 1981; 80: 254–258.

97. Rombeau JL, Takala J. Summary of round table conference: gut dysfunction in critical illness. Intensive Care Med 1997; 23: 476–479.

98. Valles J, Artigas A, Rello J et al. Continuous aspiration of subglottic secretions in preventing ventilator-associated pneumonia. Ann Intern Med 1995; 122: 179–186.

99. Gutmann L. Critical illness neuropathy and myopathy. Arch Neurol 1999; 56: 527–528.

100. Hund E. Myopathy in critically ill patients. Crit Care Med 1999; 27: 2544–2547.

101. Rocker GM, Mackenzie MG, Williams B, Logan PM. Noninvasive positive pressure ventilation: successful outcome in patients with acute lung injury/ARDS. Chest 1999; 115: 173–177.

102. Carmichael LC, Dorinsky PM, Higgins SB et al. Diagnosis and therapy of acute respiratory distress syndrome in adults: an international survey. J Crit Care 1996; 11: 9–18.

103. Feihl F, Perret C. Permissive hypercapnia. How permissive should we be? Am J Respir Crit Care Med 1994; 150: 1722–1737.

104. Hickling KG, Henderson SJ, Jackson R. Low mortality associated with low volume pressure limited ventilation with permissive hypercapnia in severe adult respiratory distress syndrome. Intensive Care Med 1990; 16: 372–377.

105. Slutsky AS. Mechanical ventilation. American College of Chest Physicians' Consensus Conference. Chest 1993; 104: 1833–1859.

106. Stewart TE, Meade MO, Cook DJ et al. Evaluation of a ventilation strategy to prevent barotrauma in patients at high risk for acute respiratory distress syndrome. Pressure- and Volume-Limited Ventilation Strategy Group. N Engl J Med 1998; 338: 355–361.

107. Brower RG, Shanholtz CB, Fessler HE et al. Prospective, randomized, controlled clinical trial comparing traditional versus reduced tidal volume ventilation in acute respiratory distress syndrome patients. Crit Care Med 1999; 27: 1492–1498.

108. Brochard L, Roudot-Thoraval F, Roupie E et al. Tidal volume reduction for prevention of ventilator-induced lung injury in acute respiratory distress syndrome. The Multicenter Trail Group on Tidal Volume reduction in ARDS. Am J Respir Crit Care Med 1998; 158: 1831–1838.

109. Amato MB, Barbas CS, Medeiros DM et al. Effect of a protective-ventilation strategy on mortality in the acute respiratory distress syndrome. N Engl J Med 1998; 338: 347–354.

110. ARDS Network. Ventilation with lower tidal volumes as compared with traditional tidal volumes for acute lung injury and the acute respiratory distress syndrome. The Acute Respiratory Distress Syndrome Network. N Engl J Med 2000; 342: 1301–1308.

111. Hebert PC, Wells G, Blajchman MA et al. A multicenter, randomized, controlled clinical trial of transfusion requirements in critical care. Transfusion Requirements in Critical Care Investigators, Canadian Critical Care Trials Group. N Engl J Med 1999; 340: 409–417.

112. Pepe PE, Hudson LD, Carrico CJ. Early application of positive endexpiratory pressure in patients at risk for the adult respiratory-distress syndrome. N Engl J Med 1984; 311: 281–286.

113. Marcy TW, Marini JJ. Inverse ratio ventilation in ARDS. Rationale and implementation. Chest 1991; 100: 494–504.

114. Krishnan JA, Brower RG. High-frequency ventilation for acute lung injury and ARDS. Chest 2000; 118: 795–807.

115. Carlon GC, Howland WS, Ray C et al. High-frequency jet ventilation. A prospective randomized evaluation. Chest 1983; 84: 551–559.

116. Broccard A, Shapiro RS, Schmitz LL et al. Prone positioning attenuates and redistributes ventilator-induced lung injury in dogs. Crit Care Med 2000; 28: 295–303.

117. Chatte G, Sab JM, Dubois JM et al. Prone position in mechanically ventilated patients with severe acute respiratory failure. Am J Respir Crit Care Med 1997; 155: 473–478.

118. Pelosi P, Brazzi L, Gattinoni L. Prone position in acute respiratory distress syndrome. In: Evans TW, Griffiths MJD, Keogh B, ed. European Respiratory Monograph: ARDS. Copenhagen: International Publishers; 2002: (in press).

119. Lamm WJ, Graham MM, Albert RK. Mechanism by which the prone position improves oxygenation in acute lung injury. Am J Respir Crit Care Med 1994; 150: 184–193.

120. Germann P, Poschl G, Leitner C et al. Additive effect of nitric oxide inhalation on the oxygenation benefit of the prone position in the adult respiratory distress syndrome. Anesthesiology 1998; 89: 1401–1406.

121. Langer M, Mascheroni D, Marcolin R, Gaffinoni L. The prone position in ARDS patients. A clinical study. Chest 1988; 94: 103–107.

122. Curley MA. Prone positioning of patients with acute respiratory distress syndrome: a systematic review. Am J Crit Care 1999; 8: 397–405.

123. Payen DM. Inhaled nitric oxide and acute lung injury. Clin Chest Med 2000; 21: 519–529, ix.

124. Manktelow C, Bigatello LM, Hess D, Hurford WE. Physiologic determinants of the response to inhaled nitric oxide in patients with acute respiratory distress syndrome. Anesthesiology 1997; 87: 297–307.

125. Puybasset L, Rouby JJ, Mourgeon E et al. Factors influencing cardiopulmonary effects of inhaled nitric oxide in acute respiratory failure. Am J Respir Crit Care Med 1995; 152: 318–328.

126. Papazian L, Roch A, Bregeon F et al. Inhaled nitric oxide and vasoconstrictors in acute respiratory distress syndrome. Am J Respir Crit Care Med 1999; 160: 473–479.

127. Cuthbertson BH, Dellinger P, Dyar OJ et al. UK guidelines for the use of inhaled nitric oxide therapy in adult ICUs. American–European Consensus Conference on ALI/ARDS. Intensive Care Med 1997; 23: 1212–1218.

128. Radermacher P, Santak B, Wust HJ et al. Prostacyclin for the treatment of pulmonary hypertension in the adult respiratory distress syndrome: effects on pulmonary capillary pressure and ventilation-perfusion distributions. Anesthesiology 1990; 72: 238–244.

129. Dellinger RP. Inhaled nitric oxide in acute lung injury and acute respiratory distress syndrome. Inability to translate physiologic benefit to clinical outcome benefit in adult clinical trials. Intensive Care Med 1999; 25: 881–883.

130. Gregory TJ, Steinberg KP, Spragg R et al. Bovine surfactant therapy for patients with acute respiratory distress syndrome. Am J Respir Crit Care Med 1997; 155: 1309–1315.

131. Anzueto A, Baughman RP, Guntupalli KK et al. Aerosolized surfactant in adults with sepsis-induced acute respiratory distress syndrome. Exosurf Acute Respiratory Distress Syndrome Sepsis Study Group. N Engl J Med 1996; 334: 1417–1421.

132. Gerlach H. Extracorporeal ventilatory support. In: Evans TW, Griffiths MJD, Keogh B, ed. European Respiratory Monograph: ARDS. Copenhagen: International Publishers; 2002: (in press).

133. Haitsma J, Lachmann B. Partial liquid ventilation in ARDS. In: Evans TW, Griffiths MJD, Keogh B, ed. European Respiratory Monograph: ARDS. Copenhagen: International Publishers; 2002: (in press).

134. Hirschl RB, Pranikoff T, Wise C et al. Initial experience with partial liquid ventilation in adult patients with the acute respiratory distress syndrome. JAMA 1996; 275: 383–389.

135. Simmons RS, Berdine GG, Seidenfeld JJ et al. Fluid balance and the adult respiratory distress syndrome. Am Rev Respir Dis 1987; 135: 924–929.

136. Mitchell JP, Schuller D, Calandrino FS, Schuster DP. Improved outcome based on fluid management in critically ill patients requiring pulmonary artery catheterization. Am Rev Respir Dis 1992; 145: 990–998.

137. Hayes MA, Timmins AC, Yau EH et al. Elevation of systemic oxygen delivery in the treatment of critically ill patients. N Engl J Med 1994; 330: 1717–1722.

138. Gattinoni L, Brazzi L, Pelosi P et al. A trial of goal-oriented hemodynamic therapy in critically ill patients. SvO2 Collaborative Group. N Engl J Med 1995; 333: 1025–1032.

139. Gadek JE, DeMichele SJ, Karlstad MD et al. Effect of enteral feeding with eicosapentaenoic acid, gamma-linolenic acid, and antioxidants in patients with acute respiratory distress syndrome. Enteral Nutrition in ARDS Study Group. Crit Care Med 1999; 27: 1409–1420.

140. Beale RJ, Bryg DJ, Bihari DJ. Immunonutrition in the critically ill: a systematic review of clinical outcome. Crit Care Med 1999; 27: 2799–2805.

141. Barnes PJ. Molecular mechanisms of glucocorticoid action in asthma. Pulmon Pharmacol Ther 1997; 10: 3–19.

142. Lazrak A, Samanta A, Venetsanou K et al. Modification of biophysical properties of lung epithelial Na(+) channels by dexamethasone. Am J Physiol Cell Physiol 2000; 279: C762–C770.

143. Bernard GR, Luce JM, Sprung CL et al. High-dose corticosteroids in patients with the adult respiratory distress syndrome. N Engl J Med 1987; 317: 1565–1570.

144. Luce JM, Montgomery AB, Marks JD et al. Ineffectiveness of high-dose methylprednisolone in preventing parenchymal lung injury and improving mortality in patients with septic shock. Am Rev Respir Dis 1988; 138: 62–68.

145. Kehrer JP, Klein-Szanto AJ, Sorensen EM et al. Enhanced acute lung damage following corticosteroid treatment. Am Rev Respir Dis 1984; 130: 256–261.

146. Meduri GU, Headley AS, Golden E et al. Effect of prolonged methylprednisolone therapy in unresolving acute respiratory distress syndrome: a randomized controlled trial. JAMA 1998; 280: 159–165.

147. Chabot F, Mitchell JA, Gutteridge JM, Evans TW. Reactive oxygen species in acute lung injury. Eur Respir J 1998; 11: 745–757.

148. Pacht ER, Timerman AP, Lykens MG, Merola AJ. Deficiency of alveolar fluid glutathione in patients with sepsis and the adult respiratory distress syndrome. Chest 1991; 100: 1397–1403.

149. Walsh TS, Lee A. N-acetylcysteine administration in the critically ill (editorial). Intensive Care Med 1999; 25: 432–434.

150. Bone RC, Slotman G, Maunder R et al. Randomized double-blind, multicenter study of prostaglandin E1 in patients with the adult respiratory distress syndrome. Prostaglandin E1 Study Group. Chest 1989; 96: 114–119.

151. Abraham E, Baughman R, Fletcher E et al. Liposomal prostaglandin E1 (TLC C-53) in acute respiratory distress syndrome: a controlled, randomized, double-blind, multicenter clinical trial. TLC C-53 ARDS Study Group. Crit Care Med 1999; 27: 1478–1485.

152. Williams JG, Maier RV. Ketoconazole inhibits alveolar macrophage production of inflammatory mediators involved in acute lung injury (adult respiratory distress syndrome). Surgery 1992; 112: 270–277.

153. ARDS Network. Ketoconazole for early treatment of acute lung injury and acute respiratory distress syndrome: a randomized controlled trial. JAMA 2000; 283: 1995–2002.

154. Abraham E. Lisofylline versus placebo for ALI and ARDS. Am J Respir Crit Care Med 2000; 161: A379.

155. Sartori C, Lipp E, Duplain H et al. Prevention of high-altitude pulmonary edema by beta-adrenergic stimulation of the alveolar transepithelial sodium transport. Am J Respir Crit Care Med 2000; 161: A415.

156. Mason RJ, McCormick-Shannon K, Rubin JS et al. Hepatocyte growth factor is a mitogen for alveolar type II cells in rat lavage fluid. Am J Physiol 1996; 271: L46–L53.

157. Abel SJ, Finney SJ, Brett SJ et al. Reduced mortality in association with the acute respiratory distress syndrome (ARDS). Thorax 1998; 53: 292–294.

158. Milberg JA, Davis DR, Steinberg KP, Hudson LD. Improved survival of patients with acute respiratory distress syndrome (ARDS): 1983–1993. JAMA 1995; 273: 306–309.

159. Krafft P, Fridrich P, Pernerstorfer T et al. The acute respiratory distress syndrome: definitions, severity and clinical outcome. An analysis of 101 clinical investigations. Intensive Care Med 1996; 22: 519–529.

160. Artigas A. Epidemiology and prognosis of acute respiratory distress syndrome. In: Evans TW, Griffiths MJD, Keogh B, ed. European Respiratory Monograph: ARDS. Copenhagen: International Publishers; 2002: (in press).

161. Davidson TA, Caldwell ES, Curtis JR et al. Reduced quality of life in survivors of acute respiratory distress syndrome compared with critically ill control patients. JAMA 1999; 281: 354–360.

162. McHugh LG, Milberg JA, Whitcomb ME et al. Recovery of function in survivors of the acute respiratory distress syndrome. Am J Respir Crit Care Med 1994; 150: 90–94.

29 Iatrogenic respiratory disease

Philippe Camus and G John Gibson

Key points

- Adverse reactions to drugs need to be included in the differential diagnosis of several respiratory conditions, including parenchymal disease (interstitial pneumonitis, pulmonary eosinophilia, organising pneumonia, pulmonary fibrosis), pleural thickening/effusion, pulmonary oedema, alveolar haemorrhage and pulmonary hypertension.

- Amiodarone, cytotoxic agents, antibiotics and non-steroidal anti-inflammatory drugs (NSAIDs) are the most common drugs causing infiltrative lung disease.

- The likelihood of cytotoxic drugs causing lung toxicity is increased by use of combinations of drugs, and by concurrent or later use of radiotherapy or oxygen.

- NSAIDs and beta-blockers are the drugs that most frequently cause asthmatic attacks. Such attacks may be severe or even fatal.

- Classical radiation pneumonitis and fibrosis are typically limited to the area of lung irradiated but radiation therapy can also cause migratory foci of organising pneumonia.

- Up-to-date information on the long list of potentially pneumotoxic drugs is available at http://www.pneumotox.com.

Drug-induced reactions in the respiratory system are believed to account for approximately 7% of all drug-induced reactions.[1] Like other adverse reactions to drugs, most have been recognised relatively recently. Indeed, most of the information on this topic has been published since the 1960s,[2] at which time only a limited number of clinical patterns and causative drugs were known. Since then, accrual of information has been relentless, and the following general conclusions can be drawn.

- The number of causative drugs has increased progressively and stands at 342 as of May 2002.[3,4] The reader is invited to consult the *Pneumotox* website[4] for further referencing.

- The clinical pictures of adverse reactions to drugs are manifold, with about 50 distinctive clinical–radiographic patterns.[4] In addition to the classic drug-induced interstitial lung diseases, other infiltrative lung diseases and diseases of pleura or pulmonary circulation have been described.[5]

- Several substances of therapeutic interest, in addition to drugs, may also cause lung disease. Examples include interferons,[6] immunoglobulins (IVIG),[7] anti-thymocyte globulin,[8] granulocyte- and granulocyte–monocyte-colony-stimulating factors (G-CSF/GM-CSF),[9] cytokines,[10] components of blood or fractionated plasma,[11,12] vaccines[13] and dietary compounds or herbs.[14,15] Accordingly, history-taking should also include these possibilities.

- In addition, medical devices (e.g. catheters,[16,17] pacemaker leads[18]) and medical,[19] radiographic[20] or surgical procedures (e.g. surgery in distant sites,[21] acupuncture,[22] bone marrow,[23] stem cell,[24] cord blood[25] or lung transplantation[26]) can cause distinctive lung problems. These may be due to various combinations of the underlying disease, graft-*versus*-host disease and therapy, including drugs, radiation and other modalities such as colony stimulating factors (CSFs) or investigational therapies. Consequently, the term *iatrogenic respiratory disease* now seems more appropriate than the more traditional and restrictive *drug-induced lung disease*.

- Associations of pneumotoxic compounds (concomitantly or in sequence) have been recognised as more toxic than each taken separately.[27–32] Examples include combinations of chemotherapeutic agents, or of chemotherapeutic agents and radiation therapy to either the chest or whole body. Of note, systemic anticancer chemotherapy given even months after irradiation of the chest may lead to reactivation of the process within the radiation field ('recall pneumonitis'),[27,33,34] and this is sometimes associated with *en face* radiation dermatitis. Similarly, oxygen therapy may potentiate or exacerbate the toxicity of such drugs as amiodarone,[35] bleomycin[36] or anticancer agents, although this is debated.[31] Prudence is therefore required if such combined therapeutic approaches are planned.

- Routes of drug administration other than conventional oral and parenteral routes may also lead to pulmonary toxicity. These include intrathecal,[37] ocular,[38] peri/retrobulbar,[39] intravesical,[40,41] vaginal,[42] and possibly transdermal administration.

- The rate at which novel offending drugs are being identified renders any publication on this topic rapidly out of date. The free, monthly updated *Pneumotox*® website gives up-to-date information on the list of drugs that may cause respiratory disease and on the clinical patterns resulting from exposure.[4]

- Some drug-induced respiratory diseases have reached the proportions of mini-epidemics.[43] This has resulted in the formation of groups of patients who now seek compensation for drug-induced disability.

- The present chapter is devoted to iatrogenic respiratory diseases and encompasses asthma-like, parenchymal infiltrative (including pulmonary oedema and alveolar haemorrhage), bronchial, pleural and vascular reactions, as well as 'radiotherapy lung', respiratory problems in illicit drug users, and miscellaneous other iatrogenic lung problems. It should also be remembered that steroid-induced[44-46] or chemotherapy-induced[47] respiratory infections are an important differential diagnosis of drug-induced lung disease, but these are outwith the province of this chapter. The heart can also be damaged by drugs, via either adverse inotropic effects or toxic/immunological mechanisms,[48] all of which can lead to heart failure and pulmonary oedema; these effects are not reviewed here.

- Knowledge of iatrogenic diseases is important to all respiratory specialists and intensivists because drugs will often provide an explanation for a variety of acute or chronic lung diseases. Furthermore, withdrawal of the causative drug will often lead to improvement or even resolution of the respiratory illness. Hence, early recognition of drug-induced lung disease and prompt cessation of the drug (which should be done carefully, as the underlying disease may flare up following drug withdrawal) should, at least theoretically, translate into shorter illness and better prognosis.

- The diagnosis of iatrogenic respiratory disease should be as firm as practicable (see Diagnostic criteria, below), and can only be accepted after other causes (mainly inhalational and infectious) have been carefully considered and excluded. If the clinical situation permits, steroids should be avoided, at least for a while, in order to assess the effects of drug withdrawal on the course of the illness.

- Symptoms common to many forms of iatrogenic disease include dyspnoea, dry cough, fever, chest pain and, in some cases, respiratory failure. Extrapulmonary manifestations (e.g. changes in liver chemistry, cutaneous rash or systemic symptoms) may also be evident. The severity of symptoms (from mild to life-threatening) and their time to onset (from seconds, in drug-induced bronchospasm or anaphylaxis, to years in lung disease due to amiodarone,

chemotherapy or radiation) vary according to drug, clinical picture and patient, and are often difficult to foresee.

- Some drugs tend to cause a consistent type of pulmonary reaction. For instance, methotrexate, minocycline, busulfan and ergot derivatives typically induce acute hypersensitivity pneumonitis, eosinophilic pneumonia, pulmonary fibrosis and pleural thickening or effusion, respectively. For these drugs, a class effect is plausible. By contrast, other drugs can induce a wide range of clinicopathological patterns. For example, amiodarone can cause asymptomatic radiographic opacities, multiple lung nodules, pulmonary eosinophilia, the adult respiratory distress syndrome (ARDS) or pulmonary fibrosis. The reasons for this disparity are unclear.

Epidemiology

Estimating the epidemiology of iatrogenic respiratory disease is difficult because:

- widely accepted criteria are lacking
- tools available for diagnosis (e.g. chest radiography, computed tomography – CT – scans, changes in pulmonary function, changes in bronchoalveolar lavage – BAL – cell numbers or differential), have different sensitivities
- patients receiving pneumotoxic drugs or undergoing potentially pneumotoxic procedures are often cared for in non-pulmonary settings. For instance, methotrexate can be prescribed by family practitioners or physicians in haematology, oncology, rheumatology or gastroenterology. It is possible that recognition of the iatrogenic aetiology of a respiratory condition varies among these specialities, as would probably be the case for recognition of non-respiratory iatrogenic effects by respiratory physicians
- in clinical settings such as (haemato-)oncology, adverse reactions are common. Patients are submitted to a wide array of drugs and procedures in sequence, many of which may induce lung disease with varying latency. The cumulative effect of these toxic factors may ultimately lead to a pattern of late interstitial pneumonitis/fibrosis with little residual specificity, a phenomenon known as late or delayed pulmonary toxicity syndrome.[29,49-51] In this setting, the respective role of each drug or factor is difficult to define.

The frequency of adverse pulmonary effects from any given drug can be estimated approximately from the number of published reports (see 'four-star drugs' on the *Pneumotox* website[4] and Table 29.1). Judged in this way, amiodarone, angiotensin-converting-enzyme (ACE) inhibitors, bleomycin, methotrexate, nitrofurantoin, non-steroidal anti-inflammatory drugs (NSAIDs) and mineral oil emerge as common offenders, with 100–1000 reported cases each. For all other drugs, the number of available reports ranges from a few cases (e.g. azathioprine, flecainide; the 'one-star' drugs on the *Pneumotox* website[4] and Table 29.1), to a few dozen (e.g. minocycline, sulfasalazine, nitrosoureas or methotrexate; see 'two-' and 'three-star' drugs on the *Pneumotox* website[4] and Table 29.1). It should be noted, however, that the number of publications on the adverse effects from a given drug

Table 29.1 Adverse effects from drugs in the respiratory system

Drug	Clinical pattern observed	Frequency	Drug	Clinical pattern observed	Frequency
Abacavir	X a	+	Blood transfusion	I c; II a; VIII a	++++
Abciximab	III a	+	Bromocriptine	I g; V a, c	+++
Acebutolol	I b, d; V a, b, c, d	++	Bucillamine	I c; IV d	+
Acetylcysteine	IVa	+	Bumetanide	XI b	++
Acetylsalicylic acid (aspirin)	I c; II a, b; III a; IV a, b; VId; VIIb; Xa	+++	Buprenorphine	IIa	+
Acrylate	VI a	++	Busulphan	I e, g; IV c; VI c	+++
Acyclovir	I b; V a, b, c	+	Cabergoline	V a, c	+
Adenosine and derivatives	IV a; XI b	+	Camptothecin-11	I c	+
Adrenaline (epinephrine)	II a	+	Captopril	I b, c, f; IV d; VIII a	++++
Albumin	II a	+	Carbamazepine	I a, b, c, d, k; II a; IIIa; IV a; V d; VII a, b; Xa	+++
Allopurinol	VI d	+	Carbimazole	VI d	+
Almitrine	XI d	+	Carmustine (BCNU)	I b, I g; II b; V a, f; VIc	+++
Aminoglutethimide	I c	+	Celiprolol	I a	+
Aminoglycoside antibiotics	IX a	++	Cephalosporins	I c, d; IV a, b	+
Aminorex (*recalled in early 1970s*)	VI b	++++	Chlorambucil	I b	++
			Chloroquine	I c	++
			Chlorozotocin (DCNU)	I g	++
Amiodarone	I b, c, d, g, k; II b; III a; IV a, b; V a, c, d	++++	Chlorpromazine	I c; IIa; V d; VI a	+
			Chlorpropamide	I c; Xa	+
Amitriptyline	II a, b	+	Ciprofloxacin	IV b	+
Amphotericin B	I d; II a, b; IV a	++	Cisapride	IV a	+
Ampicillin	I b, c	+	Clindamycin	I c	+
Amrinone	I b	+	Clofazimine	I h	+
ACE inhibitors	I b, c; IV a, b, d; V d; VIII a	++++	Clofibrate	I c; V d	+
Antazoline	I b	+	Clomiphene	II a, b; V a; VI a	++
Anti-thymocyte globulin	I g; II a	++	Clonidine	V d	+
Aprotinin	VI a	+	Clozapine	I b; V a, b; XI b	++
L-asparaginase	IV a, b; VI a	+	Colchicine	II a; Xa	+
Aspirin, see Acetylsalicylic acid			Contraceptives (oral)	V d; VI b, c	+++
ATRA (all-trans-retinoic acid) *see* Retinoic acid			Cotrimoxazole	I a, b, c; II a; VII a	++
			Cromoglycate	I a, b	+
			Curare-like drugs	IV a, b	+++
Aurothiopropano-sulfonate (gold salt)	I a, b, c, d, g; IV c	++++	Cyclophosphamide	I g; II a; IV a, b. V a; XI e	+++
			Cyclosporin	I b, j; II a; III a; VI b	++
Azapropazone	I b	+	Cytarabine (cytosine arabinoside; ara-C)	II b; III a	++
Azathioprine	I b; III a; IV b	++			
Azithromycin	I c; VI d	+	Danazol	I g	+
BCG therapy (intravesical)	I b; XI e	++	Dantrolene	V b	+
			Dapsone	I c; V a; X a; XI a	++
Barbiturates	I d	+	Daunorubicin	V a; XI b	+
Beclometasone	I c	++	Deferoxamine (desferrioxamine)	II a, b; VI a; XI e	++
Betahistine	IV a	+			
Betaxolol	I d; V c	+	Desipramine	I c; IV a	++
Bepridil	I g	+	Dexamethasone	II a	++
β-agonists (*administered i.v. as tocolytic*)	II a	+++	Dextran	II a; III a; IV b	++
			Diclofenac	I c, IV a	++
Bicalutamide	I b, c	+	Diflunisal	I c; VI d	+
			Dihydralazine see Hydralazine		++
Bleomycin	I b, c, d, g, k; II b; V f, VI c; VII a; XI b	++++	Dihydro-5-azacytidine	XI b	++
			Dihydroergocristine	V a, c	+
			Dihydroergocryptine	I b, d; V c	++

Continued

Table 29.1 Adverse effects from drugs in the respiratory system (*cont'd*)

Drug	Clinical pattern observed	Frequency	Drug	Clinical pattern observed	Frequency
Dihydroergotamine	I d; V a	+	Hydrochlorothiazide	I b, c; II a, b	+ + +
Dimethyl sulfoxide (DMSO)	IV b	+	Hydrocortisone	IV b	+
			Hydroxyquinoline	I b	+
Diltiazem	II a	+	Hydroxycarbamide (hydroxyurea)	I b	+ +
Docetaxol	I a, b; V a	+ +			
L-dopa	V d; VII b; IX b	+ +	Ibuprofen	I c; II a; IV a	+
Dothiepin	I b, g	+	Ifosfamide	I b; XI a	+
Doxorubicin	XI b	+	Imipramine	I c	+ +
Enalapril	IV d; VIII a	+ +	Immunoglobulins (IVIG)	II a; IV b	+ +
Epoprostenol see Prostacyclin	II a		Indinavir	II b	+
			Indometacin	IV b	+
Ergometrine	IV a	+	Insulin	II a	+ +
Ergotamine	I b, g; V a	+ +	Interferon (alpha)	I b, d, e; IV a; VII e	+ +
Erythromycin	I c; II a, b; IV a, b; VI d	+ +	Interferon (beta)	I d; VII a, e	+ +
Ethambutol	I c	+	Interferon (gamma)	VII f	+
Ethchlorvynol	II a; V a	+	Interleukin-2	I c; II a, b; IV a, d; V a; VI b (transient)	+ +
Etoposide	I b; XI b (due to coronary spasm)	+ + +	Irinotecan	I b	+
Etretinate	II b?	+	Itraconazole	V c	+
Febarbamate	I c	+	Isoflurane	IV d	+ +
Fenbufen	I c, VII a	+	Isoniazid	I c; V d	+ +
Fenfluramine/ dexfenfluramine	I a, b, c; V b; VI b	+ + +	Isotretinoin	I c, IV a; V b, c	+ +
			Itraconazole	V c	+
Fenoprofen	I c	+	Ketamine	II a	+
Fibrinolytics (including rTPA)	III a	+ +	Ketorolac	IV a	+
			Labetalol	I c, g; V d	+
FK506	I d	+	Leuprorelin	I g; II b; V e	+
Flecainide	I b	+	Levomepromazine	VIII a	+ +
Fludarabine	I a; II b; III a?	+	Lidocaine (lignocaine)	II a; IV b	+
Fluorescein	II a	+	Lipids (intralipid, soya)	II b; VI b	+ +
5-fluorouracil	I g	+	Lisinopril	VIII a	+ +
Flurbiprofen	IV a	+	Lisuride	V a, c	+
Fluoxetine	I b	+ +	Lomustine (CCNU)	I g, VIc	+ +
Flutamide	I g	+	Losartan	IV a, b, d	+
Fluticasone	XI f	+ +	Loxoprofen	I c; IV a	+
Fluvastatin	II b; V d	+	Maprotiline	I b, c	+
Fosinopril	I c	+	Mazindol	VI b	+
Fotemustine	I g	+	Mecamylamine (discontinued)	I d	+ +
Gemcitabine	I b; II b; IV b	+ +			
Glibenclamide	I b; III a; Xa	+	Medroxyprogesterone	I g; II a, b	+
Gliclazide	V b	+	Mefloquine	I b	+
G(M)-CSF	I b, c; II b; VI e; V a	+ + +	Melphalan	I g; IV a	+ +
Gold, see Aurothiopropano- sulfonate			Mephenesin	I c	+
			Mephenytoin	VII a	+ +
			6-mercaptopurine	I b; XI e	+
Gonadotrophin	V g	+ + +	Mesalamine	I c, d; IV a; XI b	+ +
Haloperidol	II b	+	Metapramine	I b	+
Heroin	I b; II a; IV a	+ + + +	Metformin	I b	+
Heparin	II b	+	Methadone	II a	+
Hexamethonium (discontinued)	I d, g	+ + +	Methotrexate	I a, b, c, g; II a, b; III a; IV b, d; V a; XI b; XI e	+ + + +
Hydralazine	I b; III a; V a, d; VI b	+ +	Methyldopa	V d; VII b; XI b	+ +

Table 29.1 Adverse effects from drugs in the respiratory system (*cont'd*)

Drug	Clinical pattern observed	Frequency	Drug	Clinical pattern observed	Frequency
Methylphenidate	I c	++	Parenteral nutrition	VI a, b	+
Methylprednisolone	IV a	+	Paroxetine	IVd, VIII a	+
Methysergide	I b, g; V a, c; VIId, XI b	++	Penicillamine	I b, c, d, g; III a, b; IV a, c; V a, c	+++
Metoclopramide	IV a	+			
Metoprolol	IV a; VI b	+	Penicillins	I c; IV a, b; VI d; VII a, b	+
Metronidazole	I c	+	Pentamidine	I c; IV a	+
Miconazole	II b	+	Pergolide	V a, c	+
Midazolam	IV a	+	Perindopril	I c	+
Minocycline	I c, d, k; V d; VII a; Xa; XI b, c	+++	Phenylbutazone	I c; II a; VII a; Xa	++
			Phenytoin	I b, c, d, f, k; III a; V a, c, d; VI a, d; VII a, b	++++
Minoxidil	V a	+			
Mitomycin C	I b, g; II b, c; III a; VI b, f	+++	Phenylephrine	II a	+
Mitoxantrone (mitozantrone)	I b	+	Pindolol	I g; V d	+
			Piroxicam	I c	+
Montelukast	I c	+	Pituitary snuff	I b	+
Moxalactam	III a	+	Plasma (fresh frozen)	II a	++
Mycophenolate mofetil	I g; II b; IV d	+	Polyethylene glycol	II b; IV a	+
			Practolol (*recalled*)	I b, g; V b, c	+++
Nadolol	I b	+	Praziquantel	V a	+
Naftidrofuryl	IV a	+	Procainamide	I b; V a; d; VI a	+++
Nalbuphine	II a	++	Procarbazine	I a, b, c	++
Nalidixic acid	I c; V d	+	Propafenone	IV a	+
Naloxone	II a	++	Propoxyphene	II a	+
Naproxen	I c, IV a	+	Propranolol	I c; IV a; V a, d; VI b	++
Nevirapine	V a; X a	+	Propylene-glycol	IV a	+
Nicergoline	V a, c; XI b	++	Propylthiouracil	I b, c, k; II b; III a; V a, b; VI d	+++
Niflumic acid	I c	+			
Nilutamide	I a, b, c, d	+++	Prostacyclin	II a	++
Nitric oxide (NO)	III a?; XI a	+	Prostaglandin $F_{2\alpha}$	IV a	+
Nitrofurantoin	I a, b, c, d, e, g; II b; III a; IV a, b; V a, d; VI d; VIII b; Xa; XI b, c	++++	Protamine	II a, b; IV b; VI b	++
			Pyrimethamine–dapsone	I c; Xa	+
Nitroglycerin	II a	++	Pyrimethamine–sulfadoxine	I b, c; II a	+
Nitrosoureas	I b, I g, VI c	+++			
Nomifensine	I b, c; VI d	+	Quinidine	I b; III a; V d; VI d	++
NSAIDs	I c; IV a; Xa	+++	Radiation	I b, d, g; II b; V a, c, f; VI c; VII d; IX a	++++
Noramidopyrine (metamizole)	II a	+			
Oestrogens	VI a	+++	Radiographic contrast media	I c, j; II a, b; III a; IV a, b	++++
OKT3	II b	+			
Olsalazine	V d	+	Raltitrexed	I b	+
Opioids (morphine agonist/antagonist)	II a; IV d; IX a	+++	Retinoic acid	I b; II a, b; V f; VI a	++
			Rifampicin	I c; IV a	+
Oxprenolol	Ib, IV a; V a, c	+	Risperidone	IV b	+
Oxyphenbutazone	I b	+	Ritodrine	II a	++
Paclitaxel	I b; IV a	++	Rituximab	I e	+
Para(4)-aminosalicylic acid (PAS)	I c; II a	++	Roxithromycin	I c; VI d	+
			Salbutamol	II a; IV a; XI d	++++
Paracetamol (acetominophen)	I c, IV a	+	Sertraline	I c	+
			Sirolimus	I b	++
Paraffin (mineral oil)	I j	++++	Sodium cromoglicate	I b, c	+
			Sotalol	I d; IV a	+

Table 29.1 Adverse effects from drugs in the respiratory system (*cont'd*)

Drug	Clinical pattern observed	Frequency	Drug	Clinical pattern observed	Frequency
Steroids	IV d; VI a; VII c; IX a; XI e	++++	Tricyclic antidepressants	II a	+++
Streptokinase	IIb; III a; IV a, d	++	Trimethoprim–sulfamethoxazole see Co-trimoxazole		
Streptomycin	I c	++			
Sulfamides–sulphonamides	I b, c; II a, b; IV a, b; V a d; VI d; VII b	+++	Trimipramine	I c; V b, f	++
Sulphasalazine	I b, c, e, g; II a; V b, d; VI d	+++	Troglitazone	II a; V a	+
Sulindac	I c; Xa	+	L-tryptophan (*recalled*)	I c; IV d; V a; VI b, d	++++
Tacrolimus	VI f	+	D-tubocurarine, see Curare-like drugs	IV a, b	+++
Tamoxifen	I g; II a; IV a; VI a	+			
Tenidap	I c	+	Urokinase	III a; IV a	+
Terbutaline	II a	++	Valproate (valproic acid)	III a; V b	+
Tetracycline	I c; V d	+	Valsartan	I b; IV b; X b	++
Thiopentone	IV b	++	Vancomycin	IV b	+
Ticlopidine	I d	+	Vasopressin	II a	+
Tiopronin	I b; IV c	+	Venlafaxine	I c	+
TNF-α	II a; III a	++	Vinblastine	I k; II b; IV a, b	+++
Tocainide	I b, g	+	Vindesine	I b, IV a, b	++
Tolazamide	I c	+	Vinorelbine	II a; IV a	+
Tolfenamic acid	I c	+	Vitamin D	I i	+
Topiramate	VI b, d	+	Warfarin	III a; V e; VIIIb	+++
Tosufloxacin	I c	+	Zafirlukast	VI d	++
Tramadol	IX a	+	Zanamivir	IV a	++
Trazodone	I c	+	Zomepirac	IV a	+
Triazolam	II a	+			

For further and continuously updated references, consult www.pneumotox.com

Key to clinical patterns
I = Interstitial lung disease: a, acute hypersensitivity pneumonitis and respiratory failure; b, subacute cellular interstitial pneumonitis; c, pulmonary infiltrates and eosinophilia; d, organising pneumonia ± bronchiolitis obliterans; e, desquamative interstitial pneumonia; f, lymphocytic interstitial pneumonia; g, pulmonary fibrosis; h, subclinical cytological changes in bronchoalveolar lavage cell profile; i, diffuse pulmonary calcification; j, mineral oil pneumonia with basal or more diffuse chronic lung changes; k, lung nodules. **II = Pulmonary oedema:** a, acute pulmonary oedema; b, acute permeability oedema with or without acute respiratory distress syndrome (ARDS); c, acute permeability oedema, ARDS and the haemolytic–uraemic syndrome. **III = Pulmonary haemorrhage:** a, alveolar haemorrhage; b, Goodpasture-like syndrome. **IV = Airway disease:** a, bronchospasm; b, bronchospasm ± laryngeal oedema and anaphylactic shock; c, irreversible bronchiolitis obliterans; d, lone cough. **V = Pleural changes:** a, pleural effusion; b, eosinophilic pleural effusion; c, pleural/pericardial thickening or effusion; d, pleural/pericardial thickening or effusion and positive antinuclear/antihistone antibodies – the drug-induced lupus syndrome; e, haemothorax; f, pneumothorax / pneumomediastinum; g, pleural effusion and ascites. **VI = Vascular changes:** a, thromboembolic disease; b, pulmonary hypertension (some are transient); c, pulmonary venoocclusive disease; d, vasculitis–angiitis; e, fat embolism; f, haemolytic–uraemic syndrome ± pulmonary hypertension. **VII = Mediastinal changes:** a, enlarged hilar/mediastinal lymph nodes; b, angioimmunoblastic-lymphadenopathy-like syndrome; c, mediastinal fatty deposits (lipomatosis); d, sclerosing mediastinitis; e, pseudosarcoidosis; f, enlarged thymus. **VIII = Major airway involvement:** a, upper airway obstruction from laryngeal oedema; b, upper airway obstruction from peritracheal mediastinal haemorrhage. **IX = Muscle and nerves:** a, abnormal (reduced) force generation; b, disordered breathing or respiratory movements (respiratory dyskinesia). **X = Constitutional/systemic symptoms:** a, systemic hypersensitivity syndrome with a combination of skin rash, eosinophilia, changes in liver function tests and mental disturbances; b, drug-induced antisynthetase syndrome. **XI = Miscellaneous effects:** a, methaemoglobinaemia, cyanosis, elevated blood nitrates; b, chest pain; c, chest pain in association with allergic interstitial pneumonitis; d, metabolic acidosis and dyspnoea; e, opportunistic infective pneumonia (including viral, bacterial, tuberculosis, *Pneumocystis carinii*); f, opportunistic airway infection (including mycotic)

Key to frequency
+, one or very few cases described (awaiting confirmation); ++, less than 10–15; +++, up to 100; ++++, more than 100.

tends to diminish with time (this is known as the 'β effect'), to a minimum, which can be so low that the condition may be unrecognised by younger specialists.[2]

Only for widely prescribed drugs that cause a significant rate of adverse effects can epidemiological data be inferred. With amiodarone, for example, the reported frequency has ranged between 0.003% and more than 40%, depending on the doses used. The likelihood of methotrexate pneumonitis in rheumatoid arthritis patients has been estimated to be 3.2%, or 1 per 50 patient-years.[52] The classically quoted frequency of bleomycin pneumonitis is '10%, of which 10% are fatal'. However, recent studies have shown that the frequency can be as high as 33%,[53] with an average mortality rate of 2.3%, increasing with advanced age and with impaired renal function.[54] When multidrug preconditioning of chemotherapy regimens are used for bone-marrow transplantation or for the treatment of breast cancer, the prevalence of lung toxicity may reach up to two-thirds of the exposed population and represent a limiting attrition rate.[51,55,56]

Risk factors

A few adverse effects are gender-specific, e.g. tocolytic-induced pulmonary oedema[57] and the ovarian hyperstimulation syndrome[58] in women and nilutamide-induced pneumonitis in men with prostate cancer.[59] Pulmonary complications of some chemotherapy regimens may be somewhat related to gender[32,60] but the association seems weak.

Ethnicity may also play a role. Indeed, the Japanese seem at greater risk of developing interstitial lung disease from nilutamide[59,61] and possibly other drugs.[62] In this context it should be noted that halothane hepatitis was reported to be more prevalent in whites than in black Africans.[63] Differences in activation/detoxication systems and in helper T-cell activity may explain the variable toxicological and hypersensitivity response among patients of different ethnic groups as well as between individuals of the same ethnic group.

Unstable or severe asthma is usually considered as a risk factor for bronchoconstriction precipitated by NSAIDs or aspirin,[64] probably because asthma in sensitive patients is intrinsically more severe. Many cases of drug-induced bronchospasm or anaphylaxis, however, are totally unexpected.[65,66] Smoking, pre-existing lung disease, advanced age and such underlying diseases as rheumatoid arthritis may expose the patient to greater risk of developing adverse respiratory effects from drugs. Renal failure increases the risk of developing bleomycin toxicity, via increased blood levels.[54] Exposure to asbestos has been shown to increase the likelihood of developing pleural thickening/effusion from ergot drugs.[67] Respiratory infections may increase the risk of, or trigger, analgesic-induced bronchospasm[68] and possibly also amiodarone-induced pneumonitis (unpublished observations).

As stated above, drug interactions (e.g. in multidrug chemotherapy regimens,[69] particularly the association of cyclophosphamide and nitrosoureas[51]) or association of anticancer chemoltherapy drugs and radiation[30] are likely to increase the risk of pulmonary toxicity. It often remains difficult to determine which drug in a multidrug regimen is the toxic one[49,70]

unless the clinical pattern is distinctive (e.g. the effect of methotrexate as opposed to other chemotherapeutic agents).

Prior irradiation of the chest may prime the lung for future injury from doses of chemotherapeutic agents normally considered to be safe.[71] Likewise, concomitant administration of chemotherapy with radiation,[71] or with total body irradiation[55] also increases the risk of lung toxicity. There is still controversy as to whether oxygen therapy[31] or G/GM-CSF[72] actually increases the risk of pulmonary toxicity from such drugs as bleomycin, other chemotherapy or amiodarone. In practice, however, it is wise to err on the safe side and to use oxygen or G/GM-CSF in such patients only if necessary and in the lowest possible doses.

Only with a few drugs have higher doses been associated with greater likelihood of pulmonary toxicity. This is considered likely for nitrosoureas, with a threshold of 475–600 mg/m^2,[29,32,73] above which unacceptable toxicity may develop. A dose–toxicity relation also exists for radiation therapy,[30] for which port size and dose delivered both influence toxicity.[51] A definite, but looser, dose–toxicity relation prevails for amiodarone and bleomycin. This conclusion is, however, potentially misleading, as several indisputable cases of pulmonary toxicity have been reported after low doses of these drugs.[74-76] Therefore, no dose should be considered completely safe, and the diagnosis of lung toxicity should not be rejected on this basis. With some drugs, pneumonitis emerges within a relatively narrow time frame (approximately 2 weeks for minocycline;[62] within 6 months for nilutamide[59]) but such a characteristic is distinctly unusual. For all other drugs, no consistent role of drug dose or duration on the likelihood of developing adverse pulmonary effects has been shown.

Diagnostic criteria

Recognition of iatrogenic respiratory disease depends on the conjunction of clinical, imaging and pathological information, as well as careful analysis of the temporal relation between exposure to the drug(s) and development of the adverse effect. While only a positive rechallenge would definitely establish the drug-induced nature of the condition, this is rarely performed, because of uncertainties regarding risks (particularly of a 'booster phenomenon'), dose to be used, duration of exposure and time to recurrence which may be as long as months.[77] The discriminant role of in-vitro tests as diagnostic tools remains unclear.

Five criteria should be evaluated, in order to support the diagnosis of iatrogenic respiratory disease with a reasonable degree of confidence, and hasten the diagnosis.

- **There should have been definite exposure to the drug prior to the onset of the respiratory condition.** Obviously, any drug taken only after the onset of the respiratory problem is ruled out as a causative agent. A few drugs induce adverse respiratory effects almost instantly after intake, reinforcing the strength of a cause-and-effect relationship. This holds true for NSAIDs, aspirin, anaphylaxis-inducing drugs[66] and hydrochlorothiazide,[78] which can induce catastrophic bronchoconstriction, respiratory failure or pulmonary oedema, respectively. Affected patients may have been exposed to the drug only once and very shortly (minutes) before the onset of the reaction.[66] For drugs other than these, medium-to-long-term exposure is required, before the adverse effect develops. Accordingly, patients who experience a pulmonary event very shortly after exposure to any drug other than those mentioned above are unlikely to have drug-induced respiratory disease. Occasionally, the onset of the adverse respiratory effect will be delayed by weeks or months (amiodarone), to years (cyclophosphamide, nitrosoureas) after cessation of the drug.[49,79–84] History-taking should therefore also include exposure to drugs in the remote past. In patients who have been exposed to chemotherapy or radiation in childhood (e.g. nitrosoureas for childhood brain tumours, cyclophosphamide, or chest irradiation for Hodgkin's disease), clinical symptoms of therapy-related lung disease may be discovered only in adolescence, possibly because of increased respiratory needs at that time or because of chemotherapy-related disturbances in lung growth, or both.[85]

- **The clinical picture should be consistent with what is known in the literature following exposure to the drug in question.**[4] While the possibility exists for any clinician to be confronted by the first case of an adverse effect to a particular drug,[77] inevitably this is rare.[86] The extent of the data now available in the medical literature and via the Internet[4] allows the question to be answered appropriately and satisfactorily in most instances, and a database should incorporate earlier relevant literature. Overlooking earlier literature, especially when older drugs are reintroduced for diagnostic or therapeutic purposes, has led to tragic events.[87,88]

- **A careful search for alternative explanations for the respiratory problem should be made.** Indeed, most clinical–radiographic patterns resulting from exposure to drugs are identical to those from other causes, or which occur idiopathically.[5] Among alternative causes, inhalation of noxious or immunogenic substances, infections and pulmonary manifestations of the disease for which the drug was being given are at the forefront. For example, diuresis should be attempted if there is the slightest doubt of pulmonary congestion or left heart dysfunction. If, following this therapeutic trial, radiographic pulmonary opacities persist, even attenuated, a workup for infiltrative lung disease should be pursued. Of note, the administration of diuretics for a few days may partially clear the radiographic density of interstitial pneumonitis and, therefore, pulmonary oedema as a diagnosis should be accepted only if complete clearing has occurred. It is of the utmost importance to remember that opportunistic infections (e.g. by *Pneumocystis carinii*) are common in patients receiving chemotherapy, immunosuppression or long-term steroids (oral and, possibly, inhaled).[86] The picture of drug-induced infection is often indistinguishable clinically and by imaging from drug toxicity, and prompt diagnosis and treatment is required. The confident diagnosis of iatrogenic disease in

this situation depends on confident exclusion of an infective cause. Accordingly, a careful history, together with smears and cultures of sputum, BAL fluid and blood, and extensive serological testing, should be performed as routine. The possible respiratory manifestations of the underlying illness for which the suspected drug was being given should also be considered. This is particularly relevant for chemotherapeutic agents, immunosuppressives, NSAIDs, gold, sulfasalazine and amiodarone, *versus* the underlying cancer, leukaemia or lymphoma,[89] autoimmune disease, rheumatoid arthritis,[90,91] inflammatory bowel disease[92] and left heart failure, respectively. Nevertheless, in some cases, sorting out the respective role of one drug among others, and of drug(s) *versus* the underlying illness may be extremely difficult, if not impossible.

- **Improvement of symptoms should occur once the drug is discontinued.** This is usually apparent in patients after recovery from drug-induced bronchoconstriction/anaphylaxis, or from parenchymal reactions characterised by a predominantly inflammatory, cellular or fluid overload pattern (e.g. drug-induced interstitial pneumonias, pulmonary eosinophilia or pulmonary oedema). Authentic drug-induced respiratory reactions may, however, fail to show this behaviour on cessation of exposure to the drug, either because the condition is fibrotic in nature and therefore irreversible (e.g. pulmonary fibrosis, bronchiolitis obliterans, pulmonary hypertension), or because the drug-induced process may require several months (e.g. amiodarone pneumonitis) or even years to improve or clear (e.g. ergot-induced pleural thickening). In some cases of severe drug-induced pulmonary inflammation (e.g. acute interstitial pneumonia, hypersensitivity pneumonitis, eosinophilic pneumonia), withdrawal of the drug may lead to no detectable improvement until a few days have elapsed, or steroids (which are often required in such situations) have been given. A notable exception to the rule of improvement upon drug withdrawal is amiodarone pneumonitis, presumably because retention of the drug in lung tissue is prolonged[93] and it does not clear from the lung until several months after cessation of treatment. Furthermore, the possible consequences of drug withdrawal should be balanced against the possible recurrence or exacerbation of the underlying disease.

- **Symptoms should recur if the drug is readministered.** In addition to ethical problems, rechallenge raises several issues concerning potential risks, dose to be used and ways to monitor recurrence (chest radiograph? CT scan? BAL?). Also, the effects of rechallenge in many drug-induced diseases have a long latency (e.g. fibrosing processes affecting the parenchyma, pleura, bronchi or vessels). These are likely to be difficult to interpret, and may add a further burden of irreversible lesions. In general, rechallenge for diagnostic purposes is not recommended and should be strictly restricted to cases where the drug is essential to the patient and no alternative is available. Often, 'indirect rechallenge' is proposed, which consists of the sequential readministration of all drugs taken by the patient, apart from the most likely culprit.

Drug-induced asthma

Asthma induced by therapeutic drugs is usually seen against a background of pre-existing asthma. Less commonly, it occurs de novo, when, rarely, it may persist after exposure has ceased.

The gravity of drug-induced bronchoconstriction resides in its unpredictability, the severity of the asthmatic attack and the consequent respiratory failure, which may lead to death or irreversible neurological damage.

A non-specific bronchial irritant effect is sometimes seen with inhalation of drugs used in the treatment of asthma. This may be related to the temperature, osmolality, pH, or tonicity of the carrier agent, or to the mode of delivery. For example, exacerbation of asthma by earlier chlorofluorocarbons (CFCs) probably accounts for the acute bronchoconstriction that has been described following inhalation of salmeterol, as the therapeutic effect of this agent has a slower onset than short-acting beta-stimulants, allowing a bronchoconstrictor effect of the carrier to become apparent.[94] Inhaled corticosteroids and cromolyn can lead to similar bronchoconstrictor effects. The potential of the newer non-CFC carriers to provoke a similar effect is as yet uncertain. Nebulised bronchodilator solutions have also been reported occasionally to provoke bronchoconstriction due either to the tonicity of the solution or to added preservatives.[95] Nebulised antibiotics[96] or pentamidine[97] may have similar bronchoconstrictor effects. N-acetylcysteine administered by inhalation or via a fiberoptic bronchoscope may also induce severe bronchospasm.[98]

Occasionally, asthma develops during the manufacture of drugs such as antibiotics,[99] or biological detergents,[100] when inhalation sensitises the airways of a previously non-asthmatic individual and causes occupational asthma (see Chapter 48.13).

Exacerbation of asthma resulting from more specific drug actions may be either a predictable consequence of the pharmacological properties of the drug concerned or an idiosyncratic response.

Pharmacological effects

Bronchoconstriction results predictably from use of cholinergic agents via a direct action on bronchial smooth muscle. This underlies the effects of systemic agents such as carbachol and also of the ophthalmic preparation of pilocarpine. Provocation of asthma may also result from the cholinergic effect of the cholinesterase inhibitor pyridostigmine, used in the treatment of myasthenia gravis.[101] Predictably, the bronchoconstrictor prostaglandin $PGF_{2\alpha}$, used to induce labour or abortion, is potentially hazardous in patients with asthma.

Non-specific inhibitors of ACE are well recognised to cause chronic disabling cough,[102,103] an effect that has been attributed to inhibition of breakdown of bradykinin and substance P. This effect is usually unrelated to asthma and is avoided by using the newer specific angiotensin-II-receptor antagonists, such as losartan or candesartan, even in asthmatics.[104] The latter drugs do not affect catabolism of kinins. Occasional reports of cough while taking angiotensin-II inhibitors deserve attention, however.[105] Although most individuals affected by ACE-inhibitor-induced cough have no features of asthma, occasionally deterioration of pre-existing asthma has been reported,[106] although a true association has been questioned.[107]

Beta-blockers

Despite publicity over many years, exacerbation of asthma by β-adrenergic drugs remains relatively common and even death from asthma still occurs.[108] The frequency of reactions is due to the widespread use of beta-blockers in the treatment of both hypertension and ischaemic heart disease and also as eyedrops in the treatment of glaucoma.[38] Although rarely given to patients with recognised asthma, beta-blockers are not infrequently used inadvertently in patients whose asthma has not previously been recognised. While, in some instances, a catastrophic asthmatic attack is triggered immediately,[65] in others asthma may deteriorate insidiously over a longer period. Thus, weaning from a beta-blocker should be considered in symptomatic patients, even if initially they appeared to tolerate the drug. Late catastrophic events have occasionally been reported in patients on beta-blockers who are exposed to radiographic contrast media or insect stings. Also, beta-blockers complicate the treatment of such incidents, because the response of patients to β_2-stimulants or adrenaline (norepinephrine) is sluggish. Beta-blockers should be used with great caution in any patient with a history of anaphylaxis.

The more selective β_1-blockers, such as metoprolol and atenolol, are less dangerous than non-selective drugs such as propranolol but the degree of selectivity is relative and none of these agents is completely safe in asthma.[109]

The mechanism of bronchoconstriction is presumed to be antagonism of β_2-adrenoreptors but the site of the receptors involved is unclear, as human bronchial smooth muscle has no significant direct sympathetic innervation. It is usually assumed that circulating catecholamines have a tonic smooth-muscle-relaxing effect in asthma and that this is inhibited by beta-blockers. However, the concentration of circulating catecholamines in resting subjects is very low and other mechanisms may be involved. One suggestion is that propranolol acts on bronchial smooth muscle via the parasympathetic nervous system by causing blockade of inhibitory presynaptic β_2-adrenoreptors on cholinergic nerves.[110]

Even a single therapeutic dose of a non-selective beta-blocker can cause life-threatening or fatal asthma.[65] Observational studies have also suggested that previously mild asthma may become more difficult to control after exposure to a beta-blocker.[111] The likelihood of an adverse reaction depends on both the selectivity of the drug and its plasma concentration and the bronchoconstrictor effects may be minimised by use of a slow-release drug-delivery system, giving a stable concentration,[112] but the usual advice is to avoid these drugs in asthma unless essential. In the treatment of systemic hypertension, several other classes of effective drugs are available, but recent evidence on the benefits of treatment with beta-blockers after myocardial infarction has reopened debate on whether in individuals with mild asthma the benefit of a selective agent may outweigh its acknowledged risks.

The non-selective beta-blocker timolol is widely used as eyedrops for the treatment of glaucoma, and several reports have highlighted it as a cause of exacerbations of asthma.[113] The potential adverse effect of eyedrops is more easily over-looked than that of tablets, but intraocular administration allows rapid access to the systemic circulation via the naso-lacrimal duct and the nasal mucosa, and even one drop of a 0.5% solution of timolol gives measurable plasma levels.[114] Also of relevance is the age at which glaucoma usually occurs, as it is well recognised that asthma is relatively underdiagnosed in elderly individuals. In patients with suspected asthma, viable alternatives for treatment of glaucoma include the selective β_1-antagonist betaxolol and the adrenaline (epinephrine) precursor dipivefrin, which is effective without any risk of bronchoconstriction.[113]

Idiosyncratic effects

Acute anaphylaxis or a non-immunologically-mediated anaphy-lactoid reaction has been reported following administration of several agents, with penicillin[115] and other antibiotics among those more frequently reported.[66] Anaphylactoid reactions are also a recognised hazard during anaesthesia, where they may be associated either with volatile agents such as althesin or with muscle relaxants such as suxamethonium and other curare-like drugs.[116] Usually, although not always, such reactions occur in patients with pre-existing asthma. The reaction is characterised by severe acute bronchoconstriction, angioneurotic oedema, hypotension and loss of consciousness, leading to irreversible neurological damage or death unless treated promptly.[66] Evaluation by skin testing may be helpful in patients who give a history of earlier allergic or anaphylactic reactions.

The most important therapeutic agent for acute anaphylaxis is adrenaline (epinephrine) given in small doses (0.5 mg in adults) *intramuscularly*.[66,117] Intravenous administration is potentially hazardous and runs the risk of provoking a hyper-tensive crisis, stroke, myocardial infarction or acute pulmonary oedema.[66] Supplementary treatment includes oxygen, plus intramuscular or intravenous antihistamine (chlorphenamine/chlorpheniramine) corticosteroid (hydrocortisone)[117] and some-times mechanical ventilation.

Intravenous *N*-acetylcysteine, used in treatment of paraceta-mol poisoning, occasionally provokes an exacerbation of asthma; the mechanism is unknown.[98]

Asthma induced by non-steroidal anti-inflammatory drugs

The sensitivity of certain asthmatic subjects to aspirin and other NSAIDs is well recognised[118,119] but its prevalence varies appre-ciably in different series, depending on diagnostic criteria. Estimates based on history alone suggest sensitivity in 1–3% of all asthmatic subjects but if challenge tests are performed the prevalence increases appreciably. Clinically evident sensitivity is also much higher among subjects prone to acute severe asthma. It has been apparent for many years that the pathogenesis of aspirin-induced asthma is related to metabolism of prosta-glandins,[120] as the agents provoking asthma all inhibit cyclo-

oxygenase (COX), the enzyme responsible for prostaglandin synthesis (see Chapter 48.2). Although the precise mechanism remains uncertain, the picture has been clarified with increased understanding of the interactions between prostaglandins and leukotrienes (LTs) and the discovery of two isoforms of COX (COX1 and COX2).

It appears that the most important bronchoconstrictors in aspirin-induced asthma are the cysteinyl-leukotrienes, in parti-cular LTC_4.[121] Expression of the enzyme LTC_4 synthase in bronchial biopsy specimens from asthmatic subjects with aspirin sensitivity has been shown to correlate with bronchial respon-siveness to inhaled lysine aspirin and, in one study,[122] subjects with aspirin sensitivity had many more cells (mainly eosinophils) expressing this enzyme in the airway than either non-sensitive asthmatics or normal subjects. Furthermore, one particular form of the LTC_4-synthase gene promoter associated with greater expression of LTC_4 synthase has been shown to be more frequent in aspirin-sensitive than non-sensitive asthmatic subjects.[123]

Following local bronchial challenge with lysine aspirin, aspirin-sensitive individuals show marked suppression of syn-thesis of the bronchodilator prostaglandin PGE_2 without inhi-bition of other prostanoids, whereas, in aspirin-tolerant subjects, synthesis of other prostaglandins is also reduced.[124] It has, therefore, been proposed that PGE_2 normally acts as a 'brake' on the effects of the bronchoconstrictor leukotrienes and when this 'brake' is removed by NSAIDs, greater amounts of leukotrienes are produced.[125] In sensitive individuals, inhibi-tion of PGE_2 synthesis by NSAIDs may be a 'trigger', resulting in the unopposed action of bronchoconstrictor leukotrienes, which are present in greater amounts in such individuals,[122] possibly because of a particular polymorphism of the LTC_4-synthase gene.[123] This hypothesis does not, however, com-pletely explain aspirin-sensitive asthma, as some patients do not possess the predisposing variant of the LTC_4 synthase gene and antileukotriene drugs do not prevent NSAID-induced asthma.

Clinical features

Typically, patients with aspirin-sensitive asthma develop asthma in adult life, although sensitivity also occurs occasionally in childhood.[126] Aspirin-sensitive asthma is more common in women than men, in a ratio of about 2:1, and approximately 60% of the patients have nasal polyps.[127] Rhinitis and rhinor-rhoea usually precede the development of asthma, with aspirin sensitivity becoming apparent subsequently.[127] It has been esti-mated that, of the total population of subjects with nasal polyps, about 20% have overt aspirin sensitivity[128] but, in the absence of a suggestive clinical history, only a small minority of individuals with polyps are likely to be aspirin-sensitive. The prevalence of positive skin tests to common allergens is similar in subjects with and without aspirin sensitivity.[129] Patients with aspirin sen-sitivity often have 'difficult to manage' asthma, with about 50% requiring regular treatment with oral corticosteroids.[130] It is also noteworthy that these individuals represent an important pro-portion of patients subject to life-threatening attacks: in one series one-quarter of patients requiring assisted ventilation for acute asthma were sensitive to aspirin.[64] At its most dramatic, the response to a single tablet of aspirin or other NSAID is anaphylactoid, with shock, life-threatening bronchoconstriction, severe nasal symptoms and oedema of the upper airway, leading to a choking sensation and rapid loss of consciousness. Less sensitive individuals show more gradual development of rhinitis and asthma. Slowly developing symptoms, over a couple of hours, may be less readily attributable to the provoking drug, and are usually less severe. The imaging pattern is similar to that of asthma from other causes, and the chest radiograph will show hyperinflation.

In many subjects, the history is sufficiently clear for further investigation to be unnecessary, other than that required to assess the overall severity of asthma. When the association is less definite or when treatment with an NSAID is desirable, carefully controlled challenge tests are justified. These can be performed by bronchial challenge, using inhaled lysine aspirin, which is safe and more rapid than oral challenge, although a little less sensitive.[131] A simpler alternative is nasal challenge with lysine aspirin, but this is rather less reliable for confident exclusion of sensitivity.[132]

Treatment

Patients with a clear history of intolerance to aspirin should be advised to avoid all aspirin-containing products and other NSAIDs. Early data on the selective COX-2 antagonists suggest that they are likely to be safer.[133] Paracetamol (acetaminophen) is a very weak inhibitor of COX and is safe in normal therapeutic doses in most patients with NSAID sensitivity, but large doses produce reactions in a sizeable minority.[134] The likely pathogenetic mechanisms of NSAID-induced asthma would suggest that drugs that inhibit leukotrienes or antagonise their effects might be useful. Some protection has been shown in single-exposure challenges and in a double-blind study of the 5-lipoxygenase inhibitor zileuton.[135] However, severe sensitivity may not be countered by leukotriene inhibitors[136] and it is not clear whether subjects with NSAID sensitivity derive greater benefit from these agents than do those with non-sensitive asthma.

Desensitisation to aspirin is practised in some centres, with well-documented good results in selected patients. The observation that a single NSAID challenge results in a refractory period, which can last for up to 5 days,[137] led to desensitising schedules using gradually increasing doses followed by regular treatment. This is required to maintain the refractory state as otherwise sensitivity returns in a few days.[138] If desensitisation to aspirin is achieved, there is tolerance to other NSAIDs as well.[138] No more than 2 days without the drug should be allowed, if tolerance is to be maintained.

Occasional patients with aspirin sensitivity react adversely to intravenous hydrocortisone sodium succinate.[139,140] This effect appears to be related to the succinate ester and may be avoided by using hydrocortisone sodium phosphate or a different corticosteroid.

Drug-induced infiltrative lung diseases

In addition to drug-induced/iatrogenic interstitial lung diseases, infiltrative lung diseases encompass alveolar diseases, pulmonary oedema and pulmonary haemorrhage.[5] The term 'infiltrative' is preferred because, in addition to 'pure' interstitial lung diseases (e.g. 'non-specific interstitial pneumonia', according to the newer pathological classification; eosinophilic pneumonia; pulmonary fibrosis), drugs can also induce mixed interstitial/alveolar reactions (e.g. amiodarone pneumonitis, organising pneumonia), or predominantly alveolar reactions (e.g. desquamative interstitial pneumonia, lipoid pneumonia, pulmonary oedema or alveolar haemorrhage). Also, the radiographic distinction between severe interstitial and alveolar disease may be difficult.[5]

Drug-induced interstitial pneumonitides

Various drug-induced conditions are encompassed by this heading, with diverse clinical, imaging, BAL and histopathological appearances. Several subtypes of drug-induced interstitial pneumonitis have been described, depending on clinical severity, extent and distribution of involvement, histopathology, or results of BAL.

Drug-induced infiltrative lung diseases usually develop in patients who have received the causative agent for at least weeks and up to years. In most cases, the drug is still being taken at the time of onset of the lung disease. As stated above, exceptions include nitrosoureas,[81,82] amiodarone,[84] radiotherapy[141] and, less commonly, methotrexate,[80] in which the therapy may have been discontinued before the onset of pneumonitis, the longest lag times having been observed with nitrosoureas and radiation therapy.

The chest radiograph generally shows symmetrical infiltrates of variable extent and density. Severity may range from subclinical involvement, as detected by changes in BAL cell differential, or on the basis of minor opacities visible only on CT (as reported in patients exposed to amiodarone, bleomycin or chemotherapy),[142-147]· to a pattern indistinguishable from ARDS.[72,148-152] Usually, a restrictive defect of lung function is present, along with severely diminished transfer factor for carbon monoxide. In addition to drug withdrawal (where possible), steroids are required in patients with severe lung involvement, provided that infection has been considered and reasonably ruled out. Dose and duration of steroid treatment should be titrated against the clinical, radiographic and functional response, and weaning from steroids should be prudent and gradual, in order to minimise the likelihood of uncontrollable recurrence, especially with amiodarone or chemotherapy.

The patterns of drug-induced pneumonitis are presented in approximate order of frequency.

Non-specific or cellular interstitial pneumonia

This is probably the most common pattern of drug-induced infiltrative lung disease. Typical drugs causing this syndrome include beta-blockers, gold, methotrexate, nilutamide and nitrofurantoin, but about 80 other drugs are capable of causing the condition, plus anecdotal reports incriminating other drugs (see one- and two-star drugs in Table 29.1). The range of cumulative doses received by patients varies with the compound; for instance, methotrexate pneumonitis has been shown to develop following doses spanning a 1600-fold range and durations of treatment ranging from a few days to years.[153] The range of total doses is 10-fold narrower for such drugs as nilutamide or gold, and affected patients usually develop the disease within the first 3–6 months of treatment.

The onset of the pneumonitis ranges from subacute (gold, nilutamide) to rapid or abrupt (methotrexate). With nearly all causes, no other triggering factor is identifiable. Usually, the lung is the only organ involved, but a skin rash or concomitant liver involvement have occasionally been reported. The latter association has been reported particularly with the use of nitro drugs.[154-156] The respiratory presentation is with dyspnoea and cough. An associated fever may exceed 40°C. Rarely, patients develop severe systemic symptoms, associated multiorgan failure[157] or extrapulmonary involvement, as with the hypersensitivity syndrome seen with some anticonvulsants.[158] The clinical severity of drug-induced interstitial pneumonitis is variable: for instance, methotrexate pneumonitis is usually severe and may run a stormy course,[37] often with full-blown ARDS. Other drugs (e.g. nilutamide) induce a milder, self-limiting condition.[59]

Bilateral infiltrates are usually present on the chest radiograph. They are approximately symmetrical and may predominate in the bases, apices or midfields of the lung, depending more on the individual patient than the causative drug (Figs 29.1 & 29.2). Severe cases show diffuse infiltrates and reduced lung volumes (Fig. 29.2). Associated pleural effusion or mediastinal/hilar adenopathy is occasionally seen (methotrexate). The BAL fluid is usually rich in inflammatory cells, predominantly lymphocytes of the CD8+ or, less often, the CD4+ phenotype.

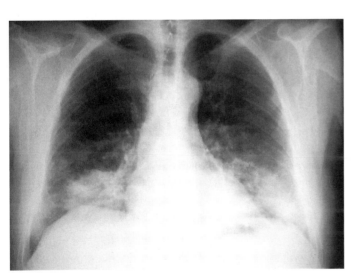

Fig. 29.1 Bibasal shadowing in a patient with drug (nilutamide)-induced pneumonitis. For a given drug, the extent and distribution of shadowing with classical interstitial pneumonitis are almost unpredictable. (With permission from Pfitzenmeyer et al 1992,[59] courtesy of Dr P Fargeot.)

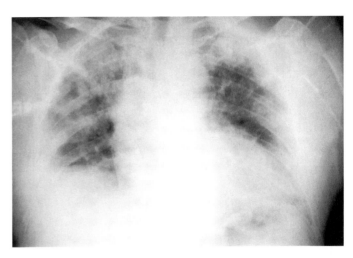

Fig. 29.2 Diffuse radiographic shadowing and marked volume loss in a patient taking the beta-blocker acebutolol long-term. The shadowing cleared progressively over a few weeks and recurred following inadvertent rechallenge with the drug. This radiographic picture usually corresponds to a histopathological pattern of florid nonspecific cellular interstitial pneumonia. This type of disease can result from exposure to many drugs, including methotrexate and gold salts.[4] (With permission from Lombard et al 1993.[77])

Patients with methotrexate pneumonitis may have a CD8+ lymphocytosis, pure CD4+ lymphocytosis or, less commonly, neutrophilia in their BAL.[159-161] The in-vitro proliferative response of peripheral cells challenged with the drug, and drug-related inhibition of leucocyte migration, have been demonstrated in some cases, but the significance of these tests is unclear.[162-164]

Careful investigation of BAL fluid for possible infection is necessary, particularly in patients with acute and extensive infiltrates developing while receiving chemotherapy or immunosuppressive regimens; the main differential diagnosis being infective pneumonia (Fig. 29.3). Varicella-zoster virus, *Pneumocystis carinii*, *Cryptococcus neoformans*, *Nocardia asteroides*, *Histoplasma capsulatum* and cytomegalovirus are among the opportunistic agents capable of inducing infective pneumonia in patients on methotrexate or other immunosuppressive agents.[165,166]

Although a lung biopsy would definitively rule out infection or other causes and support the histopathological diagnosis of nonspecific interstitial pneumonia, the procedure is rarely performed as it may be risky, especially in patients with respiratory failure. Transbronchial lung biopsy is also not free from risks and may give too small a specimen for definitive diagnosis. Video-assisted thoracoscopic lung biopsy may be the method of choice, should histology be required. Lung sections typically demonstrate a dense mononuclear interstitial infiltrate in alveolar walls, along with some intervening interstitial or alveolar oedema (Fig. 29.4). Alveolar spaces may be partially filled with packed mononuclear cells, in the pattern of a desquamative interstitial pneumonia (Fig. 29.5). Interstitial fibrosis, usually low-grade, may also be present and in this context does not seem to imply an ominous prognosis. Some cases show well-formed granulomata (Fig. 29.6) but this remains a distinctly unusual finding, which has been

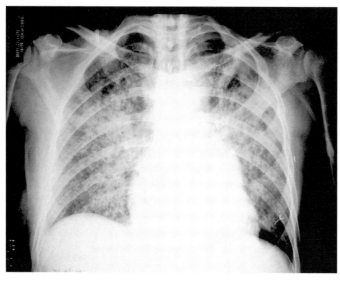

Fig. 29.3 In the diagnostic work-up of almost any patient with drug-induced lung disease, it is crucial to rule out infection. This patient developed extinsive tuberculosis following chemotherapy for breast cancer, and the imaging picture resembles that of drug-induced pneumonitis.

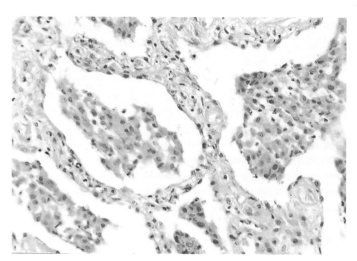

Fig. 29.5 Histopathological appearances of moderately severe drug-induced cellular interstitial pneumonia This section shows a more extensive infiltrate than in Figure 29.4, with several layers of mononuclear cells within the interstitium and packed alveolar macrophages in the alveolar spaces (a desquamative-interstitial-pneumonia-like pattern). In this case, there were extensive radiographic shadows and the pneumonitis was due to the beta-blocker acebutolol. (Courtesy of Dr K. Scully.)

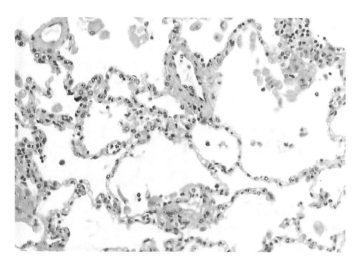

Fig. 29.4 Histopathological appearances in mild drug-induced interstitial pneumonia (cellular type). This section shows a discrete interstitial incellular infiltrate in a patient with methotrexate pneumonitis. (Courtesy of Professor F. Piard.)

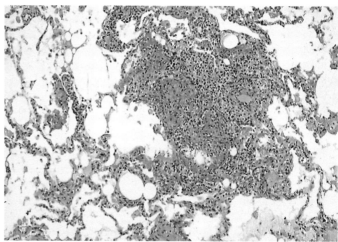

Fig. 29.6 Non-caseating granulomata with giant cells is a distinctly unusual finding in drug-induced lung disease. Methotrexate (as in the present case), intravesical *Bacillus* Calmette–Guérin and interferons are among the drugs that can cause this pattern. (Courtesy of Professor F. Piard.)

reported following the use of methotrexate, *Bacillus* Calmette–Guérin (BCG), interferons, antiretroviral therapy and, more rarely, bleomycin, fluoxetine, 6-mercaptopurine and sulfasalazine.

The overall prognosis is favourable, with improvement within a few days or weeks. Mortality is low (about 1%), provided the diagnosis is established early. Pulmonary function normalises progressively over several weeks but may take up to a year. According to a few reports, BAL fluid lymphocytosis returns towards normal within 2–8 weeks. Although the beneficial role of steroids is not firmly established, these drugs seem to have an adjunctive role and to hasten recovery. In our view, they are not necessary in the patient with mild disease, as spontaneous recov-

ery is likely on withdrawal of the drug and steroids will obscure proper evaluation of the role of drug withdrawal in the clinical picture. In contrast, steroids are strongly recommended in patients with extensive infiltrates impacting on gas exchange, in an attempt to shorten the duration of respiratory failure and, possibly, to avoid mechanical ventilation. It should be noted that oral steroids in conventional clinical doses do not prevent drug-induced interstitial pneumonitis from developing.[167] Long-term sequelae are distinctly unusual, with very few reports of chronic pulmonary fibrosis.

Drug-induced pulmonary eosinophilia

Collectively, drugs are a common cause of pulmonary eosinophilia (also known as eosinophilic pneumonia or pulmonary infiltrates with eosinophilia, PIE). The condition has few distinctive features and resembles pulmonary eosinophilia from other causes (e.g. parasitic, idiopathic). Obviously, other aetiological factors need be carefully analysed before the diagnosis of drug-induced pulmonary eosinophilia can be accepted. This is particularly important in relation to parasitic causes, which may be seriously aggravated if steroids are used.[168,169]

Patients present with the non-specific symptoms of cough, wheezing and constitutional upset (moderate fever, night sweats and malaise). The chest radiograph typically shows biapical subpleural opacities, known as 'the photographic negative of pulmonary oedema' (Fig. 29.7), but, in about half the cases, the distribution of opacities is random or diffuse[62,170] (Fig. 29.8). The hallmark of the condition is the presence of eosinophils in the peripheral blood, BAL fluid, lung tissue or any combination thereof.[62] Of note, blood or BAL eosinophilia may be lacking, and eosinophils may only be present in lung tissue.[62] On histology, interstitial infiltrates of mononuclear cells and eosinophils are present, with cells aggregating around small pulmonary vessels[62] (Fig. 29.9). Recently, cases of eosinophilic pneumonia plus angiitis, fulfilling the criteria for the Churg–Strauss syndrome, have been reported in patients receiving leukotriene-antagonist drugs[171,172] (see Iatrogenic diseases of the pulmonary circulation, below).

Pulmonary eosinophilia can be caused by several dozens of chemically unrelated drugs.[4] Classical causative agents include antibiotics, NSAIDs, salicylate, ACE inhibitors and the antidepressants imipramine and desipramine. Anecdotally, the con-

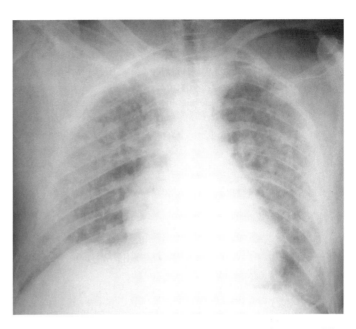

Fig. 29.8 Diffuse infiltrates in severe eosinophilic pneumonia. This young patient developed acute respiratory failure following minocycline treatment for *acne vulgaris*.[62] (Courtesy of Professor F. de Blay.)

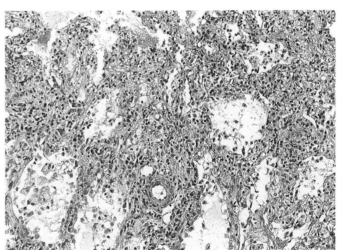

Fig. 29.9 Histopathological appearances of pulmonary eosinophilia, caused in this case, by minocycline (transbronchial lung biopsy). There is a dense interstitial infiltrate of mononuclear cells and eosinophils.[62] (Courtesy of Dr Roignot.)

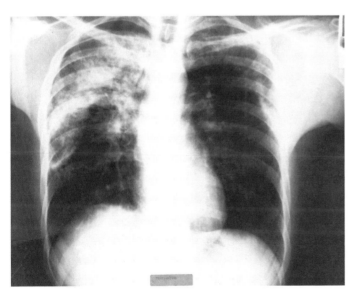

Fig. 29.7 Chest radiograph showing biapical subpleural alveolar shadows typical of eosinophilic infiltrates (the 'photographic negative of pulmonary oedema'), caused in this case by minocycline.[62] (Courtesy of Dr P. Ravier.)

dition has been reported after the use of other drugs.[4] The condition is often self-limiting and the outcome after simple withdrawal of the drug is generally favourable. In some cases, possibly as a result of delayed diagnosis or delayed drug withdrawal, severe acute eosinophilic pneumonia with associated respiratory failure may develop[62,158,173] (Fig. 29.8). Steroids are generally quite effective in drug-induced eosinophilic pneumonia and should be used liberally in documented cases with extensive radiographic involvement, significant symptoms or respiratory failure.

In the past, intake of a specific brand of the dietary supplement L-tryptophan, containing a trace amount of a contaminant, led to a distinctive pattern of 'eosinophilia–myalgia syndrome'.[174,175] Patients presented with severe constitutional symptoms, fever, blood eosinophilia, eosinophilic pneumonia, scleroderma-like skin changes and involvement of liver, heart and nervous system. Many patients showed chronic immune stimulation and suffered persistent disabling systemic or organ-specific symptoms in spite of withdrawal of the drug. In some, irreversible pulmonary hypertension (PHT) had developed. L-tryptophan-containing dietary compounds were recalled following this epidemic, but patients may continue to experience disabling symptoms years after cessation of exposure.[175]

Amiodarone pneumonitis – 'amiodarone lung'

Amiodarone very commonly causes lung disease. The iodine-containing drug is used in refractory arrhythmias, and amiodarone pneumonitis has been known since 1980.[176] Several hundreds of cases have been reported worldwide and mortality is substantial. Amiodarone pneumonitis has distinctive clinical and imaging features, which deserve special consideration.[177,178] The differential diagnosis is also distinctive, in that patients on amiodarone are at risk of left heart failure and of pulmonary embolism. On the other hand, withdrawal of amiodarone may expose the patient to the risk of fatal recurrence of arrhythmias, a possible cause of death in this context. Consequently, the diagnosis of amiodarone pneumonitis must be established as early, and reliably, as possible.

It is not clear whether patients with previously impaired lung function have an increased risk of developing amiodarone pneumonitis. The condition mostly affects men and, on average, the risk of developing lung toxicity ranges between 1% and 5% of the treated population. A relationship with daily dose is likely, amiodarone pneumonitis being less common (about 2%) in patients taking 200 mg daily or less. In contrast, the prevalence may exceed 50% in patients treated with high (> 1200 mg) daily doses. The duration of treatment before the onset of pneumonitis is inversely related to the daily dose. On average, patients with amiodarone pneumonitis who have taken 200 mg amiodarone or less daily develop the disease within 2.5 years, whereas it takes about 1.5 years in patients treated with 200–400 mg, and less than 1 year in those treated with more than 400 mg daily.[179] This information is useful for planning appropriate respiratory follow-up of patients taking amiodarone.

Although the shortest reported time to pneumonitis is 8 days, it is unusual for amiodarone pneumonitis to develop after less than 1–2 months of treatment, the longest recorded time being 14 years. While the threshold range of dose above which amiodarone pneumonitis is more likely to develop is 140–230 g, it should be remembered that, in the individual patient, there is no real safe dose.[180] Whether previous treatment with amiodarone in the recent past increases the likelihood of amiodarone pneumonitis, and whether remote treatment with the drug is a risk factor for pulmonary fibrosis later in life, is uncertain but possible.[181]

Although occasionally amiodarone pneumonitis can be detected by routine radiological follow-up of patients taking the drug, in most it is the onset of respiratory symptoms that leads to diagnosis. It is relatively uncommon for the patient with amiodarone lung to experience other adverse effects of the drug.[182] Typically, the onset of pneumonitis is gradual and insid-

ious, with dyspnoea on exertion, moderate fever, weight loss, constitutional symptoms and an increased erythrocyte sedimentation rate. Dyspnoea and crackles on auscultation are nearly always present. Patients are often seen after several weeks of disabling symptoms, and earlier diagnosis is desirable.

The chest radiograph shows various patterns, the most common being bilateral, asymmetrical, interstitial or alveolar opacities (Fig. 29.10). Others include unilateral consolidation (Fig. 29.11), lobar/segmental consolidation or masse(s) (Figs 29.12 & 29.13), multiple migratory (sub)segmental opacities corresponding to bronchiolitis obliterans and organising pneumonia (see Organising pneumonia, below), bibasal roughly symmetrical shadows (Fig. 29.14) and sometimes 'white lungs' with the features of ARDS. Pleural effusion is relatively common, but is rarely seen as the sole abnormality. On CT imaging (Figs 29.15 & 29.16), opacities often cross fissures, contain air bronchograms and may exhibit high density, thought to result from the presence of iodine in the amiodarone molecule. Contralateral diminutive foci of amiodarone pneumonitis should be looked for; they are helpful adjuncts to the diagnosis (Figs 29.16 & 29.17). CT seems more sensitive than the plain chest radiograph in this respect.[144,147,177] Small infiltrates may also be found at CT in patients on amiodarone who are asymptomatic and have a normal chest radiograph. These infiltrates correspond histologically to small foci of amiodarone pneumonitis.[144,147,177] Increased density of the liver, where storage of amiodarone also takes place, is common.[183] An unusual pattern of amiodarone pneumonitis on CT is represented by multiple bilateral 'shaggy' nodules (Fig. 29.18). A few patients present with rapidly migrating segmental or lobar opacities correspon-

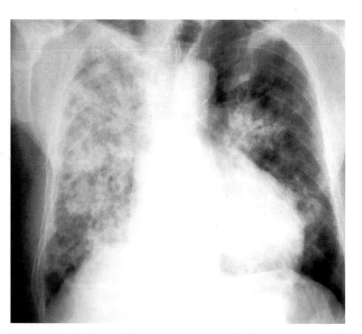

Fig. 29.10 Radiographic appearances in amiodarone pneumonitis are manifold. Most often, the changes are bilateral and asymmetrical, with no definite lobar distribution. They may range from barely visible opacities, best seen on computed tomography, to a picture of diffuse involvement with the features of acute respiratory distress syndrome. (Courtesy of Dr M. Fraison.)

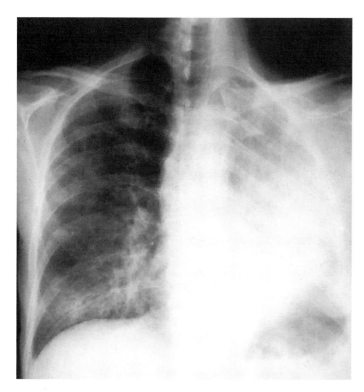

Fig. 29.11 Amiodarone pneumonitis: opacification of the entire left lung and more limited shadowing at the right lung base.

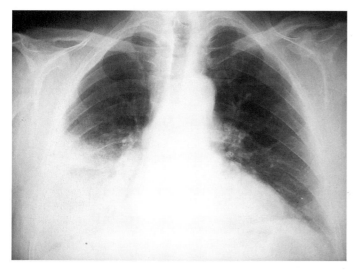

Fig. 29.12 Amiodarone pneumonitis: predominant opacification of the right lower lobe and part of the right upper lobe (same patient as in Figs 29.16 and 29.17).

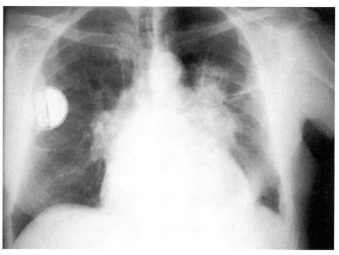

Fig. 29.13 Amiodarone pneumonitis with the appearance of an isolated mass.

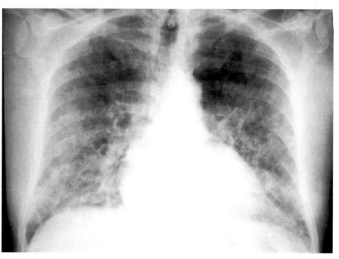

Fig. 29.14 Bilateral, approximately symmetrical involvement in amiodarone pneumonitis.

ding histologically to amiodarone-induced bronchiolitis obliterans and organising pneumonia (BOOP)[184,185] (see Organising pneumonia, below).

Pulmonary function tests in amiodarone pneumonitis typically show a restrictive ventilatory defect, with decreased transfer factor for carbon monoxide. In some cases, lung volumes remain normal. Coexisting airway obstruction may result from earlier exposure to tobacco smoke. Gas exchange is often severely impaired, as exemplified by significant arterial hypoxaemia.

The BAL pattern is variable, with approximately 25% of patients showing each of neutrophilia, lymphocytosis and a mixed lymphocytic and neutrophilic pattern, and the remainder having a normal cell differential.[186] Many patients exhibit lipid-laden macrophages, thought to reflect amiodarone-induced disturbance in phospholipid metabolism[186] (Fig. 29.19). Other than to rule out infection, BAL is not a reliable diagnostic tool in amiodarone pneumonitis. The ratio of CD4+ to CD8+ lymphocytes in the BAL has often been found to be decreased, but the diagnostic value of this finding is unclear. Patients with a lymphocytic BAL pattern have usually developed the condition within a shorter period of time.[179] Otherwise, there is no clear relation between the BAL cell pattern and the outcome of amiodarone pneumonitis, in particular in terms of risk of developing pulmonary fibrosis.[186]

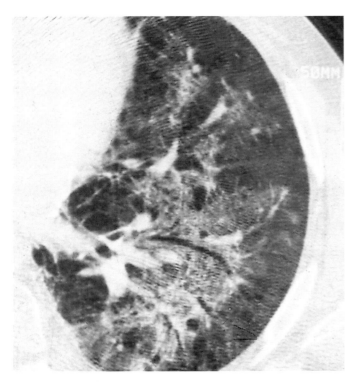

Fig. 29.15 The computed tomography scan in amiodarone pneumonitis usually shows opacities with no segmental or lobar distribution.

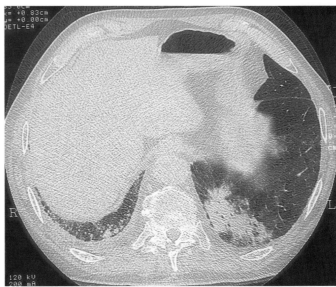

Fig. 29.17 The finding of contralateral minor foci of shadowing is helpful for diagnosis of amiodarone pneumonitis (same patient as in Figs 29.12 and 29.16).

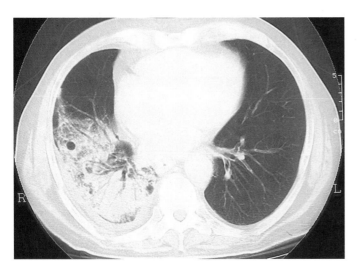

Fig. 29.16 Lobar consolidation corresponding to amiodarone pneumonitis. Like other forms of amiodarone pneumonitis, such foci show little change on serial chest radiographs, apart from when steroids are given (same patient as in Figs 29.12 and 29.17).

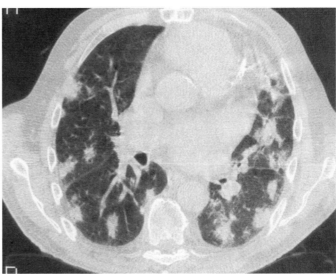

Fig. 29.18 Occasional patients with amiodarone pneumonitis show multiple 'shaggy' nodules on computed tomography.

Since withdrawing amiodarone may expose the patient to fatal recurrence of arrhythmias, careful differential diagnosis is crucial. Left ventricular failure usually shows a different radiographic picture and will usually respond to diuretic treatment. Echocardiography and, possibly, measurement of pulmonary capillary wedge pressure may be required in selected cases, in order to differentiate cardiac failure from amiodarone pneu-

monitis. Measurement of CO factor, which may be more severely impaired in amiodarone pneumonitis than in left heart failure, and gallium-67 scanning may help in difficult cases.[187] The distinction between pulmonary infarction and amiodarone pneumonitis may also be difficult, because a lung perfusion scan will show a reduction of perfusion in the areas of amiodarone pneumonitis. A single report warned that pulmonary angiography might be dangerous in patients on amiodarone[188] but no further reports have appeared, in particular about use of contrast-enhanced CT.

In difficult cases, e.g. when valve replacement or heart transplantation is planned, histological examination of the lung may be

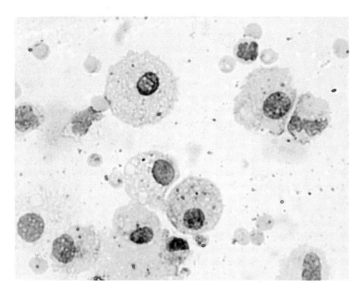

Fig. 29.19 In amiodarone pulmonary toxicity, bronchoalveolar lavage fluid often shows numerous phospholipid-laden macrophages, presumably of alveolar origin (see also Fig. 29.20a).

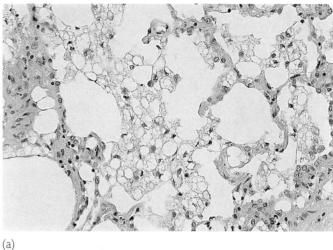

(a)

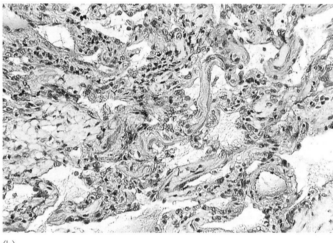

(b)

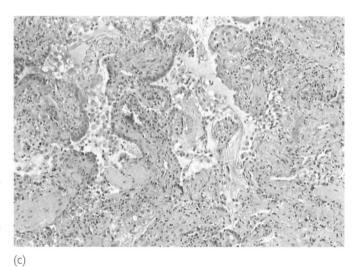

(c)

required to confirm the diagnosis, to rule out alternative diagnoses such as bronchioloalveolar carcinoma or pulmonary lymphoma, and to monitor amiodarone treatment appropriately. Histopathology shows a combination of changes that, collectively, are very suggestive of amiodarone pneumonitis.[189-191] These include the presence of packed, foamy, lipid-laden macrophages within the alveolar spaces (Fig. 29.20a), lipid infiltration of endothelial and type II cells, reflecting a generalised disturbance of pulmonary phospholipid turnover (Fig. 29.20b), septal thickening by an infiltrate of mononuclear cells (Fig. 29.20A & B), and some interstitial fibrosis (Fig. 29.20b). In a small proportion of patients (about 10%), extensive fibrosis is present in the form of dense fibrotic areas on chest radiograph, CT scanning (Fig. 29.21), and at histology (Fig. 29.20c). In a few cases, organising pneumonia is found, in the form of numerous buds of connective tissue within distal airspaces[184] (see below).

The outcome of amiodarone pneumonitis is favourable in approximately 80% of cases. Resolution of symptoms and radiographic opacities is usually slow and may take months to complete. The mortality rate is about 10–15%, with early deaths resulting from uncontrollable, steroid-resistant respiratory failure in fragile patients, pulmonary fibrosis, recurrence of ventricular dysrhythmias or sudden cardiac death. Late deaths are related to progressive pulmonary fibrosis and to complications of long-term steroids. Sequelae in the form of radiographic abnormalities and/or persistent impairment of lung function, CO transfer or gas exchange remain in a sizeable proportion of patients.

Once the diagnosis of amiodarone pneumonitis is established, steroids are recommended, in an attempt to hasten recovery and, presumably, to diminish the likelihood of developing pulmonary fibrosis. In our experience (and in contrast to other drugs), persistent amiodarone pneumonitis appears to carry a significant risk of irreversible pulmonary fibrosis. After some time, it may be necessary to increase the dose of steroids, should

Fig. 29.20 Histopathological appearances in amiodarone pneumonitis, with (a) the pattern of phospholipid-laden macrophages in alveolar spaces and slight interstitial thickening, (b) the commonest pattern of moderate pulmonary fibrosis with lipid-laden cells within alveolar spaces, and (c) extensive irreversible pulmonary fibrosis.

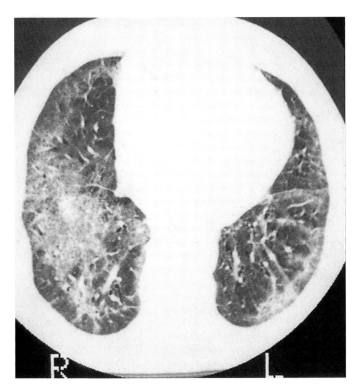

Fig. 29.21 In a small proportion of patients with amiodarone pneumonitis, pulmonary opacities may persist indefinitely, despite drug withdrawal and steroid treatment. These foci correspond to irreversible amiodarone-induced fibrosis. (The corresponding histopathology in this patient is shown in Fig. 29.20c.)

clinical and imaging features of amiodarone pneumonitis fail to show a definite response to the usual doses, e.g. 0.75 mg/kg of prednisolone or equivalent. Steroids are generally required for 6 months to 1 year, in tapering dosage, to avoid recurrences related to the prolonged retention of amiodarone in the lung.[192–194] Prolonged treatment with steroids requires careful follow-up, in order to detect adverse effects. Severe opportunistic infections can develop in patients treated with steroids long-term.

If patients were rechallenged with amiodarone, recurrence of the pneumonitis would ensue in the great majority and the time to the second episode would be shorter.[179] In patients who are in great need of amiodarone for arrhythmias, a compromise may be achieved by reducing (e.g. halving) the dose of amiodarone, at the same time treating with moderate doses of oral steroids (0.5 mg/kg, decreasing subsequently). This may enable both the resolution of the pulmonary opacities and continuation of the drug.

Patients taking amiodarone who undergo coronary bypass grafting may develop extensive postoperative bilateral radiographic opacities culminating in ARDS.[195] High perioperative concentrations of oxygen may act as a precipitating factor. The histological appearance is that of acute interstitial pneumonia, ± diffuse alveolar damage superimposed on the baseline histopathological features of amiodarone pneumonitis. The prognosis is poor.[196]

Drug-induced organising pneumonia

Organising pneumonia (otherwise bronchiolitis obliterans organising pneumonia, BOOP), is a pattern of lung response seen with a limited number of drugs, mainly amiodarone,[184,185] beta-blockers,[197] bleomycin,[198–200] gold,[201] interferons,[6,202] mesalazine,[92] nitrofurantoin,[203] statins,[204] sulfasalazine[92] and following radiation therapy for breast cancer in women.[205,206]

The clinical picture is usually of progressive breathlessness with cough and moderate fever. Physical examination may show crackles or a friction rub, or may remain normal. Clinical–radiographic patterns are manifold. The most typical is of migratory infiltrates evolving in a manner not dissimilar from that of idiopathic BOOP (Fig. 29.22), occasionally associated with intense chest pain. Intervening periods of progressive clearing or of complete radiographic resolution may separate exacerbations of pulmonary opacities. In the presence of this pattern, and now that these clinical imaging features are well-known, a lung biopsy is not systematically performed, and drug withdrawal is attempted. If steroids are given and the drug-related aetiology is not recognised, infiltrates may recur at relatively high steroid doses in the face of continuing use of the causative drug.

Other patterns include diffuse organising pneumonia (Fig. 29.23), 'white lungs' with attendant respiratory failure,[207] non-migratory infiltrates, solitary masses and pseudometastatic nodules (e.g. in patients exposed to amiodarone, bleomycin or minocycline;[208–210] Fig. 29.24). The latter pattern of multiple rounded opacities may simulate pulmonary metastases. However, the opacities will usually resolve slowly upon cessation of bleomycin, leaving inert residual fibrotic foci or no trace at all of their earlier presence. In patients having received bleomycin, a lung biopsy may be required for definitive exclusion of neoplastic nodules.[211]

Of note, the inflammatory-bowel-disease (IBD)-modifying drugs mesalazine and salicylazosulfapyridine can elicit organising pneumonia but the same condition can also occur in the untreated course of IBD.[92] It may thus be difficult to delineate the role of drugs as opposed to the underlying disease. Prudent continuation of the drug in a lower dose, or stepwise rechallenge if the drug was withdrawn initially, may be considered, to evaluate the role of the drug as opposed to the underlying IBD.

On histology, buds of connective tissue are present within distal air passages and alveoli (Fig. 29.25a), with the shape of bludgeons or butterflies.[184] Nodular organising pneumonia from bleomycin shows a distinctive histopathological stellar pattern (Fig. 29.25b). Buds, as a prominent histological pattern, should be distinguished from the occasional buds found on histology of classic interstitial pneumonitis or of eosinophilic pneumonia, which can be misleading on a small transbronchial lung biopsy specimen, on which a bud can appear prominently.

The prognosis of drug-induced organising pneumonia is favourable in many cases. Steroids seem to promote improvement, as with organising pneumonia from other causes (see Chapter 42). Steroids are required in patients with severe involvement or relapsing episodes. The duration of treatment depends on the causative drug: a few weeks will be sufficient in

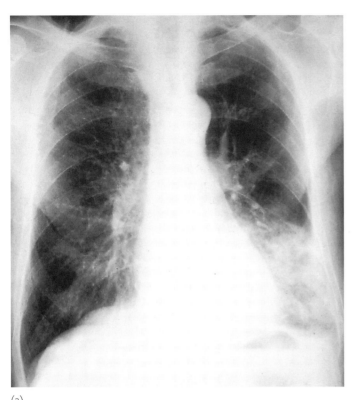

(a)

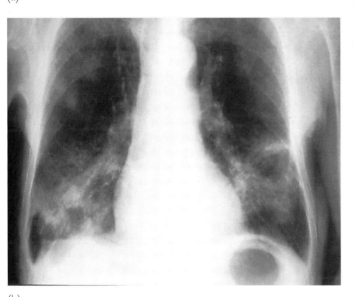

(b)

Fig. 29.22 Drug-induced organising pneumonia: sequential chest radiographs taken several weeks apart in a patient with organising pneumonia (BOOP) linked to treatment with amiodarone. Wandering opacities were noted for 18 months before the amiodarone was eventually withdrawn, following which no further opacities developed. (Courtesy of Prof. P. Pfitzenmeyer.)

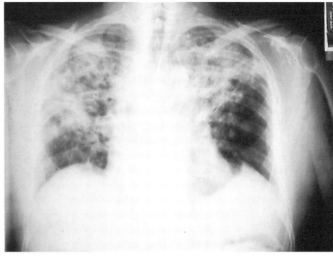

Fig. 29.23 Drug-induced organising pneumonia: chest radiograph showing bilateral fixed and patchy infiltrates 1 month after initiation of nilutamide. Organising pneumonia was evidenced on transbronchial lung biopsy. Drug discontinuation and steroids led to complete clearing of the opacities. (With permission from Pfitzenmeyer et al 1992.[59])

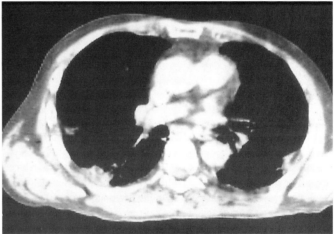

Fig. 29.24 Computed tomography scan of nodular organising pneumonia caused by bleomycin. Pleural-based or parenchymal nodules represent one very distinctive pattern of lung injury by bleomycin. The differential diagnosis may include pulmonary metastases. (Courtesy of Professor P. Romanet.)

most cases due to drugs other than amiodarone. With amiodarone, steroids should be given for several months, in order to avoid recurrences. Unfortunately, in a few cases (especially patients with rheumatoid arthritis receiving disease-modifying drugs), the condition goes out of control despite steroids or immunosuppressives.[207]

Pulmonary fibrosis – 'chemotherapy lung'

'Drug-induced pulmonary fibrosis' (see also Pulmonary complications of radiation therapy, below) is most often due to prolonged treatment with chemotherapeutic agents (busulfan, bleomycin, cyclophosphamide, nitrosoureas),[29,51,56,212,213] amiodarone[79,214,215] and, less commonly, nitrofurantoin,[216] gold[217,218] or sulfasalazine.[219]

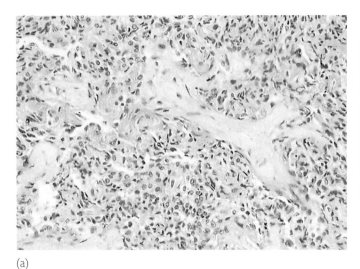

(a)

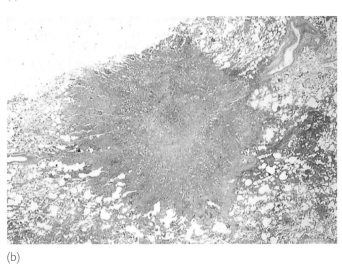

(b)

Fig. 29.25 (a) Histopathological appearances of drug-induced organising pneumonia showing obliteration of distal airspaces (bronchioles, alveolar ducts, alveoli) by buds of young connective tissue (video-assisted lung biopsy).[184] (Courtesy of Professor F. Piard.) (b) Histopathological appearances of nodular organising pneumonia from bleomycin. A low-power view shows a stellate focus of organising pneumonia. The lung parenchyma at the periphery of the nodule remains little affected. (Courtesy of Dr B. Coudert and Professor F. Piard.)

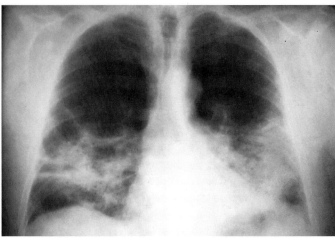

Fig. 29.26 Chest radiograph in drug (busulphan)-induced pulmonary fibrosis. Interstitial, sometimes confluent opacities tend to localise at the bases but may be diffuse. (Courtesy of Professor R. Putelat.)

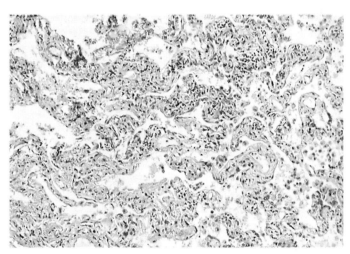

Fig. 29.27 Lung section showing drug-induced pulmonary fibrosis. Regardless of the causative drug, the interstitium appears thickened by bland, paucicellular fibrosis. Large, atypical type II pneumocytes (not present in this section) are classically associated with fibrosis from chemotherapeutic agents or radiation therapy. (Courtesy of Professor F. Piard.)

The onset is progressive over months, with dyspnoea, cough, low-grade fever and weight loss. Finger clubbing is inconstant.

The chest radiograph shows patchy alveolar and interstitial shadowing, which tend to have a bibasal distribution (Fig. 29.26). Later, or terminally, opacities tend to involve the lungs diffusely. On CT, there are areas of ground-glass attenuation, along with interstitial opacities. Honeycombing is infrequently observed.[212,220]

Pulmonary function shows a restrictive ventilatory defect, often with severe hypoxaemia.

The BAL usually shows neutrophilia and occasionally mild lymphocytosis, along with dysplastic type II pneumocytes,[51] a feature suggestive of chemotherapy lung or radiation-induced pulmonary damage (see below), among other causes.[221,222]

Histological appearances show a combination of bland fibrosis, loose and sparse mononuclear interstitial infiltrate, interstitial pulmonary oedema, alveolar filling by proteinaceous exudate or by alveolar macrophages, and lining with hyaline membranes and bizarre dysplastic alveolar type II cells (Fig. 29.27). A proteinosis-like pattern has been described in some patients taking busulfan.[223]

The overall prognosis of drug-induced pulmonary fibrosis resembles that of fibrosis from other causes. The condition of some patients will apparently stabilise on treatment with steroids, while others progress to terminal respiratory failure within months, in spite of withdrawal of the offending drug and addition of steroids or immunosuppressives.[156,224,225] The fibrotic lungs are prone to infection, which requires prompt recognition and treatment to avoid significant and sometimes irreversible deterioration of lung function. A few cases of drug-induced lung fibrosis have come to successful lung transplantation.

A peculiar form of pulmonary fibrosis developing after sequential cytotoxic chemotherapy has merited the name 'chemotherapy lung', or '(delayed) pulmonary toxicity syndrome'.[49,51] The syndrome is seen mostly following long-term cytotoxic chemotherapy for breast cancer, or after conditioning regimens for bone-marrow transplantation. The term 'chemotherapy lung' includes interstitial pneumonitis and fibrosis, along with diffuse alveolar damage of variable severity and vascular changes. Many combinations of chemotherapeutic agents have been reported to cause the syndrome, the most frequently implicated being bleomycin, cyclophosphamide, melphalan, mitomycin, nitrosoureas, and also radiation therapy or total body irradiation.[29,49,51,70,212,213,226] The possible aetiological role of 5-fluorouracil, platinum salts, vindesine and doxorubicin is questionable.[227] Newer drugs such as docetaxel and gemcitabine can also cause the syndrome.[56,72,228,229] It is important to look for such possible triggering factors as infection, exposure to high concentrations of oxygen, administration of CSFs or radiotherapy. The pattern of radiographic involvement tends to be bibasal or diffuse (see Fig. 29.26). Response to steroids is, as in other forms of fibrosis, difficult to predict but some patients will respond favourably to these agents, at least temporarily.

Miscellaneous infiltrative lung disease

Nitrofurantoin seems the only drug reported capable of reproducing the histopathological pattern of desquamative interstitial pneumonia.[230] Distinctive features include bilateral opacities (Fig. 29.28) and a rather sharply demarcated mosaic

pattern on CT (Fig. 29.29). On histology (Fig. 29.30), there is extensive alveolar filling by alveolar macrophages, along with mild or moderate fibrosis of the alveolar walls and interstitium. Prognosis is favourable upon withdrawal of nitrofurantoin and institution of steroids, but fibrotic sequelae are possible.

Mineral oils used as laxative agents in the elderly or debilitated, as well as nose or throat drugs in a lipid vehicle, may spread into the bronchial tree and lung, or be aspirated, especially during the night. This leads to typical basal opacities seen on the chest radiograph and CT (Fig. 29.31). The clinical pattern ranges from radiographic opacities with slight impact on lung functions to acute respiratory failure.[231,232] Often, the

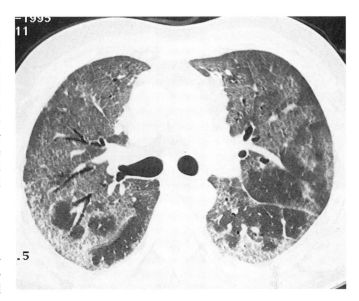

Fig. 29.29 A sharply demarcated pattern of involvement is a CT feature of desquamative interstitial pneumonia. (Same patient as in Figs 29.28 and 29.30.)

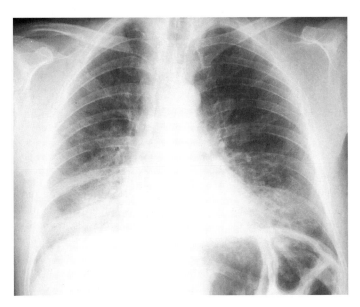

Fig. 29.28 Drug (nitrofurantoin)-induced desquamative interstitial pneumonia (corresponding lung section shown in Fig. 29.30). (Courtesy of Dr D. Lacroix.)

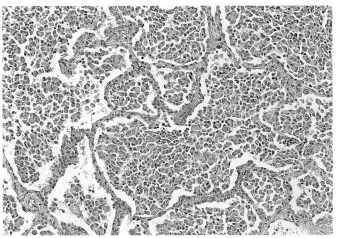

Fig. 29.30 Histopathological appearances of desquamative interstitial pneumonia, with the characteristic accumulation of macrophages in the alveolar lumena. The interstitium shows mild fibrotic changes. (Courtesy of Professor F. Piard.)

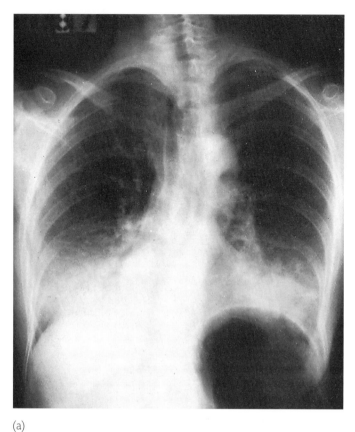

(a)

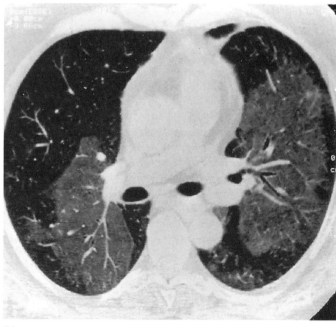

(b)

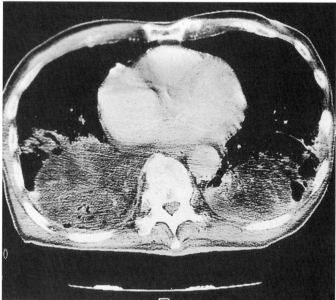

(c)

Fig. 29.31 (a) Chest radiograph in a patient with mineral oil (paraffin) pneumonia showing bibasal localisation. (b) & (c) Typical computed tomography appearances of exogenous lipoid pneumonia, showing non-segmental, mosaic-shaped alveolar shadows (b) and bibasal shadows of lipid density (c). (Courtesy of Professor J. C. Dalphin.) For further imaging data, see Gondouin et al 1996.[232]

chronic intake of oils is overlooked on history taking, and patients may undergo unnecessary biopsy. Opacities of lipid density may be seen on CT or magnetic resonance imaging[232,233] (Fig. 29.31b & c). Spontaneous visualisation of the pulmonary vasculature has also been described with unenhanced CT.[234]

Examination of sputum or BAL is useful, as it shows macrophages typically laden with mineral lipid droplets which stain positive with Sudan black or oil red O.[232,235] These droplets differ, morphologically and on lipid stains, from those seen in the BAL of patients with amiodarone pneumonitis. The diagnosis may also be confirmed by chromatography of BAL fluid on silica plates, where paraffin can be identified.[236] Lung biopsy is not required but would show alveolar filling by oil and lipid-laden macrophages.[232] Steroids seem to offer little benefit and the consolidative foci tend to persist for prolonged periods. Some patients may develop irreversible lung fibrosis, mycobacterial superinfection or malignancy.[232]

Several drugs have been reported to cause 'transient pulmonary infiltrates', which are benign pulmonary opacities of uncertain histological nature (possibly mild pulmonary oedema or transient angiitis; Fig. 29.32). Nitrofurantoin, hydrochlorothiazide, novel anticancer agents, CSFs and anti-thymocyte globulin have been cited.[4,8,237–243] The prognosis is favourable but recurrence is likely on resumption of the drug.

Drug-induced pulmonary oedema

Criteria for the diagnosis of drug-induced pulmonary oedema include a close temporal relation between drug administration and the onset of symptoms (which generally develop shortly (minutes to hours) following the administration of the drug), intake of a compatible drug and consistent imaging features. In one study, the average time between the administration of hydrochlorothiazide (Fig. 29.32) and onset of respiratory symptoms was 44 minutes.[244]

A relation to the dose received has been reported for cytosine arabinoside and neuroleptics. Indeed, pulmonary oedema with or without ARDS is a well-known complication of overdoses of opiate or tricyclic antidepressants in attempted suicide.[245]

Pulmonary oedema is also a classical complication of heroin addiction or overdose.[246] Historically, episodes of pulmonary oedema were reported in psychotic patients deliberately submitted to insulin-induced hypoglycaemia.[247]

Among the drugs used in clinical practice that can generate pulmonary oedema are:

- β_2-agonists in parturients[57,248]
- hydrochlorothiazide[78,249]
- transfusions of blood (especially from multiparous women)[12,250] or of blood fractions (the 'TRALI' syndrome)
- salicylate[251–253]
- opiates[254]
- vinorelbine.[255,256]

Other relevant causes include desferrioxamine, contrast media, naloxone, cytosine arabinoside, methotrexate, streptokinase and prostacyclin.[257] Occasional reports have also cited anti-thymocyte globulin,[258] intravenous immunoglobulins[7] and cytokines.[10,259,260] Also, local anaesthesia, ophthalmological and neurological surgery may lead to pulmonary oedema (see below).[261]

Clinically, respiratory distress develops rapidly, with cough, often productive of pink and frothy sputum, and crackles and wheezes on auscultation. The chest radiograph shows bilateral alveolar opacities (Fig. 29.33). Some cases of pulmonary oedema may be difficult to differentiate clinically from rapid-onset hypersensitivity pneumonitis, or from acute interstitial pneumonia, but evidence of pulmonary congestion such as enlarged lobular septae, thickened minor/major fissures or pleural effusion, which are absent in interstitial lung disease, helps to distinguish the two conditions.

Drug-induced pulmonary oedema is generally non-cardiogenic in nature, as pulmonary capillary wedge pressure and

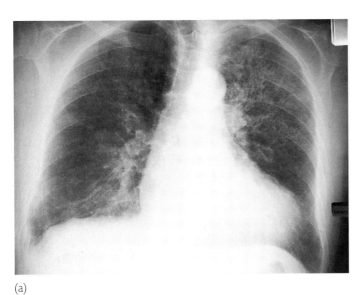

(a)

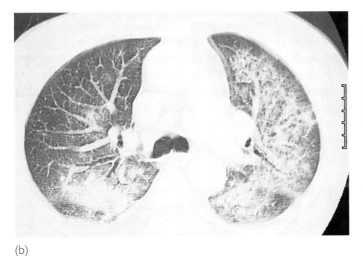

(b)

Fig. 29.32 Chest radiograph taken at admission (a) and computed tomography scan (b) of a patient with acute respiratory distress due to exposure to hydrochlorothiazide. Oral intake of the drug was closely followed (within minutes) by respiratory distress and fever. A similar episode had occurred 6 months earlier but was missed at history taking. No advice had been given on avoidance of the drug. (Courtesy of Dr D. Kandhouche.)

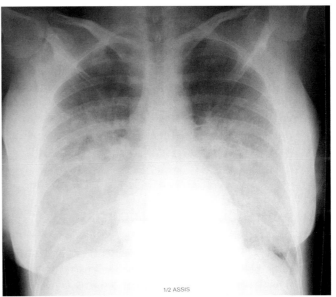

Fig. 29.33 Extensive bilateral alveolar shadowing developing shortly *post-partum* in a young woman exposed to intravenous beta-agonists to retard labour.

echocardiography are normal. Histological evidence is rarely obtained but, when it is, it shows a combination of alveolar flooding by proteinaceous fluid and occasional hyaline membranes or haemorrhage, while the interstitium appears little affected. Late cases with unfavourable outcome may show a histological picture similar to that of ARDS, with inflammation, atelectasis and fibrosis. In most cases, however, the prognosis is favourable, with symptoms and radiographic opacities resolving within a few hours or days in mild cases; the minority of more severe cases progress to respiratory failure,[57] irreversible ARDS,[253] with definite mortality.[262]

Drug-induced alveolar haemorrhage

Some degree of 'non-specific' alveolar haemorrhage may accompany severe cases of interstitial pneumonitis (e.g. due to nitrofurantoin or gold).[263,264] Most commonly, alveolar haemorrhage results from exposure to oral anticoagulants and the risk does not correlate well with the prothrombin level or the INR.[265] Oral anticoagulants lead to other haemorrhagic problems in the chest (see 'Miscellaneous adverse effects of drugs and related substances', below). Fibrinolytics, even when administered locally, can also induce alveolar haemorrhage.[266,267] Pulmonary haemorrhage may also complicate drug-induced hepatic failure or thrombocytopenia.[268]

Penicillamine has been associated with the development of a Goodpasture-like syndrome.[269] Patients on rather high doses of the drug presented with diffuse alveolar haemorrhage and renal failure. Antiglomerular basement membrane antibodies were lacking. Immunosuppression and plasmapheresis have been shown to improve prognosis.[270] The drug is much less used nowadays.

Cases of alveolar haemorrhage with pulmonary angiitis, lung nodules and p-ANCA, have been reported as a complication of the anti-thyroid drug propylthiouracil.[271-274] Diffuse alveolar haemorrhage has also been reported with the use of valproate,[275] and recently following hepatitis B immunisation.[13]

Patients present with shortness of breath, and haemoptysis is not always a feature, even if massive alveolar bleeding has occurred. Typically, the chest radiograph shows a 'bat's wing', 'butterfly'[270] or diffuse distribution of alveolar shadowing.[276] The BAL fluid is stained with blood and contains iron-stainable macrophages. Resolution usually follows withdrawal of the causative drug but early diagnosis is encouraged to avoid diffuse irreversible coagulation in the alveolar spaces and end-stage lung.

Drug-induced bronchiolitis obliterans

Bronchiolitis obliterans has been associated particularly with penicillamine treatment of rheumatoid arthritis in women.[277] More rarely, chrysotherapy was thought to be causative.[278] Bronchiolitis obliterans has also been reported after bone marrow[279] and lung transplantation[280] and, in rare instances, following blood-transfusion-induced microchimerism.[25]

Rapidly progressive and, most often, irreversible airflow obstruction develops in a few months, with forced expiratory volume in 1 second usually less than 1 litre. The chest radiograph and CT scan may remain normal or show a discrete mosaic pattern. Although lung biopsy is not necessary to the diagnosis, which is strongly suggested by the results of pulmonary function tests, histology would show diffuse narrowing of small airways by endoluminal plugs of granulation tissue or by fibrotic and concentric narrowing of airway walls.[281] In bronchiolitis obliterans induced by the dietary supplement *Sauropus androgynus* in Taiwan, associated necrosis of bronchiolar walls has also been reported.[15,282]

There is almost no improvement of the airflow obstruction following administration of bronchodilators or steroids. Although most cases of iatrogenic bronchiolitis obliterans are irreversible, early diagnosis and withdrawal of the drug,[283] or augmented immunosuppression in transplantees,[280] has been followed by stabilisation or improvement in some cases. Lung transplantation has sometimes been required in patients with *Sauropus*-induced bronchiolitis obliterans.[284]

Drug-induced pleural disease

In addition to non-specific pleural effusions, which may accompany classic drug-induced pneumonitides (e.g. amiodarone pneumonitis), specific pleural disease has been attributed to drugs.

■ A group of drugs is well-known to induce the lupus syndrome (e.g. ACE inhibitors, α-methyldopa, beta-blockers, captopril, hydralazine, isoniazid, procainamide, quinidine, sulfasalazine, to mention but a few[285]). The drug-induced lupus syndrome is characterised by constitutional symptoms (arthralgias, fever), along with pleural and/or pericardial effusion or constriction (Fig. 29.34), which may

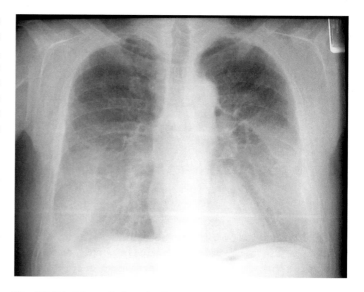

Fig. 29.34 Bilateral pleural effusions in drug-induced lupus erythematosus. Positive antinuclear antibodies and slow resolution on cessation of the drug are typical.

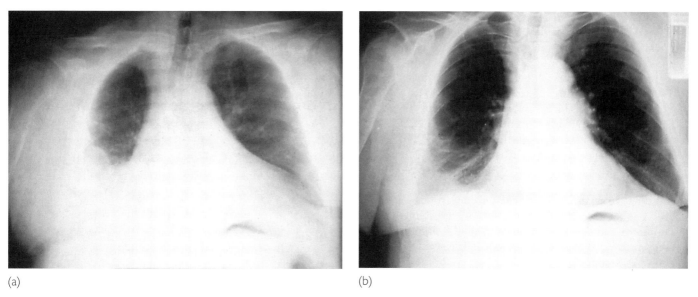

(a)   (b)

Fig. 29.35 (a) Chest radiograph showing pleuropericardial effusion and thickening in a patient treated long-term with an ergot drug. (b) Cessation of exposure to the drug was followed by slow and incomplete resolution. Four years elapsed between (a) and (b).

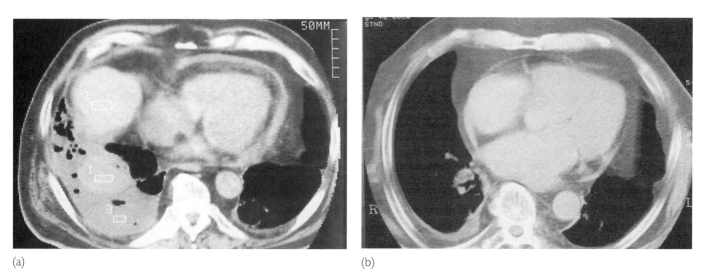

(a)   (b)

Fig. 29.36 Computed tomography scans of the patient shown in Figure 29.35, demonstrating (a) pleuropericardial thickening/effusion and (b) incomplete resolution with time (four years).

be the presenting and most prominent features. Pleural effusion may mimic empyema. Parenchymal pulmonary manifestations are less common and range from discrete infiltrates to ARDS.[286] Antinuclear and antihistone antibodies are typically found in serum, whereas anti-DNA antibodies are rare. Moderate eosinophilia may be an associated feature.[287] Antibody levels tend to diminish or disappear a few weeks or months after drug withdrawal. A few cases of the drug-induced lupus syndrome have been complicated by pulmonary thromboembolism.[288,289]

■ Exudative pleural effusions/thickening without other features of drug-induced lupus have been reported following the use of the ergot-like drugs: bromocriptine, cabergoline,

ergotamine, dihydroergotamine, lisuride, methysergide, pergolide and dopamine agonists (Fig. 29.35).[290] Patients develop slowly progressive dyspnoea and chest tightness, along with an elevated erythrocyte sedimentation rate. Bilateral pleural thickening and/or effusions are visible on the chest radiograph and on CT (Fig. 29.36). Pleural thickening and subpleural areas of rounded parenchymal atelectasis,[59] along with pericardial thickening/effusion, are better seen on CT scanning (Fig. 29.36). The differential diagnosis includes asbestos-related pleural disease, which produces similar radiographic and CT appearances, although calcification is not usually seen in the drug-related condition. Asbestos seems to be a promoting factor, as ergot-induced pleural disease was found to be more prevalent in persons previously exposed to asbestos.[67] There is whitish pleural thickening at thoracoscopy, and histology shows bland pleural fibrosis with little or no cellular infiltrate.[290] This adverse effect improves following discontinuation of the drug (Figs 29.35 & 29.36 (a) vs. (b)). Systemic symptoms clear rapidly but the pleural lesions take months or years to recover and some pleural thickening usually persists indefinitely (Figs 29.35b and 29.36b).[290]

- A few compounds such as dantrolene,[291] propylthiouracil[292] and sulfasalazine[293] have been reported to cause eosinophilic pleural effusion.
- A distinctive syndrome of generalised congestion, pleural effusions and sometimes ascites, along with systemic symptoms, can develop in women of child-bearing age receiving ovarian hyperstimulation.[58,294] The syndrome is known as 'the ovarian hyperstimulation syndrome' and ARDS may follow in some instances.
- A few patients receiving high-dose methotrexate have been reported to develop intense chest pain due to pleuritis.[295]
- Medial or lateral chest pain has been reported after sclerotherapy of oesophageal or gastric varices.[296] This corresponds to mediastinal or pleural irritation following the procedure.

Drug-induced pulmonary vascular disorders

(See also Adverse pulmonary effects of illicit drug use, below.)

Drug-induced pulmonary hypertension (PHT)

Apart from PHT due to illicit intravenous injection of pills intended for oral use, drug-induced PHT is similar in symptoms and course to primary PHT.[43] The onset is usually gradual, with dyspnoea and occasionally substernal chest pain on exertion. There is progressive enlargement of pulmonary arteries on the chest radiograph and ultimately right heart failure may develop. A perfusion lung scan does not show clearly defined perfusion defects.

Drugs reported to cause PHT include anorectic agents and, less often, contraceptive pills. The first causative agent identified was the anorectic drug aminorex,[297] which has not been generally available since the early 1970s, except following private synthesis.[298] Pulmonary hypertension has also been reported with use of the newer anorectics fenfluramine and dexfenfluramine,[299,300] and PHT appears to be a class effect of the anorectic agents. These drugs have now been recalled. Anecdotal reports of PHT following treatments with phendimetrazine, phenformin and L-tryptophan have also been published.[4]

Most cases of PHT induced by anorectics behave like primary PHT, with intractable right heart failure, and death in many cases. Although pulmonary vasodilators, including prostacyclin, may offer transient benefit in some cases, transplantation appears to be the only effective long-term treatment.[43] Very few reports have shown that anorectic-induced PHT can regress following discontinuation of the drug, with recurrence following rechallenge.

A few cases of sudden, catastrophic pulmonary hypertension associated with systemic hypotension have been reported following infusion of protamine to reverse heparin anticoagulation.[301]

The drug-induced haemolytic–uraemic (thrombotic microangiopathic) syndrome

Mitomycin and, less often, cis-platinum or combination therapy for cancer, lymphoma or leukaemia, are known to induce the syndrome of thrombocytopenia, haemolytic anaemia, renal failure and sometimes alveolar haemorrhage known as haemolytic–uraemic syndrome.[302–305] The syndrome resembles the idiopathic form of the haemolytic–uraemic syndrome.

Patients present with a combination of bilateral lung infiltrates,[306] pulmonary hypertension and sometimes alveolar haemorrhage,[307] with respiratory and renal failure requiring support. Schizocytes and helmet cells typical of microangiopathic haemolysis are present in the peripheral blood. Transfusion of red blood cells may exacerbate the syndrome and should be avoided as much as possible. On histological investigation, fibrin thrombi are present within the pulmonary and renal vessels. Of note, the syndrome can develop at any time during treatment with mitomycin and up to several months after termination of treatment.[308]

The syndrome has recently been described in a patient receiving the immunosuppressant tacrolimus.[309]

Drug-induced pulmonary veno-occlusive disease

Pulmonary veno-occlusive disease is rare but may be under-recognised. It results from the generalised development of organised thrombi and endoluminal fibrosis in pulmonary venules. Pulmonary veno-occlusive disease has been reported mainly in patients treated months to years previously for various solid tumours or haematological malignancies with chemotherapeutic agents such as carmustine (BCNU), bleomycin, mitomycin and vinca alkaloids, radiotherapy or bone-marrow transplantation.[310–314]

The disease is difficult to diagnose in life. Patients present with progressive dyspnoea and ill-defined interstitial radiographic infiltrates with Kerley B lines. The picture evolves towards refractory postcapillary pulmonary hypertension and right-sided heart failure. Of note, pulmonary veno-occlusive disease has been described in Hodgkin's disease treated with radiotherapy only, in untreated Hodgkin's disease and following bone-marrow transplantation. At this time, the responsibility of drugs remains unclear in many cases.[315]

Drug-induced pulmonary embolism

Patients present with dyspnoea of recent onset. Typical findings on perfusion scanning, angiography or contrast-enhanced CT may be absent if emboli are discrete.

In addition to the classic causative contraceptive pills and oestrogens,[316,317] other causative drugs include clozapine,[318] desferrioxamine,[319] L-asparaginase,[320] intravenous immunoglobulin;[321]

intravenous lipids,[322] *trans*-retinoic acid,[323] fibrinolytic therapy for venous thrombosis[324] and illicit drugs.[325]

In addition to drugs, procedures such as the occlusion of oesophageal varices,[326,327] sclerotherapy of leg varices, intra-articular injections,[328] endovascular obliteration of brain vascular malformations or fistulae,[329] orthopaedic surgery[330] and liposuction[331] can cause pulmonary embolism (Table 29.2).

A few cases of the drug-induced lupus syndrome with circulating lupus anticoagulant and pulmonary thromboembolism have been reported.[288] The clue to diagnosis is the intake of a lupus-inducing drug (procainamide and chlorpromazine have been the only drugs implicated to date), along with the presence of antinuclear or anticardiolipin antibodies in blood.

Drug-induced angiitis

Propylthiouracil has been shown to induce a picture of pulmonary angiitis, with round or cavitating lung nodules, accompanied by circulating cANCA of myeloperoxidase specificity.[274,350] Alveolar haemorrhage or ARDS may be associated features.

In anecdotal reports, exposure to macrolide antibiotics, carbamazepine and aspirin, or vaccination against hepatitis B has been associated with development of the Churg–Strauss syndrome[351-354] (Fig. 29.37a & b)

More recently, cases with eosinophilic pneumonia with constitutional symptoms, evidence of angiitis and possible extrapulmonary (heart) involvement, also Churg–Strauss syndrome,

have been reported following the use of the newer leukotriene-antagonist drugs.[172,355-357] Although initially thought due to the tapering of steroids concomitant with the initiation of these drugs, the Churg–Strauss syndrome can develop after treatment with antileukotrienes alone.[172]

Miscellaneous iatrogenic disease of the pulmonary circulation

Increased cell trafficking may plug the pulmonary microcirculation, and this has emerged as a novel iatrogenic pulmonary vascular complication:

■ Colony stimulating factors may promote plugging by young neutrophils, resulting in pulmonary infiltrates or oedema[9]
■ trans-retinoic acid may promote plugging by myelomonocytic cells, resulting in pulmonary oedema or ARDS[358-361]
■ the first course of chemotherapy for leukaemias with high circulating cell counts can be complicated by lung damage resulting from the lysis of malignant cells within the pulmonary circulation; ARDS may ensue[362,363] as well as multiple organ dysfunction[363]
■ recently, a new pulmonary complication of haemopoietic stem cell transplantation has been reported. Patients presented 2–3 months post-transplantation with fever and

Table 29.2 Respiratory complications of procedures, and non-pharmaceutical agents.

Causative procedure	Clinical pattern	References
Blood and derivatives	Pulmonary oedema ('TRALI' syndrome)	11
Catheters, pacemakers	Pneumothorax, pulmonary infection, pulmonary embolism, pulmonary air embolism, loss or fragmentation of catheter, valve damage, endocarditis, aneurysms and fistulae	332–334
Assisted ventilation, CPAP	Pneumothorax, pneumomediastinum, pneumopericardium, upper airway obstruction, negative pressure pulmonary oedema	335, 336
Pulmonary function testing	Pneumothorax	337
Pleural drainage	Reexpansion pulmonary oedema	338
Transoesophageal echocardiography	Oesophageal rupture and mediastinitis	339
Acupuncture	Pneumothorax, haemothorax, haemopericardium	22, 340
Coronary bypass surgery	Persistent pleural effusions, diaphragmatic palsy	341
Oesophageal/gastric variceal sclerotherapy	Pleuritic chest pain, mediastinitis, pulmonary embolism	296, 342, 343
Distant interventional radiology	Pulmonary embolism	20
Local anaesthesia	Pulmonary oedema	39, 344
Insertion of transjugular portosystemic shunt	Pulmonary oedema	345
Intravesical therapy for cancer	Pulmonary embolism, interstitial pneumonitis and fibrosis, mycobacterial disemination infection	40, 346, 347
Orthopaedic surgery	Bronchospasm, pulmonary embolism of methacrylate cement	330, 348
Haemodialysis (chronic)	Diffuse pulmonary calcinosis	349

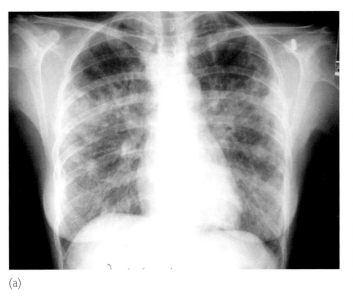

(a)

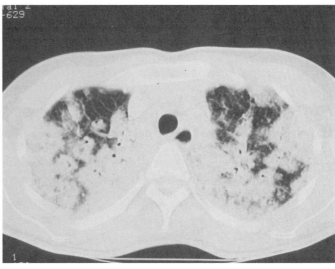

(b)

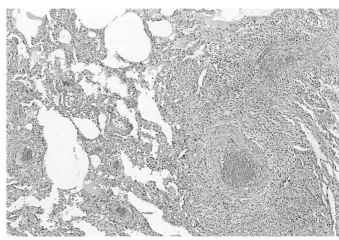

(c)

Fig. 29.37 Diffuse alveolar opacities (a), some being angiocentric (b), which, together with respiratory failure and extensive cutaneous rash, developed a few days after starting treatment with penicillin. Lung biopsy (c) showed eosinophilic angiitis (Churg–Strauss syndrome). (Courtesy of Dr d'Arlhac.)

pulmonary nodules on chest imaging that corresponded to pulmonary cytolytic thrombi.[364,365] Biopsy of the pulmonary nodules showed necrotic, basophilic thromboemboli with amorphous material suggestive of cellular breakdown products. Immunohistochemistry showed entrapped leukocytes and disrupted endothelium, with no evidence of infectious organisms. The prognosis has been favourable in only two-thirds of the patients[365]

Miscellaneous adverse effects of drugs and related substances

A few patients have been described with upper airway obstruction while taking oral anticoagulants, as the result of sublingual haematoma[366] or via the development of asphyxiating tracheal compression from peritracheal mediastinal haemorrhage/ haematoma.[367]

Long-term warfarin has been proposed as a cause of tracheal ring calcification in elderly persons[368] in a single study.

Mediastinal lymph node enlargement, sometimes containing giant-cell granulomata, has been described in patients treated with penicillin, phenytoin, sulfasalazine and methotrexate or after vaccinations.[369-373] A sarcoidosis-like picture has also been described following treatment with phenytoin or with chemotherapy for malignant lymphoma but a cause-and-effect relationship is uncertain.[370,371,374-379]

Drugs have even been suggested to induce various types of lymphoma.[380-384] Recently, patients receiving interferons for haematological or hepatic disorders,[373,385,386] or highly active anti-retroviral retrotherapy for HIV-related conditions,[387-389] have been shown to develop drug-related granulomatosis in mediastinal lymph nodes or in extrathoracic organs.

Compressive cervical lymphadenopathy with vascular erosion has been described following BCG immunotherapy for bladder carcinoma.[390]

Chronic exposure to steroids is associated with the development of mediastinal lipomatosis, which may cause diagnostic confusion. The condition is seen on chest radiography or on CT scanning, when its characteristic low density is diagnostic.[391]

Very rarely, it may compress airways or mediastinal structures. Cough and mediastinal haemorrhage have been reported in this context.[392,393]

Self-induced respiratory disease

Some patients suffer from self-induced lung problems. These result from the self-administration of compounds via various routes, with the idea of improving health status or in the context of the Munchausen syndrome. They include:

- the ingestion of dietary herbs and supplements, which may induce bronchospasm, interstitial pneumonitis[14] or severe bronchiolitis obliterans[284]
- the long term inhalation of abrasive powders, which may lead to acute silicosis,[394] of talc, which has been associated with refractory wheezing,[395] of crack cocaine laced with an anticoagulant rodenticide,[396] resulting in a severe haemorrhagic diathesis
- the autoinjection of liquid metallic mercury, leading to characteristic and durable opacification of the pulmonary circulation on the chest radiograph and in the right ventricular chamber,[397] along with possible systemic toxicity from the mercury
- the autoinjection of olive oil,[398] leading to lipoid pneumonia, or of domestically synthesised recreational chemicals.[298]

Other iatrogenic lung diseases

Among the late complications of the treatment of Hodgkin's disease by chemo- or radiotherapy in young persons, cancers of the lung[399] or pleura[400] can develop within the radiation fields. In one series, the incidence reached 7.7% and was associated with a poor prognosis.[399] Long-term survivors should, therefore, be discouraged from smoking.

In addition to drugs, medical, radiographic or surgical procedures may lead to acute, and/or painful problems in the chest. Currently recognised iatrogenic respiratory complications of this type are listed in Table 29.2.

Practical management of respiratory diseases induced by drugs

Predicting iatrogenic respiratory disease

Routine monitoring of patients to detect drug-induced lung disease is unrewarding in most cases,[401–406] because of its low incidence and the unreliability of predictive tests.

Sometimes, tests of pulmonary function may even be misleading. For example, patients taking bleomycin often show a decrease in lung volumes regardless of whether or not they develop overt toxicity,[401] and muscle weakness may be the explanation. Prospective pulmonary function testing has been unsuccessful in detecting the adverse pulmonary effects of methotrexate.[407,408] Similarly, although CO transfer factor is abnormal in established bleomycin lung, it does not seem to be capable of detecting early bleomycin toxicity.[409] Nonetheless, targeted follow-up assessment may be useful in patients taking drugs that commonly induce adverse pulmonary effects (e.g. amiodarone, chemotherapeutic agents, bleomycin) or for which a threshold dose is known to exist.[73] Pretreatment measurement of lung function and chest radiography may be helpful as 'baseline' information, should adverse effects develop.[406]

Attributing responsibility to particular drugs

Determining which is the causative agent in patients exposed to several potentially pneumotoxic drugs may be difficult. However, establishing the exact responsibility of drugs is important, in order not to rechallenge the patient inadvertently with the causative drug and not to deprive the patient of a potentially useful drug. In this context, it is important to relate the clinical picture in the patient, with what has been reported in the literature concerning each of the drugs to which the patient was exposed.[4] Often, the clinical pattern is sufficiently distinctive to point to the agent responsible. It is, for instance, usually possible to differentiate bleomycin lung from methotrexate pneumonitis in patients who have received both drugs in combination.

An indirect way to sort out the respective responsibilities of different drugs is to perform sequential rechallenges with the drug(s) that appear less likely responsible for the respiratory event, provided this is justified in the patient in question, under close medical supervision.

Withdrawing the causative drug

This should also be done cautiously. In many cases, the drug can be withdrawn without harm to the patient. However, stopping treatment with such drugs as amiodarone given for refractory ventricular dysrhythmias, chemotherapy in cancer, anti-inflammatory drugs in rheumatoid arthritis or disease-modifying drugs in inflammatory bowel disease may result in severe or fulminating exacerbation of the underlying disease which may prove difficult to control. In such instances, drug withdrawal dictates either replacement of the offending drug by another agent, which should be non-toxic to the lung, or alternative therapeutic choices (e.g. insertion of an automatic defibrillator, in the case of amiodarone pneumonitis). In situations where the underlying disease is potentially life-threatening (e.g. patients with amiodarone pneumonitis and arrhythmia), treatment with the offending drug at a lower dose has been proposed, together with oral steroids, in an attempt to minimise the adverse effects.

Rechallenge

Rechallenge should be considered only when:

- there is no alternative therapeutic choice
- cases of negative rechallenge have been reported with the drug in question in the literature. In this situation, and provided the drug is really necessary, prudent rechallenge

with minute doses is justified. The dose is increased progressively each day or every 2 days but the drug should be withdrawn definitively at the earliest sign of intolerance. Such rechallenges have enabled patients with rheumatoid arthritis with aspirin or NSAID intolerance to continue these drugs harmlessly but daily intake is required for the tolerance to be maintained[410–412] and after a few days without regular treatment the risk of bronchoconstriction recurs as before.

Although apparently safe rechallenge has been described in patients following pneumonitis from amiodarone, minocycline, NSAIDs, sulfasalazine, nilutamide and methotrexate, relying on these observations can be misleading. Indeed, there is substantial mortality rate following the reintroduction of methotrexate, for instance.[413] The outcome of rechallenges reported in the literature is also likely to be biased, because troublesome or fatal re-exposures may not have been published. Rechallenge for diagnostic purposes is not justified.

Adverse pulmonary effects of radiation

The lungs are subjected to direct irradiation in the treatment not only of primary lung tumours but also of cancers of the breast, spine, thymus and oesophagus. Part of the lungs is also included with 'mantle' irradiation of mediastinal, cervical and axillary nodes in patients with lymphoma. Occasionally, the whole lung is included, in total body irradiation or in the treatment of multiple secondary deposits from an osteosarcoma or germ cell tumour, or prior to bone-marrow or stem-cell transplantation. The effects of radiation on the lungs may be early (acute lung injury spreading outside the radiation ports), intermediate (classical radiation pneumonitis) or delayed (radiation fibrosis, BOOP).[414]

Estimates of the overall frequency of adverse effects of therapeutic radiation on the lungs vary considerably. The best estimates of symptomatic 'acute' radiation pneumonitis suggest a frequency of 7–8%, while the overall frequency of radiographic changes is much higher, around 40%.[415] The prevalence of lung injury is higher than suggested by earlier reports and very late effects of radiation damage may be seen many years after treatment. Some of these late respiratory manifestations (pulmonary oedema, pleural effusion) result from long-term effects on the heart.[416]

Radiation pneumonitis and fibrosis

The pulmonary effects of radiation are traditionally separated into the 'acute' phase of radiation pneumonitis and later radiation fibrosis. The former is, however, more appropriately considered as a subacute reaction as it tends to develop over several weeks and rarely produces clinical problems within 2 months of radiotherapy, except in rare cases of extensive lung injury, especially if hazardous combined therapy is employed, e.g. radiation plus chemotherapy and/or oxygen.

Pathogenesis

Studies in experimental animals show demonstrable injury within 24 hours of irradiation, with the main effects seen in the type II pneumocytes and pulmonary endothelial cells. A likely mechanism by which ionising radiation damages tissues is by the generation of free radicals, which damage cell membranes and DNA. Studies in animal models have shown that the effects are reduced by antioxidants (oxygen radical scavengers) and increased by hyperoxia. The cell injury results in exudation of protein-rich fluid into the alveolar spaces. Macrophages release cytokines, including transforming growth factor (TGF)-β, which is known to stimulate fibroblast proliferation and may contribute to fibrosis. The delayed onset of the clinical features of 'acute' radiation pneumonitis has been attributed to the turnover time of endothelial cells. Radiation induces genetic changes in these cells and it is suggested that the integrity of the endothelium is maintained until later generations of damaged cells develop. Alveolar lavage in animals shows an increase in phospholipids shortly after irradiation, resulting from increased production of surfactant by hyperplastic type II pneumocytes. This may reflect a reaction to the exudation of protein.[417] If corticosteroids (which have a beneficial effect on acute radiation pneumonitis) are administered, this phospholipid production increases further.

Alveolar lavage in human subjects following irradiation shows an increased proportion of lymphocytes, irrespective of whether the patient subsequently develops clinically evident radiation pneumonitis.[418] Even if only one lung has been irradiated, these changes occur in both lungs,[419] suggesting that immunological mechanisms may also be involved, particularly in those who develop pneumonitis or organising pneumonia (see below) outside the irradiated field. Nevertheless, the risk of developing clinically evident radiation lung injury is related to the total dose of radiation[420] and also to the fractionation pattern.[415] With unilateral irradiation using fractionated treatment schedules, total doses of less than 30 Gy (3000 rads) usually have little clinical effect, while radiographic changes are seen variably after doses between 30 and 40 Gy and are usual with doses exceeding 40 Gy.[421] A daily fraction size above 2.67 Gy is particularly likely to result in radiation pneumonitis.[415] The likelihood of lung injury is increased with simultaneous use of cytotoxic drugs.[422]

The phenomenon of 'recall' pneumonitis is also increasingly recognised.[33,423] This occurs when chemotherapy following radiotherapy leads to the development of pneumonitis in the areas previously irradiated. A further factor that may precipitate radiation-induced changes is withdrawal of corticosteroids.[422] A recent study has suggested that continuing smoking reduces the likelihood of radiation pneumonitis.[424] The parallel finding in extrinsic allergic alveolitis (hypersensitivity pneumonitis – see Chapter 55) again suggests the possible involvement of immunological mechanisms in radiation lung injury.

Pathology

Early changes in human lung include oedema and thickening of the alveolar walls, with hyperplasia, atypia and desquamation

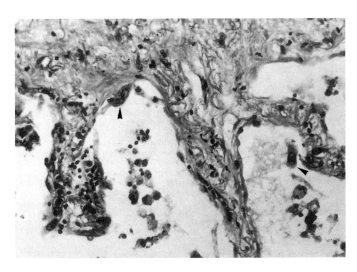

Fig. 29.38 Lung section obtained at post-mortem examination from a patient with radiation fibrosis, showing extensive deposition of collagen with large, atypical pneumocytes (arrowed). (Courtesy of Dr T. Ashcroft.)

of type II pneumocytes together with thrombosis of small pulmonary vessels. After a few months, there may be progressive interstitial and intra-alveolar fibrosis (Fig. 29.38), with a marked reduction in vasculature and sclerosis of vessels. The fibrosis can increase for up to 12 months and thrombosed vessels may show recanalisation.

Clinical features

With extensive radiation pneumonitis, a troublesome non-productive cough, shortness of breath and occasionally fever occur, usually 2–3 months after injury. Earlier symptoms portend a more serious reaction.[422] Occasionally, a generalised acute reaction is seen following local irradiation, presumably caused by hypersensitivity. Such reactions can be very severe, occasionally resulting in ARDS.[425] Withdrawal of steroids during a course of radiation therapy has been blamed in some cases.[426]

In many patients the acute response subsides spontaneously or after treatment with corticosteroids. Shortness of breath is likely to persist in those with severe pneumonitis or with pre-existing impairment of lung function. The chest radiograph typically shows hazy shadowing within the first 2–3 months (Fig. 29.39a), progressing to more dense consolidation, often with an air bronchogram. Later, as fibrosis develops, streaky linear shadowing with contraction and distortion of lung architecture is seen (Fig. 29.39b), and a characteristic feature of the radiographic shadowing is its sharp margin versus normally aerated lung, due to the limitation to the irradiated field. The portal arrangements differ in breast versus lung cancer or intrathoracic lymphomas, and this will influence both the extent and the shape of pulmonary opacities related to radiation pneumonitis.[427] Sometimes, the shadowing spreads outside the field, either early as a result of fulminant lung injury, or later because of distortion by fibrosis. Computed tomography[427] and magnetic resonance imaging[428] are more sensitive than plain chest radiography, showing postradiother-

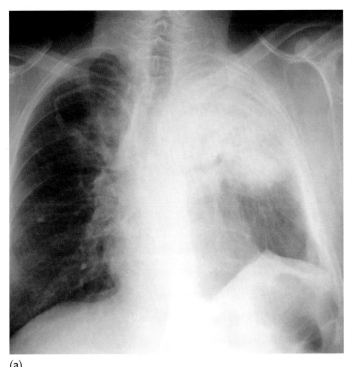

(a)

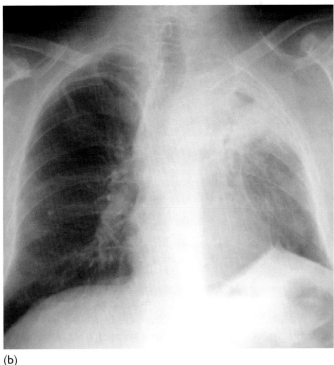

(b)

Fig. 29.39 Chest radiographs of a patient with classical radiation pneumonitis confined to the radiation portal. Hazy shadowing is typically seen within the first months (a), progressing to more dense consolidation with contraction and distortion of the lung architecture (b).

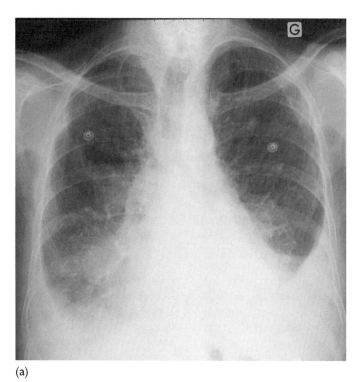

(a)

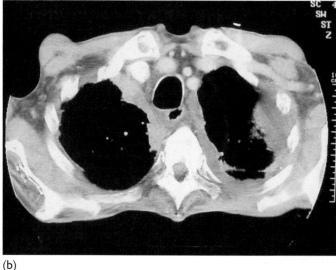

(b)

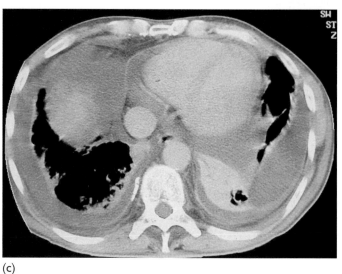

(c)

Fig. 29.40 Chest radiograph and computed tomography scans of a patient with late radiation-induced changes associated with respiratory and cardiac failure following radiation therapy to the mediastinum for Hodgkin's disease 35 years earlier. Sharply demarcated mediastinal fibrosis is visible in (b) and bilateral pleural transudative effusions related to haemodynamically proven cardiac failure (without valvular damage) in (a) and (b). A pericardial effusion is also present (c), presumably radiation-induced.

apy changes with greater frequency and at an earlier stage of the reaction, and associated changes (Fig. 29.40). Later, retractile fibrosis develops in the form of a mass, which can result in necrosis, cavitation, colonisation with *Aspergillus* or haemoptysis. Other radiation-induced thoracic damage may manifest by mediastinal widening, increase in cardiac size related to valvular dysfunction heart failure or pericarditis,[429] pleural effusions from cardiac dysfunction, pulmonary vein stenosis or chylothorax.

The effects on respiratory function are dependent on the extent of lung affected. With localised radiation damage, there may be no detectable functional loss but, when the abnormality is more generalised, there is a reduction in lung volume and carbon monoxide transfer factor.[422] Reduced perfusion of the affected area following an initial transient increase is a relatively early finding, often preceding other changes and sometimes persisting and causing diagnostic confusion.[430]

The most common problem of differential diagnosis is from recurrent tumour. A sharp margin to radiographic shadowing is usually helpful and CT scanning may aid further, although

confident diagnosis sometimes remains difficult. Occasionally, particularly after supraclavicular irradiation, apical shadowing is seen that resembles pulmonary tuberculosis.[427]

Treatment

In most cases, no treatment is required. When radiation pneumonitis causes extensive changes and troublesome symptoms, corticosteroids are usually used. Although no controlled studies are available, there is a strong clinical impression of their efficacy in radiation pneumonitis.[422] No treatment has been shown to be effective once fibrosis has developed.

Organising pneumonia

(See also Drug-induced organising pneumonia, above)
There have been several reports of organising pneumonia following radiotherapy.[431,432] This reaction is different from both acute pneumonitis and chronic radiation fibrosis. It may develop in an area of lung previously irradiated but frequently it affects

lung beyond the irradiated field and it can develop as long as several months after treatment. Reports have been almost exclusively in women who have received radiotherapy following surgery for breast cancer. The clinical presentation, radiographic and pathological appearances are similar to those in cryptogenic organising pneumonia (see Chapter 54). In the largest series of patients with organising pneumonia in the non-irradiated lung, the average time from symptoms to diagnosis was 18 weeks.[431] Patients characteristically present with cough, shortness of breath and fever and the chest radiograph shows peripheral alveolar shadowing with a migratory pattern. The erythrocyte sedimentation rate is typically elevated and the response to corticosteroid therapy is usually very good although, as with cryptogenic organising pneumonia, relapses frequently occur following too early steroid withdrawal.[432]

Miscellaneous effects

Late complications of thoracic irradiation include pleural effusion or thickening, localised bronchiectasis[421] and occasionally spontaneous pneumothorax,[433] cavitation of fibrotic foci with aspergilloma formation,[434] phrenic nerve palsy,[435] or chylothorax.[436] Telangiectasia of the overlying skin is common; similar changes affect the airways within the irradiated field and occasionally give rise to haemoptysis. Unhealed rib fractures caused by bone necrosis are sometimes seen and, in children, hypoplasia of the thoracic skeleton occurs occasionally after extensive thoracic irradiation.[437]

Radionuclide injury

The radioactive isotopes uranium-238 and thorium-232 occur naturally in rocks and soil. Spontaneous decay of uranium releases other radioactive isotopes, including gaseous radon-222 and its further decay products or 'daughters'. Miners in certain industries

have consequently been exposed to radioactivity above normal environmental levels and increased risks of lung cancer have been shown in those who have mined fluorospar,[438] uranium[439] and tin.[440]

Therapeutic use of radioactive isotopes has occasionally been reported to cause bilateral radiation pneumonitis, particularly after treatment of metastatic thyroid malignancy with iodine-131[441] (for illustrations, see Lin 1994[442]).

Adverse pulmonary effects of illicit drug use

A large range of adverse respiratory effects of illicit or 'street drugs' has been described, particularly when the drugs are taken by inhalation or crushed tablets are injected intravenously. Interpretation of the precise causes and mechanisms of pulmonary toxicity is frequently complicated by difficulties in history taking, use of more than one agent, by impurities in the drugs used and by interactions with the effects of tobacco or possible HIV infection. Consequently, much of the evidence in the literature is circumstantial and uncontrolled.

The more commonly described effects of inhaled illicit drugs are listed in Table 29.3. The largest literature relates to the effects of inhaling freebase or 'crack' cocaine.[443,444] A productive cough with characteristically black sputum is commonly reported. The sputum is produced within a short time of inhalation and the colour is attributed to carbon residue from hydrocarbon or alcohol-soaked cotton sponges used to ignite the cocaine.[450] Exacerbation of asthma after inhalation is also well recognised,[451] and recent evidence suggests that cocaine use may be a more frequent risk factor than previously recognised, at least in some communities: two reports[452,453] of patients admitted to inner city Emergency Departments in the

Table 29.3   Respiratory effects of inhaled illicit drugs

Agent	Effects	References
Cocaine ('crack')	Productive cough with black sputum	443, 444
	Exacerbation of asthma	451
	Chest pain	443
	Barotrauma	443, 445
	Haemoptysis	446
	Pulmonary haemorrhage	447
	Non-cardiogenic pulmonary oedema	448
	'Crack lung'	455
Cannabis (marijuana)	Acute bilateral non-infections inhalation pneumonitis	
	Chronic bronchitis	458
	Squamous metaplasia	461
	? Lung cancer	
Opiates	Exacerbation of asthma	449
	Non-cardiogenic pulmonary oedema	444
	Respiratory depression	

USA with acute severe asthma showed positive urine tests for cocaine metabolites in a sizeable minority. Chest pain is another symptom frequently reported by crack users; in a small minority this is due to barotrauma, which may manifest as pneumothorax, pneumomediastinum or pneumopericardium. Barotrauma in this context is attributed to forceful deep inhalation through a narrow pipe, followed by a Valsalva manoeuvre (which allegedly increases the euphoria).[443] Haemoptysis is also well recognised after cocaine inhalation and is usually presumed due to rupture of a small bronchial vessel. Less commonly, alveolar haemorrhage occurs.[454] This is notably common at autopsy in the lungs of subjects who have died after cocaine use. Various other alveolar reactions have been described, including non-cardiogenic pulmonary oedema and pulmonary eosinophilia. The latter is sometimes reported as 'crack lung', characterised by diffuse radiographic infiltrates, sometimes associated with fever and pulmonary and systemic eosinophilia and developing within 48 hours of heavy cocaine smoking.[455] Cases of tracheal thermal injury have also been reported.[456,457]

Regular smokers of cannabis (marijuana) develop a chronic productive cough similar to that of tobacco smokers.[458] A recent longitudinal study has, however, suggested that, unlike tobacco smoking, habitual cannabis smoking does not accelerate the decline in FEV_1 with age.[459] However, the smoke from cannabis contains similar constituents (apart from nicotine) to tobacco smoke and, indeed, the tar from the smoke contains greater concentrations of carcinogens such as benzpyrenes than the tar in tobacco smoke.[460] Not surprisingly, therefore, chronic use of cannabis is associated with the development of squamous metaplasia of the bronchial epithelium.[461] Several case reports have further suggested a relation between cannabis smoking and cancer of the upper airway. As yet there is no definite evidence of an increased risk of bronchial carcinoma, but clearly the potential exists and appropriate epidemiological studies are required.

Opiate drugs are well-recognised as potentially exacerbating asthma or causing non-cardiogenic pulmonary oedema and both have also been described after inhalation. Depression of respiration is a further predictable consequence, which may exacerbate the situation.

Illicit drugs taken by mouth are much less likely to have serious respiratory consequences than those taken by inhalation. However, amphetamine and its derivatives, including the 'designer drug' MDMA (Ecstasy), have occasionally been reported to cause fatal asthma or pulmonary oedema.[462] Similar stimulant drugs in long-term use are recognised to cause pulmonary hypertension (see Chapter 65).[298,463–465]

Users of intravenous drugs, in particular opiates[466] and methylphenidate[467] sometimes develop an unusual form of premature emphysema affecting mainly the lower lobes and associated with talcosis. The effect is probably due to particle embolisation rather than to the drugs themselves.

Occlusion of small pulmonary vessels may eventually lead to pulmonary hypertension. Thrombophlebitis or right-sided endocarditis due to intravenous drug abuse can result in septic pulmonary emboli, infarction and cavitation[468] (see Chapter 64).

Therapeutic principles

- Acute anaphylaxis or anaphylactoid reactions require immediate but cautious treatment with intramuscular adrenaline (epinephrine) supplemented by oxygen, antihistamine, parenteral corticosteroid and nebulised bronchodilator.

- In suspected drug-induced lung disease, rechallenge is usually inadvisable unless the drug is absolutely essential for the patient.

- Corticosteroid treatment is indicated for drug- or radiation-induced pneumonitis or organising pneumonia:
  - only if an infectious cause has carefully been excluded
  - when reduction or withdrawal of the relevant drug is not effective
  - in symptomatic or hypoxaemic patients
  - in patients with extensive disease.

- If required in patients with amiodarone pneumonitis, steroids should be administered for an extended period because of the prolonged retention of this drug in lung tissue.

? Unresolved questions

- The epidemiology of drug-induced respiratory disease is imprecise

- The mechanisms by which either non-steroidal anti-inflammatory drugs or beta blockers (and other asthma-inducers) provoke asthma remain uncertain.

- The mechanisms (metabolic activation, hypersensitivity) of drug-induced pneumonitis and the reasons for variable individual susceptibility (genomic differences in drug metabolism/detoxication, or reactivity of the immune system) are unclear.

- Optimal strategies for minimising the risk of lung injury from potentially toxic drugs and for monitoring patients on treatment have not been clearly defined.

- Assessing the true relevance of illicit drug use to acute asthma requires further study.

References

1. Hartmann K, Koller Doser A, Kuhn M. Postmarketing safety information: how useful are spontaneous reports? Pharmacoepidemiol Drug Safety 1999; 8: S65–S71.
2. Camus P. Respiratory disease induced by drugs. Eur Respir J 1997; 10: 260–264.
3. Foucher P, Biour M, Blayac JP et al. Drugs that may injure the respiratory system. Eur Respir J 1997; 10: 265–279.
4. http://www.pneumotox.com: 'Pneumotox on the Web'. Producers: Foucher P, Camus P. Last update: July 2001.

 читатель

5. Camus P, Foucher P, Bonniaud P, Ask K. Drug-induced infiltrative lung disease. Eur Respir J Suppl 2001; 32: 93s–100s.
6. Ferriby D, Stojkovic T. Bronchiolitis obliterans with organizing pneumonia during interferon β-1a treatment. Lancet 2001; 357: 751.
7. Rizk A, Gorson KC, Kenney L, Weinstein R. Transfusion-related acute lung injury after the infusion of IVIG. Transfusion 2001; 41: 264–268.
8. Maillard N, Foucher P, Caillot D et al. Transient pulmonary infiltrates during treatment with anti-thymocyte globulin. Respiration 1999; 66: 279–282.
9. Ruiz-Argüelles GJ, Arizpe-Bravo D, Sanchez-Sosa S et al. Fatal G-CSF-induced pulmonary toxicity. Am J Hematol 1999; 60: 82–83.
10. White RL, Schwartzentruber DJ, Guleria A et al. Cardiopulmonary toxicity of treatment with high dose interleukin-2 in 199 consecutive patients with metastatic melanoma or renal cell carcinoma. Cancer 1994; 74: 3212–3222.
11. Wallis JP. Transfusion-related acute lung injury. Transfusion Med 2000; 10: 92–93.
12. Popovsky MA, Davenport RD. Transfusion-related acute lung injury: femme fatale? Transfusion 2001; 41: 312–315.
13. Guo XQ, Gopalan R, Ugbarugba S et al. Hepatitis B-related polyarteritis nodosa complicated by pulmonary hemorrhage. Chest 2001; 119: 1608–1610.
14. Mizushima Y, Oosaki R, Kobayashi M. Clinical features of pneumonitis induced by herbal drugs. Phytother Res 1997; 11: 295–298.
15. Wang JS, Tseng HH, Lai RS et al. *Sauropus androgynus*-constrictive obliterative bronchiolitis/bronchiolitis. Histopathological study of pneumonectomy and biopsy specimens with emphasis on the inflammatory process and disease progression. Histopathology 2000; 37: 402–410.
16. Madhavi P, Jameson R, Robinson MJ. Unilateral pleural effusion complicating central venous catheterisation. Arch Dis Child 2000; 82: F248–F249.
17. Thanigaraj S, Panneerselvam A, Yanos J. Retrieval of an IV catheter fragment from the pulmonary artery 11 years after embolization. Chest 2000; 117: 1209–1211.
18. Müller P, Wertenbruch R. Endocarditic vegetations in the right heart after pacemaker implantation as a cause of a round pulmonary infiltrate. Dtsch Med Wschr 1998; 123: 766–770.
19. Pang WW, Chang DP, Lin CH, Huang MH. Negative pressure pulmonary oedema induced by direct suctioning of endotracheal tube adapter. Can J Anaesth 1998; 45: 785–788.
20. Diez JJ, Iglesias P. Pulmonary thromboembolism after inferior petrosal sinus sampling in Cushing's syndrome. Clin Endocrinol 1997; 46: 777.
21. Browne J, Murphy D, Shorten G. Pneumomediastinum, pneumothorax and subcutaneous emphysema complicating MIS herniorrhaphy. Can J Anaesth 2000; 47: 69–72.
22. Peuker ET, White A, Ernst E et al. Traumatic complications of acupuncture. Therapists need to know human anatomy. Arch Fam Med 1999; 8: 553–558.
23. Shankar G, Cohen DA. Idiopathic pneumonia syndrome after bone marrow transplantation: the role of pre-transplant radiation conditioning and local cytokine dysregulation in promoting lung inflammation and fibrosis. Int J Exp Pathol 2001; 82: 101–113.
24. O'Hearn DJ, Leiferman KM, Askin F, Georas SN. Pulmonary infiltrates after cytokine therapy for stem cell transplantation. Massive deposition of eosinophil major basic protein detected by immunohistochemistry. Am J Respir Crit Care Med 1999; 160: 1361–1365.
25. Ohnuma K, Toyoda Y, Ishida Y et al. Fatal obstructive lung disease after haploidentical sibling cord blood transplantation. Bone Marrow Transplant 1998; 21: 939–941.
26. Arcasoy SM, Kotloff RM. Lung transplantation. N Engl J Med 1999; 340: 1081–1091.
27. Schweitzer VG, Juillard GJF, Bajada CL, Parker RG. Radiation recall dermatitis and pneumonitis in a patient treated with paclitaxel. Cancer 1995; 76: 1069–1072.
28. Berkman N, Goldstein RH, Breuer R. Bleomycin-induced lung injury is enhanced by interferon-alpha. Life Sci 1997; 60: Pl415-Pl421.
29. Rubio C, Hill ME, Milan S et al. Idiopathic pneumonia syndrome after high dose chemotherapy for relapsed Hodgkin's disease. Br J Cancer 1997; 75: 1044–1048.
30. Segawa Y, Takigawa N, Kataoka M et al. Risk factors for development of radiation pneumonitis following radiation therapy with or without chemotherapy for lung cancer. Int J Radiation Oncol Biol Phys 1997; 39: 91–98.
31. Donat SM, Levy DA. Bleomycin associated pulmonary toxicity: is perioperative oxygen restriction necessary? J Urol 1998; 160: 1347–1352.
32. Alessandrino EP, Bernasconi P, Colombo A et al. Pulmonary toxicity following carmustine-based preparative regimens and autologous peripheral blood progenitor cell transplantation in hematological malignancies. Bone Marrow Transplant 2000; 25: 309–313.
33. Thomas PS, Agrawal S, Gore M, Geddes DM. Recall lung pneumonitis due to carmustine after radiotherapy. Thorax 1995; 50: 1116–1118.
34. Fogarty G, Ball D, Rischin D. Radiation recall reaction following gemcitabine. Lung Cancer 2001; 33: 299–302.
35. Saussine M, Colson P, Alauzen M, Mary H. Postoperative acute respiratory distress syndrome. A complication of amiodarone associated with 100 percent oxygen ventilation. Chest 1992; 102: 980–981.
36. Ingrassia TSI, Ryu JH, Trastek VF, Rosenow ECIII. Oxygen-exacerbated bleomycin pulmonary toxicity. Mayo Clin Proc 1991; 66: 173–178.
37. Dai MS, Ho CL, Chen YC et al. Acute respiratory distress syndrome following intrathecal methotrexate administration: a case report and review of literature. Ann Hematol 2000; 79: 696–699.
38. Prakash UBS. Pulmonary complications from ophthalmic preparations. Mayo Clin Proc 1990; 65: 521–529.
39. Kwinten FA, de Moor GP, Lamers RJ. Acute pulmonary edema and trigeminal nerve blockade after retrobulbar block. Anesth Analg 1996; 83: 1322–1324.
40. Wilhelms E, Criée CP, Neubauer H, Neuhaus KL. Lungengerüsterkrankung nach Instilllation von Mitomycin C in die Harnblase. Dtsch Med Wschr 1986; 111: 1564–1566.
41. Mooren FC, Lerch MM, Ullerich H et al. Systemic granulomatous disease after intravesical BCG instillation. Br Med J 2000; 320: 219.
42. Donlan CJ Jr, Scutero JV. Transient eosinophilic pneumonia secondary to use of a vaginal cream. Chest 1975; 67: 232–233.
43. Simonneau G, Fartoukh M, Sitbon O et al. Primary pulmonary hypertension associated with the use of fenfluramine derivatives. Chest 1998; 114: 195S-199S.
44. Hernandez-Cruz B, Sifuentes-Osornio J, Rosales SP et al. *Mycobacterium tuberculosis* infection in patients with systemic rheumatic diseases. A case-series. Clin Exp Rheumatol 1999; 17: 289–296.
45. Leav BA, Fanburg B, Hadley S. Invasive pulmonary aspergillosis associated with high-dose inhaled fluticasone. N Engl J Med 2000; 343: 586.
46. La Civita L, Battiloro R, Celano M. Nocardia pleural empyema complicating anti-Jo1 positive polymyositis during immunoglobulin and steroid therapy. J Rheumatol 2001; 28: 215–216.
47. Rolston KVI. The spectrum of pulmonary infections in cancer patients. Curr Opin Oncol 2001; 13: 218–223.
48. Feldman AM, McNamara D. Myocarditis. N Engl J Med 2000; 343: 1388–1398.
49. Wilczynski SW, Erasmus JJ, Petros WP et al. Delayed pulmonary toxicity syndrome following high-dose chemotherapy and bone marrow transplantation for breast cancer. Am J Respir Crit Care Med 1998; 157: 565–573.
50. Kantrow SP, Hackman RC, Boeckh M et al. Idiopathic pneumonia syndrome – changing spectrum of lung injury after marrow transplantation. Transplantation 1997; 63: 1079–1086.
51. Bhalla KS, Wilczynski SW, Abushamaa AM et al. Pulmonary toxicity of induction chemotherapy prior to standard or high-dose chemotherapy with autologous hematopoietic support. Am J Respir Crit Care Med 2000; 161: 17–25.
52. Cottin V, Tebib J, Massonne B et al. Pulmonary function tests in patients receiving long-term low-dose methotrexate. Presse Med 1997; 26: 404–406.
53. Saxman SB, Nichols CR, Einhorn LH. Pulmonary toxicity in patients with advanced-stage germ cell tumors receiving bleomycin with and without granulocyte colony stimulating factor. Chest 1997; 111: 657–660.
54. Simpson AB, Paul J, Graham J, Kaye SB. Fatal bleomycin pulmonary toxicity in the west of Scotland 1991–95: a review of patients with germ cell tumours. Br J Cancer 1998; 78: 1061–1066.
55. Chen CI, Abraham R, Tsang R et al. Radiation-associated pneumonitis following autologous stem cell transplantation: predictive factors, disease characteristics and treatment outcomes. Bone Marrow Transplant 2001; 27: 177–182.
56. Mileshkin L, Prince HM, Rischin D, Zimet A. Severe interstitial pneumonitis following high-dose cyclophosphamide, thiotepa and docetaxel: two case reports and a review of the literature. Bone Marrow Transplant 2001; 27: 559–563.
57. Pisani RJ, Rosenow ECI. Pulmonary edema associated with tocolytic therapy. Ann Intern Med 1989; 110: 714–718.
58. Roden S, Juvin K, Homasson JP, Israel-Biet D. An uncommon etiology of isolated pleural effusion. The ovarian hyperstimulation syndrome. Chest 2000; 118: 256–258.
59. Pfitzenmeyer P, Foucher P, Piard F et al. Nilutamide pneumonitis: a report on eight patients. Thorax 1992; 47: 622–627.
60. Lund MB, Kongerud J, Boe J et al. Cardiopulmonary sequelae after treatment for Hodgkin's disease: increased risk in females? Ann Oncol 1996; 7: 257–264.
61. Akaza H, Aso Y, Niijima T et al. Clinical study of RU 23908 (nilutamide) in prostatic cancer. Acta Urol Jpn 1991; 37: 407–420.

62. Sitbon O, Bidel N, Dussopt C et al. Minocycline pneumonitis and eosinophilia: a report on 8 patients. Arch Intern Med 1994; 154: 1633–1640.

63. Voigt M D, Workman B, Lombard C, Kirsch R E. Halothane hepatitis in a South African population. Frequency and the influence of gender and ethnicity. S A Med J 1997; 87: 882–885.

64. Marquette CH, Saulnier F, Leroy O, et al. Long-term prognosis of near-fatal asthma. A 6-year follow-up study of 145 asthmatic patients who underwent mechanical ventilation for a near-fatal attack of asthma. Am Rev Respir Dis 1992; 146: 76–81.

65. Williams IP, Millard FJC. Severe asthma after inadvertent ingestion of oxprenolol. Thorax 1980; 35: 160.

66. Pumphrey RSH. Lessons from management of anaphylaxis from a study of fatal reactions. Clin Exp Allergy 2000; 30: 1144–1150.

67. De Vuyst P, Pfitzenmeyer P, Camus P. Asbestos, ergot drugs and the pleura. Eur Respir J 1997; 10: 2695–2698.

68. Nakagawa H, Yoshida S, Nakabayashi M et al. Possible relevance of virus infection for development of analgesic idiosyncrasy. Respiration 2001; 68: 422–424.

69. Ngan HYS, Liang RHS, Lam WK, Chan TK. Pulmonary toxicity in patients with non-Hodgkin's lymphoma treated with bleomycin-containing combination chemotherapy. Cancer Chemother Pharmacol 1993; 32: 407–409.

70. Trisolini R, Lazzari Agli L, Tassinari D et al. Acute lung injury associated with 5-fluorouracil and oxaliplatinum combined chemotherapy. Eur Respir J 2001; 18: 243–245.

71. Ooi GC, Kwong DL, Ho JC et al. Pulmonary sequelae of treatment for breast cancer: a prospective study. Int J Radiation Oncol Biol Phys 2001; 50: 411–419.

72. Briasoulis E, Froudarakis M, Milionis H et al. Chemotherapy-induced noncardiogenic pulmonary edema related to gemcitabine plus docetaxel combination with granulocyte colony-stimulating factor support. Respiration 2000; 67: 680–683.

73. Aronin PA, Mahaley MSJ, Rudnick SA et al. Prediction of BCNU pulmonary toxicity in patients with malignant gliomas: an assessment of risk factors. N Engl J Med 1980; 303: 183–188.

74. Foresti V, Parisio E, Pepe R et al. Adverse effects of amiodarone at low doses. 1989; 95: 254–255.

75. Real E, Roca MJ, Vinuales A et al. Life threatening lung toxicity induced by low doses of bleomycin in a patient with Hodgkin's disease. Haematologica 1999; 84: 667–668.

76. Alliot C, Tabuteau S, Desablens B et al. Fatal pulmonary fibrosis after a low cumulated dose of bleomycin: role of alpha1-antitrypsin deficiency? Am J Hematol 1999; 62: 198–199.

77. Lombard JN, Bonnotte B, Maynadié M et al. Celiprolol pneumonitis. Eur Respir J 1993; 9: 588–591.

78. Almoosa KF. Hydrochlorothiazide-induced pulmonary edema. South Med J 1999; 92: 1100–1102.

79. Esinger W, Schleiffer T, Leinberger H et al. Steroidrefraktäre Lungenfibrose durch Amiodaron. Klinik und Morphologie nach einem amiodaronfreien Intervall von 3 Monaten. Dtsch Med Wschr 1988; 113: 1638–1641.

80. Elsasser S, Dalquen P, Soler M, Perruchoud A. Methotrexate-induced pneumonitis: appearance four weeks after discontinuation of treatment. Am Rev Respir Dis 1989; 140: 1089–1092.

81. Limper AH, McDonald JA. Delayed pulmonary fibrosis after nitrosourea therapy. N Engl J Med 1990; 323: 407–409.

82. Hasleton PS, O'Driscoll BR, Lynch P. Late BCNU lung: a light and ultrastructural study on the delayed effect of BCNU on the lung parenchyma. J Pathol 1991; 164: 31–36.

83. Willenbacher W, Mumm A, Bartsch HH. Late pulmonary toxicity of bleomycin. J Clin Oncol 1998; 16: 3205.

84. Wilhelm JM, Thannberger P, Derragui A. Interstitial pneumonia 2 months after discontinuing amiodarone. Presse Med 1999; 28: 2040.

85. O'Driscoll BR, Hasleton PS, Taylor PM,. Active lung fibrosis up to 17 years after chemotherapy with carmustine (BCNU) in childhood. N Engl J Med 1990; 323: 378–382.

86. Ward MM, Donald F. Pneumocystis carinii pneumonia in patients with connective tissue diseases. The role of hospital experience in diagnosis and mortality. Arthritis Rheum 1999; 42: 780–789.

87. Ramsay S. Johns Hopkins takes responsibility for volunteer's death. Lancet 2001; 358: 213.

88. McLellan F. 1966 and all that – when is a literature search done? Lancet 2001; 358: 646.

89. Poletti V, Salvucci M, Zanchini R. The lung as a target organ in patients with hematologic disorders. Haematologica 2000; 85: 855–864.

90. Marie I, Hatron PY, Hachulla E. Pulmonary involvement in polymyositis and in dermatomyositis. J Rheumatol 1998; 25: 1336–1343.

91. Keane MP, Lynch JP. Pleuropulmonary manifestations of systemic lupus erythematosus. Thorax 2000; 55: 159–166.

92. Camus P, Piard F, Ashcroft T. The lung in inflammatory bowel disease. Medicine (Baltimore) 1993; 72: 151–183.

93. Camus P, Coudert B, d'Athis P. Pharmacokinetics of amiodarone in the isolated rat lung. J Pharmacol Exp Ther 1990; 254: 336–343.

94. Wilkinson JRW, Roberts JA, Bradding P. Paradoxical bronchoconstriction in asthmatic patients after salmeterol by metered dose inhaler. Br Med J 1992; 305: 931–932.

95. Asmus MJ, Sherman J, Hendeles L. Bronchoconstrictor additives in bronchodilator solutions. J Allergy Clin Immunol 1999; 104: S53–S60.

96. Erjavec Z, Woolthuis GMH, de Vries-Hospers HG. Tolerance and efficacy of amphotericin B inhalations for prevention of invasive pulmonary aspergillosis in haematological patients. Eur J Clin Microbiol Infect Dis 1997; 16: 364–368.

97. Shelton MJ, Minor JR. Aesosolized pentamidine in AIDS patients with asthma. Am J Hosp Pharm 1991; 48: 556–557.

98. Mant TG, Tempowski JH, Volans GL, Talbot JC. Adverse reactions to acetylcysteine and effects of overdose. Br Med J 1984; 289: 217–219.

99. Sastre J, Quirce S, Novalbos A et al. Occupational asthma induced by cephalosporins. Eur Respir J 1999; 13: 1189–1191.

100. Cullinan P, Harris JM, Taylor AJN et al. An outbreak of asthma in a modern detergent factory. Lancet 2000; 356: 1899–1900.

101. Shale DJ, Lane DJ, Davis CJF. Airflow limitation in myasthenia gravis. Am Rev Respir Dis 1983; 128: 18–621.

102. Sebastian JL, McKinney WP, Kaufman J, Young MJ. Angiotensin-converting enzyme inhibitors and cough: prevalence in an outpatient medical clinic population. Chest 1991; 99: 36–39.

103. Israili ZH, Hall WD. Cough and angioneurotic edema associated with angiotensin-converting enzyme inhibitor therapy. Ann Intern Med 1992; 117: 234–242.

104. Tanaka H, Teramoto S, Oashi K et al. Effects of candesartan on cough and bronchial hyperresponsiveness in mildly to moderately hypertensive patients with symptomatic asthma. Circulation 2001; 104: 281–285.

105. Conigliaro RL, Gleason PP. Losartan-induced cough after lisinopril therapy. Am J Health-Syst Pharm 1999; 56: 914–915.

106. Lunde H, Hedner T, Samuelsson O et al. Dyspnoea, asthma and bronchospasm in relation to treatment with angiotensin convertin enzyme inhibitors. Br Med J 1994; 308: 18–21.

107. Inman WHW, Pearce G, Wilton L, Mann RD. Angiotensin converting enzyme inhibitors and asthma. Br Med J 1994; 308: 593–594.

108. Fallowfield JM, Marlow HF. Propranolol is contraindicated in asthma. Br Med J 1996; 313: 1486.

109. Chafin CC, Soberman JE, Demerkan K, Self T. Beta blockers after myocardial infarction: do benefits ever outweigh risks in asthma? Cardiology 1999; 92: 99–105.

110. Myers JD, Higham MA, Shakur BH, Wickremasinghe PW. Attenuation of propranolol-induced bronchoconstriction by frusemide. Thorax 1997; 52: 861–865.

111. Anderson EG, Calcraft B, Jariwalla AG, Al-Zaiback M. Persistent asthma after treatment with beta-blocking drugs. Br J Dis Chest 1979; 73: 407–408.

112. Bauer K, Kaik G, Kaik B. Osmotic release of oral drug delivery system of metoprolol in hypertensive asthmatic patients. Pharmacodynamic effects on β_2 adrenergic receptors. Hypertension 1994; 24: 339–346.

113. Diggory P, Franks WA. Glaucoma therapy may take your breath away. Age Ageing 1997; 26: 63–67.

114. Passo MS, Palmer E , Van Buskirk EM. Plasma timolol in glaucoma patients. Ophthalmology 1984; 91: 1361–1363.

115. Idsoe O, Guthe T, Wilcox RR, Weck AL. Nature and extent of penicillin side reactions with particular reference to fatalities from anaphylactic shock. Bull WHO 1968; 38: 159–188.

116. Stoelting RK. Allergic reactions during anesthesia. Anesth Analg 1983; 62: 341–356.

117. Project Team of the Resuscitation Council (UK). Emergency medical treatment of anaphylactic reactions. J Accident Emerg Med 1999; 16: 243–247.

118. Hailemeskel B, Namanny MD, Metzger SD. Severe asthmatic reaction to contraindicated anti-inflammatory drug. Am J Health-Syst Pharm 1997; 54: 199–200.

119. Stevenson DD. Adverse reactions to nonsteroidal anti-inflammatory drugs. Immunol Allergy Clin North Am 1998; 18: 773–798.

120. Anonymous. Analgesics and asthma. Br Med J 1973; 3: 419–420.

121. Israel E, Fischer AR, Rosenberg MA. The pivotal role of 5 lipoxygenase products in the reaction of aspirin sensitive asthmatics to aspirin. Am Rev Respir Dis 1993; 148: 1447–1451.

122. Cowburn AS, Sladek K, Soya J. Overexpression of leukotriene C4 synthase in bronchial biopsies from patients with aspirin intolerant asthma. J Clin Invest 1998; 101: 834–846.

123. Sanak M, Simon HU, Szczeklik A. Leukotriene C-4 synthase promoter polymorphism and risk of aspirin-induced asthma. Lancet 1997; 350: 1599–1600.

124. Szczeklik A, Sladek K, Dworski R et al. Bronchial aspirin challenge causes specific eicosanoid response in aspirin-sensitive asthmatics. Am J Respir Crit Care Med 1996; 154: 1608–1614.

125. Sestini P, Armetti L, Gambaro G et al. Inhaled PGE(2) prevents aspirin-induced bronchoconstriction and urinary LTE(4) excretion in aspirin-sensitive asthma. Am J Respir Crit Care Med 1996; 153: 572–575.

126. Fischer TJ, Guilfoile TD, Kesarwala HH et al. Adverse pulmonary responses to aspirin and acetaminophen in chronic childhood asthma. Pediatrics 1983; 71: 313–318.

127. Szczeklik A, Nizankowska E, Duplaga M. Natural history of aspirin-induced asthma. Eur Respir J 2000; 16: 432–438.

128. Larsen K. The clinical relationship of nasal polyps to asthma. Allergy Asthma Proc 1996; 17: 243–249.

129. Kalyoncu AF, Kisacik G, Sahin AA, Baris YI. Prevalence of cross-sensitivity with acetaminophen and other nonsteroidal antiinflammatory drugs in asthmatic patients. J Allergy Clin Immunol 1996; 98: 713.

130. Szczeklik A, Sanak M. Genetic mechanisms in aspirin-induced asthma. Am J Respir Crit Care Med 2000; 161: S142–S146.

131. Nizankowska E, Bestynska-krypel A, Cmiel A, Szczeklik A. Oral and bronchial provocation tests with aspirin for diagnosis of aspirin induced asthma. Eur Respir J 2000; 15: 863–869.

132. Milewski M, Mastalerz L, Nizankowska E, Szczeklik A. Nasal provocation test with lysine-aspirin for diagnosis of aspirin-sensitive asthma. J Allergy Clin Immunol 1998; 101: 581–586.

133. Szczeklik A, Nizankowska E, Bochenek G et al. Safety of a specific COX-2 inhibitor in aspirin-induced asthma. Clin Exp Allergy 2001; 31: 219–225.

134. Settipane RA, Shrank PJ, Simon RA et al. Prevalence of cross sensitivity with acetaminophen in aspirin asthmatics. J Allergy Clin Immunol 1995; 96: 480–485.

135. Dahlen B, Nizankowska E, Szczeklik A. Benefits from adding the 5-lipoxygenase inhibitor zileuton to conventional therapy in aspirin tolerant asthmatics. Am J Respir Crit Care Med 1998; 157: 1187–1194.

136. Enrique E, Garcia-Ortega P, Gaig P, San Miguel MM. Failure of montelukast to prevent anaphylaxis to diclofenac. Allergy 1999; 54: 529–530.

137. Van Arsdel PPJ. Aspirin idiosyncrasy and tolerance. J Allergy Clin Immunol 1984; 73: 431–434.

138. Pleskow WW, Stevenson DD, Mathison DA et al. Aspirin desensitisation in aspirin sensitive asthmatic patients clinical manifestations and characterisation of the refractory period. J Allergy Clin Immunol 1982; 69: 11–19.

139. Partridge MR, Gibson GJ. Adverse bronchial reactions to intravenous hydrocortisone in two aspirin-sensitive asthmatic patients. Br Med J 1978; 1: 1521–1522.

140. Dajani BM, Sliman NA, Shubair KS, Hamzeh YS. Bronchospasm caused by intravenous hydrocortisone sodium succinate (solu cortef) in aspirin sensitive asthmatics. J Allergy Clin Immunol 1981; 68: 201–204.

141. Rodriguez-Garcia JL, Fraile G, Moreno MA et al. Recurrent massive pleural effusion as a late complication of radiotherapy in Hodgkin's disease. 1991; 100: 1165–1166.

142. Finley TN, Aronow A, Cosentino AM, Golde DW. Occult pulmonary hemorrhage in anticoagulated patients. Am Rev Respir Dis 1975; 112: 23–29.

143. Van Rooij WJ, van der Meer SC, van Royen EA et al. Pulmonary gallium-67 uptake in amiodarone pneumonitis. J Nucl Med 1984; 25: 211–213.

144. Standertskjöld-Nordenstam CG, Wandtke JC, Hood WJ Jr et al. Amiodarone pulmonary toxicity. Chest radiography and CT in asymptomatic patients. Chest 1985; 88: 143–145.

145. Garbes ID, Henderson ES, Gomez GA et al. Procarbazine-induced interstitial pneumonitis with a normal chest X-ray: a case report. Med Pediatr Oncol 1986; 14: 238–241.

146. Gaetani P, Silvani V, Butti G et al. Nitrosourea derivatives induce pulmonary toxicity in patients treated for malignant brain tumors. Early subclinical detection and its prevention. Eur J Cancer Clin Oncol 1987; 23: 267–271.

147. Kuhlman JE, Scatarige JC, Fishman EK, Siegelman SS. CT demonstration of high attenuation pleural-parenchymal lesions due to amiodarone therapy. J Comput Assist Tomogr 1987; 11: 160–162.

148. Niitsu N, Iki S, Muroi K et al. Interstitial pneumonia in patients receiving granulocyte colony-stimulating factor during chemotherapy: survey in Japan 1991–96. Br J Cancer 1997; 76: 1661–1666.

149. Dooren MC, Ouwehand WH, Verhoeven AJ et al. Adult respiratory distress syndrome after experimental intravenous gamma-globulin concentrate and monocyte-reactive IgG antibodies. Lancet 1998; 352: 1601–1602.

150. Hein KD, Wechsler ME, Schwartzstein RM, Morris DJ. The adult respiratory distress syndrome after dextran infusion as an antithrombotic agent in free TRAM flap breast reconstruction. Plastic Reconstruct Surg 1999; 103: 1706–1708.

151. Lucas GF, Leach M. Transfusion-related acute lung injury. Transfusion Med 2000; 10: 91–92.

152. De Lavigerie B, Joasson JM. Adult respiratory distress syndrome after antineoplastic chemotherapy: probable effect of gemcitabine. Presse Med 2001; 30: 851–854.

153. Imokawa S, Colby TV, Leslie KO, Helmers RA. Methotrexate pneumonitis: review of the literature and histopathological findings in nine patients. Eur Respir J 2000; 15: 373–381.

154. Lingenfelser T, Pfohl M, Grauer W et al. Nitrofurantoin-induzierte Hepatitis und Pneumonitis. Münch Med Wschr 1991; 133: 495–498.

155. Reinhart HH, Reinhart E, Korlipara P, Peleman R. Combined nitrofurantoin toxicity to liver and lung. Gastroenterology 1992; 102: 1396–1399.

156. Schattner A, Von der Walde J, Kozak N et al. Nitrofurantoin-induced immune-mediated lung and liver disease. Am J Med Sci 1999; 317: 336–340.

157. Mulberg AE, Bell LM. Fatal cholestatic hepatitis and multisystem failure associated with nitrofurantoin. J Pediatr Gastroenterol Nutr 1993; 17: 307–309.

158. De Vriese ASP, Philippe J, Van Renterghem DM et al. Carbamazepine hypersensitivity syndrome: report of 4 cases and review of the literature. Medicine (Baltimore) 1995; 74: 144–150.

159. Akoun GM, Mayaud CM, Touboul JL, Denis M. Methotrexate induced pneumonitis: diagnostic value of bronchoalveolar lavage cell data. Arch Intern Med 1986; 146: 804–805.

160. Schnabel A, Richter C, Bauerfeind S, Gross WL. Bronchoalveolar lavage cell profile in methotrexate induced pneumonitis. Thorax 1997; 52: 377–379.

161. Salaffi F, Manganelli P, Carotti M et al. Methotrexate-induced pneumonitis in patients with rheumatoid arthritis and psoriatic arthritis: report of five cases and review of the literature. Clin Rheumatol 1997; 16: 296–304.

162. Holland P, Mauer AM. Drug-induced in-vitro stimulation of peripheral lymphocytes. J Pediatr 1965; 1: 1368–1369.

163. Walzer RA, Feinstein R, Shapiro C, Einbinder J. Severe hypersensitivity reaction to gold. Positive lymphocyte transformation test. Arch Dermatol 1972; 106: 231–234.

164. Fujimori K, Yokoyama A, Kurita Y et al. Paclitaxel-induced cell-mediated hypersensitivity pneumonitis. Diagnosis using leukocyte migration test, bronchoalveolar lavage and transbronchial lung biopsy. Oncology 1998; 55: 340–344.

165. Starzl TE. Infectious pulmonary disease in patients receiving immunosuppressive therapy for organ transplantation – introduction. Rev Med Virol 1999; 9: 3–5.

166. Starzl TE. Infectious pulmonary disease in patients receiving immunosuppressive therapy for organ transplantation – commentary. Rev Med Virol 1999; 9: 10–14.

167. Schrijvers D, Catimel G, Highley M et al. KW-2149-induced pulmonary toxicity is not prevented by corticosteroids: a phase I and pharmacokinetic study. Anticancer Drugs 1999; 10: 633–639.

168. Setoyama M, Fukumaru S, Takasaki T et al. SLE with death from acute massive pulmonary hemorrhage caused by disseminated strongyloidiasis. Scan J Rheumatol 1997; 26: 389–391.

169. Kinjo T, Tsuhako K, Nakazato I et al. Extensive intra-alveolar haemorrhage caused by disseminated strongyloidiasis. Int J Parasitol 1998; 28: 323–330.

170. Benzaquen-Forner H, Dournovo P, Tandjaoui-Lambiotte H et al. Pneumopathie hypoxémiante sous traitement par IEC. Rev Mal Respir 1998; 15: 804–810.

171. Pedvis S, Anastakis D, Inman R. Churg–Strauss syndrome associated with zafirlukast. J Rheumatol 1999; 26: 1630.

172. Tuggey JM, Hosker HSR. Churg–Strauss syndrome associated with montelukast therapy. Thorax 2000; 55: 805–806.

173. Coëtmeur D, Guivarch G, Briens E, Lopes C. Pneumopathie éosinophilique aiguë. Rôle possible de la chloroquine. Rev Mal Respir 1998; 15: 657–660.

174. Kilbourne EM, Philen RM, Kamb ML, Falk H. Tryptophan produced by Showa Denko and epidemic eosinophilia–myalgia syndrome. J Rheumatol 1996; 23: 81–88.

175. Pincus T. Eosinophilia–myalgia syndrome: patient status 2–4 years after onset. J Rheumatol 1996; 23(Suppl 46): 19–24.

176. Rotmensch HH, Liron M, Tupilsky M, Laniado S. Possible association of pneumonitis with amiodarone therapy. Am Heart J 1980; 100: 412–413.

177. Adams PC, Gibson GJ, Morley AR et al. Amiodarone pulmonary toxicity: clinical and subclinical features. Q J Med 1986; 59: 449–471.

178. Zitnik RJ. Drug-induced lung disease: antiarrhythmic agents. J Respir Dis 1995; 17: 254–270.

179. Lombard JN. Pneumopathies de l'amiodarone. Medical Thesis, Université de Bourgogne, Dijon; 1990.

180. Vorperian VR, Havighurst TC, Miller S, January CT. Adverse effects of low dose amiodarone: a meta-analysis. J Am Coll Cardiol 1997; 30: 791–798.

181. Camus P. Drug history and remote exposure to drugs. A cause of lung disease? Eur Respir J 2000; 16: 381–384.

182. Chuang CL, Chern MS, Chang SC. Amiodarone toxicity in a patient with simultaneous involvement of cornea, thyroid gland, and lung. Am J Med Sci 2000; 320: 64–68.

183. Hopper KD, Potock PS. Hepatic and pulmonary accumulation of amiodarone. Am J Roentgenol 1994; 162: 1149–1450.

184. Camus P, Lombard JN, Perrichon M et al. Bronchiolitis obliterans organising pneumonia in patients taking acebutolol or amiodarone. Thorax 1989; 44: 711–715.

185. Aranda EA, Basanez RA, Jimenez YL. Bronchiolitis obliterans organising pneumonia secondary to amiodarone treatment. Neth J Med 1998; 53: 109–112.

186. Coudert B, Bailly F, André F et al. Amiodarone pneumonitis: bronchoalveolar lavage findings in 15 patients and review of the literature. Chest 1992; 102: 1005–1012.

187. Zhu YY, Botvinick E, Dae M et al. Gallium lung scintigraphy in amiodarone pulmonary toxicity. Chest 1988; 93: 1126–1131.

188. Wood DL, Osborn MJ, Rooke J, Holmes DR Jr. Amiodarone pulmonary toxicity: report of two cases associated with rapidly progressive fatal adult respiratory distress syndrome after pulmonary angiography. Mayo Clin Proc 1985; 60: 601–603.

189. Myers JL, Kennedy JI, Plumb VJ. Amiodarone lung: pathologic findings in clinically toxic patients. Hum Pathol 1987; 18: 349–354.

190. Bedrossian CW, Warren CJ, Ohar J, Bhan R. Amiodarone pulmonary toxicity: cytopathology, ultrastructure, and immunocytochemistry. Ann Diagn Pathol 1997; 1: 47–56.

191. Leonard A, Corris P, Parums D. Amiodarone pulmonary toxicity. Authors did not emphasise typical radiological and histological features sufficiently. Br Med J 1997; 314: 1831–1832.

192. Manresa F, Dorca J, Rodriguez Sanchon B et al. Recurrent form of amiodarone-induced pneumonitis. Chest 1984; 86: 944.

193. Scardi S, Ciani F, Pandullo C, Pivotti F. Alveolite ricorrente da amiodarone. G Ital Cardiol 1986; 16: 177–180.

194. Parra O, Ruiz J, Ojanguren I et al. Amiodarone toxicity: recurrence of interstitial pneumonitis after withdrawal of the drug. 1989; 2: 905–907.

195. Ashrafian H, Davey P. Is amiodarone an underrecognized cause of acute respiratory failure in the ICU? Chest 2001; 120: 275–282.

196. Donaldson L, Grant IS, Naysmith MR, Thomas JS. Acute amiodarone-induced lung toxicity. Intensive Care Med 1998; 24: 626–630.

197. Faller M, Quoix E, Popin E et al. Migratory pulmonary infiltrates in a patient treated with sotalol. Eur Respir J 1997; 10: 2159–2162.

198. Zucker PK, Khouri NF, Rosenshein NB. Bleomycin-induced pulmonary nodules: a variant of bleomycin pulmonary toxicity. Gynecol Oncol 1987; 28: 284–291.

199. Trump DL, Bartel E, Pozniak M. Nodular pneumonitis after chemotherapy for germ cell tumors. Ann Intern Med 1988; 109: 431–432.

200. Weyl Ben Arush M, Roguin A, Zamir E et al. Bleomycin and cyclophosphamide toxicity simulating metastatic nodules to the lungs in childhood cancer. Pediatr Hematol Oncol 1997; 14: 381–386.

201. Morley TF, Komansky HJ, Adelizzi RA, Giudice JC. Pulmonary gold toxicity. Eur J Respir Dis 1984; 65: 627–632.

202. Ogata K, Koga T, Yagawa K. Interferon-related bronchiolitis obliterans organizing pneumonia. Chest 1994; 106: 612–613.

203. Fawcett IW, Ibrahim NBN. BOOP associated with nitrofurantoin. Thorax 2001; 56: 161.

204. Nizami IY, Kissner DG, Vissher DW, Dubaybo BA. Idiopathic bronchiolitis obliterans with organizing pneumonia. An acute and life-threatening syndrome. Chest 1995; 108: 271–277.

205. Crestani B, Kambouchner M, Soler P et al. Migratory bronchiolitis obliterans organizing pneumonia after unilateral radiation therapy for breast carcinoma. Eur Respir J 1995; 8: 318–321.

206. Bayle J, Nesme P, Bejui-Thivolet F et al. Migratory organizing pneumonitis 'primed' by radiation therapy. Eur Respir J 1995; 8: 322–326.

207. Cohen AJ, King TE Jr, Downey GP. Rapidly progressive bronchiolitis obliterans with organizing pneumonia. Am J Respir Crit Care Med 1994; 149: 1670–1675.

208. Glasier CM, Siegel MJ. Multiple pulmonary nodules: unusual manifestation of bleomycin toxicity. AJR 1981; 137: 155–156.

209. Patel P, Honeybourne D, Watson RD. Amiodarone-induced pulmonary toxicity mimicking metastatic lung disease. Postgrad Med J 1987; 63: 393–394.

210. Piperno D, Donné C, Loire R, Cordier JF. Bronchiolitis obliterans organizing pneumonia associated with minocycline therapy: a possible cause. Eur Respir J 1995; 8: 1018–1020.

211. Steyerberg EW, Keizer HJ, Messemer JE et al. Residual pulmonary masses after chemotherapy for metastatic nonseminomatous germ cell tumor: prediction of histology. Cancer 1997; 79: 345–355.

212. Sostman HD, Putman CE, Gamsu G. Diagnosis of chemotherapy lung. AJR 1981; 136: 33–40.

213. Kreisman H, Wolkove N. Pulmonary toxicity of antineoplastic therapy. Semin Oncol 1992; 19: 508–520.

214. Bowers PN, Fields J, Schwartz D et al. Amiodarone induced pulmonary fibrosis in infancy. PACE 1998; 21: 1665–1667.

215. Lengyel C, Boros I, Varkonyi T et al. Amiodarone-induced pulmonary fibrosis. Orv Hetil 1996; 137: 1759–1762.

216. Robinson BWS. Nitrofurantoin-induced interstitial pulmonary fibrosis. Med J Austr 1983; 1: 72–76.

217. Geddes DM, Brostoff J. Pulmonary fibrosis associated with hypersensitivity to gold salts. Br Med J 1976; 1: 1444.

218. Chastzigiannis I, Schmidt KL, Stambolis C. Tödliche Lungenfibrose durch Gold Therapie? Z Rheumatol 1984; 43: 49–58.

219. Williams T, Eidus L, Thomas P. Fibrosing alveolitis, bronchiolitis obliterans, and sulfasalazine therapy. Chest 1982; 81: 766–768.

220. Tucker AS, Newman AJ, Alvorado C. Pulmonary, pleural and thoracic changes complicating chemotherapy. Radiology 1977; 125: 805–809.

221. Camus P, Reybet-Degat O, Justrabo E, Jeannin L. D-penicillamine-induced severe pneumonitis. Chest 1982; 81: 376–378.

222. Beskow CO, Drachenberg CB, Bourquin PM et al. Diffuse alveolar damage. Morphologic features in bronchoalveolar lavage fluid. Acta Cytol 2000; 44: 640–646.

223. Aymard JP, Gyger M, Lavallee R et al. A case of pulmonary alveolar proteinosis complicating chronic myelogenous leukemia. A peculiar pathologic aspect of busulfan lung? Cancer 1984; 53: 954–956.

224. Van der Veen MJ, Dekker JJ, Dinant HJ et al. Fatal pulmonary fibrosis complicating low dose methotrexate therapy for rheumatoid arthritis. J Rheumatol 1995; 22: 1766–1768.

225. Malik SW, Myers JL, DeRemee RA, Specks U. Lung toxicity associated with cyclophosphamide use. Two distinct patterns. Am J Respir Crit Care Med 1996; 154: 1851–1856.

226. Chap L, Shpiner R, Levine M et al. Pulmonary toxicity of high-dose chemotherapy for breast cancer: a non-invasive approach to diagnosis and treatment. Bone Marrow Transplant 1997; 20: 1063–1067.

227. Salvucci M, Zanchini R, Molinari A L et al. Lung toxicity following fludarabine, cytosine arabinoside and mitoxantrone (FLAN) treatment for acute leukemia. Haematologica 2000; 85: 769–770.

228. Dunsford ML, Mead GM, Bateman AC et al. Severe pulmonary toxicity in patients treated with a combination of docetaxel and gemcitabine for metastatic transitional cell carcinoma. Ann Oncol 1999; 10: 943–947.

229. Linskens RK, Golding RP, van Groeningen CJ, Giaccone G. Severe acute lung injury induced by gemcitabine. Neth J Med 2000; 56: 232–235.

230. Bone RC, Wolfe J, Sobonya RE et al. Desquamative interstitial pneumonia following long-term nitrofurantoin therapy. Am J Med 1976; 60: 697–701.

231. Soloaga ED, Beltramo MN, Veltri MA et al. Acute respiratory failure due to lipoid pneumonia. Medicina (B Aires) 2000; 60: 602–604.

232. Gondouin A, Manzoni P, Ranfaing E et al. Exogenous lipid pneumonia: a retrospective multicentre study of 44 cases in France. Eur Respir J 1996; 9: 1463–1469.

233. Carrillon Y, Tixier E, Revel D, Cordier JF. MR diagnosis of lipoid pneumonia. J Comput Assist Tomogr 1988; 12: 876–877.

234. Guichenez G, Polderman B, Durand G, Savin D. Signe de l'angiogramme positif: apport au diagnostic de pneumopathie huileuse exogène chez une personne âgée. Rev Pneumol Clin. 1999; 55: 51.

235. Bandla HPR, Davis SH, Hopkins NE. Lipoid pneumonia: a silent complication of mineral oil aspiration. Pediatrics 1999; 103: E191-E194.

236. Dongay G, Levade T, Caratero A et al. Etude biochimique et cytologique du liquide de lavage alvéolaire dans 4 cas de pneumopathies huileuses. Presse Med 1986; 15: 1863–1868.

237. Baillie J. Sulfasalazine and pulmonary infiltrates. Am J Gastroenterol 1984; 79: 77.

238. Pusateri DW, Muder RR. Fever, pulmonary infiltrates, and pleural effusion following acyclovir therapy for herpes zoster ophthalmicus. Chest 1990; 98: 754–756.

239. Takimoto CH, Lynch D, Stulbarg MS. Pulmonary infiltrates associated with sulindac therapy. Chest 1990; 97: 230–232.

240. Heyll A, Aul C, Gogolin F et al. Granulocyte colony-stimulating factor (G-CSF) treatment in a neutropenic leukemia patient with diffuse interstitial pulmonary infiltrates. Ann Hematol 1991; 63: 328–332.

241. Ramanathan RK, Belani CP. Transient pulmonary infiltrates: a hypersensitivity reaction to Paclitaxel. Ann Intern Med 1996; 124: 278.

242. Verlag GT. ACE-blocker associated interstitial infiltrates in the lungs. Dtsch Med Wschr 1996; 121: 81.

243. Jedynak U, Ciezarek M, Kopinski P. Pulmonary infiltrates with masto- and lymphocytosis in BALF associated with Arechine. Pol J Pathol 1997; 48: 63–67.

244. Biron P, Dessureault J, Napke E. Acute allergic interstitial pneumonitis induced by hydrochlorothiazide. Can Med Assoc J 1991; 145: 28–34.

245. Varnell RM, Godwin JD, Richardson ML, Vincent JM. Adult respiratory distress syndrome from overdose of tricyclic antidepressants. Radiology 1989; 170: 667–670.

246. Louria DB, Hensle T, Rose J. The major medical complications of heroin addiction. Ann Intern Med 1967; 67: 1–22.

247. Nielsen JM, Ingham SD, von Hagen KO. Pulmonary edema and embolism as complications of insulin shock in the treatment of schizophrenia. JAMA 1938; 111: 2455–2458.

248. Samet A, Bayoumeu F, Longrois D, Laxenaire MC. Acute pulmonary edema associated with use of beta-adrenergic agonists in tocolytic therapy. Ann Fr Anesth Reanim 2000; 19: 35–38.

249. Bernal C, Patarca R. Hydrochlorothiazide-induced pulmonary edema and associated immunologic changes. Ann Pharmacother 1999; 33: 172–174.

250. Palfi M, Berg S, Ernerudh J, Berlin G. A randomized controlled trial of transfusion-related acute lung injury: is plasma from multiparous blood donors dangerous? Transfusion 2001; 41: 317–322.

251. Heffner JE, Sahn SA. Salicylate-induced pulmonary edema: clinical features and prognosis. Ann Intern Med 1981; 95: 405–409.

252. Liebman RM, Katz HM. Pulmonary edema in a 52 year-old woman ingesting large amounts of aspirin. JAMA 1981; 246: 2227–2228.

253. Gonzolez ER, Cole T, Grimes MM et al. Recurrent ARDS in an 39-year-old woman with migraine headaches. Chest 1998; 114: 919–922.

254. Stadnyk A, Grossman RF. Nalbuphine-induced pulmonary edema. Chest 1986; 90: 773–774.

255. Vaylet F, Plotton C, Algayres JP et al. Oedème aigu du poumon après vinorelbine. Presse Med 1996; 25: 1259–1260.

256. Cattan CE, Oberg KC. Vinorelbine tartrate-induced pulmonary edema confirmed on rechallenge. Pharmacotherapy 1999; 19: 992–994.

257. Palmer SM, Robinson LJ, Wang AD et al. Massive pulmonary edema and death after prostacyclin infusion in a patient with pulmonary veno-occlusive disease. Chest 1998; 113: 237–240.

258. Sirventvon-Bueltzingsloewen A, Gratecos N, Legros L et al. Antithymocyte-associated reticulonodular pneumonitis during a conditioning regimen of reduced intensity for genoidentical bone marrow transplantation. Bone Marrow Transplant 2001; 27: 891–892.

259. Oldham RK, Brogley J, Braud E. Contrast medium 'recalls' interleukin-2 toxicity. J Clin Oncol 1990; 8: 942–943.

260. Hotton KM, Khorsand M, Hank J A et al. A phase Ib/II trial of granulocyte-macrophage-colony stimulating factor and interleukin-2 for renal cell carcinoma patients with pulmonary metastases. A case of fatal central nervous system thrombosis. Cancer 2000; 88: 1892–1901.

261. Taylor I, Watters M. Pulmonary oedema after ophthalmic regional anaesthesia in an unfasted patient undergoing elective surgery. Anaesthesia 2001; 56: 444–446.

262. Gertz MA, Lacy MQ, Bjornsson J, Litzow MR. Fatal pulmonary toxicity related to the administration of granulocyte colony-stimulating factor in amyloidosis: a report and review of growth factor-induced pulmonary toxicity. J Hematother Stem Cell Res 2000; 9: 635–643.

263. Averbuch SD, Yungbluth P. Fatal pulmonary hemorrhage due to nitrofurantoin. Arch Intern Med 1980; 140: 271–273.

264. Noseworthy TW, Davey RS, Percy JS, King EG. Hypoxemic respiratory failure in rheumatoid arthritis: gold related? Crit Care Med 1983; 11: 761–762.

265. Barnett VT, Bergmann F, Humphrey H, Chediak J. Diffuse alveolar hemorrhage secondary to superwarfarin ingestion. Chest 1992; 102: 1301–1302.

266. Cuellar Obispo E, Torrado Gonzalez E, Alvarez Bueno M et al. Spontaneous pulmonary hemorrhage following thrombolytic therapy in an acute myocardial infarct. Rev Esp Cardiol 1992; 45: 421–424.

267. Masip J, Vecilla F, Paez J. Diffuse pulmonary hemorrhage after fibrinolytic therapy for acute myocardial infarction. Int J Cardiol 1998; 63: 95–97.

268. Alperin JB, de Groot WJ, Cimo PL. Quinidine-induced thrombocytopenia with pulmonary hemorrhage. Arch Intern Med 1980; 140: 266–267.

269. Louie S, Gamble CN, Cross CE. Penicillamine associated pulmonary hemorrhage. J Rheumatol 1986; 13: 963–966.

270. Lauque D, Courtin JP, Fournie B et al. Syndrome pneumo-rénal induit par la D-pénicillamine: syndrome de Goodpasture ou polyartérite microscopique? Rev Med Interne 1990; 11: 168–171.

271. Ohtsuka M, Yamashita Y, Doi M, Hasegawa S. Propylthiouracil-induced alveolar haemorrhage associated with antineutrophil cytoplasmic antibody. Eur Respir J 1997; 10: 1405–1407.

272. Harper L, Cockwell P, Savage COS. Case of propylthiouracil-induced ANCA associated small vessel vasculitis. Nephrol Dialysis Transplant 1998; 13: 455–458.

273. Dhillon SS, Singh D, Doe N et al. Diffuse alveolar hemorrhage and pulmonary capillaritis due to propylthiouracil. Chest 1999; 116: 1485–1488.

274. Morita S, Ueda Y, Eguchi K. Anti-thyroid drug-induced ANCA-associated vasculitis: a case report and review of the literature. Endocrine J 2000; 47: 467–470.

275. Sleiman C, Raffy O, Roue C, Mal H. Fatal pulmonary hemorrhage during high-dose valproate monotherapy. Chest 2000; 117: 613.

276. Kalra S, Bell MR, Rihal CS. Alveolar hemorrhage as a complication of treatment with abciximab. Chest 2001; 120: 126–131.

277. Camus P. Manifestations respiratoires associées aux traitements par la D-pénicillamine. Rev Fr Mal Respir 1982; 10: 7–20.

278. Schwartzman KJ, Bowie DM, Yeadon C et al. Constrictive bronchiolitis obliterans following gold therapy for psoriatic arthritis. Eur Respir J 1995; 8: 2191–2193.

279. Clark JG, Crawford SW, Madtes DK, Sullivan KM. The clinical presentation and course of obstructive lung disease after allogeneic marrow transplantation. Ann Intern Med 1989; 111: 368–376.

280. Boehler A, Kesten S, Weder W, Speich R. Bronchiolitis obliterans after lung transplantation. A review. Chest 1998; 114: 1411–1426.

281. Yokoi T, Hirabayashi N, Ito M et al. Broncho-bronchiolitis obliterans as a complication of bone marrow transplantation: a clinicopathological study of eight autopsy cases. Virchows Arch 1997; 431: 275–282.

282. Chang YL, Yao YT, Wang NS, Lee YC. Segmental necrosis of small bronchi after prolonged intakes of Sauropus androgynus in Taiwan. Am J Respir Crit Care Med 1998; 157: 594–598.

283. Le Loet X, Ozenne G, Pinel B, Deshayes P. Atteinte bronchiolaire réversible au cours d'une polyarthrite rhumatoïde traitée par D-pénicillamine. Rhumatologie 1983; 35: 19–21.

284. Hsu H, Chang H, Goan Y. Intermediate results in Sauropus androgynus bronchiolitis obliterans patients after single-lung transplantation. Transplant Proc 2000; 32: 2422–2423.

285. Skaer TL. Medication-induced systemic lupus erythematosus. Clin Ther 1992; 14: 496–506.

286. Stridhar MK, Abdulla A. Fatal lupus-like syndrome and ARDS induced by fluvastatin. Lancet 1998; 352: 114.

287. Khosla R, Butman AN, Hammer DF. Simvastatin-induced lupus erythematosus. South Med J 1998; 91: 873–874.

288. Asherson RA, Zulman J, Hugues GRV. Pulmonary thromboembolism associated with procainamide-induced lupus syndrome and anticardiolipin antibodies. Ann Rheum Dis 1989; 48: 232–235.

289. Roche-Bayard P, Rossi R, Mann JM et al. Left pulmonary artery thrombosis in chlorpromazine-induced lupus. Chest 1990; 98: 1545.

290. Pfitzenmeyer P, Foucher P, Dennewald G et al. Pleuropulmonary changes induced by ergoline drugs. Eur Respir J 1996; 9: 1013–1019.

291. Miller DH, Haas LF. Pneumonitis, pleural effusion and pericarditis following treatment with dantrolene. J Neurol Neurosurg Psychiatry 1984; 47: 553–554.

292. Middleton KL, Santella R, Couser JI Jr. Eosinophilic pleuritis due to propylthiouracil. Chest 1993; 103: 955–956.

293. Farre JM, Perez T, Hautefeuille P et al. Pleurésie à éosinophiles induite par la salazosulfapyridine. Presse Med 1989; 18: 987–988.

294. Abramov Y, Elchalal U, Schenker JG. Pulmonary manifestations of severe ovarian hyperstimulation syndrome: a multicenter study. Fertil Steril 1999; 71: 645–651.

295. Urban C, Nirenberg A, Caparros B et al. Chemical pleuritis as the cause of acute chest pain following high-dose methotrexate treatment. Cancer 1983; 51: 34–37.

296. Bacon BR, Bailey-Newton RS, Connors AF Jr. Pleural effusion after endoscopic variceal sclerotherapy. Gastroenterology 1985; 88: 1910–1914.

297. Gurtner HP. Pulmonary hypertension, 'plexogenic pulmonary arteriopathy' and the appetite depressant drug aminorex: post or propter? Bull Eur Physiopathol Respir 1979; 15: 897–923.

298. Gaine SP, Rubin LJ, Kmetzo JJ et al. Recreational use of Aminorex and pulmonary hypertension. Chest 2000; 118: 1496–1500.

299. Abenhaim L, Moride Y, Brenot F et al, Group at IPPHS. Appetite-suppressant drugs and the risk of primary pulmonary hypertension. N Engl J Med 1996; 335: 609–616.

300. Delcroix M, Kurz X, Walckiers D et al. High incidence of primary pulmonary hypertension associated with appetite suppressants in Belgium. Eur Respir J 1998; 12: 271–276.

301. Lowenstein E, Zapol WM. Protamine reactions, explosive mediator release, and pulmonary vasoconstriction. Anesthesiology 1990; 73: 373–375.

302. McCarthy JT, Staats BA. Pulmonary hypertension, hemolytic anemia, and renal failure. A mitomycin-associated syndrome. Chest 1986; 89: 608–611.

303. Lesesne JB, Rotschild N, Erickson B et al. Cancer-associated hemolytic–uremic syndrome: analysis of 85 cases from a National Registry. J Clin Oncol 1989; 7: 781–789.

304. Montes A, Powles TJ, O'Brien MER et al. A toxic interaction between mitomycin C and tamoxifen causing the haemolytic uraemic syndrome. Eur J Cancer 1993; 29: 1854–1857.

305. Van der Heijden M, Ackland SP, Deveridge S. Haemolytic uraemic syndrome associated with bleomycin, epirubicin and cisplatin chemotherapy – a case report and review of the literature. Acta Oncol 1998; 37: 107–109.

306. Linette DC, McGee KH, McFarland JA. Mitomycin-induced pulmonary toxicity: case report and review of the literature. Ann Pharmacother 1992; 26: 481–484.

307. Torra R, Poch E, Torras A et al. Pulmonary hemorrhage as a clinical manifestation of hemolytic–uremic syndrome associated with mitomycin C therapy. Chemotherapy 1993; 39: 453–456.

308. Boven E, Pinedo HM. Mitomycin C: interstitial pneumonitis and haemolytic–uraemic syndrome. A report of two cases and review of the literature. Neth J Med 1983; 26: 153–156.

309. Schmidt RH, Lenz T, Gröne H-J et al. Haemolytic-uraemic syndrome after tacrolimus rescue therapy for cortisone-resistant rejection. Nephrol Dial Transplant 1999; 14: 979–983.

310. Joselson R, Warnock M. Pulmonary veno-occlusive disease after chemotherapy. Hum Pathol 1983; 14: 88–91.

311. Rose AG. Pulmonary veno-occlusive disease due to bleomycin therapy for lymphoma. SA Med J 1983; 64: 636–638.

312. Capewell SJ, Wright AJ, Ellis DA. Pulmonary veno-occlusive disease in association with Hodgkin's disease. Thorax 1984; 39: 554–555.

313. Lombard CM, Churg A, Winokur S. Pulmonary veno-occlusive disease following therapy for malignant neoplasms. Chest 1987; 92: 871–876.

314. Kramer MR, Estenne M, Berkman N et al. Radiation-induced pulmonary veno-occlusive disease. Chest 1993; 104: 1282–1284.

315. Vansteenkiste JF, Bomans P, Verbeken EK et al. Fatal pulmonary veno-occlusive disease possibly related to gemcitabine. Lung Cancer 2001; 31: 83–85.

316. Zreik TG, Odunsi K, Cass I et al. A case of fatal pulmonary thromboembolism associated with the use of intravenous estrogen therapy. Fertility Sterility 1999; 71: 373–375.

317. Parkin L, Skegg DCG, Wilson M et al. Oral contraceptives and fatal pulmonary embolism. Lancet 2000; 355: 2133–2134.

318. Maynes D. Bilateral pulmonary embolism in a patient on clozapine therapy. Can J Psychiatry 2000; 45: 296–297.

319. Cianciulli P. Pulmonary embolism and intravenous high-dose desferrioxamine. Haematologica 1992; 77: 368–369.

320. Barbui T, Rodeghiero F, Meli S, Dini E. Fatal pulmonary embolism and antithrombin III deficiency in adult lymphoblastic leukaemia during L-asparaginase therapy. Acta Hematol 1983; 69: 188–191.

321. Alliot C, Rapin JP, Besson M et al. Pulmonary embolism after intravenous immunoglobulin. J Roy Soc Med 2001; 94: 187–188.

322. Kitchell CC, Balogh K. Pulmonary lipid emboli in association with long-term hyperalimentation. Hum Pathol 1986; 17: 83–85.

323. Jiménez-Yuste V, Martin MP, Canales M et al. Pulmonary embolism in a patient with acute promyelocytic leukemia treated with all-trans retinoic acid. Leukemia 1997; 11: 1988–1989.

324. Smits HFM, Vanrijk PP, Vanisselt JW et al. Pulmonary embolism after thrombolysis of hemodialysis grafts. J Am Soc Nephrol 1997; 8: 1458–1461.

325. Tomashefski JF Jr, Hirsch CS, Jolly PN. Microcrystalline cellulose pulmonary embolism and granulomatosis: a complication of illicit intravenous injections of pentazocine tablets. Arch Pathol Lab Med 1981; 105: 89–93.

326. Tsokos M, Bartel A, Schoel R et al. Tödliche Lungenarterienembolie nach endoskopischer Embolisation einer 'Downhill-Varize' des Ösophagus. Dtsch Med Wschr 1998; 123: 691–695.

327. Roesch W, Rexroth G. Pulmonary, cerebral and coronary emboli during bucrylate injection of bleeding fundic varices. Endoscopy 1998; 30: S89–S90.

328. Famularo G, Liberati C, Sebastiani GD, Polchi S. Pulmonary embolism after intra-articular injection of methylprednisolone and hyaluronate. Clin Exp Rheumatol 2001; 19: 355.

329. Pelz DM, Lownie SP, Fox AJ, Hutton LC. Symptomatic pulmonary complications from liquid acrylate embolization of brain arteriovenous malformations. Am J Neuroradiol 1995; 16: 19–26.

330. Padovani B, Kasriel O, Brunner P, Peretti-Viton P. Pulmonary embolism caused by acrylic cement: A rare complication of percutaneous vertebroplasty. Am J Neuroradiol 1999; 20: 375–377.

331. De Mey A. Surgical treatment of lipodystrophies. Rev Med Brux 1996; 17: 240–243.

332. Kannan S, Morrow B, Furness G. Tension pneumothorax and pneumomediastinum after nasogastric tube insertion. Anaesthesia 1999; 54: 1012–1013.

333. Nolan RL, McAdams HP. Bronchopericardial fistula after placement of an automatic implantable cardioverter defibrillator: radiographic and CT findings. AJR 1999; 172: 365–368.

334. Rumi MN, Schumann R, Freeman RB et al. Acute transjugular intrahepatic portosystemic shunt migration into pulmonary artery during liver transplantation. Transplantation 1999; 67: 1492–1494.

335. McEachern RC, Patel RG. Pneumopericardium associated with face-mask continuous positive airway pressure. Chest 1997; 112: 1441–1443.

336. Devys JM, Balleau C, Jayr C, Bourgain JL. Biting the laryngeal mask: an unusual cause of negative pressure pulmonary edema. Can J Anaesth 2000; 47: 176–178.

337. Carbognani P, Solli P, Rusca M et al. Pneumomediastinum following Politzer's manoeuvre. Thorax 1996; 51: 1169.

338. Iqbal M, Multz AS, Rossoff LJ, Lackner RP. Reexpansion pulmonary edema after VATS successfully treated with continuous positive airway pressure. Ann Thorac Surg 2000; 70: 669–671.

339. Badaoui R, Choufane S, Riboulot M et al. Perforation de l'oesophage après échocardiographie transoesophagienne. Ann Fr Anesth Réanim 1994; 13: 850–852.

340. Ritter HG, Tarala R. Pneumothorax after acupuncture. Br Med J 1978; 2: 602–603.

341. Areno JP, McCartney JP, Eggerstedt J et al. Persistent pleural effusions following coronary bypass surgery. Chest 1998; 114: 311–314.

342. Althoff M, Schoenemann J, Wienhold ST, Spitz P. Mediastinal abscess following sclerotherapy of oesophageal varices. Endoscopy 1995; 27: 630.

343. Hwang SS, Kim HH, Park SH et al. N-butyl-2-cyanoacrylate pulmonary embolism after endoscopic injection sclerotherapy for gastric variceal bleeding. J Comput Assist Tomogr 2001; 25: 16–22.

344. Sullivan M. Unilateral negative pressure pulmonary edema during anesthesia with a laryngeal mask airway. Can J Anaesth 1999; 46: 1053–1056.

345. Willoughby PH, Beers RA, Murphy KD. Pulmonary edema after transjugular intrahepatic portosystemic shunt. Anesth Analy 1996; 82: 895–896.

346. Reinert KU, Sybrecht GW. T helper cell alveolitis after bacillus Calmette–Guérin immunotherapy for superficial bladder tumor. J Urol 1994; 151: 1634–1635.

347. Talbot EA, Perkins MD, Silva SFM, Frothingham R. Disseminated Bacille Calmette–Guérin disease after vaccination: case report and review. Clin Infect Dis 1997; 24: 1139–1146.

348. Nimmagadda U, Salem MR. Acute bronchospasm associated with methylmethacrylate cement. Anesthesiology 1998; 89: 1290–1291.

349. Matsuo T, Tsukamoto Y, Tamura M et al. Acute respiratory failure due to 'pulmonary calciphylaxis' in a maintenance haemodialysis patient. Nephron 2001; 87: 75–79.

350. Choi HK, Merkel PA, Cohen-Tervaert JW et al. Alternating antineutrophil cytoplasmic antibody specificity. Drug-induced vasculitis in a patient with Wegener's granulomatosis. Arthr Rheum 1999; 42: 384–388.

351. Orriols R, Munoz X, Ferrer J et al. Cocaine-induced Churg–Strauss vasculitis. Eur Respir J 1995; 9: 175–177.

352. Josefson D. Asthma drug linked with Churg–Strauss syndrome. Br Med J 1997; 315: 330.

353. Kränke B, Aberer W. Macrolide-induced Churg–Strauss syndrome in patient with atopy. Lancet 1997; 350: 1551–1552.

354. Katz RS, Papernik M. Zafirlukast and Churg–Strauss syndrome. JAMA 1998; 279: 1949.

355. Schmitz Schumann M, Palca A, Simon U, Blaser K. Aspirin-induced asthma and Churg–Strauss-syndrome. Eur J Clin Invest 1998; 28(Suppl 1): A49.

356. Vanoli M, Gambini D, Scorza R. A case of Churg–Strauss vasculitis after hepatitis B vaccination. Ann Rheum Dis 1998; 57: 256–257.

357. Villena V, Hidalgo R, Sotelo MT, Martin-Escribano P. Montelukast and Churg–Strauss syndrome. Eur Respir J 2000; 15: 626.

358. Frankel SR, Eardley A, Lauwers G et al. The 'retinoic acid syndrome' in acute promyelocytic leukemia. Ann Intern Med 1992; 117: 292–296.

359. Maloisel F, Petit T, Kessler R, Oberling F. Cytologic examination of broncho-alveolar fluid during the retinoic acid syndrome. Eur J Haematol 1996; 56: 319–320.

360. Van de Loodsdrecht AA, van Imhoff GW. All-trans-retinoic acid related pulmonary syndrome. Neth J Med 1999; 54: 131–132.

361. Raanani P, Segal E, Levi I et al. Diffuse alveolar hemorrhage in acute promyelocytic leukemia patients treated with ATRA – a manifestation of the basic disease or the treatment? Leukemia Lymphoma 2000; 37: 605–610.

362. Tryka AF, Godleski JJ, Fanta CH. Leukemic cell lysis pneumopathy. A complication of treated myeloblastic leukemia. Cancer 1982; 50: 2763–2770.

363. Marenco JP, Nervi A, White AC. ARDS associated with tumor lysis syndrome in a patient with non-Hodgkin's lymphoma. Chest 1998; 113: 550–552.

364. Gulbahce HE, Manivel JC, Jessurun J. Pulmonary cytolytic thrombi – a previously unrecognized complication of bone marrow transplantation. Am J Surg Pathol 2000; 24: 1147–1152.

365. Woodard JP, Gulbahce E, Shreve M et al. Pulmonary cytolytic thrombi: a newly recognized complication of stem cell transplantation. Bone Marrow Transplant 2000; 25: 293–300.

366. Cohen AF, Warman SP. Upper airway obstruction secondary to warfarin-induced sublingual hematoma. Arch Otolaryngol 1989; 115: 718–720.

367. Reussi C, Schiavi J E, Altman R et al. Unusual complications in the course of anticoagulant therapy. Am J Med 1969; 46: 460–463.

368. Moncada RM, Venta LA, Venta ER et al. Tracheal and bronchial cartilaginous rings: warfarin sodium-induced calcification. Radiology 1992; 184: 437–439.

369. Hartstock RJ. Postvaccinal lymphadenitis. Hyperplasia of lymphoid tissue that stimulates malignant lymphoma. Cancer 1968; 21: 632–649.

370. Brown JM. Drug-associated lymphadenopathies with special reference to the Reed–Sternberg cell. Med J Aust 1971; 58: 375–378.

371. Sorell TC, Forbes IJ. Phenytoin sensitivity in a case of phenytoin-associated Hodgkin's disease. Austr NZ J Med 1975; 5: 144–147.

372. Lafeuillade A, Bolla G, Horschowski N et al. Lymphadénopathies sous sulfasalazine au cours d'une polyarthrite rhumatoïde. Presse Med 1989; 18: 1709.

373. Bobbio-Pallavicini E, Valsecchi C, Tacconi F et al. Sarcoidosis following beta-interferon therapy for multiple myeloma. Sarcoidosis 1995; 12: 140–142.

374. Olmer J, Paillas J, Roger J et al. Manifestations ganglionnaires au cours de traitements par la méthyl-3-phenyl éthyl-5-hydantoïne. Presse Med 1952; 11: 1748–1750.

375. Gams RA, Neal JA, Conrad FG. Hydantoin-induced pseudo-pseudolymphoma. Ann Intern Med 1968; 69: 557–568.

376. Trump DL, Ettinger DS, Feldman MJ, Dragon LH. 'Sarcoidosis' and sarcoid-like lesions. Their occurrence after cytotoxic and radiation therapy for testis cancer. Arch Intern Med 1981; 141: 37–38.

377. Swinburn CR. Pulmonary infiltration and lymphadenopathy in association with fenbufen. Hum Toxicol 1988; 7: 35–36.

378. Yonemaru M, Mizuguchi Y, Kasuga I et al. Hilar and mediastinal lymphadenopathy with hypersensitivity pneumonitis induced by penicillin. Chest 1992; 102: 1907–1909.

379. Merchant TE, Filippa DA, Yahalom J. Sarcoidosis following chemotherapy for Hodgkin's disease. Leukemia Lymphoma 1994; 13: 339–347.

380. Saltzstein SL, Ackerman LV. Lymphadenopathy induced by anticonvulsant drugs and mimicking clinically and pathologically malignant lymphomas. Cancer 1959; 12: 164–182.

381. Hymen GA, Sommers SC. The development of Hodgkin's disease and lymphoma during anticonvulsant therapy. Blood 1966; 28: 416–427.

382. Li FP, Willard DR, Goodman R, Vawter G. Malignant lymphoma after diphenylhydantoin (Dilantin) therapy. Cancer 1975; 36: 1359–1362.

383. Rosenthal CJ, Noguera CA, Coppola A, Kapelner SN. Pseudolymphoma with mycosis fungoides manifestations, hyperresponsiveness to diphenylhydantoin, and lymphocyte dysregulation. Cancer 1982; 49: 2305–2314.

384. Yates P, Stockdill G, McIntyre M. Hypersensitivity to carbamazepine presenting as pseudolymphoma. J Clin Pathol 1986; 39: 1224–1228.

385. Vander Els NJ, Gerdes H. Sarcoidosis and IFN-alpha treatment. Chest 2000; 117: 294.

386. Krehmeier H. Sarcoidosis after interferon-alpha in hepatitis-C. Dtsch Med Wschr 2001; 126: 460.

387. Blanche P, Passeron A, Gombert B et al. Sarcoidosis and HIV infection: influence of highly active antiretroviral therapy. Br J Dermatol 1999; 140: 1185.

388. Naccache JM, Antoine M, Wislez M et al. Sarcoid-like pulmonary disorder in human immunodeficiency virus-infected patients receiving antiretroviral therapy. Am J Respir Crit Care Med 1999; 159: 2009–2013.

389. Wohlrab JL, Read CA, O'Donnell AE. Granulomatous interstitial lung disease in patients with human immunodeficiency virus on highly active antiretroviral therapy. Chest 2000; 118: 288S.

390. Geldmacher H, Taube C, Markert U, Kirsten DK. Nearly fatal complications of cervical lymphadenitis following BCG immunotherapy for superficial bladder cancer. Respiration 2001; 68: 420–421.

391. Teates CD. Steroid-induced mediastinal lipomatosis. Radiology 1970; 96: 501–502.

392. Sorhage F, Stover DE, Mortazavi A. Unusual etiology of cough in a woman with asthma. Chest 1996; 110: 852–854.

393. Taille C, Fartoukh M, Houel R et al. Spontaneous hemomediastinum complicating steroid-induced mediastinal lipomatosis. Chest 2001; 120: 311–313.

394. Järveläinen H, Vainionpää H, Kuopio T, Lehtonen A. A woman with nodules in her lungs. Lancet 1998; 351: 494.

395. Egan AJM, Tazelaar HD, Myers JL, Abell-Aleff PC. Munchausen syndrome presenting as pulmonary talcosis. Arch Pathol Lab Med 1999; 123: 736–738.

396. Waien SA, Hayes DJ, Leonardo JM. Severe coagulopathy as a consequence of smoking crack cocaine laced with rodenticide. N Engl J Med 2001; 345: 700–701.

397. Gutiérrez F, Leon L. Elemental mercury embolism to the lung. N Engl J Med 2000; 342: 1791.

398. Bhagat R, Holmes IH, Kulaga A et al. Self-injection with olive oil. A cause of lipoid pneumonia. Chest 1995; 107: 875–876.

399. Munker R, Grützner S, Hiller E et al. Second malignancies after Hodgkin's disease: the Munich experience. Ann Hematol 1999; 78: 544–554.

400. Neugut AI, Ahsan H, Antman KH. Incidence of malignant pleural mesothelioma after thoracic radiotherapy. Cancer 1997; 80: 948–950.

401. Lewis BM, Izbicki R. Routine pulmonary function tests during bleomycin therapy. Tests may be ineffective and potentially misleading. JAMA 1980; 243: 347–351.

402. Mason JW. Prediction of amiodarone-induced pulmonary toxicity. Am J Med 1987; 86: 2–3.

403. Horowitz LN. Detection of amiodarone pulmonary toxicity: to screen or not to screen, that is the question! J Am Coll Cardiol 1988; 12: 789–790.

404. Kerin NZ, Rubenfire M. Detection of amiodarone pulmonary toxicity. J Am Coll Cardiol 1989; 13: 261–262.

405. Vrobel TR, Miller PE, Mostow ND, Rakita L. A general overview of amiodarone toxicity: its prevention, detection and management. Progr Cardiovasc Dis 1989; 31: 393–426.

406. Ulrik CS, Aldershvile J. Early diagnosis of amiodarone-induced pulmonary toxicity: are repeated lung function tests of any value? Ugeskr Laeger 1996; 158: 3445–3447.

407. Carroll GJ, Thomas R, Pathouros CC et al. Incidence, prevalence and possible risk factors for pneumonitis in patients with rheumatoid arthritis receiving methotrexate. J Rheumatol 1994; 21: 51–54.

408. Cottin V, Tébib J, Massonnet B et al. Pulmonary function in patients receiving long-term low-dose methotrexate. Chest 1996; 109: 933–938.

409. Bell MR, Meredith DJ, Gill PG. Role of carbon monoxide diffusing capacity in the early detection of major bleomycin-induced pulmonary toxicity. Austr NZ J Med 1985; 15: 235–240.

410. Simon M, Seiger RS. Aspirin desensitization in aspirin-sensitive asthmatic patients: clinical manifestations and characterization of the refractory period. J Allergy Clin Immunol 1982; 69: 11.

411. Schaefer OP, Gore JM. Aspirin sensitivity: the role for aspirin challenge and desensitization in postmyocardial infarction patients. Cardiology 1999; 91: 8–13.

412. Szczeklik A, Stevenson DD. Aspirin-induced asthma: advances in pathogenesis and management. J Allergy Clin Immunol 1999; 104: 5–13.

413. Kremer JM, Alarcon GS, Weinblatt ME et al. Clinical, laboratory, radiographic, and histopathologic features of methotrexate-associated lung injury in patients with rheumatoid arthritis. Arthr Rheum 1997; 40: 1829–1837.

414. Logan PM. Thoracic manifestations of external beam radiotherapy. AJR 1998; 171: 569–577.

415. Roach M, Gandara DR, Yuo HS et al. Radiation pneumonitis following combined modality therapy for lung cancer: analysis of prognostic factors. J Clin Oncol 1995; 13: 2606–2612.

416. Veinot JP, Edwards WD. Pathology of radiation-induced heart disease. A surgical and autopsy study of 27 cases. Hum Pathol 1996; 27: 766–773.

417. Roswit B, White DC. Severe radiation injuries of the lung. AJR 1977; 129: 127–136.

418. Martin C, Romero S, Sanchez-Paya J et al. Bilateral lymphocytic alveolitis: a common reaction after unilateral thoracic irradiation. Eur Respir J 1999; 13: 727–732.

419. Roberts CM, Foulcher E, Zaunders JJ et al. Radiation pneumonitis: a possible lymphocyte-mediated hypersensitivity reaction. Ann Intern Med 1993; 118: 696–700.

420. Kwa SLS, Lebesque JV, Theuws JCM et al. Radiation pneumonitis as a function of mean lung dose: an analysis of pooled data of 540 patients. Int J Radiation Oncol Biol Phys 1998; 42: 1–9.

421. Davis SD, Yankelevitz DF, Henschke CI. Radiation effects on the lung: clinical features, pathology, and imaging findings. AJR 1992; 159: 1157–1164.
422. Movsas B, Raffin TA, Epstein AH, Link CJ. Pulmonary radiation injury. Chest 1997; 111: 1061–1076.
423. Ma LD, Taylor GA, Wharam MD, Wiley JM. Recall pneumonitis: Adriamycin potentiation of radiation pneumonitis in two children. Radiology 1993; 187: 465–467.
424. Johansson S, Bjermer L, Franzen L, Henriksson R. Effects of ongoing smoking on the development of radiation-induced pneumonitis in breast cancer and oesophagus cancer patients. Radiother Oncol 1998; 49: 41–47.
425. Byhardt RW, Abrams R, Almagro U. The association of adult respiratory distress syndrome (ARDS) with thoracic irradiation (RT). Int J Radiat Oncol Biol Phys 1988; 50: 1441–1446.
426. Castellino RA, Glatstein E, Turbow MM et al. Latent radiation injury of lung or heart activated by steroid withdrawal. Ann Intern Med 1974; 80: 593–599.
427. Park KJ, Chung JY, Chun MS, Suh JH. Radiation induced lung disease and the impact of radiation methods on imaging features. Radiographics 2000; 20: 83–98.
428. Glazer HS, Lee JKT, Levitt RG et al. Radiation fibrosis: differentiation from recurrent tumour by MR imaging. Radiology 1985; 156: 721–726.
429. Zinzani PL, Gherlinzoni F, Piovaccari G et al. Cardiac injury as late toxicity of mediastinal radiation therapy for Hodgkin's disease patients. Haematologica 1996; 81: 132–137.
430. Freedman GS, Lofgen SB, Kligerman MM. Radiation-induced changes in pulmonary perfusion. Radiology 1974; 112: 435–437.
431. Crestani B, Valeyre D, Roden S et al. Bronchiolitis obliterans organizing pneumonia syndrome primed by radiation therapy to the breast. Am J Respir Crit Care Med 1998; 158: 1929–1935.
432. Arbetter KR, Prakash UBS, Tazelaar HD, Douglas WW. Radiation-induced pneumonitis in the 'nonirradiated' lung. Mayo Clin Proc 1999; 74: 27–36.
433. Rowinsky EK, Abeloff MD, Wharam MD. Spontaneous pneumothorax following thoracic radiation. Chest 1985; 88: 703–708.
434. Ward MJ, Davies D. Pulmonary aspergilloma after radiation therapy. Br J Dis Chest 1982; 76: 361–364.
435. De Vito EL, Quadrelli SA, Montiel GC, Roncoroni AJ. Bilateral diaphragmatic paralysis after mediastinal radiotherapy. Respiration 1996; 63: 187–190.
436. Lee YC, Tribe AE, Musk AW. Chylothorax from radiation-induced mediastinal fibrosis. Austr NZ J Med 1998; 28: 667–668.
437. Jochelson MS, Tarbell NJ, Weinstein HJ. Unusual thoracic radiographic findings in children treated for Hodgkin's disease. J Clin Oncol 1986; 4: 874–882.
438. Morrison HI, Semeciw R, Mao Y, Wigle DT. Cancer mortality among a group of fluorspar miners exposed to radon progeny. Am J Epidemiol 1988; 128: 1266–1275.
439. Wagoner JK, Archer VE, Lundin FE et al. Radiation as a cause of lung cancer among uranium miners. N Engl J Med 1965; 273: 181.
440. Hodgson JT, Jones RD. Mortality of a cohort of tin miners 1941–86. Br J Ind Med 1990; 47: 665–676.
441. Rall JE, Alpers JB, Lewallen CG et al. Radiation pneumonitis and fibrosis: a complication of radioiodine treatment of pulmonary metastases from cancer of the thyroid. J Clin Endocrinol Metab 1957; 17: 1263–1276.
442. Lin M. Radiation pneumonitis caused by Yttrium-90 microspheres: radiologic findings. AJR 1994; 162: 1300–1302.
443. Albertson TE, Walby WF, Derlet RW. Stimulant-induced pulmonary toxicity. Chest 1995; 108: 1140–1149.
444. Cruz R, Davis M, O'Neil H et al. Pulmonary manifestation on inhaled street drugs. Heart Lung 1998; 27: 297–305.
445. Seaman ME. Barotrauma related to inhalational drug abuse. J Emerg Med 1990; 8: 141–149.
446. Tashkin DP, Khalsa ME, Gorelick D et al. Pulmonary status of habitual cocaine smokers. Am Rev Respir Dis 1992; 145: 92–100.
447. Bailey M, Fraire A, Greenberg S et al. Pulmonary histopathology in cocaine abusers. Hum Pathol 1994; 25: 203–207.
448. Hoffman K, Goodman PC. Pulmonary edema in cocaine smokers. Radiology 1989; 172: 463–465.
449. Hughes S, Calverley PMA. Heroin inhalation and asthma. Br Med J 1988; 297: 1511–1512.
450. Klinger JR, Bensadoun E, Corrao WM. Pulmonary complications from alveolar accumulation of carbonaceous materials in a cocaine smoker. Chest 1992; 101: 1171–1173.
451. Rubin R, Neugarten J. Cocaine-associated asthma. Am J Med 1990; 88: 438–439.
452. Osborn HH, Tang M, Bradley K, Duncan BR. New onset bronchospasm or recrudescence of asthma associated with cocaine abuse. Acad Emerg Med 1997; 4: 689–692.
453. Rome LA, Lippmann ML, Dalsey WC et al. Prevalence of cocaine use and its impact on asthma exacerbation in an urban population. Chest 2000; 117: 1324–1329.
454. Perez GMGR, Bragado FG, Gil AMP. Pulmonary hemorrhage and antiglomerular basement membrane antibody-mediated glomerulonephritis after exposure to smoked cocaine (crack): a case report and review of the literature. Pathol Int 1997; 47: 692–697.
455. Forrester JM, Steele AW, Waldron JA, Parsons PE. Crack lung: an acute pulmonary syndrome with a spectrum of clinical and histopathological findings. Am Rev Respir Dis 1990; 142: 462–467.
456. Taylor RF, Bernard GR. Airway complications from free-basing cocaine. Chest 1989; 95: 476–477.
457. Haim DY, Lippmann ML, Goldberg SK, Walkenstein MD. The pulmonary complications of crack cocaine. A comprehensive review. Chest 1995; 107: 233–240.
458. Tashkin DP, Coulson AH, Clark VA et al. Respiratory symptoms and lung function in habitual heavy smokers of marijuana alone, smokers of marijuana and tobacco, smokers of tobacco alone and non-smokers. Am Rev Respir Dis 1987; 135: 205–216.
459. Tashkin DP, Simmons MS, Sherril DL, Coulson AH. Heavy habitual marijuana smoking does not cause an accelerated decline in FEV$_1$ with age. Am J Respir Crit Care Med 1997; 155: 141–148.
460. Ashton CH. Adverse effects of cannabis and cannabinoids. Br J Anaesth 1999; 83: 637–649.
461. Hall W. The respiratory risks of cannabis smoking. Addiction 1998; 93: 1461–1463.
462. Dowling G, McDonough E, Bost R. Eve and Ecstasy. A report of five deaths associated with the use of MDEA and MDMA. JAMA 1987; 257: 1615–1617.
463. Albertson TE, Walby WF. Respiratory toxicities from stimulant use. Clin Rev Allergy Immunol 1997; 15: 221–241.
464. Kleerup EC, Wong M, Marques Magallanes JA et al. Acute effects of intravenous cocaine on pulmonary artery pressure and cardiac index in habitual crack smokers. Chest 1997; 111: 30–35.
465. Lemoine R, Dusmet M. Pulmonary granulomas in an intravenous drug user. N Engl J Med 2000; 343: 1312.
466. Paré JAP, Coté G, Fraser RS. Long-term follow-up of drug abusers with intravenous talcosis. Am Rev Respir Dis 1989; 139: 233–241.
467. Ward S, Heyneman LE, Reittner P et al. Talcosis associated with IV abuse of oral medications: CT findings. AJR 2000; 174: 789–793.
468. Hecht SR, Berger M. Right-sided endocarditis in intravenous drug users. Prognostic features in 102 episodes. Ann Intern Med 1992; 117: 560–566.

30 Toxic lung injury: inhaled agents

David J Hendrick

 Key points

- The major sites of inhalation injury depend on the nature of the exposure agent (highly soluble gases are chiefly deposited proximally, small particles distally) and its dose – high dose levels leading to more widespread involvement.

- The effects are largely non-specific, reflecting direct damage (largely through alkaline, acidic, thermal or oxidant reactions) and the inflammatory and healing responses that follow.

- The wide range of effects can conveniently be classified by time of onset into acute, subacute and chronic categories.

- Although most severe events are occupational in origin, many may occur in domestic or recreational environments or in the general environment – usually as a consequence of accidents.

A large variety of inhaled agents can produce a variety of toxic reactions in the lungs, both acute and chronic. The chronic effects may be consequences of the acute effects (generally the result of an unpredictable accident) or the more predictable consequence of regular ongoing exposure that has no detectable adverse effect following exposure over a single day. These effects are not always readily distinguished from those brought about by 'non-toxic' processes including allergy, autoimmunity, autonomic reflexes, barotrauma, haemodynamic disruption and infection. This reflects the limited spectrum of response available at each level of pulmonary tissue when exposure occurs to environmental or endogenous insults. Some 'toxic' agents are of course microbial in origin, and their effects may not be sensibly distinguished from those of infection, and some toxic chemicals additionally behave has allergens. The pattern of response may therefore be complex and may vary widely between individuals according to differences in susceptibility and differences in exposure 'dose'. The spectrum ranges from mild mucosal irritation at one extreme to severe parenchymal disruption and death at the other.

There is generally an acute inflammatory response, which may be followed by a destructive or distorting fibrotic process or even malignant transformation, the clinical consequences of which are determined largely by the major site of involvement. This, in turn, depends on solubility and the ensuing pH (for gases, vapours and certain chemical dusts), particle size (for aerosols such as dusts, fog, fumes, mists, smog and smoke) and on whether toxic molecules become adsorbed on to the surface of inhaled particles. These various physical forms in which respirable environmental agents may be encountered are defined in Table 30.1. The greater the solubility and the greater the particle size, the more proximal are the major effects. Particles 10 mm or more in diameter are generally deposited in the nose and throat, as are most particles of 5–10 mm in diameter. Most deposition in the intrathoracic airways occurs over a particle diameter range of 1–10 mm, whereas the optimal size for particles to be retained in the gas-exchanging tissues is 0.05–5 mm.

The major site of involvement is not necessarily the only site, particularly for gases and vapours or particles of respirable size (i.e. aerodynamic diameter sufficiently small to allow penetration to the alveoli). Different levels within the respiratory tract may consequently be affected by a given exposure, and some overlap in the nature of the effects is to be expected – especially if the exposure is prolonged and there is greater opportunity to involve different levels.

Potency and dose provide the two other determinants of critical importance, assuming host susceptibility is similar among different subjects. Such an assumption, a fundamental characteristic that usually distinguishes toxicity from hypersensitivity and idiosyncrasy, is not fully valid and the severity of response in a population exposed apparently uniformly to a toxic atmosphere may cover a wide range. Some of this variability may be attributed to pre-existing airway obstruction or mucus hypersecretion, which, in turn, influence dose retention and site of deposition. Some can be attributed to differences in host response. The levels of antiproteases and the generation of antioxidants, for example, may be critical in limiting the

Table 30.1 Definitions of respirable agents by physical form

Gas	A formless compressible fluid in which all molecules of the agent move freely at room temperature (25°C) and standard pressure (760 mmHg) to fill the space available
Vapour	Gaseous state of an agent which is normally liquid or solid at room temperature and standard pressure
Aerosol	Dispersion of solid or liquid particles of microscopic size in a gaseous medium. The following are examples:
Dust	Dispersion of solid particles. Those of respirable size are not readily seen with the naked eye unless they are bathed in bright light
Fog	Dispersion of liquid particles generated by condensation from the vapour state
Fume	Dispersion of solid particles generated by condensation from the vapour state
Mist	Dispersion of liquid particles generated by condensation or mechanical means (e.g. nebulisation). The droplets are generally larger than those of a fog and may be visible individually to the naked eye
Smog	Mixture of smoke and fog – the former being the result of industrial pollution, the latter of natural climatic factors
Smoke	Dispersion of small particles (usually less than 0.1 μm diameter) resulting from incomplete combustion of organic substances

harmful effects of the inflammatory response, just as α_1-protease inhibition protects the lung from the effects of tobacco smoke. Much has still to be explained but it is probable that mechanistic pathways are shared by a number of apparently separate disease processes.

Nevertheless, toxicity implies that all members of an exposed population will produce similar end-organ effects given sufficient degrees of exposure. For the lung, exposure involves two principal routes: the airways and the vasculature. Only the airway route will be considered in this chapter, first with regard to the clinical effects that may ensue acutely or chronically at different levels within the respiratory tree, and second with regard to the more important specific agents involved. The dose actually delivered to the airways will depend on the quantity released into the environment, its dilution in ambient air and the period of exposure. Accidents in confined environments therefore pose substantially greater risks than those in the open or in circumstances of brisk ventilation, particularly if escape is impeded or there are few immediate symptoms to identify the hazard.

Some varieties of inhalant lung injury brought about (or partially brought about) by toxic agents are recognised as distinct disease entities: chronic bronchitis and emphysema from tobacco smoke; pneumoconiosis from certain mineral dusts; pneumonitis or oedema/fibrosis from drugs, environmental pollutants, radiation, drowning and gastric aspiration; bronchial carcinoma from tobacco smoke, asbestos, a variety of chemicals and radiation; and mesothelioma from asbestos. Other effects of inhaled toxic agents are systemic or involve target organs beyond

the lung itself (e.g. poisoning from carbon monoxide and lead fumes). Those described in other chapters are not reviewed in detail here.

Acute effects

The potential for serious inhalation injury is much greater in certain occupational settings than outside the workplace but such settings are relatively few in number. In a review of acute symptomatic episodes of inhalation injury that were evaluated in the San Francisco 'Poison Centre' the majority (62%) were the result of non-occupational incidents.[1] Within the occupational setting, in the UK, inhalation accidents accounted for about 9% of over 24 000 newly recognised cases of occupational lung disease reported to the SWORD (surveillance of work-related and occupational respiratory disease) scheme over the 8 years 1990–97.[2] Although most incidents involve only a few (or single) victims, occasional accidents may involve many and so overwhelm the available medical facilities – e.g. the Bhopal disaster with methyl isocyanate or the rupture of a derailed chlorine-containing rail tank.[3,4]

Tracheitis and bronchitis

The initial pulmonary effects of highly soluble irritant gases or reactive aerosols are seen in the trachea and bronchi, and these are likely to be associated with irritation of the exposed mucous membranes of the eyes, nose and throat. Given a threshold level of dose, there will be reflex-mediated cough followed by an acute inflammatory response if the affected subject is unable to withdraw immediately from exposure. Depending on severity there may be cellular infiltration, oedema, exudation, ulceration, bleeding and sloughing of the mucosa. There may also be widespread bronchoconstriction, subjects with pre-existing hyper-responsive airways no doubt being at greater risk. Wheezing, chest tightness and breathlessness may therefore accompany any cough and the latter may be associated with the expectoration of bloody or mucopurulent sputum and mucosal debris. Hoarseness provides a warning that significant inflammation has occurred in the upper airway, and stridor signifies the potential for life-threatening obstruction of the central airway. Thermal injury involves the upper respiratory tract and major airways disproportionately, because heat exchange occurs rapidly as air passes down the tracheobronchial tree to the gas-exchanging tissues.

The most commonly encountered gases and vapours of high solubility that are likely to induce acute tracheitis and bronchitis are acetic acid, ammonia, hydrogen chloride, formaldehyde and sulphur dioxide. Ammonia exerts its toxic effects principally through its alkaline properties, whereas acetic acid, hydrogen chloride and sulphur dioxide act as acids. Chlorine has intermediate solubility and acts as an oxidant. It may certainly produce effects in the upper and major airways, although it has greater potential to penetrate more distally. This is true also for other gases of intermediate solubility such as hydrogen sulphide and methyl isocyanate.

Bronchiolitis, pneumonitis and adult respiratory distress syndrome

Acute tracheobronchitis occurs in isolation following exposure to highly soluble toxic gases only if the exposure dose is comparatively mild. The greater the level of exposure, the more distal is the extent of involvement. Bronchioles and alveoli become inflamed as well and a bronchiolitis and pneumonitis result, usually with pulmonary oedema. This more life-threatening effect then dominates the clinical picture, which is essentially identical for all toxic respirable agents inhaled in sufficient dose.

When the toxic agent is more readily deposited distally than proximally or when there are few immediate effects to curtail ongoing exposure, the gas-exchanging tissues provide the major site of involvement from the outset. Poorly soluble toxic gases such as ozone, phosgene and the oxides of nitrogen may consequently be tolerated for relatively long periods (even hours, pending on concentration) and almost 2000 times as much ozone can be inhaled than ammonia for similar amounts to be dissolved in the mucosal fluids of the trachea and bronchi.[5] A number of toxic metals (their fumes or some of their compounds) may similarly be deposited dominantly in the gas-exchanging tissues rather than the airways, the most prominent being cadmium, manganese, mercury, nickel and zinc. The agents known to cause acute pneumonitis if inhaled in sufficient dose are listed in Table 30.2.

The clinical effects themselves are non-specific and depend chiefly on severity. In mild cases there is a dry irritating cough and impaired exercise tolerance only, symptoms subsiding after 24–48 hours. In more severe cases damage from derangements in pH, oxidant injury or other chemical reactions and the ensuing inflammatory cellular responses with cytokine release lead to permeability of the epithelial lining, air-space filling, ventilation–perfusion mismatching, hypoxaemia, breathlessness, constitutional upset and even death. The presence of bronchiolitis, essentially a histological diagnosis, is not easily detected clinically in such circumstances but can be assumed. A mosaic pattern (some exudative alveolar filling and some air-trapping from bronchiolar obstruction) is characteristic on computed tomographic (CT) scanning, particularly in expiration. It usually resolves spontaneously together with the acute inflammatory effects at other levels of the respiratory tree, but it is occasionally complicated by widespread bronchiolar fibrosis (bronchiolitis obliterans), with or without a distinctive organising intrabronchiolar and intraalveolar exudate (bronchiolitis obliterans organising pneumonia, BOOP).[6,7] Depending on extent and severity, this may lead to a crippling impairment of lung function (a mixture of small-airway obstruction, ventilatory restriction and ventilation–perfusion mismatching) and survival of only weeks or months.

The acute toxic effects may also be complicated by the adult respiratory distress syndrome and secondary infection. The former reflects the severity of the ensuing inflammatory response and may depend on the uncontrolled effects of oxidant activity. Secondary infection reflects the damage to normal defensive barriers and the often difficult eradication of infection attests to a more widespread derangement in antimicrobial defences. It may be the immediate cause of death when recov-

ery is delayed beyond 24–48 hours from the period of toxic exposure, in which circumstances multiple organisms (usually from the oropharynx) are likely to be involved.

In the absence of severe secondary infection, survival from these acute toxic effects on the lungs is usually (but not invariably) accompanied by full recovery. The popular belief that war gases such as chlorine and phosgene commonly caused permanent respiratory disability is unfounded.[8,9] There are sporadic reports of chronic sequelae, however, which include chronic airways obstruction, bronchiectasis and bronchiolitis obliterans. It is also recognised that a major toxic insult to the airways may

Table 30.2 Agents known to cause toxic pneumonitis

Chemical gases/vapours/aerosols	Acetic acid (and other organic acids)
	Aldehydes (e.g. acetaldehyde, formaldehyde, acrolein)
	Ammonia
	Chloramines
	Chlorine
	Chromic acid
	Hydrazine
	Hydrogen chloride
	Hydrogen fluoride
	Hydrogen sulphide
	Methyl isocyanate
	Mustard gas
	Oxides of nitrogen
	Ozone
	Paraquat
	Phosgene (carbonyl chloride)
	Sulphur dioxide
	Tear gas (orthochlorobenzylidenemalonitrile, chloroacetophenone)
	Toluene diisocyanate (and other volatile diisocyanates)
Metals	Beryllium
	Cadmium
	Hydrides of boron, lithium, arsenic and tin
	Manganese
	Mercury
	Nickel carbonyl
	Osmium dioxide
	Selenium dioxide
	Titanium tetrachloride
	Uranium hexafluoride
	Vanadium pentoxide
	Zinc chloride
	Zinc oxide
	Zirconium tetrachloride
Smoke	Fire smoke
	Plastic pyrolysis products
Microbes	Fungal mycotoxins

occasionally cause asthma that continues to be active for months or years, even indefinitely.[10] This has been termed the reactive airways dysfunction syndrome (RADS) or irritant asthma. Neither is a fully satisfactory term. The former may disguise the fact that the ongoing clinical disorder is asthma, with all the other characteristics of asthma irrespective of cause; the latter suggests that mere irritation rather than toxicity is the causal factor. This is by no means certain, although there is some suspicion of it.

Inhalation fever and organic dust toxic syndrome

Inhalation of toxic agents of widely different origins and even certain allergens (e.g. avian protein, chemical polymers, dusts from cotton, grain and wood, metal fumes and microbial toxins) may produce an acute benign feverish illness that characteristically begins within a few hours of exposure onset, lasts for no more than 24–48 hours and leaves no obvious persisting damage. Immunological hypersensitivity is not a feature in most cases and this febrile reaction may occur following the initial exposure. In one celebrated example, 55 of 67 (82%) participants were affected at a college fraternity gathering where exposure occurred to mouldy straw.[11]

Inhalation fever is dominated by an influenza-like illness, with malaise, aches and pains in muscles and joints, fever, anorexia, nausea and headache. Respiratory symptoms are less prominent and may be absent, and it is not always possible to demonstrate a pyrexia. They include cough (generally dry), chest discomfort or tightness, wheezing and breathlessness. They reflect toxic responses in either the airways or the lung parenchyma, or both, but the initiating event may generate non-specifically the release from the lung of proinflammatory cytokines (principally interleukins 6 and 8, and tumour necrosis factor) without clear evidence of any pulmonary toxicity.[12–14] The precise mechanism is unknown, but the reaction is usually associated with a transient neutrophil response in peripheral blood and alveolar fluid. The chest radiograph is typically normal but minor degrees of airway obstruction may be observed and there may be mild decrements in gas transfer. These effects may be associated with wheezes and crackles on physical examination, but auscultation is more commonly unremarkable. Rarely, more serious and disabling reactions occur.

The lung evidently makes a critical aetiological contribution since metal fume fever occurs only following inhalation. It does not occur after the gastrointestinal or intravenous administration of similar 'doses' of zinc oxide, which is the major cause of metal fume fever.[15] This condition is generated readily when zinc coated (galvanised) steel is welded or heat-cut ('burned'), although it is also associated with other vaporised metals and their condensation products. The vapour from heating cadmium-containing alloys is importantly more hazardous. It readily causes a life-threatening toxic pneumonitis rather than a benign inhalation fever. Metal fume fever differs from other inhalation fevers only by the commonly associated 'metal taste'. 'Monday fever' in cotton workers is equally well recognised within the cotton industry and is identical to 'grain fever' in grain workers and 'humidifier fever' in those exposed to microbially contaminated humidifiers or air conditioners[16,17] (see Chapter 32). 'Polymer fume fever' is associated particularly with the fluorine-containing polymer polytetrafluoroethylene (Teflon®), although not exclusively so.[18]

When organic dust is the causal agent of inhalation fever the epithet 'organic dust toxic syndrome' is commonly used. This convention was advocated at an international symposium in 1986 that considered inhalation fevers in farm workers.[19] This syndrome is associated particularly with animal husbandry and raising large numbers of animals in confined environments.[20,21] The causal agents are derived predominantly from microbial contaminants of bedding material and their products, chiefly bacterial endotoxin and fungal mycotoxin, although ammonia and hydrogen sulphide are additional agents of probable aetiological significance. Similar microbial contamination occurs in stored vegetable produce generally and the syndrome is not uncommon in farmers who store grain or hay (even fruit)[22] and in wood or forestry workers exposed to contaminated wood and wood products (especially wood dust and chippings).[23] Such exposure to mouldy wood chippings or compost may also occur in domestic settings and, with repeated exposure at less 'toxic' levels, there is the potential for allergic sensitisation and the development of extrinsic allergic alveolitis This too is characterised in its acute form by the features of inhalation fever, so it may be difficult to distinguish the two (Table 30.3).

Subacute and chronic effects

Although full recovery is the rule following survival from acute heavy (i.e. accidental) exposures to toxic agents, chronic exposure at dose levels unassociated with obvious immediate effects may produce permanent derangement with some agents in some subjects. Such exposures, which are usually occupational, generally extend over many years before the effect becomes detectable. With some agents, however, the latent period may be no more than a few weeks or months, resulting in a rare group of disorders that are subacute in nature. Example include:

- sprayed polymeric Acramin paint causing the 'Ardystil syndrome'[24,25]
- respirable silica in high concentration causing acute silicoproteinosis[26]
- trimellitic anhydride and pyromellitic dianhydride causing the pulmonary haemorrhagic syndrome[27,28]
- oil aerosols causing lipoid pneumonia[29]
- respirable fragments of nylon causing nylon flock worker's lung.[30,31]

Furthermore, the effect may be manifested in a minority only of the exposed population, indicating that differences in deposition characteristics or host susceptibility play important roles. These features imply that extensive and costly epidemiological studies may be required before a suspected effect can be confirmed and quantified, or excluded. It is therefore inevitable that some controversy and much uncertainty remain.

Table 30.3 Characteristic similarities and differences between nitrogen dioxide pneumonitis (silo filler's disease), organic dust toxic syndrome and acute allergic alveolitis

	Nitrogen dioxide pneumonitis	Organic dust toxic syndrome	Acute extrinsic allergic alveolitis
Susceptibility in smokers	Unknown	Unknown	Decreased
Relation to time of harvest	Recent	Distant	Distant
Microbial decomposition of harvest product	Little	Marked	Variable
Confined exposure space	+ + +	+	+
Previous episodes	–	–	+ +
Symptoms			
Dry cough	+ +	+ +	+ +
Breathlessness	+ +	+ +	+ +
Wheeze	–	–	–
Systemic upset	+	+	+ +
Signs			
Basal crackles	+	+	+
Fever	+	+	+
Time of onset after beginning exposure (hours)	1–10	1–10	1–10
Duration	Hours–days	Hours–days	Hours–days
Investigations			
Leukocytosis	+	+	+
Radiograph – small irregular opacities, alveolar shadows	+	+	+
Restricted ventilation	+	+	+
Reduced gas transfer	+	+	+
Hypoxia	+	+	+
Fungi from secretions/biopsy	–	+ + +	+
Methaemoglobin	+	–	–
Serum precipitins	–	–	+ (? in smokers)
Response to steroids	+	–	+ +
Life-threatening	Not uncommonly	Occasionally	Rarely

Chronic bronchitis, chronic obstructive pulmonary disease and asthma

The greatest uncertainty lies proximally, in the conducting airways. Although the chronic obstructive (i.e. irreversible chronic obstructive pulmonary disease, COPD) and chronic bronchitic (i.e. mucus hypersecretion) effects of tobacco smoke have been widely recognised for several generations, the possibility of parallel effects associated with a variety of unrelated environmental, largely industrial, agents has only recently been appreciated. This is perhaps surprising because the chronic obstructive effect associated with cotton dust exposure (now known as byssinosis grade 3) was described in the 19th century. It is inherently improbable that such a common effect would occur with only two of a great variety of atmospheric pollutants. The problem, of course, has lain with the confounding effect of tobacco smoke at a time when cigarette smoking was the rule in most workforces in industrialised countries.

Nevertheless, it is now clear that, in a number of industrial populations, airway obstruction and productive cough are more prevalent and more severe than can be accounted for by smoking alone. Compared with smokers, habitual non-smokers are less commonly and less severely affected, especially with regard to airway obstruction, and smoking is almost invariably the more important factor when both factors coexist. The effect of the industrial agent is usually additive or even multiplicative. In a longitudinal study of workers manufacturing isocyanates, however, similar excess declines in ventilatory function over time were noted from either smoking or high levels of isocyanate exposure, but no additional effect was noted in workers expressing both risk factors.[32] A similar outcome has been reported in grain handlers.[33] As with cigarette smoke alone, the bronchitic effect and the obstructive effect of these airway toxins may occur independently – the one not necessarily predicting the development of the other.

Occupational agents most prominently associated with these airway effects are cotton and grain dusts, isocyanates, mineral dusts and welding fumes (see below), although the relationships have not been without controversy.[34–39] Less definite associations have been recorded with chlorine, oxides of nitrogen, phosgene and sulphur dioxide.[40–44] Grain dust and isocyanates are also associated with asthma, and the question arises whether the chronic obstructive effect is simply a consequence of long-standing asthma. This does not seem to have been the case with isocyanates, because an observed excess mean decline in ventilatory function over a period of 5 years was not diminished by excluding those with obvious asthma.[32] The evidence in grain workers for a chronic obstructive effect independent of asthma is reasonably persuasive also.[33]

With mineral dusts (particularly from silica and coal) and welding fumes, there is no major confounding influence from occupational asthma but it has proved difficult to obtain satisfactory control populations and so to allow fully for the influence of smoking and other variables of possible relevance. It has also proved difficult over the long time intervals involved (20–40 years) to take full account of probable selection biases from 'healthy worker' and 'survivor' effects. It seems increasingly likely that significant risks of chronic airway obstruction are experienced from all of these agents, but the mean effect may be small even after long periods of exposure and not readily detected. Whether the mean loss of ventilatory function is usually a consequence of most exposed subjects experiencing trivial losses or of a few suffering severe (and disabling) losses is not yet clear.

Asthma is usually a hypersensitivity rather than a toxic effect but antibody responses are not commonly demonstrated in asthma induced by industrial chemicals and the precise mechanism is unclear in most cases (see Chapter 48.13). Furthermore, acute massive (i.e. accidental) exposures to a variety of inhaled toxic agents occasionally lead to persistent asthma when all other evidence of acute toxicity has subsided. Such a development, which may persist for months, years or indefinitely, is most commonly known as RADS (see above). It accounts for about 5% of all cases of asthma of occupational origin. There may be an important pathogenic parallel in that asthma starting acutely in members of the population at large sometimes does so immediately after a viral infection – a naturally occurring acute toxic injury to the airways. It would appear that RADS itself may follow any severe exposure of the airways to a toxic chemical and so each reported (or potential) cause is not specifically identified later in this chapter when the particular effects of individual occupational toxins are discussed. Although it is a rare consequence of toxic exposure and hence is generally observed only sporadically, it has been reported in as many as four of 44 hospital employees exposed to moderate or high doses of acetic acid following a major spill in a laboratory.[45] Other common causes include sulphuric acid, chlorine, ammonia, a number of household and industrial cleaning agents (which may release chlorine, ammonia or various acid aerosols) and fire smoke.[46,47]

As airway inflammation, a cardinal feature of active asthma, might plausibly be induced by many respirable irritants at more modest dose levels than those associated with accidents and RADS, it is reasonable to consider whether asthma might arise through toxic mechanisms from repeated low-level exposures. There is some evidence for this.[48] In the case of nitrogen dioxide and ozone, both asthmatic reactions and increases in non-specific airway responsiveness have been observed with human inhalation provocation studies.[49,50] Although there is no evidence to date that occupational exposure to these oxidant gases was primarily responsible for the development of asthma in previously unaffected subjects, both have been shown to provoke airway inflammation, bronchial hyper-responsiveness and airway obstruction in previously healthy dogs.[51]

Bronchiectasis

This is a rare complication of acute chemical toxicity. Ammonia is the most prominent cause, possibly because of its high solubility and alkalinity, although sulphur dioxide and fire smoke have also been implicated.[52,53]

Bronchiolitis obliterans

Histological evidence of chronic airway obstruction/obliteration distal to the bronchi (i.e. bronchiolitis obliterans) has been reported in association with a number of toxic agents, particularly ammonia, chlorine, nitrogen dioxide and sulphur dioxide.[54–59] It appears to occur only as a consequence of an acute massive exposure and then only rarely. Less specifically it has been reported following exposure to heated trichloroethylene, to gases released from cleansing agents and to mould toxins.[60–62] Whether bronchiolitis obliterans arising in such circumstances is usually associated with organising pneumonia (BOOP) is less clear, but the characteristics of BOOP have been reported with some cases – particularly those with the Ardystil syndrome.[24,25,63]

Emphysema

In addition to intrinsic disease of the airways themselves, chronic obstruction may result from destruction of the parenchymal and interstitial supporting tissue of the lungs (emphysema) and loss of elastic recoil. Cigarette smoking is by far the most common cause, but cadmium (which, interestingly, is a minor component of cigarette tobacco) and mineral dusts have also been implicated.[64] Whether chronic exposure to low levels of cadmium is a true cause of emphysema has been disputed, although one study provided strongly supportive evidence from lung function measurements and chest radiographs.[65] Emphysema and airway obstruction are also characteristic of complicated pneumoconiosis.

Lipoid pneumonia/pneumonitis

A chronic pneumonitis, almost invariably of the lower lobes, may result from recurrent regular aspiration of mineral and vegetable oils. This was commonly observed in the elderly when it was customary to take paraffin as nasal drops or as an aperient, and it has been reported in workers exposed habitually to oil mists and to burning fat.[66] A lipoid pneumonia follows, the degree of inflammation and hence associated pneumonitis depending on the irritant properties of the lipid material and the dose retained. It can be recognised by demonstrating lipid in sputum, bronchoalveolar fluid or resected tissue and by its appearance on CT scanning.[67–71] Bronchoalveolar lavage in the acute phase has been reported to be beneficial.[72] Ultimately there may be fibrosis and irreversible loss of volume, and complicating infection is not uncommon.

Recurrent localised aspiration may produce a clearly demarcated host response so that tumour is simulated – a 'paraffinoma'.

Pulmonary fibrosis

With ongoing exposure to low levels of atmospheric toxins, deposition at alveolar level is relatively trivial compared to that in the airways unless the agent is poorly soluble and particle size is largely confined to the 0.05–5 mm diameter range. Chronic parenchymal disease is consequently rare unless the toxic agent is retained for long periods. In these circumstances a much larger cumulative dose is able to exert its effects after latencies of up to 30 years. Such agents must be particulate in nature, largely insoluble and relatively unreactive. In practice they comprise minerals generated from mining or refining, metals or their oxides, other particulate products of combustion or pyrolysis and, perhaps, synthetic mineral fibres. They are responsible for the pneumoconioses.

The interstitial nodular fibrosis from, for example, coal (see Chapter 26) and silica (see Chapter 25) and the more widespread interstitial and alveolar fibrosis/alveolitis from asbestos (see Chapter 27) are discussed fully elsewhere. A more obviously toxic effect of silica deserves mention here, because it illustrates a rather different form of pulmonary response. When continual massive exposures occur from, for example, drilling, sand-blasting (Fig. 30.1) and the use of explosives in driving tunnels through siliceous rock without adequate respiratory protection, there is the risk of both alveolar and interstitial inflammation, which produces not only a rapidly progressive fibrosis but also cellular desquamation and the exudation of proteinaceous material into the air spaces (Fig. 30.2). It closely resembles idiopathic alveolar proteinosis and so is known as acute or subacute silicoproteinosis. It is generally considered to be unresponsive to therapeutic bronchoalveolar lavage, although this is being re-examined,[73,74] and death usually supervenes within 1–3 years. In one reported case, an unusual response was obtained from corticosteroid therapy but this proved to be no more than temporary.[75]

Occasionally acute silicoproteinosis is associated with features of systemic sclerosis (as may more conventional manifestations of silicosis), which is a complication of considerable

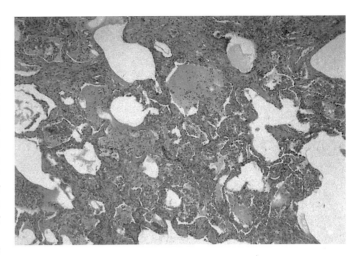

Fig. 30.2 Acute silicoproteinosis in a rock driller. The alveoli are filled with proteinaceous material and desquamated pneumocytes; there is a cuboidal metaplasia of pneumocytes and the interstitium shows inflammation and fibrosis. Haematoxylin and eosin stain. (Courtesy of Dr D. E. Banks.)

interest in view of the tendency of subjects with silicosis to produce a variety of autoantibodies. Here, toxic and immunological responses appear to interact to produce autoimmune disease – not simply in the target organ receiving the toxic insult but systemically. The sarcoidosis-like granulomatous inflammation following chronic exposure to airborne beryllium might also be mentioned in this context, although here the initial insult to the lungs is generally thought to be immunological (cellular hypersensitivity) rather than toxic.

Secondary infection

The apparent overstimulation by silica of immunological defence mechanisms is particularly notable in light of the impaired ability of silicotic lungs to resist mycobacterial infection. The explanation appears to lie with the macrophage, which acts as the primary phagocytic cell for silica particles and normally plays a major early role in controlling mycobacterial proliferation. The ingested silica profoundly disrupts this role and provides a further example of primary toxicity (even of low degree) encouraging secondary infection.

Vasculitis

The vascular compartment of the lung parenchyma is rarely the major site of a toxic response to airborne insults. One interesting example associated with the inhalation route has been vasculitis and pulmonary hypertension (together with pneumonitis and fibrosis) in blackfat tobacco smokers living in Guyana.[76] The habit of adulterating poor-quality (usually commercially rejected) tobacco with various mineral oils improves the flavour. The cost in health may be extreme in the heavier consumers, progressive pulmonary hypertension and fibrosis leading to premature death from cor pulmonale.

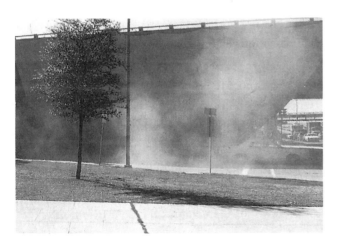

Fig. 30.1 Photograph of dust cloud generated by sand blasting a New Orleans bridge before repainting. The workers are invisible within the cloud, and not all were using protective respirators.

Malignancy

The effect of malignant transformation may be observed throughout the airways, parenchyma and pleural coverings of the lung. Tobacco smoke and asbestos constitute the greatest threat, the risk of bronchial carcinoma approaching an astonishing and tragic 100% when both are experienced in high cumulative dose (see Chapter 27). Passive smoking, arsenic, chromates, chloroethers, coal gasification, coking fumes, tetrachlorodibenzo-para-dioxin, mustard gas, radiation (and radon-releasing mineral ores), silica and sulphuric acid are among a number of less influential causes in epidemiological terms, asbestos being in turn far less important than tobacco smoke.[77-84]

Asbestos (and the similar fibrous mineral erionite) is, however, unique in inducing pleural mesothelioma and a variety of non-malignant pleural effects – unique, that is, if exposure is limited to the inhalation route. With direct instillation into the pleural cavities of experimental animals, glass fibre has also been shown to induce mesothelioma.[85] Physical properties facilitating penetration may therefore be more relevant than chemical constitution.

Aetiological agents

Air pollutants

Of the many components of air pollution, those thought to pose the greatest threat to the lungs comprise aeroallergens, smoke particles, volatile aromatic hydrocarbons, nitrogen dioxide, sulphur dioxide and ozone. The toxic (i.e. non-allergenic) components are considered separately and in more detail below, but the overall effects of air pollution are considered briefly here.

Although aeroallergens and hypersensitivity mechanisms have certainly been responsible for some seasonal, even epidemic, exacerbations of asthma (e.g. the dramatic epidemic days in Barcelona attributable to the release of soy bean dust[86]), there is increasing evidence that irritant air pollutants and toxic mechanisms may play a more important role.[87,88] Their effects may extend beyond exacerbating asthma, because additional associations have been reported between air-pollution peaks on the one hand and acute respiratory infections, exacerbations of COPD and even mortality on the other. Such peak levels have not always exceeded statutory limits and there is speculation that long-term low levels of pollution may play a role in causing as well as exacerbating airway obstruction.

The particulate component of air pollution has attracted special attention over recent years, a number of studies demonstrating that respirable particles (i.e. those with diameters less than 10 μm, PM_{10}s) can be related to mortality – principally from cardiopulmonary disease and lung cancer – and to various measures of morbidity (e.g. pneumonia, exacerbations of asthma, childhood lung function, coronary events and heart failure).[89-91] PM_{10} levels in ambient air are expressed gravimetrically as micrograms per cubic metre. Average levels over periods of 1–4 days are associated consistently with mortality on the following day, independently of season, global site and smoking habit, although the effect is stronger in winter and cities are necessarily more polluted (and hence more affected) than rural areas. The effect appears to be independent also of the level of gaseous pollution but PM_{10} concentrations tend to be closely correlated with sulphur dioxide levels and the effect of the one is not always readily distinguished from that of the other.

The 16-year surveillance study of six US cities showed a 26% increase in mortality in the most polluted city compared with the least after adjustment for confounding factors, and particulate pollution was associated with similar excess mortality in the 17-year prospective study of 0.5 million adults followed by the US Cancer Society.[89,90] Not surprisingly, the elderly are unduly vulnerable (partly but not entirely because death for some is likely to be imminent anyway), and for them a 10 μg/m³ increase in PM_{10} causes an increase in mortality of about 1%, compared with an average for the whole population of about 0.7%.[91] Mean annual PM_{10} levels in the USA vary over the range 18–50 μg/m³ from rural to urban areas but may reach peaks of 100–300 μg/m³ in cities when averaged over 24 hours.

Most PM_{10}s are sulphates and products of fuel combustion but in some areas particles derived from the earth's crust provide an important, although probably less hazardous, contribution. More relevant, perhaps, are the molecules adsorbed on to the surfaces and the degree of any acidity. The former include ammonium ions, aliphatic carbons, carbonyl carbons and organonitrates.[91] The smaller the particles, the greater is the relative surface, and the stronger is the association with intravascular coagulation/sequestration (hence coronary events).[92] This may reflect greater potency, greater alveolar deposition (about 10% for particle diameters of 5 μg, 30% for 0.1 μg and 50% for 0.05 μg[91]) and a greater proportion of particles originating from combustion. Thus, quantification of $PM_{2.5}$ levels, which depend dominantly on gaseous photochemical reactions, may prove to be a more useful index of particulate pollution than PM_{10} for clinical purposes.

While PM_{10}s are more concentrated in outdoor than indoor environments, very fine particles (PM_1s) are distributed more evenly and so contribute, with nitrogen dioxide (largely from gas cookers and heaters) and tobacco smoke, to indoor air pollution, which is also being linked increasingly with acute respiratory disorders. Children appear to be most affected and asthma, intercurrent infections and impaired development of lung function are said to be the major manifestations.[87,88,93]

Aldehydes

Acetaldehyde, acrylic aldehyde (acrolein) and formaldehyde are three irritant low-molecular-weight aldehydes used widely in the chemical and plastics industries. They are also found in the combustion products of diesel oil and petrol, and so contribute to the irritant properties of urban pollution. In high doses, all three may produce an acute pneumonitis and pulmonary oedema, but their immediate and profound irritant effects (particularly of acrolein) on the mucous membranes generally guard against a continuing dangerous level of exposure. Acetaldehyde (a liquid) and formaldehyde (a water-soluble gas) are also used as disinfectant/sterilising agents and may be encountered in the health-care industry. The former has an additional narcotic effect, while formaldehyde occasionally produces skin rashes, rhinitis and/or asthma – probably through hypersensitivity mechanisms.[94]

Investigation in rodents of the chronic effects of continual exposure to formaldehyde has also revealed an alarming potential to induce nasal carcinomas.[95] However, the dose levels encountered by these obligate nose-breathing animals were unrealistically high in comparison to human experiences, and it is reassuring that no convincing evidence of formaldehyde-induced malignancy has emerged from surveys in humans.

Ammonia

Ammonia is both highly irritating and highly soluble. These properties in a gas that is extensively used in industry as a 'building brick' for nitrogenous products (fertilisers, explosives, plastics) carry considerable potential for lung toxicity. Typical acute inflammatory reactions occur readily throughout the airways and parenchyma but are particularly marked in the eyes, nose and throat initially. The greater the level of exposure, the greater is the risk of rapid death from suffocation as the upper airway becomes obstructed by secretions and oedema. With lesser exposures, the threat to life rests more with parenchymal disruption and secondary infection, and is delayed from a matter of minutes to one of hours or days. Survival usually brings full recovery but bronchiectasis, bronchiolitis obliterans and fixed airway obstruction have been described.[53,55,56]

Carbon monoxide

Carbon monoxide is not strictly a cause of toxic lung injury (the lung provides a portal of entry for toxicity centred in other organs) but it may contribute importantly to morbidity, even mortality, when toxic lung injury rises from other exposures – particularly when organic materials, chemicals or fuels are subjected to heat or combustion and oxygen is not freely available. The metabolism of absorbed methylene chloride (an organic solvent used widely as paint stripper and degreasing agent) provides a further source in intoxicated individuals, one that is poorly recognised.

The danger of carbon monoxide (a gas without warning odour, taste or colour, and without immediate mucosal irritation) is a consequence of it binding with haemoglobin with considerably greater avidity than oxygen. This displaces oxygen from blood, diminishes its delivery and causes tissue hypoxia. It additionally shifts the oxygen dissociation curve to the left and so reduces tissue delivery even more. The major clinical effects are manifested in the central nervous system and the heart and there is particular danger to the unborn fetus. For a given hazardous level of exposure there is also particular danger from heavy exertion in heavy smokers, since equilibrium (and toxicity) is reached more quickly.

With mild to moderate intoxication characterised by carboxyhaemoglobin levels of 10–30%, there is headache, fatigue, dizziness, nausea, tiredness and possibly diminished intellectual capability. Greater levels of intoxication cause vomiting, weak-ness, irritability, impaired judgement, syncope on exertion and impaired consciousness and are associated with hypertension, flushing and tachycardia. Coma and convulsions are increasingly likely at carboxyhaemoglobin levels exceeding 50% and respiratory depression and death are to be expected at levels of 60–80%.[96] Survival following coma is commonly complicated by loss of intellectual function, extrapyramidal disablement and other 'neuropsychiatric' disturbances, and there is increasing concern that neuropsychiatric upset may complicate less obvious episodes of intoxication when consciousness is not affected. Difficulty in assessment arises from a delayed onset of such effects after an initial period of apparent full recovery.

Management requires prompt cessation of exposure, supportive and intensive care according to need, and the use of supplemental oxygen in high concentration. Controversy has attended the use of hyperbaric oxygen, and in practice this is generally restricted to subjects with coma. It remains unclear whether any benefits in survival and long-term sequelae outweigh the added risks that attend management in a sealed chamber.

Chlorine

Chlorine is a highly reactive oxidant gas whose chief use is in the chemical industry. It and volatile toxic chloramines may be encountered in the home if bleaching or cleaning chemicals are mixed with acids or alkalis. It is transported in bulk under pressure as a liquid, which carries the risk of major environmental pollution with accidents that cause container rupture.[4] Heavy exposure in such circumstances or in war has proved to be fatal from a combination of asphyxia and acute airway/parenchymal toxicity before rescue services could be mounted. Pulmonary oedema has been common in early survivors with moderate exposures, and may be delayed in its onset for many hours. In long-term survivors, parenchymal function generally recovers fully, but some controversy attends the outcome in the airways.[97] Most investigations have not shown a chronic obstructive effect beyond that to be expected from attendant tobacco smoking alone, although occasional cases of bronchiolitis obliterans have been reported.[9,40,98]

A chronic obstructive effect has, however, been postulated when there are repeated accidental gassings of modest, but not necessarily massive, degree in environments where chlorine is used regularly. Such exposures are met in the chemical manufacturing industry and in pulp mills/paper manufacture. In the latter, unusually, a chronic obstructive effect (which was of mild degree only but appeared to be related to chlorine) was seen most clearly in the absence of smoking.[99,100] Advantage is taken of the familiar properties of chlorine in swimming pools and in the home but in such circumstances exposure levels rarely pose any hazard. It may occasionally stimulate attacks of bronchoconstriction non-specifically in subjects already suffering from asthma.

Illicit drugs

A number of illicit drugs are taken by the respiratory route and a number of toxic effects may result. Most prominent are cannabis and cocaine, and in the USA some 10 million individuals are estimated to use marijuana regularly and 5 million to use cocaine regularly. Although the initial use of marijuana produces mild bronchodilatation, tolerance may develop to this effect and it may be succeeded by mild chronic obstruction and by chronic bronchitis.[101] The latter is more common with smokers of hashish, a separate derivative of the cannabis plant. Fungal contamination of marijuana has led occasionally to rather more serious respiratory complications, namely infection and hypersensitivity. In one interesting case allergic bronchopulmonary aspergillosis is thought to have been a consequence.[102]

The potential effects of cocaine are far more diverse and disabling, although not unduly common. When prepared as the alkaloid base ('cocaine freebase') it is sufficiently heat-stable to be active after smoking, and its use in this fashion has led to pneumothorax, pneumomediastinum, hypersensitivity pneumonitis, pulmonary eosinophilia, pulmonary haemorrhage, obliterative bronchiolitis, asthma and pulmonary oedema[103–105] (see Chapter 29).

Metals and metalloids

A number of elemental metals/metalloids, their oxides or their salts (usually as fume or nebulised solutions) may produce acute mucosal irritation and even pneumonitis/oedema within the lungs. They include: antimony pentachloride; beryllium and some of its compounds; cadmium oxide; chromic acid; cobalt; hydrides of arsenic, boron (diborane) and lithium; manganese dioxide; mercury; nickel carbonyl; osmium tetroxide; selenium dioxide and anhydride; titanium tetrachloride; uranium fluoride; vanadium pentoxide; zinc chloride; and zirconium tetrachloride.[106–111]

Chronic effects, particularly the pneumoconioses, are generally seen with less chemically reactive metals. Cobalt, chromium, nickel and vanadium have all been reported to cause asthma; nickel to cause Loeffler's syndrome (with asthma); and arsenic, beryllium, cadmium, chromium and nickel to cause lung cancer.[83,112–116]

Cobalt is also responsible for 'hard-metal disease' a fibrosing alveolitis associated with the preparation of tungsten carbide drills and cutting tools.[117] During the manufacturing (heating) phase, cobalt acts as binder or solvent for the tungsten. A similar clinical picture has been noted with zinc fumes[106] and in vineyard workers as a result of spraying copper sulphate (an antifungal agent) on the vines.[118] Beryllium and some of its compounds are unique in producing a sarcoidosis-like picture through hypersensitivity mechanisms.

Methyl isocyanate

Methyl isocyanate became an instantly notorious pulmonary toxin as a result of a single catastrophic accident when 15 tonnes were released into the atmosphere of the Indian city of Bhopal on the night of 3 December 1984.[3] An estimated 2000–2500 inhabitants died within hours or days from pneumonitis/pulmonary oedema/secondary infection, and many more are feared to have become permanently maimed from ocular or respiratory disorders. It has been claimed that the respiratory disorders included airway obstruction, bronchiolitis obliterans and pulmonary fibrosis but major logistical problems existed in mounting a fully comprehensive survey, in obtaining unbiased population samples for investigation and in assessing the extent of these disorders before the accident. As a result, no consensus has yet been reached from the evidence currently available for analysis.[119,120]

There was much confusion during the earlier hours of the disaster as to whether cyanide poisoning coexisted (or even was the primary problem) and hence whether there was a place for specific therapy with dicobalt edetate and sodium nitrite/thiosulphate.[121] In practice, the medical services were overwhelmed and there was little hope for most of the early casualties. The most obvious implications for the future lie with prevention and the wisdom of manufacturing highly toxic chemicals in densely populated locations. When specific local risks do exist the sharing of relevant toxicological knowledge between management and local authorities would appear to be essential.

Mineral oils/petroleum

In addition to its effects in blackfat tobacco smokers, mineral oil may produce an intense pneumonitis when aspirated (shipwrecked sailors) or inhaled (fire-fighters). More chronic exposure to respirable oil mists, generated when lubricant and cooling fluids are subjected to high speed or pressure in the mechanical engineering industry, may cause a chronic pneumonitis/fibrosis or asthma.[29,66,122]

The most commonly inhaled components/products of petroleum are the short-chain hydrocarbon gases (e.g. propane), which are liquefied under pressure for use as domestic fuels, and the medium-chain hydrocarbon liquid distillates such as petrol (gasoline, C_{4-12}) and paraffin (kerosene, C_{10-16}), which are used as motor, aviation and domestic fuels. The gases have negligible pulmonary toxicity and produce their adverse effects chiefly as asphyxiants and central-nervous-system depressants. The volatile liquids such as petrol may induce these effects when vapour is 'sniffed'. If there is repeated exposure to the vapour of leaded 'antiknock' petrol, characteristic features of chronic lead poisoning may arise from the cumulative lead burden. With the substitution of unleaded petrol this problem has fortunately become vanishingly rare.

Petrol and paraffin do occasionally provoke acute inflammatory responses in the lungs but the dose encountered from vapour alone is rarely (petrol) or never (paraffin) sufficient for this to pose clinical problems. However, severe pulmonary toxicity in the form of a diffuse, sometimes haemorrhagic, pneumonia or localised pneumonia is not infrequently seen following inadvertent ingestion (e.g. children taking drinks from unlabelled bottles, siphoning accidents), especially if this is complicated by vomiting and aspiration. It has been argued that intubation and gastric lavage are contraindicated in managing such accidents for fear of inducing aspiration but a multicentre collaborative study provided no supportive evidence for this.[123] Also, it did not demonstrate any benefit, although it did find evidence of toxic pneumonitis in the apparent absence of aspiration (or intubation), suggesting that blood-borne dissemination of absorbed hydrocarbon was responsible.

Nitrogen dioxide

Nitrogen dioxide is met in a variety of settings, including the chemical industry, mining (nitro explosives), fires (domestic gas cookers/heaters) and the accidental combustion of nitrocellulose in radiograph films,[124] diesel fumes and welding. Perhaps the most celebrated is the agricultural silo, where decomposing grain or silage releases nitrogen dioxide into the confined and poorly ventilated space immediately above the level of the stored produce. Being denser than air it disperses slowly and may reach sufficiently high concentrations to cause asphyxia. It is not readily soluble and may have little immediate effect on the mucous membranes of the upper respiratory tract, thus allowing dangerous levels of exposure to accumulate while further work filling the silo continues without much discomfort. Silo-filler's lung, a toxic pneumonitis/pulmonary oedema associated with constitutional upset, may then follow several hours later. Although readily preventable, the disorder is distressingly common and often fatal. A review from New York State suggested an annual incidence of 5 cases per 100 000 workers at risk, and a mortality rate of 20%.[125]

Remarkably, life-threatening pulmonary oedema may recur during the 2–8 weeks following an episode of nitrogen dioxide toxicity for reasons that are not fully understood. Such a recurrence is uncommon and unpredictable. Fortunately, it is readily prevented with the prophylactic use of corticosteroids. Whether short-term corticosteroid treatment also reduces the long-term risk of bronchiolitis obliterans (which is remote anyway) is not clear.

In contrast to these well-recognised effects of accidental exposure to moderate or high levels of nitrogen dioxide (i.e. hundreds of parts per million), it has been suggested that chronic ambient exposure to levels of the order 0.05–0.5 ppm may cause a reduction in flow rates and an increase in intercurrent respiratory illnesses in children. Such levels may occur in homes using gas rather than electricity for cooking/heating and in cities with high levels of air pollution.[93,126,127] Even with marked pollution, concentrations in non-industrial settings are almost invariably less than 1 ppm and these probably pose little airway risk to adults unless asthma is already present. When asthma is present, however, nitrogen dioxide may be the constituent most responsible for exacerbations provoked by air pollution.[128]

Organic dust/manure

Toxicity from fungal contamination of ingested food (mycotoxicosis) is widely recognised; that from inhaled fungal toxins less so. Reported initially in Russia in 1960, it was not until 1975 that pulmonary mycotoxicosis was described in the English language literature.[129] Those affected were farm workers engaged in unloading (decapping), rather than filling, storage silos. To impede aerobic microbial growth and trap the chemical products of initial decomposition so that these were able to 'pickle' the remainder of the crop, plastic sheeting had been used to cover the main crop within the silos. This had then been secured by the weight of a further layer of silage, which was able to decompose more freely. Exposures of an hour or so to this mouldy layer,

when the silos were decapped many months later, led to an acute febrile influenza-like illness after a few hours. It was accompanied by irritation of the mucous membranes of the eyes, nose and throat, and by cough and shortness of breath. In some cases, but not all, auscultation showed crackles (but not wheezes), the chest radiograph diffuse interstitial changes and the peripheral blood neutrophilia. Lung biopsy was performed in one affected subject and revealed a multifocal acute pneumonitis affecting bronchioles, alveoli and interstitium. Culture produced a profuse growth of several fungi but no bacteria. Full recovery followed without the use of antimicrobial or corticosteroid therapy.

This interesting disorder was discussed at an international workshop in 1986, when the less explicit term 'organic dust toxic syndrome' was recommended for its future identification instead of pulmonary mycotoxicosis.[19] Its clinical features share much in common with nitrogen dioxide toxicity (silo filler's disease) and the acute form of farmer's lung, all three disorders presenting with a wide spectrum of severity depending on exposure dose. In practice, nitrogen dioxide toxicity is more prevalent during silo filling and during aerobic decomposition (days or weeks), and involves exposure to gas in circumstances of minimum ventilation in the confined atmosphere of the silo.

Farmer's lung, on the other hand, requires exposure to dust laden with microbial particles (spores). The number tends to increase, not dissipate, with time. The more massive and the more prolonged the exposure to such dust, the more likely is a resulting acute pneumonitis to be caused by toxic rather than by hypersensitivity mechanisms, especially if the history does not suggest previous similar episodes and if there are no serum-precipitating antibodies to the dust concerned. Farmer's lung is not, however, invariably associated with a precipitin response to the relevant provoking dust (especially if the exposed subject is a smoker)[130] and it may not always be easy to distinguish the one disorder from the other. More sophisticated immunological investigations, possibly using the products of bronchoalveolar lavage, may prove to be useful in this respect.[131,132]

The more important clinical and laboratory features of nitrogen dioxide toxicity, organic dust toxic syndrome and extrinsic allergic alveolitis are compared and contrasted in Table 30.3. From the therapeutic viewpoint, all three disorders are usually self-limiting, although each can be life-threatening. Corticosteroids are indicated for nitrogen dioxide toxicity and for the more severe episodes of farmer's lung, but may encourage fungal growth and tissue invasion if used in high doses for prolonged periods. Figure 30.3 illustrates the post-mortem findings in a 10-year-old boy who spent several hours playing in mouldy hay/straw, only to develop acute pneumonitis some hours later. Initial progress following treatment with oxygen, antibiotics and increasing doses of corticosteroids was fluctuating and unsatisfactory, and was succeeded by inexorable deterioration. The lungs proved to be widely invaded by replicating *Aspergillus* sp. A companion was less severely affected and recovered without specific treatment within 48 hours.

A similar range of outcomes has been reported following inhalational exposure to a rather different type of organic waste – liquid manure. A farmer partially drained then entered an underground storage tank in an attempt to recover the lid, which had been kicked inside by a cow. He quickly lost con-

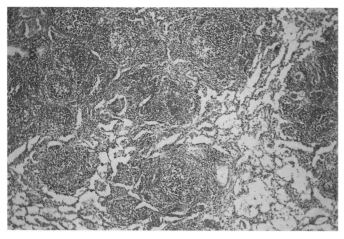

(a)

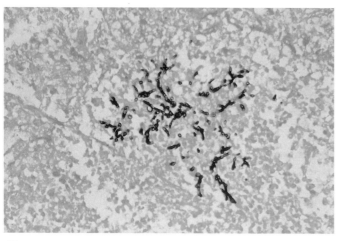

(b)

Fig. 30.3 Histology of fatal *Aspergillus* pneumonia following heavy exposure of a previously healthy young boy who played in mouldy hay/straw for several hours. a. Haematoxylin and eosin stain showing multiple microabscesses. b. Grocott stain showing branching fungal hyphae of *Aspergillus fumigatus*.

sciousness, as did a series of unfortunate would-be rescuers. Among a mixture of toxic and asphyxiant gases (which included methane, carbon monoxide, carbon dioxide and ammonia), hydrogen sulphide was considered to be primarily responsible for fatal intoxication and pulmonary oedema in one 'rescuer' who showed no post-mortem evidence of aspiration. With two further fatalities there was evidence of aspiration after loss of consciousness, while in a survivor aspiration and pneumonitis were followed by infection with multiple organisms.[133] Hydrogen sulphide was considered to have played a double role because of its inhibitory effect at cellular level of cytochrome oxidase (resembling cyanide poisoning) and its toxic effect to mucosal surfaces and the alveolar capillary membrane.

Ozone

Ozone occurs naturally in the atmosphere, especially at altitudes above 3000 metres. It may also reach levels of clinical import-

ance as a constituent of ground-level air pollution, particularly when products of petroleum combustion drift from urban centres to elevated and sunlit rural areas. Urban reactions between ozone and nitric oxide diminish ozone levels and produce nitrogen dioxide but the reaction is reversed with ultraviolet radiation. In the workplace ozone is used as a bleaching agent and to mask unpleasant odours, and it is evolved as an unwanted by-product in welding. It is a powerful oxidant (more so than nitrogen dioxide) and, like nitrogen dioxide, may provoke both delayed acute effects in the lung parenchyma and chronic effects in the airways. It is rarely encountered in very high concentrations (above 1 ppm) and its low solubility allows irritative and oxidative effects to accumulate in the gas-exchanging tissues. When severe, these result in pneumonitis and pulmonary oedema, with a fatal outcome in some cases.

Rather more interest has centred in recent years on the effects of ozone on the airways – in both humans and experimental animal models. Levels of exposure of 0.3–0.5 ppm cause inflammation and an increase in non-specific airway responsiveness.[50] High levels may also provoke asthmatic reactions, although frequently repeated exposures soon lead to tolerance.[134] The full clinical significance of these discoveries is not yet clear, and occupational asthma attributable to ozone alone has not been described. As ozone is often encountered with other irritant pollutants, the possibility of interactive effects is not easily excluded. Indeed, evidence already exists that interactions of clinical significance do occur with nitrogen dioxide and sulphur dioxide.

Phosgene (carbonyl chloride)

The use of phosgene as a First World War poison was attributable to three major properties: it is highly toxic (more so than chlorine), heavy (and so disperses only slowly) and not readily soluble in water. As a result, hazardous cumulative exposure doses may be absorbed before symptoms arise and before any danger is appreciated. Death from pneumonitis and pulmonary oedema was consequently distressingly common. Today, phosgene is encountered in the chemical industry as a means of chlorination, and where there are combustion products of chlorinated hydrocarbons (e.g. fires and welding metal that has been degreased with these compounds). A particular example is methylene chloride, which is often used as a paint-stripping solvent. If heat is applied after application, especially in a poorly ventilated environment, toxic concentrations of phosgene may result.[135] When methylene chloride itself is absorbed its metabolism leads to the production of carbon monoxide, a feature that may increase its toxicity. The readily measured carboxyhaemoglobin level may help to quantify cumulative exposure.

Smog

Smog (i.e. smoke, fog and air pollution), coupled with unusually low temperatures and a 5-day temperature inversion, conspired to produce a calamitous excess of respiratory illness and death in London during December 1952.[136] This disaster, which caused approximately twice as many deaths as the Bhopal disaster, was but one of a series of incidents in Europe and North America. At a time of stable high barometric pressure (and hence little lateral air dispersion), a layer of dense, cold air caused a temperature inversion immediately overlying an industrial area, temporarily preventing the dilution and upward dispersion of the polluted surface atmosphere. Those most affected in the London incident were individuals already afflicted with respiratory or cardiac disease. Intercurrent viral infection is likely to have played a contributory role and bronchitis was the most commonly certified cause of death. This brief epidemic illustrates the potential interactive danger when different respiratory toxins (and probably microorganisms) are encountered together in high concentration by an unduly susceptible population.

The major pollutants were derived primarily from industrial and domestic discharges of smoke. It is probable that acidic aerosols were prominent among them, and these have attracted much interest subsequently. Both animal experiments and epidemiological investigations indicate an adverse effect on airway responsiveness, which may particularly affect children, and there may be increased susceptibility to infection.[88,93]

Smoke

The hazards from smoke from accidental fires depend not only on the level of exposure but also on the degree of combustion and the nature of the burning materials. Those that contain chlorine and isocyanate (e.g. polyvinyl chloride, polyurethane) are particularly hazardous because they may yield chlorine, hydrogen chloride, phosgene, isocyanates and hydrogen cyanide – blood concentrations of the last in some fatal cases exceeding the usual lethal level. Limited availability of oxygen results in incomplete combustion and products of greater toxicity (e.g. aldehydes and carbon monoxide). Injuries to the airways and parenchyma appear to be chemical rather than thermal, and often occur in the absence of burns to the skin. When burns are extensive, however, there may be considerable loss of body fluids and plasma proteins, thereby enhancing the risk of pulmonary oedema, systemic infection and the adult respiratory distress syndrome.

The immediate threat to life comes from hypoxaemia, which may be seriously augmented by both carbon monoxide poisoning and, if nitrogen-containing plastics are involved, hydrogen cyanide poisoning. High blood levels of either would be an indication for intensive care and, possibly, the use of hyperbaric oxygen or nitrites; however, the hydrogen cyanide content can rarely be measured quickly enough to be of practical value. Fortunately it correlates with the carboxyhaemoglobin level, and this can be used as a marker for both toxins when fires are known to have involved nitrogenous plastics.[137] A more comprehensive method of identifying high risks of mortality and the need for special care uses carboxyhaemoglobin level, age and the percentage of surface burn in a prediction equation derived from a stepwise linear logistic regression analysis.[138] Seven clinical features (fire in an enclosed space, black sputum, perioral burns, altered consciousness, altered voice, symptoms and signs of respiratory distress) quantified by a 0–7 score were found to improve the predictive value of

the equation when substituted for the carboxyhaemoglobin level. This level, together with the arterial blood gas tensions and the chest radiograph appearances, offered no additional benefits if retained in the equation together with the clinical score.

In survivors there are rarely permanent sequelae, although diffuse bronchoconstriction associated with the induction of airway hyper-responsiveness may occur.[139,140] Very occasionally there is persisting asthma. Bronchorrhoea may also be prominent, the secretions being characteristically discoloured by black pigment from the smoke itself. Persisting diffuse airway obstruction, tracheo- or bronchostenosis and bronchiectasis have been described in a few individual survivors, and 2 years after a catastrophic fire in a London underground station a mild obstructive effect in the small (but not large) airways has been reported.[141] The evidence for a disabling chronic obstructive effect in subjects exposed repeatedly to smoke (i.e. firefighters) is not, however, convincing. Chronic ambient exposure to smoke particulates in Britain (from burning domestic coal) before the Clean Air Act of the late 1950s was, however, associated with chronic airway obstruction – possibly because of sulphur dioxide adsorbed on to the surfaces of respirable particles.

Sulphur dioxide

Advantage is taken of the toxic properties of sulphur dioxide in its use as a fumigant. It is also encountered extensively in the paper industry, where it is used as a bleaching agent, and in the chemical industry. It evolves as a pollutant when sulphur-bearing coal is burned or when sulphur-bearing ore is refined. It is highly reactive and with water generates sulphurous acid. More commonly it is reacted with water to produce sulphuric acid, having first been oxidised to sulphur trioxide over a vanadium catalyst. Its high solubility ensures that mild-to-medium levels of exposure are quickly recognised by their irritant effects on the mucosal surfaces of the eyes and upper respiratory tract. This 'alarm' generally protects the subject from more dangerous prolonged exposures. Accidental exposures to high levels have caused death within minutes, post-mortem findings revealing extensive sloughing of the airway mucosa and a haemorrhagic alveolar exudation.[142]

With less serious levels of accidental exposure, airway obstruction has been observed, and in a few cases this has been progressive. The relevance of sulphur dioxide in polluted cities has consequently been the subject of much study. Correlations have been noted between atmospheric concentrations of sulphur dioxide on the one hand and asthma, other acute respiratory illnesses (particularly in children) and acute exacerbations of chronic obstructive pulmonary disease on the other. Although sulphur dioxide may act as a marker for more relevant pollutants, correlations have generally been less strong with other constituents – apart from the particulates. It has been suggested that the latter could absorb sulphur dioxide, allowing it to penetrate more deeply into the airways and the lung parenchyma – a possible mechanism of interaction of considerable interest in many environmental diseases of the lung.

Tear gas

Two types of 'tear gas' are in common use for controlling unruly crowds or violent individuals – orthochlorobenzylidenemalonitrile (CS) and chloroacetophenone (CN). They produce immediate and intense irritation of the ocular mucosa, which generally provokes immediate withdrawal and hence cessation of ongoing exposure. They have proved generally to be safe but their irritating properties become toxic properties if prompt withdrawal is not possible and there is concern that they may additionally be allergenic. Prolonged exposure in confined environments may be particularly hazardous and both pneumonitis and RADS have been reported.[143-145]

Volcanic emissions

The celebrated volcanic eruption in May 1980 of Mt St Helens in the state of Washington, USA, removed 3–4 km^3 of mountain, reduced the height of the summit by 400 m and deposited dense clouds of smoke, ash and powdered rock (most of it respirable) as far as 1600 km away (e.g. Denver, Colorado). It caused only 30–40 immediate deaths, however, and was a relatively minor eruption by global standards. In Colombia just 5 years later some 15 000 inhabitants died following a volcanic eruption, while the notorious Krakatoa (Java) eruption of 1883 dispatched an entire island (and 5 cubic miles of rock) into the heavens and the sea, and caused 36 000 deaths and 2.5 days of local darkness.

The Mt St Helens eruption nevertheless led to the most detailed study of the respiratory consequences of volcanic emissions. The immediate threat to life came from blast injury and the inhalation of hot, oxygen-depleted air that was heavily contaminated with respirable ash and toxic gases. Acute respiratory death was thus the result of thermal and chemical injury coupled with suffocation. The risks of lung disease in the substantially greater population exposed to the cooled respirable particles at distances of 16 km or more were assumed to lie chiefly with the crystalline silica (about 6%) and amorphous silicate (65%) contents, because the remainder (largely oxides of aluminium, calcium and iron, and carbonates of potassium and sodium) are not recognised to be hazardous. At such a range the threat from toxic and asphyxiant gases is removed by the process of diffusion and hence dilution.

Reports so far in local children and forestry loggers are encouraging and have not demonstrated any appreciable acute, subacute or chronic respiratory effects.[146-148] Furthermore, exposure studies in laboratory animals have shown the volcanic ash to have far less inflammatory and fibrogenic properties than equal quantities of quartz.[148] Significant pathological effects were, however, noted in these animals and it remains to be seen whether sufficient quantities of ash have been retained in exposed human populations to induce pneumoconiosis or airway disease in the years to come. At present this appears unlikely.

Welding fumes

Like smoke from fires, welding fumes (and fumes from burning, i.e. cutting and gouging, metal) are likely to contain a variety of different toxic agents. These derive from the parent metal, any coating materials (e.g. paints, degreasing agents, zinc galvanisation), the consumable rod/electrode, atmospheric nitrogen and oxygen, and any heating gas. Their effects might therefore be predictable, depending on the precise exposures involved. In practice, any one welder will work under many different conditions in a lifetime, and a single day's exposure will rarely lead to acute toxic effects unless very high concentrations develop in confined spaces and the welder is not adequately protected with a respirator. A notable exception is fume derived from cadmium-containing alloys, which may readily cause a life-threatining pneumonitis.

Metal-fume fever is the most common acute effect, particularly when galvanised metal and zinc fume are involved (see Inhalation fever, above). Non-specific acute toxicity in the lung itself from welding fumes could be induced by nitrogen dioxide, ozone, manganese, combustion products of the coatings or even the trace metals. Chromium is especially prominent in stainless steels, and in this setting has been associated with occupational asthma. It is conceivable that nickel and the oxidant gases nitrogen dioxide and ozone could also be relevant in this respect but no confirmatory evidence for this has yet been found. Evidence is, however, emerging that welding fume may have a mild adverse effect on non-specific airway responsiveness, even at exposure levels complying with current regulatory limits and after periods as short as 5 years.[38,149] It is conceivable, therefore, that heavy and prolonged exposures in the past have caused asthma in some welders.

Other chronic effects on the airways include bronchitis (which is not uncommon) and, probably, COPD. Examination of the effect of welding fume on the development of fixed airway obstruction has been bedevilled by the confounding effect of cigarette smoking. Most investigations have failed to demonstrate a welding fume effect, although there have been exceptions. Most recently, cross-sectional and longitudinal investigation of shipyard welders in the north-east of England has shown more convincing evidence of fixed airway obstruction, but it was not marked (it was possibly partially masked by survivor bias) and it appeared to depend on interactions with both smoking and atopy.[36,37] The effect was largely confined to older welders with heavy cumulative exposures, often in confined environments without adequate ventilation or extraction. Such exposures are not commonly encountered today.

Siderosis (welder's lung) is not infrequent after a lifetime's work. This is a benign, non-fibrogenic, type of pneumoconiosis and is recognised from a fine mottling of small rounded opacities on the chest radiograph, which are a consequence of iron deposits in alveolar macrophages, lymphatic channels and alveolar walls.[150]

An excess of lung cancer among welders has been a source of particular concern and welding fumes have been classified as possibly carcinogenic by the International Agency for Research on Cancer.[151] Coincidental exposure to asbestos may account for most or all the excess, as might tobacco smoke, since welders tend to smoke more heavily than other occupational groups. Welders are, however, additionally exposed to other recognised carcinogens, such as chromium, nickel and thorium (incorporated into some tungsten electrodes), which might additionally contribute to the observed excess incidence.

Management

Acute effects

The acute effects of toxic agents on the lung are largely those of non-specific inflammation and so there is rarely a role for specific antidotes. Treatment is directed essentially to supportive measures designed to maintain life and alleviate discomfort until inflammation subsides and healing occurs, coupled with the obvious need to prevent further exposure and ensure that toxic agents do not continue to contaminate skin or clothing. The greatest threats are posed by upper-airway obstruction and failure of gas exchange, leading to severe hypoxaemia. Monitoring the arterial blood gas pressures is consequently essential when serious accidents occur, implying the need for hospital admission and close clinical and radiological surveillance. This normally involves intensive care. Since the onset of life-threatening responses to some inhaled toxic agents may be delayed for up to 24 hours and since the specific agents involved are often unclear or unknown, any seemingly serious exposure should provoke close hospital observation for at least this period. Ongoing close surveillance is necessary if pulmonary toxicity is then evident, since its course is often unpredictable.

Oxygen-enriched humidified air will be required in many cases, although high tensions may exacerbate the harmful effect of inflammatory oxidants. It may be best simply to ensure there is adequate oxygenation rather than normal oxygenation in cases of severe toxicity. Secretions and laryngeal oedema may produce stridor, especially following exposure to highly irritant agents that have high solubilities, and this may require emergency tracheal intubation or even tracheotomy. More diffuse airway obstruction may benefit from treatment with bronchodilators and corticosteroids, especially if RADS becomes evident. As severity increases, gas exchange worsens, the lungs become stiffer and exhaustion adds a further burden to ventilation. These signal the need for mechanical ventilatory support.

These emergency measures will often preserve life, but shock, pain, anxiety and chemical burns to the skin may require additional critical care. Systemic corticosteroid treatment is likely to moderate the harmful effects of the inflammatory response and should be used in these circumstances, although its value has provoked controversy in some situations, e.g. mineral oil aspiration.[152] In the case of nitrogen dioxide, at least, such treatment should be continued for 6–8 weeks to prevent a recurrent episode of pulmonary oedema, and if bronchiolitis obliterans or BOOP ensues corticosteroid treatment is usually needed for at least 6 months. The early use of corticosteroids may lessen the risk of such complications but there are currently insufficient data on this issue. The use of corticosteroids does not have confirmed benefit in managing the adult respiratory distress syndrome. Many authorities recommend prophylactic antibiotic treatment in addition, but this could encourage the emergence of a dominant resistant organism and it may be preferable to await clinical evidence of infection. Sputum microscopy and laboratory culture should then provide the most rational choice of antibiotic(s).

Progression in spite of these supportive measures implies a very grave prognosis and merits more desperate intervention. Bronchoscopy may help to clear secretions from the major airways and bronchoalveolar lavage may improve patency in the more distal airways. Finally, the justification for temporary extracorporeal cardiopulmonary support or even for lung transplantation may need to be considered.

With a few toxic agents certain specific complications may arise for which there are specific antidotes. Methaemoglobinaemia, for example, may be a manifestation of oxidant toxicity, although this occurs most commonly as a result of alimentary rather than inhalational poisoning. It may, however, complicate nitrogen dioxide toxicity, exaggerating the apparent cyanosis of respiratory failure and reducing oxygen transport within the blood. If severe it can be treated with the reducing agent methylthionium chloride (methylene blue), but this is rarely necessary. Similarly, the use of the chelating agent ethylenediamine tetraacetic acid has been advocated for acute cadmium toxicity, although its value is disputed. With smoke inhalation involving hydrogen cyanide, the immediate use of inhaled amyl nitrite followed by intravenous sodium nitrite and sodium thiosulphate may prove life-saving, as may intravenous replacement of fluids and the use of topical antibiotics and grafts, if it is accompanied by severe burns to the skin.

Subacute and chronic effects

Prevention requires reliable epidemiological data from which effective but realistic exposure standards can be determined. Where these cannot be achieved by measures of hygiene control, areas of persisting hazard must be clearly identified and adequate respiratory protection equipment provided. It may not be easy, however, to obtain satisfactory worker co-operation in using uncomfortable or inconvenient respiratory equipment to eliminate a poorly perceived risk of disease developing decades in the future. Education and understanding provide the best solution, coupled with firm direction from management.

Where the risks are greatest, a programme of surveillance should allow adverse effects to be detected before serious disability arises. Subjects with undue susceptibility can thus be removed from further exposure. Where there is the possibility of serious accidental exposure, ready communication, first aid and rapid transportation facilities are the key to minimising the risk of death.

Therapeutic principles

- Prompt cessation of exposure, with care to avoid ongoing exposure from contaminated clothing.

- Care that rescuers are adequately protected from hazardous levels of exposure, particularly when operating in a confined environment.

- Urgent assessment of airway patency and oxygenation, and rapid transportation of serious cases to appropriate medical facilities.

- Supportive care including, where necessary, intensive care.

- Surveillance for a minimum of 24 hours of all cases with potentially life-threatening exposures.

- Administration of specific antidotes when (rarely) such exist (e.g. for cyanide poisoning, methaemoglobinaemia)

- Steroid administration for 6–8 weeks following acute pneumonitis induced by nitrogen dioxide.

- Risk assessment and evaluation of measures to prevent subsequent incidents.

? Unresolved questions

- How often are inhalation accidents complicated by obstructive bronchiolitis or bronchiolitis obliterans organising pneumonia?

- What are the risks of chronic obstructive pulmonary disease, pulmonary fibrosis and lung cancer from a single major exposure to irritant or toxic dusts and gases compared with those from ongoing low levels of exposures?

- What are the role and mechanisms of differences in susceptibility?

- What are the best preventive and management strategies for adult respiratory distress syndrome and secondary infection?

References

1. Blanc PD, Galbo M, Hiatt P, Olson KR. Morbidity following acute irritant inhalation in a population-based study. JAMA 1991; 266: 664–669.
2. Ross DJ. Ten years of the SWORD project. Clin Exp Allergy 1999; 29: 750–753.
3. Anonymous. Calamity at Bhopal. Lancet 1984; 2: 1378–1379.
4. Jones RN, Hughes JM, Glindmeyer H, Weill H. Lung function after acute chlorine exposure. Am Rev Respir Dis 1986; 134: 1190–1195.
5. Morgan M, Frank R. Uptake of pollutant gases in the respiratory system. In: Brain J, Proctor D, Reid L, ed. Respiratory defence mechanisms, part I. New York: Marcel Dekker; 1977.
6. Epler GR, Colby TV, McLoud TC et al. Bronchiolitis obliterans organizing pneumonia. N Engl J Med 1985; 312: 152–158.
7. Epler GR. Bronchiolitis obliterans organizing pneumonia: definition and clinical features. Chest 1992; 102(1 suppl): 2S–6S.
8. Gilchrist HL, Matz PB. The residual effects of warfare gases: the use of chlorine gas, with report of cases. Med Bull Vet Admin 1933; 9: 229–270.
9. Pennington AH. War gases and chronic lung disease. Med J Austr 1954; 1: 510–516.
10. Brooks SM, Weiss MA, Bernstein IL. Reactive airways dysfunction syndrome (RADS): persistent asthma syndrome after high level irritant exposures. Chest 1985; 88: 376–384.
11. Brinton WT, Vastbinder EE, Greene JW et al. An outbreak of organic dust toxic syndrome in a college fraternity. JAMA 1987; 258: 1210–1212.
12. Fine JM, Gordon T, Chen LC et al. Metal fume fever. J Occup Environ Med 1997; 39: 722–726.
13. Blanc PD, Boushey HA, Wong H et al. Cytokines in metal fume fever. Am Rev Respir Dis 1993; 147: 134–138.
14. Kuschner WG, D'Alessandro A, Wong H, Blanc PD. Early pulmonary cytokine responses to zinc oxide fume formation. Environ Res 1997; 75: 7–11.
15. McMillan G. Welding: In Hendrick DJ, Burge PS, Beckett WS, Churg A, ed. Occupational disorders of the lung. London: WB Saunders; in press.
16. Mamolen M, Lewis DM, Blanchet MA et al. Investigation of an outbreak of 'Humidifier Fever' in a print shop. Am J Ind Med 1993; 23: 483–490.
17. Pal TM, de Monchy JG, Groothoff JW, Post D. The clinical spectrum of humidifier disease in synthetic fiber plants. Am J Ind Med 1997; 31: 682–692.
18. Shusterman DJ. Polymer fume fever and other fluorocarbon pyrolysis-related syndromes. Occup Med 1993; 8: 519–531.
19. DoPico GA. International Workshop on Health Effects of Organic Dusts in the Farm Environment, Skokloster, Sweden. Am J Ind Med 1986; 10: 261–265.
20. Vogelzang PFJ, van der Gulden JWJ, Folgering H, van Schayck CP. Organic dust toxic syndrome in swine confinement farming. Am J Ind Med 1999; 35: 332–334.
21. Simpson JCG, Niven RM, Pickering CAC et al. Prevalence and predictors of work related respiratory symptoms in workers exposed to organic dusts. Occup Environ Med 1998; 55: 668–672.
22. Cormier Y, Fournier M, Laviolette M. Farmer's fever. Chest 1993; 103: 632–634.
23. Wintermeyer SF, Kuschner WG, Wong H et al. Pulmonary responses after wood chip mulch exposure. J Occup Environ Med 1997; 39: 308–314.
24. Moya C, Antó JM, Newman Taylor AJ, the Collaborative Group for the Study of Toxicity in Textile Aerographic Factories. Outbreak of organising pneumonia in textile printing sprayers. Lancet 1994; 343: 498–502.
25. Ould Kadi F, Mohammed-Brahim B, Fyad A et al. Outbreak of pulmonary disease in textile dye sprayers in Algeria. Lancet 1994; 344: 962–963.
26. Banks DE, Bauer MA, Castellan RM, Lapp NL. Silicosis in surface coal mine drillers. Thorax 1983; 38: 275–278.
27. Grammer LC, Shaughnessy MA, Zeiss CR et al. Review of trimellitic anhydride (TMA) induced respiratory response. Allergy Asthma Proc 1997; 18: 235–237.
28. Kaplan V, Baur X, Czuppon A et al. Pulmonary hemorrhage due to inhalation of vapor containing pyromellitic dianhydride. Chest 1993; 104: 644–645.
29. Glynn KP, Gale NA. Exogenous lipoid pneumonia due to inhalation of spray lubricant (WD-40 lung). Chest 1990; 97: 1265–1266.
30. Kern DG, Crausman RS, Durand KTH et al. Flock worker's lung: chronic interstitial lung disease in the nylon flocking industry. Ann Intern Med 1998; 129: 261–272.
31. Eschenbacher WL, Kreiss K, Lougheed MD et al. Nylon flock-associated interstitial lung disease. Am J Respir Crit Care Med 1999; 159: 2003–2008.
32. Diem JE, Jones RN, Hendrick DJ et al. Five-year longitudinal study of workers employed in a new toluene diisocyanate manufacturing plant. Am Rev Respir Dis 1982; 126: 420–428.
33. Chan-Yeung M, Enarson DA, Kennedy SM. The impact of grain dust on respiratory health. State of the art. Am Rev Respir Dis 1992; 145: 476–487.
34. DoPico GA, Reddan W, Flaherty D et al. Respiratory abnormalities among grain handlers. A clinical, physiologic, and immunologic study. Am Rev Respir Dis 1977; 115: 915–927.
35. Rogan JM, Attfield MD, Jacobsen M et al. Role of dust in the working environment in development of chronic bronchitis in British coal miners. Br J Ind Med 1973; 30: 217–226.
36. Cotes JE, Feinmann EL, Male VJ et al. Respiratory symptoms and impairment in shipyard welders and caulker/burners. Br J Ind Med 1989; 46: 292.
37. Chiun DJ, Stevenson IC, Cotes JE. Longitudinal respiratory survey of shipyard workers: effects of trade and atopic status. Br J Ind Med 1990; 47: 83.
38. Sferlazza SJ, Beckett WS. State of the art: the respiratory health of welders. Am Rev Respir Dis 1992; 143: 1134–1148.
39. Cowie R, Mafena SK. Silicosis, chronic airflow limitation, and chronic bronchitis in South African gold miners. Am Rev Respir Dis 1992; 143: 80–84.
40. Chester EH, Kaimal J, Payne CB, Kohn PM. Pulmonary injury following exposure to chlorine gas. Possible beneficial effects of steroid treatment. Chest 1977; 72: 247–250.
41. Becklake MR, Goldman HI, Bosman AR, Freed CC. The long-term effects of exposure to nitrous fumes. Am Rev Tuberc 1957; 76: 398–409.
42. Galdston M, Luetscher JA, Longcope WT, Ballich NL. A study of the residual effects of phosgene poisoning in human subjects. 1. After acute exposure. J Clin Invest 1947; 26: 145–168.

43. Snyder RW, Mishel HS, Christensen GC. Pulmonary toxicity following exposure to methylene chloride and its combustion product, phosgene. Chest 1992; 102: 1921.

44. Harkonen H, Nordman H, Korhonen O, Winblad I. Long-term effects of exposure to sulfur dioxide. Am Rev Respir Dis 1983; 128: 890–893.

45. Kern DG. Outbreak of the reactive airways dysfunction syndrome after a spill of glacial acetic acid. Am Rev Respir Dis 1991; 144: 1058–1064.

46. Alberts WM, do Pico GA. Reactive airways dysfunction syndrome. Chest 1996; 109: 1618–1626.

47. Stenton SC, Kelly CA, Walters EH, Hendrick DJ. Induction of bronchial hyperresponsiveness following smoke inhalation injury. Br J Dis Chest 1988; 82: 436–438.

48. Kipen HM, Blume R, Hutt D. Asthma experience in an occupational and environmental medicine clinic. Low-dose reactive airways dysfunction syndrome. J Occup Med 1994; 36: 1133–1137.

49. Orehek J, Massari JP, Gayrard P et al. Effect of short term, low level nitrogen dioxide exposure on bronchial sensitivity of asthmatic patients. J Clin Invest 1976; 57: 301–307.

50. Golden JA, Nadel JA, Boushey HA. Bronchial hyperirritability in healthy subjects after exposure to ozone. Am Rev Respir Dis 1978; 118: 287–294.

51. Walters EH, O'Byrne PM, Graf PD et al. The responsiveness of airway smooth muscle in vitro from dogs with airway hyper-responsiveness in vivo. Clin Sci 1986; 71: 605–611.

52. Kass I, Zamel N, Dobry CA, Holzer M. Bronchiectasis following ammonia burns of the respiratory tract. A review of two cases. Chest 1972; 62: 282–285.

53. Bates DV, Macklem PT, Christie RV. Respiratory function in disease. Toronto: WB Saunders; 1971: 392–394.

54. Sobonya R. Fatal anhydrous ammonia inhalation. Hum Pathol 1977; 8: 293–299.

55. Leduc D, Gris P, Lheureux P et al. Acute and long term respiratory damage following inhalation of ammonia. Thorax 1991; 47: 755–757.

56. McAdams AJ, Krop S. Injury and death from red fuming nitric acid. JAMA 1955; 158: 1022–1024.

57. Fleming GM, Chester EH, Montenegro HD. Dysfunction of small pulmonary airways following pulmonary injury due to nitrogen dioxide. Chest 1979; 75: 720–721.

58. Woodford DM, Coutu RE, Gaensler EA. Obstructive lung disease from acute sulfur dioxide exposure. Respiration 1979; 38: 238–245.

59. Charan NB, Myers CG, Laksminarayan S, Spencer TM. Pulmonary injuries associated with acute sulfur dioxide inhalation. Am Rev Respir Dis 1979; 119: 555–560.

60. Sjögren B, Plato N, Alexandersson R et al. Pulmonary reactions caused by welding-induced decomposed trichloroethylene. Chest 1991; 99: 237–238.

61. Murphy DMF, Fairman RP, Lapp NL, Morgan WKC. Severe airway disease due to inhalation of fumes from cleansing agents. Chest 1976; 69: 372–376.

62. Bates C, Read RC, Morice AH. A malicious mould. Lancet 1997; 349: 1598.

63. Douglas WW, Colby TV. Fume-related bronchiolitis obliterans. In: Epler GR, ed. Diseases of the bronchioles. New York: Raven Press; 1994: 187–213.

64. Bonnell JA, Kazantzis G, King F. A follow up of men exposed to cadmium oxide fume. Br J Ind Med 1959; 16: 135.

65. Davison AG, Fayers PM, Newman Taylor AJ et al. Cadmium inhalation and emphysema. Thorax 1986; 41: 714.

66. Cullen MR, Balmes JR, Robins JM, Walker Smith GJ. Lipoid pneumonitis caused by oil mist exposure from a steel rolling tandem mill. Am J Ind Med 1981; 2: 51–58.

67. Corrin B, Crocker PR, Hood BJ et al. Paraffinoma confirmed by infrared spectrophotometry. Thorax 1987; 42: 389.

68. Penes MC, Vallon JJ, Sabot JF, Vallon C. Gas chromatography and mass spectroscopy detection of paraffin in a case of lipoid pneumonia following occupational exposure to oil spray. J Anal Toxicol 1990; 14: 372–374.

69. Silverman JF, Turner RC, West RL, Dillard TA. Bronchoalveolar lavage in the diagnosis of lipoid pneumonia. Diagn Cytol 1989; 5: 3–8.

70. Levade T, Salvayre R, Dongay G et al. Chemical analysis of the bronchoalveolar lavage washing fluid in the diagnosis of liquid paraffin pneumonia. J Clin Chem Clin Biochem 1987; 25: 45–48.

71. Lee JS, Im J-G, Song KM et al. Exogenous lipoid pneumonia: high resolution CT findings. Eur Radiol 1999; 9: 287–291.

72. Chang H-Y, Chen C-W, Chen C-Y et al. Successful treatment of diffuse lipoid pneumonitis with whole lung lavage. Thorax 1993; 48: 947–948.

73. Wilt JL, Banks DE, Weissman DN et al. Reduction of lung dust burden in pneumoconiosis by whole-lung lavage. J Occup Environ Med 1996; 38: 619–624.

74. Zhang H, Li Q, Yao R, Guo N. Experimental studies on the therapeutic effects of lung lavage with large volume saline on silicosis. Wel Sheng Yen Chiu/J Hyg Res 1997; 26: 77–79.

75. Goodman GB, Kaplan PD, Stachura I et al. Acute silicosis responding to corticosteroid therapy. Chest 1992; 101: 366–370.

76. Miller GJ, Ashcroft MT, Beadnell HMSG et al. The lipoid pneumonia of blackfat smokers in Guyana. Q J Med 1971; 40: 457–470.

77. Finkelstein MM. Clinical measures, smoking, radon exposure, and risk of lung cancer in uranium miners. J Occup Environ Med 1996; 53: 697–702.

78. Davies JM, Easton DF, Bistrup PL. Mortality from respiratory cancer and other causes in United Kingdom chrome production workers. Br J Ind Med 1991; 48: 299.

79. Weiss W, Moser RL, Auerbach O. Lung cancer in chloromethyl ether workers. Am Rev Respir Dis 1979; 120: 1031.

80. Enterline PE, Henderson VL, Marsh GM. Exposure to arsenic and respiratory cancer. Am J Epidemiol 1987; 125: 929.

81. Dong MH, Redmond CK, Mazumdar S, Costantino JP. A multistage approach to the cohort analysis of lifetime lung cancer risk among steel workers exposed to coke oven emissions. Am J Epidemiol 1988; 128: 860.

82. Blot WJ. Lung cancer and occupational exposures. In: Mixell M, Correa P, ed. Lung cancer causes and prevention. Deerfield, FL: Verlag Chemical International; 1985: 47.

83. Gong N, Christiani DC. Lung cancer: In: Hendrick DJ, Burge PS, Beckett WS, Churg A, ed. Occupational disorders of the lung. London: WB Saunders; 2001

84. International Agency for Research on Cancer. An evaluation of carcinogenic risk to humans. Overall evaluation of carcinogenicity: an updating of IARC monographs Vols 1–42, 440pp Suppl. 7. Lyon: IARC; 1987.

85. Stanton MF, Layard M, Tegeris A et al. Carcinogenicity of fibrous glass: pleural response in the rat in relation to fiber dimension. J Natl Cancer Inst 1977; 58: 587.

86. Sunyer J, Anto JM, Sabria J et al. Risk factors of soybean epidemic asthma. The role of smoking and atopy. Am Rev Respir Dis 1992; 145: 1098.

87. Report of the ATS Workshop on the health effects of atmospheric acids and their precursors. Am Rev Respir Dis 1991; 144: 464.

88. Britton J. Pollution and respiratory morbidity: how much do we accept? Thorax 1992; 47: 391.

89. Dockery DW, Pope CA III, Xu X et al. An association between air pollution and mortality in six US cities. N Engl J Med 1993; 329: 1753–1759.

90. Pope CA III, Thun MJ, Nanboodiri MM et al. Particulate air pollution as a predictor of mortality in a prospective study of US adults. Am J Respir Crit Care Med 1995: 151: 669–674.

91. Bates DV. Particulate air pollution. Thorax 1996; 51(suppl 2): 53–58.

92. Seaton A, Soutar CA, Crawford V et al. Particulate air pollution and the blood. Thorax 1999; 54: 1027–1032.

93. Diskstra L, Houthuijs D, Brunekreef B et al. Respiratory health effects of the indoor environment in a population of Dutch children. Am Rev Respir Dis 1990; 142: 1172.

94. Hendrick DJ, Lane DJ. Occupational formalin asthma. Br J Ind Med 1977; 34: 11.

95. Hendrick DJ. The formaldehyde problem – a clinical appraisal. Immunol Allergy Pract 1983; 5: 97.

96. Encyclopaedia of occupational health and safety. Geneva: International Labour Office; 1983: 395–399.

97. Schwartz D, Smith D, Lakshminarayan S. The pulmonary sequelae associated with accidental inhalation of chlorine gas. Chest 1990; 97: 820–825.

98. Weill H, George R, Schwarz M, Ziskind M. Late evaluation of pulmonary function after acute exposure to chlorine gas. Am Rev Respir Dis 1969; 99: 374.

99. Kennedy SM, Enarson DA, Janssen RG, Chan-Yeung M. Lung health consequences of reported accidental chlorine gas exposures among pulpmill workers. Am Rev Respir Dis 1991; 143: 74.

100. Toren K, Blanc PD. The history of pulp and paper bleaching: respiratory-health effects. Lancet 1997; 349: 1316–1321.

101. Glassroth J, Adams G, Scholl S. The impact of substance abuse on the respiratory system. Chest 1987; 91: 595.

102. Llamas R, Hart DR, Schneider NS. Allergic bronchopulmonary aspergillosis associated with smoking marijuana. Chest 1978; 73: 871.

103. Ettinger N, Albin R. A review of the respiratory effects of smoking cocaine. Am J Med 1989; 87: 664.

104. Patel RC, Dutta D, Schonfeld SA. Free-base cocaine use associated with bronchiolitis obliterans organizing pneumonia. Ann Intern Med. 1987; 107: 186–187.

105. Haim DY, Lippmann ML, Goldberg SK, Walkenstein MD. The pulmonary complications of crack cocaine. A comprehensive review. Chest 1995; 107: 233–240.

106. Amelle J, Brechot JM, Brochard P et al. Occupational hypersensitivity pneumonitis in a smelter exposed to zinc fumes. Chest 1992; 101: 862.

107. Kanluen S, Gottlieb CA. A clinical pathologic study of four adult cases of acute mercury inhalation toxicity. Arch Pathol Lab Med 1991; 115: 6–60.

108. Fernandez MA, Sanz P, Palomar M et al. Fatal chemical pneumonitis due to cadmium fumes. Occup Med 1996; 46: 372–374.

109. Liles R, Miller A, Lerman Y. Acute mercury poisoning with severe chronic pulmonary manifestations. Chest 1985; 88: 306–309.

110. Levin M, Jacob J, Polos PG. Acute mercury, poisoning and mercurial pneumonitis from gold ore purification. Chest 1988; 94: 554–556.

111. Rowens B, Guerrero-Betancourt D, Gottlieb CA et al. Respiratory failure and death following acute inhalation of mercury vapor. A clinical and histologic perspective. Chest 1991; 99: 185–190.

112. Gheysens B, Auwerx J, Van-den-Eeckhout A, Demedts M. Cobalt induced bronchial asthma in diamond polishers. Chest 1985; 88: 740.

113. Williams CW. Asthma related to chromium compounds. NC Med J 1969; 30: 482.

114. Block GT, Yeung M. Asthma induced by nickel. JAMA 1982; 247: 1600.

115. Musk AW, Tees JG. Asthma caused by occupational exposure to vanadium compounds. Med J Austr 19821: 183.

116. Enterline PE. Respiratory cancer among chromate workers. J Occup Med 1974; 16: 523.

117. Davison AG, Haslam PL, Corrin B et al. Interstitial lung disease and asthma in hard-metal workers: bronchoalveolar lavage, ultrastructural, and analytical findings and results of bronchial provocation tests. Thorax 1983; 38: 119.

118. Villar TG. Vineyard sprayers' lung. Am Rev Respir Dis 1974; 110: 545.

119. Cullinan P, Acquilla S, Ramana Dhara N. Respiratory morbidity 10 years after the Union Carbide Gas leak at Bhopal: a cross sectional survey. Br Med J 1997; 314: 338–343.

120. Nemery B. Late consequences of accidental exposure to inhaled irritants : RADS and the Bhopal disaster. Eur Respir J 1996; 9: 1973–1976.

121. Meredith TJ, Vale JA, Proudfoot AT. Poisoning caused by inhaled agents. In: Weatherall DJ, Ledingham JGG, Warrell DA, ed. Oxford textbook of medicine. Oxford: Oxford University Press; 1987: 6.56.

122. Robertson AS, Wieland GA, Burge PS. Occupational asthma due to oil mists. Thorax 1986; 41: 250.

123. Subcommittee on Accidental Poisoning, American Academy of Pediatrics. Evaluation of gastric lavage and other factors in the treatment of accidental ingestion of petroleum distillate products. Cooperative kerosene poisoning study. Pediatrics 1962; 29: 648.

124. US Chemical Warfare Service. Proceedings of a board appointed for the purpose of investigating conditions incident to the disaster at the Cleveland Hospital Clinic, Cleveland, Ohio, on May 15th 1929. Washington, DC: US Government Printing Office; 1929.

125. Zwemer FL Jr, Pratt DS, May JJ. Silo filler's disease in New York State. Am Rev Respir Dis 1992; 146: 650.

126. Melia RJW, Florey C du V, Altman DG et al. Association between gas cooking and respiratory disease in children. Br Med J 1977; 2: 149.

127. Speizer FE, Ferris B, Bishop YMM et al. Respiratory disease rates and pulmonary function in children associated with nitrogen dioxide exposure. Am Rev Respir Dis 1980; 121: 3.

128. Rossi OVJ, Kinnula VL, Tienari J, Huhti E. Association of severe asthma attacks with weather, pollen, and air pollutants. Thorax 1993; 48: 244.

129. Emmanuel DA, Wenzel FJ, Lawton BR. Pulmonary mycotoxicosis. Chest 1975; 67: 293.

130. Morgan DC, Smyth JT, Lister RW, Pethybridge RJ. Chest symptoms and farmer's lung: a community survey. Br J Ind Med 1973; 30: 259.

131. May JJ, Stallones L, Darrow D, Pratt DS. Organic dust toxicity (pulmonary mycotoxicosis) associated with silo unloading. Thorax 1986; 41: 919.

132. Lecours R, Laviolette M, Cormier Y. Bronchoalveolar lavage in pulmonary mycotoxicosis (organic dust toxic syndrome). Thorax 1986; 41: 924.

133. Osbern LN, Crapo RO. Dung lung: a report of toxic exposure to liquid manure. Ann Intern Med 1981; 95: 312.

134. Folinsbee LJ, Bedi JF, Horvath SM. Respiratory responses to humans repeatedly exposed to low concentrations of ozone. Am Rev Respir Dis 1980; 121: 431.

135. Synder RW, Mishel HS, Christensen GC III. Pulmonary toxicity following exposure to methylene chloride and its combustion product, phosgene. Chest 1992; 101: 860.

136. Anonymous. Mortality and morbidity during the London fog of December 1952. Report on Public Health and Medical Subjects, 95. London: HMSO; 1954.

137. Clark CJ, Campbell D, Reid WH. Blood carboxyhaemoglobin and cyanide levels in fire survivors. Lancet 1981; 1: 1332.

138. Clark CJ, Reid WH, Gilmour WH, Campbell D. Mortality probability in victims of fire trauma: revised equation to include inhalation injury. Br Med J 1986; 292: 1303.

139. O'Hickey SP, Pickering CAC, Jones PE, Evans JD. Manchester air disaster. Br Med J 1987; 294: 1663.

140. Stenton SC, Kelly CA, Walters EH, Hendrick DJ. Induction of bronchial hyperresponsiveness following smoke inhalation injury. Br J Dis Chest 1988; 82: 436.

141. Fogarty PW, George PJM, Solomon M et al. Longterm effects of smoke inhalation in survivors of the King's Cross underground station fire. Thorax 1991; 46: 914.

142. Charan NB, Myers CG, Lakshminaryan S, Spencer TM. Pulmonary injuries associated with acute sulfur dioxide inhalation. Am Rev Respir Dis 1979; 119: 555.

143. Hill AR, Silverberg NB, Mayorga D, Baldwin HE. Medical hazards of the tear gas CS. A case of persistent, multisystem, hypersensitivity reaction and review of the literature. Medicine 2000; 79: 234–420.

144. Breakell A, Bodiwala GG. CS gas exposure in a crowded night club: the consequences for an accident and emergency department. J Accid Emerg Med 1998; 15: 56–64.

145. Fraunfelder FT. Is CS gas dangerous? Current evidence suggests not but unanswered questions remain. Br Med J 2000; 320: 458–459.

146. Johnson KG, Loftsgaarden DO, Gideon RA. The effects of Mount St Helens volcanic eruption on the pulmonary function of 120 elementary school children. Am Rev Respir Dis 1982; 126: 1066.

147. Buist AS, Bernstein RS, Johnson LR, Vollmer WM. Evaluation of physical health effects due to volcanic hazards: human studies. Am J Pub Health 1986; 76(suppl): 66.

148. Martin TR, Wehner AP, Butler J. Pulmonary toxicity of Mt St Helens volcanic ash. A review of experimental studies. Am Rev Respir Dis 1983; 128: 158.

149. Beach JR, Dennis JH, Avery AJ et al. An epidemiologic investigation of asthma in welders. Am J Respir Crit Care Med 1996; 154: 1394–1400.

150. Morgan WKC, Kerr HD. Pathologic and physiologic studies of welder's siderosis. Ann Intern Med 1963; 58: 293.

151. International Agency for Research on Cancer. IARC monographs on the evaluation of carcinogenic risks to humans. Vol 49, Chromium, nickel and welding. Lyon: IARC; 1990.

152. Steele RW, Canklin RH, Mark M. Corticosteroids and antibiotics for the treatment of fulminant hydrocarbon aspiration. JAMA 1972; 219: 1434.

31 Toxic lung injury: ingested agents

Peter G Blain

Key points

- The human lung is susceptible to damage from ingested toxic chemicals.

- Ingested chemicals may be directly toxic to the lung or may be converted to a toxic metabolite.

- Specific lung cells are responsible for local intracellular metabolism of compounds and susceptibility to toxic effects.

- Animal-based investigations have identified many compounds with the potential to damage human lungs and the possible toxic mechanisms, but data in humans are limited.

The main route by which the lungs are exposed to toxins is inhalation but they are vulnerable also to the toxic effects of compounds ingested or produced by metabolism in other organs and present in blood passing through the pulmonary circulation. These toxic compounds may be drugs (see Chapter 29), toxic metabolites, food contaminants or chemicals ingested, intentionally or accidentally, at home, in the workplace or in the general environment.

Metabolism of exogenous compounds

Most toxic exogenous compounds (xenobiotics) are metabolised, reducing their potential toxicity and facilitating elimination from the body. Compounds that are rapidly absorbed into the body are usually lipophilic and, therefore, likely to be retained. Consequently, they must be converted into a form that is more easily eliminated from the body before they can be excreted.

The liver is the most important organ for xenobiotic metabolism (biotransformation), although other organs such as the skin, lungs, kidney and skeletal muscle may have a significant capability, but at a lower level of activity than the liver (Table 31.1). Occasionally, detoxification does not occur or, paradoxically, toxicity may be enhanced (activated) as a result of metabolic changes (e.g. procarcinogens, some organophosphate pesticides).

Metabolism of xenobiotics is carried out mainly by a group of relatively non-specific enzymes that are classified as mixed function oxidases. One specific family of isoenzymes has a characteristic peak in the reduced form at 450 nm in a carbon monoxide adduct difference spectrum and are, therefore, called the cytochromes P450. The active site of cytochrome P450 contains an iron atom that can switch between divalent and trivalent oxidation states. This combines with a substrate and molecular oxygen as part of a process by which the substrate is oxidised. The enzyme requires an electron (e^-) transport chain for its reduction.

The cytochromes P450 are abundant in the liver, which is the body's primary site of defence against systemic poisons,

Table 31.1 Comparative capability for biotransformation

Organ	Approximate comparative capability for biotransformation of foreign agents (% relative to activity of liver)
Liver	100
Adrenal cortex	75
Lungs	30
Kidney	30
Testes	20
Skin	10
Gastrointestinal tract	10
Spleen	5
Heart muscle	3
Skeletal muscle	1

but also occur in other organs such as the lungs, kidney, ovaries, placenta, testes and olfactory mucosa. The presence of the enzyme in the lungs, skin, placenta and gastrointestinal tract may reflect a defensive role of these organs against toxic exogenous compounds.

The cytochromes have differing and overlapping specificities and at least eight gene families have been identified. The cytochrome P450 nomenclature (CYP) is based on gene structure, the first number designating the gene family, the capital letter the subfamily and the second number the specific protein. The P450 isoenzymes share some structural similarities and it has been estimated that there are some 200 different P450 isoenzymes in most mammalian species. Related enzymes isolated from lung and liver within a species appear to be similar in structural characteristics but the regulation of enzyme expression varies considerably among tissues. As a group the isoenzymes exhibit broad substrate specificity and are capable of metabolising many diverse compounds, although individually they may exhibit unique substrate specificities. Some of the P450 isoenzymes are inducible by exposure to environmental chemicals. Phenobarbital, 3-methylcholanthrene (3MC) and 2,3,7,8-tetrachlorodibenzodioxin (TCDD) are well-recognised inducers of hepatic P450 isoenzymes in animals and humans.

Mixed function oxidase activity is associated with cellular smooth endoplasmic reticulum and, when tissues such as the liver are homogenised, the endoplasmic reticulum is broken down to form small vesicles known as microsomes. Microsomes are the fraction collected from the centrifugation of tissue homogenate at about 100 000 g and, essentially, contain the rough and smooth endoplasmic reticulum and Golgi apparatus. The microsomal enzymes are associated with lipid membranes and are lipid-dependent. Sonic vibration, or the use of hypotonic solutions, fails to solubilise them, whereas treatment of microsomes with deoxycholic acid, which solubilises lipid membranes, destroys the activity of oxidative enzymes.

Phases of biotransformation

Biotransformation of xenobiotics usually consists of two phases:

- **Phase 1**: oxidation (via the cytochrome P450-dependent mixed function oxygenases), reduction or hydrolysis of the parent compound
- **Phase 2**: conjugation of the metabolite to glucuronic acid, glutathione, glycine sulphate or other endogenous compound.

In phase 1 a polar reactive group is introduced into the molecule, which increases water solubility and makes the compound suitable for phase 2. In phase 2 reactions the functional groups on a molecule (e.g. carboxyl, amino, hydroxyl or sulphydryl groups) are conjugated with endogenous compounds or sugars to form water-soluble, polar derivatives that can be excreted more readily and are usually less toxic. The reduction in lipid solubility also decreases back-diffusion across membranes.

Conjugation with glucuronic acid is the most important and most common mechanism in phase 2 metabolism. The enzyme UDPglucuronyltransferase catalyses the transfer of glucuronic acid from uridine diphosphate glucuronic acid. Glucuronide conjugation products are classified by the site of binding: a hydroxyl functional group forms an ether glucuronide, a carboxyl acid group an ester glucuronide. Glucuronides may be attached directly to nitrogen as the linking atom (e.g. aniline glucuronide) or through an intermediate oxygen atom such as occurs in the conjugation product N-hydroxyacetylaminoglucuronide, but this, paradoxically, is a more potent carcinogen than the parent compound, N-hydroxyacetylaminofluorene.

Glutathione, a tripeptide of glutamic acid, cysteine and glycine, is another endogenous compound utilised in phase 2 reactions. The thiol (SH) groups in glutathione form covalent bonds with the xenobiotic. Glutathione conjugates may be excreted directly or after further metabolism to mercapturic acids (compounds with N-acetylcysteine attached). The enzyme glutathione transferase is required for the conjugation process and is found in multiple forms throughout the body.

Sulphate conjugates are completely ionised and, therefore, are highly efficient for eliminating xenobiotics in the urine. The compounds that form sulphate conjugates are alcohols, phenols and arylamines.

Most compounds undergo both metabolic transformation and conjugation but, occasionally, only the first of these reactions occurs because biotransformation produces a metabolite that is sufficiently water-soluble to be easily excreted without conjugation. Alternatively, the compound already possesses groups that are easily conjugated, so that phase 1 metabolism is not required.

The principal effect of biotransformation is to facilitate the elimination of a xenobiotic by its conversion to a more polar (water-soluble) metabolite and it is therefore usually a detoxification mechanism. In some cases the intermediate metabolites, or final products, may be more toxic than the parent compound (i.e. there is entoxification or activation). These metabolites may be systemically toxic or, because they are produced locally by an organ (such as in the lung), have direct toxic effects on the tissues where biotransformation is occurring. Most cells, and especially hepatocytes, have protective biochemical systems to prevent damage to vital cell processes from locally produced toxic metabolites.

Pulmonary biotransformation of xenobiotics

More than 40 histologically different cell types have been identified in lung tissue. The susceptibility of an individual cell to toxic compounds, or their metabolites, in blood depends in part on the specific metabolic functions of that cell.[1] For many compounds the lungs appear to be a target organ for toxicity and, in some cases, there is selective toxicity to a specific type of lung cell (e.g. naphthol is a specific Clara-cell toxin). The level of metabolic activity of a cell depends on its degree of specialisation and the nature of the enzyme substrates. The lung is capable of metabolising many xenobiotics by both phase 1 and phase 2 reactions.

The characterisation of pulmonary P450 isoenzymes and their role in xenobiotic metabolism is complicated by the diversity of cell types within the lung and the relatively low activity of P450 isoenzymes in lung tissue. Studies of microsomal enzyme activities have shown that the lung contains fewer P450 isoenzymes than the liver. The average concentration of P450 isoenzymes in lung tissue is low (about 10% of that found in liver measured per gram of microsomal protein) but some P450 isoenzymes appear to be concentrated in specific lung cell types. Measurement of P450 activity in whole lung microsomes tends to underestimate the capacity of lung because P450 activity in specific cells is diluted by inactive cells.

The non-ciliated bronchiolar (Clara) cell is metabolically the most active lung cell and has a high activity of mixed-function oxidases. Localisation of P450 isoenzymes shows the highest concentrations in pulmonary Clara cells and type II epithelial cells; this distribution may determine the role of the lung as a target organ for certain toxic xenobiotics.

Relatively detailed information about cytochrome P450 (CYP) isoenzymes is available for animal lungs but the individual isoenzymes have not been well characterised in human lung, although it has been shown to contain much lower levels of cytochrome P450 isoenzymes than the lungs of other species. Thus, the levels of total cytochromes P450 in human lung microsomes are approximately 5% of those in rat lung and less than 1% of those in rabbit lung microsomes. Cytochrome P450 1A1 (CYP1A1) has been identified in human lung cells and this correlates well with 7-ethoxyresorufin O-deethylase (EROD) activity in lung samples. An oligonucleotide probe specific for the CYP1A1 gene has demonstrated expression in human lung. CYP1A1 mRNA has been detected in lung tissue from cigarette smokers but not from non-smokers. The amount of CYP1A1 mRNA expressed in smokers correlates with the levels of cytochrome P450 1A1 reflected as EROD activity in lung tissue from smokers. Immunoblot analysis of lung microsomes using antibodies cross-reacting with human liver P450 isoenzymes showed no evidence of CYPs 1A2, 2C, 2D and 3A. Studies have suggested that CYP2B may be a major P450 in rodent and human lung, capable of activating organophosphate pesticides and naphthalene, and lung-specific P450s CYP4B, CYP2J and CYP2F have also been identified.

Other components of the mono-oxygenase system, including cytochrome P450 reductase and cytochrome b_5, are present also in human lung microsomes. Cytochrome P450 reductase has been localised to bronchiolar epithelial cells, including the Clara cell and type II alveolar cells, in parallel with P450 localisation. Cytochrome-P450-mediated metabolic reactions, including CYP1A1 activation of polyaromatic hydrocarbon carcinogens, have been measured in adult human lung. Cultured bronchial cells metabolise benzo[a]pyrene and 7,12-dimethylbenzo-anthracene to reactive intermediates that bind to DNA. The ultimate carcinogen, benzo[a]pyrene-7,8-dihydrodiol-9,10-oxide, has been isolated from bronchial explants after exposure to benzo[a]pyrene.

Ethoxycoumarin-O-deethylase (ECOD) activity has been detected in the human lung and is a cytochrome-P450-catalysed reaction that reflects the metabolic contributions of several isoenzymes. Arylhydrocarbon hydroxylase (AHH) activity is also present. The addition of benz[a]anthracene to cultured human bronchial cells produces a threefold increase in AHH activity and an increase in binding of reactive benzo[a]pyrene metabolites to DNA. Pulmonary ECOD activity is induced by rifampicin, and environmental pollutants, such as polyaromatic hydrocarbons, also affect pulmonary xenobiotic metabolism.

Activation of polyaromatic hydrocarbons, such as benzo-[a]pyrene, to a carcinogen involves transformation by cytochrome P450-1A1-dependent mono-oxygenases and epoxide hydrolase. Many studies have established the role of CYP1A1 in mutagenesis and initiation of carcinogenesis, so it might be expected that even minimum levels of this isoenzyme in human lung microsomes would be significant (higher levels are found in smokers). However, this must be seen in the context of the other metabolic pathways for activation and detoxication, and also DNA repair mechanisms. DNA repair rates are considerably higher in type II cells than in Clara cells, so that the overall balance of metabolic enzymes and repair enzymes is probably a more important factor in the risk of carcinogenesis than the individual contribution of specific enzymes.

A genetic predisposition to AHH induction (Ah receptor polymorphism) has been suggested as influencing the susceptibility of an individual to lung cancer. AHH may also serve as a prognostic indicator for recovery from lung cancer. Similarly an elevation of specific glutathione transferases has been observed in pulmonary lavage from lung cancer patients and may serve as an early marker for lung neoplasia. It appears, however, that the prediction of individual susceptibility to environmental carcinogens must again take into account the balance between activation and detoxication enzymes, as well as the confounding effects of other environmental chemicals.

Carbon tetrachloride is a recognised hepatotoxin, producing fatty degeneration and centrilobular necrosis of the liver. Biotransformation of carbon tetrachloride takes place in the liver and toxicity is believed to be linked to the production of $CCl^{\cdot-}_3$ radical, which causes lipid peroxidation and irreversible damage to membrane systems. Although the liver is the target organ of toxicity for this chemical, damage to the metabolically active Clara cells, as well as types I and II alveolar epithelial cells and pulmonary endothelial cells, has been reported. Focal atelectasis and haemorrhages with ultrastructural changes in type II cells, including a decrease in lamellar bodies, have been found,[2] suggesting damage to the pulmonary surfactant system. Carbon tetrachloride probably also has direct toxic effects on lung phospholipids, because the main route of elimination of unchanged carbon tetrachloride is via the breath. Carbon tetrachloride hepatotoxicity has been shown to affect lipoprotein synthesis in the liver of hyper β-lipoproteinaemic rats. Defective, or modified, lipoproteins may be subsequently actively phagocytosed by blood monocytes which then transform into foamy *lipid-ingested* monocytes or giant foamy lipid-ingested monocytes and result in the development of pulmonary foam cells and, possibly, pulmonary embolism.[3]

Mechanisms of specific pulmonary cell toxicity

The profile of isoenzymes of cytochrome-P450-dependent mono-oxygenases in the lung cells is important for understanding the toxicity of substances that undergo metabolic activation. The heterogeneity of cellular distribution and the high levels of enzyme activity in certain cells can explain specific cell toxicity for some compounds (such as ipomeanol for the Clara cell) but it is not so clear why other toxins (e.g. butylated hydroxytoluene and trialkylphosphorothioates) are specifically toxic to type I alveolar epithelial cells. Butylated hydroxytoluene appears to be species-specific in causing murine lung damage and, in spite of extensive human safety evaluation, the potential of butylated hydroxytoluene in food to cause toxic lung damage in humans has not been demonstrated. The trialkylphosphorothioates, occurring as impurities in many organophosphorus thionates manufactured for use as pesticides (e.g. malathion), may be environmental causes of cell-specific lung damage in humans.

Type I alveolar epithelial cells do not demonstrate significant cytochrome P450 isoenzyme activity and, consequently, their potential for xenobiotic biotransformation is unknown. It is possible that there is metabolic activation in another cell type and transport of the toxic metabolite to the type I cell. Type I cells are derived from type II cells, which do have demonstrable drug-metabolising capability. However, in vitro the total enzyme activities of a lung preparation cannot be accounted for by the sum of just the Clara and type II cells. The other enzyme systems that may be involved in the activation of toxins in the lung include pulmonary flavins (flavin adenine dinucleotide, FAD), mono-oxygenases (Clara and alveolar type II cells) and pulmonary prostaglandin H synthase, which is capable of activating chemicals by co-oxidation with prostaglandin precursors. This pathway, in particular, could be relevant to the pulmonary toxicity of α-naphthylthiourea and N-methylthiobenzamide (see below). The latter compound has a similar toxicity profile to α-naphthylthiourea and has been shown to be metabolised by a pulmonary FAD-dependent mono-oxygenase. α-naphthyl-thiourea produces severe, non-haemorrhagic, pulmonary oedema with fibrin-rich pleural effusions in animals and has been used as an animal model for the study of the pathophysiology of pulmonary oedema. Pulmonary prostaglandin-H-synthase-mediated co-oxygenation has been shown to activate procarcinogens such as benzo[a]pyrene and aflatoxin B₁.

The role of glutathione (GSH) in pulmonary detoxification has been investigated for ipomeanol and naphthalene, both of which selectively damage Clara cells in mice. GSH and glutathione S-transferase concentrations are lower in the lungs than in liver and the cellular distribution is unclear, although there appears to be more activity in the Clara cells than in type II cells. Consequently, the protective detoxification mechanisms of the lungs are less effective than those of the liver. Low glutathione transferase activity in the lung compared with aryl hydroxylase activity has been associated with the increased risk of lung cancer in tobacco smokers.

The lung is a target organ for many other toxic compounds. Some of the mechanisms involved in systemic lung toxicity have been identified in animal toxicity models. Administration of paraquat to animals causes lung fibrosis, the herbicide entering the type I and II lung cells by a selective active uptake process. Hydrazine given intraperitoneally in mice can produce lung tumours, and chlorphentermine, after chronic oral dosing, accumulates in the fatty tissue of the lung (and the adrenals) and causes a phospholipidosis. Polycyclic aromatic hydrocarbons may be metabolically activated in the lung or metabolised elsewhere and transported to the lungs. There are significant species differences in susceptibility to the toxic effects of butylated hydroxy-

toluene, the trialkylphosphorothioates, α-naphthylthiourea, ipomeanol and paraquat. The pulmonary toxicity of these and other specific compounds will be reviewed in more detail.

Specific environmental chemicals

Paraquat

Paraquat (1,1′-dimethyl-4,4′-dipyridylium dichloride) is a contact herbicide that has been widely used throughout the world for more than 30 years and has proved to be safe in normal application. It was originally used as a redox indicator (methylviologen) in chemistry laboratories and only later were its herbicidal properties fully appreciated.

Most of the reported human deaths with paraquat have resulted from accidental or intentional poisoning with the concentrated commercial product (Gramoxone®). Paraquat sprayers do not appear to be at risk of absorption through the skin or by inhalation when exposed to the diluted formulation.[4] In the poisoned patient, the mode of death is most commonly from hypoxaemia secondary to progressive and severe lung damage.

Animal models of toxicity

The rat is a good animal model for studying the toxic mechanisms of paraquat in the human lung. In rat lung the toxic damage occurs in two phases. There is an initial destructive phase during which the alveolar epithelium (type I and II epithelial cells) is damaged. At this stage an extensive alveolitis may develop with infiltration by neutrophil polymorphonuclear cells into the alveolar tissue (Fig. 31.1). Progressive pulmonary oedema occurs that can be severe enough to cause early death. The second phase is a consequence of the alveolitis and epithelial cell damage. Extensive intra-alveolar and interalveolar fibro-

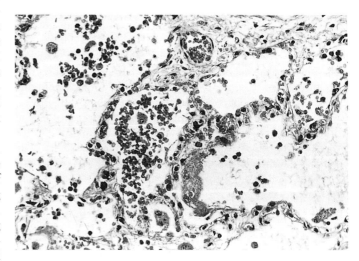

Fig. 31.1 Early pulmonary paraquat toxicity: there is diffuse alveolar damage with congestion, alveolar haemorrhage and hyaline membrane formation. Haematoxylin and eosin stain. (Courtesy of Dr T. Ashcroft.)

sis develops, which may be severe enough to destroy the alveolar architecture and critically reduce any effective gaseous exchange. The resultant intractable hypoxaemia ends in death. In mice, radiolabelled paraquat accumulates principally in the type II alveolar epithelial cells. This has been confirmed histologically since these alveolar epithelial cells are damaged initially by paraquat.[5]

Toxic mechanisms

The mechanism of paraquat toxicity has been extensively investigated. There is no evidence that paraquat is metabolised: ingested paraquat is ultimately excreted unchanged in the urine. Absorption is rapid following ingestion and, although it does not appear to take place in the stomach, the actual site of absorption in humans is unknown. It is well established that, once paraquat has entered the systemic circulation, it is accumulated into lung tissue via a time-dependent process.[6–7] Of all organs, the lung and kidney have the highest tissue concentrations and, not surprisingly, are quickly and selectively damaged by paraquat. A three-compartment pharmacokinetic model has been described following ingestion of tracer doses, including a 'deep' compartment for active pulmonary accumulation.[8] A more widespread picture of general organ toxicity is seen following the ingestion of large volumes of the concentrated formulation.

Accumulation by lung tissue in vitro has been shown to be an energy-dependent process that obeys saturation kinetics. Lung tissue from many animal species will accumulate paraquat and, in most, this occurs by active uptake through an endogenous cellular membrane transport system for diamine and polyamine compounds such as putrescine, cadaverine, spermidine and spermine.[9] There is a structural similarity between the dipyridyl molecule of paraquat and several of these diamines and polyamines (Fig. 31.2). It has been suggested also that the distance (about 0.6–0.7 nm) between the quaternary nitrogen atoms of the paraquat molecule is the critical factor in enabling paraquat to act as a substrate for this active transport system and, therefore, for its active accumulation in the lung cells.[10] The normal function of this naturally occurring polyamine uptake system has not been determined: the polyamines may have a role in the regulation of cell growth and division. Diquat, a herbicide with a similar chemical structure to paraquat but a smaller intramolecular diameter, is not accumulated by the lung cells and is less toxic to the lung.

Inside a type II epithelial cell, the primary mechanism of toxicity is a consequence of the ability of the paraquat molecule

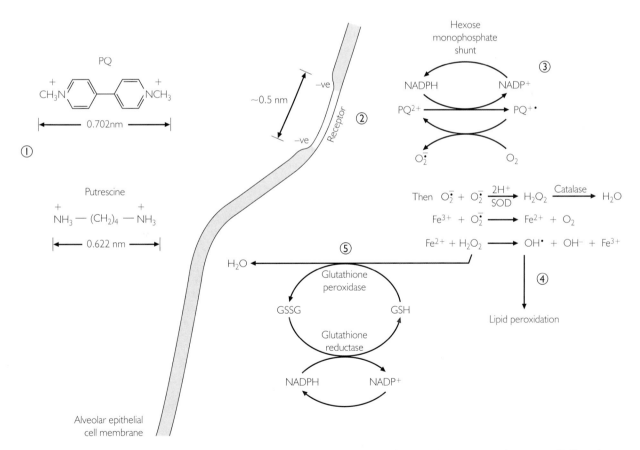

Fig. 31.2 Proposed mechanism of pulmonary toxicity of paraquat. (1) Comparison of molecular structure of paraquat (PQ) and putrescine. (2) Putative polyamine membrane receptor. (3) Redox cycling of paraquat. (4) Oxygen-derived free radical generation and lipid peroxidation. (5) Depletion of nicotinamide adenine dinucleotide phosphate (NADPH), in addition to (3). SOD, superoxide dismutase. (Adapted with permission from a diagram prepared by Dr L. L. Smith, ICI plc.)

to undergo continuous redox cycling between its oxidised and reduced forms. Under anaerobic conditions the paraquat cation can be reduced by nicotinamide adenine dinucleotide phosphate (NADPH) and a flavoprotein to the reduced radical. This may react with molecular oxygen to reform oxidised paraquat, but with the resultant production of a superoxide anion ($O_2^{\cdot-}$). If there is a continuous supply of electrons to the paraquat molecule, and oxygen is present, the paraquat molecule will undergo continuous redox cycling. This has been found to occur in microsomal preparations from the lung, liver and kidney.

There are two possible consequences of redox spinning. The first is that the superoxide anion damages all cell membranes by lipid peroxidation.[11] The rate of lipid peroxidation in vitro is increased but there is no direct evidence that this occurs in vivo. It has been suggested that the delayed increase in lipid peroxidation in the lung is a result of phagocytic macrophages rather than toxic cell injury.[12] The second consequence is that accumulation of high concentrations of paraquat within a cell reduces the concentration of reducing equivalents (such as NADPH) and prevents the cell from carrying out the many vital biochemical processes that depend upon a continuous supply of such cofactors. The ratio of NADPH to $NADP^+$ in lungs from rats given paraquat is decreased suggesting oxidation of this reduced nucleotide. NADPH will be consumed also in the detoxification of the hydrogen peroxide formed by the action of the enzyme superoxide dismutase on the superoxide anion. Hydrogen peroxide is converted to water by catalase and via glutathione peroxidase and glutathione reductase. This enzyme couple requires NADPH (Fig. 31.2)

The cytotoxic drug bleomycin can undergo redox cycling in a manner similar to paraquat. Bleomycin is capable of binding also to Fe_2^+ and to DNA. The reduced iron reacts with hydrogen peroxide to form a hydroxyl ($OH^{\cdot}$) radical, which could damage DNA.

Nitrofurantoin can also produce pulmonary damage by redox cycling but, as it is not selectively accumulated by the lung, very large doses of the drug are required to produce lung toxicity.

Paraquat poisoning in man

Paraquat is safe when used in an appropriately diluted solution as a non-selective contact herbicide. There is little evidence of absorption by inhalation or through the skin. The droplets generated during mechanised agricultural spraying appear to be too large to be inhaled and the skin acts as an impermeable barrier to diluted paraquat.[13,14] Nose-bleeds and throat irritation have been reported following inhalation of the spray. Paraquat concentrate is a strong irritant, which can produce inflammation, blistering and necrosis on contact with mucous membranes and epithelia.

Paraquat is highly toxic to humans following oral ingestion. Most cases follow intentional self-poisoning with the concentrated commercial product and as little as a mouthful of concentrate may be fatal. Social factors are involved in the use of paraquat for suicide: clusters of cases often follow media reports of a fatality.

The clinical features that occur almost immediately after paraquat ingestion are nausea, vomiting and diarrhoea. A large dose (> 50 ml) of the concentrated formulation may result in death, within a few hours, from a combination of multiorgan toxic failure, metabolic acidosis, depression of myocardial and respiratory function with pulmonary oedema, and widespread depression of the central nervous system.

Ingestion of a smaller dose (e.g. 1.5–2 sachets of the domestic granules, Weedol®) initially produces painful ulceration of the mouth and pharynx followed by dysphagia, dysphonia and cough. After 3–5 days there may be evidence of mild hepatocellular damage and acute renal failure, with tubular necrosis, may become apparent. However, it is the progressive breathlessness, and subsequent appearance of pulmonary opacities on the chest radiograph, that heralds death from rapidly progressive pulmonary fibrosis within a few days or weeks (Fig. 31.3). Death is miserable, with progressive respiratory failure over a period of several days in a fully conscious patient. Management of these patients should be humane and not heroic.

Plasma paraquat concentration can be measured by a quantitative radioimmunoassay. A rapid qualitative colorimetric screening test for the presence of paraquat in the urine is available. Some prediction of the probable outcome for a patient can be made by reference to a graph comparing the plasma paraquat concentrations at specific times after ingestion and the reported outcomes (Fig. 31.4). The evolution of the pulmonary changes can be monitored by serial chest radiographs and pulmonary function tests (including measurement of carbon monoxide transfer factor, $T_L CO$).

Treatment

There is no effective antidote or specific treatment for paraquat poisoning.[15] An emetic is included in some of the commercial formulations and research by the manufacturers is progressing on specific agents that will prevent absorption from the gas-

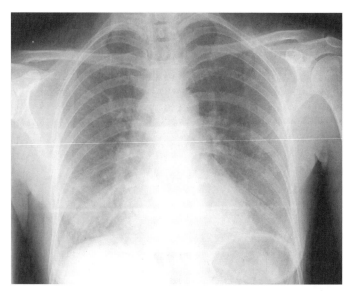

Fig. 31.3 Chest radiograph of a 44-year-old woman who had intentionally ingested paraquat a week earlier. She died 10 days later. Five months later her husband also died after ingesting paraquat.

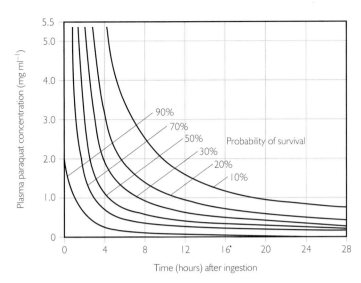

Fig. 31.4 Relationship of plasma paraquat concentration, time from ingestion and probability of survival. (Adapted with permission from a diagram prepared by Dr L. L. Smith, ICI plc.)

trointestinal tract or antagonise the active uptake by lung cells. In most cases, several hours will have elapsed between ingestion of paraquat and admission to hospital, so that most of the paraquat will have been absorbed by the time the patient is seen by a physician.

Plasma paraquat concentrations in humans rise rapidly and peak about 2 hours after ingestion, before declining exponentially. Most of the paraquat is absorbed within 12 hours of dosing. The plasma profile in humans is similar to that found in dogs, whereas in the rat absorption of paraquat is much slower. The rapid absorption in humans indicates that any treatment aimed at removing paraquat from the gastrointestinal tract (emesis, gastric lavage or whole gut lavage) or preventing its absorption (administration of adsorbents) must be initiated within a few hours of ingestion. Bentonite or Fuller's earth may be given orally in an attempt to bind paraquat in the gut and slow down absorption. Ordinary soil may provide sufficient adsorbents to be an emergency oral treatment when the paraquat-poisoned patient lives in an remote location far from hospital facilities.

Failure to prevent the absorption of paraquat into the systemic circulation has led to the use of forced diuresis, haemodialysis or haemoperfusion to increase the clearance of paraquat from the blood and reduce the amount available for uptake into the lung. Renal function is often compromised in paraquat poisoning so that haemodialysis or haemoperfusion may be more effective than forced diuresis. It is suggested that the low mortality rates observed in one study resulted from the prompt use of haemodialysis,[16] but other factors such as the severity of poisoning or the use of pulsed methylprednisolone may have been important. Unfortunately, the plasma profile of paraquat absorption and the active uptake mechanisms in the lung require that these measures must be initiated as soon as possible after ingestion. In many cases, by the time the patient reaches hospital it is unlikely that these treatments will significantly reduce the amount of paraquat taken up by the lungs.

However, a favourable outcome in two patients when haemodialysis was initiated quite late after ingestion suggests that this treatment should always be considered when there is some probability of survival. It is doubtful that there is any role for repeated haemoperfusion.[17]

Other therapeutic approaches might be used to prevent or inhibit the uptake of paraquat by the lung or to prevent the redox cycling of paraquat in pulmonary cells. Several polyamine analogues, which inhibit the active uptake mechanism, have been synthesised but all are too toxic for administration to humans. D-propranolol has been given to compete with paraquat for uptake by the lung, but with little success. Increasing the concentration of superoxide dismutase in lung cells, either by direct aerosol inhalation or bronchial lavage with a solution of the enzyme, is another theoretical method for reducing the activity of the superoxide anion, but again this has not proved effective in clinical practice. The administration of low oxygen concentrations to poisoned patients is a reasonable action to reduce redox cycling, but the reaction between paraquat and oxygen is so avid that only complete absence of oxygen would have any effect! Prophylactic inhaled administration of α-tocopherol in liposomes confers some protection against paraquat-induced lung damage in the rat[18] but has no postexposure treatment potential. Pre-exposure induction of pulmonary metallothionein similarly protects against the lung toxicity of paraquat but has no therapeutic value.[19]

Most patients with paraquat poisoning die from the extensive pulmonary fibrosis that follows an initial alveolitis. Consequently, large doses of steroids have been given with the aim of reducing the alveolitis and preventing development of fibrosis. Steroids have not been effective in cases of poisoning with large doses of paraquat but they may be crucial if the lung damage is close to that likely to cause death. A combination of steroids and cyclophosphamide has been tried in an attempt to reduce the infiltration by polymorphonuclear cells into the lung and so diminish the alveolitis and fibrosis. However, the drugs appear to have no effect on the necrosis of alveolar epithelial cells and the extensive damage to lung architecture, so that the early claims of success have not been confirmed. Similarly, radiotherapy has been unsuccessful in the prevention of pulmonary fibrosis.

The possible benefit of nitric oxide inhalation was reported in a patient who had ingested a solution of paraquat and diquat and developed adult respiratory distress syndrome and pulmonary fibrosis.[20] The predicted probability of survival was 30% and although other treatments, including oral Fuller's earth, forced diuresis, haemofiltration, N-acetylcysteine, methylprednisolone, cyclophosphamide, vitamin E and colchicine, were given, treatment with continuous nitric oxide inhalation is suggested as the critical therapy since the patient recovered and pulmonary function was subsequently normal.

The increased opportunity for organ transplantation suggests that a patient with extensive pulmonary fibrosis from paraquat toxicity but recoverable damage to other organs might survive with a lung transplant. Regrettably, in those few instances where this has been attempted, there was uptake of residual paraquat in other organs by the transplanted lung, with subsequent lung toxicity.[21]

In the management of the paraquat-poisoned patient the outlook is inevitably grim. If a patient is admitted to hospital within a few hours of paraquat ingestion there is a strong case for intensive care, administration of adsorbents and haemoperfusion. The patient with a plasma paraquat concentration on the borderline of a predicted fatal outcome may benefit from steroid administration. Most patients appreciate an open discussion of the probable outcome and a sensitive, compassionate approach to possible terminal care.

Spanish toxic oil syndrome

A new multisystem disease appeared in 1981 as an epidemic in Spain. Over 20 000 people were affected and around 380 have since died from the disease. The development of this syndrome was associated with the use of unlabelled cooking oil sold by travelling salesmen. Subsequent analysis of suspect oil, presumed to have been obtained from affected families, showed that it contained varying proportions of several vegetable oils and animal fats and frequently had some evidence of contamination with aniline.

This particular toxic oil syndrome had two phases. In the acute phase, a fever developed with interstitial pneumonitis, eosinophilia, myalgia, arthralgia, pruritus and an exanthematous rash. At this stage there were a few deaths from respiratory failure. Of the survivors, some progressed to a chronic phase with neuromyopathies, liver dysfunction and a scleroderma-like illness with some features of a collagen vascular disease. The pneumonic component had a favourable outcome; only 5% of patients went into acute respiratory distress and died. Some 10% of patients had moderate hypoxaemia with a normal chest film. Transbronchial biopsies in these cases showed severe endothelial lesions and some had clinical signs of pulmonary hypertension. This was moderate and did not improve with oxygen or vasoactive agents. The neurological damage was progressive and led to severe neuromuscular atrophy, sometimes accompanied by alveolar hypoventilation. Up to one year after onset there was still a reduction in lung volumes and T_LCO. Some patients had permanent residual neuromyopathies and severe scleroderma-like lesions of the skin.[22]

Computer-assisted gallium-67 scanning and bronchoalveolar lavage in patients with persistently abnormal T_LCO failed to show significant differences from controls. A rise in IgA and IgG concentrations and falls in the α_1-antiprotease and transferrin concentrations were demonstrated. However, phospholipid and lecithin concentrations and alveolar macrophage function were normal.[23]

The main pathological findings were generalised endothelial lesions, septal oedema, mild inflammatory mononuclear infiltrates and hydropic degeneration of type I and II pneumocytes with desquamation of type I pneumocytes. Histological investigation of the lung in the acute phase showed an endovasculitis with features consistent with adult respiratory distress syndrome. Post-mortem histology of the elastic pulmonary arteries showed pronounced intimal proliferation with oedema and accumulation of large vacuolated cells within the media and loss of vascular smooth muscle. In the muscular pulmonary arteries there was pronounced medial hypertrophy and intimal proliferation, sometimes causing almost complete occlusion.

Foamy cells were found in the intima and there was muscularisation of the walls of the pulmonary arterioles.[24]

The source and nature of this oil has not been conclusively determined. Olive oil adulterated with denatured rape seed oil, an industrial oil contaminated with aniline or a pesticide have all been suspected. Toxicological databases for petroleum refinery products, such as mineral oils, potential contaminants and additives, were reviewed to determine whether the clinical findings in human poisoning with an adulterant in the oil could suggest the cause of the unusual symptomatology characterising the syndrome.[25]

More than 70 chemicals and mixtures were reviewed but none had been reported to produce adverse toxic effects resembling the specific collection of symptoms and progression that characterised the toxic oil syndrome. No chemical, refinery product, additive or contaminant was associated with the vasculitis, thrombotic episodes and immunological effects, such as T-lymphocyte activation and cytokine release, that are considered to be the cellular basis of the syndrome.

The World Health Organization (WHO) initiated an investigation into the cause of this toxic epidemic but failed to reach a conclusion.

Miscellaneous potential toxins

α-Naphthylthiourea[26] is a selective rodenticide (a phenylthiourea) effective in killing rats at low dosage but relatively safe for humans (i.e. it has a high safety index). However, its use as a pesticide has been largely superseded by newer rodenticides. Although there is a substantial degree of interspecies and intraspecies variation in toxicity and tolerance for the thioureas, α-naphthylthiourea has been used as a model toxin for studying the pathogenesis of chemical-induced pulmonary oedema in animals. The specific toxic effects of α-naphthylthiourea on the lungs are of theoretical interest as a mechanistic model for human lung toxicity: cases of human poisoning are rare.

Administration of α-naphthylthiourea to rats produces a massive, non-haemorrhagic pulmonary oedema in which there are invariably pleural effusions with a high fibrin concentration. The pulmonary oedema is present 2 hours after parenteral administration and reaches a maximum clinical effect at around 4 hours. This is then followed by almost equally rapid clinical resolution in the rats that survive. Death occurs between 8 and 10 hours after exposure but survivors have reabsorbed the exudate by 24 hours.

Ipomeanol[27] is a mycotoxin produced by a fungus, *Fusarium solani*, which grows on sweet potatoes. Cattle develop toxic pulmonary effects after consuming sweet potatoes spoiled with this mould. Intraperitoneal administration of pure ipomeanol produces pulmonary damage in a number of animal species. The gross toxic effects include pulmonary oedema with congestion and haemorrhages, which are probably secondary changes resulting from the primary lesion: the cause of death is usually pulmonary oedema. Several natural products have been isolated from sweet potatoes but the pulmonary toxin was identified as ipomeanol, a furanosesquiterpene.

The most obvious pathological finding in the lungs is a selective primary necrosis of Clara cells, ipomeanol being covalently bound to these specific target cells. Ipomeanol has not been associated with human poisoning, although a theoretical risk of human lung damage does exists in view of the recognised effects in other mammals.

The movement of cattle on to new pasture may be associated with a different pulmonary toxicity syndrome. The cause of this disease is 3-methylindole, which is produced from tryptophan by ruminal *Lactobacillus* spp. The bacteria overgrow in the bovine stomach as a result of a sudden improvement in the quality of vegetation consumed. Activation by a cytochrome P450 (CYP2F) of 3-methylindole is required for its toxicity and Clara cells and alveolar epithelial cells are the specific target for the toxic metabolite.

Fumonisin B1[28] is a mycotoxin, produced by *Fusarium moniliforme* growing on corn, that causes death from pulmonary oedema in pigs. On histological examination, the porcine pulmonary macrophages are found to contain large amounts of a membranous material. Although the exact toxic mechanism is not known, this material may be the result of altered sphingolipid metabolism in the liver.

Butylated hydroxytoluene[29] is a widely used antioxidant additive in food. It is an inhibitor of free radicals and is used, therefore, to reduce oxidative damage to food. At high oral or intravenous doses it can cause lung damage in mice. Female mice developed both hyperplasia and hypertrophy of alveolar epithelial cells, with maximal thickening of the alveolar epithelium between 2 and 5 days after intraperitoneal administration of 250 mg/kg butylated hydroxytoluene. Alveolar type I cell damage, with alveolar oedema, was noted first, the type II epithelial cells and the endothelial cells being unaffected initially. After 3–4 days the type II cells began to proliferate. However, they had returned to normal about 9 days after dosing. There was some proliferation of endothelial cells and subsequent development of a mild fibrosis. It is suggested that the type II cells proliferated to replace the damaged type I cells. Butylated hydroxytoluene does not affect rat lung at comparable doses.

The situation in humans is unknown but long-term oral studies in mice have provided some evidence for hepatic carcinogenicity and suspicions of a carcinogenic effect on the lung.[30] Concern persists that the risk to humans from butylated hydroxytoluene have not been conclusively assessed.

Trialkylphosphorothioates are contaminants of many commercial formulations containing organophosphate pesticides. The lung appears to be the main target organ of toxicity and the pathological features in rat lung are similar to the butylated-hydroxytoluene-induced lung lesion in mice: there is selective destruction of type I alveolar epithelial cells within 24–48 hours, accompanied by hypertrophy and hyperplasia of type II alveolar epithelial cells and massive interstitial thickening. Inflammatory cells infiltrate the alveolar interstitium and alveolar oedema develops with the presence of numerous alveolar macrophages. There is little evidence of endothelial cell damage and, if the animal survives, the alveolar oedema resolves with a decrease in the thickening of the alveolar walls. The lung morphology returns to normal in 14 days, apart from some focal areas of interstitial thickening and leukocyte infiltration. At the bronchiolar level there is some evidence of significant damage to the Clara cells and raised lactate dehydrogenase activity in lavage fluid. Accidental

exposure to trialkylphosphorothioates, as contaminants in phosphorothionate pesticides, can cause direct lung damage in humans or may, by enzyme interaction, affect the susceptibility of the lung to the toxic effects of other compounds.

Pyrrolizidine alkaloids

The pyrrolizidine group of alkaloids is found in a variety of plant species (e.g. *Crotalaria* and *Senecio* spp.) and the clinical effects of poisoning have been reported in grazing animals and in humans[31-33] when the plants have been used for 'medicinal' uses. Pyrrolizidine alkaloids have been identified in comfrey (*Symphytum officinale*), used in herbal remedies.[34]

Pulmonary hypertension is produced in animals grazing on various plants belonging to the species *Crotalaria* and *Senecio*. The pulmonary toxicity results from the pyrrolizidine alkaloids undergoing bioactivation to alkylating agents. This activation is mediated by CYP3A2, which is predominantly present in liver. It is probable that monocrotaline (a pyrrolizidine alkaloid) is bioactivated to a pyrrol in the liver and transported by the systemic circulation to the lungs. Other studies suggest that hepatic formation of reactive glutathione conjugates from monocrotaline may also play a role in the toxicity of this pyrrolizidine alkaloid.

The lung lesion is identifiable in animals several days after systemic administration of a pyrrolizidine alkaloid such as monocrotaline.[35] The major site of damage is the endothelial cells lining pulmonary blood vessels. Thrombi appear on the surface of the cells and there is increased permeability, resulting in intra-alveolar and interstitial oedema, and pleural effusions. A focal necrosis of the alveolar wall occurs, accompanied by damage to interstitial cells, endothelial and alveolar cell proliferation, medial thickening and intimal hyalinosis of arteries. These changes may lead to pulmonary hypertension with right ventricular hypertrophy. A dose–response relationship in intoxication by the pyrrolizidine alkaloid monocrotaline has been reported.[36]

The normal active uptake of biogenic amines (e.g. 5-hydroxytryptamine) by pulmonary endothelial cells is inhibited following pyrrolizidine alkaloid administration. Monocrotaline inhibits noradrenaline (norepinephrine) uptake, which may contribute to the development of pulmonary hypertension. Pulmonary angiotensin-converting enzyme (ACE) activity (located in the pulmonary endothelial cells) is decreased following pyrrolizidine alkaloid administration.

The doses required to produce pulmonary damage are higher than those needed for liver damage. Administration of antioxidants may reduce the extent of damage to the lungs. There is evidence that a active toxic metabolite is produced in the liver and transported in blood to the lungs so that the initial toxic damage is directly to pulmonary endothelial cells.

A major review of the toxicity profile of pyrrolizidine alkaloids was published by a WHO working group in 1988.[37]

Sauropus androgynus

Sauropus androgynus (katuk) is a perennial green vegetable that is widely grown in Asia, especially Malaysia, Borneo, India and Taiwan. *Sauropus* may grow to a height of 6 m but when grown

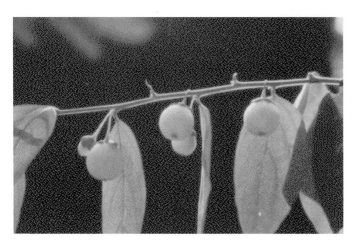

Fig. 31.5 *Sauropus androgynus.* (Photograph courtesy of Katetsart University, Bangkok, http://www.ku.ac.th/AgrInfo/plant/plant2/p045.html.)

as a vegetable crop it is pruned to 1–2 m (Fig. 31.5). The leaves and stem tips of the plant have a pleasant, slightly nutty taste, similar to fresh garden peas. They are eaten raw in salads or steamed and added to stir-fry, rice, soups or casseroles and served in restaurants as *sayor manis*. The flowers and small fruits of the plant are also eaten.

In 1995 an outbreak of a poorly defined respiratory illness (a form of bronchiolitis obliterans) was observed in southern Taiwan that appeared to be related to the ingestion of the leaves of *Sauropus androgynus*, which was then a popular ingredient of a weight-control regimen.[38,39] The most common form was prepared as an extract with fruit juice. The development of a constrictive bronchiolitis obliterans in patients ingesting *Sauropus androgynus* juice had not been previously reported.

The clinical findings were of a rapidly progressive obstructive lung disease that developed up to 40 days after consumption ceased. The individuals who had ingested high levels of *Sauropus* appeared to be the worst affected, especially those consuming the plant as the uncooked extract. The toxic effects were believed, initially, to be caused by the alkaloid papaverine, but this compound had not been previously associated with such a level of toxicity.

Lung biopsies showed bronchiolitis obliterans that proved unresponsive to conventional treatment with steroids and bronchodilators. Some patients died and many developed chronic respiratory failure. Single-lung transplantation was performed in four patients. The excised lungs had focal fibromuscular sclerosis and obliteration of bronchial arteries in the walls of large bronchi (diameter 4–5 mm) with segmental necrosis of smaller bronchi (diameter 2–4 mm). The bronchi proximal to the necrotic zone had fibrosis, with atrophy of cartilage, bronchial glands and smooth muscle cells. The distal bronchioles showed obstruction or dilatation. Bronchi with a diameter larger than 5 mm, the pulmonary vessels, the small bronchioles and alveoli were little affected. The pathological changes were consistent with segmental ischaemic necrosis of bronchi at the watershed zone of the bronchial and pulmonary circulation.

More detailed histopathological investigations were performed on open lung biopsies from four patients with *Sauropus-androgynus*-associated constrictive bronchiolitis obliterans.[40] The changes ranged from slight bronchiolar inflammation and fibrosis to marked submucosal fibrosis causing complete obliteration of the lumen. A dense eosinophil infiltrate was noted in the bronchiolar submucosa or fibrotic tissue of the completely obliterated bronchioles in two patients. Immunohistochemical studies showed a lymphocytic infiltrate consisting mainly of T lymphocytes in all patients. Immunofluorescent stains for immunoglobulins (IgG, IgA, IgM), C1q, C3 and C4 were negative. Electron microscopy showed no immune complex deposition in the specimens examined. The finding of predominant T-lymphocytic infiltrates suggests that a T-cell-mediated immune response is involved in the pathogenesis of the disease. The lymphocytic infiltrates in many bronchioles, without significant collagen deposition, suggests that lymphocyte infiltration may precede the tissue fibrosis. The dense eosinophil infiltration may combine with lymphocytes and other immunological and mesenchymal cells to promote antigen-specific stimulation of lymphocytes and the induction of fibrosis.

Therapeutic chemicals

Many of the adverse effects on the lungs that are associated with the systemic administration of drugs are single-case reports. An adverse effect can either be predicted from knowledge of the pharmacology of the drug (type A adverse reaction) or be idiosyncratic and totally unpredictable (type B adverse reaction). Many of the toxic pulmonary side effects of systemic drugs appear to be unpredictable type B adverse reactions. The clinical aspects of the pulmonary adverse reactions of therapeutic agents are detailed in Chapter 29. Consequently, only the toxic mechanisms of some of these adverse effects will be reviewed.

Antineoplastic drugs

Many antineoplastic drugs can produce pulmonary fibrosis. The most significant include carmustine (BiCNU), bleomycin, cyclophosphamide, busulfan, mitomycin C and methotrexate. There are many histological features common to the pulmonary toxicity associated with each drug, the principal difference being the duration of administration before the toxic effects become apparent.

Bleomycin initially damages type I alveolar epithelial cells, although electron microscopy may reveal abnormal and proliferating type II cells and pulmonary endothelial cell damage. There is accumulation of a proteinaceous fluid in the alveoli, metaplasia of the alveolar epithelium and fibroblastic proliferation with interstitial oedema, but relatively little evidence of inflammation. A similar picture is seen with busulfan and carmustine. Busulfan can also cause pulmonary ossification and dystrophic calcification.

Pulmonary clearance of ^{99m}Tc-DTPA has been used for monitoring the permeability of lung epithelium during bleomycin therapy.[41] Carbon monoxide transfer factor does not appear to be a good predictor of whether or not any bleomycin toxicity has clinical significance.[42] Some of the bleomycin lung damage may be reversed by aggressive treatment with azathioprine and corticosteroids.[43] Animals that are resistant to bleomycin-induced lung damage possess an enzyme (bleomycin hydrolase) that is lacking in bleomycin-sensitive species. The combination of bleomycin and cisplatin appears to increase the risk of pulmonary toxicity.[44]

Lung and bladder injury may occur as adverse side effects of treatment with cyclophosphamide. In the rat, cyclophosphamide produces septal and intra-alveolar haemorrhages, together with endothelial and type I cell damage. Around 4 days after administration, the type II cells become damaged and there may be hyaline membrane formation. The alveoli then undergo re-epithelialisation but with an increase in collagen deposition, characteristic of fibrosis. Acrolein, a potential metabolite of cyclophosphamide, produces similar changes in the lungs. Mixed-function oxidases can metabolise cyclophosphamide to reactive species, although inhibitors of these enzymes have no effect on the toxicity of this drug to the lung. Unrelated biochemical pathways can also metabolise cyclophosphamide, so mixed-function-oxidase-mediated activation may not be essential for the development of lung toxicity.[45] Inhibitors of prostaglandin H synthase have been shown to reduce the severity of lung toxicity with cyclophophamide.[46]

Methotrexate-induced pulmonary fibrosis is rare and differs from that of the other antineoplastic agents in that an inflammatory response is predominant, with interstitial infiltration by mononuclear and eosinophilic cells and nodular aggregates of multinucleated giant cells. Its effects are partly reversible.[47]

Other antineoplastic drugs causing pulmonary fibrosis include mitomycin C and chlorambucil.[48] High concentrations of oxygen may increase the risk of antineoplastic-drug-induced lung damage, as may ionising radiation. Other factors include the patient's age, the total dose administered and the coadministration of other antineoplastic drugs (see Chapter 29).

Amiodarone

Amiodarone treatment may be associated with pulmonary fibrosis and a phospholipidosis. Prophylactic niacin and taurine can protect against this toxic effect in laboratory animals, as they do for bleomycin.[49] An interstitial pneumonitis is the most serious long-term toxic effect of amiodarone but this may be dependent on an individual's genetic susceptibility.[50] The clinical and pathological manifestations of amiodarone lung toxicity are reviewed in Chapter 29.

Phospholipid storage disorders of the lung

Drugs that are amphipathic and cationic are associated with the induction of pulmonary phospholipidosis. This is a histological and biochemical diagnosis: there are often minimal clinical findings. The drugs that are capable of causing phospholipid changes

in animals include chlorphentermine, imipramine, amiodarone and chloroquine.

Large phospholipid-containing cells (foam cells) are seen on histological examination of the alveolar wall about 24 hours after the administration of chlorphentermine to rats. Electron microscopy of the cells demonstrated the presence of myelinoid bodies, believed to be lysosomal in origin. They may be storage vesicles, rich in phospholipids from membranes, whose metabolism has been inhibited by the administration of the drug. The drugs may be inhibiting lysosomal phospholipases, since their toxicity can be reduced by the prior administration of inducers of the mixed-function-oxidase system.

Conclusion

The lungs are directly exposed to inhaled toxic compounds but there is growing evidence that they are also susceptible to ingested toxic chemicals present in the pulmonary circulation. In addition, it appears that certain cells in the lungs are capable of local intracellular metabolism of specific ingested compounds to toxic metabolites. Animal-based investigations have identified several of these exogenous chemicals and the toxic mechanisms involved, but there are limited data for humans. Nevertheless, the possibility of localised pulmonary metabolism of xenobiotics to toxic metabolites must be considered a risk in humans, in addition to the direct toxicity of ingested compounds themselves to the lungs.

Therapeutic principles

- Treatment for toxic lung damage is largely symptomatic.
- Interactions may occur with administered drugs as a result of induction or inhibition of enzymes responsible for metabolising ingested agents.
- The lung has a low capacity for metabolising toxic chemicals compared to the liver.
- Primary prevention of exposure is the optimum for therapeutic management followed by removal from further exposure.

? Unresolved questions

- How is the risk of damage to human lung from ingested agents best assessed?
- How applicable to humans are animal toxicity data?
- How effective are lung protective and repair mechanisms in humans?
- How can the best treatment regime be identified?

Further reading

Glatt HR. An overview of bioactivation of chemical carcinogens. Biochem Soc Trans 2000; 28: 1–6.

Indulski JA, Lutz W. Metabolic genotype in relation to individual susceptibility to environment carcinogens. Int Arch Occup Environ Health 2000; 73: 71–85.

Kehrer JP, Kacew S. Systematically applied chemicals that damage lung tissue. Toxicology 1985; 35: 251.

Smith BR, Brain WR. The role of metabolism in chemical-induced pulmonary toxicity. Toxicol Pathol 1991; 19: 470.

Wheeler CW, Guenthert TM. Cytochrome p450 dependent metabolism of xenobiotics in human lung. J Biochem Toxicol 1991; 6: 163.

References

1. Sorokin SP. The cells of the lungs. In: Nettesheim P, Hanna MG, Deatherage JW, ed. Conference on Morphology of Experimental Carcinogenesis. USA: Atomic Energy Commission; 1970: 3.
2. Gould VE, Smuckler EA. Alveolar injury in acute carbon tetrachloride intoxication. Arch Intern Med 1971; 128: 109.
3. Shibuya K, Tajima M, Yamate J et al. Carbon tetrachloride-induced hepatotoxicity enhances the development of pulmonary foam cells in rats fed a cholesterol-cholic acid diet. Toxicol Pathol 1997; 25: 487.
4. Howard JK, Sabopathy NN, Whitehead PA. Study of the health of Malaysian plantation workers with particular reference to Paraquat spraymen. Br J Ind Med 1981; 38: 110.
5. Onyeama HP, Oehme FW. A literature review of paraquat toxicity. Vet Hum Toxicol 1984; 26: 494.
6. Rose MS, Smith LL, Wyatt I. Evidence for energy-dependent accumulation of Paraquat into rat lung. Nature 1974; 252: 314.
7. Rose MS, Lock EA, Smith LL, Wyatt I. Paraquat accumulation: tissue and species specificity. Biochem Pharmacol 1976; 25: 119.
8. Bismuth-C, Garnier-R, Baud-F-J et al. Paraquat poisoning. An overview of the current status. Drug Safety 1990; 54: 243.
9. Smith LL. The identification of an accumulation system for diamines and polyamines into the lung and its relevance to Paraquat toxicity. Arch Toxicol 1982; 5(suppl.): 1.
10. Smith LL, Lewis CP, Wyatt I, Cohen GM. The importance of epithelial uptake systems in lung toxicity. Environ Health Perspect 1990; 85: 25.
11. Fairshter RD. Paraquat toxicity and lipid peroxidation. Arch Intern Med 1981; 141: 1121.
12. Ogata T, Manabe S. Correlation between lipid peroxidation and morphological manifestation of paraquat-induced lung injury in rats. Arch Toxicol 1990; 64: 7.
13. Hidy GM. Aerosols: an industrial and environmental science. London: Academic Press; 1984.
14. Scott RC, Walker M, Dugard PH. A comparison of the in vitro permeability of human and some laboratory animal skins. Int J Cosmetic Sci 1986; 8: 189.
15. Meredith TJ, Vale JA. Treatment of paraquat poisoning in man: methods to prevent absorption. Hum Toxicol 1987; 6: 49.
16. D'Avila K, Salum FA, Rodrigues CIS et al. Analysis of the evolution, hemodialysis response and survival in paraquat poisoning. Rev Bras Med 1998; 55: 711
17. Hampson EC, Effeney DJ, Pond SM. Efficacy of single or repeated hemoperfusion in a canine model of paraquat poisoning. J Pharmacol Exp Ther 1990; 254: 732
18. Suntres ZE, Hepworth SR, Shek PN. Protective effect of liposome-associated alpha-tocopherol against paraquat-induced acute lung toxicity. Biochem Pharmacol 1992; 44: 1811.
19. Satoh M, Naganuma A, Imura N. Effect of preinduction of metallothionein on paraquat toxicity in mice. Arch Toxicol 1992; 66: 145.
20. Eisenman A, Armali Z, Raikhlin-Lisehkraft B et al. Nitric oxide inhalation for paraquat-induced lung injury. J Toxicol Clin Toxicol 1998; 36: 575
21. Bismuth C, Gamier K, Baud FJ et al. Paraquat poisoning: an overview of the current status. Drug Safety 1990; 54: 243.
22. Phelps RG, Fleischmajer R. Clinical, pathological and immunopathologic manifestations of the toxic oil syndrome. Analysis of fourteen cases. J Am Acad Dermatol 1988; 18: 313.
23. De la Cruz JL, Oteo LA, Lopez C et al. Toxic-oil syndrome. Gallium-67 scanning and bronchoalveolar lavage studies in patients with abnormal lung function. Chest 1985; 88: 398.
24. Fernandez-Segoviano P, Esteban A, Martinez-Cabruja R. Pulmonary vascular lesions in the toxic oil syndrome in Spain. Thorax 1983; 38: 724.
25. Hard GC. Short-term adverse effects in humans of ingested mineral oils, their additives and possible contaminants – a review. Hum Exp Toxicol 2000; 19: 158.
26. Scott AM, Powell GM, Upshall DG, Curtis CG. Pulmonary toxicity of thioureas in the rat. Environ Health Perspect 1990; 85: 43.
27. Boyd MR, Burka LT, Wilson BJ, Sasame HA. In vitro studies on the metabolic activation of the pulmonary toxin 4-ipomeanol by rat lung and liver microsomes. J Pharmacol Exp Ther 1978; 207: 677.
28. Haschek WM, Motelin G, Ness DK et al. Characterization of fumonisin toxicity in orally and intravenously dosed swine. Mycopathologia 1992; 117: 83.
29. Marino AA, Mitchell JT. Lung damage in mice following intraperitoneal injection of butylated hydroxytoluene. Proc Soc Exp Biol Med 1972; 140: 122.
30. BIBRA Working Group. Butylated hydroxytoluene. Toxicity profile. London: British Industrial Biological Research Association; 1988.
31. Huxtable RJ. Problems with pyrrolizidines. Trends Pharmacol Sci 1980; 1 : 299.
32. McLean EK. The toxic actions of pyrrolizidine (Senecio) alkaloids. Pharmacol Rev 1970; 22: 429.
33. Schoental R. Health hazards by pyrrolizidine alkaloids: a short review. Toxicol Lett 1982; 10: 323.
34. Couet CE, Crews C, Hanley AB. Analysis, separation, and bioassay of pyrrolizidine alkaloids from comfrey (Symphytum officinale). Nat Toxins 1996; 4: 163
35. Shubat PJ, Hubbard AK, Huxtable RJ. Dose–response relationship in intoxication by the pyrrolizidine alkaloid monocrotaline. J Toxicol Environ Health 1989; 28: 445.
36. Shubat PJ, Hubbard AK, Huxtable RJ. Dose–response relationship in intoxication by the pyrrolizidine alkaloid monocrotaline. J Toxicol Environ Health 1989; 28: 445
37. WHO Working Group. Pyrrolizidine alkaloids. Environ Health Criteria 1988; 80.
38. Chang YL, Yao YT, Wang NS, Lee YC. Segmental necrosis of small bronchi after prolonged intakes of Sauropus androgynus in Taiwan. Am J Respir Crit Care Med 1998; 157: 594.
39. Ger LP, Chiang AA, Lai RS et al. Association of Sauropus androgynus and bronchiolitis obliterans syndrome: a hospital-based case-control study. Am J Epidemiol 1997; 145: 842.
40. Chang H, Wang JS, Tseng HIT et al. Histopathological study of Sauropus androgynus associated constrictive bronchiolitis obliterans: a new cause of constrictive bronchiolitis obliterans. Am J Surg Pathol 1997; 21: 35
41. Ugur O, Caner B, Balbay MD et al. Bleomycin lung toxicity detected by technetium-99m diethylene triamine penta-acetic acid aerosol scintigraphy. Eur J Nucl Med 1993; 20: 114.
42. McKeage J, Evans BD, Atkinson C et al. Carbon monoxide diffusing capacity is a poor predictor of clinically significant bleomycin lung. J Clin Oncol 1990; 8: 779.
43. Maher J, Daly PA. Severe bleomycin lung toxicity: reversal with high dose corticosteroids. Thorax 1993; 48: 92.
44. Rabinowits M, Souhami L, Gil RA et al. Increased pulmonary toxicity with bleomycin and cisplatin chemotherapy combinations. Am J Clin Oncol 1990; 13: 132.
45. Smith RD, Kehrer JP. Cooxidation of cyclophosphamide as an alternative pathway for its bioactivation and lung toxicity. Cancer Res 1991; 51: 542.
46. Kanekal S, Kehrer JP. Evidence for peroxidase-mediated metabolism of cyclophosphamide. Drug Metab Dispos 1993; 21: 37.
47. McKenna-KE, Burrows-D. Pulmonary toxicity in a patient with psoriasis receiving methotrexate therapy. Clin Exp Dermatol 2000; 25: 24.
48. Giles FJ, Smith MP, Goldstone AH. Chlorambucil lung toxicity. Acta Haematol 1990; 83: 156.
49. Wang Q, Hollinger MA, Giri SN. Attenuation of amiodarone-induced lung fibrosis and phospholipidosis in hamsters by taurine and/or niacin treatment. J Pharmacol Exp Ther 1992; 266: 127.
50. Roca J, Heras M, Kodriguez-Koisin R et al. Pulmonary complications after long term amiodarone treatment. Thorax 1992; 47: 372.

32 Humidifier fever

P Sherwood Burge

Clinical features

Humidifier fever occurs in workers exposed to microbiological
aerosols. The common sources are humidification systems,
coolant oil/water emulsions and perhaps cotton spinning. It is
an acute illness, usually starting 4–8 hours after the start of a
working shift, most frequently on the first day of work after a
weekend. Symptoms are often worse after return from a longer
period off work.[1] The full syndrome includes fever, sweats,
headache, aches in the limbs, cough, breathlessness and general
malaise. The symptoms usually resolve in 24–48 hours despite
continuing exposure. Sometimes the illness is milder, consisting
of headache, malaise and joint pains with a similar periodicity.
There may be confusion with the sick building syndrome,
where headache and lethargy are common. Sick building syndrome is more common in humidified buildings[2] but is not associated with raised levels of precipitating antibodies to
humidifier extracts.[1] During the acute illness, crackles may be
audible in the lung fields. Sometimes there is associated
wheeze (although this feature may be a manifestation of the
additional diagnosis of occupational asthma). Lung function
tests may show a restrictive defect and reduced gas transfer in
the more severe cases.

Environmental circumstances and relationship to other disorders

The attack rate for similarly exposed workers is often in the
range of 5–30%. Other workers similarly exposed may develop
occupational asthma[3] or occasionally extrinsic allergic alveolitis.[4,5]
Extrinsic allergic alveolitis is relatively common when the humidifiers contain warm water, supporting the growth of thermophilic
Actinomyces,[6] but it is rare with cold-water humidifiers, which
are the type usually found in central air-conditioning plants. The
distinction between extrinsic allergic alveolitis and humidifier
fever is unclear. The clinical features and results of investigations
are identical in the acute phase of both diseases. However,
humidifier fever improves with continuing exposure whereas
extrinsic allergic alveolitis usually deteriorates with continuing
exposure. So far there have been no recorded patients with radiological changes during humidifier fever; in particular, no patient
has developed fibrotic pulmonary disease, features which are relatively common in extrinsic allergic alveolitis.[7]

The pathogenesis of humidifier fever is unknown. It is
unclear why the same antigen sometimes causes extrinsic allergic alveolitis, with progressive disease, and sometimes humidifier fever, with improvement despite continued exposure. It is
possible that humidifier fever is due predominantly to endotoxins produced by bacteria. Tolerance to endotoxins is known to
occur. Some of the features that may help to distinguish
between humidifier fever, acute allergic alveolitis, organic dust
toxic syndrome, occupational asthma and silo filler's disease are
shown in Table 32.1.

The microbiology of humidifier fever

Cold water humidifiers using recirculating water readily become
contaminated with micro-organisms, most of which find their

Table 32.1 Clinical and laboratory features in humidifier fever, extrinsic allergic alveolitis, organic dust toxic syndrome, occupational asthma and silo filler's disease*

	Humidifier fever	Acute extrinsic allergic alveolitis	Organic dust toxic syndrome	Occupational asthma	Silo filler's disease
Acute systemic reaction with sweating, joint aches and lassitude	+	+	+	Rare	?
Reduced D_LCO and hypoxia	+	+	+	–	?
Airways obstruction	Sometimes	Sometimes	?	+	–
Precipitating IgG antibodies	+	+	Sometimes	–	–
Improvement with continuing exposure	+	–	?	–	–
Incomplete recovery without further exposure	–	Common	?	Common	Common

* Extrinsic allergic alveolitis is dealt with in Chapter 55, organic dust toxic syndrome in Chapter 30, occupational asthma in Chapter 48.13, and silo filler's disease in Chapter 30.

way into the system via either the incoming water or the incoming air. Many of the outbreaks have occurred in printing works,[8] perhaps because of the necessity for humidification and perhaps also because paper dust, which finds its way into the return air passing through the humidifier, provides a substrate for bacterial growth. Investigation of the water has failed to show any one organism responsible for the disease. In most carefully investigated outbreaks large numbers of different bacteria, fungi and unicellular organisms are identified. Whether the reaction is due to bacterial or fungal antigens or to endotoxin is unresolved. Individual outbreaks have been attributed to acanthamoebae, pullularia, flavobacteria, *Bacillus subtilis*, pseudomonads and *Sporothrix schenckii*. However, positive results on bronchial provocation testing have never been found to be limited to a single organism; the most appropriate antigen to use for the investigation of an outbreak is an extract prepared from the uncultured contaminated water.[9] There is substantial antigenic cross-reaction between acanthamoebae and other humidifier antigens (which may be partially due to ingestion of bacteria by the acanthamoebae), and this adds to the difficulty of determining the specific cause.

Diagnosis and investigation

The diagnosis rests on the history and is confirmed by precipitin tests or other tests of specific IgG antibodies. All patients who have developed humidifier fever have strongly positive precipitating antibodies to antigens prepared from extracts of humidifier water. Many of the outbreaks have common antigens but the antigens between different outbreaks do not always cross-react. Precipitins to humidifier antigens correlate with the length and degree of exposure to contaminated aerosols and also inversely to cigarette smoking.[9–11] The immunosuppressive effect of cigarette smoking on precipitin levels seems to wane after stopping smoking.[10] Precipitating antibodies are usually found in a large proportion of exposed asymptomatic workers. Their presence

denotes exposure rather than disease.[12] Bronchial provocation testing has occasionally been used to elucidate the nature of an outbreak or of illness in an individual (Fig. 32.1) but it is not recommended as a standard element in the investigation.

Prevention

It is often not necessary to humidify the air in the first place. There are many office buildings with humidifiers that are out of use with no apparent detriment to the quality of air in the building.[13] However some industrial activities, in particular printing, require that a relatively high humidity be maintained. It has been found to be impossible to keep heavily contaminated humidifiers clean with regimens including cleaning and biocides. Several outbreaks have been stopped by replacing cold-water spray humidifiers with steam humidification where there is no recirculation of water. It is important to avoid pooling of water from condensation in ductwork. It is also theoretically possible that antigen may accumulate in chiller units, although as yet no cases of humidifier fever have been attributed to these. Once steps have been taken to eliminate exposure, the effectiveness of control can be monitored biologically by serial estimations of precipitating antibodies in affected workers.[14] It is also possible to measure antigen in the air, although this is time-consuming and expensive.[15]

Pontiac fever

Air-conditioning systems may occasionally be contaminated with *Legionella pneumophila* serotype 1. This organism does not grow in cold water but requires water above about 35°C such as occurs in heating systems and in evaporative condensers. Vapour drift from evaporative condensers may enter air-conditioning systems. Exposure of healthy workers to such contaminated air-conditioning systems leads to an illness similar to humidifier fever but with a very high attack rate, reaching 95% of those

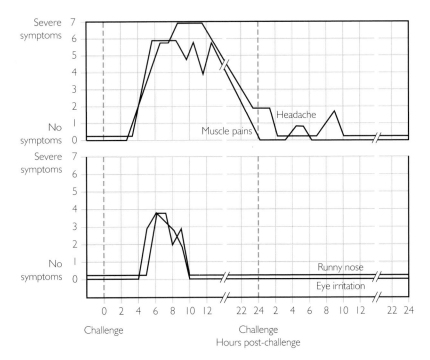

Fig. 32.1 Symptom scores during bronchial provocation testing with an extract from a contaminated humidifier, which caused no reaction in unexposed asthmatic subjects. The same challenge was repeated on two consecutive days, during which diary cards were filled in every hour, monitoring headache, muscle pains, runny nose and eye irritation. After the first exposure, symptoms started at 4 hours and were at their peak at 8 hours. A similar challenge on the second day resulted in a much reduced reaction, showing that tolerance had developed.

exposed in the original Pontiac outbreak.[16,17] In the 1985 outbreak in Stafford District General Hospital, 80% of the nurses working daily in the wards supplied by the contaminated air-conditioning system developed precipitating antibodies to *Legionella pneumophila* at 1:16 or greater, compared with 30% of nurses working daily in wards supplied by the neighbouring air-conditioning unit. There was an association between positive precipitating antibodies and an acute febrile illness without clinical pneumonia.[18] Other outbreaks of similar disease have been attributed to *Legionella anisa*[19] and *Legionella micdadei*.[20]

Therapeutic principles

■ Humidifier fever resolves with no specific treatment and no long-term health consequences.

? Unresolved questions

■ Is the disease due to specific bacteria (or fungi) or to soluble products from them?

■ Is humidification needed for working environments, particularly for worker comfort?

■ Do biocides added to prevent bacterial growth cause occupational asthma and other symptoms?

References

1. McSharry CP, Anderson K, Speekenbrink A et al. Discriminant analysis of symptom pattern and serum antibody titres in humidifier related disease. Thorax 1993; 48: 496–500.
2. Burge PS, Hedge A, Wilson S et al. Sick building syndrome; a study of 4373 office workers. Ann Occup Hyg 1987; 31: 493–504.
3. Burge PS, Finnegan M, Horsfield N et al. Occupational asthma in a factory with a contaminated humidifier. Thorax 1985; 40: 248–254.
4. Robertson AS, Burge PS, Wieland GA, Carmalt MHB. Extrinsic allergic alveolitis caused by a cold water humidifier. Thorax 1987; 42: 32.
5. Pal TM, De Monchy JG, Groothoff JW, Post D. The clinical spectrum of humidifier disease in synthetic fiber plants. Am J Ind Med 1997; 31: 682–692.
6. Pickering CAC. Humidifier fever. Eur J Respir Dis 1982; 63(suppl. 123): 104–107.
7. Pal TM, De Monchy JG, Groothoff JW, Post D. Follow up investigation of workers in synthetic fibre plants with humidifier disease and work related asthma. Occup Environ Med 1999; 56: 403–410.
8. Jost M, Lehmann M. Humidifier syndrome as occupational disease in Switzerland [in German]. Schweiz Rundsch Med Prax 1990; 79: 797–803.
9. Baur X, Richter G, Pethran A et al. Increased prevalence of IgG-induced sensitization and hypersensitivity pneumonitis (humidifier lung) in nonsmokers exposed to aerosols of a contaminated air conditioner. Respiration 1992; 59: 211–124.
10. Finnegan MJ, Pickering CAC, Davies PS, Austwick PKC. Factors affecting the development of precipitating antibodies in workers exposed to contaminated humidifiers. Clin Allergy 1985; 15: 281–292.
11. Finnegan MJ, Little S, Gordon DJ et al. The effect of smoking on the development of allergic disease and specific immunological responses in a factory work force exposed to humidifier contaminants. Br J Ind Med 1991; 48 : 30–33.
12. Anderson K, McSharry CP, Clark C et al. Sump bay fever: inhalational fever associated with a biologically contaminated water aerosol. Occup Environ Med 1996; 53: 106–111.
13. Burge PS, Jones P, Robertson AS. Sick Building Syndrome; environmental comparisons of sick and healthy buildings. Indoor Air 90 1990; 1: 479–483.
14. Perdrix A, Lascaud D, Dell'Accio P et al. Humidifier fever in an industrial setting, results of three years control using precipitin measurements. Bronches 1979; 29: 53–63.

15. Harrison J, Pickering CAC, Faragher EB et al. An investigation of the relationship between microbial and particulate air pollution and the sick building syndrome. Respir Med 1992; 86: 225–235.
16. Glick TH, Gregg MB, Berman B et al. Pontiac fever. Am J Epidemiol 1978; 107: 149–160.
17. Kaufmann AF, McDade JE, Patton CM et al. Pontiac fever; isolation of the etiologic agent (*Legionella pneumophila*) and demonstration of its mode of transmission. Am J Epidemiol 1981; 114: 337.
18. Badenoch J. First report of the committee of enquiry into the outbreak of legionnaires' disease in Stafford in April 1985. Cmd 9772. London: HMSO; 1986: 1.
19. Fenstersheib MD, Miller M, Diggins C et al. Outbreak of Pontiac fever due to *Legionella anisa*. Lancet 1990; 336: 35–37.
20. Goldberg DJ, Wrench JG, Collier PW. Lochgoilhead fever: outbreak of non-pneumonic legionellosis due to *Legionella micdadei*. Lancet 1989; 1: 316–318.

33 Respiratory problems in adverse environments

David M Denison

 Key points

- Atmospheric pressure and inspired P_{O_2} fall exponentially with altitude, halving every 5.5 km (18 000 ft).

- In healthy individuals there are no significant effects of breathing ambient air up to an altitude of 10 000 feet.

- Compression (e.g. during descent in water) can be rapid but decompression must be slow to avoid decompression sickness.

- Diving should cease at least 12 hours before a flight.

- Commercial aircraft are pressurised to an equivalent cabin altitude of about 8000 feet (2.4 km), which in a healthy subject gives an inspired P_{O_2} of about 108 mmHg (14.4 kPa) and P_aO_2 of about 55 mmHg (7.3 kPa).

- Potential problems for patients with respiratory disease at altitude (including flight) can result from hypoxia, reduced ambient pressure or low humidity.

This chapter concerns respiratory aspects of climbing, flying, diving and living in poorly ventilated spaces. Also discussed are the pulmonary problems of escaping from aircraft and submarines and the effects of respiratory disease on 'fitness to fly' and 'fitness to dive'. These fields are covered in detail in four excellent books.[1–4]

Geographical constraints

Almost three-quarters of the Earth's surface is covered by water (Fig. 33.1). Close to the shore, over the continental shelf, the sea is less than one-third of a kilometre deep; elsewhere it is up to 10 km deeper. The great majority of animals in the sea are confined to the upper 200–300 m; lack of light and plants are the main obstacles to animals living at greater depth. The ambient pressure in water increases linearly by one atmosphere for every 10 m (33 ft) of descent. The upper seas are well stirred and equilibrated with the oxygen in air at sea level, so there are no great changes of its partial pressure with depth. At great depths the P_{O_2} falls but some active fish survive, even in the deepest trenches.

Most of the dry land is just above sea level but the tallest peak rises nearly 9 km. Almost all mammals live below an altitude of 1.5 km. Cold and lack of oxygen are the principal barriers to living much higher. In air, ambient pressure falls exponentially with ascent, halving every 5.5 km (18 000 ft). The lower atmosphere is well stirred by meteorological variations and has a uniform oxygen concentration (20.93 vol%); thus ambient P_{O_2} also halves with every 5.5 km of ascent. The atmosphere has not always contained this amount of oxygen. Life began in an almost oxygen-free environment, where the production of oxygen by blue–green algae presented a profound threat to evolution, detectable in responses to hypoxia and hyperoxia today.[5,6]

Physiological constraints

The narrow vertical range of the biomass (1.5 km above to 0.3 km below sea level) contains a 60-fold variation of ambient pressure (Fig. 33.2). The majority of animal life is aquatic and the majority of aquatic animals live at a pressure of about 5 atmospheres (505 kPa), with an ambient P_{O_2} of 0.2 ATA (Fig. 33.2). Humans, like other animals with high aerobic capacities, evolved in air at sea level and cannot stray from it easily. Remarkably, in 1978 Reinhold Messner and Peter Habeler reached the summit of Everest without additional oxygen, but they had to descend almost immediately. Several climbers have done so since but, 15 years earlier and more surprisingly, the respiratory physiologist Tom Hornbein and colleagues survived overnight without oxygen at an altitude of about 8500 m. If balloonists and aviators breathe pure oxygen at ambient pressure they remain alert and energetic to an altitude of 12 km but quickly lose consciousness if they go any higher.

Going in the opposite direction, most humans can only breath-hold dive to 10–30 m. They are limited by breath-holding

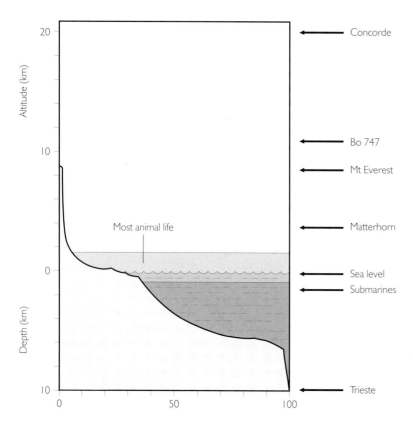

Fig. 33.1 Cumulative frequency histogram of the altitudes and depths of Earth's rock surface, from the top of Mount Everest to the bottom of the Challenger Deep. Most animal life is confined between the two horizontal bars (dotted area). The arrows on the right indicate the levels at which *Concorde*, most commercial jets (Boeing 747), most submarines and the research submarine *Trieste* operate. Space vehicles go very much higher but the aeromedical problems in them and in high-performance jet fighters are very similar.

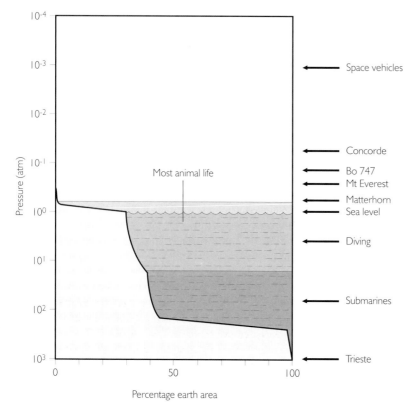

Fig. 33.2 Cumulative frequency histogram of the absolute pressure that humans can reach unaided or in various vehicles. Most animal life is confined between the two horizontal bars.

time. The current world records for breath-hold dives are held by Umberto Pelizzari, who can descend to 80 m unaided and to 150 m with the help of a concrete sled to descend and an inflated balloon to return to the surface. If swimmers take a supply of air with them they can dive safely to 50 m for prolonged periods but if they go deeper nitrogen narcosis develops. If the nitrogen in air is replaced by helium it is possible to dive to 300–600 m. Below this depth distortion of nerve membranes by ambient pressure causes unacceptable hyperexcitability, manifest initially as tremor and eventually as convulsions. This condition is known as the high-pressure nervous syndrome.

Within these extended limits of survival (12 km above to 0.6 km below sea level), precautions have to be taken if individuals are subjected to changes in ambient pressure. In general, compression can be rapid, but decompression should be slow. If there is a need to move up and down further or faster, it is necessary to travel in a pressure-resistant shell, which presents several problems if the vessel is poorly ventilated or its walls fail (Fig. 33.3).

The respiratory system is vulnerable to changes of gas pressure and composition for many reasons (Fig. 33.4).[7] The airways are easily irritated and narrow or close when stimulated. The lung walls rupture at transmural pressures of about one-10th of an atmosphere (10 kPa). The muscles of the chest wall fatigue if transmural pressures exceed one-20th of an atmosphere (5 kPa) for more than a few minutes. The respiratory surface of the lung is vast (100 m²), very thin (1–2 μm) and passive. It cannot prevent the rapid indiscriminate absorption of inhaled gases. It

comes in contact with almost all of the circulating blood volume every minute or less. The transport medium (haemoglobin) is readily denatured by certain common gases so the entire circulation can be poisoned in a short time. Blood quickly carries inhaled gases to tissues, which require precise gas levels for many vital tasks. Excess oxygen can be as damaging as too little (see Chapter 13), and nerve function depends upon the inert gas content of the neurilemma, and on local pH, which is set by local P_{CO_2}. Hence, tissues can rapidly be disabled by changes in inspired gas composition or pressure.

The speed with which individual elements of tissue can be affected by changes in the gases breathed depends in part on the ratio of tissue blood flow to tissue volume. More precisely, the gas tensions of blood and tissue equilibrate with each other, with time constants that are proportional to the volume of the tissue element and the solubility of the gas in the tissue, and are inversely proportional to local blood flow and the solubility of the gas in blood (Fig. 33.5). These factors determine how gas accumulates and empties from tissues as the pressure or composition of the inhalate changes.

The behaviour of oxygen is different from that of most gases because it is metabolised. Oxygen is handled almost entirely by enzymes, of which there may be many different ones within a single cell. The most obvious (cytochrome oxidase) uses oxygen as the final electron sink in oxidative phosphorylation. This process has an extremely high affinity for oxygen and continues without faltering until the local P_{O_2} falls below 3 mmHg (0.4 kPa) or so. Many other oxygen-consuming reactions con-

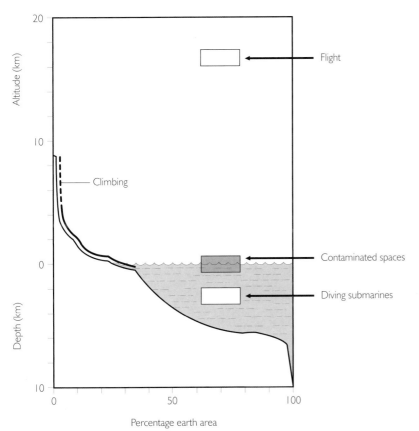

Fig. 33.3 Cumulative frequency histogram of the altitudes and depths of the Earth's rock surface. The heavy curve indicates the range that humans can invade without the help of specialised breathing mixtures and/or pressure-resistant vehicles. The broken ends of the curve show extremes that can be reached transiently.

(a)

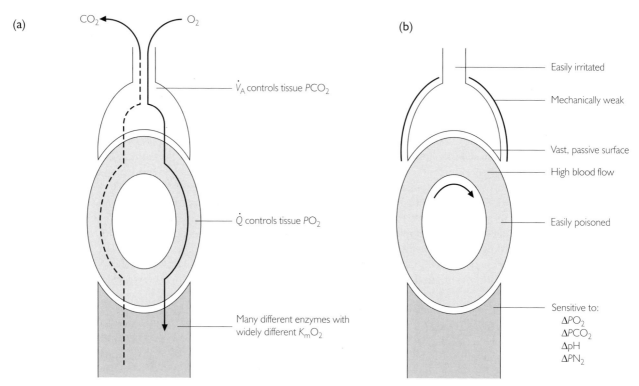

(b)

Fig. 33.4 (a) An elementary model of respiration comprising lungs (upper element), circulation (middle) and tissues (lower) and emphasising that : alveolar ventilation ($\dot{V}_A$) controls tissue carbon dioxide pressure; local blood flow ($\dot{Q}$) determines tissue oxygen pressure; and oxygen is metabolised in many ways, which vary in their sensitivity to hypoxia and hyperoxia. (b) Another view of the same model to indicate its principal areas of vulnerability. The bold curves around the lungs represent the thoracoabdominal wall.

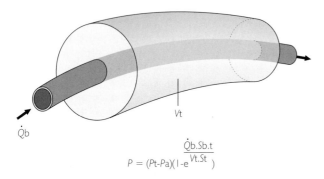

$$P = (Pt\text{-}Pa)(1\text{-}e^{\frac{\dot{Q}b.Sb.t}{Vt.St}})$$

Fig. 33.5 A conceptual tissue element served by a single capillary. Gas exchange between the element and the blood in the capillary is governed by the equation shown, in which P, the instantaneous gas pressure in the tissue, depends upon the initial tissue (P_t) and arterial (P_a) gas tensions, blood flow ($\dot{Q}_b$), the solubility of the gas in blood (S_b), the volume of tissue (V_t) and the solubility of the gas in the tissue (S_t).

cerned, for example, with the production and destruction of neural transmitters, have lower affinities and are much more vulnerable to hypoxia and hyperoxia. Such reactions represent about 10% of resting metabolism. The biochemistry of oxygen is complex. Its exceptionally high affinity for electrons leads to the formation of toxic free radicals in many reactions. Normally these are inactivated by antioxidant defences and rarely escape

from reaction sites but this leakage is considerably increased in hypoxia and hyperoxia.[8] Radicals released by endothelium, inflammatory cells and platelets injure extravascular tissues, particularly in the lung. This damage can be initiated or augmented by ischaemia. On the return of blood flow inflammatory cells are activated, releasing more free radicals (reperfusion injury).

If, in the elementary model of respiration shown in Figure 33.4, it is assumed that the lungs are healthy, the circulatory compartment is filled with blood of normal characteristics and the tissues largely impose an oxygen demand and carbon dioxide output on the cardiopulmonary system, the following important features of respiration emerge. Tissue oxygenation is determined mainly by local blood flow and haemoglobin content and is almost independent of ventilation. Tissue carbon dioxide tensions are set by ventilation and are almost entirely independent of blood flow. Put crudely, local blood vessels are employed to set tissue P_{O_2} and the lungs set tissue P_{CO_2}. The potential competition between tissues for the most appropriate level of P_aCO_2 is dominated by the brain and spinal cord, which normally require a P_{CO_2} of 40 mmHg (5.3 kPa) for the preservation of local pH.

Such a model accurately predicts that any increase in ambient P_{CO_2} will be met by an increase in ventilation, with little response from blood flow. Any fall in ambient P_{O_2} will be countered initially by an increase in blood flow, which costs much energy but can be deployed very rapidly. Later, this is offset by a modest hyperventilation, which in energetic terms is less expensive. The pace at which acceptable hyperventilation develops is set by renal excretion of bicarbonate, which maintains brain pH. In the longer term these responses to hypoxaemia are superseded by increases in haemoglobin content and capillarity, which are even more economical but take time to engineer. The model also correctly forecasts that exercise, which increases the demand for oxygen and the production of carbon dioxide, will lead to linear increases in ventilation (for carbon dioxide elimination) and blood flow (for the provision of oxygen), again maintaining P_ACO_2 at 40 mmHg (5.3 kPa), which preserves brain pH.

Breathing apparatus

Successful living in hostile respiratory environments depends on the design and performance of appropriate breathing equipment. Ventilation via breathing apparatus is compromised by the composition, delivery and ease of exhalation of the mixture provided. There are four types of equipment. The first blows a continuous stream of fresh inspirate into a through-flow cavity such as an aircraft cabin or a diver's helmet. It is simple to design and breathe from but wasteful, because it requires a large supply of gas. Delivery pressure is set by inflow and the characteristics of the outlet valve.

In the second technique, gas is delivered from some substantial source, often via a lengthy umbilical tube, but is presented to a demand valve, so-called because it provides inspirate only on demand, and is therefore more economical (Fig. 33.6). As it depends on the user developing a negative pressure in the cavity to establish the demand, it is commonly fitted to an oronasal mask or a mouthpiece. The important features of the system are the opening and closing pressures of the demand valve, the characteristics of the exhalation valve and the integrity of the cavity from which the subject breathes. Often the demand valve is set to operate at a slight positive pressure relative to the environment (*safety pressure*) to ensure that any leaks are outboard. Such oronasal masks usually require a soft reflected edge to seal on the face, the delivery pressure of the demand valve has to be fed to the external surface of the expiratory valve to prevent gas blowing away (a *compensated outlet valve*) and the exoskeleton and harness of the mask have to be carefully designed to avoid the mask tilting and leaking as the over-pressure develops.

In the third method, the subject takes a restricted gas supply with him/her ('*scuba*' = self-contained breathing apparatus) to avoid the problems of being tethered by an umbilical line. The subject is then limited in addition by the organisation and volume of the finite gas supply. Often it is divided into twin cylinders with a manifold so that it cannot all be lost by accident at one time. Finally, there are *closed circuit breathing systems* or '*rebreathers*', in which expired air is scrubbed of carbon dioxide, refreshed with oxygen and recycled. These are discussed below under 'Sealed spaces'.

All these systems allow access to environments which could not otherwise be invaded but they impose some physiological penalties when they are operating as designed and there may be catastrophic consequences if they fail. When accidents occur in flying, fire-fighting or diving, it is important to impound all respiratory apparatus and breathing mixtures as often the causes of the accidents are in one of these and are only detected on specialised investigation.

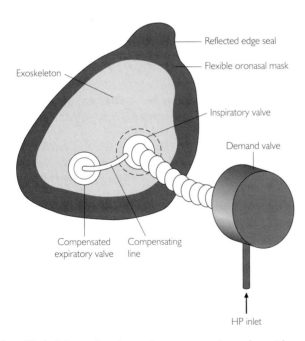

Fig. 33.6 Schematic view of an oronasal mask, with a soft, reflected edge to hold 'safety pressure', a hard exoskeleton to keep the soft mask in place, a demand valve to conserve a high-pressure gas supply, an inspiratory valve to seal off inward gas flow during expiration and a demand-valve delivery pressure compensation expiratory valve to permit expiration while maintaining safety pressure.

Flying

In the late 19th century balloonists were capable of ascending to the height of the Everest in an hour or two. Many studies on such flights confirmed and extended the early work of Boyle, Torricelli, Pascal, Priestley and Lavoisier. It was shown, for example, that atmospheric pressure did fall exponentially with altitude, halving every 5.5 km (18 000 ft); that the oxygen concentration was constant; and therefore that its partial pressure also fell at the same exponential rate. These studies also showed that oxygen was essential to life and consciousness. Almost all that is now known about altitude physiology was established and understood by Paul Bert in the 1870s at the time of the first deaths from aviation hypoxia.[9]

Propellor-driven aircraft were invented at the beginning of the 20th century. As they require dense air to pull on, they are limited to a ceiling altitude of 30 000 feet (9 km; conventionally all altitudes relevant to aviation are cited in feet rather than metres). Jet aircraft move forward by reaction to a stream of hot exhaust gases pumped backwards. They fly best at altitudes of 20 000–60 000 feet (6–18 km), where air resistance is less, but they cannot rise much higher because their engines need sufficient ambient oxygen to ignite the fuel.

Modem fighters can ascend to this ceiling in a minute or two. Rockets carry oxidants with them, operate best in a vacuum and can reach the stratosphere within a minute. Aircraft introduced fresh respiratory problems into aviation medicine which had not been experienced in 'open-basket' ballooning.[4,10] Altitude hypoxia, however, remained the principal problem.[11]

Effects of flying on normal subjects

Studies of hypoxia in humans have a long and distinguished international history. For operational reasons, some of the most elegant recent work has been done in the UK.[12] Most small private aircraft have, and almost all aircraft of the past had, unpressurised cabins. Thousands of experiences during the Second World War and many experimental studies since have shown there are no marked physiological effects of breathing ambient air during flight at heights up to 10 000 feet (3000 m) for a few hours at a time. Above that altitude, mental deterioration becomes progressively more marked. This results entirely from hypoxia and is reversed completely by oxygen administration. Decisions become unreliable, awareness is reduced and physical strength is limited. Consciousness is grossly impaired at 20 000 feet (6 km) and lost within a few minutes at 25 000 feet (7.5 km). Abrupt exposures to higher altitudes show that the time of useful consciousness falls progressively, to a minimum of 15 seconds at 40 000 feet (12 km). This minimum period represents the sum of the lung-to-brain circulation time (8 s) and the additional few seconds needed to use up oxygen dissolved in cerebral tissue.

Unpressurised aircraft are therefore generally limited to an altitude ceiling of 10 000 feet, unless they carry supplemental oxygen. If this were available in abundance, such aircraft could be taken up to 40 000 feet, with the crew breathing pure oxygen. If, however, ambient pressure falls more rapidly than the nitrogen previously dissolved in tissues can diffuse away, the nitrogen aggregates as bubbles, which deform cells, block vessels and initiate a train of inflammatory events that together produce altitude decompression sickness. This can occur at altitudes as low as 15 000 ft (4.5 km)and is a serious risk above 25 000 feet.[13-16] It can be avoided by prolonged oxygen breathing beforehand (denitrogenation), but this has its own disadvantages. It is corrected by returning to ground level.

Normally, commercial jet aircraft are pressurised to keep the cabin 'altitude' below 8000 feet (2.4 km; cabin pressure = 565 mmHg). Such aircraft climb gradually to their actual cruise altitudes of 30 000–60 000 feet. At the maximum cabin altitude of 8000 feet, the oxygen tension in moist inspired air is 108 mmHg (14.4 kPa), alveolar Po_2 (P_AO_2) is about 65 mmHg (8.6 kPa), and blood leaving healthy lungs has a Po_2 (arterial Po_2, P_aO_2) close to 55 mmHg (7.3 kPa), so that it remains almost completely saturated with oxygen (S_aO_2 approximately 90%). Most flight stages at this cabin altitude last no more than a few hours. Such exposure may be mildly tiring and does have measurable effects on psychomotor performance, but there have been no satisfactory demonstrations that they have functional consequences. There is a reduction in night vision, which is of no practical significance, and gradual and just detectable hyperventilation. Millions of healthy people have flown in these circumstances without physical ill effect.

Medical problems associated with flying

Physicians face four problems concerned with aviation:

- Is this patient fit to fly?
- How should this emergency be dealt with in flight?
- Is this candidate acceptable for aircrew training?
- Is this experienced person fit to continue as aircrew?

In brief, the answers to these questions are simple. Almost all patients can be flown if necessary and all the major airlines have highly competent medical departments to assist in this. Most medical emergencies during commercial flights have to be dealt with by common sense, oxygen, radioing ahead for ambulance reception and little else. Diverting the flight can be very expensive and disruptive, and should only be considered as a last resort. Aircrew are extremely costly to train, therefore they have to be selected with special care. Once trained, that investment and their livelihoods have to be protected by returning them to flying duties wherever possible.

Effects on patients with respiratory disease

On average 1 in 6.4 million passengers dies in flight, 1 in 10 000 commercial flights is diverted for medical reasons and serious medical emergencies arise in approximately 1 in 1000 flights. If hyperventilation is excluded, few of these emergencies are respiratory.

Patients with chest disease are at three disadvantages in flight: the drop in barometric pressure might expand and burst a poorly ventilated space in the lung; the fall in ambient oxygen pressure could make patients more hypoxaemic than at ground level; and the low humidity of the cabin atmosphere may lead to drying of some secretions and provoke bronchial responses to evaporative cooling. It is often stated that bullae themselves may be a problem because they are 'non-communicating' and could burst. Bullae must, however, communicate with an airway to remain inflated. Truly sealed and tense spaces are rare in chest disease, because gas in any closed cavity tends to be resorbed (absorption atelectasis).

A vast number of people with gross chronic chest disease have flown safely in commercial aircraft. With the exception of patients with chest trauma or existing pneumothoraces, there is little, if any, evidence of anyone developing pulmonary barotrauma or air embolism in routine flight. In the rare event of a survivable loss of cabin pressure at high altitude, patients with chest disease are at greater risk of lung rupture but this probability is so low that it is usually ignored. Pulmonary embolism is a commonly cited hazard for middle-aged and elderly passengers on long-haul flights, but its true incidence is unknown. This illustrates the general problem of obtaining good epidemiological data on the health of passengers after flights. Arriving at their destination, and again on returning home, passengers leave the airport rapidly and disperse widely. Also it could well be that several conditions, such as aircraft-acquired infections and pulmonary embolism, are under-recognised as complications of commercial flight. These topics have been discussed in detail very recently by the British Thoracic Society and in a House of Lords inquiry.[17,18]

There is no doubt that patients with diseased lungs, who are hypoxaemic at ground level, will become more so on ascent to 8000 feet, although the fall in P_aO_2 will not be as great as the 42 mmHg (5.6 kPa) fall in ambient oxygen pressure.[19] In many, who are only mildly hypoxaemic at normal pressure, the fall in P_aO_2 will pass unremarked at rest, but such patients might be slightly more dyspnoeic walking about when the aircraft is at cruise altitude. For others, in whom hypoxaemia is more severe, ground-level conditions can be restored in flight by oxygen from an oronasal mask. Raising the inspired oxygen concentration to 28% is sufficient for this purpose. If airline medical services are notified beforehand they will provide an additional oxygen supply for the journey and are very used to such requests. On long-distance flights, it is wise to check the altitude of any intermediate stops and ensure that oxygen is available there also. Similarly, a small humidifier and mask can cope with problems, such as drying of a tracheostomy, created by the low ambient humidity.

Problems associated with military flight

Large military aircraft are organised along similar lines to commercial passenger aircraft but there are more provisions for escape and survival, because damage in flight is more probable. Small fighters need to be faster and more manoeuvrable and cannot accept the weight penalty of a cabin pressurised to 8000 feet. They are usually fitted with a lightweight compartment in which the crew breathe oxygen-rich mixtures as the cabin altitude rises to a maximum of 25 000 feet. Such aircraft turn at speed by banking sharply, using the flat wing areas to force the change in direction. As a result, the crew experience a caudal force several times that of normal gravity. This drives blood from the apices to the bases of the lung, resulting temporarily in gross ventilation–perfusion inequality. This is exaggerated by distortion and transient blocking of airways, trapping highly soluble oxygen in the alveoli beyond. This leads to absorption atelectasis, seen as linear shadows on the chest radiograph. Effective shunts of 25% or more of the cardiac output are common and increase the risk of loss of consciousness in subsequent high-G turns.[20] This problem is responsible for the loss of several high-performance aircraft each year. The atelectasis can usually be reversed by deep inspirations after each turn. Modern fighter aircraft are much more agile than hitherto, and are capable of sustaining higher G forces for longer periods of time, making G-induced loss of consciousness more likely. Fighter pilots prefer to sit upright to retain the clearest possible all-round view of events outside. In principle, the pilot who can retain consciousness for even a few seconds longer than his opponent is likely to win the dog-fight. However, if pilots could fly in a recumbent position they could pull higher G levels with safety. In future aircraft this conflict may be resolved, because the advent of laser weapons may force aircraft designers to protect their aircrew by dispensing with transparent cockpits altogether. In that case the pilot could be positioned anywhere in the vehicle and adopt any comfortable posture.

Chest disease in aircrew

Commercial and military aircrew are responsible for expensive equipment, critical decisions and many lives, so they are subject to rigorous criteria of fitness to fly, laid down by International Aviation Authorities[21] and the Armed Services respectively. Assessments for this purpose are conducted only by authorised medical examiners. In principle, candidates with any history of spontaneous pneumothorax are rejected unless they have had a pleurectomy or pleurodesis, because of the high recurrence rate ipsilaterally (20–50%) and contralaterally (10%). Recurrence rates after pleurodesis or pleurectomy are very low. Similarly, candidates with any history of asthma are rejected because of its liability to recur. Evidence of other obstructive pulmonary disease, or any radiographic abnormality of the lungs is a bar to training as professional crew but asymptomatic sarcoidosis or previous limited surgery for benign lung tumours is not. Sarcoidosis is, however, of particular concern because of the risk of sudden death from myocardial involvement, so extensive cardiological tests are required before such a patient can be accepted.

When established aircrew develop chest disease, the criteria are slightly less stringent. They are allowed, for example, to return to flying duties 3 trouble-free months after pleurodesis or pleurectomy for a spontaneous pneumothorax. Aircrew with well-controlled asthma can continue to fly, preferably with inhaled corticosteroid prophylaxis. As methyl xanthines irritate the central nervous system they are unsuitable treatment in this situation. Usually, asthmatic aircrew are expected to fly with a co-pilot and are not allowed to drive high-performance jets because of the risk of inducing an attack by bronchial irritation during high-G turns. Regulations for private pilots are not as strict. Current details can be obtained from the Civil Aviation Authorities, who maintain a panel of physicians to conduct medical examinations on their behalf.

Escape from aircraft

Military aircrew are trained to bring back aircraft that have been badly damaged in flight, wherever possible, and to escape from them where not. With modern high-performance vehicles these are not simple tasks. As an example, consider the pilot of a single-seat fighter getting into difficulties at an altitude of 60 000 feet (18 km). He will have been breathing oxygen at a cabin altitude of 25 000 feet (7.5 km; 282 mmHg). The pressure outside the aircraft will be 54 mmHg. If he has not lost cabin pressure already, he will choose to dump it slowly (over several seconds) to avoid the risk of explosive decompression later. This will involve an approximately fivefold expansion of lung gas over the same timescale. He will choose to expire to residual volume to minimise this. At the same time, however, an automatic oxygen supply regulator, sensing the fall in local pressure will operate to maintain his alveolar pressure at 141 mmHg (18.8 kPa), to keep P_AO_2 at 65 mmHg (8.6 kPa). As this overpressure of 141 − 54 = 87 mmHg (11.8 kPa) is more than the bursting pressure of the lung or the sustained mechanical ability of the chest wall, the same breathing pressure will be used to inflate a pressure jerkin that encloses his thoracoabdominal wall. However, this in turn will pressurise his trunk at the expense of his head and limbs, obstructing peripheral venous return. The breathing pressure will be used again to inflate leggings, sleeves and the interior of a sealed helmet to prevent this. If the helmet visor is not already sealed, the rise in breathing pressure will automatically close that too. Remarkably, a single device the size of a matchbox, mounted on the pilot's chest or the side of his ejection seat, is able to sense and execute all these tasks, and maintain him in relative safety. The pilot has then to return the unpressurised aircraft to base at the lowest altitude possible. This may still be quite high, particularly if the aircraft is short of fuel, because of the increased air resistance close to ground. Thus, the pilot of a plane damaged in mid-Atlantic might have to remain in an unpressurised cabin, above 20 000 feet for some hours.

Sometimes aircrew have to leave their vessel in flight, within a second or less. The principal problems then are rapid decompression, blast injury, rapid acceleration to get clear of the tailplane and survival of the subsequent descent. Where cabin pressure has not been lost already, and there is no time to jettison the canopy, spikes on the ejection seat and detonating cord in the canopy destroy the canopy as the seat leaves. The pilot will have done his best to exhale to residual volume in the half second required to operate the seat trigger. His chest-mounted regulator will sort out the immediate problems of the decompression. Automatically operated wires attached to the pilot's helmet, gloves and boots draw his head and limbs close to the seat to prevent blast injury as he enters the high-speed air stream. Once clear of the tailplane, the seat will freefall to an altitude of 10 000 feet to minimise time spent in the extremely cold and hypoxic air. During this time the pilot will breathe oxygen, at a gradually reducing over-pressure from a small cylinder mounted on the seat. At 10 000 feet a barometric sensor will release him from the heavy seat and allow his parachute to deploy.

Climbing and living at high terrestrial altitudes

There are many differences between life at sea level and in mountains, where winds are stronger, the air is cooler, the sun fiercer, diurnal swings in climate greater and the diet, work patterns and ethnic backgrounds of the inhabitants distinct from those below.[3,22-25] There is therefore no simple way of comparing highlanders and lowlanders, or of distinguishing hypobaric from other causes of differences between the two. One in seven people live above 1000 m (3500 ft) and 1 in 20 above 3000 m (about 10 000 ft). Many communities, especially in South America, live above 5000 m (16 000 ft) and work up to 5500 m (18 000 ft). A large number of mountaineers have climbed above 6000 m (20 000 ft) and several have scaled Everest (8748 m, 28 700 ft) without oxygen. There do not seem to be any genetic adaptations to hypoxia in humans. Acclimatisation gives these mountain dwellers and climbers access to altitudes that would prove severely damaging or fatal to lowlanders on acute exposure.

The principal adaptations are progressive hyperventilation, which develops over several days, and increased red-cell mass, which develops over several weeks. These are accompanied by some increases in mitochondrial and capillary density, which augment the surface areas and reduce the diffusion path lengths for oxygen transfer. The ability to develop new capillaries is maximal in utero and may account for much of the advantage shown by people who were carried and born at altitude; it diminishes rapidly with age.

High-altitude disorders appear if exposure profiles exceed these slowly developing changes, or if the responses become deranged.

Acute mountain sickness can present within a few hours of a quick ascent to above 3400 m (11 000 ft). The affected individual becomes lethargic and may be breathless, but can sleep only fitfully, waking with mild ataxia and a marked headache that is commonly occipital. In most people the symptoms regress over a few days without descent or recourse to oxygen, probably because of the slowly progressive hyperventilation. In some they progress to (high-altitude) pulmonary and/or cerebral oedema, which can be fatal. Reasons for the wide variability in individual responses are not clear but may be related to variation in ventilatory and fluid balance responses. Those individuals who hyperventilate and develop a diuresis on ascent do well, compared to those who ventilate less and retain fluid. The conditions can be prevented by avoiding rapid ascent and cured by descent or administration of oxygen. Furosemide (frusemide) helps to limit pulmonary oedema, and acetazolamide, which increases respiratory drive, prevents or reduces the cerebral oedema if used at an early stage. Retinal hyperperfusion and haemorrhages are common even in asymptomatic climbers. Dexamethasone may prevent and cure retinal and cerebral oedema. Although the mechanisms of these disorders are not yet clear, it is certain that they are direct responses to moderate prolonged hypoxia. It is possible that generalised hypoxic pulmonary vasoconstriction plays a part but studies of the effect of hypoxaemia on red-cell flexibility suggest this may have a larger role in obstructing capillary beds than was hitherto suspected.[26,27]

After some weeks' exposure at high altitude, polycythaemia may be sufficient in some individuals to promote venous thrombosis, pulmonary emboli, ventilation–perfusion mismatching in the lung and metabolism–perfusion mismatching in the systemic vascular bed. After exposures of several years most people show a slight rise in pulmonary artery pressure and a few may show an exaggerated increase, leading to high-altitude cor pulmonale (chronic mountain sickness). This is associated with marked polycythaemia and characteristic modifications of pulmonary vessel histology. Such changes appear to be determined by the amount of muscle initially present in the pulmonary vascular bed. For example, most lowland cattle have vigorous muscles in pulmonary vessels, and respond badly to altitude (brisket disease). Highland species, such as the yak and llama, have flimsy coats of muscle in their lung vessels and do well. These variations are genetic and so are true adaptations. Sui and colleagues have described a subacute infantile version of this disease, affecting children born at low altitudes and brought almost immediately to high altitudes. They almost always die within a few months.[28]

Diving

Good, recent and comprehensive books on diving medicine are readily available.[1,4,29,30] Humans have breath-hold dived since ancient times. The diving women of Korea and Japan descend to 10–20 m to collect seaweeds, sea urchins, abalone and pearl. Greek sponge divers go to similar depths. Polynesian pearl divers go somewhat deeper (30–35 m). Modern spear fishers commonly breath-hold dive to the same depths. The current world record for a breath-hold dive, mentioned earlier, is to a depth of 150 m (500 ft). All these people face much the same respiratory problems, namely those of buoyancy, breath-hold times, profound hypoxia developing suddenly on ascent, and some risk of decompression sickness on repetitive dives.

Buoyancy is very important but easily overlooked. At full inspiration an unclothed man in water is some 2.5 kg positively buoyant. The 2.5 kg above water usually includes his nose and mouth. If any other part of the body is raised above water, the nose and mouth descend. At residual volume, the same person is 2.5 kg negatively buoyant. The maximum thrust a swimmer can develop is about 5 kg, so at the surface he would require half his aerobic capacity to swim away from the surface. This is why it is much more practicable to swing several kilograms of leg into the air to get under way. On leaving the surface, ambient pressure increases by one atmosphere for every 10 m of descent. This is transmitted directly to alveolar gas by the chest wall, which can only sustain transmural pressures equivalent to 1–2 m of sea water.

The gas in the lungs compresses according to Boyle's law, i.e. to half its original volume at 10 m and to a quarter of its original volume (equivalent to residual volume) at 30 m. At this depth the breath-hold diver is 2.5 kg heavy and will need his aerobic capacity to reach the surface. During the descent P_AO_2 increases as the lungs are compressed. As the diver works on the bottom P_AO_2 falls progressively. On ascent, which can be physically demanding, P_AO_2 drops abruptly as the lungs decompress. If P_AO_2 falls below 40 mmHg (5.3 kPa) the diver is likely to lose consciousness before or immediately after reaching the surface. This is more probable if the diver hyperventilates before descent, which reduces body carbon dioxide levels and prolongs breath-holding but does nothing for tissue oxygenation generally and actively promotes brain hypoxia by inducing cerebral vasoconstriction. These phenomena account for most deaths in breath-hold divers (the 'taravana' syndrome occurring in pearl divers). In addition, if breath-hold dives are packed close together it is possible to accumulate sufficient nitrogen in tissues to suffer decompression sickness on the later ascents, but this is rare. Marine mammals are able to breath-hold dive frequently to much greater depths (300–600 m), because the reinforced small airways of their lungs allow alveoli to empty completely early in the dive.

The future of deep diving is in considerable doubt, because of its expense and logistic complexity. It is certain that remotely operated vehicles with sensors and manipulators will take over many of the tasks currently performed by divers. Almost all commercial and military diving is carried out with free-flow or demand breathing systems at the end of an umbilical line or with self-contained gas supplies. The principal additional respiratory problems are inert gas narcosis, oxygen toxicity, the high-pressure nervous syndrome, a much greater risk of decompression sickness, pulmonary barotrauma and substantial respiratory heat loss.

On descent, gas is normally delivered at ambient pressure so, for example, on full inspiration at 30 m, the diver's lungs contain the sea-level equivalent of four total lung capacities of air. The nitrogen pressure will therefore be approximately 2500 mmHg (333 kPa). Carried to the tissues, dissolving mainly in fat, this nitrogen deforms nerve membranes, leading to inert gas narcosis.[31] Because of this phenomenon, the greatest depth at which air can be breathed with safety is 50 m. It is not practicable to replace the nitrogen in air with oxygen, because oxygen is toxic to the lungs when P_AO_2 exceeds 0.5 ATA and leads to widespread damage elsewhere when P_AO_2 rises above 2 ATA (oxygen toxicity).[32,33] Convulsions occur within minutes when it exceeds 4 ATA. For that reason, nitrogen is replaced with helium, to permit divers to go deeper. Unfortunately, this does not prevent direct compression of the nerve sheath and the membrane becomes more excitable as the dive deepens (the high-pressure nervous syndrome),[34] which is an important barrier to dives below 300–500 m. Various mixtures of hydrogen, helium and nitrogen are being tried, with some success, to overcome this problem.

It used to be supposed that inhalational anaesthetics exerted their effects by generalised solution in nerve membranes. Although this does occur and may very well be the source of the massive eruptions of gas seen by Francis et al[35] in decompressed nervous tissue, the elegant studies of Franks & Lieb[36] suggest that inhalational anaesthetics, and by presumption inert gases, exert their effects by selective deformation of proteins lining ligand-gated ion channels of nerve membranes in or close to synapses.

Mixtures of gases for diving have to be designed and delivered with care, because the PO_2 at the operating depth should not exceed 0.5 ATA. Thus at a depth of 150 m (where the pressure is 16 ATA = 15 ATA of water + 1 ATA of air), the desirable mixture contains only 3% O_2. A diver will, however, become dangerously hypoxic if he breathes this 'desirable' mixture at depths less than 50 m. For this reason diving supervisors have to keep careful watch, during the course of any deep dive, on a diver's actual, as opposed to 'intended', depth. At depths below 30 m the work of breathing rises progressively as gas density increases. This can sometimes lead to hypercapnia and panic.

There is some evidence that exposure to cold water can precipitate systemic hypertension, left heart failure and pulmonary oedema in some individuals.[37] Typically, symptoms come on a few minutes into the dive when the subject is descending or exercising at the bottom. He or she produces copious frothy white sputum tinged with blood. Symptoms regress rapidly on getting out of the water. This syndrome may be under-recognised and may explain some sudden deaths underwater currently attributed to drowning. It is not clear how frequently it occurs.

On ascent the diver faces two further problems. The first of these, which has been touched on briefly above is, decompression sickness. It is one of the most obdurate problems in environmental pathophysiology. Many experiments, beginning with those of Paul Bert in the late 19th century, and Haldane at the turn of the 20th, have established that, with an abrupt change in alveolar inert gas pressure, gas accumulates in or diffuses out of tissues at an approximately exponential rate, at times determined by the tissue's fat content and local blood flow. Any ascent must be slow enough to allow all tissues to decant their enriched inert gas stores without significant bubble formation. After long dives this can take several days. In spite of this knowledge, we are little better at preventing or treating decompression sickness than we were 50 years ago. The literature on this subject is massive.[38,39] Until recently, practical experience suggested that safe dive profiles could be computed using a body model consisting of four or five compartments with time constants ranging from 5 minutes to 24 hours. Recent experience with the brief profound compressions of submarine escape, however, suggests that some tissue elements may have time constants of a minute or less.[40] It is possible that arterial blood itself bubbles en route to tissues during very rapid ascents.[41]

The solution of gases in liquids and solids, and the formation and growth of bubbles, are not straightforward. Gases dissolve in interstices in liquids. In a highly structured fluid like water, in which hydrogen bonding draws water molecules together, interstices are few and gas solubility is low. In hydrocarbons, which are less cohesive, there is more room. In fluorocarbon liquids, which are very loosely held together, gas solubility is high.[42] In addition, in most fluids there are microscopic bubbles that were included at their formation or have been produced by cavitation since. It is these bubble nuclei, for instance, that allow a column of water to fracture when drawn above about 10 m, although the true tensile strength of water is much greater.

Once formed, especially in biological fluids, bubbles acquire a complex structure. They attract and denature proteins and other amphiphilic molecules on their surface. In blood, they also adsorb platelets and precipitate many inflammatory cascades. This shell of material modifies gas exchange between the bubble and surrounding fluids, and opposes its complete solution. On ascent from a dive, arterial blood is in equilibrium with alveolar gas and does not form bubbles unless the ascent is extremely rapid. Venous blood is in equilibrium with tissues and may, in addition, cavitate on its way round the circulation. Once formed, bubbles resist deformation from spherical shapes, and tend to coalesce and to exchange gas by diffusion from smaller to bigger bubbles, even though they are not in direct contact. As ascent continues they expand according to Boyle's law, and they may continue to grow by accumulation of dissolved gas for some time after arrival at sea level.

At present the only practicable form of treatment is immediate recompression, usually to about 50 m, with careful use of oxygen to accelerate inert gas excretion. Several investigators are studying the possible use of fluorocarbon infusions to hasten bubble resorption, but no studies have yet been performed in humans.

It is now widely agreed that it is often impossible to decide whether symptoms following decompression are the result of the eruption of bubbles from gas dissolved in blood or other tissues or of the escape of gas into the circulation from a rupture in the lung. Rather than presume, i.e. guess at, a mechanism, it is thought that all such conditions should be described as *decompression illness*, further defined by its site, severity and rate of evolution.[43]

In practice, the most common forms of decompression sickness are mild skin itching (formication); a pulmonary form believed to be linked to arrival of bubbles in the lung's capillary bed ('the chokes'); main joint problems that are sometimes associated with necrosis of articular surfaces ('the bends'); and neurological involvement, which can be catastrophic and appears to involve the spinal cord more commonly than the brain. Symptoms usually appear many minutes to several hours after arrival at the surface.[44] As the manifestations of decompression sickness are so protean, it is usual to regard any abnormal sign or symptom developing in this time after a dive of suspect duration as decompression sickness.

Some of the neurological cases are the result of bubbles in central venous blood passing through a patent foramen ovale, which is found in about 20% of healthy subjects. The opening of the foramen would be promoted by the Valsalva manoeuvre divers use to clear their ears, by the rise in apparent intrathoracic pressure during rapid ascents and by the rise in pulmonary arterial pressure secondary to the arrival of cascades of microbubbles in the pulmonary capillary bed.[45-48] It may be that people who suffer from migraine with aura are at particular risk.[49] Although there is no doubt that people with decompression disorders display an unusually high percentage of patent foramen ovale, it is not clear whether this is cause or effect. One school of thought holds that the decompression disorders result from otherwise silent (asymptomatic) bubbles passing through the septal perforation to cause symptomatic damage on the systemic side of the circulation. Others believe that the accumulation of asymptomatic bubbles in the lung leads to pulmonary and thus right atrial hypertension, opening up a previously 'sealed' foramen ovale. Careful studies are needed before sensible advice can be given to would-be divers.

Patients with decompression illness who have only an itchy skin and/or very mild limb pains are observed closely and treated by oxygen inhalation at sea level alone. All those with other symptoms or signs are treated by recompression at the earliest time possible. Divers who fly at altitudes above 3000 feet within 12 hours of a dive are liable to develop symptoms after dives that would have been safe had they stayed at sea level. All divers, amateur and professional, should be instructed to stop diving at least 12 hours before a flight.

Respiratory decompression sickness ('the chokes') is rare but occurs in divers, aircrew and caisson workers who are decompressed very rapidly. It is believed to result from widespread embolisation of the lung by bubbles from systemic veins. In subclinical cases the bubbles trapped in the small vessels of the lung slowly evaporate and the dyspnoea and hypoxaemia they cause disappear. In severe cases dyspnoea and hypoxaemia progress and can be fatal.

At the beginning of an ascent, the diver's lungs contain gas at close to ambient pressure. As he/she rises and ambient pressure falls this gas will expand unless it vents freely. If the transmural pressure of any part of the lung exceeds about 75 mmHg (10 kPa) (equivalent to 1 m of water), it is believed the lung will burst.[50] Subpleural rupture is very rare in pulmonary barotrauma but leads to a pneumothorax, which will expand rapidly as the ascent continues. Peribronchial rupture is much more common and results in mediastinal emphysema, extending into the neck as the ascent progresses. Internal rupture is more common still and leads to arterial gas emboli, which in upright divers most often travel to the brain where they lodge at prearteriolar levels. Symptoms appear within minutes of arrival at the surface, and usually progress rapidly. The sole treatment is early recompression with careful oxygenation.[51] This form of pulmonary barotrauma is the most common cause of serious accidents in diving. It occurs frequently in amateur divers who panic and hold their breath on ascent, when something goes wrong with their equipment. It also occurs in professional divers who are inadvertently pulled or swept towards the surface, faster than they can vent their lungs. Usually, in survivors, the lung heals quickly, and without scarring. Treated rapidly, the neurological symptoms are often reversed substantially, although not completely. After any delay, the results can be tragic. There is also some evidence that any recurrence in a subsequent dive is more severe than the first event.

The physiology of lung rupture in diving is by no means fully understood. For example, post-mortem studies of underwater blast injuries during the Second World War showed gross tearing of internal tissue but no pneumothoraces in those dying immediately. Pneumothoraces appeared in those surviving a few hours. There is no evidence that primary spontaneous pneumothorax associated with apical bullae is more prevalent underwater, although its consequences are more damaging. Common sense suggests that obstructive lung disease would be the most important cause of lung rupture, but there are many examples of people with severe airway obstruction who have dived regularly without ill effect. Contrary to expectation, a recent survey of spirometric indices in 1000 trainee submariners showed that the 12 who suffered probable barotrauma in buoyant ascents had a normal ratio of forced expiratory volume in 1 second to forced vital capacity (FEV_1/FVC) but a low FVC.[52] Colebatch et al[53] studied 16 divers, of whom six had suffered barotrauma up to 2 years previously. The six had smaller, stiffer lungs than the remainder. These observations suggest that shear stresses may be more important than overinflation, and contrast with the observation that fibrotic lungs empty more fully and rapidly than normal lungs do.

Most lung ruptures that are not due to breath-holding on ascent do not have an obvious cause. I believe that many of these are due to divers taking unwisely deep breaths at depth, e.g. by 'skip-breathing' to conserve air. Evidence for this view is largely anecdotal and further large-scale studies are needed to refute or support the contention, which relates to a relatively rare event.[43]

There is some evidence that asymptomatic divers who have not been known to suffer from decompression illness display unexpected areas of infarction in the retina, brain and spinal cord.[54,55] These observations have raised fears that diving, perhaps through the generation of silent bubbles, may cause cumulative damage to the central nervous system that may only become apparent long after the subjects have retired from diving. The consensus view at present is that this is unlikely, but the matter is not resolved. Cumulative bubble-induced damage to long bones is well documented.[56,57] Prolonged diving, e.g. in saturation dives, appears to enlarge the lung and to reduce carbon monoxide transfer.[58-60] These effects gradually reverse at the end of the dive but the time courses of development and regression are unknown. Thus it is possible that the effects of repeated saturation dives may be cumulative. This is now being investigated in several centres.

Living in sealed spaces

Many more people work at high pressures in caissons than dive. Excellent accounts of their circumstances are given elsewhere.[61,62] They generally follow the same pressure profiles as divers and are particularly subject to bone necrosis. Their working conditions are governed in the UK by the voluntary Medical Code of Practice, which is brief and very clearly written.[63] Caissons are ventilated by external air. Other people work in submarines, space vehicles and similar enclosed vessels at normal pressures. In such closed-circuit breathing systems, oxygen has to be replaced and carbon dioxide adsorbed to maintain acceptable conditions. Usually the inspired Po_2 is held between 100 and 350 mmHg (13–46.5 kPa) and inspired Pco_2 below 5 mmHg (0.7 kPa). The fire risk rises sharply with Po_2 over that range and is somewhat reduced if there is also a hyperbaric Pn_2. A wide range of metabolic and industrial contaminants that accumulate in sealed spaces have to be resorbed. Strict concentration limits have been set for very many of these toxins. The long-term respiratory health effects of hyperbaric exposure have been reviewed in detail elsewhere.[64,65]

Escape from submarines

Submarines contain up to 180 crew. Should one sink while over the continental shelf, it would come to rest at a depth of up to 300 m. Attempts would be made to lock a deep submergence rescue vehicle on to the sunken vessel to transfer several men at a time to the surface, under near-normobaric conditions. If time ran out, the crew would be obliged to escape beforehand. It would be hoped that a surface rescue fleet had been deployed by that stage. The preferred escape technique is that submariners enter an escape compartment, one or two at a time. They wear loose immersion suits with a transparent hood attached to a pipe with a self-sealing bayonet fitting. In the compartment they attach this pipe to a demand valve fitted to a compressed air supply. They then compress themselves to ambient pressure by opening a flood valve. This has to be done very rapidly to limit their exposure to compressed gas. Typically the pressure doubles every few seconds until ambient pressure is reached. The demand valve must sense and deliver gas to the individual very precisely to avoid crushing injuries or lung rupture. Once the pressure has equalised, the hatched roof of the compartment opens automatically, allowing the submariners to float to the surface, by the buoyancy of their suit, hood and lungs, at a limiting velocity of about 3 m/s. During the ascent the hood vents freely, so that for practical purposes their lungs are at ambient pressure throughout the ascent. It is essential that the submariner exhales throughout this time. On arrival at the surface, the escaper unzips the hood to breathe fresh air. Many years ago, and again in 1987 off the coast of Norway, British Royal Navy volunteers successfully escaped from a submarine about 180 m (600 ft) below the surface. The pressure at that depth is almost 20 ATA.

During the compression phase and for most of the ascent (which together form the 'acquisition phase'), the escaper may absorb sufficient nitrogen to develop decompression sickness at the surface, even though the whole escape has lasted only a couple of minutes. The early stages of bubble formation up to capillary dimensions of a few micrometres are rapid, occurring perhaps within a second. Subsequent expansion can continue for minutes or hours. During the ascent the submariner may fail to vent his/her lungs sufficiently, which can lead to cerebral arterial gas embolism, as mentioned above. Recompression facilities would be needed at the surface to treat people with these conditions. Hyperventilation before escape may limit the accumulation of nitrogen and so reduce the risk of bubble formation in cerebrospinal tissue, but this would have no influence on the development of bubbles in arterial blood proposed by Omhagen et al[41] and may well be opposed by the exertion of escaping. There is also some evidence to suggest that submariners could minimise the accumulation of unwanted inert gas by switching to a very insoluble inspirate (carbon tetrafluoride) immediately before escaping. In general it is not wise to hyperventilate before diving, because it causes mental confusion and permits dangerously long breath-holds that culminate in severe hypoxaemia on ascent.

Fitness to dive

Professional divers in the UK are required to have an annual chest radiograph and 'fitness to dive' examination. In general, any radiographic abnormality, history of serious chest disease, current trivial respiratory disease or evidence of obstructive ventilatory function is taken as a bar to recertification. Some see these standards as unnecessarily conservative. If a commercial diver disagrees with the withholding of a certificate on such grounds, he/she has the right to appeal to a Health and Safety Executive tribunal, who refer appellants to chest physicians specialising in diving medicine, for advice. It only seems ethical to bar someone from employment when he/she possesses a relevant defect. Determining what is relevant is, however, not straightforward, as the pulmonary factors contributing to lung rupture are not clear and the ventilatory function of working divers differs from that of the general population in ways that may be the result of self-selection as well as of their employment. I currently use the following rules: full (inspiratory and expiratory) spirometry, absolute lung volumes and airway resistance (by whole-body plethysmography), and carbon monoxide transfer are measured in each subject. Quite commonly FEV_1/FVC ratio is low but the FVC is normal or supernormal, a pattern that is well-recognised in uncommonly fit people and by itself is no bar to diving. If there is any evidence of a true but mild obstructive or restrictive disorder (e.g. raised airway resistance, significant concavity of the maximum expiratory flow–volume curve or a definite (> 12%) shortfall of the 10-second helium dilution

volume (V_A) compared with plethysmographic total lung capacity), serial computed tomographs are taken of the lung (10 mm slice width at 10 mm intervals) in full inspiration to look for scars (abnormal opacities), and again in full expiration to look for areas of defective lung emptying (abnormal lucencies). This technique can detect small lesions and, if the scan is normal, we suggest that the person is fit to dive and review him/her and the diving history in a year's time.

If there is evidence of more than mild obstructive or restrictive disease, certification is withheld, without recourse to a scan. Patients referred following suspected or proved pulmonary barotrauma commonly have absolutely normal lung function and scans. In such cases, if it is a first event, they are judged to be fit to dive 3 months after injury. Where there is any functional or tomographic abnormality, or history of previous lung rupture, they are refused a certificate and advised not to dive again. Many amateur divers are referred for assessment because of asthma. If the asthma is mild and stable, and they have a clear understanding of the risks of emergency ascents and of only diving when the asthma is well controlled we suggest that they are fit to dive but their condition is reviewed 1 year later.

Medical assessments of fitness to dive are discussed in more detail elsewhere.[4,65] Wider aspects of adverse environments are discussed in *Life at the Extremes: the Science of Survival*.[66]

Therapeutic principles

- Decompression sickness is treated by oxygen if very mild, otherwise urgent recompression is indicated.

- With appropriate notice, low flow oxygen is readily available on most commercial flights and allows even patients with advanced respiratory disease and consequent hypoxaemia to fly safely.

? Unresolved questions

- What are the reasons for the marked individual susceptibility to acute mountain sickness?

- At what level of P_aO_2 should supplemental oxygen be advised during flight?

- What is the true incidence of, and best prophylactic treatment against, pulmonary embolism during long haul flights?

References

1. Bennett PB, Elliott DH, ed. The physiology and medicine of diving, 4th ed. London: WB Saunders; 1993.
2. Ernsting J, Nicholson AN, Rainford DJ, ed. Aviation medicine, 3rd ed. London: Butterworths; 1999.
3. West JB. High life: a history of high altitude physiology and medicine. Oxford: Oxford University Press; 1998.
4. Lundgren CEG, Miller JN, ed. The lung at depth. New York: Marcel Dekker; 1999.

5. Wayne RP. Chemistry of atmospheres, 3rd ed. Oxford: Oxford University Press; 2000.

6. Autor AP, ed. Pathology of oxygen. New York: Academic Press; 1982.

7. Denison DM. Physiological principles. In: Parkes WR, ed. Occupational lung disorders, 3rd ed. Oxford: Butterworth Heinemann; 1994: 18.

8. Halliwell B, Gutteridge JMC. Free radicals in biology and medicine, 3rd ed. Oxford: Oxford University Press; 1999.

9. Bert P. La pression atmospherique. Recherches de physiologie experimentale. Paris: Masson et Cie; 1878. (Also available in translation by Hitchcock MA, Hitchcock FA. Columbus, OH: College Book Co; 1943.)

10. Denison DM, Bagshaw M. Aerospace medicine. In: Warrell DA, Cox TM, Firth JD, ed. Oxford textbook of medicine, 4th ed. Oxford: Oxford University Press; in press.

11. Ernsting J. Prevention of hypoxia: acceptable compromises. Aviat Space Environ Med 1978; 49: 495.

12. Harding RM, Gradwell DP. Hypoxia and hyperventilation. In: Ernsting J, Nicolson AN, Rainford DJ, ed. Aviation medicine, 3rd ed. London: Butterworths; 1999.

13. Macmillan AJF. Decompression sickness and hyperbaric therapy. In: Ernsting J, Nicholson AN, Rainford DJ, ed. Aviation Medicine. London: Butterworths; 1999.

14. Van Liew HD, Burkard ME. Simulation of gas bubbles in hypobaric decompressions: roles of O_2, CO_2 and H_2O. Aviat. Space Environ Med 1995; 66: 50–55.

15. Webb JT, Balldin UI, Pilmanis AA. Prevention of decompression sickness in current and future aircraft. Aviat Space Environ Med 1993; 64: 1048–1050.

16. Kumar VK, Billica RD, Waligora JM, Utility of Doppler-detectable microbubbles in the diagnosis and treatment of decompression sickness. Aviat Space Environ Med 1997; 68: 151–158.

17. Coker RD, ed. Managing passengers with lung disease planning air travel: British Thoracic Society recommendations. Thorax 2002; in press.

18. House of Lords Inquiry. Air travel and health. London: The Stationery Office; 2001.

19. Reeves JT, Welsh CH, Wagner PD. The heart and lungs at extreme altitude. Thorax 1994; 49: 63l.

20. Burton RR, Cohen MM, Guedry FE Jr, ed. G-induced loss of consciousness. Aviat Space Environ Med 1988; 59: 1.

21. Joint Aviation Authorities. Joint aviation requirements: flight crew medical requirements. (JAR/FCL/Part 3 – Medical). Cheltenham, Glos: Westwood Digital; 2001.

22. Baker PT, ed. The biology of high altitude peoples. Cambridge: Cambridge University Press; 1978.

23. Heath D, Williams DR. High altitude medicine and pathology. London: Butterworths; 1989.

24. Ward MP, Milledge JS, West JB. High altitude medicine and physiology. London: Chapman & Hall; 1989.

25. Rennie D. Diseases of high terrestrial altitudes. In: Ledingham JGG, Warrell DA, ed. Concise Oxford Textbook of Medicine. Oxford: Oxford University Press; 2000; 1908.

26. Hakim TS, Macek AS. Role of erythrocyte deformability in the acute hypoxic pressor response in the pulmonary vasculature. Respir Physiol 1988; 72: 95.

27. Hakim TS, Malik AB. Hypoxic vasoconstriction in blood- and plasma-perfused lungs. Respir Physiol 1988; 72: 109.

28. Sui GJ, Liu YH, Cheng IS et al. Subacute infantile mountain sickness. J Pathol 1988; 155: 161.

29. Edmonds C, Lowry C, Pennefather J, ed. Diving and subaquatic medicine, 3rd ed. Oxford: Butterworth-Heinemann; 1993.

30. Bove AA, ed. Diving medicine, 3rd ed. Philadelphia, PA: WB Saunders; 1997.

31. Bennett PB. Inert gas narcosis. In: Bennett PB, Elliott DH, ed. The physiology and medicine of diving, 4th ed. London: WB Saunders; 1993: 170.

32. Beers MF, Fisher AB. Oxygen toxicity. In: Carlson RW, Geheb MA, ed. The principles and practice of medical intensive care. Philadelphia, PA: WB Saunders; 1994.

33. Clark JM. Oxygen toxicity. In: Bennett PB, Elliott DH, ed. The physiology and medicine of diving, 4th ed. London: WB Saunders; 1993: 121.

34. Bennett PB, Rostain JC. The high pressure nervous syndrome. In: Bennett PB, Elliott DH, ed. The physiology and medicine of diving, 4th ed. London: WB Saunders; 1993: 194.

35. Francis TJR, Griffin JL, Homer LD et al. Bubble-induced dysfunction in acute spinal cord decompression sickness. J Appl Physiol 1990; 68: 1368.

36. Franks NP, Lieb WR. Molecular and cellular mechanisms of general anaesthesia. Nature 1994; 367: 607.

37. Wilmshurst PT, Nuri M, Crowther A, Webb-Peploe MM. Cold-induced pulmonary oedema in SCUBA divers and swimmers and subsequent development of pulmonary hypertension. Lancet 1989; 1: 62.

38. Hempleman HV. History of decompression procedures. In: Bennett PB, Elliott DH, ed. The physiology and medicine of diving, 4th ed. London: WB Saunders; 1993: 342.

39. Vann RD, Thalmann ED. Decompression physiology and practice. In: Bennett PB, Elliott DH, ed. The physiology and medicine of diving, 4th ed. London: WB Saunders; 1993: 376.

40. Denison DM, Bridgewater B, Deam R, Savage A. The role of hyperventilation in submarine escape. Institute of Naval Medicine Report. London: Ministry of Defence; 1994.

41. Ornhagen H, Carlioz M, Muren A. Could fast ascents create arterial bubbles? Proceedings of the 14th Meeting of the European Undersea Medical Society, Aberdeen; 1988: 1.

42. Bridgewater BJM. Perfluorocarbon emulsions and bubble related disease. University of London: PhD Thesis, 1994.

43. Francis TJR, Smith DJ. Describing decompression illness. Proceedings of the 43rd Workshop of the Undersea and Hyperbaric Medicine Society. 79 (DECO) 15/5/91, Bethesda, MA; 1991.

44. Francis TJR, Pearson RR, Robertson AG et al. Central nervous system decompression sickness: I. The latency of 1070 human cases. Undersea Biomed Res 1988; 15: 403.

45. Moon RE, Camporesi EM, Kislo JA. Patent foramen ovale and decompression sickness. Lancet 1989; 1: 513.

46. Wilmshurst PT, Byrne JC, Webb-Peploe MM. Relation between arterial shunts and decompression sickness in divers. Lancet 1989; 1302.

47. Parker EC, Survanishi SS, Massell PB, Weathersby PK. Probabilistic models of the role of oxygen in human decompression sickness. J Appl Physiol 1998; 84: 1096–1102.

48. Schwerzmann M, Seller C, Lipp E et al. Relation between directly detected patent foramen ovate and ischaemic brain lesions in sports divers. Ann Intern Med 2001; 134: 21–24.

49. Wilmshurst P, Nightingale S. Relationship between migraine and cardiac and pulmonary right-to-left shunts. Clin Sci 2001; 100: 215–220.

50. Francis TJ, Denison DM. Pulmonary barotrauma. In: Lundgren CEG, Miller JN, ed. The lung at depth. New York: Marcel Dekker; 1999: 295.

51. Moon RE, Gorman DF. Treatment of the decompression disorders. In: Bennett PB, Elliott DH, ed. The physiology and medicine of diving, 4th ed. London: WB Saunders; 1993: 506.

52. Benton PJ, Woodfine JD, Francis TJR. A review of spirometry and UK submarine escape training tank incidents (1954–1993) using objective diagnostic criteria INM Report R94011. Alverstoke, Hants: Institute of Naval Medicine; 1994.

53. Colebatch HJH, Smith MM, Ng CKY. Increased elastic recoil as a determinant of pulmonary barotrauma in divers. Respir Physiol 1973; 26: 55.

54. Polkinghorne PJ, Sehmi K, Cross MR et al. Ocular fundus lesions in divers. Lancet 1988; 2: 1381.

55. Palmer AC, Calder IM, Yates PO. Cerebral vasculopathy in divers. Neuropath Appl Neurobiol 1992; 18: 113.

56. Elliott DH, Moon RE. Longterm health effects of diving. In: Bennett PB, Elliott DH, ed. The physiology and medicine of diving, 4th ed. London: WB Saunders; 1993: 585–604.

57. Medical Research Council Decompression Sickness Panel. Long term health effects of diving. London: Medical Research Council; 1990.

58. Lanphier EH, Camporesi EM. Respiration and exertion. In: Bennett PB, Elliott DH, ed. The physiology and medicine of diving, 4th ed. London: WB Saunders; 1993: 77.

59. Segedal K, Gulsvik A, Nicolayson G. Respiratory changes with deep diving. Eur Respir J; 1990; 3: 101.

60. Thorsen E, Reed JW, Elliott C et al. The contribution of hyperoxia to reduced pulmonary function after deep saturation dives. J Appl Physiol 1993; 75: 657.

61. Kindwall EP. Compressed air work. In: Bennett PB, Elliott DH, ed. The physiology and medicine of diving, 4th ed. London: WB Saunders; 1993: 1.

62. Walder DN. The compressed air environment. In: Bennett PB, Elliott DH, ed, The physiology and medicine of diving, 3rd ed. London. Baillière Tindall; 1993: 15.

63. Walder DN. Medical code of practice for work in compressed air. London: Butterworths; 1989.

64. Elliott DH, ed. Medical assessment of fitness to dive. Ewell, Surrey: Biomedical Seminars; 1995.

65. Hope A, Lund D, Elliott DH et al, ed. Long term health effects of diving. Bergen: NUTEC; 1993.

66. Ashcroft F. Life at the extremes: the science of survival. London: Harper Collins; 2000.

34 Near drowning

Mark Harries

 Key points

- Complete recovery is possible even following more than 1 hour's submersion.

- Those recovered from swimming pools may also have suffered a dislocated cervical spine.

- Facilities for extracorporeal rewarming should be available.

- Resuscitation should not be abandoned while the patient is still cold.

Prolonged immersion in a fluid results in drowning if the victim asphyxiates, but in near drowning should he survive. The clinical picture is usually one of asphyxiation, often with pulmonary oedema caused by water inhalation, in a profoundly cold subject. Complete recovery after 40 minutes' submersion has been documented.[1] The resuscitation and subsequent management of near-drowned victims differs from all other emergencies in which cardiopulmonary arrest is a feature.

Incidence

The incidence of near drowning is unknown but that of drowning ranges from 0.4 to 9.0 deaths per 100 000 per year, being highest in the warmer and less developed countries. Overall, male deaths outnumber female by 4:1. In the age range 1–14 years, only road traffic accidents and cancers account for more deaths. Two-thirds die in fresh water, chiefly because the opportunity to drown in unguarded inland waters is greater than in the sea.[2] Between 25% and 50% of adults who drown show evidence of recent alcohol ingestion.[3]

Pathophysiology

Death following submersion is by asphyxiation, but a person who survives receives a thermal challenge if the water is below body temperature, lung injury if water is inhaled and brain injury if the resulting hypoxaemia is not treated promptly.

Effects of cold

Both the specific heat and thermal conductivity of water are significantly greater than air, and so body cooling is much faster in water than in air at the same temperature. Sudden immersion of an unacclimatised subject in ice-cold water results in reflex hyperventilation and tachycardia – often with supraventricular ectopic beats and hypertension, a response known as 'cold shock'.[4] Drowning may occur at this early stage unless a buoyancy aid is used, enabling the airway to be held above the surface of the water. A clothed adult immersed in water below 5°C can be expected to lose consciousness in less than an hour. Without a correctly inflated life jacket, water will then enter the unprotected airway. Cold water also severely limits swimming ability, as a result of loss of synchrony between stroke and breathing.[5]

Post-immersion collapse

Head-out upright immersion in water at body temperature results in a 32–66% increase in cardiac output caused by the pressure exerted by the surrounding water, an effect similar to wearing a gravity suit. On leaving the water the assistance to circulation is removed and, in addition, there is gravitational venous pooling. In normal individuals with intact homoeostatic responses, these changes are compensated for by baroreceptor reflexes. The result is an increase in heart rate, cardiac output and vascular smooth muscle tone. Following prolonged immersion in cold water these responses are compromised. It is likely that post-immersion circulatory collapse is the cause of death among those found conscious in cold water wearing a life jacket but who perish within minutes of rescue. A mean increase in heart rate of 16% during vertical lifting from water compared with lifting the victim in a horizontal or sitting position has been reported.[6]

Asphyxiation

Infants show the apnoeic phase of the 'diving response' when thrown into water, but this reflex tends to wane by the toddler stage.[7] After infancy, submersion beyond the breath-hold breaking point ends in involuntary gasps and aspiration.

Post-mortem measurements of lung weight show that between 10% and 18% of those who drown inhale very little water, hence the term 'dry drowning'.[8] Failure of water to enter the lungs has been attributed to laryngospasm. However, the trachea and bronchial tree form a blind-ending tube and filling may well not occur if, for example, the victim is submersed face down or head down. Doubtless there is a gradation from asphyxiation with very little water in the lungs to lungs that fill completely.

Recovery from asphyxia following long periods of submersion occurs in circumstances that favour rapid cooling, such as those arising when a small child or infant is submerged in ice-cold water, typically below 5°C.[9] It seems probable that circulatory arrest occurs well after the head is immersed so that cerebral perfusion continues during the cooling process. Experience in children undergoing open heart surgery shows that, with hypothermia, circulation can be arrested for at least 30 minutes.

The survival advantage bestowed by submersion in ice-cold water is exemplified by the unique set of circumstances surrounding a young female skier. She was with friends when she fell down a water-filled gully and became trapped beneath an ice sheet. She struggled for 40 minutes while attempts were made to extract her before all movements ceased. Her body was recovered through a hole cut in the ice 1 hour and 19 minutes later. Though she was clinically dead, cardiopulmonary resuscitation was administered throughout the air-ambulance flight to hospital, where her core temperature was 13.7°C. She was resuscitated by means of an extracorporeal membrane oxygenator and then spent a further 35 days on a ventilator. At 5 months, her faculties had recovered sufficiently to allow her to return to work as a hospital doctor[10] (Table 34.1).

Fluid-electrolyte effects

Much higher death rates follow immersion in fresh water than in the sea. However, this has little to do with the salinity of the water but derives from the quality of the rescue services, which are sparse on inland waters by comparison with the coast. Experiments with dogs suggest that fresh water instilled into the trachea produces more lung injury than either isotonic or hypertonic saline.[11] In humans, fresh water washes out surfactant, causing atelectasis and intrapulmonary shunting. By contrast, salt-water aspiration appears to be associated with very little alveolar–capillary damage.[12] Earlier claims that red-cell haemolysis gives rise to hyperkalaemia have been refuted. On the con-

Table 34.1 Essential factors concerning the immersion incident

Length of time submerged	Favourable outcome associated with submersion for less than 5 min
Quality of immediate resuscitation	Favourable outcome if heart beat can be restored at once
Temperature of the water	Favourable outcome associated with immersion in ice-cold water (below 5°C), especially infant victims
Shallow water	Consider fracture/dislocation of cervical spine
A buoyancy aid being used by the casualty	Likely to be profoundly hypothermic. Victim may not have aspirated water. See post-immersion collapse
Nature of the water (fresh or salt)	Ventilation/perfusion mismatch from fresh-water inhalation more difficult to correct. Risk of infection from river water high. Consider leptospirosis

trary, hypokalaemia is seen after both fresh- and salt-water aspiration. The volume of water that would have to be inhaled to cause clinically significant red cell haemolysis is greatly in excess of that which can produce irreversible pulmonary damage.[13] Ventricular fibrillation following immersion is predominately a complication of hypothermia and not of electrolyte imbalance. The electrolyte changes that are seen probably result from absorption of ingested fluid from the stomach rather than from the lungs. High serum sodium and magnesium levels may be seen after immersion in sea water but seldom require treatment. Water intoxication causing convulsions in infants has been described rarely.

Emergency management

Swimmers recovered unconscious from shallow water should be assumed to have suffered fracture or dislocation of the cervical spine, particularly if there is injury to the face or head. Care must be taken not to overextend the neck during expired air resuscitation. The head and neck must be immobilised during transport to hospital. Rupture of the liver or spleen may have occurred if the victim has entered the water from a height.

After removal from the water the subject should be laid prone and cardiopulmonary resuscitation should be carried out in all other respects in the usual way.[14] The quality of the resuscitation procedure is the single most important factor that determines outcome. The subject's prognosis is transformed if the heart can be restarted at once. Simcock reported that around 70% of subjects arriving in the emergency room of a hospital apnoeic but with a pulse could be expected to survive, compared with only 8% in whom the heart was not restarted outside hospital.[15] It may be necessary to continue chest compression for an hour or more, and attempts at resuscitation should not be abandoned while the subject remains cold. Pragmatic advice on the management of hypothermia in the field is available from the Medical Commission on Accident Prevention.[16]

Regurgitation of gastric contents during resuscitation occurs in nearly all unconscious victims. The airway should therefore be secured with an endotracheal tube as early as possible and high-concentration oxygen given. The pulse may be slow and of low volume, making assessment very difficult. An added dilemma is that bradyarrhythmias may be converted to ventricular fibrillation by chest compression in profoundly cold subjects. For this reason, great care is needed in assessing the carotid pulse. Palpation for at least 10 seconds is recommended.

Management in hospital

Near drowning is a medical emergency. At worst the subject may present deeply unconscious with acidosis and profound hypothermia. Pulmonary oedema is an early complication. Cerebral oedema and septicaemia may develop later and are life-threatening.

Early measures

Subjects who appear to be completely well should be kept under observation for 6 hours in case of delayed-onset pulmonary oedema (secondary drowning). They may then be discharged provided there is no cough or lung crackles, the chest radiograph shows no shadows and the respiratory rate and arterial oxygen level are normal with the subject breathing air. Anyone who has inhaled water is at risk of infection and should be followed up with a chest radiograph. Unconscious or apnoeic subjects require intubation and positive-pressure ventilation with a high concentration of oxygen. Venous access through a central line is essential both for monitoring pressure and for giving fluids or drugs. An electrocardiogram may reveal bradyarrhythmias or ventricular fibrillation in those who appear to be pulseless. Blood should be drawn for both aerobic and anaerobic culture. Broad-spectrum antibiotics effective against Gram-negative organisms should be given (Table 34.2).

Arterial blood gases

A low P_aO_2 in a subject breathing air provides an early indication that water has been inhaled and suggests pulmonary oedema or atelectasis with shunting. Arterial gases and pH should be measured in all subjects, including those who are conscious and apparently well on arrival in hospital. Modern analysers assume a normal body temperature of 37°C. Failure to enter a low core temperature in those who are hypothermic will result in a falsely high arterial oxygen reading. Differences become significant when core temperature is as little as 1°C below normal. As, in practice, recordings around 30°C are not unusual, this correction is essential. An initial arterial pH of 7 or less is a poor prognostic sign.

Electrocardiography

In immersion victims, abnormalities of cardiac rhythm are the result of hypothermia coupled with hypoxia rather than of

Table 34.2 Essential early measures

Tracheal intubation for unconscious victims	Secures the airway in the event of regurgitation
Electrocardiogram	Pulseless patient may have bradyarrhythmias or ventricular fibrillation
Nasogastric tube	Decompresses the stomach, thereby assisting ventilation. Reduces the risk of regurgitation
Rectal temperature	Use low-reading thermometer. Insert the probe at least 10 cm
Arterial blood gases	Low P_aO_2 breathing air is a marker for pulmonary oedema or atelectasis with shunting. A pH less than 7 associated with poor prognosis
Chest X-ray	Shows aspirated fluid examination. Early indication of pulmonary oedema
Central venous line	Essential for monitoring level of positive end-expiratory pressure respiration
Culture blood for both aerobic and anaerobic organisms	Septicaemia common. Consider 'exotic' organisms. Brain abscess a late complication

changes in serum electrolytes. Sinus or nodal bradycardia is common, making the carotid pulse very difficult to find in some cases. Nevertheless circulation may still be adequate, so early monitoring of the electrocardiogram is essential to establish cardiac activity. Ventricular dysrhythmias induced by hypothermia do not respond to direct-current cardioversion; once established, the treatment of fibrillation is to support the circulation with chest compression until the temperature of the myocardium (deep body) exceeds 28°C.

Venous pressure and intravenous drugs

A central venous line provides access and allows pressure measurement. This becomes important in the event of pulmonary oedema, when its use to monitor the optimum level of positive end-expiratory pressure (PEEP) may be critical. Central venous pressure is often low initially and plasma expansion is indicated. Acidosis is managed with mechanical hyperventilation; sodium bicarbonate is seldom needed. The use of systemic corticosteroids has not been convincingly shown to prevent the development of pulmonary oedema or to influence its course, and is not recommended.[17] Antibiotics should be given after first obtaining a blood culture.

Hypothermia

A fully conscious subject may be hypothermic and yet not shiver, underlining the importance of rectal temperature readings. Hypothermic subjects must be rewarmed and their rectal temperature measured with a low-reading thermometer. The probe should be placed at least 10 cm beyond the anal sphincter to avoid erroneously low readings from the cooler periphery. Aspiration of stomach contents by nasogastric tube prevents further absorption of water or salt and removes the risk of regurgitation. Rewarming in bath water at 40°C is most satisfactory. If not possible, then passive rewarming is achieved by insulation in thick woollen blankets, after first cutting off wet clothing. A short-lived fall in core temperature, commonly seen as rewarming commences and known as the 'after-drop', is caused by continued loss of heat through conduction from the core to the cooler peripheral tissues. It occurs independently of blood supply and is not a risk factor.[18]

Active rewarming by heating the blood with extracorporeal bypass can be life-saving for those found unconscious with profound hypothermia.[19] Bolte and colleagues[20] used this technique to revive a child who had been submerged in ice-cold water for 66 minutes, Letsou et al[21] reviewed the clinical course of five subjects, each presenting with a rectal temperature below 26°C, all of whom were rewarmed on bypass. Three survived to be discharged with normal mental scores. Over several years, Swiss mountain rescue teams have recovered the bodies of 46 victims of avalanche or incarceration in ice; all were sent to one of three major centres in Switzerland with extracorporeal blood rewarming facilities. Out of 32 people rewarmed in this way, 15 have survived[22] (Table 34.3).

Pulmonary oedema

Pulmonary oedema occurs only in those who have inhaled water and usually within 4 hours of aspiration.[23] It is believed to be the result of a plasma leak through a damaged alveolar–capillary membrane and not of fluid overload. Left atrial pressure remains normal throughout, a picture similar to adult respiratory distress syndrome.

The earliest sign of impending pulmonary oedema is a falling P_aO_2, and may precede any changes seen on the chest radiograph. Respiratory distress should be treated promptly by assisted ventilation and with PEEP. The pressure setting is that which maintains the P_aO_2 above 10 kPa with a F_1O_2 that ideally should not exceed 0.6. Pressures above 2.0 kPa may be needed to obtain satisfactory arterial oxygenation following fresh water aspiration but are poorly tolerated because of impairment of cardiac output.

Table 34.3 Further measures

- Measure arterial gases: ensure low temperature correction
- In case of hypothermia raise core temperature above 28°C before defibrillation
- Consider plasma expanders and prophylactic antibiotics
- Rewarm in bath water at 40°C
- Remove wet clothing if casualty can be sheltered
- Actively rewarm with extracorporeal bypass if necessary

Cerebral oedema

Cerebral oedema is the result of hypoxaemia and contributes further to any damage the hypoxia may already have induced. There was a vogue for more aggressive treatment in children with prolonged hypothermia by means of barbiturate-induced coma. However, no improvement in outcome has been demonstrated, so the technique has been abandoned, and with it the need to monitor intracranial pressure.[24] Reducing the P_aCO_2 by mechanical hyperventilation induces cerebral vasoconstriction and may be useful. Early use of diuretics such as mannitol may also help.

Septicaemia

Lung infection is common following near drowning. Septicaemia and brain abscess have also been reported suggesting that arterial embolisation of infected material occurs, possibly as a result of pulmonary barotrauma. As well as common pathogens, exotic organisms have been described, including *Pseudomonas putrifaciens*,[25] *Pseudomonas pseudomallei*,[26] *Aspergillus fumigatus*,[27] lactose-positive *Vibrio* sp.[28] and *Petriellidium boydii*.[29] Leptospirosis is a hazard well recognised in inland waters. Victims of such immersion should be warned of fever developing within a few days of the accident and offered short-term follow-up.

Therapeutic principles

- Plasma expansion using colloid.
- Positive end-expiratory pressure ventilation for hypoxia.
- Intravenous antibiotics effective against Gram-negative organisms.
- Follow-up chest X-ray in outpatients.

References

1. Siebke H, Rod T, Breivik H, Lynd B. Survival after 40 minutes submersion without cerebral sequelae. Lancet 1975; 1: 1276.
2. Home Office Report. Report of the Working Party on Water Safety. London: HMSO; 1977.
3. Howland J, Hinson R. Alcohol as a risk factor for drownings: a review of the literature (1950–1985). Accid Anal Prev 1988; 20: 19.
4. Tipton MJ. The initial responses to cold-water immersion in man. Clin Sci 1989; 77: 581.
5. Tipton MJ, Golden FStC. Immersion in cold water: effects on performance and safety. In: Harries M, Micheli LJ, Stannish WD, William C, ed. Oxford textbook of sports medicine, 2nd ed. Oxford: Oxford University Press; 1998.
6. Golden FStC, Hervey GR, Tipton MJ. Circum-rescue collapse: collapse, sometimes fatal, associated with rescue of immersion victims. J Roy Nav Med Serv 1991; 77: 139.
7. Daly M de B, Angell-James JE, Elsner R. Role of carotid-body chemoreceptors and their reflex interactions in bradycardia and cardiac arrest. Lancet 1987; 1: 764.
8. Copeland AR. An assessment of lung weights in drowning cases. The Metro Dade County experience from 1978 to 1982. Am J Forens Pathol 1985; 6: 301.
9. Orlowski JP. Drowning, near-drowning and ice-water submersions. Pediatr Clin North Am 1987; 34: 75.
10. Gilbert, M. et al. Resuscitation from accidental hypothermia of 13.7°C with cardiac arrest. Lancet 2000, 355: 375–376.

11. Orlowski JP, Abulliel MM, Phillips JM. Effects of tonicities of saline solutions on pulmonary injury in drowning. Crit Care Med 1987; 1:126.

12. Cohen DS, Matthay MA, Cogan MG, Murray JF. Pulmonary edema associated with salt water near drowning: new insights. Am Rev Respir Dis 1992; 146: 794.

13. Modell JH, Graves SA, Ketover A. Clinical course of 91 consecutive near-drowning victims. Chest 1976; 70: 231.

14. Evans TR, ed. ABC of resuscitation. London: British Medical Journal; 1990.

15. Simcock AD. Treatment of near drowning – a review of 130 cases. Anaesthesia 1986; 41: 643.

16. Medical Commission on Accident Prevention. Report of the working party on out of hospital management of hypothermia. London: Medical Commission on Accident Prevention; 1992: 35–43.

17. Bernard GR, Luce LM, Sprung CL et al. High dose corticosteroids in patients with Adult Respiratory Distress Syndrome. N Engl J Med 1987; 317: 1565.

18. Golden FStC, Hervey GR. The after-drop and death after rescue from immersion in cold water. In: Adam JA, ed. Hypothermia ashore and afloat. Aberdeen: Aberdeen University Press; 1981.

19. Norberg WJ, Agnew RF, Brunsvold R et al. Successful resuscitation of a cold water submersion victim with the use of cardiopulmonary bypass. Crit Care Med 1992; 20: 1355.

20. Bolte RG, Black PG, Bowers RS et al. The use of extracorporeal rewarming in a child submerged for 66 minutes. JAMA 1988; 260: 377.

21. Letsou GV, Kopf GS, Elefteriades JA et al. Is cardiopulmonary bypass effective for treatment of hypothermic cardiac arrest due to drowning or exposure? Arch Surg 1992; 127: 525.

22. Walpoth BH, Walpoth-Aslan BN, Mattle HP et al. Outcome of survivors of accidental deep hypothermia and circulatory arrest treated with extracorporeal blood warming. N Engl J Med 1997; 337: 1500–1505

23. Pratt FD, Haynes BE. Incidence of 'secondary drowning' after saltwater submersion. Ann Emerg Med 1986; 15: 1084.

24. Bohn DJ, Biggar DW, Smith CR et al. Influence of hypothermia, barbiturate therapy and intracranial pressure monitoring on morbidity and mortality after near-drowning. Crit Care Med 1986; 14: 529.

25. Rosenthal SL, Zuger JH, Apollo E. Respiratory colonisation with *Pseudomonas putrefaciens* after near-drowning in sea water. Am J Clin Pathol 1975; 64: 382.

26. Lee N, Wu JL, Lee CH, Tsai WC. *Pseudomonas mallei* infection from drowning: the first reported case in Taiwan. J Clin Microbiol 1985; 22: 352.

27. Vieira DF, Van Saene HK, Miranda DR. Invasive pulmonary aspergillosis after near-drowning. Intens Care Med 1984; 10: 203.

28. Kelley MT, Avery DM. Lactose-positive *Vibrio* in sea water: a cause of pneumonia and septicaemia in a drowning victim. J Clin Microbiol 1980; 11: 278.

29. Fisher JF, Shadomy S, Teabeaut R et al. Near-drowning complicated by brain abscess due to *Petriellidium boydii*. Arch Neurol 1982; 39: 511–513.

35 Pneumonia and other acute respiratory infections

John T Macfarlane and Anne Thomson

Infections of the respiratory tract are very common and are associated with significant morbidity and mortality. This chapter deals with upper respiratory tract infections, infections of the airways and the different types of pneumonia. Important specific respiratory pathogens are described in detail.

Infections of the upper respiratory tract

Infections of the sinuses

Acute maxillary sinusitis is a common upper respiratory tract condition that causes significant morbidity to the patient but is often ignored or managed badly by the physician.[1,2]

Pathophysiology and anatomy

As the maxillary sinus is conical in shape, with a narrow ostium, situated superiorly (Fig. 35.1), drainage is inefficient. Factors predisposing to sinusitis include congenital factors such as ciliary abnormalities, bony abnormalities, cystic fibrosis and dental problems. More commonly, sinusitis is secondary to an upper respiratory tract infection or allergic rhinitis. With repeated infections, chronic inflammation of the antral mucosa occurs, resulting in mechanical obstruction of the ostium.

Aetiology

In studies of adult community-acquired sinusitis where cultures have been obtained by sinus puncture, *Streptococcus pneumoniae* and uncapsulated *Haemophilus influenzae* have been implicated in over half of the cases, viruses in 15% and anaerobic bacteria, Gram-positive bacteria (such as *Staphylococcus aureus*) and Gram-negative bacteria in around 10% each. *Pseudomonas aeruginosa* and *S. aureus* are most frequently found in those with cystic fibrosis or primary ciliary dyskinesia.

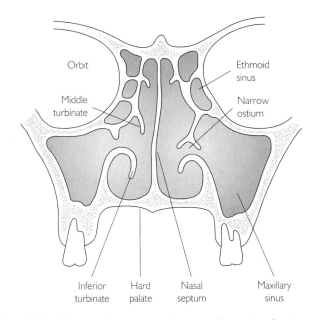

Fig. 35.1 The maxillary antrum in coronal section showing the relationship to the nasal cavity, teeth and orbit. Note the position of the maxillary ostium that produces inefficient drainage.

Clinical features

These include fever, malaise, blocked nose, purulent nasal discharge, facial pain and pain on chewing.

Therapy

Antibiotics need to cover both *S. pneumoniae* and *H. influenzae*, and amoxicillin and its derivatives, such as co-amoxiclav, or fluoroquinolones are appropriate, probably best given for up to 10 days.

Chronic sinusitis

After repeated acute attacks of sinusitis, irreversible damage occurs to the sinus mucosa, with hypertrophy and polyposis, together with loss of effective ciliary action and mucus clearance because of blockage of the ostium. Anaerobes and polymicrobial isolates are more frequently found than in acute sinusitis. Computed tomography (CT) scanning and nasoendoscopy may be helpful investigations. Topical steroids and prolonged antibiotic courses are often used, but drainage surgery may be necessary.[3]

Pharyngitis

The pathogens vary according to age.[4,5] In the first few years of life most cases are caused by viruses, whereas, during the school years, group A streptococci are the most frequently identified agents, with a peak incidence at 5–10 years of age. In young adults the incidence of streptococcal sore throats declines but other infections such as herpes virus and *Mycoplasma pneumoniae* occur. In the case of recurrent tonsillitis, β-haemolytic streptococci are less frequently isolated from resected tonsillar tissue than *H. influenzae* (62%) and *S. aureus* (40%), which are often found in mixed culture.[6]

Clinical features

The hallmark is a sore throat, often associated with cervical lymphadenopathy, fever and malaise. Deciding aetiology on clinical appearances is misleading.

Management

A throat swab should be taken before any antibiotic therapy, if this is practical. The decision to prescribe antibiotics is primarily made on the clinical state of the patient and is particularly appropriate if marked constitutional features are present. Penicillin or a macrolide is preferred to amoxicillin because of the risk of a glandular fever rash with the latter. In the case of recurrent tonsillitis, a β-lactamase-stable antibiotic should be used.

Epiglottitis

This condition is well recognised in children,[7] but can also affect previously healthy adults.[1,8]

Aetiology

H. influenzae type B is the most common pathogen found, followed by *S. pneumoniae*. Other organisms, such as group A β-haemolytic streptococcus and *Moraxella catarrhalis*, can also cause epiglottitis.

Epidemiology

Acute epiglottitis has become rare in paediatric practice following the great success of *H. influenzae* type b (Hib) conjugate vaccine. The peak incidence of epiglottitis was in children aged 2–5 years, with Hib accounting for over 90% of childhood cases.

The introduction of an effective vaccine was followed by a reduction in incidence of epiglottitis of over 90% in Sweden from a rate of 20.9 per 100 000 in 1997 to 0.9 per 100 000 children in 1996.[7] The introduction of Hib vaccine in the UK was followed by a prospective study of vaccine efficacy. The overall efficacy was 98.1%, with only 10 cases of epiglottitis in the UK occurring in vaccinated children over a 3-year period.[9] Consequently, many paediatricians now complete their training without ever seeing a case of epiglottitis.

Pathogenesis

The organisms reach the upper airway via the blood stream rather than by spread along the mucosal surfaces. Epiglottitis is always therefore part of a septicaemia. Infection of the epiglottis causes a local inflammatory response, with the oedematous so-called 'cherry-red' epiglottis, but also involvement of the arytenoid surfaces, including the aryepiglottic folds. There is surface mucosal ulceration and there may be microabscesses.

Clinical features

Paediatric
The characteristic features are the abrupt onset of high fever, sore throat and mild cough. This quickly proceeds to stridor, which is soft and low-pitched, along with some dysphagia. Characteristically, the child is anxious, drooling, unable to swallow their secretions, propped forward with the chin extended and neck hyperextended to maintain their airway. Most importantly they look septicaemic.

Adult
Clinical features may range from a sore throat and dysphagia to rapidly increasing symptoms of upper airway obstruction. Findings include fever, hoarse voice, tenderness in the neck and pooling of saliva in the throat. Acute respiratory obstruction is less likely in adults than in children because of the shape of the epiglottis.

Management

Paediatric
The most important part of management is to establish a stable artificial airway as early as possible. Crying and agitation increase upper airway obstruction. The parents should therefore be asked to administer oxygen near the child while an experienced paediatric anaesthetist is called. On no account should the traditional lateral X-ray of the neck be performed as putting the child in the position to obtain good quality radiographs has a high risk of inducing complete obstruction.

An inhalational anaesthetic is given and the diagnosis is made at laryngoscopy. Once an artificial airway is in place, specimens for diagnosis, including blood culture, can be obtained and intravenous lines for antibiotics can be inserted. It is important to know the emergency management for sudden complete obstruction, which can occur at any time. The first emergency manoeuvre is mandibular traction to try and reopen the airway. A Heimlich manoeuvre is sometimes also successful. Rarely, an emergency tracheostomy is required.

Antibiotic therapy should cover penicillinase-producing *H. influenzae* and group A streptococci. A third-generation cephalosporin such as cefotaxime or ceftriaxone is the drug of choice. Once the septicaemia is treated there is a prompt decrease in the oedematous swelling of the epiglottis and extubation is usual within 24–48 hours.

Adult

Management is the same as for children, using a β-lactamase-stable cephalosporin. There are no clinical data to support the routine use of steroids. Less than a quarter of the cases in the reported literature have needed tracheotomy or intubation; however, careful monitoring of the airways is essential.

Laryngotracheobronchitis (croup) in children

Epidemiology and aetiology

Croup is an inflammatory response of the upper and lower airways to viral infection. It is most common between the ages of 6 months and 5 years, with a peak occurring in the second year of life. Up to 15% of children may experience an episode of croup. Although croup can occur as a consequence of infection with any of the common respiratory viruses, parainfluenza virus is the most common isolate. In a prospective study over a 20-year period of 1429 children. where nasal washes were used to obtain viral specimens in all children with febrile upper or lower respiratory tract illnesses, parainfluenza virus was responsible for 64% of the cases of croup in illnesses identified with a positive viral culture.[10] Parainfluenza virus 1 and 2 are more likely to be associated with croup than parainfluenza virus 3 and 4 but parainfluenza virus 3 is a more ubiquitous organism that is frequently isolated in children with respiratory symptoms and so numerically it contributes most to the burden of croup.[10,11]

Pathology

In response to the virus there is marked oedema in the lamina propria, submucosa and mucosa with a cellular infiltrate consisting of histiocytes, lymphocytes, plasma cells and neutrophils. This is most prominent in the subglottic airway.

Clinical features

Classically, the child has rhinorrhoea with a sore throat and mild fever for 24–48 hours and then, often during the night, wakes with a barking cough, hoarseness, inspiratory stridor and a low-grade fever. In mild cases the child has a barking cough but audible stridor only when upset or excited, and has no other clinical features of respiratory distress. In severe cases, the child has dramatic airway obstruction during inspiration with gross intercostal, subcostal, suprasternal and tracheal indrawing, and requires intubation to protect the airway. A number of 'croup scores' have been drawn up based on clinical features such as degree of stridor and retractions along with features such as restlessness and cyanosis (or oxygen saturation). The simplest Fox score has acceptable interobserver agreement[12] (Table 35.1).

Table 35.1 The clinical Croup score

Clinical feature		Score
Stridor	None	0
	Only on crying/exertion	1
	At rest	2
	Severe (biphasic)	3
Retractions	None	0
	Only on crying/exertion	1
	At rest	2
	Severe (biphasic)	3

Management

Mild – first aid

The classical history of croup in a child waking at night, appearing to have difficulty in breathing and making an unusual noise is very alarming to parents. The traditional therapy is for the child to breathe in a warm, misty atmosphere produced by running the hot tap or by steaming a kettle. However, the benefits of warm mist have not been demonstrated in controlled trials.[13] Crying and agitation exacerbate the stridor: a quiet calm atmosphere with minimal disturbance is helpful.

Moderate

The management of moderate to severe croup has changed over the past 10 years, with firm evidence that the use of high-dose steroid therapy is effective. A meta-analysis in 1989[14] demonstrated efficacy in hospitalised children and since then a number of studies have examined the strength of dose, mode of delivery and groups suitable for treatment. A series of elegant studies[12,15,16] showed that oral dexamethasone in a dose of 0.15 mg/kg was as effective as higher doses in children hospitalised with croup,[12] that both oral dexamethasone and inhaled budesonide were effective in reducing symptoms and duration of hospitalisation in children with croup, and that both treatments showed an effect within 1 hour.[15] A single oral dose of dexamethasone 0.15 mg/kg was also demonstrated to be effective in the management of mild croup presenting to a paediatric emergency department.[16] In addition, it was demonstrated that steroid therapy reduced the duration of intubation and the need for re-intubation for children intubated for croup.[17]

A recent review[18] of 24 studies involving 2221 patients concluded that glucocorticoid treatment improved the croup severity score at 6 hours but that this was no longer significant at 24 hours. There was a decrease in the core interventions with a decrease of 9% (95% CI 2–16%) in the number of adrenaline (epinephrine) treatments in patients treated with budesonide and a decrease of 12% (95% CI 4–20%) in those treated with dexamethasone. There was a decrease in the length of time spent in accident and emergency departments (–11 hours, 95% CI –18–4 hours) and for inpatients hospital stay was reduced by

16 hours (95% CI 31–1 hour). A single dose of 0.15 mg/kg of dexamethasone (or 1 mg/kg prednisolone) is easy to give, cheap and effective. Children with mild to moderate croup may be treated with steroids in the community provided that appropriate arrangements are made for clinical review of the child within a few hours.

Severe croup

A child presenting with severe croup should be given oral or intramuscular steroids and nebulised adrenaline (epinephrine) in an attempt to improve the airway while the steroids take effect. The adrenaline should be nebulised with oxygen and the child should be closely monitored. Despite these measures, some children will require intubation. Inhalational anaesthetic and intubation should be performed by an experienced paediatric anaesthetist. Steroid therapy has reduced the number of children needing intubation, the duration of intubation and the total days of paediatric intensive care used for croup.[16,17] The average duration of intubation of children with croup treated with steroids is 3–4 days.[17] Recognised complications include blockage of the intratracheal tube with secretions and the development of granulation tissue in the subglottic area secondary to intubation.

Role of nebulised adrenaline (epinephrine)

Racemic adrenaline (epinephrine) has been widely used for many years in North America for the treatment of moderate and severe croup. It is thought to stimulate α-adrenergic receptors in the subglottic mucosa, producing vasoconstriction and hence decreasing hyperaemia and oedema and increasing airway diameter. When given by nebuliser, it is effective within 30 minutes, but the effect lasts for only approximately 2 hours. A double-blind placebo-controlled trial[19] demonstrated that racemic adrenaline was significantly better than placebo in terms of improvement in a total croup score and on inspiratory stridor, retractions and air entry on clinical examination. A prospective randomised double blind study compared racemic adrenaline (epinephrine) with the more readily available L-adrenaline. The patients showed significant clinical improvement transiently after both nebulised treatments and there were no differences found between treatments.[20]

Both types of adrenaline (epinephrine) have a transient effect that has largely gone by 2 hours.[20] Although the treatment may be repeated with good effect, it should be considered a first-aid measure in severe croup while waiting for steroid treatment to take effect. A child requiring repeated doses should be closely monitored, preferably in a paediatric intensive care unit as intubation may be required.

Spasmodic croup

This term is used to describe the sudden onset of symptoms at night in a child who has previously been well. Such children are usually afebrile but the symptoms are otherwise identical to those of viral croup, although usually at the mild end of the spectrum. Recurrent attacks are common. Spasmodic croup is thought to be an allergic reaction to antigen (perhaps viral) and is most common in children with a personal or family history of atopy.[21]

Bacterial tracheitis

Aetiology and clinical features

Bacterial tracheitis presents as severe upper airway obstruction. There is a diffuse inflammatory process in the larynx, trachea and bronchi with a mucopurulent exudate forming a semiadherent pseudomembrane of neutrophils and cellular debris. The clinical features are similar to those of severe viral croup but there is usually a high fever and the child appears toxic. *S. aureus* is the most common organism isolated but *H. influenzae*, *S. pneumoniae* and *Klebsiella pneumoniae* have also been reported.

Management

Steroids and nebulised adrenaline (epinephrine) are not effective and intubation is necessary to relieve the obstruction. Frequent suction and careful tracheal toilet are needed to prevent debris blocking the endotracheal tube. The infection responds to high-dose antibiotics but intubation is often needed for 7 days or more.

Diphtheria

This disease is exceptionally rare in Western countries but should be considered where a child has not been immunised against *Corynebacterium diphtheriae*. The child presents with stridor, cervical lymphadenopathy and a pseudomembrane over the tonsils or pharyngeal wall. There may also be a serosanguinous nasal discharge.

Infectious mononucleosis

Acute upper airway obstruction in an older child may be secondary to the massive lymphadenopathy seen in glandular fever.

Infections of the lower respiratory tract

This term relates to infection below the larynx and includes bronchial infections and the various forms of pneumonia. Such infections are commonly also grouped under the loose term 'chest infection' or as lower respiratory tract infection. The incidence of lower respiratory tract infections is around 40 per 1000 population per year but is considerably higher in very young and elderly people. It is important for hospital-based doctors to appreciate that the vast majority of lower respiratory tract illness and infection is managed by general practitioners and that those admitted to hospital are the tip of the iceberg[22,23] (Fig. 35.2).

Bronchial infections

Acute bronchitis in adults

Acute bronchitis is a common condition often occurring at the time of or shortly after an upper respiratory infection, when the patient complains that 'the cold has gone on to the chest'.

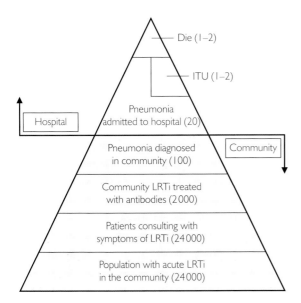

Fig. 35.2 The layers of the iceberg of lower respiratory tract illness, lower respiratory tract infection and pneumonia seen in the community and in hospital. The numbers in parentheses are estimates of the relative proportions of patients in each category. ITU, intensive care unit. Redrawn with permission from Macfarlane 1999.[56]

Aetiology

In the absence of chronic bronchopulmonary disease, the aetiological agents causing acute bronchitis are very similar to those causing community-acquired pneumonia.[23-26]

Clinical features

These include cough, sputum production and wheeze, often associated with a slight fever and symptoms of an associated upper respiratory infection. The chest radiograph is normal.

Management

The condition is usually managed outside hospital. About three-quarters of adults with bronchitis are prescribed antibiotics, although a meta-analysis demonstrated that they confer no overall benefit.[27,28] The decision to use antibiotics is based on several considerations, including duration of symptoms, purulence of the sputum, pre-existing medical condition, clinical features such as focal chest signs, patient expectations and social factors. Recurrent attacks of acute bronchitis in a previously healthy person are unusual and other conditions, particularly asthma, must be considered.

Complications

Pneumonia is the main complication. Bronchial hyperresponsiveness can also develop.

Acute exacerbation of chronic bronchitis in adults

Acute exacerbations are common in winter. They are characterised by an increase in cough, dyspnoea, sputum purulence, volume and thickness, and difficulty in expectoration.

Aetiology

H. influenzae (40%), *S. pneumoniae* (20%) and *M. catarrhalis* (17%) are most commonly isolated.[23,29]

Investigation

Sputum culture is not necessary unless the presentation is unusual or the patient is seriously ill.

Treatment

Overall, antibiotics confer little benefit unless there is worsening dyspnoea, sputum purulence or increased sputum volume.[30] Any associated problems of airflow obstruction, respiratory failure and cor pulmonale will require treatment. Annual influenza vaccination and pneumococcal vaccination are recommended for those with chronic lung disease. Antibiotic prophylaxis is still occasionally used, but at the expense of introducing side effects.

Bronchial infections in children

In children the aetiology is almost exclusively viral, with the exception of *Bordetella pertussis* infection (whooping cough). Antibiotics are not indicated and resolution is normally within 2–3 weeks.

Whooping cough
Epidemiology

Whooping cough remains a relatively common and important infectious illness despite near universal infant immunisation in the UK. A recent report from general practice of serological or culture-positive cases in patients presenting with spasmodic cough (greater than 3 weeks duration) gave an equivalent annual incidence of 330 per 100 000 population,[31] nearly 100 times the statutory England and Wales notification rates. US data indicate an increasing incidence in adolescents and adults.[32]

Aetiology

Whooping cough is classically due to *Bordetella pertussis* but other *Bordetella* species such as *B. parapertussis* and *B. cholmesii* can cause a similar clinical picture.

Clinical features

The intubation period is 10–14 days. The illness starts with coryzal features – nasal discharge, dry cough and mild pyrexia. After a few days the cough becomes more prominent and paroxysmal. The child starts a spasm of coughing, going red in the face or occasionally becoming cyanosed. The coughing spasm is often terminated by either a vomit or the classical 'whoop'. The whoop is produced by a rapid inspiration from residual volume through a partially opened glottis. The child becomes exhausted by repeated coughing spasms. Vomiting may be responsible for weight loss and failure to thrive. The illness is less severe in older children and adults but young children are frequently hypoxic during coughing episodes and need hospital care. The acute phase of the illness lasts several weeks, with gradual decrease in frequency and severity of cough episodes. The cough generally lasts for about 3 months with exacerbations if any respiratory viral infection is encountered. Previously immunised children and adults generally have a milder picture with a cough lasting 4–8 weeks and less than 10% have a classic whoop. Parapertussis causes a similar but generally milder illness.

Diagnosis

Diagnosis is easy when the full clinical picture is present but is often not considered in older children, adults and those known to be fully vaccinated. *B. pertussis* can be cultured from nasopharyngeal aspirates in the first 2 weeks of the illness. Later diagnosis is by serology. A lymphocytosis (greater than 70%) on the peripheral blood count is supportive evidence. With severe pertussis the lymphocyte count can exceed 80 000.

Complications

There is diffuse inflammation of the larynx, trachea and bronchi with semiadherent pseudomembranes consisting of mucus, neutrophils and cellular debris.

Petechiae of the face, neck and trunk are common, as are subconjunctival haemorrhages. Common respiratory complications include apnoea and bradycardia, particularly in young infants, and bronchopneumonia. Neurological complications can be severe and are related to the hypoxia developed during coughing spasms. Deaths are still reported, especially in infants less than 3 months of age.[33] Rarely, a whooping cough encephalitis can occur, with devastating consequences.

Treatment

Antibiotics, particularly erythromycin, decrease infectivity and thereby limit spread of the infection but do not modify the illness unless given at the coryzal stage. Erythromycin should therefore be given to all young contacts as well as the index case. Treatment is otherwise supportive, consisting of oxygen, suction and nutritional support. There is no convincing evidence that either sedatives or steroids are effective and salbutamol has been shown to be ineffective.[34]

Prevention

Vaccination provides protection against clinical disease (80–95%) and amelioration in those not fully protected.[35] Vaccine-related immunity wanes with time and booster immunisation of school children and adults is being considered.

Acute bronchiolitis

Acute bronchiolitis is the most common lower respiratory tract infection in infancy. It occurs in winter epidemics each year and between 80% and 90% of cases are caused by respiratory syncytial virus (RSV). Other viruses, including parainfluenza virus, adenovirus and influenza virus, can cause a similar clinical picture.

Epidemiology of RSV bronchiolitis

Respiratory syncytial virus is an RNA virus with two major subtypes (A and B) subdivided into six and three subgroups respectively. Both types are present during an epidemic. Natural immunity is not fully protective and reinfection is common. It can occur within a single season and with the same type and subgroup. Passively acquired maternal antibody may provide some protection in the first 4–6 weeks of life. Around 70% of infants acquire RSV in the first year of life. RSV is spread by infected droplets. The infection can vary in severity from mild upper respiratory tract symptoms and cough to severe bronchiolitis and pneumonia. Subsequent infections are usually less severe but reinfection continues in adult life and RSV has been implicated in significant respiratory morbidity in the elderly.[36]

Pathology and pathogenesis

The virus infection causes a predominantly neutrophilic inflammatory response in the airways with resultant interleukin-8 cytokine production, mucosal oedema and exudation. There has been considerable interest in the immunological response to RSV but to date there is no definite evidence that host response is responsible for disease severity.

Clinical features

The illness starts with a coryzal illness and mild fever (temperature less than 38.°C), progressing after 2–3 days to a dry, repetitive cough and tachypnoea. The infant finds it difficult to feed. On examination there is hyperinflation of the chest with subcostal and intercostal recession and tachypnoea. Auscultation reveals the widespread fine crepitations characteristic of the disease with additional respiratory wheeze present in many. Hypoxemia indicates severe disease and some infants progress to respiratory failure. Apnoea is common in very young infants and those born prematurely. In these, apnoea may be the first sign of RSV infection. The illness progresses in severity over 4–5 days, then plateaus for several days before it resolves. There may be a residual cough for a subsequent 10–14 days.

Diagnosis

Diagnosis is confirmed by isolation of virus from nasopharyngeal secretions. Rapid diagnostic kits using indirect immunofluorescence or enzyme immunoassay are readily available and have been used for near-patient testing. No other investigation is necessary. A chest X-ray should only be performed if the child is severely ill or there is an unexpected deterioration.

Risk

Groups at increased risk of severe disease are infants born prematurely, those with pre-existing cardiac or lung disease and those with immunodeficiency. Parental smoking is associated with a higher risk of hospital admission.

Management

Most infants are managed at home with small, frequent feeds. Infants who are unable to feed and those with severe respiratory distress are admitted to hospital for careful monitoring, correction of hypoxemia, provision of adequate fluids and respiratory support. There is little evidence that any drug is of benefit.[37–40] Ribovarin, the first specific antiviral agent, achieved some popularity in high-risk infants but its trials have so far lacked sufficient power.[41] A few infants require respiratory support for either recurrent apnoea or respiratory failure. Continued positive airway pressure may be sufficient to prevent ventilation, particularly in those infants presenting with apnoea. When full ventilation is needed, a permissive hypercarbic strategy is generally used, keeping peak pressures at the minimum required to achieve acceptable oxygenation without acidosis.

Outcome

Outcome is good even in infants who have had severe disease. The small residual mortality is in high-risk infants.[42] There is, however, a residual morbidity, with 40–60% of infants having recurrent episodes of wheeze with subsequent respiratory virus infection.

Prevention

It is important to prevent spread of the disease in hospital, where strategies such as cohort nursing and careful attention to hand washing are effective.[43] In recent years, two strategies for immunoprophylaxis in the high-risk infant have been developed. Intravenous immunoglobulin containing high titres of RSV-specific antibodies is effective in preventing lower respiratory tract infection but high cost and monthly infusions are considerable drawbacks and such treatment is contraindicated in infants with cyanotic congenital heart disease.[44] The alternative is a humanised monoclonal antibody directed against the F (fusion) protein given by monthly intramuscular injection. This has also been shown to be safe and effective in the prevention of serious RSV illness in preterm infants and those with bronchopulmonary dysplasia.[45] However, 17 infants need to be treated to prevent one hospital admission and costs are high.[46] Attempts continue to develop an effective vaccine against RSV.

Pneumonia

Pneumonia is one of the leading causes of morbidity and death worldwide, particularly in developing countries, where pneumonia is the most common cause of hospital attendance in adults and where pneumonia mortality in children is very high. It is

Table 35.2 A sensible clinical classification of pneumonia allows a logical approach to likely aetiology and management

Community-acquired pneumonia
Hospital-acquired (nosocomial) pneumonia
Aspiration and anaerobic pneumonia (including lipoid pneumonia)
Pneumonia in the immunocompromised host
AIDS-related pneumonia
Recurrent pneumonia
Pneumonias peculiar to specific parts of the world

estimated that 4 million children under the age of 5 years die of pneumonia each year in developing countries. A useful and practical classification of the types of pneumonia includes reference to clinical and environmental features (Table 35.2).

Community-acquired pneumonia

Community-acquired pneumonia may be primary and random, secondary to a predisposing condition (e.g. chronic lung disease, age, diabetes, etc.) or secondary to some epidemiological or environmental factor (e.g. viral epidemic, zoonosis such as psittacosis or Q fever, environmental source of *Legionella*).

Incidence

The annual incidence of community-acquired pneumonia is 5–11 per 1000 adult population, accounting for 5–12% of all cases of adult lower respiratory tract infection managed by general practitioners. Each general practitioner in the UK deals with about 10 adults and 12 children with primary pneumonia each year. The proportion of community-acquired pneumonia patients requiring hospitalisation is 1–4 per 1000 population. Between 22% and 42% of adults with community-acquired pneumonia are admitted to hospital in the UK, and 5–10% of these require intensive therapy. Mortality in the community is very low, less than 1%. In hospital, mortality is 6–12%, being as high as 50% for those requiring intensive care.[47–51] Mortality in children is very low in developed countries.

The costs associated with community-acquired pneumonia are high, estimated to be $8.4 billion per year in the USA and about £500 million in the UK, mostly associated with inpatient care costs.[52]

Epidemiology

A knowledge of the epidemiology of community-acquired infections is very helpful for management. Some pathogens have characteristic seasonal patterns[53] (Fig. 35.3). The incidence of respiratory infections and pneumonia rises dramatically during the first quarter of the year, associated with the peak of influenza virus infection, when bacterial infections are much commoner. In contrast, *Legionella* pneumonia is more common in the summer and rhinovirus and respiratory syncytial virus appear in early and mid-winter.

Mycoplasma infection is unusual in occurring in large epidemics throughout the world every 3–4 years with only sporadic

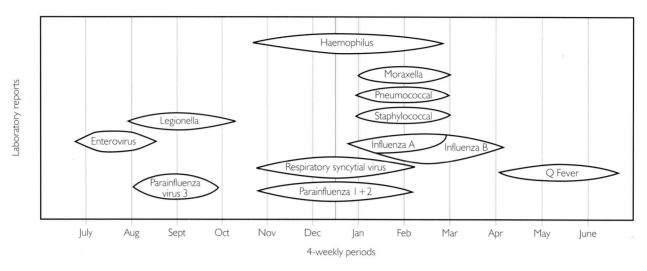

cases at other times[54] (Fig. 35.4). The last epidemic was in 1998. An unexpected clustering of two or more cases of a less usual pneumonia, such as psittacosis, Q fever or *Legionella* infection, should point to the need for an epidemiological study to investigate the source of the local epidemic.

Aetiology in adults

The knowledge that only a few pathogens cause most community-acquired pneumonia is the key to logical treatment[54] (Table 35.3). Bacteria are the cause in 60–80% of cases, atypical agents such as *Mycoplasma* in 10–20% and viruses in 10–15%. By far the most common pathogen is *S. pneumoniae* and it is probably also the cause of most cases in which no pathogen can

be identified. Prior antibiotics and incomplete specimen collection account for underdiagnosis in many cases.

Chlamydia pneumoniae and *M. pneumoniae* are the next most common pathogens. When there is a cyclical *Mycoplasma* epidemic, this organism can account for up to 23% of cases.[49,55] *H. influenzae*, the next pathogen in order of frequency, is usually associated with chronic lung disease. Influenza virus is the most frequent viral pathogen encountered, and is usually complicated by secondary bacterial pneumonia. Psittacosis and *Legionella* pneumonia each account for between 2% and 5% of cases. There is marked geographical variation in the reported incidence of *Legionella* pneumonia, depending on whether the studies are community- or hospital-based.[23,56] Infections with other bacteria such as *M. catarrhalis*, Gram-negative enteric bacillary infec-

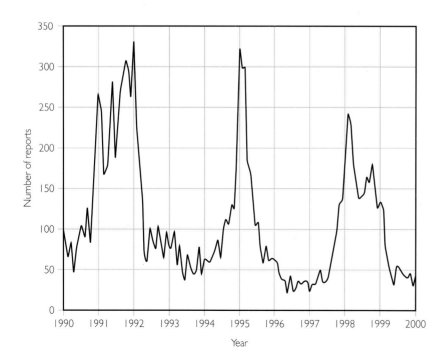

Fig. 35.4 Laboratory reports to the Communicable Disease Surveillance Centre of *Mycoplasma* infections: England and Wales, 1990–2000 (4-weekly). Data obtained from the Public Health Laboratory Service website, www.phls.co.uk/seasonal/mycoplasma.

Table 35.3 Community-acquired pneumonia studies conducted in hospital in different parts of the world, including studies of severe pneumonia conducted on intensive care units (ICU). Data from Macfarlane et al 2001[54]

Where managed	UK Hospital Mean %	ICU Mean %	Rest of Europe Hospital Mean %	ICU Mean %	Australia + New Zealand Hospital Mean %	North America Hospital Mean %
n	1137	185	6026	1148	453	1306
Streptococcus pneumoniae	39	22	19	22	38	11
Haemophilus influenzae	5	4	4	5	9	6
Legionella spp.	4	18	5	5	7	5
Moraxella catarrhalis	2	?	1	7	3	1
Staphylococcus aureus	2	9	1	4	3	4
Gram-negative Enterobacteriaceae	1	2	3	9	5	5
Mycoplasma pneumoniae	11	3	6	2	15	4
Chlamydia pneumoniae	13	?	6	7	3	6
Chlamydia psittaci	3	2	1	1	1	0
Coxiella burnetii	1	0	1	1	0	2
Viruses	13	10	9	4	11	9
Influenza A and B	11	5	5	2	6	6
Mixed infections	14	6	6	5	20	8
Other	2	5	2	8	4	8
None	31	32	51	43	32	41

tions and *S. aureus* are very uncommon. However the last occurs in association with influenza epidemics and is important because of its high mortality, even in previously fit individuals.

The findings in the UK are broadly similar to those in Sweden,[57] Australia[58] and New Zealand[59] but some studies from North America have more frequently reported Gram-negative enteric bacillary infection, aspiration and staphylococcal infection, probably because debilitated patients, substance abusers and those at risk of HIV infection form a higher proportion of the patients studied and also because of different diagnostic criteria.[60,61]

Aetiology in the elderly

The pneumococcus is again the most important pathogen, followed by *H. influenzae*. Atypical pathogens and *Legionella* pneumonia are uncommon in elderly people, apart from *Chlamydia pneumoniae*.[50,54,62] North American hospital and nursing home studies show more Gram-negative enteric bacillary infection in elderly people than in the UK.[63] Tuberculosis must never be forgotten as a possible pathogen in this population.

Aetiology in the child

Studies of the aetiology of community-acquired pneumonia in children are complicated by the difficulty in obtaining appropri-

ate samples. A pathogen is not identified in between 20% and 60% of cases. Viruses alone account for between 14% and 35% of community-acquired pneumonia in childhood. *S. pneumoniae* is the most common bacterial cause of pneumonia. In 8–30% of cases there is a mixed viral and bacterial infection. Age is a good predictor of likely pathogen, with viral infections (especially RSV) found more commonly in younger children and *Mycoplasma* and *Chlamydia pneumoniae* more common in school-age children.[64,65]

Pathogenesis

This varies according to the pathogen. Infection may arise from aspiration of endogenous organisms resident in the nasopharynx (e.g. pneumococcal infection), inhalation of infected droplets from another patient (e.g. viral infections), inhalation of infected particles from animals (e.g. psittacosis, Q fever) or inhalation of infected droplets from the environment (e.g. water droplets contaminated with *Legionella* organisms).

Clinical features in adults

Men are affected two to three times more commonly than women. General symptoms include those of any infection, i.e. malaise, anorexia, sweating, rigors, myalgia, arthralgia and headache. There may be a preceding history of upper respiratory tract symptoms, particularly with viral and mycoplasmal infections. Patients with bacteraemic pneumonia may become critically ill within hours and, in contrast, some patients with mycoplasmal pneumonia may have had symptoms for 2–3 weeks.

Sometimes, non-respiratory symptoms can dominate the picture and mask the diagnosis. Marked confusion is seen in patients with any severe pneumonia but is also a peculiar feature of *Legionella* and psittacosis pneumonia. Lower lobe pneumonia may mimic an acute abdominal or urinary problem, and chest examination and a chest radiograph are essential in the investigation of anyone with an 'acute abdomen'. This is particularly evident at extremes of age. In elderly people the classic symptoms and signs of pneumonia may be absent, the only indications being a raised pulse and respiratory rate and a deterioration in physical or mental state.[54]

Respiratory symptoms vary, but classically they include cough in nearly all patients, shortness of breath in over two-thirds, pleural pain in 60%, new sputum production in over half and haemoptysis in 15%. In the early stages of pneumonia, sputum is usually mucoid, scanty or absent, particularly with atypical and *Legionella* pneumonias, becoming purulent later.

Physical signs in adults

High fever and rigors are particularly common in young patients and in those with pneumococcal and *Legionella* infection. Little or no fever may be seen in elderly or seriously ill patients. Herpes labialis is seen in about a third of pneumococcal cases. Classic signs of lobar consolidation with dullness to percussion and bronchial breathing are less common than focal inspiratory crackles.

Upper abdominal tenderness is not unusual, particularly with lower lobe pneumonia or if there is hepatitis. A rash is usually the result of antibiotic therapy but various skin manifestations have been reported occasionally with mycoplasmal and psittacosis and uniformly with chickenpox pneumonia.

Differential diagnosis in adults

The most common diagnostic dilemma is that of distinguishing pneumonia from pulmonary infarction or atypical pulmonary oedema. Careful physical examination and interpretation of investigations are usually helpful but, on occasion, the distinction is very difficult and treatment may have to be given to cover more than one condition until the situation becomes clearer. Less common conditions that enter the differential diagnosis include pulmonary eosinophilia, acute allergic or cryptogenic alveolitis and primary or metastatic lung tumours. Disease below the diaphragm such as hepatic abscess, appendicitis, pancreatitis or perforated ulcer can mimic lower lobe pneumonia, and vice versa.

Clinical features and signs in children

In young children a respiratory rate greater than or equal to 50/min and/or chest indrawing are indicators of radiologically proven pneumonia (positive predictive value 43%) and their absence makes consolidation unlikely (negative predictive value

Table 35.4 Clinical features of bacterial and viral pneumonia in children

Bacterial infection
Fever >38.5°C
Respiratory rate >50 breaths/min
Chest recession
Clinical and radiological signs of consolidation rather than collapse

Viral infection
Wheeze
Fever <38.5°C
Hyperinflation
Respiratory rate normal or raised
Radiograph shows hyperinflation and patchy collapse

83%).[66] In another study a respiratory rate greater than 70/min in infants predicted hypoxaemia ($p = 0.001$, sensitivity 63%, specificity 89%).[67] Over the age of 3 years, tachypnoea and chest recession are not sensitive signs: crackles and bronchial breathing are more helpful. Wheeze is a feature of viral infection and in a young child it makes a primary bacterial pneumonia unlikely; in an older child *Mycoplasma* infection should be considered. Abdominal pain may be referred from the diaphragm in lower lobe pneumonia and neck pain and stiffness from an upper lobe pneumonia (Table 35.4).

Investigations in adults

The diagnostic value of various microbiological tests is summarised in the following paragraph. The tests to be performed depend on how ill the patient is. For patients with mild pneumonia responding well to treatment, no particular investigations are required except for a chest radiograph after clinical recovery to confirm resolution and identify any underlying lung disease. This is important. In one radiographic study, previously unsuspected malignant disease was surprisingly common, being present in 7% of pneumonia cases, including 17% of smokers over the age of 60 years.[47] For patients who are ill, the aim is to assess severity and discover the aetiology of pneumonia as speedily as possible.

Microbiological tests in adults

- **Sputum Gram stain.** Confirms that specimen is sputum, not saliva. Low sensitivity (10%). High specificity if positive (70–80%). Important, as gives a rapid indication of possible pathogen in those with severe pneumonia.
- **Sputum culture.** Oropharyngeal contamination and effect of prior antibiotics a problem. Only available in 50–66% patients with community-acquired pneumonia on admission. Washing or diluting sputum before culture is helpful. Should be obtained if available, and can be of value in those who have not received prior antibiotics.
- **Blood culture.** It is important to obtain this before starting antibiotics. Positive in only 20–25% of bacterial pneumonias but relates to aetiology and prognosis.

- **Pleural fluid**. Essential to sample for stain/culture/pH if present to exclude empyema or complicated parapneumonic effusion.
- **Serological tests for acute disease and follow-up**. For diagnosis of viral, atypical and *Legionella* pathogens, usually retrospectively. Most laboratories only test paired samples. Only of practical value in management if first titre is high. Useful for aetiology research studies.
- **Cold agglutinins**. Positive in over 50% of patients with mycoplasmal pneumonia. Can be detected by bedside agglutination test, in which a few drops of blood are added to a citrated tube and placed in a 4°C refrigerator for a few minutes.
- **Antigen detection**. Particularly useful for pneumococcal infection. Sputum positive in 80%; urine in 36–45%; serum in 9–23%. Not routine in most laboratories. New bedside slide agglutinin test kits for pneumococcal and *Legionella* antigen detection in urine are available and are being evaluated (see section on pneumococcal infection later in this chapter).

Invasive tests in adults

In patients who are seriously ill or who present a diagnostic problem, invasive techniques should be considered for obtaining uncontaminated lower respiratory secretions or lung biopsies. Close liaison between the clinician and the microbiologist is essential to ensure that appropriate testing is arranged. This is particularly important because not all laboratories have facilities for quantitative microbiology and immunofluorescent staining for a full range of respiratory pathogens. Fibreoptic bronchoscopy, allows bronchoalveolar lavage and the introduction of a protected brush catheter. Percutaneous needle aspiration gives good results in experienced hands but at the risk of pneumothorax. Lung biopsy is rarely performed for pneumonia, except where the diagnosis is unclear. The specimens obtained can be cultured and examined by Gram stain, direct fluorescent antibody stain (for *Legionella*, viruses and *Pneumocystis*) and fungal stains.[68]

General investigations in adults

- **Oxygen assessment**. Oximetry should be performed on all adults admitted to hospital with pneumonia and arterial blood gases checked in those who have an S_aO_2 of 92% or less or features of severe disease.
- **White blood cell count (WBC)**. The total count is over $15.0 \times 10^9/l$ in most patients with pneumococcal and *H. influenzae* pneumonias, marginally raised with *Legionella* infections (WBC $< 15 \times 10^9/l$) and variable with staphylococcal pneumonia.[69,70] In patients with atypical or viral pneumonia not complicated by bacterial superinfection a near-normal white cell count is usual.[71] Marked leukopenia (WBC $< 4 \times 10^9/l$) and leukocytosis (WBC $> 30 \times 10^9/l$) are seen in those with severe infection and indicate a poor prognosis.
- **Biochemistry**. Abnormal liver function tests are not unusual in patients with bacterial pneumonia, particularly if bacteraemic.

Raised blood urea, hypokalaemia, hypoalbuminaemia, proteinuria, haematuria and hyponatraemia can be seen with any severe pneumonia, the last being particularly common in *Legionella* infection. Biochemical features of multisystem involvement are less usual with mycoplasmal pneumonia. C reactive protein (CRP) is usually over 100 mg/l in adults with bacterial pneumonia but high levels do not reliably exclude viral or atypical pathogens.[72]

Specific microbiological tests in children

It is important to attempt a microbiological diagnosis in children admitted to hospital with pneumonia.

- **Blood cultures** should be performed in all children suspected of having a bacterial pneumonia but are positive in less than 10%.
- **Nasopharyngeal aspirate**. Virus antigen detection is sensitive (approximately 80%) and highly specific for RSV, parainfluenza virus, adenovirus and influenza virus. Rapid viral diagnosis is particularly useful for segregating infected children during outbreaks. Viruses can also be cultured from nasopharyngeal samples but the result is generally retrospective.
- **Serum** obtained on admission should be saved and a convalescent sample taken if a microbiological diagnosis is not reached during the acute illness. Methods for the serological diagnosis of pneumococcal disease are improving but are still poor in the very young.[73]
- **Pleural fluid**, if present, should be aspirated for diagnostic purposes. In a large series comprising 840 pleural fluid samples from children aged 1–12 years, bacteria were cultured in 17.7% and antigen detection tests (at least two of three positive) provided further evidence of aetiology in another 41%.[74]

General investigations in children

- **Pulse oximetry** provides a non-invasive estimate of arterial oxygenation and should be performed in all children admitted to hospital with pneumonia.
- **Acute phase reactants** such as white blood cell count, CRP and ESR are generally performed to distinguish viral from bacterial pneumonia and help decide whether to prescribe antibiotics, but recent studies suggest that they do not reliably distinguish between viral and bacterial infection in children.[75,76] Routine measurement of acute phase reactants is not recommended.
- **Biochemical tests**. Urea and electrolytes should be performed if the child is severely ill or shows evidence of dehydration.

Radiological features

Homogeneous lobar or segmental opacification is more common than patchy shadows in bacterial pneumonia but is also seen in over half of patients with atypical pneumonia. Small pleural effusions are detectable in about a quarter of cases. Cavitation is infrequent in community-acquired pneumonia except with staphylococcal and pneumococcal serotype 3 pneumonia.

Spread of lung shadowing to more than one lobe is a feature of severe infection but is also seen with *Legionella* and sometimes mycoplasmal pneumonia, in spite of apparently appropriate antibiotic therapy.[77]

The rate of radiological clearance of shadows can be surprisingly slow, lagging considerably behind clinical recovery. Speed of resolution is affected by the age of the patient, the presence of any underlying chronic lung disease and the pathogen involved. *Legionella* pneumonia and bacteraemic pneumococcal pneumonia are peculiar in showing very slow clearance rates over many months, in contrast to atypical pneumonias, which normally clear within 2–3 months (Fig. 35.5).

Clinical differentiation of the cause of the pneumonia

Unfortunately, none of the pathogens has a clinical, laboratory or radiological pattern sufficiently characteristic to enable a confident diagnosis when the patient is first seen. Comparative features of some of the common causes of community-acquired pneumonia are shown in Tables 35.5 and 35.6. The term 'atypical' pneumonia is misleading and should be abandoned as it implies incorrectly a characteristic 'typical' and 'atypical' clinical presentation that allows an aetiology to be deduced by the clinician.

Prognostic factors and identifying severe infection in adults

It is important to identify early those patients with severe pneumonia as this is crucial to management, picking out those patients

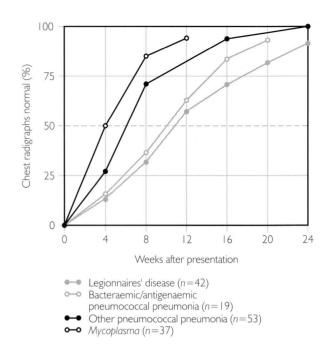

Fig. 35.5 Rates of resolution of radiographic shadowing for adults with various forms of community-acquired pneumonia. Redrawn with permission from Macfarlane et al 1984.[77]

who may require intensive observation and therapy. Prognosis is related to the pathogen, the host and the relationship between the two. Generally, patients with atypical pathogens do well and deaths are uncommon. The mortality rate of community-

Table 35.5 Comparative features of adults with different types of community acquired pneumonia seen in hospital

Nature	Pneumococcal (n = 83) Staphylococcal (n = 61)		Legionella (n = 79) Mycoplasma (n = 62)	
Mean age (years)	52	53	47	34
Pre-existing chronic disease (%)	59	35	49	19
Mortality (%)	18	16	30	0
Mean symptom duration (days)	5	7	7	13
Upper respiratory symptoms (%)	21	14	41	40
Productive cough (%)	69	41	70	73
Pleural pain (%)	72	36	50	38
Confusion (%)	25	43	22	2
Bronchial breathing (%)	37	22	25	29
White cell count $> 15 \times 10^9/l$ (%)	60	14	41	13
White cell count $< 10 \times 10^9/l$ (%)	15	40	36	51
Abnormal liver function (%)	34	59	55	16
Abnormal renal function (%)	55	60	52	16
Hyponatraemia (%)	23	55	21	5

Table 35.6 Comparative radiographic features of adults with different types of community acquired pneumonia seen in hospital

Feature	Pneumococcal (n = 91)	Mycoplasma (n = 46)	Legionella (n = 49)	Psittacosis (n = 10)
Mainly homogenous shadows (%)	74	82	50	60
Mainly patchy shadows (%)	26	18	50	40
Pleural effusion (%)	33	24	20	20
Some pulmonary collapse (%)	25	37	26	20
Hilar lymphadenopathy (%)	0	0	22	0
Cavitation of lung (%)	5	2	0	10
Radiographic deterioration after hospital admission (%)	35	65	25	0
Weeks after presentation for half of radiographs to show resolution (%)	8 (approx.)	11	4	4

acquired *Legionella* pneumonia is 5–15%. Bacteraemia signifies a poor prognosis, increasing the mortality two- to threefold. Pulmonary infections with *S. aureus*, *H. influenzae* or Gram-negative enteric bacilli also carry a poor prognosis. Mortality and morbidity rise progressively with increasing age and the presence of chronic disease. Other factors shown to be pointers to severe pneumonia are given in Table 35.6. Various prediction models have been developed to identify on admission those who have a poor prognosis, but they are an aid rather than a substitute for clinical judgement.[54]

The modified BTS rule

Three studies have reported that the presence of two or more of the following is associated with a high risk of death: new mental confusion; respiratory rate ≥ 30/min; diastolic blood pressure ≤ 60 mmHg; and blood urea > 7 mmol/l (sensitivity 83%; specificity 70%; negative predictive value 97%; positive predictive value 26%).[54] With such a high negative predictive value, absence of these features makes severe pneumonia and death very unlikely.[78]

The pneumonia severity index

This more complicated risk equation stratifies patients into six risk categories[79,80] and has been validated in large cohorts of patients in North America. It has not found favour in routine clinical practice in Europe because of the need to document multiple features to calculate the index. However, identifying those in risk category I, in whom the mortality is less than 0.5%, is simple, requiring only clinical data, and may allow recognition of those who do not need hospital admission. An algorithm for identifying those with both a low risk of death and high risk of death from pneumonia is outlined in Figure 35.6.

Management of community-acquired pneumonia in adults

Guidelines for the investigation and management of pneumonia have been published recently by the British Thoracic Society.[54] A plan of management is summarised in Figure 35.7 and the 'Ten Commandments' of management are listed in Table 35.7.

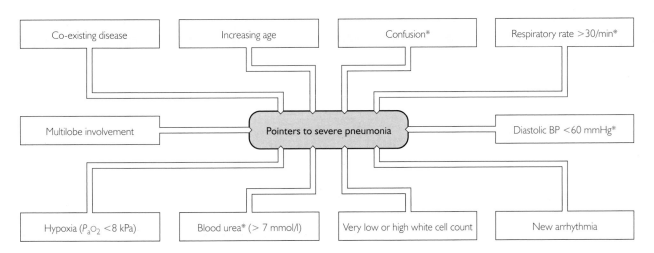

Fig. 35.6 Factors associated with poor prognosis in adult community acquired pneumonia. Redrawn with permission from Macfarlane et al 2001.[54]

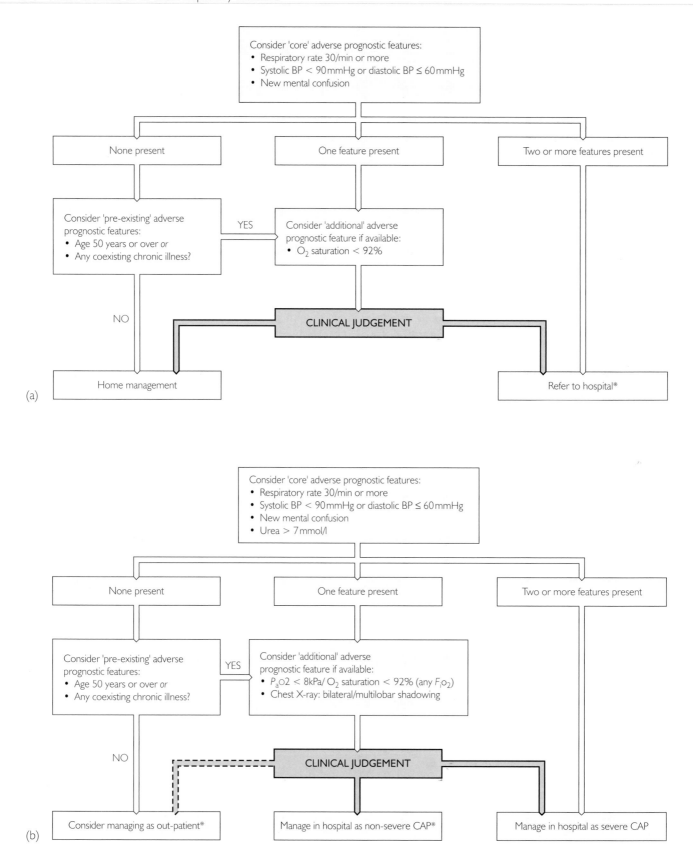

Fig. 35.7 Algorithm for identifying adults who are at low risk of death and may be managed in the community (a) and those at intermediate and high risk of death who will probably need hospital admission or intensive management (b). *Also consider social circumstances, patient and GP wishes. Redrawn with permission from Macfarlane et al 2001.[54]

Table 35.7 The 'ten commandments' for managing community-acquired pneumonia

---

All infections

Only a few pathogens are involved

Always cover *Streptococcus pneumoniae* – the most common cause

Consider epidemiology, patient's age and prior health

Remember *Mycoplasma* during epidemics, *Staphylococcus aureus* in flu season

Do not delay starting antibiotics

Severe infections

Assess prognostic factors and identify severe infection early

Establish aetiology quickly

Adequate oxygen, hydration and nutrition essential

Careful monitoring – transfer high-risk patients early to intensive treatment unit

Initial antibiotics must cover all the likely pathogens

General management in adults

The general management of a patient with pneumonia is important but often neglected. Patients should rest in bed, take plenty of fluid and be strongly encouraged not to smoke. Aspirin or a non-steroidal anti-inflammatory drug will often relieve pleural pain and fever.

Adequate oxygen therapy is essential for patients with moderate or severe pneumonia and those recognised as having severe infection are best observed in an intensive care unit, which has facilities for assisted ventilation. Cardiorespiratory failure can appear rapidly and early assisted ventilation can be life-saving, gaining time for specific antibiotics to work. As a rule of thumb, if a previously fit adult cannot maintain a P_aO_2 of 8 kPa (60 mmHg), with or without supplemental oxygen, assisted ventilation is probably required. The danger period is the first 3–4 days after hospital admission, during which time seriously ill patients should be monitored closely.[81] Ventilation may be required for many days or weeks.

Antibiotics commonly used for respiratory tract infections

Penicillins

Amoxicillin is a popular oral antibiotic, being well absorbed and having a well-known side-effect profile.

Augmentation of amoxicillin by adding clavulanic acid (co-amoxiclav), which inactivates β-lactamase, extends the cover to β-lactamase-producing organisms such as *S. aureus*, some strains of *H. influenzae* and *M. catarrhalis*. Co-amoxiclav is best taken at the start of a meal to reduce gastrointestinal upset, which occurs twice as commonly as with amoxicillin. Flucloxacillin provides effective cover for *S. aureus* but at the expense of reduced activity against other Gram-positive cocci such as *S. pneumoniae*.

Cephalosporins

Oral cephalosporins are generally not used for pneumonia because of their variable absorption, poor lung penetration and intestinal side effects. Parenteral preparations are useful for severe pneu-monia but are associated with the risk of *Clostridium difficile* enteropathy.[82]

Trimethoprim

This has not established itself as a popular choice for respiratory infections but is likely to be effective in mild cases.

Tetracyclines

As a result of reduced use over the last decade, the prevalence of tetracycline-resistant organisms has declined and there is a resurgence of interest in using them for mild community-acquired pneumonia. They also have a role in treating atypical pathogens and also methicillin-resistant *S. aureus* (MRSA) infections. Doxycycline is a popular choice: being lipid-soluble it penetrates lung white cells and macrophages and consequently is effective against intracellular atypical respiratory pathogens and *Legionella*. Tetracyclines act on bacterial ribosomes to inhibit bacterial protein synthesis. However, toxicity is a problem. There is a high incidence of gastrointestinal side effects, probably resulting part from a chemical effect and part from an effect on the bowel flora, which may result in secondary candidal infection. Photosensitivity may be encountered in sunny climates, while tetracyclines are contraindicated in children and pregnant women because of teeth discoloration. They may also cause hepatic and renal damage, particularly in elderly people.

Macrolides

Over the last 40 years, erythromycin has gained a reputation as a reliable alternative to β-lactam agents for the treatment of bacterial and atypical respiratory tract infections. Macrolides accumulate in lung cells, resulting in a high tissue:plasma antibiotic concentration, and are effective for intracellular atypical pathogens. Oral erythromycin is cheap but is associated with dose-related gastrointestinal disturbance (mainly nausea and vomiting), which can affect up to 20% of patients. Another important limitation of erythromycin is its poor activity against *H. influenzae*, which precludes its empirical use in patients with chronic lung disease

Newer macrolides such as clarithromycin and azithromycin have several advantages, including improved acid stability, greater absorption, considerably fewer side effects and longer elimination half-lives, permitting less frequent and lower dosing regimens. They are also more active against *H. influenzae*. They can be regarded as an alternative if a patient is intolerant of erythromycin.

Fluoroquinolones

Fluoroquinolones are highly active in vitro against a range of Gram-negative organisms including *H. influenzae*, *M. catarrhalis*, enteric bacilli and *Legionella* spp. Ciprofloxacin also has acceptable in vitro activity against *Pseudomonas aeruginosa*, the only oral agent that has. Currently, the only fluoroquinolones licensed for respiratory tract infections in the UK are levofloxacin, ciprofloxacin and ofloxacin. The latter two have questionable in vitro activity against *S. pneumoniae*, which is partially compensated by the high levels achieved in the lung. However, this discourages their use as first-line treatment for community-acquired lower respiratory tract infections. Levofloxacin is the first of a series of new-generation fluoroquinolones that have enhanced activity against pneumococci. Others are shortly to be licensed, or have been launched and then withdrawn because of unacceptable side effects. They are well absorbed after oral administration, resulting in peak serum levels close to those achieved after parenteral delivery, and they have relatively long half-lives in serum, allowing for once- or twice-daily administration. They penetrate lung tissue and bronchial mucosa and accumulate within cells, producing high concentrations. All these features make them excellent oral agents.

Adverse reactions to currently available fluoroquinolones are notably rare. Mild gastrointestinal disturbance, skin photosensitivity, headaches and dizziness are the most frequent. Seizures have also been reported. The most important interaction is with ciprofloxacin and theophylline, and the resulting toxicity is well recognised. As with all new oral antibiotics, fluoroquinolones are relatively expensive.

Current fluoroquinolones have a place as alternative choice in the oral therapy of Gram-negative enteric bacillary nosocomial pneumonias and for infective exacerbations of chronic obstructive airway disease where ampicillin-resistant *H. influenzae* is a possibility, or where treatment with preferred agents such as amoxicillin has failed. They also have a low propensity to cause *C. difficile* enteropathy and therefore have a place in institutions where this problem is endemic and is associated with excess β-lactam antibiotic use.

Antibiotic treatment of community-acquired pneumonia in adults

The few causes of community-acquired pneumonia make an initial, empirical and logical antibiotic choice relatively easy.[54] The antibiotic chosen must provide effective cover against pneumococcal infection, which is by far the most common cause. The decision whether to use oral or parenteral antibiotics is dictated largely by the severity of the illness and the patient's ability to swallow. Most patients with mild or moderate pneumonia can be managed with oral therapy but an understanding of the spectrum of activity, side-effect profile and pharmacokinetics is important.

Mild community-acquired pneumonia
Amoxicillin, taken orally, is well tolerated and effective. A macrolide is a sensible alternative in penicillin-allergic patients and is particularly appropriate if atypical or *Legionella* infection is suspected. For those requiring admission to hospital, a combination of macrolide and aminopenicillin provides appropriate empirical therapy. A fluoroquinolone with effective pneumococcal cover is an alternative choice. Additional antistaphylococcal agents, such as flucloxacillin, must be considered during influenza epidemics.

Severe community-acquired pneumonia
Initial antibiotics must cover all probable pathogens until the results of laboratory tests are available.[51,83] This includes pneumococcal, *Legionella*, staphylococcal (particularly during influenza epidemics) and *Haemophilus* pneumonias, as well as the atypical infections. A parenteral β-lactamase-stable penicillin (e.g. co-amoxiclav) or cephalosporin (e.g. cefuroxime, cefotaxime) together with a macrolide provide good initial cover for these pathogens. An additional antistaphylococcal agent such as flucloxacillin should be considered as well during periods of

influenza, or rifampicin added if *Legionella* is seriously considered. The antibiotics are adjusted appropriately depending on clinical response or if investigations identify a specific pathogen. The widespread use of parenteral cephalosporins has been linked to *C. difficile* antibiotic-associated enteropathy in many hospitals,[82] which has led to newer fluoroquinolones being used as alternative choices for community-acquired pneumonia. However, more experience is required before recommending newer fluoroquinolones alone: most clinicians add parenteral penicillin initially.

Response to treatment

The duration of therapy is usually 7–10 days, as guided by clinical improvement. Patients on parenteral therapy can usually be switched to oral antibiotics 24 hours after the temperature settles, providing absorption is considered satisfactory. Prolonged therapy is required if there is cavitation.

If recovery is unsatisfactory, a number of possibilities should be considered (Fig. 35.8).

Complications

Lung abscess and empyema are uncommon, occurring in around 1–5% of pneumonias. A sterile, high-protein, sympathetic effusion develops in up to a quarter of cases. It should always be sampled to exclude an empyema but usually resolves without other intervention.

The vast majority of patients recover completely but some degree of focal lung scarring or more diffuse fibrosis may follow severe pneumonia.

Management of community-acquired pneumonia in children

Severity assessment
Children with mild to moderate respiratory symptoms can be managed safely at home. Those with signs of severe disease should be admitted to hospital (Table 35.9).

A key indication for admission is hypoxaemia as demonstrated by oxygen saturation levels below 92%. Other indicators for admission to hospital are clinical signs of severe disease or a family incapable of appropriate observation and supervision of the child (Table 35.10).

General management in the community
Families of children who are well enough to be cared for at home need information on managing pyrexia, preventing dehydration and identifying any deterioration. The general practitioner should review the situation if the child is deteriorating or not improving after 48 hours treatment.

General management in hospital
Oxygen therapy should be given by nasal cannulae, headbox or face mask to maintain S_aO_2 above 92%. It is important to remember that agitation in children may be a sign of hypoxia. Severely affected children may be unable to maintain fluid intake. If a nasogastric tube is necessary, the smallest tube should be chosen and it should be passed up the narrower nostril. If intravenous fluids are needed, they should be given at 80% basal levels and

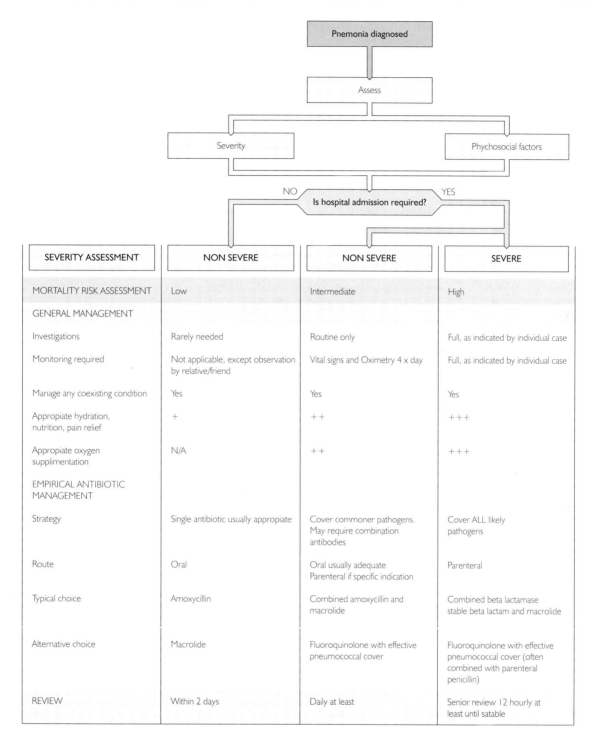

Fig. 35.8 A schema for the management of adult community acquired pneumonia.

serum electrolytes monitored as inappropriate ADH secretion is a recognised complication in severe pneumonia. Antipyretics and analgesics should be used for comfort and to permit coughing. Chest physiotherapy is not beneficial.

Transfer to intensive care
This should be considered when:

- The child is failing to maintain an oxygen saturation greater than 92% in F_iO_2 greater than 0.6;
- The child is in shock;

- There is a rising respiratory and rising pulse rate with clinical evidence of severe respiratory distress and exhaustion with or without a raised arterial P_{CO_2};
- There is recurrent apnoea or slow irregular breathing.

Antibiotic treatment

The above general discussion on antibiotic therapy applies equally to children and adults but there are some specific considerations in children.

Table 35.8 Factors to consider when a patient's response to initial therapy is poor (Adapted with permission from Macfarlane JT. In: Weatherall DJ et al, ed. Oxford textbook of medicine, 2nd ed. Oxford: Oxford University Press; 1986)

Factors	Action
Improvement expected too soon	Continued therapy – review again (common in elderly or debilitated)
Diagnosis of infective pneumonia incorrect	Review history, examination and data Consider differential diagnosis (e.g. pulmonary infarction)
Unexpected pathogen involved or pathogen resistant to antibiotic	Review history (e.g. ?travel abroad, seasonal factors, avian contact) Review microbiological data Consider alternative or invasive tests
Complicating lung disease (e.g. bronchial obstruction, bronchiectasis)	Review recent and past chest radiographs Consider bronchoscopy
Complicating generalised disease (e.g. primary or acquired immune deficiency, diabetes	Appropriate tests
Local intrathoracic complication (e.g. pleural effusion, empyema, lung abscess	Repeat chest radiograph Aspirate any pleural fluid
Metastatic infective complications (e.g. arthritis, meningitis, endocarditis)	Detailed clinical examination and appropriate tests
Persistent cause for pneumonia (e.g. aspiration, bacteraemia from distant focus)	Review history Repeat blood cultures
Secondary complications (e.g. intravenous cannula-related infection, venous thrombosis)	Detailed clinical examination
General factors (e.g. dehydration, nutrition, hypoxia)	Manage appropriately
Allergic reaction to antibiotics (often after several days of therapy)	Look for rash and recurrence of fever Consider stopping/changing antibiotic
Patient not actually receiving or taking the antibiotic	Check

Table 35.9 Features of severe pneumonia in children

		Mild	Severe
Infant		Temperature < 38.5°C	Temperature > 38.5°C
		Respiratory rate < 50	Respiratory rate > 70
		Mild recession	Moderate–severe recession
		Taking full feeds	Nasal flaring Cyanosis Intermittent apnoea Grunting respiration Not feeding
Older child		Temperature < 38.5°C	Temperature > 38.5°C
		Respiratory rate < 50	Respiratory rate > 50
		Mild breathlessness	Severe breathing difficulty
		No vomiting	Nasal flaring Cyanosis Grunting respiration Signs of dehydration

■ **Whether to give an antibiotic.** Much lower respiratory infection in children is viral and antibiotic therapy is of no benefit. Bacterial resistance to antibiotics is increasing and a factor contributing to this is overuse of antibiotics. A randomised controlled trial of antibiotics versus placebo in children aged less than 6 years with mild infection found no difference in outcome.[84] It is reasonable practice to avoid antibiotic treatment in young children with mild symptoms.

■ **Which antibiotic.** As treatment is almost invariably started before an organism is identified the choice of drug aims to select one that is effective against the majority of pathogens, well tolerated and cheap. Amoxicillin fulfils these criteria in young children. A macrolide would be an equally good choice in the school-age child, when atypical organisms are more prevalent.

■ **Which route.** In a large, adequately powered trial that compared intramuscular penicillin to oral amoxicillin in ambulatory patients, no difference in outcome was idenitifed.[85] The parenteral route should be reserved for cases where the child is severely ill or, where there are concerns about oral absorption (e.g. vomiting), the child should be switched to oral therapy when there is clear evidence of improvement.

Failure to improve and complications in children

If the child remains pyrexial and unwell 48 hours after admission to hospital, re-evaluation is necessary with consideration given to the following questions:

- Is the drug appropriate and the dosage adequate? There has been concern that the increasing prevalence of penicillin-resistant *S. pneumoniae* will lead to failure of treatment. However, a recent study provided no support for this: it was found that the serum concentration of penicillin or ampicillin achieved with standard intravenous dosages is much greater then the minimum inhibitory concentration (MIC) for most penicillin-resistant strains.[86]
- Are 'atypical' pathogens covered?
- Has the pneumonia been complicated by empyema or lung abscess? Parapneumonic effusions develop in approximately 40% of bacterial pneumonias admitted to hospital. Persistent pyrexia despite adequate antibiotic treatment should always lead the clinician to suspect the development of an empyema. Pleural fluid is evident on plain radiographs and the amount is best estimated by ultrasound. Any pleural effusion should be drained if pyrexia persists. Lung abscess is a rare complication in children. Suspicious features evident on plain chest radiographs may be confirmed by CT scan. Prolonged intravenous antibiotic therapy may be required but it is rare for other interventions to be necessary.
- Is there metastatic infection? This may develop in children, particularly with *S. aureus* infections, when osteomyelitis or septic arthritis should be considered.
- Is there immunodeficiency or suppression or coexistent disease such as cystic fibrosis?

Hospital-acquired pneumonia

Definition

Hospital-acquired pneumonia is one that develops 2 or more days after admission and was not incubating at the time of admission.

Incidence

In North America, hospital-acquired pneumonia occurs in 0.5–5% of hospitalised patients, accounts for 10–15% of all hospital-acquired infections and ranks third behind urinary tract infection and wound infection in order of frequency but first in terms of morbidity and mortality.[87-89]

Aetiology in adults and in children

The spectrum of pathogens encountered in nosocomial pneumonia is different from that in community-acquired cases but is affected by how soon after admission the pneumonia develops, any complicating factors and the severity of the infection[87] (Table 35.10).

In paediatric practice nosocomial viral transmission, particularly of RSV, is a major problem in open wards in winter. Scrupulous attention to hand-washing and segregation of patients are important preventative strategies. Gram negative

Table 35.10 Indications that a child with pneumonia needs to be admitted to hospital

Infants	Older children
$S_aO_2 \leq 92\%$, cyanosis	$S_aO_2 \leq 92\%$, cyanosis
Respiratory rate > 70/min	Respiratory rate > 50/min
Difficulty breathing	Difficulty breathing
Intermittent apnoea, grunting	Grunting
Not feeding	Signs of dehydration
Family not able to provide appropriate observation or supervision	Family not able to provide appropriate observation or supervision

organisms, particularly *Pseudomonas aeruginosa*, are responsible for most cases of ventilator-associated pneumonia.

Pathogenesis

Infection can arise in three ways: the aspiration of infected nasopharyngeal secretions, the inhalation of bacteria from contaminated respiratory equipment and haematogenous spread (Table 35.11). Broadly, there are three distinct steps in the pathogenesis of nosocomial pneumonia:

- The incidence of colonisation of the nasopharynx by aerobic Gram-negative bacilli increases dramatically in patients who are hospitalised, chronically ill or who have had recent broad-spectrum antibiotics.[90]
- There are several factors that increase the chance of microaspiration of nasopharyngeal or oesophageal secretions.[91,92]
- The physical and immunological defences of the lung are often impaired in hospitalised patients.[93]

Clinical features in adults

Hospital-acquired pneumonia usually presents with fever, purulent bronchopulmonary secretions, raised WBC and the appearance of new patchy opacification on the chest radiograph. Abscess formation can result from some Gram-negative enteric bacillary and anaerobic infections. Foul-smelling sputum or empyema fluid suggests anaerobic infection.

Investigations in adults

Finding the cause of the pneumonia is often difficult.[94,95] If blood, sputum and pleural fluid cultures are unhelpful, invasive techniques may be necessary to obtain useful lower respiratory secretions. Appropriate tests for *Legionella* pneumonia should be considered, if this infection is known to be a local problem.

Treatment in adults

Guidelines from North America[87,96] provide a logical approach to management but it is not known how applicable these are to

Table 35.11 Spectrum of pathogens and management to consider in adults with hospital-acquired pneumonia (HAP). (Adapted from American Thoracic Society Guidelines.[97])

(a) Non-severe HAP with no unusual risk factors and early-onset severe HAP

'Core' pathogens	'Core' antibiotics
Gram-negative Enterobacteriaceae	2nd- or 3rd-generation cephalosporins
Escherichia coli	*or*
Klebsiella spp.	beta-lactam + beta-lactamase inhibitor (e.g. co-amoxiclav)
Proteus spp.	*together with*
Serratia marcescens	if penicillin-allergic, fluoroquinolone
Enterobacter spp.	
'Usual' community pathogens	
Haemophilus influenzae	
Streptococcus pneumoniae	
Staphylococcus aureus (methicillin-sensitive)	

(b) Non-severe HAP with additional risk factors

Core pathogens plus:		Core antibiotics plus:
Pathogens	**Risk factor**	**Antibiotics**
Anaerobes	Recent thoracoabdominal surgery	Clindamycin
	Impaired swallowing	*or*
	Witnessed aspiration	beta-lactam + beta-lactamase inhibitor
	Dental sepsis	
Staphylococcus aureus	Coma	Consider adding vancomycin if
	Head trauma	methicillin-resistant *S. aureus* possible
	Neurosurgery	
	Diabetes mellitus	
	Renal failure	
Legionella spp.	High-dose corticosteroids	Erythromycin
	Organism endemic in hospital	± rifampicin
		± fluoroquinolone
Pseudomonas aeruginosa	Prior antibiotics	Treat as severe HAP (see below)
	High-dose corticosteroids	
	Prolonged ICU stay	
	Structural lung disease (e.g. bronchiectasis)	

(c) Severe HAP

Core pathogens plus:	Antibiotics
Pseudomonas aeruginosa	*Combination of:*
Acinetobacter spp.	aminoglycoside or ciprofloxacin
Methicillin-resistant *S. aureus* in some	*plus one of:*
hospitals – if early-onset, see **(a)**	antipseudomonal beta-lactamase stable beta-lactam antibiotic
	meropenem
	± vancomycin

hospital-acquired pneumonia in other countries. Antibiotic therapy is directed at the 'core' pathogens, as well as any 'additional' pathogens that may be present (see Table 35.10). Physiotherapy is important in clearing respiratory secretions, both prophylactically in those patients at risk and also once nosocomial pneumonia has developed.

Prevention[97]

Important preventive measures include cessation of smoking before the operation, early postoperative mobilisation, scrupulous care of respiratory equipment, use of disposable endotracheal tubes and suction catheters, elimination of unnecessary instrumentation of the respiratory tract, and strict attention to hospital staff hygiene, including hand-washing between patients.[98,99] Judicious use of antibiotics throughout the hospital and monitoring of infection control in high-risk areas, such as intensive care units, are also important. Local selective decontamination of the upper respiratory and gastrointestinal tracts has been successfully used to reduce colonisation with Gram-negative enteric bacilli. Meta-analyses of randomised controlled trials indicate that selective decontamination reduces infection rates, but no definite effect on mortality rates was reported.[100,101]

Aspiration and anaerobic pneumonia

The most frequent conditions associated with aspiration pneumonia are impaired consciousness and dysphagia. Problems can include aspiration of solid material, gastric juice, lipid and bacteria.

Bacteriology

Aspiration contaminates the lower respiratory tract with a complex bacterial flora. In community cases, multiple anaerobes from the oropharynx and teeth crevices are the principal pathogens in over two-thirds of cases and pure aerobic infections occur in less than 10% of cases. Anaerobic infection is rare in edentulous patients.[102,103] In contrast, in hospital-acquired infections anaerobes are the sole pathogen in only 17–22% of cases, around half are mixed infections and in a quarter to a third only aerobic bacteria are present, principally Gram-negative enteric bacilli and *P. aeruginosa*, both related to nasopharyngeal colonisation. The important anaerobes include the Gram-positive anaerobic cocci *Peptostreptococcus* and *Peptococcus* spp. and Gram-negative bacilli of *Fusobacteroides* and *Bacteroides* spp., the latter often being penicillin-resistant.

Clinical features

In the presence of aspiration pneumonia the clinical picture may be dominated by the features of acid inhalation causing pulmonary oedema or particulate matter causing airway obstruction or infection. Where anaerobic infection is predominant four types of pleuropulmonary syndromes can be seen: anaerobic bacterial pneumonia, necrotising pneumonia (Fig. 35.9), lung abscess and empyema.

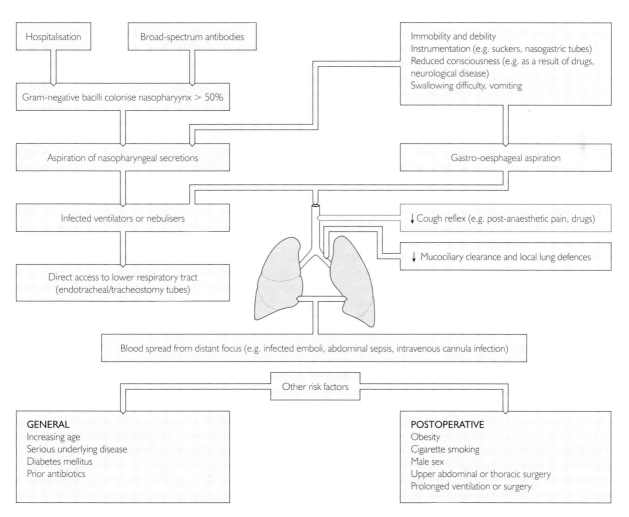

Fig. 35.9 Factors involved in the pathogenesis of hospital acquired pneumonia. Reproduced with permission from Macfarlane JT. Med Int 1986; 36: 1498–1506.

Diagnosis

There are usually clues to the diagnosis, including some predisposition to aspiration, poor dental hygiene, subacute onset, foul sputum, abscess or empyema formation, or infection developing beyond a bronchial carcinoma or in previously damaged or bronchiectatic lung. The presence of multiple Gram-positive cocci and Gram-negative bacilli in sputum or pleural fluid that is sterile on aerobic culture is also suggestive.[104]

Management

For community-acquired cases of aspiration or anaerobic infection, combined parenteral penicillin and metronidazole, or clindamycin monotherapy, is appropriate.

For hospital-acquired cases it is essential also to cover for Gram-negative enteric bacilli by adding an aminoglycoside, a third-generation cephalosporin or a fluoroquinolone. Prolonged therapy is often necessary.

Prognosis

The mortality can be high, often reflecting the severity of the predisposing disease.

Lipoid (lipid) pneumonia

This is a form of aspiration pneumonia, whereby inhaled lipid incites lung inflammation. It is uncommon as the usual agent, liquid paraffin, is now rarely used as a laxative.

Recurrent pneumonia

Recurrent pneumonia is defined as three or more separate attacks of pneumonia in one patient. Pneumonia recurring in one part of the lung suggests a localised bronchopulmonary abnormality; when it recurs in different sites a more generalised disorder is likely. In the former a local bronchial obstruction or local bronchopulmonary disease (e.g. pulmonary sequestration, localised bronchiectasis, carnified lung from chronic pneumonia) should be suspected. When pneumonia recurs in different sites a more generalised disorder is likely, such as bronchiectasis, cystic fibrosis, primary ciliary dyskinesia, chronic sinusitis with postnasal drip, recurrent aspiration due to neuromuscular and oesophageal problems (Fig. 35.10) and immunodeficiency states. Repeated pulmonary emboli may present as a recurrent pneumonia.

Pneumonias peculiar to specific geographical areas

Specific bacterial, viral, fungal and protozoal infections have to be considered in patients who have visited or live in certain parts of the world. Examples include typhoid pneumonia in the tropics, histoplasmosis in the USA,[105] paragonomiasis[106] or melioidosis in the Far East[107] and tularaemia in the USA, Scandinavia and central Europe. Details of some of these can be found later in this chapter.

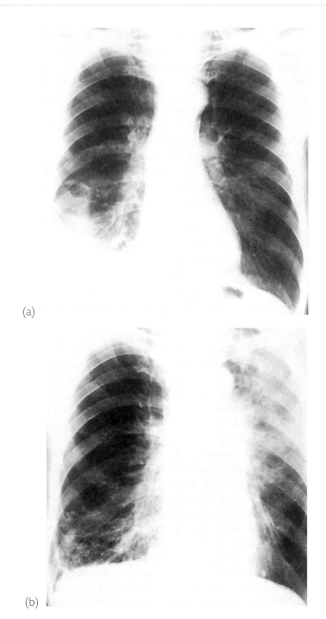

(a)

(b)

Fig. 35.10 (a) Chest radiograph of a 60-year-old man presenting with an anaerobic right lower lobe pneumonia. *Streptococcus milleri* was isolated from his bronchial aspirate. (b) Six months later, he presented with left upper lobe pneumonia. A subsequent barium swallow showed gastro-oesophageal reflux and silent aspiration. There were no further pneumonias after gastric fundoplication.

Specific respiratory pathogens

This section provides specific details of commoner respiratory bacterial, atypical and viral pathogens. Details of fungal, mycobacterial, protozoal and parasitic infections will be found elsewhere in this book.

Common bacterial pathogens

These include Gram-positive cocci and Gram-negative cocci and bacilli.

Gram-positive cocci

Streptococcus pneumoniae

This is the most common bacterium to cause pulmonary infection in adults and is still associated with significant morbidity and mortality in spite of apparently effective antibiotics.

Microbial characteristics

The growth requirements are best met by blood agar at pH 7.4 in an enriched carbon dioxide medium. Virulent strains form glistening, dome-shaped colonies with characteristic umbilicated centres. Pneumococci can be differentiated from other viridans streptococci by their sensitivity to Optochin and lysis in the presence of bile. The Quellung reaction, sometimes employed for rapid identification, depends on the fact that the capsule swells when mixed with specific antisera – a reaction that can be identified quickly on a slide under oil immersion.

So far, at least 90 serotypes of pneumococci have been recognised, on the basis of the specific antigenic composition of the pneumococcal polysaccharide capsule. However, only a small proportion are involved in most infections.

Epidemiology

The human nasopharynx is the natural habitat of the pneumococcus. There is no recognised animal or environmental reservoir and spread is by droplet. Both carriage and clinical disease peak in the winter and early spring months in temperate climates but in tropical countries are most frequent during the hot dry time of the year. Viral infections increase the carriage rate of pneumococci.[108] Carriage rates of up to 50% can be found in healthy individuals. Most disease is sporadic, occurring in asymptomatic carriers whose local defence mechanisms are impaired for some reason, but outbreaks occur in overcrowded living areas.[109]

Pathology

The initial response to pneumococci dividing in the alveolar spaces is capillary congestion and an outpouring of protein-rich fluid followed by neutrophils filling the affected alveoli. This is the stage of red hepatisation described by Laennec in 1834. Later, the congestion subsides and fibrin in the alveoli contracts so that the lung is soft and lemon-yellow and exudes purulent fluid on cutting. This is the stage of grey hepatisation. Remarkably, the affected lobe can recover completely, both anatomically and functionally.

Pathogenicity

The polysaccharide capsule is the main determinant of pathogenicity (Fig. 35.11). The capsule impairs phagocytosis, which is in any case very dependent on the appearance of anticapsular antibodies to aid opsonisation after 5–7 days of infection. Those with impaired antibody production or complement activation, such as patients with hypogammaglobulinaemia, lymphoma or hyposplenia, are at particular risk of pneumococcal infection.

Clinical features

The onset of illness is abrupt, with rigors, high fever, malaise, tachycardia and tachypnoea, and a cough that is dry or productive of sticky pink sputum developing over a few hours. Focal crackles are more common than bronchial breathing. Herpetic cold sores are seen in over a third of cases. This classic pattern is less commonly seen now than 100 years ago when described by Sir William Osler. Today, the illness may be modified into a less acute presentation resulting from partially effective antibiotics.

Diagnostic tests

The diagnosis of pneumococcal pneumonia can be confidently made if pneumococci are detected in the blood, pleural fluid or lung secretions of a patient with pneumonia. In practice, however, lung secretions or pleural fluid may not be available and blood cultures are only positive in 20% of cases. If sufficient pneumococci are present in a good sputum sample to show up as the predominant organism in a Gram stain, this is highly specific for pneumococcal pneumonia, but the sensitivity is low, at 10%. A positive sputum culture has less specificity but can be taken as reasonable evidence of pneumococcal infection in a patient with pneumonia.

Pneumococcal capsular polysaccharide antigen can be detected readily in biological samples, even after antibiotics, by simple immunological tests such as countercurrent immunoelectrophoresis and latex agglutination[110,111] and, if present in

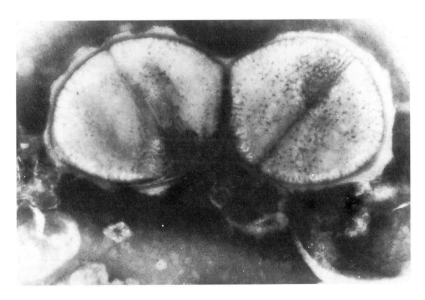

Fig. 35.11 Negatively stained preparation (1% phosphotungstic acid) of pairs of *Streptococcus pneumoniae*, showing their prominent capsules. Courtesy of Dr TSJ Elliot.

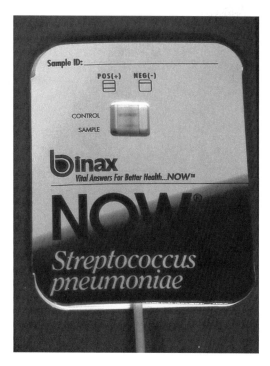

Fig. 35.12 A clear precipitation line shows up in the test window 15 minutes after priming the 'bedside' test kit with urine from a patient with pneumococcal pneumonia and test reagent. The diagnosis was confirmed subsequently by blood culture.

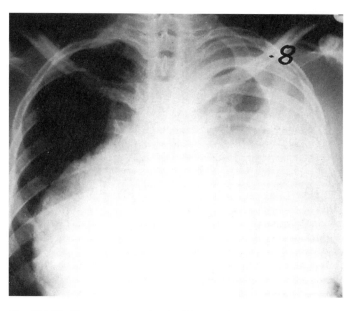

Fig. 35.13 Chest radiograph of a 20-year-old man who presented with acute pneumonia and the signs of tamponade. Pneumococci were cultured from the 2 litres of pus drained from the pericardial sac and left pleural effusion.

serum, urine and pleural fluid, provides firm evidence of active infection. Few laboratories offer antigen testing by countercurrent immunoelectrophoresis because it is time-consuming, but new bedside slide agglutination kits using urine are promising aids to early diagnosis (Fig. 35.12).

General diagnostic tests

The white blood cell count is raised in most patients. In over three-quarters of cases, the chest radiograph reveals homogeneous consolidation and in up to a third of cases a pleural effusion is present. Two or more lobes are involved in a third of cases at presentation. Spread of the consolidation may occur despite apparently effective therapy, particularly in severe disease.

Complications

Extrapulmonary spread of the infection to the pleura, pericardium, meninges, joints, peritoneum and endocardium is occasionally seen (Fig. 35.13). Type 3 infection is sometimes associated with abscess formation or lung scarring.

Treatment

Most strains are very sensitive to penicillin, with MICs of 0.02 mg/l or less, and the response of patients with pneumococcal pneumonia to penicillin is often dramatic. However there have been worrying developments, with clinical isolates of *S. pneumoniae* showing decreased penicillin sensitivity and, in many cases, multiple antibiotic resistance being reported worldwide. There is wide geographical variation, with intermediate (MIC 0.1–1 mg/l) and high (MIC > 1 mg/l) resistance being reported frequently in North America and countries of Mediterranean and eastern Europe.[112-115]

Assessment of the situation in the UK is dependent on isolates reported by the public health laboratories. The level of intermediate and high resistance in 1998 was around 2% for penicillin, similar for tetracycline and over 10% for macrolides.[54] Much higher levels of macrolide resistance are reported in other countries, especially France.

Reported experience suggests that infections caused by pneumococci with intermediate resistance respond normally to penicillin, although higher doses may be needed. For highly-resistant pneumococci, cefotaxime, ceftriaxone and vancomycin are recommended.[114-116]

Cephalosporins and erythromycin are effective alternatives in penicillin-hypersensitive patients, although 8–15% of such patients will also show cross-sensitivity to cephalosporins and erythromycin resistance is an increasing problem. All pneumococci are resistant to aminoglycosides .

Prevention

The available 23-valent pneumococcal vaccine covers nearly 90% of adult types, nearly 100% of types causing severe illness in children and 85% of strains involved in otitis media. The efficacy of pneumococcal immunisation has been proved conclusively in studies of healthy individuals with a high incidence of pneumococcal disease in South African gold mines and also in New Guinea.[117,118] However, for those at increased risk of pneumococcal infection and its complications, the evidence is less convincing.[119] Current recommendations in the UK suggest that immunisation should be offered to all those over the age of 2 years in whom pneumococcal infection is likely to be common and/or dangerous. These include homozygous sickle-cell disease patients (often together with penicillin prophylaxis), before planned splenectomy, a month or so after unplanned splenectomy and in those with impaired splenic function, chronic renal disease, immunodeficiency or immunosuppression due to disease or treatment, including HIV infection, chronic cardio-respiratory disease, chronic liver disease and diabetes.

Immunisation is given subcutaneously or preferably intra-muscularly as a single injection and appears to be safe, causing a mild localised reaction in most, a systemic reaction in 1% and a severe reaction rarely. Protection appears to last for several years in healthy adults but for shorter periods in patients with poor immune function. Re-immunisation is not normally advised and is contraindicated within 3 years. There is no impairment of antibody response when given at the same time as influenza immunisation.[120]

Streptococcus pyogenes

Epidemiology and pathogenesis
Infection occurs in the winter from spread by droplets from the nasopharynx in crowded conditions, often following viral infection. It is most common in children and young adults.[121] A number of enzymes, toxins and haemolysins are produced, which enhance pathogenicity and lead to bronchopneumonia with reddening and ulceration of the entire respiratory tract, microabscess formation and characteristic early pleural involvement.

Clinical features
The onset is usually rapid with rigors, cough, bloody sputum, pleural pain and pneumonia. The striking characteristic is early empyema formation, which is initially serous but rapidly becomes purulent, fibrinous and difficult to drain.

Diagnostic tests
Diagnosis depends on isolation of group A β-haemolytic strepto-cocci from sputum, blood (only 12% of cases) or pleural fluid. Most patients have a raised antistreptolysin O titre at a later stage.

Treatment
High-dose parenteral penicillin or a cephalosporin is necessary. Tube drainage of the purulent empyema is usually required.

Staphylococcus aureus

Microbial characteristics
Staphylococci are catalase-producing, Gram-positive cocci that cluster, like bunches of grapes. They grow well on solid medium and are subdivided into *S. aureus* and the less patho-genic *S. epidermidis*.

Epidemiology
Although *S. aureus* causes less than 5% of all pneumonia its importance exceeds this in view of the high mortality and mor-bidity even in previously healthy individuals. The organism infects humans primarily, infection occurring by autoinoculation in carriers or spread of infection to others. Around 30% of adults carry *S. aureus* in their anterior nares.

Pathogenicity
The production of toxins and aggressins results in extensive tissue necrosis and abscess formation. Necrosis is aided by small-vessel thrombosis. Most patients with overwhelming staphylo-coccal infection have an obvious pre-existing acute (e.g. influenza virus infection) or chronic defect of host defence.

Clinical features
In children, staphylococcal pneumonia normally follows mild viral respiratory illness with rapid deterioration over a few days, associated with tachypnoea and cyanosis. Empyema and pneu-mothorax are common and pneumatoceles may be apparent on the chest radiograph.

In adults staphylococcal pneumonia usually follows influenza virus infection at a time when the patient appears to be improv-ing from influenza. There may be very rapid onset of fever, toxaemia, confusion and respiratory distress. Associated staphy-lococcal skin lesions may sometimes be seen. Those with chronic cardiopulmonary disease are especially at risk. The chest radiograph usually shows scattered patchy infiltrates with pneu-matoceles and abscess formation in a quarter and empyema in around 10% (Fig. 35.14).

Staphylococcal pneumonia may also occur secondary to a bacteraemia from a distant site, sometimes related to infected intravenous cannulae, intravenous drug abuse or right-sided endocarditis.

Diagnostic tests
At least 25% of cases have positive blood cultures. Sputum smear showing many large, round, Gram-positive cocci in clus-ters, with some intracellular organisms, is highly suggestive and can be helpful in over two-thirds of cases. Pleural fluid should always be sampled because the effusion is more often than not infected.

Treatment
Penicillinase-producing strains are now nearly universal, so stan-dard initial therapy for staphylococcal pneumonia is with β-lactamase-resistant penicillins such as flucloxacillin. Fusidic acid, rifampicin and cephalosporins also have good activity. MRSA strains are increasingly encountered in hospital-associated staphylococcal infection and should also be considered in those

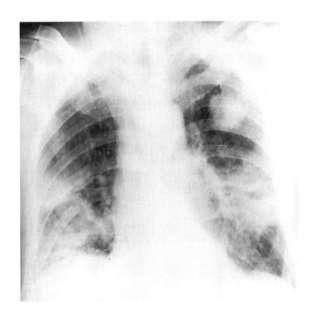

Fig. 35.14 Chest radiograph of a 70-year-old man with staphylococcal pneumonia, showing multifocal consolidation and abscess formation.

admitted from nursing homes. Vancomycin is the treatment of choice for most MRSA strains.

The mortality rate remains high, at around 30% but up to 70% in the presence of bacteraemia. The response to antibiotics is often slow, partly as a result of reduced antibiotic penetration into avascular and necrotic areas so that cultures from clinical specimens can remain positive for several days after treatment starts.[122] This suggests that treatment should continue for longer than is usual for pneumonia, probably for 2–4 weeks.

Prevention
Good hygiene and hand-washing strategies are easy, cheap and effective at reducing *S. aureus* cross-infection. Efforts to reduce carriage by using local nasal antibiotics are usually unsuccessful.

Gram-negative bacteria

Moraxella catarrhalis

This organism was formerly called *Branhamella* or *Neisseria catarrhalis* and is now recognised as the third most common bacterial cause of sinusitis, otitis media (especially in children) and bronchitis in adults, but falling considerably behind *S. pneumoniae* and *H. influenzae* in frequency.

Microbial characteristics
The organisms are Gram-negative diplococci that are sometimes seen within sputum leukocytes. The best growth is obtained with selective media and some laboratories do not report positive cultures as being significant.

Epidemiology
One large survey found that, in healthy adults, the carrier rate was 5% compared with 50% in children and 26% in people older than 60 years.[123] Infection is more common in winter. Nosocomial outbreaks of infection are well recognised, especially in wards dealing with patients with chronic lung disease.

Clinical features
The typical clinical picture is that of purulent tracheobronchitis or patchy lower lobe pneumonia in an elderly patient with underlying chronic obstructive pulmonary disease, malignancy or immunosuppression who has not improved with an aminopenicillin.[124,125] The appreciable mortality is partly related to the pre-existing disease.

Diagnostic tests
The diagnosis is usually made by a combination of a positive sputum Gram stain and culture using dilution techniques. Pleural fluid and blood cultures are rarely positive.

Treatment
Most strains are now ampicillin-resistant and treatment with co-amoxiclav, cephalosporins, macrolides or quinolones is required.

Haemophilus influenzae

H. influenzae is an uncommon cause of bacterial pneumonia in adults.

Microbial characteristics
The organisms are small, Gram-negative, pleomorphic rods, which can vary from coccobacilli to long filamentous rods.

Pathogenic strains are usually encapsulated and divided into six serological types (a–f). Type b is the most frequent cause of epiglottitis, bacteraemia, meningitis and pneumonia in children, and non-capsulated types usually cause bronchopulmonary disease in adults.

Epidemiology
Non-capsulated *H. influenzae* is frequently recovered from the upper respiratory tract of healthy individuals and in over half of specimens of mucoid sputum from patients with chronic simple bronchitis.

Pathogenesis
Infection occurs by either aspiration of organisms from the upper respiratory tract or by inhalation of infected droplets from a carrier. Resistance to infection depends on effective bronchopulmonary defences and specific antibody.

Clinical features
In the bacteraemic form it presents as a severe infection with a significant mortality in previously debilitated people. Non-typable strains more commonly cause patchy bronchopneumonia, which may present in a subacute manner with persistent purulent sputum, fevers and malaise.[126]

Diagnostic tests
A confident diagnosis requires isolation of the organism from blood, pleural fluid, transtracheal or lung aspirate. Sputum culture may be misleading because of the high incidence of carriage. A positive Gram stain is more convincing.[127]

Treatment
Ampicillin derivatives are the drug of choice for susceptible strains. However, there is increasing ampicillin resistance as a result of plasmid-mediated β-lactamase production. The incidence of resistant strains in the UK reported in 1999 varied widely (2–17%) and is higher in other parts of Europe.[112,113] Other effective agents include quinolones, co-amoxiclav and cephalosporins.

Legionella pneumophila

The outbreak of a severe pneumonic illness among the Pennsylvanian branch of the American Legion in July 1976 led to the description of legionnaires' disease. Subsequently a Gram-negative bacillus was isolated from the lung of a legionnaire and named *Legionella pneumophila*. It has subsequently been shown to be a significant cause of both community- and hospital-acquired infections, both sporadically and in epidemics.[54]

Microbial characteristics
Legionella pneumophila is a short, flagellated bacillus that takes Gram counterstain very poorly and does not grow on ordinary media, requiring specific buffered charcoal yeast extract agar with growth appearing in 2–4 days. Numerous serogroups of *L. pneumophila* have now been identified but most infections are caused by serogroup 1. In addition, numerous other *Legionella* spp. have been identified. Of these *L. micdadei*, *L. bozemanni* and *L. dumoffii*, among others, sometimes cause pneumonia.

Epidemiology
Legionella organisms are ubiquitous in water. They have been isolated from almost every water system that has been tested,

including such diverse sites as rivers, lakes, muddy pools, thermal springs, under ice, in tropical rain forests, irrigation sprinklers, industrial coolant fluids and circulating water in both large buildings and domestic systems. The organism is sensitive to drying but can survive in tap water at room temperature for longer than a year. There is no human or animal reservoir, although algae or free-living amoebae may act as hosts.

Epidemic and endemic infections have been particularly associated with new buildings such as hospitals and hotels.[129] A chain of events is necessary before *Legionella* infection is likely to occur. First, there must be an environmental reservoir where the legionellae live. This is most commonly hot water systems or cooling towers. Second, there must be amplification factors such as stagnation, dirt and sludge, which allow legionellae to grow from low to high concentrations at a temperature ideally between 20°C and 45°C. Fan-assisted cooling systems, defective air-conditioning systems, showers, respiratory therapy equipment and possibly spray taps can then all nebulise and disseminate infected droplets, which may be inhaled in sufficient quantity into the alveoli of a susceptible host, where pathogenic bacteria can lead to infection.

Legionella pneumonia appears in three forms: as explosive epidemics, as endemic infection or most commonly as sporadic cases. Epidemics and endemics are commonly associated with specific buildings but, in contrast, sporadic cases have been reported throughout the world. Such cases are much more common during the summer months, which is only part explained by increased foreign travel and hotel holidays.[130]

Pathogenesis

The organisms are facultative intracellular pathogens and are engulfed by macrophages in the lung alveoli, where they resist destruction by releasing secretory enzymes and toxins, and multiply intracellularly with subsequent destruction of the macrophage when bacteria and toxic products are released and further cellular invasion occurs (Fig. 35.15).

Clinical features

Legionella infection manifests itself in two forms, either as Pontiac fever or as *Legionella* pneumonia (legionnaires' disease).[131,132] It is not known why different forms occur but they probably reflect the differing virulence of *Legionella* strains and also host factors. Pontiac fever, named after an outbreak in Pontiac, Michigan, in 1968, is characterised by an acute, self-limiting, flu-like illness without pneumonia. The incubation period is only 24–48 hours and the attack rate of those exposed is over 90%. This type of illness, which is rarely diagnosed, may explain the seropositivity found in population screening.

Legionella pneumonia is the more usual form. It is three times more common in men than in women, with the highest incidence in 40–70-year-olds. People at special risk include smokers, alcoholics, diabetics and those on immunosuppressive drugs. The incubation period is up to 14 days. A wide spectrum of clinical presentation exists, from a mild respiratory illness to fulminating pneumonia.[133] Typically, the illness starts abruptly with high fever, rigors, malaise and myalgia and often trivial cough. Severe headache, confusion and delirium occur in more than half of the patients and can dominate the clinical picture, masking the true diagnosis of pneumonia. Focal neurological,

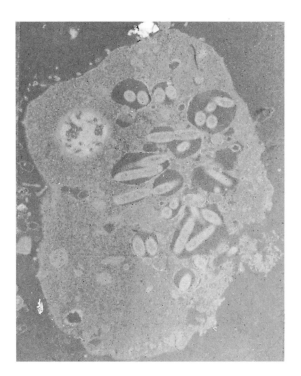

Fig. 35.15 Ultrathin section of a neutrophil containing numerous *Legionella pneumophila* bacteria intact within vacuoles where they can multiply, protected from antimicrobial agents. Courtesy of Dr TSJ Elliott.

particularly cerebellar, signs are well described; amnesia on recovery is common. Some patients have marked diarrhoea, abdominal pain or a tender liver.

The white count is usually less than 15.0×10^9/l. Features of multisystem involvement are found in about 50% of cases, with hyponatraemia, abnormal liver function tests, hypoalbuminaemia, raised blood urea, raised muscle enzymes, haematuria and proteinuria. Initial blood and sputum Gram stain and cultures are negative.

Radiological shadowing is usually homogeneous and unilobar on presentation. But deterioration often occurs after treatment has started with increasing opacification, both within the same lung and to the opposite lung (Fig. 35.16). Clearance in survivors is particularly slow, with only 60% being clear by 3 months (see Fig. 35.5).

Diagnostic tests

The diagnosis has traditionally been made by detecting a rise in specific antibodies by the indirect fluorescent antibody test, by direct fluorescent antibody staining of the organism in lower respiratory secretions and lung tissue, and by culture. Rapid urine antigen tests for soluble *Legionella* antigen are increasingly available and are extremely useful and can provide an answer within a short time. Soluble antigen is excreted in the urine for 1–3 weeks during the acute pneumonia, and longer in immunocompromised patients, and its detection has a high specificity and sensitivity, particularly for *L. pneumophila* serogroup 1.[134,135] Although not all laboratories offer these tests routinely, they should be requested in all patients with severe pneumonia and where there is the possibility of *Legionella* infection from epidemiological evidence.

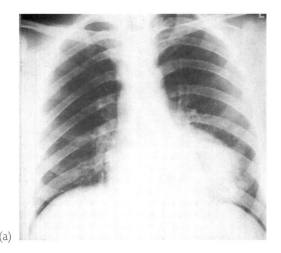

(a)

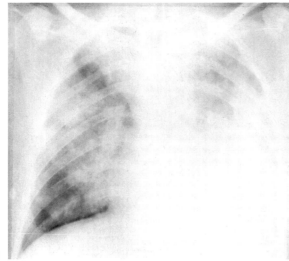

(b)

Fig. 35.16 (a) Admission chest radiograph of a previously fit 31-year-old man with *Legionella pneumophila* serogroup 1 pneumonia. Reproduced with permission from Macfarlane JT. Legionnaires' disease. Practitioner 1983; 227: 1707–1718. (b) Four days later – marked radiographic deterioration in spite of intravenous erythromycin. The patient required mechanical ventilation but recovered well.

Treatment

Suitable antibiotics must be capable of penetrating the alveolar macrophages and neutrophils where the organisms are dividing (see Fig. 35.15). There are no controlled clinical trials but reported experience suggests that macrolides, fluoroquinolones and rifampicin are the best antibiotics.[54,136,137] Respiratory failure is not infrequent with *Legionella* pneumonia, and assisted ventilation and intensive care management can be life-saving.

Prevention

The diagnosis of two or more cases together should prompt seeking expert epidemiological help from the local Public Health Department to investigate a possible source. Implicated water systems should be thoroughly cleaned and sterilised as far as possible with hyperchlorination and heating. Good engineer-

ing design and maintenance are essential to prevent legionellae from multiplying in water systems.

Complications

A large number of complications have been reported (Table 35.12).[133]

Gram-negative enteric bacillary infections

Aerobic Gram-negative enteric bacillary infections are frequently the cause of hospital-acquired respiratory infections, particularly in those who are debilitated. The bacteria usually involved include *P. aeruginosa*, *Acinetobacter calcoaceticus* and Enterobacteriaceae.[138] The latter family includes *Klebsiella pneumoniae*, *Escherichia coli*, *Enterobacter* spp., *Proteus* spp. and *Serratia marcescens*, and are normal commensals in the bowel. They all cause similar disease in similar situations.

Table 35.12 Some reported complications of *Legionella* pneumonia

Respiratory	Acute respiratory failure	+++
	Lung cavitation	++
	Lung fibrosis	++
Cardiovascular	Pericarditis + effusion	++
	Myocarditis	++
	Endocarditis	+
	Arteriovenous fistula infection	+
Neurological	Encephalomyelitis	++
	Cerebellar involvement	+++
	Guillain–Barré syndrome	++
	Motor neuropathy	++
Musculoskeletal	Myositis	+++
	Rhabdomyolysis	++
	Arthropathy	+
Renal	Acute renal failure	++
	Interstitial nephritis	+
	Glomerulonephritis	+
Gastrointestinal	Focal gut infection	+
	Paralytic ileus	+
	Jaundice	+
	Pancreatitis	+
Others	Skin rashes	+
	Pancytopenia	+
	Thrombocytopenia	++
	Lymph node involvement	+

+++, several reports; ++ uncommon; +, very rare.

Pseudomonas aeruginosa

This is a common cause of hospital-acquired pneumonia in neutropenic patients or those with severe pneumonia or on an intensive care unit, but is uncommon in community cases.

Microbial characteristics

P. aeruginosa is a Gram-negative, non-sporing, motile bacillus that produces two pigments, which are responsible for the blue-green colour of pus and cultures. A number of bacterial enzymes are produced that are important in pathogenesis and the cell wall is protected by a polysaccharide slime layer.

Epidemiology

The organism is ubiquitous in the environment, particularly in water, vegetation and soil. Humans are not a major habitat but almost any loss of health is associated with increased carriage. The organism also thrives in damp environments and is usually part of the hospital flora. Spread among patients occurs primarily from the hands of hospital personnel.

Pathogenesis

Infection usually reaches the lung by aspiration from the upper respiratory tract but may be secondary to bacteraemia from an extrapulmonary focus. Histologically, there is colonisation of arterial walls leading to vasculitis, thrombosis and necrosis as well as pneumonic consolidation.

Clinical features

Pseudomonas pneumonia presents with an acute toxic illness, often with abscess formation (Fig. 35.17) or a complicating effusion or empyema. Ecthyma gangrenosum may be seen in bacteraemic cases. Sometimes the infection is limited to the tracheobronchial tree, just causing a purulent bronchial infection, particularly in those on assisted ventilation or with cystic fibrosis or bronchiectasis.

Treatment

Standard treatment usually includes a combination of an aminoglycoside and an antipseudomonal penicillin or cephalosporin (e.g.

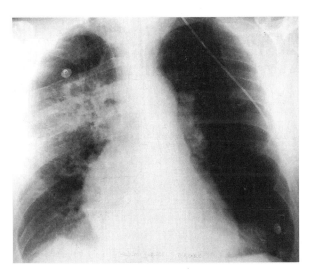

Fig. 35.17 Acute cavitating right upper lobe pneumonia caused by *Pseudomonas aeruginosa* developing in a man being ventilated on an intensive care unit.

piperacillin or ceftazidime), or ciprofloxacin. Single-agent therapy is associated with the emergence of resistance. Ciprofloxacin has the advantage of oral administration, but the emergence of resistance is a problem.

Acinetobacter spp.

This Gram-negative, non-motile, coccobacillary organism is commonly found in soil, fresh water, on the skin and occasionally in the throat. All pulmonary infections are nosocomial and are the result of *Acinetobacter calcoaceticus* var. *antitratus*, particularly in patients on ventilators. The chest radiograph usually shows multilobed infiltrates. Bacteraemia is infrequent and diagnosis is made on repeated positive sputum or tracheal cultures.

The organism is usually resistant to cephalosporins, ampicillin and chloramphenicol but a combination of an aminoglycoside and an antipseudomonal penicillin is normally used initially.

Enterobacteriaceae

Epidemiology and clinical features

These Gram-negative enteric bacilli have similar epidemiological and clinical features. They are usually associated with pneumonia acquired in hospital. Debilitated patients are at risk, as are alcoholics, diabetics and those with chronic lung disease. *E. coli* and *Proteus* spp. may also arise from urinary sepsis. *K. pneumoniae* also causes community acquired pneumonia and is reported to be the most frequent cause of severe community adult pneumonia in South Africa.

All tend to cause a lobar pneumonia that not infrequently cavitates.

Treatment

This should be guided by sensitivity patterns, but Enterobacteriaceae are usually sensitive to cephalosporins, aminoglycosides, the broad-spectrum carbapenems and quinolones, although an empirical choice will depend on the local prevalence of resistant strains.

Less usual bacteria

The following section describes features of bacterial infections that are unusual either because they are encountered only in specific areas of the world or because the respiratory tract may sometimes be affected but only as part of the overall illness.

Melioidosis

Infection with *Burkholderia pseudomallei* is widespread in the Far East.[107,139,140] It was first described in 1912 in Rangoon by Whitmore and Krishnaswami. The motile, Gram-negative rod grows well on most media and shows characteristic bipolar staining properties.

Epidemiology

The infection is endemic in humid tropical climates. The organism is a natural saprophyte in stagnant water and infection is acquired by inhalation, abrasion or ingestion, with no intermediate hosts. Asymptomatic infection is very common and clinical disease may appear many years later. Antibodies have been found in over a quarter of asymptomatic subjects in Thailand and up to 7% of US servicemen returning from south-east Asia. It is the commonest cause of severe community pneumonia in Singapore.[107]

Clinical features

Melioidosis can present abruptly as an acute septicaemic illness with high fever, cavitating pneumonia and abscesses throughout the body (Fig. 35.18). Subacute or chronic melioidosis is more common than the acute disease and presents typically as an unresolving pneumonia, which may closely resemble pulmonary tuberculosis. The condition should be considered in patients from south-east Asia in whom tuberculosis cannot be identified in the sputum. The chest radiograph usually shows widespread nodules with early cavitation.

Diagnostic tests and treatment

Sputum, pus and blood cultures are frequently positive but the bacteriologist should be warned of the possibility of melioidosis. Serological tests are helpful if there is a fourfold rise in antibody level but levels may remain high for many years, thus complicating later interpretation. Treatment is guided by sensitivities but tetracyclines, sulphonamides, chloramphenicol, co-trimoxazole and third-generation cephalosporins are generally appropriate. Prolonged therapy for 2–4 months is usually necessary, initially with two drugs, but relapses occur.

Pasteurella multocida

This is a small Gram-negative bacillus that is part of the normal flora of the upper respiratory tract of many domestic and wild animals. Local infection in humans, which is sometimes severe, can occur at the site of a bite or scratch. The organism has also been isolated from the respiratory tract of patients with established lung disease, such as bronchiectasis. It can be difficult to decide if the organism is acting as a commensal or as a pathogen, although definite infections with lung abscess and empyema

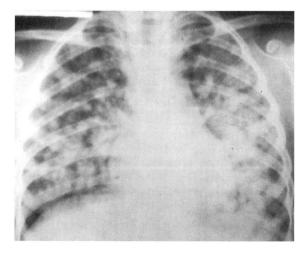

Fig. 35.18 Chest radiograph of a Thai girl admitted with shock and severe pneumonia. *Burkholderia pseudomallei* was grown from her blood cultures. Courtesy of Dr S Looareesuwan.

formation are well recorded.[141] It is usually sensitive to penicillins, cephalosporins and tetracyclines.

Tularaemia

Tularaemia is common in parts of northern Europe and North America. It was first described in 1907 by Martin, who observed five patients with disease attributable to skinning and dressing wild rabbits.

Microbial characteristics

Francisella tularensis is a small, pleomorphic, Gram-negative, non-motile, obligate anaerobe that appears as short rods or coccobacilli.

Epidemiology

F. tularensis is widely distributed throughout North America, central Europe, Japan and Scandinavia.[142] About 200 cases of tularaemia are reported each year in the USA. Infection is common in mammals, especially rabbits, squirrels, hares, voles and mice. Ticks, fleas and flies act as arthropod vectors – hence the old term 'deerfly fever'. Infection is acquired by handling infected animals or their carcasses or from animal or vector bites. Hunters are particularly at risk when skinning and eating infected animals. Two strains are recognised. Jellison type A is highly virulent and found only in North America whereas the less virulent Jellison type B is the main cause of tularaemia in Europe.

Pathogenesis

Infection may enter by the skin, eyes, mouth, intestine or by inhalation. In the lung, a granulomatous reaction develops, with necrosis of alveolar walls.

Clinical features

Infection may present as an ulcer at the entry site on the skin or the eye, sometimes with associated lymphadenopathy. There is also a typhoidal type of presentation and an intestinal type with abdominal pain, diarrhoea and vomiting. Pneumonia may develop through blood spread from any of these types. The patient presents with myalgia, fevers and a dry cough, and subsequently produces mucoid or bloody sputum. The chest radiograph shows bronchopneumonia, sometimes with hilar lymphadenopathy.

Diagnostic tests

A contact history is often helpful. Culturing is difficult and hazardous. Diagnosis is usually made serologically and retrospectively by the bacterial agglutination technique.

Treatment

Streptomycin is the treatment of choice. Tetracyclines and chloramphenicol are probably less effective. Vaccines can afford up to 5 years' protection from the disease and are useful for those likely to be exposed in the field or the laboratory.

Actinomycosis

This infection by *Actinomyces israelii* is rare but can present as cervicofacial, pulmonary or abdominal disease. Another organism, *Arachnia propionica*, can present in a similar way. It has also been reported in immunocompromised individuals and responds to prolonged penicillin therapy.

Microbial characteristics and epidemiology
Formerly thought to be a fungus, the organism is now classed as a Gram-positive, branching, anaerobic bacterium. The characteristic sulphur granules seen on culture are masses of tangled Gram-positive filaments cemented together by a polysaccharide protein. *A. israelii* is a normal commensal of the mouth and lower gut and infection is invariably endogenous. It is found in nearly all dental plaques. In the chest, the organism is aspirated into a relatively anaerobic, atelectatic area and a pneumonia develops with chronic inflammation, suppuration, necrosis and fibrosis with local spread to the rib and chest wall. *A. israelii* is almost never found in pure culture in actinomycotic lesions and is usually mixed with other bacteria, both aerobic and anaerobic.

Clinical features
A subacute presentation is usual, with low-grade fever, sweats, weight loss, purulent or bloody sputum and subsequent empyema, rib involvement and subcutaneous abscesses.

The chest radiograph may show local infiltrates, consolidation, abscesses, pleural effusions, and bone involvement with lytic or blastic changes in the ribs or vertebrae can occur.

Diagnosis and treatment
Diagnosis is difficult and less than 10% of cases are diagnosed on initial presentation. The organism can be identified and cultured from pus or biopsy material. Treatment of choice is high-dose intravenous penicillin (10–20 MU per day) given for 4 weeks, followed by oral penicillin for a further 6 months or so. Prolonged courses of erythromycin and tetracycline have been successful in situations where penicillin cannot be used.

Nocardia spp.

Nocardia spp., among which *N. asteroides* is the usual pathogen, have several similarities to *Actinomyces* spp. but they are aerobic and non-acid-fast. They grow slowly on routine media. They are normal inhabitants of the soil, not normally carried by humans and acquired by inhalation.

After entry into the lung a pneumonia develops with subsequent necrosis, abscess formation and direct spread to the pleura and chest wall. Blood vessels are invaded and metastatic abscesses occur. The presentation is usually subacute.

Diagnosis is made by culture of the organism but slow growth can be a problem.

Therapy is with a sulphonamide or co-trimoxazole. Treatment may be needed for several months to prevent relapse. Abscesses should be drained.

Atypical pathogens

The term 'atypical pathogen' is used here to describe infections with *M. pneumoniae, Chlamydia* spp. and *Coxiella burnetii* (Q fever). These intracellular pathogens are usually associated with community-acquired respiratory infections and respond to antibiotics that penetrate lung cells, such as macrolides, quinolones and tetracyclines, but not to β-lactam antibiotics, which do not.

The term 'atypical pneumonia' is misleading and should be abandoned as it incorrectly suggests a characteristic clinical pattern associated with these pathogens

Mycoplasma pneumoniae

This pathogen produces illness in humans ranging from mild upper respiratory infections to severe pneumonia, which occasionally can be fatal. On occasions, potentially serious extrapulmonary manifestations may dominate the picture.

Microbial characteristics
M. pneumoniae does not have a rigid cell wall, relying on a three-layered membrane. Antibiotics acting on bacterial cell walls, such as penicillin, are therefore ineffective. Growth is very slow.

Epidemiology
Infection is transmitted by aerosol in close communities such as families, schools and barracks. The incubation period is 14–21 days. The usual age range is 5–25 years and it is uncommon in young children and in people over 65. Infection occurs in epidemics every 3–4 years throughout the world, with occasional sporadic cases in between (see Fig. 35.4).

Pathogenesis
The organism is extracellular but it impairs mucosal cells and ciliary action. Bronchiolar inflammation is seen and in pneumonic cases there is mononuclear alveolar and interstitial cellular infiltration. The organism is shed from the respiratory tract for many weeks after infection, in spite of antibiotics. Specific antibody confers resistance to infection but reinfection can occur. It has been suggested that immune responses play a part in some of the features of the illness, being less common in immunosuppressed animal models and humans.

Clinical features
Symptoms are common from the upper respiratory tract and bronchial tree, and pneumonia develops in only up to a quarter of cases. Myringitis is sometimes seen. The onset of symptoms is gradual. A wide variety of non-respiratory manifestations has been reported[143,144] (Table 35.13). Mixed infections can occur with respiratory viruses and bacterial pneumonias.

The illness is associated with moderate morbidity but a low mortality, except in debilitated patients or those with sickle-cell disease.

Diagnostic tests
The chest radiograph shows patchy shadowing in half the cases (Fig. 35.19) but lobar consolidation may also be seen. Hilar lymphadenopathy is reported. The white count is usually normal, being raised in about 20% of cases.

The diagnosis is normally made by the complement-fixing antibody test. Some laboratories are able to detect *Mycoplasma*-specific IgM, which also aids an early and specific diagnosis.

Cold agglutinins, which are IgM antibodies that bind to the erythrocyte I antigen, are present in over half the cases, especially during the second and third week of illness.

Treatment
Tetracyclines and macrolides are recommended but neither is effective in eradicating the organism from the respiratory tract.

Table 35.13 Extrapulmonary manifestations of *Mycoplasma pneumoniae* infections

Cardiac	Pericarditis, myocarditis, conduction defects
Neurological (usually in first 2 weeks)	Encephalitis, aseptic meningitis, transverse myelitis, Guillain–Barré syndrome, cranial and peripheral neuropathy, cerebellar ataxia
Gastrointestinal	Hepatitis, pancreatitis, salivary gland enlargement
Haematological (usually after second week)	Haemolytic anaemia, disseminated intravascular coagulation
Skin lesions (up to 25% of cases)	Various rashes including erythema nodosum and multiforme; Stevens–Johnson syndrome
Musculoskeletal (in first 2 weeks)	Polyarthritis of large joints
Miscellaneous	Upper respiratory tract symptoms
	Myringitis
	Immune-complex-related interstitial or glomerulonephritis
	Splenomegaly
	Generalised lymphadenopathy

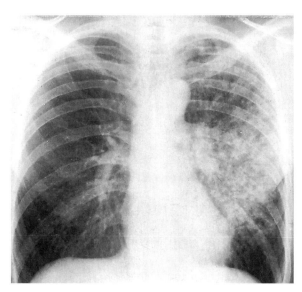

Fig. 35.19 *Mycoplasma* pneumonia: chest radiograph shows patchy diffuse left lung shadowing with hilar lymphadenopathy.

Quinolones should also be effective. Corticosteroids have been used for some of the severe complications.

Mortality and morbidity

Tracheobronchial clearance and defects of lung function may persist for many months and rarely progressive diffuse interstitial fibrosis has been reported. Deaths occur,[49] those with hypoglobulinaemia and sickle-cell disease being particularly at risk.

Chlamydial infections

The genus *Chlamydia* comprises three species: *C. trachomatis*, *C. psittaci* and *C. pneumoniae*. *C. trachomatis* is the cause of trachoma, sexually transmitted disease and infantile pneumonia. Infection with the other two species causes acute respiratory infections in adults and will be considered here.

Microbial characteristics

Chlamydia spp. are small, intracellular bacteria that are dependent on the host cell for energy production. They divide by binary fission, producing the characteristic inclusion bodies within the host cell.

Epidemiology

C. psittaci is endemic in avian species including psittacine birds, canaries, finches, pigeons and poultry. Birds are frequently asymptomatic carriers and stress associated with transport, illness or overcrowding can cause excretion of the organism. It is transmitted to humans by inhalation from bird handling or contact with feathers, faeces or cage dust, and occasionally through pecks. Pet-shop owners, veterinarians and zoo workers are at particular risk. Person-to-person transmission has been well reported in the hospital environment. In one outbreak, 11 people contracted the disease from a patient who died in hospital from psittacosis. Second attacks can occur. Psittacosis appears to be responsible for 2–5% of community-acquired pneumonias in the UK, Europe and Egypt. It is rare in children.

In 1986 a new species, C. *pneumoniae*, was described. Seroepidemiological studies have shown that infection with C. *pneumoniae* is widespread, with half of the young adult population being seropositive, implying that many infections are subclinical or lead to only a mild, self-limiting illness. Studies in which C. *pneumoniae* has been sought suggest that it accounts for 6–10% of cases of community-acquired pneumonia . An association has also been shown between both coronary artery disease and wheezing, and serological evidence of C. *pneumoniae* infection. Humans are the only known reservoir of C. *pneumoniae* and person-to-person spread is the probable mode of acquisition.[145]

Pathogenesis

This is best understood for psittacosis. After inhalation the organism passes from the respiratory tract to the reticuloendothelial system of the liver and spleen, where it multiplies. After an incubation period of 10–14 days, haematogenous spread occurs to the lung and elsewhere, causing the symptoms. A patchy lymphocytic interstitial pneumonia occurs, alveolar macrophages are seen with characteristic cytoplasmic inclusions and there is desquamation of alveolar lining cells resulting in the name 'alveolar cell pneumonia'.

Clinical features

For psittacosis, there is a varied presentation from mild flu-like illness with bronchitis through to a fulminating toxic state with multiple organ failure.[146,147] Common symptoms include high fever, rigors, backache, headache and photophobia, severe myalgia, a dry unproductive cough and confusion. A macular rash (Horden's spots) has been described and diarrhoea occurs in a quarter of cases. The patient is often confused and toxic. The chest may sound relatively clear on examination but the liver and spleen can be palpable.

The white count is normal in over three-quarters of cases and the sputum Gram stain reveals a few leukocytes but no predominant bacterial pathogens. Liver function tests may well be abnormal. The chest radiograph shows no specific pattern but opacification usually starts in the lower lobes with patchy changes. Clearance may take several weeks.

The clinical features of C. pneumoniae are not distinctive, although sore throat and dry cough are common. Primary infection can cause mild pneumonia or prolonged bronchitis in young adults, presenting in a similar clinical way to Mycoplasma infection. In older adults, reinfection can be associated with co-pathogens, particularly S. pneumoniae, making the relative importance of each pathogen difficult to ascertain.

Complications
The pattern is probably similar to those recorded for mycoplasmal pneumonia.

Diagnosis and treatment
For psittacosis the usual method of diagnosis is by serology with fourfold or more rise in complement-fixing antibodies. There are no trials of therapy but clinical experience suggests that tetracycline for 14–21 days is the antibiotic of choice, with macrolides, rifampicin and chloramphenicol being alternatives. Defervescence occurred in over 90% of 135 proven cases within 48 hours of starting tetracyclines in one study.[146] The patient should be regarded as potentially infectious initially. Doxycycline therapy has been used to protect close contacts of index cases.

When a specific bird, aviary or pet shop is implicated in the infection, veterinary advice should be sought: the destruction of infected birds is usually recommended.

C. pneumoniae is usually diagnosed serologically and isolation is very difficult.[54,148,149] The usual method is the microimmunofluorescence test using elementary body antigen of one or more strains looking for changes in IgM and IgG. In addition, an enzyme immunosorbent assay has been developed to detect C. pneumoniae antigen in sputum samples. For treatment, in vitro studies and clinical experience support the use of macrolides, especially clarithromycin and also tetracyclines. Empirical observations suggest that therapy should be given for 2–3 weeks.[150]

Prevention
Psittacosis is not a major public health problem in terms of numbers of cases reported, although these have been rising steadily in the UK in the last few years, 300–400 cases being reported each year recently. Most countries have import regulations to prevent psittacosis whereby imported captive birds are quarantined for a month or so and in some cases are also treated prophylactically with tetracycline-medicated seed.

Q fever

Q fever was first described in 1935 in nine Australian abattoir workers and the responsible organism, Coxiella burnetii, was subsequently isolated by Cox and Davis from ticks in Montana. It is a systemic illness manifested usually in its acute form by fever and variable involvement of the lungs and liver, and in a chronic form as subacute bacterial endocarditis.[151,152]

Epidemiology
Coxiella spp. are ubiquitous rickettsial zoonotic parasites with a high frequency of asymptomatic infection in domestic animals. Apparently healthy but infected animals can shed enormous numbers of organisms in milk, urine, faeces and particularly products of conception. Person-to-person transmission can occur. The organism is extremely resistant to drying and can persist for months in soil, straw, machinery and clothing. Air currents can disseminate infection widely and contact with livestock may then become very indirect and inapparent. About 130 cases of infection, including about 10 cases of endocarditis, are noted each year in England and Wales each year. It is more common in rural areas, with a peak incidence during calving and lambing periods in spring. In Nova Scotia, Q fever accounted for 20% of all cases of pneumonia studied in regional hospitals in 1983. The trapping of snowshoe hares was found to be an important factor in one study, with human illness presenting very like tularaemia.

Pathogenesis
Following inhalation or ingestion there is a long incubation period of 3 weeks, followed by a systemic illness with involvement of many organs, often including the lung. Granulomas are sometimes seen.

Clinical features
Q fever presents with a flu-like illness with a dry cough, a relatively clear chest, an enlarged liver and inflamed throat and conjunctivae. The chest radiograph usually shows multiple segmental opacities, which clear rapidly, normally within a month of therapy. Complications have been reported from many systems. They include ocular disease, arthritis, thrombophlebitis, arteritis, pericarditis, myocarditis and chronic endocarditis, particularly of the aortic valve.

Diagnostic tests
The diagnosis is normally made by serological means but interpretation of complement-fixing antibody titres requires understanding of the different antigenic phases. Antibodies to the phase II strain are found within 4 weeks in nearly all cases of acute infection, whereas antibodies to phase I strains are found only in those with chronic disease, such as endocarditis.

Treatment
Most cases of Q fever pneumonia have a self-limiting and benign nature but doxycycline results in a more rapid defervescence when compared with erythromycin. Success has also been reported with clarithromycin and quinolones.[153]

Respiratory viruses

Respiratory viral illnesses are caused by a large number of serologically distinct viruses belonging to seven major virus families. They are spread by small-particle aerosols, by large droplets requiring close contact or by hand-to-hand or hand-to-fomite transfer. A very small inoculum is needed to infect the ciliated columnar epithelial cells of the respiratory tract, which are progressively destroyed at the time of virus shedding during the symptoms and signs of the respiratory illness.[154]

The relative importance of viruses as a cause of respiratory infection varies with the setting. Cytomegalovirus is the principal pathogen in the immunocompromised patient. By contrast, the specific viral pathogens identified in 12 recent adult community-acquired pneumonia studies included influenza virus A (146), influenza virus B (48), parainfluenza virus type 3 (28), type 2 (10), type 1 (4), cytomegalovirus (28), respiratory syncytial virus (25), adenovirus (11), varicella zoster virus (2), rhinovirus (2) and other viruses (2). Details of the clinical syndromes produced by some of the viruses are given below.

Influenza

The word 'influenza' is said to have originated in Florence during the 15th century. Influenza is an acute epidemic viral infection characterised by fever, headache, myalgia, sore throat and cough. It is usually self-limiting but can be complicated by severe and fatal primary viral or secondary bacterial pneumonia.

Aetiology

The term influenza or 'flu' is often used to describe any self-limiting respiratory tract infection. True influenza is caused by the influenza virus, which belongs to the Orthomyxoviridae family. There are three types (A, B, C), determined by their internal nuclear protein.

Epidemiology

The influenza virus, in particular type A, has remarkable ability to undergo spontaneous antigenic changes in the haemagglutinin and neuraminidase) surface glycoproteins, resulting in minor 'antigenic drifts' and major 'antigenic shifts'. Minor antigenic drifts result in sporadic infections but major antigenic shifts result in pandemic disease where there is little or no immunity in the population. Such pandemics have occurred in 1890, 1918, 1929, 1946, 1957, 1968 and 1977. In 1957 there was an antigenic shift of both surface glycoproteins, resulting in severe disease. Strains are designated according to the type/place isolated/year/(antigenic properties), e.g. A/Hong Kong/68(H_3N_2).

Influenza epidemics occur in the winter months, particularly in the first part of the year in the northern hemisphere and in May to September in the southern hemisphere. The infection normally starts in children and then spreads to the working population and then elderly people. There is a corresponding rise in absences from work and school, hospital admissions for chest infections and increased reported mortality from pneumonia and influenza. Average attack rates are variable but in the order of 10–20%. During pandemics, the infection spreads rapidly from a single focus along major travel routes to all parts of the country. The attack rate is very high and all ages are affected.

Type B is much more stable antigenically and so the annual incidence remains fairly stable. Type C results in mild upper respiratory infections and has not been associated with any large-scale outbreaks.

Pathogenesis

The virus is spread in respiratory secretions which are infectious for 1–2 days after the onset of the illness. Virus from infected droplets penetrates columnar epithelial cells, resulting in necrosis and denudation of the ciliated epithelium of the tracheobronchial tree. There is associated hyperaemia and haemorrhage. If the infection reaches as far as the alveoli, there is alveolar oedema and leukocyte exudation with capillary thrombosis.

Clinical features

After an incubation period of 1–2 days, there is an onset of abrupt high fever, rigors, malaise, myalgia, headaches, dry cough and nasal discharge. These normally resolve within 3 days but there is a residual cough and malaise for 1–3 weeks.[155]

Complications

The potentially lethal complication of influenza infection is pneumonia. This can be a primary influenza virus pneumonia or a secondary bacterial pneumonia. If a direct extension of the viral infection occurs, cough, dyspnoea and cyanosis appear as a part of the influenza illness. Crackles are heard in the lung and a chest radiograph shows diffuse progressive bilateral infiltrates. There is usually a leukocytosis but no bacterial pathogens are found in the sputum and there is no response to antibiotics. Death from haemorrhagic pneumonia is frequent. At particular risk are those with heart disease or chronic illness, and women in the last trimester of pregnancy.[156,157]

Diagnostic tests

The diagnosis is normally suggested on epidemiological grounds. Virus can be identified by immunofluorescent staining or isolated from throat and nasal swabs in the first 2 days and a serological diagnosis can be made retrospectively by complement fixation or haemagglutination inhibiting antibody tests.

Treatment

Treatment is largely supportive. Amantadine has been shown to reduce the duration of uncomplicated influenza A infection but side effects reduce its usefulness for prophylaxis during epidemics.[158] Ribavirin therapy has also been tried.[159] Recently, neuraminidase inhibitor drugs have been shown to reduce the duration of influenza symptoms if taken by inhalation within 2 days of symptom onset. Their role in management is still not clear.[160]

Prevention

Whole vaccine containing type A and B subtypes and strains isolated from the previous winter's influenza season and grown in eggs is available for use in adults. A subvirion vaccine is used for children. Efficacy rates in preventing outbreaks vary from 60% to 90%, with protection lasting for 6 months. The antibody response to the vaccine is reduced in elderly people and the vaccine may not protect them against the development of upper respiratory tract symptoms. However, there is substantial protection from lower respiratory complications, the need for hospitalisation and death.[161,162] It is normally recommended for people at increased risk of complications or death from influenza, such as those with chronic disease, everyone over 65 years of age and also those in essential community service posts.

The only contraindication to immunisation is a history of hypersensitivity to eggs. Reactions to the vaccine commonly include local pain, erythema and swelling at the site of administration and occasionally systemic effects, such as fever and myalgia.[163]

Bacterial infection following viral infections

Secondary bacterial pneumonia has been reported following both viral and atypical respiratory infections.[164] However, it is usually associated with influenza virus infection.

Microbial aetiology

The bacteria most commonly implicated include *S. pneumoniae*, *H. influenzae* and *S. aureus*. Patterns of the secondary bacterial infections after influenza vary. Necropsy studies show that the principal bacterial pathogen during the 1919 influenza epidemic was *H. influenzae*, whereas during 1957 it was *S. aureus* and in 1969 *S. pneumoniae*. Initial influenza virus infection is mainly responsible for the large rise in reported cases of severe bacterial pneumonias during the early part of each year. In seven recent studies of community pneumonia where dual influenza virus and bacterial infection were described, 34 had *S. pneumoniae*, seven *H. influenzae*, six *S. aureus* and six other bacterial pathogens.

Pathogenesis

The main impact of influenza virus infection is on the ciliated respiratory epithelium which desquamates, reducing mucociliary clearance and increasing bacterial adherence to mucosal cells.[142,165] In addition to these defects in physical defence mechanisms, abnormalities of humoral and cellular immunity occur. There is impaired chemotaxis for human neutrophils following influenza and impaired monocyte and macrophage phagocytic function and reduced circulating T lymphocytes during the incubation period of acute respiratory viral infections. Surfactant probably has an important role in phagocytosis in the alveoli and its production is reduced when type II pneumocytes are destroyed during influenza virus infection.

The maximum suppression of macrophage function appears at around 7 days in experimental models at a time when virus shedding is falling dramatically. It has been suggested that, at this time, the lung macrophages have phagocytosed viral antigen from the bronchial epithelial debris and that these macrophages then become the target of the antiviral immune response, reducing the phagocytic potential of the lung.

Clinical features

Secondary bacterial pneumonia following influenza typically occurs 3 or more days after the illness as the patient is improving. There is a recurrence of fever, cough and purulent sputum and even previously fit adults may deteriorate over a few hours. In about a third of cases there is no biphasic course to the illness and pulmonary symptoms and signs blend with the initial influenzal illness.

Treatment

Patients who develop symptoms or signs of pneumonia during or shortly after an influenzal illness require prompt therapy with antibiotics that will cover the three likely bacterial pathogens, pending the results of sputum and blood cultures. A combination of a β-lactam antibiotic and flucloxacillin is appropriate. Early consideration should be given to hospital admission if the patient is toxic or unwell, because even previously fit adults can deteriorate very quickly, particularly with staphylococcal infection.

Respiratory syncytial virus infections

Respiratory syncytial virus is the major viral respiratory pathogen in infants and is now also recognised as an important pathogen in the elderly, where it can present either as a bronchial infection or as pneumonia, particularly in those with underlying chronic disease. High fever, intense cough and airway obstruction are common features. The white cell count is usually normal but the C-reactive protein is raised in over three-quarters of cases. Staff working in paediatric wards are also at risk.[166]

Herpes virus infections

These include varicella-zoster virus, herpes simplex virus, Epstein–Barr virus and cytomegalovirus.[167]

Varicella-zoster infection

This is a highly contagious infection, primarily of children. Pneumonia is rare in childhood unless due to bacterial superinfection. Most cases of varicella pneumonia occur in adults, with 75% of cases occurring in 20–30 year olds. Disseminated varicella-zoster disease is sometimes associated with pneumonia but only in the presence of immunosuppression. Smoking and pregnancy may be risk factors for developing pneumonia.

The incubation period is up to 21 days and symptomatic pneumonia usually develops early in the course of the illness particularly in those with severe skin involvement. Cough, dyspnoea and chest pain develop and the chest radiograph shows progressive bilateral fluffy infiltrates (Fig. 35.20). Calcification can develop months and years later and appears to be more common in smokers.

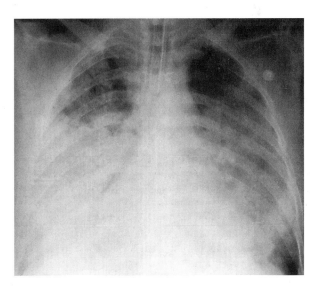

Fig. 35.20 Chest radiograph of a 24-year-old previously well man who, 3 days previously, had developed chickenpox caught from his daughter, showing widespread shadowing. He required mechanical ventilation and vidarabine therapy but made a complete recovery. Reproduced with permission from Macfarlane JT, Smith FD, Finch R. Vidarabine in fulminating chickenpox pneumonia. Thorax 1982; 37: 226–227.

The clinical diagnosis is usually obvious but can be confirmed by isolating virus from vesicles and by serological means.

Pneumonia is a serious complication of chickenpox in adults, with a reported mortality rate of up to 20% before the availability of specific antiviral therapy such as acyclovir, which is indicated for patients with primary varicella-zoster pneumonia. Assisted ventilation may be required.

Cytomegalovirus

A mild pneumonia is reported to occur in 6% of normal people developing cytomegalovirus mononucleosis, but it remains the most common viral pathogen in immunocompromised patients, particularly following bone-marrow transplantation. In such circumstances, the pathogenicity of the pneumonia is thought to be less than that of infection and more the result of T-cell cytotoxicity against viral antigens on infected cells in the lung.

Infections of the chest wall

These can include infections of the skin such as shingles, infection and inflammation of the intercostal muscles (Bornholm disease), and infectious causes of costochondritis (Tietze's syndrome).

Herpes zoster infection

The diagnosis is rarely in doubt when the characteristic dermatomal rash of shingles appears, but it can occasionally cause a diagnostic dilemma when the patient presents with fever and localised lateral chest pain in the pre-eruptive phase of the illness.

Bornholm disease

Other terms for this condition include epidemic pleurodynia, epidemic myalgia, the 'Devil's grip' and dry pleurisy. Although descriptions of the condition can be found as far back as the 18th century, the name derives from a description by Sylvest in the 1930s of 93 cases of epidemic myalgia in Denmark, in Copenhagen and on the island of Bornholm.

The condition mainly affects children and younger adults in the summer and early autumn. It can occur in epidemics or within families, although a third of cases are sporadic.[168] The condition is characterised by a sudden onset of severe chest wall and abdominal pain, fever and headaches. Cough can occur in a third of cases and a pleural rub is present in a proportion, together with some chest wall tenderness. Young children more commonly present with abdominal pain, which may mimic appendicitis. Investigations are usually normal. Treatment is symptomatic and most patients recover within a week, although relapses and lingering after-effects, including tiredness and weakness, are reported.

Complications include pericarditis, aseptic meningitis and orchitis. The diagnosis can be difficult to make with confidence without having excluded other causes of the symptoms, except during epidemics. The usual causative organism, Coxsackie B virus, can be isolated from stools during the early phase of the illness. It is thought to spread by the oral route and one report described an epidemic caused by contamination of a common drinking water container used by a football team.[169]

Tietze's syndrome

This syndrome was first described by a surgeon, Alexander Tietze, in 1921, as a benign but sometimes long-lived, painful, localised swelling of a costosternal, costochondral or sternoclavicular joint. Some attempt has been made to differentiate Tietze's syndrome from costochondritis, with the latter affecting several joints and not being associated with swelling.[170] Infection has been postulated as one of the initiating factors in Tietze's syndrome and occasionally ongoing infection is discovered.[171] In the large majority of cases no aetiological agent is discovered and treatment is symptomatic. Some patients derive benefit from local application of non-steroidal anti-inflammatory creams, or infiltration with local anaesthetic and steroid preparation at the site of maximum tenderness and swelling.

References

1. Ellis ME, McArthur P. Upper respiratory tract infections. In: Ellis ME, ed. Infectious diseases of the respiratory tract. Cambridge: Cambridge University Press; 1997: 453–485.
2. Winther B, Gwaltney JM. Acute and chronic sinusitis. In: Pennington JE, ed. Respiratory infections: diagnosis and management, 3rd edn. New York: Raven Press; 1994: 125–136.
3. Evans FO, Sydner JB, Moore WED, Moore GR. Sinusitis of the maxillary sinus. N Engl J Med 1995; 293: 735–739.
4. Editorial. Bacterial pharyngitis. Lancet 1987; 1: 1241.
5. Ellis ME. Viral lower respiratory tract infections. In: Ellis ME, ed. Infectious diseases of the respiratory tract. Cambridge: Cambridge University Press; 1997: 148–170.
6. Gaffney RJ, Freeman DJ, Walsh MA, Cafferkey MT. Differences in tonsillar core bacteriology in adults and children: a prospective study of 262 patients. Respir Med 1991; 85: 383–388.
7. Garpenholt O, Hugosson S, Fredlund H et al. Epiglottitis in Sweden before and after introduction of vaccination against Haemophilus influenzae type b. Pediatr Infect Dis J 1999; 18: 490–3.
8. Tveteras K, Kristensen S. Acute epiglottitis in adults: bacteriology and therapy. Clin Otolaryngol 1987; 12: 337–343.
9. Booy R, Heath PT, Slack MP et al. Vaccine failures after primary immunisation with Haemophilus influenzae type-b conjugate vaccine without booster Lancet 1997; 349: 1197–1202.
10. Reed G, Jewett PH, Thompson J et al. Epidemiology and clinical impact of parainfluenza virus infections in otherwise healthy infants and young children < 5 years old. J Infect Dis 1997; 175: 807–13.
11. Laurichesse H, Dedman D, Watson JM, Zambon MC. Epidemiological features of parainfluenza virus infections: laboratory surveillance in England and Wales, 1975–1997. Eur J Epidemiol 1999; 15: 475–84.
12. Geelhoed GC, Macdonald WB. Oral and inhaled steroids in croup: a randomized, placebo-controlled trial. Pediatr Pulmonol 1995; 20: 355–61.
13. Henry R. Moist air in the treatment of laryngotracheitis. Arch Dis Child 1983; 58: 577.
14. Kairys SW, Olmstead EM, O'Connor GT. Steroid treatment of laryngotracheitis: a meta-analysis of the evidence from randomized trials. Pediatrics 1989; 83: 683–93.
15. Geelhoed GC, Macdonald WB. Oral dexamethasone in the treatment of croup: 0.15 mg/kg versus 0.3 mg/kg versus 0.6 mg/kg. Pediatr Pulmonol 1995; 20: 362–8.
16. Geelhoed GC, Turner J, Macdonald WB. Efficacy of a small single dose of oral dexamethasone for outpatient croup: a double blind placebo controlled clinical trial. Br Med J 1996; 313: 140–142.
17. Tibballs J, Shann FA, Landau LI. Placebo-controlled trial of prednisolone in children intubated for croup. Lancet 1992; 340: 745–748.

18. Ausejo M, Saenz A, Pham B et al. Glucocorticoids for croup.(Cochrane Review) in : The Cochrane Library,Issue 4, 2000. Oxford :Update software.

19. Kristjansson S, Berg-Kelly K, Winso E. Inhalation of racemic adrenaline in the treatment of mild and moderately severe croup. Clinical symptom score and oxygen saturation measurements for evaluation of treatment effects. Acta Paediatr 1994; 83: 1156–1160.

20. Waisman Y, Klein BL, Boenning DA et al. Prospective randomized double-blind study comparing L-epinephrine and racemic epinephrine aerosols in the treatment of laryngotracheitis (croup). Pediatrics 1992; 89: 302–306.

21. Cohen B, Dunt D. Recurrent and non-recurrent croup: an epidemiological study. Austr Paediatr J 1988; 24: 339–42.

22. Macfarlane JT, Holmes WF, Macfarlane RM. Do hospital physicians have a role in reducing antibiotic prescribing in the community? Thorax 2000: 55: 2: 153–158.

23. Macfarlane JT. An overview of community acquired pneumonia with lessons learned from the British Thoracic Society study. Sem Respir Inf 1994: 9: 153–165

24. Macfarlane JT, Holmes WF, Macfarlane RM et al. A prospective study of the incidence, aetiology and outcome of lower respiratory tract illness in previously well adults in the community. Thorax 2001; 56: 109–114.

25. Rea HH, Wells AU. Chronic airflow obstruction, acute and chronic bronchitis and bronchiectasis. In: Ellis ME, ed. Infectious diseases of the respiratory tract. Cambridge: Cambridge University Press; 1997: 554–580.

26. Macfarlane JT, Colville A, Guion A et al. Prospective study of aetiology and outcome of adult lower respiratory tract infections in the community. Lancet 1993; 341: 511–514.

27. Macfarlane JT, Holmes WF, Macfarlane RM, et al. Contemporary use of antibiotics in 1089 adults presenting with acute lower respiratory tract illness in general practice in the UK: implications for developing management guidelines. Respir Med 1997; 91: 427–434.

28. Fahey T, Stocks N, Thomas T. Quantitative systematic review of randomised controlled trials comparing antibiotic with placebo for acute cough in adults. Br Med J 1998; 316: 906–910.

29. Hosker H, Cooke N, Hawkey P. Antibiotics in obstructive pulmonary disease Br Med J 1994; 308: 871–872.

30. The COPD Guidelines Group of the Standards of Care Committee of the British Thoracic Society. BTS guidelines for the management of chronic obstructive pulmonary disease. Thorax 1997; 52: 55–28

31. Miller E, Fleming DM, Ashworth LA et al. Serological evidence of pertussis in patients presenting with cough in general practice in Birmingham . Commun Dis Public Health 2000; 3: 132–134.

32. Guris D, Strebel PM, Bardenheier B et al. Changing epidemiology of pertussis in the United States: increasing reported incidence among adolescents and adults, 1990–1996. Clin Infect Dis 1999; 28: 1230–1237.

33. Ranganathan S, Tasker R, Booy R et al. Pertussis is increasing in unimmunized infants: is a change in policy needed? Arch Dis Child 1999; 80: 297–299.

34. Krantz I, Norrby SR, Trollfors B. Salbutamol vs. placebo for treatment of pertussis. Pediatr Infect Dis 1985; 4: 638–640.

35. Onorato IM, Wassilak SG, Meade B. Efficacy of whole-cell pertussis vaccine in preschool children in the United States . JAMA 1992; 267: 2745–2749.

36. Fleming DM, Cross KW. Respiratory syncytial virus or influenza? Lancet 1993; 342: 1507–1510.

37. Bulow SM, Nir M, Levin E et al. Prednisolone treatment of respiratory syncytial virus infection: a randomized controlled trial of 147 infants. Pediatrics 1999; 104: e77.

38. Cade A, Brownlee KG, Conway SP et al. Randomised placebo controlled trial of nebulised corticosteroids in acute respiratory syncytial viral bronchiolitis. Arch Dis Child 2000; 82: 126–130.

39. Kellner JD, Ohlsson A, Gadomski AM, Wang EE. Bronchodilators for bronchiolitis.(Cochrane Review) in : The Cochrane Library,Issue 4, 2000. Oxford :Update software.

40. Henry RL, Milner AD, Stokes GM. Ineffectiveness of ipratropium bromide in acute bronchiolitis. Arch Dis Child 1983; 58: 925–926.

41. Randolph AG, Wang EE. Ribavirin for respiratory syncytial virus infection of the lower respiratory tract. (Cochrane Review) in : The Cochrane Library,Issue 4, 2000. Oxford :Update software.

42. Navas L, Wang E, de Carvalho V, Robinson J. Improved outcome of respiratory syncytial virus infection in a high-risk hospitalized population of Canadian children. Pediatric Investigators Collaborative Network on Infections in Canada. J Pediatr 1992; 121: 348–354.

43. Isaacs D, Dickson H, O'Callaghan C et al. Handwashing and cohorting in prevention of hospital acquired infections with respiratory syncytial virus. Arch Dis Child 1991; 66: 227–231.

44. Groothuis JR, Simoes EA, Levin MJ et al. Prophylactic administration of respiratory syncytial virus immune globulin to high-risk infants and young children. The Respiratory Syncytial Virus Immune Globulin Study Group. N Engl J Med 1993; 329: 1524–1530.

45. IMpact-RSV Study Group. Palivizumab, a humanized respiratory syncytial virus monoclonal antibody, reduces hospitalization from respiratory syncytial virus infection in high-risk infants. Pediatrics 1998; 102: 531–537.

46. Joffe S, Ray GT, Escobar GJ et al. Cost-effectiveness of respiratory syncytial virus prophylaxis among preterm infants Pediatrics 1999; 104: 419–427.

47. Woodhead MA, Macfarlane JT, McCracken JS et al. Prospective study of the aetiology and outcome of pneumonia in the community. Lancet 1987; 1: 671–674.

48. Jokinen ENC, Heiskanen L, Juvonen H et al. Incidence of community acquired pneumonia in the population of four municipalities in Eastern Finland. Am J Epidemiol 1993; 137: 977–988.

49. British Thoracic Society. Community acquired pneumonia in adults in British hospitals in 1982–1983: a survey of aetiology, mortality, prognostic factors and outcome. Q J Med 1987; 239: 195–220.

50. Lim WS, Macfarlane JT, Boswell TCJ et al. Study of the causes of adult community acquired pneumonia – SCAPA: implications for management guidelines. Thorax 2001; in press.

51. British Thoracic Society Research Committee and Public Health Laboratory Service. The aetiology, management and outcome of severe community-acquired pneumonia on the intensive care unit. Respir Med 1992; 86: 7–13.

52. Guest JF, Morris A. Community-acquired pneumonia: the annual cost to the National Health Service in the United Kingdom. Eur Respir J 1997; 10: 1530–1534.

53. Macfarlane JT. Community acquired pneumonia. Br J Dis Chest 1987; 81: 116–127.

54. Macfarlane JT, Boswell T, Douglas G et al. The British Thoracic Society guidelines for the management of community acquired pneumonia in adults. Thorax 2001; in press.

55. Kurashi NY, Al-Hamdan SJ, Ibrahim EM et al. Community acquired acute bacterial and atypical pneumonia in Saudi Arabia. Thorax 1992; 47: 115–118 .

56. Macfarlane J. Lower respiratory tract infection and pneumonia in the community. Sem Respir Inf 1999; 14.2: 155–162.

57. Holmberg H. Aetiology of community acquired pneumonia in hospital treated patients. Scand J Infect Dis 1987; 19: 491–501 .

58. Lim I, Shaw DR, Stanley DP et al. A prospective hospital study of the aetiology of community acquired pneumonia. Med J Austr 1989; 151: 87–91.

59. Karalus NC, Cursons RT, Leng RA et al. Community acquired pneumonia: aetiology and prognostic index evaluation. Thorax 1991; 46: 413–418.

60. Marrie TJ, Durant H, Yates L. Community acquired pneumonia requiring hospitalisation: 5 year prospective study. Rev Infect Dis 1989; 11: 586–599.

61. Fang G, Fine M, Orloff J et al. New and emerging aetiologies for community acquired pneumonia with implications for therapy. Medicine 1990; 69: 307–316.

62. Lieberman D, Schlaeffer F, Boldur I et al. Multiple pathogens in adult patients admitted with community-acquired pneumonia: a one year prospective study of 346 consecutive patients. Thorax 1996; 51: 179–184.

63. Verghese A, Berk SL. Bacterial pneumonia in the elderly. Medicine 1983; 62: 271–285.

64. Heiskanen-Kosma T, Korppi M, Jokinen C et al. Etiology of childhood pneumonia: serologic results of a prospective, population-based study. Pediatr Infect Dis J 1998; 17: 986–991.

65. Wubbel L, Muniz L, Ahmed A et al. Etiology and treatment of community-acquired pneumonia in ambulatory children. Pediatr Infect Dis J 1999; 18: 98–104.

66. Harari M, Shann F, Spooner V et al. Clinical signs of pneumonia in children. Lancet 1991; 338: 928–930.

67. Smyth A, Carty H, Hart CA. Clinical predictors of hypoxaemia in children with pneumonia. Ann Trop Paediatr 1998; 18: 31–40.

68. Grossman RF, Fein A. Evidence-based assessment of diagnostic tests for ventilator-associated pneumonia. Chest 2000; 117: S177–S181.

69. Helms CM, Viner JP, Sturm RH et al. Comparative features of pneumococcal, mycoplasmal and legionnaires' disease pneumonias. Ann Intern Med 1979; 90: 543.

70. Woodhead MA, Macfarlane JT. Comparative clinical and laboratory features of legionella with pneumococcal and mycoplasma pneumonia. Br J Dis Chest 1987; 81: 133–139.

71. Ponka A, Sarna S. Differential diagnosis of viral, mycoplasma and bacteraemic pneumococcal pneumonia on admission to hospital. Eur J Respir Dis 1983; 64: 360–368.

72. Smith RP, Lipworth BJ, Cree IA et al. C-reactive protein. A clinical marker in community-acquired pneumonia. Chest 1995; 108: 1288–1291.

73. Korppi M, Heiskanen-Kosma T, Jalonen E et al. Aetiology of community-acquired pneumonia in children treated in hospital. Eur J Pediatr 1993; 152: 24–30.

74. Requejo HI, Guerra ML, Dos Santos M, Cocozza AM. Immunodiagnoses of community-acquired pneumonia in childhood. J Trop Pediatr 1997; 43: 208–212.

75. Korppi M, Heiskanen-Kosma T, Leinonen M. White blood cells, C-reactive protein and erythrocyte sedimentation rate in pneumococcal pneumonia in children. Eur Respir J 1997; 10: 1125–1129.

76. Nohynek H, Valkeila E, Leinonen M, Eskola J. Erythrocyte sedimentation rate, white blood cell count and serum C-reactive protein in assessing etiologic diagnosis of acute lower respiratory infections in children. Pediatr Infect Dis J 1995; 14: 484–490.

77. Macfarlane JT, Miller AC, Smith WHR et al. Comparative radiographic features of community acquired legionnaires' disease, pneumococcal pneumonia, mycoplasma pneumonia and psittacosis. Thorax 1984; 39: 28–33.

78. Lim WS, Lewis, Macfarlane JT. Severity prediction rules in community acquired pneumonia – a validation study. Thorax 2000; 55: 219–223.

79. Fine MJ, Smith MA, Carson CA et al. Prognosis and outcomes of patients with community-acquired pneumonia. A meta-analysis. JAMA 1996; 275: 134–141.

80. Ewig S, Bauer T, Hasper E et al. Prognostic analysis and predictive rule for outcome of hospital-treated community-acquired pneumonia. Eur Respir J 1995; 8: 392–397.

81. Woodhead MA. Management of pneumonia. Respir Med 1992; 86: 459–469.

82. Wilcox MH. Respiratory antibiotic use and *Clostridium difficile* infection – is it the drugs or is it the doctors? Thorax 2000; 55: 633–634.

83. Hirani NA, Macfarlane JT. Impact of management guidelines on the outcome of severe community acquired pneumonia. Thorax 1997; 52: 17–21.

84. Friis B, Andersen P, Brenoe E et al. Antibiotic treatment of pneumonia and bronchiolitis. A prospective randomised study. Arch Dis Child 1984; 59: 1038–1045.

85. Tsarouhas N, Shaw KN, Hodinka RL, Bell LM. Effectiveness of intramuscular penicillin versus oral amoxicillin in the early treatment of outpatient pediatric pneumonia. Pediatr Emerg Care 1998; 14: 338–341.

86. Deeks SL, Palacio R, Ruvinsky R et al. Risk factors and course of illness among children with invasive penicillin-resistant *Streptococcus pneumoniae* .The *Streptococcus pneumoniae* Working Group. Pediatrics 1999; 103: 409–413.

87. American Thoracic Society. Hospital-acquired pneumonia in adults: diagnosis, assessment of severity, initial antimicrobial therapy and preventive strategies. A consensus statement. Am J Respir Crit Care Med 1996; 153: 1711–1725.

88. Dal Nogare AR. Nosocomial pneumonia in the medical and surgical patient. Risk factors and primary management. Med Clin North Am 1994; 78: 1081–1090.

89. Rello J, Cabello H, Torres A. Epidemiology, risk and prognostic factors of nosocomial pneumonia. Eur Respir Monograph 1997; 3: 82–100.

90. Johanson WG Jr, Pierce AK, Sanford JP, Thomas GD. Nosocomial respiratory infections with Gram-negative bacilli. The significance of colonization of the respiratory tract. Ann Intern Med 1972; 77: 701–706.

91. Estes RJ, Medurie GU. The pathogenesis of ventilator-associated pneumonia: I. Mechanisms of bacterial transcolonization and airway inoculation. Intens Care Med 1995; 21: 365–383.

92. Rello J, Ausina V, Castella J et al. Nosocomial respiratory tract infections in multiple trauma patients. Influence of level of consciousness with implications for therapy. Chest 1992; 102: 525–529.

93. Niederman MS. The pathogenesis of airway colonization: lessons learned from the study of bacterial adherence. Eur Respir J 1994; 7: 1737–1740.

94. Brun-Buisson C. Nosocomial pneumonia during mechanical ventilation: problems with diagnostic criteria. Thorax 1995; 50: 1128–1130.

95. Pingleton SK, Fagon JY, Leeper KV Jr. Patient selection for clinical investigation of ventilator-associated pneumonia. Criteria for evaluating diagnostic techniques. Chest 1992; 102: S553–S556.

96. Mandell LA, Marrie TJ, Niederman MS. Initial antimicrobial treatment of hospital acquired pneumonia in adults: a conference report. Can J Infect Dis 1993; 4: 317–321.

97. Vincent JL. Prevention of nosocomial bacterial pneumonia. Thorax 1999; 54: 544–549.

98. Pittet D, Hugonnet S, Harbarth S et al. Effectiveness of a hospital-wide programme to improve compliance with hand hygiene. Lancet 2000; 356: 1307–1312.

99. Lim WS, Macfarlane JT. Hospital acquired pneumonia. J R Coll Phys Lond 2001; in press.

100. Selective Decontamination of the Digestive Tract Trialists' Collaborative Group. Meta-analysis of randomised controlled trials of selective decontamination of the digestive tract. Br Med J 1993; 307: 525–532.

101. D'Amico R, Pifferi S, Leonetti C et al. Effectiveness of antibiotic prophylaxis in critically ill adult patients: systematic review of randomised controlled trials. Br Med J 1998; 19: 273–278.

102. Bartlett JG, Finegold SM. Anaerobic bacterial infections of the lung. Am Rev Respir Dis 1974; 110: 56–77.

103. Finegold SM. Aspiration pneumonia, lung abscess and empyema. In: Pennington JE, ed. Respiratory infections: diagnosis and management, 3rd edn. New York: Raven Press; 1994: 311–322.

104. Tobin MJ. Diagnosis of pneumonia: techniques and problems. Clin Chest Med 1987; 8: 513–527.

105. Davies S. Histoplasma capsulation pneumonia. In: Pennington JE, ed. Respiratory infections: diagnosis and management, 3rd edn. New York: Raven Press; 1994: 599–606.

106. Singh TS, Mutum SS, Razaque MA. Pulmonary paragonimiasis: clinical features, diagnosis and treatment of 39 cases in Maniput. Trans R Soc Trop Med Hyg 1986; 80: 967–971.

107. Lim TK. Emerging pathogens for pneumonia in Singapore. Ann Acad Med Singapore 1997; 26: 651–658.

108. Kim PE, Musher DM, Glezen WP et al. Association of invasive pneumococcal disease with season, atmospheric conditions, air pollution, and the isolation of respiratory viruses. Clin Infect Dis 1996; 22: 100–106.

109. Hoge CW, Reichler MR, Dominguez EA et al. An epidemic of pneumococcal disease in an overcrowded, inadequately ventilated jail. N Engl J Med 1994; 331: 643–648.

110. Venkatesan P, Macfarlane JT. Role of pneumococcal antigen in the diagnosis of pneumococcal pneumonia. Thorax 1992; 47: 329–331.

111. Farrington M, Rubenstein D. Antigen detection in pneumococcal pneumonia. J Infection 1991; 23: 109–116.

112. Felmingham D, Washington J. Trends in the antimicrobial susceptibility of bacterial respiratory tract pathogens – findings of the Alexander Project 1992–1996. J Chemother 1999; 11(Suppl 1): 5–21.

113. Johnson AP. Antibiotic resistance among clinically important gram-positive bacteria in the UK. J Hosp Infect 1998; 40: 17–26.

114. Pallares R, Linares J, Vadillo M et al. Resistance to penicillin and cephalosporin and mortality from severe pneumococcal pneumonia in Barcelona, Spain. N Engl J Med 1995; 333: 474–480.

115. Klugman K, Feldman C. The clinical relevance of antibiotic resistance in the management of pneumococcal pneumonia. Infect Dis Clin Pract 1998; 7: 180–184.

116. Pallares R, Viladrich PF, Linares J et al. Impact of antibiotic resistance on chemotherapy for pneumococcal infections. Microb Drug Resist 1998; 4: 339–347.

117. Smit P, Oberholzer D, Hayden–Smith S et al. Protective efficacy of pneumococcal polysaccharide vaccines. JAMA 1977; 238: 2613–2616.

118. Riley ID, Parr PI, Andrews M et al. Immunisation with a polyvalent pneumococcal vaccine. Lancet 1977; 1: 1338–1341.

119. Fine MJ, Smith MA, Carson CA et al. Efficacy of pneumococcal vaccination in adults: a meta-analysis of randomized controlled trials. Arch Intern Med 1994; 154: 2666–2677.

120. Pneumococcal vaccine. In: Immunisation against infectious diseases. London: HMSO; 1996: 167–172.

121. Basiliere JL, Bistrang HW, Spencer WF. Streptococcal pneumonia: recent outbreaks in military recruit population. Am J Med 1968; 44: 580–589.

122. Woodhead MA, Macfarlane JT. Staphylococcal pneumonia. Q J Med 1987; 64: 783–790.

123. Vaneechoutte M, Varschraegen G, Glaeys G et al. Respiratory tract carrier rates of *Moraxella catarrhalis* in adults and children and interpretation of the isolation of *M. catarrhalis* from sputum. J Clin Microbiol 1990; 28: 2674–2680.

124. Wright PW, Wallace RJ, Shepherd R. A descriptive study of 42 cases of *Branhamella catarrhalis* pneumonia. Am J Med 1990; 88(Suppl 5A): 5–8.

125. Hagar H, Verghese A, Alvarez S, Berk SL. *Branhamella catarrhalis* respiratory injections. Rev Infect Dis 1987; 9: 1140–1149.

126. Woodhead MA, Macfarlane JT. *Haemophilus influenzae* pneumonia in previously fit adults. Eur J Respir Dis 1987; 70: 218–220.

127. Martin SJ, Hoganson DA, Thomas ET. Detection of *Streptococcus pneumoniae* and *Haemophilus influenzae* type of antigens in acute non-bacterial pneumonia. J Clin Microbiol 1987; 25: 248–250.

128. Joseph CA, Dedman D, Birtles R et al. Legionnaires' disease surveillance: England and Wales, 1993. Commun Dis Rep 1994; 4: 109–111.

129. Joseph CA, Harrison TG, Ilijic-Car D, Bartlett CL. Legionnaires' disease in residents of England and Wales: 1998. Commun Dis Rep 1999; 8: 280–284.

130. Joseph CA, Harrison TG, Ilijic-Car D, Bartlett CL. Legionnaires' disease in residents of England and Wales: 1998. Commun Dis Rep 1999; 8: 280–284.

131. Watson J, Macfarlane JT. Legionella infections. In: Ellis M, ed. Infectious diseases of the respiratory tract. Cambridge: Cambridge Univ Press; 1998: 237–244.

132. Miller AC. Early clinical differentiation between Legionnaires' disease and other sporadic pneumonias. Ann Intern Med 1979; 90: 526–528.

133. Woodhead MA, Macfarlane JT. The protean manifestations of legionnaires' disease. J R Coll Phys Lond 1985; 19: 224–230.

134. Joseph CA, Harrison TG, Ilijic-Car D, Bartlett CL. Legionnaires' disease in residents of England and Wales: 1996. Commun Dis Rep 1997; 7: 153–159.

135. Birtles RJ, Harrison TG, Samuel D, Taylor AG. Evaluation of urinary antigen ELISA for diagnosing *Legionella pneumophila* serogroup 1 infection. J Clin Path 1990; 43: 685–690.

136. Schulin T, Wennersten CB, Ferraro MJ et al. Susceptibilities of *Legionella* spp. to newer antimicrobials in vitro. Antimicrob Agents Chemother 1998; 42: 1520–1523.

137. Edelstein PH. Antimicrobial chemotherapy for Legionnaires disease: time for a change. Ann Intern Med 1998; 129: 328–330.

138. Eisenstadt J, Crane LR. Gram negative bacillary pneumonias. In: Pennington JE, ed. Respiratory infections: diagnosis and management, 3rd edn. New York: Raven Press; 1994: 369–406.

139. Everett ED, Nelson RA. Pulmonary melioidosis. Am Rev Respir Dis 1975; 112: 331–340.

140. Leelarasamee A, Bovornkitti S. Melioidosis: review and update. Rev Infect Dis 1989; 11: 413–425.

141. Weber DJ, Wolfson JS, Swartz MN, Hooper DC. *Pasteurella multocida* infections. Medicine 1984; 63: 133–154.

142. Parry CM, Harries AD. Respiratory infections and foreign travel. In: Ellis ME, ed. Infectious diseases of the respiratory tract. Cambridge: Cambridge University Press; 1997: 486–508.

143. Levine DP, Lerner AM. The clinical spectrum of *Mycoplasma pneumoniae* infections. Med Clin North Am 1978; 62: 961–978.

144. Murray HW, Masur H, Senterfit LB et al. The protean manifestations of *Mycoplasma pneumoniae* infection in adults. Am J Med 1975; 58: 229–241.

145. Hammerschlag MR. *Chlamydia pneumoniae* and the lung. Eur Respir J 2000; 16: 1001–1007.

146. Yung AP, Grayson ML. Psittacosis – a review of 135 cases. Med J Austr 1988; 148: 228.

147. Crosse BS. Psittacosis: a clinical review. J Infect 1990; 21: 251.

148. Sillis M, Wreghitt TG, Paul ID, Caul EO. Chlamydial respiratory infections. Don't get bogged down by differentiating species. Br Med J 1993; 307: 62–63.

149. Kutlin A, Tsumura N, Emre U et al. Evaluation of *Chlamydia* immunoglobulin M (IgM), IgG, and IgA rELISAs Medac for diagnosis of *Chlamydia pneumoniae* infection. Clin Diag Lab Immunol 1997; 4: 213–216.

150. Grayston JT. *Chlamydia pneumoniae*, Strain TWAR. Chest 1989; 95: 664–669.

151. Sobradillo V, Ansola P, Baranda F, Corral C. Q fever pneumonia: a review of 164 community acquired cases in the Basque country. Eur Respir J 1989; 2: 263–266.

152. Sawyer LA, Fishbein DB, McDade JE. Q fever: current concepts. Rev Infect Dis 1987; 9: 935–946.

153. Sobradillo V, Zalacain R, Capelastegui A et al. Antibiotic treatment in pneumonias due to Q fever. Thorax 1992; 47: 276–278.

154. Douglas RG. Pathogenic mechanisms in viral respiratory tract infections. In: Sande MA, Hudson LD Root RK, eds. Respiratory infections. Contemporary issues in infectious diseases vol 5. New York: Churchill Livingstone; 1986: 25–33.

155. Kauffman RS. Viral pneumonia. In: Pennington JE, ed. Respiratory infections: diagnosis and management, 3rd edn. New York: Raven Press; 1994: 515–532.

156. Nguyen-van-Tam JS, Nicholson KG. Influenza deaths in Leicestershire during the 1989–90 epidemic: implications for prevention. Epidemiol Infect 1992; 108: 537–545.

157. Ashley J: Smith T, Dunnell K. Deaths in Great Britain associated with the influenza epidemic of 1989–90. Population Trends 1991; 65: 16–20.

158. Jackson GG, Stanley ED. Prevention and control of influenza by chemoprophylaxis and chemotherapy. JAMA 1976; 235: 2739–2748.

159. Creticos CM, Jackson GG, Bernstein JM et al. Oral ribavirin treatment of influenza A and B. Antimicrob Agents Chemother 1987; 31: 1285–1287.

160. Hayden FG, Osterhaus A, Treanor JJ et al. Efficacy and safety of the neuraminidase inhibitor zanamivir in the treatment of influenza virus infections. N Engl J Med 1997; 337: 874–880.

161. Gross PA, Hermogenes AW, Sacks HS et al. The efficacy of influenza vaccine in elderly persons. A meta-analysis and review of the literature. Ann Intern Med 1995; 123: 518–527.

162. Palache AM, Beyer WEP, Luchters G et al. Influenza vaccines: the effect of vaccine dose on antibody response in primed populations during the ongoing interpandemic period. A review of the literature. Vaccine 1993; 11: 892–908.

163. Govaert TME, Dinant GJ, Aretz K et al. Adverse reactions to influenza vaccine in elderly people: randomised double blind placebo controlled trial. Br Med J 1993; 307: 988–990.

164. Rose RM, Pinkston P, O'Donnell C, Jensen WA. Viral infections of the lower respiratory tract. Clin Chest Med 1987; 8: 405–418.

165. Wilson R, Alton E, Rutman A et al. Upper respiratory tract viral infection and mucociliary clearance. Eur J Respir Dis 1987; 70: 272–279.

166. Montagne JR. RSV pneumonia, a community acquired infection in adults. Lancet 1997; 349: 149–150.

167. Ruben FL, Nguyen MLT. Viral pneumonitis. Clin Chest Med 1991; 12: 223–235.

168. Finn JJ, Weller TH, Morgan HR. Epidemic pleurodynia: clinical and aetiological studies based on 114 cases. Arch Intern Med 1949; 83: 305–313.

169. Ikeda RM, Kondracki SF, Drabkin PD et al. Pleurodynia among football players at a high school. An outbreak associated with coxsackievirus B1. JAMA 1993; 270: 2205–2206.

170. Aeschlimann A, Kahn MF. Tietze's Syndrome: a critical review. Clin Exp Rheumatol 1990; 8: 407–412.

171. Massie JD, Sebes JI, Cowles SJ. Bone scintigraphy and costochondritis. J Thorac Imaging 1993; 8: 137–141.

36.1 Pulmonary complications of HIV infection

Giovanni Guaraldi, Elisa Busi Rizzi and Cesare Saltini

 Key points

- The interaction between the human immunodeficiency virus (HIV) and the host immune system dictates the establishment of chronic HIV infection and the decline of CD4$^+$ cell counts. This, in turn, is the major determinant of the risk of respiratory opportunistic infections.

- Pulmonary tuberculosis, bacterial pneumonia and Kaposi's sarcoma are seen with CD4+ cell counts below 500/mm^3; *Pneumocystis carinii* pneumonia, disseminated histoplasmosis and coccidioidomycosis, miliary or extrapulmonary tuberculosis, and toxoplasmosis with counts below 200/mm^3; *Mycobacterium avium* complex and cytomegalovirus diseases with counts below 50/mm^3.

- The use of 'highly active antiretroviral therapy' (HAART) has changed the natural history of HIV infection and the rate of HIV-associated opportunistic infections, which has declined impressively with 0.5–5-fold reduction of the rates of *Pneumocystis carinii* pneumonia, pulmonary tuberculosis and *M. avium* complex.

- Conversely, some new syndromes are now being observed at the inception of HAART, including the paradoxical response to tuberculosis treatment, exacerbation of cryptococcosis and *M. avium* complex lymphadenitis.

Human immunodeficiency virus and respiratory disease

Since the first cases of human immunodeficiency virus (HIV) infection were recognised nearly 20 years ago, the acquired immunodeficiency syndrome (AIDS) epidemic continues to be one of the major world health problems, with an estimated 5.8 million new cases a year, 2.3 million deaths in 1998 and a worldwide prevalence of 33.4 million.[1,2] Moreover, in the developing countries the concurrence of AIDS with the pulmonary tuberculosis (TB) epidemic makes the AIDS threat deadlier.[3]

Although respiratory disease remains a major cause of HIV-associated morbidity and mortality, the advent of combined antiretroviral treatments, currently called 'highly active antiretroviral therapy' (HAART), in which at least three drugs are used, has changed the natural history of HIV infection in those countries where advanced therapy is widely available;[4] thus, this chapter will focus on the changing pattern of clinical presentation of lung infections in the so called 'HAART era' as well as on the progress in diagnosing, managing and preventing the pulmonary complications of HIV disease.

Replication of HIV-1 may lead to the production of more than 10 billion particles of HIV-1 in an infected individual:[5,6] measurable blood levels of HIV-1 are the result of a dynamic equilibrium between the continuous replication and production of HIV in lymphoid tissues and the clearance of the virus by the immune system. The interaction between the virus and the host immune system dictates the establishment of chronic HIV infection. Hence, the occurrence of opportunistic infections is the final result of the destruction of CD4$^+$ cells following HIV-1 replication within the cells of the immune system. Thus, careful monitoring of both virological (plasma viral load) and immunological (blood CD4 counts) parameters in HIV patients can predict disease progression and the risk of pulmonary complications. Some authors think that the level of plasma viral RNA during the course of primary HIV infection, a key phase in the immunopathogenesis of the disease, can predict both the disease pattern and the rate of progression to AIDS and may be used as an indicator of the likelihood of developing AIDS.[7,8]

In clinical practice, with the availability of an increasing number of antiretroviral agents of proven efficacy (Table 36.1.1), it has become possible to dampen viral replication, lower HIV viral load and arrest disease progression in HIV-infected persons. Aggressive treatments using combinations of drugs can thus be instigated with the goal of bringing plasma viral load to undetectable levels.[9]

Table 36.1.1   Antiretroviral drugs of current use in HIV infection

Type	International non-proprietary name	Abbreviation
Nucleoside reverse transcriptase inhibitors	Zidovudine	AZT
	Didanosine	DDI
	Stavudine	D4T
	Zalcitabine	DDC
	Lamivudine	3TC
	Abacavir	ABC
Non-nucleoside reverse transcriptase inhibitors	Nevirapine	NVP
	Efavirenz	EFV
	Delavirdine	DLV
Protease inhibitors	Indinavir	IDV
	Nelfinavir	NFV
	Ritonavir	RTV
	Saquinavir hard gel	SQV HG
	Saquinavir soft gel	SQV SG
	Lopinavir	ABT378

While quantitative virology has become indispensable for the monitoring of antiretroviral therapy, the CD4$^+$ cell count is still the best clinical marker with which to stage the disease, establish the risk of specific HIV-associated complications, determine the need for prophylaxis against opportunistic infection and assess the clinical response to antiretroviral therapy. HIV patients may have persistent generalised lymphadenopathy at any disease stage and female patients may have recurrent or severe *Candida albicans* vaginitis in the earlier phases of HIV infection. However, patients with CD4$^+$ T-cell counts in the normal range (> 500/mm^3) are usually asymptomatic (Table 36.1.2).

Pulmonary TB, bacterial pneumonia, Kaposi's sarcoma and systemic non-Hodgkin's lymphoma occur more frequently when the CD4$^+$ cell count falls below 500/mm^3, although they may occur at all stages. Patients with CD4$^+$ cell counts between 200 and 500/mm^3 are at risk for herpes zoster, oral thrush, cervical intraepithelial neoplasia, idiopathic thrombocytopenic purpura and anaemia. Some AIDS-defining conditions such Kaposi's sarcoma, non-Hodgkin's lymphoma, recurrent pneumonia, TB and invasive cervical carcinoma may occur at this stage. Most opportunistic infections occur after the CD4$^+$ count has fallen below 200/mm^3. These include *Pneumocystis carinii* pneumonia (PCP), disseminated herpes simplex virus infection, disseminated histoplasmosis and coccidioidomycosis, miliary or extrapulmonary TB, and cryptosporidiosis. Toxoplasmosis and cryptococcosis require even greater immunosuppression, typically occurring at CD4$^+$ cell counts below 100/mm^3, and disseminated *Mycobacterium avium* complex (MAC) and cytomegalovirus diseases are usually restricted to patients with CD4$^+$ cell counts less than 50/mm^3.

Epidemiology

There is a wide geographical variation in the epidemiology of opportunistic infections and other pulmonary complications of the HIV infection. The probability of developing a given disease depends on the risk of exposure to potential pathogens, the virulence of the pathogens, the level of immunosuppression of the patient and the patient's access to effective antiretroviral treatment. From 1996, with the new antiretroviral drug treatments in the 'HAART era', the incidence of HIV-associated opportunistic infections has dropped impressively, as has the rate of AIDS-associated deaths.[10] Several studies have shown that the incidence of nearly all AIDS-defining illnesses significantly decreased between 1992 and 1998[11,12] (Fig. 36.1.1).

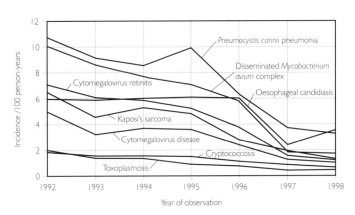

Fig. 36.1.1   The trends for opportunistic infections in HIV-infected adults and adolescents, ASD (Adult and Adolescent Spectrum of Disease) Project, 1992–98 are standardised to the population of AIDS cases reported nationally in the same years by age, sex, race, HIV exposure mode, country of origin and CD4$^+$ T lymphocyte count. Since the median CD4$^+$ T lymphocyte count of reported patients with AIDS is between 100 and 110 per litre, rates indicate the incidence of opportunistic infections among persons with CD4$^+$ counts in this range. The numbers of subjects included in the analysis are 10 441, 11 589, 11 276, 10 048, 9250, 8897 and 8074 respectively for the years 1992–98. (Adapted and updated from Jones et al.[13])

Table 36.1.2 Complications of HIV infection in relation to CD4$^+$ cell counts

CD4$^+$ cell count (cells/mm^3)	Organism	Common manifestations
More than 500	HIV HIV HIV	Primary HIV infection Persistent generalised lymphadenopathy Aseptic meningitis
Less than 500	S. pneumoniae, H. influenzae M. tuberculosis Candida species Herpes simplex virus Varicella-zoster virus Epstein–Barr virus Cryptosporidium parvum HHV-8 (KSHV)	Community-acquired pneumonia Pulmonary tuberculosis Mucosal candidiasis Orogenital herpes Varicella Oral hairy leukoplakia, non-Hodgkin's lymphoma Self-limiting diarrhoea Kaposi's sarcoma
Less than 200	P. carinii C. parvum	Pneumonia Chronic diarrhoea
Less than 100	T. gondii Microsporidia Candida species C. neoformans M. tuberculosis Herpes simplex virus Varicella-zoster virus Epstein–Barr virus M. avium complex Cytomegalovirus HIV	Encephalitis Diarrhoea Esophagitis Meningitis Disseminated tuberculosis Disseminated herpes Disseminated zoster Primary central nervous system lymphoma Disseminated M. avium complex Retinitis, encephalitis Wasting syndrome, dementia, myelopathy

With regard to opportunistic lung infections, the incidence of PCP declined by 21.5% per year between 1996 and 1998, compared with a 3.4% decline per year between 1992 and 1995. The incidence of disseminated MAC disease declined by 39.9% per year between 1996 and 1998, compared to a 4.7% decline per year between 1992 and 1995.[14] The risk of TB has declined among HIV patients taking HAART from 0.79 per 100 person-years to 0.16 for double combination therapy and 0.08 for triple combination therapy compared with no therapy or monotherapy.[15] This may be attributed partly to the availability of effective antiretroviral treatments and partly to improvements in specific measures for prevention of opportunistic infections. However, as the spectrum and relative frequencies of opportunistic infections have not changed appreciably since the beginning of the AIDS epidemic and PCP, candidal oesophagitis and MAC disease continue to be the most common infections in persons with CD4$^+$ T lymphocyte counts in the AIDS range, it seems reasonable to attribute to the new antiretroviral treatments the major role in reducing the frequency of opportunistic infection.

Conversely, some new syndromes are now being observed in the first months of combination antiretroviral therapy: these include paradoxical responses to treatment of TB,[16] exacerbation of cryptococcosis,[17] cytomegalovirus vitritis[18] and MAC lymphadenitis.[19] These syndromes, which have been termed 'reversal syndromes', frequently occur in the setting of an increasing CD4$^+$ T lymphocyte count. It has been hypothesised that they may represent either the unmasking of an undiagnosed opportunistic infection or an exacerbation of an already diagnosed opportunistic infection whereby the restoration of the patient immune function favours the development of the infection immunopathology.

While the incidence of Kaposi's sarcoma is decreasing, not all HIV-associated respiratory conditions follow the same trend. There is accumulating evidence that successful suppression of HIV RNA may not necessarily translate into decreased incidence rates of tumours such as immunoblastic lymphoma, Hodgkin's lymphoma and Burkitt's lymphoma, suggesting that the neoplastic complications of HIV infection will become relatively more frequent in the future. However, measures for preventing opportunistic infection remain important in the 'HAART era'. Certainly, they are still particularly important for those who do not have access to HAART, are not willing to take HAART, are poorly compliant with HAART or are infected with resistant strains of HIV.

Pathogenesis of the immune abnormalities of the HIV-infected lung

The key immune alterations caused by HIV penetration and replication of the virus within CD4$^+$ immune cells, i.e. the helper inducer T-cells, dendritic cells and macrophages are:

- deterioration of CD4$^+$ T-cell function
- the progressive depletion of CD4 T-cell numbers
- the progressive impairment of the antigen presenting function of macrophages and dendritic cells.

The virus enters the lung during the early phases of HIV infection and attacks alveolar macrophages. The virus has been isolated both from lung tissues and from bronchoalveolar lavage (BAL) cells.[20,21] Current concepts are that the virus is carried to the lung by tissue-bound blood mononuclear phagocytes and by infected CD4$^+$ T-cells.[22,23] In addition, the virus may itself cross the alveolar capillary barrier and then infect lung cells.

Bronchoalveolar lavage studies have shown that the early phases of HIV infection are characterised by a CD8$^+$ T-cell alveolitis[24] that is paralleled by the infiltration of the lung interstitium by mononuclear cells, mainly CD8$^+$ T-cells and plasma cells.[25] The immune responses of lung CD4$^+$ T-cells have not been studied as thoroughly as those of the blood CD4$^+$ T-cells, which have been shown to display impaired responses to soluble antigens, impaired TH1 cytokine production and reduced ability to expand clonally. CD8$^+$ T-cells have been shown to play a central role in anti-HIV defences. The studies of Pantaleo and Fauci have indicated that the activation of CD8$^+$ T-cells associated with the expansion of anti-HIV CD8$^+$ cytotoxic T-cell clones plays a beneficial role in retarding disease progression.[26] On the other hand, CD8$^+$ T-lymphocyte expansion and activation within the lung may be followed by the development of HIV-associated lymphocytic interstitial pneumonia, an immune disorder that precedes the deterioration of the patient's immune function and the appearance of opportunistic lung infections.[27]

It has been shown that the HIV isolates grown from mononuclear phagocytes can more readily infect macrophages than blood isolates.[28] As the macrophage is relatively resistant to the cytopathic effect of the virus, infected lung macrophages may represent an important reservoir of HIV.[29]

In HIV-infected patients, alveolar macrophages represent the first line of defence for the containment of bacterial infections. After phagocytosis, macrophages undergo activation, i.e. produce proinflammatory cytokines and chemokines, whose main role is to contain the spread of pathogens by recruiting peripheral lymphocytes and monocytes to the site of inflammation, and express surface cytokine and chemokine receptors. However, in the case of a concomitant HIV infection, these signals strongly enhance susceptibility to viral infection, at the level of both viral entry and viral replication. Under these conditions, viral expansion extends beyond tissue macrophages to T cells and vice versa, according to the emerging viral phenotype.

Pulmonary macrophages are susceptible to viral attack through several routes:

- phagocytosis
- binding to the CD4 receptor
- binding to the chemokine receptors.

Chemokine receptors represent a family of molecules mediating a variety of important leukocyte functions. Some of these receptors have recently been shown to function as HIV receptors. The CXCR4 and CCR5 receptors have been shown to bind the majority of clinical HIV isolates: importantly, 'non-syncytium-inducing' viruses (called R5 variants) use the CCR5 receptor to enter macrophages and CD4$^+$ T-cells while 'syncytium-inducing' viruses (called X4 variants) use the CXCR4 receptor to attack CD4$^+$ T-cells. Some HIV strains (called 'dual tropic' or R5X4) use both receptors and may also use additional receptors (including CCR2β, CCR3, CCR8 and X3CR1). Interestingly, while R5 viruses represent the dominant population in the early stages of infection, X4 and R5X4 strains emerge later in the course of infection. Importantly, the expression of these receptors on the macrophage is upregulated upon stimulation with microbial products such as lipopolysaccharide or mycobacterial products both in vitro and in vivo, thus suggesting a precise role for chronic lung infections such as TB in accelerating viral replication and the progression of HIV infection.[30-32]

It has been known for a long time that patients affected by both HIV infection and pulmonary TB have a markedly reduced percentage of CD4$^+$ alveolar lymphocytes relative to peripheral blood, impaired alveolar macrophage function and decreased lymphoproliferative responses against *Mycobacterium tuberculosis* antigens when compared with control subjects with either HIV infection or pulmonary TB. Macrophage dysfunction due to HIV infection may play an important role in susceptibility to infection.

Cigarette smoking and lung immune responses

Smoking has been associated with a relative decrease in CD4$^+$ and CD8$^+$ lymphocytes in BAL fluid and reduced levels of inflammatory cytokines, interleukin-1α and tumour necrosis factor-α[33] and it has been suggested that HIV-infected smokers may have impaired local lung defences and may therefore be more susceptible to lung disease than non-smokers. However, not all studies would support a greater susceptibility to rapid progression to AIDS in HIV-infected cigarette smokers.[34]

Respiratory infections

Pneumocystis carinii pneumonia

Epidemiology

Pneumocystis carinii pneumonia was the most common opportunistic infection associated with HIV disease during the first decade of the AIDS epidemic in Europe and the USA: the infection occurred in approximately 80% of all HIV-infected patients, up to 50 000 cases per year in the USA, with a mortality rate of 10–20%.[35]

Although the sources of *P. carinii* infection have not been identified yet, animal and environmental studies suggest airborne transmission of *P. carinii* from environmental reservoirs. Most humans are infected with *P. carinii* early in life, and the frequency of primary PCP in infants with perinatally acquired HIV is consistent with this notion.[36] Although it is generally thought that new PCP cases represent new episodes of infection rather than reactivation of latent infection, colonisation is thought to be possible.[37] In clinical practice, most experts recommend isolation of active PCP cases from other immunosuppressed individuals, although respiratory isolation, such as for TB, is not deemed necessary.

Pathogenesis

P. carinii is a difficult organism that cannot be cultured in vitro and was originally classified as a protozoon on the basis of morphology and susceptibility to antiprotozoal drugs. Recent genetic studies have suggested that *P. carinii* is more closely related to fungi.[38] The organism is 1.5–5.0 μm in size and its life cycle is characterised by three stages: the trophozoite, the most numerous stage, when small clusters of Giemsa-stained organisms are seen; the intermediate stage of 'precyst' and the cyst stage. Cysts are large inclusions containing as many as eight daughter bodies.

In the experimentally CD4⁺-depleted mouse, local inflammation driven by neutrophils and activated CD8⁺ T cells in BAL fluid leads to severe pulmonary damage with decreased lung function and hypoxaemia. This indicates that the host reaction, chiefly the CD8⁺ T lymphocytes, plays a role in the pathogenesis of the disease.[39]

In man, the trophozoite of *P. carinii* attaches to type I alveolar pneumocytes and does not invade the lung tissue but, in the absence of an effective cell-mediated immunity, proliferates as an extracellular parasite within the alveolar space, leading to the filling of the alveolar spaces with ensuing marked hypoxaemia.

Most commonly, patients present with dyspnoea, non-productive cough and fever. At physical examination they show tachypnoea, cyanosis, tachycardia and rales. Typically, chest radiography and computed tomography (CT) scans demonstrate diffuse bilateral interstitial infiltrates (Figs 36.1.2 & 36.1.3). Pulmonary function testing demonstrates reduced total lung capacity and reduced diffusing capacity. Blood gases show hypoxaemia with alkalosis. Laboratory testing shows elevated serum lactate dehydrogenase. Occasionally, however, the chest radiograph may be atypical and demonstrate unilateral infiltrates, cavities, nodules, pleural effusions, pneumothorax and pneumomediastinum (Fig. 36.1.4). As the Multicenter AIDS Cohort Study has shown,[40] PCP is most common after the CD4⁺ cell count falls below 200/mm³.

Diagnosis

Microscopic examination of induced sputum samples, the standard method for obtaining respiratory secretions from suspect PCP patients, has a sensitivity ranging between 30% and 90%, depending upon the proficiency of the laboratory. Microscopic examination of BAL samples has a higher sensitivity, of about 98–100%. Pulmonary biopsies may be used to diagnose PCP, with 90–95% sensitivity, when the other procedures have failed. To identify the organism, Wright–Giemsa or Papanicolaou stains are performed for rapid diagnosis followed by a confirmatory stain using methenamine silver staining or immunofluorescence.

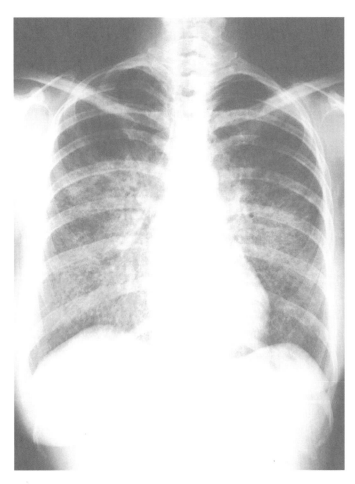

Fig. 36.1.2 The chest radiograph of an AIDS patient presenting with *Pneumocystis carinii* pneumonia shows diffuse profusion of interstitial markings, mainly micronodules.

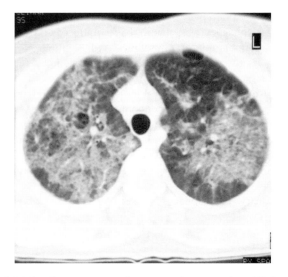

Fig. 36.1.3 Chest computed tomography scan of an AIDS patient with *Pneumocystis carinii* pneumonia. This upper lung slice shows diffuse ground-glass opacities with enhancement of the vascular aspects, indicative of *Pneumocystis carinii* alveolitis. Also seen are bullae and blebs.

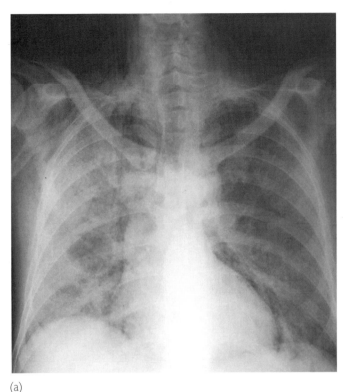

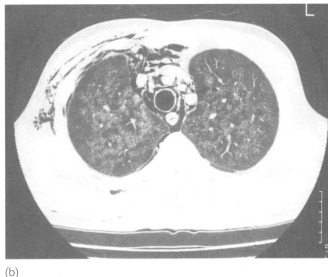

(a)

(b)

Fig. 36.1.4 Pneumomediastinum complicating *Pneumocystis carinii* pneumonia in an AIDS patient presenting with severe dyspnoea and subcutaneous emphysema. (a) The posteroanterior chest radiograph shows diffuse interstitial pneumonitis. Air is seen in the mediastinal pleura, as indicated by the marked hyperlucency of the heart and vessel contours. (b) In the apical computed tomography scan, diffuse ground-glass opacities are seen along with subpleural bullae, pneumomediastinum and subcutaneous emphysema.

Treatment

A number of drugs have shown efficacy for the treatment of PCP and six are now recommended by most authorities (Table 36.1.3). Trimethoprim-sulfamethoxazole (co-trimoxazole) remains the mainstay of treatment as newer drugs, such as atovaquone and trimetrexate–leucovorin, show lower toxicity but are far less effective. The emergence of resistance against co-trimoxazole, a drug inhibiting the key folate metabolism enzyme dihydropteroate synthase, is due to mutations in the dihydropteroate synthase gene that are thought to arise from the use of co-trimoxazole prophylaxis. The observation that these mutations may be present in patients without prior co-trimoxazole treatment has suggested person-to-person transmission.[41a]

Adjunctive therapy with corticosteroids

Adjunctive corticosteroids for the treatment of PCP have been recommended for patients with risk factors such as arterial oxygen concentration lower than 60 mmHg and BAL neutrophilia above 10%. In fact a large prospective study has shown that, in a group of patients with a P_aO_2 between 50 and 70 mmHg and BAL neutrophilia above 10%, those who received steroids had a mortality rate of only 4% compared with 50% in those who did not.[41b]

Preventive therapies for *P. carinii* infection

Four drugs are recommended for PCP prophylaxis: co-trimoxazole, dapsone, aerosolised pentamidine and atovaquone. A critical review of 35 independent studies comparing co-trimoxazole with dapsone or aerosolised pentamidine showed that co-trimoxazole provides better protection against PCP, although is does not improve survival.[42]

The frequency of adverse drug reactions leading to discontinuation of therapy with co-trimoxazole is as high as 25–50%. Side effects are dose-related and time-dependent. Intermittent therapy (three times a week) has been attempted and appears to be effective. Adverse effects with dapsone are seen in 25–40% of treated individuals. Atovaquone is usually better tolerated. In patients showing intolerance to co-trimoxazole, dapsone 100 mg once daily or nebulised pentamidine 300 mg monthly are frequently used as second-line alternatives. Discontinuation of PCP prophylaxis is now thought to be safe in patients receiving HAART, after CD4+ lymphocyte counts have risen above 200×10^3.[43,44]

Tuberculosis

Epidemiology

A number of epidemiological studies have shown that the annual rate of TB disease among untreated, tuberculin-skin-test (PPD)-

Table 36.1.3 Drugs and protocols for the treatment of *P. carinii* pneumonia

Drug	Route and dosage	Duration	Side effects
Trimethoprim–sulfamethoxazole (co-trimoxazole)	15 mg/kg (trimethoprim dose) per day p.o. or i.v. in 3–4 divided doses	21 days	Rash, Stevens–Johnson syndrome, neutropenia, hepatitis and gastrointestinal toxicity; occasionally, seizures, confusion or agitation
Pentamidine	3–4 mg/kg per day i.v.	21 days	Renal toxicity, hypotension, hypoglycaemia, neutropenia, cardiac arrhythmias, diabetes (20% of cases)
Dapsone–trimethoprim	Trimethoprim, 15 mg/kg per day p.o. or i.v. Dapsone, 100 mg per day p.o.	21 days	Rash and haemolytic anaemia, production of methaemoglobin; with increased hypoxaemia
Clindamycin–primaquine	Clindamycin 600 mg i.v. t.i.d. or 300–450 mg p.o. q.i.d. Primaquine 30 mg p.o. per day	21 days	Mild fever or rash; haemolytic anaemia in patients with G6PD deficiency, pseudomembranous colitis
Atovaquone	750 mg of suspension p.o. b.i.d. with meals	21 days	Rash, fever, elevated liver function tests
Trimetrexate–leucovorin	Trimetrexate 45 mg/m² i.v. per day Leucovorin 20 mg/m² p.o. or i.v. q.i.d.	??	Bone marrow suppression, particularly neutropenia

positive, HIV-infected persons ranges from 1.7 to 7.9 cases of TB per 100 person-years not taking preventive therapy.[45–49]

Both in-vitro studies and epidemiological data from both the developing and the industrialised world, including three cohort studies from Europe, indicate that active TB accelerates the progression of HIV infection.[50–54] In addition, HIV-seropositive patients have a significantly higher rate of resistance, compared with HIV-seronegative patients, to first-line antituberculosis drugs including isoniazid, both isoniazid and rifampicin (multidrug-resistant TB) and rifampicin monoresistance (TB resistant to rifampicin only). This is thought to be due to the higher risk among HIV-seropositive subjects of acquiring *M. tuberculosis* infection.[55,56] In this regard, the sizeable number of outbreaks of nosocomially transmitted multidrug-resistant TB affecting AIDS patients that have been reported in the literature demonstrates the increased risk of disease associated with airborne transmission of drug-resistant strains of *M. tuberculosis*.[57–63] The mortality of TB in the HIV-infected is higher than in the non-infected. The results of the treatment of TB disease in HIV-infected patients depend upon the person's degree of immunosuppression and the response to the appropriate anti-tuberculosis therapy. The overall 1-year mortality rate for HIV-related TB ranges from 20% to 35%, i.e. several times greater than for HIV-negative TB and shows little variation between industrialised and developing countries.[64–67] The cause of death is, however, largely attributable to AIDS complications other than TB.[68]

Clinical presentation

The symptoms and signs of TB in HIV-infected patients vary significantly with the progression of the immunodeficiency.[69]

Sentinel symptoms include cough, fever, weight loss and night sweats. Extrapulmonary disease is three to five times more common among the HIV-infected than the non-infected, with the ensuing symptoms resulting from liver, bone marrow, central nervous system or lymphatic involvement predominating. Chest radiographs less frequently show the typical upper-lobe lesions and may be normal in up to 10% of patients. When immunodeficiency is severe, miliary infiltrates and mediastinal or hilar adenopathy are common (Fig. 36.1.5). Thus, although the majority of patients present with clinical and radiographic pictures reminiscent of TB, such as infiltrates, cavities, enlarged lymph nodes and pleural effusions (Fig. 36.1.6), no single chest radiographic presentation rules out TB.[70,71] In this regard, in a retrospective evaluation of 118 HIV patients admitted to the Spallanzani Hospital in Rome with a bacteriologically confirmed diagnosis of pulmonary TB, diffuse miliary nodules were present in 33%, middle–lower-lobe infiltrates in 23%, with cavitation in 11%, and 32% had typical upper-lobe infiltrates. No chest radiographic abnormalities were seen in 12% (unpublished).

In consideration of the risk of airborne transmission, respiratory isolation is the top priority at admission of a HIV patient with suspected TB. Clinical, laboratory and radiographic criteria for isolation are listed in Table 36.1.4.

Paradoxical reactions to concurrent antiretroviral therapy and tuberculosis therapy

The appearance of paradoxical reactions after the initiation of chemotherapy in non-immunocompromised patients has been known for a long time and has been attributed to the reaction to antigens released from killed *M. tuberculosis*. A similar

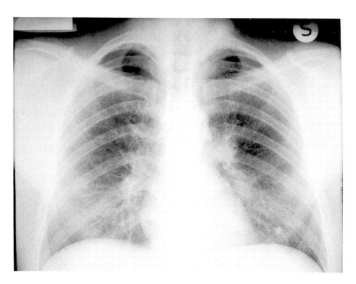

Fig. 36.1.5 Chest radiograph of an AIDS patient with tuberculosis. Notable are the diffuse micronodular infiltrate and the enlargement of the hilar lymph nodes.

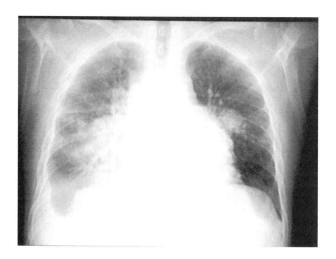

Fig. 36.1.6 Chest radiograph of an AIDS patient with tuberculosis. A diffuse bilateral micronodular infiltrate, hilar lymph node enlargement and right-sided pleural effusion are seen.

phenomenon has been described in HIV patients undergoing TB treatment (especially those with CD4+ cell counts lower than 200/mm³), concurrently with the drop in viral load occurring after the initiation of HAART. The most frequently described manifestations of paradoxical reactions during TB treatment are: fever, lymphadenopathies, worsening of chest radiographic abnormalities with the appearance of diffuse infiltrates, pleural effusions, and cavitations without a corresponding increase in the numbers of acid-fast organisms in sputum. According to published series, paradoxical reactions were more prevalent among patients with HIV-related TB who received TB treatment and combination antiretroviral therapy (36%) than among non-HIV patients receiving antituberculosis chemotherapy (2%) and HIV-infected patients during the pre-zidovudine era (7%).[47]

Table 36.1.4 Criteria for respiratory isolation of tuberculosis suspects

- Positive AFB stains obtained prior to admission
- Chest radiographic abnormalities suggesting tuberculosis
- Cough and fever in the presence of chest radiographic abnormalities of any kind
- Cough persisting for at least 15 days
- Bloody sputum
- Fever persisting for at least 7 days
- Weight loss
- Night sweats
- A history of previous attacks of tuberculosis or of tuberculosis infection (positive PPD skin test)
- Close contact with TB patients

Potential causes for an unfavourable disease course, such as treatment failure, drug resistance, non-adherence to therapy and allergic reaction to drugs, were ruled out in the above study and TB was eventually cured without modification of the chemotherapy regimen. Paradoxical reactions are in fact self-limiting and last 10–40 days. The administration of prednisolone for 4–8 weeks has been recommended. After the initiation of HAART, PPD conversions may also occur in previously PPD-negative HIV patients.

Because exacerbation of TB signs and symptoms in patients with HIV-related TB can occur soon after combination anti-retroviral therapy is initiated, clinicians should always conduct a thorough investigation to eliminate other aetiologies before making a diagnosis of paradoxical treatment reaction. For these patients, a change in antituberculosis or antiretroviral therapy is not recommended.

Diagnosis

For a detailed discussion of procedures and protocols for the diagnosis of TB the reader is referred to Chapter 38.2. In the HIV-infected TB patient, *M. tuberculosis* may affect almost any organ of the body; however, TB of the lungs is the most frequently observed and respiratory specimens are most frequently examined in the diagnosis of TB. Sputum can be spontaneously produced or can be induced with aerosols of ultrasonically generated hypertonic mists. With spontaneously produced sputum, adequate specimen collection is of utmost importance, since not all samples may contain respiratory secretions coming from the affected lobe(s). Three morning sputum samples need to be collected and examined on three consecutive days. In addition, it is advisable to send to the laboratory three blood cultures for mycobacteria on three separate days.

The sensitivity of stains for acid-fast bacilli (AFBs) on sputum smears, with a lower limit of detection of $0.5–1 \times 10^4$ bacteria/ml varies from 49–94% in immunocompetent to 21–83% in immuno-compromised patients and may be lower on BAL smears.[73] The specificity of AFBs in smears depends on specimen type, the geographical location and the HIV status of the patient. Thus, the use of amplification tests on AFB-positive samples is required to discriminate *M. tuberculosis* from non-tuberculous mycobacteria. According to the recommendations of the American Thoracic Society, a positive direct amplification test indicates TB with greater than 95% probability, requiring immediate isolation, anti-tuberculosis treatment and contact identification.[73] Thus, in patients with positive AFBs on respiratory samples, it is recommended to perform a direct amplification test, in addition to conventional and radiometric cultures. Finally, drug sensitivity testing of all *M. tuberculosis* isolates is recommended.

Serological tests do not have the sensitivity and specificity one would like to see in a test for the diagnosis of a contagious disease. However, since antibody responses are better conserved in HIV-infected subjects than skin delayed hypersensitivity reactions, antibody tests may be used for the identification of individuals infected with *M. tuberculosis*.[74,75]

Radiological examination of the HIV-infected patient with suspected TB may require the use of contrast CT scan to confirm the presence of enlarged hilar or mediastinal lymph nodes whose presence may have been suggested by an abnormal chest radiograph or an abnormal bronchoscopy. In addition, high-resolution CT may be indicated in HIV patients with negative chest radiographs to diagnose an unexplained persistent fever.

Treatment

The most recent recommendations for TB treatment of HIV-infected patients are that short-course (6-month) regimens should be used for the treatment of HIV-related pansusceptible TB (i.e. susceptible to all first-line antituberculosis drugs), whenever directly observed therapy protocols can be implemented and the response to antituberculosis drugs monitored, thus limiting the use of lengthier multidrug antituberculosis therapies to the minimum possible number of patients with TB and HIV. Because the risk of TB treatment failure is higher among patients with AIDS, some experts recommend longer duration of therapy. The available data do not permit a definitive recommendation regarding this issue. In this context, indicators of risk of treatment failure (lack of compliance with TB therapy, delayed conversion of *M. tuberculosis* sputum cultures beyond the second month and delayed clinical response) need to be carefully monitored.

Drug interactions have been described between the rifamycins used for TB treatment (rifampicin, rifabutin, and rifapentine) and antiretroviral drugs commonly used for HIV therapy, protease inhibitors (saquinavir, indinavir, ritonavir and nelfinavir) and non-nucleoside reverse transcriptase inhibitors (nevirapine, delavirdine and efavirenz). They are the result of changes in the rate of metabolism in the liver by the cytochrome CYP450 enzyme system of both the rifamycins and the antiretroviral drugs, as CYP450 is inhibited by the antiprotease drugs and induced by the rifamycins.[76] TB treatment in HIV patients under antiretroviral drug medication thus requires the use of a regimen including rifabutin (a less potent CYP450 inducer) instead of rifampicin. Alternatively, regimens including ethambutol and streptomycin may be adopted, without the need to stop antiretroviral therapy. In this regard, the result of a 'classic' large, randomised, controlled clinical trial in Hong Kong, evaluating six treatment regimens including streptomycin, isoniazid and pyrazinamide either daily, twice a week or three times a week for 6 or 9 months on 404 patients,[77] showed that 86–94% of treated patients converted within 3 months of therapy and that those treated for 9 months had a 30-month post-treatment relapse rate similar to that observed with rifampicin-based treatments (5–6%). However, as these treatment regimens were assessed in HIV-negative patients their efficacy in the HIV-positive needs to be tested.

Treatment of TB latent infection

Treatment for HIV-infected persons who are PPD positive i.e., latently infected with M. tuberculosis is an important part of a global strategy of TB control among HIV positive patients.[78–79]

In addition to the isoniazid based, 6 to 12 months preventive therapy regimens, several studies have evaluated the usefulness of combination preventive treatments. A multicenter, randomized TB prevention study conducted from 1993/1995[80] including a 6 month isoniazid arm versus a 3 month rifampin and isoniazid or pyrazinamide, rifampin and isoniazid arms showed identical protection for the three groups. Similar adverse effects were observed among persons in the rifampin plus pyrazinamide group compared to the isoniazide group, in addition, the individuals in the two and three drug groups were more likely to complete treatment, since treatment lasted for only 3 months. A recent placebo-controlled trial in Zambia demonstrated comparable protection from 3 months of rifampin and pyrazinamide versus 6 months of isoniazid[81]. In a Haiti study[82] comparing preventive treatment with rifampin and pyrazinamide twice a week for 2 months to isoniazid twice a week for 6 months; both administered by DOT, no differences were found in mortality in the two arms. Thus, short-course multidrug regimens including two drugs, rifampin and pyrazinamide for 2–3 months are effective for the prevention of active TB in HIV-patients.

The use of three drug regimens for preventive therapy, cannot be recommended for the high rate of toxicity[80], and the use of a 3-month regimen of rifampin and isoniazid is not recommended, in consideration for the risk of multi-drug-resistant TB.

To the contrary, preventive therapy with isoniazide of PPD-negative, anergic HIV seropositive persons, is not cost-effective in preventing TB[80,83] and cannot be recommended. However, some Authors recommend primary prophylaxis of PPD negative HIV infected patients when they are exposed to M. tuberculosis in institutions (hospices, prisons, shelters) to prevent *M. tuberculosis* infection.

Treatment of drug-resistant tuberculosis

Tuberculosis cases resistant to isoniazid only are generally treated with a standard short-course regimen (rifampicin or rifabutin, pyrazinamide and ethambutol) for 6–9 months or for 4 months after culture conversion. Isoniazid is generally withdrawn when resistance to $1.0\,\mu g/ml$ of isoniazid is discovered. When resistance is low-level (to $0.2\,\mu g/ml$ of isoniazid but not to $1.0\,\mu g/ml$), some authors suggest continuing isoniazid. However, since these cases could develop acquired rifamycin resistance, which would then result in multi-drug-resistant TB, these patients should be carefully supervised and managed by means of sputum microscopy, culture and nucleic acid amplification examination, chest radiography and high-resolution CT.

Tuberculosis cases resistant to rifampicin only should be generally treated with a 9-month regimen including isoniazid, streptomycin, pyrazinamide and ethambutol. Because the development of acquired isoniazid resistance would result in multi-drug-resistant TB, these patients should also be carefully supervised.

Patients with multi-drug-resistant TB (i.e. resistant to two or more than drugs, including isoniazid and rifampicin) should be managed in highly specialised centres with experience in the treatment of this type of TB.

Multi-drug-resistant TB requires an aggressive treatment with appropriate regimens to prevent mortality.[84] Drug regimens used to treat it include an aminoglycoside (streptomycin, kanamycin, amikacin) and a fluoroquinolone. Clofazimine, ethionamide and cycloserine, which are no longer in use in the standard treatment of TB because of their relatively poorer potency/toxicity ratio, are also used. Treatment of multi-drug-resistant TB in HIV-infected patients should be continued 24 months after culture conversion. Directly observed treatment should be used in all patients. Post-treatment follow-up visits every 4 months for 24 months are recommended.

Mycobacterium avium complex and other non-tuberculous mycobacterial infections

Mycobacterium avium complex is the most common non-tuberculous mycobacterial infection occurring in patients with AIDS. It presents as disseminated disease. Lung infection may be demonstrated in 50% of cases by BAL and 80% by transbronchial biopsy. Treatment usually involves rifampicin, ethambutol and ciprofloxacin. Macrolide antibiotics such as clarithromycin and azithromycin have been used instead of clofazimine and amikacin.[85,86]

Several studies have shown that rifabutin is quite effective in preventing MAC dissemination in HIV patients with CD4+ cell counts lower than 200/mm³. However, the occurrence of rifabutin-related cases of uveitis has imposed caution upon the use of this drug for preventive therapy for MAC. Clarithromycin has also been reported to be effective in MAC prevention and may result in improved survival of these patients.

In addition to MAC, which usually manifests with nodular diffuse infiltrates, hilar adenopathies (Fig. 36.1.7) and cavities, a number of non-tuberculous species of mycobacteria have been isolated from the lower respiratory tract of HIV-infected patients. *Mycobacterium kansasii* is the second most commonly found non-tuberculous mycobacterium in HIV-infected patients. In patients infected with *M. kansasii*, chest radiographs typically show thin-walled cavities and reticular nodular infiltrates. Treatment includes isoniazid, rifampicin and ethambutol.

Bacterial pneumonia

Bacterial pneumonia has been recognised as an AIDS-case-defining condition. In fact, community-acquired pneumonia is the most frequent pulmonary manifestation in HIV-infected patients. The annual rate of infection with *Streptococcus pneu-*

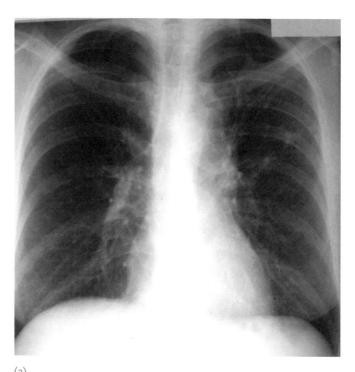

(a)

(b)

Fig. 36.1.7 (a) Chest radiograph of an AIDS patient with pulmonary *Mycobacterium avium–intracellulare* disease, posteroanterior view. A nodular infiltrate is present in the upper left lobe, with prominent homolateral hilar node enlargement. (b) Nodules and hilar lymph nodes are clearly seen on the computed tomography scan.

moniae is the highest (five times that in the general population), followed by *Haemophilus influenzae*, *Staphylococcus aureus*, *Legionella* spp., *Chlamydia pneumoniae*, *Klebsiella* spp. and *Pseudomonas aeruginosa*. Bacterial pneumonias in HIV-infected patients are more severe than in non-infected individuals and recur more often. In addition to community-acquired pneumonia, nosocomial pneumonia caused by *S. aureus*, *P. aeruginosa* and Gram-negative organisms is also common in HIV-infected patients.[87,88]

Nocardia asteroides, a rare cause of pneumonia in the immunocompetent subject, has been described as the cause of pneumonia in patients with AIDS. *N. asteroides* pneumonia mimics postprimary TB. Patients present with fever, cough, dyspnoea and chest pain. Upper-lobe infiltrates with cavitation are most frequently seen in the chest radiograph. Pleural effusions and hilar adenopathy may also occur. Sputum or BAL microscopic examination show Gram-positive, weakly acid-fast organisms presenting with branching, beaded, filamentous morphology. Penicillins are the antibiotic of choice; culture and sensitivity tests should be used to confirm the diagnosis and guide the choice of antibiotic. Treatment should last at least 6 months.

Rhodococcus equi pneumonia affects patients with AIDS and severe immunodeficiency. Patients present with a history of fever, cough, fatigue, chest pain and dyspnoea. On the chest radiograph dense infiltrates with cavitation are seen (Fig. 36.1.8); effusions may also be seen. Cultures of sputum, BAL, pleural effusion or a lung biopsy are required for the diagnosis and for sensitivity tests.[89]

Viral infections

Disseminated cytomegalovirus infection is common in patients with AIDS. Patients with pulmonary cytomegalovirus infection present with diffuse interstitial infiltrates. Definite diagnosis requires the demonstration of characteristic intranuclear inclusions on histology of lung parenchyma obtained by transbronchial biopsy. The diagnosis of cytomegalovirus pneumonia is difficult, however, because the infection is often associated with PCP. Evidence of pulmonary involvement should prompt antiviral treatment with ganciclovir or foscarnet, although it may not be effective.[90]

Herpes virus infection may cause pneumonia in patients with AIDS, although uncommonly. The diagnosis of herpes simplex pneumonia requires histological evidence of pulmonary infection in the absence of other causes.

The diagnosis of varicella-zoster pneumonia requires the demonstration of diffuse, bilateral pulmonary infiltrates in patients with disseminated varicella infection. Aciclovir and foscarnet are used to treat both herpes simplex and varicella-zoster pneumonia.

Fungal infections

Fungal infections are among the most common complications in patients with HIV infection and AIDS and may frequently be the first sign of immunodeficiency. Although the lungs are affected less frequently than the gastrointestinal tract and the brain, virtually all major fungal pathogens cause disease in HIV-positive patients. A number of fungal infections are endemic, such as histoplasmosis in mid-western USA, coccidioidomycosis in south-western USA and northern Mexico, and penicilliosis in south-east Asia; therefore, they represent frequent complications of AIDS for patients living in these regions as well as for patients who have lived in or travelled through them.

Cryptococcosis

Cryptococcus neoformans is an encapsulated fungus measuring 4–6 μm that is surrounded by a polysaccharide capsule. It is a soil organism with a worldwide distribution. Airborne transmission is thought to occur, with subsequent respiratory infection and dissemination in HIV-infected patients in the absence of cell-mediated responses. About 5% of HIV-infected patients develop disseminated cryptococcosis; most cases are seen in patients with CD4+ cell counts lower than 50/mm³. The

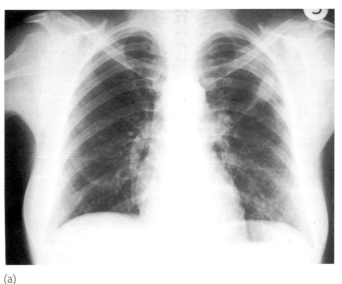
(a)

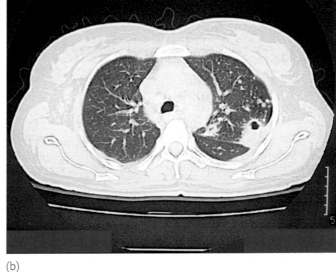
(b)

Fig. 36.1.8 *Rhodococcus equi* pneumonia. (a) A dense infiltrate is seen in the upper left lung zone. (b) The computed tomography scan demonstrates a pneumonic infiltrate surrounding a thin-walled cavity. The reactive pleural effusion can also be seen.

incidence of infection has fallen in recent years with the use of azole antifungal drugs and the advent of combination antiretroviral therapy.[91]

The most common presentation of cryptococcal infection is meningitis. Pneumonia is described in 10–30% of patients. The presentation of lung infection is characterised by cough and dyspnoea and by abnormal chest radiographs demonstrating focal or diffuse interstitial infiltrates. Cavitary lesions, pleurisy and adenopathies may also be present. Patients with lung involvement usually have disseminated infection; thus, the demonstration of the organism in respiratory secretions is an indication for thorough evaluation for cryptococcal meningitis.[92] Serological testing is recommended, as high antibody titres against cryptococcal polysaccharide antigens in serum are diagnostic of *C. neoformans* infection. The drugs of choice for cryptococcal pneumonia are amphotericin B and fluconazole.[93]

Histoplasmosis

Histoplasma capsulatum is a common cause of lung infection in AIDS patients from endemic areas, where the mycelial form of *Histoplasma* is found in the soil. The clinical presentation of lung infection is characterised by bilateral nodular infiltrates with or without adenopathy (Fig. 36.1.9). Bronchoscopy is diagnostic in most pulmonary cases, while bone marrow or blood cultures have a better yield in disseminated cases. Amphotericin B is the antifungal drug of choice for the acute episode, but itraconazole has also been used successfully. Relapses are common and mortality is high.

Coccidioidomycosis

Coccidioides immitis is found in the soil of endemic areas of the south-western USA, Mexico, and Central and South America. In these areas disseminated coccidioidomycosis is

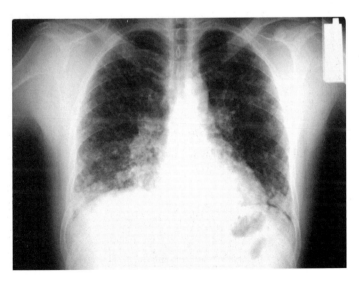

Fig. 36.1.9 Histoplasmosis. The chest radiograph of an AIDS patient shows a diffuse bilateral micronodular infiltrate with prominent hilar adenopathies.

relatively common and the lungs are involved in 60–80% of patients, who present with diffuse reticulonodular or focal infiltrates with hilar adenopathy. Pleural effusions have been described. The diagnosis is obtained by isolating the fungus from pulmonary specimens, lymph nodes, blood, urine and skin. In addition, antibody tests turn out positive in more than 90% of cases. Amphotericin B is the drug of choice; ketoconazole and fluconazole are also useful for treatment and prophylaxis. Patients with diffuse lung involvement have a very poor prognosis.

Penicilliosis

Penicilliosis is caused by the dimorphic fungus *Penicillium marneffei* in endemic areas of south-eastern Asia, where the fungus is believed to be a soil organism. The diagnosis, in the areas at risk, is based upon a clinical history of fever, weight loss and anaemia, in the presence of lung infiltrates.

Aspergillosis

Aspergillus species infection is common among patients with AIDS with low CD4+ counts, neutropenia and a history of previous pneumonia, of having received corticosteroids and of treatment with broad-spectrum antibiotics. The most common presentations of *Aspergillus* infection are lung disease and central nervous system involvement. Patients with pulmonary aspergillosis present with cough, dyspnoea, fever, chest pain and bloody sputum. The chest radiograph shows localised or diffuse nodular infiltrates with cavitation.

The diagnosis of invasive aspergillosis of the lung requires the demonstration of fungal invasion in a tissue sample. The diagnosis may, however, be established empirically upon the appearance of radiographic abnormalities together with the identification of the fungus in cultures of respiratory secretions.[94]

Candidiasis

Mucosal *Candida* infection is the most common complication of AIDS, while systemic infection is a rather rare event. Although cultures obtained at bronchoscopy frequently grow *Candida* species, the diagnosis of pulmonary candidiasis requires the histological demonstration of invasive fungal forms in the lung tissue. Pulmonary candidiasis is always associated with disseminated candidiasis, and mortality is high. The drugs of choice are amphotericin B, ketoconazole or fluconazole.

Fungal infections in the era of highly active antiretroviral therapy

The use of effective combinations of antiretroviral drugs has led to a remarkable reduction in the incidence of opportunistic fungal infections in HIV patients.[95] As for pulmonary TB, cases suggestive of an immune reconstitution illness have been described in patients with a history of cryptococcal meningitis in whom the reappearance of meningitis and lymphadenitis has been observed shortly after the initiation of HAART.[96] US guidelines state that, since an insufficient number of patients has been evaluated so far, recommendations to discontinue antifungal prophylaxis cannot be issued yet.

Protozoal infections

Toxoplasmosis rarely occurs outside endemic areas, with a general incidence of 1–3% among AIDS patients. The most common site of infection is the central nervous system, where the infection manifests as necrotising encephalitis. Pneumonia, which may also occur in the absence of central nervous system involvement, presents with nodular infiltrates or consolidations. The diagnosis requires the demonstration of the parasite by Wright or Giemsa stains of tissue material. The drug of choice are sulfadiazine and pyrimethamine.

Pulmonary disease is seen in HIV patients with gastrointestinal *Strongyloides* and *Cryptosporidium* infestation. Pulmonary microsporidiasis is seen in HIV patients with gastrointestinal infestation with *Encephalitozoon hellem* and *Septata intestinalis*.

Non-infectious complications

Kaposi's sarcoma

Kaposi's sarcoma is a common complication of AIDS, usually presenting with lesions of the skin and the oral mucosa as well as with lymphatic and gastrointestinal tract involvement. It affects the lung in 30% of cases, representing about 10% of the pulmonary complications of AIDS. The typical manifestations of pulmonary Kaposi's sarcoma are fever and weight loss. Wheezing, chest pain and bloody sputum may be present. Stridor suggests stenosis of the trachea. Radiological findings include bilateral interstitial or alveolar infiltrates. Nodules are sometimes present (Fig. 36.1.10).

Open lung biopsy is required for a definitive diagnosis of Kaposi's sarcoma. However, the finding of the macular or plaque-like cherry-red lesions of Kaposi's sarcoma in the trachea or bronchi by fibreoptic bronchoscopy is deemed diagnostic in AIDS patients with Kaposi's sarcoma involving other sites.[97]

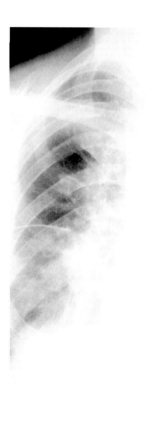
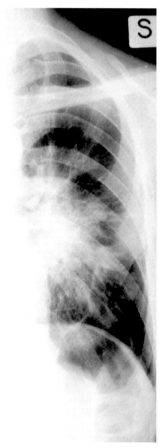

(a)

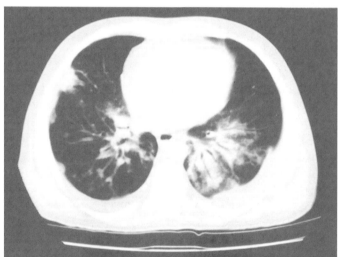

(b)

Fig. 36.1.10 Kaposi's sarcoma in AIDS. (a) The chest radiograph shows marked thickening of the peribronchial–perivascular interstitium. Lower right-lobe consolidation and pleural effusion may also be seen. (b) The computed tomography scan shows the infiltration of the peribronchial interstitium in greater detail.

Lymphoma

Non-Hodgkin's lymphoma associated with HIV is highly malignant and usually disseminated at the time of diagnosis. Lung disease is not common.

Hodgkin's lymphoma is frequent in HIV-infected patients. Endothoracic disease is not common.

Lymphoid interstitial pneumonitis

Lymphoid interstitial pneumonitis typically occurs in paediatric AIDS patients but may be seen in adults. It is characterised by the presence of mononuclear cell infiltrates comprising CD8+ T-cells and B-cells. The disease is associated with HLA-DR5 in blacks and with HLA-DR6 in whites.

The disease course is characterised by dyspnoea, cough, fever and weight loss. Adenopathies, hepatosplenomegaly and parotid enlargement may be seen at patient examination. Chest radiography reveals lower-lobe interstitial or reticulonodular infiltrates bilaterally. Because of its rarity, the diagnosis of lymphocytic interstitial pneumonia is difficult and requires transbronchial or lung biopsies.[98]

> **? Unresolved questions**
>
> - While is widely accepted that *Pneumocystis carinii* pneumonia and toxoplasmosis prophylaxis can be discontinued after immune restoration following 'highly active antiretroviral therapy', the evidence for the discontinuation of prophylaxis for mycotic and mycobacterial infections is not yet deemed to be sufficient.
>
> - The emergence of resistance to co-trimoxazole in *Pneumocystis carinii* pneumonia, attributed to the wide prophylactic use of this drug, has brought to light the lack of tools for the rapid assessment of resistance and of effective substitute drugs.
>
> - Adjunctive corticosteroids in severe *Pneumocystis carinii* pneumonia have been shown to be effective in reducing mortality; it has been suggested that this treatment may favour the activation of other opportunistic infections such as cytomegalovirus.

References

1. WHO/UNAIDS. Report on the global HIV/AIDS epidemic. Geneva: World Heath Organization; 1998.
2. WHO/UNAIDS. AIDS epidemic update. Geneva: World Health Organization; 1998.
3. Girardi E, Raviglione NC, Antonucci G et al. Impact of the HIV epidemic on the spread of other diseases: the case of tuberculosis. AIDS 2000; 14(Suppl. 3): S47–S56.
4. Forrest DN, Seminari E, Hogg RS et al. The incidence and spectrum of AIDS-defining illnesses in persons treated with anti retroviral drugs. Clin Infect Dis 1998; 27: 1379–1385.
5. Ho DD, Neumann AU, Perelson AS. Rapid turnover of plasma virions and CD+ lymphocytes in HIV-1 infection. Nature 1995; 373: 123–126.
6. Wei X, Ghosh SK, Taylor NE et al. Viral dynamics in human immunodeficiency virus type 1 infection. Nature 1995; 373: 117–122.
7. Mellors JW, Rinaldo CR, Gupta P et al. Prognosis in HIV infection predicted by the quantity of viruses in plasma. Science 1996; 272: 1167–1170.
8. Mellors JW, Munoz A, Giorgi JV et al. Plasma viral load and CD4+ lymphocytes as prognostic markers of HIV-1 infection. Ann Intern Med 1997; 126: 946–954.
9. Carpenter CC, Cooper DA, Fischl MA et al. Antiretroviral therapy in adults: updated recommendations of the International AIDS Society – USA Panel. JAMA 2000; 283: 381–390.
10. Palella FJ Jr, Delaney KM, Moorman AC et al. Declining morbidity and mortality among patients with advanced human immunodeficiency virus infection. N Engl J Med 1998; 338: 853–860.
11. Mocroft A, Vella S, Benfield TL et al. Changing patterns of mortality across Europe in patients infected with HIV-1. Lancet 1998; 352: 1725–1730.
12. Chiesi A, Mocroft A, Dally LG et al. Regional survival differences across Europe in HIV-positive people: the EuroSIDA study. AIDS 1999; 13: 2281–2288.
13. Jones JL, Hanson DL, Dworkin MS et al. Surveillance for AIDS-defining opportunistic illnesses, 1992/1997. In: CDC Surveillance Summaries. Morbidity Mortality Wkly Rep 1999; 48: 122.
14. Kaplan JE Hanson D, Dworkin MS et al. Epidemiology of human immunodeficiency virus associated opportunistic infections in the United States in the era of highly active antiretroviral therapy. Clin Infect Dis 2000; 30: S5–S14.
15. Girardi E, Antonucci G, Vanacore P et al. Impact of combination antiretroviral therapy on the risk of tuberculosis among persons with HIV infection. Gruppo Italiano di Studio Tubercolosi e AIDS. AIDS 2000: 14: 1985–1991.
16. Narita M, Ashkin D, Hollender ES, Pitchenick AE. Paradoxical worsening of tuberculosis following antiretroviral therapy in patients with AIDS. Am J Respir Crit Care Med 1998; 158: 157–161.
17. Woods ML, MacGinley R, Eisen DP, Allworth AM. HIV combination therapy: partial immune restitution unmasking latent cryptococcal infection. AIDS 1998; 12: 1491–1494.
18. Jacobson MA, Zegans M, Pavan PR et al. Cytomegalovirus retinitis after initiation of highly active antiretroviral therapy. Lancet 1997; 349: 1443–1445.
19. Race EM, Adelson-Mitty J, Kriegel GR et al. Focal mycobacterial lymphadenitis following initiation of protease-inhibitor therapy in patients with advanced HIV-1 disease. Lancet 1998; 351: 252–255.
20. Jeffrey AA, Israel Biet D, Andrieu JM et al. HIV isolation from pulmonary cells derived from bronchoalveolar lavage. Clin Exp Immunol 1991; 84: 488–492.
21. Clarke JR, Williamson JD Mitchell DM. Comparative study of the isolation of human immunodeficiency virus from the lung and peripheral blood of AIDS patients. J Med Virol 1993; 39: 196–199.
22. Agostini C, Trentin L, Zambello R, Semenzato G. HIV-1 and the lung. Infectivity, pathogenic mechanisms, and cellular immune responses taking place in the lower respiratory tract. Am Rev Respir Dis 1993; 147: 1038–1049.
23. Agostini C, Chilosi M, Zambello R et al. Pulmonary immune cells in health and disease: lymphocytes. Eur Respir J 1993; 6: 1378–1401.
24. Venet A, Clavel F, Israel-Biet D et al. Lung in acquired immune deficiency syndrome: infectious and immunological status assessed by bronchoalveolar lavage. Bull Eur Physiopathol Respir 1985; 21: 535–543.
25. Solal-Celigny P, Couderc U, Herman D et al. Lymphoid interstitial pneumonitis in acquired immunodeficiency syndrome-related complex. Am Rev Respir Dis 1985; 131: 956–960.
26. Haynes BF, Pantaleo G, Fauci AS. Toward an understanding of the correlates of protective immunity to HIV infection. Science 1996; 271: 324–328.
27. Autran B, Plata F, Guillon JM et al. HIV-specific cytotoxic T lymphocytes directed against alveolar macrophages in HIV-infected patients. Res Virol 1990; 141: 131–136.
28. Popovic M, Gartner S. Isolation of HIV-1 from monocytes but not T lymphocytes [letter]. Lancet 1987; 2: 916.
29. Meltzer MS, Kornbluth RS, Hansen B et al. HIV infection of the lung. Role of virus-infected macrophages in the pathophysiology of pulmonary disease. Chest 1993; 103(2 Suppl.): 103S–108S.
30. Mancino G, Placido R, Bach S et al. Infection of human monocytes with Mycobacterium tuberculosis enhances human immunodeficiency virus type 1 replication and transmission to T cells. J Infect Dis 1997; 175: 1531–1535.
31. Goletti D, Weissman D, Jackson RW et al. Effect of Mycobacterium tuberculosis on HIV replication. Role of immune activation. Immunology 1996; 157: 1271–1278.
32. Friaziano M, Cappelli G, Santucci M et al. Expression of CCR5 is increased in human monocyte-derived macrophages and alveolar macrophages in the course of in vivo and in vitro Mycobacterium tuberculosis infection. AIDS Res Hum Retroviruses 1999; 15: 869–874.

33. Wewers MD, Diaz PT, Wewers ME et al. Cigarette smoking in HIV infection induces a suppressive inflammatory environment in the lung. Am J Respir Crit Care Med 1998; 158: 1543–1549.

34. Nieman RB, Fleming J, Coker RJ et al. The effect of cigarette smoking on the development of AIDS in HIV-1-seropositive individuals. AIDS 1993; 7: 705–710.

35. Dohn MN, Baughman RP, Vigdorth EM, Frame DL. Equal survival for first, second and third episodes of Pneumocystis carinii pneumonia in AIDS patients. Arch Intern Med 1992; 152: 2465–2470.

36. Hoover D, Graham N, Bacellar H et al. Epidemiologic patterns of upper respiratory illness and Pneumocystis carinii pneumonia in homosexual men. Am Rev Respir Dis 1991; 144: 756–759.

37. Nevez G, Raccurt C, Jounieaux V et al. Pneumocystosis versus pulmonary Pneumocystis carinii colonization in HIV-negative and HIV-positive patients. AIDS 1999,13: 535–536.

38. Edman JC, Kovacs JA, Masur H et al. Ribosomal RNA sequences shows Pneumocystis carinii to be member of fungi. Nature 1988; 334: 519–522.

39. Wright TW, Gigliotti F, Finklestein JT et al. Immune mediated inflammation directly impairs pulmonary function, contributing to the pathogenesis of Pneumocystis carinii pneumonia. J Clin Invest 1999,104: 1307–1317.

40. Phair J, Munoz A, Detels R et al. The risk of Pneumocystis carinii pneumonia among men infected with human immunodeficiency virus type 1. N Engl J Med 1990; 322: 161–165.

41a. Helweg-Larson J, Benfield JL, Eugen-Olsen J, Lundgren B. Effects of mutations in Pneumocystis carinii dihydropteroate synthase gene on outcome of AIDS-associated P. carinii pneumonia. Lancet 1999; 354: 1347–1351.

41b. Gagnon S, Boota AM, Fischl MA, Baier H, Kirksey OW, La Voie L. Corticosteroids as adjunctive therapy for severe Pneumocystis carinii pneumonia in the acquired immunodeficiency syndrome. A double-blind, placebo-controlled trial. N Engl J Med 1990; 323: 1444–50.

42. Ioannidis J, Cappelleri J, Skolnik P et al. A meta-analysis of the relative efficacy and toxicity of Pneumocystis carinii prophylactic regimens. Arch Intern Med 1996; 156: 177–188.

43. Furrer H, Egger M, Opravil M et al for the Swiss HIV Cohort Study. Discontinuation of primary prophylaxis against I pneumonia in HIV-1 infected adults treated with combination antiretroviral therapy. N Engl J Med 1999, 340: 1301–1306.

44. Schneider MME, Borleffs JCC, Stolk RP et al. Discontinuation of prophylaxis for Pneumocystis carinii pneumonia in HIV-1 infected patients treated with highly active antiretroviral therapy. Lancet 1999; 353: 201–203.

45. Selwyn PA, Hartel D, Lewis VA et al. A prospective study of the risk of tuberculosis among intravenous drug users with human immunodeficiency virus infection. N Engl J Med 1989; 320: 545–550.

46. Daley CL, Hahn JA, Moss AR et al. Incidence of tuberculosis in injection drug users in San Francisco: impact of anergy. Am J Respir Crit Care Med 1998; 157: 19–22.

47. Markowitz N, Hansen NI, Hopewell PC et al. Incidence of tuberculosis in the United States among HIV-infected persons. Ann Intern Med 1997; 126: 123–132.

48. Antonucci G, Girardi E, Armignacco O et al. Tuberculosis in HIV infected subjects in Italy: a multicentre study. Gruppo Italiano di Studio Tubercolosi e AIDS. AIDS 1992; 6: 1007–1013.

49. Girardi E, Antonucci G, Armignacco O et al. Tuberculosis and AIDS: a retrospective, longitudinal, multicentre study of Italian AIDS patients. Italian group for the study of tuberculosis and AIDS. J Infect 1994; 28: 261–269.

50. Braun MM, Badi N, Ryder RW et al. A retrospective cohort study of the risk of tuberculosis among women of childbearing age with HIV infection in Zaire. Am Rev Respir Dis 1991; 143: 501–504.

51. Whalen C, Horsburgh CR, Hom D et al. Accelerated course of human immunodeficiency virus infection after tuberculosis. Am J Respir Crit Care Med 1995; 151: 129–135.

52. Leroy V, Salmi LR, Dupon M et al. Progression of human immunodeficiency virus in patients with tuberculosis disease. A cohort study in Bordeaux, France, 1988–1994. Am J Epidemiol 1997; 145: 293–300.

53. Perneger TV, Sudre P, Lundgren JD, Hirschel B. Does the onset of tuberculosis in AIDS predict shorter survival? Results of a cohort study in 17 European countries over 13 years. Br Med J 1995; 311: 1468–1471.

54. Tacconelli E, Tumbarello M, Ardito F, Cauda R. Tuberculosis significantly reduces the survival of patients with AIDS. Int J Tuberc Lung Dis 1997; 1: 582–584.

55. Small PM, Hopewell PC, Singh SP et al. The epidemiology of tuberculosis in San Francisco. A population-based study using conventional and molecular methods. N Engl J Med 1994; 330: 1703–1709.

56. Alland D, Kalkut GE, Moss AR et al. Transmission of tuberculosis in New York City. An analysis by DNA fingerprinting and conventional epidemiologic methods. N Engl J Med 1994; 330: 1710–1716.

57. Frieden TR, Sherman LF, Maw KL et al. A multiinstitutional outbreak of highly drug-resistant tuberculosis. Epidemiology and clinical outcomes. JAMA 1996; 276: 1229–1235.

58. Daley CL, Small PM, Schecter GF et al. An outbreak of tuberculosis with accelerated progression among persons infected with the human immunodeficiency virus. An analysis using restriction-fragment-length polymorphisms. N Engl J Med 1992; 326: 231–235.

59. Edlin BR, Tokars JI, Grieco MH et al. An outbreak of multidrug-resistant tuberculosis among hospitalized patients with the acquired immunodeficiency syndrome. N Engl J Med 1992; 326: 1514–1521.

60. Pearson ML, Jereb JA, Frieden TR et al. Nosocomial transmission of multidrug-resistant Mycobacterium tuberculosis: a risk to patients and health care workers. Ann Intern Med 1992; 117: 191–196.

61. Angarano G, Carbonara S, Costa D, Gori A. Drug-resistant tuberculosis in human immunodeficiency virus infected persons in Italy. The Italian Drug-Resistant Tuberculosis Study Group. Int J Tuberc Lung Dis 1998; 2: 303–311.

62. Di Perri G, Cruciani M, Danzi MC et al. Nosocomial epidemic of active tuberculosis among HIV-infected patients. Lancet 1989; 2: 1502–1504.

63. Moro ML, Gori A, Errante I et al. An outbreak of multidrug-resistant tuberculosis involving HIV-infected patients of two hospitals in Milan, Italy. Italian Multidrug-Resistant Tuberculosis Outbreak Study Group. AIDS 1998; 12: 1095–1102.

64. Nunn P, Brindle R, Carpenter L et al. Cohort study of human immunodeficiency virus infection in patients with tuberculosis in Nairobi, Kenya. Am Rev Respir Dis 1992; 146: 849–854.

65. Stoneburner R, Laroche E, Prevots R et al. Survival in a cohort of human immunodeficiency virus-infected tuberculosis patients in New York City. Implications for the expansion of the AIDS case definition. Arch Intern Med 1992; 152: 2033–2037.

66. Kassim S, Sassan-Morokro M, Ackah A et al Two-year follow-up of persons with HIV-1- and HIV-2-associated pulmonary tuberculosis treated with short-course chemotherapy in West Africa, AIDS 1995; 9: 1185–1191.

67. Perriens JH, Colebunders RL, Karahunga C et al. Increased mortality and tuberculosis treatment failure rate among human immunodeficiency virus (HIV) seropositive compared with HIV seronegative patients with pulmonary tuberculosis treated with 'standard' chemotherapy in Kinshasa, Zaire. Am Rev Respir Dis 1991; 144: 750–755.

68. Chaisson RE, Schecter GF, Theuer CP et al. Tuberculosis in patients with the acquired immunodeficiency syndrome. Clinical features, response to therapy, and survival. Am Rev Respir Dis 1987; 136: 570–574.

69. Jones BE, Young SM, Antoniskis D et al. Relationship of the manifestations of tuberculosis to CD4 cell counts in patients with human immunodeficiency virus infection. Am Rev Respir Dis 1993; 148: 1292–1297.

70. Theuer CP, Hopewell PC, Elias D et al. Human immunodeficiency virus infection in tuberculosis patients. J Infect Dis 1990; 162: 8–12.

71. Pitchenik AE, Rubinson HA. The radiographic appearance of tuberculosis in patients with the acquired immune deficiency syndrome (AIDS) and pre-AIDS. Am Rev Respir Dis 1985; 131: 393–396.

72. Saltini C, Vezzani V. Tuberculosis and non tuberculous mycobacteria infection. In: Brambilla C, Costabel U, Grassi C et al, ed. Pulmonary diseases. McGraw-Hill Clinical Medical Series. London: McGraw Hill; 1999: 151–163.

73. Diagnostic standards and classification of tuberculosis in adults and children. Official statement of the American Thoracic Society and the Centers for Disease Control and Prevention. Am J Respir Crit Care Med 2000; 161: 1376–1395.

74. Saltini C, Amicosante M, Girardi E et al. Early abnormalities of the antibody response against M. tuberculosis in HIV infection. J Infect Dis 1993; 168: 1409–1414.

75. Amicosante M, Richeldi L, Monno L et al. Serological markers predicting tuberculosis in HIV-infected patients. Int J Tuberc Lung Dis 1997; 1: 435–440.

76. Tseng AL, Foisy MM. Management of drug interactions in patients with HIV. Ann Pharmacother 1997; 31: 1040–1058.

77. Hong Kong Chest Service/British Medical Research Council. Controlled trial of 6-month and 9-month regimens of daily and intermittent streptomycin plus isoniazid plus pyrazinamide for pulmonary tuberculosis in Hong Kong. Results up to 30 months. Am Rev Respir Dis 1977; 115: 727–735.

78. O'Brien R, Perriens JH. Preventive therapy for tuberculosis in HIV infection: the promise and the reality. AIDS 1995; 9: 665–673.

79. Sawert H, Girardi E, Antonucci G et al. Preventive therapy for tuberculosis in HIV-infected persons: analysis of policy options based on tuberculin status and CD4+ cell count. Gruppo Italiano di Studio Tubercolosi e AIDS (GISTA). Arch Intern Med 1998; 158: 2112–2121.

80. Whalen CC, Johnson JL, Okwera A et al. A trial of three regimens to prevent tuberculosis in Ugandan adults infected with the human immunodeficiency virus. N Engl J Med 1997; 337: 801–808.

81. Mwinga A, Hosp M, Godfrey-Faussett P et al. Twice weekly tuberculosis preventive therapy in HIV infection in Zambia. AIDS 1998; 12: 2447–2457.

82. Halsey NA, Coberly JS, Desormeaux J et al. Randomised trial of isoniazid versus rifampicin and pyrazinamide for prevention of tuberculosis in HIV-1 infection. Lancet 1998; 351: 786–792.

83. Gordin FM, Matts JP, Miller C et al. A controlled trial of isoniazid in persons with anergy and human immunodeficiency virus infection who are at high risk for tuberculosis. N Engl J Med 1997; 337: 315–320.

84. Park MM, Davis AL, Schluger NW et al. Outcome of MDR-TB patients, 1983–1993. Prolonged survival with appropriate therapy. Am J Respir Crit Care Med 1996; 153: 317–324.

85. Hoy J, Mijch A, Sandland M et al. Quadruple-drug therapy for *Mycobacterium avium–intracellulare* bacteremia in AIDS patients. J Infect Dis 1990; 161: 801–805.

86. Masur H. Recommendations on prophylaxis and therapy for disseminated *Mycobacterium avium* complex disease in patients infected with the human immunodeficiency virus. Public Health Service Task Force on Prophylaxis and Therapy for *Mycobacterium avium* Complex. N Engl J Med 1993; 329: 898–904.

87. Janoff EN, Breiman RF, Daley CL, Hopewell PC. Pneumococcal disease during HIV infection. Epidemiologic, clinical, and immunologic perspectives. Ann Intern Med 1992; 117: 314–324.

88. Hirschtick RE, Glassroth J, Jordan MC et al. Bacterial pneumonia in persons infected with the human immunodeficiency virus. Pulmonary Complications of HIV Infection Study Group. N Engl J Med 1995; 333: 845–851.

89. Harvey RL, Sunstrum JC. *Rhodococcus equi* infection in patients with and without human immunodeficiency virus infection. Rev Infect Dis 1991; 13: 139–145.

90. Wallace JM, Hannah J. Cytomegalovirus pneumonitis in patients with AIDS. Findings in an autopsy series. Chest 1987; 92: 198–203.

91. Chuck SL, Sande NA. Infections with *Cryptococcus neoformans* in the acquired immunodeficiency syndrome. N Engl Med 1989; 321: 794–799.

92. Driver JA, Saunders CA, Heinze-Lacey B, Sugar AM. Cryptococcal pneumonia in AIDS: is cryptococcal meningitis preceded by clinically recognizable pneumonia? J AIDS Hum Retrovirol 1995; 9: 168–171.

93. Van der Horst CM, Saag MS, Cloud GA et al. Treatment of cryptococcal meningitis associated with the acquired immunodeficiency syndrome. National Institute of Allergy and Infectious Diseases Mycoses Study Group and AIDS Clinical Trials Group. N Engl J Med 1997; 337: 15–21.

94. Lortholary O, Meyohas MC, Dupont B et al. Invasive aspergillosis in patients with acquired immunodeficiency syndrome: report of 33 cases. French Cooperative Study Group on Aspergillosis in AIDS. Am J Med 1993; 95: 177–187.

95. Centers for Disease Control and Prevention. Update: trends in AIDS incidence 1996. Morbidity Mortality Wkly Rep 1997; 46: 861–867.

96. Lanzafame M, Trevenzoli M, Carretta G et al. Mediastinal lymphadenitis due to cryptococcal infection in HIV-positive patients on highly active antiretroviral therapy. Chest 1999; 116: 848–849.

97. Garay S, Belenko M, Fazzini S, Schinella R. Pulmonary manifestations of Kaposi's sarcoma. Chest 1987; 81: 39–43.

98. Semenzato G, Agostini C. HIV-related interstitial lung disease. Curr Opin Pulm Med 1995; 1 : 383–391.

36.2 Respiratory disease in the immunocompromised host: non-AIDS

Rudolf Speich

 Key points

- With respect to the practical clinical approach to the non-AIDS immunocompromised host the following patient categories have to be considered:
  - The solid-organ transplant recipient
  - The cancer patient with treatment-induced neutropenia
  - The haematopoietic stem-cell transplant recipient (formerly referred to as bone-marrow transplant recipient)
  - The patient suffering from primary immunodeficiency syndromes
  - The patient affected by various secondary immune deficiencies induced by drugs, infections and diseases other than HIV

- Infections are the major complications in the immunocompromised host. However various other immune or inflammatory, disease- or drug-related, indirectly or completely unrelated disease processes may occur and even coexist. The clinical approach should consider all these possibilities but completely differs among the abovementioned patient categories.

The term 'immunocompromised host' describes patients with defects of the innate and/or acquired immune defence mechanisms (see Chapter 3). This includes any condition, congenital or acquired, temporary or chronic, in which the response of the host to a foreign antigen is subnormal. These patients are at increased risk of infection with a variety of microorganisms, including those with no pathogenicity for healthy individuals (opportunistic agents). A useful approach to infections in the immunocompromised host is the recognition of the major predisposing defence defect (i.e. phagocyte, cellular, humoral or complement dysfunction) and the awareness of the microorganisms associated with a specific defect. However, specific defence defects often overlap in an individual patient and non-immune problems from disruption of skin and mucosal barriers, intravascular devices and surgical procedures may predominate.

Therefore, from the practitioner's point of view it is more convenient to group patients according to their circumstance of immunocompromise, i.e. solid-organ transplant recipients, cancer patients with treatment-induced neutropenia, haematopoietic stem-cell transplant recipients (formerly referred to as bone-marrow transplant recipients), patients suffering from primary immunodeficiency syndromes and those affected by various secondary immune deficiencies induced by drugs, infections and diseases other than human immunodeficiency virus (HIV). This approach allows a pragmatic, comprehensive and rapid management in these often very complex clinical situations.[1-5]

With an immunocompromised host suffering from pulmonary disease, different categories of problem have to be considered (Table 36.2.1).[6] Besides infectious complications, various other

Table 36.2.1 Categories of pulmonary disease in the immunocompromised host

- Opportunistic and non-opportunistic infections
- Opportunistic neoplasms (lymphoproliferative disorders, Kaposi's sarcoma)
- Recurrence of the underlying disease process involving the lungs (leukaemia, lymphoma, recurrence of disease after lung transplantation)
- Immune-mediated disorders (acute rejection after lung transplantation, obliterative bronchiolitis after lung and allogeneic haematopoietic stem-cell transplantation)
- Unusual complications of the disease or its treatment (veno-occlusive disease, alveolar haemorrhage, alveolar proteinosis, etc.)
- Non-specific inflammation (diffuse alveolar damage, organising pneumonia)
- Drug-induced pulmonary disease
- Unrelated or indirectly related disorders (cardiogenic pulmonary oedema, pulmonary embolism, acute respiratory distress syndrome)
- Combinations of two or more of the above

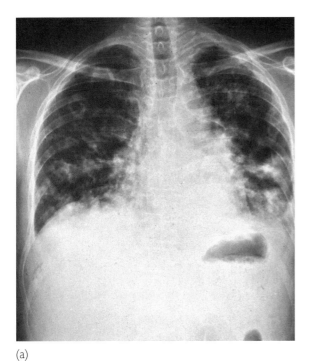
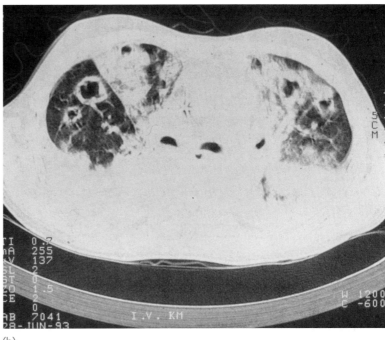

(a) (b)

Fig. 36.2.1 This patient achieved complete remission after chemotherapy for Hodgkin's disease. One year later he presented with bilateral cavitating thick-walled infiltrates on chest radiograph (a) and computed tomography (b). Nocardiosis was detected by broncho-alveolar lavage. Despite adequate treatment the patient died of progressive respiratory failure. Autopsy confirmed nocardiosis but additionally revealed angiotrophic Hodgkin's disease as the main cause of the cavitating infiltrates.

immune or inflammatory, disease- or drug-related, indirectly related or completely unrelated disease processes may occur and even coexist (Fig. 36.2.1). It is important always to consider all these possibilities.

The solid-organ transplant recipient

Spectrum of disease

Solid organ transplantation has become a therapeutic option for many diseases. One-year survival among recipients of livers, kidneys, kidney/pancreas (including islet cells), heart and lungs now reaches 80–90% in many transplant centres. This success is mainly due to careful selection of patients, improved surgical techniques, organ preservation and sophisticated postoperative management. However, the solid-organ transplant recipient is still endangered by chronic rejection and infections, interplaying in various ways. Chronic rejection may lead to over-immuno-suppression and organ dysfunction, which can propagate infection. On the other hand, it has been demonstrated for all organ transplants that cytomegalovirus (CMV) infection is a risk factor for the development of chronic rejection. Moreover, many infections can exert an immunosuppressing effect that can propagate opportunistic infections.

Pulmonary complications, predominantly of infectious origin, are the most important cause of morbidity and mortality of solid-organ transplant recipients.[1,7–10] The risk of infection, particularly opportunistic infection, varies between the different organ transplant recipients (Table 36.2.2) and is largely determined by three factors: the net state of immunosuppression, the epidemiological exposures the patient encounters and the consequences of the invasive procedures to which the patient is subjected. Most of these considerations also apply to the haematopoietic stem-cell transplant recipient (see below).

The net state of immunosuppression is determined by three factors. First, the dose, duration and temporal sequence of immunosuppressive drugs administered have to be considered. Most of these agents depress cell-mediated immunity (see below). However, besides a decreased phagocytic function induced by corticosteroids, these drugs may also result in blunted antibody responses and leukopenia. Second, metabolic factors such as protein-caloric malnutrition, uraemia and hyper-glycaemia, and breaches to the integrity of the mucocutaneous barriers are important factors. And third, infections with immunomodulating viruses such as CMV and Epstein–Barr virus (EBV) may contribute to the net state of immunosuppression.

Important epidemiological exposure of the solid-organ transplant recipient may occur within the community or within the hospital. The former environment includes *Mycobacterium tuberculosis*, the geographically restricted systemic mycoses, *Strongyloides stercoralis* and community-acquired respiratory viruses. The latter consists of environmental exposure to *Aspergillus* or *Legionella* species, and of person-to-person spread of *Pseudomonas* spp. and other highly resistant Gram-negative bacilli, azole-resistant *Candida*

Table 36.2.2 Incidence of infectious diseases in solid-organ transplant recipients

Type of infection	Incidence (%)				
	Liver	Kidney	Heart	Lung/heart–lung	Pancreas/kidney–pancreas
Bacterial	33–68	47	21–30	33–66	35
Cytomegalovirus	22–29	8–32	9–35	53–75	50
Herpes simplex virus	3–14	53	1–42	10–18	6
Varicella-zoster virus	5–10	4–12	1–12	8–15	9
Candida species	1–26	2	1–5	10–16	32
Mycelial fungi	2–4	1–2	3–6	3–19	3
Pneumocystis carinii	4–11	5–10	1–8	15	

Data are from large studies of patients not on prophylaxis in a variety of transplantation centres and are adapted from Patel & Paya.[9]

spp., methicillin-resistant staphylococci and vancomycin-resistant enterococci.

Technical aspects are of great importance in determining the risk of infection. Surgical problems (devitalised tissue, anastomotic disruptions, undrained fluid collections), vascular access devices, endotracheal tubes and drainage catheters markedly predispose the patient to potentially lethal infections.

There is a timetable or stereotypical pattern according to which different infections occur after solid-organ transplantation (Fig. 36.2.2). In other words, although a complication such as pneumonia can occur at any point in the post-transplant course, its aetiology will be very different at the different time points. The post-transplant timetable can be divided into three different time periods. During the first month post-transplant more than 95% of the complications are caused by bacterial pneumonias, bacterial or candidal infections of the surgical wound, vascular access or drainage catheters. Heart transplant recipients are at risk for mediastinitis and infection at the aortic

suture line, with resultant mycotic aneurysm, and lung transplant recipients may suffer from disruption of the bronchial anastomoses. Of special concern is the possibility of an early occurrence of herpes simplex virus (HSV) pneumonia in lung transplant recipients due to reactivation of the virus in preoperatively seropositive patients. The prophylactic use of aciclovir during this period has, however, significantly reduced the incidence of this devastating infection. Transmission of HSV by the transplant is very rare and may cause disseminated disease. Only occasional cases of human herpesvirus-6 (HHV-6) pneumonia with an onset 2–4 weeks post-transplant have been described.

During the period from the second to the sixth month post-transplant, the infections 'classically' associated with transplantation become manifest: those due to the immunomodulatory viruses such as CMV, EBV and (rarely) adenovirus, and those due to opportunistic pathogens such as *Aspergillus* and *Nocardia* spp., *M. tuberculosis*, *Pneumocystis carinii*, *Listeria monocytogenes* and *Toxoplasma gondii*. Because of the unique epidemiology of *T.*

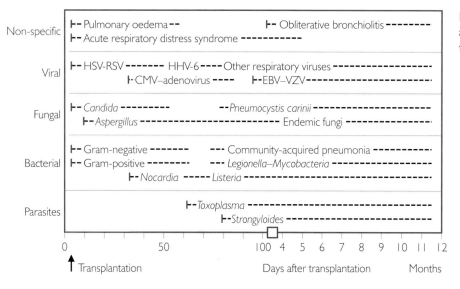

Fig. 36.2.2 Scheme of types of infection and time of occurrence after solid-organ transplantation.

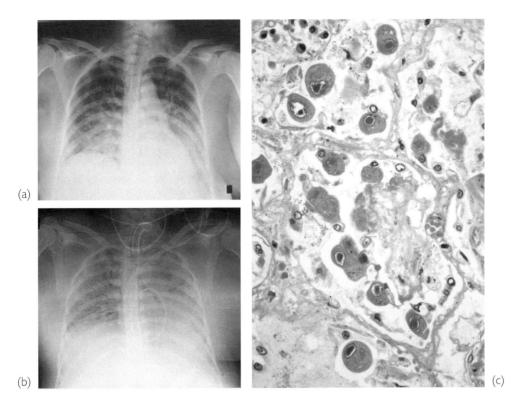

Fig. 36.2.3 Renal transplant recipient presenting with acute respiratory failure due to bilateral hazy airspace consolidations and 120/250 000 peripheral leukocytes positive for cytomegalovirus pp65 antigen (a). Despite treatment with intravenous ganciclovir the infiltrates were progressive (b) and transbronchial lung biopsy showed typical cytomegalic cells with intranuclear and intracytoplasmic viral inclusions, interstitial inflammation and alveolar haemorrhage (c).

gondii cyst formation within muscles, primary toxoplasmosis is virtually always limited to heart- and heart–lung- transplant recipients. Prophylaxis with pyrimethamine for 6 weeks has almost completely abolished this complication in susceptible subjects, i.e. seronegative recipients of a seropositive organ. Trimethoprim–sulfamethoxazole may be equally effective.

The infectious agent that dominates the second time period after solid-organ transplantation is CMV (Fig. 36.2.3).[11] Its incidence varies among the different organ transplantations, ranging from 8–32% in kidney- up to 53–75% in lung transplant recipients (Table 36.2.2). Serious disease usually occurs in seronegative recipients of organs from seropositive donors, except in lung transplant recipients, among whom seropositive recipients are also at risk. CMV disease may occur as early as 8 days postoperatively but more commonly appears after 4–5 weeks.

In the late period more than 6 months post-transplant the patient population can be divided into three subgroups. More than two-thirds of transplant patients have had a good result from transplantation and are primarily at risk from community-acquired respiratory bacteria and viruses. Some 10–15% of the patients suffer from recurrent acute rejection episodes resulting in temporarily augmented immunosuppression and recurrent infections with immunomodulatory viruses. During this time period these patients are especially susceptible to the above-mentioned infectious agents. Finally, there are the remaining 5–10%, who suffer from chronic rejection, receive excessive amounts of immunosuppression and have relatively poor allo-graft function. This subgroup is at the greatest risk of opportunistic infection, particularly with such organisms as *Aspergillus* spp., *P. carinii*, *Cryptococcus neoformans* and *L. monocytogenes*.

The utility of this timetable is threefold. First, it assists in the formulation of a differential diagnosis for the individual patient with an infectious disease syndrome. Second, it is useful as a tool for infection control, since the identification of an exception to the timetable usually connotes an excessive environmental hazard. And finally, it is the basis of a cost-effective infection control strategy (Tables 36.2.3 & 36.2.4).

Diagnostic approach

The diagnostic approach, treatment and prevention of complications after solid organ transplantation are strongly inter-related, since there are three modes in which antimicrobial agents can be prescribed. Prophylactic treatment, in which an entire population is prescribed antimicrobial therapy in order to prevent an infection that is common enough and important enough to justify such a commitment, is by far the preferred strategy (Table 36.2.3).[12] The second approach is pre-emptive treatment, in which antimicrobial therapy is prescribed before clinical infection is present to a subgroup of patients who have been shown to be at especially high risk of clinical infection on the basis of a clinico-epidemiological characteristic or laboratory marker (Table 36.2.4). And, lastly, in the therapeutic approach antimicrobial therapy is prescribed to treat clinically overt infection.

Table 36.2.3 Major pathogens and recommended prophylactic and preventive regimens in solid-organ transplant recipients

Type of infection	Prophylactic regimen
Pneumocystis carinii	Trimethoprim–sulfamethoxazole, one single-strength per day or three double-strength per week for 6 months; in all patients beyond 6 months if enhanced immunosuppression or recipient of a lung transplant. Prophylaxis is also effective for Nocardia asteroides, Listeria monocytogenes and possibly Toxoplasma gondii
Cytomegalovirus	Oral ganciclovir 1 g three times per day for at least 4 months in all seropositive recipients of liver, kidney/pancreas (including islet cells), heart and lung transplants or of seropositive organs, and seronegative recipients of seropositive kidneys
Herpes simplex virus	Valaciclovir 500 mg three times per day in long transplant recipients not receiving prophylactic ganciclovir
Varicella-zoster virus	Active immunisation of seronegative patients before transplantation
Influenza	Yearly administration of influenza vaccine at the appropriate season
Streptococcus pneumoniae	Multivalent pneumococcal polysaccharide vaccine, booster every 2–3 years
Mycobacterium tuberculosis	Isoniazid for 9–12 months in all tuberculin (PPD)-positive patients, beginning after transplantation when the immunosuppressive regimen has been stabilised
Toxoplasma gondii	Pyrimethamine in seronegative recipients of seropositive heart and heart–lung transplants; trimethoprim–sulfamethoxazole may be sufficient

Table 36.2.4 Pre-emptive therapy of selected pulmonary pathogens in solid-organ transplant recipients

Pathogen	Indication	Prophylactic regimen
Cytomegalovirus	Augmented immunosuppression (ALG/ATG or OKT-3), or 'high' level antigenaemia, or 'high' level PCR	Ganciclovir 5 mg/kg i.v. twice daily for 3 weeks, or ganciclovir 5 mg/kg i.v. twice daily for 1 week, followed by oral ganciclovir 1 g three times a day for 1 month
Aspergillus sp.	Detection in endobronchial specimens in lung transplant recipients	Itraconazole 200 mg twice daily and/or inhaled amphotericin B 5–20 mg three times a day
Azole-resistant Candida sp.	Detection in endobronchial specimens in lung transplant recipients	Amphotericin B 1 mg/kg i.v. per day immediately post-transplant; subsequently inhaled amphotericin B 5–20 mg three times a day

Besides bacterial infections CMV is the most important infectious agent in solid-organ transplant recipients.[12] Most centres monitor their patients by regular analysis of either CMV antigenaemia or PCR levels. Sensitivity and specificity for CMV disease of the presence of more than 25 antigen-positive cells per 250 000 leukocytes in the peripheral blood are 95% and 67% respectively.[13] If there are more than 100 or more than 250 antigen-positive cells detectable, specificity is 82% and 94% respectively. Thus, pre-emptive treatment may be indicated if more than 25 antigen-positive cells are present (Table 36.2.4).

The differential diagnosis of pulmonary complications in the solid-organ transplant recipient is mainly guided by the radiological pattern and the rate of progression of illness (Table 36.2.5). In patients presenting with classical signs of bacterial pneumonia such as acute onset, sputum purulence, high fevers, chills or chest pain, empirical antimicrobial treatment guided by sputum bacteriological cultures is a reasonable option. In most patients, however, a more aggressive diagnostic approach using bronchoalveolar lavage (BAL) is preferred. With respect to P. carinii it is important to remember that in solid-organ transplant recipients the sensitivity of diagnosis by sputum analysis is very low because of the low burden of microorganisms in contrast to HIV-infected patients. The sensitivity of BAL is also only about 80% in non-AIDS[14] but it may be increased if two segments are lavaged.[15] Bronchoscopy and BAL are particularly helpful in the diagnosis of bacterial infections, including tuberculosis (Fig. 36.2.4), legionellosis and nocardiosis, as well as non-infectious diseases such as alveolar haemorrhage. The detection of CMV or Aspergillus sp. in the BAL fluid is strongly indicative but not sufficient for the diagnosis of lung disease by these organisms. Thus, all patients with a non-diagnostic BAL should undergo transbronchial lung biopsy. Its sensitivity with respect to distinct disease is only about 50%[16] but it reaches 90% for the detection of lung transplant rejection, CMV disease (Fig. 36.2.3) and P. carinii pneumonia.[17,18] However, the rate of non-specific results can be substantial, and further evaluation of such cases by surgical lung biopsy is crucial.[19] The yield of this procedure is about 80% – significantly higher than in other categories of

Table 36.2.5   Differential diagnosis of fever and pulmonary infiltrates in solid-organ transplant recipients, based on radiographic abnormalities and rate of progression of symptoms

Abnormality on chest radiograph	Aetiology according to rate of progression of illness	
	Acute	Subacute or chronic
Consolidation	Bacterial pneumonia *Legionella pneumophila* Herpes simplex virus Pulmonary embolism Pulmonary oedema	Invasive aspergillosis Nocardiosis Tuberculosis *Pneumocystis carinii* Lymphoproliferative disorders
Diffuse bilateral infiltrates	Acute respiratory distress syndrome Cardiogenic pulmonary oedema Hypersensitivity pneumonitis Lung-transplant rejection (early)	Viral pneumonia (CMV, HSV) *P. carinii* Tuberculosis Hypersensitivity pneumonitis Non-herpes respiratory viruses
Nodular infiltrates	Bacterial pneumonia Pulmonary embolism	Invasive aspergillosis Tuberculosis, nocardiosis *Bartonella henselae* *P. carinii* (granulomatous) Lymphoproliferative disorders Kaposi's sarcoma
Pleural effusion	Bacterial pneumonia Lung-transplant rejection (early) Pulmonary embolism	Invasive aspergillosis Tuberculosis, nocardiosis

CMV, cytomegalovirus; HSV, herpes simplex virus.

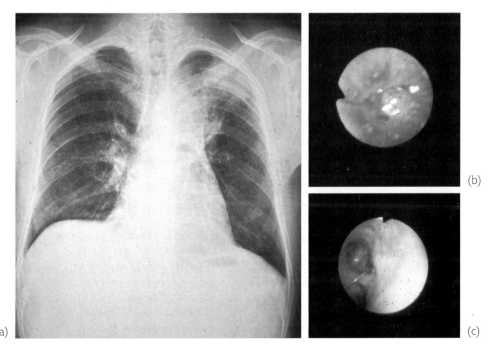

(a)

(b)

(c)

Fig. 36.2.4   (a) Liver transplant recipient presenting with an infiltrate of the left upper lobe with partial atelectasis. (b) Bronchoscopy revealed almost complete occlusion of the left upper-lobe bronchus due to endobronchial tuberculosis. (c) The lesion resolved after 9 months of antituberculosis treatment).

immunosuppressed patients.[20,21] Computed tomography of the chest often adds differential diagnostic information with respect to the various patterns of diesases[22] and may guide the biopsy procedure. Moreover it may detect pulmonary thromboembolism, which is not rare in solid-organ transplant recipients.

Treatment

Preventive measures and prophylactic treatment are the mainstay of the management of the solid-organ transplant recipient (Table 36.2.4). Trimethoprim–sulfamethoxazole should be offered to every patient for at least 6 months, and possibly lifelong in lung transplant recipients. Prophylaxis should be resumed in every case of augmented immunosuppression. Besides *P. carinii*, trimethoprim–sulfamethoxazole covers many other pathogens, such as *Legionella*, *Listeria* and *Nocardia* spp. and possibly *T. gondii*. Moreover, it protects against urinary tract infections, especially in kidney transplant recipients.

The second most important prophylactic treatment is ganciclovir, which has been shown to reduce the incidence of CMV infection and disease in large trials of liver and heart transplant recipients, and several case series of lung transplant patients. Considering the influence of CMV on the development of chronic rejection in all solid-organ transplants, besides improved immunosuppressive regimens, prophylaxis with ganciclovir appears to be the most important advance of the past 10 years in solid organ transplantation.

Treatment of infectious complications in solid-organ transplant recipients follows internationally accepted guidelines. Pre-emptive therapy is the preferred mode in many situations (Table 36.2.5). As mentioned above, a specific diagnosis should always be attempted. Empirical antibiotic therapy with high-dose trimethoprim–sulfamethoxazole may be an option in cases with non-diagnostic findings, since, besides *P. carinii* and *T. gondii*, it covers most bacterial pathogens including *Legionella*, *Listeria* and *Nocardia* sp. However, the possibility of an infection due to CMV, *Aspergillus* sp. or *M. tuberculosis* should always be kept in mind.

Kidney transplantation

An analysis of the literature about pulmonary complications after kidney transplantation including about 1500 patients reveals an incidence of pulmonary complications of 18–24%.[7,23] Up to 50% of these complications were fatal and almost half of the mortality after kidney transplantation was attributable to pulmonary disease. During the past years the incidence of these complications has decreased for various reasons. The rate of postoperative pneumonia now is about 4–9%.[24]

About one-third of pulmonary disease in kidney transplant recipients is of non-infectious origin. Pulmonary oedema occurs in 2%, most often within the first few postoperative weeks. Usually it is caused by overhydration in patients with postoperatively impaired renal function. Although the incidence of venous thromboembolism is reduced in uraemic patients, this complication causes about two-thirds of all non-infectious pulmonary problems and up to 16% of all pulmonary complications after kidney transplantation.[23]

The most important infectious disorders are nosocomial bacterial pneumonias. The incidence of CMV disease has dramatically decreased by the use of prophylactic or pre-emptive treatment with ganciclovir. Invasive aspergillosis has also become rare but may be seen in patients over-immunosuppressed because of recurrent acute or chronic rejection.

Liver transplantation

Most complications after liver transplantation occur within the first 2 postoperative months and are largely due to postoperative problems. Because the operation is very long and difficult, operation time and the occurrence of operative complications such as severe haemorrhage are the most important predictors of the subsequent course. Non-infectious problems such as pulmonary oedema, atelectasis, right-sided pleural effusion and acute respiratory distress syndrome cause at least half of the pulmonary complications in liver transplant recipients.[7,25,26] The latter occurs in 5–18% of patients and has a mortality of up to 80%. Aetiological factors are prolonged hypotension, hypertransfusion and sepsis. A rare but distinct complication are ectopic soft-tissue calcifications, which most often affect the lungs. Their cause is unknown but potential pathogenetic factors include hyperparathyroidism, calcium administered during and following surgery, renal failure, acid–base changes and citrate in fresh frozen plasma. Diagnosis may be made by technetium-99m scintigraphy.

The most important infectious complications after liver transplantation are bacterial pneumonias.[27] The major pathogens are *Staphylococcus aureus*, *Pseudomonas aeruginosa* and the Enterobacteriaceae. Invasive aspergillosis still is a problem in over-immunosuppressed patients. The occurrence of CMV disease has been virtually eliminated by the use of prophylactic or pre-emptive treatment with ganciclovir.[26]

Heart transplantation

The spectrum of non-infectious complications after heart transplantation resembles that of other cardiac surgical procedures.[7] Atelectasis occurs in 60–90% of patients and pleural effusion in up to 80%. The incidence of postoperative acute respiratory distress syndrome resulting from prolonged cardiopulmonary bypass times has been reduced by improvements in surgical and anaesthetic techniques. Acute cardiac rejection episodes leading to cardiogenic pulmonary oedema have become rare. Post-transplant pulmonary hypertension and right heart failure, however, still remain the most serious postoperative complication after heart transplantation. Preoperative testing with and perioperative use of vasodilators may improve the outcome in patients with preoperatively elevated pulmonary vascular resistance.

The spectrum of infectious complications after heart transplantation corresponds to those seen after other solid-organ transplantation.[28] Their overall incidence and severity resembles the infections occurring after liver transplantation (Table 36.2.2).

Lung transplantation

Pulmonary complications after lung transplantation are dealt with in Chapter 12.

Cancer and treatment-induced neutropenia

Spectrum of disease

Neoplastic diseases and their treatment result in specific immune defects that predispose to serious infections.[29,30] The predominant disorder is a phagocytic defect due to neutropenia, but T-cell and B-cell defects or splenectomy may additionally lead to specific infectious complications. Moreover, defects of the skin and mucous membranes as a result of the tumour or its treatment, gastrointestinal disorders, malnutrition and catheter placement also predispose to infections. The risk of infection is dependent on the degree and duration of the neutropenia. The infection rate is increased if the neutrophil count falls below 1.0×10^9/l. Severe infection is probable if the neutrophil numbers decrease to less than 0.1×10^9/l, at which level 25% of the patients get an infection within 1 week and 100% are infected within 6 weeks. It is well known that if the neutropenia lasts less than 7–10 days the risk of infection is low, whereas if the neutropenia persists for longer than 10 days the risk of infection is very high and there may be multiple and recurrent new infections. Patients treated for leukaemia and recipients of allogeneic haematopoietic stem-cell transplants usually have a neutrophil count below 0.1×10^9/l for 14–28 days, whereas patients undergoing chemotherapy for solid tumours have a neutropenia lasting less than 10 days. This distinction, however, may not be valid today, since patients with solid tumours also now and then undergo aggressive chemotherapy with stem cell rescue. Besides the level and duration of neutropenia, the risk of infection is also related to the rapidity of the decline in cell numbers. Thus, the infection rate in patients with chronic neutropenia, such as occurs in severe aplastic anaemia or idiopathic neutropenia, is lower than in patients with rapidly decreasing neutrophil counts.

In only about one-quarter of the patients with long-standing severe neutropenia can an infection be microbiologically documented. Another quarter of the patients exhibit obvious clinical signs of infection without isolation of a pathogen, i.e. they suffer from clinically documented infections. The rest of the patients have fever of unknown origin. However, because clinical signs of infection such as sputum production or pulmonary infiltrates may be absent because of the low neutrophil counts, it is estimated that more than 90% of neutropenic patients with fever in fact have an infection, with the remaining 10% having fever caused mainly by drugs, tumour or transfusions.

Most infections in these patients are derived from the patients' endogenous flora (skin, gastrointestinal tract, lungs) and approximately half are nosocomial. During recent years, the spectrum of bacteria involved has shifted from mainly Gram-negative to mainly Gram-positive organisms. Nowadays about two-thirds of infections are caused by Gram-positive bacteria, including *Staphylococcus epidermidis*, *S. aureus* and viridans streptococci. The remaining third of infections are caused by Gram-negative pathogens including *Escherichia coli*, *Klebsiella pneumoniae*, *Enterobacter* spp., *Serratia* spp. and *P. aeruginosa*. The most serious infections in profoundly neutropenic patients, however, are invasive fungal infections, primarily caused by *Aspergillus* and *Mucor* spp.

Management

During the last few decades considerable progress has been made in the management of patients with fever and neutropenia, which has resulted in improved survival rates.[30] While the mortality rates in the seventies reached 25%, the overall mortality now ranges between 5% and 10%.[31] The cornerstone of management is a pragmatic approach using empirical broad-spectrum antibiotic therapy (Fig. 36.2.5).[30–32] In a patient with neutropenia (defined by a neutrophil count below 0.5×10^9/l or below 1.0×10^9/l with predicted decline to 0.5×10^9/l or less) and fever (defined as a single oral temperature reading of more than 38.3°C or 38.0°C or more for at least 1 hour) cultures of blood (peripheral and catheter), urine and diarrhoeal stools, and a chest radiograph, should be performed.

Immediate empirical therapy with an extended-spectrum penicillin, carbapenems or a third-generation cephalosporin appropriate for coverage of *P. aeruginosa* should be initiated. If the patient is critically ill, an aminoglycoside is added (or ciprofloxacin in patients with severely impaired kidney function). In patients with persisting fever for 5–7 days, empirical antifungal therapy with amphotericin B is begun. If there are risk factors for invasive aspergillosis such as corticosteroid therapy, underlying lung disease or suspected fungal disease during a previous episode of neutropenia, amphotericin B should be given earlier. The same applies if there is a focal abnormality on auscultation of the lungs, pleuritic chest pain, haemoptysis or a pulmonary infiltrate on chest radiograph. Conventional chest radiographs are not very sensitive for the detection of early lesions of invasive aspergillosis. Therefore, if suspicion is high, high-resolution computed tomography should be performed, which is much more sensitive.[22] The presence of a single or multiple pulmonary nodules with a surrounding halo of ground-glass attenuation or patchy areas of consolidation and nodules with air crescents is almost pathognomonic of the presence of invasive aspergillosis (Fig. 36.2.6). Any patient with upper respiratory tract symptoms, maxillary sinus tenderness and necrotic or ulcerated areas in the nose should undergo computed tomography of the paranasal sinuses and diagnostic as well as therapeutic sinus lavage for *Aspergillus* or *Mucor* sp.

There is no established value for the serological diagnosis of invasive fungal infections. The sensitivity of microbiological sputum analysis is very low. The same applies to BAL, which has a sensitivity of less than 50%. On the other hand, if *Aspergillus* sp. is found in a respiratory specimen of a neutropenic patient, the specificity for the presence of invasive disease is more than 90%, in contrast to other immunosuppressed patients, in whom the respective specificity is very low.

In our opinion, bronchoscopy and BAL should be performed only in patients with diffuse pulmonary infiltrates and persisting fever despite appropriate empirical therapy, since the possibility of other opportunistic infections such as *P. carinii* pneumonia is extremely low in this patient group, except in patients with lymphatic neoplasias. Surgical lung biopsies are performed only exceptionally in patients with persisting infiltrates despite

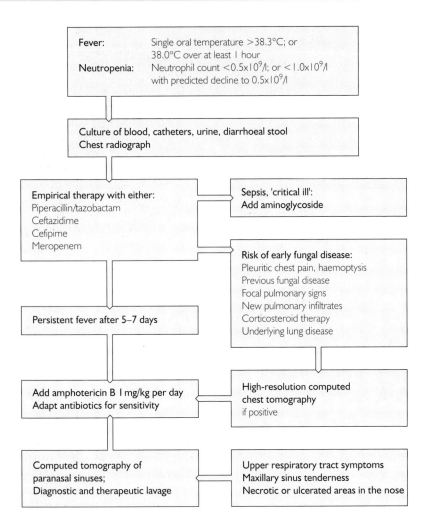

Fig. 36.2.5 Management of the patient with fever and neutropenia.

adequate treatment and negative results of BAL, or in the presence of large cavitating lesions and haemoptysis.

Using this empirical approach mortality of severely neutropenic patients has markedly decreased. Antimicrobial therapy is usually stopped at neutrophil counts above 0.5×10^9/l. The use of antiviral drugs, colony-stimulating factors or routine antibiotic or antifungal prophylaxis in afebrile neutropenic patients is not indicated. In low-risk neutropenic patients (duration of neutropenia <10 days) ambulatory oral antibiotic treatment with ciprofloxacin (750 mg twice daily) plus amoxicillin–clavulanate (625 mg three times daily) has been proven to be effective and safe.[33]

The haematopoietic stem-cell transplant recipient

Spectrum of disease

Haematopoietic stem-cell transplantation has become an accepted therapeutic option for various haematological malignancies, haemoglobinopathies and immunodeficiency disorders as well as solid tumours. Allogeneic and autologous haemato-

poietic stem-cell transplantation should be distinguished with respect to pulmonary complications.[34] In autologous haematopoietic stem-cell transplantation, neutropenia is the primary immune defect and the spectrum of infectious pulmonary diseases is comparable to that discussed in the previous section.[1] Allogeneic haematopoietic stem-cell transplantation, however, leads to a broader range of immune defects and therefore includes a high risk of CMV disease and various non-infectious disorders. Pulmonary complications occur in 40–60% of transplant patients. Their incidence depends on various factors such as the type and duration of the immunological defect produced by the underlying disease and its treatment, the presence of graft-versus-host disease and its treatment, and the conditioning regiments employed. The spectrum of pulmonary complications includes infectious and non-infectious conditions. As in solid organ transplantation, they follow a distinct timetable and are classified as early or late according to whether they occur before or after 100 days post-transplant (Fig. 36.2.7). Early complications include pulmonary oedema (incidence 0–50%), alveolar haemorrhage (0–20%), bacterial, fungal and viral pneumonias (30–40%) and the idiopathic pneumonia syndrome (0–20%). Late complications comprise pneumonias (20–30%), idiopathic pneumonia syndrome (10–20%) and obliterative bronchiolitis (10–20%).

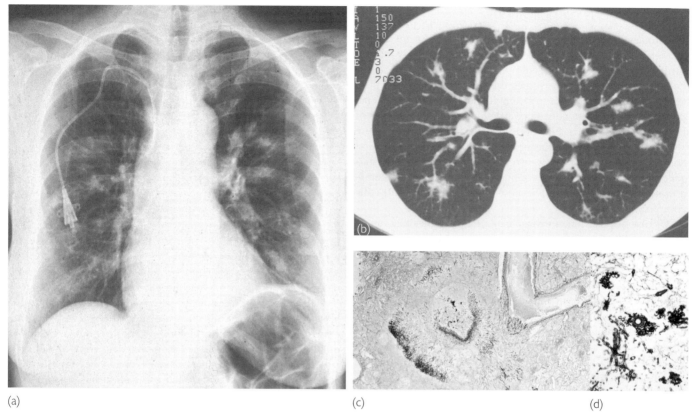

(a)   (c)   (d)

Fig. 36.2.6 This patient with prolonged neutropenia due to chemotherapy for acute myeloid leukaemia and persistent fever despite adequate antibiotic treatment showed bilateral infiltrates on chest radiograph (a). (b) Computed tomography revealed the characteristic multiple pulmonary nodules in the bronchovascular bundle with a surrounding halo of ground-glass attenuation and patchy areas of consolidation. Open lung biopsy was performed because of lack of response to antifungal therapy and demonstrated the typical vascular invasion and thrombosis (c) leading to haemorrhagic infarction by the typical narrow, septate hyphae with acute angle branching of *Aspergillus fumigatus* (d).

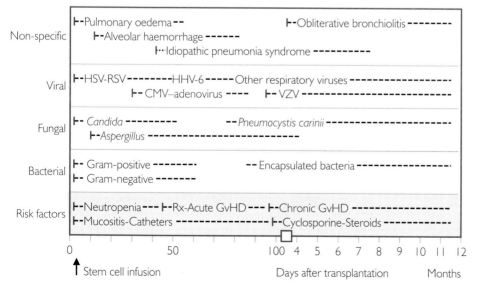

Fig. 36.2.7 Scheme of types of infection and time of occurrence after allogeneic haematopoietic stem cell transplantation.

Non-infectious complications

Pulmonary oedema is one of the earliest complications and its incidence varies greatly between centres. The aetiology may be cardiogenic or non-cardiogenic or a combination of both. Echocardiography usually shows dilated ventricles with poor function. This may be due to a combination of cardiac and renal dysfunction from previous chemotherapy and the infusion of large volumes of fluids. However, increased permeability of the alveolar–capillary membrane as a result of chemotherapy, total body irradiation and sepsis often contributes to the pathogenesis of pulmonary oedema. Thorough fluid balance and early diuretic therapy, however, almost completely prevents this complication.

Diffuse alveolar haemorrhage clinically resembles pulmonary oedema and is characterised by sudden onset of progressive dyspnoea, non-productive cough, fever and hypoxaemia. Haemoptysis is rare. The syndrome typically occurs about 10–14 days after transplantation and coincides with the time of neutrophil engraftment (take). The chest radiograph shows diffuse consolidations and BAL characteristically demonstrates progressively bloody lavage fluid without any microorganisms. Early diagnosis of diffuse alveolar haemorrhage is crucial since the administration of high doses of corticosteroids may significantly reduce the reported high mortality rates of 50–80%.

Idiopathic pneumonia syndrome is defined as a diffuse lung injury histologically characterised by an interstitial mononuclear infiltrate associated with diffuse alveolar damage in the absence of an infectious aetiology.[35] The incidence is about 10% and the onset around 40 days after transplantation, but the disease may occur as early as 14 days and as late as several months after transplantation. Risk factors are higher doses of total body irradiation and the presence of graft-versus-host disease. The diagnosis of this syndrome is usually one of exclusion. There is a gradual onset of dyspnoea, fever, non-productive cough, hypoxaemia, restrictive pulmonary function abnormality and diffuse radiographic infiltrates (Fig. 36.2.8). BAL is usually sufficient for the exclusion of an infectious aetiology. No specific therapy is available for idiopathic pneumonia syndrome but a subgroup of patients might respond to corticosteroids. The mortality rate is about 70% and lung transplantation could be an option for these patients.

The development of chronic obstructive airway disease as a result of **obliterative bronchiolitis** is a serious problem after allogeneic haematopoietic stem-cell transplantation, affecting 2–13% of patients. The disease resembles obliterative bronchiolitis in lung transplant recipients and by analogy is believed to be the result of an immunological injury to the airways secondary to graft-versus-host disease, but viral infections and other pathogenetic factors as discussed in lung transplant obliterative bronchiolitis may be relevant. The diagnosis of obliterative bronchiolitis is based on the typical clinical picture including progressive dyspnoea, irreversible obstructive ventilatory defect and hyperinflation on chest radiograph without infiltrates (Fig. 36.2.9). The initial symptoms of obliterative bronchiolitis often resemble those of an upper respiratory tract infection and may be mistakenly treated as such. In the appropriate clinical context histological diagnosis is not necessary in most cases if an infectious aetiology is excluded by BAL.

Single cases of **pulmonary veno-occlusive disease** after allogeneic haematopoietic stem cell transplantation are reported, and they may respond to corticosteroid therapy.

Infectious complications

Bacterial and fungal infections represent the most important infectious complication after allogeneic haematopoietic stem-cell transplantation. The management of patients with respect to these infections is the same as in other neutropenic patients (see above). However, it should be emphasised that there is a second period of increased risk of infection with these micro-

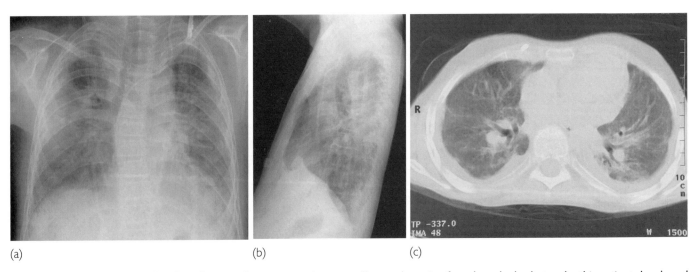

(a)   (b)   (c)

Fig. 36.2.8 (a), (b) Ten months after allogeneic haematopoietic stem-cell transplantation for adrenoleukodystrophy this patient developed progressive bilateral infiltrative lung disease. (c) Computed tomography showed bilateral ground-glass opacities, and surgical lung biopsy confirmed idiopathic pneumonia syndrome. Two years later the patient underwent successful bilateral lung transplantation.

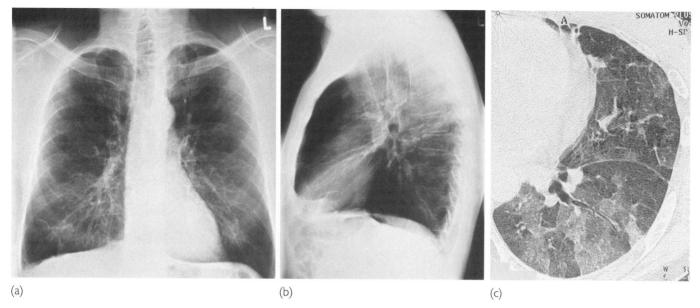

(a)   (b)   (c)

Fig. 36.2.9 This patient developed progressive dyspnoea on exertion 2 years after allogeneic haematopoietic stem-cell transplantation for aplastic anaemia. Chest radiographs showed clear lung fields (a) and severe overinflation (b). (c) High-resolution computed tomography demonstrated the characteristic mosaic perfusion pattern suggestive of obliterative bronchiolitis.

organisms after haematopoietic stem-cell transplantation in patients suffering from graft-versus-host disease and receiving immunosuppressive treatment with ciclosporin, corticosteroids and other agents.

With the use of pre-emptive ganciclovir therapy, the frequency of **CMV pneumonia** has decreased dramatically. Before, CMV pneumonia occurred in about 10–40% of allogeneic haematopoietic stem-cell transplant recipients with an onset 6–12 weeks post-transplant and a mortality rate of up to 85%. Most infections represented reactivation of latent endogenous virus but, in up to one-third of patients, CMV was acquired by infusion of a CMV-seropositive bone stem-cell transplant or by blood product transfusions. The clinical features of CMV pneumonia resemble those of the disease in solid-organ transplant recipients. The presence of clinical disease and detection of the virus in either the blood, urine, throat swab or BAL suffices for the diagnosis of CMV pneumonia in the context of allogeneic haematopoietic stem cell transplantation. Nowadays, regular monitoring for antigenaemia or PCR is performed at most centres. In the presence of any detectable viral antigen or nucleic acids, immediate pre-emptive treatment with intravenous ganciclovir is advisable.

Other viral infections include HSV, which usually presents as gingivitis or stomatitis but rarely causes severe pneumonia within the first week after transplantation. There are several cases with documented HHV-6 infection and idiopathic pneumonitis. However, the pathogenetic role of the virus is not yet clear. All patients with pneumonia should also be evaluated for other respiratory viruses such as respiratory syncytial virus, parainfluenza virus and adenovirus.

The introduction of prophylaxis has resulted in a significant reduction in the incidence of *P. carinii* pneumonia in haematopoietic stem-cell transplant recipients. It is found in only single

cases who cannot tolerate trimethoprim–sulfamethoxazole or inhaled pentamidine prophylaxis.

Primary immunodeficiency syndromes

The primary immunodeficiency syndromes are a heterogeneous group of diseases that often affect children but may also be diagnosed in adults, as is the case for the common variable immunodeficiency disease.[36–38]

The host defences against infection are classified as either innate or acquired. Innate immunity refers to all host defences that do not exhibit specificity or memory. The phagocytes, the complement system and the mucociliary apparatus of the respiratory epithelium are the major components of the innate immune system. Defects of acquired immunity are caused primarily by primary humoral and combined immunodeficiencies. Insights in the pathogenesis, diagnosis and treatment of these disorders progress rapidly, and many diseases can now be cured by haematopoietic stem-cell transplantation or gene therapy. This review includes only disorders that may involve the respiratory tract. An overview on the diagnostic procedures is given in Table 36.2.6.

Defects of innate immunity

The **phagocytic disorders** usually present in infancy or early childhood with infections of the umbilical cord, skin abscesses, periodontitis, osteomyelitis and recurrent pneumonia or sepsis due to bacteria and fungi. In **chronic granulomatous diseases**, neutrophils lack normal respiratory burst to kill ingested microbes efficiently due to mutations or absence of molecules of

Table 36.2.6 Evaluation of the patient with suspected immune deficiency

Type of immune defect	Diagnostic procedure
Cellular immune defect	Total lymphocyte count Lymphocyte subpopulation (flow cytometry) Delayed-type hypersensitivity (Multitest Mérieux) (In-vitro studies of T-cell function)
Humoral immune defect	Serum immunoglobulins and immunoglobulin G subclasses Specific antibody titre in response to immunisation (Tetanus and diphtheria toxoid, *H. influenzae* type B)
Phagocytic immune defect	Neutrophil count and morphology Flow cytometry (CD18) Nitroblue tetrazolium test or chemiluminescence assay Immunoglobulin E
Complement deficiency	Tests for humoral immune defect Total haemolytic complement (CH50)
Asplenia	Howell–Jolly bodies

For most primary immunodeficiencies genetic testing is available; see references.

the NADPH oxidase system. The most common form is X-linked and the other forms are inherited in an autosomal recessive fashion. Chronic granulomatous diseases usually presents within the first few years of life. Besides the respiratory tract, the skin and the gastrointestinal tract are most often involved. Because the bacteria are phagocytosed but not killed, they may be carried to the regional lymph nodes or the reticuloendothelial system, causing lymphadenopathy and hepatosplenomegaly.

Such infections are most commonly caused by *S. aureus*, Gram-negative bacteria and *Aspergillus* spp. Often bacteria with low virulence such as *Serratia marcescens* are involved. Chronic antibiotic (trimethoprim–sulfamethoxazole) and antifungal (itraconazole) prophylaxis and the administration of gamma-interferon (IF-γ) have improved the prognosis in these patients.

Leukocyte adhesion deficiency is caused by a failure of the production of the CD18 receptor on leukocyte surfaces, which leads to impaired endothelial adhesion of the leukocytes to intercellular adhesion molecule-1. The most common infections are omphalitis, defects in wound healing, severe periodontitis and, in patients with a less severe defect who survive the first years of life, chronic otitis media, chronic sinusitis and pneumonia due to *S. aureus*, Gram negative organisms and fungi.

Hyperimmunoglobulin E syndrome is characterised by recurrent bacterial infections, primarily by *S. aureus*, and mucocutaneous candidiasis during the first 5 years of life. A few patients have been diagnosed in adulthood. Characteristically, patients present with recurrent pneumonias and subsequent pneumatoceles, which may enlarge progressively and cause atelectasis by compression of the normal lung. Prophylactic antibiotic treatment and immunoglobulins in cases with deficiencies of IgG or IgA are indicated.

In **myeloperoxidase deficiency** there is a lack of enzymes found in the azurophilic granules of neutrophils and monocytes. Despite the fact that these granules are powerfully microbicidal, most patients are clinically normal and do not suffer from recur-

rent infections. The prevalence is as high as 1/1400 and is noteworthy only because the machines performing automated leukocyte differential counts rely on myeloperoxidase activity and leukocytes are therefore counted as 'large unstained cells'.

Chédiak–Higashi syndrome presents with recurrent pyogenic infections of the respiratory tract and the skin in the first years of life, partial albinism and multiple neurological abnormalities. Bizarre-appearing giant-granule-containing leukocytes and platelets in the peripheral blood are pathognomonic. After about 10 years patients may develop massive lymphohistiocytic infiltration of virtually all organ systems, which results in pancytopenia and even more profound immunodeficiency.

Deficiencies of various proteins of the **complement system** lead to recurrent bacterial pneumonias and skin infections. Affected patients have difficulty in coping with *Neisseria gonorrhoeae* and *N. meningitidis* infections. This results in a high incidence of meningococcal sepsis, which however has a less aggressive course than in normal hosts. Moreover, many complement defects result in autoimmune disease, especially lupus erythematosus.

There is a multitude of disorders of the ciliary apparatus, now referred to as **primary ciliary dyskinesia**. Kartagener's syndrome (situs inversus, bronchiectasis, chronic sinusitis and male infertility) is a subset of these disorders. Patients usually have a history of recurrent upper and lower airway infections since childhood and develop bronchiectasis in adult life (see Chapter 49).

Asplenia is a rare congenital abnormality that places the host at a considerable risk of overwhelming sepsis during the first years of life, caused primarily by *S. pneumoniae*. Other microorganisms involved are *Babesia microfti*, *Capnocytophaga canimorsus*, *Haemophilus influenzae* and *N. meningitidis*. Much more frequent is acquired asplenia, due either to splenectomy or impaired splenic function in patients with sickle-cell disease.

Defects of acquired immunity

Predominantly humoral immune defects lead to recurrent infections with encapsulated organisms such as *H. influenzae* and *S. pneumoniae*. They present with otitis media, sinusitis and pneumonia. **X-linked agammaglobulinaemia** (Bruton) is a rare inherited disorder that affects infants within the first year of life. The most important primary immunodeficiency syndrome, however, is **common variable immunodeficiency**.[39] Its incidence varies between 1/20 000 and 1/200 000 and males and females are equally affected. The disease usually presents during the second or third decade of life with recurrent bacterial infections of the upper and lower respiratory tract, which often lead to generalised bronchiectasis (Fig. 36.2.10). The disease is characterised by decreased serum IgG and IgA levels and generally, but not invariably, decreased serum IgM. Other causes of hypogammaglobulinaemia such as chronic lymphocytic leukaemia should be excluded. The specific defect of the disease has not been characterised yet. The majority of patients have normal numbers of B-cells. Abnormalities in T-cell number and function have been described. About half the patients develop autoimmune disease and there is an increased risk of malignancy (lymphoma, gastrointestinal cancers). Treatment consists of replacement therapy with intravenous immune globulins (0.5 mg/kg of body weight every 2–4 weeks, aiming at a serum IgG level over 5 g/l).

Selective IgA deficiency is found in up to 1/400 of the general population. Most of these subjects, however, remain asymptomatic throughout their life. Rarely, a syndrome comparable to common variable immunodeficiency develops. These patients occasionally develop antibodies to IgA in transfused blood products and are at risk of anaphylactic transfusion reaction.

Idiopathic CD4⁺ T-lymphocytopenia syndrome is an extremely rare disorder defined by an absolute CD4⁺ T-lymphocyte count below 0.3×10^9/l or less than 20% of total T-cells and the absence of a infection with any of the human T-cell lymphocytotrophic viruses.[40] The clinical presentation of the disorder resembles AIDS; however, immunoglobulin levels are often normal or decreased, and many of the patients remain stable over years.

There are a vast number of combined immunodeficiencies. **Severe combined immunodeficiency (SCID)** is a rare, most commonly X-linked disorder and presents during the first few months of life with severe pneumonia and respiratory failure due to *P. carinii* pneumonia. Children may also present with failure to thrive, persistent oral thrush, other opportunistic infections and chronic diarrhoea. The diagnosis is made by the presence of absolute lymphopenia, which, however, is often overlooked, because the lower normal limit of the lymphocyte count during the first 6 months of life is 4.0×10^9/l. **Adenosine deaminase deficiency** presents like SCID but may occur in young adults. Sinopulmonary infections, including tuberculosis resulting in bronchiectasis, predominate. The disease can be treated by enzyme replacement.

Wiskott–Aldrich syndrome is a rare X-linked disease presenting in early childhood with low numbers of small platelets,

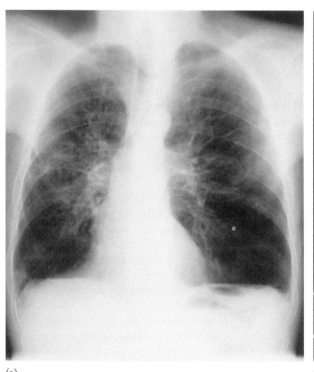

(a)

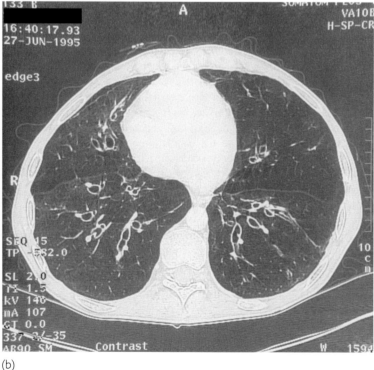

(b)

Fig. 36.2.10 This adult male patient suffered from recurrent pneumonia. (a) Chest radiography showed bilateral reticular shadows and hyperinflation. (b) Computed tomography confirmed the presence of bilateral bronchiectasis. The diagnosis of common variable immunodeficiency was made by the demonstration of severely decreased serum IgG and IgA levels.

eczema, abnormal antibody response to polysaccharide antigens and recurrent bacterial infections. The risk of lymphoproliferative disorders is increased.

Secondary immune deficiency induced by drugs, infections and diseases other than HIV

In addition to their use in transplantation and cancer chemotherapy, immunosuppressive drugs are administered for many diseases such as rheumatic disorders, autoimmune diseases and vasculitis syndromes.[41] As with the primary immunodeficiency syndromes, immunosuppressive drugs lead to an increased incidence of infection and malignancy. The spectrum of complications largely depends on the kind of immune defect induced by these drugs.

Drugs

Glucocorticosteroids are routinely used for a broad range of inflammatory disorders, as adjuncts to cancer chemotherapy and for common disorders such as chronic obstructive pulmonary disease. Their ability to induce a profound immune deficient state is often underestimated. Moreover, they are often used inappropriately. Glucocorticosteroids bind an intracellular receptor, resulting in translocation of the complex to the nucleus, where it interacts directly or indirectly with specific DNA sequences and other transcription factors such as IκBα, which negatively regulate nuclear factor kappa B (NFκB).[42] These interactions lead to increased or decreased transcription of the downstream genes. Most cytokines, such as granulocyte–macrophage-colony-stimulating factor, interleukin-1, 2, 3, 4, 6 and 8, tumour necrosis factor and IF-γ are inhibited resulting in a powerful immunomodulatory effect. Moreover, glucocorticosteroids cause a reduction in all circulating leukocytes except the neutrophils. The latter are increased in number by demargination. This effect hinders the ability of these cells to leave the circulation and enter sites of infection. Furthermore, the bactericidal capacity of all phagocytes is markedly impaired. The most important factors for the development of infectious complications in patients treated with glucocorticosteroids are the daily dose and the overall cumulative dose.[43] While the overall relative risk of infection is only about 1.6, it may be up to 40-fold for opportunistic infections. The main pulmonary infections related to glucocorticosteroid administration are due to bacteria (S. aureus and others), fungi (Aspergillus spp., P. carinii) and the herpesviruses.

Ciclosporin and tacrolimus bind to a series of intracellular proteins, which leads to an interruption of the lymphocyte-signalling pathway by inhibiting calcineurin. This results in a profound T-cell defect and an increased risk of infection with Mycobacterium spp., Nocardia spp., endemic fungi, P. carinii and the herpesviruses. Rapamycin acts synergistically with the calcineurin inhibitors. Antilymphocyte antibodies (OKT3, ATG, ALG) severely affect the cellular immune response and especially propagate infections with CMV and EBV. Azathioprine and mycophenolate inhibit DNA synthesis, leading to suppressed lymphocyte proliferation and neutropenia. Alkylating agents such as cyclophosphamide additionally affect the humoral immune response. Methotrexate inhibits nucleotide synthesis by arresting dihydrofolate reductase and may result in profound haematopoietic stem-cell suppression and a cellular as well as humoral immune defect. The incidence of pneumonia with P. carinii, CMV and Nocardia spp. is increased. Since most of the above mentioned drugs are given in combination with glucocorticosteroids, the risk of infectious complications is further enhanced. The occurrence of invasive aspergillosis is of special concern.

Infections

Many infections apart from HIV suppress the immune system by various mechanisms. Measles induces global immune suppression, leading to severe infections with bacteria and other viruses, especially in infants suffering from malnutrition. The herpesviruses are regularly associated with transient depression of the cell-mediated immunity. Other infections that negatively affect the immune system are the mycobacterioses, malaria, trypanosomiasis and leishmaniasis.

There are some systemic diseases that adversely affect the immune response of the host. In **diabetes mellitus** the phagocytic defence is impaired in direct correlation to the level of hyperglycaemia. The incidence of pneumonias (S. aureus, P. aeruginosa), rhinopulmonary mucormycosis and disseminated candidiasis is markedly increased. In patients receiving **haemodialysis** there is a significant cellular immune defect (cutaneous anergy), diminished antibody production and neutrophil dysfunction. If the underlying disease is associated with a **nephrotic syndrome**, loss of immunoglobulins and complement further increases the risk of bacterial infection. **Cirrhosis of the liver** may lead to high levels of endogenous glucocorticosteroids. In addition, shunting of portal blood reduces the ability of hepatic Kupffer cells to clear opsonised particles, and hypocomplementaemia further reduces serum opsonic activity. The most common infectious complications of severe cirrhosis are bacterial pneumonias and sepsis. **Malnutrition** results in decreased levels of circulating T cells, diminished T-cell mitogen responses and decreased phagocytic cell function. Serum immunoglobulin levels are normal or increased; however, specific antibody responses are impaired.

Iron and its binding proteins affect the immune system in various ways, including a decreased antibody-mediated and mitogen-stimulated phagocytosis by monocytes and macrophages, alterations in T-lymphocyte subsets and modification of lymphocyte distribution in different compartments of the immune system, affecting the cellular immune response. In patients with **haemochromatosis** there is an increased risk for several peculiar infectious complications, including sepsis with E. coli, Yersinia spp., Pasteurella spp., L. monocytogenes and Vibrio vulnificus. The most serious complication, however, is fulminant rhinocerebral or pulmonary mucormycosis in patients undergoing desferrioxamine treatment.

Infection is a major cause of morbidity and mortality in **systemic lupus erythematosus** and it is the main cause of death in about one-third of patients. Besides the immunosuppressive treatment with glucocorticosteroids, ciclosporin, cyclophosphamide and others, there is a defect in virtually every component of innate and acquired immune defence, including a CD4$^+$ T-cell lymphopenia, a decreased T-cell response, decreased production of cytokines, such as interleukin-2 and IF-γ, diminished numbers of natural killer cells and impaired cytotoxicity, treatment-induced or autoimmune neutropenia, diminished capacity for phagocytosis and antigen presentation, and dysgammaglobulinaemias. Frequent pathogens cover the entire microbial spectrum and include *S. aureus*, *E. coli*, *P. aeruginosa*, *S. enteritidis*, *S. pneumoniae*, *N. meningitidis*, *L. monocytogenes*, *M. tuberculosis*, varicella-zoster virus, *C. albicans*, *C. neoformans*, *P. carinii*, and *T. gondii*.

Therapeutic principles

- Prophylaxis with trimethoprim–sulfamethoxazole and ganciclovir is the most important measure in the solid-organ transplant recipient. A diagnosis has to be attempted in each patient presenting with a pulmonary complication.

- The approach to the cancer patients with treatment-induced neutropenia is largely empirical. Immediate antibiotic treatment and addition of amphotericin B in cases with characteristic pulmonary infiltrates or persistence of fever for more than 5–7 days is crucial.

- The haematopoietic stem-cell transplant recipient combines both above mentioned approaches; however with respect to ganciclovir a pre-emptive strategy is preferred.

References

1. Bowden RA, Ljungman P, Paya CV, ed. Transplant infections. Philadelphia: Lippincott-Raven; 1998.
2. Pizzo PA. Fever in immunocompromised patients. N Engl J Med 1999; 341: 893–900.
3. Rubin RH, Young LS, ed. Clinical approach to infection in the compromised host, 3rd ed. New York: Plenum; 1994.
4. Shelhamer JH, Pizzo PA, Parrillo JE, Masur H, ed. Respiratory disease in the immunosuppressed host. Philadelphia: JB Lippincott; 1991.
5. Shelhamer JH, Toews GB, Masur H et al. Respiratory disease in the immunosuppressed patient. Ann Intern Med 1992; 117: 415–431.
6. Levine SJ. An approach to the diagnosis of pulmonary infections in immunosuppressed patients. Semin Respir Infect 1990; 7: 81–95.
7. Ettinger NA, Trulock EP. Pulmonary considerations of organ transplantation. Am Rev Respir Dis 1991; 143: 1386–405; 144: 213–23, 433–451.
8. Fishman JA, Rubin RH. Infection in organ-transplant recipients. N Engl J Med 1998; 338: 1741–1751.
9. Patel R, Paya CV. Infections in solid-organ transplant recipients. Clin Microbiol Rev 1997; 10: 86–124.
10. Rubin RH, ed. Infection in transplantation. Infect Dis Clin North Am 1995; 9: 811–1074.
11. Sia IG, Patel R. New strategies for prevention and therapy of cytomegalovirus infection and disease in solid-organ transplant recipients. Clin Microbiol Rev 2000; 13: 83–121.
12. Patel R, Snydman DR, Rubin RH et al. Cytomegalovirus prophylaxis in solid organ transplant recipients. Transplantation 1996; 61: 1279–1289.
13. Van den Berg AP, van der Bij W, van Son WJ et al. Cytomegalovirus antigenemia as a useful marker of symptomatic cytomegalovirus infection after renal transplantation – a report of 130 consecutive patients. Transplantation 1989; 48: 991–995.
14. Stover DE, Zaman MB, Hajdu SI et al. Bronchoalveolar lavage in the diagnosis of diffuse pulmonary infiltrates in the immunocompromised host. Ann Intern Med 1984; 101: 1–7.
15. Grebski E, Russi E, Hess T et al. The role of two segment bronchoalveolar lavage in the diagnosis of pulmonary infection. Chest 1994; 106: 414–420.
16. Schulman LL, Smith CR, Drusin R et al. Utility of airway endoscopy in the diagnosis of respiratory complications of cardiac transplantation. Chest 1988; 93: 960–967.
17. Boehler A, Vogt P, Zollinger A et al. Prospective study of the value of transbronchial lung biopsy after lung transplantation. Eur Respir J 1996; 9: 658–662.
18. Pomerance A, Madden B, Burke MM, Yacoub MH. Transbronchial biopsy in heart and lung transplantation: clinicopathologic correlations. J Heart Lung Transplant 1995; 14: 761–773.
19. Nishio JN, Lynch JP. Fiberoptic bronchoscopy in the immunocompromised host: the significance of a 'nonspecific' transbronchial biopsy. Am Rev Respir Dis 1980; 121: 307–312.
20. Miller R, Burton NA, Karwande SV et al. Early, aggressive open lung biopsy in heart transplant recipients. J Heart Transplant 1987; 6: 96–99.
21. Waltzer WC, Sterioff S, Zincke H et al. Open lung biopsy in the renal transplant recipient. Surgery 1980; 88: 601–610.
22. Primack SL, Muller NL. High-resolution computed tomography in acute diffuse lung disease in the immunocompromised patient. Radiol Clin North Am 1994; 32: 731–744.
23. Ramsey PG, Rubin RH, Tolkoff-Rubin NE et al. The renal transplant patient with fever and pulmonary infiltrates: etiology, clinical manifestations an management. Medicine 1980; 59: 206–222.
24. Hesse UJ, Fryd DS, Chatterjee SN et al. Pulmonary infections: the Minnesota randomized prospective trial of cyclosporine vs azathioprine–antilymphocyte globulin for immunosuppression in renal allograft recipients. Arch Surg 1986; 121: 1056–1060.
25. Jensen WA, Rose RM, Hammer SM et al. Pulmonary complications of orthotopic liver transplantation. Transplantation 1986; 42: 484–490.
26. Singh N, Gayowski T, Wagener MM, Marino IR. Pulmonary infiltrates in liver transplant recipients in the intensive care unit. Transplantation 1999; 67: 1138–1144.
27. Winston DJ, Emmanouilides C, Busuttil RW. Infections in liver transplant recipients. Clin Infect Dis 1995; 21: 1077–1089.
28. Miller LW, Naftel DC, Bourge RC et al. Infection after heart transplantation: a multiinstitutional study. Cardiac Transplant Research Database Group. J Heart Lung Transplant 1994; 13: 381–392.
29. Hildebrand FL Jr, Rosenow EC, Habermann TM, Tazelaar HD. Pulmonary complications of leukemia. Chest 1990; 98: 1233–1239.
30. Pizzo PA. Management of fever in patients with cancer and treatment-induced neutropenia. N Engl J Med 1993; 328: 1323–1332.
31. Klastersky J. Treatment of neutropenic infection: trends towards monotherapy? Support Care Cancer 1997; 5: 365–370.
32. Hughes WT, Armstrong D, Bodey GP et al. 1997 guidelines for the use of antimicrobial agents in neutropenic patients with unexplained fever. Infectious Diseases Society of America. Clin Infect Dis 1997; 25: 551–573.
33. Kern WV, Cometta A, De Bock R et al. Oral versus intravenous empirical antimicrobial therapy for fever in patients with granulocytopenia who are receiving cancer chemotherapy. International Antimicrobial Therapy Cooperative Group of the European Organization for Research and Treatment of Cancer. N Engl J Med 1999; 341: 312–318.
34. Soubani AO, Miller KB, Hassoun PM. Pulmonary complications of bone marrow transplantation. Chest 1996; 109: 1066–1077.
35. Kantrow SP, Hackman RC, Boeckh M et al. Idiopathic pneumonia syndrome: changing spectrum of lung injury after marrow transplantation. Transplantation 1997; 63: 1079–1086.
36. Primary immunodeficiency diseases. Report of an IUIS Scientific Committee. International Union of Immunological Societies. Clin Exp Immunol 1999; 118 (Suppl. 1): 1–28.
37. Conley ME, Notarangelo LD, Etzioni A. Diagnostic criteria for primary immunodeficiencies. Representing PAGID (Pan-American Group for Immunodeficiency) and ESID (European Society for Immunodeficiencies). Clin Immunol 1999; 93: 190–197.
38. Rosen FS, Cooper MD, Wedgwood RJ. The primary immunodeficiencies. N Engl J Med 1995; 333: 431–440.
39. Cunningham-Rundles C, Bodian C. Common variable immunodeficiency: clinical and immunological features of 248 patients. Clin Immunol 1999; 92: 34–48.
40. Smith DK, Neal JJ, Holmberg SD. Unexplained opportunistic infections and CD4$^+$ T-lymphocytopenia without HIV infection. An investigation of cases in the United States. The Centers for Disease Control Idiopathic CD4$^+$ T-lymphocytopenia Task Force. N Engl J Med 1993; 328: 373–379.
41. Lynch JP III, McCune WJ. Immunosuppressive and cytotoxic pharmacotherapy for pulmonary disorders. Am J Respir Crit Care Med 1997; 155: 395–420.
42. Newton R. Molecular mechanisms of glucocorticoid action: what is important? Thorax 2000; 55: 603–613.
43. Stuck AE, Minder CE, Frey FJ. Risk of infectious complications in patients taking glucocorticosteroids. Rev Infect Dis 1989; 6: 954–963.

37 Lung abscess

John Moore-Gillon and Susannah J Eykyn

Key points

- There are many causes of cavitating lesions in the lung, an abscess being just one of them.

- Careful review of thoracic imaging may be necessary to distinguish an intrapulmonary lung abscess from an empyema.

- Most lung abscesses are secondary to aspiration of oropharyngeal secretions.

- It is important to exclude malignancy or other cause of endobronchial obstruction, so bronchoscopy is usually necessary.

- A single microbe is unusual unless abscesses have developed after a bacterial pneumonia. More commonly, there is a mixed growth, including anaerobes.

Table 37.1 Causes of lung abscess

- Aspiration from the oropharynx
- Bronchial obstruction
- Pneumonia
- Blood-borne infection
- Infected pulmonary infarct
- Trauma
- Transdiaphragmatic spread

Table 37.2 Principal differential diagnoses of lung abscess

- Cavitated tumour
- Infected bulla or bronchial cyst
- Localised saccular bronchiectasis
- Aspergilloma
- Wegener's granulomatosis
- Hydatid cyst
- Coal workers' pneumoconiosis
  - Progressive massive fibrosis
  - Caplan's syndrome
- Cavitated rheumatoid nodule
- Gas–fluid level in oesophagus, stomach or bowel

Definition and causes

A lung abscess is a cavitated, infected, necrotic lesion of the lung parenchyma. Some authorities distinguish between multiple small abscesses less than 2 cm in diameter (calling this 'necrotising pneumonia') and larger lesions, which they regard as true lung abscesses.[1,2] Both small and large abscesses are considered here as different manifestations of the same disorder, in some patients merely representing stages in the progression of their illness. Table 37.1 shows the main conditions predisposing to lung abscess and Table 37.2 the principal differential diagnoses.

Aspiration from the oropharynx is the most common cause of lung abscess.[3,4] The factors predisposing to aspiration are shown in Table 37.3; in some individuals more than one factor may be present. Bronchial obstruction may be the result of tumour, usually malignant, or foreign body. Pneumonia may result in lung abscess and *Mycobacterium tuberculosis* is among the most common responsible organisms, although the clinical course of this infection is chronic and distinctive, and the lesions are not usually regarded as lung abscesses. Pneumonias caused by *Staphylococcus aureus* and *Klebsiella* spp. usually cavitate, as may the occasional neglected *Streptococcus pneumoniae* infection. *Pseudomonas aeruginosa* does so less frequently. It must be stressed that almost any bacterial or fungal pneumonia may cavitate, although causative agents other than those listed here are rare. Furthermore, the increasing numbers of individuals with acquired immunodeficiency syndrome (AIDS) has led to the occurrence of cases of lung abscess caused by hitherto virtually unknown opportunistic organisms, such as *Rhodococcus equi*.[5]

Table 37.3 Principal causes of oropharyngeal aspiration

- Impaired consciousness
  - Alcohol
  - Drug abuse
  - Epilepsy
  - Anaesthesia
- Impaired innervation/musculature
  - Pharynx
  - Larynx
  - Oesophagus
- Nasal
  - Sinus disease
- Oral
  - Dental caries, gingival disease
- Pharyngeal
  - Pouch
- Laryngeal
  - Tumour
- Oesophageal
  - Stricture
  - Hiatus hernia
  - Achalasia

Blood-borne infection resulting in lung abscess occurs most commonly with *S. aureus*. Intravenous drug abusers may develop metastatic abscesses in association with tricuspid valve endocarditis. Uncommon, but probably much underdiagnosed in spite of its almost unmistakable clinical features, is necrobacillosis, the disease resulting from *Fusobacterium necrophorum* infection.[6] Typically, young, fit adults develop a severe sore throat followed by a septicaemic illness with lung abscesses, often proceeding to empyema, renal and hepatic dysfunction, and occasionally to osteomyelitis and infection elsewhere.

Non-septic embolism to the lungs may result in a pulmonary infarct which, if secondarily infected, may cavitate to form a lung abscess.

Trauma is uncommon as a cause of lung abscess; penetrating injuries may implant infected material, or a haematoma within the lung parenchyma may become infected via the bronchial tree. Transdiaphragmatic spread can occur with subphrenic or hepatic abscesses. These may be pyogenic, amoebic or infected hydatid cysts. The last of these should be suspected in any patient who has ever lived in an area where hydatid disease is or was endemic.

A malignant tumour should be strongly suspected in all middle-aged and elderly smokers presenting with a cavitated lesion on the chest radiograph. It was suggested 50 years ago that, in patients over 45 years of age ,about one-third of lung abscesses were associated with malignancy, and that figure is likely to be higher now.[7] About two-thirds of cavitated lesions associated with malignancy are the result of liquefaction in the necrotic centre of the tumour, and about one-third are true abscesses distal to bronchial obstruction by the tumour.[7] By the strict definition given above, infected bullae and bronchogenic cysts are not lung abscesses because necrosis is usually not present, but their presentation and clinical management are in many instances

exactly the same as those of a true lung abscess. An air–fluid level in a hiatus hernia, or bowel herniating through the diaphragm, may be mistaken for a lung abscess. Wegener's granulomatosis, hydatid disease, rheumatoid lung and coalworkers' pneumoconiosis may all be associated with necrotic parenchymal lesions showing cavitation. These conditions are discussed in detail elsewhere, as are aspergilloma and saccular bronchiectasis.

Clinical features

The most common abscesses, those resulting from oropharyngeal aspiration, cause general malaise, weight loss and fever, and these features are often present for several weeks before the patient seeks medical advice. When the lung abscess is associated with pneumonia or blood-borne infection, the onset is more abrupt, the duration of illness much shorter and the patient is usually very ill.

Cough, often productive of copious purulent sputum, is common. In abscesses resulting from aspiration the patient will, if specifically questioned, often say that the sputum tastes foul. Chest pain may be present and can be pleuritic in nature or a less precisely located aching sensation. There may be blood-streaking of the sputum or frank haemoptysis, which can be profuse.[8]

The clinical history is important. If an abscess is suspected, an attempt should be made to elicit features that are suggestive of one or more of the predisposing conditions outlined in Tables 37.1 and 37.3. Physical examination is often unhelpful. Finger clubbing is an unreliable guide to malignancy because it may occur within weeks of the development of lung abscess without underlying malignancy. No physical sign in the chest is specific for lung abscess. Dullness to percussion and bronchial breathing may be found over a large abscess, particularly when it is close to the pleural surface. If there is an associated empyema the signs are those of pleural effusion.

Investigations

Radiology

The plain chest radiograph usually raises the possibility of lung abscess (Figs 37.1 & 37.2). Occasionally, a lesion appears solid on the plain film but cavitation is seen on computed tomography (CT). It can be difficult to distinguish a pleural from an intrapulmonary collection of pus, and some abscesses may not be identified on conventional chest radiography at all.[9] If the lateral chest radiograph shows a D-shaped opacity, the posterior chest wall being the vertical part of the D, the lesion is more likely to be an empyema than a lung abscess.[10] CT scanning will almost always enable an experienced thoracic radiologist to distinguish between an empyema and an abscess. Abscesses typically have an irregular wall and, by comparison with empyemas, an indistinct outer margin, have an oval or round rather than a lenticular shape, make an acute rather than an obtuse angle with the chest wall, and show no evidence of compression of adjacent lung.[11] Computed tomography of an apparently single abscess

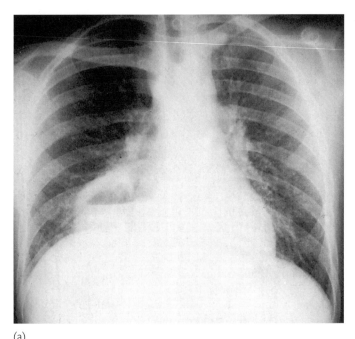

(a)

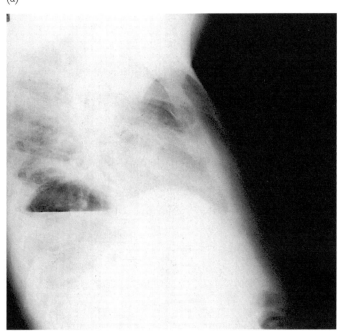

(b)

Fig. 37.1 (a) Posteroanterior and (b) right lateral chest radiographs of a 19-year-old man with an ependymoma of the fourth cerebral ventricle and chronic aspiration of oropharyngeal contents. The pus from the large right lower-lobe abscess grew three different aerobic and six different anaerobic organisms.

may reveal further lesions, and also show adjacent abnormal pleura, which is important when planning percutaneous drainage.[12] What appears to be an abscess may be stomach or bowel herniating through the diaphragm; CT scanning, or appropriate barium studies, will establish the correct diagnosis. The value of magnetic resonance imaging in the investigation of lung abscess is not established.

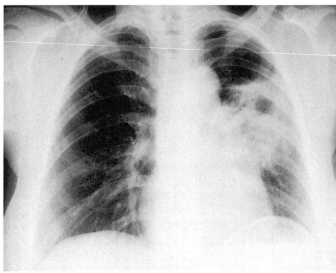

Fig. 37.2 Posteroanterior chest radiograph of a 40-year-old woman with 3 months of cough and malaise. Extensive parenchymal infiltration is seen as well as an abscess cavity. The pus grew *Streptococcus milleri* and seven different anaerobes. No obvious predisposing cause; complete recovery.

Blood

There is usually a neutrophil leukocytosis with a raised erythrocyte sedimentation rate and C-reactive protein. If the abscess is chronic, anaemia may be present. When abscesses occur in association with pneumonia or are secondary to blood-borne infection, the responsible organism can often be isolated from the blood. Serological tests may establish the diagnosis of hydatid and amoebic disease.

Microbiological sampling techniques

The microbiological investigation of the respiratory tract is considered in detail elsewhere and only those aspects directly relevant to lung abscess will be dealt with here. Investigation is often bedevilled by the lack of a suitable specimen. If the patient is coughing copious sputum and the specimen reaches the laboratory promptly then reliable results are likely but in such cases it is essential that the laboratory staff are specifically requested to set up anaerobic cultures, as these are not routinely done on expectorated sputum. Invasive techniques for collection of specimens reduce the likelihood of contamination by upper respiratory tract flora. Such techniques include bronchoscopy and occasionally transtracheal aspiration.[13] Bacteriologically, the most satisfactory specimen is that obtained by percutaneous transthoracic aspiration performed under radiological screening,[14,15] ultrasonography[16] or CT control.

Bronchoscopy

The role of bronchoscopy in the investigation of a lung abscess is to obtain microbiological specimens and to help exclude tumour, foreign bodies and other differential diagnoses.[17] Most patients with a lung abscess should undergo bronchoscopy except those with multiple blood-borne abscesses of known bacterial aetiology. The use of bronchoscopy in the treatment of lung abscess is considered later.

Microbiology

In the preantibiotic era, lung abscess was seen more frequently than today and cultures of specimens obtained at surgery or post-mortem examination provided ample opportunity to study its microbiology. These studies established the important role of anaerobic bacteria in lung abscess, although their taxonomy and laboratory techniques for their isolation were often inadequate by today's standards so these early data are of limited value. Invasive sampling techniques and a renewed interest in anaerobes have enabled a more accurate assessment of the microbiology of lung abscess.

The smell of the specimen will often provide an immediate clue to the microbial aetiology. Pus from both aerobic and anaerobic infections may look foul, but only anaerobic pus smells foul. Specimens should be cultured both aerobically and anaerobically, and the latter plates should be incubated for at least 5 days to allow the more fastidious anaerobes to grow, particularly when presumptive fusobacteria have been detected on a Gram-stained smear. Limited speciation of anaerobes (to genus level) should be possible in a routine laboratory.

The microbiology of lung abscess reflects the mechanism by which the abscess has arisen. Organisms associated with pneumonias have been outlined earlier. More common are those resulting from aspiration of oropharyngeal contents and in these cases anaerobes are the predominant pathogens. Two major studies that used invasive sampling methods reported anaerobes in two-thirds or more of lung abscesses, usually in mixed culture with aerobes.[18–20] Several anaerobes are usually isolated concomitantly from a lung abscess but their differentiation is likely to tax the resources of a non-specialist laboratory and is of no clinical importance. All isolates should be tested for their susceptibility to antibiotics so that an appropriate regimen can be devised. The commonest anaerobes in lung abscesses are *Prevotella* spp., *Porphyromonas* spp. and the anaerobic Gram-positive cocci. *Bacteroides fragilis* was formerly thought to be common, but may have been misidentified. When a single anaerobe is isolated it is usually a fusobacterium.

Aspiration is also the mechanism by which aerobic organisms such as the *milleri* group of streptococci, *S. pneumoniae* and *Haemophilus influenzae* reach the lung. Of these, the milleri group is probably the most common microbe, aerobic or anaerobic, found in lung abscess.[21,22] A range of other aerobes may also be found, including coliforms and pseudomonads. In contrast to anaerobes, when aerobes alone are isolated from a lung abscess a single species is the norm. *S. aureus* is seldom acquired by aspiration but is classically described as occurring with concomitant influenza infection. In practice, staphylococcal lung abscesses are very rare even during influenza epidemics.

Abscesses occurring as a result of blood-borne spread of infection are characteristically multiple and contain whatever microbe was in the blood. In addition to those mentioned earlier, less common organisms include gastrointestinal aerobes, such as *Escherichia coli*, and gut-specific anaerobes. Bacteria isolated from lung abscesses that arise in conjunction with bronchial tumours or other lung pathology are similar to those isolated from abscesses occurring in previously normal lung.

Treatment

Lung abscess is uncommon and few doctors gain extensive experience in its management. Antibiotics alone will not produce a satisfactory outcome unless the pus can drain from the abscess cavity. In most patients, spontaneous drainage occurs via the bronchial tree, with the production of copious purulent sputum. This may be helped greatly by postural drainage.

Antibiotics

The initial choice of antibiotics is usually made in the absence of definitive bacteriology, but a reasoned guess can be made on the basis of the underlying clinical features and on the smell of the pus and its appearance on Gram staining. As most lung abscesses contain milleri group streptococci and anaerobes, an antibiotic or combination of antibiotics active against these organisms should be selected. There are many possible initial regimens; penicillins including co-amoxiclav, cephalosporins, macrolides, chloramphenicol and clindamycin have all been used. The use of ampicillin or amoxicillin alone should be avoided because some anaerobes are resistant. In spite of the frequency of β-lactamase-producing organisms in lung abscess, in practice the combination of amoxicillin and metronidazole works well and has fewer side effects than some of the other drugs. It can be given orally, unless the patient is very ill or unable to swallow, while awaiting definitive culture results. A macrolide such as erythromycin, clarithromycin or azithromycin should be substituted for amoxicillin in patients with a history of hypersensitivity to penicillin.

The decision to change the initial antibiotics when culture results become available is primarily a clinical one. If the patient is clearly doing well then no change is necessary, but if not then laboratory reports on sensitivities may be of value in selecting a different regimen. Although lung abscesses are often treated with antibiotics for about 6 weeks, there is no clinical trial evidence to support this and shorter periods may be sufficient in those patients where the pus has drained adequately via the bronchial tree, with cessation of sputum production and disappearance of the air–fluid level on the chest radiograph. Antibiotics need not be continued until complete radiological clearing of parenchymal shadowing, which may take many weeks (see below).

Drainage

Some patients fail to respond to antibiotics and physiotherapy, and further measures must then be considered. The timing of such intervention depends upon the patient. It may occasionally be needed within days in a critically ill individual in whom there is no spontaneous drainage via the bronchial tree. In less sick individuals, fever continuing for longer than 2 weeks in spite of appropriate antibiotics and physiotherapy suggests that spontaneous drainage is inadequate and measures to improve it should be considered.

The abscess may be approached either via the bronchial tree or percutaneously. In the former technique the abscess cavity is entered directly by the fibreoptic bronchoscope or by a catheter passed through it, which may be left in place[10,23] The narrow suction channel of the fibreoptic bronchoscope is not able to aspirate large volumes of pus rapidly, which may thus spill into normal lung and critically impair gas exchange. Accordingly, endobronchial drainage is potentially hazardous if carried out via a fibreoptic bronchoscope in a conscious patient; general anaesthesia with an endotracheal tube or rigid bronchoscope in place may reduce the risk.

The percutaneous approach is preferred.[24,25] The exception is with abscesses associated with malignancy when there is an increased risk of a permanent fistula; in such cases endobronchial drainage should be considered. Percutaneous drainage is usually unhelpful with multiple small abscesses, and in these individuals there may also be a higher risk of complications such as pneumothorax and bronchopleural fistula.[2]

In the past, fluoroscopic screening has been the conventional technique for catheter placement[26] but ultrasonography allows more precise spatial localisation, is free of radiation hazard and – like fluoroscopy but unlike CT at present – gives real-time images.[27] CT is widely used.[25] It does have the advantage of better visualisation of other intrathoracic structures, and many operators have extensive experience of CT-guided biopsy of other intrathoracic lesions, which may be of value on the relatively infrequent occasions when a lung abscess is encountered. Furthermore, real-time 'CT fluoroscopy' is within the capabilities of the new-generation scanners now in development.[28]

Surgical resection

By comparison with the preantibiotic era, surgical resection of abscesses is now seldom required, but it may still be necessary if there is severe haemoptysis or the abscess is associated with malignancy. In the latter case, resection should only be attempted if the tumour itself is operable by the usual criteria, with no evidence of metastatic tumour spread, mediastinal involvement, inadequate lung function or other coexisting serious medical conditions. To these two major indications for resection may be added 'chronic abscess with persisting symptoms', particularly when other attempts to drain the abscess have failed. Chronicity may be defined temporally or pathologically, chronic abscesses being associated with granulation tissue and subsequently with fibrous tissue.[18] The temporal definition is a matter for debate, but an abscess that is still producing systemic symptoms (other than sputum production) 6 weeks after presentation, in spite of attempted endobronchial or percutaneous drainage, should be considered for surgical resection.

Progress, complications and sequelae

Successful treatment of a lung abscess is indicated first by the resolution of fever, second (and much more slowly) by closure of the cavity, and finally by radiological clearing of parenchymal infiltration.[18,19]

Fever usually disappears within days; persistence beyond 2 weeks is unusual and suggests inadequate drainage. About 50% of cavities will close in a month and the remainder within the subsequent 4–8 weeks. A falling C-reactive protein, and a patient who is feeling better and gaining weight are encouraging signs at all stages of the management of a lung abscess. Radiological infiltration may persist for 3 months or more and should not give rise to concern provided the patient's progress is otherwise good and the possibility of malignancy has been thoroughly investigated.

Complications and long-term sequelae are now seen less frequently than in the preantibiotic era but lung abscess is still associated with significant morbidity and mortality.[29,30] The commonest complication of a lung abscess is the development of an empyema; indeed, the patient may not present to the doctor until this has already occurred.[18] As the abscess enlarges, it may erode blood vessels and give rise to haemoptysis. Rarely, but particularly in immunosuppressed patients, there may be rapid spread of necrosis through the lung.

An abscess that has drained and been sterilised with the use of antibiotics may form a persistent cavity. Initially lined by granulation tissue, this is replaced by fibrous tissue and subsequently squamous or ciliated epithelium. Such a cavity may become reinfected or colonised by *Aspergillus* spp. When the original abscess formed in relation to a bronchus, rather than to the smaller airways, destruction of the bronchial wall followed by epithelialisation may give rise to local saccular bronchiectasis. Spread of infection into pulmonary veins can result in embolic cerebral abscess, but this complication is now very rare.

Therapeutic principles

- Drainage via the bronchial tree usually occurs, and a skilled respiratory therapist can help this process.
- If the abscess is large, or spontaneous drainage does not occur, percutaneous needle drainage or catheter placement may be necessary.
- The initial antibiotic regimen should include anaerobic cover where oropharyngeal aspiration is suspected as an underlying cause.
- A change in antibiotic regimen when culture results are available is unnecessary if clinical progress is good.
- Antibiotics need not be continued until complete radiological clearing of parenchymal shadowing.

References

1. Bartlett JG, Finegold SM. Anaerobic infections of the lung and pleural space. Am Rev Respir Dis 1974; 110: 56–77.
2. Hoffer FA, Bloom DA, Collin AA, Fishman SJ. Lung abscess versus necrotizing pneumonia: implications for interventional therapy. Pediatr Radiol 1999; 29: 87–91.

3. Perlman LV, Lerner E, D'Esopo N. Clinical classification and analysis of 97 cases of lung abscess. Am Rev Respir Dis 1969; 99: 390–398.
4. Bartlett JG. Anaerobic bacterial infections of the lung and pleural space. Clin Infect Dis 1993; 16 (Suppl. 4): S248–S255.
5. Shapiro JM, Romney BM, Weiden MD et al. *Rhodococcus equi* endobronchial mass with lung abscess in a patient with AIDS. Thorax 1992; 47: 62–63.
6. Moore-Gillon JC, Eykyn SJ, Phillips I. Necrobacillosis – a forgotten disease. Br Med J 1984; 288: 1526–1527.
7. Brock RC. Lung abscess. Oxford: Blackwell Scientific; 1952.
8. Philpott NJ, Woodhead MA, Wilson AG, Millard FJ. Lung abscess: a neglected cause of life threatening haemoptysis. Thorax 1993; 48: 674–675.
9. Groskin SA, Panicek DM, Ewing DK et al. Bacterial lung abscess: a review of the radiographic and clinical features of 50 cases. J Thorac Imaging 1991; 6: 62–67.
10. Le Roux BT, Mohlala ML, Odell JA, Whitton ID. Suppurative diseases of the lung and pleural space. Part 1: Empyema thoracis and lung abscess. Curr Probl Surg 1986; 23: 1–89.
11. Armstrong P, Dee P. Infections of the lungs and pleura. In: Armstrong P, Wilson AG, Dee P, ed. Imaging of diseases of the chest. Chicago: Year Book; 1990: 242–248.
12. Van Sonnenberg E, D'Agostino HB, Casola G et al. Lung abscess: CT-guided drainage. Radiology 1991; 178: 347–351.
13. Henriquez AH, Mendoza J, Gonzalez PC. Quantitative culture of bronchoalveolar lavage from patients with anaerobic lung abscesses. J Infect Dis 1991; 164: 414–417.
14. Irwin RS, Garrity FL, Erickson AD et al. Sampling lower respiratory tract secretions in primary lung abscess: a comparison of the accuracy of four methods. Chest 1981; 79: 559–565.
15. Pena Grinan N, Munoz Lucena F, Vargas Romero J et al. Yield of percutaneous needle lung aspiration in lung abscess. Chest 1990; 97: 69–74.
16. Yang PC, Luh KT, Lee VC et al. Lung abscesses: ultrasound examination and ultrasound-guided transthoracic aspiration. Radiology 1991; 180: 171–175.
17. Sosenko A, Glassroth J. Fiberoptic bronchoscopy in the evaluation of lung abscess. Chest 1985; 87: 489–494.
18. Neild JE, Eykyn SJ, Phillips I. Lung abscess and empyema. Q J Med 1985; NS 57: 875–882.
19. Bartlett JG, Gorbach SL, Tally FP, Finegold SM. Bacteriology and treatment of primary lung abscess. Am Rev Respir Dis 1974; 109: 510–518.
20. Hammond JM, Potgieter PD, Hanslo D et al. The etiology and antimicrobial susceptibility patterns or microorganisms in acute community acquired lung abscess. Chest 1995; 108: 937–941.
21. Shinzato T, Saito A. The *Streptococcus milleri* group as a cause of pulmonary infection. Clin Infect Dis 1995; 21(Suppl. 3): S238–S243.
22. Wong CA, Donald F, Macfarlane JT. *Streptococcus milleri* pulmonary disease: a review and clinical description of 25 patients. Thorax 1995; 50: 1093–1096.
23. Schmitt GS, Ohar JM, Kanter KR, Naunheim KS. Indwelling transbronchial catheter drainage of pulmonary abscess. Ann Thorac Surg 1988; 45: 43–47.
24. Klein JS, Schultz S, Heffner JE. Interventional radiology of the chest: image-guided percutaneous drainage of pleural effusions, lung abscess, and pneumothorax. AJR 1995; 164: 581–588.
25. Erasmus JJ, McAdams HP, Rossi S, Kelley MJ. Percutaneous management of intrapulmonary air and fluid collections. Radiol Clin North Am 2000; 38: 385–393.
26. Parker LA, Melton JW, Delany DJ, Yankasas BC. Percutaneous small bore catheter drainage in the management of lung abscess. Chest 1987; 92: 213–218.
27. Yang PC. Ultrasound-guided transthoracic biopsy of peripheral lung, pleural and chest-wall lesions. J Thorac Imaging 1997; 12: 272–284.
28. White CS, Meyer CA, Templeton PA. CT fluoroscopy for thoracic interventional procedures. Radiol Clin North Am 2000; 38: 303–322.
29. Hirsberg B, Sklair-Levi M, Nir-Paz R et al. Factors predicting mortality of patients with lung abscess. Chest 1999; 115: 746–750.
30. Mwandumba HC, Beeching NJ. Pyogenic lung infections: factors for predicting clinical outcome of lung abscess and thoracic empyema. Curr Opin Pulm Med 2000; 6: 234–239.

38.1 Epidemiology of tuberculosis

Hans L Rieder

Key points

- Exposure to *M. tuberculosis* remains the most important factor determining the continued prevalence of tuberculosis

- Incidence and prevalence of subclinical infection determine the dynamics of the tuberculosis epidemic in a community

- The risk factors of greatest public health importance for tuberculosis include recently acquired tuberculous infection, co-infection with HIV and the presence of fibrotic lung parenchymal lesions resulting from previous spontaneously healed tuberculosis

- The most important risk factor for death from tuberculosis in low-incidence countries is failure to include it in the differential diagnosis of persons ill with compatible signs and/or symptoms

A workable model of the epidemiology of tuberculosis needs to be as simple as possible, yet it has to be sufficiently complex to capture all the elements needed for understanding the dynamics of tuberculosis in a community. Such a model as proposed here follows the pathogenesis of tuberculosis.[1] It distinguishes four major components: exposure to *Mycobacterium tuberculosis*; subclinical, latent infection with *M. tuberculosis*; clinically manifest tuberculosis; and death from tuberculosis. Epidemiologically, each of these four distinct stages can be analysed aetiologically, descriptively, and predictively.

Aetiological epidemiology identifies risk factors that promote progression from one step to the next; descriptive epidemiology aims at determining the magnitude of the problem; and predictive epidemiology attempts to make projections on the future course based on available, historically collected data.[2]

The perspective adopted here is from a public health point of view, i.e. it addresses the epidemiology of tuberculosis in relation to the priorities for control[3] and elimination[4] of tuberculosis.

Exposure to *Mycobacterium tuberculosis*

Exposure to *M. tuberculosis* complex is defined here as occurring if a susceptible person is in relevant contact with a case of tuberculosis. Because *M. tuberculosis* is the most frequent and important transmissible agent for tuberculosis among the various species of the genus *Mycobacterium* and the subspecies within the *M. tuberculosis* complex, the discussion here is limited to airborne exposure to, infection with, disease and death from *M. tuberculosis*. Hence, in this context, relevant exposure might be defined as exposure to air that contains a sufficient number of viable *M. tuberculosis* bacilli to make subsequent inhalation of one or more infectious particles a distinct, measurable probability. As there is no tool to measure exposure to *M. tuberculosis*, it is not possible to make inferences about the risk for individuals of becoming exposed during a specified period of time. Nevertheless, as no tuberculous infection can be acquired without exposure, concepts related to its aetiological role are useful and important to consider.

Aetiological epidemiology

Obviously, without incident cases of tuberculosis capable of transmitting tubercle bacilli, no relevant exposure will occur. Yet, given a fixed incidence of infectious tuberculosis, exposure risk might still vary greatly in different situations, as two major modifiers are important. The first modifier of exposure risk is the duration of infectiousness of a potential source case. Depending on the rapidity with which transmissible tuberculosis is identified and rendered permanently non-transmissible through adequate chemotherapy, the number of persons that can become exposed will vary. Second, the number of possible contacts between a source of transmission and susceptible individuals per unit of time will also differ depending on the setting. It is apparent that, for example, the number of persons exposed to a given incident case per unit of time is likely to be much higher in crowded urban, compared to sparsely populated rural settings. The age at which incident cases of tuberculosis tend to occur will also influence the age group that has the highest risk of exposure. This is because intragenerational contacts frequently predominate over intergenerational contacts, although there are exceptions, as in child-raising age groups.[5] Another important factor influencing the frequency and type of social interactions, and thus exposure risk, is gender. All these factors are crucial in determining the risk of becoming exposed, and thus the risk of becoming infected with *M. tuberculosis*.

Infection with *M. tuberculosis*

Infection is defined in the epidemiological context as the sub-clinical, latent infection with viable *M. tuberculosis* that is the prerequisite for clinical tuberculosis. Epidemiological control strategies in tuberculosis thus aim at reducing the incidence of tuberculous infection (through case-finding and chemotherapy) or, in certain settings, embarking on an elimination strategy, to reduce the prevalence of tuberculous infection in a community (through preventive therapy programmes targeting groups at particularly high risk of progression to tuberculosis).

Aetiological epidemiology

Factors determining the risk of becoming infected with *M. tuberculosis* are overwhelmingly (but not solely) exogenous in nature. In simple terms, the risk for an individual of becoming infected depends on the density of tubercle bacilli in the ambient air and the length of time for which this person is exposed to that air. The density of tubercle bacilli in the air is determined by the characteristics of the source case and the volume of air into which bacilli are expelled. To be transmissible, tubercle bacilli must be contained in particles of a size that allows them to remain suspended in the air.[6] Thus, the source case must be capable of producing droplets that can evaporate to the size of droplet nuclei sufficiently small to be carried by the air currents and capable of reaching an alveolus of a susceptible person. Patients with respiratory tuberculosis have the ability to produce such infectious droplets, which evaporate to infectious droplet nuclei of the relevant size. If, in addition to the natural production of droplets during speaking, such

patients also cough, a highly efficient mechanism of aerosolising tubercle bacilli results.[7,8] Not all forms of respiratory tuberculosis have equal potential to generate droplets containing tubercle bacilli. The most important (because of its high frequency) is tuberculosis of the lung parenchyma and, in particular, cavitary disease, as the number of bacilli in cavity linings is particularly large.[9] Microscopic sputum smear examination is not a very sensitive method for diagnosis of pulmonary tuberculosis, because large numbers of bacilli must be present for them to be detectable.[10] However, it has long been shown that direct microscopy identifies the most efficient transmitters with a high sensitivity.[11-13] In a study carried out in British Columbia and Saskatchewan, sputum smear microscopy identified only 58% of culture-confirmed cases of pulmonary tuberculosis, but they were the sources of 92% of the infections in childhood contacts.[12] Thus, this very old technique[14] retains its value for tuberculosis control. Nevertheless, it is well recognised that culture-positive-only cases are able to transmit tubercle bacilli as well,[12,15] although to a much lesser extent than patients found to have tubercle bacilli on direct examination of sputum.

Descriptive epidemiology

It is estimated that approximately one-third of the world population is infected with *M. tuberculosis*.[16] However, the distribution of infection varies greatly in different populations,[2] by age, sex and other factors. The observed differences in age are due to differences in the population pyramids and the secular trends in the risk of successive birth cohorts becoming infected with tubercle bacilli. The highest ever recorded risks of becoming infected with *M. tuberculosis* were in Alaska in the middle[17] and in Europe at the beginning of the 20th century.[18] An example of secular trends in the annual risk of becoming infected with tubercle bacilli is shown in Figure 38.1.1.[18-20] The examples are somewhat arbitrarily chosen from four different areas of the world with reasonably high-quality data to demonstrate the key issue.

The Netherlands is an exemplar of the situation most probably prevailing in much of the industrialised world. The annual risk of tuberculous infection was probably as large as 10% in the

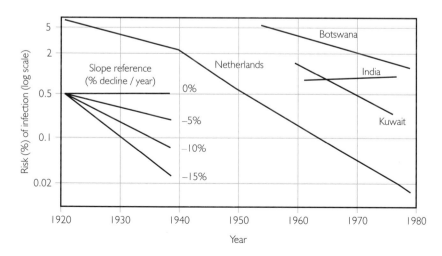

Fig. 38.1.1 Change in the annual risk of infection with *M. tuberculosis* over time in four selected countries. Data from Styblo,[18] Styblo et al[19] and Cauthen et al.[20]

early 20th century and declined before the introduction of any medical intervention by about 5% annually. With the pasteurisation of milk, progress in eradication of bovine tuberculosis and chemotherapy, the decline accelerated to more than 10% annually.[18] The annual risk of tuberculous infection is now as low as 10 per 100 000 population per year in much of western Europe.

Kuwait represents the progress that is being made in most of the eastern Mediterranean region, with a decline of about 5–10% annually, but progress is about 15 years behind that observed in the Netherlands. Because of the slower decline in the former, this gap is likely to be widening further.

Botswana is an example from sub-Saharan Africa showing that, before the HIV epidemic, some progress was being made, but the average annual decline was less than 5%.

India represents a situation that is thought to be prevailing in many high-burden countries:[21] the level of risk of infection is not very high but no decline, or even an increase, in the risk of infection can be observed.

Predictive epidemiology

These observations have profound implications for the future dynamics of tuberculosis. Analogous to compound interest, the slope (interest on interest in banking terms) is of much greater importance than the intercept (the absolute level of infection risk, or initial capital in banking terms). In western Europe, the oldest generation is likely to have a prevalence of tuberculous infection that exceeds 90%. First, they were born at a time when the annual risk of infection was large and second, they had a cumulatively long period of probability of becoming infected[2]. However, each successive cohort passing away is being replaced by cohorts with less and less infection. As a result, young adults (and children even more so) are virtually free of tuberculous infection. This has a bearing on the impact HIV is likely to have on the emergence of tuberculosis in these populations. In contrast, countries like those in sub-Saharan Africa or the Indian subcontinent with large young populations and a barely declining risk of infection have cohorts of young adults of whom half may be infected with *M. tuberculosis*.

Tuberculous infection is also unevenly distributed within societies. Men tend to have a higher prevalence of tuberculous infection than women,[22,23] urban populations a higher prevalence than rural populations,[24,25] and the poor a higher prevalence than the more affluent.[26,27] All these factors will greatly influence the future occurrence of tuberculosis.

Tuberculosis

A frequently cited figure is the estimate that the lifetime risk of tuberculosis following infection in childhood might approximate 10%[28] if no other risk factors that promote progression from latent infection to clinically overt disease supervene. However, numerous such risk factors have been identified,[2] some of which are important from a public health point of view because they are highly prevalent while others are mere medical curiosities, important for the individual concerned yet of minor significance for the global situation.

Aetiological epidemiology

Perhaps the most important risk factor is the recent acquisition of infection with *M. tuberculosis*. An individual who has acquired infection within the past year has an approximately 10-fold increased risk of progression to tuberculosis compared with a person infected more than 7 years previously.[2] This is an important factor because a large proportion of patients with infectious tuberculosis are discovered only after considerable delay, both in industrialised[29,30] and low-income countries,[31,32] so that they are likely to have infected one or more other individuals before transmissibility is curtailed.

The strongest risk factor yet identified for clinical tuberculosis among persons with tuberculous infection is HIV infection.[33] HIV infection may impact on the tuberculosis situation in three ways.[34] In populations with a high prevalence of tuberculous infection, the most frequent sequence is probably the situation where tuberculous infection occurs first, with HIV infection superimposed. The annual risk of progression to clinical disease in this situation is estimated to be around 5–10%.[33,35] The second mechanism is the inverse sequence of these events. The magnitude of the risk in this situation has not been quantified precisely, but it is likely to be considerable if no functioning immune mechanism remains to contain unrestrained multiplication of tubercle bacilli. The consequent great potential for tuberculosis morbidity has been shown, anecdotally at least, in nosocomial outbreaks among HIV-infected patients.[36] Finally, to these two direct effects is added the indirect effect, in that transmission of *M. tuberculosis* to the general population may increase as a result of excess source cases resulting from either of the two direct effects. This theoretical potential is becoming tangibly measurable and is apparently emerging in some countries of sub-Saharan Africa.[37]

In Europe, with a large elderly population many of whom were born long before the introduction of effective chemotherapy, the prevalence of persons with fibrotic residual disease resulting from spontaneously healed tuberculosis might be considerable. Patients with such fibrotic lesions are at high risk of developing tuberculosis again, a risk estimated to be some 0.3% per year.[38]

Numerous other risk factors have been identified; among the more important ones are diabetes,[39] silicosis,[40] low body weight[41] and possibly smoking.[42,43] Other factors, such as jejunoileal bypass, gastrectomy, certain rare types of malignancy and others, are of importance to the individual but have little bearing on the overall epidemiological situation.[2]

Descriptive epidemiology

The global magnitude of tuberculosis is difficult to estimate because of the inconsistency and lack of quality in notification data, globally but also even in Europe.[44] A working group of the World Health Organization has estimated that approximately 8 million cases of tuberculosis emerge each year and that 80% of these are found in just 22 countries[16]. In Europe, the Russian Federation is among these countries.

Of most concern is the impact that HIV infection has exerted on the global tuberculosis situation. As might be expected from estimates of the underlying prevalence of tuberculous infection in the age groups most susceptible to HIV infection, the impact in Europe thus far has been remarkably small. In contrast, it has been huge in many parts of sub-Saharan Africa, with exponential increases in some countries, and intermediate to nil in many other parts of the world, depending on the extent of the HIV epidemic.[2]

Predictive epidemiology

The prospects for the global tuberculosis epidemic are excellent for most industrialised countries but grim for many of the poorest countries in the world, particularly those where HIV infection is rampant or in which the relatively inexpensive first-line drugs have become ineffective, largely because of poor management.[45]

One of the most fruitful insights in epidemiological thinking about tuberculosis has been the observation by the Norwegian physician Andvord.[46] He recognised that the usual cross-sectional approach to the analysis of tuberculosis mortality data (equally applicable to morbidity data) was insufficient to convey the entire picture of the dynamics of tuberculosis in a community. Cross-sectional data are presented as, for example, age-specific morbidity rates reported during a specified calendar year. In contrast, the cohort-contour approach proposed by Andvord analyses the age-specific morbidity rates within each birth cohort. Cohort- and age-specific rates can be derived from cross-sectional data if two conditions are met. Regular cross-sectional data need to be available, e.g. every decade, and these data need to be detailed enough for age-specific data, e.g. 10-year age groups, to be matched with birth cohort years.

Härö has used the extensive data from Finland to construct the experience of tuberculosis morbidity in birth cohorts from available cross-sectional data in order to extrapolate from these the expected tuberculosis morbidity rates for future years. From these projections he was able to reconstruct expected cross-sectional age-specific morbidity rates for the years 2000 and 2010 (Fig. 38.1.2).[47] While observations of notification data will be required to prove the validity of this model, the data are judged to be sufficiently valid to demonstrate that tuberculosis

is likely to move towards self-elimination in Finland. This scenario is most probably generalisable to the indigenous population of most of Europe.

Death from tuberculosis

Aetiological epidemiology

Case fatality from tuberculosis is determined by the site and form of disease and the timeliness of intervention. If left untreated, tuberculous meningitis is the most fatal form of tuberculosis but, in terms of public health importance, pulmonary tuberculosis is the leading manifestation. Individuals with untreated sputum-smear-positive tuberculosis had a cumulative 10-year fatality of about 80% in the prechemotherapy era in Europe.[48-50] Case fatality from sputum-smear-negative tuberculosis is comparatively of much less significance.[51] Chemotherapy has fundamentally changed the outcome of tuberculosis, yet as tuberculosis has become increasingly uncommon in most European countries, unrecognised tuberculosis leading to death is occurring with disturbing frequency.[52]

Descriptive epidemiology

Accurate estimation of global tuberculosis mortality is even more demanding than estimating disease incidence. It had been estimated that as many as one quarter of all avoidable deaths among adults are attributable to tuberculosis.[53] Yet, these estimates were most probably exaggerated. A more recent estimate by the World Health Organization working group arrived at a probably more realistic estimated toll of about 1.9 million deaths per year.[16]

Predictive epidemiology

Tuberculosis deaths are declining in the industrialised world, with tuberculosis becoming increasingly uncommon and with the availability of medication that is capable of curing virtually every patient. Perhaps the most relevant remaining problem is the failure to include tuberculosis in the differential diagnosis as

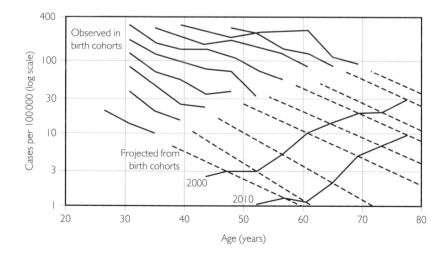

Fig. 38.1.2 Projection of tuberculosis morbidity in Finland. Data from Härö,[47] reproduced with the permission of the International Union Against Tuberculosis and Lung Disease from Rieder.[2]

other infectious diseases and medical conditions presenting with similar signs and symptoms become relatively more frequent. The prospects for the global toll that tuberculosis takes are much more gloomy, with population growth, rising case numbers and the continued failure to achieve global effective action to address this inherently curable, and to a large extent preventable, condition. This inaction implies that, even 50 years after the introduction of effective and cost-effective therapeutic agents, this controllable disease is permitted to continue its drain on humanity, as it has done for centuries before.

> **? Unresolved questions**
>
> ■ The extent to which the global tuberculosis epidemic will remain out of control in countries where the incidence of HIV infection continues unabated
>
> ■ The extent to which global tuberculosis control will be successful in areas where first-line antituberculosis medications have become ineffective

References

1. Rieder HL. Opportunity for exposure and risk of infection: the fuel for the tuberculosis pandemic (editorial). Infection 1995; 23: 1–4.
2. Rieder HL. Epidemiologic basis of tuberculosis control. Edition 1. Paris: International Union Against Tuberculosis and Lung Disease; 1999.
3. Enarson DA, Rieder HL, Arnadottir T, Trébucq A. Tuberculosis guide for low income countries , 4th ed. Paris: International Union Against Tuberculosis and Lung Disease; 1996.
4. Clancy L, Rieder HL, Enarson DA, Spinaci S. Tuberculosis elimination in the countries of Europe and other industrialized countries. Based on a workshop held at Wolfheze, Netherlands, 4–9 March 1990, under the joint auspices of the IUATLD (Europe region) and WHO. Eur Respir J 1991; 4: 1288–1295.
5. Rieder HL. Socialization patterns are key to transmission dynamics of tuberculosis (editorial). Int J Tuberc Lung Dis 1999; 3: 177–178.
6. Wells WF. On air-borne infection. Study II. Droplets and droplet nuclei. Am J Hyg 1934; 20: 611–618.
7. Loudon RG, Roberts RM. Droplet expulsion from the respiratory tract. Am Rev Respir Dis 1966; 95: 435–442.
8. Loudon RG, Spohn SK. Cough frequency and infectivity in patients with pulmonary tuberculosis. Am Rev Respir Dis 1969; 99: 109–111.
9. Canetti G. The J. Burns Amberson lecture. Present aspects of bacterial resistance in tuberculosis. Am Rev Respir Dis 1965; 92: 687–703.
10. European Society for Mycobacteriology. Manual of diagnostic and public health mycobacteriology. Edition 2. London: Bureau of Hygiene and Tropical Medicine; 1991.
11. Shaw JB, Wynn-Williams N. Infectivity of pulmonary tuberculosis in relation to sputum status. Am Rev Tuberc 1954; 69: 724–732.
12. Grzybowski S, Barnett GD, Styblo K. Contacts of cases of active pulmonary tuberculosis. Bull Int Union Tuberc 1975; 50: 90–106.
13. Van Geuns HA, Meijer J, Styblo K. Results of contact examination in Rotterdam, 1967–1969. Bull Int Union Tuberc 1975; 50: 107–121.
14. Bishop PJ, Neumann G. The history of the Ziehl–Neelsen stain. Tubercle 1970; 51: 196–206.
15. Behr MA, Warren SA, Salamon H et al. Transmission of *Mycobacterium tuberculosis* from patients smear-negative for acid-fast bacilli. Lancet 1999; 353: 444–449.
16. Dye C, Scheele S, Dolin P et al. Global burden of tuberculosis. Estimated incidence, prevalence, and mortality by country. JAMA 1999; 282: 677–686.
17. Comstock GW, Philip RN. Decline of the tuberculosis epidemic in Alaska. Publ Health Rep 1961; 76: 19–24.
18. Styblo K. Epidemiology of tuberculosis, 2nd ed. The Hague: Royal Netherlands Tuberculosis Association; 1991.
19. Styblo K, Meijer J, Sutherland I. The transmission of tubercle bacilli – its trend in a human population. Tuberculosis Surveillance Research Unit report no. 1. Bull Int Union Tuberc 1969; 42: 1–104.
20. Cauthen GM, Pio A, ten Dam HG. Annual risk of infection. World Health Organization Document; WHO/TB/88.154: 1–34. Geneva: WHO; 1988.
21. Kochi A. The global tuberculosis situation and the new control strategy of the World Health Organization (leading article). Tubercle 1991; 72: 1–6.
22. Groth-Petersen E, Knudsen J, Wilbek E. Epidemiological basis of tuberculosis eradication in an advanced country. Bull World Health Organ 1959; 21: 5–49.
23. National Tuberculosis Institute Bangalore. Tuberculosis in a rural population of South India: a five-year epidemiological study. Bull World Health Organ 1974; 51: 473–488.
24. Ministry of Health and Social Affairs, Korean Institute of Tuberculosis, Korean National Tuberculosis Association. Report on the 3rd tuberculosis prevalence survey in Korea – 1975. Seoul: Korean Institute of Tuberculosis, 1976.
25. Roelsgaard E, Iversen E, Bløcher C. Tuberculosis in tropical Africa. An epidemiological study. Bull World Health Organ 1964; 30: 459–518.
26. D'Arcy Hart P. The value of tuberculin tests in man, with special reference to the intracutaneous test. Med Res Council Special Series 1932; 164: 5–132.
27. Kuemmerer JM, Comstock GW. Sociologic concomitants of tuberculin sensitivity. Am Rev Respir Dis 1967; 96: 885–892.
28. Comstock GW, Livesay VT, Woolpert SF. The prognosis of a positive tuberculin reaction in childhood and adolescence. Am J Epidemiol 1974; 99: 131–138.
29. Rao VK, Iademarci EP, Fraser VJ, Kollef MH. Delays in the suspicion and treatment of tuberculosis among hospitalized patients. Ann Intern Med 1999; 130: 404–411.
30. Sherman LF, Fujiwara PI, Cook SV et al. Patient and health care system delays in the diagnosis and treatment of tuberculosis. Int J Tuberc Lung Dis 1999; 3: 1088–1095.
31. Salaniponi FML, Harries AD, Banda HT et al. Care seeking behaviour and diagnostic process in patients with smear-positive pulmonary tuberculosis in Malawi. Int J Tuberc Lung Dis 2000; 4: 327–332.
32. Long NH, Johansson E, Diwan VK et al. Longer delays in tuberculosis diagnosis among women in Vietnam. Int J Tuberc Lung Dis 1999; 3: 388–393.
33. Selwyn PA, Hartel D, Lewis VA et al. A prospective study of the risk of tuberculosis among intravenous drug users with human immunodeficiency virus infection. N Engl J Med 1989; 320: 545–550.
34. Sutherland I. The epidemiology of tuberculosis and AIDS. British Communicable Disease Report 1990; 10: 3–4.
35. Narain JP, Raviglione MC, Kochi A. HIV-associated tuberculosis in developing countries: epidemiology and strategies for prevention. Tuberc Lung Dis 1992; 73: 311–321.
36. Di Perri G, Cruciani M, Danzi MC et al. Nosocomial epidemic of active tuberculosis among HIV-infected patients. Lancet 1989; 2: 1502–1504.
37. Odhiambo JA, Borgdorff MW, Kiambih FM et al. Tuberculosis and the HIV epidemic: increasing annual risk of tuberculous infection in Kenya, 1986–1996. Am J Public Health 1999; 89: 1078–1082.
38. International Union Against Tuberculosis Committee on Prophylaxis. Efficacy of various durations of isoniazid preventive therapy for tuberculosis: five years of follow-up in the IUAT trial. Bull World Health Organ 1982; 60: 555–564.
39. Kim SJ, Hong YP, Lew WJ et al. Incidence of pulmonary tuberculosis among diabetics. Tuberc Lung Dis 1995; 76: 529–533.
40. Cowie RL. The epidemiology of tuberculosis in gold miners with silicosis. Am J Respir Crit Care Med 1994; 150: 1460–1462.
41. Tverdal A. Body mass index and incidence of tuberculosis. Eur J Respir Dis 1986; 69: 355–362.
42. Lowe CR. An association between smoking and respiratory tuberculosis. Br Med J 1956; 2: 1081–1086.
43. Edwards JH. Contribution of cigarette smoking to respiratory disease. Br J Prev Soc Med 1957; 11: 10–21.
44. Brown JS, Wells F, Duckworth G et al. Improving notification rates for tuberculosis. Br Med J 1995; 310: 974.
45. Pablos-Méndez A, Raviglione MC, Laszlo A et al. Global surveillance for antituberculosis-drug resistance, 1994–1997. N Engl J Med 1998; 338: 1641–1649.
46. Andvord KF. Hvad kan vi lære ved å folge tuberkulosens gang fra generasjon til generasjon? (What can we learn by studying tuberculosis by generation?) Norsk Magasin Laegevidenskap 1930; 91: 642–660.
47. Härö AS. Tuberculosis in Finland. Past – present – future. Tuberc Respir Dis Yearb. 1988; 18: 1–109.
48. Berg G. The prognosis of open pulmonary tuberculosis. A clinical-statistical analysis. Lund, Sweden: Håkan Ohlson, 1939.
49. Thompson BC. Survival rates in pulmonary tuberculosis. Br Med J 1943; 2: 721.

50. Buhl K, Nyboe J. Epidemiological basis of tuberculosis eradication. 9. Changes in mortality of Danish tuberculosis patients since 1925. Bull World Health Organ 1967; 37: 907–925.

51. Krebs W. Die Fälle von Lungentuberkulose in der aargauischen Heilstätte Barmelweid aus den Jahren 1912–1927. Beitr Klin Tuberk 1930; 74: 345–79.

52. Naalsund A, Heldal E, Johansen B et al. Deaths from pulmonary tuberculosis in a low-incidence country. J Intern Med 1994; 236: 137–42.

53. Murray CJL, Styblo K, Rouillon A. Tuberculosis in developing countries: burden, intervention and cost. Bull Int Union Tuberc Lung Dis 1990; 65: 2–20.

38.2 Clinical features and management of tuberculosis

Lawrence Peter Ormerod

Key points

- Short-course chemotherapy for 6 months, with a fourth drug in the initial phase for those at higher risk of isoniazid resistance, is the evidence-based treatment for respiratory tuberculosis.

- Inactivity of tuberculosis is shown by three negative sputum cultures and failure of any lesion seen on chest radiograph to progress.

- The chest radiograph shows the extent of disease but culture of respiratory secretions shows activity.

- All reasonable attempts should be made to obtain culture confirmation.

- In patients with coexistent HIV infection there are significant tensions between optimum tuberculosis treatment and optimum antiviral (highly active antiretroviral treatment, HAART) treatment.

- Patients with suspected multi-drug-resistant tuberculosis should be isolated in appropriate facilities and the diagnosis should be confirmed/refuted as soon as possible by genetic probes applied to microscopy- or culture-positive material.

- The outcome of a local tuberculosis programme should be regularly monitored using agreed international criteria.

This chapter covers the clinical features, diagnosis and treatment of tuberculosis (TB) caused by the *Mycobacterium tuberculosis* complex (*M. tuberculosis, Mycobacterium bovis, Mycobacterium africanum*). Infection by other types of mycobacterium can simulate tuberculosis but treatment and management are different (see Chapter 39).

Although the incidence of tuberculosis in developed countries fell progressively throughout the 20th century, particularly after chemotherapy became available, in many of these coun-

tries tuberculosis incidence rose again in the 1980s and 1990s. This was usually because of very high rates in immigrant subgroups from countries of high prevalence, who now make up an increasing proportion of cases, currently 65% of the 6000 new cases per annum in England and Wales.[1] In developed countries, tuberculosis is now increasingly confined to some geographical areas and ethnic minority groups, leading to delayed diagnosis by clinicians, who may see little of the disease. Paradoxically, in developing countries the lack of funding, social and population pressures and, in sub-Saharan Africa and soon increasingly in south-east Asia, the human immunodeficiency virus (HIV) pandemic are all factors driving up the incidence of the disease and threatening tuberculosis control programmes. The World Health Organization estimates that there are 7.9 million new clinical cases each year (95% confidence limit 6.3–11.1), 1.8 million (1.4–2.8) deaths each year and 1.8 billion persons infected in the world.[2]

History of disease and treatment

Evidence of bone tuberculosis has been found in both Egyptian and pre-Columbian mummies in South America, which, together with descriptions of pulmonary disease as 'consumption' in ancient Indian texts and as 'phthisis' in Hippocratic ones, show tuberculosis to have been widespread in antiquity. It remained so throughout the centuries, but its peak incidence in the UK and the rest of northern Europe was in the late 18th and early 19th centuries, when the poor social conditions of the Industrial Revolution provided an ideal amplification mechanism for the disease.[3] This in turn was exported round the world in the 19th century by the process of colonisation.[4] The causative agent, *M. tuberculosis* was only identified in 1882 by Robert Koch.

The incidence in Europe and North America declined in the late 19th and early 20th centuries, mainly because of social improvements in housing, nutrition and working conditions.

Prior to the chemotherapy era, treatment was largely empirical. Improved nutrition and rest allowed the disease to 'arrest' in some cases, and was formalised in the sanatorium movement.[3] Removal of infectious cases to sanatoria may also have reduced transmission opportunities. Collapse therapy by artificial pneumothorax, pneumoperitoneum with or without phrenic crush, was tried extensively between 1920 and 1950, and worked in some cases by causing closure of cavities. Pleural effusion and empyema were complications of artificial pneumothorax and its use was sometimes also limited by pleural adhesions, although these could be divided by thoracoscopy. Surgical attempts to cure tuberculosis were either by 'collapse' of the upper lung by synthetic materials put into the extrapleural space – plombage or lucite balls (Fig. 38.2.1) – or by resecting the upper thoracic ribs, varying from four to more than eight, to form a flap (thoracoplasty), collapsing the underlying lung but causing mutilation (Fig. 38.2.2). Long-term survivors of this operation have a significant morbidity from late respiratory failure.[5]

The discovery of the activity of streptomycin (1944), para-amino-salicylic acid (PAS; 1946) and isoniazid (1952) against tuberculosis brought in the chemotherapy era. Initially given alone or as an adjunct to surgery, it took some time for it to be realised that drug treatment alone was able to cure the disease. By the mid-1950s Crofton had shown that, with the combination of streptomycin, isoniazid and PAS for 3 months followed by isoniazid and PAS for a further 15 months, cure was obtainable in close to 100% of cases. Surgical treatments then largely stopped and this regimen was the 'standard' treatment until the 1970s.

Ambulatory rather than prolonged hospital treatment was then feasible and was shown to be equally effective.

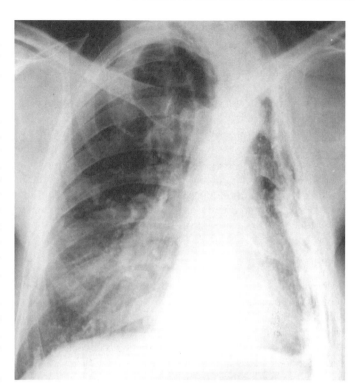

Fig. 38.2.2 Full left thoracoplasty (note also extensive left-sided pleural calcification).

The discovery of rifampicin and a re-appraisal of the role of pyrazinamide, mainly through the pioneering work of the British Medical Research Council TB Unit led by Fox,[6] allowed highly effective 6-month 'short-course' regimens to be developed, and these have been the gold standard since the early 1980s. The World Health Organization is promoting treatment by directly-observed therapy short-course (DOTS) as the main tool to combat the global emergency in tuberculosis that it identified in 1995. The emergence of drug resistance, and particularly of multi-drug-resistant organisms (MDR-TB),[7] together with the amplifying factor of TB–HIV coinfection are causing pressure on TB control programmes, particularly in the developing world, as non-standard drug regimens are needed.

Pathology and natural history

Primary tuberculosis

Nearly all primary infections are asymptomatic, even in close household contacts of sputum-microscopy-positive disease, the only marker being the development of a positive tuberculin skin test. The development of such tuberculin conversion takes 3–6 weeks from original infection and is mediated by activated T-lymphocytes. Although usually asymptomatic, some complications can occur, leading to symptoms and detection. Particularly in small children, the local hilar lymphadenopathy that is part of the primary complex can com-

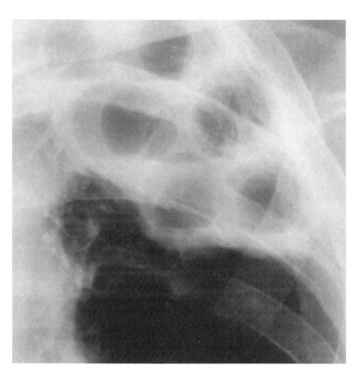

Fig. 38.2.1 Chest radiograph showing left upper-zone plombage with lucite balls.

press segmental or lobar bronchi. This can lead to extrinsic pressure on the airway, bronchostenosis or even discharge from the nodes of caseous material into the bronchial tree. Such obstructing nodes or localised airway stenoses can set up a 'ball-valve' effect, leading to lobar overinflation. A late consequence of such airway effects is development of bronchiectasis in the distal lung, the middle lobe because of its anatomy being particularly prone to such changes.[8] A transient ipsilateral pleural effusion may also occur. As part of the immune response, in some cases, high levels of circulating immune complexes may occur, leading to the development of erythema nodosum, and in developing countries phlyctenular conjunctivitis. The former usually occurs within 2 months of initial infection[9] and the latter within 12 months.

Miliary tuberculosis

Miliary tuberculosis results from tubercle bacilli spreading acutely through the blood stream after traversing vessel walls and reaching the intima. The lung is invariably involved, with other organs variably so. Microscopically the miliary lesion (Latin *milia* = seed), consists of epithelioid cells and lymphocytes containing acid-fast bacilli, Langhans giant cells and sometimes central caseation. In high-prevalence areas most cases follow soon after primary infection. In contrast, in low-prevalence areas cases occur mainly in elderly persons and represent reactivation. In the elderly and in immunocompromised patients, a non-reactive version is described with necrotic lesions containing many acid-fast bacilli but little if any cellular reaction.

Postprimary tuberculosis

Postprimary tuberculosis is the most important form, as it is much more common and such cases represent sources of continuing infection in a community. Postprimary tuberculosis can develop in a number of ways:

Reactivation of quiescent primary disease
The local primary infection in the lung is usually contained within the lung by the local immune responses, and is said to be 'arrested'. This may or may not be radiographically detectable but is marked by tuberculin skin conversion. In such 'arrested' areas, whether or not radiographically visible, tubercle bacilli can remain sequestered and dormant within macrophages or scar tissue for many years, from which they can sometimes be recovered on culture.[10] If the efficacy of local defences is impaired by increasing age, immunosuppression by drugs or HIV coinfection, or other intercurrent illnesses, e.g. diabetes or cancer, such dormant bacilli may become active and clinical disease may develop. In the white population of the UK this is thought to be the main mechanism of development of tuberculosis, since over 50% of cases occur in people aged more than 55 years,[1] representing reactivation of disease acquired initially in childhood when exposure to tuberculosis was much commoner.

Haematogenous spread to the lung
Symmetrical upper-zone shadowing of diffuse punctate type is thought, but not proved, to result from this mechanism, by dissemination from a primary complex via the blood stream.

Direct progression of primary disease
If the local immune response is insufficient to contain the primary infection at its site in the lung, progression to caseation and cavitation may occur, with progression from primary to postprimary disease over a very short time. Direct extension to the pleura as an effusion or an empyema or direct haematogenous spread may occur. The interaction of various factors, such as the dose of the infecting organism, the intensity and speed of the local immune response, the modulating effect of other diseases, e.g. HIV coinfection, and prior bacillus Calmette–Guérin (BCG) vaccination can all affect the likelihood of this occurring.

Exogenous reinfection
This mechanism was thought to be uncommon in the days before DNA fingerprinting of tubercle bacilli (RFLP typing) was available. It was held that it was very unlikely that exogenous reinfection would occur in a tuberculin-positive individual and that endogenous reactivation (as above) was the usual cause of disease. Before the advent of genetic technology, since most tubercle bacilli were (and are) still fully susceptible to first-line drugs, exogenous reinfection could only be proved by drug-resistance patterns with resistance to drugs not received by the patient.[11] If isolates are available from the initial and subsequent episodes of tuberculosis, DNA fingerprinting can be performed. Exogenous reinfection still appears to be uncommon, except in areas of high prevalence or in persons who are unusually susceptible, such as those with HIV coinfection.[12]

Clinical features

Primary tuberculosis

Primary tuberculosis is usually asymptomatic and marked by tuberculin conversion. This is why it is important particularly to screen by tuberculin-testing infants and children who are new immigrants from high-prevalence countries or close contacts of respiratory cases (Chapter 38.3). With endobronchial involvement, local signs may be present if there is segmental/lobar inflammation, so called 'epituberculosis', or a 'ball-valve' effect leading to overinflation. Physical signs and symptoms are otherwise few unless erythema nodosum or phlyctenular conjunctivitis occurs. The latter is rare in developed countries and few cases of erythema nodosum are now tuberculous, sarcoidosis, inflammatory bowel disease and streptococcal infection being commoner causes. Its association with leprosy should not be overlooked.

Miliary tuberculosis

The symptoms of miliary tuberculosis are usually insidious in onset, include fever, weight loss, malaise and anorexia, and are seen in both the 'classical' acute and cryptic miliary forms.

Acute miliary tuberculosis
Although there are systemic symptoms, respiratory symptoms and signs are few. Headache from associated tuberculous meningitis not infrequently occurs and this is sufficiently common for

lumbar puncture to be advised in 'classical' miliary tuberculosis, as central nervous system involvement requires a longer duration of chemotherapy.[13] Choroid tubercles may occur and lymph node, liver or splenic enlargement is found in a small percentage of cases.[14] In this variant, diagnosis is usually easy because of the chest X-ray appearances. Bacteriological confirmation comes from microscopy and culture of sputum, bronchoalveolar washings or cerebrospinal fluid (CSF), and urine culture. In addition to meningitis, acute respiratory distress syndrome can occur, in which event widespread diffuse or ground-glass chest radiographic changes obscure the miliary pattern.[15]

Cryptic miliary tuberculosis

This form occurs in ethnic minority groups and in the elderly white population, where it has a high mortality.[16] Apart from the systemic symptoms, focal symptoms and signs are uncommon. The chest radiograph is normal and the tuberculin skin test often negative. Blood dyscrasias of various types have been described. In such cases, bone-marrow aspirate may yield both acid-fast bacilli on culture and granulomas on microscopy. Liver biopsy has the highest diagnostic yield, with up to 75% of cases showing granulomas. The main differential diagnosis is disseminated carcinomatosis but the diagnosis is not infrequently made post-mortem.[16] The fever usually responds to treatment within 7–10 days, with clinical improvement occurring in 4–6 weeks. Where diagnostic facilities do not exist, or if the patient is unwilling to undergo invasive tests, or if all tests are negative but the patient is deteriorating, a trial of antituberculosis treatment should be considered.

Postprimary tuberculosis

The symptoms of postprimary respiratory tuberculosis can be divided into those that are systemic and non-specific and those that are respiratory. The general symptoms include malaise, anorexia, fever and weight loss. The fever is usually low-grade but can become hectic, along with increasing weight loss and night sweats, as disease progresses. Cough is the commonest respiratory symptom, sputum being mucoid or purulent with some haemoptysis. The haemoptysis is often light but can occasionally be major if a bronchial artery erodes into a cavity. Dull chest pain can be associated with mediastinal lymphadenopathy, or pleuritic pain may accompany parenchymal disease. Dyspnoea is often a late symptom, occurring only if significant lung disease, or pleural effusion, has developed. The time course of disease can vary from insidious over months to a short history simulating a pneumonia, with tuberculosis being in the differential diagnosis of a non-resolving pneumonia. Physical signs also can be respiratory or non-specific. There may be fever, evidence of weight loss or anaemia. Finger clubbing occurs only in long-standing or extensive disease. Clinical signs from the lung are found only in moderate/extensive disease with upper zone crackles or consolidation. A localised wheeze is sometimes heard in endobronchial disease. Tracheal deviation occurs, towards the side of greatest damage, in chronic disease. Evidence of extrapulmonary tuberculosis is found in up to 10% of cases in the UK, particularly in patients originating from the Indian subcontinent.[17] The usual association is of combined cervical and mediastinal lymphadenopathy

A higher proportion of HIV-coinfected cases also have disease at two or more sites.

Differential diagnosis is discussed below, along with the appropriate radiographic pattern, under Radiological diagnosis and features.

Complications can be divided into early or late. Early complications include:

- **Fever**. This usually resolves within 2 weeks of starting treatment but can occasionally be prolonged in extensive disease or with effusion. Hypersensitivity reactions to drugs need to be excluded. Corticosteroids (prednisolone 1.0 mg/kg) may be needed to suppress fever.
- **Pleurisy** may accompany pulmonary infiltration and be associated with a rub on auscultation.
- **Pleural effusion** usually occurs within 12 months of primary infection[9] but can occur as a reactivation phenomenon in the elderly.
- **Empyema**. This develops as a result of exudative lung lesions secreting acid-fast bacilli into pleural fluid. The pus may be directly positive on microscopy for acid-fast bacilli. A pyopneumothorax can occur occasionally as a result of cavity rupture, in which case management is by intercostal drainage and antituberculosis chemotherapy. Pulmonary decortication is occasionally required.
- **Laryngitis**. With extensive or long-standing sputum-smear-positive disease, laryngeal involvement can occur, causing painful hoarseness. This symptom usually responds within 2–3 weeks of starting therapy and continuing symptoms should raise the possibility of coexisting laryngeal carcinoma.
- **Alimentary spread**. Sputum containing acid-fast bacilli may be swallowed and cause associated alimentary or orificial tuberculosis.
- **Poncet's arthropathy** is a fleeting polyarthritis associated with tuberculosis, thought to be immunologically mediated. Resolution occurs within 2 months of treatment, the diagnosis being one of exclusion
- **Death**. Tuberculosis still has a high mortality, causing an estimated 1.8 million deaths per year[2] globally. In developed countries there is still an appreciable mortality. In the UK a mortality of between 6%[18] and 12%[19] has been reported for respiratory disease. Increasing age, sputum microscopy positivity, cavitation and radiographic extent of disease, but not sex or ethnic group, are all independent predictors of mortality.[18] The death rate is more than 10 times that of age- and sex-matched controls.[20] Nasogastric or parenteral feeding, parenteral antituberculosis medication, supplemental oxygen and blood transfusions may all be needed in severely ill patients. Corticosteroids may also give survival benefit in such cases and are recommended.[13]

Late complications include:

- **Airflow obstruction**. Endobronchial fibrosis may lead to airflow obstruction. Increasing age, smoking and increasing extent of disease are all factors associated with airflow obstruction.[21] One factor approximately doubles and two quadruple the proportion of patients with airflow obstruction. Chronic cough and sputum can occur and simulate chronic obstructive pulmonary disease. Occasionally, severe damage occurs endobronchially, leading to bronchiectasis.

■ **Severe lung damage**. Extensive fibrosis with or without airflow obstruction can lead to right heart failure as a late effect. The left lung is more likely than the right to suffer extensive damage. Respiratory failure due to the late effects of thoracoplasty[5] or calcified empyema, the so called 'lung *en curaisse*', can occur.

■ **Aspergilloma**. Chronic healed cavities may become colonised with *Aspergillus fumigatus*. Haemoptysis, which can occasionally be fatal, can occur. In those cases with good lung function and unilateral disease, resection may be possible. The majority of patients are unfit for surgery because of the degree of parenchymal damage. This can progress to respiratory failure. For recurrent significant haemoptysis, intracavitary treatments, radiotherapy and selective bronchial artery embolisation procedures have all been used.

■ **Amyloidosis** is seen rarely with chronic tuberculous empyema or aspergilloma.

■ **Carcinoma of the lung**. Anecdotal reports of 'scar' carcinomas are not supported by studies. Although tuberculosis and carcinoma are common in smokers, sometimes concurrently, detailed epidemiological studies show no more than a chance association.[22]

■ **Acute respiratory distress syndrome** is described with cavitary tuberculosis as well as with miliary disease.

Radiological diagnosis and features

A whole spectrum of radiographic changes are possible with TB. None is absolutely diagnostic but some patterns are highly suggestive of TB, although other diseases can be mimicked (Figs 38.2.5–38.2.19).

Pulmonary tuberculosis – primary disease

The chest radiograph may show no detectable abnormality, hilar lymphadenopathy without a Ghon focus, or a full primary complex with both a Ghon focus and hilar lymphadenopathy (Fig. 38.2.3). Calcification occurs later and may be the only radiographic sign of primary infection detected years later. In children, hilar lymphadenopathy may cause segmental or lobar shadowing (epituberculosis; Fig. 38.2.4) by rupture endo-bronchially, or unilateral overinflation/gas trapping, best shown on an expiratory film.

Postprimary disease

With this form of disease there is a marked upper-lobe predilec-tion with a tendency for the posterior segments to be affected. Disease occurring in the lower lobes tends to be in the apical seg-ments.[23] Bilateral upper-zone disease is common, initially as a nodular or patchy infiltrate, cavitation developing as the infiltra-tion becomes confluent. Long-standing disease results in signs of

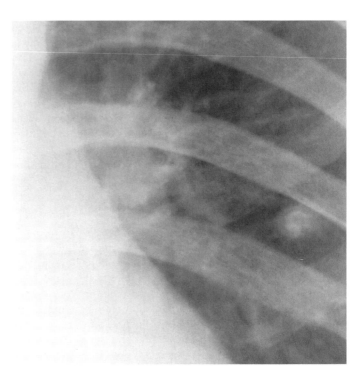

Fig. 38.2.3 Primary tuberculosis. Calcified Ghon focus in left mid zone with left hilar adenopathy. Found on contact tracing from sputum-microscopy-positive parent.

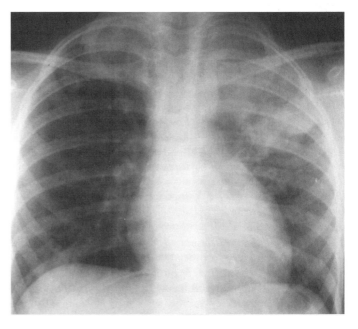

Fig. 38.2.4 Epituberculosis in left upper zone of 8-year-old contact of sputum-microscopy-positive parent.

volume loss and fibrosis, with elevation of the hila and contraction of the upper lobes, with tracheal and/or mediastinal deviation in predominantly unilateral disease. Occasionally, the chest radio-graph is normal, even in the presence of a positive culture or sputum microscopy, caused by either endobronchial disease or a

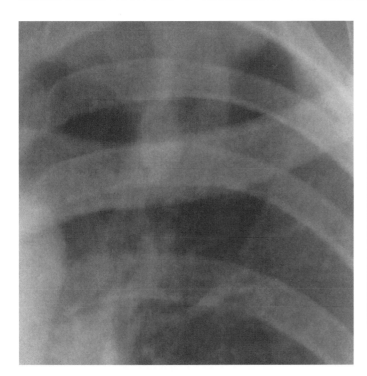

Fig. 38.2.5 Early tuberculous infiltration in the left upper zone.

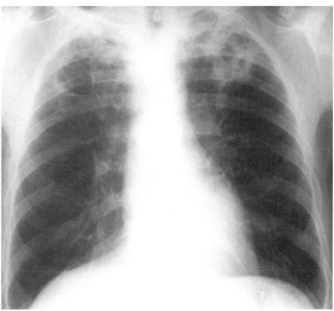

Fig. 38.2.7 Early cavitation in both apices due to tuberculosis.

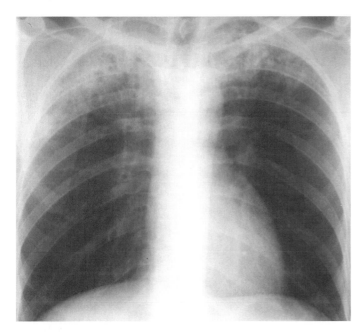

Fig. 38.2.6 Bilateral apical infiltration due to tuberculosis with early cavitation in the right apex.

node eroding into a bronchus and discharging tuberculous material. Calcification may develop in treated or 'arrested' disease.

'Activity' of disease cannot be assessed by a chest radiograph or other radiology. Inactivity of a lesion is shown by three negative sputum cultures *and* failure of a particular lesion to change with time or treatment. Activity of disease is much better assessed by microscopy and culture of respiratory samples and from associated clinical features. The usual radiographic pattern

of TB, often with sputum-microscopy-positive or smear-negative culture-positive disease, varies in two circumstances. Immigrants from the Indian subcontinent presenting with TB in developed countries have higher rates of isolated mediastinal lymphadenopathy and pleural effusion (see below) and smear- and culture-negative disease, but lower rates of smear-positive and culture-positive disease.[24] HIV coinfection, particularly but not exclusively in sub-Saharan Africa, results in a similar pattern of radiographic appearances.[25] This has had an important impact in resource-poor countries by making diagnosis harder and reducing the proportion who show positive results on sputum microscopy, which may be the only diagnostic test available.

The main differential diagnoses, for different patterns on plain radiography, are as follows.

Bilateral infiltration

Sarcoidosis can cause upper-zone infiltration but usually has a negative or only weakly positive tuberculin test. In persons who have been resident or having visited some areas of North or South America or parts of Africa, fungal illness due to histoplasmosis or coccidiomycosis have to be considered. Appropriate serological tests should confirm, but transbronchial lung biopsy may be needed.

Unilateral infiltration

Segmental or lobar pneumonic shadowing, particularly if in the upper zones, can mimic tuberculosis. Pneumonic symptoms are usually of shorter duration and symptoms more pronounced than in tuberculosis. Failure of an radiograph to improve after 3 weeks should lead to examination of sputum for tubercle bacilli.

Bilateral upper-zone fibrosis

Similar changes can occur in the later stages of sarcoidosis, chronic extrinsic allergic alveolitis and allergic bronchopulmonary aspergillosis. Calcification favours tuberculosis. In sarcoido-

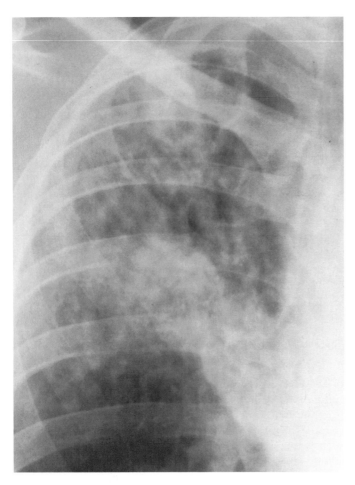

Fig. 38.2.8 More extensive tuberculous infiltration in the right mid and upper zones.

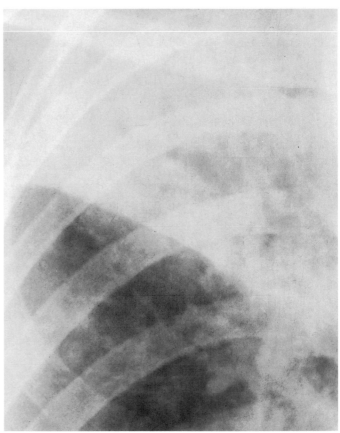

Fig. 38.2.9 Consolidation and air bronchogram in the right upper lobe. A 'non-resolving' pneumonia. No endobronchial lesion, but microscopy of bronchial washings obtained at bronchoscopy was positive for acid-fast bacilli.

sis the tuberculin test is usually negative or only weakly positive. Allergic aspergillosis or extrinsic allergic alveolitis can be diagnosed by specific tests for RAST (radioallergosorbent test) specific IgE or precipitins to the extrinsic allergen respectively.

Solitary cavitary lesions

Cavitary tuberculosis is usually sputum-microscopy-positive. If three separate negative sputum smears are obtained, the diagnosis of tuberculosis is much less likely. Cavitating lung cancer (usually squamous) is the main differential diagnosis in older persons. Bronchoscopy may be needed. Acute lung abscess due to *Staphylococcus pyogenes* and cavitating pneumonia due to *Klebsiella pneumoniae* are usually acute in onset with marked systemic symptoms and are easily confirmed by blood or sputum culture. More chronic lung abscesses due to aspiration and caused by *Bacteroides* species or *Streptococci* can be more difficult to distinguish from tuberculosis. Pulmonary infarction may cavitate but the radiographic features tend to change much more rapidly than in tuberculosis.

Bilateral cavitary lesions

The same comment about sputum-smear-positivity applies as above. *S. pyogenes* pneumonia can be a severe fulminant illness, often following influenza, and is usually readily diagnosed from blood and/or sputum cultures. Wegener's granulomatosis may have nasal or renal symptoms and signs, and is accompanied by

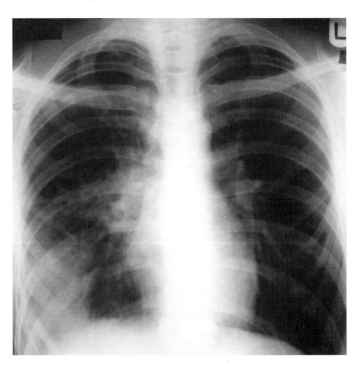

Fig. 38.2.10 Tuberculosis affecting right lower zone on postero-anterior chest radiograph.

anterior →

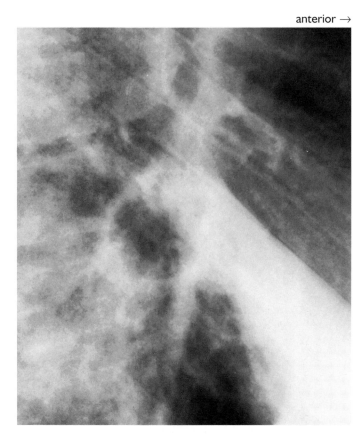

Fig. 38.2.11 Lateral film, same patient as Figure 38.2.10, showing cavitation at the root of the right lower lobe and right middle lobe collapse resulting from endobronchial disease.

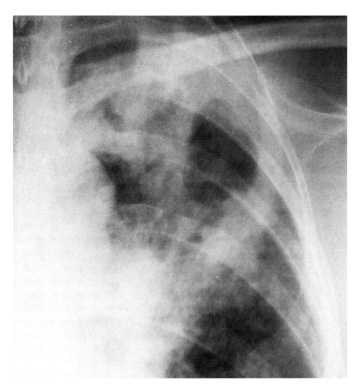

Fig. 38.2.12 Extensive left-sided tuberculosis with large left apical cavity.

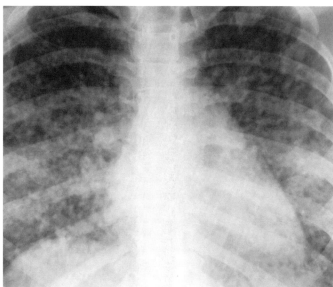

Fig. 38.2.13 Diffuse nodular tuberculosis in a 24-year-old Asian immigrant. Positive culture on bronchoscopy washings.

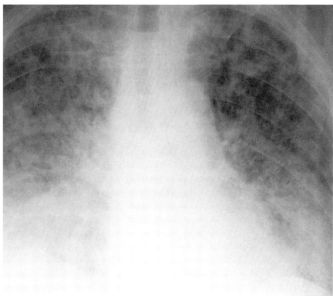

Fig. 38.2.14 Diffuse tuberculous bronchopneumonia.

a positive anticytoplasmic antibody test (ANCA) in the majority of cases. Progressive massive fibrosis on the background of coal miner's pneumoconiosis may cavitate and is usually diagnosed by the occupational history.

Miliary tuberculosis

The typical chest radiograph shows a diffuse, but even, distribution of uniform 1–2 mm nodules throughout all the lung fields. There is sometimes evidence of a primary complex or other lesion to suggest reactivation disease. The early changes of miliary disease are subtle and may be missed, particularly on an overpenetrated film. In suspected cases high-resolution CT of the thorax

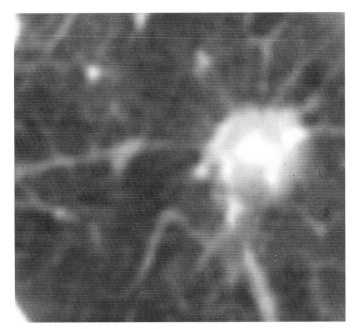

Fig. 38.2.15 Computed tomography scan of left upper zone nodule in a smoker. Some calcification is evident and a tuberculoma was confirmed on biopsy.

has a higher sensitivity and may also pick up associated mediastinal lymphadenopathy (see below). A rare variant with reticular shadowing due to lymphatic involvement is described.[26]

Mediastinal lymphadenopathy

Isolated mediastinal lymphadenopathy due to TB occurs in primary disease and is a common finding in ethnic-minority and HIV-coinfected patients. In the non-immunocompromised the tuberculin test is usually strongly positive. It is negative or only weakly positive in sarcoidosis and in lymphoma, the main differential diagnoses. In TB there may be evidence of associated lung infiltration also. Very bulky mediastinal lymphadenopathy is likely to be due to lymphoma but is occasionally seen with TB. CT scanning may help. Typically, lymph nodes enlarged as a result of TB, if larger than 2.0 cm, have a hypodense centre due to caseation and show peripheral 'ring' enhancement after contrast.[27]

Pleural effusion

There are no specific radiographic features to distinguish tuberculous pleural effusions from the many other causes, unless there are associated features of either mediastinal lymphadenopathy (as above) or infiltration. Aspiration for cytology and culture and biopsy for histology and culture are much more important than the radiographic features. Tuberculous pleural effusion is accompanied by a positive tuberculin test in the immunocompetent and the pleural fluid is a lymphocyte-rich exudate. Positive cultures are obtained in up to 50% of cases, with inoculation in a BACTEC system increasing the yield.[28] A raised level of adenosine deaminase in

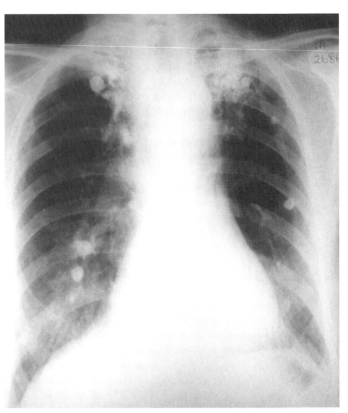

Fig. 38.2.16 Calcified 'arrested' tuberculosis in an elderly man. Sputum culture was positive despite radiographic appearances.

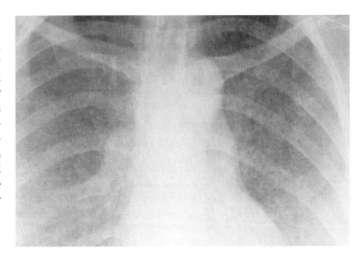

Fig. 38.2.17 Miliary tuberculosis with positive culture of bronchial washings.

the pleural fluid is not as specific as was previously thought, with an appreciable overlap with other causes of pleural effusion.[29] Multiple pleural biopsies increase the diagnostic yield;[30] thoracoscopy also increases the positive biopsy rate as this is done under direct vision and the distribution of pleural lesions is non-uniform.

Pleural effusion (and mediastinal lymphadenopathy) in high-prevalence countries, and in immigrant groups from such high-

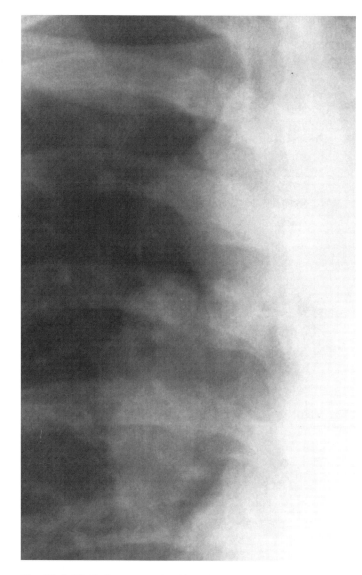

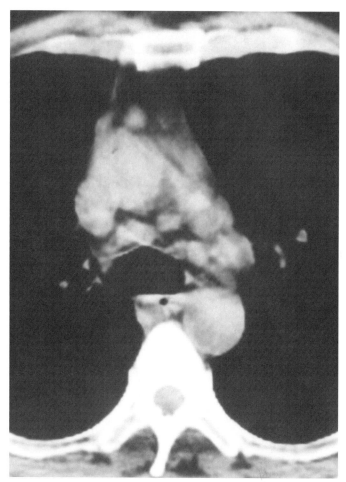

Fig. 38.2.19 Computed tomography thorax of a patient with right paratracheal tuberculous lymph nodes showing the hypodense centre representing caseation.

Fig. 38.2.18 Right paratracheal lymphadenopathy in a 17-year-old Asian girl recently returned from Asia. The tuberculin test was positive and the abnormality resolved after treatment for tuberculosis.

prevalence countries living in developed countries, should have tuberculosis as the working diagnosis, and appropriate investigations should be carried out.

Bacteriology including molecular probes

Most members of the genus *Mycobacterium* are free-living saprophytes readily isolated from the environment. Most of these do not infect humans, but some do; these are covered in Chapter 39. Those mycobacteria that are obligate pathogens causing human disease (with the exception of *Mycobacterium leprae*) are known as the '*M. tuberculosis* complex'. This consists of *M. tuberculosis*, which makes up the vast bulk of cases, *M. africanum* and *M. bovis*. *Mycobacterium microti* and the

bacillus Calmette–Guérin (BCG) vaccine strain, while strictly members of the tuberculosis 'complex', only cause disease under special circumstances.

Mycobacterium tuberculosis is an aerobic organism that grows optimally at 37°C, but slowly (its generation time is measured in hours)compared with most bacteria. Its cell wall is much thicker than most bacteria and has a high lipid content. This cell-wall structure leads to resistance to acids and alkalis and detergents, properties that lead to the 'acid-fastness' of staining of the cell wall with dyes. The organism is, however, easily destroyed by heat and ultraviolet light. Scrupulous laboratory technique is needed for work with tuberculosis. False-positive results can be obtained by contamination with environmental organisms, and false-negative results occur if sample decontamination also kills the tubercle bacilli. In developed countries, work with tuberculosis organisms and material is carried out in special facilities within the laboratory[31] to prevent laboratory-acquired infection.

Sputum microscopy

For developing countries, sputum microscopy using the Ziehl–Neelsen method is the mainstay of diagnosis. Standards and

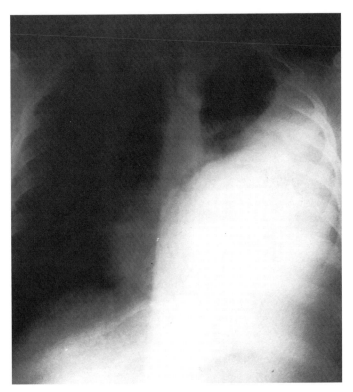

Fig. 38.2.20 Large left tuberculous effusion. Lymphocytic exudate and positive on culture at 6 weeks.

recommendations are made by the World Health Organization (WHO) and the International Union against Tuberculosis and Lung Disease (IUATLD). In developed countries screening of samples is now more commonly done with a fluorescence microscopy technique using a auramine–rhodamine stain. To exclude false-positive results, a confirmatory Ziehl–Neelsen stain is also done on any positive sample. Microscopy, however, does not differentiate between mycobacteria of the tuberculosis complex and other opportunistic mycobacteria. Care has to be taken that neither the sample, e.g. bronchoscopic washings, or laboratory reagents are contaminated by such opportunistic mycobacteria.[32]

Culture

The absolute confirmation of the diagnosis of tuberculosis is by the pure growth of *M. tuberculosis* in culture. Culture can be either on solid or in liquid media. The Lowenstein–Jensen solid medium, one tube using glycerol and one using sodium pyruvate, should be used.[33] Sodium glycerol encourages the growth of *M. bovis*, which may be missed without its use. A liquid medium such as Middlebrook 7H9 broth can also be used, and when coupled with an automatic sampling system such as BACTEC 460 or BACTEC MGIT 960, gives a faster and higher culture positive yield than solid media. On solid media, cultures are usually obtained in 2–3 weeks in microscopy-positive samples and between 4–6 weeks in microscopy-negative ones. Using a liquid medium significantly shortens both these durations.

Drug susceptibility testing

All isolated mycobacteria require testing for susceptibility to first-line antituberculosis drugs in a specialised laboratory, a service provided in the UK by the Public Health Laboratory Service. The isolated bacteria are incubated in a drug free medium and in increasing concentrations of the first-line agents. Pyrazinamide sensitivity testing is technically demanding. The susceptibility or resistance to the drugs tested is usually assessed by either the resistance ratio or modal resistance method. Resistance for the purposes of treatment is usually taken as a resistance ratio of 4 or greater. Susceptibility testing for second-line or reserve drugs (see later) is carried out for those mycobacteria showing resistance to one or more first-line drugs. Using an automated system, e.g. BACTEC, for susceptibility testing usually allows a turn-round time of 2 weeks for positive cultures. Other methods, e.g. phaB assays, are being assessed to see if more rapid results are possible. The diagnosis of *M. bovis* is a bacteriological rather than a clinical diagnosis.

Molecular methods

These are increasingly being used in a number of areas of tuberculosis diagnosis.

Speciation

Specific molecular probes are available for rapid identification of the species of mycobacteria, which may be crucial in some patients, such as those with acquired immunodeficiency syndrome (AIDS). Probes using specific target DNA hybridisation can identify within a few hours whether the organism is of the tuberculosis complex or one of the opportunist mycobacteria.[34] These tests, however, can only be performed on microscopy- or culture-positive material as they require significant amounts of target DNA.

Drug resistance

The mutation for rifampicin resistance is a stable one in the *rpoB* gene and this can be detected with 95% accuracy by a polymerase chain reaction (PCR) technique.[35] This also can be done on microscopy- or culture-positive material. Since isolated rifampicin resistance is uncommon,[13] rifampicin resistance is a marker for MDR-TB in over 90% of cases. Where such MDR-TB is suspected, molecular methods should be used,[13] with treatment[13] and isolation as for MDR-TB[36] in those with a positive result for rifampicin resistance pending full standard drug susceptibility data.

Diagnosis

Polymerase chain reaction, using amplification of DNA sequences in vitro, has been studied in microscopy-negative disease to see if it would enhance or speed up diagnosis. Using, usually the IS*6110* insertion sequence, as few as 10–1000 organisms of *M. tuberculosis*, well below the microscopy detection rate, can be identified.[37] The sensitivity, specificity and positive predictive value of PCR compared with culture in some studies are high, at 83.5%, 99% and 94.2% respectively.[38] There are, however, problems with false-positive and false-negative results, interlaboratory variability and the presence of inhibitors.[39] These techniques have not yet replaced culture, and results should be interpreted with caution, being used only as one of the pieces of evidence influencing the decision as to whether to start treatment.

Other investigations

Tuberculin skin test

The tuberculin skin test is only occasionally helpful in making a diagnosis of clinical tuberculosis. It does not differentiate between infection (exposure) and disease, particularly in subjects over the age of 35 years. It is much more useful in epidemiological work and contact screening (Chapter 38.3). The tuberculin test may be falsely negative, being suppressed in some cases with extensive pulmonary or miliary disease and in those with HIV coinfection, where, because of reduced CD4+ cell counts, 'anergy' to tuberculin can occur in those with active disease or a history of prior infection.[40] A strongly positive tuberculin test indicates infection but is unhelpful on its own in the presence of a normal examination and chest radiograph, unless in the context of a contact or new immigrant screening investigation (Chapter 38.3)

Bronchoscopy

Where tuberculosis is strongly suspected but either sputum is negative on microscopy or none can be produced, fibreoptic bronchoscopy is a proven technique with a significant yield.[41] Bronchial washings and brushing[42] and bronchoalveolar lavage[43] all give useful yields and are superior to techniques such as gastric lavage. Transbronchial biopsy combined with bronchoscopy may increase the yield.[44] Care must be taken both with sterilisation of the bronchoscope so as not to transmit tuberculosis and with infection control measures so that tuberculosis is not transmitted by the aerosol route, particularly with immunosuppressed patients.[36]

Serology

While various tests against a variety of mycobacterial antigens have been studied, sometimes with moderate results, the sensitivity and specificity of these tests is less than nuclear amplification techniques, especially PCR, and conventional bacteriology and they are not routinely used in clinical practice.[45]

Other blood tests

Elevation of erythrocyte sedimentation rate (ESR) or C-reactive protein (CRP), a normochromic anaemia, a modestly elevated gamma-globulin and reduced serum sodium all occur in tuberculosis and, while associated with disease severity,[46] none is specific to tuberculosis. Modest elevations of hepatic transaminases may also occur in miliary or extensive pulmonary disease.[13]

Diagnosis of tuberculosis

The diagnosis of tuberculosis is made from a combination of suspicion of the possibility and confirmation by the appropriate investigations, crucially bacteriology. A risk assessment is needed for all possible cases, bearing in mind known risk factors such as HIV coinfection, ethnicity, recent residence in a high-prevalence country and other copathology. Clinical suspicion is harder to maintain in a low-incidence setting than in an area or population group with a high incidence. After carrying out appropriate bacteriological tests, it is sometimes appropriate to commence a trial of full antituberculosis therapy pending the results of culture, with monitoring of the response. In some ethnic minority groups, up to 30% of respiratory tuberculosis is both sputum-microscopy- and culture-negative.[1,17]

Scientific basis for short-course chemotherapy

The first-line antituberculosis drugs vary in their capacity to kill bacteria, to sterilise lesions and to prevent the emergence of drug resistance. Isoniazid is the most powerful bactericidal drug and kills more than 90% of bacilli within 7 days, acting principally on metabolically active bacilli. It is also quite effective in preventing the emergence of drug resistance.

Rifampicin is also a good bactericidal drug with good ability to prevent the emergence of drug resistance. In addition to acting on rapidly dividing bacilli, it kills so called 'persisters', bacilli that remain inactive for long periods with occasional metabolic spurts. This effect, with only a short drug exposure, is crucial to its sterilising ability.

Pyrazinamide, although bactericidal, is used mainly for its sterilising effect. It is particularly effective in killing intracellular bacilli sequestered inside macrophages in an acid environment.[47]

Ethambutol and streptomycin are less potent drugs, ethambutol probably being bactericidal only at high concentrations. These two agents are less good than rifampicin and isoniazid at preventing the emergence of drug resistance. They are included in the regimen when there is a chance of significant primary drug resistance, particularly to isoniazid. Ethambutol is usually added to the initial phase of treatment in countries where there is significant isoniazid resistance, which in practice is most of the developing world, and in certain minority groups, usually foreign born or ethnic minority groups, in developed countries.

Many trials of short-course chemotherapy in sputum-smear-positive and sputum-smear-negative tuberculosis have defined the principles of chemotherapy, the roles of various drugs and the efficacy of treatment, so that they allow highly specific recommendations to be made.[6,48] Regimens based on rifampicin, isoniazid and pyrazinamide convert more than 90% of patients with sputum-smear-positive disease to culture-negative at 2 months, with cure rates exceeding 95% and relapse rates less than 5%. Treatment of smear-positive cases for less than 6 months gives unacceptably high relapse rates[49] in developed countries. Pyrazinamide is only of use in the initial 2 months of therapy, but if it cannot be tolerated or is not included, then a 9-month regimen with initial ethambutol is needed.[50]

Six-month short-course chemotherapy is equally effective whether the dosing schedule is daily throughout, daily initially with an intermittent continuation phase, or intermittent throughout.[6,48] If rifampicin is not included in the continuation phase, 6-month regimens produce inadequate sterilisation and hence high relapse rates. A longer continuation phase is then needed. Although there are small differences in dosage between fixed-dose combination tablets and the drugs given individually, providing that the combination tablets are of proven bioavailability there are no significant differences in practice.[48] With sputum-smear-negative tuberculosis there is some evidence that shorter 4-month regimens can give good results,[48] but most authorities recommend the 6-month regimen for all pulmonary tuberculosis irrespective of the sputum status.[13]

Chemoprophylaxis (preventive therapy)

Among individuals who are tuberculin positive, indicating infection, but without evidence of clinical disease, or with small, non-progressive lesions on radiography, a proportion are thought to harbour a small number of potentially viable tubercle bacilli. If antituberculosis drug(s) are given successfully to such persons to kill the bacilli and sterilise any lesions, this will reduce the possibility of later reactivation and clinical disease. Preventive therapy is occasionally primary, i.e. given to a person exposed but not yet infected, usually a neonate or young child (see Chapter 38.3), but is usually secondary, i.e. given to persons already infected as judged by a positive tuberculin skin test. In placebo-controlled trials in primary contacts,[48,51] isoniazid for 6 months has been shown significantly to reduce the incidence of clinical disease both during and after treatment. The multicentre IUATLD study[52] showed that, for small radiographic lesions (< 2 cm), 6 months of treatment with isoniazid was as effective as 12 months, and for larger lesions (> 2 cm) 6 months of isoniazid provided considerable protection.

Compliance with prophylaxis is a problem in asymptomatic individuals, which, together with some concerns about possible isoniazid hepatotoxicity,[51] has led to shorter regimens of chemoprophylaxis being sought. Rifampicin and pyrazinamide, as stated earlier, have better sterilisation properties than isoniazid. Data are available on shorter regimens of 3 months of rifampicin/isoniazid in HIV-negative, high-risk adults,[53] in children[54] and in HIV-infected persons,[55] and for regimens of 2 months of rifampicin/pyrazinamide in HIV-positive individuals.[56] In the UK the Joint Tuberculosis Committee recommends 3 months of rifampicin/isoniazid (3HR) as an alternative to 6 months of isoniazid (6H) as a chemoprophylaxis regimen.[57] This recommendation is based on the equivalence of efficacy of 3HR with rifampicin/pyrazinamide for 2 months (2RZ), on the better tolerance of 3HR compared with 2RZ, and on the availability of HR combination tablets. On the basis of the same data, the American Thoracic Society recommends 2RZ as an alternative to 6H.[58]

Secondary prophylaxis (isoniazid or rifampicin/isoniazid) is indicated for:

- children (< 16 years) with strongly positive tuberculin tests (Heaf grades 2–4 or Mantoux > 5 mm if no prior BCG or Heaf grades 3–4 (Mantoux ≥ 15 mm) if prior BCG)
- those in whom recent tuberculin conversion is documented
- HIV-infected contacts of smear-positive pulmonary disease.

The question is sometimes asked why three or four drug combinations are used for treatment of disease but only one or two drugs for prophylaxis, and whether this increases the chance of drug resistance developing. The chance of spontaneous mutation occurring leading to resistance to a single drug is of the order of $1/10^6$. In persons with active disease, particularly smear-positive pulmonary disease, the organism burden is greater than 10^{10}. Hence monotherapy would inevitably lead to resistance and multiple drug regimens are therefore used. In persons requiring chemoprophylaxis, animal studies suggest that only some 10^3–10^4 viable organisms may be present and hence single-drug prophylaxis is associated with an extremely low risk of acquired drug resistance.

Clinical pharmacology of tuberculosis drugs

First-line drugs

Isoniazid

Isoniazid is a bactericidal drug that inhibits mycolic acid synthesis in the cell wall of *M. tuberculosis*. Absorption is complete in the fasted state but reduced after food. Substantial first-pass metabolism in the gut and the liver reduces bioavailability. The drug is widely distributed and crosses the blood–brain barrier. The main enzyme catalysing its metabolism is an acetyl transferase, which has variable expression, causing wide variation in half-life.

Adverse effects

Because of interference with vitamin B_6 metabolism, a mixed sensorimotor peripheral neuropathy can occur. Hepatitis can occur in 0.5–1.0% of cases, being commoner in females and with increasing age.[48] Acne can be worsened.

Interactions

Isoniazid increases serum levels of phenytoin, carbamazepine, warfarin and diazepam; its serum level is decreased by prednisolone.

Rifampicin

Rifampicin is bactericidal by interfering with the β subunit of the ribosomal ribonucleic acid (RNA) polymerase.[59] It is well absorbed orally but the timing of its maximum blood level is delayed and is reduced by food. The formulation is critical to its bioavailability and only individual or combination tablets of proven bioavailability should be used. Rifampicin is metabolised, mainly in the liver, to more water-soluble active metabolites, some of which are excreted in bile and urine. Urine, sweat and tears can be coloured orange or red for several hours after ingestion and contact lenses may become stained.

Adverse effects

Some side effects are more common with intermittent than with daily administration. Hepatitis occurs in between 1.5% and 3.0% of cases. Rashes can also occur. With intermittent treatment two or three times weekly, antibodies to rifampicin can occur, which lead to a 'flu-like' syndrome with fever, chills and headache. More rarely, thrombocytopenic purpura, haemolysis, shock and acute renal failure can occur. In the event of these latter reactions, rifampicin should be stopped immediately and not reintroduced.[13,48]

Interactions

Rifampicin is a major enzyme inducer and reduces the serum levels of many drugs, including warfarin, sulphonylureas, corticosteroids, oral contraceptives, phenytoin, cyclosporin, opiates and some anti-HIV drugs, particularly protease inhibitors.[60] Its serum level is reduced by concurrent use of ketoconazole.

Pyrazinamide

Pyrazinamide is bactericidal, particularly to subpopulations of organisms that are sequestered intracellularly, but its precise mode of action is not yet worked out. It is metabolised by pyrazinamidase to pyrazinoic acid, its main active metabolite. Oral absorption is complete; the drug is approximately 50% protein-bound and is widely distributed, including in the CSF, which it penetrates well, reaching levels equivalent to those in plasma.[61]

Adverse effects

Pyrazinamide can cause hepatitis in its own right, in up to 2% of cases, but the frequency of drug-induced hepatitis does not increase when it is added to isoniazid and rifampicin.[48] Self-limiting facial flushing can occur in the first few days. Pruritus and a widespread erythematous or papular rash can also occur. Arthralgia can occur in up to 10%; hyperuricaemia occurs but is seldom symptomatic.

Interactions

The serum level of pyrazinamide is increased by probenecid.

Ethambutol

Ethambutol is bacteriostatic when used in a dose of 15 mg/kg, but may be weakly bactericidal at 25 mg/kg. It acts to inhibit cell-wall synthesis by interfering with arabinogalactan biosynthesis.[62] It is well absorbed orally and is distributed to most body fluids, but CSF penetration, even in meningitis, is not good. It is cleared largely unchanged in urine, with a half-life of 10–15 hours. Significant accumulation can occur in renal impairment.

Adverse effects

Dose related optic neuritis occurs. At 15 mg/kg with normal renal function this is very rare, but at doses of 25 mg/kg it occurs in 3% of individuals.[63] Visual acuity should be shown to be normal before its use[64] and the patient should be warned to stop the drug and report in the event of any visual change. Optic neuritis is usually, but not invariably, reversible on withdrawal of the drug.

Interactions

The serum level of ethambutol is reduced by aluminium hydroxide administration.

Streptomycin

Streptomycin is an aminoglycoside with weak bactericidal activity resulting from interference with ribosomal proteins that block protein synthesis. It requires intramuscular injection as it has no significant oral absorption. Approximately 50% is protein-bound, with a fairly wide distribution but poor CSF penetration. It is not significantly metabolised and is excreted unchanged in the urine, with a half-life of 3 hours. Renal impairment can greatly prolong its excretion, leading to toxicity.

Adverse effects

The most severe is concentration-dependent damage to the vestibular portion of the eighth cranial nerve, causing dizziness, the risk increasing with age and with reduced renal function. Mild hypersensitivity with fever is common but not frequently severe. Renal impairment due to the drug can occasionally occur. It should be avoided in pregnancy as it can damage the eighth cranial nerve of the fetus.

Interactions
None of note.

Reserve drugs

These drugs should only be used if there is significant toxicity from first-line drugs requiring a non-standard regimen, or as part of a multidrug regimen for MDR-TB. They all have lower efficacy against tuberculosis and increased toxicity compared with first-line drugs. Brief details will be given of action, adverse effects and toxicity. For more detail, manufacturers' data and pharmacological textbooks should be consulted.

Capreomycin

Capreomycin is weakly bactericidal and is used where there is resistance to streptomycin, with which there is usually no cross-resistance. It is not an aminoglycoside. It is given intramuscularly in a dose of 15 mg/kg. It should be used with caution and reduced dosage in renal impairment.

Adverse effects are as for streptomycin.

Kanamycin and amikacin

These agents have similar activity and action to streptomycin, with which there is often cross-resistance, less so with amikacin than with kanamycin. They should only be used if susceptibility of the organism has been shown. Dosage and adverse effects are as for streptomycin.

Ethionamide or prothionamide

These drugs inhibit mycolic acid synthesis by a different action from that of isoniazid. They are weakly bactericidal, moderately good at preventing resistance emerging, but have little sterilising efficacy. There is no cross-resistance with isoniazid but there is with thiacetazone. They are well absorbed orally and distributed widely, including the CSF at levels similar to serum. Metabolism is by the liver with excretion in the urine, renal impairment impairing excretion.

Adverse effects include gastrointestinal upset, hepatitis and rash.

Cycloserine

Cycloserine is an analogue of the amino acid alanine, the uptake of which it inhibits, thereby interfering with cell-wall peptido-glycan production. It has only weak sterilising and resistance-preventing properties. Having a molecular weight of only 99, it is well absorbed orally and penetrates all fluids well, including CSF. It is excreted largely unchanged in the urine and may accumulate in renal impairment. Adverse effects include depression, psychosis and convulsions. It should be avoided in epilepsy. Cycloserine potentiates alcohol, impairs phenytoin metabolism and may interact with ofloxacin.

Macrolides (clarithromycin/azithromycin)

Macrolides have some bactericidal activity against mycobacteria, including *M. tuberculosis*. They are well absorbed from the gut but have reduced bioavailability resulting from first-pass metabolism. The drugs and their metabolites are renally cleared, and raised levels can occur in renal impairment.

Adverse effects include gastrointestinal upset and hepatitis. Uveitis may occur in HIV-positive patients in conjunction with rifabutin. There may also be interactions with warfarin, carbamazepine, cyclosporin and aminophylline.

Fluoroquinolones (ciprofloxacin/ofloxacin)

These have bactericidal activity against mycobacteria by their inhibition of the DNA gyrase system. Different quinolones have different MICs; sparfloxacin, which has a good MIC, is limited by heliosensitivity. Absorption orally is good with a wide distribution. Metabolism is predominantly hepatic, but with renal clearance.

Adverse effects include rash, photosensitivity and hepatitis. The levels of fluoroquinolones some are decreased by antacids; they increase the serum level of theophylline and warfarin.

Rifabutin

Rifabutin is another rifamycin similar to rifampicin. Because there is a high level of cross-resistance with rifampicin it should not be used to treat rifampicin-resistant organisms unless susceptibility to rifabutin has been confirmed. Metabolism, mode of action and adverse effects are as for rifampicin.

Rifabutin is a less potent enzyme inducer than rifampicin, and so has fewer interactions with drugs, particularly with protease inhibitors used in the treatment of HIV infection. Some advocate its use for the treatment of TB and HIV coinfection (see Treatment, HIV-positive patients, below).

Clofazimine

Clofazimine is an antileprosy drug that has some activity against *M. tuberculosis*. Oral absorption is incomplete and very formulation-dependent. Clofazimine is widely distributed, is lipophilic and penetrates peripheral nerves. It crosses the placenta and enters breast milk. Adverse effects include skin staining and pigmentation, and gastrointestinal upset.

Thiacetazone

Thiacetazone is a thiosemicarbazone that probably acts on mycolic acid synthesis, a conclusion inferred by the frequent cross-resistance encountered to ethionamide. Thiacetazone is good at preventing resistance emerging but has little sterilising ability. It is well absorbed orally and metabolism is largely hepatic. Adverse effects include gastrointestinal upset, hepatitis and rashes. The rash can be severe in HIV-positive patients, with 10% developing Stevens–Johnson syndrome and 1% mortality.[65] The drug should not be given to patients known to be or suspected of being HIV-positive.

Interactions: aminoglycosides may be displaced from protein-binding, increasing toxicity.

Para-amino-salicylic acid

Para-amino-salicylic acid (PAS) was one of the original antituberculosis drugs, with some chemical similarity to aspirin. It acts by competing with para-amino benzoic acid for mycobacterial dihydropterorate synthetase. It is well absorbed orally but may need to be taken after food because of gastric upset (absorption is not affected). It is widely distributed, reaching high levels in pleural fluid and caseous tissue. It is cleared renally after acetylation. Adverse effects include nausea, abdominal pain, diarrhoea, goitre, fever and rashes.

Treatment of tuberculosis

As set out earlier, the scientific basis of chemotherapy allows highly evidence-based criteria to be used for the treatment of tuberculosis. The recommendations for respiratory tuberculosis are based on multiple clinical trials, and are therefore an 'A'-grade recommendation.[66] In the UK, a 6-month regimen of rifampicin, isoniazid, pyrazinamide and ethambutol for the initial 2 months followed by rifampicin and isoniazid for a further 4 months is recommended as standard treatment for both adults and children with respiratory tuberculosis (including isolated pleural effusion and mediastinal lymphadenopathy), irrespective of the bacteriological status of the sputum.[13] The fourth drug (ethambutol) can only be omitted in patients with a low risk of isoniazid resistance on the basis of national resistance data[67] – in other words, previously untreated patients of white ethnic origin who are known to be or thought likely to be HIV-negative on risk assessment and who are not contacts of known drug-resistant organisms. Individuals who are known or suspected to be HIV-positive, who are from other ethnic groups or who have had previous treatment, and recent arrivals such as immigrants and refugees of any ethnic group, are at significant higher risk of infection by organisms resistant to isoniazid and other drugs, and should be treated initially with the four-drug combination unless there are very strong contraindications to the use of one of these drugs.

The same regimens are recommended for all forms of non-pulmonary tuberculosis, with the exception of central nervous system disease,[13] when the same initial phase should be used but with the continuation phase of rifampicin and isoniazid prolonged to 10 months.[13] The European Respiratory Society/World Health Authority also advises a four-drug regimen for those with sputum-smear-positive respiratory disease and in those with extensive smear-negative tuberculosis.[68] The American Thoracic Society advises a three-drug initial phase, with the addition of ethambutol in areas or groups where the isoniazid resistance rate is equal to or greater than 4%.[69] If initial pyrazinamide is not used or cannot be tolerated, the duration of treatment in adults and children should be extended to 9 months, with ethambutol given for the initial 2 months. Routine daily pyridoxine is not required but should be given to those at increased risk of peripheral neuropathy, such as diabetic, alcoholic or HIV-positive patients and those with chronic renal failure or malnutrition. A dose of 10 mg daily prevents peripheral neuropathy. Dosages of drugs for daily or intermittent use are given in Table 38.2.1.

Pretreatment screening

Liver function should be checked in clinical cases before treatment and renal function in those being treated with either ethambutol or streptomycin. Ethambutol in the dose of 15 mg/kg rarely causes toxic effects on the eye (optic neuritis) but it is recommended that visual acuity is tested using a Snellen chart before ethambutol is taken.[64] For its safe use, patients should have reasonable visual acuity and be able to appreciate and report symptoms. The patient should be told to stop the drug immediately if visual symptoms occur and report this to the physician. This information should also be recorded in the clinical notes. In those with language difficulties or in smaller children, ethambutol should be given when appropriate, with the above advice given to family members and parents. Family doctors and patients should be informed about possible side effects, together with indications for stopping treatment and seeking advice. Where possible this should be given to patients in their own language. Regular monitoring of liver function is not required in cases with no evidence of pre-existing liver disease and normal pretreatment liver function. However, liver function should be checked, and treatment stopped if appropriate, if fever, malaise, unexplained deterioration, vomiting or jaundice occur.[13]

Special situations

Diabetes

Diabetics have both an increased incidence of tuberculosis and more extensive pulmonary disease.[70] Standard treatment should be given, but rifampicin reduces the efficacy of sulphonylureas, which may require dosage adjustment or change to insulin therapy.

Liver disease

Rifampicin, isoniazid and pyrazinamide are all potentially hepatotoxic, but the addition of pyrazinamide to regimens of rifampicin and isoniazid does not increase the frequency of hepatotoxicity.[71] Patients with known chronic liver disease such as alcoholism, chronic active hepatitis or cirrhosis, or known carriers of hepatitis B or C, require both baseline and regular liver function monitoring. Weekly liver function tests for the first 2 weeks followed by 2-weekly tests for the first 2 months are recommended.[72]

Table 38.2.1 Recommended doses of standard antituberculosis drugs

| Drug | Daily dosage | | | Intermittent dosage | | |
| | Children | Adults | | Children | Adults | |
		Weight	Dose		Weight	Dose
Isoniazid	5 mg/kg (maximum 300 mg)	–	300 mg	15 mg/kg 3 times weekly	–	15 mg/kg 3 times weekly (maximum 900 mg)
Rifampicin	10 mg/kg (maximum 600 mg)	<50 kg >50 kg	450 mg 600 mg	15 mg/kg 3 times weekly	–	600–900 mg 3 times weekly
Pyrazinamide	35 mg/kg	<50 kg >50 kg	1.5 g 2.0 g	50 mg/kg 3 times weekly 75 mg/kg 2 times weekly	<50 kg >50 kg <50 kg >50 kg	2.0 g 3 times weekly 2.5 g 3 times weekly 3.0 g 2 times weekly 3.5 g 2 times weekly
Ethambutol*	15 mg/kg	–	15 mg/kg	30 mg/kg 3 times weekly 45 mg/kg 2 times weekly	–	30 mg/kg 3 times weekly 45 mg/kg 2 times weekly

* Accurate calculation is required to reduce the risk of toxicity

Pregnancy

Pregnancy occurring while taking rifampicin is not an indication for termination. None of the first-line drugs has been shown to be teratogenic in humans but ethionamide and prothionamide may be teratogenic and are best avoided. Streptomycin and other aminoglycosides may be ototoxic to the fetus and should be avoided in pregnancy. Standard treatment should be given to pregnant women. Patients may breast-feed normally while taking antituberculosis drugs.

Renal disease

Isoniazid, rifampicin and pyrazinamide can be given in standard doses in renal impairment. If streptomycin or ethambutol are used, because they are virtually entirely renally excreted, reduced doses should be used and serum concentrations should be monitored. Dialysis in patients with chronic renal failure affects the clearance of drugs and requires modifications of dose.[73]

Silicosis

Patients with underlying silicosis complicated by tuberculosis need longer then standard treatment because they have pulmonary macrophage dysfunction that both makes them substantially more likely to develop tuberculosis and slows the immune response required to help clear the disease. Studies by the British Medical Research Council[74] showed that extension of the continuation phase of treatment to 6 months (8 months' treatment in total) is required to give acceptably low relapse rates.

Unconscious patients

Standard therapy should be given to unconscious patients. Isoniazid and rifampicin can be administered either as syrup via a nasogastric tube or by once-daily intravenous infusion. Isoniazid can also be administered by intramuscular injection. Pyrazinamide can be administered either as crushed tablets or syrup via a nasogastric tube. Streptomycin is given intramuscularly. Ethambutol should be avoided as visual acuity cannot be tested.

HIV-positive patients

Patients who are HIV-positive should be given the standard four-drug regimen unless MDR-TB is suspected. Coinfected patients who have low CD4+ lymphocyte counts are more likely to have disseminated tuberculosis. Small clinical studies suggest that tuberculosis in HIV-positive patients responds just as rapidly as in those who are HIV-negative.[75] Overall, however, HIV-coinfected persons with tuberculosis have a higher mortality than HIV-negative tuberculosis patients.[76,77]

Drug reactions are much commoner in HIV-positive patients and life-threatening adverse events can occur with any antimycobacterial regimen. Thiacetazone should be avoided because severe Stevens–Johnson syndrome occurs in 10% of cases so treated, with a mortality rate of 1–2%.[65] Ketoconazole can inhibit rifampicin absorption if taken at the same time, which can lead to

treatment failure.[78] Rifampicin and isoniazid can interact with other azole antifungal drugs, reducing serum concentrations of fluconazole and itraconazole to subtherapeutic levels.[79,80]

There are potential interactions, particularly between rifampicin and classes of antiretroviral drugs which may be given to HIV-positive in multiple combinations (highly active antiretroviral therapy, HAART). These result from the induction of the CYP3A P450 enzyme by rifampicin, through which system some antiretroviral drugs, particularly protease inhibitors, are metabolised.[60] Protease-inhibitor drug levels can be severely decreased, leading to loss of antiretroviral effect.[81] There are therefore tensions between the treatment required for tuberculosis and that for HIV in dually infected persons.[60] In individuals taking protease inhibitors or in whom they are being considered there are three main options:

- Discontinue protease inhibitors and use alternative antiretroviral drugs until the tuberculosis has been treated.
- Use indinavir as the protease inhibitor and substitute rifabutin in reduced dosage for rifampicin.[82]
- Omit rifampicin from the regimen and extend treatment to 18 months.

The first option is recommended whenever possible.[13,60]

In addition to these problems, significantly immunosuppressed HIV patients who begin HAART at the same time as, or after, drug therapy for TB can experience a florid immune response to TB, due to the immune reconstitution syndrome.[83]

Non-compliance

Vagrants, alcohol or drug abusers and patients with mental illness are unlikely to be compliant with self-administered drug therapy. Such persons, anyone having retreatment and anyone found to be non-compliant during therapy should be treated with a fully supervised regimen. An intermittent three-times-weekly regimen with rifampicin, isoniazid, pyrazinamide and streptomycin/ethambutol for the 2-month initial phase and rifampicin and isoniazid for the 4-month continuation phase is recommended.[13]

To help patient compliance, directly observed therapy (DOT), where every drug ingestion is monitored, has been promoted by the WHO. Cohort studies compared with historical controls have shown increased cure rates and reduced drug resistance rates and relapses[84,85] but in one semi-structured study DOT was outperformed by self-supervision.[86] The US Centers for Disease Control recommend that DOT be considered for all patients but accepts that, if more than 90% of the patients in an area are completing self-administered treatment, selective DOT in unreliable patients (as set out above) is an alternative.[87] Decision analyses, however, support universal or selective DOT strategies over self-medication.[88,89] In the UK, selective DOT is advised.[13] There are conflicts between civil liberty (the patient's right to chose) and public health (the population's right to prevent/treat disease). In the UK, compulsory admission and detention under the Public Health Act are possible but compulsory treatment is not allowed. The balance between the rights of the patient and those of the general public varies from country to country.

Corticosteroids

There is evidence to support the addition of corticosteroids to antituberculosis drugs for endobronchial disease in children[90] and there may be a place for them in pleural effusion,[91] in patients with extensive pulmonary disease[92] and to suppress hypersensitivity reactions to antituberculosis drugs.[92] Because of enzyme induction the maintenance dose of corticosteroid taken for other conditions should be doubled if rifampicin is used.[93]

Management of drug reactions

All drugs can cause adverse reactions (set out above) but most are minor and self-limiting gastrointestinal upsets. Treatment has to be temporarily or permanently changed with drug withdrawal in 5–10% of cases.[19] The most serious reactions are those involving hepatitis caused by pyrazinamide, rifampicin and isoniazid; rashes occur mainly with pyrazinamide but also with rifampicin and streptomycin; vestibular damage occurs with streptomycin and optic neuritis with ethambutol. Detailed advice on the management of hepatic reactions has recently been published.[13,72] Alternative treatment will be needed if the patient is still potentially infectious.[13] If a drug (or drugs) has to be withdrawn permanently, there will be the need for an individually tailored drug regimen to which the organism is known, or thought likely, to be susceptible. Occasionally, reserve drugs have to be used when the potential hepatotoxicity of ethionamide/prothionamide and the macrolides have to be considered. If the choice of agents is limited, e.g. in drug-resistant cases, desensitisation and reintroduction of the offending drug, under cover of other drugs and using conventional protocols, may be needed.[13] Peripheral neuropathy from isoniazid can be prevented by administration of pyridoxine, vitamin B_6, in a dose of 10 mg/day. This is only required for those at higher risk of peripheral neuropathy such as those with diabetes, malnutrition, renal failure or HIV positivity.[13]

Management of drug resistance

Because of the increasing proportion of cases in the UK and in other developed countries coming from ethnic minority groups with higher rates of drug resistance, and involving persons with a possible history of prior treatment or HIV coinfection, it is essential to confirm the diagnosis bacteriologically whenever possible. This also allows drug susceptibility tests. In patients with respiratory disease unable to produce sputum, confirmation may involve fibreoptic bronchoscopy and bronchial washings and lavage, or gastric lavage in children. Such samples, and biopsies from respiratory (mediastinal gland, pleura or endobronchial) or extrapulmonary sites (e.g. lymph nodes) sent for TB culture must not be placed in formalin or similar agents. Risk factors for drug resistance in the UK are a history of prior treatment or of HIV positivity, both independent of ethnic group, and ethnicity, particularly those of Indian subcontinent or black African ethnic origin.[94]

Isolated resistances

Streptomycin resistance

In ethnic minority groups in particular, some of the drug resistance seen is to streptomycin alone. The efficacy of the standard recommended regimen is not affected by this and standard treatment can be given without modification.[13]

Isoniazid resistance

In ethnic minority patients and in those who are HIV-positive, higher rates of isoniazid resistance are found. In the UK these are in the order of 4–6%,[1,94] whereas isoniazid resistance is uncommon (< 2%) in previously untreated white patients.[1,94] If isoniazid resistance is known before treatment commences, a fully supervised regimen of 2 months of rifampicin, pyrazinamide, ethambutol and streptomycin, followed by rifampicin and ethambutol for 7 months more gives good results.[95] Although there is some evidence that the standard regimen may be effective in isoniazid resistance,[96] in developed countries it is considered safer to stop the isoniazid and alter the regimen.[13] Ethambutol (15 mg/kg) and rifampicin should be given together for a minimum of 12 months, together with pyrazinamide for 2 months.[13]

Pyrazinamide resistance

Mycobacterium bovis is genetically resistant to pyrazinamide. If the infecting organism is *M. bovis* without other resistance, a regimen of rifampicin and isoniazid for 9 months supplemented by 2 months' initial ethambutol should be used.[13] Isolated resistance of *M. tuberculosis* to pyrazinamide is rare but should be treated with the same regimen as for *M. bovis*.

Ethambutol resistance

This isolated resistance is uncommon. It can be treated with the 6-month regimen of rifampicin and isoniazid supplemented by 2 months' initial pyrazinamide.[13]

Rifampicin resistance

Isolated rifampicin resistance is uncommon. In the UK rifampicin resistance is a marker for MDR-TB in over 90% of cases[13] and cases showing rifampicin resistance, particularly if shown on molecular probes,[97,98] should be treated and isolated as for MDR-TB until the full susceptibility pattern is known. The molecular probes used to determine rifampicin resistance on positive sputum microscopy smear or positive culture have approximately 95% accuracy when compared with conventional drug susceptibility testing.[97,98] Tests for rifampicin resistance in primary specimens are becoming available[99] but should be used only as a guide, a rifampicin-based regimen being used with two or three additional drugs added until full conventional drug susceptibility results are available.[13]

If true isolated rifampicin resistance is confirmed, treatment should be modified to an 18-month regimen of isoniazid and ethambutol, supplemented by an initial 2 months of pyrazinamide.[13]

Combined resistances other than multi-drug-resistant tuberculosis

Combined resistance to isoniazid and streptomycin is the commonest dual resistance; management as for isolated isoniazid resistance found after initiation of treatment is recommended but with treatment fully supervised throughout.[13] Other non-MDR-TB dual resistances are uncommon and need an individual regimen planned with advice from experienced clinicians based on wider drug susceptibility test results.[13]

Multidrug-resistant tuberculosis

This is defined as high-level resistance to rifampicin and isoniazid with or without resistance to additional drugs. It is very serious, as the main killing drug (isoniazid) and the main sterilising drug (rifampicin) are lost. Treatment of such cases is difficult for both physician and patient, complex and prolonged. It is recommended by the British Thoracic Society and supported by the ERS/WHO,[68] that such cases should be managed:

- *only* by physicians with substantial experience in managing complex drug resistant cases
- *only* in hospitals with appropriate negative-pressure isolation facilities
- only in close collaboration with mycobacteriology services.

If the first two criteria are not met the patient should be transferred to a unit where they are. Treatment has to be planned on an individual basis[100,101] and needs to include reserve drugs. These drugs include:

- Capreomycin, kanamycin, amikacin or streptomycin
- Ciprofloxacin or ofloxacin
- Cycloserine
- Ethionamide or prothionamide
- Rifabutin*
- Clarithromycin or azithromycin
- Thiacetazone
- Clofazimine
- PAS sodium

(*not advised unless full susceptibility confirmed).

Initial treatment should be with five or more drugs, including an injectable agent where possible, to which the organism is, or is thought likely to be, susceptible, and continued until sputum cultures become negative. Drug treatment should then continue with a minimum of three drugs to which the organism has been proved to be susceptible for a minimum of 9 further months.[13] Cultures should be persistently negative for at least this period, and treatment may be needed for up to or beyond 24 months, depending on the drug susceptibility pattern, the drugs available and the patient's HIV status.[101] Sometimes, for localised unilateral disease, surgical resection under drug cover is an option.[101] Because of the greater side-effect profile of many 'reserve' drugs, but particularly to prevent the emergence of any further acquired resistance, full compliance is essential, and so *all* treatment, both inpatient and outpatient, should be directly observed throughout. Different infection control procedures also apply.[36,57]

Such cases have a much worse prognosis than those involving fully susceptible organisms, particularly if the patient is HIV-positive,[102] but some patients survive following scrupulous treatment and monitoring.[103] Follow-up after completion of treatment should be indefinite.[13]

The management of close contacts of MDR-TB who fulfil the criteria for chemoprophylaxis (see above) is contentious. There

are no good data on which to base advice. If the drug susceptibility pattern is not known, giving pyrazinamide with ciprofloxacin or ofloxacin has been suggested.[104] The US Centers for Disease Control suggest this combination or ethambutol or pyrazinamide.[105] Such regimens may not be possible because of either drug toxicity or inappropriateness in the light of the drug susceptibility pattern. In the UK close clinical monitoring and follow-up without chemoprophylaxis is recommended until more data are available.[13]

Monitoring and compliance assessment during treatment

Each case should be notified to the proper authorities both for statistical and epidemiological purposes but also so that appropriate contact tracing (Chapter 38.3) can be undertaken.[13,106] Most patients do not require admission to hospital and can be treated and supervised as outpatients. If an HIV-negative patient is admitted to hospital and sputum is microscopy-positive for acid-fast bacilli, segregation for reasons of infectivity is generally only required for 2 weeks. Such patients become non-infectious within 2 weeks of treatment.[13,48] Different criteria apply in the control of infection in HIV-positive patients and those with MDR-TB.[36,57]

In individuals infected with HIV, tuberculosis, pulmonary and non-pulmonary, is an AIDS-defining illness. HIV testing, with informed consent and counselling, should be considered in all cases of tuberculosis, especially if a risk assessment suggests the patient to be from an area or background with an increased risk of coinfection.[13]

Liver function tests only need to be performed in those with pre-existing liver disease or if symptoms develop suggesting hepatitis – sudden deterioration, jaundice or vomiting. Patients taking ethambutol should be advised to report any change in vision.

Compliance with the drug regimen is the major determinant of outcome.[107] Specialist TB nurses or health visitors have vital roles in monitoring patient compliance with treatment, detecting possible side effects and confirming the accuracy and continuity of prescribing. If DOT is not being used, tablet checks and random urine tests should be carried out at least monthly throughout treatment.[13] If combination tablets are used for both initial and continuation phases, the rifampicin component can be used as the marker for treatment compliance. Non-compliance with self-medication detected during monitoring should lead to a switch to a fully supervised regimen.

Clinical follow-up should be at least monthly initially and then 2-monthly, with the early follow-up being used to reinforce patient education. Sputum microscopy and culture should be done monthly if the patient is producing sputum, and definitely 2 months prior to the planned treatment cessation if the clinical progress is unsatisfactory or there are compliance doubts. Failure during chemotherapy in patients prescribed an effective regimen is almost invariably due to poor compliance, which may also have induced drug resistance. A single drug must never be added to a failing regimen, as such an addition in the presence of regimen failure is only likely to add sequential additional drug resistance. It must be assumed that failure during chemotherapy is due, at least in part, to acquired resistance to some/all drugs. Repeat cultures and drug susceptibility tests should be performed and molecular probes for rifampicin resistance considered. If rifampicin resistance is reported, treatment and isolation should be as for MDR-TB until full susceptibility data are available.

Re-treatment after treatment failure should follow a recommended re-treatment regimen[68] or be with an appropriate regimen for susceptible or resistant organisms[13] based on drug susceptibility data. Treatment should be fully supervised throughout for any re-treatment regimen.

Outcome/programme monitoring

In the UK, when the recommended regimen has been given to patients with fully susceptible organisms, relapse is uncommon (0–3%) if there has been good compliance. If compliance has been good and there are no residual clinical problems, follow-up after cessation of treatment is not necessary. The patient and family practitioner should be advised of the need for re-referral should symptoms recur. Follow-up is only required for:

- patients with residual clinical problems
- patients with doubts about compliance
- patients with drug resistant organisms (excluding isolated streptomycin resistance), who should be followed up for at least 12 months.[13] In those with MDR-TB, particularly if HIV-positive, follow-up should be long-term.[13]

Therapeutic principles

- Short-course chemotherapy for 6 months is the standard evidence-based treatment.

- Pretreatment liver function should be measured; renal function and visual acuity should be checked if ethambutol is to be used.

- First-line drugs vary in their killing ability, sterilising ability and ability to prevent the emergence of drug resistance.

- Combination tablets rather than individual drugs should be used whenever possible to aid compliance and avoid monotherapy for disease.

- Standard treatment can be given in pregnancy.

- Patients should be informed of potential side-effects and there should be an action plan for implementation if these develop.

- Standard regimens should be varied only in cases with drug intolerance or resistance.

- Multi-drug-resistant tuberculosis should be treated only in appropriate isolation facilities, by someone experienced in treating such cases and with an individualised regimen.

- Different regimens are used in treatment and prophylaxis because of the different bacterial loads and the potential risks of development of drug resistance.

The overall effectiveness of a local/unit TB programme should be monitored. Recently, outcome criteria have been agreed for Europe.[108] Definite pulmonary cases are those confirmed on sputum microscopy or culture; those 'other than definite' are those where a clinician feels that the patient's clinical and/or radiological signs and/or symptoms are compatible with TB and the patient is treated with a full course of chemotherapy. Definitions of treatment outcome are as follows.[68,108]

For cases confirmed by sputum microscopy:

- **Cured**: sputum smears negative on two occasions during the continuation phase of treatment
- **Treatment completed**: documented treatment completion but no sputum-smear microscopy available at the end of treatment
- **Treatment failure**: sputum smears remaining or becoming positive again after 5 months or more of treatment.

For cases confirmed only by sputum culture:

- **Cured**: documented conversion of culture during the continuation phase
- **Treatment completed**: documented treatment completion but no documented culture conversion
- **Treatment failure**: culture remaining or becoming positive again after 5 months or more of treatment.

For both microscopy-confirmed and culture-confirmed cases

- **Death**: death of the patient irrespective of the cause at any time before the envisaged end of treatment
- **Treatment interrupted**: patient off treatment for 2 or more months, failure to complete treatment within 9 months for a 6-month regimen or within 12 months for a 9-month regimen, or drug intake less than 80%
- **Transfer out**: patient referred to another clinician/unit for treatment for whom information on treatment outcome cannot be obtained.

The sum of cases cured and completing treatment represent cases 'treated successfully'. Some authors have suggested that, in a monitored programme if treatment success rates do not exceed 90%, a switch to a universal DOT strategy should be made.[84]

? Unresolved questions

- Can a regimen of less than 6 months' duration be used in smear- and culture-negative disease with an acceptably low relapse rate (< 5%)?

- What should the exact role of polymerase chain reaction technology be in the diagnostic algorithm?

- What proportion of patients should be treated with directly observed therapy: should its use be universal or selective?

- What is the best regimen for chemoprophylaxis (preventive therapy)?

References

1. Rose AMC, Watson JM, Graham C et al. Tuberculosis at the turn of the century: results of a national survey. Thorax 2001; 56: 173–179.
2. Dye C, Scheele S, Dolin P et al. Consensus statement. Global burden of tuberculosis: estimated incidence, prevalence and mortality by country. World Health Organization Global Surveillance and Monitoring Project. JAMA 1999; 18: 677–686.
3. Dormandy T. The white death – a history of tuberculosis. London: Hambledon Press; 1999.
4. Davies PDO. Tuberculosis and migration. In: Clinical tuberculosis, 2nd edn. London: Chapman & Hall; 1998: 365–382.
5. Phillips MS, Kinnear WJM, Schneerson JM. Late sequelae of tuberculosis treated by thoracoplasty. Thorax 1987; 42: 445–451.
6. Fox W, Mitchison DA. Whither short course chemotherapy? Bull Int Union Tuberc 1981; 56: 135–155.
7. Pablos-Mendez A, Raviglione MC, Laszlo A et al. Global surveillance for antituberculosis drug resistance, 1994–97. N Engl J Med 1998; 338: 1641–1649.
8. Brock RC. Post-tuberculous bronchostenosis and the middle lobe syndrome. Thorax 1950; 5: 5–39.
9. Wallgren A. The timetable of tuberculosis. Tubercle 1948; 29: 245–251.
10. Blacklock JWS. Tuberculous disease in children: its pathology and bacteriology. Medical Research Council, Special Report Series 172. London: HMSO; 1932.
11. Ormerod LP, Skinner C. Reinfection tuberculosis: two cases in the family of a patient with drug resistant disease. Thorax 1980; 42: 986–987.
12. Godfrey-Fausett P, Githui W, Batchelor B et al. Recurrence of HIV-related tuberculosis in an endemic area may be due to relapse or re-infection. Tuberc Lung Dis 1994; 75: 199–202.
13. Joint Tuberculosis Committee of the British Thoracic Society. Chemotherapy and management of tuberculosis in the United Kingdom: recommendations 1998. Thorax 1998; 53: 536–548.
14. Sahn SA, Neff TA. Miliary tuberculosis. Am J Med 1974; 56: 495–505.
15. Heap MJ, Bion JF, Hunter KR. Miliary tuberculosis and the adult respiratory distress syndrome. Respir Med 1989; 83: 153–156.
16. Sime PJ, Chilvers ER, Leitch AG. Miliary tuberculosis in Edinburgh – a comparison between 1984–92 and 1954–67. Respir Med 1994; 88: 609–611.
17. Kumar D, Watson JM, Charlett A et al. Tuberculosis in England and Wales in 1993: results of a national survey. Thorax 1997; 52: 1060–1067.
18. Ormerod LP, Bentley C. The management of pulmonary tuberculosis in England and Wales in 1993. J R Coll Phys Lond 1997; 31: 662–665.
19. Humphries MJ, Byfield SP, Darbyshire JH et al. Deaths occurring in newly notified patients with pulmonary tuberculosis in England and Wales. Br J Dis Chest 1984; 78: 149–158.
20. Cullinan P, Meredith SK. Deaths in adults with notified pulmonary tuberculosis 1983–5. Thorax 1991; 46: 347–350.
21. Snider GL, Doctor L, Demas TA et al. Obstructive airway disease in patients with treated pulmonary tuberculosis. Am Rev Respir Dis 1971; 103: 625–640.
22. Sternitz R. Pulmonary tuberculosis and carcinoma of the lung: a survey from two population based disease registers. Am Rev Respir Dis 1965; 92: 758–766.
23. Chang SC, Lee PY, Perng RP. Lower lung field tuberculosis. Chest 1987; 91: 230–232.
24. Medical Research Council Tuberculosis and Lung Diseases Unit. National survey of tuberculosis notifications in England and Wales 1983; characteristics of disease. Tubercle 1987; 68: 19–32.
25. Harries AD. Tuberculosis and HIV infection in developing countries. Lancet 1990; 335: 387–390.
26. Price M. Lymphangitis reticularis tuberculosa. Tubercle 1968; 49: 377–384.
27. Im JG, Itoh H, Shim YS et al. Pulmonary tuberculosis: CT findings – early active disease and sequential change with antituberculosis therapy. Radiology 1993; 186: 653–660.
28. Maartens G, Bateman ED. Tuberculous pleural effusions: increased culture yield with bedside innoculation of pleural fluid and poor diagnostic yield. Thorax 1991; 46: 96–99.
29. Ocana I, Martinez-Vazquez JM, Segura RM et al. Adenosine deaminase in pleural fluid: test for diagnosis of tuberculous pleural effusion. Chest 1983; 84: 51–53.
30. Mungall IPF, Cowen PN, Cooke NT et al. Multiple pleural biopsy with the Abrams needle. Thorax 1981; 35: 600–602.
31. DHSS. A code of practice for the prevention of infection in clinical laboratories. Department of of Health and Social Security. London: HMSO; 1978.
32. Shears P, Rhodes LE, Syed Q, Watson J. A pseudo outbreak of tuberculosis. Commun Dis Rev 1994; 4: R9–10.
33. Zaher F, Marks J. Methods and medium for the culture of tubercle bacilli. Tubercle 1977 58: 143–145.
34. Body BA, Warren NG, Spicer A et al. Use of Gen-Probe and BACTEC for rapid isolation and identification of mycobacteria. Correlation of probe results with growth index. Am J Clin Pathol 1990; 93: 415–420.
35. De Beenhonwer H, Lhiang Z, Jannes G et al. Rapid detection of rifampicin resistance in sputum and biopsy specimens from tuberculosis patients with PCR and line probe assay. Tuberc Lung Dis 1995; 76: 425–430.
36. Interdepartmental Working Group on Tuberculosis. The prevention and control of tuberculosis in the United Kingdom. UK guidance on the prevention and control of transmission of 1. HIV related tuberculosis 2. Drug-resistant, including multiple drug-resistant, tuberculosis. London: Department of Health, Scottish Office, Welsh Office; September 1998.
37. Brisson-Noel A, Gicguel B, Lecossier D et al. Rapid diagnosis of tuberculosis by amplification of mycobacterial DNA in clinical samples. Lancet 1989; 2: 1069–1071.
38. Clarridge JE, Shawar RM, Shinnick TM, Plikaytis BB. Large scale use of polymerase chain reaction for detection of *Mycobacterium tuberculosis* in a routine Mycobacteriology laboratory. J Clin Microbiol 1993; 31: 2049–2056.
39. Shaw RJ, Taylor GM. Polymerase chain reaction: applications for diagnosis drug sensitivity and strain identification of *M. tuberculosis* complex. In: Davies PDO, ed. Clinical tuberculosis, 2nd ed. London: Chapman & Hall; 1998: 97–110.
40. Joint Tuberculosis Committee of the British Thoracic Society. Guidelines on the management of tuberculosis and HIV infection in the United Kingdom. Br Med J 1992; 304: 1231–1233.
41. Willcox PA, Benatar SR, Potgeiter PD. Use of the flexible fibreoptic bronchoscope in the diagnosis of sputum negative pulmonary tuberculosis. Thorax 1982; 37: 598–601.
42. Funahashi A, Lohaus GH, Politis J et al. Role of fibreoptic bronchoscopy in the diagnosis of mycobacterial diseases. Thorax 1983; 38: 267–270.
43. De Garcia J, Curull V, Vidal R et al. Diagnostic value of bronchoalveolar lavage in suspected pulmonary tuberculosis. Chest 1988; 93: 329–332.
44. Wallace JM, Deutsch AL, Harrell JM et al. Bronchoscopy and transbronchial biopsy in the evaluation of patients with suspected acute tuberculosis. Am J Med 1981; 70: 1189–1194.
45. Wilkins EGL. Antibody detection in tuberculosis. In: Davies PDO, ed. Clinical tuberculosis, 2nd ed. London: Chapman & Hall; 1998: 81–96.
46. Morris CDW, Bird AR, Nell H. Haematological and biochemical changes in severe pulmonary tuberculosis. Q J Med 1989; 73: 1151–1159.
47. Jindani A, Aber VR, Edwards EA, Mitchison DA. The early bactericidal activity of drugs in patients with pulmonary tuberculosis. Am Rev Respir Dis 1980; 121: 139–148.
48. Ormerod LP. Chemotherapy of tuberculosis. Eur Respir Monograph 1997; 2 (monograph 4): 273–297.
49. Singapore Tuberculosis Service/British Medical Research Council. Clinical trial of 6-month and 4-month regimens of chemotherapy in the treatment of pulmonary tuberculosis. Am Rev Respir Dis 1979; 119: 579–585.
50. British Thoracic Association. Short course chemotherapy in pulmonary tuberculosis. Lancet 1980; 1: 1182–1183.
51. Ferebee SH. Controlled chemoprophylaxis trials in tuberculosis: a general review. Adv Tuberc Res 1969; 17: 29–106.
52. Thompson NJ. Efficacy of various durations of isoniazid preventive therapy in tuberculosis: 5 years of follow-up in the IUATLD trial. Bull WHO 1982; 60: 555–564.
53. Hong Kong Chest Service, Tuberculosis Research Centre Madras and British Medical Research Council. A double-blind placebo-controlled clinical trial of three antituberculosis chemoprophylaxis regimens in patients with silicosis in Hong Kong. Am Rev Respir Dis 1992; 145: 36–41.
54. Ormerod LP. Rifampicin and isoniazid prophylactic therapy for tuberculosis. Arch Dis Child 1998; 78: 169–171.
55. Mwinga A, Hosp M, Godfrey-Faucett P et al. Twice weekly tuberculosis preventive therapy in HIV infection in Zambia. AIDS 1998; 12: 2447–2457.
56. Halsey NA, Coberly JS, Desormeaux J et al. Randomized trial of isoniazid versus rifampicin and pyrazinamide for prevention of tuberculosis in HIV-1 infection. Lancet 1998; 351: 786–792.
57. Joint Tuberculosis Committee of the British Thoracic Society. Control and prevention of tuberculosis in the United Kingdom: Code of Practice 2000. Thorax 2000; 55: 887–901.
58. American Thoracic Society and Centers for Disease Control and Prevention. Targeted tuberculin testing and treatment of latent tuberculosis infection. Am J Respir Crit Care Med 2000; 161: S221–S249.

59. Jin D, Gross C. Mapping and sequencing of mutations in the *Escherichia coli* *rpoB* gene that lead to rifampicin resistance. J Mol Biol 1988; 202: 45–58.

60. Pozniak A, Miller R, Ormerod LP. The treatment of tuberculosis in HIV-infected persons. AIDS 1999; 13: 435–445.

61. Ellard GA, Humphries MJ, Gabriel M, Teoh R. Cerebrospinal fluid and serum levels of pyrazinamide and rifampicin in patients with TB meningitis. Curr Ther Res 1987; 42: 235–242.

62. Telenti A, Philipp WJ, Sreevatsan S et al. The *emb* operon, a gene cluster of *Mycobacterium tuberculosis* involved in resistance to ethambutol. Nat Med 1997; 3: 567–570.

63. Liebold JE. The ocular toxicity of ethambutol and its relation to dose. Ann NY Acad Sci 1966; 135: 904–909.

64. Citron KM, Thomas GO. Ocular toxicity from ethambutol. Thorax 1986; 41: 737–739.

65. Nunn P, Kibuya D, Gathua S et al. Cutaneous hypersensitivity reaction due to thiacetazone in HIV seropositive patients treated for tuberculosis. Lancet 1991; 337: 627–630.

66. Petrie JG, Barnwell E, Grimshaw J on behalf of the Scottish Intercollegiate Guidelines Network. Clinical guidelines: criteria for appraisal for national use. Edinburgh: Royal College of Physicians; 1995.

67. Public Health Laboratory Service Communicable Disease Surveillance Centre database/website.

68. Task Force of the European Respiratory Society, World Health Organization and the Europe Region of the International Union against Tuberculosis and Lung Disease. Tuberculosis management in Europe. Eur Respir J 1999; 14: 978–992.

69. American Thoracic Society. Treatment of tuberculosis and tuberculosis infection in adults and children. Am J Respir Crit Care Med 1994; 149: 1359–1374.

70. Hendy M, Stableforth DE. The effect of established diabetes mellitus on the presentation of infiltrative pulmonary tuberculosis in the immigrant Asian community of an inner city area of the United Kingdom. Br J Dis Chest 1983; 77: 87–89.

71. British Thoracic Association. A controlled trial of 6-months chemotherapy in pulmonary tuberculosis. First report: results during chemotherapy. Br J Dis Chest 1981; 75: 141–153.

72. Ormerod LP, Skinner C, Wales JM. Hepatotoxicity of antituberculosis drugs. Thorax 1996; 51: 111–113.

73. Burn R, Ashley C, ed. The renal drug handbook. Oxford: Radcliffe Medical Press. 1999: 147.

74. Hong Kong Chest Service/Tuberculosis Research Centre Madras/British Medical Research Council. A controlled clinical comparison of 6 and 8 months of antituberculosis chemotherapy in the treatment of patients with silicotuberculosis in Hong Kong. Am Rev Respir Dis 1991; 143: 262–267.

75. Perriens JH, St Louis ME, Yiadiul B et al. Pulmonary tuberculosis in HIV-infected patients in Zaire. N Engl Med J 1995; 332: 779–784.

76. Grosset JH. Treatment of tuberculosis in HIV infection. Tuberc Lung Dis 1992; 73: 378–383.

77. Ackah AN, Coulibaly D, Digbeu H et al. Response to treatment, mortality and CD4 lymphocyte counts in HIV-infected persons with tuberculosis in Abidjan, Cote D'Ivoire. Lancet 1995; 345: 607–610.

78. Englehard D, Sutman HR, Marks MI. Interaction of ketoconazole with rifampicin and isoniazid. N Engl J Med 1994; 311: 1681–1683.

79. Lazar JD, Wilner KD. Drug interactions with fluconazole. Rev Infect Dis 1990; 12(suppl. 3): S327–S333.

80. Heyden R, Miller R. Adverse effects and drug interactions of medications commonly used in the treatment of adult HIV positive patients. Genitourin Med 1996; 72: 237–246.

81. Heyden R, Miller R. Adverse effects and drug interactions of medications commonly used in the treatment of adult HIV positive patients: part 2. Genitourin Med 1997; 73: 5–11.

82. McGregor MM, Olliaro P, Wolramans L et al. Efficacy and safety of rifabutin in the treatment of patients with newly diagnosed pulmonary tuberculosis. Am J Respir Crit Care Med 1996; 154: 1462–1467.

83. Kunimoto DY, Chiu L, Nobert E, Houston S. Immune mediated 'HAART' attack during treatment for tuberculosis. Int J Tuberc Lung Dis 1999; 3: 944–947.

84. Morse DI. Directly observed therapy for tuberculosis. Br Med J 1996; 312: 719–720.

85. China Tuberculosis Control Collaboration. Results of directly observed short-course chemotherapy in 12,842 Chinese patients with smear-positive tuberculosis. Lancet 1996; 347: 358–362.

86. Zwarenstein M, Schoeman JH, Vundule C et al. Randomised controlled trial of self-supervised and directly observed treatment for tuberculosis. Lancet 1998; 352: 1340–1343.

87. Centers for Disease Control. Initial therapy for tuberculosis in the era of multidrug resistance: recommendations of the advisory council for the elimination of tuberculosis. Morbidity Mortality Wkly Rep 1993; 42: RR-7.

88. Miller B, Plamer CS, Halpern MT et al. Decision model to assess the cost-effectiveness of DOT for tuberculosis. Tuberc Lung Dis 1996; 77(suppl. 2): 74–75.

89. Moore RD, Chaulk CP, Griffiths R et al. Cost effectiveness of directly observed therapy versus self administered therapy for tuberculosis. Am J Respir Crit Care Med 1996; 154: 1013–1019.

90. Toppet M, Malfroot A, Derde MP et al. Corticosteroids in primary tuberculosis with bronchial obstruction. Arch Dis Child 1990; 65: 1222–1226.

91. Lee CH, Wang WJ, Lan RS et al. Corticosteroids in the treatment of tuberculosis pleurisy. A double blind, placebo controlled, randomised study. Chest 1988; 94: 1256–1259.

92. Horne NW. A critical evaluation of corticosteroids in tuberculosis. Adv Tuberc Res 1966; 15: 1–54.

93. Edwards OM, Courtney-Evans RJ, Galley JM et al. Changes in cortisol metabolism following rifampicin therapy. Lancet 1974; 2: 549–551.

94. Hayward AC, Bennett DE, Herbert J et al. Risk factors for drug resistance in patients with tuberculosis in England and Wales 1993–4. Thorax 1996; 51(suppl, 3): S32.

95. Babu Swai O, Alnoch JA, Githui WA et al. Controlled clinical trial of a regimen of two durations for the treatment of isoniazid resistant tuberculosis. Tubercle 1988; 69: 5–14.

96. Mitchison DA, Nunn AJ. Influence of initial drug resistance on the response to short course chemotherapy in pulmonary tuberculosis. Am Rev Respir Dis 1986; 133: 423–430.

97. Telenti A, Imboden P, Marchesi F et al. Detection of the rifampicin-resistance mutation in *Mycobacterium tuberculosis*. Lancet 1993; 341: 647–650.

98. Drobniewski FA, Pozniak AL. Molecular diagnosis, detection of drug resistance and epidemiology of tuberculosis. Br J Hosp Med 1996; 56: 204–208.

99. Goyal M, Shaw RJ, Banerjee DK et al. Rapid detection of multidrug-resistant tuberculosis. Eur Respir J 1997; 10: 120–124.

100. Goble M, Iseman M, Madsen LA et al. Treatment of 171 patients with pulmonary tuberculosis resistant to isoniazid and rifampin. N Engl J Med 1993; 328: 527–532.

101. Iseman M. Treatment of multidrug-resistant tuberculosis. N Engl J Med 1993; 328: 784–790.

102. Centres for Disease Control. Nosocomial transmission of Multidrug Resistant Tuberculosis among HIV-infected persons – Florida and New York, 1988–1991. Morbidity Mortality Wkly Rep 1991; 40: 585–590.

103. Drobniewski FA. Is death inevitable with multiresistant tuberculosis plus HIV infection? Lancet 1997; 328: 71–72.

104. Gallagher CT, Passannante MR, Reichman LB. Preventive therapy for multidrug resistant tuberculosis (MDR tuberculosis): a Delphi survey. Am Rev Respir Dis 1992; 145: abstract.

105. Anonymous. Management of persons exposed to multidrug resistant tuberculosis. Morbidity Mortality Wkly Rep 1992; 41: 61–71.

106. Ormerod LP, Watson JM, Pozniak A et al. Notification of tuberculosis: an updated code of practice for England and Wales. J Roy Coll Phys Lond 1997; 31: 299–303.

107. Ormerod LP, Prescott R. Inter-relations between relapses, drug regimens and compliance with treatment in tuberculosis. Br J Dis Chest 1991; 85: 239–242.

108. Veen J, Raviglione MC, Reider HL et al. Standardised outcome monitoring in Europe: recommendations of a Working Group of the WHO and IUATLD (Europe Region). Eur Respir J 1998; 12: 505–510.

38.3 The control of tuberculosis

Peter D O Davies

 Key points

Control of tuberculosis requires

- Effective treatment of disease in clinically affected patients
- Active case finding in high-risk groups:
  - Contacts of cases
  - Immigrants from high-incidence countries
  - The homeless and substance abusers
  - HIV-positive individuals
  - Subjects with predisposing conditions, e.g. renal failure, diabetes
- Preventive treatment of infected individuals
- Protection by BCG (where in accordance with national policy)
- Education of the community regarding relevant symptoms

There is an interesting divergence across the world in the of control of tuberculosis. In the developing world health-care systems are being strained to breaking point by the increase in cases of tuberculosis due to a combination of factors, principally population increase, human immunodeficiency virus (HIV), poverty and a breakdown of national tuberculosis programmes.[1-3] These nations are struggling to treat even infectious, smear-positive cases. On the other hand, many developed nations are also experiencing an increase in case-load, mainly because of immmigration from developing countries.[4,5] Here, where resources are good and case-finding and cure are the rule, the emphasis is now on elimination by giving preventive treatment to those with latent tuberculosis infection.[6] Those at increased risk of infection, such as immigrants from developing countries, are being screened and preventive therapy is being given to those who are tuberculin positive.[6] In terms of cost-effectiveness, the cure of patients in their country of origin to control disease there is likely to prove cheaper than preventive therapy to many who might never develop disease.

The reason for the disparity is evident from Table 38.3.1, which shows rates of disease increasing in most areas except western Europe, where they are estimated to remain steady or decline.

Principles of disease control

There are three principal methods of controlling tuberculosis in the community:

- The identification and treatment of patients with the disease
- The screening of individuals with a high risk of developing disease and giving preventive therapy to selected individuals with latent infection
- The protection from infection of the rest of the community by screening and immunisation as appropriate.

Exactly what measures are used to carry out these steps will depend on the resources available and the overall prevalence of the disease in the community or country concerned. In a developed country adequate resources should be available and the prevalence of disease is likely to be low. The younger indigenous population is unlikely to be infected and only elderly people are at any appreciable risk of disease, resulting from a recrudescence of endogenous infection incurred many years previously. Within a developed country there are likely to be minority groups at high risk of disease, such as the homeless or ethnic minorities, and services may need to be targeted at such groups. In a developing country, resources may be very limited and the prevalence of disease so high that individuals are likely to incur infection in the first or second decades of life and develop disease in childhood or early adulthood. Here the emphasis should be on completion of treatment of cases, particularly those who are sputum-smear-positive and therefore likely to be infectious.

Control of disease in a low-prevalence country

Guidelines have been issued by the thoracic societies of the UK (BTS),[7] Europe (ERS)[8] and the USA (ATS),[6,9-13] which are appropriate for disease control in the relevant mainly low-prevalence countries.

Table 38.3.1 Estimated number of cases and rates of tuberculosis world-wide

Region	1990		1995		2000		2005	
	Cases (thousands)	Rate*	Cases (thousands)	Rate*	Cases (thousands)	Rate*	Cases (thousands)	Rate*
Southern Asia	3106	237	3499	241	3952	247	4454	256
Western Pacific†	1839	136	2045	140	2255	144	2469	151
Africa	992	191	1467	242	2079	293	2849	345
Eastern Mediterranean	641	165	745	168	870	168	987	170
Americas‡	569	127	606	123	645	120	681	114
Eastern Europe§	194	47	202	47	210	48	218	49
Western Europe and others¶	196	23	204	23	211	24	217	24
All regions	**7537**	**143**	**8768**	**152**	**10222**	**163**	**11 875**	**176**
Percentage increase since 1990			16.3		35.6		57.6	

* Crude incidence rate per 100 000 population. † Includes all countries of the World Health Organization (WHO) Western Pacific region except Japan, Australia and New Zealand. ‡ Includes all countries of the WHO American region except the USA and Canada. § Includes all independent states of the former Union of Soviet Socialist Republics. ¶ Western Europe and the USA, Canada, Japan, Australia and New Zealand.

Identification of patients with disease

Methods of diagnosis and treatment are covered in Chapter 38.2. There are two important factors that may improve the speed with which patients with disease present to the appropriate tuberculosis services (passive case finding). These are: first, an awareness by individuals within a population that they may have tuberculosis, so that they present early for treatment; and second, the readiness of the primary health-care system, to which patients usually present, to consider the possibility of tuberculosis, to carry out the relevant investigations and to refer appropriately. The recent publicity that tuberculosis has received in many countries may help to improve public and professional awareness alike.

Notification

It is a statutory duty in the UK for a doctor who 'believes a patient to be suffering from tuberculosis' to notify that patient to the proper officer, usually the Consultant in Communicable Disease Control (CCDC) of the local authority in which the patient is normally resident.[14] Most developed countries have similar systems but definitions of what constitutes a 'case' of tuberculosis may vary. The purpose of notification is first to provide surveillance data of disease in an area and second to instigate contact tracing

Infectivity and isolation of patients

Only patients with sputum-smear-positive pulmonary tuberculosis are likely to be infectious and infectivity declines rapidly with treatment. If nursed in hospital, patients suspected or shown to be infectious should be kept in a side room with their own washing and toilet facilities until they have been on treatment for 2 weeks. No specific nursing procedures such as barrier nursing are required and no special cleaning of utensils is required beyond normal washing procedures.

As treatment rapidly renders the patient non-infectious, treating the patient at home exposes family contacts to negligible further risk of infection.

Patients with smear-negative or extrapulmonary disease do not need segregation.

Patients with infectious or non-infectious tuberculosis should not be allowed to come in contact with those who may be immunocompromised, particularly if HIV-seropositive. These individuals should be separated from cases of tuberculosis. Patients known to have, or at risk of having drug-resistant tuberculosis, especially multi-drug-resistant disease, require special segregation. Advice in the UK guidelines states that these persons should be nursed in a negative-pressure isolation room and that staff should be required to wear special tight fitting masks (PFR95).[7] Where such facilities are not available, exposure of room air to ultraviolet light offers a fairly effective alternative.

Risk to staff

Risk of infection and disease among health-care workers is variable. In the UK, microbiology technicians, mortuary attendants and ward carers have been shown to be at increased risk in different studies.[15–17] Evidence from developing countries, particularly Africa, suggests that health-care workers may be at considerable risk.[18]

The policy in the UK is for all staff to have pre-employment screening. Only those with suggestive symptoms need have a chest radiograph. If the worker has good evidence of previous bacillus Calmette–Guérin (BCG) vaccination, no further action is taken. If there is no history of having had BCG and no scar is present the worker has a tuberculin test and is offered BCG if this is negative. Workers who may be at risk because they have acquired HIV should be advised not to work in contact with patients with tuberculosis.

Staff in regular contact with cases of tuberculosis should be advised to obtain a chest X-ray if they develop symptoms that might be due to tuberculosis such as a chronic cough or weight loss.

Screening those at greatest risk

Individuals at greatest risk of tuberculosis include:

- Contacts of patients with active disease
- Recent immigrants from countries with a high prevalence of the disease
- Recent tuberculin converters
- Young children with a strongly positive tuberculin test
- Immunocompromised individuals, especially those infected with HIV
- Patients with certain medical conditions (Table 38.3.2)[6]
- Intravenous drug users.

Contact screening

Once a patient is notified, it is usually the responsibility of the public health authorities (in the UK this is the responsibility of the CCDC) to undertake contact tracing. This is usually carried out by a specialist tuberculosis health visitor in conjunction with the local respiratory service, where screening is carried out. It is important that personnel involved in screening are fully trained. Adequate screening requires not only a thorough knowledge of the disease by those involved but also good personal skills and tact to persuade potentially reluctant contacts to attend for screening.

Only those contacts of patients found to have acid-fast bacilli in a direct smear of the sputum (sputum-smear-positive disease) are at appreciable risk of infection and disease. Five contact studies in the UK, which included a total of 22 971 contacts, showed that up to 10% of tuberculosis cases were diagnosed by contact tracing and that disease is identified in about 1% of contacts. It is usually found at the first screening visit in unvaccinated, close contacts of smear-positive cases.

When a patient is notified the tuberculosis health visitor or other appropriately trained individual must first compile a list of

Table 38.3.2 Relative risk* for developing active tuberculosis, by selected clinical conditions

Clinical condition	Relative risk
Silicosis	30.0[37,38]
Diabetes mellitus	2.0–4.1[42–44]
Chronic renal failure/haemodialysis	10.0–25.3[39–41]
Gastrectomy	2.0–5.0[45–47]
Jejunoileal bypass	27.0–63.0[48,49]
Solid organ transplantation	
Renal	37.0[50]
Cardiac	20.0–74.0[51,52]
Carcinoma of head or neck	16.0[53]
* Relative to control population; independent of tuberculin-test status.	

contacts of the (index) patient. These may be divided into close contacts (defined as those sharing a kitchen or bathroom or closely associating with the index case, or others who may have been in close and frequent contact, usually those of the same household) and casual contacts, such as those at the same place of work or education. Each contact should then be offered an appointment to attend the relevant clinic. Where an index case has a large number of potentially relevant contacts the principle of the 'stone in the pond' in tracing can be employed.[24] By this method a relatively small number of casual contacts who are the most likely to have been infected are screened first. If these prove to be clear of disease no further screening is undertaken. If, however, some are shown to have evidence of recent infection or disease, contact tracing is widened.

For adults with smear-negative pulmonary disease or extrapulmonary disease, contact tracing is not usually required. However, contact tracing of children who have primary disease, including pleural or meningeal disease or erythema nodosum, should be undertaken to identify a possible source case.[25]

Screening procedure

In countries where BCG vaccination is undertaken routinely, all adults and teenagers who have received BCG vaccine should have a chest radiograph. Children, whether or not they have received previous BCG immunisation, should have a tuberculin test. This is most conveniently carried out using a Heaf multipuncture test. Alternatively, the Mantoux test can be used (see below).

Children with a strongly positive tuberculin test (Fig. 38.3.1) should have a chest radiograph. In the UK it is advised that those with a negative or weakly positive test (grade I Heaf) should receive BCG vaccine, or be tested 6 weeks later if their most recent contact with the untreated index case has been within 6 weeks of the test. Children with a strongly positive tuberculin test (Heaf grade IV) but normal chest radiograph should be considered for preventive therapy. Children from a high-risk group with a grade III or IV reaction, or a grade II reaction with no prior history of BCG immunisation, should also be considered for preventive therapy.

Children under the age of 2 years who are close contacts of a sputum-smear-positive case should receive preventive therapy as soon as the index case is diagnosed. Adults or children found to have tuberculosis on chest radiography should be treated with 6 months of chemotherapy in the usual fashion (Chapter 38.2).

Screening of recent immigrants

Successive notification surveys of tuberculosis in England and Wales have shown Asian immigrants and other ethnic minorities to have considerably higher rates of disease than native white individuals.

A survey of notifications of tuberculosis in England and Wales in 1998 showed that, with respect to the rate of disease in whites, those of African origin had rates more than 30 times greater, those of Indian ethnic origin rates 20 times greater and those of West Indian origin rates six times greater.[26]

All subjects entering a low-prevalence country from a high-prevalence country (the latter defined arbitrarily as a country

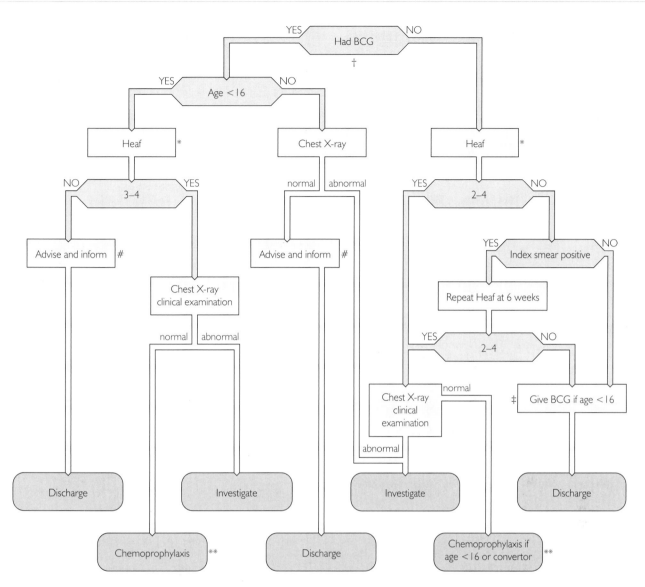

† Previous BCG cannot be accepted as evidence of immunity in HIV-positive subjects

* Negative test in immunocompromised subjects does not exclude tuberculous infection

Advise patient of tuberculosis symptoms, inform general practitioner of contact

** Persons eligible for, but not given, chemoprophylaxis should have follow up chest x-rays at 3 and 12 months

‡ See text

Figure 38.3.1 Examination of close contacts of pulmonary tuberculosis. Contacts of non-pulmonary tuberculosis need not usually be examined. Note: children under 2 who have not had bacillus Calmette–Guérin (BCG) vaccination who are close contacts of a smear-positive index patient should receive prophylaxis irrespective of tuberculin status.

with an incidence greater than 40/100 000 per annum) should be specifically screened for tuberculosis on, or as soon as possible after, arrival in the host country. This would include immigrants from most Asian and African countries. All such adults should have a chest radiograph and all children and teenagers should have a tuberculin test. Action should be as for close contacts. It is probably unproductive to continue to screen immigrants after the initial chest radiograph but health services and the individuals themselves should be advised that immigrants have an increased risk of disease for many years after migration

has taken place and that the diagnosis of tuberculosis should be considered if the patient presents with any symptoms that might be due to the disease.[27]

In the UK, children with a negative tuberculin test are offered BCG.

Tuberculin testing

The three principal methods for tuberculin testing are the Mantoux, Heaf and tine tests.

Mantoux test

For the Mantoux test, 0.1 ml of solution containing a known number of tuberculin units (TU) of purified protein derivative (PPD) of tuberculin is injected intradermally and the diameter of the induration is read 48–72 hours later. In the UK, PPD is supplied at three dilutions giving the number of international units per 0.1 ml injections as follows:

- 1:100   (1000 TU/ml)   100 TU/0.1 ml
- 1:1000   (100 TU/ml)   10 TU/0.1 ml
- 1:10 000   (10 TU/ml)   1 TU/0.1 ml.

The usual dose for tuberculin testing is 10 TU, i.e. 0.1 ml of 1:1000. In other countries, 5 TU is usually used for standard Mantoux testing.

Heaf test

The Heaf test is performed with a spring-loaded gun with a magnetic disposable head. After cleaning the skin on the volar surface of the forearm the Heaf gun is used to puncture through a drop of undiluted PPD (100 000 TU/ml), thus injecting the PPD into the dermis.

The reaction is read at 3–10 days as follows:

- Grade I: four or more discrete papules
- Grade II: confluent papules forming a ring
- Grade III: a disc of induration up to 10 mm in diameter.
- Grade IV: a disc of induration greater than 10 mm in diameter and/or vesiculation of the disc (Fig. 38.3.2).

The Heaf test is not recommended in several countries but remains the most convenient method of screening a large number of individuals at one time. The tine test is no longer recommended.

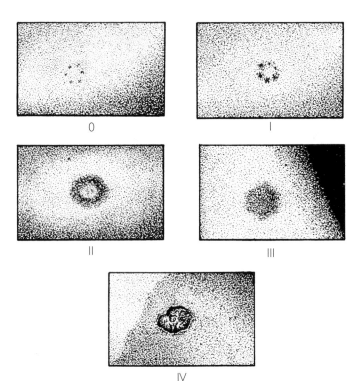

Figure 38.3.2 Results of Heaf multiple puncture test read at 3–10 days.

Interpretation of the tuberculin test

Heaf (or Mantoux) testing of a population of schoolchildren can be expected to provide a continuum of reactions. Approximately 90% may be expected to have a grade 0 or I reaction (equivalent to 9 mm of induration to 10 TU PPD by the Mantoux test). Only 5–6% will have grade III or IV Heaf (> 15 mm of induration to 10 TU), which in the UK is regarded as indicating infection by *Mycobacterium tuberculosis*.

Bacillus Calmette–Guérin vaccine can be expected to convert most (80%) individuals to Heaf grade I or II. Those who have had BCG vaccine with grade III or IV reactions should still be regarded as having infection by *M. tuberculosis*, although the proportion in these categories after BCG immunisation may be slightly increased (10%).

The cut-off point for a positive test (i.e. indicating infection with *M. tuberculosis*) may vary from country to country because tuberculin reactions are affected by exposure to environmental mycobacteria.

In the USA, where 5 TU of PPD is used in the standard Mantoux test, a differential cut-off point is used depending on the relative risk of the patient (Table 38.3.3).

Other groups at risk

Children who have had a pre-BCG tuberculin test and who have a significantly positive result (grade III or IV) should be screened. Those who have a grade II Heaf and no history of BCG immunisation do not require further follow-up (chest radiograph or chemotherapy) unless they are from a high-risk group.

Screening of close contacts of children with a grade IV reaction on pre-BCG testing should be considered, especially if the child is from a high-risk group.

Immunocompromised patients

Patients known to be immunocompromised as a result of HIV infection are at increased risk of becoming infected with the tubercle bacillus and, once infected, of progressing rapidly to disease.[28] All HIV-seropositive individuals should be tuberculin-tested. In low prevalence countries the tuberculin-postive HIV-positive patient should receive preventive therapy. From a series of trials, the usefulness of preventive therapy in the tuberculin-negative HIV-positive individual is less clear-cut. In a high-prevalence area where reinfection is likely the benefit of a limited course of preventive therapy is also less clear.[29-35]

High-risk institutions

Evidence from the USA suggests that residents of homes for elderly people are at increased risk of tuberculous infection and disease,[36] whereas evidence from the UK suggests that such individuals are not at increased risk.[37] Residents of prisons, common lodging houses and psychiatric hospitals have been found to have increased risk of disease. A survey of chest radiographs of individuals living rough in London who were admitted to sleep in communal accommodation showed that 12 of 642 had active disease.[38] The abandonment of mass miniature radiography in the UK has made screening of such individuals

Table 38.3.3 Criteria for tuberculin positivity, by risk group. Adapted from Centers for Disease Control and Prevention. Screening for tuberculosis and tuberculosis infection in high-risk populations: recommendations of the Advisory Council for the Elimination of Tuberculosis. MMWR 1995; 44 (No. RR-11): 19–34.

Reaction ≥ 5 mm of induration	Reaction ≥ 10 mm of induration	Reaction ≥ 15 mm of induration
Human-immunodeficiency-virus-positive persons Recent contacts of tuberculosis patients Fibrotic changes on chest radiograph consistent with prior tuberculosis Patients with organ transplants and other immunosuppressed patients (receiving the equivalent of 15 mg/d of prednisolone or more for 1 month or more[†]	Recent immigrants (i.e. within the last 5 years) from high-prevalence countries Injection drug users Residents and employees* of the following high-risk congregate settings: prisons and jails, nursing homes and other long-term facilities for the elderly, hospitals and other health-care facilities, residential facilities for patients with acquired immunodeficiency syndrome and shelters for the homeless Mycobacteriology laboratory personnel Persons with the following clinical conditions that place them at high risk: silicosis, diabetes mellitus, chronic renal failure, some haematological disorders (e.g. leukaemias and lymphomas), other specific malignancies (e.g. carcinoma of the head and neck or lung), weight loss of 10% or more of ideal body weight, gastrectomy and jejunoilieal bypass Children younger than 4 years of age, or infants, children and adolescents exposed to adults at high risk	Persons with no risk factors for tuberculosis

* For persons who are otherwise at low risk and are tested at the start of employment, a reaction ≥ 15 mm induration is considered positive.
† Risk of tuberculosis in patients treated with corticosteroids increases with higher dose and longer duration.

more difficult. One cheap, effective way of screening individuals who may have active, infectious disease is by direct smear of a sputum sample.

In the UK, the risk of disease in such institutions is not currently considered high enough to undertake regular screening but this policy should receive regular review.

Preventive therapy

Preventive therapy, formerly called chemoprophylaxis, is defined as primary when it is given to uninfected tuberculin-negative individuals, e.g. young children in contact with a mother with infectious pulmonary disease for whom separation from the mother is undesirable, to prevent infection.

Secondary preventive therapy refers to the use of antituberculosis drugs in infected (tuberculin-test-positive) individuals with no evidence of disease, to prevent its emergence. There is a wide variety of regimens recommended in the various guidelines summarised in Table 38.3.4.

Clinical follow-up to determine the development of possible adverse effects of the drugs is required. Routine biochemical

Table 38.3.4 Treatment regimens for preventive therapy. H, isoniazid; R, rifampicin; Z, pyrazinamide; E, ethambutol; Ofl, ofloxacin. Number before letter indicates number of months of therapy; subscript after letter indicates number of times a week by directly observed therapy.

Country	Recommended regimen
UK	6H 3HR
Europe	≥ 6H
USA	6 or 9H 6 or 9H_2 2RZ 2–3R_2Z_2 4R
For contacts of multi-drug-resistant tuberculosis	6–12ZE or ZOfl

Table 38.3.5 Groups recommended for preventive treatment

Category	UK[7]	Europe[8]	USA[6]
Human-immunodeficiency-virus (HIV)-infected persons	As for HIV-negative individuals		≥ 5 mm*
Contacts of cases	Age < 16 years[†]	Not specified	Any age
	Age < 2 years[‡]	≥ 15 mm*	≥ 15 mm*
Immigrants	> 40/100 000[§]	Not specified	Not specified
	Age < 16[†]		
	16–34[†] should be considered		

* Millimetres of induration in Mantoux test to 5 TU.
† Grade 3 or 4 Heaf test.
‡ Whether Heaf positive or negative.
§ Rate of disease in country of origin.

monitoring of liver and renal function is only required in cases where there is a particular risk.

Rifampicin is contraindicated in HIV-positive individuals receiving antiviral therapy. In such individuals, rifampicin may be substituted with rifabutin, which can be safely used with indinavir, nelfinavir, amprenavir, ritonavir and efavirenz.[6]

Who should be given preventive therapy depends on the relative risk of tuberculosis developing in the individuals concerned. Table 38.3.5 summarises the recommendations from the different guidelines.[6–8] In addition to individuals in the groups specified in Table 38.3.5, those with medical conditions giving increased risk should also be considered for preventive therapy (see Table 38.3.2.)

Multi-drug-resistant tuberculosis

The emergence of multi-drug-resistant strains of tuberculosis has meant that preventive therapy with first-line drugs such as isoniazid and/or rifampicin may not be appropriate for certain groups, such as health-care workers in contact with patients harbouring these organisms. Protection with BCG immunisation would therefore seem the best means of providing protection (see below).

Prevention of infection in uninfected individuals

BCG immunisation

Although there has been much dispute internationally about the efficacy of BCG immunisation, several British studies have shown that, given to children aged 13 years, it provides 75% protection for up to 15 years.[39] The progressive decline in the incidence of tuberculosis in the age group protected (15–30-year-olds) has meant that, by 1989, 3600 immunisations were required to prevent a single case. It was therefore proposed that BCG immunisation at the age of 13 should be abandoned.[40] However, as a result of the recent increase in tuberculosis in many countries and the cessation of decline in notifications in Britain,[41] the decision has been made to continue immunisation for the time being.[42] National policy is therefore to continue to vaccinate all tuberculin-negative children at the age of 13 and to offer vaccination to neonates of high-risk groups.[43]

The consistent efficacy of BCG immunisation in the UK is in contrast to equivocal results reported from elsewhere, particularly the USA and South India.[44] These inconsistencies may be explained by a number of factors, including differences in the potency of the vaccine, immunisation technique, the age of those immunised, genetic make-up, nutrition and infection with environmental mycobacteria, although none of these provides a satisfactory explanation.

High-risk groups
In addition to national policy outlined above, vaccination with BCG should be considered for the following high-risk groups, who may have missed the schools programme:

- Hospital workers – all those in care institutions who may come into contact with patients with tuberculosis or with the tubercle bacillus in the laboratory or the mortuary
- Travellers to areas of high prevalence
- Contacts of patients with disease (see above)
- Immigrants from high-prevalence countries who are tuberculin-negative.

Technique
Tuberculin testing should be undertaken before immunisation except in the newborn. Those with Heaf grade 0 or I or whose Mantoux reaction to 10 TU is less than 6 mm of induration then receive BCG vaccine. Freeze-dried vaccine is used. A dose of 0.1 ml should be injected intradermally (0.05 ml for infants) over the site of the insertion of the deltoid muscle into the humerus. Subcutaneous injection may cause ulceration or abscess.

The patient should be warned that a blister or small ulcer may form but that the site should not be covered.

Adverse reactions

Ulcers, abscesses or local lymphadenopathy may occur, usually as a result of faulty vaccination technique. Although isoniazid has been used in the treatment of these reactions, there is no good evidence that it is effective. Very rarely, a disseminated BCG reaction has been reported when immunisation is given inadvertently to an immunocompromised individual.

Bacillus Calmette–Guérin and human immunodeficiency virus infection

The World Health Organization advises that BCG immunisation should not be given to an individual with AIDS. In the developing world, BCG immunisation may be given to asymptomatic HIV-seropositive individuals because the risk of infection with the tubercle bacillus is considered to be high. However, the protective efficacy of BCG in the presence of HIV infection is not currently known. BCG vaccine should not be given to a HIV-seropositive person if the risk of infection with tuberculosis is low, as is likely in most developed countries.

Control of disease in high-prevalence countries

The basic principles of disease control apply to developing as well as to developed countries, namely the identification and treatment of patients with disease, particularly sputum-smear-positive patients, the screening of individuals at greatest risk of developing disease and the provision of protection to the rest of the community. As a result of the high rates of disease and the relative poverty of resources, the great bulk of control measures must necessarily go towards case finding and treatment.

The rapid increase of disease in many countries has meant that fresh initiatives in programmes of disease control have had to be undertaken. International bodies such as the International Union Against Tuberculosis and Lung Disease and the World Health Organization are now active in organising national programmes in many developed countries, with funding from the World Bank. A recent study has suggested that money spent on tuberculosis control in developing countries is the most cost-effective way of using money for health care because it targets the young adult population, those who are most economically productive.[45]

Directly observed therapy

Tuberculosis control programmes aim to cover 75% of all cases in a developing country and provide 85% cure. Many varied resources need to be organised to provide an effective tuberculosis control programme. Any person or service treating tuberculosis should know its success rates (Fig. 38.3.3)

The World Health Organization has recommended that directly observed therapy be mandatory to ensure that medication is taken, the patient being observed to swallow the tablets by a trained overseer. A number of different provisions must be in place for a successful control programme.[45]

First, agreement must be reached at national and local government level to provide the necessary staff of doctors, nurses, clerical staff and assistants. A national programme of health education should be undertaken to encourage all those who think that they may have the disease to present early to the health services. This will include the use of television and radio, national and local press, school talks and even street theatre. The basis of passive case finding is by smear examination of sputum from any individual who has had a cough for more than 3 weeks. Good microbiological services with well-maintained equipment and trained, motivated staff are vital.

Short-course (6-month) chemotherapy should be given, supervised by direct observation of the patient as the medication is taken. Intermittent, three-times-weekly regimens are useful for this. Alternatively, hospital admission may be required.

Regular contact with the patient at home to 'chase up' possible defaulters will be required. The person 'chasing' defaulters will need special skills to persuade a patient who feels better to complete the full course of treatment or to attend the clinic for further treatment. Meticulous records must be kept to ensure that the programme is running smoothly and that the results are audited. Clinics treating tuberculosis should be required to submit returns every 3 months and annually to audit the proportion of patients being cured and make improvements where necessary. A secure drug supply is needed. If a programme is to be started, at least 6 months of drug supplies should be available and adequate stocks laid in if there are likely to be seasonal transport problems. Staff will need regular retraining and motivation as the programme progresses.

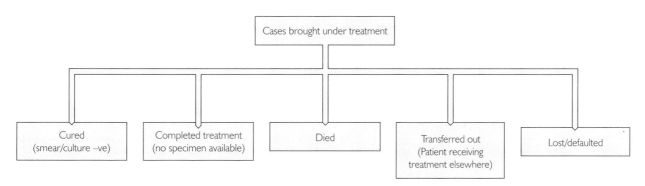

Figure 38.3.3 Possible outcomes of tuberculosis treatment.

Screening of family contacts of sputm-smear-positive patients is likely to be productive but priority should be given to ensure that patients complete medication.

Immunisation of infants with BCG should be undertaken, as protection against disseminated disease is highest in early childhood.

Conclusions

In the long term, the development of a new vaccine, much more effective than BCG, probably offers the best hope of tuberculosis control. Recent research in this area has moved from the development of recombinant BCG DNA to isolating smaller segments of the bacterial DNA to detect sections that, it is hoped, will provide better enhancement of host immunity.

The fact that developed countries are seeking the elimination of tuberculosis within their own borders by ever more aggressive policies of preventive therapy for latent infection, while many developing countries are sinking beneath an increasing case-load suggests a curious lack of world-wide co-operation. To achieve elimination of tuberculosis, a word-wide strategy is essential.[47] It would be more cost-effective to invest in treatment of tuberculosis in the developing world, where at least 98% of tuberculosis transmission takes place, than to spend resources on preventive therapy in developed countries. Recent acknowledgement of the problem by the G8 nations is perhaps a good first step down this road.

> **? Unresolved questions**
>
> ■ How to achieve a global strategy for elimination of tuberculosis
>
> ■ Development of more effective immunisation
>
> ■ Development of inexpensive molecular techniques for accurate early detection of infection

References

1. Clancy L, Rieder HL, Enarson DA, Spinachi S. Tuberculosis elimination in the countries of Europe and other industrialised countries. Eur Respir J 1991; 4: 1283–1295.
2. Udwadia ZF. India. In: Davies PDO, ed. Clinical tuberculosis, 2nd ed. London: Chapman & Hall; 1998: 592–606.
3. Mwinga A. Africa. In: Davies PDO, ed. Clinical tuberculosis, 2nd ed. London: Chapman & Hall; 1998: 619–630.
4. Rieder HL, Zellweger JP, Raviglione MC et al. Tuberculosis control in Europe and international migration. Eur Respir J 1994; 7: 1545–1553.
5. www.phls.co.uk/facts/TB/index.htm.
6. Targeted tuberculin testing and treatment of Latent Tuberculosis Infection. ATS CDC Am Rev Respir Crit Care 2000; 161: S220–S247.
7. Joint Tuberculosis Committee of the British Thoracic Society. Control and prevention of tuberculosis in the UK. Code of practice 2000. Thorax 2000; 55: 887–901.
8. Migliori GB, Raviglione MC, Schaberg T et al. Tuberculosis management in Europe. Eur Respir J 1999: 978–992.
9. American Thoracic Society. Diagnostic standards and classification of tuberculosis in adults and children. Am J Respir Crit Care Med 2000; 161: 1376–1395.
10. American Thoracic Society. Treatment of tuberculosis and tuberculosis infection in adults and children. Am J Respir Crit Care Med 1994; 149: 1359–1374.
11. Joint Tuberculosis Committee of the British Thoracic Society. Chemotherapy and management of tuberculosis in the UK: recommendations 1998. Thorax 1998; 53: 536–548.
12. Centers for Disease Control and Prevention. Essential components of tuberculosis control and prevention program: recommendations of the Advisory Council for the Elimination of Tuberculosis. MMWR 1995; 44(No. RR-11): 1–16.
13. Centers for Disease Control and Prevention. Prevention and treatment of tuberculosis among patients infected with human immunodeficiency virus: principles of therapy and revised recommendations. MMWR 1998; 47 (No. RR-20): 36–42.
14. Ormerod LP, Watson JM, Pozniac A et al. Notification of tuberculosis: an updated code of practice for England and Wales. J R Coll Phys Lond 1997; 31: 299–303.
15. Lunn JA, Mayho V. Incidence of pulmonary tuberculosis by occupation of hospital employees in the National Health Service in England and Wales 1980–84. J Soc Occup Med 1989; 39: 30–32.
16. Meredith S, Watson JM, Citron KM et al. Are health-care workers in England and Wales at increased risk of tuberculosis? Br Med J 1996; 313: 522–525.
17. Cockcoft A, Chapman S, InsallC et al. Tuberculin reactivity in new employees in a London health district. Thorax 1988; 43: 834.
18. Fennelly KP, Iseman MD. Health-care workers and tuberculosis: the battle of the century (editorial). Int J Tuberc Lung Dis 1999; 3: 363–364.
19. Hussain SF, Watura R, Cashman B et al. Tuberculosis contact tracing – are the British Thoracic Society Guidelines still appropriate? Thorax 1992; 47: 984–985.
20. Leitch AG. Audit of tuberculosis contact tracing procedures in South Gwent. Respir Med 1992; 86: 173.
21. Teale C, Cundall DB, Peaarson SB. Time of development of tuberculosis in contacts. Respir Med 1991; 85: 475–77.
22. Ormerod LP. Tuberculosis contact tracing. Blackburn 1982–90. Respir Med 1992; 87: 127–131.
23. Kumar S, Innes JA, Skinner C. Yield from tuberculosis contact tracing in Birmingham. Thorax 1992; 47: 875.
24. Veen J. Tuberculosis in a low prevalence country: a wolf in sheep's clothing. Bull Int Union Tuberc Lung Dis 1991; 66: 203.
25. Wales JM, Buchan AR, Cookson JB et al. Tuberculosis in a primary school: the Uppingham outbreak. Br Med J 1985; 291: 1039.
26. Rose AMC. 1998 National TB Survey in England and Wales: final results. Thorax 1999: 54(Suppl 3); A5.
27. Ormerod LP. Is immigrant screening for tuberculosis still worthwhile? J Infect 1998; 37: 269–271.
28. Selwyn PA, Hartel D, Lewis VA et al. A prospective study of the risk of tuberculosis among intravenous drug users with human immunodeficiency virus infection. N Engl J Med 1989; 320: 546.
29. Pape JW, Jean SS, Ho JL et al. Effect of isoniazid prophylaxis on incidence of active tuberculosis and progression of HIV infection. Lancet 1993; 342: 268–272.
30. Whalen CC, Johnson JL, Okwera A et al. A trial of three regimens to prevent tuberculosis in Ugandan adults infected with the human immunodeficiency virus. N Engl J Med 1997; 338: 801–808.
31. Hawken MP, Meme HK, Elliot LC et al. Isoniazid preventive therapy for tuberculosis in HIV-I infected adults: results of a randomized controlled trial. AIDS 1997; 11: 875–882.
32. Mwinga AM, Hosp P, Godfrey-Faussett M et al. Twice weekly tuberculosis preventative therapy in HIV infection in Zambia. AIDS 1998; 12: 2447–2457.
33. Gordin FM, Matts JP, Miller C et al. A controlled trial of Isoniazid in persons with anergy and human immunodeficiency virus infection who are at high risk for tuberculosis. N Engl J Med. 1997; 337: 315–320.
34. Halsey NA, Coberly JS, Desormeaux J et al. Rifampin and pyrazinamide vs. Isoniazid for prevention of tuberculosis in HIV-1 infected persons: an international randomised trial. Lancet 1998; 351: 786–792.
35. Gordin FM, Chaisson RE, Matts JP et al. An international, randomized trial of Rifampin and pyrazinamide versus Isoniazid for prevention of tuberculosis in HIV-infected persons. JAMA 2000; 283: 1445–1450.
36. Stead WW, Lofgren JP, Warren E, Thomas C. Tuberculosis as an endemic and nosocomial infection among the elderly in nursing homes. N Engl J Med 1985; 312: 1483.
37. Nisar M, Williams CSD, Ashby D, Davies PDO. Tuberculin screening of residential homes for the elderly. Thorax 1993; 48: 1257–1260.
38. Kumar D, Citron KM, Leese J, Watson JM. Tuberculosis among the homeless at a temporary shelter in London: report of a chest X-ray screening programme. J Epidemiol Community Health 1995; 49: 629–363.
39. Sutherland I, Springett VH. Effectiveness of BCG vaccination in England and Wales in 1983. Tubercle 1987; 68: 81.
40. Springett VH, Sutherland I. BCG vaccination of school children in England and Wales. Thorax 1990; 45: 83.
41. Watson JM. Tuberculosis in Britain today. Br Med J 1993; 306: 221.

42. Citron KM. BCG vaccination against tuberculosis: international perspectives. Br Med J 1993; 306: 222.

43. Department of Health. Immunisation against infectious disease. London: HMSO, 1992: 76.

44. Smith PG, Fine PEM. BCG vaccination. In: Davies PDO, ed. Clinical tuberculosis, 2nd ed. London: Chapman & Hall; 1998: 417–434.

45. Murray CJL, Styblo K, Rouillon A. Tuberculosis in developing countries; burden, intervention and cost. Bull Int Union Tuberc Lung Dis 1990; 65.

46. Kumaresan J. Control in high-prevalence countries. In: Davies PDO, ed. Clinical tuberculosis, 2nd ed. London: Chapman & Hall; 1998: 451–468.

47. Enarson DA. Why not the elimination of tuberculosis? Mayo Clin Proc 1994; 69: 85–86.

39 Opportunistic mycobacterial infections

Ian A Campbell and Peter A Jenkins

Key points

- Opportunistic mycobacteria are ubiquitous in the environment and are low-grade pathogens

- They cause at least 5% of all mycobacterial pulmonary disease in the UK. It may be difficult to distinguish casual contamination from disease.

- Symptoms, signs and radiographic appearances do not allow differentiation between species nor from *M. tuberculosis*.

- Special culture techniques are required to distinguish between species. Molecular biology methods are becoming helpful.

- Results of in-vitro sensitivity tests do not predict clinical response, except for *M. kansasii*.

This chapter is concerned with pulmonary disease caused by mycobacteria that do not belong to the *Mycobacterium tuberculosis* complex, which comprises *M. tuberculosis* and its geographical variants, *Mycobacterium bovis*, *Mycobacterium africanum*, bacillus Calmette–Guérin (BCG) and *Mycobacterium microti*. The other mycobacteria have been variously called anonymous, atypical, environmental, non-tuberculous or mycobacteria other than tubercle bacilli (MOTT). None of these is totally acceptable and the authors prefer the term 'opportunistic', as they usually require either pre-existing lung damage or an immunological defect before they can cause infection.[1]

The opportunistic mycobacteria are ubiquitous in the environment and exposure to them is unavoidable. The infections that they cause are indistinguishable both clinically and radiologically from those caused by *M. tuberculosis* and it is only when the laboratory has isolated and identified the organism that the clinician becomes aware that he/she is dealing with an opportunistic mycobacterial infection rather than classic tuberculosis. Acid-fast bacilli can be detected in sputum by direct microscopy of a Ziehl–Neelsen-stained smear in around 60% of

patients.[2] However, the morphology of the bacilli in such a preparation is similar to that of *M. tuberculosis* and it would be unwise for the microbiologist to suggest that what has been seen is an opportunistic mycobacterium. The clinical significance of an isolate can be doubtful because the ubiquity of these mycobacteria means that they can be present in a specimen as casual contaminants. At what point, therefore is it reasonable to initiate treatment? The isolation of the same opportunistic mycobacterium from specimens taken 7 days apart, together with radiographic appearances suggestive of a mycobacterial infection, would in the authors' view constitute grounds for chemotherapy. If, in addition, symptoms suggestive of pulmonary infection are present, treatment is clearly indicated.

The opportunistic mycobacteria that most commonly cause pulmonary disease are:

- *Micobacterium kansasii*, *Micobacterium xenopi*, *Micobacterium malmoense* and a group referred to as the MAIS complex – *Micobacterium avium*, *Micobacterium intracellulare*, *Micobacterium scrofulaceum*.
- *Micobacterium szulgai*, *Micobacterium simiae*, *Micobacterium fortuitum* and *Micobacterium chelonae* subspecies *abscessus* have been reported as causing pulmonary disease but the number of cases worldwide is very small.[3–5]
- *Micobacterium gordonae*, *Micobacterium terrae*, *Micobacterium triviale*, *Micobacterium nonchromogenicum* and *Micobacterium gastri* are generally taken to be saprophytes but very occasionally have been identified as the cause of genuine infections.[6,7]

Isolation and cultural characteristics

The isolation of opportunistic mycobacteria presents the same problems as the isolation of *M. tuberculosis*. As mycobacteria grow slowly other bacteria have to be eliminated from the specimen by prior treatment with acid or alkali. Solid media such as Lowenstein–Jensen egg or Middlebrook 7H10/7H11 agar are the most commonly used and if mycobacteria are present colonies will appear after 2–6 weeks' incubation. Some species, particularly the MAIS complex and *M. malmoense*, grow more quickly in a liquid medium such as Middlebrook 7H12 broth as used in the Bactec 460 system (Becton Dickinson, Oxford). Growth of *M. malmoense* is even more successful in the Bactec medium used for assessing the sensitivity of *M. tuberculosis* to pyrazinamide: this medium (PZA test medium) has a pH of 6.0 compared with 7.0 in the standard vial (Bactec 12B).

Most opportunistic mycobacteria that are met in clinical practice can be assigned to species or groups by the use of a small number of simple biochemical and cultural tests. These involve temperature range, pigment production, oxygen preference and the ability to hydrolyse Tween 80. Together with the drug sensitivity pattern, these tests are sufficient to identify a strain as far as is clinically necessary.[8] If further tests are required, e.g. for difficult strains or epidemiological purposes, then techniques such as thin-layer chromatography of surface lipids, high-pressure liquid chromatography, gas–liquid chromatography or serotyping are available.[9,10] However, these techniques are only undertaken in specialised reference laboratories. DNA probes are now available that can identify some species in a few hours. The probe hybridises with specific target DNA and the hybridisation product is detected with a chemiluminescent marker. Probes are available for the *M. tuberculosis* complex, the MAIS complex, *M. kansasii* and *M. gordonae* (Accuprobe®, Gen-probe, San Diego CA).

Amplification techniques targeting specific DNA sequences will eventually supersede the classical cultural and biochemical methods.

The foremost of these amplification methods are:

- polymerase chain reaction (Roche Molecular Systems)
- Gen-probe amplification assay (Gen-Probe)
- strand displacement amplification (Becton Dickinson DNA Diagnostics).

It is not possible to predict when one or more of these will become routinely available.

One outcome of the use of these new techniques has been the discovery of unique nucleotide sequences of 16S rRNA and as a result many new species of mycobacteria have been discovered. Most of these have been non-pathogenic or have been isolated from a single patient.[11] The species listed at the beginning of this chapter remain the most common opportunistic mycobacteria causing pulmonary disease and their cultural characteristics are shown in Table 39.1. *M. kansasii* is a photochromogen (produces pigment only when exposed to light) that grows better at 37°C than at 25°C. The MAIS group grow at 25°C and 37°C but are variable in their ability to grow at 45°C. They are microaerophilic and do not hydrolyse Tween 80. *M. scrofulaceum* is scotochromogenic (produces pigment in both the light and the dark). *M. malmoense* is similar to the MAIS complex but is variable in its ability to hydrolyse Tween 80. Its sensitivity pattern differs from that of the MAIS complex and, when such strains are isolated, lipid analysis is the most accurate method of confirming the identity of a strain.[12] *M. xenopi* is a thermophile, growing better at 45°C than at 37°C and not at all at 25°C. It tends to be scotochromogenic but the pigment is often faint.

Epidemiology

Opportunistic mycobacteria can be isolated from a wide variety of environmental sources. For example, *M. kansasii* has been isolated from tap water,[13,14] the MAIS complex from water and soil[15,16] and *M. xenopi* from the toad (*Xenopus laevus*)[17] and water.[14] To date, perhaps because of inadequacies of technique, *M. malmoense* has not been isolated from the environment except for one report of *M. malmoense* isolated from the soil in 1973 in Zaire.[18] Animals also provide a reservoir in that the lymph nodes of pigs and cattle frequently contain opportunistic mycobacteria.[19] *M. malmoense* is occasionally isolated from the sputum on a single occasion only, when it may be regarded as not clinically significant. This suggests that it has established itself in the environment in such a way that it can enter the sputum as a casual contaminant.

The true incidence of infections caused by opportunistic mycobacteria is difficult to determine. Systems for notification

Table 39.1 Cultural characteristics of clinically important opportunistic mycobacteria

Species	Temperature range			Pigment produced		Oxygen preference	Tween hydrolysis
	25°C	37°C	45°C	Light	Dark		
M. kansasii	+	+	–	+	–	A	P
M. avium	+	+	V	–	–	M	N
M. intracellulare	+	+	V	–	–	M	N
M. scrofulaceum	+	+	V	+	+	M	N
M. malmoense	+	+	–	–	–	M	V
M. xenopi	–	+	+	+	+	M	N

A, aerobic; M, microaerophilic; P, positive; N, negative; V, variable.

of cases vary from country to country and it is probable that none of them is accurate. In England and Wales since 1981 laboratories have been asked to notify the Communicable Disease Surveillance Centre (CDSC) of the Public Health Laboratory Service of all new cases of clinically significant disease caused by opportunistic mycobacteria. The figures presented in Table 39.2 are certainly underestimates as it is known that not all laboratories are diligent in notifying cases. A conservative estimate would be that in England and Wales 5% of all mycobacterial pulmonary disease is caused by opportunistic mycobacteria.

In Cleveland, Ohio, isolates of the MAIS complex outnumbered those of *M. tuberculosis* in 1985 and this was attributed to mycobacterial disease in patients with acquired immunodeficiency syndrome (AIDS).[20]

In English and Welsh patients who do not have AIDS, *M. kansasii* and *M. malmoense* give rise to pulmonary disease more commonly than other opportunist mycobacterial pathogens. In other parts of the world the relative frequencies vary considerably. It can be seen in Table 39.2 that the figures for *M. kansasii* and *M. xenopi* have risen gradually but there has been a much steeper rise in the incidence of infection caused by the MAIS complex. As in the USA, this has been attributed to infections in patients with AIDS.[20-22] The true incidence of infections caused by the MAIS complex could be twice the number reported to the CDSC. For example, in 1986 the Mycobacterium Reference Unit in Cardiff knew of 72 cases, 39 of which were in patients with a positive human immunodeficiency virus (HIV) test, but only 37 of the 72 were reported to the CDSC.

In 1987 in London, 23% of 92 AIDS patients developed mycobacterial pulmonary infection and over half of these were with opportunistic mycobacteria, mainly the MAIS complex (R. Shaw 1987, personal communication) Since the introduction of highly active antiretroviral therapy (HAART), the incidence of mycobacterial disease in England, Wales and Northern Ireland as an AIDS-defining illness has fallen from 237 cases in 1994 (40% due to opportunist mycobacteria) to 116 in 1999, 30% of which were caused by opportunist mycobacteria (B. Evans 2001, personal communication). Infections with *M. kansasii*, *M. xenopi* and *M. malmoense* have all been reported in AIDS patients but the numbers are small. It is not understood why the MAIS complex, and in particular *M. avium*, should be more virulent than the other opportunistic mycobacteria for this group of patients.

The reported rise in the incidence of infections caused by *M. malmoense* is not the result of AIDS but is more likely to be related to cultural techniques.[23] On primary isolation the organism grows very slowly – one report quotes a mean of 54 days (range 31–87 days) before growth was detected. For all other mycobacteria the mean was 30 days (range 10–84 days).[24] It is likely that a number of factors are involved, including quality of the medium and the severity of the decontamination procedure.

Infectivity

The opportunistic mycobacteria are low-grade pathogens and as such do not constitute a threat to most people. More importantly, they do not constitute a threat to the close contacts of infected patients even when the sputum of such patients is positive for acid-fast bacilli on direct smear. There is, as far as we know, only one report of a person-to-person transmission of opportunistic mycobacterial infection and that was between a father and son and involved *M. kansasii*.[25]

Table 39.2 Incidence of infection with opportunistic mycobacteria as reported to the Communicable Disease Surveillance Centre of the UK Public Health Laboratory Service

	M. kansasii	**MAIS complex**	*M. malmoense*	*M. xenopi*
1989	65	64	35	25
1990	42	81	36	24
1991	39	96	44	33
1992	57	106	28	12
1993	60	195	67	23
1994	80	171	87	29
1995	69	195	92	39
1996	66	255	113	33
1997	77	342	87	39
1998	109	295	137	47
1999	110	303	118	62

MAIS, *Mycobacterium avium–intracellulare–scrofulaceum*.

Sensitivity testing

The slow growth of most mycobacteria means that the normal disc method of sensitivity testing is not appropriate. Instead it is usual to determine either the proportion of the population that is resistant to a critical concentration of a drug or a resistance ratio by titrating the test strain and comparing its end-point with that of a standard strain. The use of a single standard strain can lead to difficulties[26] and a more effective method is to use the 'mode' of resistance of a number of wild strains of *M. tuberculosis* isolated from patients who have never been treated.[27] This concept of 'modal resistance' works very well for *M. tuberculosis* because strains are relatively homogeneous and the end-points in titrations do not vary much from strain to strain. When resistance develops as a result of inadequate chemotherapy or erratic compliance, the strain will exhibit a level of resistance at least eight times that of the mode, and it is generally accepted that the drug involved is no longer of benefit to the patient.

The extension of this principle to the opportunistic mycobacteria provides the sensitivity patterns shown in Table 39.3. The sensitivity of *M. kansasii* to rifampicin and ethambutol accords well with the clinical response to treatment with these drugs.[28] For the others the situation is less clear. A strain within the MAIS complex, for example, is composed of at least three different cell types, which give rise to different colony forms. The relative proportion of these cell types varies from strain to strain and even within the same strain, depending on growth conditions. This lack of homogeneity causes considerable interstrain variation and makes it difficult to interpret the results of sensitivity tests.

Retrospective studies have shown a lack of correlation between the in-vitro sensitivity results and the response to treatment.[29-31] The recent prospective trial conducted by the British Thoracic Society (BTS) has confirmed this finding.[2] This may be the result of the limitations of applying a technique of sensitivity testing developed for *M. tuberculosis* to the opportunistic mycobacteria. Further work has suggested that there is a degree of synergy between rifampicin and ethambutol. When strains of the MAIS complex, *M. xenopi* and *M. malmoense* were tested against these two drugs individually, most were resistant but, when the two drugs were combined, 31% of the MAIS strains,

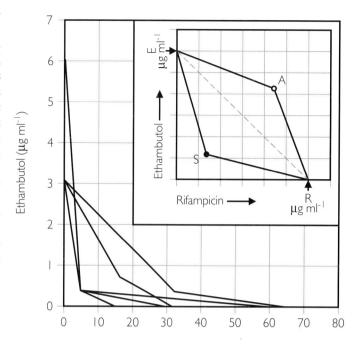

Fig. 39.1 Isobolograms for strains of *Mycobacterium malmoense* tested against ethambutol combined with rifampicin. The lines connect the lowest concentrations of the two agents that inhibit growth of the five strains tested. The plot shows evidence of synergy between rifampicin and ethambutol. **Inset.** If the two drugs were neither synergistic nor antagonistic in antimycobacterial activity the plot would be a straight line (X). If there was synergy the line would be curved downwards (S) towards lower concentrations when the drugs are used in combination. If there was antagonism the line would be curved upwards (A). (With permission from Banks & Jenkins 1987.[32])

86% of the *M. xenopi* strains and 100% of the *M. malmoense* strains were sensitive (Fig. 39.1).[32]

The meaning of in-vitro sensitivity results to the newer drugs such as the fluoroquinolones (ciprofloxacin, sparfloxacin, etc.), the macrolides (clarithromycin, azithromycin) and rifabutin is subject to the same qualifications and reservations. Some species appear to be sensitive and others resistant, but how this relates to clinical response is not known. The antileprosy drug

Table 39.3   Sensitivity of opportunistic mycobacteria to individual antituberculosis drugs in vitro

Species	Strepto-mycin	Isoniazid	Rifampicin	Etham-butol	Ethionamide*	Capreo-mycin	Cyclo-serine	Clarithro-mycin	Cipro-floxacin
M. kansasii	B	R	S	S	S	B	S	S	V
MAIS complex	R	R	R	R	S	R	S	S	R
M. malmoense	R	R	V	V	S	R	S	S	S
M. xenopi	S	R	V	R	S	S	S	S	S

Pyrazinamide is tested by a different technique but all opportunistic mycobacteria are resistant.
*Prothionamide has the same profile as ethionamide.
B, borderline; MAIS, *Mycobacterium avium–intracellulare–scrofulaceum*; R, resistant; S, sensitive; V, variable.

clofazimine and even amikacin have also been suggested for treatment but again their efficacy is unproven.

Clinical features and radiological appearances

The clinical features and radiological appearances of infection do not differ much among the four main species and they will be described together.

Clinical features

Except for MAIS, where the balance between the genders tends to be even,[33] most patients are male and in the middle-aged to elderly age groups.[34-36] Over half have pre-existing lung disease, predominantly chronic obstructive pulmonary disease (COPD) and some have old, healed tuberculosis.[28-31,33-40] Peptic ulcer, previous gastroduodenal surgery and conditions associated with impaired immunoresponsiveness are present in a number of patients but whether or not these are true associations has not been clearly established.[28,31,39,40]

Symptoms and signs

Cough, sputum, haemoptysis, weight loss, malaise and increasing breathlessness are the most common complaints but between 10% and 40% of patients may be asymptomatic.[28,30,31,37,39,41-43] When present, symptoms tend to have developed gradually so that the picture is one of a subacute or chronic illness rather than an acute one. Besides fever, the physical signs are usually those associated with underlying COPD.

Chest radiology

The appearances on the chest radiograph are much like the infiltrates and cavities of *M. tuberculosis* infection (Fig. 39.2). It is not possible to distinguish between the various opportunistic species by looking at the chest radiograph.[44] In *M. kansasii* infection the disease was noted to be unilateral in 70% in one report[28] and 50% in another.[34] In the latter series disease was confined to the upper zones in 30% while 45% of the patients had disease in three zones or more. Multiple, large cavities (2 cm or more in diameter) were present in 45% of pretreatment radiographs. Pleural effusion is rare with *M. kansasii*.[45] With infection by the MAIS complex, Yeager & Raleigh[43] found unilateral disease in the majority, as did Engbaek et al.,[42] but Etzkorn et al[46] found bilateral disease in 80%. In the recent prospective study by the BTS, bilateral disease was evident in 44% and three or more lung zones were involved in a little less than one-third. Cavitation was noted in 61%, most having at least one cavity of 2 cm or more in diameter.[33]

With the advent of computerised tomography it has been suggested that particular patterns of bronchiectasis are associated with MAIS[47,48] but further work is needed to confirm the association.

Unilateral changes have been reported in between 50% and 80% of patients with *M. malmoense*.[31,49] In a recent BTS study[35] the figure was 52% and three-quarters of the patients had cavitation, with larger cavities again predominating. Three zones or more were involved in 26%.[35] With *M. xenopi*, cavitation has been reported in 73–100%,[30,36,37,50] although Costrini et al found it in only half of their 19 patients.[41]

Treatment

Treatment of *M. kansasii* infection

Rifampicin was used in all 30 of the patients described by Banks et al. and in 26 (87%) ethambutol was also included in the regimen.[28] The duration of chemotherapy ranged from 3 to 24 months. There was 100% cure with no relapses after a mean follow-up period of 5 years. From this retrospective study the authors suggested that therapy with rifampicin and ethambutol should be given for 15 months, advising as a counsel of perfection the inclusion of ethionamide until the organisms' sensitivity to rifampicin and ethambutol was confirmed.

The BTS has completed a prospective study of ethambutol and rifampicin given for 9 months to patients with *M. kansasii* pulmonary infection. Most patients also received a third or fourth drug (isoniazid and/or pyrazinamide) for the first 2–3 months because treatment had usually started before the nature of the mycobacterium had been established. Of the 173 patients, 11% had positive sputum cultures after 3 months' treatment but only one patient (a poor complier) had positive cultures when tested at two of the last 3 months of treatment. Two-thirds of the patients consistently showed satisfactory progress during and after treatment and, of the remainder, in only 20% was unsatisfactory progress attributed to *M. kansasii*. Of the 68 patients with a complete series of follow-up radiographs, 86% showed radiographic 'healing' within 3 years of completing chemotherapy. Although a quarter of the patients died during the period of the study, none did so because of *M. kansasii* infection. In the 51-month follow-up period after the end of chemotherapy, 10% again developed two or more positive cultures: probable underlying factors could be identified in half of these, e.g. non-compliance with therapy, severe malnourishment, severe bronchiectasis, steroid treatment. In another quarter the radiographic appearances suggested reinfection rather than relapse, leaving 2–3% as relapses for which no reason was apparent. All responded satisfactorily to re-treatment.[34]

In summary, 9 months' treatment with rifampicin and ethambutol was associated with a 10% relapse/reinfection rate. *M. kansasii* is a ubiquitous, low-grade pathogen: those who develop disease may well have a predisposition to mycobacterial disease, a factor that would increase the probability of reinfection. Thus one practical option is to treat with ethambutol and rifampicin for 9 months, using prothionamide in cases of ethambutol or rifampicin resistance, and accept that 10% or so will develop disease again and require re-treatment. Alternatively, chemotherapy could be given to all patients for 15–24 months.[28]

Treatment of infection with the MAIS complex

Many reports testify to the difficulty of treating patients infected with this complex. Yeager & Raleigh[43] used five or six drugs and obtained only a 43% response rate, 11% dying from MAIS-complex infection and 20% relapsing after treatment. Ahn et al.[51]

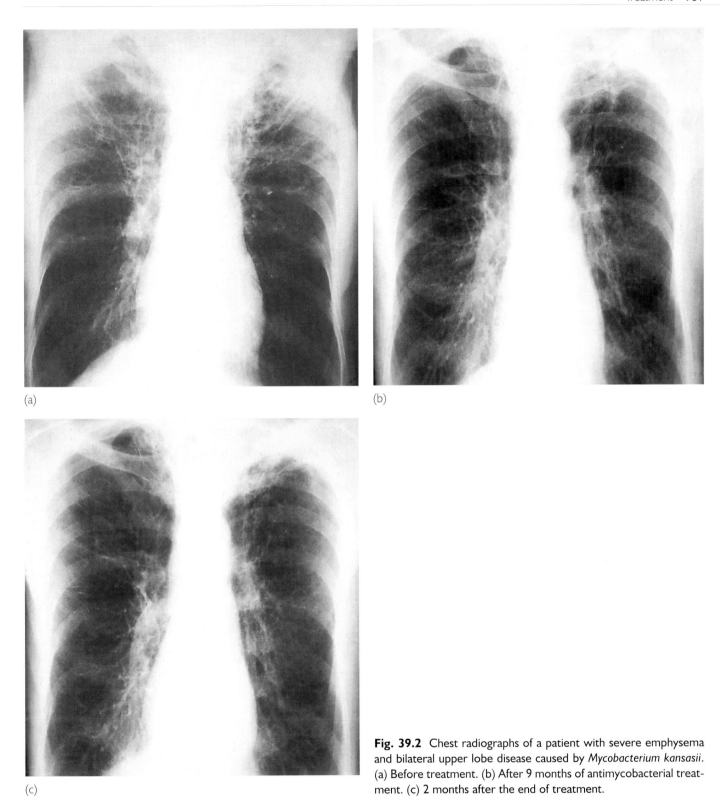

(a)

(b)

(c)

Fig. 39.2 Chest radiographs of a patient with severe emphysema and bilateral upper lobe disease caused by *Mycobacterium kansasii*. (a) Before treatment. (b) After 9 months of antimycobacterial treatment. (c) 2 months after the end of treatment.

found a similar relapse rate. Dutt & Stead[52] found that 80% showed an initial bacteriological response to a multiple drug regimen but later relapse was common: only 46% were culture-negative after 3–8 years. Subtotal gastrectomy seemed to be associated with failure of treatment or relapse. Etzkorn et al[46] found no significant difference in terms of sputum conversion rate among regimens containing three, four or five drugs, and noted

that conversion could take up to 1 year. Hunter et al[29] confirmed that symptomatic patients who were left untreated were likely to die. Asymptomatic patients often had 'benign' disease but some developed progressive disease. When isoniazid, rifampicin and streptomycin, or isoniazid, rifampicin and ethambutol, were given for between 9 and 24 months, 84% showed satisfactory clinical, radiological or bacteriological response but 14% relapsed within a year of the end of treatment. Three of the four patients who did not respond to treatment died. When second- or third-line drugs, or regimens with four or more drugs, were used, toxicity and non-compliance became significant problems.

In the study by the BTS, rifampicin and ethambutol or rifampicin, ethambutol and isoniazid were given for 2 years: by the end of 5 years 36% of the 75 patients had died but in only three was death thought to be directly attributable to the disease and damage caused by the organism. Deaths in the group on triple therapy exceeded those who received only rifampicin and ethambutol. Twenty-one patients (28%) either had positive cultures at the end of treatment or relapsed bacteriologically after treatment, more doing so in the group receiving rifampicin and ethambutol. Despite the eventually high death, failure of treatment and relapse rates, the physician deemed clinical progress as satisfactory on nearly 90% of the reviews performed during the trial. Only 31% of the patients were known to be alive and cured at 5 years, some 20% or so of the original 75 having defaulted from follow-up before the end of 5 years.[33]

Taking the results of all of these studies, it would seem appropriate to treat with 2 years of rifampicin and ethambutol, adding one or more of isoniazid, clarithromycin, ciprofloxacin, streptomycin or one of the newer rifamycins when patients fail to respond. The ongoing second BTS study will give sound information on the roles of clarithromycin, ciprofloxacin and immunotherapy with M. vaccae.

There seems to be no advantage in using toxic, second- or third-line drugs or more than four drugs. In non-responders who are fit enough, resection of the affected lobe and continuation of chemotherapy might achieve cure.[29]

Treatment of M. malmoense infection

Ethambutol and rifampicin are the key drugs in treatment. In two retrospective studies it was apparent that patients treated for 18–24 months with regimens including ethambutol and rifampicin did better than patients in whom other regimens, or shorter durations, were used.[31,39] When streptomycin, pyrazinamide or second-line drugs such as ethionamide, prothionamide, cycloserine or capreomycin were included or formed the basis of the regimen, therapy was poorly tolerated and the results of treatment were poor. A randomised, prospective comparison has been made of 2 years of rifampicin and ethambutol versus 2 years of rifampicin, ethambutol and isoniazid in 106 patients: after 5 years 34% had died, 42% were known to be alive and cured while 10% had either failed to convert to culture-negative during treatment or had relapsed. There was no difference in efficacy between the two regimens.[35] In patients with unsatisfactory responses to chemotherapy, resection of the affected lobe has been of benefit.[31] Chemotherapy should be continued after surgery, probably for at least 18 months. Sadly, surgery is often precluded by poor respiratory function. The outlook is often dictated by the age and poor physical condition of the patient and by other coexisting disease. Four of 19 patients in one series died but in none of these was death the result of mycobacterial infection.[39] Two of the 34 patients described in the other report died because of unrelated causes whereas three died because of their M. malmoense infection.[31] Delay in presentation and in start of treatment was an important factor in these deaths. In the BTS

trial, although a third of the patients died, only four of these 36 deaths were thought to have been directly attributable to the mycobacterial lung disease. Despite the high all-cause death rate, clinical progress was classed by the physicians as satisfactory on 90% of the observations made over 5 years.[35] On the evidence available to date treatment with rifampicin and ethambutol for 2 years is as effective as other regimens, with fewer side-effects. Ciprofloxacin and clarithromycin are often effective in vitro but their benefit in vivo is not yet adequately documented.

Treatment of M. xenopi infection

Using various regimens, usually containing isoniazid and ethambutol, Costrini et al[41] described a 50% response rate. Smith & Citron[37] considered that eight of 11 patients given chemotherapy for between 8 and 24 months were cured (follow-up extending for a minimum of 3 years). One patient died in spite of treatment. In another series the authors could define only 23% as cured after chemotherapy. The disease progressed in 10% of patients in spite of chemotherapy; 26% showed an initial response and then relapsed; and 16% died from their infection with M. xenopi. Regimens based on rifampicin and isoniazid, plus ethambutol or streptomycin as a third drug, appeared preferable to those based on second- or third-line drugs. Four patients underwent resection because of poor response or relapse, and chemotherapy was continued or reinstituted; all of these were cured. Four patients received no treatment and the disease progressed in all. Again, multiple drug therapy including second- or third-line drugs conferred no advantage in the treatment of this condition.[30]

In the BTS study 42 patients were treated for 2 years either with rifampicin and ethambutol or with those two drugs plus isoniazid and were followed up for 3 years after the end of chemotherapy. Three patients still had positive sputum cultures after 2 years and two patients relapsed after the end of chemotherapy, giving a failure of treatment/relapse rate of 12%. The death rate (69%) was higher than those reported for M. kansasii,[34] MAIS[33] and M. malmoense[35] but, as with those studies, only a small minority (7%) died directly because of the mycobacterial disease. Despite the high death rate, clinical progress was reported by the physicians as satisfactory at over 80% of the reviews during the trial. By the end of 5 years only 17% of the patients were known to be alive and cured. Neither regimen proved superior to the other.[36]

In the present state of knowledge it would appear prudent to give ethambutol and rifampicin, or ethambutol, rifampicin and isoniazid, for 2 years, using streptomycin as well if necessary. Again, the roles of ciprofloxacin and clarithromycin or the newer rifamycins are not clear. In those who fail to respond or who relapse, surgery should be employed where possible.[53]

Treatment of opportunistic mycobacterial pulmonary infection in patients with AIDS

Response to treatment in patients with AIDS, as in other immunocompromised groups, is likely to depend as much on the degree of immunosuppression as on the antimycobacterial therapy. Infection is rarely confined to the lung and is frequently associated with bacteraemia, diagnosis often being made on

Table 39.4 Suggested chemotherapy and duration

	Rifampicin (R)	Ethambutol (E)	Isoniazid (H)	Streptomycin (S)	Prothionamide
M. kansasii	9–15 months	9–15 months	–	–	Add if RE insufficient
MAIS complex	18–24 months	18–24 months	Add if RE insufficient	Add if REH insufficient	–
M. malmoense	18–24 months	18–24 months	–	Add if RE insufficient	–
M. xenopi	18–24 months	18–24 months	–	Add if RE insufficient	–

MAIS, *Mycobacterium avium–intracellulare–scrofulaceum*.

blood culture. Until recently, in contrast to *M. tuberculosis*, the response, if any, to chemotherapy has usually been transient and the prognosis was dismal.[54] But with the advent of HAART this poor outlook has been considerably improved.

In the current state of knowledge it would appear logical to treat those with *M. kansasii* infection with ethambutol and rifampicin, plus or minus prothionamide, for 2 years or until the sputum has been negative on culture for 12 months.[55,56] Symptomatic infection by the MAIS complex, *M. malmoense* or *M. xenopi* should be treated with rifampicin, ethambutol and clarithromycin (or azithromycin).[55] Therapy should be continued indefinitely because discontinuation often results in recurrence of disease and bacteraemia.[57] Ciprofloxacin, streptomycin or amikacin can be tried as reserve drugs. It should be remembered that the clinical response to an individual antimycobacterial drug does not relate to the results of the in-vitro sensitivity tests in the same way that it does with *M. tuberculosis*. In addition, drug interactions between macrolides, rifamycins and protease inhibitors further complicate the choice of antimycobacterial regimen.

In HIV-positive patients who have not yet developed AIDS, prophylaxis against disseminated MAIS-complex disease should be started when the CD4 count falls below 50 cells/mm³: daily clarithromycin or weekly azithromycin are preferable to the rifamycins.[55]

Superficial lymph node infections

Opportunistic mycobacteria can cause cervical lymphadenopathy, most frequently in children. The MAIS complex is the most frequent cause, followed by *M. malmoense*. As with pulmonary disease, the true incidence is difficult to ascertain but 153 cases caused by the MAIS complex and 44 caused by *M. malmoense* were reported to the CDSC during the period 1996–99. The nodes are unilateral and may be 'hot' or 'cold'. There is little systemic upset and the chest radiograph is clear. Routine haematological investigations and the Mantoux test are unhelpful. Histological appearances are indistinguishable from those caused by *M. tuberculosis*. A differential skin test comparing reactions to antigens prepared from the appropriate opportunistic mycobacteria can sometimes be more helpful.[58] Treatment is by total excision of the affected nodes.[59] Antimycobacterial chemotherapy is not indicated unless disease recurs, surgical excision is incomplete/impossible or chemical debulking is necessary in order to allow excision. Aspiration of the node should be avoided because it can leave

a discharging sinus, which can persist for many months and sometimes leads to ugly scarring.

Conclusion

Although clinical tuberculosis may eventually be eliminated in developed countries, this is unlikely to be the case with the opportunistic mycobacteria, which are ubiquitous and thus likely to continue to cause disease in humans. For pulmonary disease caused by *M. malmoense* and *M. xenopi*, chemotherapy for 18 months to 2 years with rifampicin and ethambutol would, in the present state of knowledge, seem to be the initial treatment of choice (Table 39.4). For the MAIS complex the addition of isoniazid should be considered for those who are not responding satisfactorily. Streptomycin and/or possibly clarithromycin and/or ciprofloxacin are sensible reserve drugs for all these species, with the more toxic antimycobacterial drugs being very much third reserves. The current BTS trial should clarify the places of clarithromycin, ciprofloxacin and immunotherapy with *M. vaccae*. *M. kansasii* should be treated for 9–15 months with rifampicin and ethambutol. For those with AIDS and opportunistic mycobacterial infection the restoration of immunocompetence with HAART may permit antimycobacterial therapy to be curative rather than just palliative.

Therapeutic principles

- The key drugs are rifampicin and ethambutol, which, in combination, act synergistically.

- The duration of treatment necessary is longer than for *M. tuberculosis*. *M. kansasii*: 9 months; other species: 2 years.

- Isoniazid has a limited therapeutic role (MAIS). Second- and third-line antituberculosis drugs are of limited value because of side effects. Streptomycin can be helpful.

- In HIV patients, highly active antiretroviral treatment has reduced the incidence of disease and improved prognosis.

- In children with infected lymph nodes, resection is preferable to chemotherapy.

References

1. Marks J. Nomenclature of the mycobacteria. Am Rev Respir Dis 1964; 90: 278.
2. BTS Research Committee. First randomised trial of treatments for pulmonary disease caused by M. avium intracellulare, M. malmoense and M. xenopi in HIV negative patients: rifampicin, ethambutol and isoniazid versus rifampicin and ethambutol. Thorax 2001; 56: 167–172.
3. Schaefer WB, Wolinsky E, Jenkins PA, Marks J. Mycobacterium szulgai: a new pathogen. Am Rev Respir Dis 1973; 108:1320.
4. Rose HD, Dorff GJ, Louwasser M, Sheth NK. Pulmonary and disseminated Mycobacterium simiae infection in humans. Am Rev Respir Dis 1982; 126:1110.
5. Wallace RJ Jr, Swenson JM, Silcox VA, Good RC, Tschen JA, Stone MS. Spectrum of disease due to rapidly growing mycobacteria. Rev Infect Dis 1983; 5: 657.
6. Clague H, Hopkins CA, Roberts C, Jenkins PA. Pulmonary infection with Mycobacterium gordonae in the presence of bronchial carcinoma. Tubercle 1985; 66: 61.
7. Tsukamura M, Kita N, Otsuka W, Shimoide H. A study of the taxonomy of the Mycobacterium nonchromogenicum complex and report of six cases of lung infection due to Mycobacterium nonchromogenicum. Microbiol Immunol 1983; 27: 219.
8. Marks J. Classification of mycobacteria in relation to clinical significance. Tubercle 1972; 53: 259.
9. Jenkins PA. Lipid analysis for the identification of mycobacteria: an appraisal. Rev Infect Dis 1981; 3: 862.
10. Heifets LB, Jenkins PA. Speciation of mycobacteria in clinical laboratories. In: Gangadharam PRJ, Jenkins PA, ed. Mycobacteria I. Basic aspects. New York: International Thomson Publishing; 1998: 308.
11. Goodfellow M, Magee JG. Taxonomy of mycobacteria. In: Gangadharam PRJ, Jenkins PA, ed. Mycobacteria I. Basic aspects. New York: International Thomson Publishing; 1998: 1.
12. Jenkins PA, Tsukamura M. Infections with Mycobacterium malmoense in England and Wales. Tubercle 1979; 60: 71.
13. Joynson DM. Water: the natural habitat of Mycobacterium kansasii. Tubercle 1979; 60: 77.
14. McSwiggan DA, Collins CH. The isolation of M. kansasii and M. xenopi from water systems. Tubercle 1974; 55: 291.
15. Paull A. An environmental study of the opportunist mycobacteria. Med Lab Technol 1973; 30: 11.
16. Brooks RW, Parker BC, Gruft H, Falkinham J III. Epidemiology of infection by nontuberculous mycobacteria. V. Numbers in eastern United States soils and correlation with soil characteristics. Am Rev Respir Dis 1984; 130: 630.
17. Schwabacher H. A strain of mycobacterium isolated from skin lesions of a cold blooded animal Xenopus laevus and its relation to atypical bacilli occurring in man. J Hyg (Lond) 1959; 57: 57.
18. Portaels F, Larsson L, Jenkins PA. Isolation of Mycobacterium malmoense from the environment in Zaire. Tubercle Lung Dis 1995; 76: 160–162.
19. Meissner G, Anz W. Sources of Mycobacterium avium complex infection resulting in human disease. Am Rev Respir Dis 1977; 116: 1057.
20. Woods GL, Washington JA II. Mycobacteria other than Mycobacterium tuberculosis: review of microbiologic and clinical aspects. Rev Infect Dis 1987; 9: 275.
21. Centers for Disease Control, US Department of Health and Human Services. Diagnosis and management of mycobacterial infection and disease in persons with human immuno-deficiency virus infection. Ann Intern Med 1987; 106: 254.
22. Jenkins PA. AIDS and the lung (letter). Br Med J 1987; 295: 331.
23. Jenkins PA. Mycobacterium malmoense. Tubercle 1985; 66: 193.
24. Ispanhani P, Baker M. Mycobacterial culture: how long? Lancet 1988; 1: 305.
25. Penny ME, Cole RB, Gray J. Two cases of Mycobacterium kansasii infection occurring in the same household. Tubercle 1982; 63: 129.
26. Leat JL, Marks J. Improvement of drug-sensitivity tests on tubercle bacilli. Tubercle 1970; 51: 68.
27. Marks J. The design of sensitivity tests on tubercle bacilli. Tubercle 1961; 42: 314.
28. Banks J, Hunter AM, Campbell IA et al. Pulmonary infection with Mycobacterium kansasii in Wales, 1970–9: review of treatment and response. Thorax 1983; 38: 271.
29. Hunter AM, Campbell IA, Jenkins PA, Smith AP. Treatment of pulmonary infections caused by mycobacteria of the Mycobacterium avium-intracellulare complex. Thorax 1981; 36: 326.
30. Banks J, Hunter AM, Campbell IA et al. Pulmonary infection with Mycobacterium xenopi: review of treatment and response. Thorax 1984; 39: 376.
31. Banks J, Jenkins PA, Smith AP. Pulmonary infection with Mycobacterium malmoense – a review of treatment and response. Thorax 1985; 66: 197.
32. Banks J, Jenkins PA. Combined versus single anti-tuberculosis drugs on the in vitro sensitivity patterns of nontuberculous mycobacteria. Thorax 1987; 42: 838.
33. BTS Research Committee. Pulmonary disease caused by Mycobacterium avium-intracellulare in HIV negative patients: five year follow-up of patients receiving standardised treatment. Int J Tuberc Lung Dis, in press.
34. BTS Research Committee. Mycobacterium kansasii infection: a prospective study of the results of 9 months treatment with rifampicin and ethambutol. Thorax 1994; 49: 442.
35. BTS Research Committee. Pulmonary disease caused by M. malmoense in HIV negative patients: five year follow-up of patients receiving standardised treatment. Submitted for publication.
36. BTS Research Committee. Pulmonary disease caused by M. xenopi in HIV negative patients: five year follow-up of patients receiving standardised treatment. Eur Resp J, in press.
37. Smith MJ, Citron KM. Clinical review of pulmonary disease caused by Mycobacterium xenopi. Thorax 1983; 38: 373.
38. British Thoracic and Tuberculosis Association. Opportunist mycobacterial pulmonary infection and occupational dust exposure: an investigation in England and Wales. Tubercle 1975; 56: 295.
39. France AJ, McLeod DT, Calder MA, Seaton A. Mycobacterium malmoense infections in Scotland: an increasing problem. Thorax 1987; 42: 593.
40. Rosenzweig DY. Pulmonary mycobacterial infections due to Mycobacterium intracellulare-avium complex. Chest 1979; 75: 115.
41. Costrini AM, Mahler DA, Gross WM et al. Clinical and roentographic features of nosocomial pulmonary disease due to Mycobacterium xenopi. Am Rev Respir Dis 1981; 123: 104.
42. Engbaek HC, Vergmann B, Bentzon MW. Lung disease caused by Mycobacterium avium-intracellulare. Eur J Respir Dis 1981; 62: 72.
43. Yeager H, Raleigh JW. Pulmonary disease due to Mycobacterium intracellulare. Am Rev Respir Dis 1973; 108: 547.
44. Christensen EE, Dietz GW, Ahn CH et al. Initial roentgenographic manifestations of pulmonary Mycobacterium tuberculosis, M. kansasii and M. intracellulare infections. Chest 1981; 80: 132.
45. Evans SA, Colville A, Evans AJ et al. Comparison of the clinical features of pulmonary infections with Mycobacterium kansasii and Mycobacterium tuberculosis. Thorax 1992; 47: 876.
46. Etzkorn ET, Aldarondo S, McAllister CK et al. Medical therapy of Mycobacterium avium-intracellulare pulmonary disease. Am Rev Respir Dis 1986; 134: 442,
47. Kennedy TP, Weber DJ. Nontuberculous mycobacteria: an underappreciated cause of geriatric lung disease. Am J Respir Crit Care Med 1994; 149: 1654.
48. Lynch DA, Simone PM, Fox MA et al. CT features of pulmonary mycobacterium avium complex infection. J Computer Assisted Tomogr 1995; 19: 353.
49. Evans AJ, Crisp AJ, Colville A et al. Pulmonary infection caused by Mycobacterium malmoense: radiographic features compared with Mycobacterium tuberculosis. AJR 1993; 161: 733.
50. Contreras MA, Cheung OT, Sanders DE et al. Pulmonary infection with non-tuberculous mycobacteria. Am Rev Respir Dis 1988; 137: 149.
51. Ahn CH, Ahn SS, Anderson RA et al. A four-drug regimen for initial treatment of cavitary disease caused by Mycobacterium avium complex. Am Rev Respir Dis 1986; 134: 438.
52. Dutt AK, Stead WW. Long-term results of medical treatment in Mycobacterium intracellulare infection. Am J Med 1979; 67: 449.
53. Parrot RG, Gross AJH. Post-surgical outcome of 57 patients with Mycobacterium xenopi pulmonary infection. Tubercle 1988; 69: 47.
54. Hawkins CC, Gold JWM, Whimbey E et al. Mycobacterium avium complex infections in patients with the acquired immunodeficiency syndrome. Ann Intern Med 1986; 105: 184.

55. British Thoracic Society. Management of opportunist mycobacterial infections: Joint Tuberculosis Committee Guidelines 1999. Thorax 2000; 55: 210.

56. Pozniak AC, Miller R, Ormerod LP. The treatment of tuberculosis in HIV-infected persons. AIDS 1999; 13: 435.

57. Kemper CA, Havlir D, Bartock AE et al. Transient bacteraemia due to *Mycobacterium avium* complex in patients with AIDS. J Infect Dis 1994; 170: 488.

58. Stanford JL. Newer tuberculins – profile in developing countries. In: Seth V, ed. Essentials of TB in children. 1997; 58–72.

59. White MP, Bangash H, Goel KM, Jenkins PA. Non-tuberculous mycobacterial lymphadenitis. Arch Dis Child 1986; 61: 368.

40 Bronchopulmonary aspergillosis

Douglas Robinson and Patrick Flood-Page

 Key points

1 Allergic bronchopulmonary aspergillosis

- Allergic bronchopulmonary aspergillosis (ABPA) occurs almost exclusively in atopic individuals with underlying asthma or cystic fibrosis.
- Pathology results from the host immune response to persistent *Aspergillus* colonisation of the airways.
- ABPA is characterised by:
  - pulmonary eosinophilia
  - mucus plugging with pulmonary, lobar or segmental collapse
  - central bronchiectasis
  - *Aspergillus*-specific IgE and IgG.
- ABPA should be excluded in asthmatics with unexplained deterioration or irreversible airway obstruction.

2 Aspergilloma

- Aspergillomas represent fungal growth in existing lung cavities.
- Pathology results from a combination of direct damage by the fungus itself and the host immune response.
- *Aspergillus* precipitins are usually positive.
- Computed tomography is frequently diagnostic.
- Massive haemoptysis is a common complication.

3 Invasive aspergillosis

- Invasive aspergillosis is predominantly a disease of the immunocompromised, especially neutropenic patients.
- Pathology results primarily from direct damage caused by *Aspergillus* organisms.
- Diagnosis may be by computed tomography and/or serology.
- Prognosis is poor, particularly if treatment is delayed.

Aspergillosis, a collective name for conditions caused by members of the genus *Aspergillus*, was one of the first mycoses to be recognised in humans.[1] It was not until published reports in the 1950s, however, that the importance of these mycoses was fully appreciated. *Aspergillus fumigatus* is by far the most common cause of pulmonary aspergillosis, but other species (*Aspergillus clavatus*, *Aspergillus flavus*, *Aspergillus nidulans*, *Aspergillus niger*, *Aspergillus niveus*, *Aspergillus oryzae* and *Aspergillus terreus*) can cause disease of the lungs and nasal sinuses.

Aspergillus species are ubiquitous in our environment, found typically in moist areas of decaying organic matter such as hay and compost. However, they can also be cultured from such indoor sources as house dust and air-conditioning units. *Aspergillus* spores are 2–3 mm in diameter and are readily respirable, deposition occurring principally in the proximal large airways. The humidity and temperature of 37°C here are the optimal growth conditions for *Aspergillus fumigatus* and this may be part of the reason why airway colonisation occurs so readily with this species.

There are three main types of pulmonary disease caused by *Aspergillus*:

- allergic reactions to *Aspergillus* species: here the pathology results from the host immune response to the organism
- colonising aspergillosis: fungal growth in pre-existing scars or cavities
- invasive and disseminated aspergillosis: pathology caused by unchecked fungal growth.

The vast majority of disease states within these three categories occur in patients with pre-existing bronchial, bronchopulmonary or systemic diseases (e.g. bronchial asthma, cystic fibrosis, bronchopulmonary cavitation caused by tuberculosis and other diseases, and immunodeficiency states).

Pathogenesis

The pathogenesis of fungal disease is not well understood. While the association between invasive aspergillosis and granulocyte dysfunction, between asthma and allergic bronchopulmonary aspergillosis (ABPA) and between cavitary lung disease and aspergilloma is clear, the cellular mechanisms underlying these disorders are less certain. The pathological features of all these diseases result, in part, from the damage caused by the fungus itself and, in part, from the often unsuccessful attempts of the host immune system to clear it. The relative contribution of these two features in a given setting determines the appearances seen.

Aspergillus-related tissue damage

Mucociliary factors

Epithelial damage appears to be a common feature connecting asthma and cystic fibrosis, both of which predispose to ABPA. Similarly, individuals with chronic obstructive pulmonary disease (COPD), sarcoidosis and other chronic lung disorders are at higher risk of invasive aspergillosis, while underlying disruption of lung architecture is a prerequisite for aspergilloma formation. It may be that factors that damage the airway and interfere with fungal clearance allow colonisation and immune activation, and are thus important in the pathogenesis of ABPA in particular but also in other *Aspergillus*-related diseases.

Culture filtrates of clinical isolates of *A. fumigatus* have been shown to slow ciliary beat frequency and to damage human respiratory epithelium in vitro.[2] This effect is in part mediated by gliotoxin produced by *Aspergillus*, which is toxic to the bronchial epithelium at low concentrations, but may involve other *Aspergillus* toxins and as yet uncharacterised high-molecular-weight *Aspergillus* proteins. Thus, *Aspergillus* colonisation may further impair mucociliary clearance and predispose to chronic fungal colonisation and progression of underlying pathology such as cystic fibrosis.

Interference with phagocyte function

Cell-mediated immunity and activation of the alternative complement pathway play a crucial role in the host defence against fungal pathogens. Alveolar macrophages and polymorphonuclear cells cooperate in the control and elimination of the fungus in the airways. Several fungal metabolites, including gliotoxin and aflatoxin, have been shown to interfere with macrophage adherence and phagocytosis and with intracellular killing.[3] Henwick found that *A. fumigatus* bound fewer complement molecules than did less pathogenic species.[4] A fungus-derived complement inhibitory factor has been described that has been shown to decrease binding of the key complement component, C3b, to fungal surfaces.[5] This protein is not expressed by less pathogenic species.

In addition, gliotoxin has been shown to inhibit T-cell proliferation, cytotoxic T-cell activation and monocyte and fibroblast function. This immunosuppressive action of gliotoxin and aflatoxin and other toxins produced by *A. fumigatus*, including fumagillin and the ribotoxin restitocin, are thought to be important factors facilitating fungal colonisation of the airways.[6]

Adhesion

Adhesion of *A. fumigatus* to the bronchial epithelium may be a crucial step allowing fungal colonisation and the development of ABPA in susceptible individuals. Adhesion of *A. fumigatus* has been described to extracellular matrix, serum proteins and other subepithelial components exposed after tissue damage, in particular, laminin, fibronectin, collagen and fibrinogen.[6] *A. fumigatus* binds more strongly to fibronectin and to the basal lamina than other *Aspergillus* species,[7] while only pathogenic *Aspergillus* species, including *A. fumigatus*, bind to fibrinogen.[8]

Tissue damage

Aspergillus species produce a large variety of extracellular enzymes, including nucleases, phosphatases, peptidase and proteases. These degrade macromolecules to provide nutrients for the fungus but the tissue damage they cause at the same time may be important in the pathogenesis of *Aspergillus*-related disease.[6]

Elastase activity has been associated with *A. fumigatus* virulence in mice.[9] Antibodies against AFA1P, the major elastinolytic protease produced by *A. fumigatus*, protected immunocompetent mice against fatal infection.[10] In addition, in immunocompetent hosts, fungal proteases may induce local airway inflammation through the recruitment of inflammatory cells following activation of epithelial cells.[11]

The importance of *Aspergillus* proteases in the pathogenesis of fungal infections, however, has not always been confirmed by other studies.

Host immunological factors

Effective phagocyte function is an essential component of the host defences against fungal infection. Macrophage and, in particular, neutrophil dysfunction is the principal immunological defect underlying the majority of cases of invasive aspergillosis, either through a reduction in absolute numbers of granulocytes, as in the pre-engraftment phase of bone-marrow transplant, or through a specific neutrophil defect such as the impaired intracellular killing underlying myeloperoxidase deficiency and chronic granulomatosis. Corticosteroid treatment and human immunodeficiency virus (HIV) infection are risk factors for invasive aspergillosis and are also associated with impaired neutrophil function.

T-cell function is also important, particularly in the more chronic forms of invasive aspergillosis.[12] Individuals with severe combined immunodeficiency and those taking ciclosporin and other immunosuppressive agents that depress T-cell function – after organ transplant, for example – are also at relative risk of invasive aspergillosis. An interaction between neutrophil dysfunction and T-helper (Th) cells via interleukin (IL)-4 has been observed in experimental models of invasive aspergillosis.[12] Impaired Th2 cell responses in IL-4 knockout mice have been associated with resistance to invasive aspergillosis.[13] Conversely, interferon (IFN)-γ knockout mice are more susceptible to disease.

In profoundly immunocompromised individuals with invasive fungal infection, lesions are associated with minimal tissue response and the necrosis seen in such lesions is primarily related to fungal proteolytic enzymes and other toxic metabolites capable of tissue damage. In those with lesser degrees of immunocompromise, and seen most dramatically in the setting of neutrophil recovery following bone-marrow transplant, there may be a florid tissue response with extensive local tissue damage. The risk of vascular invasion and life-threatening haemorrhage in this setting may be a major management problem.

By contrast, in ABPA and aspergilloma, although fungal metabolites may exacerbate inflammation[11] there is little evidence that these are central to the pathogenesis of ABPA and it is more likely that the immunological response to the presence of Aspergillus antigen in the airways is more important.

One prominent feature of the immune response to Aspergillus that has received much attention is the intense polyclonal antibody response to the high antigen load resulting from Aspergillus colonisation of the airways. Total and specific immunoglobulin (Ig)E, IgG and IgA levels are elevated in disease. During exacerbation of ABPA and persistently in the majority with aspergilloma, titres may reach extremely high levels. These may drop to normal levels after treatment with oral steroids. There is evidence that IgE and IgA specific to A. fumigatus, but not IgG, is produced locally in the airways.[14]

It has been suggested that the locally high concentrations of antigen and specific antibody leads to a local immune-complex deposition and a type III immunological response that underlies the pathological changes seen in ABPA and may be responsible for local damage surrounding aspergilloma. Although there is some evidence that the presence of both IgE and IgG precipitating antibody are necessary for the development of ABPA in a monkey model,[15] local immune-deposition is not a prominent pathological feature of ABPA and moreover the same pathological studies show little evidence of the vasculitis and neutrophilic infiltrate that would normally be expected in a type III reaction.[16,17]

One striking feature in the majority of individuals with ABPA is the elevated level of both non-specific and Aspergillus-specific IgE. A role for a type I reaction to the pathogenesis of ABPA has been proposed with mast cell degranulation and the release of, in particular, histamine, leukotrienes, IL-4, IL-5 and other cytokines. ABPA has, however, been reported in individuals

with a negative immediate cutaneous reaction to Aspergillus antigen,[18] not all individuals with ABPA have elevated IgE levels[19] and mast cells are not a prominent feature of the disease.[16] Certainly, Aspergillus sensitisation may occur in isolation in asthmatics, without ABPA, and here Aspergillus-specific IgE may contribute to immediate symptoms. The role of environmental fungi in allergic asthma is not well defined, though it is of note that at least one study suggested that fungal sensitisation (to Alternaria species) contributed to a seasonal increase in asthma deaths in the mid-western USA.[20]

More recent work has looked at the importance of T-cell-mediated inflammation in ABPA. Histopathological studies have shown a spectrum of appearances. Asthmatic individuals may show features of predominately Th2-related inflammation, with prominent submucosal inflammation, abundant eosinophils and subepithelial fibrosis. Non-asthmatics, by contrast, may have features more typical of a Th1 inflammation, with multinucleated giant cells and granulomata formation. Most, however, show varying combination of these features with eosinophils and granulomata being usual findings.[16,17]

Chauhan and co-workers found that the majority of Aspergillus-antigen-specific T-cell clones in three asthmatics with ABPA produced a typical Th1 profile in the presence of whole antigen.[21] Murali, however, found a mixed pattern of cytokine production in peripheral mononuclear cells.[22] In response to stimulation with two Aspergillus antigens (the 35 kDa antigen and heat shock protein (HSP)-1, they found an increase in IFN-γ, IL-2 and IL-5 but no increase in either IgE or IL-4. One possible factor predisposing to ABPA in asthma is the Th2-type 'environment' of the airway, where the protective Th1 response to Aspergillus colonisation may be reduced relative to non-asthmatic individuals.

One difficulty with the current understanding of ABPA pathogenesis is that it does not address why some individuals with asthma or other conditions develop ABPA while the vast majority of others do not. Chauhan and co-workers observed that, in individuals with ABPA, the majority of T-cells responded to antigen only in association with specific HLA-DR subtypes. The extension of these findings to a larger group identified six HLA-DR subtypes that accounted for most cases of ABPA.[21] This potentially important finding ties in with the idea of a T-cell-driven process favoured by some and discussed above.

Grunig et al found that IL-10 knockout mice were markedly more susceptible to lung pathology induced by A. fumigatus proteins.[23] This model may mimic ABPA and offers an opportunity to explore the relative roles of host immunogenetics (and class II major histocompatibility complex, MHC, in recognition of Aspergillus antigens) and the failure of regulatory T-cell responses to suppress potentially pathological T-cell activation. These possibilities are shown in Figure 40.1.

Allergic reactions to *Aspergillus* species in asthma

Up to 25% of asthmatic individuals have a positive skin-prick test to A. fumigatus extract, indicating the presence of specific

Asthmatic   **Non-asthmatic**

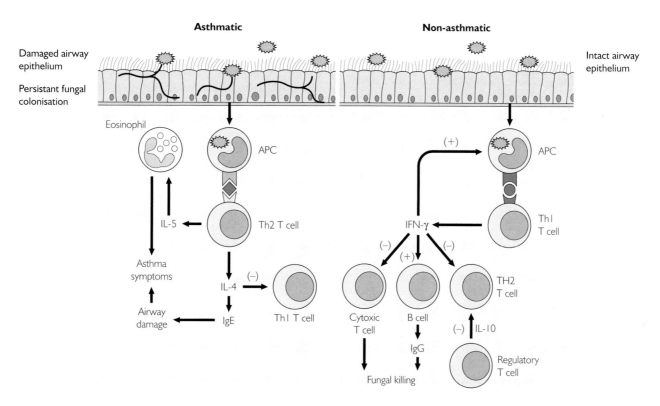

Fig. 40.1 Pathogenesis of allergic bronchopulmonary aspergillosis. In the non-asthmatic epithelium there is a predominantly Th1-type inflammatory response to the presence of *Aspergillus* with clearance of the fungus from the airways. In the asthmatic individual the impaired epithelial integrity facilitates persistent fungal colonisation. A predominantly Th2-type inflammatory response to the presence of *Aspergillus* leads to persistent airways inflammation, which fails to clear the fungus, perpetuating the cycle of continuing fungal colonisation, inflammation, worsening asthma symptoms and ultimately airway damage. APC, antigen presenting cells; IFN, interferon; Ig, immunoglobulin; IL, interleukin; Th, T-helper.

IgE. In these individuals experimental exposure to inhaled *Aspergillus* can cause an early and late airway response that resembles exposure to other allergens, e.g. house dust mite.[24] It is likely, therefore, that exposure to *Aspergillus* spores in the environment is contributory to asthmatic symptoms in these individuals. Most have evidence of immediate cutaneous hypersensitivity to other common allergens and the vast majority of asthmatics with skin-test evidence of hypersensitivity to *A. fumigatus* have asthma that is not clinically distinguishable from that in other atopic asthmatics with perennial symptoms. It is not understood why only a small proportion of individuals go on to develop ABPA.

Allergic aspergillosis

Allergic aspergillosis can be subdivided into three main groups:

- ABPA
- allergic *Aspergillus* sinusitis
- allergic alveolitis.

Allergic bronchopulmonary aspergillosis

Allergic bronchopulmonary aspergillosis, first described in 1952, is caused by hypersensitivity reactions to *A. fumigatus* involving

the bronchial wall and peripheral parts of the lung. It is characterised by intermittent or continuous colonisation of the bronchi by vegetative *A. fumigatus* elements along with immunological evidence of body tissue reactions to this fungus. In the vast majority of cases it is associated with asthma, but the incidence of ABPA is higher in all individuals with atopic disorders[25] and in those with cystic fibrosis and pre-existing idiopathic bronchiectasis.[26] There are also isolated reports of ABPA-like syndromes associated with other *Aspergillus* species as well as the other fungi, *Curvularia*, *Candida*, *Dreschlera* and *Stemphylium*.[27]

There is no generally accepted prevalence for ABPA. Studies have used different criteria in different populations but the prevalence of ABPA in a general asthmatic population is probably between 1% and 2%,[28] and 7–14% in patients with corticosteroid-dependent asthma.[29]

Allergic bronchopulmonary aspergillosis complicates cystic fibrosis in about 8–10% of cases.[26]

In one series, 50% of patients with 'pulmonary eosinophilia' were subsequently shown to have ABPA.[30]

Pathology

Because the diagnosis of ABPA has been made largely by clinical evaluation and laboratory testing, lung biopsies are seldom performed in this setting and there are few published studies of the pathology of ABPA.

There are two apparently distinct pathological processes.[16,17]

■ Dense eosinophilic infiltration of the lung parenchyma is responsible for the fleeting peripheral radiological shadows characteristic of this disease. Histological examination of lesions of this type has shown a form of eosinophilic pneumonia. It is not clear whether or not this eosinophilic infiltration of the interstitial parts of the lung produces permanent pathological sequelae.

■ Macroscopically, there is often occlusion of bronchi by mucus plugs which may be associated with distal collapsed lung. Associated with this there may be bronchiectasis, often proximal and in the upper lobes.

Histologically, the findings in most individuals resemble asthma, with epithelial damage, a prominent eosinophilic and mononuclear infiltrate and subepithelial collagen deposition. Non-asthmatics show few of these features, although eosinophil inflammation tends to remain prominent. In addition, in both asthmatics and non-asthmatics there are usually granulomata, often displaying central necrosis and multinucleate giant cells. Bronchi contain mucus and often Curschmann's spirals, Charcot–Leyden crystals (eosinophil degradation products) and fungal hyphae, which are not seen to invade the bronchial wall. There may be bronchial-wall thickening and fibrosis and other microscopic features of bronchiectasis.

Bronchocentric granulomatosis

The inflammation in ABPA is bronchocentric, perhaps reflecting the inhaled antigen, and in one study 15 of 18 subjects had histological features resembling bronchocentric granulomatosis.[16] Bronchocentric granulomatosis is thought of as a distinct clinical entity consisting of chronic symptoms of malaise, cough, fever, breathlessness, chest pain and haemoptysis in association with a focal lesion on chest radiograph or computed tomography (CT). Other clinical features of ABPA are not seen and Aspergillus precipitins are often negative. The lesions tend to be peripheral and usually contain Aspergillus hyphae. The relationship to ABPA is uncertain. One possibility is that this represents localised ABPA, or a similar immune response to other foreign antigens.

Bronchocentric granulomatosis and its pathological features are discussed in more detail later in this book.

Clinical features

Allergic bronchopulmonary aspergillosis occurs predominantly in patients with pre-existing asthma. It has been reported in infants but is most often found in adults. It is a relatively common complication of cystic fibrosis (see below) and it can rarely present with lobar or segmental pulmonary collapse in atopic but non-asthmatic individuals.[31]

Fever, breathlessness, cough productive of bronchial casts and worsening of asthmatic symptoms can all be manifestations of ABPA, but an acute exacerbation of ABPA in asthmatic individuals may be asymptomatic[32] and occasionally the diagnosis is suggested by abnormalities on incidental chest radiographs of patients whose asthmatic symptoms are no worse than usual. When repeated episodes of ABPA have been responsible for the development of bronchiectasis, the symptoms and complications of that disease often overshadow those of asthma, and the clinical manifestations of bacterial bronchopulmonary infection may be difficult to distinguish from episodes of ABPA.

Allergic bronchopulmonary aspergillosis has been classified into five stages: I (acute), II (remission), III (exacerbation), IV (corticosteroid-dependent asthma) and V (fibrotic end stage), in an attempt to aid diagnosis and management.[33]

Individuals without radiological evidence of bronchiectasis but with other features consistent with ABPA have been termed seropositive ABPA (ABPA-S) and those with central bronchiectasis, ABPA-CB.[34] Whether these represent different stages of disease or separate clinical patterns is uncertain, as therefore is any strategy to prevent progression of ABPA-S to ABPA-CB. Thus such classification is of limited clinical relevance.

Diagnosis

Allergic bronchopulmonary aspergillosis is suspected on clinical grounds but the diagnosis is confirmed by serological and radiological findings. There are no internationally agreed guidelines for the diagnosis of ABPA but most authors' diagnostic criteria include the following.

In the USA the first five group A criteria are considered essential and one of group B is normally also required to make a firm diagnosis.[35] While most of the criteria tend to be present during acute exacerbations of ABPA (stages I and III),[36] they are rarely all present at the same time between exacerbations (stages II and V) or while taking oral steroids (stage IV). Using these guidelines, therefore, there may be a delay of some years before a certain diagnosis is established. Authors in the UK have suggested less stringent diagnostic criteria requiring only a positive skin-prick test, with positive serum precipitins and/or evidence of Aspergillus in sputum together with the presence of, or clear history of, an infiltrate on chest radiograph.[37] While this second approach may be more useful in practice, none of the group A criteria are specific for ABPA and, as uncomplicated asthma may have some or occasionally all of these criteria, it may be more difficult to distinguish these asthmatic individuals from those with ABPA and a normal or near-normal chest radiographic appearance at the time of the examination. To some extent the distinction is academic, unless clearly effective strategies to prevent disease progression are agreed.

Skin-prick tests

Skin-prick tests use commercially prepared standardised extracts of A. fumigatus and detect specific IgE, a positive weal and flare being apparent within 15 minutes. The maximum diameter of the weal should be measured and reactions of 3 mm or more than the negative control should be regarded as positive.

A positive reaction is seen in practically all cases of ABPA and a negative test effectively excludes the diagnosis. Variation in the quality of Aspergillus extract composition has been cited as a potential reason for earlier reports of negative reactions in individuals with ABPA.[38] Using modern standardised allergen extracts within a defined shelf-life, these problems can largely be avoided.

In addition, isolated cases when other clinical features are consistent with ABPA, skin-prick tests, serology or sputum culture may suggest another fungal species as the causative agent.

While the skin-prick test is a very sensitive screening tool it is not particularly specific for ABPA; up to 25% of uncomplicated asthmatics have positive tests.[28]

Serum IgE

Total serum IgE levels in ABPA are generally markedly above the normal range and higher than those found in uncomplicated asthma.[39] This is mainly caused by a non-specific increase in IgE. As for skin-prick tests (which also detect specific IgE), the absence of A.-fumigatus-specific IgE makes the diagnosis of ABPA unlikely. Although A.-fumigatus-specific IgE and IgG levels are also higher in ABPA than in A.-fumigatus-sensitised asthmatic patients, there is considerable overlap. Because of this, most radioallergosorbent tests (RAST) and enzyme-linked immunosorbent assays (ELISA) to specific IgE and IgG have not been found useful in clinical practice – they add little to the skin-prick tests but are equally non-specific. There is evidence, however, that different Aspergillus proteins are expressed depending on the growth environment that the fungus is found in[40] and more recent studies have attempted to use proteins expressed preferentially in ABPA as the basis for immunological testing. Using the purified Aspergillus protein Asp f2 [41] as the basis for an ELISA and RAST and using recombinant Asp f4 and Asp f6 [42] protein as the basis for a skin-prick test, these tests have been found to be more specific for ABPA. Both trials, however, used selected populations. Neither test has been proven as yet in clinical practice but may show promise for the future.

Serum precipitins

Precipitating antibody of IgG type to A. fumigatus is present in the serum of 70% of patients. Concentration of the serum increases the number of positive precipitin reactions to more than 90%.[43] Although less sensitive than the skin-prick test it is more specific for ABPA but, even so, precipitins have been found in 3% of healthy office workers, 12% of patients with atopic asthma and 27% of patients with farmer's lung.[44] These antibodies are detected using a double gel diffusion technique (Fig. 40.2).

Mycological examination of sputum

The visualisation of Aspergillus hyphae in sputum from patients with asthma indicates fungal colonisation of the bronchial wall and provides strong confirmation of a diagnosis of ABPA. Sputum culture using mycological media is positive in around 60% of patients with ABPA,[45] rising to around 80% during exacerbation.[18] Sputum containing A. fumigatus is produced only intermittently by patients with allergic aspergillosis. A single negative sputum sample on microscopy and culture cannot therefore be used as evidence to exclude a diagnosis of ABPA.

The clinical and laboratory features of ABPA are summarised in Table 40.1.

Chest radiograph changes

The chest radiograph may be normal.

Abnormalities on chest radiograph can be subdivided into transient and permanent.

Transient radiological abnormalities

Transient changes may be diffuse non-segmental pulmonary infiltrates (Fig. 40.3) or whole-lung, lobar or segmental collapse, depending on the underlying pathology.

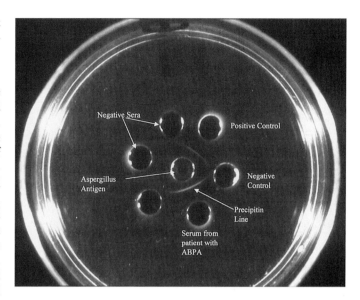

Fig. 40.2 Aspergillus precipitins – double gel diffusion technique. A. fumigatus antigen is placed in the central well and the test serum in the surrounding wells. An arc of antibody/antigen complex precipitates when the test serum contains IgG against A. fumigatus. When the titre is high, in individuals with aspergilloma for example, multiple precipitin arcs may form.

Pulmonary, lobar or segmental collapse are usually caused by bronchial occlusion without prominent pulmonary infiltration (Fig. 40.4). This is demonstrated by the almost immediate clearing of radiological abnormality that occurs after bronchoscopic removal of mucus plugs. It is likely, however, that persisting occlusion of major bronchi is responsible for permanent bronchopulmonary damage, which, in turn, is the cause of the fixed radiological abnormalities.

Diffuse pulmonary infiltrates are non-segmental and represent the eosinophilic infiltrative process seen histologically. They may be bilateral but are rarely as extensive and uniformly distributed as those seen in cryptogenic eosinophilic pneumonia. These infiltrates are characteristically transient or fleeting and are usually accompanied by a marked elevation of the peripheral blood eosinophil count. Perihilar infiltrates may simulate hilar lymphadenopathy.

Permanent radiological abnormalities

The range of radiological changes seen in 111 cases of ABPA has been reviewed and described in detail.[49] Chronic changes of bronchiectasis are common and usually favour the upper lobe. Tramline or parallel-line shadows may be visible. These extend out from the hilum in the anatomical direction of the larger bronchi and represent the combination of bronchial wall thickening and dilatation of bronchiectasis. There may also be evidence of ring shadows caused by dilated bronchi seen in cross-section and the cysts of proximal saccular bronchiectasis. These changes may be isolated or may merge with more generalised lung fibrosis with volume contraction.

When mucus impaction in a large and dilated bronchus does not result in collapse of the distal segments, the impacted bronchus may be clearly outlined, giving a 'gloved-finger', 'tooth-

Table 40.1 The clinical and laboratory features of allergic bronchopulmonary aspergillosis (ABPA)

	ABPA (%)	Asthma (%)	Cystic fibrosis (%)
ABPA	–	1–2[28]	8–10[26]
Cutaneous immediate reaction	±100	25[28]	47–53[26]
Specific IgE	±100	NR	20[26]
Total IgE >1000 ng/ml	64 /95[34‡]	50[46]	22[26]
Serum precipitins	70–90[44*]	10[28]	31–51[26,47]
Sputum *Aspergillus*	58/83[18,45†‡]	NR	9–25[26,47]
Blood eosinophilia	35/94[48‡]	40[46]	18[26]
Asthma	96[46]	–	27[26]

* 90% after concentration. †Sputum on three consecutive days. ‡ In remission/during exacerbation. NR, not recorded.

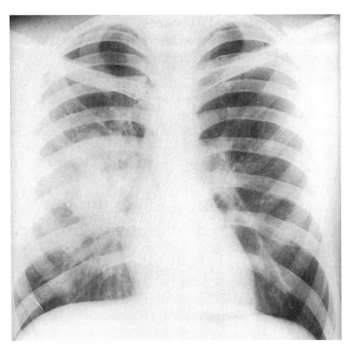

Fig. 40.3 Radiograph showing peripheral pulmonary shadowing in a patient with allergic bronchopulmonary aspergillosis. This patient had repeated episodes of fleeting pulmonary shadowing associated with worsening of asthmatic symptoms.

paste' or 'rabbits ear' appearance (Fig. 40.5). Mucus may be expectorated in the form of bronchial casts and these radiological abnormalities disappear. Although for this reason these radiological shadows can be transient, they differ from the fleeting pulmonary opacities described above in that they are associated with permanent distortion of bronchial architecture, whereas this is not necessarily the case with fleeting peripheral pulmonary infiltrates.

Upper lobe abnormalities are common in ABPA but similar radiological changes are seen in tuberculosis, sarcoidosis, allergic alveolitis and cystic fibrosis.

It is important to emphasise that an inconspicuous radiological abnormality such as a parallel-line shadow may be evidence of extensive bronchopulmonary damage, and also that the chest radiograph may be normal in the presence of extensive bronchiectasis.

Computed tomography

As CT scanning technology has improved and experience with ABPA has increased, CT scanning has emerged as a key imaging modality in the diagnosis of ABPA.

High-resolution CT is considerable more sensitive than chest radiography for the detection of bronchiectasis.[50] This feature is seen in between 80%[50] and 95%[51] of cases of ABPA defined using the clinical group A criteria above. It tends to favour the upper lobes, except in advanced disease where it may be more widespread. The bronchiectasis is classically central in distribution and this is the most common pattern seen (Fig. 40.6). A predominantly central pattern is, however, seen in up to 35% of cases of bronchiectasis of other causes, and this feature is therefore not diagnostic.[52]

Mucoid impaction is also a prominent CT feature, frequently seen as branching structures, most commonly in the upper lobes.[53] Mucoid impaction may be seen on chest radiograph but, again, CT is more sensitive, detecting more subtle changes, some with atelectasis distally. Centrilobular nodules, thought to be mucus impaction seen in cross-section, were reported in 93% of individuals in one study.[51]

Pulmonary infiltrates are seen most commonly as areas of consolidation affecting the mid-zones but may have a mass-like appearance. Pathologically, these areas represent the eosinophilic infiltration of acute ABPA and may be migratory. There may be pleural thickening.

None of these CT features is diagnostic of ABPA. The differential diagnosis of each individual feature is wide but the coincidence of fleeting consolidation with central bronchiectasis and other features is highly suggestive of ABPA.

The separation of skin-prick-positive asthma from ABPA as noted above is a frequent diagnostic problem. A recent study comparing the CT appearances of these two groups found that

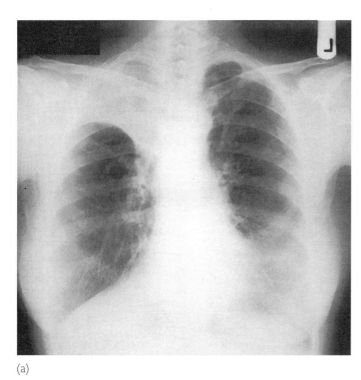

(a)

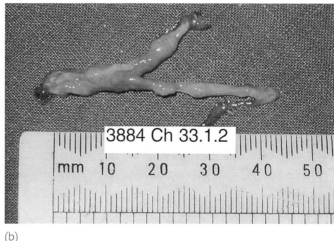

(b)

Fig. 40.4 (a) Radiograph showing collapse of the right upper lobe due to mucoid impaction in a patient with allergic bronchopulmonary aspergillosis. The upper lobe did not aerate with intensive medical treatment and the mucus plug had to be removed at bronchoscopy. (b) A bronchial cast (mucus plug) extracted at bronchoscopy from a patient with allergic bronchopulmonary aspergillosis who presented with lobar collapse.

bronchiectasis affecting more than three lobes, centrilobular nodules and mucus impaction were highly suggestive of ABPA.[51] The correct diagnosis was made by both observers in more than 90% of cases. Although this study was undertaken in a tertiary referral centre and may therefore reflect a more severe spectrum of disease, modern CT techniques may well prove useful in this difficult area in the future.

Lung function tests

Lung function abnormalities in acute and chronic ABPA are variable and are not diagnostic. Acute exacerbations may not alter lung function tests, may cause further airway obstruction in asthma or may lead to a restrictive defect with reduced gas transfer. Worsening airway obstruction in chronic asthma, particularly when difficult to reverse, should prompt a search for evidence of ABPA. Lung function monitoring is often used to guide therapy in chronic ABPA, with some evidence that oral corticosteroid therapy can reduce progressive decline.

An approach to the diagnosis of ABPA is outlined in Figure 40.7.

Treatment

Treatment of ABPA has three aims:

- acute therapy to control exacerbations
- maintenance therapy to prevent recurrences and to limit progressive lung damage
- control of the predisposition lung condition (asthma or cystic fibrosis).

There are two approaches to treatment: the suppression of inflammation with systemic steroids and the reduction of the allergen load with antifungals.

Management of the acute exacerbation

The principal drug used in the management of ABPA remains a systemic corticosteroid.

Corticosteroids, typically prednisolone at 0.5 mg/kg rapidly clear the pulmonary infiltrate and associated symptoms of an acute ABPA exacerbation. Lobar, segmental or subsegmental collapse caused by bronchial occlusion does not always respond to such treatment and, if evidence of major bronchial obstruction persists after a week of intensive bronchodilator therapy, vigorous physiotherapy and high-dose corticosteroid treatment, bronchoscopy should be undertaken to remove impacted mucus.[46]

In theory, reducing the amount of *Aspergillus* allergen in the bronchi with antifungal medication will reduce antigenic stimulation to some extent, with a reduction in the inflammatory response. Most of the published studies have focused on the use of these drugs in chronic ABPA. Although an effect on acute exacerbations has been reported in one study using itraconazole,[54] others have noted that acute exacerbations occurring during studies of chronic disease were not cleared by itraconazole, although the frequency of exacerbation was reduced.[55]

Chronic disease

While the role of systemic corticosteroids in the acute exacerbation is well established, the use of these agents in long-term prophylaxis with the aim of preventing exacerbation and reducing the decline in lung function is less clear.

There are reports from retrospective studies that patients treated with long-term oral corticosteroids fare better than those who receive this form of treatment intermittently.[56,57] Many episodes of radiological relapse are not associated with symptoms and, because of concern that treatment limited to symptomatic episodes might allow permanent lung damage to take place unnoticed, maintenance oral steroids have been recommended by some for all patients with frequent pulmonary

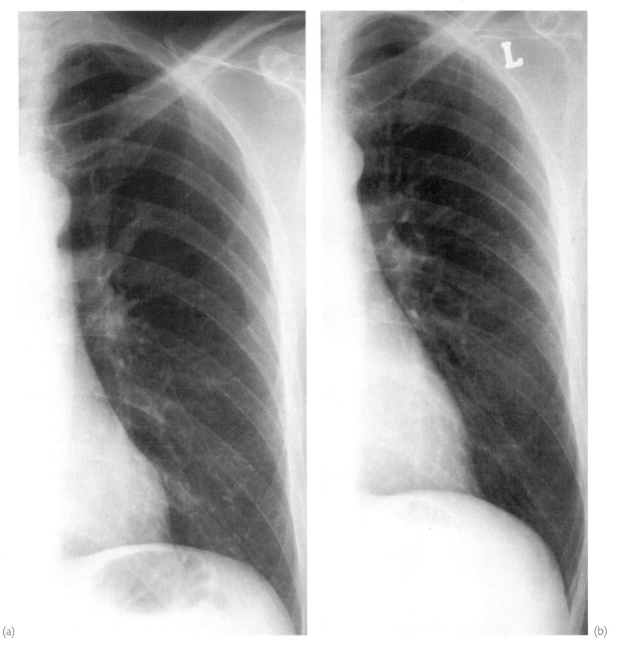

(a)

(b)

Fig. 40.5 Gloved-finger abnormality and central bronchiectasis. (a) Chest radiograph showing gloved-finger abnormality affecting the left upper lobe. (b) Chest radiograph 6 weeks later with clearance revealing the underlying bronchiectasis.

infiltrates.[56] There is some evidence that a rising IgE level predicts subsequent ABPA exacerbation.[34] By regularly monitoring IgE levels and obtaining a chest radiograph when the levels rise two- to threefold it may be possible to identify radiological relapse, which may be associated with increased airflow obstruction and reduced carbon monoxide transfer factor (T_LCO) and/or restrictive changes. Some authors have recommended this approach to identify and treat asymptomatic ABPA exacerbations[37] in the hope that this would help prevent lung function decline. Further prospective studies are required, but this approach seems reasonable on current evidence if rising specific IgE and X-ray changes are associated with deterioration in lung function.

However, only a minority of patients with ABPA are at risk of progressive lung damage and the evidence for long-term benefit comes from retrospective uncontrolled studies, while the long-term side effects of systemic steroids are well known and include a small risk of invasive aspergillosis.[58]

Until there is more evidence defining the precise role of systemic steroids in the long-term management of ABPA, many authors would restrict its use to two groups of patients – those with frequent symptomatic exacerbations and those with evidence of progressive lung damage.[46] In the remainder, once symptoms have improved and with radiological clearance, the oral steroids should be tailed off over the next month. Some authors, however, recommend 3 months of treatment with

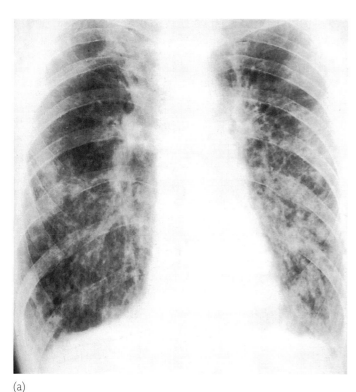

(a)

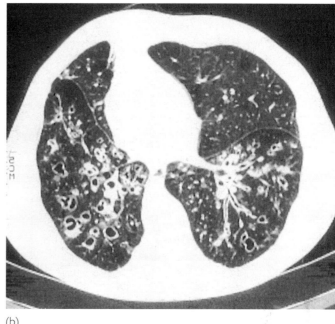

(b)

Fig. 40.6 Bronchiectasis associated with allergic bronchopulmonary aspergillosis.

withdrawal over the subsequent 3 months.[37] Because of concerns that even relatively short courses of oral steroids can increase the risk of bone loss and fracture, this approach should probably be reserved for those with an early relapse following a shorter course.

Inhaled corticosteroids help to control the symptoms of asthma but are not thought to prevent exacerbations of ABPA or progression of lung damage, although there have been no studies directed towards these specific areas.

The problems with systemic steroids have led to a search for alternative therapies. Studies of treatment with various inhaled and oral antifungal agents have shown variable results. Those showing benefit were uncontrolled and improvements may have represented the episodic nature of the disease process. Recently, a randomised controlled study using itraconazole showed a small but significant benefit in terms of a combined lung function, symptom score, IgE concentration and radiological resolution endpoint after 16 weeks, with additional benefit during a following-on open-label period.[55] The benefit in the relatively short blinded phase was modest and the significance of the open-label phase is unproven, although the results were largely in keeping with other uncontrolled studies using itraconazole.[59] The results of longer-term controlled studies are awaited.

While these and other studies have found itraconazole to be well tolerated, there remains a concern with liver toxicity during long-term therapy and liver function should be monitored.

Control of environmental exposure

There is some evidence that exposure to high concentration of *A. fumigatus* in the environment may be associated with exacerbation either of ABPA or of underlying asthma.[60] Removal of the source of *Aspergillus* in one household was not associated with

improvement in 13 ABPA patients in one study.[45] Although acute exposure to environments likely to have high levels of *Aspergillus*, e.g. compost, should be avoided, it is not known whether chronic low-level exposure is important and whether life-style changes, e.g. movement from damp housing, should be recommended.

Optimal control of underlying disease

Adequate treatment of airflow obstruction is much more important in ABPA than in patients with uncomplicated asthma. Retention of mucus and formation of bronchial casts are more likely to occur in narrowed airways than in bronchi of normal calibre; hence every attempt should be made to achieve as good control of asthmatic symptoms as is possible. This will, in most cases, require an inhaled corticosteroid as well as, in some, maintenance oral treatment, together with bronchodilators. Inhaled corticosteroids do not prevent pulmonary infiltrates but improve asthma control without encouraging fungal growth within the lungs.[32] Good control of cystic fibrosis is important for the same reasons.

Allergic bronchopulmonary aspergillosis in cystic fibrosis

Some 8–10% of patients with cystic fibrosis develop ABPA; these patients are almost always atopic. It is not clear whether ABPA causes progression of the underlying cystic fibrosis bronchiectasis but this seems likely, and the condition has implications for suitability for lung transplantation. Thus diagnosis and treatment of ABPA in cystic fibrosis is important.

Diagnosing ABPA in cystic fibrosis can present considerable difficulties. Symptoms may be similar to those of an infective

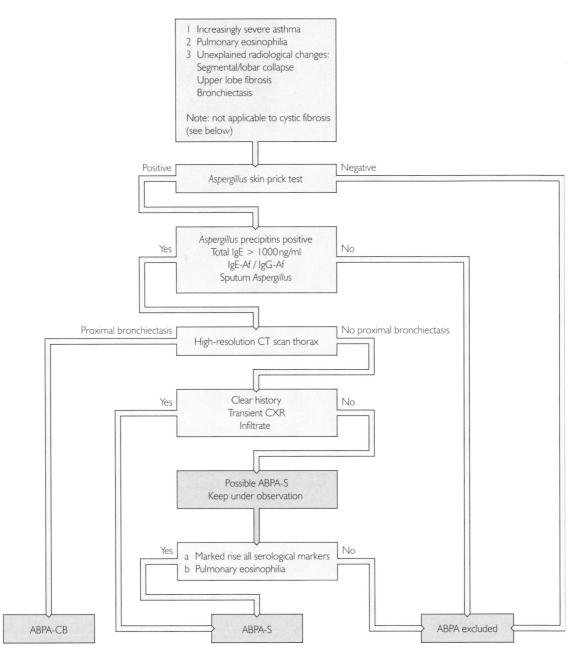

Fig. 40.7 A diagrammatic approach to the diagnosis of allergic bronchopulmonary aspergillosis (ABPA). CT, computed tomography; CXR, chest radiograph; ABPA-S, Allergic bronchopulmonary aspergillosis–seropositive; ABPA-CB, Allergic bronchopulmonary aspergillosis–with sentral bronchietasis.

exacerbation of cystic fibrosis bronchiectasis. The CT findings of ABPA may all be seen in cystic fibrosis alone, skin-prick tests and precipitins may often be positive in the absence of ABPA, and colonisation of the bronchi by *Aspergillus* is common. Pulmonary infiltrates on chest radiograph, in cystic fibrosis, are unusual with bacterial exacerbation of bronchiectasis and should raise a strong clinical suspicion of ABPA (Fig. 40.8). Diagnosis may therefore depend on the resolution of pulmonary infiltrates following steroid therapy.

Aspergillus colonisation of the airways in cystic fibrosis raises potential problems for transplantation. The Royal Brompton cystic fibrosis unit adopts the following policy: if a patient has *Aspergillus* in sputum cultures in the pretransplant assessment,

further samples are sent for culture. If two or three positive samples occur, oral itraconazole and nebulised amphotericin are given and this is continued for 1 month post-transplant. The same treatment is given if patients develop sputum cultures positive for *Aspergillus* after lung transplantation.

Aspergilloma is a relative contraindication to transplant, although some patients have been transplanted successfully.

Allergic *Aspergillus* sinusitis

Sinusitis with histological features similar to those of ABPA is now recognised and has been named allergic *Aspergillus* sinusitis.[61] Clinical presentation is usually with sinusitis that is

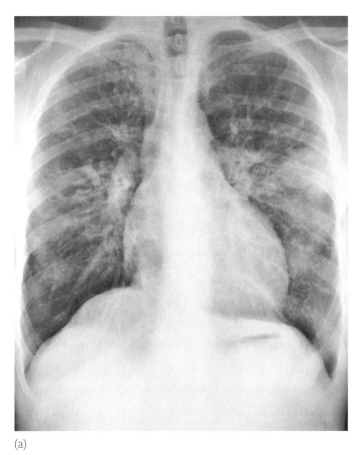

(a)

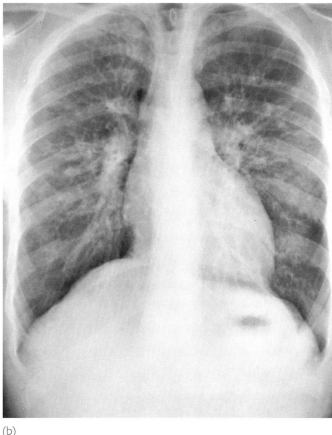

(b)

Fig. 40.8 Allergic bronchopulmonary aspergillosis in cystic fibrosis. Chest radiography sequence showing clearance of left mid-zone consolidation after oral corticosteroid therapy.

unresponsive to medical treatment. Many patients also have nasal polyps. Conventional radiographs show opaque nasal sinuses and computed tomography may show soft-tissue densities filling the sinuses but without evidence of bone abnormality. Allergic *Aspergillus* sinusitis may coexist with ABPA.[62] Skin tests and serological findings are similar to those in ABPA. Multiple surgical procedures are frequently performed on these patients before the diagnosis is realised. Early diagnosis and treatment with oral steroids is effective and reduces the need for surgical intervention, although an initial debridement may be required.[63]

Allergic alveolitis

Extrinsic allergic alveolitis has many causes. The basic immunological mechanisms, clinical features and treatment are described in Chapter 55. The most common *Aspergillus* species associated with extrinsic allergic alveolitis is *A. clavatus*, seen in maltworkers.[64] Extrinsic allergic alveolitis has also been described in a young man exposed to *A. fumigatus* in vegetable compost.[65]

Colonising aspergillosis

A. fumigatus is by far the most common causative organism of this condition in which colonisation of abnormal cavities or spaces in the bronchi, lungs and pleural space occurs leading to

the formation of a mass or ball of fungus (aspergilloma). *A. niger* is responsible for aspergillomas much more frequently in the USA than in the UK. Other species have been occasionally implicated, e.g. *A. flavus* and *A. nidulans*, and other fungi reported to cause fungus balls include *Pseudallescheria*, *Sporotrichum*, *Torulopsis*, *Candida* and *Streptomyces* spp.[66]

Aspergillomas form in abnormal tissue spaces in the lungs produced by other diseases. The most common predisposing disease is tuberculosis, but any cavity-forming disease, such as suppurative pneumonia, lung abscess, sarcoidosis, pulmonary infarction, pneumoconiosis, carcinoma, fibrosing alveolitis and upper lobe fibrosis associated with ankylosing spondylitis and histoplasmosis, can produce cavities or cysts in communication with the atmosphere that fungus can colonise, subsequently forming an aspergilloma. Aspergillomas in tuberculosis usually form in 'healed' cavities but can be found in sputum-positive disease. Aspergillomas can form in ABPA in the bronchiectatic cavities produced by the same organism. Occasionally, an aspergilloma can develop in an empyema space and in the presence of a bronchopleural fistula. Aspergillomas can also occur in paranasal sinuses and the orbit.

The vast majority of aspergillomas arise from colonisation of pre-existing bronchopulmonary cavities, but fungal ball formation has been described without parenchymal cavitation – 'primary aspergilloma' – as an acute complication of invasive aspergillosis in immunocompromised patients.[66]

Aspergilloma is underdiagnosed. The British Thoracic and Tuberculosis Association reported radiological features consistent with aspergilloma in 17% of patients with post-tuberculous cavities[67], this study before the widespread use of CT scanning. Aspergilloma has been found in 7% of patients with ABPA.[68]

The absolute incidence of aspergilloma in the general population is decreasing in the UK with the falling numbers of individuals from the pre-antibiotic era with untreated cavitary tuberculous disease.

Pathology

Aspergillomas most commonly occur in the upper lobes because this is the site most frequently affected by pulmonary tuberculosis. They are brownish-yellow or green in colour and bounded by a fibrous wall. The centre of the fungal ball contains fibrin, debris, inflammatory cells and a felted network of fungal hyphae. The cavity wall is rarely invaded by fungus but invasion and destruction of the wall and surrounding lung occurs in those patients in whom invasive aspergillosis develops. Squamous carcinoma has been reported to have developed in the wall of a chronic aspergilloma cavity.[69]

Clinical features

Aspergillomas are often asymptomatic and detected on routine chest radiographs. Many patients have symptoms of the underlying disease process that has resulted in cavitation and allowed the fungus ball to develop. Sputum production is common but may also be a consequence of the underlying condition.

Haemoptysis is common. In a review of 10 series reporting the frequency of haemoptysis, this symptom was found to occur at some stage in 74% of patients.[66] Haemoptysis is usually minor but massive haemoptysis is not uncommon, and more than 150 ml of expectorated blood over a 24 hour period has been reported in 20–55% of patients.[70,71] Massive haemoptysis is often recurrent and may be fatal in 5–10% of patients.[67]

Systemic symptoms of fever, malaise and weight loss are well recognised but are less common than haemoptysis.

Investigation

The diagnosis of intracavitary aspergilloma is often suggested by the chest radiograph and confirmed by CT scanning. The diagnosis is supported by the presence of precipitating antibodies against A. fumigatus in the serum and by mycological examination of the sputum.

Radiological features

Chest radiographs taken before the development of the fungus ball may show a cavity or cystic space. Classically, the aspergilloma appears as a new solid, usually spherical opacity within the cavity, associated with a rim or halo of air. More commonly, however, these radiological changes are obscured by the fibrotic lung tissue that often surrounds aspergilloma or by the features of the underlying disease process. In addition, the ball and halo sign is not specific for aspergilloma and has been reported in a number of conditions, including invasive aspergillosis, bronchogenic carcinoma, haematoma, chronic abscess and pulmonary haemangioma. Using the fibrotic thickening of the lateral cavity wall as a marker for the presence of aspergilloma, one study reported an improvement of chest radiograph sensitivity to 62% with a specificity of 93% when compared with CT.[72]

Although the diagnosis may be strongly suspected radiologically, determination of the number and location of aspergilloma is often not possible using a conventional chest radiograph.

Computed tomography is more accurate than chest radiograph for the evaluation of aspergilloma and is accepted by many as the diagnostic gold standard.[72] It has superseded linear tomography.

Computed tomography usually shows clearly the spherical mass within a cavity, with a surrounding crescent-shaped air collection between the non-dependent surfaced of the mass and the cavity wall (Fig. 40.9). In addition, the cavity is often thick-walled and may compress the surrounding tissue, forming a 'pseudowall'. Classically, the fungal ball is mobile within the cavity and sequential scans show movement of the mass with patient position. Fronds of fungal tissue may attach the ball to the cavity wall and movement may not be seen or the mass may completely fill the cavity. In addition immature, forming aspergillomata may be seen. Fronds of fungal tissue form within the cavity lumen initially, intersecting to form an irregular spongiform network. These fronds eventually coalesce to form the mature fungal ball but may remain a spongiform mass (Fig. 40.10). Calcification within the fungus ball is seen only rarely.

While the CT appearance may often be diagnostic of aspergilloma, CT assessment is often also of value in planning management. The feasibility of surgery and the procedure to be undertaken are influenced by the number and location of the aspergillomas.

Serum antibodies to *Aspergillus fumigatus*

Precipitating antibodies to A. fumigatus are present in at least 95% of patients.[66] Multiple precipitin arcs are usually seen when double-diffusion or immunoelectrophoretic techniques are used in contrast to less strongly positive reactions in other types of aspergillosis (Fig. 40.2). Occasionally, serum precipitins are absent in immunosuppressed patients.

Liquefaction and disappearance of the fungus ball is mirrored by decrease in and later disappearance of serum precipitins. Similarly, quantitative measurement of A. fumigatus using an IgG-ELISA has been used to monitor activity of disease.[73] Specific A. fumigatus IgE antibodies may be detected in sera of patients with aspergillomas and in particular those who have developed fungus balls in bronchiectatic cavities caused by ABPA. These individuals also have a positive skin-prick test to Aspergillus antigen.

Mycological examination of sputum

Most patients who develop aspergillomas produce sputum. Unlike bronchopulmonary aspergillosis, in which expectoration of sputum containing fungal elements is intermittent, hyphae tend to be present consistently in sputum from patients with aspergillomas. Hyphae are scanty, however, and may not yield a positive culture because they are often non-viable. Culture was positive in only 58% of individuals in one large series,[66] although the collection of a large volume of sputum over 24 hours may improve sensitivity.[74] Specimen contamination with colonising

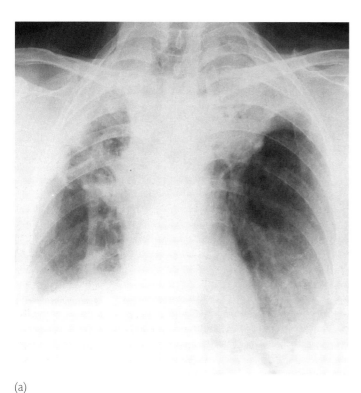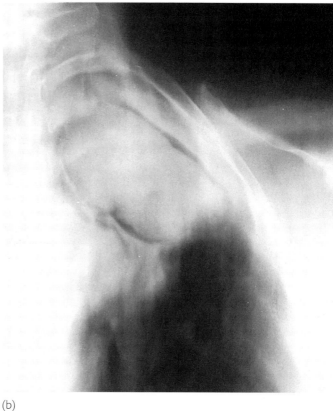

(a)   (b)

Fig. 40.9 Aspergilloma. (a) Chest radiograph of an elderly female patient who had been treated for extensive pulmonary tuberculosis. There is gross abnormality in both upper zones but the presence of an aspergilloma in the apparently uniform density in the left upper lobe is not immediately apparent. (b) Computed tomography scan from the same patient showing multiple cavities with several aspergillomas lying within them.

Aspergillus may confuse the picture, although on microscopic examination *Aspergillus* hyphae in sputum samples from aspergilloma patients have a different shape and structure compared with hyphae seen in sputum from patients with other forms of aspergillosis and it may be possible to confidently suggest a diagnosis of aspergilloma on this basis.[74]

Aspergillus skin tests

Immediate skin test reactivity to *Aspergillus* antigens has been reported in 30–75% of patients with aspergillomas, depending on methods of patient selection.[75] Skin tests are therefore of little diagnostic value in aspergilloma.

Treatment

The management of aspergilloma is controversial. There is a lack of controlled randomised data on which patients require intervention and which treatment should be offered.

Surgical management

Surgery is the only curative treatment. It is most commonly offered to patients with recurrent or uncontrolled haemoptysis but also to those with persistent and distressing systemic symptoms.

The technique used depends on the nature of the lesion and the preoperative condition of the individual patient.

In simple and single, thin-walled lesions a segmentectomy may be possible but more commonly a lobectomy is required. In more complex and thick-walled lesions, bilobectomy or even pneumonectomy may be necessary.

Substantial surrounding tissue may be affected by the aspergilloma and the residual lung parenchyma may be insufficiently compliant to fully expand to fill the pleural cavity. Under these circumstances a thoracoplasty may need to be performed.

Those with limited respiratory reserve or coexisting medical or surgical conditions may be unfit for lobectomy. In these patients a cavernostomy can be performed, if necessary under local or regional anaesthesia. This involves removal of the aspergilloma with obliteration of the residual cavity using a muscle flap mobilised from latissimus dorsi.

There has been a perception that surgery carries a very high risk of complications and a high mortality. Some studies have shown mortality rates of up to 24.5%.[76] However, improvements in surgical technique and careful patient selection have improved operative outcomes over the past 30 years and surgery is increasingly being offered to asymptomatic, fit individuals who have simple or localised aspergillomas.[77]

Overall operative mortality, however, remains high – between 5–10% in most series[77–79] – although considerably less in those individuals at low risk with simple forms.[77,80]

Haemorrhage, incomplete lung expansion, empyema and bronchopleural fistula are the most commonly encountered postoperative complications. Complications are seen in between 15% and 35% of cases,[77,80] although studies have shown rates of up to 60%.[76]

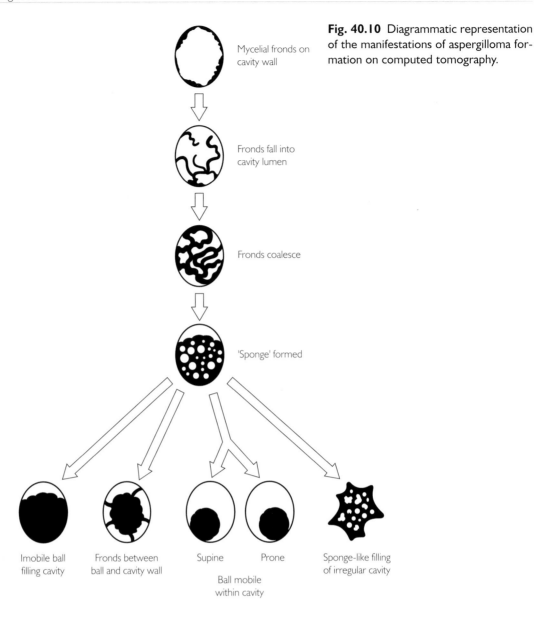

Mycelial fronds on cavity wall

Fronds fall into cavity lumen

Fronds coalesce

'Sponge' formed

Imobile ball filling cavity

Fronds between ball and cavity wall

Supine

Prone

Ball mobile within cavity

Sponge-like filling of irregular cavity

Fig. 40.10 Diagrammatic representation of the manifestations of aspergilloma formation on computed tomography.

Medical management

Systemic antifungal treatment has been found to be of limited value in the management of aspergilloma, although there has been more recent promising but uncontrolled data suggesting a resolution of haemoptysis, cough and systemic symptoms in up to 40% of cases using itraconazole.[81]

Endobronchial or intracavitary instillation of antifungal agents has been attempted with mixed success. Non-retention of antifungal agents necessitating multiple treatments has been a disadvantage. Studies have used a gelatinous preparation of amphotericin that solidifies at body temperature. In the largest of these studies, albeit uncontrolled, haemoptysis ceased in every case and a complete resolution of aspergilloma was seen in 26 of 40.[82] Most centres, however, have found this treatment difficult and impractical to perform and it is not routinely offered.

While the precise role of medical treatment remains to be established, the principal disadvantage is that the cavity remains, with a risk of recurrence at a later date.

Haemoptysis, sputum production and systemic symptoms of fever, malaise and weight loss may respond to corticosteroid treatment.[83] Steroids are associated with the small but well-recognised risk of invasive aspergillosis and treatment should be monitored closely.

Control of major haemoptysis

The principal life-threatening complication of aspergilloma and the most common indication for surgery is massive or recurrent haemoptysis.

When haemoptysis is life-threatening, bronchial artery embolisation can be attempted, but the results may be poorer than in haemoptysis from other causes because the cavity wall often has more than one feeding artery and the collateral blood supply may come from both systemic and pulmonary circulations.[84] Even if bronchial artery embolisation is initially effective, the haemoptysis usually recurs and embolisation should only be used as a temporising measure unless surgery is contraindicated. The risk of anterior spinal artery occlusion and of transverse myelitis have been overstated in the past.[85] Preoperative embolisation of the bronchial circulation has been recommended but the results are variable. Radiotherapy has been reported to be successful in one patient.[86]

Prognosis

The overall mortality rate for individuals with aspergilloma rate is high. The British Thoracic and Tuberculosis Association reported a rate of 6% per annum,[67] although these individuals frequently have multiple pathology and not all deaths are directly attributable to the aspergilloma – around one-third in one study.[70]

Invasive aspergillosis

This is an uncommon but serious form of pulmonary mycosis in which fungal infection spreads throughout the lungs producing granulomata, necrotic and/or suppurative lesions.

There are three principal patterns of pulmonary involvement:

- angioinvasive aspergillosis
- airway-invasive aspergillosis (*Aspergillus* tracheobronchitis)
- chronic necrotising aspergillosis.

Angioinvasive and airway-invasive aspergillosis are more rapidly progressive and can cause extensive pulmonary damage and death within a few days. Fulminating invasive aspergillosis can be accompanied terminally by blood-borne dissemination of fungal infection. Chronic necrotising aspergillosis is a more indolent form of this disease in which pulmonary invasion happens slowly over weeks, months or even years. Invasive aspergillosis is found most often in immunocompromised patients or in those with chronic debilitating disease such as diabetes mellitus, although it can occur in previously healthy patients.[87] In some the underlying source of infection is an aspergilloma. Over 90% of cases are caused by *A. fumigatus*. *A. terreus*, *A. flavus*, *A. niger* and *A. nidulans* account for most of the remainder.[88]

The incidence of invasive aspergillosis in unselected individuals at autopsy in European tertiary-care hospitals in the 1990s was around 4%.[89,90] There has been a substantial increase in this figure over the past 20 years. One study showed a 14-fold increase over the years 1978–92.[89] The principal reason for the increase has been the marked increase in the numbers of individuals with profound and, in particular, neutropenic immunocompromise, in particular with:

- the development of chemotherapeutic regimes for both haematological and solid tumours
- increasing use of bone-marrow transplantation
- an increase in the number of organ-transplant recipients
- the use of immunosuppressive regimens for autoimmune and other disorders
- the advent of AIDS.

Epidemiology

Invasive aspergillosis occurs predominantly in the setting of profound immunocompromise and in particular in individuals with granulocytopenia. The incidence increases progressively with the number of granulocytopenic days. One study documented a plateau of 70% among patients with granulocytopenia for more than 34 days.[91]

The incidence varies considerably from centre to centre; approximate incidences for different patient groups are shown in Table 40.2.

The routine provision of laminar air flow and hepafiltration in some centres may reduce the exposure of high-risk individuals to environmental sources of *Aspergillus*.[94]

Nosocomial invasive aspergillosis in immunosuppressed patients is well-documented. Recognised sources of infection include building and road construction sites,[95] contaminated dietary pepper[96] and pot-plants.[97]

Pathology and pathophysiology

Neutrophils and macrophages are the two principal cells involved in host defence against *Aspergillus* infection. T-cell function is also important and dysfunction of these three factors underlies the majority of disease. Which cells are most affected and the degree of dysfunction may also in part determine the pattern of disease in the lungs.

Angioinvasive aspergillosis

Angioinvasive disease is the most common form of invasive aspergillosis and is seen predominantly in individuals with severe neutropenia.

The characteristic pathological lesion is an angiocentric nodular area of pulmonary infarction containing fungal hyphae radiating into a surrounding area of haemorrhage (sunray colonies[98]). The area of haemorrhage corresponds to the halo seen on CT scan.[99] These lesions usually present during the first 2 weeks of infection. Some lesions remain stable but, characteristically, 2–3 weeks later, with the recovery of neutrophil numbers, others progress to larger pulmonary consolidations with infarction and cavitation.[100] As neutrophils resorb the

Table 40.2 Incidence of invasive aspergillosis[92]

Condition	Range (%)
Chronic granulomatous disease	19–26
Acute leukaemia	5–24
Bone-marrow transplantation (overall)	5.7–19.1[93]*
Acute immunodeficiency syndrome (AIDS)	0–12
Liver transplantation	1.5–10
Heart and lung or lung transplantation	5–26†
Severe combined immunodeficiency	approximately 3.5
Heart and renal transplantation	0.5–10
Severe burns	1–7

* Incidence higher in allogenic and unmatched-donor than in autologous transplants. †Distinguishing colonisation from disease is difficult.

necrotic tissue, retraction occurs from the adjacent viable lung parenchyma, leaving the air crescent seen on later CT scans.[101]

Airway invasive disease (*Aspergillus* tracheobronchitis)

This is less common than the angioinvasive form, approximately 10–34% of cases.[102] Individuals with this form are less likely to be neutropenic; it is proportionally more common in lung-transplant recipients[103] and in those individuals with HIV[104] infection, although invasive aspergillosis is an uncommon complication of this condition. Some 25% of affected individuals are not apparently immunocompromised.[104]

The lesions are bronchocentric, containing *Aspergillus* organisms invading deep to the basement membrane with a predominantly neutrophilic infiltrate.[102] The affected airway is surrounded by a variably sized zone of haemorrhage and/or organising pneumonia.[102]

If disease affects proximal airways, the accumulation of necrotic and fungal debris can lead to luminal obstruction. Occasionally, perforation of the trachea or bronchus may occur.

Chronic necrotising aspergillosis (semi-invasive aspergillosis)

This uncommon form of invasive aspergillosis characteristically occurs in individuals with milder degrees of immunocompromise – chronic granulomatous disease, alcoholism, diabetes – or corticosteroid therapy in those with underlying lung disease, e.g. COPD, sarcoid and pulmonary fibrosis.[105] Many individuals, however, do not have recognised immune dysfunction.

The lesion is focal, often cavitating and evolves slowly over time. Mycetoma may form within areas of cavitation. Histologically, hyphae tend to be scarce and there are often abundant granulomata. A spectrum of histological patterns has been described from lesions resembling angioinvasive disease to those resembling bronchocentric granulomatosis.[106]

Clinical features

Symptoms are non-specific and may be absent in up to a third of patients.

Early symptoms include fever and an often unproductive cough. There may be dull, sometimes pleuritic chest pain and dyspnoea may be a feature of more diffuse disease. Haemoptysis is uncommonly a presenting feature but in the later stages of disease it is seen in around 30% of cases, is frequently massive and may be fatal.[107] Pneumothorax is an occasional presenting feature in neutropenic patients and in this setting is highly suggestive of invasive aspergillosis.

Individuals with the airway-invasive form may develop a wheeze or stridor reflecting luminal obstruction with necrotic material.

Diagnosis

Despite advances in the treatment of invasive aspergillosis, 30% of cases remain undiagnosed and untreated at death.[89,90] Early diagnosis of invasive aspergillosis has been shown to have a major impact on disease outcome. One study showed that, while the mortality was in excess of 90% when treatment was started more than 10 days after the first clinical or radiological evidence of disease, this fell to around 40% when treatment was started

early.[108] Over the past 5 years there have been two key advances in this area: early CT scanning and improvement in antigen detection techniques.

Radiology

The chest radiographic appearance at presentation may show nodular opacities, infiltrates or consolidation but these are non-specific and the chest radiograph is normal in approximately 25% of subsequently proved invasive aspergillosis.[109] CT is more sensitive and specific than conventional radiology for the diagnosis of early disease[110] and allows localisation of disease for direction of bronchoscopic examination or fine needle aspiration if required. The characteristic lesion in angioinvasive disease is a haemorrhagic mass represented on CT as a nodule or area of consolidation surrounded by a halo of ground-glass attenuation. Later in the course of disease these nodules may cavitate, resulting in a characteristic air crescent (Fig. 40.11). The appearance of this sign is thought to coincide with the recovery of the neutrophil count.[111]

Although the halo sign can be seen surrounding a haemorrhagic nodule of any aetiology, in the appropriate setting it is highly suggestive of early invasive aspergillosis. In one study it was seen in 72% of individuals with subsequently proved invasive aspergillosis when performed within 10 days of the appearance of the first symptom or sign but in only 23% if the examination was performed after this time.[110] In another 92% of scans performed within 5 days showed this sign.[107] In both studies the patients were primarily neutropenic haematology patients.

The air-crescent sign can be seen in other cavitating lung diseases.[112] In larger lesions, this cavitation may look like an aspergilloma and show up on plain radiograph (Fig. 40.12). This lesion has been called a mycotic lung sequestrum.[113] Less commonly, pleurally based consolidation develops, representing the

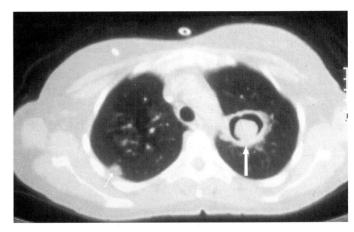

Fig. 40.11 Computed tomography appearances in invasive aspergillosis (angioinvasive type) – halo and air-crescent signs. Thoracic scan showing a nodule surrounded by ground-glass shadowing in the right lung (halo sign – small arrow) with a large cavitating lesion in the left lung (air-crescent sign – large arrow). The perihilar location of the cavitating lesion is associated with a high risk of catastrophic pulmonary haemorrhage and is an indication for emergency surgery.

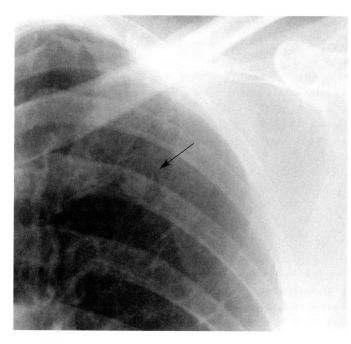

Fig. 40.12 Cavitating lesion of invasive aspergillosis in the left upper zone resembling an aspergilloma.

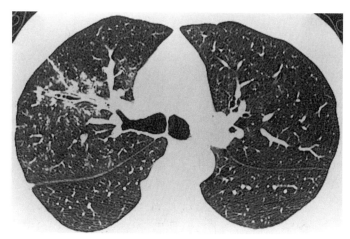

Fig. 40.13 Thoracic computed tomography scan showing the peribronchial nodules and consolidation of airway invasive aspergillosis.

involvement of pulmonary vessels with infarction of distal lung parenchyma.[100]

Airway-invasive aspergillosis appears as peribronchial nodular opacities or areas of peribronchial consolidation[102] (Fig. 40.13). These findings are non-specific and are seen in other infections and in patients with bronchiolitis obliterans organising pneumonia, but in the context of immunocompromise are suspicious of invasive aspergillosis.

In addition to the above features, non-specific infiltrates and areas of consolidation are common and in some cases may be the only findings. CT findings resembling bronchopneumonia or diffuse interstitial pneumonitis have also been reported.[114]

In chronic suppurative aspergillosis, CT findings are non-specific areas of peripheral consolidation, typically involving the apex of the lung and surrounded by thickening of adjacent pleura and distortion of surrounding lung architecture. There may be cavitation and mycetoma formation, and features of an underlying precipitant disease process may be apparent[115] (Fig. 40.14).

Serology

The recent development of an ELISA test against the (1→5)-β-D-galactofuranoside side-chain of galactosammon, an *Aspergillus* antigen, represents a potentially major advance in the early detection of invasive aspergillosis. The earlier latex agglutination tests to galactosammon were specific but were hampered by low sensitivity (detection threshold around 15 ng/ml, resulting in the detection of serum galactosammon only at late stages of disease. The ELISA detects galactosammon at a lower threshold of 0.5 ng/ml and, performed as a screening test in high-risk haematology patients it has been shown to be highly effective in detecting invasive aspergillosis[116] with a sensitivity of 92.6%

and specificity of 95.4%. Importantly, antigenaemia was detected on average 6–13 days before the formal diagnosis was made by other means. Other studies have shown lower sensitivity and specificity[117] but lacked histological confirmation of the diagnosis.

Some foods containing galactosammon can lead to false-positive results and the test can also occasionally be falsely positive where cytotoxic agents or graft versus host disease have damaged the gut wall. To reduce these false-positive results the test is performed on two consecutive days and is considered positive if both tests detect antigen.

Although potentially a valuable investigation in the early detection of invasive aspergillosis, particularly if used in conjunction with CT imaging, more studies are needed to confirm the findings of the above studies in larger numbers and in non-haematology patients, and, in particular, to show improved

Polymerase chain reaction may be of value in the future. In one study results were similar to the ELISA in terms of sensitivity and specificity and early diagnosis.[118]

Aspergillus precipitins and other antibody tests are generally unhelpful in the context of acute disease but are frequently positive in chronic suppurative aspergillosis.[88]

Mycological examination

Cough is usually non-productive in the early stages of invasive aspergillosis. Sputum examination, although often positive in the later stages of disease, is rarely useful in early diagnosis.

The diagnostic value of bronchoalveolar lavage (BAL) depends on the underlying pattern of disease in the chest. It is more likely to be positive in the less common airway-invasive pattern than in angioinvasive disease, 80% and 20% respectively in one study,[119] and more likely to be positive in diffuse than focal disease. Although the sensitivity of BAL and sputum examination is generally low for the identification of *Aspergillus* in the airways in invasive aspergillosis, when *Aspergillus* is found this has a high positive predictive value for invasive disease in the immunocompromised, except in the setting of lung transplantation or in chronic lung diseases, where *Aspergillus* colonisation is common.

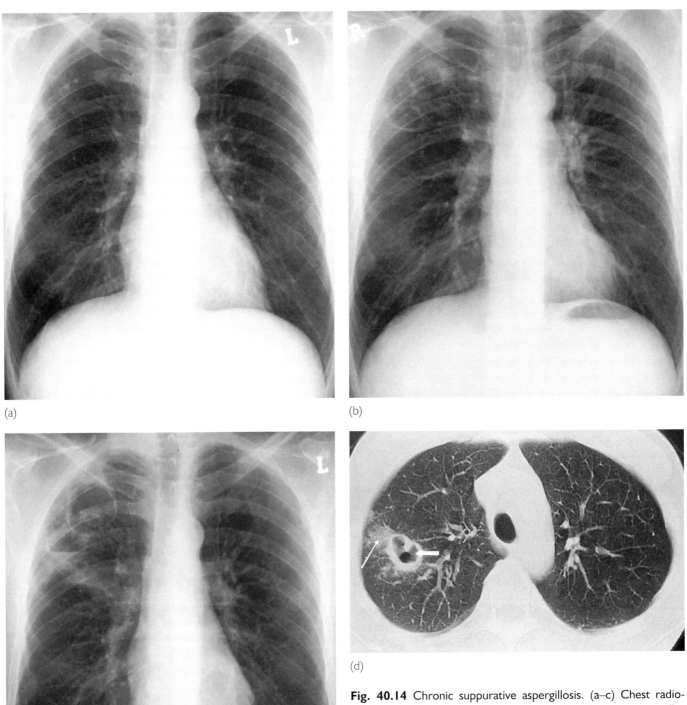

(a)

(b)

(c)

(d)

Fig. 40.14 Chronic suppurative aspergillosis. (a–c) Chest radiograph series of a patient with allergic bronchopulmonary aspergillosis on oral corticosteroid therapy, showing progressive enlargement of right upper-lobe lesions over a 6-month period. (d) Thoracic computed tomography scan in the same patient through the inferior area of cavitation seen on chest radiograph (large arrow). Note ground-glass shadowing (small arrow) corresponding to a focus of angioinvasion. A right upper lobectomy was performed, confirming the diagnosis of invasive aspergillosis.

Planning of investigations

The combination of a halo sign on CT scan and evidence of *Aspergillus* antigenaemia in a high-risk patient may be sufficient for the diagnosis to be made without additional histological evidence.[120] Empirical antifungal therapy is often started while investigations are performed, particularly in the neutropenic and in those with unexplained chest radiograph shadowing.

When these investigations are not conclusive bronchoscopy, fine-needle aspiration and thoracotomy can be considered.

In practice some patients, around 25% in one study,[121] are either too unwell to undergo invasive investigation or have refractory disease with a poor prognosis where further invasive procedures are felt to be inappropriate.

A diagnostic pathway for invasive aspergillosis in the immunosuppressed is outlined in Figure 40.15.

Treatment

Acute invasive aspergillosis is rapidly fatal in almost all cases if untreated and empirical treatment must be considered if there is a delay in diagnosis and preliminary investigations are consistent with the diagnosis. In practice, the neutropenic patient is often started on antifungal treatment if there has been no response after 4–5 days treatment with broad-spectrum antibiotics.[121]

Medical treatment

Amphotericin is the first-line therapy in invasive aspergillosis. Because of adverse reactions to conventional amphotericin, most commonly nephrotoxicity, many units now use only the less toxic lipid-associated amphotericin.

Itraconazole has been used to prevent relapse after remission has been induced by amphotericin[122] however it is being used increasingly as initial therapy in those able to take medication orally and initial response rates have been reported in excess of 60–70%.

Flucytosine has an additive effect when used in conjunction with amphotericin and has been used as an amphotericin sparing agent to reduce toxicity. It has been largely replaced by the less toxic amphotericin regimens.

The rate of response to treatment depends on the degree of immunocompromise. Initial response rate may be up to 68%[105] but between 33% and 54%[92,105] will subsequently relapse. The response rate is significantly worse in those with prolonged neutropenia.

After initial remission is achieved, consolidation therapy with itraconazole may be required for up to 6 months after haematological recovery.[122] Relapse occurs even after months of therapy if patients remain immunocompromised[88] and treatment may be required indefinitely in this group or in those likely to require further cytotoxic therapy.

The overall prognosis for medically treated patients remains extremely poor, with an overall mortality of about 65%. In bone-marrow transplant populations[56] when neutropenia is prolonged, and, for reasons that are not clearly understood, in liver transplant recipients[124], the mortality is much worse, approaching 95% in most series. In other populations, e.g. in renal or heart transplant patients, where neutropenia is less marked,

mortality may be better. The outcome for airway-invasive disease and angioinvasive disease is similar.[102] The outcome for chronic necrotising invasive aspergillosis may be better.

Surgery

Surgical treatment was first established as an emergency procedure for severe haemoptysis. The risk of massive haemoptysis is greatest in central lesions close to major vessels[122] and is most likely to happen as neutrophil recovery occurs.[107]

For this reason, early surgery before neutrophil recovery was adopted in those with lesions on CT scan suggesting angioinvasive aspergillosis to prevent life-threatening haemorrhage.[121] In addition, others have performed surgery later for persistent disease after neutrophil recovery.[125]

The published studies involve a majority of haematology patients. The overall 30-day mortality of 17.2% with fungal relapse in 7.5% compared very favourably with the outcome in medically treated patients.[126] These studies, however, were all uncontrolled, used different selection criteria and in many the data was collated retrospectively.

Most surgeons offer urgent surgery for those with haemoptysis and CT lesions suggesting angioinvasive disease or where these lesions are either enlarging or are close to major vessels, when there is a high risk of catastrophic haemorrhage.[121] Many would also offer surgery for persistent focal disease following neutrophil recovery and despite medical therapy, in order to prevent a relapse of invasive aspergillosis where further immunosuppression is necessary for the treatment of the underlying disorder.[121] Diffuse disease without features of angioinvasion is treated with medical therapy alone unless there are separate indications for surgery.

One group, treating invasive aspergillosis in acute leukaemia with a combination of early CT, serology, azole therapy and from 50% to 17% over 6 years.[122]

Prevention and prophylaxis

Measures to reduce environmental exposure to *Aspergillus* in high-risk individuals, such as the use of hepafiltration and laminar air flow, has reduced the incidence of invasive aspergillosis in certain haematology units.[94] Other measures such as isolation from construction work and avoiding contact with pepper and pot-plants are also thought to be of some importance.[127]

Prophylaxis with itraconazole is associated with partial protection in high-risk groups.[128] Nebulised amphotericin has had variable results.

Cytokine therapy

Treatment of immunosuppressed patients with bone-marrow growth factors is of theoretical value both in the prophylaxis and treatment of invasive aspergillosis. Granulocyte–macrophage-colony-stimulating factor (GM-CSF) is routinely used in neutropenic haematology patients and has been shown to reduce the duration of neutropenia.[129] Although there are isolated reports of *Aspergillus* infection in the immunosuppressed responding to GM-CSF,[130] more studies are need to establish the value of this and other growth factors in invasive aspergillosis.

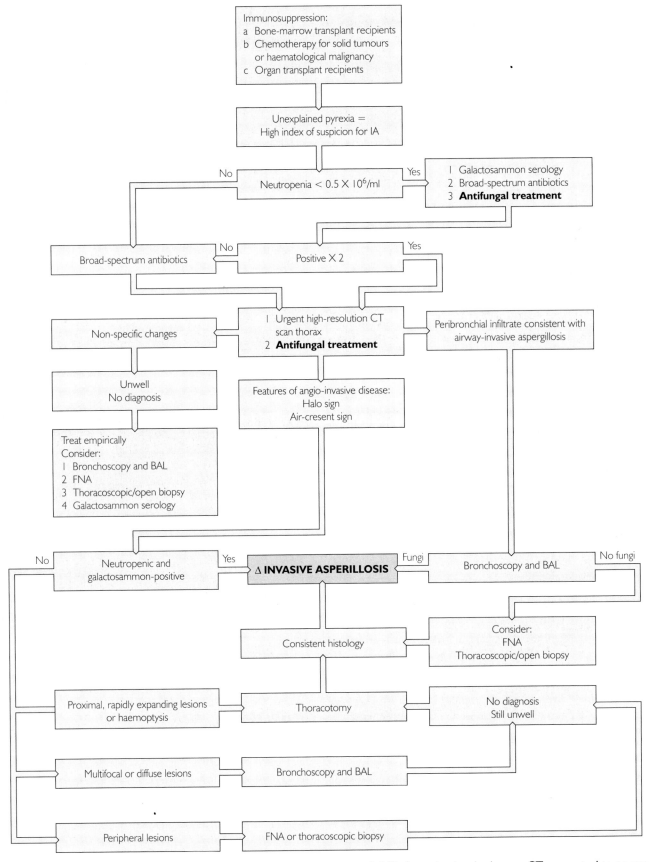

Fig. 40.15 Diagnosis of invasive aspergillosis (IA) in the immunocompromised. BAL, bronchoalveolar lavage; CT, computed tomography; CXR, chest radiograph; FNA, fine-needle aspiration.

Therapeutic principles

1 Allergic bronchopulmonary aspergillosis

- Oral corticosteroids are indicated for:
  - acute exacerbations (with pulmonary infiltrates and/or airflow obstruction)
  - chronic deteriorating airflow obstruction.

- Inhaled corticosteroids are used mainly for control of underlying asthma.

- Antifungals (imidazoles) may reduce exacerbations of chronic disease.

2 Aspergilloma

- Acute haemoptysis may require bronchial artery embolisation or surgery.

- Surgery is the only effective way of controlling recurrent major haemoptysis.

- Aspergilloma is a relative contraindication to lung transplantation.

3 Invasive aspergillosis

- Intravenous amphotericin is often given early on the basis of clinical suspicion.

- Early diagnosis and treatment improve outcome.

- Surgery may be useful for localised disease or for persistent and progressive disease in patients in whom future myelosuppressive treatment is planned.

? Unresolved questions

1 Allergic bronchopulmonary aspergillosis

- Do inhaled corticosteroids prevent disease progression?
- Do antifungals have a place in chronic disease management?

2 Aspergilloma

- What is the value of prophylactic surgery in otherwise healthy individuals to avoid future haemoptysis and lung fibrosis?
- How safe and effective are conservative surgical procedures in patients unfit for major procedures?
- What is the place of oral or intracavitary antifungal treatment?

3 Invasive aspergillosis

- Is serum antigen detection useful for early diagnosis?
- How effective are oral antifungals as initial therapy for invasive aspergillosis or as prophylaxis in the immunocompromised?
- Does surgery improve the outcome?
- Does GM-CSF or other cytokine therapy improve the outcome?

References

1. Bristowe JS. Trans Pathol Soc Lond 1854; 5: 38.
2. Amitani R, Sato A, Matsui Y et al. Effects of *Aspergillus* species culture filtrates on human respiratory ciliated epithelium in vitro (abstract). Am Rev Respir Dis 1992; 145: A548.
3. Mullbacher A, Waring P, Eichner RD. Identification of an agent in cultures of *Aspergillus fumigatus* displaying anti-phagocytic and immunomodulating activity in vitro. J Gen Microbiol 1985; 131: 1251–1258.
4. Henwick S, Hetherington SV, Patrick CC. Complement binding to *Aspergillus* conidia correlates with pathogenicity. J Lab Clin Med 1993; 122: 27–35.
5. Washburn RG, Hammer CH, Bennett JE. Inhibition of complement by culture supernatants of *Aspergillus fumigatus*. J Infect Dis 1986; 154: 944–951.
6. Tomee JF, Kauffman HF. Putative virulence factors of *Aspergillus fumigatus*. Clin Exper Allergy 2000; 30: 476–484.
7. Wasylnka JA, Moore MM. Adhesion of *Aspergillus* species to extracellular matrix proteins: evidence for involvement of negatively charged carbohydrates on the conidial surface. Infect Immun 2000; 68: 3377–3384.

8. Bouchara JP, Bouali A Tronchin G et al. Binding of fibrinogen to the pathogenic *Aspergillus* species. J Med Vet Mycol 1998; 26: 327–334.

9. Kothary MH, Chase TJ, Macmillan JD. Correlation of elastase production by some strains of *Aspergillus fumigatus* with ability to cause pulmonary invasive aspergillosis in mice. Infect Immun 1984; 43: 320–325.

10. Frosco MB, Chase TJ, Macmillan JD. The effect of elastase-specific monoclonal and polyclonal antibodies on the virulence of *Aspergillus fumigatus* in immunocompromised mice. Mycopathologia 1994; 125: 65–76.

11. Tomee JF, Wierenga AT, Hiemstra PS, Kauffman HK. Proteases from *Aspergillus fumigatus* induce release of proinflammatory cytokines and cell detachment in airway epithelial cell lines. J Infect Dis 1997; 176: 300–303.

12. Cenci E, Perito S, Enssle KH et al. Th1 and Th2 cytokines in mice with invasive aspergillosis. Infect Immun 1997; 65: 564–570.

13. Cenci E, Mencacci A, Del Sero G et al. Interleukin-4 causes susceptibility to invasive pulmonary aspergillosis through suppression of protective type I responses. J Infect Dis 1999; 180: 1957–1968.

14. Greenberger PA, Smith LJ, Hsu CC et al. Analysis of bronchoalveolar lavage in allergic bronchopulmonary aspergillosis: divergent responses of antigen-specific antibodies and total IgE. J Allergy Clin Immunol 1988; 82: 164–170.

15. Slavin RG, Fischer VW, Levine EA et al. A primate model of allergic broncho-pulmonary aspergillosis. Int Arch Allergy Appl Immunol 1978; 56: 325–333.

16. Bosken CH, Myers JL, Greenberger PA, Katzenstein AL. Pathologic features of allergic bronchopulmonary aspergillosis. Am J Surg Pathol 1988; 12: 216–222.

17. Slavin RG, Bedrossian CW, Hutcheson PS et al. A pathologic study of allergic bronchopulmonary aspergillosis. J Allergy Clin Immunol 1988; 81: 718–725.

18. Rosenberg M, Patterson R, Mintzer R et al. Clinical and immunologic criteria for the diagnosis of allergic bronchopulmonary aspergillosis. Ann Intern Med 1977; 86: 405–414.

19. Maiz L, Cuevas M, Quirce S et al. Allergic bronchopulmonary aspergillosis with low serum IgE levels in a child with cystic fibrosis. J Allergy Clin Immunol 1997; 100: 431–432.

20. O'Hollaren MT, Yunginger JW, Offord KP et al. Exposure to an aeroallergen as a possible precipitating factor in respiratory arrest in young patients with asthma. N Engl J Med 1991; 324: 359–363.

21. Chauhan B, Knutsen A, Hutcheson PS et al. T cell subsets, epitope mapping, and HLA-restriction in patients with allergic bronchopulmonary aspergillosis. J Clin Invest 1996; 97: 2324–2331.

22. Murali PS, Kurup VP, Bansal NK et al. IgE down regulation and cytokine induction by *Aspergillus* antigens in human allergic bronchopulmonary aspergillosis. J Lab Clin Med 1998; 131: 228–235.

23. Grunig G, Corry DB, Leach MW et al. Interleukin-10 is a natural suppressor of cytokine production and inflammation in a murine model of allergic bronchopulmonary aspergillosis. J Exper Med 1997; 185: 1089–1099.

24. Pepys J, Riddell RW, Citron KM et al. Clinical and immunological significance of *Aspergillus fumigatus* in the sputum. Am Rev Respir Dis 1959; 80: 167

25. Grammer LC, Greenberger PA, Patterson R. Allergic bronchopulmonary aspergillosis in asthmatic patients presenting with allergic rhinitis. Int Arch Allergy Appl Immunol 1986; 79: 246–248.

26. Laufer P, Fink JN, Bruns WT et al Allergic bronchopulmonary aspergillosis in cystic fibrosis. J Allergy Clin Immunol 1984; 73: 44–48.

27. Greenberger PA. Allergic bronchopulmonary aspergillosis. In: Allergy. Principles and practice, 4th ed. CV Mosby; 1993: 1395–1415.

28. Schwartz HJ, Citron KM, Chester EH et al. A comparison of the prevalence of sensitization to *Aspergillus* antigens among asthmatics in Cleveland and London. J Allergy Clin Immunol 1978; 62: 9–14.

29. Basich JE, Graves TS, Baz MN et al. Allergic bronchopulmonary aspergillosis in corticosteroid-dependent asthmatics. J Allergy Clin Immunol 1981; 68: 98–102.

30. Chapman BJ, Capewell S, Gibson R et al. Pulmonary eosinophilia with and without allergic bronchopulmonary aspergillosis. Thorax 1989; 44: 919–924.

31. Glancy JJ, Elder JL, McAleer R. Allergic bronchopulmonary fungal disease without clinical asthma. Thorax 1981; 36: 345–349.

32. Crompton GK. Inhaled beclomethasone dipropionate in allergic bronchopulmonary aspergillosis. Report to Research Committee of British Thoracic Association. Br J Dis Chest 1979; 73: 349

33. Patterson R, Greenberger PA, Radin RC, Roberts M. Allergic bronchopulmonary aspergillosis: staging as an aid to management. Ann Intern Med 1982; 96: 286–291.

34. Ricketti AJ, Greenberger PA, Patterson R. Varying presentations of allergic bronchopulmonary aspergillosis. Int Arch Allergy Appl Immunol 1984; 73: 283–285.

35. Greenberger PA, Patterson R. Diagnosis and management of allergic bronchopulmonary aspergillosis. Ann Allergy 1986; 56: 444–448.

36. Greenberger PA, Patterson R. Allergic bronchopulmonary aspergillosis and the evaluation of the patient with asthma. J Allergy Clin Immunol 1988; 81: 646–650.

37. Wang JL, Patterson R, Roberts M, Ghory AC. The management of allergic bronchopulmonary aspergillosis. Am Rev Respir Dis 1979; 120: 87–92.

38. American Academy of Allergy. AaI. Position statement. The use of standardized allergen extracts. J Allergy Clin Immunol 1997; 99: 583–586.

39. Patterson R, Fink JN, Pruzansky JJ et al. Serum immunoglobulin levels in pulmonary allergic aspergillosis and certain other lung diseases, with special reference to immunoglobulin E. Am J Med 1973; 54: 16–22.

40. Borga A. Allergens of *Aspergillus fumigatus*. PhD thesis, Karolinska Institute, Stockholm; 1990.

41. Banerjee B, Kurup VP, Greenberger PA et al. Purification of a major allergen, Asp f 2 binding to IgE in allergic bronchopulmonary aspergillosis, from culture filtrate of *Aspergillus fumigatus*. J Allergy Clin Immunol 1997; 99: 821–827.

42. Hemmann S, Menz G, Ismail C et al. Skin test reactivity to 2 recombinant *Aspergillus fumigatus* allergens in *A. fumigatus*-sensitized asthmatic subjects allows diagnostic separation of allergic bronchopulmonary aspergillosis from fungal sensitization. J Allergy Clin Immunol 1999; 104: 601–607.

43. Ghory AC, Patterson R, Greenberger P, Roberts M. Extended evaluation of allergic bronchopulmonary aspergillosis. Int Arch Allergy Appl Immunol 1980; 62: 285–291.

44. Pepys J. Hypersensitivity diseases of the lungs due to fungi and organic dusts. Monogr Allergy 1969; 4: 1–147.

45. McCarthy DS, Pepys J. Allergic broncho-pulmonary aspergillosis. Clinical immunology. 2. Skin, nasal and bronchial tests. Clin Allergy 1971; 1: 415–432.

46. Wardlaw A, Geddes DM. Allergic bronchopulmonary aspergillosis: a review. J R Soc Med 1992; 85: 747–751.

47. Mroueh S, Spock A. Allergic bronchopulmonary aspergillosis in patients with cystic fibrosis. Chest 1994; 105: 32–36.

48. Leser C, Kauffman HF, Virchow CS, Menz G. Specific serum immunopatterns in clinical phases of allergic bronchopulmonary aspergillosis. J Allergy Clin Immunol 1992; 90: 589–599.

49. McCarthy DS, Simon G, Hargreave FE. The radiological appearances in allergic broncho-pulmonary aspergillosis. Clin Radiol 1970; 21: 366–375.

50. Angus RM, Davies ML, Cowan MD et al. Computed tomographic scanning of the lung in patients with allergic bronchopulmonary aspergillosis and in asthmatic patients with a positive skin test to *Aspergillus fumigatus*. Thorax 1994; 49: 586–589.

51. Ward S, Heyneman L, Lee MJ et al. Accuracy of CT in the diagnosis of allergic bronchopulmonary aspergillosis in asthmatic patients. AJR 1999; 173: 937–942.

52. Reiff DB, Wells AU, Carr DH et al. CT findings in bronchiectasis: limited value in distinguishing between idiopathic and specific types. AJR 1995; 165: 261–267.

53. Logan PM, Muller NL. CT manifestations of pulmonary aspergillosis. Crit Rev Diagn Imaging 1996; 37: 1–37.

54. Germaud P, Tuchais E. Allergic bronchopulmonary aspergillosis treated with itraconazole (letter). Chest 1995; 107: 883

55. Stevens DA, Schwartz HJ, Lee JY et al. A randomized trial of itraconazole in allergic bronchopulmonary aspergillosis. N Engl J Med 2000; 342: 756–762.

56. Middleton WG, Paterson IC, Grant IW, Douglas AC. Asthmatic pulmonary eosinophilia: a review of 65 cases. Br J Dis Chest 1977; 71: 115–122.

57. Safirstein BH, D'Souza MF, Simon G et al. Five-year follow-up of allergic bronchopulmonary aspergillosis. Am Rev Respir Dis 1973; 108: 450–459.

58. Riley DJ, Mackenzie JW, Uhlman WE, Edelman NH. Allergic bronchopulmonary aspergillosis: evidence of limited tissue invasion. Am Rev Respir Dis 1975; 111: 232–236.

59. Salez F, Brichet A, Desurmont S et al. Effects of itraconazole therapy in allergic bronchopulmonary aspergillosis. Chest 1999; 116: 1665–1668.

60. Stevens EA, Hilvering C, Orie NG. Inhalation experiments with extracts of *Aspergillus fumigatus* on patients with allergic aspergillosis and aspergilloma. Thorax 1970; 25: 11–18.

61. Katzenstein AL, Sale SR, Greenberger PA. Allergic *Aspergillus* sinusitis: a newly recognized form of sinusitis. J Allergy Clin Immunol 1983; 72: 89–93.

62. Sher TH, Schwartz HJ. Allergic *Aspergillus* sinusitis with concurrent allergic bronchopulmonary *Aspergillus*: report of a case. J Allergy Clin Immunol 1988; 81: 844–846.

63. Waxman JE, Spector JG, Sale SR et al. Allergic *Aspergillus* sinusitis: concepts in diagnosis and treatment of a new clinical entity. Laryngoscope 1987; 97: 261

64. Grant IW, Blackadder ES, Greenberg M, Blyth W. Extrinsic allergic alveolitis in Scottish maltworkers. Br Med J 1976; 1: 490–493.

65. Vincken W, Roels P. Hypersensitivity pneumonitis due to *Aspergillus fumigatus* in compost. Thorax 1984; 39: 74–75.

66. Glimp RA, Bayer AS. Pulmonary aspergilloma. Diagnostic and therapeutic considerations. Arch Intern Med 1983; 143: 303–308.

67. Anonymous. British Thoracic and Tuberculosis Association Report: Aspergilloma and residual tuberculosis cavities: the result of a re-survey. Tubercle; 51: 227–245.

68. Sugar AM, Olek EA. *Aspergillus* syndromes, mucormycosis, and pulmonary candidiasis. In: Fishman AP, ed. Pulmonary diseases and disorders, 2nd ed. New York: McGraw-Hill, 1997: 2265–2287.

69. Andrew SM, Bhattacharjee M, Keenan DJ, Reid H. Squamous cell carcinoma occurring in the wall of a chronic aspergilloma. Thorax 1991; 46: 542–543.

70. Jewkes J, Kay PH, Paneth M, Citron KM. Pulmonary aspergilloma: analysis of prognosis in relation to haemoptysis and survey of treatment. Thorax 1983; 38: 572–578.

71. Karas A, Hankins JR, Attar S et al. Pulmonary aspergillosis: an analysis of 41 patients. Ann Thorac Surg 1976; 22: 1–7.

72. Sansom HE, Baque-Juston M, Wells AU, Hansell DM. Lateral cavity wall thickening as an early radiographic sign of mycetoma formation. Eur Radiol 2000; 10: 387–390.

73. Tomee JF, van der Werf TS, Latge JP et al. Serologic monitoring of disease and treatment in a patient with pulmonary aspergilloma. Am J Respir Crit Care Med 151: 199–204.

74. Milne LJR. Direct microscopical examination. In: Evans EGV, ed. Medical mycology: a practical approach. London: IRL Press; 1989.

75. McCarthy DS, Pepys J. Pulmonary aspergilloma – clinical immunology. Clin Allergy 1973; 3: 57–70.

76. Daly RC, Pairolero PC, Piehler JM et al. Pulmonary aspergilloma. Results of surgical treatment. J Thorac Cardiovasc Surg 1986; 92: 981–988.

77. Chen JC, Chang YL, Luh SP et al. Surgical treatment for pulmonary aspergilloma: a 28 year experience. Thorax 1997; 52: 810–813.

78. El Oakley R, Petrou M, Goldstraw P. Indications and outcome of surgery for pulmonary aspergilloma. Thorax 1997; 52: 813–815.

79. Babatasi G, Massetti M, Chapelier A et al. Surgical treatment of pulmonary aspergilloma: current outcome. J Thorac Cardiovasc Surg 2000; 119: 906–912.

80. Regnard JF, Icard P, Nicolosi M et al. Aspergilloma: a series of 89 surgical cases. Ann Thorac Surg 2000; 69: 898–903.

81. Pulmonary Aspergilloma Study Group. Multicentre clinical trial of itraconazole in the treatment of pulmonary aspergilloma. Kekkaku 1997; 72: 557–564.

82. Giron J, Poey C, Fajadet P et al. CT-guided percutaneous treatment of inoperable pulmonary aspergillomas: a study of 40 cases. Eur J Radiol 1998; 28: 235–242.

83. Hilvering C, Stevens EA, Orie NG. Fever in *Aspergillus* mycetoma. Thorax 1970; 25: 19–24.

84. Remy J, Arnaud A, Fardou H et al. Treatment of hemoptysis by embolization of bronchial arteries. Radiology 1977; 122: 33–37.

85. McDermott VG, Payne CS, Smith TP. Angiographic techniques in the evaluation and management of suspected pulmonary disease. In: Fishman AP, ed. Fishman's pulmonary disease and disorders, 3rd ed. New York: McGraw-Hill; 1998.

86. Shneerson JM, Emerson PA, Phillips RH. Radiotherapy for massive haemoptysis from an aspergilloma. Thorax 1980; 35: 953–954.

87. Hovenden JL, Nicklason F, Barnes RA. Invasive pulmonary aspergillosis in non-immunocompromised patients. Br Med J 1991; 302: 583–584.

88. Denning DW. Invasive aspergillosis. Clin Infect Dis 1998; 26: 781–803.

89. Groll AH, Shah PM, Mentzel C et al. Trends in the postmortem epidemiology of invasive fungal infections at a university hospital. J Infect 1996; 33: 23–32.

90. Vogeser M, Wanders A, Haas A, Ruckdeschel G. A four-year review of fatal aspergillosis. Eur J Clin Microbiol Infect Dis 1999; 18: 42–45.

91. Gerson SL, Talbot GH, Hurwitz S et al. Prolonged granulocytopenia: the major risk factor for invasive pulmonary aspergillosis in patients with acute leukemia. Ann Intern Med 1984; 100: 345–351.

92. Denning DW. Therapeutic outcome in invasive aspergillosis. Clin Infect Dis 1996; 23: 608–615.

93. Ho PL, Yuen KY. Aspergillosis in bone marrow transplant recipients. Crit Rev Oncol Hematol 2000; 34: 55–69.

94. Sherertz RJ, Belani A, Kramer BS et al. Impact of air filtration on nosocomial *Aspergillus* infections. Unique risk of bone marrow transplant recipients. Am J Med 1987; 83: 709–718.

95. Lentino JR, Rosenkranz MA, Michaels JA et al. Nosocomial aspergillosis: a retrospective review of airborne disease secondary to road construction and contaminated air conditioners. Am J Epidemiol 1982; 116: 430–437.

96. De Bock R, Gyssens I, Peetermans M, Nolard N. *Aspergillus* in pepper (letter). Lancet 1989; 2: 331–332.

97. Staib F. Ecological and epidemiological aspects of aspergilli pathogenic for man and animal in Berlin (West). Zblatt Bakteriol Mikrobiol Hygiene A 1984; 257: 240–245.

98. Spencer H. Pathology of the lung, 4th ed. Oxford: Pergamon Press; 1985.

99. Hruban RH, Meziane MA, Zerhouni EA et al. Radiologic-pathologic correlation of the CT halo sign in invasive pulmonary aspergillosis. J Computer Assisted Tomogr 1987; 11: 534–536.

100. Herbert PA, Bayer AS. Fungal pneumonia (Part 4): invasive pulmonary aspergillosis. Chest 1981; 80: 220–225.

101. Kuhlman JE, Fishman EK, Burch PA et al. CT of invasive pulmonary aspergillosis. AJR 50: 1015–1020.

102. Logan PM, Primack SL, Miller RR, Muller NL. Invasive aspergillosis of the airways: radiographic, CT, and pathologic findings. Radiology 1994; 193: 383–388.

103. Kramer MR, Denning DW, Marshall SE et al. Ulcerative tracheobronchitis after lung transplantation. A new form of invasive aspergillosis. Am Rev Respir Dis 1991; 144: 552–556.

104. Kemper CA, Hostetler JS, Follansbee SE et al. Ulcerative and plaque-like tracheobronchitis due to infection with *Aspergillus* in patients with AIDS. Clin Infect Dis 1993; 17: 344–352.

105. Denning DW, Stevens DA. Antifungal and surgical treatment of invasive aspergillosis: review of 2,121 published cases . Rev Infect Dis 1990; 12: 1147–1201.

106. Yousem SA. The histological spectrum of chronic necrotizing forms of pulmonary aspergillosis. Hum Pathol 1997; 28: 650–656.

107. Albelda SM, Talbot GH, Gerson SL et al. Pulmonary cavitation and massive hemoptysis in invasive pulmonary aspergillosis. Influence of bone marrow recovery in patients with acute leukemia. Am Rev Respir Dis 1985; 131: 115–120.

108. Von Eiff M, Zuhlsdorf M, Roos N et al. Pulmonary fungal infections in patients with hematological malignancies – diagnostic approaches. Ann Hematol 1995; 70: 135–141.

109. Klein DL, Gamsu G. Thoracic manifestations of aspergillosis. AJR 1980; 134: 543–552.

110. Blum U, Windfuhr M, Buitrago-Tellez C et al. Invasive pulmonary aspergillosis. MRI, CT, and plain radiographic findings and their contribution for early diagnosis. Chest 1994; 106: 1156–1161.

111. Gefter WB, Albelda SM, Talbot G et al. New observations on the role of significance of the air crescent in invasive aspergillosis (abstract). Radiology 1984; 153: 136.

112. Thompson BH, Stanford W, Galvin JR, Kurihara Y. Varied radiologic appearances of pulmonary aspergillosis. Radiographics 1995; 15: 1273–1284.

113. Kibbler CC, Milkins SR, Bhamra A et al. Apparent pulmonary mycetoma following invasive aspergillosis in neutropenic patients. Thorax 1988; 43: 108–112.

114. Pennington JE. *Aspergillus* lung disease. Med Clin North Am 1980; 64: 475–490.

115. Aquino SL, Kee ST, Warnock ML, Gamsu G. Pulmonary aspergillosis: imaging findings with pathologic correlation. AJR 1994; 163: 811–815.

116. Maertens J, Verhaegen J, Demuynck H et al. Autopsy-controlled prospective evaluation of serial screening for circulating galactomannan by a sandwich enzyme-linked immunosorbent assay for hematological patients at risk for invasive Aspergillosis. J Clin Microbiol 1999; 37: 3223–3228.

117. Sulahian A, Tabouret M, Ribaud P et al. Comparison of an enzyme immunoassay and latex agglutination test for detection of galactomannan in the diagnosis of invasive aspergillosis. Eur J Clin Microbiol Infect Dis 1996; 15: 139–145.

118. Williamson EC, Leeming JP, Palmer HM et al. Diagnosis of invasive aspergillosis in bone marrow transplant recipients by polymerase chain reaction. Br J Haematol 2000; 108: 132–139.

119. Brown MJ, Worthy SA, Flint JD, Muller NL. Invasive aspergillosis in the immunocompromised host: utility of computed tomography and bronchoalveolar lavage. Clin Radiol 1998; 53: 255–257.

120. Ascioglu S, De Pauw B, Bennett JE et al. Analysis of definitions used in clinical research on invasive fungal infections (IFI): consensus proposal for new, standardised definitions. Interscience Conference on Antimicrobial Agents and Chemotherapy, San Francisco, September 1999: Abstract.

121. Yeghen T, Kibbler CC, Prentice HG et al. Management of invasive pulmonary aspergillosis in hematology patients: a review of 87 consecutive cases at a single institution. Clin Infect Dis 2000; 31: 859–868.

122. Caillot D, Casasnovas O, Bernard A et al. Improved management of invasive pulmonary aspergillosis in neutropenic patients using early thoracic computed tomographic scan and surgery. J Clin Oncol 1997; 15: 139–147.

123. Denning DW, Lee JY, Hostetler JS et al. NIAID Mycoses Study Group multicenter trial of oral itraconazole therapy for invasive aspergillosis. Am J Med 1994; 97: 135–144.

124. Kusne S, Torre-Cisneros J, Manez R et al. Factors associated with invasive lung aspergillosis and the significance of positive *Aspergillus* culture after liver transplantation. J Infect Dis 1992; 166: 1379–1383.

125. Baron O, Guillaume B, Moreau P et al. Aggressive surgical management in localized pulmonary mycotic and nonmycotic infections for neutropenic patients with acute leukemia: report of eighteen cases. J Thorac Cardiovasc Surg 115: 63–68.

126. Reichenberger F, Habicht J, Kaim A et al. Lung resection for invasive pulmonary aspergillosis in neutropenic patients with hematologic diseases. Am J Respir Crit Care Med 158: 885–890.

127. Vargas S, Hughes WT, Giannini MA. *Aspergillus* in pepper (letter). Lancet 1990; 336: 881

128. Nucci M, Biasoli I, Akiti T et al. A double-blind, randomized, placebo-controlled trial of itraconazole capsules as antifungal prophylaxis for neutropenic patients. Clin Infect Dis 2000; 30: 300–305.

129. Goldstone AH, Khwaja A. The role of haemopoietic factors in bone marrow transplantation. Leukemia Res 1990; 14: 721–729.

130. Catalano L, Fontana R, Scarpato N et al. Combined treatment with amphotericin-B and granulocyte transfusion from G-CSF-stimulated donors in an aplastic patient with invasive aspergillosis undergoing bone marrow transplantation. Haematologica 1997; 82: 71–72.

41 Infections due to dimorphic pathogenic fungi – *Histoplasma*, *Coccidioides*, *Blastomyces*, *Paracoccidioides* and *Penicillium marneffei*

Roderick J Hay

The dimorphic fungal pathogens are organisms that are found in the environment and can cause disease in man or animals after inhalation. The majority of those exposed do not develop signs of infection; however, in susceptible patients, clinical illness can result after primary exposure or following re-activation.

Histoplasmosis

Histoplasmosis has a wide distribution. Most infections are either subclinical or self-limiting.

Aetiology

Histoplasma capsulatum is a dimorphic fungus that grows as a mould fungus in its natural habitat[1] or on primary isolation in culture at 23–25°C. The infective propagules are microconidia (2–5 μm in diameter); macroconidia (8–14 μm in diameter) are also produced in mould cultures. If incubated at temperatures above 35°C on enriched media, or when causing human or experimental infections, *H. capsulatum* grows in a yeast phase, producing round or oval cells, 2–3 × 3–4 μm in diameter.

Epidemiology

Apart from Europe, the distribution of histoplasmosis is worldwide, but the areas with highest prevalence of exposure are the valleys of the Mississippi and Ohio Rivers in the USA. However the infection is also seen in other parts of the USA and Canada, central and south America, Africa, India and south-east Asia.[2] Within such endemic regions, *H. capsulatum* appears to be associated with certain locations, e.g. microfoci on river banks, in wooded areas, large parks, caves or under the eaves of houses – indeed, in any area where there are accumulations of birds or bats. The growth of *H. capsulatum* is greatly enhanced in soils by the presence of bird or bat excreta; in acute outbreaks activities that are liable to generate an aerosol from soil have been associated with infections.

Pathogenesis and pathology

After entry of the microconidia into the lung the organisms develop into a yeast phase, a transformation accompanied by the production of a fungal heat-shock protein (HSP 70). The organism has a number of different virulence determinants such as catalase and the presence of intramural melanin, but in most normal hosts the infection is controlled by the development of a T-lymphocyte-mediated response about 10–14 days after infection. In the presence of a large inoculum the symptoms may be augmented by an immune-complex-mediated inflammation with arthralgia, uveitis and erythema multiforme. Although the activated macrophages are fungicidal, some yeasts may be able to survive intracellularly. Where there is serious impairment of cell-mediated immune capability, as in the acquired immunodeficiency syndrome (AIDS), the infection may progress.[3] In addition, reactivation from an internal source may occur as a consequence of immunosuppression such as occurs with lymphoma or solid organ transplantation. Patients who have compromised pulmonary defences, such as those with chronic obstructive pulmonary disease (COPD), are vulnerable to persistent pulmonary infection.

The histopathological response is granulomatous and typically non-caseating, with an infiltrate of lymphocytes, monocytes and fibroblasts. Necrosis may mimic abscess formation and the opposite extreme, extensive fibrosis, may also occur. In immunocompromised patients, granulomas are poorly formed and histiocytes containing numerous yeasts predominate.

Clinical manifestations

Most patients develop no symptoms or signs following exposure. The only evidence of exposure is a positive histoplasmin test. However, clinical disease is seen in about 1% of persons, with dissemination or chronic pulmonary infection in about 0.05% and chronic fibrosing disease in about 0.02%.[2,4]

Acute (epidemic) pulmonary histoplasmosis

This is an acute self-limiting illness that begins with symptoms of an upper respiratory tract infection and substernal pain. Patchy or micronodular pulmonary infiltrates are commonly found on radiological examination (Fig. 41.1); pleural effusions are present in about 5% of patients. With heavy exposures, acute respiratory insufficiency may be associated with a diffuse micronodular pattern of pulmonary disease.

Enlargement of the mediastinal lymph nodes is usual in acute histoplasmosis and may be so marked that pulmonary obstruction and compression of the major vessels and other mediastinal structures results. If the lymphadenitis progresses to necrosis of the mediastinal nodes, fistulae with neighbouring structures may form. Immune-complex-related symptoms such as arthralgia and arthritis, with or without erythema multiforme or nodosum, may occur

as part of the acute disease in about 10% of patients. These are typically self-limiting and relieved by non-steroidal anti-inflammatory agents, but there may be relapses. Pericarditis without fungal invasion also occurs in about 10% of patients; anti-inflammatory drugs are effective in reducing symptoms and antifungal drugs are seldom necessary and may precipitate immune-complex-mediated symptoms such as erythema multiforme.[5]

Chronic pulmonary histoplasmosis

Chronic pulmonary histoplasmosis occurs mainly in patients with chronic obstructive pulmonary disease This form is slowly progressive and presents with malaise, fatigue, chest pain, sweats and inconstant, but low-grade, fever. Productive cough is associated with upper lobe infiltration, cavitation,[6] pleural thickening, calcification and hilar retraction.

In addition, in some otherwise healthy patients there are uniform, rounded, calcified opacities scattered throughout the lung fields. These lesions represent sites of earlier, unsuspected acute lung involvement and are not symptomatic (Fig. 41.2).

Disseminated histoplasmosis

Disseminated histoplasmosis may occur in immunocompetent people but is mainly seen in infants, the elderly and the immunosuppressed The clinical and laboratory manifestations of dissemination are non-specific: fever, loss of weight, hepatomegaly, splenomegaly and haematological abnormalities all occur.[4] Pulmonary and mediastinal disease may be seen on the chest radiograph. The central nervous system, usually presenting with meningitis, is involved in 20% of patients with disseminated disease.[4]

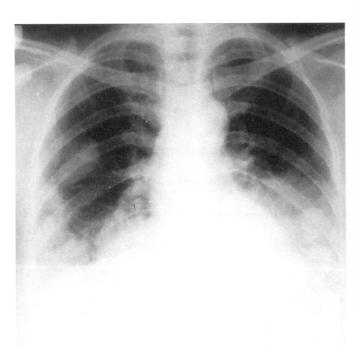

Fig. 41.1 Chest radiograph of a patient with acute histoplasmosis. Bilateral pulmonary infiltrates are maximal at the bases and there is mediastinal widening consistent with lymphadenopathy

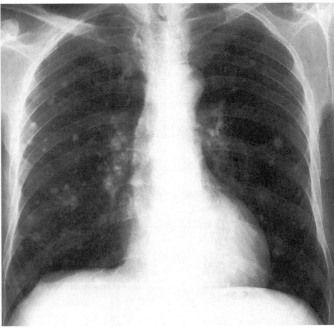

Fig. 41.2 Histoplasmosis: chest radiograph of a patient with incidental disease. The patient, from an endemic area in Canada, was known to have had an abnormal chest radiograph for 30 years. The Mantoux test was negative but he had a positive histoplasmin skin test.

In as many as 20% of patients with histoplasmosis complicating AIDS, the disease is accompanied by positive blood cultures.[3] Except for their greater severity, the clinical signs do not differ greatly from those in other patients, although progression is more rapid.

Chronic disseminated histoplasmosis in immunocompetent individuals often evolves slowly over periods of as long as 20 years.[2,4] Half of the patients have intermittent fever and loss of weight, oropharyngeal ulcerations appear in two-thirds, and up to 10% will develop other complications such as meningitis, endocarditis or Addison's disease.

Mediastinal fibrosis following chronic inflammatory histoplasmosis may cause obstruction of some, or all, of the mediastinal contents.[7]

Diagnosis

Definitive proof of the diagnosis is by culture of *H. capsulatum*. In disseminated disease, e.g. in AIDS patients, as many as 70% of blood cultures and 80% of bone-marrow cultures will yield *H. capsulatum*. Up to 70% of lung, 33% of liver and 30% of urine cultures are also positive. However, in all forms of disease, 2–6 weeks may pass before identification is possible. In the acute pulmonary form, only about 10% of the cases can be diagnosed by culture and in the chronic pulmonary diseases repeated attempts at culture may be necessary.[6] The yield is higher with specimens collected from relevant regions of the lung by bronchoscopy.

Examination of biopsy specimens stained with methenamine silver (Fig. 41.3) is highly suggestive of the diagnosis in about 70% of patients with disseminated disease and the same is true in up to 90% of lung, 50% of marrow and 30% of liver biopsies. Wright-stained peripheral blood smears may contain recognisable *H. capsulatum* cells (Fig. 41.4).

Skin testing with histoplasmin should not be used for diagnosis because it merely reflects exposure (often asymptomatic).[2] Many patients with disseminated disease have negative skin tests and, furthermore, skin testing may induce antibody forma-

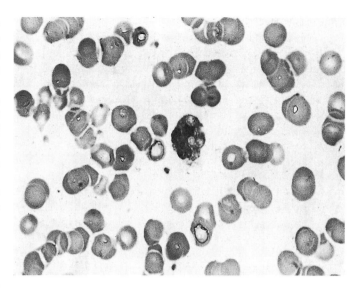

Fig. 41.4 Yeast-like forms of *Histoplasma capsulatum* inside a polymorphonuclear leukocyte in the peripheral blood. Wright stain.

tion, making it difficult to interpret serological tests. Serological tests are useful, especially in disseminated disease;[1,2,4] there is nearly a 100% positive response rate for specific antibody in the immunocompetent and about 80% in immunosuppressed patients. Over 90% of patients with chronic cavitary disease are seropositive. The complement fixation test is widely used employing both mycelial and yeast phase antigens. A single titre of 1:32 or more is significant, although a fourfold rise in titre in sequential specimens of serum is ideal proof of active infection. Other tests include immunodiffusion (useful to confirm a low titre by complement fixation), radioimmunoassay and enzyme-linked immunosorbent assays (ELISA). IgG antibodies persist for many years, limiting the diagnostic value of a single test. Also, there is cross-reactivity with other fungal diseases in as many as 50% of patients.

Radioimmunoassay may detect a glycoprotein antigenic component of *H. capsulatum* in blood, urine, cerebrospinal fluid and bronchoalveolar lavage specimens. It is useful in patients with disseminated histoplasmosis (particularly those who are HIV-positive), but of less diagnostic value for chronic pulmonary disease.[1] A new test using an inhibition ELISA is also useful, shows little cross-reactivity with other endemic mycoses and can be used for monitoring treatment; it cannot be used on urine samples.[8]

Prognosis

Patients with the acute, self-limiting syndromes (pulmonary, rheumatological, pericarditis) recover completely, albeit slowly, without specific therapy. Untreated disseminated disease is generally fatal after a course that may be as long as 20 years.[1,2] Chronic cavitary histoplasmosis, if untreated, will be progressive in about half the patients.[6]

Treatment

Specific antifungal treatment is not necessary in acute histoplasmosis, except in patients who have respiratory insufficiency.

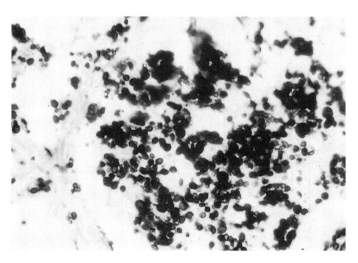

Fig. 41.3 Yeast-like forms of *Histoplasma capsulatum* in a biopsy specimen of lung from the same patient as Figure 41.1 Methenamine silver stain.

Itraconazole 200 mg daily for 4–6 weeks or amphotericin B given over 2 weeks usually suffices.[1,2]

All patients with disseminated histoplasmosis should be treated[2] and, whether immunosuppressed or not, more than 90% are cured with intravenous amphotericin B. Patients with AIDS are exceptions in that all relapse within a year after normally curative therapy;[3] hence, chronic suppressive therapy should follow the initial course of treatment, usually with an oral azole derivative – itraconazole. Itraconazole (200–400 mg/day) is well tolerated and is usually effective as primary treatment. However intravenous amphotericin B (0.75 mg/kg body weight twice weekly) is an alternative; amphotericin B may also be used particularly in those who are severely ill. Fluconazole (200 or 400 mg as a single dose, daily) may also be used. Long-term follow-up is necessary.

About half the patients with *Histoplasma* meningitis relapse after treatment with amphotericin B (dosage as for disseminated disease). Intrathecal treatment may be given, along with intravenous therapy.[2] Although the course of chronic cavitary histoplasmosis is slow and the outcome may be favourable without specific therapy, itraconazole (200–400 mg/day) is effective in many patients and may be preferred for initial treatment because it is better tolerated than amphotericin B. Amphotericin B (dosage as for disseminated disease) can also be used, curing more than 80% of patients.[6] There is no place for surgical intervention in the treatment of chronic pulmonary histoplasmosis.

Although treatment with amphotericin B or itraconazole may be helpful in some patients with mediastinal lymphadenitis, excisional surgery is contraindicated because of high morbidity and poor results. The course of fibrosing mediastinitis is not influenced by chemotherapy or surgery.[7]

Prevention

The accumulated epidemiological experience clearly implicates mechanical disturbance of or close exposure to soils and sites rich in bird and bat excrement as antecedents to epidemics of histoplasmosis.[1,2] If such activities are unavoidable, decontamination of foci with formalin may be preventive. In addition, public warning signs can be posted at known danger areas, e.g. caves.

Coccidioidomycosis

Coccidioidomycosis is an infectious disease caused by *Coccidioides immitis*, a dimorphic, saprophytic fungus that can be isolated from soils of semi-arid regions of the Americas. As with other dimorphic fungal infections, inhalation of arthroconidia usually results in sensitisation without disease but in some may cause fatal illness.[9]

Aetiology

In its normal habitat in the soil, and laboratory culture media, C. *immitis* grows as a mould with septate hyphae.[9] Certain hyphae form thick-walled, barrel-like, 2–5 mm arthroconidia, which are extremely resistant to drying and easily dispersed on air currents. Inhaled arthroconidia that survive phagocytosis grow as

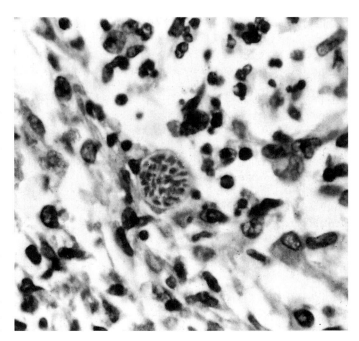

Fig. 41.5 Coccidioidal spherule in a biopsy specimen of lung tissue. Haematoxylin and eosin stain.

spherules – reproductive structures 50–100 mm in diameter (Fig. 41.5) that, on maturation, release endospores (individually 2–3 mm in diameter). Surviving endospores mature to form new spherules, often within host cells.

Epidemiology

Coccidioides immitis is found in certain soils in a region extending from about 40°N, 120°W in California to about 40°S, 65°W in Argentina. Its favoured habitat is a semi-desert climate with low rainfall; irrigation projects appear to diminish the risk of infection. Areas in the USA where this disease is endemic include parts of California, Arizona, Texas, New Mexico and other dry regions. The endemic zone extends to Mexico, Guatemala, Colombia and Venezuela, as well as northern Argentina and Uruguay. Upsurges of infection may follow changes in climatic conditions, such as dust storms, that release arthroconidia from soil into the air. This may affect both residents and those passing through an endemic area, including visitors and military personnel. The disease can affect laboratory personnel working with cultures.

Black, Filipino and, perhaps, other Asian people are more likely to develop coccidioidal disease, extrapulmonary dissemination, meningitis and death than white people. Pregnant women are more susceptible than men, but men are more susceptible than non-pregnant women.

Pathogenesis and pathology

The initial neutrophil reaction to inhaled arthroconidia gives way, after a few days, to progression to a granulomatous reaction.[9,10] Caseation may occur but calcification is rare. Initially, the process is endobronchiolar and it is variable in extent and location.

Chest radiographs may show a patchy bronchopneumonia, often with ipsilateral hilar adenopathy and pleural effusion.

In most exposed individuals there is complete healing without residual damage. However in 2–5% there is focal pulmonary necrosis or abscesses that may progress to cavitation.

Haematogenous dissemination of endospores may lead to extrapulmonary disease in lymph nodes, spleen, skin, liver, kidneys, bones, meninges, adrenal glands and myocardium. The meningitis is primarily basilar, may lead to hydrocephalus and, rarely, is associated with arteritis in the brain or spinal cord.[11]

Both humoral and cell-mediated immune responses may be detected.[9,10] Although serial assessment of antibody titres in the serum is diagnostically and prognostically useful, it is the development of cell-mediated immunity that is essential to recovery. A more destructive disease process may develop in HIV-positive individuals.

Clinical manifestations

Infection with C. immitis is asymptomatic in about 80% of those exposed, the only evidence being a positive skin test (coccidioidin). When disease occurs, non-productive cough is the usual initial manifestation. Chills without rigors, night sweats and pleuritic chest pain, along with headache, malaise and myalgia, are also seen. Patients may develop symptoms due to immune complex formation such as a toxic erythema, erythema multiforme, or erythema nodosum associated with arthralgia and iritis in about a third of the patients. Spontaneous self-cure occurs in most of these patients.

More persistent pulmonary disease may be apparent as the development of non-cavitary infiltrates or nodules or cavitary forms in 25% of symptomatic patients. Intrapulmonary fungal balls may also develop. Progressive pulmonary infection is a feature of the infection in the severely immunocompromised.

Disseminated coccidioidomycosis may also develop. Manifestations of extrapulmonary coccidioidomycosis include widespread dissemination with multiorgan disease and proliferating granulomata of the skin, arthritis, osteomyelitis (Fig. 41.6) or meningitis.

Diagnosis

In endemic areas, the clinical findings may be highly suggestive of the diagnosis. However, demonstration of spherules in biopsy specimens or aspirated materials (pus, exudates or cerebrospinal fluid) as well as sputum is necessary.

Culture of C. immitis may be hazardous. The mycelial growth is not specific and unsuspecting laboratory personnel may inhale an infecting inoculum simply by raising the lid of a Petri dish. Thus, it is important that the clinician warn laboratory personnel if C. immitis is suspected. Confirmation that a mould is C. immitis requires documentation of conversion of arthroconidia to spherules. While originally this was done by experimental infection of mice or on special media (Converse's medium) nowadays the mould-form cultures may be identified as C. immitis by the reaction of antigens, extracted from the agar medium, with specific anticoccidioidal antiserum – exoantigen test.

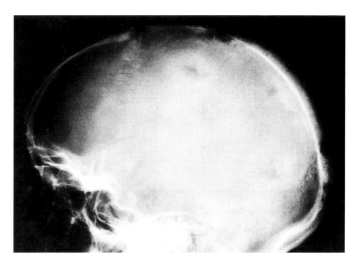

Fig. 41.6 Lateral radiograph of the skull showing several foci of osteomyelitis causing destruction of the external table of the skull. Culture was positive for *Coccidioides immitis*.

As with histoplasmosis the coccidioidin skin test confirms cell-mediated immunity but gives no clue as to the presence of infection. Newly infected people become skin-test-reactive 3 days to 3 weeks after the onset of symptoms; those with erythema multiforme or erythema nodosum may be highly reactive and, in these, coccidioidin diluted to 1:10 000 is appropriate to start testing. A substantial proportion of those with chronic pulmonary or disseminated coccidioidomycosis have negative skin tests.[9,10]

Starting in the first week of illness, anticoccidioidal IgM may be detected in the serum by immunodiffusion. Asymptomatic individuals are not usually immunodiffusion-positive. Detection of IgG by complement fixation testing has been the standard serodiagnostic method,[12] although immunodiffusion has increased sensitivity.[13] Most patients with coccidioidomycosis develop complement fixation antibodies 6–10 weeks after the onset of symptoms; with recovery, the titre usually drops and many apparently cured patients have titres of 1:8 or less for life. Rising titres (e.g. above 1:32) may signal dissemination, whereas falling titres indicate a favourable course.

Progress

Over 80% of patients exposed to C. immitis either do not develop disease at all or show resolution of a trivial respiratory illness[9,10] without specific therapy. By contrast, patients with disseminated infections or meningitis may die of the infection.[11] Survival in all forms of coccidioidomycosis is increased by treatment with amphotericin B;[14,15] however, cure of coccidioidal meningitis remains elusive.

Treatment

As with histoplasmosis, the choice of treatment depends on the type of disease. The treatment of progressive forms of coccidioidomycosis is often particularly difficult and there are no well-established regimens based on comparative clinical trials. In many cases azoles are now used even although there is little comparative data. Of the presently available drugs, only fluconazole enters urine, eyes and cerebrospinal fluid in therapeutic concentrations.[9] However, usage supports the value of either itraconazole or fluconazole in some patients, particularly those with uncomplicated primary infections and those at potential risk from dissemination, e.g. Filipinos. Likewise, for the first-line treatment of cavitary disease or disseminated infections of slow onset, an azole is used. The initial treatment of coccidioidal meningitis is usually fluconazole (400 mg daily), even although there has been no comparative study versus amphotericin B. Itraconazole in doses of 400 mg daily may also be used but there is less experience in meningeal disease. Generally, in AIDS patients, long-term suppressive therapy with itraconazole or fluconazole is used after an initial course of amphotericin B.

Amphotericin B is usually given for rapidly progressing disease or where serious complications are imminent, e.g. progressive pneumonia. It may also be used as initial therapy in HIV-positive patients. It may be difficult to decide if treatment with amphotericin B is needed for a patient with acute, pulmonary disease caused by *C. immitis*. Drug side effects have to be weighed against the possibility of development of either persistent pulmonary or disseminated disease. Factors such as ethnic background, pregnancy and underlying diseases, i.e. immunocompetence, must be considered. Amphotericin B must be given intravenously in a daily dose per injection of 0.75–1.0 mg/kg body weight. Such regimens require 2–3 months for completion, a duration dependent on the relatively slow rate of replication of *C. immitis* and the toxicity of amphotericin B. As a result of the poor penetration of amphotericin B from the blood into the central nervous system and cerebrospinal fluid, the drug may have to given via an intraventricular reservoir in coccidioidal meningitis.

Prevention

Avoidance of inhalational exposure to air-borne soil dust that contains coccidioidal arthroconidia is advisable; although specific measures, other than the commonsensical, such as winding up car windows in a dust storm in endemic areas, are difficult to implement. Attempts to develop a specific form of immunisation using an antigen of *C. immitis*, spherulin, was not successful.

Blastomycosis

Blastomycosis is a systemic mycosis which follows inhalation and is caused by *Blastomyces dermatitidis*. Recognised most often in North America, blastomycosis also occurs in Africa and very rarely elsewhere, e.g. in India and the Middle East.

Aetiology

Blastomyces dermatitidis is dimorphic.[16] In tissue, it grows as a yeast (8–15 mm diameter), is thick-walled (nearly 1 mm) and reproduces by budding, characteristically with a wide base between mother and daughter cell. On culture media, and presumably in nature, *B. dermatitidis* grows as mycelium (2–3 mm in diameter), from which project special, slender hyphae (conidiophores) that bear conidia, the infective agents.

Epidemiology

Blastomyces dermatitidis is difficult to isolate from the environment. It appears in sandy, acid soils or wood debris.[17] First described in Baltimore, MD, most cases continue to be reported from the south-eastern USA.[18] Yet, the disease also occurs in the Mississippi and Ohio River basins of the USA, in Quebec, Ontario and the maritime provinces of Canada, in the Middle East and in widely scattered areas in Africa.[16]

Men are affected about 10 times more often than women. Among non-human animals, dogs, particularly hunting breeds, are infected most frequently. Cases have also been documented in horses, sea lions and African lions;[16–18] there is no evidence to support transmission from dogs to humans. While the ecological niche of *Blastomyces* remains unknown, epidemiological data from human and dog infection in the USA suggest that the disease is acquired most often close to waterways or areas subject to flooding. These may be some distance from urban areas.

Pathogenesis and pathology

Humans acquire blastomycosis by inhaling conidia; as with other dimorphic infections most of those exposed do not develop the disease. The average incubation period is 45 days; the range of 21–106 days reflects variations in host defence capabilities and the intensity of exposure.

The initial reaction is an acute neutrophil response; if the proliferating yeast-phase fungi are not contained, an area of pneumonia forms from which infection may extend to the hilar lymph nodes. In the later stages, and with T-cell recruitment, granulomas form, often around a neutrophil cluster. Yeast-phase *B. dermatitidis* can be seen in pus and biopsy specimens with appropriate stains (e.g. periodic-acid–Schiff). With an adequate cellular immune response the infection is usually confined to the lungs and hilar nodes. Interestingly, despite the evidence for a key role for T cells, blastomycosis is not often seen in AIDS patients.[19]

Clinical manifestations

Although the lung is the usual portal entry of *B. dermatitidis*, the manifestations of pulmonary infection may not be clinically dominant.[16,18,20,21] In addition, because there is no reliable skin-test antigen, it is difficult to understand the frequency of asymptomatic disease after exposure. However, pulmonary blastomycosis is both frequent and important, and may be disabling. In some patients, productive cough, pleurisy and haemoptysis herald the onset of pulmonary disease; at the other extreme, a chance chest film (as may be obtained during investigation of an epidemic) may reveal pulmonary infection in an asymptomatic person. There may be slow progression with fever, night sweats, malaise, anorexia and loss of weight. The physical findings are often sparse. There is no typical or diagnostic radiological pattern as the spectrum extends from a scant localised infiltrate to acute respiratory distress syndrome (ARDS). Pleural effusion is uncommon, as are solitary pulmonary nodules. Occasionally, cavities form; calcification is quite uncommon.[16,18,19]

In disseminated blastomycosis, skin lesions appear either individually or at multiple sites. They start as subcutaneous nodules, evolve with necrosis, becoming plaques that are typically raised, verrucous, weeping–crusting, painless and non-pruritic. Regional nodes are not involved. The vertebrae and ribs are the usual sites of blastomycosis affecting bone. The meningitis of blastomycosis is chronic and may be difficult to distinguish from meningitic tuberculosis or of cryptococcosis. The prostate is the usual site of genitourinary blastomycosis, with the epididymis the next most frequently affected; the enlarged gland is slightly tender and may cause urinary obstruction.[18,19]

Diagnosis

Yeast-phase *B. dermatitidis* cells (8–10 mm), which can be found by microscopic examination of sputum and pus, is the most rapid and perhaps still the best method of diagnosis.[16,18] The thick, refractile wall, the single daughter cell attached on a broad base and the size are characteristic. However, specimens should be cultured. Expectorated sputum is a reliable specimen because contamination by other similar-appearing fungi, even *Candida* spp., is rare. Pus, biopsy specimens, and scrapings from skin and mucosal lesions are satisfactory for culture.

In tissue sections, *B. dermatitidis* yeasts are the same size as *Cryptococcus neoformans* but lack a capsule and do not stain with mucicarmine.[16] The yeast forms of *B. dermatitidis* are usually larger than the yeast form of *H. capsulatum*, although rarely *B. dermatitidis* produces small yeast cells. Although *Histoplasma duboisii* is about the same size as *B. dermatitidis* (the two fungi may coexist as causes of disease in Africa), the broad-based buds of *B. dermatitidis* cells enable differentiation.[16–19] The blastomycin skin test is of no value in diagnosis. None of the several methods used to test for humoral antibodies is clinically useful because of cross-reactivity with other dimorphic fungi;[22] however, a positive serological test, e.g. immunodiffusion, in a patient with an appropriate history and signs should be treated with suspicion.

Prognosis

It is likely that some patients with blastomycosis recover without antifungal therapy,[21] although how common this is not clear. The course of the disease is unpredictable, varying from slow progression to spontaneous remissions of lesions. Specific antifungal therapy will influence the outcome in patients with progressive pneumonia.

Treatment

Blastomyces dermatitidis is susceptible to several antifungal agents. As a result of the occurrence of spontaneous remissions of lesions, it is possible that not every patient requires specific therapy.[16,21] However as blastomycosis responds well to triazoles such as itraconazole, current practice is to treat all patients

including those with acute respiratory infections. If a decision to withhold treatment is made it is important to follow the patient for 1–2 years to ensure that there is no recurrence.

The antifungal azole drugs are active against *B. dermatitidis* and may be preferred for initial therapy for mild-to-moderate pulmonary blastomycosis and non-life-threatening extrapulmonary disease. Oral itraconazole is recommended (200–400 mg/day, given in two equal doses, 12-hourly) for such cases; ketoconazole 200–400 mg daily is an alternative. Fluconazole is relatively untried.

However, for severe cases amphotericin B is usually given. The usual dose is 1 mg/kg body weight daily, although doses of 0.60–0.75 mg/kg given intravenously on alternate days to a total dose of 30 mg/kg can be given.[16] Amphotericin B should always be used to treat meningeal blastomycosis and severe forms of pulmonary blastomycosis.

Prevention

No preventive measures have proved to be of value.

Paracoccidioidomycosis

Paracoccidioidomycosis (South American blastomycosis) is caused by the dimorphic fungus, *Paracoccidioides brasiliensis*.[23] Growth is thought to be mycelial in the natural environment and when cultured at 28°C. The organism is a yeast in tissue and when cultured at 35–37°C. The development of the yeast phase is partially controlled by an oestrogen receptor in the cytosol and infections in women are rare. The yeast has a characteristic mode of budding, with multiple cells forming around the periphery of the mother yeast. The tropical and subtropical forested regions of Latin America between latitudes 23°N and 34°S are endemic for *P. brasiliensis*. Most cases originate from Colombia, Venezuela, Brazil and Argentina. However, the natural habitat of *P. brasiliensis* is unknown.

Typically, young adults are affected, with a self-limiting infection of the respiratory tract.[21] Reactivation of quiescent lesions may occur years later and result in progressive pulmonary disease,[24] with or without dissemination to involve virtually other organs (particularly skin or mucocutaneous junctions, lymph nodes, adrenal glands).[23,24] A 'juvenile' form corresponds to the widely disseminated type of infection seen with infections due to other dimorphic fungi.

Diagnosis depends on:

- detection of characteristic yeast-like forms in clinical specimens
- isolation of *P. brasiliensis* from clinical specimens by the use of selective culture media
- detection of a specific antibody response (immunodiffusion, complement fixation test or ELISA). There is an antigen detection system also, which appears to be useful in following treatment responses.[25]

Itraconazole is a highly effective treatment in most cases, although ketoconazole is an alternative. Amphotericin B is used in severe infections or where there is no response to itraconazole. There are no preventive measures.

Infections due to *Penicillium marneffei*

Penicillium marneffei is a dimorphic fungal pathogen that causes infection after inhalation.[26] Its natural habitat is unknown, although in endemic areas of south-east Asia it also affects bamboo rats. It is seen in Thailand, southern China, Vietnam, Laos, Malaysia, Myanmar (Burma) and Assam. However, cases have also been diagnosed in Hong Kong and Taiwan and in travellers returning to Europe or the USA from the endemic area. At room temperature, *P. marneffei* forms a mould with a red to black pigment and conidia, but in tissue it is a yeast-like cell that divides by transverse fission rather than budding. The disease shows a higher incidence after the rainy season.[27]

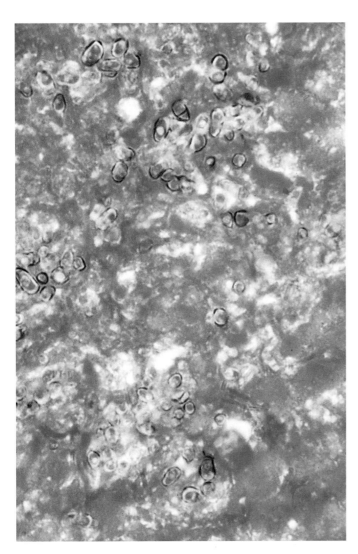

Fig. 41.7 Yeast-phase *Penicillum marneffei* in tissue showing cells divided by septa. Methenamine silver stain.

While it can affect otherwise healthy patients, the infection is mainly associated with AIDS and, indeed, is a clinical marker for AIDS in the endemic areas.

Clinically, the pulmonary signs are usually few compared to the systemic features, such as hepatosplenomegaly, bone-marrow infiltration, multiple skin lesions (in 70% of AIDS patients) and gastrointestinal infiltration. However, pulmonary changes range from diffuse infiltrates to mass or cavitating lesions.[26,28,29]

The diagnosis is made by:

- demonstration of the organisms, with the characteristic division and septal formation between cells, in biopsies, bone marrow or blood films
- culture of the organism (Fig. 41.7).

At present there is no commercial serological test, although western blots and an ELISA have been used. The organism cross-reacts serologically with *Aspergillus* spp.

Severely ill patients receive amphotericin B but itraconazole is also effective and can also be used for long-term suppression of recurrence in AIDS patients.[26]

References

1. Deepe GS. Histoplasma capsulatum. In: Mandell GL, Bennett JE, Dolin R, ed. Principles and practice of infectious diseases, 5th ed. Philadelphia, PA: Churchill Livingstone; 2000: 2718
2. Sarosi GA, Davies SF, ed. Fungal diseases of the lung. New York: Grune & Stratton, 1986: 43.
3. Wheat LJ, Conolly-Stringfield PA, Baker RL et al. Disseminated histoplasmosis in the acquired immune deficiency syndrome: clinical findings, diagnosis and treatment, and review of the literature. Medicine 1990; 69: 361.
4. Sathapatayavons B, Batteiger BE, Wheat LJ et al. Clinical and laboratory features of disseminated histoplasmosis during two large urban outbreaks. Medicine 1983; 69: 263.
5. Wheat LJ, Stein L, Corya BC et al. Pericarditis as a manifestation of histoplasmosis during two large urban outbreaks. Medicine 1983; 62: 110.
6. Wheat LJ, Wass JL, Norton JA et al. Cavitary histoplasmosis occurring during two large urban outbreaks. Medicine 1984; 63: 201
7. Godwin RA, Nickell JA, Des Prez AM. Mediastinal fibrosis complicating healed primary histoplasmosis and tuberculosis. Medicine 1972; 51: 227.
8. Gomez BL. Figueroa JI. Hamilton AJ et al. Detection of the 70-kilodalton *Histoplasma capsulatum* antigen in serum of histoplasmosis patients: correlation between antigenemia and therapy during follow-up. J Clin Microbiol 1999; 37: 675.
9. Kirkland TN, Fierer J. Coccidioidomycosis: a reemerging infectious disease. Emerg Infect Dis 1996; 2: 192.
10. Drutz DJ, Catanzaro A. Coccidioidomycosis. Am Rev Respir Dis 1978; 117: 559, 727.
11. Bouza E, Dreyer JS, Hewitt WL, Meyer RD. Coccidioidal meningitis: An analysis of thirty-one cases and review of the literature. Medicine 1981; 60: 139.
12. Smith CE, Saito MT, Simmons SA. Pattern of 39,500 serologic tests in coccidioidomycosis. JAMA 1956; 160: 546
13. Pappagianis D, Zimmer BL. Serology of coccidioidomycosis. Clin Microbiol Rev 1990; 3: 247.
14. Oldfield EC, Bone WD, Martin CR et al. Prediction of relapse after treatment of coccidioidomycosis. Clin Infect Dis 1997; 25: 1205.
15. Kafka JA, Catanzaro A. Disseminated coccidioidomycosis in children. J Pediatr 1981; 98: 355.
16. Bradsher RW. A clinician's view of blastomycosis. Curr Topics Med Mycol 1993: 5: 181.
17. Klein BS, Vergeront JM, Weeks RJ et al. Isolation of *Blastomyces dermatitidis* in soil associated with a large outbreak of blastomycosis in Wisconsin. N Engl J Med 1986; 314: 529.
18. Bradsher RW. Clinical features of blastomycosis. Semin Respir Infect 1997; 12: 229.
19. Davies SF, Sarosi GA. Clinical manifestations and management of blastomycosis in the compromised patient. In: Warnock DW, Richardson MD, ed. Fungal

infection in the compromised patient, 2nd ed. New York, John Wiley & Sons; 1991: 215.

20. Davies SF, Sarosi GA Epidemiological and clinical features of pulmonary blastomycosis. Semin Respir Infect 1997; 12: 229

21. Sarosi GA, Davies F, Phillips JR. Self-limited blastomycosis: a report of 39 cases. Semin Respir Infect 1986; 1: 40.

22. Davies SF, Sarosi GA. Role of serodiagnostic tests and skin tests in the diagnosis of fungal diseases. Clin Chest Med 1987; 8: 135.

23. Londero AT, Severo LC. The gamut of progressive pulmonary paracoccidioidomycosis. Mycopathologia 1981; 75: 65.

24. Franco M, Lacaz CS, Restrepo A, del Negro G, ed. Paracoccidioidomycosis. Boca Raton, FL: CRC Press; 1994.

25. Gomez B, Figueroa JI, Hamilton AJ et al. Antigenemia in paracoccidioidomycosis: detection of the 87 kDa determinant in patients during and after antifungal therapy. J Clin Microbiol 1998; 36: 3309

26. Supparatpinyo K, Khamwan C, Baosoung V et al. Disseminated *Penicillium marneffei* infection in southeast Asia. Lancet 1994; 344: 110.

27. Chariyalertsak S, Sirisa nthana T, Supparatpinyo K, Nelson KE. Seasonal variation of disseminated *Penicillium marneffei* infections in northern Thailand: a clue to the reservoir? J Infect Dis 1996 173: 1490.

28. McShane H. Tang CM. Conlon CP. Disseminated *Penicillium marneffei* infection presenting as a right upper lobe mass in an HIV-positive patient. Thorax 1998; 53: 905.

29. Sekhon AS, Stein L, Garg AK et al. Pulmonary penicilliosis marneffei: report of the first imported case in Canada. Mycopathologia 1994; 128: 3

42 Parasitic diseases

Nicholas Roche and Gerard Huchon

Key points

- Knowledge of the geographical distribution of the main parasites involved in lung diseases and of their mode of transmission allows adequate suspicion of possible diagnoses (Table 42.2).

- Depending on the parasites involved, several tools can be used to confirm the diagnosis (Table 42.4), leading to administration of the appropriate treatment (Table 42.5).

- Prevention is based on pharmacological agents only for malaria, the choice of the prophylaxis depending on the geographical area and its resistance profile.

- Other parasitic diseases can be prevented by adequate life-style measures adapted to the geographical area and the mode of transmission of the corresponding parasite (Table 42.1).

Parasites involved in lung diseases

In Western countries parasitic diseases of the lung mainly affect travellers and immigrants. The majority of parasites can infest and cause clinical manifestations in non-immunocompromised hosts (although disease prevalence and severity are greater in immunocompromised subjects), while some become pathogenic only in patients with impaired cellular immunity (e.g. *Cryptosporidium* spp.; Table 42.1). Suspicion of a parasitic lung disease is based on knowledge of the geographical distribution and life-cycle of the parasite.

Classification, geographical distribution

Parasites involved in human respiratory diseases belong to three families: protozoa, nematodes and platyhelminths, the last category being divided into trematodes and cestodes (Table 42.1). Most parasitic diseases are predominantly found in tropical or subtropical areas, although each species has a specific geographical distribution (Table 42.2).

Humans as part of parasitic life-cycles and transmission

Humans are accidental intermediate hosts for a variety of parasites. As shown in Table 42.2, the mode of transmission is variable: mosquito bite for malaria (Fig. 42.1), dirofilariasis and tropical pulmonary eosinophilia; transcutaneous penetration for schistosomiasis (Fig. 42.2); ingestion of contaminated water or food for other parasites (e.g. *Echinococcus* spp.; Fig. 42.3). Interhuman transmission is highly infrequent, being reported only for amoebiasis in homosexual men.

Protozoa

Toxoplasmosis

Epidemiology and pathogenesis

Toxoplasmosis[5] is a worldwide infection with a varying prevalence, ranging from 14% in the USA to 81% in France. Transmission to humans occurs in three main ways: transplacental, oral (e.g. by eating undercooked or raw 'steak tartare') and faeco-oral.

Clinical presentation and diagnosis

Symptoms and signs are absent in a high proportion of cases in immunocompetent patients and when present they are very variable. They include fever, headache, lymphadenopathy, myalgia, arthralgia, a rash and hepatosplenomegaly. Hilar and mediastinal lymphadenopathy may be present. Retinochoroiditis and neonatal infections are well documented.

Diagnosis depends on histological investigation of infected tissue and serology. In the immunocompetent host, specific IgG are present within 2–3 weeks and persist for life. The presence of IgM suggests infection within the last year. Post-mortem examinations in adults have shown interstitial pneumonia, focal hepatitis, pancreatitis, myocarditis, myositis and encephalitis associated with the parasite.

Table 42.1   Agents of parasitic pneumonia, classified according to the immunological status of the host (Adapted from Huchon & Roche 1999.)

	Mainly in non-immunocompromised hosts	Both in immunocompromised and normal hosts	Mainly in immunocompromised hosts
Protozoa			
	Entamoeba histolytica (amoebiasis)	*Toxoplasma gondii*	*Cryptosporidium* spp.
	Plasmodium sp. (malaria)		
Nematodes			
	Trichinella spiralis	*Strongyloides stercoralis*	
	Ascaris		
	Hookworm (*Ancylostoma* spp. and		
	Necator americanus)		
	Toxocara canis (visceral larva migrans)		
	Dirofilaria immitis		
	Gnathostoma spinigerum		
	Wucheria bancrofti, Brugia malayi		
	(tropical eosinophilia)		
Platyhelminths			
Trematodes	*Paragonimus* sp.		
	Schistosoma sp.		
Cestodes	*Echinococcus* sp.		

Table 42.2   Geographical distribution and mode of transmission of the main parasites involved in lung diseases

Parasites (diseases)	Geographical distribution	Mode of transmission
Protozoa		
Toxoplasma gondii (toxoplasmosis)	Worldwide	Transplacental, oral, faeco-oral
Entamoeba histolytica (amoebiasis)	West and southern Africa, south and south-east Asia, South America and Mexico	Contaminated food or water
Plasmodium spp. (malaria)	Tropical and subtropical areas	Mosquitoes
Trichinella spiralis (trichinosis)	Worldwide	Improperly cooked meat of wild animals or domestic pigs
Nematodes		
Ascaris lumbricoides (ascariasis)	Africa, Asia, Central and South America	Oral
Ancylostoma spp. and *Necator americanus* (ancylostomiasis)	Tropical and subtropical areas of Africa, Asia and America	Skin penetration
Strongyloides stercoralis (strongyloidiasis)	Tropical and subtropical areas	Skin penetration
Toxocara canis (visceral larva migrans)	Worldwide	Oral (canine species/soil)
Dirofilaria immitis (dirofilariasis)	Tropical and subtropical areas	Mosquitoes
Gnathostoma spinigerum (gnathostomiasis)	Asia (Thailand and Japan)	Raw or undercooked flesh of fish, frog or snake
Wucheria bancrofti	India, south-east Asia, Africa Pacific islands, Caribbean	Mosquitoes
Brugia malayi (tropical pulmonary eosinophilia)	South India, south-east Asia, the Philippines, China and South Korea	
Trematodes		
Paragonimus spp. (paragonimiasis)	South-east Asia, Indian subcontinent, Central and South America and Africa	Insufficiently cooked crabs or crayfish
Schistosoma spp. (schistosomiasis)	Egypt, west and east Africa, Brazil, the Philippines and the Yangtze valley in China (Table 42.3)	Skin penetration in water
Cestodes		
Echinococcus spp. (hydatidosis)	Worldwide	Oral

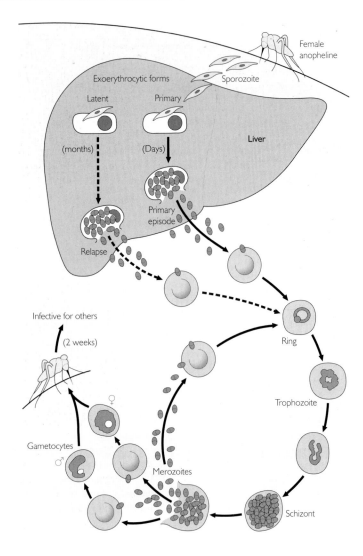

Fig. 42.1 Life cycle of plasmodia in humans. (Adapted from Wyler 1992.[2])

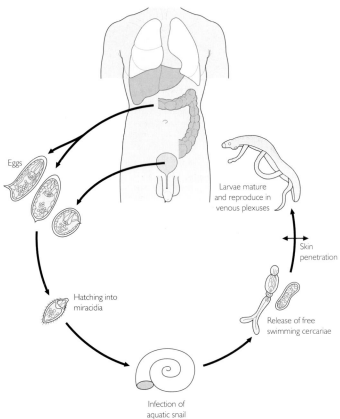

Fig. 42.2 Life cycle of *Schistosoma* spp. (Adapted from King & Mahmoud 1992.[3])

Treatment

Treatment is not necessary in immunocompetent hosts with mild clinical presentation. When required, treatment is with sulfadiazine and pyrimethamine for 4–6 weeks or longer.

Amoebiasis

Epidemiology and pathogenesis

Entamoeba histolytica is a protozoon with a cystic and a trophozoite stage that is endemic in west and southern Africa, south and south-east Asia, South America and Mexico. The disease[6,7] is transmitted by contaminated food or water. Following the ingestion of cysts, trophozoites develop in the small intestine and are carried in the faecal stream into the caecum. The pathogenicity of different strains of *E. histolytica* varies: some are

invasive whereas others cause only asymptomatic infections. The initial lesion is a small focus of necrosis in the large intestine, which develops into a characteristic undermined and sharply defined ulcer found anywhere from the caecum to the rectum. Trophozoites in the crater of the ulcer may enter the portal venous system and give rise to an amoebic abscess in the liver, whence they may infect the pleural cavity or lung by direct extension across the diaphragm. Less commonly, the organisms may enter the systemic circulation directly via the rectal venous plexus. Pleuropulmonary complications occur in less than 5% of patients with intestinal infection but in up to 50% of patients with liver abscesses, and can be due to either direct extension from the liver or haematogenous dissemination.

Clinical presentation and diagnosis

Intestinal symptoms range from diarrhoea and abdominal cramps to dysentery or even intestinal perforation resulting from mucosal ulceration. Symptoms of pleuropulmonary amoebiasis include cough, dyspnoea, pleuritic chest pain (typically right-sided), fever and rigors, diaphoresis, and weight loss. Rupture into the pleura leads to an amoebic effusion (Fig. 42.4), whereas rupture into the lung results in consolidation, abscess or, rarely, a hepatobronchial fistula, in which case amoebic pus may be expectorated. This is a mixture of blood

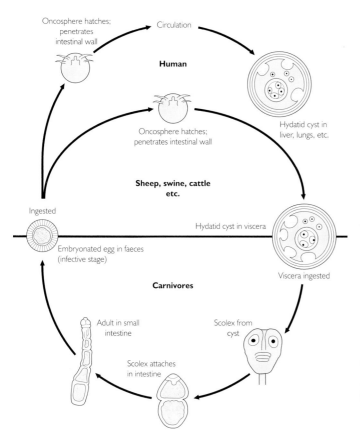

Fig. 42.3 Life cycle of *Echinococcus granulosus*. (Adapted from Willms 1992.[4])

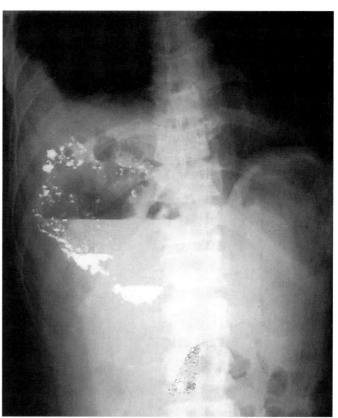

Fig. 42.4 Amoebiasis: thoracoabdominal radiograph of a 50-year-old Thai man showing a liver abscess that has ruptured into the pleural cavity (abscess cavity outlined by contrast). Liver abscess aspiration obtained 'anchovy sauce' pus, which was negative for *Entamoeba histolytica* trophozoites. Three days after admission he developed a cough with expectoration of 'anchovy sauce' sputum.

and necrotic material devoid of leukocytes and characteristically is not foul-smelling. The chest radiograph may show elevation of the right hemidiaphragm, pleural effusion, atelectasis, lung consolidation (usually affecting the right lower lobe) or lung abscess. Amoebic abscesses in the lung or liver and pleural empyema can be imaged by contrast radiography (Fig. 42.4), ultrasonography (Fig. 42.5) or computed tomography (CT). Pericardial involvement may be observed. In about 3% of patients secondary infection develops and the pus turns creamy-white or yellow.

The diagnosis can be made by serology, which has a high sensitivity (up to 95%) and specificity in invasive disease. Antigen detection may be performed in pleural fluid, respiratory secretions or faeces. In the rare instances when amoebae are seen in pus, they are to be found in the terminal portion of the aspirated fluid. Microscopic examination of stools has a poor sensitivity (less than 30%). Finally, needle aspiration of lung or liver abscesses may be necessary in a few cases.

Treatment

The drug of choice for the treatment of invasive amoebiasis is metronidazole (750 mg three times a day during 5–10 days) associated with agents active against intraluminal protozoa, such as diloxanide (500 mg t.i.d. for 10 days), iodoquinol or paromomycin.

Malarial lung disease

Epidemiology and pathogenesis

Malaria remains one of the most widespread parasitic diseases in the world, with half of the global population still at risk. Imported malaria is becoming an appreciable problem in developed countries. Malignant tertian malaria is a medical emergency because it passes very rapidly from a mild infection – the treatment of which is simple – to a catastrophic fatal illness.

The incubation period varies from 10 to 20 days, with most cases in developed countries seen within a month of return from an endemic area. Of the four species that infect humans, the only one of importance as far as the lungs are concerned is *Plasmodium falciparum*.

Clinical presentation and diagnosis

Malignant tertian malaria can present in a mundane fashion, with fever and symptoms and signs suggestive of influenza or viral hepatitis. On the other hand, one or more of the following severe manifestations can occur, especially if a delay in diagno-

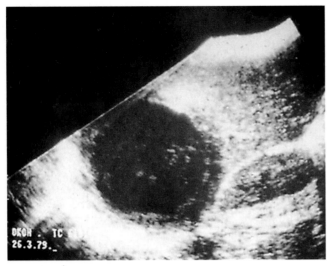

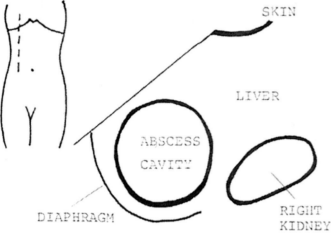

Fig. 42.5 Ultrasonic image and diagram of a large amoebic abscess. (Courtesy of Dr A. Bryceson.)

sis has occurred: cerebral malaria, severe anaemia, jaundice, renal failure, fluid and electrolyte disturbances, hyperthermia, hypoglycaemia, circulatory collapse, haemoglobinuria, septicaemia, bleeding and blood clotting disturbances and lung involvement. Non-severe respiratory involvement is probably underdiagnosed and may affect up to 20% of patients with *falciparum* malaria; it is characterised by mild cough associated to pleural effusion, lung consolidation or interstitial infiltrates. Severe respiratory involvement is due to lung oedema and pleural effusion; it presents as acute respiratory distress syndrome (ARDS) and is associated with cerebral involvement and high parasitaemia. It can also occur at day 3–4, when parasitaemia has decreased following antimalarial treatment. The diagnosis relies on blood smears.

Treatment

In addition to supportive and respiratory care, treatment of severe disease requires intravenous quinine. Other antimalarial agents may be necessary, depending on resistance profiles in the area of contamination. Exchange transfusion may be required in

the most severe cases. Despite these measures, prognosis for the malarial lung remains poor.

Nematodes

Trichinosis

Epidemiology and pathogenesis

Trichinosis is caused by the tissue nematode *Trichinella spiralis* and is acquired from eating improperly cooked meat of wild animals or domestic pigs. The disease has a worldwide distribution and the severity of the illness is usually related to the intensity of infection, i.e. to the number of larvae per gram of muscle.

Clinical presentation and diagnosis

The disease is characterised mainly by fever, gastrointestinal symptoms, myositis, swollen eyelids and eosinophilia. Involvement of the respiratory muscles may cause dyspnoea and very occasionally respiratory failure. The penetration of the larvae into muscle cells initiates a strong inflammatory response, with pain and tenderness affecting the diaphragm and other muscles, reaching its peak between the second and fourth weeks of infection.

A variety of serological tests can be used for diagnosis, e.g. bentonite flocculation test or enzyme-linked immunosorbent assay (ELISA). Often, these are not positive until 3–4 weeks after the onset of symptoms. Levels of muscle enzymes are often raised. Alternatively, the larvae may be found on muscle biopsy.

Treatment

Treatment involves the use of corticosteroids to control the acute symptoms and antihelminthics to remove the adult worms from the intestine. Prednisolone 40–60 mg daily should be given until the fever and signs subside. Mebendazole 20 mg/kg 6-hourly for 2 weeks is thought to kill some migrating larvae. For prevention, pork must be thoroughly cooked, especially if it is from a wild animal. Freezing for 3 weeks at –15°C also kills larvae.

Pulmonary ascariasis

Epidemiology and pathogenesis

Infection with the large roundworm nematode *Ascaris lumbricoides* affects up to one-quarter of the world's population. Endemic areas include Africa, Asia, Central and South America. Transmission occurs throughout the year in the moist tropical regions but only seasonally in countries with dry climates. Autochthonous infections in Europe are nowadays uncommon and pneumonic manifestations very rare. The normal habitat of the adult worm is the jejunum; infection follows ingestion of embryonated eggs, which liberate larvae in the small intestine; penetration of the intestinal wall is followed by migration through blood or lymph vessels. In the lung,[8-10] the embryo reaches capillaries and penetrates into the alveoli (Fig. 42.6). It is then cleared

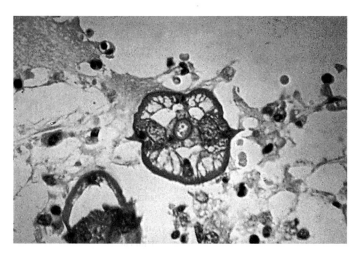

Fig. 42.6 Ascariasis: section of *Ascaris* larva in the lung.

to the throat via the tracheobronchial tree before being swallowed again. Maturation and copulation then occur in the small intestine. Migration through the lungs may be responsible for *Ascaris* pneumonia (20% of cases), a self-limiting disease that occurs 4–16 days after ingestion, lasts 10 days to several weeks and is due to both worm burden and host immune response.

Clinical presentation and diagnosis

Lung ascariasis presents as a Löffler-like syndrome with cough (and sometimes haemoptysis), wheezing, dyspnoea, chest pain (substernal burning) and fever. Fatal respiratory obstruction by worms blocking the trachea or main bronchi has been described. Cutaneous reactions (urticaria, angioneurotic oedema) and gastrointestinal symptoms (abdominal pain, nausea and vomiting, hepatomegaly) may occur simultaneously. Chest radiograph demonstrates patchy peribronchial alveolar migratory infiltrates. Eosinophilia and sometimes IgE elevation are found on blood examination. Sputum analysis reveals eosinophils, Charcot–Leyden crystals and sometimes larvae. The diagnosis is usually made by finding the characteristic eggs in the faeces, although stool examination may be negative at this early stage of ascariasis. Serology is useless because of cross-reactions with other nematode infections.

Treatment

Bronchodilators and corticosteroids may be useful when a bronchospasm is present. Antihelminthic therapy is necessary to eradicate intestinal adult worms. At least four effective drugs are available : levamisole is considered by many to be the drug of choice. It is given by mouth in a single dose of 3 mg/kg. Alternatives are mebendazole 100 mg twice a day for 1 day, pyrantel in a single oral dose of 10 mg/kg and albendazole in a single oral dose of 400 mg.

Ancylostomiasis

Ancylostomiasis, or hookworm infection, may be due to three nematodes, *Ancylostoma duodenale*, *Necator americanus* and *Ancylostoma ceylonicum*. *N. americanus* is the dominating hookworm in North America and has its highest prevalence in the south-eastern USA. Humans are infested after skin penetration by the larvae.[11] Pulmonary manifestations are similar to but less frequent and less intense than those of ascariasis.[9] Mebendazole 100 mg orally twice a day for 3 days is now considered the drug of choice but pyrantel 20 mg/kg in a single oral dose or albendazole 400 mg, also as a single oral dose, are also very effective.

Strongyloidiasis

Epidemiology and pathogenesis

Strongyloides stercoralis is endemic in tropical and subtropical areas but the prevalence of strongyloidiasis[12] is lower than that of ascariasis and ancylostomiasis. The life-cycle of the parasite is unique in that all stages can develop in humans, so that autoinfection is common and may lead to the hyperinfection syndrome in debilitated patients.[13]

Contamination occurs via skin penetration followed by migration through the lungs to the small intestine.

Clinical presentation and diagnosis

The disease may be asymptomatic or limited to a Löffler-like syndrome that occurs during migration of the parasite through the lungs and may be associated with abdominal symptoms. Hypereosinophilia is common. The hyperinfection syndrome or disseminated strongyloidiasis is characterised by abdominal, respiratory and general manifestations, which can be as severe as ileus or ARDS.[13] It can be accompanied by a Gram-negative septicaemia, pneumonia and meningitis. The diagnosis can be made by examination (string test) of sputum, stools, duodenal or pleural aspiration. Serological techniques may be used in chronic cases with negative string test.

Treatment

The preferred treatment is thiabendazole (25 mg/kg body weight) or albendazole (400 mg) given twice daily over 2–3 days and usually repeated 1 week later. Ivermectin may also be used. Longer durations of treatment may be administered in disseminated disease.

Visceral larva migrans

Epidemiology and pathogenesis

Human visceral larva migrans,[14-16] also called systemic toxocariasis, is due to the roundworms *Toxocara canis* and, less frequently, *Toxocara catis*. The disease has a worldwide distribution and the prevalence of the infection in dogs is about 3%. Transmission to humans occurs by ingestion of infective ova from animals harbouring the adult worms, or by ingestion of eggs in contaminated soil by children or subjects with geophagia. Larvae migrate through lymphatic and blood vessels and reach the liver, the lungs or, less frequently, the brain or heart. They induce an eosinophilic IgE-mediated host response.

Clinical presentation and diagnosis

The clinical features depend on the intensity of infection and the organs affected. Ophthalmic, hepatic, pulmonary and cerebral lesions occur, although in many cases infection is asymptomatic. Initial infection in children sometimes causes fever, cough, malaise and hypereosinophilia. A common presentation is for a child to lose the sight of one eye. Larval invasion of the liver causes tender hepatomegaly and eosinophilia whereas encephalitis with convulsions occurs when the brain is involved. Clinically, pulmonary involvement may present as bronchiolitis, pneumonia that may cause acute respiratory failure, or cough and wheezing. Abnormalities may be seen on chest radiograph in one-third to one-half of patients with respiratory symptoms, and usually consist of mild migratory infiltrates. Pulmonary nodules corresponding to granulomata can also be observed. The diagnosis can be made by serology or histological examination of invaded tissues.

Treatment

In mild cases, the disease is self-limiting and requires no specific treatment. In more severe cases, treatment is with thiabendazole (25 mg/kg b.i.d. for 7 days repeated 1 month later) or diethylcarbamazine (3 mg/kg t.i.d. for 3 weeks). Corticosteroids may improve the prognosis.

Dirofilariasis

Epidemiology and pathogenesis

Human dirofilariasis[17–20] is the consequence of infestation by the nematode *Dirofilaria immitis*, which is a dog-heart parasite transmitted by mosquitoes in both temperate and tropical/subtropical areas of the world. In rare cases, larvae injected by mosquitoes into humans do not die in subcutaneous tissues and are transported by blood vessels to the pulmonary circulation, where they can cause thrombosis, infarction and subsequent granulomatous reaction.

Clinical presentation and diagnosis

Clinical signs (cough, haemoptysis, chest pain, fever) are infrequent. Chest radiograph can show peripheral nodules, which may calcify ('coin lesion'); such aspects are the most frequent mode of diagnosis. Peripheral eosinophilia may be found in a few cases. The diagnosis can be made by serology or histological examination of surgically resected lung tissues. Histological investigation shows a dead immature worm occluding a pulmonary artery in the centre of a necrotic focus.

Treatment

Dirofilariasis is a self-limiting disease that does not require any specific treatment.

Gnathostomiasis

Epidemiology and pathogenesis

Gnathostomiasis[21] has been reported mainly from Asia and particularly from Thailand and Japan. *Gnathostoma spinigerum*, a tissue nematode, only rarely causes infection of the human lung. Humans acquire the infection when consuming raw or undercooked flesh of fish, frogs or snakes containing the encysted third-stage infective larvae of the nematode worm.

Clinical presentation and diagnosis

The early manifestations of larval gnathostomiasis are migratory subcutaneous swellings and an abdominopulmonary hypereosinophilic syndrome consisting of fever, abdominal pain, tender hepatomegaly, pleurisy or pneumonitis, and hypereosinophilia. Occasionally, haemoptysis and spontaneous pneumothorax may occur. The patients reported with respiratory tract gnathostomiasis had a history of previous attacks of migratory swellings; the worms were expelled by violent and frequent coughing.

The diagnosis is difficult and usually depends on recovering the immature worm from the lungs. A purified *G. spinigerum* antigen used in an indirect ELISA is sensitive and specific.

Treatment

There is no available effective treatment.

Tropical pulmonary eosinophilia

Epidemiology and pathogenesis

Tropical pulmonary eosinophilia[14,22–25] is related to infection with *Wucheria bancrofti* and *Brugia malayi*, which are lymphatic-dwelling filaria found in tropical and subtropical areas. *W. bancrofti* occurs most frequently in India, south-east Asia, Africa and the Pacific islands; there are, however, pockets of infection in the Caribbean, Egypt and South America. *B. malayi* has a more restricted global distribution, occurring in south India, south-east Asia, the Philippines, China and South Korea. Transmission is due to mosquitoes, which ingest microfilaria and inject larvae when they bite humans. Tropical eosinophilia affects men in 80% of cases and involves the lungs in more than 90% of cases. Pulmonary manifestations are the consequence of hypersensitivity reactions following the discharge of microfilaria into the circulation by gravid female filariae.

Clinical presentation and diagnosis

Symptoms are both respiratory (cough, wheezing and dyspnoea) and general (fever, weakness, anorexia, weight loss). Chest radiography demonstrates bilateral basal interstitial infiltrates, increased bronchovascular markings or diffuse miliary mottling (Fig. 42.7).[26] Hypereosinophilia may reach very high levels and is associated with high levels of blood IgE. Diagnosis relies upon serology or antigen detection in circulating blood. If warranted, lung biopsy may be undertaken and is generally specific.

Treatment

The standard treatment is diethylcarbamazine, 10 mg/kg body weight in three daily doses for 5 days to 3 weeks. Alternatives are mebendazole and levamisole. An antiallergic agent (i.e. an antihistamine or corticosteroids) may be necessary, as well as

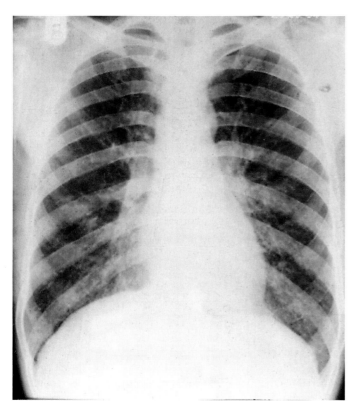

Fig. 42.7 Tropical pulmonary eosinophilia: transient nodular shadows in the lungs of a young Indian man caused by infection by filarial worms. (Courtesy of Dr A. Bryceson.)

repeated courses of treatment. Response to treatment is less dramatic in patients with a long duration of symptoms.[14]

Trematodes

Paragonimiasis

Epidemiology and pathogenesis

Paragonimus spp.[21,27-29] are hermaphrodite flukes that are endemic in south-east Asia, the Indian subcontinent, Central and South America and Africa. Many give rise to pulmonary manifestations. The most common species responsible for respiratory disease are *Paragonimus westermani, Paragonimus szechuanensis* group, *P. westermani ichunensis* and *Paragonimus tuanshanensis*. Transmission to humans occurs by ingestion of insufficiently cooked crabs or crayfish that contain the encysted parasite. The disease may also be acquired by eating the meat of a temporary host, such as a wild boar, that has been infected by eating crabs or crayfish. After excystation in the small intestine, the larvae reach the lung through the intestinal wall, peritoneal cavity, diaphragm and pleura.

Clinical presentation and diagnosis

The first symptoms may occur during migration from the intestine to the lung and include abdominal pain, diarrhoea,

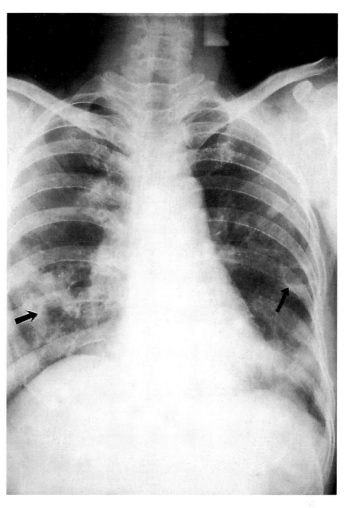

Fig. 42.8 Paragonimiasis: chest radiograph of a 23-year-old Thai woman who gave a history of haemoptysis for 1.5 years and admitted to eating raw crabs, shrimps and fish. It shows a 'signet ring' shadow in the left mid-zone and non-specific shadowing elsewhere, compatible with paragonimiasis. The sputum was positive for *Paragonimus* eggs but negative for acid-fast bacilli.

hypersensitivity reactions (urticaria, eosinophilia, fever). In most cases, however, there are no symptoms until the adult parasite begins to produce eggs in the lung (i.e. 6–10 days after infection), which induces fever, night diaphoresis, chest pain, dyspnoea, cough and haemoptysis with jelly-like, brownish-red sputum that may contain eggs. There may also be subcutaneous nodules, abdominal signs and symptoms and central nervous system involvement. Chest radiography usually shows cloudy infiltrates or nodular shadows, which may convert to cavities surrounded by a thin infiltrate ('ring cysts'; Fig. 42.8). Areas of fibrosis, bronchiectasis, pleural effusions and pleural thickening that may calcify can be observed in long-lasting untreated disease. Finally, many cases are asymptomatic, with a normal chest radiograph in up to 20% of cases. The diagnosis is based on the demonstration of eggs in bronchial secretions, pleural fluid or faeces. Several serological techniques may be used when direct microbiological diagnosis is negative.

Table 42.3   Pathogenic species of Schistosoma and their target organs and treatment. (Adapted from Huchon & Roche 1999.[1])

Species	Area	Venous plexuses in which mature parasites develop
S. mansoni	Arabia, Africa, South America, Caribbean	Inferior mesenteric veins
S. japonicum	China, Japan, Philippines	Superior mesenteric plexus
S. haematobium	Africa, Middle East	Vesical plexus

Treatment

The preferred treatment is praziquantel (25 mg/kg body weight t.i.d. for 3 days), which cures most cases. Bithionol (40 mg/kg body weight every other day for 2 weeks) is less effective.

Schistosomiasis

Epidemiology and pathogenesis

Several species of *Schistosoma* (*Schistosoma haematobium*, *Schistosoma mansoni* and *Schistosoma japonicum*) may be pathogenic for humans, and large endemic foci of schistosomiasis[30-32] are found in Egypt, west and east Africa, Brazil, the Philippines and the Yangtze valley in China. The geographical distribution and target organs of the various species are shown in Table 42.3. The schistosome cercariae thrive in fresh water and penetrate the skin to transform into immature parasites, which are transported by blood vessels to mature in venous plexuses, where they reproduce (Fig. 42.2). Eggs deposited in the intestine or bladder induce local granulomatous reactions and may migrate to the liver, causing portal hypertension; migration to the lung is then possible by portosystemic collaterals. Pulmonary lesions are arterial (endarteritis obliterans; Fig. 42.9) and parenchymal (extravascular granulomata and scarring; Fig. 42.10).

Clinical presentation and diagnosis

Symptoms depend on the stage of the disease. During the stage of migration from the skin to their final habitat in the human body, severe toxaemia with fever, cough, wheezing, arthralgia, hepatosplenomegaly and marked eosinophilia develop. The chest radiograph may show pulmonary mottling. This syndrome, which occurs with all three species of schistosomes, is known as 'Katayama fever' and is an early manifestation of the disease. The most frequent pulmonary manifestation is pulmonary hypertension, which occurs in the chronic stages of infection with *S. mansoni* or *S. japonicum*. The direct diagnosis may be

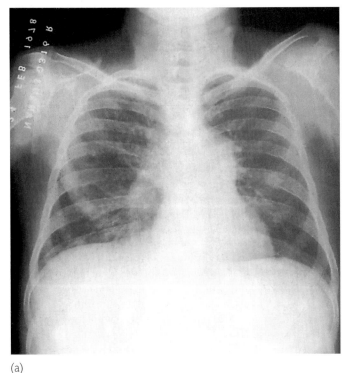

(a)

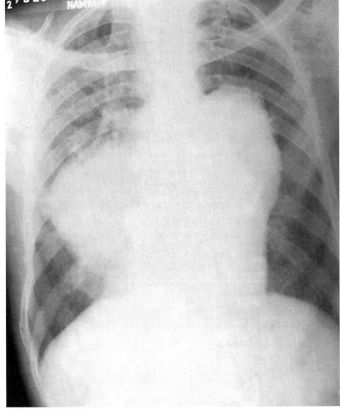

(b)

Fig. 42.9 Cor pulmonale caused by schistosomiasis. (a) Early stage showing dilatation of central pulmonary arteries. (b) Late stage showing gross aneurysmal dilatation. (Courtesy of Dr Z. Farid.)

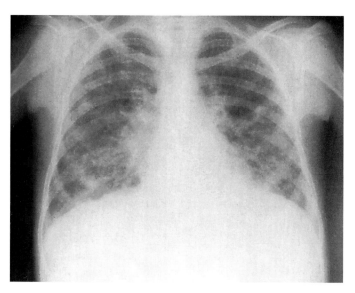

Fig. 42.10 Bronchopulmonary schistosomiasis: chest radiograph showing diffuse pulmonary mottling caused by widespread granuloma formation. (Courtesy of Dr Z. Farid.)

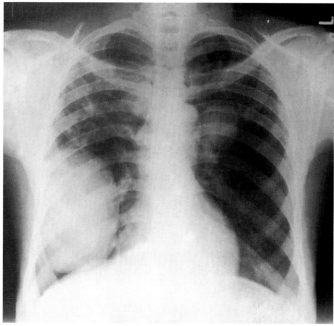

Fig. 42.11 Chest radiograph showing multiple hydatid cysts of lung.

based on stool (Kato thick smear), sputum or urine examination, or on rectal biopsies. Several serological techniques are available.

Treatment

Treatment of pulmonary hypertension with or without cardiac failure is similar to that of other forms of cor pulmonale. Antischistosomal therapy will not reverse the chronic pathology but is still worth giving because it will arrest further progress of the disease. Praziquantel 40 mg/kg in a single oral dose is the drug of choice.

Cestodes (tapeworms)

Hydatidosis

Epidemiology and pathogenesis

Hydatid disease[33-35] is caused by larvae of the platyhelminths *Echinococcus granulosus* (which causes cystic hydatid disease) and *Echinococcus multilocularis* (which causes alveolar hydatid disease). Humans become infested through ingestion of eggs. The parasite is then transported to the liver and the lungs by blood or lymphatic vessels. Humans are a blind alley in the parasite life cycle, which occurs in dog and sheep: dogs eat scoleces contained in the organs of dead sheep; in the small intestine, these scoleces develop into adult worms, which produce eggs; when these eggs are eaten by sheep, they in turn give rise to hydatid cysts containing scoleces. Cystic hydatid disease (90% of human cases of hydatid disease) is the manifestation of the slow growth of larvae into hydatid cysts, producing space-occupying lesions, while alveolar hydatid disease is due to persisting proliferating and destructive parasites. Respiratory involvement is more frequent in cystic hydatid disease.

Clinical presentation and diagnosis

Most cases of pulmonary cystic hydatid disease are asymptomatic and usually discovered on routine chest radiograph. Symptoms may be related to compression of adjacent structures, rupture or secondary infection. They include chest pain, dyspnea, cough, expectoration of cyst contents (i.e. daughter cysts and watery fluid), hemoptysis, or even respiratory distress. Rupture may also lead to dissemination of cysts in the lungs, urticaria and anaphylactic shock or pleural effusion.[36] Eosinophilia is common. The chest radiograph shows rounded, well-defined, uniformly dense opacities nicknamed 'cannon balls', the borders of which may calcify (Fig. 42.11). If the cyst communicates with a bronchus, a cap of air may be seen above the cyst, whereas if the cyst ruptures and the laminated membrane collapses, the membrane floating on the residual fluid produces the characteristic 'lily pad' appearance. Computed tomography exhibits sharply limited cysts that may themselves contain smaller 'daughter' cysts. In alveolar hydatid disease, pulmonary masses are less well-defined and have necrotic centres. The diagnosis is based on the aspect of lung lesions, the presence of associated hepatic cysts, serological tests (although these are poorly specific) and rarely the presence of cyst contents in sputum. In difficult cases, immunodiagnostic tests that detect immune complexes or circulating antigen can be carried out in specialised reference centres. Aspiration of the cyst contents should be avoided to prevent dissemination and hypersensitivity reactions.

Treatment

The treatment of choice of compressive cysts is surgical resection followed by albendazole to prevent recurrence from spillage.[37-42] When surgery is not indicated or is contraindicated,

Table 42.4   Summary of clinical presentation and diagnostic methods of lung parasitic diseases

Parasites (diseases)	Presentation	Diagnosis
Protozoa		
Toxoplasma gondii (toxoplasmosis)	Fever, headache, lymphadenopathy (which may be hilar/mediastinal), myalgia, arthralgia, rash, hepatosplenomegaly, retinochoroiditis	Histology Serology
Entamoeba histolytica (amoebiasis)	Intestinal symptoms Fever and rigors, diaphoresis, weight loss Pleural effusion, atelectasis, lung consolidation or abscess	Serology Antigen detection Direct examination of pus Stool microscopic examination
Plasmodium spp. (malaria)	Signs of tertian malaria Pleural effusion, lung consolidation or interstitial infiltrates Pulmonary oedema/ARDS	Blood smears
Trichinella spiralis (trichinosis)	Fever, gastrointestinal symptoms, myositis, swollen eyelids, eosinophilia, dyspnoea (respiratory muscle involvement)	Serology Muscle biopsy
Nematodes		
Ascaris lumbricoides (ascariasis)	Löffler-like syndrome Cutaneous reaction Gastrointestinal symptoms Hypereosinophilia	Stool examination
Ancylostoma spp. and *Necator americanus* (ancylostomiasis)	See Ascariasis	
Strongyloides stercoralis (strongyloidiasis)	See Ascariasis Hyperinfection syndrome (see text)	Examination (string test) of sputum, stools, duodenal or pleural aspiration Serology
Toxocara canis (visceral larva migrans)	Ophthalmic, hepatic, pulmonary and cerebral lesions Hypereosinophilia	Serology Histology
Dirofilaria immitis (dirofilariasis)	Cough, haemoptysis, chest pain, fever Coin lesions on chest radiograph	Serology Histology
Gnathostoma spinigerum (gnathostomiasis)	Fever, abdominal pain, tender hepatomegaly, pleurisy or pneumonitis, hypereosinophilia, rarely haemoptysis and spontaneous pneumothorax	Examination of respiratory secretions Serology
Wucheria bancrofti, Brugia malayi (tropical pulmonary eosinophilia)	Respiratory and general symptoms Hypereosinophilia, high IgE levels	Serology Antigen detection in blood Lung biopsy
Trematodes		
Paragonimus sp. (paragonimiasis)	Intestinal symptoms, hypersensitivity reactions, fever, dyspnoea, cough, haemoptysis with jelly-like brownish-red sputum Ring cysts on chest radiograph	Demonstration of eggs in bronchial secretions, pleural fluid or faeces Serology
Schistosoma spp. (schistosomiasis)	Katayama fever (see text) Pulmonary hypertension	Stool (Kato thick smear), sputum or urine examination Rectal biopsies Serology
Cestodes		
Echinococcus spp. (hydatidosis)	Chest pain, dyspnea, cough, expectoration of cyst contents, hemoptysis, respiratory distress, eosinophilia, allergic reactions Characteristic chest and liver radiographic appearances (see text)	Serology Examination of respiratory secretions Antigen detection

ARDS, acute respiratory distress syndrome.

Continued

Table 42.5 Treatment of lung parasitic diseases in the non-immunocompromised host. See text for details of treatment modalities

Parasites (diseases)	First-line treatment	Alternatives
Protozoa		
Toxoplasma gondii (toxoplasmosis)	Sulfadiazine and pyrimethamine	
Entamoeba histolytica (amoebiasis)	Metronidazole + diloxanide	Metronidazole + iodoquinol or paromomycin
Plasmodium spp. (malaria)	Depends on disease severity and geographical area	
Trichinella spiralis (trichinosis)	Prednisolone + mebendazole	
Nematodes		
Ascaris lumbricoides (ascariasis)	Levamisole ± bronchodilators and corticosteroids	Pyrantel Albendazole
Ancylostoma spp. and *Necator americanus* (ancylostomiasis)	Mebendazole	Pyrantel Albendazole
Strongyloides stercoralis (strongyloidiasis)	Thiabendazole Albendazole	Ivermectin
Toxocara canis (visceral larva migrans)	Thiabendazole ± corticosteroids	Diethylcarbamazine
Dirofilaria immitis (dirofilariasis)	None	
Gnathostoma spinigerum (gnathostomiasis)	None	
Wucheria bancrofti, Brugia malayi (tropical pulmonary eosinophilia)	Diethylcarbamazine ± antihistamines or corticosteroids	Mebendazole
Trematodes		
Paragonimus spp. (paragonimiasis)	Praziquantel	Bithionol
Schistosoma spp. (schistosomiasis)	Praziquantel See Table 42.3 for details	
Cestodes		
Echinococcus spp. (hydatid disease)	Albendazole Surgery	

or when there is dissemination of the parasite because of the rupture of a cyst, the preferred pharmacological treatment is albendazole 400 mg b.i.d. (10–15 mg/kg body weight per day) for 4–8 weeks.[40] Treatment courses may be repeated.

References

1. Huchon GJ, Roche N. Fungal and parasitic pneumonia. In: Albert R, Spiro S, Jett J, ed. Comprehensive respiratory medicine. London: Mosby; 1999: 23.1–23.8.
2. Wyler DJ. *Plasmodium* and *Babesia*. In: Gorbach SL, Bartlett JG, Blacklow NR, ed. Infectious diseases. Philadelphia, PA: WB Saunders; 1992: 1967–1977.
3. King CH, Mahmoud AAF. *Schistosoma* and other trematodes. In: Gorbach SL, Bartlett JG, Blacklow NR, ed. Infectious diseases. Philadelphia, PA: WB Saunders; 1992: 2015–2020.
4. Willms K. Cestodes (tapeworms). In: Gorbach SL, Bartlett JG, Blacklow NR, ed. Infectious diseases. Philadelphia, PA: WB Saunders; 1992: 2021–2036.
5. Campagna AC. Pulmonary toxoplasmosis. Semin Respir Infect 1997; 12: 98–105.
6. Lyche KD, Jensen WA. Pleuropulmonary amebiasis. Semin Respir Infect 1997; 12: 106–112.
7. Mbaye PS, Koffi N, Camara P et al. [Pleuropulmonary manifestations of amebiasis]. Rev Pneumol Clin 1998; 54: 346–352.
8. Reeder MM. The radiological and ultrasound evaluation of ascariasis of the gastrointestinal, biliary, and respiratory tracts. Semin Roentgenol 1998; 33: 57–78.
9. Sarinas PS, Chitkara RK. Ascariasis and hookworm. Semin Respir Infect 1997; 12: 130–137.
10. Khuroo MS. Ascariasis. Gastroenterol Clin North Am 1996; 25: 553–577.
11. Prociv P. Pathogenesis of human hookworm infection: insights from a 'new' zoonosis. Chem Immunol 1997; 66: 62–98: 62–98.
12. Wilson CM. Respiratory distress caused by parasites. Pediatr Ann 1994; 23: 443–446.
13. Jamil SA, Hilton E. The *Strongyloides* hyperinfection syndrome. NY State J Med 1992; 92: 67–68.
14. Chitkara RK, Sarinas PS. Dirofilaria, visceral larva migrans, and tropical pulmonary eosinophilia. Semin Respir Infect 1997; 12: 138–148.
15. L'Her P, Vaylet F, Hovette P. [Pulmonary parasitoses. General aspects]. Rev Pneumol Clin 1998; 54: 321–328.
16. Vaylet F, Grassin F, Le Vagueresse R et al. [Parasitic eosinophilic lungs]. Rev Pneumol Clin 1998; 54: 329–339.
17. Flieder DB, Moran CA. Pulmonary dirofilariasis: a clinicopathologic study of 41 lesions in 39 patients. Hum Pathol 1999; 30: 251–256.
18. Hiroshima K, Iyoda A, Toyozaki T et al. Human pulmonary dirofilariasis: report of six cases. Tohoku J Exp Med 1999; 189: 307–314.
19. Narine K, Brennan B, Gilfillan I, Hodge A. Pulmonary presentation of *Dirofilaria immitis* (canine heartworm) in man. Eur J Cardiothorac Surg 1999; 16: 475–477.
20. Shah MK. Human pulmonary dirofilariasis: review of the literature. South Med J 1999; 92: 276–279.
21. Bovornkitti S. Tropical pulmonary diseases. Respirology 1996; 1: 11–21.
22. Cooray JH, Ismail MM. Re-examination of the diagnostic criteria of tropical pulmonary eosinophilia. Respir Med 1999; 93: 655–659.
23. Marshall BG, Wilkinson RJ, Davidson RN. Pathogenesis of tropical pulmonary eosinophilia: parasitic alveolitis and parallels with asthma. Respir Med 1998; 92: 1–3.

24. Sandhu M, Mukhopadhyay S, Sharma SK. Tropical pulmonary eosinophilia: a comparative evaluation of plain chest radiography and computed tomography. Australas Radiol 1996; 40: 32–37.

25. Udwadia FE. Tropical eosinophilia: a review. Respir Med 1993; 87: 17–21.

26. Kim Y, Lee KS, Choi DC et al. The spectrum of eosinophilic lung disease: radiologic findings. J Comput Assist Tomogr 1997; 21: 920–930.

27. Carre JC, Houmdaophet S. [Paragonimiasis]. Rev Pneumol Clin 1998; 54: 359–364.

28. Charoenratanakul S. Tropical infection and the lung. Monaldi Arch Chest Dis 1997; 52: 376–379.

29. Nawa Y. Re-emergence of paragonimiasis. Intern Med 2000; 39: 353–354.

30. Bethlem EP, Schettino GD, Carvalho CR. Pulmonary schistosomiasis. Curr Opin Pulm Med 1997; 3: 361–365.

31. Morris W, Knauer CM. Cardiopulmonary manifestations of schistosomiasis. Semin Respir Infect 1997; 12: 159–170.

32. Palmer PE. Schistosomiasis. Semin Roentgenol 1998; 33: 6–25.

33. Thameur H, Chenik S, Abdelmoulah S et al. [Thoracic hydatidosis. A review of 1619 cases]. Rev Pneumol Clin 2000; 56: 7–15.

34. Tor M, Atasalihi A, Altuntas N et al. Review of cases with cystic hydatid lung disease in a tertiary referral hospital located in an endemic region: 10 years' experience. Respiration 2000; 67: 539–542.

35. Pedrosa I, Saiz A, Arrazola J et al. Hydatid disease: radiologic and pathologic features and complications. Radiographics 2000; 20: 795–817.

36. Aguilar X, Fernandez-Muixi J, Maragolas R et al. An unusual presentation of secondary pleural hydatisosis. Eur Respir J 1998; 11: 243–245.

37. Aarons BJ. Thoracic surgery for hydatid disease. World J Surg 1999; 23: 1105–1109.

38. Burgos R, Varela A, Castedo E et al. Pulmonary hydatidosis: surgical treatment and follow-up of 240 cases. Eur J Cardiothorac Surg 1999; 16: 628–634.

39. Celik M, Senol C, Keles M et al. Surgical treatment of pulmonary hydatid disease in children: report of 122 cases. J Pediatr Surg 2000; 35: 1710–1713.

40. Mawhorter S, Temeck B, Chang R et al. Nonsurgical therapy for pulmonary hydatid cyst disease. Chest 1997; 112: 1432–1436.

41. Safioleas M, Misiakos EP, Dosios T et al. Surgical treatment for lung hydatid disease. World J Surg 1999; 23: 1181–1185.

42. Salih OK, Topcuoglu MS, Celik SK et al. Surgical treatment of hydatid cysts of the lung: analysis of 405 patients. Can J Surg 1998; 41: 131–135.

Index

Page numbers in *italics* indicate figures or tables.